STAFF

ice President, Planning and evelopment
innie Bowen Rose, RN, BSN, MEd

nior Publisher
tricia Dwyer Schull, RN, MSN

Director
 Hubbard

aging Editor
 w T. McPhee, RN, BSN

al Manager
. Barrow, RN, MSN, CCRN

Editor
 hohan

 mento, Ellen Newman
 , Traci A. Ginnona, Bernice
 nice Hodgson, Carol Munson,
 ewell, June Norris

ditors
 rdish Fischer, RN, BSN;
 Fries, RN, BSN, CCRN;
 hop Hendler, RN, CCRN;
 n, RN, MSN; Nancy F. Mar-
 ybeth Morrell, RN, CCRN;

Lori Musolf Neri, RN, MSN, CCRN; Carla Roy, RN, BSN; Valerie Sauler, RN, CCRN

Associate Acquisitions Editors
Betsy K. Snyder, Louise Quinn

Copy Editors
Cynthia C. Breuninger (manager), Karen Comerford, Dionne Henderson, Brenna Mayer, Beth Pitcher, Pam Wingrod

Designers
Arlene Putterman (associate art director), Matie Patterson (assistant art director)

Typographers
Diane Paluba (manager), Joyce Rossi Biletz, Phyllis Marron, Valerie Rosenberger

Manufacturing
Deborah Meiris (manager), Pat Dorshaw, T.A. Landis, Otto Mezei

Editorial Assistants
Mary Madden, Carol A. Caputo, Carrie R. Krout

Indexer
Barbara Hodgson

articles and reviews. For information, write Springhouse Corporation, 1111 Bethlehem Pike, P.O. Box 908, Springhouse, PA 19477-0908. Authorization to photocopy items for internal or personal use, or the internal or personal use of specific clients, is granted by Springhouse Corporation for users registered with the Copyright Clearance Center (CCC) Transactional Reporting Service, provided that the fee of $.75 per page is paid directly to CCC, 222 Rosewood Dr., Danvers, MA 01923. For those organizations that have been granted a photocopy license by CCC, a separate system of payment has been arranged. The fee code for users of the Transactional Reporting Service is 0874348919/98 $00.00 + $.75.

Ⓡ A member of the Reed Elsevier plc group

Printed in the United States of America.
NDH-010897
ISSN 0273-320X
ISBN 0-87434-891-9

SO-AIH-439

Drug	metoclopramide HCl	midazolam HCl	morphine sulfate	nalbuphine HCl	pentazocine lactate	pentobarbital Na	perphenazine	phenobarbital Na	prochlorperazine edisylate	promazine HCl	promethazine HCl	ranitidine HCl	scopolamine HBr	secobarbital Na	sodium bicarbonate	thiethylperazine maleate	thiopental Na
atropine sulfate	P	Y	P	Y	P	P	Y		P	P	P	Y	P				
benzquinamide HCl		Y	Y		Y	N		N				Y	N				N
butorphanol tartrate	Y	Y	Y		Y	N	Y		Y		Y		Y			Y	
chlorpromazine HCl	P	Y	P		P	N	Y		P	P	P	Y	P				N
cimetidine HCl		Y	Y	Y	Y	N			Y	Y	Y		Y	N			
codeine phosphate																	
dimenhydrinate	P	N	P		P	N	Y		N	N	N	Y	P				N
diphenhydramine HCl	Y	Y	P	Y	P	N	Y		P	P	P	Y	P				N
droperidol	P	Y	P	Y	P	N	Y		P	P	P		P				
fentanyl citrate	P	Y	P		P	N	Y		P	P	P	Y	P				
glycopyrrolate		Y	Y	Y	N	N			Y	Y	Y	Y	Y	N	N		N
heparin Na	Y		N*		N			P(5)		N							
hydromorphone HCl		Y			Y	Y			N*		Y	Y	Y			Y	
hydroxyzine HCl	P	Y	P	Y	P	N	Y		P	P	P	N	P				
meperidine HCl	P	Y	N		P	N	Y		P	P	P	Y	P				N
metoclopramide HCl	■	Y	P		P		P		P	P	P	Y	P		N		
midazolam HCl	Y	■	Y	Y		N	N		N	Y	Y	N	Y			Y	
morphine sulfate	P	Y	■		P	N*	Y		P*	P	P*	Y	P				N
nalbuphine HCl		Y		■		N			Y		N*	Y	Y			Y	
pentazocine lactate	P		P		■	N	Y		P	Y	Y	Y	Y				
pentobarbital Na		N	N*	N	N	■	N		N	N	N	N	P		Y		Y
perphenazine	P	N	Y		Y	N	■		Y	Y	Y	Y		N			
phenobarbital Na								■				N					
prochlorperazine edisylate	P	N	P*	Y	P	N	Y		■	P	P	Y	P				N
promazine HCl	P	Y	P		Y	N			P	■	P		P				
promethazine HCl	P	Y	P*	N*	Y	N	Y		P	P	■	Y	P				N
ranitidine HCl	Y	N	Y	Y	Y	N	Y	N	Y		Y	■	Y			Y	
scopolamine HBr	P	Y	P	Y	P	P	Y		P	P	P	Y	■				Y
secobarbital Na														■			
sodium bicarbonate				Y											■		N
thiethylperazine maleate	Y		Y			N					Y					■	
thiopental Na		N			Y			N		N		Y		N			■

Nursing98
DRUG
HANDBOOK®

D
M

Se
Pa

Art
Joh

Man
Andre

Clinic
Ann M

Senior
Naina

Editors
Diane A.
Feinstein
Heller, Ja
Karyn C.

Clinical E
Patricia Ka
Colleen M.
Collette Bis
Andrea Mar
tin, RN; Mar

NURSING
SPRINGHOUS
SPRINGHOUS

CONTENTS

Advisors and Clinical Consultants..**vii**
Acknowledgments .... **ix**

General Information

1. How to use *Nursing98 Drug Handbook*.................................1
2. Drug actions, reactions, and interactions....................................6
3. Drug therapy in children 13
4. Drug therapy in elderly patients 18
5. Drug therapy and the nursing process 21

Anti-infective Drugs

6. Amebicides and antiprotozoals 25
7. Anthelmintics 31
8. Antifungals..34
9. Antimalarials...45
10. Antituberculars and antileprotics 52
11. Aminoglycosides..65
12. Penicillins...75
13. Cephalosporins..105
14. Tetracyclines 136
15. Sulfonamides...146
16. Fluoroquinolones 153
17. Antivirals..166
18. Macrolide anti-infectives..191
19. Miscellaneous anti-infectives 198

Cardiovascular System Drugs

20. Inotropics 216
21. Antiarrhythmics..221
22. Antianginals 246
23. Antihypertensives...263
24. Antilipemics..312
25. Miscellaneous cardiovascular drugs.....................................322

Central Nervous System Drugs

26. Nonnarcotic analgesics and antipyretics 330
27. Nonsteroidal anti-inflammatory drugs 342
28. Narcotic and opioid analgesics 366
29. Sedative-hypnotics 390
30. Anticonvulsants..403
31. Antidepressants 423
32. Antianxiety drugs..449

33. Antipsychotics 462
34. CNS stimulants 488
35. Antiparkinsonian drugs 503
36. Miscellaneous CNS drugs 514

Autonomic Nervous System Drugs

37. Cholinergics (parasympathomimetics) 524
38. Anticholinergics 533
39. Adrenergics (sympathomimetics) 541
40. Adrenergic blockers (sympatholytics) 552
41. Skeletal muscle relaxants 556
42. Neuromuscular blockers 565

Respiratory Tract Drugs

43. Antihistamines 583
44. Bronchodilators 597
45. Expectorants and antitussives 621
46. Miscellaneous respiratory drugs 624

Gastrointestinal Tract Drugs

47. Antacids, adsorbents, and antiflatulents 642
48. Digestive enzymes and gallstone solubilizers 650
49. Antidiarrheals 656
50. Laxatives 662
51. Antiemetics 678
52. Antiulcer drugs 689

Photoguide to Tablets and Capsules

Hormonal Drugs

53. Corticosteroids 699
54. Androgens and anabolic steroids 718
55. Estrogens and progestins 729
56. Gonadotropins 756
57. Antidiabetic drugs and glucagon 761
58. Thyroid hormones 781
59. Thyroid hormone antagonists 788
60. Pituitary hormones 794
61. Parathyroid-like drugs 802

Drugs for Fluid and Electrolyte Balance

62. Diuretics 808
63. Electrolytes and replacement solutions 832
64. Acidifier and alkalinizers 847

Hematologic Drugs

65. Hematinics 851
66. Anticoagulants 857
67. Blood derivatives......866
68. Thrombolytic enzymes......874

Antineoplastic Drugs

69. Alkylating drugs......883
70. Antimetabolites 902
71. Antibiotic antineoplastic drugs 915
72. Antineoplastics that alter hormone balance 927
73. Miscellaneous antineoplastic drugs 937

Immunomodulation Drugs

74. Immunosuppressants......969
75. Vaccines and toxoids......978
76. Antitoxins and antivenins......1008
77. Immune serums 1012
78. Biological response modifiers......1022

Ophthalmic, Otic, and Nasal Drugs

79. Ophthalmic anti-infectives 1039
80. Ophthalmic anti-inflammatory drugs......1054
81. Miotics 1062
82. Mydriatics 1071
83. Ophthalmic vasoconstrictors......1078
84. Miscellaneous ophthalmics 1081
85. Otics 1096
86. Nasal drugs......1099

Topical Drugs

87. Local anti-infectives......1111
88. Scabicides and pediculicides......1132
89. Topical corticosteroids 1137

Nutritional Drugs

90. Vitamins and minerals......1156
91. Calorics 1176

Miscellaneous Drug Categories

92. Antigout drugs......1182
93. Enzymes 1189
94. Oxytocics 1192
95. Spasmolytics 1198
96. Gold salts......1203

97. Miscellaneous antagonists and antidotes 1204
98. Uncategorized drugs...1225

Appendices and Index

A. Selected local and topical anesthetics 1262
B. Cancer chemotherapy: Acronyms and protocols.................1268
C. Table of equivalents...1279
D Diagnostic skin tests...1280
E. Nomogram for estimating surface area in children.........1282
Index..1283

Nursing98 DrugDisk ....inside back cover

ADVISORS AND CLINICAL CONSULTANTS

At the time of publication, the advisors and clinical consultants held the following positions.

Advisors

Lillian S. Brunner, RN, MSN, ScD, FAAN
Nurse-Author
Lancaster, Pa.

Luther P. Christman, RN, PhD
Nurse Consultant
Chapel Hill, Tenn.

Kathleen A. Dracup, RN, DNSc, FAAN
Professor and L.W. Hassenplug Chair
University of California School of Nursing
Los Angeles

Stanley J. Dudrick, MD, FACS
Program Director
St. Mary's Hospital Department of Surgery
Waterbury, Conn.
Clinical Professor of Surgery
Yale University School of Medicine
New Haven, Conn.

Halbert E. Fillinger, MD
Forensic Pathologist and Coroner
Montgomery County
Norristown, Pa.

M. Josephine Flaherty, RN, PhD
Consultant
Ottawa, Canada

Dennis E. Leavell
Associate Professor
Mayo Medical Laboratories
Mayo Clinic
Rochester, Minn.

Ara G. Paul, PhD
Dean Emeritus and Professor of Pharmacognosy
College of Pharmacy
University of Michigan
Ann Arbor

Rose Pinneo, RN, MS
Professor Emeritus
University of Rochester (N.Y.) School of Nursing

Thomas E. Rubbert, JD, LLB, BSL
Attorney-at-Law
Pasadena, Calif.

Clinical Consultants

Thomas E. Ary, BPharm, PhD
Director of Compliance
PRACS Institute, Ltd.
Fargo, N. Dak.

David J. Blanchard, RPh, BS
Pharmacist
St. Luke's Memorial Hospital
New Hartford, N.Y.

Karen T. Bruchak, RN, MSN, MBA
Assistant Administrator, Cancer Clinical Programs
University of Pennsylvania Medical Center
Philadelphia

James Camamo, PharmD
Clinical Pharmacist, Medication Information and
Policy Development
University Medical Center
Tucson, Ariz.

Lawrence Carey, PharmD
Clinical Pharmacist Coordinator
Jefferson Home Infusion Service
Thomas Jefferson University Hospital
Philadelphia

Sandra L. Chase, PharmD, BS
Clinical Pharmacist, Drug Use Policy & Medical
Information Service
Thomas Jefferson University Hospital
Philadelphia

Nancy R. Cirone, RN,C, MSN, CDE
Clinical Development Specialist
Allegheny University Hospitals, Bucks
Warminister, Pa.

Rachael Clark-Vetri, RPh, PharmD
Clinical Assistant Professor
Temple University School of Pharmacy
Philadelphia

Patricia Drobins, RN, BSN, OCN
Clinical Research Nurse Specialist
University of Pennsylvania Cancer Center
Philadelphia

Teresa S. Dunsworth, PharmD, BCPS
Assistant Professor of Clinical Pharmacy
West Virginia University School of Pharmacy
Morgantown, W.V.

Bruce M. Frey, RPh, PharmD, BSPharm
Clinical Pharmacist in Pediatrics and Hematology
Thomas Jefferson University Hospital
Philadelphia

Douglas R. Geraets, RPh, PharmD, FCCP
Clinical Pharmacy Specialist, Ambulatory Care
VA Medical Center, Pharmacy Service
Iowa City, Iowa

Mary Jo Gerlach, RN, MSNEd
Assistant Professor Adult Nursing
Medical College of Georgia
Athens, Ga.

Martin R. Giannamore, RPh, PharmD
Assistant Professor of Clinical Pharmacy Practice
Ohio State University, College of Pharmacy
Columbus

John D. Grabenstein, MS Pharm, EdM, FASHP
Medical Service Corps, United States Army

Mary Beth Gross, PharmD, FASCP
Manager, Pharmacy
Mercy Hospital Medical Center;
Associate Professor of Pharmacy
Drake University, College of Pharmacy
Des Moines, Iowa

David W. Hawkins, PharmD
Professor and Assistant Dean of Pharmacy
University of Georgia
Athens, Ga.

James R. Hildebrand, III, PharmD
Drug Information Product Manager
SmithKline Beecham Pharmaceuticals
Philadelphia

Jeffrey W. Hui, RPh, PharmD
Drug Information Resident
Department of Pharmacy
Temple University Hospital
Philadelphia

Lori Ann Hytrek, PharmD
Drug Information Specialty Resident
University of California
San Francisco

Cary E. Johnson, PharmD
Associate Professor of Pharmacy;
Clinical Pharmacist, Pediatrics
University of Michigan, College of Pharmacy
Ann Arbor

William A. Kehoe, PharmD, MA, BCPS
Professor of Clinical Pharmacy
University of the Pacific, School of Pharmacy
Stockton, Calif.

James Allen Koestner, PharmD
Clinical Pharmacist, Trauma
Vanderbilt University Medical Center
Nashville, Tenn.

W. Greg Leader, PharmD
Assistant Professor
West Virginia University School of Pharmacy
Morgantown

Marie Maloney, PharmD
Clinical Pharmacist
University Medical Center
Tucson, Ariz.

Michael A. Mancano, RPh, PharmD, BS Pharm
Director of Drug Information
Temple University Hospital
Assistant Professor of Clinical Pharmacy
Temple University School of Pharmacy
Philadelphia

Jan E. Markind, RPh, PharmD, BS
Drug Information Specialist and Clinical Assistant
Professor
University of Illinois
Chicago

Dawna Martich, RN, MSN
Clinical Manager
University of Pittsburgh Medical Center, USO
Moon Township, Pa.

Michael K. McGuire, PharmD
Clinical Coordinator
Germantown Hospital and Medical Center
Philadelphia

Joan A.W. Mege, PharmD, RPh
Freelance Medical Writer;
Formerly Pharmacy Practice Resident,
Milton S. Hershey Medical Center
Hershey, Pa.

Steven Meisel, PharmD
Assistant Director, Pharmacy
Fairview Southdale Hospital
Edina, Minn.

William O'Hara, RPh, PharmD, BS
Clinical Pharmacist
Thomas Jefferson University Hospital
Philadelphia

Theresa R. Prosser, PharmD, BCPS
Associate Professor
St. Louis (Mo.) College of Pharmacy

Leslie N. Schechter, PharmD
Clinical Coordinator
Department of Pharmacy
Thomas Jefferson University Hospital
Philadelphia

Michelle Swartz, BS
Teacher, Upper Dublin School District
Fort Washington, Pa.

Lynda Thomson, RPh, PharmD, BS
Clinical Pharmacist, Infectious Diseases
Thomas Jefferson University Hospital
Philadelphia

Candy Tsourounis, RPh, PharmD
Assistant Clinical Professor
Drug Information Analysis Service
University of California
San Francisco

Kenneth K. Wieland, PharmD
Director of Pharmacy
Chestnut Hill Hospital
Philadelphia

Stacy A. Wiegman, RPh, PharmD, MS
Fellow
Institute for Safe Medication Practices
Warminister, Pa.

ACKNOWLEDGEMENTS

We would like to thank the following companies for granting us permission to include their drugs in the full-color photoguide.

Abbott Laboratories
Biaxin®
Depakote®
Depakote® Sprinkle
E.E.S.®
Ery-Tab®
Erythrocin Stearate Filmtab®
Erythromycin Base Filmtab®
Hytrin®
PCE®

Astra Merck
Prilosec®

Astra USA
Toprol XL™

Bristol-Myers Squibb Company
BuSpar®
Capoten®
Cefzil®
cephalexin
Duricef®
Estrace®
Pravachol®
Sumycin®
Trimox®
Veetids®

Daniels Pharmaceuticals, Inc.
Levoxyl®

Dupont/Merck
Coumadin®
Percocet®
Sinemet®
Sinemet® CR

Eli Lilly and Company
Axid®
Ceclor®
Darvocet-N® 100
Lorabid®
Prozac®

ESI/Lederle Generics
atenolol

Ethex Corporation
potassium chloride

Forest Pharmaceuticals, Inc.
Lorcet® 10/650

Glaxo Wellcome Inc.
Ceftin®
Lanoxin®
Zantac®
Zantac® EFFERdose®
Zovirax®

Goldline Laboratories, Inc.
verapamil hydrochloride

Hoechst Marion Roussel, Inc.
Altace®
Carafate®
Cardizem®
Cardizem® CD
Cardizem® SR®
DiaBeta®
Lasix®
Seldane®
Seldane-D®
Trental®

Hoffman-La Roche, Inc.
Bumex®
Klonopin®
Naprosyn®
Toradol®
Valium®

Janssen Pharmaceutical, Inc.
Hismanal®
Propulsid®

Knoll Pharmaceutical Company
E-Mycin®
ibuprofen
Synthroid®
Vicodin®
Vicodin ES®

Lederle Laboratories
Suprax®
Verelan®

Lemmon Company
acetaminophen and codeine (300 mg/30 mg)
Cotrim® D.S.

MD Pharmaceutical, Inc.
methylphenidate hydrochloride

Merck & Co., Inc.
Mevacor®
Pepcid®
Prinivil®
Vasotec®
Zocor®

Miles, Inc.
Adalat®
Cipro®

Mylan Pharmaceuticals Inc.
amitriptyline hydrochloride
cimetidine

cyclobenzaprine hydrochloride
doxepin hydrochloride
furosemide
glipizide
naproxen
propoxyphene napsylate with acetaminophen

Novopharm USA Inc., Division of Novopharm Limited
amoxicillin trihydrate

Ortho/McNeil Pharmaceutical
Floxin®
Tylenol® with Codeine No. 3
Ultram®

Pfizer Inc.
Diflucan®

Proctor and Gamble Pharmaceuticals
Macrobid®

Purepac Pharmaceutical Co.
acetaminophen and codeine (300 mg/60 mg)

Rhône-Poulenc Rorer Pharmaceuticals Inc.
Dilacor XR®
Lozol®
Slo-bid® Gyrocaps®

A.H. Robins Company
Micro-K Extencaps®

Roxane Laboratories, Inc.
Roxicet™

Rugby Laboratories, Inc.
dicyclomine hydrochloride

Sandoz Pharmaceuticals Corporation
DynaCirc®
Fiorinal® with Codeine
Pamelor®

Schein Pharmaceutical, Inc.
nortriptyline hydrochloride

Schering-Plough Corporation
Claritin®
K-Dur®
Theo-Dur®

G.D. Searle & Company
Ambien®
Calan®
Daypro®

SmithKline Beecham Pharmaceuticals
Amoxil®
Augmentin®
Compazine®
Compazine® Spansule®
Dyazide®
Paxil®
Relafen®
Tagamet®

Solvay Pharmaceuticals, Inc.
Orasone®

The Upjohn Company
Ansaid®
Deltasone®
Glynase®
Halcion®
Micronase®
Motrin®
Ogen®
Provera®
Xanax®

U.S. Pharmaceuticals Group
Pfizer Inc.
Cardura®
Glucotrol®
Glucotrol XL®
Norvasc®
Procardia XL®
Zithromax®
Zoloft®

Warner-Lambert Company
Accupril®
Dilantin®
Dilantin®
Kapseals®
gemfibrozil
Lopid®
Nitrostat®

Watson Laboratories, Inc.
hydrocodone bitartrate and
acetominophen

Wyeth-Ayerst Laboratories
Ativan®
Effexor®
Inderal®
Lodine®
Oruvail®
Premarin®

Zeneca Pharmaceuticals
Nolvadex®
Tenormin®
Zestril®

1

How to use *Nursing98 Drug Handbook*

Nursing98 Drug Handbook is meant to fill a special need. It represents a joint effort by pharmacists and nurses to provide the nursing profession with drug information that focuses on what nurses need to know. With this in mind, *Nursing98 Drug Handbook* emphasizes clinical aspects of drugs without attempting to replace detailed pharmacology texts. In addition, the information is arranged in a format designed to make it readily accessible.

Features in this edition
The 1998 edition contains several features to enhance nursing knowledge and skills:
• A "New Drug" logo before a generic drug name indicates that the drug was approved by the FDA within the past year.
• A new "New Indications" logo spotlights newly approved uses for existing drugs.
• A new "Effects on Diagnostic Tests" section details possible effects each drug might have on a wide variety of diagnostic tests.
• Adverse reactions are classified five ways to enhance patient safety. (See "Adverse Reactions" later in this chapter for details.)
• An expanded Patient Teaching section gathers all patient-oriented instructions under one heading. (See "Patient Teaching" later in this chapter for details.)
• A colorful "Alert" logo identifies situations that could jeopardize patient safety and suggests ways to avoid harm.
• *NDH98 DrugDisk* (inside back cover) lets the user take two continuing education tests (and earn 7 contact hours), learn and perform dosage calculations, and identify dangerous drug interactions.

Introductory chapters
Chapter 2 explains, in a general way, how drugs work. It also tells about adverse reactions and gives general guidelines about drug use in pregnancy and the presence of drugs in breast milk. Chapters 3 and 4 discuss the unique problems of administering drugs to children and elderly patients and offer guidelines to minimize problems in these areas. Chapter 5 discusses drug therapy as it relates to the nursing process.

Therapeutic class chapters
In chapters 6 to 98, all drugs are classified according to their approved therapeutic uses. Drugs with multiple therapeutic uses are classified according to their most common use; they are also listed (with a cross-reference to the major drug entry) in drug groups that share their secondary applications. For example, nadolol, a beta-adrenergic blocker, is described in the chapter that covers antianginals because its major therapeutic application is the management of angina pectoris. Because the drug is less commonly used to treat hypertension, it is also listed among the generic drugs grouped as antihypertensives, with a cross-reference to Chapter 22, Antianginals.

Such classification by therapeutic use offers several advantages. It helps the reader identify an unknown drug by its clinical application alone. At the same time, it automatically identifies all other drugs that share the same use and provides easy comparison of their dosages and effects. In this way, it quickly identifies potential pharmacotherapeutic alternatives for patients who cannot tolerate or fail to respond to a particular drug.

Each chapter, representing a major

therapeutic use, begins with an alphabetical list of the generic drugs described in that chapter. This is followed by a list of selected combination products in which these drugs are found. Specific information on each drug is arranged under the following headings: *How Supplied; Action; Onset, Peak, Duration; Indications & Dosage; Adverse Reactions; Interactions; Effects on Diagnostic Tests; Contraindications; Nursing Considerations;* and *Patient Teaching.*

In each drug entry, the generic name is followed by an alphabetized list of its brand names. A trade name followed by an open diamond (◊) indicates a drug available in preparations that don't need a prescription. Brands available *only* in Canada are designated with a dagger (†); those available *only* in Australia, with a double dagger (‡). A brand name with no symbol is available in the United States, Canada, and possibly Australia. The mention of a brand name in no way implies endorsement of that product or guarantees its legality.

Alcohol and Tartrazine Content
Many liquid drug preparations for oral use contain alcohol. Although the slight sedative effect that alcohol produces is not harmful in most patients—and can sometimes be beneficial—alcohol ingestion can be undesirable and even dangerous. Oral drugs that contain alcohol should be given cautiously, if at all, to patients who are:
● concomitantly taking potent CNS depressants such as barbiturates
● taking drugs that may produce a disulfiram-type reaction (such as chlorpropamide or metronidazole)
● taking disulfiram as part of a treatment program for their alcoholism.
Such patients, upon ingestion of alcohol, will exhibit severe symptoms that may include blurred vision, confusion, dyspnea, flushing, sweating, and tachycardia.

To help prevent inadvertent exposure to alcohol, the text signals alcohol content with a single asterisk (*) after each brand of a liquid preparation that may contain it. In many of the preparations so marked, the alcohol content is small. Nevertheless, these drugs should be avoided in patients susceptible to adverse effects after exposure to alcohol.

Tartrazine dye, also known as FD&C Yellow No. 5, is a common coloring agent in some foods and drugs. Usually harmless, it can provoke a severe reaction in susceptible persons. For this reason, most drug manufacturers have begun to eliminate tartrazine from their products, but many drugs still contain it.

The incidence of tartrazine sensitivity is approximately 1 in 10,000 in the general population but somewhat higher in persons with asthma or sensitivity to aspirin. Why this is so is unknown. The most common symptoms of tartrazine sensitivity are urticaria, rhinorrhea, asthma, and angioedema. Acutely sensitive persons may develop allergic vascular purpura, tachycardia, dyspnea, and chest pain. These allergic symptoms typically subside spontaneously upon discontinuation of the drug but may require treatment with antihistamines or epinephrine.

Tartrazine may be present in yellow-colored drugs and drugs of many other colors, including turquoise, green, and maroon. This text signals tartrazine content with a double asterisk (**) after each brand that may contain it. If you suspect tartrazine sensitivity in a patient receiving such a drug, inform the doctor and contact the manufacturer to determine which dosage forms contain tartrazine.

Controlled Substance Schedules
If a drug is a controlled substance, that is indicated (example: Controlled Substance Schedule II). Drugs regulated under the jurisdiction of the Controlled Substances Act of 1970 are divided into the following groups, or schedules:
● Schedule I (C-I): High abuse potential

and no accepted medical use—for example, heroin, marijuana, and LSD.
- Schedule II (C-II): High abuse potential with severe dependence liability—for example, narcotics, amphetamines, dronabinol, and some barbiturates.
- Schedule III (C-III): Less abuse potential than schedule II drugs and moderate dependence liability—for example, nonbarbiturate sedatives, nonamphetamine stimulants, and limited amounts of certain narcotics.
- Schedule IV (C-IV): Less abuse potential than schedule III drugs and limited dependence liability—for example, some sedatives, antianxiety agents, nonnarcotic analgesics.
- Schedule V (C-V): Limited abuse potential. Primarily small amounts of narcotics, such as codeine, used as antitussives or antidiarrheals. Under federal law, limited quantities of certain C-V drugs may be purchased without a prescription directly from a pharmacist if allowed under specific state statutes. The purchaser must be at least age 18 and must furnish suitable identification. All such transactions must be recorded by the dispensing pharmacist.

Pregnancy Risk Category
Each systemically absorbed drug has been assigned a pregnancy risk category based upon available clinical and preclinical information. The Pregnancy Risk Category parallels the five Pregnancy Categories (A, B, C, D, and X) assigned by the Food and Drug Administration to reflect a drug's potential to cause birth defects. Although drugs are best avoided during pregnancy, this rating system permits rapid assessment of the risk-benefit ratio should drug administration to a pregnant woman become necessary. Drugs in category A are generally considered safe to use in pregnancy; drugs in category X are generally contraindicated.
- A: Adequate studies in pregnant women have failed to show a risk to the fetus.

- B: Animal studies have not shown a risk to the fetus, but controlled studies have not been conducted in pregnant women; or animal studies have shown an adverse effect on the fetus, but adequate studies in pregnant women have not shown a risk to the fetus.
- C: Animal studies have shown an adverse effect on the fetus, but adequate studies have not been conducted in humans. The benefits from use in pregnant women may be acceptable despite potential risks.
- D: The drug may cause risk to the human fetus, but the potential benefits of use in pregnant women may be acceptable despite the risks.
- X: Studies in animals or humans show fetal abnormalities, or adverse reaction reports indicate evidence of fetal risk. The risks involved clearly outweigh potential benefits.
- NR: Not rated.

How Supplied
This section lists the preparations available for each drug (for example, tablets, capsules, solutions for injection), specifying available dosage forms and strengths. Dosage strengths available *only* in Canada are designated with a dagger (†); those available *only* in Australia, with a double dagger (‡). Preparations that do not require a prescription are marked with an open diamond (◇).

Action
This section succinctly describes the mechanism of action—that is, how the drug provides its therapeutic effect. For example, although all antihypertensives lower blood pressure, they don't all do so by the same pharmacologic process.

Onset, Peak, Duration
This section describes the onset, peak (described in terms of effect or peak blood level), and duration of drug action for each route of administration, if data are available or applicable. Values listed are for patients with normal renal func-

tion, unless specified otherwise.

Indications & Dosage

This section lists general dosage information for adults (including recommended geriatric dosages, when available) and children, as applicable. Dosage instructions reflect current clinical trends in therapeutics and can't be considered as absolute and universal recommendations. For individual application, dosage instructions must be considered in light of the patient's clinical condition.

Adverse Reactions

This section lists adverse reactions to each drug by body system. The most common adverse reactions (those experienced by at least 10% of people taking the drug in clinical trials) are in *italic* type; less common reactions are in roman type; life-threatening reactions are in *bold italic* type; and reactions that are common *and* life-threatening are in BOLD CAPITAL LETTERS.

Interactions

This section lists each drug's confirmed, *clinically significant* interactions with other drugs (additive effects, potentiated effects, and antagonistic effects); foods, with specific suggestions for avoiding dangerous drug or food interactions (for example, by reducing doses or monitoring food intake); or lifestyle (such as alcohol or tobacco use). Drug interactions are listed under the drug that is adversely affected. For example, magnesium trisilicate, an ingredient in antacids, interacts with tetracycline to cause decreased absorption of tetracycline. Therefore, this interaction is listed under tetracycline. To check on the possible effects of using two or more drugs simultaneously, refer to the interaction entry for each of the drugs in question.

Effects on Diagnostic Tests

This section lists significant interference with a diagnostic test or its result by di-

rect effects on the test itself or by systemic drug effects that lead to misleading test results.

Contraindications

This section lists any conditions, especially diseases, in which the use of the drug is undesirable.

Nursing Considerations

This section lists recommendations for cautious use, followed by other useful information, such as monitoring techniques and suggestions for prevention and treatment of adverse reactions. Also included are suggestions for patient comfort and for preparing, administering, and storing each drug. Recommendations for I.V. use are highlighted by **boldface** type.

Patient Teaching

This section focuses on explaining the drug's purpose, promoting compliance, and ensuring proper use and storage of the drug. It also includes instructions for preventing or minimizing adverse reactions.

Photoguide to tablets and capsules

To make drug identification easier for nurses and to enhance patient safety, *Nursing98 Drug Handbook* offers a full-color photoguide to the most commonly prescribed tablets and capsules. Shown in actual size, the drugs are arranged alphabetically for quick reference, along with their most common dosage strengths. Page references to the drugs appear in boldface type in the Index.

A guide to abbreviations

a.c.	before meals
ACE	angiotensin-converting enzyme
AD	right ear
ADH	antidiuretic hormone
AIDS	acquired immunodeficiency syndrome
ALT	alanine aminotransferase
AS	left ear
AST	aspartate aminotransferase
AU	both ears
AV	atrioventricular
b.i.d.	twice daily
BUN	blood urea nitrogen
cAMP	cyclic 3', 5' adenosine monophosphate
CBC	complete blood count
CHF	congestive heart failure
CK	creatine kinase
CMV	cytomegalovirus
CNS	central nervous system
COPD	chronic obstructive pulmonary disease
CSF	cerebrospinal fluid
CV	cardiovascular
CVA	cerebrovascular accident
D_5W	dextrose 5% in water
DNA	deoxyribonucleic acid
ECG	electrocardiogram
EEG	electroencephalogram
EENT	eyes, ears, nose, throat
FDA	Food and Drug Administration
g	gram
G	gauge
GFR	glomerular filtration rate
GI	gastrointestinal
GU	genitourinary
G6PD	glucose-6-phosphate dehydrogenase
H_1	histamine$_1$
H_2	histamine$_2$
HIV	human immunodeficiency virus
h.s.	at bedtime
I.D.	intradermal
I.M.	intramuscular
IND	investigational new drug
INR	international normalized ratio
IPPB	intermittent positive-pressure breathing
IU	international unit
I.V.	intravenous
kg	kilogram
M	molar
m^2	square meter
MAO	monoamine oxidase
mcg	microgram
mEq	milliequivalent
mg	milligram
MI	myocardial infarction
ml	milliliter
mm^3	cubic millimeter
Na	sodium
NaCl	sodium chloride
NSAID	nonsteroidal anti-inflammatory drug
OD	right eye
OS	left eye
OTC	over the counter
OU	both eyes
PABA	para-aminobenzoic acid
p.c.	after meals
PCA	patient-controlled analgesia
P.O.	by mouth
P.R.	by rectum
p.r.n.	as needed
PT	prothrombin time
PTT	partial thromboplastin time
PVCs	premature ventricular contractions
q	every
q.d.	every day
q.i.d.	four times daily
q.o.d.	every other day
RBC	red blood cell
RDA	recommended daily allowance
REM	rapid eye movement
RNA	ribonucleic acid
RSV	respiratory syncytial virus
SA	sinoatrial
S.C.	subcutaneous
SIADH	syndrome of inappropriate antidiuretic hormone
S.L.	sublingual
ss̄	one half
stat	at once
U	units
T_3	triiodothyronine
T_4	thyroxine
t.i.d.	three times daily
UCE	urea cycle enzymopathy
USP	United States Pharmacopeia
WBC	white blood cell

2

Drug actions, reactions, and interactions

Administration of any drug provokes a series of physicochemical events within the body. The first event, when a drug combines with cellular drug receptors, is known as the drug action. What follows as a result of this action of the drug is known as the drug effect. Depending on the number of different cellular drug receptors affected by a given drug, a drug effect can be local, systemic, or both. Obviously, a local effect follows application to the skin; however, transdermal absorption can produce systemic effects. Moreover, local effects can follow systemic absorption. For example, the antipeptic ulcer drug cimetidine acts solely by blocking histamine receptor cells in the parietal cells of the stomach. This is known as a local drug effect because the drug action is sharply limited to one area and does not spread to other parts of the body. On the other hand, diphenhydramine produces a systemic effect in that it blocks histamine receptors in widespread areas of the body. In other words, local drug effects are specific to a limited number of organ systems, whereas systemic drug effects are generalized and affect different and diverse organ systems.

Four important drug properties
1. Absorption
Before a drug can act within the body, it must be absorbed into the bloodstream—usually after oral administration, the most frequently used route. Before a drug contained in a tablet or capsule can be absorbed, the dosage form must disintegrate—that is, break into smaller particles. Then these smaller particles can dissolve in gastric juices. Only after so dissolving can a drug be absorbed. Most absorption of orally administered drugs occurs in the small intestine, where the mucosal villi provide extensive surface area. Once absorbed and circulated in the bloodstream, it is bio-available, or ready to produce a drug effect. Whether such absorption is complete or partial depends on several factors: the drug's physicochemical effects, its dosage form, its route of administration, its interactions with other substances in the GI tract, and various patient characteristics. These same factors also determine the speed of absorption. Thus, oral solutions and elixirs, which bypass the need for disintegration and dissolution, are usually absorbed more rapidly. Some tablets have enteric coatings that prevent disintegration in the acidic environment of the stomach; others may have coatings of varying thickness that delay release of the drug.

Drugs administered intramuscularly must first be absorbed through the muscle into the bloodstream. Rectal suppositories must dissolve to be absorbed through the rectal mucosa. Drugs administered intravenously, which are injected directly into the bloodstream, are completely and immediately bioavailable.

2. Distribution
After absorption, a drug moves from the bloodstream into various fluids and tissues within the body; this is distribution. Individual patient variations can greatly alter the amount of drug that is distributed throughout the body. For example, in an edematous patient, a given dose must be distributed to a larger volume than in a nonedematous patient; the amount of drug must sometimes be increased to account for this. Remember, the dose should be decreased when the edema is corrected. Conversely, in an extremely dehydrated patient, the drug will be distributed to a much smaller volume, so the dose must then be decreased. The total area to which a drug

is distributed is known as volume of distribution. Patients who are particularly obese may present another problem when considering drug distribution. Some drugs—such as digoxin, gentamicin, and tobramycin—are not well distributed to fatty tissue. Therefore, dosing based on actual body weight may lead to overdose and serious toxicity. In some cases, dosing must be based on lean body weight, which may be estimated from actuarial tables that give average weight range for height.

3. Metabolism

Most drugs are metabolized in the liver. Hepatic diseases may affect one or more of the metabolic functions of the liver. Therefore, in patients with hepatic disease, the metabolism of a drug may be increased, decreased, or unchanged. Clearly, all patients with hepatic disease must be monitored closely for drug effect and toxicity.

The rate at which a drug is metabolized varies with the individual. In some patients, drugs are metabolized so quickly that their blood and tissue levels prove therapeutically inadequate. In others, the rate of metabolism is so slow that ordinary doses can produce toxic results.

4. Excretion

The body eliminates drugs by metabolism (usually hepatic) and excretion (usually renal). Drug excretion refers to the movement of a drug or its metabolites from the tissues back into circulation and from the circulation into the organs of excretion where they are removed from the body. Although most drugs are excreted by the kidneys, some drugs can be eliminated via the lungs, exocrine glands (sweat, salivary, or mammary), liver, skin, and intestinal tract. Drugs may also be removed artificially by direct interventions, such as peritoneal dialysis or hemodialysis.

Other modifying factors

An important factor that influences a drug's action and effect is its *binding to plasma proteins,* especially albumin, and other tissue components. Because only a free, unbound drug can act in the body, such binding greatly influences effectiveness and duration of effect. Protein binding can be influenced by malnutrition, renal failure, and other protein-bound drugs. When protein binding occurs, drug dosing may need to be modified.

The *patient's age* is another important factor. Elderly patients usually have decreased hepatic function, less muscle mass, and diminished renal function. Consequently, they need lower doses and sometimes longer dosage intervals to avoid toxicity. With similar consequences, neonates have underdeveloped metabolic enzyme systems and inadequate renal function. They need highly individualized dosages and careful monitoring.

Underlying disease can also markedly affect drug action and effect. For example, acidosis may cause insulin resistance. Genetic diseases, such as G6PD deficiency and hepatic porphyria, may turn drugs into toxins with serious consequences. Patients with G6PD deficiency may develop hemolytic anemia when given sulfonamides or a number of other drugs. A genetically susceptible patient can develop an acute porphyria attack if given a barbiturate. Also, patients who have highly active hepatic enzyme systems (for example, rapid acetylators), when treated with isoniazid, can develop hepatitis from the rapid intrahepatic buildup of a toxic metabolite.

Things to consider about administration

● *Dosage forms do matter.* Some tablets and capsules are too large to be easily swallowed by very ill patients. You may then request an oral solution or elixir of the same drug, but bear in mind that because a liquid is more easily and completely absorbed, it produces higher blood levels than a tablet. When a potentially toxic drug (such as digoxin) is given, the increased amount absorbed could cause toxicity. Sometimes a change in dosage form requires a change in dosage.

• *Routes of administration are not therapeutically interchangeable.* For example, diazepam is readily absorbed orally but is slowly and erratically absorbed intramuscularly. On the other hand, gentamicin must be given parenterally because oral administration yields inadequate blood levels to treat systemic infections.

• *Improper storage can alter a drug's potency.* Most drugs should be stored in tight containers protected from direct sunlight and extremes in temperature and humidity that can cause them to deteriorate. Some may require special storage conditions, such as refrigeration.

• *The timing of drug administration can be important.* Sometimes, giving an oral drug during or shortly after mealtime decreases the amount of drug absorbed. This is not clinically significant with most drugs and may in fact be desirable with irritating drugs, such as aspirin. But penicillins and tetracyclines should not be scheduled for administration at mealtimes because certain foods can inactivate them. If in doubt about the effect of food on a certain drug, check with the pharmacist.

• *Consider the patient's age, height, and weight.* The doctor will need this information when calculating the dosage for many drugs. It should be accurately recorded on the patient's chart. This chart should also include current laboratory data, especially renal and liver function studies, so the doctor can adjust the dosage as needed.

• *Watch for metabolic changes.* Monitor for any physiologic change (depressed respiratory function, acidosis or alkalosis) that might alter drug effect.

• *Know the patient's history.* Whenever possible, obtain a comprehensive family history from the patient or his family. Ask about past reactions to drugs, possible genetic traits that might alter drug response, and the current use of other drugs. Multiple drug therapy can cause drug interactions that can dramatically change the effects of many drugs.

Drug interactions

When one drug administered in combination with or shortly after another drug alters the effect of one or both drugs, this is known as a drug interaction. Usually, the effect of one drug is increased or decreased. For instance, one drug may inhibit or stimulate the metabolism or excretion of the other, or it may release another from plasma protein-binding sites, freeing it for further action.

Combination therapy is based on drug interaction. One drug, for example, may be given to potentiate another. Probenecid, which blocks the excretion of penicillin, is sometimes given with penicillin to maintain adequate blood levels of penicillin for a longer period. Often, two drugs with similar actions are given together precisely because of the additive effect that results. For instance, aspirin and codeine, both analgesics, are often given in combination because together they provide greater pain relief than either alone.

Drug interactions are sometimes used to prevent or antagonize certain adverse reactions. Hydrochlorothiazide and spironolactone, both diuretics, are often administered in combination because the former is potassium-depleting, whereas the latter is potassium-sparing.

But not all drug interactions are beneficial. Multiple drugs can interact to produce effects that are often undesirable and sometimes hazardous. Harmful drug interactions decrease efficacy or increase toxicity. For example, in a patient taking both diuretics and lithium, the diuretics may cause an increase in serum levels of lithium, resulting in lithium toxicity. Such a drug effect is known as antagonism. Drug combinations that produce these effects should be avoided if possible. Another kind of inhibiting effect occurs when a tetracycline drug is administered with calcium- or magnesium-containing drugs or foods (such as antacids or milk). These combine with tetracycline in the GI tract and cause inadequate absorption of tetracycline.

Adverse reactions

Any drug effect other than what is therapeutically intended can be called an adverse reaction. It may be expected and benign or unexpected and potentially harmful. Mild, but *predictable,* adverse reactions are sometimes called side effects. Drowsiness caused by antihistamines is an example of this. During hay fever season, a patient may have to contend with this drowsiness to get relief from hay fever symptoms. In such a case, the dosage may be adjusted up or down to balance therapeutic effects with side effects.

An adverse reaction may be tolerated for a necessary therapeutic effect, or it may be hazardous and unacceptable and require discontinuation of the drug. Some adverse reactions subside with continued use. As an example, the drowsiness associated with paroxetine and the orthostatic hypotension associated with prazosin usually subside after several days, as the patient develops a tolerance to these effects. But many adverse reactions are dosage-related and lessen or disappear only if the dosage is reduced. Although most adverse reactions are not therapeutically desirable, an occasional one can be put to clinical use. An outstanding example of this is the drowsiness associated with diphenhydramine, which makes it clinically useful as a mild hypnotic.

Hypersensitivity, a term sometimes used interchangeably with drug allergy, is the result of an antigen-antibody immune reaction that occurs in the body when a drug is given to a susceptible patient. One of the most dangerous of all drug hypersensitivities is penicillin allergy. In its severest form, penicillin anaphylaxis can rapidly become fatal.

Rarely, idiosyncratic reactions occur. These are highly unpredictable, individual, and unusual. Probably the best known idiosyncratic drug reaction is the aplastic anemia caused by the antibiotic chloramphenicol. This reaction appears in only 1 out of 40,000 patients, but when it does, it can be fatal. A more common idiosyncratic reaction is extreme sensitivity to very low doses of a drug, or insensitivity to higher-than-normal doses.

To deal with adverse reactions correctly, you need to be alert to even minor changes in the patient's clinical status. Such minor changes may be an early warning of pending toxicity. Listen to the patient's complaints about his reactions to a drug, and consider each complaint objectively. You may be able to reduce adverse reactions in several ways. Obviously, dosage reduction often helps. But often so does a simple rescheduling of the same dose. For example, pseudoephedrine may produce stimulation that will be no problem if it's given early in the day; similarly, the drowsiness that occurs with antihistamines or tranquilizers can be totally harmless if the dose is given at bedtime. Most important, your patient needs to be told what adverse reactions to expect so he won't become worried or even stop taking the drug on his own. Of course, the patient should report any unusual or unexpected adverse reactions to the doctor.

Recognizing drug allergies or serious idiosyncratic reactions can sometimes be lifesaving. Ask each patient about drugs he is taking or has taken in the past and what, if any, unusual reactions he experienced from taking them. If a patient claims to be allergic to a drug, ask him to tell you exactly what happens when he takes it. He may be calling a harmless side effect such as upset stomach an allergic reaction, or he may have a true tendency toward anaphylaxis. In either case, you and the doctor need to know this. Of course, you must record and report any clinical changes throughout the patient's hospital stay. If you suspect a severe adverse reaction, withhold the drug until you can check with the pharmacist and the doctor.

Toxic reactions

Chronic drug toxicities are generally caused by the cumulative effect and resulting buildup of the drug in the body. These effects may be extensions of the desired therapeutic effect. For example, glyburide will normalize blood sugar when given in usual doses but can produce undesired hypoglycemia if given in larger doses.

Drug toxicities typically occur when drug blood levels rise due to impaired metabolism or excretion. For example, blood levels of theophylline rise when hepatic dysfunction impairs metabolism of the drug. Similarly, digoxin toxicity can follow impaired renal function because digoxin is eliminated from the body almost exclusively by the kidneys (via glomerular filtration). Of course, toxic blood levels also follow excessive dosage. Aspirin tinnitus is usually a sign that the safe dose has been exceeded.

Most drug toxicities are predictable and dosage-related; fortunately, most are also readily reversible upon dosage adjustment. So be sure to monitor patients carefully for physiologic changes that might alter drug effect. Watch especially for impaired hepatic and renal function. Warn the patient about signs of pending toxicity, and tell him what to do if a toxic reaction occurs. Also, be sure to emphasize the importance of taking a drug exactly as prescribed. Warn the patient about serious problems that could arise if he changes the dose or the schedule for taking it.

Drugs and pregnancy

Ever since the thalidomide tragedy of the late 1950s—when thousands of malformed infants were born after their mothers used this mild sedative-hypnotic during pregnancy—use of drugs during pregnancy has been a source of serious medical concern and controversy. To identify drugs that may cause such teratogenic effects, preclinical drug studies always include tests on pregnant laboratory animals. These tests point out gross teratogenicity but do not clearly establish safety. Because different species react to drugs in different ways, animal studies do not rule out possible teratogenic effects in humans. For example, the preliminary studies on thalidomide gave no warning of teratogenic effects, and it was subsequently released for general use in Europe.

What about the placental barrier? Once thought to protect the fetus from drug effects, the placenta isn't actually much of a barrier at all. Except for drugs with exceptionally large molecular structure, almost every drug administered to a pregnant woman crosses the placenta and enters the fetal circulation. An example of a drug with a large molecular size is heparin, the injectable anticoagulant. Theoretically, then, heparin could be used in a pregnant woman without fear of harming the fetus—but even heparin carries a warning for cautious use in pregnancy. Conversely, just because a drug crosses the placenta doesn't necessarily mean it's harmful to the fetus.

Actually, only one factor—stage of fetal development—seems clearly related to exaggerated risk during pregnancy. During two stages of pregnancy—the first and the third trimesters—the fetus is especially vulnerable to damage from maternal use of drugs. During these times, *all* drugs should be given with extreme caution.

The most sensitive period for drug-induced fetal malformation is the first trimester, when fetal organs are differentiating (organogenesis). During this time, *all* drugs, except those labeled as category A or B, should be withheld unless doing so would jeopardize the mother's health. Theoretically, during this sensitive time, even aspirin could harm the fetus. So, strongly advise your patient to avoid *all* self-prescribed drugs during early pregnancy. The other time of special fetal sensitivity to drugs is the last trimester. The reason? At birth, when separated from his mother, the neonate must rely on his own metabolism to eliminate any remaining drug. Because his detoxifying systems are not fully developed, any residual drug may take a long time to be metabolized—and thus may induce prolonged toxic reactions. Consequently, drugs should be used only when absolutely necessary during the last 3 months of pregnancy.

Of course, in many circumstances, pregnant women must continue to take certain drugs. For example, a woman with a seizure disorder that is well controlled with an anticonvulsant should continue to take the drug even during pregnancy. Similarly, a pregnant woman with a bacterial infection must receive antibiotics. In such cases, the potential risk to the fetus is outweighed by the mother's need. The relative risk to the fetus is expressed by the drug's pregnancy risk category (see Chapter 1).

Following these general guidelines can prevent indiscriminate and potentially harmful use of drugs in pregnancy:
● Before a drug is prescribed for a woman of childbearing age, she should be asked the date of her last menstrual period and whether she may be pregnant. If a drug is a known teratogen (for example, isotretinoin), some manufacturers may recommend special precautions to ensure that the drug not be given to a female of childbearing age until pregnancy is ruled out.
● Especially during the first and the third trimesters, a pregnant patient should avoid *all* drugs except those *essential* to maintain the pregnancy or maternal health.
● Topical drugs are not exempt from the warning against indiscriminate use during pregnancy. Many topically applied drugs can be absorbed in large enough amounts to be harmful to the fetus.
● When a pregnant patient needs *any* drug, the doctor should prescribe the *safest* possible drug in the *lowest* possible dose to minimize any harmful effect to the fetus.
● Every pregnant patient should check with her doctor before taking *any* drug.

Drugs and lactation
Most drugs a mother takes appear in breast milk. Drug levels in breast milk tend to be high when blood levels are high—generally, shortly after taking each dose. Therefore, the mother should be advised to breast-feed *before* taking medication, not *after*.

Nevertheless, with very few exceptions, a mother who wishes to breast-feed may continue to do so with her doctor's permission. However, breast-feeding should be temporarily interrupted and replaced with bottle-feeding when the mother must take tetracyclines, chloramphenicol, sulfonamides (during first 2 weeks postpartum), oral anticoagulants, iodine-containing drugs, or antineoplastics.

To protect her infant, a breast-feeding mother should avoid taking drugs indiscriminately. If she needs to take a drug, she should first check with her doctor to be sure of taking the safest drug at the lowest dose.

What to teach patients about proper use of drugs
The following general guidelines will help to ensure that the patient gets maximal therapeutic benefits and avoids adverse reactions, accidental overdose, or potentially harmful changes in effectiveness:
● Store drugs in their original containers, at room temperature (unless directed otherwise), in places that are not accessible to children or exposed to sunlight. Avoid storage in the bathroom medicine cabinet or the glove compartment or trunk of an automobile, where

extremes of temperature and humidity will cause them to deteriorate.

● Learn the trade name and generic name of any drug you are taking. Be sure to tell doctors, nurses, dentists, or other health care professionals you see regularly that you are taking it. Before taking any drug, be sure you have informed your doctor, nurse, or pharmacist about any unusual reactions you've had to drugs in the past and about your allergies to foods and other substances, any special medical problems, and any drugs you've taken over the last few weeks, including any OTC drugs.

● Always read the label before taking any drug, and take the drug exactly as prescribed at the recommended dosage and for the duration of treatment. Never share prescription drugs.

● When using a drug prescribed for occasional or prolonged use, check the container for an expiration date.

● To avoid potentially harmful changes in effectiveness, do not change brands of a drug without medical approval. Certain generic preparations are not precisely equivalent in effect to brand-name preparations of the same drug.

● Never mix different drugs in a single container, and don't remove any drug from its original container or remove the label. Relying on your memory to identify a drug and specific directions for its use is hazardous.

● Discard any drugs that are outdated or no longer needed.

● Before you have any surgery (including dental surgery), tell the doctor about all the drugs that you have been taking.

● Be sure to tell the doctor, nurse, or pharmacist about any adverse reactions you've experienced while taking a drug.

● If you or someone else has taken an overdose, call your doctor, poison control center, or pharmacist immediately. Keep syrup of ipecac in your home to induce vomiting, but induce vomiting only if one of these professionals advises you to do so.

● Try to have all your prescriptions filled at the same pharmacy so that the pharmacist can identify and warn against potentially harmful drug interactions. Inform the pharmacist and doctor of any OTC drugs you're taking.

● Be sure to bring ample supplies of your drugs with you when you travel.

3

Drug therapy in children

A child's absorption, distribution, metabolism, and excretion processes undergo profound changes that affect drug dosage. To ensure optimal drug effect and minimal toxicity, consider these factors when administering drugs to a child.

Absorption

Drug absorption in children depends on the form of the drug; its physical properties; other drugs or substances, such as food, taken simultaneously; physiologic changes; and concurrent disease.

● The pH of neonatal gastric fluid is neutral or slightly acidic and becomes more acidic as the infant matures. This affects drug absorption. For example, nafcillin and penicillin G are better absorbed in an infant than in an adult because of low gastric acidity.

● Various infant formulas or milk products may increase gastric pH and impede absorption of acidic drugs. So, if possible, give a child oral medications on an empty stomach.

● Gastric emptying time and transit time through the small intestine—which is longer in children than in adults—can affect absorption. Also, intestinal hypermotility (as in diarrhea) can diminish the drug's absorption.

● A child's comparatively thin epidermis allows increased absorption of topical drugs.

Distribution

As with absorption, changes in body weight and physiology during childhood can significantly influence a drug's distribution and effects. In a premature infant, body fluid makes up about 85% of total body weight; in a full-term infant, 55% to 70%; and in an adult, 50% to 55%. Extracellular fluid (mostly blood) constitutes 40% of a neonate's body weight, compared with 20% in an adult. Intracellular fluid remains fairly constant throughout life and has little effect on drug dosage.

Extracellular fluid volume influences a water-soluble drug's concentration and effect because most drugs travel through extracellular fluid to reach their receptors. Children have a larger proportion of fluid to solid body weight, so their distribution area is proportionately greater.

Because the proportion of fat to lean body mass increases with age, the distribution of fat-soluble drugs is more limited in children than adults. As a result, a drug's lipid or water solubility affects the dosage for a child.

Binding to plasma proteins

As the result of a decrease in albumin concentration or intermolecular attraction between drug and plasma protein, many drugs are less bound to plasma proteins in infants than in adults.

Furthermore, preparations that bind plasma proteins may displace endogenous compounds, such as bilirubin or free fatty acids. Conversely, an endogenous compound may displace a weakly bound drug. For example, displacement of bound bilirubin can cause a rise in unbound bilirubin, which can lead to increased risk of kernicterus at normal bilirubin levels.

Since only an unbound, or free, drug has a pharmacologic effect, any alteration in ratio of a protein-bound to an unbound active drug can greatly influence its effect.

Several diseases and disorders, such as nephrotic syndrome and malnutrition, can also decrease plasma protein and increase the concentration of an unbound drug, intensifying the drug's effect or producing toxicity.

Metabolism

A neonate's ability to metabolize a drug depends on the integrity of the hepatic enzyme system, the intrauterine exposure to the drug, and the nature of the drug itself.

Certain metabolic mechanisms are underdeveloped in neonates. Glucuronidation is a metabolic process that renders most drugs more water soluble, thereby facilitating renal excretion. This process is insufficiently developed to permit full pediatric doses until the infant is 1 month old. Because of this, the use of chloramphenicol in a neonate may cause gray syndrome, illustrating the infant's inability to metabolize the drug. Use of chloramphenicol in neonates, therefore, requires decreased dosage (25 mg/kg/day) and monitoring of blood levels.

Conversely, intrauterine exposure to drugs may induce precocious development of hepatic enzyme mechanisms, increasing the infant's capacity to metabolize potentially harmful substances.

Older children can metabolize some drugs (theophylline, for example) more rapidly than adults. This ability may come from their increased hepatic metabolic activity. Larger doses than those recommended for adults may be required.

Also, preparations given concurrently to a child may alter hepatic metabolism and induce production of hepatic enzymes. Phenobarbital, for example, can induce hepatic enzyme production and accelerate metabolism of drugs given concurrently.

Excretion

Renal excretion of a drug is the net effect of glomerular filtration, active tubular secretion, and passive tubular reabsorption. Because so many drugs are excreted in the urine, the degree of renal development or presence of renal disease can profoundly affect a child's dosage requirements.

If a child is unable to excrete a drug renally, drug accumulation and possible toxicity may result unless the dosage is reduced.

Physiologically, an infant's kidneys differ from an adult's in that they have:
● high resistance to blood flow and receive a smaller proportion of cardiac output
● incomplete glomerular and tubular development and short, incomplete loops of Henle (A child's glomerular filtration reaches adult values between ages 2½ to 5 months; his tubular secretion may reach adult values between ages 7 to 12 months.)
● low glomerular filtration rate (Penicillins are eliminated by this route.)
● decreased ability to concentrate urine or reabsorb various filtered compounds
● reduced ability of the proximal tubules to secrete organic acids.

Both children and adults have diurnal variations in urine pH that correlate with sleep-awake patterns.

Calculating and monitoring pediatric dosages

When calculating pediatric dosages, don't use formulas that modify adult dosages: A child is not a scaled-down version of an adult. Pediatric dosages should be calculated on the basis of either body weight (mg/kg) or body surface area (mg/m²).
● Reevaluate dosages at regular intervals to ensure necessary adjustments as the child develops.
● Although body surface area provides a useful standard for adults and older children, don't use it in premature or full-term infants. Use the body weight method instead.
● Don't exceed the maximum adult dosage when calculating amounts per kilogram of body weight (except with certain drugs, such as theophylline, if indicated).
● Obtain an accurate maternal drug history—prescription and nonprescription drugs, vitamins, and herbs or other health foods taken during pregnancy.

● Drugs passed through breast milk can also have adverse effects on the breast-feeding infant. Before a drug is prescribed for a breast-feeding mother, the potential effects on the infant should be investigated. For example, sulfonamides given to a breast-feeding mother for a urinary tract infection appear in breast milk and may cause kernicterus at lower-than-normal levels of unconjugated bilirubin. Also, high concentrations of isoniazid appear in breast milk. Since this drug is metabolized by the liver, an infant's immature hepatic enzyme mechanisms cannot metabolize the drug, and the infant may suffer CNS toxicity.

Oral medications
● *When giving oral medication to an infant,* administer it in liquid form if possible. For accuracy, measure and give the preparation by syringe; never use a vial or cup.
● Lift the patient's head to prevent aspiration of the medication, and press down on his chin to prevent choking.
● You may also place the drug in a nipple and allow the infant to suck the contents.
● *If the patient is a toddler,* explain how you're going to give him the medication. If possible, have the parents enlist the child's cooperation.
● Don't mix medication with food or call it "candy," even if it has a pleasant taste.
● Let the child drink liquid medication from a calibrated medication cup rather than from a spoon: It's easier and more accurate. If the preparation is available only in tablet form, crush it and mix it with a compatible syrup. (Check with the pharmacist to verify that the tablet can be crushed without compromising its effectiveness.)
● *If the patient is an older child* who can swallow a tablet or capsule by himself, have him place the medication on the back of his tongue and swallow it with water or fruit juice. Remember,

milk or milk products may interfere with drug absorption.

I.V. infusions
When administering I.V. infusions to children, note the following special considerations.

Protecting the insertion site
In infants, use a peripheral vein or a scalp vein in the temporal region for I.V. infusions. The scalp vein is safest in that the needle is not likely to be dislodged; however, the head must be shaved around the site. Temporary disfigurement may also result from the needle and infiltrated fluids. For these reasons, the scalp veins are not used as frequently today as they were in the past.

The extremities are the most accessible insertion sites; however, since patients tend to move about, take these precautions:
● Protect the insertion site to prevent catheter or needle dislodgment.
● Use a padded arm board to minimize dislodgment. Remove the arm board during range-of-motion exercises.
● Place the clamp out of the child's reach; if extension tubing is used to allow the child greater mobility, securely tape the connection.
● Restrain the child only when necessary.
● To allay anxiety, give a simple explanation to the child who must be restrained while asleep.

Maintaining flow rate and fluid balance
While administering an I.V. infusion to a child, monitor flow rate and check the patient's condition and insertion site at least hourly—more frequently if indicated.

Adjust the flow rate only while the patient is composed; crying and emotional upset can constrict blood vessels. Flow rate may vary if a pump isn't used. Flow should be adequate because some drugs (calcium, for example) can be very irritating at low flow rates. Infants, small children, and children with compromised cardiopulmonary status are particularly vulnerable to fluid overload with I.V. medication administration. To prevent this problem and help ensure that a limited amount of fluid is infused in a controlled manner, use a volume-control set (a volume-control device in the I.V. tubing) and an infusion pump or a syringe. Do not place more than 2 hours worth of I.V. fluid at a time in the volume-control set.

I.M. injections

I.M. injections are preferred when the drug cannot be given by other parenteral routes and rapid absorption is necessary.

● In children under age 2, the vastus lateralis muscle is the preferred injection site; in older children, either the ventrogluteal area or the gluteus medius muscle can be used.

● To determine correct needle size, consider the patient's age, muscle mass, and nutritional status and the drug's viscosity; record and rotate injection sites.

● Explain to the patient that the injection will hurt, but that the medication will help him. Restrain him during the injection, if needed, and comfort him afterward.

Topical medications and inhalants

● Use ear drops warmed to room temperature; cold drops can cause considerable pain and possibly vertigo.

● To administer drops, turn the patient on his side, with the affected ear up. If he is under age 3, pull the pinna down and back; if he is age 3 or over, pull the pinna up and back.

● Avoid using inhalants in very young children: obtaining their cooperation is difficult.

● Before attempting to administer medication through a metered-dose nebulizer to an older child, explain the inhaler to him. Then have him hold the nebulizer upside down and close his lips around the mouthpiece. Have him exhale, pinch his nostrils shut and, when

he starts to inhale, release one dose of medication into his mouth. Tell the patient to continue inhaling until his lungs feel full.

● Most inhaled agents are not useful if taken orally; therefore, if you doubt the patient's ability to use the inhalant correctly, don't use it.

● Use topical corticosteroids with caution because chronic steroid use in children has been associated with delayed growth. When topical corticosteroids are used on the diaper area of infants, avoid covering this area with plastic or rubber pants, which will act as an occlusive dressing and enhance systemic absorption.

Parenteral nutrition

I.V. nutrition is given to patients who can't or won't take adequate food orally and patients with hypermetabolic conditions who need supplementation. The latter group includes premature infants and children who have burns or other major trauma, intractable diarrhea, malabsorption syndromes, GI abnormalities, emotional disorders (such as anorexia nervosa), and congenital abnormalities.

Before fat emulsions are administered to infants and children, however, potential benefits must be weighed against possible risks.

Fats—supplied as 10% or 20% emulsions—are administered both peripherally and centrally. Their use is limited by the child's ability to metabolize them. An infant or a child with a diseased liver cannot efficiently metabolize fats, for example.

Some fats, however, must be supplied both to prevent essential fatty acid deficiency and to permit normal growth and development. A minimum of calories (2% to 4%) must be supplied as linoleic acid—an essential fatty acid found in lipids. In infants, fats are essential for normal neurologic development.

Nevertheless, fat solutions may decrease oxygen perfusion and may adversely affect children with pulmonary disease. This risk can be minimized by supplying only the minimum fat needed for essential fatty acid requirements and not the usual intake of 40% to 50% of the child's total calories.

Fatty acids can also displace bilirubin bound to serum albumin, causing a rise in free, unconjugated bilirubin and an increased risk of kernicterus. However, fat solutions may interfere with some bilirubin assays and cause falsely elevated levels. To avoid this complication, a blood sample should be drawn 4 hours after infusion of the lipid emulsion; or if the emulsion is introduced over 24 hours, the blood sample should be centrifuged before the assay is performed.

Drug therapy in elderly patients

If you're providing drug therapy for elderly patients, you'll want to understand physiologic and pharmacokinetic changes that may alter appropriate drug dosage or cause common adverse reactions or compliance problems in elderly patients.

Physiologic changes affecting drug action

As a person ages, gradual physiologic changes occur. Some of these age-related changes may alter the therapeutic and toxic effects of medications.

Body composition

Proportions of fat, lean tissue, and water in the body change with age. Total body mass and lean body mass tend to decrease; the proportion of body fat tends to increase.

Varying from person to person, these changes in body composition affect the relationship between a drug's concentration and distribution in the body.

For example, a water-soluble drug, such as gentamicin, is not distributed to fat. Since there's relatively less lean tissue in an elderly person, more drug remains in the blood.

GI function

In elderly patients, decreases in gastric acid secretion and GI motility slow the emptying of stomach contents and the movement of intestinal contents through the entire tract. Furthermore, research suggests that elderly patients may have more difficulty absorbing medications. This is a particularly significant problem with drugs having a narrow therapeutic range, such as digoxin, in which any change in absorption can be crucial.

Hepatic function

The liver's ability to metabolize certain drugs decreases with age. This is caused by diminished blood flow to the liver, which results from the age-related decrease in cardiac output and from the diminished activity of certain liver enzymes. When an elderly patient takes certain sleep medications, such as flurazepam, the liver's reduced ability to metabolize the drug may produce a hangover effect the next morning.

Decreased hepatic function may cause:
- more intense drug effects due to higher blood levels
- longer-lasting drug effects due to prolonged blood concentrations
- greater incidence of drug toxicity.

Renal function

Although an elderly person's renal function is usually sufficient to eliminate excess body fluid and waste, the ability to eliminate some medications may be reduced by 50% or more.

Many medications commonly used by elderly patients, such as digoxin, are excreted primarily through the kidneys. If the kidneys' ability to excrete the drug is decreased, high blood concentrations may result. Digoxin toxicity, therefore, is relatively common in elderly patients who are not receiving a reduced digoxin dosage that accommodates decreased renal function.

Drug dosages can be modified to compensate for age-related decreases in renal function. Aided by laboratory tests, such as blood urea nitrogen and serum creatinine, doctors may adjust medication dosages so the patient receives the expected therapeutic benefits without the risk of toxicity. Observe your patient for signs of toxicity. A patient taking digoxin, for example, may experience anorexia, nausea, vomiting, or confusion.

Adverse drug reactions

Compared with younger people, elderly patients experience twice as many adverse drug reactions relating to greater drug consumption, poor compliance, and physiologic changes.

Signs and symptoms of adverse drug reactions—confusion, weakness, and lethargy—are often mistakenly attributed to senility or disease. If the adverse reaction isn't identified, the patient may continue to receive the drug. Furthermore, he may receive unnecessary additional medication to treat complications caused by the original medication. This can sometimes result in a pattern of inappropriate and excessive medication use.

Although any medication can cause adverse reactions, most of the serious reactions in the elderly are caused by relatively few medications. Be particularly alert for toxicities resulting from diuretics, antihypertensives, digoxin, corticosteroids, sleeping aids, and nonprescription drugs.

Diuretic toxicity

Because total body water content decreases with age, normal dosages of potassium-wasting diuretics, such as hydrochlorothiazide and furosemide, may result in fluid loss and even dehydration in an elderly patient.

These diuretics may deplete serum potassium, causing weakness in the patient, and they may raise blood uric acid and glucose levels, complicating preexisting gout and diabetes mellitus.

Antihypertensive toxicity

Many elderly people experience light-headedness or fainting when using antihypertensive medications, partly in response to atherosclerosis and decreased elasticity of the blood vessels. Antihypertensive drugs lower blood pressure too rapidly, resulting in insufficient blood flow to the brain. This may cause dizziness, fainting, or even stroke.

Consequently, dosages of antihypertensive drugs must be carefully individualized. In elderly patients, too aggressive treatment of high blood pressure may do more harm than good, so treatment goals should be reasonable. Although bringing blood pressure down to 120/85 mm Hg may be appropriate in a young hypertensive patient, a more reasonable goal for an elderly hypertensive patient might be 150/95 mm Hg.

Digoxin toxicity

As the body's renal function and rate of excretion decline, digoxin concentrations in the blood may build to toxic levels, causing nausea, vomiting, diarrhea, and—most serious—cardiac arrhythmias. Try to prevent severe toxicity by monitoring serum levels and by observing your patient for early signs, such as appetite loss, confusion, or depression.

Corticosteroid toxicity

Elderly patients on corticosteroids may experience short-term effects, including fluid retention and psychological manifestations ranging from mild euphoria to acute psychotic reactions. Long-term toxic effects, such as osteoporosis, can be especially severe in elderly patients who have been taking prednisone or related steroidal compounds for months or even years. To prevent serious toxicity, carefully monitor patients on long-term regimens. Observe them for subtle changes in appearance, mood, and mobility, as well as for signs of impaired healing and fluid and electrolyte disturbances.

Anticoagulants

Elderly patients taking anticoagulants have an increased risk of bleeding, expecially when they take NSAIDs at the same time (many do). Observe international normalized ratios carefully, and monitor the patient for bruising and other signs of bleeding.

Sleeping aid toxicity
Sedatives or sleeping aids, such as flu-razepam, may cause excessive sedation or residual drowsiness. Keep in mind that ingestion of alcohol may exagger-ate such depressant effects, even if the sleeping aid was taken the previous evening.

Nonprescription drug toxicity
When aspirin, aspirin-containing anal-gesics, and other nonprescription NSAIDs (ibuprofen, latoprofen, naprox-en) are used in moderation, toxicity is minimal, but prolonged ingestion may cause GI irritation—even ulcers—and gradual blood loss resulting in severe anemia. Prescription NSAIDs may cause similar problems, especially in the elderly. Although anemia from chronic aspirin consumption can affect all age-groups, elderly patients may be less able to compensate because of their already reduced iron stores.

Laxatives may cause diarrhea in el-derly patients who are extremely sensi-tive to such drugs as bisacodyl. Chronic oral use of mineral oil as a lubricating laxative may result in lipid pneumonia from aspiration of small residual oil droplets in the patient's mouth.

Patient noncompliance
Poor compliance can be a problem with patients of any age. However, in elderly patients, specific factors linked to ag-ing—such as diminished visual acuity, hearing loss, forgetfulness, the common need for multiple drug therapy, and vari-ous socioeconomic factors—can com-bine to make compliance a special prob-lem. Approximately one-third of elderly patients fail to comply with their pre-scribed drug therapy. They may fail to take prescribed doses or to follow the correct schedule or they may take med-ications prescribed for previous disor-ders, discontinue medications prema-turely, or use p.r.n. medications indis-criminately. Elderly patients may also have multiple prescriptions for the same

medication and, therefore, inadvertently take an overdose.

Review your patient's medication regimen with him. Make sure he under-stands the medication amount and the time and frequency of doses. Also, ex-plain how he should take each medica-tion—that is, with food or water or by itself.

Give your patient whatever help you can to avoid drug therapy problems. Suggest that he use drug calendars, pill "sorters," or other aids to help him com-ply, and refer him to the doctor or phar-macist if he needs further information.

Drug therapy and the nursing process

The nursing process guides nursing decisions about drug administration to ensure the patient's safety and meet medical and legal standards. This five-step process provides thorough assessment, appropriate nursing diagnosis, effective planning, correct interventions, and constant evaluation.

First step: Assessment

During assessment, the nurse focuses on direct data collection by:
● obtaining a drug history from the patient, parent, spouse, or companion
● reviewing the patient's medical history
● performing a physical examination
● obtaining and interpreting relevant laboratory or diagnostic test results.

Drug history

Data collection begins at admission to the hospital or in an outpatient setting with specific questions about the patient's background, including allergies, medical history, habits, socioeconomic status, lifestyle and beliefs, and sensory deficits. These aspects of the patient's background can significantly influence drug therapy.

Allergies

The patient's allergy profile includes reactions to both drugs and food. Information about allergic reactions must specify the drug; a description of the reaction; its situation, time, and setting; and any contributing factors. Examples of contributing factors include concurrent use of stimulants, tobacco, alcohol, or illegal drugs or a significant change in nutritional patterns. Asking the patient to describe his allergic reaction is especially important to help determine whether the patient reacts adversely or simply dislikes taking the drug.

Allergies to foods can also affect drug therapy. For example, allergies to shellfish can contraindicate use of drugs that contain iodine or are by-products of shellfish. Allergies to eggs are significant in patients who are to receive vaccines, which are commonly derived from chick embryos.

Prescription drugs

The patient's drug history should explore the following:
● the reason for using the drug
● the patient's knowledge of the appropriate dosage
● the patient's knowledge about determining effectiveness of the drug (if appropriate), potential adverse effects, what to do about adverse effects, and when to contact the doctor
● route of administration
● the pattern of administration at home
● use of OTC drugs
● cognitive status.

Note any special monitoring the patient must perform, such as blood glucose monitoring before insulin administration or checking radial pulse rate before taking digoxin. Make sure the patient is performing such procedures correctly and that the results are within acceptable limits.

Discuss the effects of drug therapy with the patient and determine if new symptoms or unpredicted adverse reactions have developed. Noting the patient's pattern of administration may provide insight into why a particular drug regimen succeeds or fails.

OTC drugs

A comprehensive drug history should also list any OTC drugs the patient is taking. Many OTC drugs can inhibit or potentiate the effects of a prescribed drug. For example, aspirin potentiates the anticoagulant effects of warfarin.

OTC drugs include a wide range of products, from aspirin and nutritional supplements to various sprays and cleaning agents. The patient may not think of these as drugs, so the nurse may have to name types of products to get an accurate response.

Dosage and frequency of use are just as important as the type of OTC product. One aspirin tablet taken once a day may have no effect on concomitant drug therapy; however, a higher dosage (such as that used for arthritis) could profoundly influence therapy.

Medical history
In gathering the medical history, note any chronic diseases or disorders the patient may have and record the following information for each:
• date of diagnosis
• initial prescribed treatment
• current treatment
• the doctor in charge.

Careful attention to this part of the medical history can uncover one of the most important problems with drug therapy—conflicting and incompatible drug regimens. The patient who does not have a family doctor to oversee and coordinate all care may seek the care of several specialists who may prescribe drug treatment without knowing what other drugs the patient is taking. A carefully detailed medical history can uncover such problems. The nurse who identifies such conflicting or overlapping drug therapy must call them to the appropriate doctor's attention and then teach the patient about the importance of informing caregivers about all drugs he is taking.

Habits
Carefully consider dietary habits and the nontherapeutic use of drugs.

Certain foods can directly affect the effectiveness of many drugs. For example, a person who is taking the anticoagulant warfarin should not increase his intake of green leafy vegetables because they contain levels of vitamin K that can antagonize the drug's anticoagulant effect.

Nontherapeutic use of drugs can profoundly affect a patient's health and impair the effectiveness of drug therapy. Consider the possible use of alcohol, tobacco, caffeine, and illegal drugs, such as marijuana, cocaine, and heroin. For example, if the patient uses alcohol, note the frequency of use, the amount, and the type of alcohol consumed. Carefully document the intake of stimulants, such as caffeine, because they significantly affect a patient's cardiovascular status and nervous system. Record the type of stimulant, the frequency of intake, and the amount consumed.

For the patient who uses tobacco, document the following information:
• the number of years the patient has used tobacco
• the kind of tobacco the patient smokes (cigarettes, cigar, or pipe) or chews
• how many cigarettes or cigars the patient smokes per day or how much and how long he chews tobacco daily
• the brand of tobacco the patient smokes or chews.

Defining the patient's use of illegal drugs may be difficult. However, the nurse who suspects such use should encourage the patient to discuss it honestly, emphasizing that these drugs have profound effects that may cause serious drug interactions. If the patient admits using illegal drugs, document the drug, the amount and frequency of use, and the route of administration.

Socioeconomic status
Note the patient's age, educational level, occupation, and insurance coverage. These factors may be significant to compliance and to an effective plan of care. The patient's age, for example, can determine whom to include in the care (parents or other family members) and the level of information that is appropriate for teaching the patient.

Knowing the patient's educational background and occupation helps you select interventions at an appropriate level, plan a drug regimen that fits the patient's daily routine, and encourage compliance. Knowing the patient's insurance status may help you anticipate the need for financial assistance and counseling. Remember that noncompliance commonly results from inability to afford medications.

Lifestyle and beliefs
Support systems, marital status, child-bearing status, attitudes toward health and health care, use of the health care system, and daily patterns of activities all affect the plan of care and patient compliance. For example, an 18-year-old single parent who is a high-school dropout on medical assistance and has no family support will probably require more teaching and support to gain a commitment and compliance than a 40-year-old affluent professional who has family support, can understand why she needs the drug, and can readily pay for it.

Sensory deficits
Any sensory deficit can significantly shape an appropriate plan of care. For example, impaired vision, paralysis of one or more extremities, loss of a limb, or loss of sensation in an extremity can impair the patient's ability to administer a subcutaneous injection, break a scored tablet, or open a medication container. Color blindness may cause difficulty in distinguishing between two medications. Hearing impairment can complicate effective patient instruction. Any sensory deficit requires careful consideration in any plan of prescribed drug therapy.

Clinical status
Two other factors can profoundly influence drug therapy: the patient's cognitive status and the systemic effects of the prescribed drugs. A patient's intact cognitive abilities ensure that he can understand and implement the actions necessary for compliance. During the interview, note if the patient is alert and oriented, if he is able to interact appropriately with people, and if his conversation is appropriate. Consider whether the patient can think clearly and express his thoughts coherently. Finally, check both short-term and long-term memory because the patient needs both to follow a specified drug regimen. If such evaluation identifies a cognitive deficit, determine the probable cause, which can range from a transient drug-related effect to permanent neurologic impairment, and then determine whether or not the patient can carry out the prescribed drug regimen. If not, the nurse must find another way to ensure that the patient receives the prescribed therapy.

After completing the drug history, perform a physical examination to assess those body systems that may be affected by a particular drug the patient is taking or that may be prescribed. Every drug has a desired effect on a body system, but it may have an undesired effect on another. For example, chemotherapeutic agents destroy cancerous cells, but they also affect normal cells and typically cause the patient to experience hair loss, diarrhea, or nausea. Therefore, examine the patient for expected drug effects; also closely monitor the patient for potentially harmful adverse effects.

Second step: Formulating a nursing diagnosis
Using information gathered during assessment, define any potential or actual drug-related problems by formulating each in a relevant nursing diagnosis. The most common problem statements related to drug therapy are *Knowledge deficit; Noncompliance;* and *Health Maintenance, Altered.*

Third step: Planning
Nursing diagnoses provide the frame-

work for planning interventions and outcome criteria (patient goals).

Outcome criteria
Outcome criteria state the desired patient behaviors or responses that should result from nursing care. Such criteria should be measurable and objective, concise, realistic for the patient, and attainable by nursing management. They should also express patient behavior in terms of expectations and specify a time frame. A typical outcome statement is "Before discharge, the patient verbalizes major adverse effects related to his chemotherapy."

Fourth step: Intervention
After developing the outcome criteria, the nurse determines the interventions needed to help the patient reach the desired behavior or goals. Drug-related interventions may focus on patient teaching for a drug's action, adverse effects, scheduling, steps to avoid or treat a drug reaction, or drug administration techniques.

Appropriate interventions related to drug therapy will also include administration procedures and techniques, legal and ethical concerns, patient teaching, and any concerns related to special groups of patients (geriatric, pediatric, pregnant, or breast-feeding patients). Such interventions may be independent nursing actions, such as turning a bedridden patient every 2 hours, or may be nursing actions that require a doctor's order.

Fifth step: Evaluation
The final component of the nursing process, evaluation, is a formal and systematic process for determining the effectiveness of nursing care. This process enables the nurse to determine whether outcome criteria were met and thereby make informed decisions about subsequent interventions. For example, if the patient experienced relief of headache within 1 hour after the nurse adminis-

tered a p.r.n. analgesic, the outcome criterion was met. If the headache was the same or worse, the outcome criterion was not met and requires a new assessment. This may result in a new plan of care or may yield new data that invalidate the nursing diagnosis or suggest new nursing interventions that are more specific or more acceptable to the patient. This assessment could lead to a higher dosage, a different analgesic, or a reevaluation of the cause.

Evaluation enables the nurse to design and implement a revised plan of care, to continuously reevaluate outcome criteria, and to plan again until each nursing diagnosis is successfully completed.

6

Amebicides and antiprotozoals

atovaquone
chloroquine hydrochloride
(See Chapter 9, ANTIMALARIALS.)
chloroquine phosphate
(See Chapter 9, ANTIMALARIALS.)
iodoquinol
metronidazole
metronidazole hydrochloride
paromomycin sulfate
pentamidine isethionate

COMBINATION PRODUCTS
None.

---

atovaquone
Mepron

Pregnancy Risk Category: C

HOW SUPPLIED
Suspension: 750 mg/5 ml

ACTION
Unknown. Appears to interfere with electron transport in protozoal mitochondria, inhibiting enzymes needed for the synthesis of nucleic acids and adenosine triphosphate.

ONSET, PEAK, DURATION
Onset and duration unknown. Two peak plasma levels occur after an oral dose, suggesting enterohepatic recycling. The first occurs after 1 to 8 hours; the second occurs after 1 to 4 days.

INDICATIONS & DOSAGE
Acute, mild to moderate Pneumocystis carinii *pneumonia in patients who cannot tolerate co-trimoxazole—*
Adults: 750 mg P.O. b.i.d. with food for 21 days.

ADVERSE REACTIONS
CNS: *headache, insomnia,* asthenia,

anxiety, dizziness.
EENT: *cough,* sinusitis, rhinitis, taste perversion.
GI: *nausea, diarrhea, vomiting,* constipation, *abdominal pain,* anorexia, dyspepsia.
Skin: *rash,* pruritus, *diaphoresis.*
Other: *fever, oral monilia, pain,* hypoglycemia, hypotension.

INTERACTIONS
Rifampin, rifabutin: decreases atovaquone's steady state concentration. Avoid concurrent use.

EFFECTS ON DIAGNOSTIC TESTS
None known.

CONTRAINDICATIONS
Contraindicated in patients with hypersensitivity to the drug.

NURSING CONSIDERATIONS
● Use cautiously in breast-feeding patients. In animal studies, drug was excreted in breast milk.
● Because drug is highly bound to plasma protein (greater than 99.9%), also use cautiously with other highly protein-bound drugs.
● Because of the risk of other concurrent pulmonary infections, monitor patients closely during therapy.

☑ **PATIENT TEACHING**
● Instruct patient to take drug with meals because food enhances absorption significantly.

---

iodoquinol
(diiodohydroxyquin)
Diodoquin†, Diquinol,
Yodoquinol, Yodoxin

Pregnancy Risk Category: C

HOW SUPPLIED
Tablets: 210 mg, 650 mg
Powder: 25 g

ACTION
Unknown. It is an iodine derivative with amebicidal activity in the intestinal lumen.

ONSET, PEAK, DURATION
Unknown.

INDICATIONS & DOSAGE
Intestinal amebiasis—
Adults: 630 to 650 mg P.O. t.i.d. after meals for 20 days. Total daily dosage should not exceed 1.95 g.
Children: usual dosage is 20 to 40 mg/kg of body weight daily in two to three divided doses for 20 days.
   Additional doses should not be repeated before a resting interval of 2 to 3 weeks.

ADVERSE REACTIONS
CNS: vertigo, headache, peripheral neuropathy.
EENT: optic neuritis, optic atrophy.
GI: anorexia, vomiting, abdominal cramps, diarrhea, anal irritation and itching.
Skin: pruritus, hives, papular and pustular eruptions, urticaria, bullae.
Other: thyroid enlargement, fever, chills.

INTERACTIONS
None significant.

EFFECTS ON DIAGNOSTIC TESTS
Iodoquinol may increase protein-bound iodine levels and therefore interfere with thyroid function tests for up to 6 months after discontinuation of therapy.

CONTRAINDICATIONS
Contraindicated in patients with hypersensitivity to 8-hydroxyquinoline derivatives or iodine-containing preparations. Iodoquinol causes liver damage in such patients. Also contraindicated in patients with hepatic or renal disease or preexisting optic neuropathy.

NURSING CONSIDERATIONS
● Use cautiously in patients with thyroid diseases.
● If the patient has difficulty swallowing, crush tablets and mix with applesauce or chocolate syrup.
● Record fluid intake and output and color and amount of stools. Send warm specimens to laboratory for analysis.
● Watch for diarrhea during the first 2 or 3 days; notify the doctor if diarrhea continues.

☑ PATIENT TEACHING
● Recommend that the patient have periodic ophthalmic examinations during treatment.
● Advise the patient not to discontinue the drug prematurely. Tell him to notify the doctor if rash occurs.
● To help prevent reinfestation, teach the patient about the need for personal hygiene, especially good hand-washing technique. Encourage the patient not to prepare food for others until stools are negative.

---

metronidazole
Apo-Metronidazole†, Flagyl, Metric-21, Metrogyl‡, Metrozine‡, Neo-Metric†, Novonidazol†, PMS Metronidazole†, Protostat, Trikacide†

metronidazole hydrochloride
Flagyl I.V. RTU, Metro I.V., Novonidazol†

Pregnancy Risk Category: B

HOW SUPPLIED
Tablets: 200 mg‡, 250 mg, 375 mg, 400 mg‡, 500 mg
Oral suspension (benzoyl metronidazole): 200 mg/5 ml‡
Injection: 500 mg/100 ml ready to use
Powder for injection: 500-mg single-dose vials

ACTION
A direct-acting trichomonacide and amebicide that works at both intestinal and extraintestinal sites. It is thought to enter the cells of microorganisms that contain nitroreductase. Unstable compounds are then formed that bind to DNA and inhibit synthesis, causing cell death.

ONSET, PEAK, DURATION
Onset occurs immediately after I.V infusion, unknown after oral administration. Peak plasma levels occur immediately after I.V. infusion and within 1 to 2 hours of oral administration. Duration unknown.

INDICATIONS & DOSAGE
Amebic hepatic abscess—
Adults: 500 to 750 mg P.O. t.i.d. for 5 to 10 days.
Children: 30 to 50 mg/kg daily (in three doses) for 10 days.
Intestinal amebiasis—
Adults: 750 mg P.O. t.i.d. for 5 to 10 days.
Children: 30 to 50 mg/kg daily (in three doses) for 10 days.
   Therapy for adults or children is followed with oral iodoquinol.
Trichomoniasis—
Adults: 250 mg P.O. t.i.d. for 7 days or 2 g P.O. in single dose (may give the 2-g dose in two 1-g doses, each on the same day); 4 to 6 weeks should elapse between courses of therapy.
Children: 5 mg/kg dose P.O. t.i.d. for 7 days.
Refractory trichomoniasis—
Adults: 250 mg P.O. b.i.d. for 10 days. Alternatively, 500 mg P.O. b.i.d. for 7 days.
Bacterial infections caused by anaerobic microorganisms—
Adults: loading dose is 15 mg/kg I.V. infused over 1 hour (approximately 1 g for a 70-kg adult). Maintenance dose is 7.5 mg/kg I.V. or P.O. q 6 hours (approximately 500 mg for a 70-kg adult). First maintenance dose should be given 6 hours after loading dose. Maximum dosage not to exceed 4 g daily.
Giardiasis—
Adults: 250 mg P.O. t.i.d. for 5 to 7 days or 2 g P.O. once daily for 3 days.
Children: 5 mg/kg P.O. t.i.d. for 5 to 7 days.
Prevention of postoperative infection in contaminated or potentially contaminated colorectal surgery—
Adults: 15 mg/kg I.V. infused over 30 to 60 minutes and completed about 1 hour before surgery. Then, 7.5 mg/kg I.V. infused over 30 to 60 minutes at 6 and 12 hours after initial dose.

ADVERSE REACTIONS
CNS: vertigo, headache, ataxia, dizziness, syncope, incoordination, confusion, irritability, depression, weakness, insomnia, *seizures,* peripheral neuropathy.
CV: ECG change (flattened T wave), edema (with I.V. RTU preparation).
GI: abdominal cramping, stomatitis, epigastric distress, nausea, vomiting, anorexia, diarrhea, constipation, proctitis, dry mouth.
GU: darkened urine, polyuria, dysuria, cystitis, decreased libido, dyspareunia, dryness of vagina and vulva, vaginal candidiasis.
Hematologic: transient leukopenia, neutropenia.
Skin: flushing, rash.
Other: overgrowth of nonsusceptible organisms, especially *Candida* (glossitis, furry tongue); metallic taste; fever; thrombophlebitis after I.V. infusion; fleeting joint pains, sometimes resembling serum sickness.

INTERACTIONS
Cimetidine: increased risk of metronidazole toxicity because of inhibited hepatic metabolism. Monitor closely.
Disulfiram: acute psychoses and confusional states. Don't use together.
Ethanol: disulfiram-like reaction (nausea, vomiting, headache, cramps, flushing). Don't use together.

---

*Liquid contains alcohol.   **May contain tartrazine.   †Canada only.   ‡Australia only.   ◇OTC.

Lithium: increased lithium levels resulting in possible toxicity. Monitor serum lithium levels closely.

Oral anticoagulants: increased anticoagulant effects. Monitor closely.

Phenytoin, phenobarbital: decreased metronidazole effectiveness. Monitor closely.

EFFECTS ON DIAGNOSTIC TESTS
Metronidazole may interfere with the chemical analyses of aminotransferases and triglyceride, leading to falsely decreased values. It may flatten the T waves on an ECG or interfere with AST, ALT, lactate dehydrogenase, and glucose levels.

CONTRAINDICATIONS
Contraindicated in patients with hypersensitivity to the drug or other nitroimidazole derivatives.

NURSING CONSIDERATIONS
● Use cautiously in patients with a history of blood dyscrasia or CNS disorder and in patients with retinal or visual field changes. Use cautiously in patients with hepatic disease or alcoholism and in conjunction with hepatotoxic drugs.
● If indicated during pregnancy for trichomoniasis, be aware that the 7-day regimen is preferred over the 2-g single-dose regimen.
● Give oral form with meals.
● **I.V. use:** No preparation is necessary for RTU (ready to use). To prepare lyophilized vials of metronidazole, add 4.4 ml of sterile water for injection, bacteriostatic water for injection, sterile 0.9% sodium chloride for injection, or bacteriostatic 0.9% sodium chloride for injection. The reconstituted drug contains 100 mg/ml. Add the contents of the vial to 100 ml of D_5W, lactated Ringer's injection, or 0.9% sodium chloride for a final concentration of 5 mg/ml. The resulting highly acidic solution must be neutralized before administering. Carefully add 5 mEq sodium bicarbonate for each 500 mg metronida-

zole; carbon dioxide gas will form and may need to be vented.
Alert: Infuse drug over at least 1 hour. Don't give I.V. push.
● Don't refrigerate the neutralized diluted solution. Precipitation may occur. If Flagyl I.V. RTU is refrigerated, crystals may form. These disappear after the solution warms to room temperature.
● Observe for edema, especially in patients receiving corticosteroids; Flagyl I.V. RTU may cause sodium retention.
● Record number and character of stools when used in the treatment of amebiasis. Metronidazole should be used only after *Trichomonas vaginalis* has been confirmed by wet smear or culture or *Entamoeba histolytica* has been identified. Asymptomatic sexual partners of patients being treated for *T. vaginalis* infection should be treated simultaneously to avoid reinfection.

☑ **PATIENT TEACHING**
● Instruct patient to take oral form with food to minimize GI upset.
● Inform patient that sexual partners should be treated simultaneously to avoid reinfection.
● Instruct patient in proper hygiene.
● Tell patient to avoid alcohol and alcohol-containing medications during therapy and for at least 48 hours after therapy is completed.
● Tell patient metallic taste and dark or red-brown urine may occur.

paromomycin sulfate
Humatin

Pregnancy Risk Category: C

HOW SUPPLIED
Capsules: 250 mg

ACTION
Unknown but it acts as an intestinal amebicide. It appears to inhibit protein synthesis in susceptible bacteria at the 30S segment of the ribosome.

ONSET, PEAK, DURATION
Unknown.

INDICATIONS & DOSAGE
Intestinal amebiasis, acute and chronic—
Adults and children: 25 to 35 mg/kg daily P.O. in three doses with meals for 5 to 10 days.
Tapeworms (fish, beef, pork, dog)—
Adults: 1 g P.O. q 15 minutes for four doses.
Children: 11 mg/kg P.O. q 15 minutes for four doses.

ADVERSE REACTIONS
CNS: headache, vertigo.
EENT: ototoxicity (potential).
GI: anorexia, nausea, vomiting, epigastric pain and burning, abdominal cramps, diarrhea, increased motility, steatorrhea, pruritus ani, malabsorption syndrome.
GU: hematuria, *nephrotoxicity* (potential).
Hematologic: eosinophilia.
Skin: rash, exanthema.
Other: overgrowth of nonsusceptible organisms.

INTERACTIONS
None significant.

EFFECTS ON DIAGNOSTIC TESTS
None reported.

CONTRAINDICATIONS
Contraindicated in patients with hypersensitivity to the drug and in those with impaired renal function or intestinal obstruction.

NURSING CONSIDERATIONS
● Use cautiously in patients with ulcerative lesions of the bowel to avoid inadvertent absorption and resulting renal toxicity. Poorly absorbed orally, but will accumulate in patients with renal impairment or ulcerative lesions.
● Ask about history of sensitivity to drug before giving first dose.

● Administer with meals.
● Be aware that criterion of cure is absence of amebae in stools examined weekly for 6 weeks after treatment and thereafter at monthly intervals for 2 years. Examine stools of family members or suspected contacts.
● Be aware that patient should avoid high doses or prolonged therapy.
● Watch for signs of superinfection (continued fever and other signs of new infections, especially monilial infections).
● Notify doctor if ringing in ears, hearing impairment, or dizziness occurs.

☑ PATIENT TEACHING
● Instruct patient to take drug with meals.
● To help prevent reinfestation, teach patient about the need for personal hygiene, especially good hand-washing technique.
● Instruct patient to refrain from preparing food for others until stools are negative.

---

pentamidine isethionate
NebuPent, Pentacarinat, Pentam 300, Pneumopent

Pregnancy Risk Category: C

HOW SUPPLIED
Injection: 300-mg vial
Aerosol: 300-mg vial

ACTION
Interferes with biosynthesis of DNA, RNA, phospholipids, and proteins in susceptible organisms.

ONSET, PEAK, DURATION
Unknown except peak serum levels occur ½ to 1 hour after I.M. injection, immediately after I.V. infusion.

INDICATIONS & DOSAGE
Pneumocystis carinii pneumonia—
Adults and children: 3 to 4 mg/kg I.V. or I.M. once daily for 14 to 21 days.

Prevention of P. carinii *pneumonia in high-risk individuals—*
Adults: 300 mg by inhalation (using a Respirgard II nebulizer) once every 4 weeks.

ADVERSE REACTIONS
CNS: confusion, hallucinations, *fatigue, dizziness,* headache.
CV: *hypotension, ventricular tachycardia,* chest pain.
GI: *nausea, metallic taste, decreased appetite, pharyngitis, vomiting,* diarrhea, abdominal pain, anorexia, bad taste in mouth.
GU: *elevated serum creatinine,* **acute renal failure.**
Hematologic: leukopenia, ***thrombocytopenia,*** anemia.
Hepatic: elevated liver function tests.
Respiratory: *cough, bronchospasm, shortness of breath,* pneumothorax.
Skin: *rash,* **Stevens-Johnson syndrome.**
Other: *hypoglycemia,* hypocalcemia, *sterile abscess, pain or induration at injection site, congestion, night sweats, chills,* edema, myalgia.

INTERACTIONS
Aminoglycosides, amphotericin B, capreomycin, cisplatin, colistin, methoxyflurane, polymyxin B, vancomycin: increased risk of nephrotoxicity.

EFFECTS ON DIAGNOSTIC TESTS
BUN, serum creatinine, AST, and ALT levels may increase during pentamidine therapy. Hyperkalemia and hypocalcemia may occur. Hypoglycemia may occur initially; later, hyperglycemia may result from pancreatic cell damage.

CONTRAINDICATIONS
Contraindicated in patients with a history of an anaphylactic reaction to drug.

NURSING CONSIDERATIONS
● Use cautiously in patients with hypertension, hypotension, hypoglycemia, hypocalcemia, leukopenia, thrombocytopenia, anemia, or hepatic or renal dysfunction.
● Administer the aerosol form only by Respirgard II nebulizer. Dosage recommendations are based on the particle size and delivery rate of this device. To administer aerosol, mix the contents of one vial in 6 ml of sterile water for injection. *Do not use* 0.9% sodium chloride solution. Do not mix with other drugs.
● Do not use low-pressure (less than 20 psi) compressors. The flow rate should be 5 to 7 liters/minute from a 40- to 50-psi air or oxygen source.
● **I.V. use:** Reconstitute drug with 3 ml of sterile water for injection. Then dilute in 50 to 250 ml of D_5W. Inject over at least 60 minutes.
Alert: To minimize risk of hypotension when the drug is given I.V., infuse drug slowly with the patient lying down. Closely monitor blood pressure.
● For I.M. injection, reconstitute drug with 3 ml of sterile water for a solution containing 100 mg/ml; administer deeply. Expect pain and induration.
● Monitor blood glucose, serum calcium, serum creatinine, and BUN levels daily. After parenteral administration, blood glucose level may decrease initially; hypoglycemia may be severe in 5% to 10% of patients. This may be followed by hyperglycemia and insulin-dependent diabetes mellitus, which may be permanent.
● In patients with AIDS, be aware that pentamidine may produce less severe adverse reactions than co-trimoxazole.

☑ PATIENT TEACHING
● Instruct the patient to use the aerosol device until the chamber is empty, which may take up to 45 minutes.
● Warn the patient that I.M. injection is painful.

7
Anthelmintics

mebendazole
pyrantel pamoate
thiabendazole

COMBINATION PRODUCTS
None.

---

mebendazole
Vermox

Pregnancy Risk Category: C

HOW SUPPLIED
Tablets (chewable): 100 mg
Oral suspension: 100 mg/5 ml‡

ACTION
Selectively and irreversibly inhibits uptake of glucose and other nutrients in susceptible helminths.

ONSET, PEAK, DURATION
Onset unknown. Plasma levels peak in 2 to 5 hours. Duration varies.

INDICATIONS & DOSAGE
Pinworm—
Adults and children over 2 years: 100 mg P.O. as a single dose; repeated if infection persists 2 to 3 weeks later.
Roundworm, whipworm, hookworm—
Adults and children over 2 years: 100 mg P.O. b.i.d. for 3 days; repeated if infection persists 3 weeks later.

ADVERSE REACTIONS
GI: occasional, transient abdominal pain and diarrhea in massive infection and expulsion of worms.
Other: fever.

INTERACTIONS
Cimetidine: increased plasma concentrations of mebendazole. Monitor closely.

EFFECTS ON DIAGNOSTIC TESTS
None reported.

CONTRAINDICATIONS
Contraindicated in patients with hypersensitivity to the drug.

NURSING CONSIDERATIONS
● Be aware that tablets may be chewed, swallowed whole, or crushed and mixed with food.
● Administer the drug to all family members, as prescribed, to decrease the risk of spreading the infection.
● Know that no dietary restrictions, laxatives, or enemas are necessary.

☑ PATIENT TEACHING
● Teach the patient about personal hygiene, especially good hand-washing technique. Advise him to refrain from preparing food for others.
● To avoid reinfection, teach the patient to wash perianal area daily, to change undergarments and bedclothes daily, and to wash hands and clean fingernails before meals and after bowel movements.

---

pyrantel pamoate
Antiminth, Combantrin†, Reese's Pinworm Medicine

Pregnancy Risk Category: C

HOW SUPPLIED
Tablets: 125 mg†
Oral suspension: 50 mg/ml

ACTION
Blocks neuromuscular action, paralyzing the worm and causing its expulsion by normal peristalsis.

ONSET, PEAK, DURATION
Onset is highly variable. Plasma levels peak within 1 to 3 hours. Duration varies with GI transit time and extent of infestation.

INDICATIONS & DOSAGE
Roundworm and pinworm—
Adults and children over 2 years: 11 mg/kg P.O. as a single dose. Maximum dosage is 1 g. For pinworm, dosage should be repeated in 2 weeks.

ADVERSE REACTIONS
CNS: headache, dizziness, drowsiness, insomnia.
GI: anorexia, nausea, vomiting, gastralgia, abdominal cramps, diarrhea, tenesmus.
Hepatic: transient elevation of AST.
Skin: rash.
Other: fever, weakness.

INTERACTIONS
Piperazine salts: possible antagonism; don't give together.

EFFECTS ON DIAGNOSTIC TESTS
Pyrantel pamoate may cause transient elevations of liver function tests.

CONTRAINDICATIONS
Contraindicated in patients with hypersensitivity to the drug.

NURSING CONSIDERATIONS
● Use cautiously in patients with severe malnutrition or anemia or in patients with hepatic dysfunction.
● Be aware that no diet restrictions, laxatives, or enemas are needed.
● Be aware that drug should be given to all family members.

☑ PATIENT TEACHING
● Advise the patient that pyrantel may be taken with food, milk, or fruit juices. Shake suspension well.
● Teach the patient about personal hygiene, especially good hand-washing technique. To avoid reinfection, teach the patient to wash perianal area daily, to change undergarments and bed-clothes daily, and to wash hands and clean fingernails before meals and after bowel movements.
● Advise him to refrain from preparing food for others.

---

thiabendazole
Mintezol

Pregnancy Risk Category: C

HOW SUPPLIED
Tablets (chewable): 500 mg
Oral suspension: 500 mg/5 ml

ACTION
Unknown, but the drug appears to inhibit the helminth-specific enzyme fumarate reductase.

ONSET, PEAK, DURATION
Onset and duration unknown. Plasma levels peak in 1 to 2 hours.

INDICATIONS & DOSAGE
Cutaneous infestations with larva migrans (creeping eruption)—
Adults and children: 25 mg/kg P.O. b.i.d. for 2 to 5 days. Maximum dosage is 3 g daily. If lesions persist after 2 days, course is repeated.
Roundworm, threadworm, whipworm—
Adults and children: 25 mg/kg P.O. in two doses daily for 2 successive days.
Trichinosis—
Adults and children: 25 mg/kg P.O. in two doses daily for 2 to 4 successive days.

ADVERSE REACTIONS
CNS: impaired mental alertness, impaired coordination, numbness, seizures, *drowsiness, fatigue,* giddiness, *headache,* dizziness.
CV: *hypotension.*
EENT: tinnitus, blurry vision, dry mouth and eyes, xanthopsia.
GI: *anorexia, nausea, vomiting,* diar-

rhea, epigastric distress, cholestasis.
GU: hematuria, enuresis, crystalluria, malodorous urine.
Hematologic: leukopenia.
Hepatic: *jaundice, parenchymal liver damage.*
Skin: *rash, pruritus, erythema multiforme, Stevens-Johnson syndrome.*
Other: lymphadenopathy, fever, flushing, chills, *angioedema, anaphylaxis.*

INTERACTIONS
Theophylline: may impair hepatic metabolism of theophylline, increasing risk of toxicity. Monitor the patient closely.

EFFECTS ON DIAGNOSTIC TESTS
Transient elevations of AST levels have been reported.

CONTRAINDICATIONS
Contraindicated in patients with hypersensitivity to the drug.

NURSING CONSIDERATIONS
● Use cautiously in patients with hepatic or renal dysfunction, severe malnutrition, and anemia and in patients who are vomiting.
● Be aware that drug should be administered to all family members, as prescribed, to prevent risk of spreading infection.
● Be aware that no dietary restrictions, laxatives, or enemas are necessary. However, know that supportive therapy is indicated for anemic, dehydrated, or malnourished patients.

☑ **PATIENT TEACHING**
● Teach the patient to take drug after meals. For oral suspension, shake before measuring dose. For tablets, advise patient to chew before swallowing.
● Advise the patient to avoid hazardous activities, such as driving, because drug may cause drowsiness.
● Teach the patient about personal hygiene, especially good hand-washing technique. To avoid reinfection, teach the patient to wash perianal area daily,

change undergarments and bedclothes daily, and wash hands and clean fingernails before meals and after bowel movements. Tell him not to prepare food for others during infestation.

*Liquid contains alcohol.   **May contain tartrazine.   †Canada only.   ‡Australia only.   ◊ OTC.

8

Antifungals

amphotericin B
fluconazole
flucytosine
griseofulvin microsize
griseofulvin ultramicrosize
itraconazole
ketoconazole
miconazole
nystatin

COMBINATION PRODUCTS
None.

---

amphotericin B
Amphocin, Amphotericin B for Injection, Fungilin Oral‡, Fungizone Intravenous

Pregnancy Risk Category: B

HOW SUPPLIED
Tablets: 100 mg‡
Oral suspension: 100 mg/ml‡
Lozenges: 10 mg‡
Injection: 50-mg lyophilized cake

ACTION
Unknown. Probably acts by binding to sterol in the fungal cell membrane, altering cell permeability and allowing leakage of intracellular components.

ONSET, PEAK, DURATION
Onset is immediate and serum levels peak immediately after I.V. infusion. Onset, peak, and duration are unknown after oral administration.

INDICATIONS & DOSAGE
Systemic fungal infections (histoplasmosis, coccidioidomycosis, blastomycosis, cryptococcosis, disseminated moniliasis, aspergillosis, phycomycosis), meningitis—
Adults: initially, a test dose of 1 mg in

20 ml of D$_5$W infused I.V. over 20 to 30 minutes may be recommended. If tolerated, daily dosage is then initiated as 0.25 to 0.3 mg/kg daily by slow I.V. infusion (0.1 mg/ml) over 2 to 6 hours. Daily dosage is gradually increased to maximum 1 mg/kg daily. If drug is discontinued for 1 week or more, drug is resumed with initial dose and increased gradually.
Infections of the GI tract caused by Candida albicans—
Adults: 100 mg P.O. q.i.d. for 2 weeks.
Oral and perioral candidal infections—
Adults: 1 lozenge q.i.d. for 7 to 14 days. Lozenge should dissolve slowly.

ADVERSE REACTIONS
CNS: *headache,* peripheral neuropathy, *seizures.*
CV: hypotension, *cardiac arrhythmias, asystole,* hypertension.
EENT: hearing loss, tinnitus, transient vertigo, blurred vision, diplopia.
GI: *anorexia, weight loss, nausea, vomiting, dyspepsia, diarrhea, epigastric pain, cramping,* melena, ***hemorrhagic gastroenteritis.***
GU: *abnormal renal function with hypokalemia, azotemia, hyposthenuria, renal tubular acidosis, nephrocalcinosis;* with large doses—***permanent renal impairment,*** anuria, oliguria.
Hematologic: *normochromic, normocytic anemia,* ***thrombocytopenia,*** leukopenia, ***agranulocytosis,*** eosinophilia, leukocytosis.
Hepatic: hepatitis, jaundice, ***acute liver failure.***
Respiratory: dyspnea, tachypnea, bronchospasm, wheezing.
Skin: maculopapular rash, pruritus (without rash).
Other: arthralgia, tissue damage with extravasation, *phlebitis, thrombophlebitis, pain at injection site,* myalgia,

---

Reactions may be *common,* uncommon, *life-threatening,* or COMMON AND LIFE-THREATENING.

fever, chills, malaise, generalized pain, flushing, ***anaphylactoid reactions.***

INTERACTIONS

Corticosteroids: enhanced potassium depletion. Monitor serum potassium levels.

Digitalis glycosides: increased risk of digitalis toxicity in potassium-depleted patients. Monitor closely.

Flucytosine: synergistic effect; may cause increased toxicity of flucytosine. Monitor closely.

Other nephrotoxic drugs, such as antibiotics or antineoplastic agents: may cause additive renal toxicity. Administer cautiously.

EFFECTS ON DIAGNOSTIC TESTS

Amphotericin B therapy may increase BUN, serum creatinine, alkaline phosphatase, and bilirubin levels. The drug may also cause hypokalemia and hypomagnesemia and may decrease WBC, RBC, and platelet counts.

CONTRAINDICATIONS

Contraindicated in patients with hypersensitivity to the drug.

NURSING CONSIDERATIONS

● Use cautiously in patients with impaired renal function.

Alert: To reduce severe adverse reactions, be aware that the patient may receive premedication with antipyretics, antihistamines, antiemetics, or small doses of corticosteroids; addition of phosphate buffer and heparin to the solution; and alternate-day schedule. For severe reactions, discontinue drug and notify doctor.

● Monitor fluid intake and output; report change in urine appearance or volume. Monitor BUN and serum creatinine (or creatinine clearance) at least weekly. Kidney damage is typically reversible if drug is stopped at first sign of dysfunction.

● Obtain liver and renal function studies weekly, if ordered. Drug may be stopped if alkaline phosphatase or bilirubin levels increase. If BUN exceeds 40 mg/100 ml, or if serum creatinine exceeds 3 mg/100 ml, doctor may reduce or stop drug until renal function improves. Monitor CBC weekly.

● Monitor potassium levels closely, and report signs of hypokalemia. Check calcium and magnesium levels twice weekly, as ordered.

● **I.V. use:** Be prepared to give initial test dose as prescribed. Monitor the patient's pulse, respiratory rate, temperature, and blood pressure for at least 4 hours.

● Use an infusion pump and in-line filter with mean pore diameter larger than 1 micron. Rapid infusion may cause cardiovascular collapse.

● Choose I.V. sites in distal veins. If veins become thrombosed, alternate administration sites.

● Monitor vital signs every 30 minutes; fever, shaking chills, and hypotension may appear 1 to 2 hours after start of I.V. infusion and should subside within 4 hours of stopping drug.

● Be aware that reconstituted solution is stable for 1 week under refrigeration or 24 hours at room temperature. It has 8-hour stability in room light.

● Give antibiotics separately; don't mix or piggyback them with amphotericin B.

● Know that amphotericin B seems to be compatible with limited amounts of heparin sodium, hydrocortisone sodium succinate, and methylprednisolone sodium succinate.

● Store the dry form at 2° to 8° C (35.6° to 46.4° F). Protect from light. Reconstitute with 10 ml of sterile water only. To avoid precipitation, do not mix with solutions containing sodium chloride, other electrolytes, or bacteriostatic agents (such as benzyl alcohol). Do not use if solution contains precipitate or foreign matter.

☑ PATIENT TEACHING

● Warn the patient of possible discomfort at I.V. site and of other potential ad-

verse reactions. Instruct the patient to report signs and symptoms of hypersensitivity immediately.
● Inform patient that therapy may take several months. Stress importance of compliance and recommended follow-up.

---

fluconazole
Diflucan

Pregnancy Risk Category: C

HOW SUPPLIED
Tablets: 50 mg, 100 mg, 150 mg, 200 mg
Powder for oral suspension: 10 mg/ml, 40 mg/ml
Injection: 200 mg/100 ml, 400 mg/200 ml

ACTION
Inhibits fungal cytochrome P-450 (responsible for fungal sterol synthesis) and weakens fungal cell walls.

ONSET, PEAK, DURATION
Onset immediate with I.V. administration; unknown with oral administration. Peak serum levels occur immediately after I.V. infusion, 1 to 2 hours after oral administration. Duration unknown.

INDICATIONS & DOSAGE
Oropharyngeal candidiasis—
Adults: 200 mg P.O. or I.V. on first day, followed by 100 mg once daily. Therapy should last at least 2 weeks.
Esophageal candidiasis—
Adults: 200 mg P.O. or I.V. on the first day, followed by 100 mg once daily. Higher doses (up to 400 mg daily) have been used, depending on the patient's condition and tolerance of treatment. Patients should receive the drug for at least 3 weeks and for 2 weeks after symptoms resolve.
Systemic candidiasis—
Adults: 400 mg P.O. or I.V. on the first day, followed by 200 mg once daily.

Treatment should continue for at least 4 weeks and for 2 weeks after symptoms resolve.
Cryptococcal meningitis—
Adults: 400 mg P.O. or I.V. on the first day, followed by 200 mg once daily. Higher doses (up to 400 mg daily) may be used. Treatment should continue for 10 to 12 weeks after CSF cultures are negative.
Prevention of candidiasis in bone marrow transplant—
Adults: 400 mg P.O. or I.V. once daily. Start prophylaxis several days before anticipated agranulocytosis. Continue therapy for 7 days after the neutrophil count rises above 1,000 cells/mm^3.
Suppression of relapse of cryptococcal meningitis in patients with AIDS—
Adults: 200 mg P.O. or I.V. daily.
In patients with renal failure: If creatinine clearance is 21 to 50 ml/minute, dosage is reduced by 50%. If creatinine clearance is 11 to 20 ml/minute, dosage is reduced by 75%. Patients receiving regular hemodialysis treatment should receive the usual dose after each dialysis session.

ADVERSE REACTIONS
CNS: headache.
GI: *nausea,* vomiting, abdominal pain, diarrhea.
Hepatic: *hepatotoxicity* (rare), elevated liver enzymes.
Skin: rash, **Stevens-Johnson syndrome** (rare).
Other: *anaphylaxis.*

INTERACTIONS
Cyclosporine, phenytoin: may increase plasma concentrations of these drugs. Monitor serum cyclosporine or phenytoin levels.
Isoniazid, phenytoin, rifampin, valproic acid, oral sulfonylureas: increased incidence of elevated hepatic transaminases. Monitor closely.
Oral antidiabetic agents (tolbutamide, glyburide, glipizide): may increase plasma concentrations of these drugs. Moni-

---

tor for enhanced hypoglycemic effect.
Rifampin: enhanced metabolism of fluconazole. Monitor for lack of response.
Warfarin: increased risk of bleeding.
Monitor PT.

EFFECTS ON DIAGNOSTIC TESTS
Increased liver transaminase serum levels may occur with fluconazole.

CONTRAINDICATIONS
Contraindicated in patients with hypersensitivity to the drug.

NURSING CONSIDERATIONS
● Use cautiously in patients with hypersensitivity to other antifungal azole compounds; no information exists regarding cross-sensitivity.
● Do not remove protective overwrap from I.V. bags until just before use, to ensure product sterility. The plastic container may show some opacity from moisture absorbed during sterilization. This is normal, doesn't affect the drug, and diminishes over time.
● **I.V. use:** Administer by continuous infusion at a rate not to exceed 200 mg/hour. Use an infusion pump. To prevent air embolism, do not connect in series with other infusions. Do not add any other drugs to the solution.
● Periodically monitor liver function during prolonged therapy, as ordered. Although adverse hepatic effects are rare, they can be serious.
● If the patient develops mild rash, monitor closely. Discontinue drug if lesions progress and notify doctor.
● Be aware that the incidence of adverse reactions appears to be greater in HIV-infected patients.

☑ **PATIENT TEACHING**
● Instruct patient to take medication as directed, even after he feels better.
● Tell the patient to shake oral suspension in its container before measuring each dose.
● Instruct the patient to report adverse reactions promptly.

flucytosine (5-fluorocytosine, 5-FC)
Ancobon, Ancotil†

Pregnancy Risk Category: C

HOW SUPPLIED
Capsules: 250 mg, 500 mg

ACTION
Unknown. Appears to penetrate fungal cells and cause defective protein synthesis.

ONSET, PEAK, DURATION
Onset and duration unknown. Serum levels peak 1 to 2 hours after oral dose.

INDICATIONS & DOSAGE
Severe fungal infections caused by susceptible strains of Candida *(including septicemia, endocarditis, urinary tract and pulmonary infections) and* Cryptococcus *(meningitis, pulmonary infection, and possible urinary tract infection)—*
Adults and children weighing more than 50 kg/or more: 50 to 150 mg/kg daily P.O. in four equally divided doses q 6 hours.
Adults and children under 50 kg: 1.5 to 4.5 g/m^2/day P.O. in four divided doses.

ADVERSE REACTIONS
CNS: headache, vertigo, sedation, fatigue, weakness, confusion, hallucinations, psychosis, ataxia, hearing loss, paresthesia, parkinsonism, peripheral neuropathy.
CV: *cardiac arrest.*
GI: nausea, vomiting, diarrhea, abdominal pain, emesis, dry mouth, duodenal ulcer, *hemorrhage,* ulcerative colitis.
GU: azotemia, elevated creatinine and BUN levels, crystalluria, *renal failure.*
Hematologic: anemia, *leukopenia, bone marrow suppression, thrombocytopenia,* eosinophilia, *agranulocytosis, aplastic anemia.*

---

*Liquid contains alcohol.   **May contain tartrazine.   †Canada only.   ‡Australia only.   ◊ OTC.

Hepatic: elevated liver enzymes, elevated serum alkaline phosphatase, jaundice.
Respiratory: *respiratory arrest,* chest pain, dyspnea.
Skin: occasional rash, pruritus, urticaria, photosensitivity.
Other: hypoglycemia, hypokalemia.

INTERACTIONS
Amphotericin B: synergistic effects and possibly enhanced toxicity when used together. Monitor closely.

EFFECTS ON DIAGNOSTIC TESTS
Flucytosine causes falsely elevated creatinine values on iminohydrolase enzymatic assay. The drug may increase alkaline phosphatase, AST, ALT, BUN, and serum creatinine levels and may decrease WBC, RBC, and platelet counts.

CONTRAINDICATIONS
Contraindicated in patients with hypersensitivity to the drug.

NURSING CONSIDERATIONS
● Use with extreme caution in patients with impaired hepatic or renal function or bone marrow suppression.
● Obtain hematologic tests and renal and liver function studies, as ordered. Ensure that susceptibility tests establishing that organism is flucytosine-sensitive are on the chart.
● Administer capsules over 15 minutes to reduce adverse GI reactions.
● Monitor blood, liver, and renal function studies frequently during therapy; obtain susceptibility tests weekly, as ordered, to monitor drug resistance.
● Monitor fluid intake and output; report any marked change.
● If possible, regularly perform blood level assays of drug, as ordered, to maintain flucytosine at therapeutic level (25 to 120 mcg/ml). Higher blood levels may be toxic.

☑ **PATIENT TEACHING**
● Inform the patient that therapeutic re-

sponse may take weeks or months.
● Instruct the patient to report adverse reactions promptly.

---

griseofulvin microsize
Fulcin‡, Fulvicin-U/F, Grifulvin V, Grisactin, Grisovin‡, Grisovin 500‡, Grisovin-FP

griseofulvin ultramicrosize
Fulvicin P/G, Grisactin Ultra, Griseostatin‡, Gris-PEG

Pregnancy Risk Category: NR

HOW SUPPLIED
griseofulvin microsize
Tablets: 250 mg, 500 mg
Capsules: 125 mg, 250 mg
Oral suspension: 125 mg/5ml
griseofulvin ultramicrosize
Tablets: 125 mg, 165 mg, 250 mg, 330 mg

ACTION
Arrests fungal cell activity by disrupting its mitotic spindle structure.

ONSET, PEAK, DURATION
Onset and duration unknown. Serum levels peak 4 to 8 hours after oral dose.

INDICATIONS & DOSAGE
Ringworm infections of skin, hair, nails (tinea corporis, tinea capitis, tinea cruris) when caused by Trichophyton, Microsporum, *or* Epidermophyton—
Adults: 500 mg of microsize P.O. daily in single or divided doses. Severe infections may require up to 1 g daily. Alternatively, 330 to 375 mg ultramicrosize P.O. daily in single or divided doses.
Tinea pedis and tinea unguium—
Adults: 0.75 to 1 g of microsize P.O. daily. Alternatively, 660 to 750 mg of ultramicrosize P.O. daily in divided doses.
Children: 11 mg/kg/day of microsize P.O. Alternatively, 7.3 mg/kg/day of ultramicrosize P.O.

Reactions may be *common*, uncommon, *life-threatening*, or COMMON AND LIFE-THREATENING.

ADVERSE REACTIONS
CNS: headache (in early stages of treatment), transient decrease in hearing, fatigue with large doses, occasional mental confusion, impaired performance of routine activities, psychotic symptoms, dizziness, insomnia, paresthesias of the hands and feet after extended therapy.
GI: nausea, vomiting, flatulence, diarrhea, epigastric distress, *bleeding.*
GU: proteinuria.
Hematologic: leukopenia, *agranulocytosis,* (requires discontinuation of drug), porphyria.
Hepatic: *hepatic toxicity.*
Skin: *rash, urticaria,* photosensitivity, angioneurotic edema.
Other: oral thrush, hypersensitivity reactions (rash), menstrual irregularities, lupus erythematosus.

INTERACTIONS
Coumarin anticoagulants: decreased effectiveness. Monitor PT and INR when used concurrently.
Ethanol: may cause tachycardia, diaphoresis, and flushing. Avoid ethanol.
Oral contraceptives: decreased effectiveness. Suggest alternative methods of contraception.
Phenobarbital: decreased griseofulvin blood levels due to decreased absorption or increased metabolism. Avoid using together or administer griseofulvin t.i.d.

EFFECTS ON DIAGNOSTIC TESTS
Griseofulvin may cause proteinuria; it also may decrease granulocyte counts.

CONTRAINDICATIONS
● Contraindicated in those with hypersensitivity to drug and in those with porphyria or hepatocellular failure.
● Also contraindicated in pregnant patients or women who intend to become pregnant during therapy.

NURSING CONSIDERATIONS
● Use cautiously in penicillin-sensitive patients.
Alert: Because of potential toxicity, know that drug is used only when topical treatment fails.
● Obtain laboratory tests as ordered to confirm diagnosis. Continue drug until clinical and laboratory examinations confirm eradication.
● Be aware that because griseofulvin ultramicrosize is dispersed in polyethylene glycol, it is absorbed more rapidly and completely than microsize preparations and is effective at one-half to two-thirds the usual griseofulvin dose.
● Administer after a high-fat meal to enhance absorption and minimize GI distress.
● Assess hematologic, renal, and hepatic function periodically during prolonged therapy, as ordered.
● Keep in mind that effective treatment of tinea pedis may require concomitant use of a topical agent.

☑ PATIENT TEACHING
● Tell the patient to take drug after a high-fat meal.
● Advise him that prolonged treatment may be needed to control infection and prevent relapse, even if symptoms abate in first few days of therapy. Tell him to keep skin clean and dry and to maintain good hygiene.
● Tell him to avoid intense sunlight.

---

itraconazole
Sporanox

Pregnancy Risk Category: C

HOW SUPPLIED
Capsules: 100 mg

ACTION
Interferes with fungal cell-wall synthesis by inhibiting the formation of ergosterol and increasing cell-wall permeability that makes the fungus susceptible to osmotic instability.

ONSET, PEAK, DURATION
Unknown.

INDICATIONS & DOSAGE

Pulmonary and extrapulmonary blastomycosis; nonmeningeal histoplasmosis—
Adults: 200 mg P.O. daily. Dosage increased as needed and tolerated in 100-mg increments to a maximum of 400 mg daily. Dosages that exceed 200 mg daily should be given in two divided doses. Treatment should continue for a minimum of 3 months. In life-threatening illness, a loading dose of 200 mg t.i.d. is given for 3 days.
Aspergillosis—
Adults: 200 to 400 mg P.O. daily.
Onychomycosis (fungal nail disease) from dermatophytes of toenail—
Adults: 200 mg P.O. once daily for 12 consecutive weeks.
✳**New indication:** *Onychomycosis of the fingernail—*
Adults: initially, 200 mg P.O. b.i.d. for 1 week; after 3 weeks, dosage is repeated.

ADVERSE REACTIONS

CNS: headache, dizziness, somnolence.
CV: hypertension.
GI: *nausea,* vomiting, diarrhea, abdominal pain, anorexia.
GU: albuminuria.
Hepatic: impaired hepatic function.
Skin: rash, pruritus.
Other: edema, fatigue, fever, malaise, decreased libido, hypokalemia, impotence.

INTERACTIONS

Astemizole, cisapride, terfenadine: inhibited metabolism of these antihistamines, resulting in elevated blood levels and risk of serious cardiac toxicity. Never administer together.
Cyclosporine, digoxin: possible increased plasma levels of these drugs. Monitor plasma levels closely.
H₂-receptor antagonists, antacids, rifampin, phenytoin: possible lowered itraconazole plasma levels. Avoid concomitant use.
Isoniazid: may decrease plasma levels

of itraconazole. Monitor closely.
Oral anticoagulants: possible enhanced anticoagulant effects. Monitor PT and INR closely.
Oral antidiabetic agents: similar antifungals have caused hypoglycemia. Monitor blood glucose levels closely.

EFFECTS ON DIAGNOSTIC TESTS
None reported.

CONTRAINDICATIONS
Contraindicated in patients with hypersensitivity to the drug; in patients receiving astemizole, cisapride, or terfenadine; and in breast-feeding patients because drug is excreted in breast milk.

NURSING CONSIDERATIONS
● Use cautiously in patients with hypochlorhydria; they may not absorb drug readily. Because hypochlorhydria can accompany HIV infection, use cautiously in HIV-infected patients.
● Use cautiously in patients receiving other highly bound medications because drug and its metabolites are more than 99% bound to plasma proteins.
● Perform baseline liver function tests, as ordered, and monitor periodically.

☑ PATIENT TEACHING
● Teach the patient to recognize and report the signs and symptoms of liver disease (anorexia, dark urine, pale stools, unusual fatigue, or jaundice).
● Tell the patient to take drug with food to ensure maximal absorption.

---

ketoconazole
Nizoral

Pregnancy Risk Category: C

HOW SUPPLIED
Tablets: 200 mg
Oral suspension: 100 mg/5 ml†

ACTION
Inhibits purine transport and DNA,

RNA, and protein synthesis; increases cell-wall permeability, making the fungus more susceptible to osmotic pressure.

ONSET, PEAK, DURATION
Onset and duration unknown. Serum levels peak 1 to 2 hours after oral dose.

INDICATIONS & DOSAGE
Systemic candidiasis, chronic mucocandidiasis, oral thrush, candiduria, coccidioidomycosis, histoplasmosis, chromomycosis, and paracoccidioidomycosis; severe cutaneous dermatophyte infections resistant to therapy with topical or oral griseofulvin—
Adults and children over 40 kg: initially, 200 mg P.O. daily in a single dose. Dosage may be increased to 400 mg once daily in patients who don't respond to lower dosage.
Children 2 years and over: 3.3 to 6.6 mg/kg P.O. daily as a single dose.

ADVERSE REACTIONS
CNS: headache, nervousness, dizziness, somnolence, photophobia, *suicidal tendencies,* severe depression.
GI: *nausea, vomiting,* abdominal pain, diarrhea.
Hematologic: *thrombocytopenia,* hemolytic anemia, leukopenia.
Hepatic: elevated liver enzymes or *fatal hepatotoxicity.*
Skin: pruritus.
Other: gynecomastia with tenderness, fever, chills, impotence.

INTERACTIONS
Antacids, anticholinergics, H₂ blockers: decreased absorption of ketoconazole. Wait at least 2 hours after ketoconazole dose before administering these drugs.
Astemizole, terfenadine: may increase plasma levels of these drugs, precipitating CV events. Monitor closely.
Cisapride: may cause ventricular arrhythmias. Avoid concomitant use.
Rifampin, isoniazid: increased ketoconazole metabolism. Monitor for decreased antifungal effect.

EFFECTS ON DIAGNOSTIC TESTS
Ketoconazole has been reported to cause transient elevations of AST, ALT, and alkaline phosphatase levels. It has also been reported to cause transient alterations of serum cholesterol and triglyceride levels.

CONTRAINDICATIONS
Contraindicated in patients with hypersensitivity to the drug and in those taking terfenadine or astemizole.

NURSING CONSIDERATIONS
● Use cautiously in patients with hepatic disease and in those who are taking other hepatotoxic drugs.
● Because of the potential for serious hepatotoxicity, be aware that ketoconazole should not be used for less serious conditions, such as fungus infections of the skin or nails.
● Monitor for elevated liver enzymes and nausea that does not subside, as well as for unusual fatigue, jaundice, dark urine, or pale stools—all signs of possible hepatotoxicity.
● Keep in mind that much larger doses (up to 800 mg/day) can be used to treat fungal meningitis and intracerebral fungal lesions.

☑ PATIENT TEACHING
● Instruct the patient with achlorhydria to dissolve each tablet in 4 ml aqueous solution of 0.2 N hydrochloric acid, sip the mixture through a glass or plastic straw (to avoid contact with teeth), and end the procedure by drinking a glass of water because ketoconazole requires gastric acidity for dissolution and absorption.
● Make sure the patient understands that treatment should be continued until all tests indicate that active fungal infection has subsided. If drug is discontinued too soon, infection will recur. Minimum treatment for candidiasis is 7 to 14 days; for other systemic fungal infections, 6

---

months; for resistant dermatophyte infections, at least 4 weeks.
● Reassure patient that nausea, common early in therapy, will subside. To minimize, divide daily dosage into two doses or take it with meals.

---

miconazole
Monistat I.V.

Pregnancy Risk Category: C

HOW SUPPLIED
Injection: 10 mg/ml

ACTION
Inhibits purine transport and DNA, RNA, and protein synthesis; increases cell-wall permeability, making the fungus more susceptible to osmotic pressure.

ONSET, PEAK, DURATION
Onset immediate. Plasma levels peak immediately after I.V. infusion. Duration unknown.

INDICATIONS & DOSAGE
Systemic fungal infections (coccidioidomycosis, candidiasis, cryptococcosis, paracoccidioidomycosis), chronic mucocutaneous candidiasis—
Adults: 200 to 3,600 mg/day I.V. Dosages may vary with diagnosis and with infective agent. Daily dosage may be divided over 3 infusions, 200 to 1,200 mg per infusion. Dilute in at least 200 ml of 0.9% sodium chloride. Repeated courses may be needed because of relapse or reinfection.
Children 1 year and over: 20 to 40 mg/kg/day I.V. Do not exceed 15 mg/kg per infusion.
Fungal meningitis—
Adults: 20 mg intrathecally as adjunct to I.V. administration q 1 to 2 days if subcutaneous ventricular reservoir is used or q 3 to 7 days if reservoir is not used.

ADVERSE REACTIONS
CNS: dizziness, drowsiness.
GI: *nausea,* vomiting, diarrhea.
Hematologic: transient decrease in hematocrit, ***thrombocytopenia.***
Skin: *pruritic rash.*
Other: ***anaphylactoid reactions,*** *fever, chills,* transient decrease in serum sodium, *phlebitis at injection site.*

INTERACTIONS
Astemizole, cisapride, terfenadine: may cause serious CV effects. Never administer together.
Oral anticoagulants: enhanced anticoagulant effect. Monitor closely.

EFFECTS ON DIAGNOSTIC TESTS
Miconazole may cause a transient decrease in hematocrit and an increase or decrease in platelet counts. It frequently causes erythrocyte aggregation. Miconazole also may cause hyponatremia, hyperlipidemia, and hypertriglyceridemia; abnormalities in lipoprotein and immunoelectrophoretic patterns are from the polyoxyl 35 castor oil vehicle.

CONTRAINDICATIONS
Contraindicated in patients with hypersensitivity to the drug and in patients taking terfenadine, astemizole, or cisapride.

NURSING CONSIDERATIONS
● Use cautiously because the drug is dissolved in a vehicle containing polyoxyl 35 castor oil, a substance known to cause anaphylactoid reactions. Give the first dose under continuous medical supervision with emergency resuscitative equipment immediately available. Subsequent doses may be administered on an outpatient basis in selected patients.
● To lessen adverse GI reactions, do not administer at mealtimes.
● Know that premedication with antiemetic may lessen nausea and vomiting.
● **I.V. use:** Be aware that I.V. miconazole has been replaced largely by newer drugs that are better tolerated.

Reactions may be *common*, uncommon, ***life-threatening***, or COMMON AND LIFE-THREATENING.

• Dilute infusion with at least 200 ml of 0.9% sodium chloride solution and infuse over 30 to 60 minutes.
Alert: Rapid I.V. injection of undiluted miconazole may produce arrhythmias.
• For intrathecal use, administer drug undiluted using a subcutaneous intrathecal (Ommaya) reservoir. Alternatively, drug may be given by lumbar or cisternal puncture.
• Monitor levels of hemoglobin, hematocrit, electrolytes, and lipids regularly. Transient elevations in serum cholesterol and triglycerides may be caused by castor oil vehicle.
• In treatment of fungal meningitis and urinary bladder infections, assist with supplemental intrathecal administration and bladder irrigation, respectively.

☑ **PATIENT TEACHING**
• Inform the patient that pruritic rash, which may be controlled with diphenhydramine, may persist for weeks after drug is discontinued.
• Inform the patient that adequate therapeutic response may take weeks or months. Stress importance of compliance with drug therapy and follow-up.
• Instruct the patient to report adverse reactions promptly.
• Advise the patient to avoid performing hazardous activities if drowsiness or dizziness occurs.

---

nystatin
Mycostatin*, Nadostine†, Nilstat, Nystat-Rx, Nystex*

Pregnancy Risk Category: NR

HOW SUPPLIED
Tablets: 500,000 units
Oral suspension: 100,000 units/ml; 50, 150, 500 million units; 1, 2 billion units
Powder: 150, 250, 500 million units; 1, 2, 5 billion units
Vaginal suppositories: 100,000 units

ACTION
Unknown. Probably acts by binding to sterols in fungal cell membrane, altering cell permeability and allowing leakage of intracellular components.

ONSET, PEAK, DURATION
Not applicable; drug is not absorbed.

INDICATIONS & DOSAGE
GI infections—
Adults: 500,000 to 1 million units as oral tablets t.i.d.
Oral, vaginal, and intestinal infections caused by Candida albicans (Monilia) *and other* Candida *species—*
Adults: 400,000 to 600,000 units oral suspension q.i.d. for oral candidiasis.
Children and infants over 3 months: 250,000 to 500,000 units oral suspension q.i.d.
Neonates and premature infants: 100,000 units oral suspension q.i.d.
Vaginal infections—
Adults: 100,000 units, as vaginal tablets, inserted high into vagina, daily or b.i.d. for 14 days.

ADVERSE REACTIONS
GI: transient nausea, vomiting, diarrhea (usually with large oral dosage).

INTERACTIONS
None significant.

EFFECTS ON DIAGNOSTIC TESTS
None reported.

CONTRAINDICATIONS
Contraindicated in patients with hypersensitivity to the drug.

NURSING CONSIDERATIONS
• Keep in mind that nystatin is not effective against systemic infections.
• Know that vaginal tablets can be used by pregnant patients up to 6 weeks before term to treat maternal infection that may cause thrush in neonates.
• For treatment of oral candidiasis (thrush): After the mouth is clean of

---

food debris, have the patient hold suspension in mouth for several minutes before swallowing. When treating infants, swab medication on oral mucosa. Immunosuppressed patients are sometimes instructed by the doctor to suck on vaginal tablets (100,000 units) because this provides prolonged contact with oral mucosa.

☑ PATIENT TEACHING
● Advise the patient to continue medication for at least 2 days after symptoms disappear. Consult the doctor for exact length of therapy.
● Instruct the patient to continue therapy during menstruation.
● Explain that predisposing factors of vaginal infection include use of antibiotics, oral contraceptives, and corticosteroids; diabetes; reinfection by sexual partner; and tight-fitting panty hose. Encourage the patient to use cotton (not synthetic) underpants.
● Instruct the patient in careful hygiene for affected areas, including cleaning perineal area from front to back after defecation.
● Advise the patient to report redness, swelling, or irritation.
● Tell the patient that overusing mouthwash or wearing poorly fitting dentures, especially in older patients, may promote infection.

9

Antimalarials

chloroquine hydrochloride
chloroquine phosphate
chloroquine sulfate
doxycycline
   (See Chapter 14, TETRACYCLINES.)
hydroxychloroquine sulfate
mefloquine hydrochloride
primaquine phosphate
pyrimethamine
pyrimethamine with sulfadoxine

COMBINATION PRODUCTS
ARALEN PHOSPHATE WITH PRIMAQUINE
PHOSPHATE: chloroquine phosphate 500
mg (300-mg base) and primaquine
phosphate 79 mg (45-mg base).

---

chloroquine hydrochloride
Aralen HCl, Chlorquin‡

chloroquine phosphate
Aralen Phosphate, Chlorquin‡

chloroquine sulfate
Nivaquine‡

Pregnancy Risk Category: C

HOW SUPPLIED
chloroquine hydrochloride
Injection: 50 mg/ml (40-mg/ml base)
chloroquine phosphate
Tablets: 250 mg (150-mg base), 500 mg
(300-mg base)
chloroquine sulfate
Tablets: 200 mg (150-mg base)
Syrup: 68 mg (50-mg base)/5 ml

ACTION
Unknown. As an antimalarial, chloroquine may bind to and alter the properties of DNA in susceptible parasites.

ONSET, PEAK, DURATION
Onset and duration unknown. Peak levels occur 30 minutes after parenteral administration and within 1 to 3 hours after oral administration.

INDICATIONS & DOSAGE
Acute malarial attacks caused by Plasmodium vivax, P. malariae, P. ovale, *and
susceptible strains of* P. falciparum—
Adults: initially, 600 mg (base) P.O.,
then 300 mg at 6, 24, and 48 hours. Or
160 to 200 mg (base) I.M. initially; repeated in 6 hours p.r.n. Patient should
be switched to oral therapy as soon as
possible.
Children: initially, 10 mg (base)/kg
P.O., then 5 mg (base)/kg at 6, 24, and
48 hours (do not exceed adult dose). Or
5 mg (base)/kg I.M. initially; repeated
in 6 hours p.r.n. Do not exceed 10 mg
(base)/kg/24 hours. Patient should be
switched to oral therapy as soon as possible.
Malaria prophylaxis—
Adults and children: 5 mg (base)/kg
P.O. (not to exceed 300 mg) weekly on
the same day (begun 2 weeks before
probable exposure and continued for 4
to 6 weeks after leaving endemic area).
If treatment begins after exposure, the
initial dose is doubled (10 mg/kg) in
two divided doses P.O. 6 hours apart.
Extraintestinal amebiasis—
Adults: 1 g (600-mg base) chloroquine
phosphate P.O. daily for 2 days; then
500 mg (300-mg base) daily for 2 to 3
weeks. Treatment is usually combined
with an intestinal amebicide.
Children: 16.7 mg/kg chloroquine
phosphate (10 mg/kg base) P.O. once
daily for 2 to 3 weeks. Maximum
dosage is 500 mg chloroquine phosphate (300-mg base) daily.

ADVERSE REACTIONS
CNS: mild and transient headache, psychic stimulation, *seizures,* dizziness,

---

*Liquid contains alcohol.   **May contain tartrazine.   †Canada only.   ‡Australia only.   ◇OTC.

neuropathy.

CV: hypotension, ECG changes.

EENT: visual disturbances (blurred vision; difficulty in focusing; reversible corneal changes; typically irreversible, sometimes progressive or delayed retinal changes, such as narrowing of arterioles; macular lesions; pallor of optic disk; optic atrophy; patchy retinal pigmentation, typically leading to blindness), ototoxicity (nerve deafness, vertigo, tinnitus).

GI: anorexia, abdominal cramps, diarrhea, nausea, vomiting, stomatitis.

Hematologic: *agranulocytosis, aplastic anemia,* hemolytic anemia, *thrombocytopenia.*

Skin: pruritus, lichen planus eruptions, skin and mucosal pigmentary changes, pleomorphic skin eruptions.

INTERACTIONS

Cimetidine: decreased hepatic metabolism of chloroquine. Monitor for toxicity.

Magnesium and aluminum salts, kaolin: decreased GI absorption. Separate administration times.

EFFECTS ON DIAGNOSTIC TESTS

Chloroquine may cause inversion or depression of the T wave or widening of the QRS complex on ECG. Rarely, it may cause decreased WBC, RBC, or platelet counts.

CONTRAINDICATIONS

Contraindicated in patients with hypersensitivity to the drug and in those with retinal or visual field changes or porphyria.

NURSING CONSIDERATIONS

● Use with extreme caution in patients with severe GI, neurologic, or blood disorders.

● Use cautiously in patients with hepatic disease or alcoholism because drug concentrates in liver, and in those with G6PD deficiency or psoriasis because drug may exacerbate these conditions.

● Ensure baseline and periodic ophthalmic examinations are performed. Check periodically for ocular muscle weakness after long-term use.

● Assist patient with obtaining audiometric examinations before, during, and after therapy, especially if long-term.

● Monitor CBCs and liver function studies periodically during long-term therapy as ordered; if a severe blood disorder not attributable to the disease develops, drug may need to be discontinued.

Alert: Monitor the patient for possible overdose, which can quickly lead to toxic symptoms: headache, drowsiness, visual disturbances, cardiovascular collapse, and seizures, followed by cardiopulmonary arrest. Children are extremely susceptible to toxicity; avoid long-term treatment.

☑ PATIENT TEACHING

● To enhance compliance for prophylaxis, advise the patient to take drug immediately before or after meals on same day each week.

● Instruct the patient to avoid excessive sun exposure to prevent exacerbation of drug-induced dermatoses.

● Tell the patient to report adverse reactions promptly, especially blurred vision, increased sensitivity to light, or muscle weakness.

---

hydroxychloroquine sulfate
Plaquenil

Pregnancy Risk Category: C

HOW SUPPLIED
Tablets: 200 mg (155-mg base)

ACTION
Unknown. May bind to and alter the properties of DNA in susceptible organisms.

ONSET, PEAK, DURATION
Onset and duration unknown. Plasma

levels peak within 2 to 4½ hours.

INDICATIONS & DOSAGE
Suppressive prophylaxis of malaria attacks caused by Plasmodium vivax, P. malariae, P. ovale, *and susceptible strains of* P. falciparum—
Adults and children: for suppression—5 mg (base)/kg P.O. (not to exceed 310 mg) weekly on same day of the week (begin 2 weeks before entering endemic area and continue for 8 weeks after leaving endemic area). If not started before exposure, initial dose is doubled (10 mg/kg) in two divided doses P.O. 6 hours apart.
Acute malarial attacks—
Adults: initially, 800 mg (sulfate) P.O., then 400 mg after 6 to 8 hours, then 400 mg daily for 2 days (total 2 g sulfate salt).
Children: 13 mg/kg (sulfate) P.O., then 6.5 mg/kg 6 hours later, then 6.5 mg/kg daily for 2 days.
Lupus erythematosus (chronic discoid and systemic)—
Adults: 400 mg (sulfate) P.O. daily or b.i.d., continued for several weeks or months, depending on response. For prolonged maintenance dosage, 200 to 400 mg (sulfate) daily.
Rheumatoid arthritis—
Adults: initially, 400 to 600 mg (sulfate) P.O. daily. When good response occurs (usually in 4 to 12 weeks), dosage is cut in half.

ADVERSE REACTIONS
CNS: irritability, nightmares, ataxia, *seizures*, psychosis, vertigo, nystagmus, dizziness, hypoactive deep tendon reflexes, ataxia, lassitude, skeletal muscle weakness, headache.
EENT: visual disturbances (blurred vision; difficulty in focusing; reversible corneal changes; typically irreversible, sometimes progressive or delayed retinal changes, such as narrowing of arterioles; macular lesions; pallor of optic disk; optic atrophy; visual field defects; patchy retinal pigmentation, commonly leading to blindness), ototoxicity (irreversible nerve deafness, tinnitus, labyrinthitis).
GI: anorexia, abdominal cramps, diarrhea, nausea, vomiting.
Hematologic: *agranulocytosis, leukopenia, thrombocytopenia, hemolysis in patients with G6PD deficiency, aplastic anemia.*
Skin: pruritus, lichen planus eruptions, skin and mucosal pigmentary changes, pleomorphic skin eruptions.
Other: weight loss, alopecia, bleaching of hair.

INTERACTIONS
Cimetidine: decreased hepatic metabolism of hydroxychloroquine. Monitor for toxicity.
Magnesium and aluminum salts, kaolin: decreased GI absorption. Separate administration times.

EFFECTS ON DIAGNOSTIC TESTS
Hydroxychloroquine sulfate may cause inversion or depression of the T wave or widening of the QRS complex on ECG. Rarely, it may cause decreased WBC, RBC, or platelet counts.

CONTRAINDICATIONS
Contraindicated in patients with hypersensitivity to the drug, in long-term therapy for children, and in patients with retinal or visual field changes or porphyria.

NURSING CONSIDERATIONS
● Use with extreme caution in patients with severe GI, neurologic, or blood disorders.
● Use cautiously in patients with hepatic disease or alcoholism because drug concentrates in liver, and in those with G6PD deficiency or psoriasis because drug may exacerbate these conditions.
● Ensure baseline and periodic ophthalmic examinations are performed. Check periodically for ocular muscle weakness after long-term use.
● Assist patient with obtaining audio-

---

*Liquid contains alcohol.   **May contain tartrazine.   †Canada only.   ‡Australia only.   ◊ OTC.

metric examinations before, during, and after therapy, especially if long-term.
• Monitor CBCs and liver function studies periodically during long-term therapy, as ordered; if severe blood disorder not attributable to disease develops, drug may need to be discontinued.
Alert: Monitor the patient for possible overdose, which can quickly lead to toxic symptoms: headache, drowsiness, visual disturbances, cardiovascular collapse, and seizures, followed by cardiopulmonary arrest. Children are extremely susceptible to toxicity; long-term treatment should be avoided.

☑ **PATIENT TEACHING**
• To enhance compliance for prophylaxis, advise the patient to take hydroxychloroquine immediately before or after meals on same day each week.
• Instruct the patient to report adverse reactions promptly.

---

mefloquine hydrochloride
Lariam

Pregnancy Risk Category: C

HOW SUPPLIED
Tablets: 250 mg

ACTION
Unknown. Antimalarial activity may be related to its ability to form complexes with hemin.

ONSET, PEAK, DURATION
Onset and duration unknown. Time to peak concentrations is 7 to 24 hours.

INDICATIONS & DOSAGE
Acute malaria infections caused by mefloquine-sensitive strains of Plasmodium falciparum *or* P. vivax—
Adults: 1,250 mg P.O. as a single dose. Patients with *P. vivax* infections should receive subsequent therapy with primaquine or other 8-aminoquinolines to avoid relapse after treatment of the ini-

tial infection.
Malaria prophylaxis—
Adults: 250 mg P.O. once weekly. Prophylaxis should be initiated 1 week before entering endemic area and continued for 4 weeks after returning. If the patient returns to an area without malaria after a prolonged stay in an endemic area, prophylaxis should end after three doses.

ADVERSE REACTIONS
CNS: dizziness, syncope, headache, psychotic manifestations, hallucinations, confusion, anxiety, fatigue, vertigo, depression, *seizures.*
CV: extrasystoles.
EENT: tinnitus, visual disturbances.
GI: anorexia, vomiting, *nausea,* loose stools, diarrhea, abdominal discomfort or pain.
Skin: rash.
Other: fever, chills, myalgia.

INTERACTIONS
Quinine, chloroquine: increased risk of seizures.
Quinine, quinidine, beta-adrenergic blockers: ECG abnormalities and cardiac arrest may occur. Avoid concomitant use.
Valproic acid: decreased valproic acid blood levels and loss of seizure control at start of mefloquine therapy. Monitor anticonvulsant blood levels.

EFFECTS ON DIAGNOSTIC TESTS
Drug may cause decreased hematocrit and transient elevations of transaminases, leukopenia, and thrombocytopenia.

CONTRAINDICATIONS
Contraindicated in patients with hypersensitivity to mefloquine or related compounds.

NURSING CONSIDERATIONS
• Use cautiously in patients with cardiac disease or seizure disorders.
• Because the health risks from concomitant administration of quinine and

---

mefloquine are great, be aware that mefloquine therapy should not begin sooner than 12 hours after the last dose of quinine or quinidine.

● Keep in mind that patients with *P. vivax* infections are at high risk for relapse because the drug does not eliminate the hepatic phase (exoerythrocytic parasites). Follow-up therapy with primaquine is advisable.

● Monitor liver function tests periodically as ordered.

● In cases of suspected overdose, induce vomiting or perform gastric lavage as appropriate because of potential for cardiotoxicity. Animal studies reveal that mefloquine has cardiac actions similar to quinidine and quinine.

☑ PATIENT TEACHING

● Advise the patient to take the drug on the same day of the week when using it for prophylaxis.

● Tell the patient not to take the drug on an empty stomach and always to take it with a full glass (at least 8 oz [240 ml]) of water.

● Advise the patient to use caution when performing activities that require alertness and coordination because dizziness, disturbed sense of balance, and neuropsychiatric reactions may occur.

● Instruct the patient taking mefloquine prophylactically to discontinue the drug if signs or symptoms of impending toxicity, such as unexplained anxiety, depression, confusion, or restlessness, occur and to notify the doctor.

● Advise the patient undergoing long-term therapy to have periodic ophthalmic examinations because ocular lesions have been noted in laboratory animals.

---

primaquine phosphate

Pregnancy Risk Category: C

HOW SUPPLIED
Tablets: 7.5 mg (base)‡, 15 mg (base)

ACTION
Unknown. It may be effective because of the drug's ability to bind to and alter the properties of DNA.

ONSET, PEAK, DURATION
Onset and duration unknown. Plasma levels peak in 2 to 3 hours.

INDICATIONS & DOSAGE
Radical cure of relapsing Plasmodium vivax *malaria, eliminating symptoms and infection completely; prevention of relapse—*
Adults: 15 mg (base) P.O. daily for 14 days. (A 26.3-mg tablet provides 15 mg of base.)
Children: 0.5 mg/kg/day (0.3 mg base/kg/day; maximum 15 mg base/dose) P.O. for 14 days.

ADVERSE REACTIONS
GI: nausea, vomiting, epigastric distress, abdominal cramps.
Hematologic: leukopenia, *hemolytic anemia in G6PD deficiency*, methemoglobinemia in NADH methemoglobin reductase deficiency.

INTERACTIONS
Magnesium and aluminum salts: decreased GI absorption. Separate administration times.
Quinacrine: enhanced toxicity of primaquine. Don't use together.

EFFECTS ON DIAGNOSTIC TESTS
Decreases or increases in WBC counts and decreases in RBC counts may occur during primaquine therapy. Methemoglobinemia may occur.

CONTRAINDICATIONS
Contraindicated in patients with systemic diseases in which agranulocytosis may develop (such as lupus erythematosus or rheumatoid arthritis) and in those taking bone marrow suppressants and potentially hemolytic drugs.

NURSING CONSIDERATIONS

• Use cautiously in patients with previous idiosyncratic reaction (manifested by hemolytic anemia, methemoglobinemia, or leukopenia); in those with a family or personal history of favism; and in those with erythrocytic G6PD deficiency or NADH methemoglobin reductase deficiency.
• Administer drug with meals.
• Keep in mind that when administering the drug, a fast-acting antimalarial (such as chloroquine) is used to reduce possibility of drug-resistant strains.
• Obtain frequent blood studies and urine examinations as ordered in light-skinned patients taking more than 30 mg (base) daily, dark-skinned patients taking more than 15 mg (base) daily, and patients with severe anemia or suspected sensitivity.
• Monitor patient for sudden fall in hemoglobin concentration, erythrocyte or leukocyte count, or marked darkening of the urine, which suggests impending hemolytic reactions. Discontinue drug immediately and notify the doctor.

☑ **PATIENT TEACHING**
• Instruct patient to take drug with meals to minimize stomach upset. If stomach upset (nausea, vomiting, or stomach pain) persists, tell patient to notify doctor.
• Tell patient to stop drug therapy and notify doctor immediately if marked darkening of urine occurs.
• Stress to patient the importance of completing full course of therapy.

---

pyrimethamine
Daraprim

pyrimethamine with
sulfadoxine
Fansidar

Pregnancy Risk Category: C

HOW SUPPLIED
pyrimethamine
Tablets: 25 mg
pyrimethamine with sulfadoxine
Tablets: pyrimethamine 25 mg, sulfadoxine 500 mg

ACTION
Inhibits the enzyme dihydrofolate reductase, thereby impeding reduction of dihydrofolic acid to tetrahydrofolic acid. Sulfadoxine competitively inhibits use of PABA.

ONSET, PEAK, DURATION
Onset and duration unknown. When administered alone, pyrimethamine serum levels peak 2 to 6 hours after oral dose. When given as the combination product, serum pyrimethamine levels peak 1½ to 8 hours and sulfadoxine levels peak 2½ to 6 hours after oral dose.

INDICATIONS & DOSAGE
Malaria prophylaxis and transmission control (pyrimethamine)—
Adults and children 10 years and older: 25 mg P.O. weekly.
Children 4 to 10 years: 12.5 mg P.O. weekly.
Children under 4 years: 6.25 mg P.O. weekly.
    Needs to be continued in all age-groups 6 to 10 weeks after leaving endemic areas.
Acute attacks of malaria (Fansidar)—
Adults and children 14 years and older: 2 to 3 tablets as a single dose, either alone or in sequence with quinine or primaquine.
Children 9 to 14 years: 2 tablets.
Children 4 to 8 years: 1 tablet.
Children under 4 years: ¾ tablet.
Malaria prophylaxis (Fansidar)—
Adults and children 14 years and older: 1 tablet weekly, or 2 tablets q 2 weeks.
Children 9 to 14 years: ¾ tablet weekly, or 1½ tablets q 2 weeks.
Children 4 to 8 years: ½ tablet weekly, or 1 tablet q 2 weeks.

Children under 4 years: ¼ tablet weekly, or ½ tablet q 2 weeks.
Acute attacks of malaria (pyrimethamine)—
Adults and children 15 years and older: 25 mg P.O. daily for 2 days.
Children under 15 years: 12.5 mg P.O. daily for 2 days.

Not recommended alone in nonimmune patients; should be used with faster-acting antimalarials, such as chloroquine, for 2 days to initiate transmission control and suppressive cure.
Toxoplasmosis (pyrimethamine)—
Adults: initially, 100 mg P.O., then 25 mg P.O. daily for 4 to 5 weeks; at the same time, 1 g sulfadiazine is given P.O. q 6 hours.
Children: initially, 1 mg/kg P.O. (not to exceed 100 mg) in two equally divided doses for 2 to 4 days, then 0.5 mg/kg daily for 4 weeks, along with 100 mg sulfadiazine/kg P.O. daily, divided q 6 hours.

ADVERSE REACTIONS
GI: anorexia, vomiting, atrophic glossitis.
Hematologic: *agranulocytosis, aplastic anemia,* megaloblastic anemia, leukopenia, *thrombocytopenia, pancytopenia*.
Note: Adverse drug reactions related to sulfadiazine are similar to sulfonamides.

INTERACTIONS
Folic acid, PABA: decreased antitoxoplasmic effects. May require dosage adjustment.
Sulfonamides, co-trimoxazole, methotrexate: increased risk of bone marrow suppression. Don't use together.

EFFECTS ON DIAGNOSTIC TESTS
Pyrimethamine therapy may decrease WBC, RBC, and platelet counts.

CONTRAINDICATIONS
Pyrimethamine is contraindicated in patients with hypersensitivity to the drug and in patients with megaloblastic ane-

mia caused by folic acid deficiency. Fansidar is contraindicated in patients with porphyria.

Repeated use of Fansidar is contraindicated in patients with severe renal insufficiency, marked liver parenchymal damage or blood dyscrasias, known hypersensitivity to pyrimethamine or sulfonamides, documented megaloblastic anemia due to folate deficiency; in infants under 2 months; in pregnancy at term; and during breast-feeding.

NURSING CONSIDERATIONS
● Use cautiously in patients with impaired hepatic or renal function, severe allergy or bronchial asthma, G6PD deficiency, or seizure disorders (smaller doses may be needed) and after treatment with chloroquine.
● Obtain twice-weekly blood counts, including platelets, as ordered, for the patient with toxoplasmosis because dosages used approach toxic levels. If signs of folic acid or folinic acid deficiency develop, dosage should be reduced or discontinued while the patient receives parenteral folinic acid (leucovorin) until blood counts become normal.
● Keep in mind that, when used to treat toxoplasmosis in patients with AIDS, therapy may be lifelong.
● Know that Fansidar should be used only in areas where chloroquine-resistant malaria is prevalent and only if the traveler plans to stay longer than 3 weeks.

☑ **PATIENT TEACHING**
● Tell patient to take drug with meals.
● Inform the patient with toxoplasmosis of the importance of frequent laboratory studies and compliance with therapy. Tell the patient of potential need for long-term therapy.
● Warn the patient taking Fansidar to stop drug and notify doctor at first sign of rash.
● Tell him to take first prophylactic dose 1 to 2 days before traveling.

10

Antituberculars and antileprotics

aminosalicylate sodium
capreomycin sulfate
clofazimine
cycloserine
dapsone
ethambutol hydrochloride
ethionamide
isoniazid
pyrazinamide
rifabutin
rifampin
streptomycin sulfate
(See Chapter 11, AMINOGLYCOSIDES.)

COMBINATION PRODUCTS
RIFAMATE: isoniazid 150 mg and rifampin 300 mg.
RIFATER: isoniazid 50 mg, rifampin 120 mg, and pyrazinamide 300 mg.
RIMACTANE/INH DUAL PACK: thirty 300-mg isoniazid tablets and sixty 300-mg rifampin capsules.

---

aminosalicylate sodium (para-amino salicylate, PAS)
Nemasol Sodium†, Sodium P.A.S.

Pregnancy Risk Category: NR

HOW SUPPLIED
Tablets: 500 mg

ACTION
Unknown. Believed to suppress growth and reproduction of *Mycobacterium tuberculosis* by competitively inhibiting the formation of folic acid.

ONSET, PEAK, DURATION
Onset and duration unknown. Serum levels peak within 1 to 2 hours.

INDICATIONS & DOSAGE
Adjunctive treatment of tuberculosis—
Adults: 4 g P.O. q 8 hours, or 5 to 6 g q

12 hours. Maximum daily dosage is 12 g. Must be taken with other antituberculars.
Children: 150 mg/kg P.O. daily; alternatively, 75 mg/kg P.O. b.i.d. Maximum daily dosage is 12 g. Must be taken with other antituberculars.

ADVERSE REACTIONS
GI: *abdominal pain, nausea, vomiting, diarrhea,* anorexia.
Hematologic: hemolytic anemia, leukopenia, *agranulocytosis, thrombocytopenia.*
Hepatic: *hepatitis,* jaundice.
Skin: eruptions of various types.
Other: *hypersensitivity reactions (fever),* mononucleosis-like syndrome, goiter or myxedema (with long-term therapy), encephalopathy.

INTERACTIONS
Aminobenzoate derivatives: decreased absorption of aminosalicylate sodium from the GI tract. Avoid concomitant use.
Cyanocobalamin (vitamin B₁₂): decreased absorption of vitamin B_{12} from the GI tract. Provide parenteral supplement as ordered.
Digoxin: may cause decreased absorption of digoxin. Monitor closely.
Probenecid, sulfinpyrazone: decreased excretion of aminosalicylate sodium, resulting in toxicity. Monitor closely.
Rifampin: may impair the absorption of rifampin. Separate administration times by at least 6 hours.
Warfarin, other anticoagulants: enhanced anticoagulant effect. Monitor for bleeding.

EFFECTS ON DIAGNOSTIC TESTS
Aminosalicylate sodium may produce a false-positive test result with copper sulfate tests used for urine glucose deter-

---

Reactions may be *common,* uncommon, *life-threatening,* or COMMON AND LIFE-THREATENING.

minations; may increase serum values of ALT and AST; may produce an orange turbidity or yellow color with Ehrlich's reagent used for urine urobilinogen determinations; and may cause Schilling test results to be misinterpreted because of impaired absorption of vitamin B_{12}.

CONTRAINDICATIONS
Contraindicated in patients with hypersensitivity to the drug, other salicylates, or sulfonamides.

NURSING CONSIDERATIONS
● Use cautiously in patients with peptic ulcer or other GI disease and in patients with CHF. Also use cautiously in patients who may become pregnant because the drug may be teratogenic.

☑ PATIENT TEACHING
● Advise the patient to take the drug with meals or antacids to minimize GI adverse effects. Children may tolerate this drug better than adults.
● Tell the patient to report back pain; pain during urination; unusual bruising or bleeding; fever or sore throat; yellow eyes, sclera, or skin; or severe joint pain.
● Encourage the patient to comply with therapy, which may last several months.
● Instruct the patient to store drug away from heat, humidity, or direct sunlight. Tell the patient not to take tablets that are discolored.

---

capreomycin sulfate
Capastat Sulfate

Pregnancy Risk Category: C

HOW SUPPLIED
Injection: 1 g/vial

ACTION
Unknown.

ONSET, PEAK, DURATION
Onset and duration unknown. Plasma levels peak 1 to 2 hours after I.M. injection.

INDICATIONS & DOSAGE
Adjunctive treatment of tuberculosis—
Adults: 15 mg/kg/day up to 1 g I.M. daily injected deeply into large muscle mass for 60 to 120 days; then 1 g two to three times weekly for 18 to 24 months. Maximum dosage should not exceed 20 mg/kg/day. Must be given in conjunction with another antitubercular.

ADVERSE REACTIONS
EENT: *ototoxicity,* tinnitus, vertigo, hearing loss.
GU: *nephrotoxicity (elevated BUN).*
Hematologic: eosinophilia, leukocytosis, leukopenia, *thrombocytopenia.*
Other: *hypersensitivity reactions* (with concomitant use of other antituberculars); urticaria; maculopapular rashes; hepatotoxicity; pain, induration, excessive bleeding, and sterile abscesses at injection site; hypokalemia.

INTERACTIONS
Nephrotoxic or ototoxic drugs such as aminoglycosides, colistin, polymyxin B, or vancomycin: increased risk of additive toxicity. Avoid concomitant use.
Nondepolarizing neuromuscular blockers: Neuromuscular blockade may be enhanced by concurrent capreomycin due to a synergistic effect on myoneural function. Monitor closely.

EFFECTS ON DIAGNOSTIC TESTS
The drug's physiologic effects may decrease sulfobromophthalein (BSP) excretion. Capreomycin-induced nephrotoxicity may elevate BUN and serum creatinine levels, and increase urinary WBCs, RBCs, casts, and protein.

CONTRAINDICATIONS
Contraindicated in patients with hypersensitivity to the drug.

---

*Liquid contains alcohol.   **May contain tartrazine.   †Canada only.   ‡Australia only.   ◊ OTC.

NURSING CONSIDERATIONS

• Use with extreme caution in patients receiving other ototoxic or nephrotoxic drugs.

• Use cautiously in patients with impaired renal function, history of allergies, or hearing impairment.

• Assess patient's hearing before beginning therapy. Evaluate patient's hearing every 1 to 2 weeks afterward. Notify the doctor if the patient complains of tinnitus, vertigo, or hearing impairment.

• Assess patient's renal function before beginning therapy. Monitor renal function during therapy; notify the doctor if function diminishes. In renal impairment, dosage must be reduced.

• Be aware that capreomycin is considered a "second-line" drug in the treatment of tuberculosis and should always be administered with other antituberculars to prevent the development of resistant organisms.

• To prepare solution, add 2 ml of 0.9% sodium chloride or sterile water for injection to powder to obtain a 1-g dose; add 2.15 ml for a 350 mg/ml concentration; 2.63 ml for a 300 mg/ml concentration; 3.3 ml for a 250 mg/ml concentration; and 4.3 ml for a 200 mg/ml concentration. Wait 2 to 3 minutes for complete dissolution.

• Be aware that straw- or dark-colored solution after reconstitution does not indicate a loss in potency. Do not administer solutions that contain a precipitate. *Alert:* Give deep I.M. to minimize local reactions. Apply ice to injection site p.r.n. for pain. Know that drug is never given I.V. because this route may cause neuromuscular blockade.

• Monitor serum potassium levels regularly as ordered.

☑ **PATIENT TEACHING**

• Instruct a family member or friend how to prepare drug and administer an I.M. injection. Tell them not to use any solution that contains a precipitate. However, reassure them that straw- or dark-colored solution may be used.

• Warn the patient that injection may be painful, and suggest applying ice to injection site p.r.n. for pain.

• Instruct the patient to report adverse reactions promptly.

• Stress the importance of recommended laboratory tests to monitor for adverse reactions.

---

clofazimine
Lamprene

Pregnancy Risk Category: C

HOW SUPPLIED
Capsules: 50 mg, 100 mg

ACTION
Unknown. Thought to inhibit mycobacterial growth by binding preferentially to mycobacterial DNA. Also has anti-inflammatory effects that suppress skin reactions of erythema nodosum leprosum.

ONSET, PEAK, DURATION
Onset and duration unknown. With long-term therapy, time to peak concentration is 1 to 6 hours.

INDICATIONS & DOSAGE
Dapsone-resistant leprosy (Hansen's disease)—
Adults: 100 mg P.O. daily in combination with other antileprotics for 3 years. Then, clofazimine *alone,* 100 mg daily.
Erythema nodosum leprosum—
Adults: 100 to 200 mg P.O. daily for up to 3 months; when prolonged, concomitant corticosteroid therapy is necessary. Dosage is tapered to 100 mg daily as soon as possible. Dosages above 200 mg daily are not recommended.

ADVERSE REACTIONS
EENT: *conjunctival and corneal pigmentation, dryness, burning, itching, irritation.*
GI: *epigastric pain, diarrhea, nausea, vomiting, GI intolerance,* **bowel ob-**

Reactions may be *common,* uncommon, ***life-threatening,*** or COMMON AND LIFE-THREATENING.

struction, bleeding.
Skin: *pink to brownish black pigmentation, ichthyosis and dryness,* rash, pruritus.
Other: *splenic infarction,* discolored body fluids and excrement.

INTERACTIONS
Dapsone: impaired anti-inflammatory effects of clofazimine; no intervention appears necessary.
Isoniazid: may decrease skin levels and increase serum and urine levels of clofazimine. Monitor for decreased effectiveness.
Rifampin: decreased rifampin bioavailability. Monitor for decreased effectiveness.

EFFECTS ON DIAGNOSTIC TESTS
Clofazimine therapy can elevate blood glucose, albumin, serum bilirubin, and AST and can cause hypokalemia and eosinophilia.

CONTRAINDICATIONS
None known.

NURSING CONSIDERATIONS
● Use cautiously in patients with GI dysfunction, such as abdominal pain and diarrhea.
● Be aware that dosages exceeding 100 mg daily should be given for as short a period as possible and only under close medical supervision.
● If the patient complains of colic, burning abdominal pain, or any other GI symptom, report this to the doctor, who may reduce the dose or increase the interval between doses.

☑ PATIENT TEACHING
● Advise the patient to take the drug with meals or milk.
● Warn the patient that clofazimine may discolor skin, body fluids, and excrement. The color ranges from pink to brownish black. Reassure the patient that the unsightly skin discoloration is reversible but may not disappear until

several months or years after drug treatment ends.
● Tell the patient to apply skin oil or cream to help reverse skin dryness or ichthyosis.

---

cycloserine
Seromycin

Pregnancy Risk Category: C

HOW SUPPLIED
Capsules: 250 mg

ACTION
Inhibits cell-wall biosynthesis by interfering with the bacterial use of amino acids. Action may be bacteriostatic or bactericidal, depending on the concentration of the drug attained at the site of infection and the susceptibility of the infecting organism.

ONSET, PEAK, DURATION
Onset and duration unknown. Serum levels peak 3 to 4 hours after oral dose.

INDICATIONS & DOSAGE
Adjunctive treatment in pulmonary or extrapulmonary tuberculosis—
Adults: initially, 250 mg P.O. q 12 hours for 2 weeks; then, if blood levels are below 25 to 30 mcg/ml and no toxicity has developed, dose is increased to 250 mg q 8 hours for 2 weeks. If optimum blood levels are still not achieved and no toxicity has developed, then dose is increased to 250 mg q 6 hours. Maximum dosage is 1 g/day. If CNS toxicity occurs, drug is discontinued for 1 week, then resumed at 250 mg daily for 2 weeks. If no serious toxic effects occur, dosage is increased by 250-mg increments q 10 days until blood level of 25 to 30 mcg/ml is obtained.

ADVERSE REACTIONS
CNS: *seizures,* drowsiness, somnolence, headache, tremor, dysarthria, vertigo, confusion, loss of memory, *possi-*

---

ble suicidal tendencies, psychosis, hyperirritability, paresthesia, paresis, hyperreflexia, *coma.*
CV: sudden CHF.
Other: hypersensitivity reactions (allergic dermatitis), elevated transaminase level.

INTERACTIONS
Ethanol or ethionamide: increased risk of CNS toxicity (seizures); monitor patient closely.
Isoniazid: CNS toxicity (dizziness or drowsiness); monitor patient closely.

EFFECTS ON DIAGNOSTIC TESTS
Cycloserine may elevate serum transaminase levels, especially in patients with hepatic disease.

CONTRAINDICATIONS
Contraindicated in patients with hypersensitivity to the drug and in those with seizure disorders, depression or severe anxiety, psychosis, severe renal insufficiency, or excessive concurrent use of alcohol.

NURSING CONSIDERATIONS
● Use cautiously in patients with impaired renal function; reduced dosage is required.
● Obtain specimen for culture and sensitivity tests before therapy begins and periodically thereafter to detect possible resistance.
● Know that cycloserine is considered a "second-line" drug in the treatment of tuberculosis and should always be administered with other antituberculars to prevent the development of resistant organisms.
● Monitor serum cycloserine levels periodically as ordered, especially in patients receiving high doses (more than 500 mg daily) because toxic reactions may occur with blood levels above 30 mcg/ml.
● Monitor results of hematologic tests and renal and liver function studies.
● Observe for psychotic symptoms, hal-

lucinations, and possible suicidal tendencies.
● Administer pyridoxine, anticonvulsants, tranquilizers, or sedatives, as ordered, to relieve adverse reactions.

☑ PATIENT TEACHING
● Warn the patient to avoid alcohol, which may cause serious neurologic reactions.
● Advise the patient not to perform hazardous activities if drowsiness occurs.
● Tell the patient to report adverse reactions promptly because dosage adjustment may be necessary or other medications may be prescribed to relieve adverse reactions.

dapsone
Avlosulfon†, Dapsone 100‡

Pregnancy Risk Category: C

HOW SUPPLIED
Tablets: 25 mg, 100 mg

ACTION
Unknown. May inhibit folic acid biosynthesis in susceptible organisms.

ONSET, PEAK, DURATION
Onset and duration unknown. Plasma levels peak 4 to 8 hours after oral dose.

INDICATIONS & DOSAGE
All forms of leprosy (Hansen's disease)—
Adults: 100 mg P.O. daily, indefinitely; give with rifampin 600 mg P.O. daily for 6 months.
Children: 1.4 mg/kg P.O. daily for a minimum of 3 years.
Dermatitis herpetiformis—
Adults: 50 mg P.O. daily; increased to 300 mg daily as needed.

ADVERSE REACTIONS
CNS: insomnia, psychosis, headache, paresthesia, peripheral neuropathy, vertigo.

Reactions may be *common,* uncommon, *life-threatening,* or COMMON AND LIFE-THREATENING.

EENT: tinnitus, blurred vision.
GI: anorexia, abdominal pain, nausea, vomiting.
GU: albuminuria, nephrotic syndrome, renal papillary necrosis.
Hematologic: *hemolytic anemia (dose-related), agranulocytosis, aplastic anemia.*
Skin: lupus erythematosus, phototoxity, *exfoliative dermatitis, toxic erythema, erythema multiforme, toxic epidermal necrolysis, morbiliform and scarlatiniform reactions, urticaria, erythema nodosum.*
Other: fever, tachycardia, pancreatitis, male infertility, pulmonary eosinophilia, infectious mononucleosis-like syndrome, *sulfone syndrome (fever, malaise, jaundice* [with hepatic necrosis]*, lymphadenopathy, methemoglobinemia, hemolytic anemia).*

INTERACTIONS

Activated charcoal: may decrease dapsone's GI absorption and enterohepatic recycling. Monitor closely.
Didanosine: possible therapeutic failure of dapsone, leading to an increase in infection. Avoid concomitant use.
Folic acid antagonists, such as methotrexate: increased risk of adverse hematologic reactions. Avoid concomitant use.
PABA: PABA may antagonize the effect of dapsone by interfering with the primary mechanism of action. Monitor for lack of efficacy.
Probenecid: probenecid reduces urinary excretion of dapsone metabolites, increasing plasma concentrations. Monitor closely.
Rifampin: increased hepatic metabolism of dapsone. Monitor for lack of efficacy.
Trimethoprim: increased serum levels of both drugs may occur, possibly increasing the pharmacologic and toxic effects of each drug. Monitor closely.

EFFECTS ON DIAGNOSTIC TESTS
None reported.

CONTRAINDICATIONS
Contraindicated in patients with hypersensitivity to the drug.

NURSING CONSIDERATIONS
● Use cautiously in patients with chronic renal, hepatic, or CV disease; refractory types of anemia; and G6PD deficiency.
● Obtain baseline CBC as ordered. Monitor CBC weekly for the first month, monthly for 6 months, and semiannually thereafter.
● Be prepared to reduce or temporarily discontinue dapsone if hemoglobin falls below 9 g/dl, WBC count falls below 5,000/mm³, or RBC count falls below 2.5 million/mm³ or remains low.
● If generalized, diffuse dermatitis occurs, notify doctor and prepare to interrupt therapy.
● Administer antihistamines as ordered to combat allergic dermatitis.
● Monitor for signs and symptoms of erythema nodosum reaction, which may occur during therapy as a result of *Mycobacterium leprae* bacilli (malaise, fever, painful inflammatory induration in the skin and mucosa, iritis, and neuritis). In severe cases, therapy should be stopped and glucocorticoids given cautiously.

☑ PATIENT TEACHING
Alert: Instruct the breast-feeding patient to report cyanosis in infant, which indicates high sulfone level.
● Tell the patient to avoid prolonged exposure to sunlight or sunlamps as dapsone may cause photosensitivity.
● Inform the patient of need for long-term therapy. Stress importance of compliance with drug therapy.

---

ethambutol hydrochloride
Etibi†, Myambutol

Pregnancy Risk Category: C

HOW SUPPLIED
Tablets: 100 mg, 400 mg

ACTION
Unknown. Appears to interfere with the synthesis of one or more metabolites of susceptible bacteria, altering cellular metabolism during cell division (bacteriostatic).

ONSET, PEAK, DURATION
Onset and duration unknown. Plasma levels peak within 2 to 4 hours after oral dose.

INDICATIONS & DOSAGE
Adjunctive treatment in pulmonary tuberculosis—
Adults and children over 13 years: for patients who have not received previous antitubercular therapy, 15 mg/kg P.O. as a single dose daily.
Re-treatment: 25 mg/kg P.O. daily as a single dose for 60 days (or until bacteriologic smears and cultures become negative) with at least one other antitubercular; then decreased to 15 mg/kg/day as a single dose.

ADVERSE REACTIONS
CNS: headache, dizziness, mental confusion, possible hallucinations, peripheral neuritis (numbness and tingling of extremities).
EENT: optic neuritis (related to dose and duration of treatment).
GI: anorexia, nausea, vomiting, abdominal pain, GI upset.
Skin: dermatitis, pruritis, toxic epidermal necrolysis.
Other: *anaphylactoid reactions,* fever, malaise, bloody sputum, *thrombocytopenia,* joint pain, elevated uric acid level, precipitation of acute gout, abnormal liver function test results.

INTERACTIONS
Aluminum salts: may delay and reduce absorption of ethambutol. Separate administration times by several hours.

EFFECTS ON DIAGNOSTIC TESTS
Ethambutol may elevate serum urate levels and liver function test results.

CONTRAINDICATIONS
Contraindicated in patients with hypersensitivity to the drug, in those with optic neuritis, and in children under 13 years.

NURSING CONSIDERATIONS
● Use cautiously in patients with impaired renal function, cataracts, recurrent eye inflammations, gout, and diabetic retinopathy.
● Perform visual acuity and color discrimination tests before and during therapy.
● Obtain AST and ALT levels before therapy, and monitor these levels every 3 to 4 weeks, as ordered.
● Anticipate dosage reduction in patients with impaired renal function.
● Know that ethambutol should always be administered with other antituberculars to prevent the development of resistant organisms.
● Monitor serum uric acid level as ordered; observe the patient for signs of gout.

☑ PATIENT TEACHING
● Reassure the patient that visual disturbances will generally disappear several weeks to months after drug is stopped.
● Inform the patient that drug is administered concurrently with other antituberculars.
● Stress importance of compliance with drug therapy.

ethionamide
Trecator-SC

Pregnancy Risk Category: C

HOW SUPPLIED
Tablets: 250 mg

ACTION
Unknown. Probably inhibits peptide synthesis.

ONSET, PEAK, DURATION
Onset and duration unknown. Plasma levels peak in approximately 1.8 hours.

INDICATIONS & DOSAGE
Adjunctive treatment in pulmonary or extrapulmonary tuberculosis (when primary therapy with streptomycin or isoniazid cannot be used or has failed)—
Adults: 500 mg to 1 g P.O. daily in one to three equally divided doses. Concomitant administration of other antituberculars and pyridoxine is recommended.
Children: 15 to 20 mg/kg P.O. daily in three to four doses. Maximum dosage is 1 g daily.

ADVERSE REACTIONS
CNS: *depression, asthenia, drowsiness,* peripheral neuritis and neuropathy, olfactory disturbances, blurred vision, diplopia, optic neuritis, dizziness, headache, restlessness, psychosis.
CV: postural hypotension.
GI: *anorexia, nausea, vomiting,* metallic taste, diarrhea, stomatitis.
Hematologic: *thrombocytopenia.*
Hepatic: jaundice, *hepatitis,* elevated AST and ALT levels.
Skin: rash, acne, alopecia.
Other: gynecomastia, impotence, menorrhagia, increased difficulty managing diabetes mellitus.

INTERACTIONS
None significant.

EFFECTS ON DIAGNOSTIC TESTS
Ethionamide may cause transient elevations of liver function test results; it may decrease serum protein-bound iodine and thyroxine values.

CONTRAINDICATIONS
Contraindicated in patients with hypersensitivity to the drug or severe liver damage.

NURSING CONSIDERATIONS
● Use cautiously in patients with diabetes mellitus.
● Obtain culture and sensitivity tests, as ordered, before starting therapy.
● Remember that ethionamide should always be administered with other antituberculars to prevent the development of resistant organisms.
● Give with meals or antacids to minimize GI effects. The patient may require an antiemetic.
● Monitor hepatic function every 2 to 4 weeks.
● If rash occurs, withhold drug and notify doctor; condition may progress to exfoliative dermatitis.
● Be aware that pyridoxine may be ordered to prevent neuropathy.

☑ **PATIENT TEACHING**
● Instruct the patient to take this drug exactly as prescribed; warn against discontinuing drug without the doctor's consent.
● Tell the patient to take drug with meals or antacids to minimize stomach upset.
● Warn the patient against excessive alcohol ingestion, which may make him more vulnerable to liver damage.
● Stress importance of compliance with drug therapy.

isoniazid (isonicotinic acid hydride, INH)
Isotamine†, Laniazid, Nydrazid**, PMS Isoniazid†

Pregnancy Risk Category: C

HOW SUPPLIED
Tablets: 50 mg, 100 mg, 300 mg
Oral solution: 50 mg/5 ml
Injection: 100 mg/ml

ACTION
Unknown. Appears to inhibit cell-wall biosynthesis by interfering with lipid and DNA synthesis (bactericidal).

ONSET, PEAK, DURATION
Onset and duration unknown. Plasma levels peak within 1 to 2 hours after oral or I.M. administration.

INDICATIONS & DOSAGE
Actively growing tubercle bacilli—
Adults: 5 mg/kg P.O. or I.M. daily in a single dose, up to 300 mg/day, continued for 6 months to 2 years.
Infants and children: 10 to 20 mg/kg P.O. or I.M. daily in a single dose, up to 300 to 500 mg/day, continued long enough to prevent relapse. Concomitant administration of at least one other antitubercular is recommended.
Prevention of tubercle bacilli in those exposed to tuberculosis or those with positive skin test whose chest X-rays and bacteriologic studies are consistent with nonprogressive tuberculosis—
Adults: 300 mg P.O. daily in a single dose, continued for 6 months to 1 year.
Infants and children: 10 mg/kg P.O. daily in a single dose, up to 300 mg/day, continued for 1 year.

ADVERSE REACTIONS
CNS: *peripheral neuropathy* (dose-related and especially in patients who are malnourished, alcoholic, diabetic, or slow acetylators), usually preceded by paresthesia of hands and feet, seizures, toxic encephalopathy, optic neuritis and atropy, memory impairment, toxic psychosis.
GI: nausea, vomiting, epigastric distress.
Hematologic: *agranulocytosis,* hemolytic anemia, *aplastic anemia,* eosinophilia, *thrombocytopenia,* sideroblastic anemia.
Hepatic: *hepatitis* (occasionally severe and sometimes fatal, especially in elderly patients), jaundice, *elevated serum transaminase levels,* bilirubinemia.
Other: rheumatic and lupuslike syndromes, hypersensitivity reactions (fever, rash, lymphadenopathy, vasculitis), hyperglycemia, metabolic acidosis, pyridoxine deficiency, hypocalcemia, hypophosphatemia, gynecomastia, irritation at I.M. injection site.

INTERACTIONS
Aluminum-containing antacids and laxatives: may decrease the rate and amount of isoniazid absorbed. Give isoniazid at least 1 hour before antacid or laxative.
Benzodiazepines: isoniazid may inhibit the metabolic clearance of benzodiazepines that undergo oxidative metabolism (diazepam, triazolam), possibly increasing the activity of the benzodiazepine. Monitor closely.
Carbamazepine, halothane: increased risk of isoniazid hepatotoxicity. Use together cautiously.
Corticosteroids: may decrease therapeutic effectiveness of isoniazid. Monitor need for larger isoniazid dose.
Cycloserine, meperidine: may increase CNS adverse reactions and hypotension (meperidine only). Institute safety precautions.
Disulfiram: may cause neurologic symptoms, including changes in behavior and coordination. Avoid concomitant use.
Enflurane: in rapid acetylators of isoniazid, high-output renal failure may occur due to nephrotoxic concentrations of inorganic fluoride. Monitor renal function.
Ethanol: may be associated with increased incidence of isoniazid-related hepatitis. Avoid concomitant use.
Ketoconazole: serum concentrations of ketoconazole may be decreased. Monitor for lack of efficacy.
Oral anticoagulants: anticoagulant activity may be enhanced. Monitor PT closely.
Phenytoin, carbamazepine: increased plasma levels of these anticonvulsants. Monitor closely.

EFFECTS ON DIAGNOSTIC TESTS
Isoniazid alters results of urine glucose tests that use cupric sulfate method (Benedict's reagent or Clinitest). Elevat-

ed liver function study results occur in about 15% of patients; most abnormalities are mild and transient, but some may persist throughout treatment.

CONTRAINDICATIONS
Contraindicated in patients with acute hepatic disease or isoniazid-associated liver damage.

NURSING CONSIDERATIONS
● Use cautiously in patients with chronic non-isoniazid-associated liver disease, seizure disorders (especially in those taking phenytoin), severe renal impairment, and chronic alcoholism and in elderly patients.
● Be aware that isoniazid should always be administered with other antituberculars to prevent the development of resistant organisms.
● Keep in mind that isoniazid pharmacokinetics may vary among patients because its metabolism occurs in the liver by genetically controlled acetylation. Fast acetylators metabolize the drug up to five times as fast as slow acetylators. About 50% of blacks and whites are slow acetylators; over 80% of Chinese, Japanese, and Eskimos are fast acetylators.
● Monitor hepatic function closely for changes.
● Administer pyridoxine, as ordered, to prevent peripheral neuropathy, especially in malnourished patients.

☑ PATIENT TEACHING
● Instruct the patient to take this drug exactly as prescribed; warn against discontinuing drug without the doctor's consent.
● Advise the patient to take with food if GI irritation occurs.
● Tell the patient to notify the doctor immediately if symptoms of liver impairment occur (anorexia, fatigue, malaise, jaundice, dark urine).
● Advise the patient to avoid alcoholic beverages while taking this drug. Also tell the patient to avoid certain foods

(fish such as skipjack and tuna and tyramine-containing products such as aged cheese, beer, and chocolate) because drug has some MAO inhibitor activity.
● Encourage the patient to fully comply with treatment, which may take months or years.

---

pyrazinamide
Pyrazinamide†, Tebrazid†, Zinamide‡

Pregnancy Risk Category: C

HOW SUPPLIED
Tablets: 500 mg

ACTION
Unknown.

ONSET, PEAK, DURATION
Onset and duration unknown. Serum levels peak in 1 to 2 hours.

INDICATIONS & DOSAGE
Adjunctive treatment of tuberculosis (when primary and secondary antituberculars cannot be used or have failed)—
Adults: 15 to 30 mg/kg P.O. once daily. Maximum dosage is 2 g daily. Alternatively, when compliance is a problem, 50 to 70 mg/kg (based on lean body mass) P.O. twice weekly.

ADVERSE REACTIONS
GI: anorexia, nausea, vomiting.
GU: dysuria.
Hematologic: sideroblastic anemia, *thrombocytopenia.*
Skin: rash, urticaria, pruritis, photosensitivity.
Other: malaise, fever, porphyria, hyperuricemia and gout, interstitial nephritis, *arthralgia, myalgia, **hepatitis.***

INTERACTIONS
None significant.

EFFECTS ON DIAGNOSTIC TESTS
Pyrazinamide may interfere with urine ketone determinations. The drug's systemic effects may temporarily decrease 17-ketosteroid levels; it may increase protein-bound iodine and urate levels and results of liver enzyme tests.

CONTRAINDICATIONS
Contraindicated in patients with hypersensitivity to the drug, severe hepatic disease, or acute gout.

NURSING CONSIDERATIONS
• Use cautiously in patients with diabetes mellitus, renal failure, or gout.
• Be aware that pyrazinamide should always be administered with other antituberculars to prevent the development of resistant organisms.
• Know that drug is administered for the initial 2 months of a 6-month or longer treatment regimen for drug susceptible patients. Patients with concomitant HIV infection may require longer courses of therapy.
• Keep in mind that a reduced dosage is needed in patients with renal impairment because nearly 100% of the drug is excreted in urine.
• Question doses that exceed 35 mg/kg because they may cause liver damage.
• Monitor hematopoietic studies and serum uric acid levels, as ordered.
• Monitor liver function studies; assess for jaundice and liver tenderness or enlargement before and frequently during therapy.
• Watch closely for signs of gout and of liver impairment (anorexia, fatigue, malaise, jaundice, dark urine, and liver tenderness). Notify the doctor at once.
• When used with surgical management of tuberculosis, pyrazinamide is started 1 to 2 weeks before surgery and continued for 4 to 6 weeks postoperatively.

☑ **PATIENT TEACHING**
• Inform the patient that other antituberculars will be required concomitantly.
• Instruct the patient to report adverse reactions promptly.
• Stress importance of compliance with drug therapy. If daily therapy poses a problem for the patient, tell him to ask doctor about twice-weekly dosing.

---

rifabutin
Mycobutin

Pregnancy Risk Category: B

HOW SUPPLIED
Capsules: 150 mg

ACTION
Inhibits DNA-dependent RNA polymerase in susceptible bacteria, blocking bacterial protein synthesis.

ONSET, PEAK, DURATION
Onset and duration unknown. Plasma levels peak 1½ to 4 hours after an oral dose.

INDICATIONS & DOSAGE
Prevention of disseminated Mycobacterium avium *complex in patients with advanced HIV infection—*
Adults: 300 mg P.O. daily as a single dose or divided b.i.d.

ADVERSE REACTIONS
GI: dyspepsia, eructation, flatulence, diarrhea, nausea, vomiting, abdominal pain.
GU: discolored urine.
Hematologic: *neutropenia, leukopenia, thrombocytopenia,* eosinophilia.
Skin: *rash.*
Other: fever, myalgia, headache.

INTERACTIONS
Oral contraceptives: decreased effectiveness. Instruct patient to use nonhormonal forms of birth control.
Zidovudine, drugs metabolized by the liver: may alter serum levels of these drugs. Dosage adjustments may be necessary.

Reactions may be *common,* uncommon, *life-threatening,* or COMMON AND LIFE-THREATENING.

EFFECTS ON DIAGNOSTIC TESTS
None reported.

CONTRAINDICATIONS
Contraindicated in patients with hypersensitivity to the drug or other rifamycin derivatives (such as rifampin). Also contraindicated in patients with active tuberculosis because single-agent therapy with rifabutin increases the risk of inducing bacterial resistance to both rifabutin and rifampin.

NURSING CONSIDERATIONS
• Use cautiously in patients with preexisting neutropenia and thrombocytopenia. Perform baseline hematologic studies and repeat periodically.
• Know that high-fat meals slow the rate, but not the extent, of absorption.
• Mix with soft foods, such as applesauce, for patients who have difficulty swallowing.

☑ **PATIENT TEACHING**
• Instruct the patient to take drug for as long as prescribed, exactly as directd, even after he feels better.
• Tell the patient that drug or its metabolites may discolor urine, feces, sputum, saliva, tears, and skin brownish orange. Tell him to avoid wearing soft contact lenses because they may be permanently stained.
• Tell the patient to report photophobia, excessive lacrimation, or eye pain immediately. Rarely, the drug has caused uveitis.

rifampin (rifampicin)
Rifadin, Rifadin IV, Rimactane, Rimycin‡, Rofact†

Pregnancy Risk Category: C

HOW SUPPLIED
Capsules: 150 mg, 300 mg
Injection: 600 mg

ACTION
Inhibits DNA-dependent RNA polymerase, thus impairing RNA synthesis (bactericidal).

ONSET, PEAK, DURATION
Onset and duration unknown. Serum levels peak 2 to 4 hours after oral dose.

INDICATIONS & DOSAGE
Pulmonary tuberculosis—
Adults: 600 mg P.O. or I.V. daily in single dose 1 hour before or 2 hours after meals.
Children over 5 years: 10 to 20 mg/kg P.O. or I.V. daily in single dose 1 hour before or 2 hours after meals. Maximum dosage is 600 mg daily. Concomitant administration with other antituberculars is recommended.
Meningococcal carriers—
Adults: 600 mg P.O. or I.V. b.i.d. for 2 days, or 600 mg P.O. or I.V. once daily for 4 days.
Children 1 month to 12 years: 10 mg/kg P.O. or I.V. b.i.d. for 2 days, not to exceed 600 mg/day, or 10 to 20 mg/kg once daily for 4 days.
Neonates: 5 mg/kg P.O. or I.V. b.i.d. for 2 days.
Prophylaxis of Haemophilus influenzae type b—
Adults and children: 20 mg/kg P.O. daily for 4 days, not to exceed 600 mg/day.

ADVERSE REACTIONS
CNS: headache, fatigue, drowsiness, behavioral changes, dizziness, mental confusion, generalized numbness.
GI: epigastric distress, anorexia, nausea, vomiting, abdominal pain, diarrhea, flatulence, sore mouth and tongue, pseudomembranous colitis, pancreatitis.
GU: hemoglobinuria, hematuria, and *acute renal failure.*
Hematologic: eosinophilia, *thrombocytopenia,* transient leukopenia, hemolytic anemia.
Hepatic: *hepatotoxicity, transient abnormalities in liver function tests.*

Skin: pruritus, urticaria, rash.
Other: flulike syndrome, discoloration of body fluids, hyperuricemia, shortness of breath, wheezing, *shock,* ataxia, osteomalacia, visual disturbances, exudative conjunctivitis, porphyria exacerbation, menstrual disturbances.

INTERACTIONS

Anticoagulants, corticosteroids, cyclosporine, digitalis glycosides, quinidine, oral contraceptives, sulfonylureas, dapsone, narcotics, analgesics, methadone, barbiturates, diazepam, verapamil, beta-adrenergic blockers, clofibrate, progestins, disopyramide, mexiletine, theophylline, chloramphenicol, anticonvulsants: reduced effectiveness of these drugs. Monitor closely.
Ethanol: may increase risk of hepatotoxicity and should be avoided.
Halothane: may increase risk of hepatotoxicity of both drugs. Monitor liver function closely.
Ketoconazole, para-aminosalicylate sodium: may interfere with absorption of rifampin. Give these drugs 8 to 12 hours apart.
Probenecid: may increase rifampin levels. Use cautiously.

EFFECTS ON DIAGNOSTIC TESTS

Rifampin alters standard serum folate and vitamin B_{12} assays. The drug's systemic effects may cause asymptomatic elevation of liver function tests (14%) and serum uric acid. Rifampin may cause temporary retention of sulfobromophthalein in the liver excretion test. It may also interfere with contrast material in gallbladder studies and urinalysis based on spectrophotometry.

CONTRAINDICATIONS

Contraindicated in patients with hypersensitivity to the drug.

NURSING CONSIDERATIONS

● Use cautiously in patients with liver disease.
● Be aware that concomitant treatment

with at least one other antitubercular is recommended.
● Give 1 hour before or 2 hours after meals for optimal absorption; however, if GI irritation occurs, the patient may take rifampin with meals.
● **I.V. use:** Reconstitute vial with 10 ml of sterile water for injection to make a solution containing 60 mg/ml. Add to 100 ml of D_5W and infuse over 30 minutes, or add to 500 ml of D_5W and infuse over 3 hours. When dextrose is contraindicated, drug may be diluted with 0.9% sodium chloride for injection. Do not use other I.V. solutions.
● Monitor hepatic function, hematopoietic studies, and serum uric acid levels, as ordered.
● Watch closely for signs of hepatic impairment and, if present, report them to the doctor.
● May cause hemorrhage in neonates of rifampin-treated mothers.

☑ PATIENT TEACHING

● Instruct the patient who develops drug-induced GI upset to take drug with meals.
● Warn the patient about drowsiness and possible red-orange discoloration of urine, feces, saliva, sweat, sputum, and tears. Soft contact lenses may be permanently stained.
● Advise the patient to avoid alcoholic beverages while taking this drug.

Reactions may be *common,* uncommon, *life-threatening*, or COMMON AND LIFE-THREATENING.

11

Aminoglycosides

amikacin sulfate
gentamicin sulfate
kanamycin sulfate
neomycin sulfate
netilmicin sulfate
streptomycin sulfate
tobramycin sulfate

COMBINATION PRODUCTS
NEOSPORIN G.U. IRRIGANT: 40 mg neomycin sulfate and 200,000 units polymixin B sulfate/ml.

---

amikacin sulfate
Amikin

Pregnancy Risk Category: D

HOW SUPPLIED
Injection: 50 mg/ml, 250 mg/ml

ACTION
Inhibits protein synthesis by binding directly to the 30S ribosomal subunit. Generally bactericidal.

ONSET, PEAK, DURATION
Onset immediate after I.V. infusion; unknown after I.M. injection. Peak serum levels occur immediately after I.V. infusion, 1 hour after I.M. injection. Measurable serum levels persist for 8 to 12 hours.

INDICATIONS & DOSAGE
Serious infections caused by sensitive strains of Pseudomonas aeruginosa, Escherichia coli, Proteus, Klebsiella, Serratia, Enterobacter, Acinetobacter, Providencia, Citrobacter, Staphylococcus—
Adults and children: 15 mg/kg/day divided q 8 to 12 hours I.M. or I.V. infusion (in 100 to 200 ml of D_5W or 0.9% sodium chloride solution run in over 30 to 60 minutes).

Neonates: initially, loading dose of 10 mg/kg I.V., followed by 7.5 mg/kg q 12 hours.
Uncomplicated urinary tract infection—
Adults: 250 mg I.M. or I.V. b.i.d.
In impaired renal function—
Adults: initially, 7.5 mg/kg. Subsequent doses and frequency determined by blood amikacin levels and renal function studies.

ADVERSE REACTIONS
CNS: *neuromuscular blockade.*
EENT: *ototoxicity.*
GU: *nephrotoxicity, azotemia.*
Other: arthralgia, acute muscular paralysis.

INTERACTIONS
Cephalothin: increased nephrotoxicity. Use together cautiously.
Dimenhydrinate: may mask symptoms of ototoxicity. Use with caution.
General anesthetics, neuromuscular blockers: may potentiate neuromuscular blockade.
Indomethacin: may increase serum trough and peak levels of amikacin. Monitor serum amikacin level closely.
I.V. loop diuretics (such as furosemide): increased ototoxicity. Use cautiously.
Other aminoglycosides, acyclovir, amphotericin B, cisplatin, methoxyflurane, vancomycin: increased nephrotoxicity. Use together cautiously.
Parenteral penicillins (such as ticarcillin): amikacin inactivation in vitro. Don't mix together.

EFFECTS ON DIAGNOSTIC TESTS
Amikacin-induced nephrotoxicity may elevate BUN, nonprotein nitrogen, or serum creatinine levels, and increase urinary excretion of casts.

---

*Liquid contains alcohol.   **May contain tartrazine.   †Canada only.   ‡Australia only.   ◊OTC.

CONTRAINDICATIONS

Contraindicated in patients with hypersensitivity to the drug or other aminoglycosides.

NURSING CONSIDERATIONS

- Use cautiously in patients with impaired renal function or neuromuscular disorders, in neonates and infants, and in elderly patients.
- Obtain specimen for culture and sensitivity tests before first dose. Therapy may begin pending results.
- Evaluate patient's hearing before and during therapy. Notify the doctor if the patient complains of tinnitus, vertigo, or hearing loss.
- Weigh the patient and review renal function studies before therapy begins.
- **I.V. use:** After I.V. infusion, flush line with 0.9% sodium chloride solution or D_5W.
- Obtain blood for peak amikacin level 1 hour after I.M. injection and 30 minutes to 1 hour after infusion ends; for trough levels, draw blood just before next dose. Don't collect blood in a heparinized tube; heparin is incompatible with aminoglycosides.
- Be aware that peak blood levels above 35 mcg/ml and trough levels above 10 mcg/ml may be associated with a higher incidence of toxicity.
- Monitor renal function (output, specific gravity, urinalysis, BUN and creatinine levels, and creatinine clearance). Notify the doctor of signs of decreasing renal function.
- Watch for superinfection (continued fever and other signs of new infection, especially of upper respiratory tract).
- Keep in mind that therapy is usually continued for 7 to 10 days. If no response occurs after 3 to 5 days, therapy may be stopped and new specimens obtained for culture and sensitivity testing.

☑ PATIENT TEACHING

- Instruct patient to report adverse reactions promptly.
- Encourage adequate fluid intake.

gentamicin sulfate

Cidomycin†‡, Garamycin, Gentamicin Sulfate ADD-Vantage, Jenamicin

Pregnancy Risk Category: NR

HOW SUPPLIED

Injection: 40 mg/ml (adult), 10 mg/ml (pediatric), 2 mg/ml (intrathecal)
I.V. infusion (premixed): 40 mg, 60 mg, 70 mg, 80 mg, 90 mg, 100 mg, available in 0.9% sodium chloride solution

ACTION

Inhibits protein synthesis by binding directly to the 30S ribosomal subunit. Usually bactericidal.

ONSET, PEAK, DURATION

Onset immediate after I.V. administration, unknown after I.M. administration. Peak serum levels occur in 30 to 90 minutes. Duration unknown.

INDICATIONS & DOSAGE

Serious infections caused by sensitive strains of Pseudomonas aeruginosa, Escherichia coli, Proteus, Klebsiella, Serratia, Enterobacter, Citrobacter, Staphylococcus—
Adults: 3 mg/kg daily in divided doses I.M. or I.V. infusion q 8 hours (in 50 to 200 ml of 0.9% sodium chloride solution or D_5W infused over 30 minutes to 2 hours). For life-threatening infections, the patient may receive up to 5 mg/kg daily in three to four divided doses; this dosage should be reduced to 3 mg/kg daily as soon as clinically indicated.
Children: 2 to 2.5 mg/kg q 8 hours I.M. or by I.V. infusion.
Neonates over 1 week or infants: 7.5 mg/kg daily in divided doses q 8 hours.
Neonates under 1 week and preterm infants: 2.5 mg/kg I.V. q 12 hours.
Meningitis—
Adults: systemic therapy as above; or 4 to 8 mg intrathecally daily.
Children and infants over 3 months:

systemic therapy as above; or 1 to 2 mg intrathecally daily.

Endocarditis prophylaxis for GI or GU procedure or surgery—
Adults: 1.5 mg/kg I.M. or I.V. 30 minutes before procedure or surgery. Maximum dosage is 80 mg. Given with ampicillin (vancomycin in penicillin-allergic patients). Repeated in 8 hours.
Children: 2 mg/kg I.M. or I.V. 30 minutes before procedure or surgery. Maximum dosage is 80 mg. Given with ampicillin (vancomycin in penicillin-allergic patients). After 8 hours, half the initial dose is given.
After hemodialysis to maintain therapeutic blood levels—
Adults: 1 to 1.7 mg/kg I.M. or by I.V. infusion after each dialysis.
Children: 2 to 2.5 mg/kg I.M. or by I.V. infusion after each dialysis.

ADVERSE REACTIONS
CNS: headache, lethargy, encephalopathy, confusion, dizziness, *seizures,* numbness, peripheral neuropathy.
CV: hypotension.
EENT: *ototoxicity,* blurred vision.
GI: vomiting, nausea.
GU: *nephrotoxicity.*
Hematologic: anemia, eosinophilia, leukopenia, *thrombocytopenia,* agranulocytosis.
Respiratory: apnea.
Skin: rash, urticaria, pruritus, tingling.
Other: fever, muscle twitching, myasthenia gravis-like syndrome, *anaphylaxis,* pain at injection site.

INTERACTIONS
Cephalothin: increased nephrotoxicity. Use together cautiously.
Dimenhydrinate: may mask symptoms of ototoxicity. Use with caution.
General anesthetics, neuromuscular blockers: may potentiate neuromuscular blockade.
Indomethacin: may increase serum peak and trough levels of gentamicin. Monitor serum gentamicin levels closely.
I.V. loop diuretics (such as furosemide):

increased ototoxicity. Use cautiously.
Other aminoglycosides, acyclovir, amphotericin B, cisplatin, methoxyflurane, vancomycin: increased ototoxicity and nephrotoxicity. Use together cautiously.
Parenteral penicillins (such as ampicillin and ticarcillin): gentamicin inactivation in vitro. Don't mix together.

EFFECTS ON DIAGNOSTIC TESTS
Gentamicin-induced nephrotoxicity may elevate levels of BUN, nonprotein nitrogen, or serum creatinine, and increase urinary excretion of casts.

CONTRAINDICATIONS
Contraindicated in patients with hypersensitivity to the drug or other aminoglycosides.

NURSING CONSIDERATIONS
● Use cautiously in neonates, infants, elderly patients, and patients with impaired renal function or neuromuscular disorders.
● Obtain specimen for culture and sensitivity tests before first dose.
● Evaluate patient's hearing before and during therapy. Notify the doctor if the patient complains of tinnitus, vertigo, or hearing loss.
● Weigh the patient and review renal function studies before therapy begins.
● **I.V. use:** When giving by intermittent I.V. infusion, dilute with 50 to 200 ml of D_5W or 0.9% sodium chloride injection and infuse over 30 minutes to 2 hours. After completing I.V. infusion, flush the line with 0.9% sodium chloride solution or D_5W.
● Use preservative-free formulations of gentamicin when intrathecal route is ordered.
● Obtain blood for peak gentamicin level 1 hour after I.M. injection and 30 minutes to 1 hour after I.V. infusion; for trough levels, draw blood just before next dose. Don't collect blood in a heparinized tube; heparin is incompatible with aminoglycosides.
● Be aware that peak blood levels above

12 mcg/ml and trough levels above 2 mcg/ml may be associated with higher incidence of toxicity.
• Monitor renal function (output, specific gravity, urinalysis, BUN and creatinine levels, and creatinine clearance). Notify the doctor of signs of decreasing renal function.
• Know that hemodialysis (8 hours) removes up to 50% of drug from blood.
• Watch for superinfection (continued fever and other signs of new infection, especially of upper respiratory tract).
• Know that therapy usually continues for 7 to 10 days. If no response occurs in 3 to 5 days, therapy may be stopped and new specimens obtained for culture and sensitivity testing.

☑ **PATIENT TEACHING**
• Instruct patient to report adverse reactions promptly.
• Encourage adequate fluid intake.
• Caution patient not to perform hazardous activities if adverse CNS reactions occur.

---

kanamycin sulfate
Kanasig‡, Kantrex

Pregnancy Risk Category: D

HOW SUPPLIED
Capsules: 500 mg
Injection: 37.5 mg/ml (pediatric), 250 mg/ml, 333 mg/ml

ACTION
Inhibits protein synthesis by binding directly to the 30S ribosomal subunit. Generally bactericidal.

ONSET, PEAK, DURATION
Onset immediate after I.V. infusion, unknown after I.M. or oral administration. Peak serum levels occur immediately after I.V. infusion, 1 hour after I.M. injection. Measurable serum levels persist for 8 to 12 hours.

INDICATIONS & DOSAGE
Serious infections caused by sensitive strains of Escherichia coli, Proteus, Enterobacter aerogenes, Klebsiella pneumoniae, Serratia marcescens, Acinetobacter—
Adults and children with normal renal function: 15 mg/kg/day divided q 8 to 12 hours I.M. or I.V. Maximum daily dosage is 1.5 g.
Neonates: 15 mg/kg/day divided q 12 hours I.M. or I.V.
Adjunct treatment in hepatic coma—
Adults: 8 to 12 g P.O. daily in divided doses.
Preoperative bowel sterilization—
Adults: 1 g P.O. q 1 hour for four doses, then q 4 hours for four doses; or 1 g P.O. q 1 hour for four doses, then q 6 hours for 36 to 72 hours.
Intraperitoneal irrigation—
500 mg in 20 ml sterile distilled water instilled via catheter into wound after patient has recovered from anesthesia and neuromuscular blocker effects.
Wound irrigation—
Up to 2.5 mg/ml in 0.9% sodium chloride solution.
Aerosol treatment—
250 mg diluted with 3 ml of 0.9% sodium chloride solution via nebulizer two to four times per day.

ADVERSE REACTIONS
CNS: *neuromuscular blockade.*
EENT: *ototoxicity.*
GU: *nephrotoxicity.*
Respiratory: *apnea.*
Other: pain at injection site, acute muscular paralysis.

INTERACTIONS
Cephalothin: increased nephrotoxicity. Use together cautiously.
Dimenhydrinate: may mask symptoms of ototoxicity. Use with caution.
General anesthetics, neuromuscular blockers: may potentiate neuromuscular blockade.
I.V. loop diuretics (such as furosemide): increased ototoxicity. Use cautiously.

Reactions may be *common,* uncommon, *life-threatening,* or COMMON AND LIFE-THREATENING.

Other aminoglycosides, acyclovir, amphotericin B, cisplatin, methoxyflurane, vancomycin: increased nephrotoxicity. Don't use together.
Parenteral penicillins (such as ticarcillin): kanamycin inactivation in vitro. Don't mix together.

EFFECTS ON DIAGNOSTIC TESTS
Kanamycin-induced nephrotoxicity may elevate levels of BUN, nonprotein nitrogen, or serum creatinine, and increase urinary excretion of casts.

CONTRAINDICATIONS
Contraindicated for oral use in patients with intestinal obstruction and in treatment of systemic infection. Also contraindicated in patients with hypersensitivity to the drug or other aminoglycosides.

NURSING CONSIDERATIONS
● Use cautiously in patients with impaired renal function or neuromuscular disorders and in elderly patients.
● Obtain specimen for culture and sensitivity tests before first dose. Therapy may begin pending results.
● Evaluate the patient's hearing before and during therapy. Notify the doctor if the patient complains of tinnitus, vertigo, or hearing loss.
● Weigh the patient and review renal function studies before therapy.
● Know that darkening of vials during shelf life does not indicate loss of potency.
● **I.V. use:** Dilute 500 mg of the drug with 200 ml of 0.9% sodium chloride solution or D_5W and infuse over 30 to 60 minutes.
● For I.M. administration, inject deeply into upper outer quadrant of buttocks. Rotate injection sites.
● Obtain peak and trough levels as ordered. Know that the desirable peak serum concentration is 15 to 30 mcg/ml and trough concentration should not exceed 10 mcg/ml. Prolonged peak concentrations above 30 to 35 mcg/ml may

be associated with increased incidence of toxicity.
● Monitor renal function (output, specific gravity, urinalysis, BUN and creatinine levels, and creatinine clearance). Notify the doctor of signs of decreasing renal function.
● Watch for superinfection (continued fever and other signs of new infection, especially of upper respiratory tract).
● Know that if no response occurs in 3 to 5 days, therapy may be stopped and new specimens obtained for culture and sensitivity testing.

☑ PATIENT TEACHING
● Instruct patient to report adverse reactions promptly.
● Encourage adequate fluid intake.

neomycin sulfate
Mycifradin, Neo-fradin, Neosulf‡, Neo-Tabs

Pregnancy Risk Category: NR

HOW SUPPLIED
Tablets: 500 mg
Oral solution: 125 mg/5 ml

ACTION
Inhibits protein synthesis by binding directly to the 30S ribosomal subunit. Generally bactericidal.

ONSET, PEAK, DURATION
Onset unknown. Peak plasma levels occur in 1 to 4 hours. The drug is usually detectable in plasma for about 8 hours.

INDICATIONS & DOSAGE
Infectious diarrhea caused by enteropathogenic Escherichia coli—
Adults: 50 mg/kg daily P.O. in four divided doses for 2 to 3 days; maximum of 3 g daily is usually adequate.
Children: 50 to 100 mg/kg daily P.O. divided q 4 to 6 hours for 2 to 3 days.
Suppression of intestinal bacteria preoperatively—

Adults: 1 g P.O. q 1 hour for four doses, then 1 g q 4 hours for the balance of the 24 hours. A saline cathartic should precede therapy.
Children: 40 to 100 mg/kg daily P.O. divided q 4 to 6 hours. First dose should follow saline cathartic.
Adjunct treatment in hepatic coma—
Adults: 1 to 3 g P.O. q.i.d. for 5 to 6 days; or 200 ml of 1% solution or 100 ml of 2% solution as enema retained for 20 to 60 minutes q 6 hours.

ADVERSE REACTIONS
EENT: *ototoxicity.*
GI: nausea, vomiting, diarrhea, malabsorption syndrome, *Clostridium difficile*-associated colitis.
GU: *nephrotoxicity.*

INTERACTIONS
Cephalothin: increased nephrotoxicity. Use together cautiously.
Digoxin: decreased digoxin absorption. Monitor closely.
Dimenhydrinate: may mask symptoms of ototoxicity. Use with caution.
I.V. loop diuretics (such as furosemide): increased ototoxicity. Use cautiously.
Oral anticoagulants: inhibited vitamin K-producing bacteria; may potentiate anticoagulant effect.
Other aminoglycosides, acyclovir, amphotericin B, cisplatin, methoxyflurane, vancomycin: increased nephrotoxicity. Use together cautiously.

EFFECTS ON DIAGNOSTIC TESTS
Neomycin-induced nephrotoxicity may elevate levels of BUN, nonprotein nitrogen, or serum creatinine; it may increase urinary excretion of casts if systemic absorption occurs.

CONTRAINDICATIONS
Contraindicated in patients with hypersensitivity to other aminoglycosides and in those with intestinal obstruction.

NURSING CONSIDERATIONS
● Use cautiously in patients with im-paired renal function, neuromuscular disorders, or ulcerative bowel lesions and in elderly patients. Never administer parenterally.
● Monitor renal function (output, specific gravity, urinalysis, BUN and creatinine levels, and creatinine clearance). Notify the doctor of signs of decreasing renal function.
● Evaluate patient's hearing before and during prolonged therapy. Notify the doctor if the patient complains of tinnitus, vertigo, or hearing loss. Onset of deafness may occur several weeks after drug is stopped.
● Watch for superinfection (fever or other signs of new infection).
● In adjunctive treatment of hepatic coma, decrease the patient's dietary protein, and assess neurologic status frequently during therapy.
● For preoperative disinfection, provide a low-residue diet and a cathartic immediately before oral administration of neomycin, as ordered.
● Keep in mind that the ototoxic and nephrotoxic properties of neomycin limit its usefulness.
● Know that neomycin is nonabsorbable at the recommended dosage. However, more than 4 g/day may be systemically absorbed and lead to nephrotoxicity.
● Be aware that drug is available in combination with polymyxin B as a urinary bladder irrigant.

☑ **PATIENT TEACHING**
● Instruct patient to report adverse reactions promptly.
● Encourage adequate fluid intake.

---

netilmicin sulfate
Netromycin

Pregnancy Risk Category: D

HOW SUPPLIED
Injection: 25 mg/ml†, 50 mg/ml†, 100 mg/ml

ACTION
Inhibits protein synthesis by binding directly to the 30S ribosomal subunit. Generally bactericidal.

ONSET, PEAK, DURATION
Onset immediate after I.V. infusion, unknown after I.M. injection. Peak serum levels occur immediately after I.V. infusion, $\frac{1}{2}$ to 1 hour after I.M. injection. Measurable serum levels persist for 8 to 12 hours.

INDICATIONS & DOSAGE
Serious infections caused by sensitive strains of Pseudomonas aeruginosa, Escherichia coli, Proteus, Klebsiella, Serratia, Enterobacter, Citrobacter, Staphylococcus—
Adults and children over 12 years: 4 to 6.5 mg/kg/day by I.M. injection or I.V. infusion. May be given q 12 hours to treat serious urinary tract infections (UTIs) and q 8 to 12 hours to treat serious systemic infections.
Infants and children 6 weeks to 12 years: 5.5 to 8 mg/kg/day by I.M. injection or I.V. infusion given either as 1.8 to 2.7 mg/kg q 8 hours or as 2.7 to 4 mg/kg q 12 hours.
Neonates under 6 weeks: 4 to 6.5 mg/kg/day by I.M. injection or I.V. infusion given as 2 to 3.25 mg/kg q 12 hours.
Complicated UTIs—
Adults with normal renal function: 3 to 4 mg/kg/day by I.M. injection or I.V. infusion divided into two equal doses given q 12 hours.

ADVERSE REACTIONS
CNS: *neuromuscular blockade,* encephalopathy, *seizures,* dizziness, numbness, peripheral neuropathy.
EENT: *ototoxicity.*
GU: *nephrotoxicity.*
Respiratory: apnea.
Other: muscle twitching, myasthenia gravis-like syndrome, skin tingling.

INTERACTIONS
Cephalothin: increased nephrotoxicity. Use together cautiously.
Dimenhydrinate: may mask symptoms of ototoxicity. Use cautiously.
General anesthetics, neuromuscular blockers: may potentiate neuromuscular blockade.
I.V. loop diuretics (such as furosemide): increased ototoxicity. Use cautiously.
Other aminoglycosides, acyclovir, amphotericin B, cisplatin, methoxyflurane, vancomycin: increased nephrotoxicity. Use together cautiously.
Parenteral penicillins (such as ticarcillin): netilmicin inactivation. Don't mix together.

EFFECTS ON DIAGNOSTIC TESTS
Netilmicin-induced nephrotoxicity may elevate levels of BUN, nonprotein nitrogen, or serum creatinine, and increase urinary excretion of casts.

CONTRAINDICATIONS
Contraindicated in patients with hypersensitivity to the drug or other aminoglycosides.

NURSING CONSIDERATIONS
● Use cautiously in patients with impaired renal function or neuromuscular disorders and in neonates, infants, and elderly patients. Commercially available form contains sulfites, which may cause an allergic reaction in certain individuals.
● Obtain specimen for culture and sensitivity tests before first dose. Therapy may begin pending results.
● Weigh the patient and review renal function studies before therapy begins.
● Evaluate the patient's hearing before and during therapy. Notify the doctor if the patient complains of tinnitus, vertigo, or hearing loss. However, some studies show that this drug is less ototoxic than other aminoglycosides.
● **I.V. use:** After completing I.V. infusion, flush the line with 0.9% sodium

---

chloride solution or D_5W.
● Obtain blood for peak level 1 hour after I.M. injection and ½ to 1 hour after infusion ends; for trough levels, draw blood just before next dose. Don't draw blood in a heparinized tube because heparin is incompatible with aminoglycosides.
● Be aware that blood levels above 16 mcg/ml and trough levels above 4 mcg/ml may be associated with higher incidence of toxicity.
● Monitor renal function (output, specific gravity, urinalysis, BUN and creatinine levels, and creatinine clearance) as ordered. Notify the doctor of signs of decreasing renal function.
● Watch for superinfection (continued fever and other signs of new infection, especially of upper respiratory tract).
● Know that therapy usually continues for 7 to 10 days. If no response occurs in 3 to 5 days, therapy may be stopped and new specimens obtained for culture and sensitivity testing.

☑ **PATIENT TEACHING**
● Instruct patient to report adverse reactions promptly.
● Caution patient not to perform hazardous activities if dizziness occurs.
● Encourage adequate fluid intake.

---

streptomycin sulfate

Pregnancy Risk Category: D

HOW SUPPLIED
Injection: 1 g/2.5 ml ampules

ACTION
Inhibits protein synthesis by binding directly to the 30S ribosomal subunit. Generally bactericidal.

ONSET, PEAK, DURATION
Onset and duration unknown. Serum levels peak 1 to 2 hours after I.M. injection.

INDICATIONS & DOSAGE
Streptococcal endocarditis—
Adults: 1 g q 12 hours I.M. for 1 week, then 500 mg I.M. q 12 hours for 1 week, given with penicillin. Patients over 60 years should receive 500 mg I.M. q 12 hours for entire 2 weeks.
Primary and adjunctive treatment in tuberculosis—
Adults: 1 g or 15 mg/kg I.M. daily for 2 to 3 months, then 1 g I.M. two or three times a week.
Children: 20 to 40 mg/kg I.M. daily in divided doses injected deeply into large muscle mass. Given concurrently with other antitubercular agents, but *not* with capreomycin; continued until sputum specimen becomes negative.
Enterococcal endocarditis—
Adults: 1 g I.M. q 12 hours for 2 weeks, then 500 mg I.M. q 12 hours for 4 weeks, given with penicillin.
Tularemia—
Adults: 1 to 2 g I.M. daily in divided doses injected deep into upper outer quadrant of buttocks; continued for 7 to 14 days or until patient is afebrile for 5 to 7 days.

ADVERSE REACTIONS
CNS: *neuromuscular blockade.*
EENT: *ototoxicity.*
GI: vomiting, nausea.
GU: some nephrotoxicity (not as frequently as with other aminoglycosides).
Hematologic: eosinophilia, leukopenia, *thrombocytopenia.*
Respiratory: apnea.
Skin: *exfoliative dermatitis.*
Other: hypersensitivity reactions (rash, fever, urticaria, angioedema), *anaphylaxis.*

INTERACTIONS
Cephalothin: increased nephrotoxicity. Use together cautiously.
Dimenhydrinate: may mask symptoms of streptomycin-induced ototoxicity. Use together cautiously.
General anesthetics, neuromuscular blockers: may potentiate neuromuscular

---

Reactions may be *common*, uncommon, *life-threatening*, or COMMON AND LIFE-THREATENING.

blockade.
I.V. loop diuretics (such as furosemide): increased ototoxicity. Use together cautiously.
Other aminoglycosides, acyclovir, amphotericin B, cisplatin, methoxyflurane, vancomycin: increased nephrotoxicity. Use together cautiously.

EFFECTS ON DIAGNOSTIC TESTS
Streptomycin may cause a false-positive reaction in copper sulfate tests for urine glucose (Benedict's reagent or Clinitest). Streptomycin-induced nephrotoxicity may elevate levels of BUN, nonprotein nitrogen, or serum creatinine, and increase urinary excretion of casts.

CONTRAINDICATIONS
Contraindicated in patients with hypersensitivity to the drug or other aminoglycosides and in patients with labyrinthine disease. Never administer I.V.

NURSING CONSIDERATIONS
● Use cautiously in patients with impaired renal function or neuromuscular disorders and in elderly patients.
● Obtain specimen for culture and sensitivity tests before first dose except when treating tuberculosis. Therapy may begin pending results.
● Evaluate patient's hearing before therapy and for 6 months afterward. Notify the doctor if the patient complains of hearing loss, roaring noises, or fullness in ears.
● Protect hands when preparing because drug is irritating.
● For I.M. administration, inject deeply into upper outer quadrant of buttocks. Rotate injection sites.
● Obtain blood for peak streptomycin level 1 to 2 hours after I.M. injection; for trough levels, draw blood just before next dose. Don't use a heparinized tube because heparin is incompatible with aminoglycosides.
● Watch for signs of superinfection (continued fever and other signs of new infection).

● Be aware that in primary treatment of tuberculosis, streptomycin is discontinued when sputum becomes negative.

☑ **PATIENT TEACHING**
● Instruct patient to report adverse reactions promptly.
● Encourage adequate fluid intake.
● Emphasize the need for blood tests to monitor streptomycin levels and determine the effectiveness of therapy.

tobramycin sulfate
Nebcin

Pregnancy Risk Category: D

HOW SUPPLIED
Multi-dose vials: 80 mg/2 ml, 20 mg/ 2 ml (pediatric)
Premixed parenteral injection for I.V. infusion: 60 mg or 80 mg in 0.9% sodium chloride solution

ACTION
Inhibits protein synthesis by binding directly to the 30S ribosomal subunit. Generally bactericidal.

ONSET, PEAK, DURATION
Onset immediate after I.V. infusion, unknown after I.M. injection. Peak serum levels occur immediately after I.V. infusion, 30 to 90 minutes after I.M. injection. Measurable serum levels persist for about 8 hours after I.M. or I.V. administration.

INDICATIONS & DOSAGE
Serious infections caused by sensitive strains of Escherichia coli, Proteus, Klebsiella, Enterobacter, Serratia, Morganella morganii, Staphylococcus aureus, Pseudomonas, Citrobacter, Providencia—
Adults: 3 mg/kg I.M. or I.V. daily divided q 8 hours. Up to 5 mg/kg daily divided q 6 to 8 hours for life-threatening infections; this dosage should be reduced to 3 mg/kg daily as soon as clini-

cally indicated.
Children: 6 to 7.5 mg/kg I.M. or I.V. daily in three or four equally divided doses.

Neonates under 1 week or premature infants: up to 4 mg/kg/day I.V. or I.M. in two equal doses q 12 hours.

ADVERSE REACTIONS
CNS: headache, lethargy, confusion, disorientation.
EENT: *ototoxicity.*
GI: vomiting, nausea, diarrhea.
GU: *nephrotoxicity.*
Hematologic: anemia, eosinophilia, leukopenia, thrombocytopenia, agranulocytosis.
Other: fever, rash, urticaria, pruritus.

INTERACTIONS
Cephalothin: increased nephrotoxicity. Use together cautiously.
Dimenhydrinate: may mask symptoms of ototoxicity. Use with caution.
General anesthetics, neuromuscular blockers: may potentiate neuromuscular blockade.
I.V. loop diuretics (such as furosemide): increased ototoxicity. Use together cautiously.
Other aminoglycosides, acyclovir, amphotericin B, cisplatin, methoxyflurane, vancomycin: increased nephrotoxicity. Use together cautiously.
Parenteral penicillins (such as ticarcillin): tobramycin inactivation in vitro. Don't mix together.

EFFECTS ON DIAGNOSTIC TESTS
Tobramycin may elevate BUN, nonprotein nitrogen, or serum creatinine levels and increase urinary excretion of casts.

CONTRAINDICATIONS
Contraindicated in patients with hypersensitivity to the drug or other aminoglycosides.

NURSING CONSIDERATIONS
● Use cautiously in patients with impaired renal function or neuromuscular disorders and in elderly patients.
● Obtain specimen for culture and sensitivity tests before first dose. Therapy may begin pending results.
● Weigh the patient and review renal function studies before therapy.
● Evaluate patient's hearing before and during therapy. Notify the doctor if the patient complains of tinnitus, vertigo, or hearing loss.
● **I.V. use:** Dilute in 50 to 100 ml of 0.9% sodium chloride solution or D_5W for adults and in less volume for children. Infuse over 20 to 60 minutes. After I.V. infusion, flush line with 0.9% sodium chloride solution or D_5W.
● Obtain blood for peak level 1 hour after I.M. injection and ½ to 1 hour after infusion ends; draw blood for trough level just before next dose. Don't collect blood in a heparinized tube because heparin is incompatible with aminoglycosides.
Alert: Be aware that blood levels over 12 mcg/ml and trough levels above 2 mcg/ml may be associated with increased incidence of toxicity.
● Monitor renal function (output, specific gravity, urinalysis, BUN and creatinine levels, and creatinine clearance). Notify the doctor of signs of decreasing renal function.
● Watch for signs of superinfection (continued fever and other signs of new infection).
● Be aware that if no response occurs in 3 to 5 days, therapy may be stopped and new specimens obtained for culture and sensitivity testing.

☑ PATIENT TEACHING
● Instruct patient to report adverse reactions promptly.
● Caution patient not to perform hazardous activities if adverse CNS reactions occur.
● Encourage adequate fluid intake.

12

Penicillins

amoxicillin/clavulanate
   potassium
amoxicillin trihydrate
ampicillin
ampicillin sodium
ampicillin trihydrate
ampicillin sodium/sulbactam
   sodium
bacampicillin hydrochloride
carbenicillin indanyl sodium
cloxacillin sodium
dicloxacillin sodium
mezlocillin sodium
nafcillin sodium
oxacillin sodium
penicillin G benzathine
penicillin G potassium
penicillin G procaine
penicillin G sodium
penicillin V
penicillin V potassium
piperacillin sodium
piperacillin sodium and
   tazobactam sodium
ticarcillin disodium
ticarcillin disodium/clavulanate
   potassium

COMBINATION PRODUCTS

AUGMENTIN, CLAVULIN†: amoxicillin
250 mg and clavulanate potassium 125
mg/tablet; amoxicillin 500 mg and
clavulanate potassium 125 mg/tablet;
amoxicillin 125 mg and clavulanate
potassium 31.25 mg/chewable tablet;
amoxicillin 250 mg and clavulanate
potassium 62.5 mg/chewable tablet;
amoxicillin 125 mg and clavulanate potassium 31.25 mg/5 ml oral suspension;
amoxicillin 250 mg and clavulanate
potassium 62.5 mg/5 ml oral suspension.
POLYCILLIN-PRB: ampicillin trihydrate
3.5 g and probenecid 1 g per bottle.
PRINCIPEN WITH PROBENECID: ampicillin
trihydrate 3.5 g and probenecid 1 g per
bottle.

amoxicillin/clavulanate potassium (amoxycillin/clavulanate potassium)
Augmentin, Clavulin†

Pregnancy Risk Category: B

HOW SUPPLIED
Tablets (chewable): 125 mg amoxicillin
trihydrate, 31.25 mg clavulanic acid;
250 mg amoxicillin trihydrate, 62.5 mg
clavulanic acid
Tablets (film-coated): 250 mg amoxicillin trihydrate, 125 mg clavulanic
acid; 500 mg amoxicillin trihydrate, 125
mg clavulanic acid
Oral suspension: 125 mg amoxicillin
trihydrate and 31.25 mg clavulanic
acid/5 ml (after reconstitution); 250 mg
amoxicillin trihydrate and 62.5 mg clavulanic acid/5 ml (after reconstitution)

ACTION
An aminopenicillin that prevents bacterial cell-wall synthesis during replication. Clavulanic acid increases amoxicillin effectiveness by inactivating beta
lactamases, which destroy amoxicillin.

ONSET, PEAK, DURATION
Onset unknown. Serum levels peak in 1
to 2½ hours. Serum concentrations are
usually low or undetectable 6 to 8 hours
after oral administration.

INDICATIONS & DOSAGE
*Lower respiratory infections, otitis me-
dia, sinusitis, skin and skin-structure infections, and urinary tract infections
caused by susceptible strains of gram-
positive and gram-negative organisms—*
Adults and children 40 kg or over:
250 mg (based on the amoxicillin component) P.O. q 8 hours. For more severe
infections, 500 mg q 8 hours.

Children weighing less than 40 kg: 20 to 40 mg/kg (based on the amoxicillin component) P.O. daily in divided doses q 8 hours.

ADVERSE REACTIONS
CNS: agitation, anxiety, insomnia, confusion, behavioral changes, dizziness.
GI: *nausea,* vomiting, *diarrhea,* indigestion, gastritis, stomatitis, glossitis, black "hairy" tongue, enterocolitis, pseudomembranous colitis.
Hematologic: anemia, *thrombocytopenia,* thrombocytopenic purpura, eosinophilia, leukopenia, *agranulocytosis.*
Other: hypersensitivity reactions (erythematous maculopapular rash, urticaria, *anaphylaxis*), overgrowth of nonsusceptible organisms, vaginitis.

INTERACTIONS
Allopurinol: increased incidence of rash.
Oral contraceptives: efficacy of oral contraceptives may be decreased. Additional form of contraception recommended during penicillin therapy.
Probenecid: increased blood levels of amoxicillin and other penicillins. Probenecid may be used for this purpose.

EFFECTS ON DIAGNOSTIC TESTS
Amoxicillin/potassium clavulanate alters results of urine glucose tests that use cupric sulfate (Benedict's reagent or Clinitest). Make urine glucose determinations with glucose oxidase methods (Clinistix or Tes-Tape). Positive Coombs' tests have been reported with other clavulanate combinations. Amoxicillin may falsely decrease serum aminoglycoside concentrations.

CONTRAINDICATIONS
Contraindicated in patients with hypersensitivity to the drug or other penicillins and in those with a previous history of amoxicillin-associated cholestatic jaundice or hepatic dysfunction.

NURSING CONSIDERATIONS
● Use cautiously in patients with other drug allergies, especially to cephalosporins (possible cross-sensitivity), and in those with mononucleosis (high incidence of maculopapular rash).
● Before giving, ask the patient about any allergic reactions to penicillin. However, a negative history of penicillin allergy is no guarantee against an allergic reaction.
● Obtain specimen for culture and sensitivity tests before first dose. Therapy may begin pending results.
● Give drug at least 1 hour before bacteriostatic antibiotics.
● Observe closely. With large doses and prolonged therapy, bacterial or fungal superinfection may occur, especially in elderly, debilitated, or immunosuppressed patients.
Alert: Know that both the "250" and "500" tablets contain the same amount of clavulanic acid (125 mg). Therefore, two "250" tablets are not equivalent to one "500" tablet.
● Be aware that this drug combination is particularly useful in clinical settings with high prevalence of amoxicillin-resistant organisms.
● After reconstitution, refrigerate the oral suspension; discard after 10 days.

☑ PATIENT TEACHING
● Tell the patient to take entire quantity of drug exactly as prescribed, even after he feels better.
● Instruct him to take drug with food to prevent GI upset. If he's taking the oral suspension, tell him to keep drug refrigerated, to shake it well before administration, and to discard any remaining drug after 10 days.
● Tell the patient to call doctor if a rash occurs. A rash is a sign of an allergic reaction.

Reactions may be *common*, uncommon, *life-threatening*, or COMMON AND LIFE-THREATENING.

amoxicillin trihydrate (amoxycillin trihydrate)

Alphamox‡, Amoxil, Apo-Amoxi†, Cilamox‡, Ibiamox‡, Larotid, Moxacin‡, Novamoxin†, Nu-Amoxi†, Polymox, Trimox, Wymox

Pregnancy Risk Category: NR

HOW SUPPLIED
Tablets (chewable): 125 mg, 250 mg
Capsules: 250 mg, 500 mg
Oral suspension: 50 mg/ml (pediatric drops), 125 mg/5 ml, 250 mg/5 ml (after reconstitution)

ACTION
An aminopenicillin that inhibits cell-wall synthesis during bacterial multiplication; bacteria resist amoxicillin by producing penicillinases—enzymes that hydrolyze amoxicillin.

ONSET, PEAK, DURATION
Onset unknown. Serum levels peak within 1 to 2 hours. Serum concentrations are usually low or undetectable 6 to 8 hours after oral administration.

INDICATIONS & DOSAGE
Systemic infections, acute and chronic urinary tract infections caused by susceptible strains of gram-positive and gram-negative organisms—
Adults and children 20 kg or over: 250 to 500 mg P.O. q 8 hours.
Children under 20 kg: 20 mg/kg P.O. daily in divided doses q 8 hours; in severe infection, 40 mg/kg P.O. daily in divided doses q 8 hours or 500 mg to 1 g/m² P.O. in divided doses q 8 hours.
Uncomplicated gonorrhea—
Adults and children over 45 kg: 3 g P.O. with 1 g probenecid given as a single dose. Do not give probenecid to children under age 2.
Endocarditis prophylaxis for dental procedures—
Adults: initially, 3 g P.O. 1 hour before procedure; then 1.5 g 6 hours later.

Children: initially, 50 mg/kg P.O. 1 hour before procedure; then half the initial dose 6 hours later.

ADVERSE REACTIONS
CNS: lethargy, hallucinations, *seizures,* anxiety, confusion, agitation, depression, dizziness, fatigue.
GI: *nausea,* vomiting, *diarrhea,* glossitis, stomatitis, gastritis, abdominal pain, enterocolitis, pseudomembranous colitis, black "hairy" tongue.
GU: interstitial nephritis, nephropathy.
Hematologic: anemia, *thrombocytopenia,* thrombocytopenic purpura, eosinophilia, leukopenia, hemolytic anemia, *agranulocytosis.*
Other: hypersensitivity reactions (erythematous maculopapular rash, urticaria, *anaphylaxis*), overgrowth of nonsusceptible organisms, vaginitis.

INTERACTIONS
Allopurinol: increased incidence of rash.
Oral contraceptives: efficacy of oral contraceptives may be decreased. Additional form of contraception recommended during penicillin therapy.
Probenecid: increased blood levels of amoxicillin and other penicillins. Probenecid may be used for this purpose.

EFFECTS ON DIAGNOSTIC TESTS
Amoxicillin may alter results of urine glucose tests that use cupric sulfate (Benedict's reagent or Clinitest). Make urine glucose determinations with glucose oxidase methods (Clinistix or Tes-Tape). Amoxicillin may falsely decrease serum aminoglycoside concentrations.

CONTRAINDICATIONS
Contraindicated in patients with hypersensitivity to the drug or other penicillins.

NURSING CONSIDERATIONS
● Use cautiously in patients with other drug allergies, especially to cephalo-

sporins (possible cross-sensitivity), and in those with mononucleosis (high incidence of maculopapular rash).

● Before giving, ask the patient about allergic reactions to penicillin. A negative history of penicillin allergy is no guarantee against allergic reaction.

● Obtain specimen for culture and sensitivity tests before first dose. Therapy may begin pending results.

● Give amoxicillin at least 1 hour before bacteriostatic antibiotics.

● Observe closely. With large doses and prolonged therapy, superinfection may occur, especially in elderly, debilitated, or immunosuppressed patients.

● Store Trimox oral suspension at room temperature for up to 2 weeks. Be sure to check individual product labels for storage information.

● Keep in mind that amoxicillin generally causes diarrhea less often than ampicillin.

☑ PATIENT TEACHING
● Tell the patient to take entire quantity of medication exactly as prescribed, even after he feels better.

● Tell him to take drug with food.

● Tell the patient to call the doctor if rash, fever, or chills develop. A rash is the most common allergic reaction, especially when the patient is also taking allopurinol.

---

ampicillin
Apo-Ampi†, Novo Ampicillin†, Nu-Ampi†, Omnipen, Principen

ampicillin sodium
Ampicin†, Ampicyn Injection‡, Omnipen-N, Penbritin†, Polycillin-N, Totacillin-N

ampicillin trihydrate
Ampicyn Oral‡, D-Amp, Omnipen, Penbritin‡, Polycillin, Principen-250, Principen-500, Totacillin

Pregnancy Risk Category: B

HOW SUPPLIED
Capsules: 250 mg, 500 mg
Oral suspension: 100 mg/ml (pediatric drops), 125 mg/5 ml, 250 mg/5 ml, 500 mg/5 ml (after reconstitution)
Injection: 125 mg, 250 mg, 500 mg, 1 g, 2 g
Infusion: 500 mg, 1 g, 2 g
Pharmacy bulk package: 10-g vial

ACTION
An aminopenicillin that inhibits cell-wall synthesis during microorganism multiplication; bacteria resist ampicillin by producing penicillinases—enzymes that hydrolyze ampicillin.

ONSET, PEAK, DURATION
Onset immediate after I.V. administration, unknown after I.M. injection. Peak plasma levels occur immediately after I.V. administration, within 1 hour of I.M. administration, and within 2 hours of oral administration. Serum levels are usually low or undetectable 6 to 8 hours after oral administration.

INDICATIONS & DOSAGE
Systemic infections and acute and chronic urinary tract infections caused by susceptible strains of gram-positive and gram-negative organisms—
Adults and children 20 kg or over: 250 to 500 mg P.O. q 6 hours; or 2 to 12 g I.M. or I.V. daily, in divided doses q 4 to 6 hours.
Children under 20 kg: 50 to 100 mg/kg P.O. daily, in divided doses q 6 hours; or 100 to 200 mg/kg I.M. or I.V. daily, in divided doses q 6 hours.
Meningitis—
Adults: 8 to 14 g I.V. daily in divided doses q 3 to 4 hours.
Children: up to 300 mg/kg I.V. daily in divided doses q 3 to 4 hours.
Uncomplicated gonorrhea—
Adults and children over 45 kg: 3.5 g P.O. with 1 g probenecid given as a single dose.
Endocarditis prophylaxis for dental procedures—

Adults: 2 g I.M. or I.V. with genta-micin 30 minutes before procedure; and 1 g I.M. or I.V. 6 hours after initial dose.
Children: 50 mg/kg I.M. or I.V. with gentamicin 2 mg/kg 30 minutes before procedure; half the initial dose is given 6 hours later.

ADVERSE REACTIONS
CNS: lethargy, hallucinations, *seizures,* anxiety, confusion, agitation, depression, dizziness, fatigue.
GI: *nausea,* vomiting, *diarrhea,* glossitis, stomatitis, gastritis, abdominal pain, enterocolitis, pseudomembranous colitis, black "hairy" tongue.
GU: interstitial nephritis, nephropathy.
Hematologic: anemia, *thrombocytopenia,* thrombocytopenic purpura, eosinophilia, leukopenia, hemolytic anemia, *agranulocytosis*.
Other: hypersensitivity reactions (erythematous maculopapular rash, urticaria, *anaphylaxis*), overgrowth of nonsusceptible organisms, pain at injection site, vein irritation, thrombophlebitis, vaginitis.

INTERACTIONS
Allopurinol: increased incidence of rash.
Oral contraceptives: efficacy of oral contraceptives may be decreased. Additional form of contraception recommended during penicillin therapy.
Probenecid: increased blood levels of ampicillin and other penicillins. Probenecid may be used for this purpose.

EFFECTS ON DIAGNOSTIC TESTS
Ampicillin alters results of urine glucose tests that use cupric sulfate (Benedict's reagent or Clinitest). Make urine glucose determinations with glucose oxidase methods (Clinistix or Tes-Tape). Ampicillin may falsely decrease serum aminoglycoside concentrations.

CONTRAINDICATIONS
Contraindicated in patients with hyper-sensitivity to the drug or other penicillins.

NURSING CONSIDERATIONS
● Use cautiously in patients with other drug allergies, especially to cephalosporins (possible cross-sensitivity), or in those with mononucleosis (high incidence of maculopapular rash).
● Before giving, ask the patient about any allergic reactions to penicillin. However, a negative history of penicillin allergy is no guarantee against a future allergic reaction.
● Obtain specimen for culture and sensitivity tests before first dose. Therapy may begin pending results.
● **I.V. use:** For I.V. injection, reconstitute with bacteriostatic water for injection. Use 5 ml for the 125-mg, 250-mg, or 500-mg vials; 7.4 ml for the 1-g vials; or 14.8 ml for the 2-g vials. Give direct I.V. injections over 3 to 5 minutes for doses of 500 mg or less; over 10 to 15 minutes for larger doses. Don't exceed a rate of 100 mg/minute. Alternatively, dilute in 50 to 100 ml of 0.9% sodium chloride for injection and give by intermittent infusion over 15 to 30 minutes.
Alert: Don't mix with solutions containing dextrose or fructose because these solutions promote rapid breakdown of ampicillin.
● Use initial dilution within 1 hour. Follow manufacturer's directions for stability data when ampicillin is further diluted for I.V. infusion.
● Give I.V. intermittently to prevent vein irritation. Change site every 48 hours.
● Give the drug I.M. or I.V. only if prescribed and the infection is severe or if patient can't take oral dose.
● Give 1 to 2 hours before or 2 to 3 hours after meals. When given orally, drug may cause GI disturbances. Food may interfere with absorption.
● Give ampicillin at least 1 hour before bacteriostatic antibiotics.
● Observe closely. With large doses or

prolonged therapy, bacterial or fungal superinfection may occur, especially in elderly, debilitated, or immunosuppressed patients.

• Know that dosage should be altered in patients with impaired renal function.

• Be aware that in pediatric meningitis, ampicillin may be given concurrently with parenteral chloramphenicol for 24 hours pending cultures.

☑ PATIENT TEACHING

• Tell the patient to take entire quantity of medication exactly as prescribed, even after he feels better.

• Instruct the patient to take oral form on an empty stomach.

• Tell the patient to call the doctor if rash, fever, or chills develop. A rash is the most common allergic reaction, especially if the patient is also taking allopurinol.

• Instruct the patient to report discomfort at I.V. injection site.

---

ampicillin sodium/sulbactam sodium
Unasyn

Pregnancy Risk Category: B

HOW SUPPLIED
Injection: vials and piggyback vials containing 1.5 g (1 g ampicillin sodium with 0.5 g sulbactam sodium) and 3 g (2 g ampicillin sodium with 1 g sulbactam sodium)
Pharmacy bulk package: 15 g (10 g ampicillin sodium with 5 g sulbactam sodium)

ACTION
Ampicillin (an aminopenicillin) inhibits cell-wall synthesis during microorganism multiplication; sulbactam inactivates bacterial beta-lactamase, which inactivates ampicillin and causes bacterial resistance to it.

ONSET, PEAK, DURATION
Onset immediate after I.V. administration, unknown after I.M. injection. Peak serum levels occur immediately after I.V. administration, unknown after I.M. injection. Duration unknown.

INDICATIONS & DOSAGE
Intra-abdominal, gynecologic, and skin-structure infections caused by susceptible strains—
Adults: dosage expressed as total drug (each 1.5-g vial contains 1 g ampicillin sodium and 0.5 g sulbactam sodium)—1.5 to 3 g I.M. or I.V. q 6 hours. Maximum daily dosage is 4 g sulbactam and 8 g ampicillin (12 g of combined drugs).

ADVERSE REACTIONS
GI: *nausea,* vomiting, *diarrhea,* glossitis, stomatitis, gastritis, black "hairy" tongue, enterocolitis, pseudomembranous colitis.
Hematologic: anemia, ***thrombocytopenia,*** thrombocytopenic purpura, eosinophilia, leukopenia, ***agranulocytosis.***
Other: hypersensitivity reactions (erythematous maculopapular rash, urticaria, ***anaphylaxis***), ***overgrowth of nonsusceptible organisms,*** pain at injection site, vein irritation, thrombophlebitis.

INTERACTIONS
Allopurinol: increased incidence of rash.
Oral contraceptives: efficacy of oral contraceptives may be decreased. Additional form of contraception recommended during penicillin therapy.
Probenecid: increased levels of ampicillin. Probenecid may be used for this purpose.

EFFECTS ON DIAGNOSTIC TESTS
Ampicillin alters results of urine glucose tests that use cupric sulfate (Benedict's reagent or Clinitest). Make urine glucose determinations with glucose oxidase methods (Clinistix or Tes-Tape).

Reactions may be *common,* uncommon, ***life-threatening,*** or COMMON AND LIFE-THREATENING.

In pregnant women, transient decreases in serum estradiol, conjugated estrone, conjugated estriol, and estriol glucuronide may occur.

CONTRAINDICATIONS
Contraindicated in patients with hypersensitivity to the drug or other penicillins.

NURSING CONSIDERATIONS
● Use cautiously in patients with other drug allergies, especially to cephalosporins (possible cross-sensitivity), or in those with mononucleosis (high incidence of maculopapular rash).
● Before giving, ask the patient about any allergic reactions to penicillin. However, a negative history of penicillin allergy is no guarantee against a future allergic reaction.
● Obtain specimen for culture and sensitivity tests before first dose. Therapy may begin pending results.
● **I.V. use:** When preparing I.V. injection, reconstitute powder with any of the following diluents: 0.9% sodium chloride solution, sterile water for injection, D_5W, lactated Ringer's injection, ⅙ M sodium lactate, dextrose 5% and 0.45% sodium chloride for injection, and 10% invert sugar. Stability varies with diluent, temperature, and concentration of solution.
● After reconstitution, allow vials to stand for a few minutes for foam to dissipate. This will permit visual inspection of contents for particles.
● Give I.V. dose by slow injection (over 10 to 15 minutes), or dilute in 50 to 100 ml of a compatible diluent, and infuse over 15 to 30 minutes. If permitted, give intermittently to prevent vein irritation. Change site every 48 hours.
● When giving I.V., don't add or mix with other drugs because they might prove incompatible.
● For I.M. injection, reconstitute with sterile water for injection or 0.5% or 2% lidocaine hydrochloride injection. Add 3.2 ml to a 1.5-g vial (or 6.4 ml to a 3-g

vial) to yield a concentration of 375 mg/ml. Administer deeply.
● Give drug at least 1 hour before bacteriostatic antibiotics.
● Observe closely. With large doses and prolonged therapy, bacterial or fungal superinfection may occur, especially in elderly, debilitated, or immunosuppressed patients.
● Know that dosage should be altered in patients with impaired renal function.

☑ **PATIENT TEACHING**
● Tell the patient to report a rash, fever, or chills. A rash is the most common allergic reaction.
● Also tell the patient to report discomfort at I.V. insertion site.
● Warn the patient that I.M. injection may cause pain at injection site.

---

bacampicillin hydrochloride
Penglobet†, Spectrobid

Pregnancy Risk Category: B

HOW SUPPLIED
Tablets: 400 mg

ACTION
An aminopenicillin that inhibits cell-wall synthesis during microorganism multiplication; bacteria resist bacampicillin by producing penicillinases—enzymes that hydrolyze its active form (ampicillin) when drug is absorbed in GI tract.

ONSET, PEAK, DURATION
Onset unknown. Plasma levels peak within 30 to 90 minutes. Serum concentrations are usually low or undetectable 6 to 8 hours later.

INDICATIONS & DOSAGE
Upper respiratory tract infections and otitis media caused by streptococci, pneumococci, staphylococci, and Haemophilus influenzae; *urinary tract infections caused by* Escherichia coli,

Proteus mirabilis, *and* Enterococcus faecalis; *skin infections caused by streptococci and susceptible staphylococci—*
Adults and children over 25 kg: 400 mg P.O. q 12 hours.
Children 25 kg or less: 25 mg/kg/day P.O. in divided doses q 12 hours.
Lower respiratory tract infections; other severe infections—
Adults and children over 25 kg: 800 mg P.O. q 12 hours.
Children 25 kg or less: 50 mg/kg/day P.O. in divided doses q 12 hours.
Gonorrhea—
Adults: 1.6 g P.O. plus 1 g probenecid given as a single dose.

ADVERSE REACTIONS
GI: *nausea,* vomiting, *diarrhea,* glossitis, stomatitis, epigastric upset, black "hairy" tongue, enterocolitis, pseudomembranous colitis.
Hematologic: anemia, ***thrombocytopenia,*** thrombocytopenic purpura, eosinophilia, leukopenia, ***agranulocytosis.***
Other: hypersensitivity reactions (erythematous maculopapular rash, urticaria, ***anaphylaxis***), overgrowth of nonsusceptible organisms.

INTERACTIONS
Allopurinol: increased incidence of rash.
Disulfiram: possible disulfiram-alcohol reaction. Do not give together.
Oral contraceptives: efficacy of oral contraceptives may be decreased. Additional form of contraception recommended during penicillin therapy.
Probenecid: increased blood levels of bacampicillin or other penicillins. Probenecid may be used for this purpose.

EFFECTS ON DIAGNOSTIC TESTS
Bacampicillin alters results of urine glucose tests that use cupric sulfate (Benedict's reagent or Clinitest). Make urine glucose determinations with glucose oxidase methods (Clinistix or Tes-Tape).

Bacampicillin may falsely decrease serum aminoglycoside concentrations.

CONTRAINDICATIONS
Contraindicated in patients with hypersensitivity to the drug or other penicillins.

NURSING CONSIDERATIONS
• Use cautiously in patients with other drug allergies, especially to cephalosporins (possible cross-sensitivity), or in those with mononucleosis (high incidence of maculopapular rash).
• Before giving, ask the patient about any allergic reactions to penicillin. However, a negative history of penicillin allergy is no guarantee against an allergic reaction.
• Obtain specimen for culture and sensitivity tests before first dose. Therapy may begin pending results.
• Unlike ampicillin, administer bacampicillin with meals without fear of diminished drug absorption.
• Give bacampicillin at least 1 hour before bacteriostatic antibiotics.
• Observe closely. With large doses and prolonged therapy, bacterial or fungal superinfection may occur, especially in elderly, debilitated, or immunosuppressed patients.
• Know that diarrhea may occur less frequently with bacampicillin than with ampicillin.
• Be aware that bacampicillin is specially formulated to cause high blood levels of antibiotic when administered twice daily.

☑ PATIENT TEACHING
• Tell the patient to take entire quantity of medication as prescribed, even after he feels better.
• Inform the patient that drug may be taken with or without food.
• Tell the patient to call the doctor if rash, fever, or chills develop. A rash is the most common allergic reaction.

carbenicillin indanyl sodium
Geocillin, Geopen Oral†

Pregnancy Risk Category: B

HOW SUPPLIED
Tablets: 382 mg

ACTION
An extended-spectrum penicillin that inhibits cell-wall synthesis during microorganism multiplication; bacteria resist carbenicillin by producing penicillinases—enzymes that hydrolyze its active form.

ONSET, PEAK, DURATION
Onset unknown. Serum levels peak within 30 minutes. Serum carbenicillin concentrations are generally low or undetectable 6 hours after a dose.

INDICATIONS & DOSAGE
Urinary tract infection caused by susceptible strains of gram-negative organisms—
Adults: 382 to 764 mg P.O. q.i.d. for 10 days or longer.
Prostatitis caused by susceptible strains of gram-negative organisms—
Adults: 764 mg P.O. q.i.d. for 2 to 4 weeks or longer.

ADVERSE REACTIONS
GI: *nausea,* vomiting, *diarrhea, flatulence, abdominal cramps, unpleasant taste,* glossitis, dry mouth, furred tongue.
Hematologic: leukopenia, neutropenia, eosinophilia, *hemolytic anemia, thrombocytopenia.*
Other: hypersensitivity reactions (rash, urticaria, pruritus, *anaphylaxis*), overgrowth of nonsusceptible organisms.

INTERACTIONS
Oral contraceptives: efficacy of oral contraceptives may be decreased. Additional form of contraception recommended during penicillin therapy.

EFFECTS ON DIAGNOSTIC TESTS
Carbenicillin indanyl sodium alters results of urine glucose tests that use cupric sulfate (Benedict's reagent or Clinitest). Make urine glucose determinations with glucose oxidase methods (Clinistix or Tes-Tape). Drug causes increased serum uric acid values (cupric sulfate method) and false elevations of urine specific gravity in dehydrated patients with low urine output. Positive Coombs' tests have been reported after carbenicillin therapy; drug also interferes with some HLA antigen tests that could cause inaccurate HLA typing. Systemic effect of carbenicillin may prolong PT. It may cause transient elevations in liver function study results and transient reductions in RBC, WBC, and platelet counts. Carbenicillin may also decrease serum aminoglycoside concentrations.

CONTRAINDICATIONS
Contraindicated in patients with hypersensitivity to the drug or other penicillins.

NURSING CONSIDERATIONS
● Use cautiously in patients with other drug allergies, especially to cephalosporins (possible cross-sensitivity).
● Before giving, ask the patient about any allergic reactions to penicillin. However, a negative history of penicillin allergy is no guarantee against a future allergic reaction.
● Obtain specimen for culture and sensitivity tests before first dose. Therapy may begin pending results.
● Know that drug is used only in patients whose creatinine clearance values are 10 ml/minute or more.
● Give 1 to 2 hours before or 2 to 3 hours after meals because food may interfere with absorption.
● Observe closely. With large doses or prolonged therapy, bacterial or fungal superinfection may occur, especially in elderly, debilitated, or immunosuppressed patients.

---

*Liquid contains alcohol.   **May contain tartrazine.   †Canada only.   ‡Australia only.   ◇ OTC.

☑ **PATIENT TEACHING**
● Tell the patient to take all of the medication exactly as prescribed, even after he feels better.
● Instruct the patient to take drug on an empty stomach.
● Tell the patient to call the doctor if rash, fever, or chills develop. A rash is the most common allergic reaction.

---

cloxacillin sodium
Alclox‡, Apo-Cloxi†, Austrastaph‡, Cloxapen, Novo-Cloxin†, Nu-Cloxi†, Orbenin†, Orbenin Injection‡, Tegopen

Pregnancy Risk Category: B

HOW SUPPLIED
Capsules: 250 mg, 500 mg
Oral solution: 125 mg/5 ml (after reconstitution)

ACTION
A penicillinase-resistant penicillin that inhibits cell-wall synthesis during microorganism multiplication; bacteria resist penicillins by producing penicillinases—enzymes that convert penicillins to inactive penicillic acid. Cloxacillin resists these enzymes.

ONSET, PEAK, DURATION
Onset unknown. Plasma levels peak within 2 hours. Drug concentrations are generally low 6 hours after a dose.

INDICATIONS & DOSAGE
Systemic infections caused by penicillinase-producing staphylococci—
Adults and children over 20 kg: 250 to 500 mg P.O. q 6 hours.
Children 20 kg or under: 50 to 100 mg/kg P.O. daily, in divided doses q 6 hours.

ADVERSE REACTIONS
CNS: lethargy, hallucinations, *seizures,* anxiety, confusion, agitation, depression, dizziness, fatigue.
GI: *nausea,* vomiting, *epigastric distress, diarrhea,* enterocolitis, pseudomembranous colitis, black "hairy" tongue, abdominal pain.
GU: interstitial nephritis, nephropathy.
Hematologic: eosinophilia, anemia, *thrombocytopenia,* leukopenia, hemolytic anemia, *agranulocytosis.*
Other: hypersensitivity reactions (rash, urticaria, chills, fever, sneezing, wheezing, *anaphylaxis*), intrahepatic cholestasis, overgrowth of nonsusceptible organisms.

INTERACTIONS
Oral contraceptives: efficacy of oral contraceptives may be decreased. Additional form of contraception recommended during penicillin therapy.
Probenecid: increased blood levels of cloxacillin and other penicillins. Probenecid may be used for this purpose.

EFFECTS ON DIAGNOSTIC TESTS
Cloxacillin alters test results for urine and serum proteins; it produces false-positive or elevated results in turbidimetric urine and serum protein tests using sulfosalicylic acid or trichloroacetic acid; it also reportedly produces false results on the Bradshaw screening test for Bence Jones protein. Cloxacillin may cause transient elevations in liver function study results and transient reductions in RBC, WBC, and platelet counts. Elevated liver function test results may indicate drug-induced cholestasis or hepatitis. Cloxacillin may falsely decrease serum aminoglycoside concentrations.

CONTRAINDICATIONS
Contraindicated in patients with hypersensitivity to the drug or other penicillins.

NURSING CONSIDERATIONS
● Use cautiously in patients with other drug allergies, especially to cephalosporins (possible cross-sensitivity), or in

---

those with mononucleosis (high incidence of maculopapular rash).
● Before giving, ask the patient about any allergic reactions to penicillin. However, a negative history of penicillin allergy is no guarantee against a future allergic reaction.
● Obtain specimen for culture and sensitivity tests before first dose. Therapy may begin pending results.
● Give 1 to 2 hours before or 2 to 3 hours after meals. Drug may cause GI disturbances. Food may interfere with its absorption.
● Give cloxacillin at least 1 hour before bacteriostatic antibiotics.
● As ordered, periodically assess renal, hepatic, and hematopoietic function in patients receiving long-term therapy.
● Observe closely. With large doses and prolonged therapy, bacterial or fungal superinfection may occur, especially in elderly, debilitated, or immunosuppressed patients.

☑ **PATIENT TEACHING**
● Tell the patient to take entire quantity of medication exactly as prescribed, even after he feels better.
● Instruct the patient to take drug on an empty stomach.
● Tell the patient to call the doctor if rash, fever, or chills develop. A rash is the most common allergic reaction.
Alert: Instruct the patient to take each dose with a full glass of water, not with fruit juice or carbonated beverage because their acid will inactivate the drug.

dicloxacillin sodium
Dycill, Dynapen, Pathocil

Pregnancy Risk Category: NR

HOW SUPPLIED
Capsules: 250 mg, 500 mg
Oral suspension: 62.5 mg/5 ml (after reconstitution)

ACTION
A penicillinase-resistant penicillin that inhibits cell-wall synthesis during microorganism multiplication; bacteria resist penicillins by producing penicillinases—enzymes that convert penicillins to inactive penicillic acid. Dicloxacillin resists these enzymes.

ONSET, PEAK, DURATION
Onset unknown. Plasma levels peak within 2 hours. Drug concentrations are generally low 6 hours after a dose.

INDICATIONS & DOSAGE
Systemic infections caused by penicillinase-producing staphylococci—
Adults and children over 40 kg: 125 to 250 mg P.O. q 6 hours.
Children 40 kg or under: 12.5 to 25 mg/kg P.O. daily, in divided doses q 6 hours depending on severity.

ADVERSE REACTIONS
CNS: neuromuscular irritability, *seizures,* lethargy, hallucinations, anxiety, confusion, agitation, depression, dizziness, fatigue.
GI: *nausea,* vomiting, *epigastric distress,* flatulence, *diarrhea,* enterocolitis, pseudomembranous colitis, black "hairy" tongue, abdominal pain.
GU: interstitial nephritis, nephropathy.
Hematologic: eosinophilia, anemia, *thrombocytopenia,* eosinophilia, leukopenia, hemolytic anemia, *agranulocytosis.*
Other: hypersensitivity reactions (pruritus, urticaria, rash, *anaphylaxis*), overgrowth of nonsusceptible organisms.

INTERACTIONS
Oral contraceptives: efficacy of oral contraceptives may be decreased. Additional form of contraception recommended during penicillin therapy.
Probenecid: increased blood levels of dicloxacillin and other penicillins. Probenecid may be used for this purpose.

---

*Liquid contains alcohol. **May contain tartrazine. †Canada only. ‡Australia only. ◇ OTC.

EFFECTS ON DIAGNOSTIC TESTS

Dicloxacillin alters test results for urine and serum proteins; it produces false-positive or elevated results in turbidimetric urine and serum protein tests using sulfosalicylic acid or trichloroacetic acid; it also reportedly produces false results on the Bradshaw screening test for Bence Jones protein. Dicloxacillin may cause transient elevations in liver function study results and transient reductions in RBC, WBC, and platelet counts. Elevated liver function test results may indicate drug-induced cholestasis or hepatitis. Dicloxacillin may falsely decrease serum aminoglycoside concentrations.

CONTRAINDICATIONS

Contraindicated in patients with hypersensitivity to the drug or other penicillins.

NURSING CONSIDERATIONS

● Use cautiously in patients with other drug allergies, especially to cephalosporins (possible cross-sensitivity), or in those with mononucleosis (high incidence of maculopapular rash).
● Before giving, ask the patient about any allergic reactions to penicillin. However, a negative history of penicillin allergy is no guarantee against a future allergic reaction.
● Obtain specimen for culture and sensitivity tests before first dose. Therapy may begin pending results.
● Give 1 to 2 hours before or 2 to 3 hours after meals. Drug may cause GI disturbances. Food may interfere with absorption.
● Give dicloxacillin at least 1 hour before bacteriostatic antibiotics.
● As ordered, periodically assess renal, hepatic, and hematopoietic function in patients receiving long-term therapy.
● Observe closely. With large doses and prolonged therapy, bacterial or fungal superinfection may occur, especially in elderly, debilitated, or immunosuppressed patients.

☑ **PATIENT TEACHING**
● Tell the patient to take entire quantity of medication exactly as prescribed, even after he feels better.
● Instruct the patient to take drug on an empty stomach.
● Tell the patient to call the doctor if rash, fever, or chills develop. A rash is the most common allergic reaction.

mezlocillin sodium
Mezlin

Pregnancy Risk Category: B

HOW SUPPLIED

Injection: 1 g, 2 g, 3 g, 4 g
Pharmacy bulk package: 20 g

ACTION

An extended-spectrum penicillin that inhibits cell-wall synthesis during microorganism multiplication; bacteria resist mezlocillin by producing penicillinases—enzymes that hydrolyze mezlocillin.

ONSET, PEAK, DURATION

Onset immediate after I.V. administration, unknown after I.M. injection. Peak serum levels occur immediately after I.V. administration, within 45 to 90 minutes of I.M. injection. Duration unknown.

INDICATIONS & DOSAGE

Systemic infections caused by susceptible strains of gram-positive and especially gram-negative organisms (including Proteus *and* Pseudomonas aeruginosa)—

Adults: 200 to 300 mg/kg daily I.V. or I.M. in four to six divided doses. Usual dose is 3 g q 4 hours or 4 g q 6 hours. For very serious infections, up to 24 g daily may be administered.
Children up to 12 years: 50 mg/kg q 4 hours by I.V. infusion or direct I.V. injection.

ADVERSE REACTIONS
CNS: neuromuscular irritability, *seizures.*
GI: nausea, diarrhea, vomiting, abnormal taste sensation, pseudomembranous colitis.
GU: interstitial nephritis.
Hematologic: *bleeding* (with high doses), neutropenia, *thrombocytopenia*, eosinophilia, leukopenia, *hemolytic anemia*.
Other: hypersensitivity reactions (*anaphylaxis*, edema, fever, chills, rash, pruritus, urticaria), overgrowth of nonsusceptible organisms, *hypokalemia*, pain at injection site, vein irritation, phlebitis.

INTERACTIONS
Aminoglycoside antibiotics (such as amikacin, gentamicin and tobramycin): chemically incompatible. Don't mix together in I.V. solution. Give 1 hour apart, especially in patients with renal insufficiency.
Oral contraceptives: efficacy of oral contraceptives may be decreased. Additional form of contraception recommended during penicillin therapy.
Probenecid: increased blood levels of mezlocillin. Probenecid may be used for this purpose.

EFFECTS ON DIAGNOSTIC TESTS
Mezlocillin alters tests for urine or serum proteins; it interferes with turbidimetric methods that use sulfosalicylic acid, trichloroacetic acid, acetic acid, or nitric acid. Mezlocillin does not interfere with tests using bromphenol blue (Albustix, Albutest, MultiStix). Positive Coombs' tests have been reported in patients taking mezlocillin. Drug may prolong PT. It may also cause transient elevations in liver function study results and transient reductions in RBC, WBC, and platelet counts.

CONTRAINDICATIONS
Contraindicated in patients with hypersensitivity to the drug or other penicillins.

NURSING CONSIDERATIONS
● Use cautiously in patients with other drug allergies, especially to cephalosporins (possible cross-sensitivity), or in those with bleeding tendencies, uremia, or hypokalemia.
● Before giving, ask the patient about any allergic reactions to penicillin. A negative history of penicillin allergy, however, is no guarantee against future allergic reaction.
● Obtain specimen for culture and sensitivity tests before first dose. Therapy may begin pending results.
● **I.V. use:** Reconstitute vials with at least 10 ml/g of drug using sterile water for injection, D_5W, or 0.9% sodium chloride for injection. Solutions with a concentration not exceeding 10% may be given by direct injection over 3 to 5 minutes. Alternatively, dilute in about 50 to 100 ml of suitable I.V. solution, and give by intermittent infusion over 30 minutes.
● Give I.V. intermittently to prevent vein irritation. Change site every 48 hours.
● When giving I.M., don't give more than 2 g per injection. Inject deeply and slowly (12 to 15 seconds) into the body of a large muscle.
● Give mezlocillin at least 1 hour before bacteriostatic antibiotics.
● Check CBC and platelet counts frequently, as ordered. Drug may cause thrombocytopenia.
● Monitor serum potassium level.
Alert: Institute seizure precautions. Patients with high serum levels of this drug may have seizures.
● Observe closely. With large doses and prolonged therapy, bacterial or fungal superinfection may occur, especially in elderly, debilitated, or immunosuppressed patients.
● Be aware that dosage should be altered in patients with impaired renal function.
● Be aware that drug is almost always used with another antibiotic, such as gentamicin.

☑ **PATIENT TEACHING**
● Instruct patient to report adverse reactions promptly.
● Tell patient to alert nurse if discomfort occurs at I.V. site.
● Caution patient to limit salt intake during mezlocillin therapy because of drug's high sodium content.

---

nafcillin sodium
Nafcil, Nallpen, Unipen

Pregnancy Risk Category: B

HOW SUPPLIED
Capsules: 250 mg
Oral solution: 250 mg/5 ml (after reconstitution)
Injection: 500 mg, 1 g, 2 g
I.V. infusion piggyback: 1 g, 2 g
Pharmacy bulk package: 10 g

ACTION
A penicillinase-resistant penicillin that inhibits cell-wall synthesis during microorganism multiplication; bacteria resist penicillins by producing penicillinases—enzymes that hydrolyze penicillins. Nafcillin resists these enzymes.

ONSET, PEAK, DURATION
Onset immediate after I.V. administration, unknown after I.M. injection. Peak serum levels occur immediately after I.V. administration, within ½ to 1 hour of I.M. injection, ½ to 2 hours after oral administration. Duration unknown.

INDICATIONS & DOSAGE
Systemic infections caused by penicillinase-producing staphylococci—
Adults: 250 to 500 mg P.O. q 4 to 6 hours (more severe infections may be treated with 1 g P.O. q 4 to 6 hours); or with 2 to 12 g I.M. or I.V. daily in divided doses q 4 to 6 hours.
Children older than 1 month: 50 to 100 mg/kg P.O. daily, in divided doses q 6 hours; or 100 to 200 mg/kg I.M. or I.V. daily in divided doses q 4 to 6 hours.

ADVERSE REACTIONS
GI: *nausea,* vomiting, diarrhea.
Hematologic: transient leukopenia, neutropenia, agranulocytosis, ***thrombocytopenia*** with high doses.
Other: hypersensitivity reactions (chills, fever, rash, pruritus, urticaria, ***anaphylaxis***), vein irritation, thrombophlebitis.

INTERACTIONS
Aminoglycosides: synergistic effect; monitor closely. Chemical and physical incompatibility; do not mix together in same I.V. solution.
Oral contraceptives: efficacy of oral contraceptives may be decreased. Additional form of contraception recommended during penicillin therapy.
Probenecid: increased blood levels of nafcillin. Probenecid may be used for this purpose.
Rifampin: dose-dependent antagonism. Monitor closely.
Warfarin: increased risk of bleeding when used with I.V. nafcillin. Monitor closely.

EFFECTS ON DIAGNOSTIC TESTS
Nafcillin alters tests for urine and serum proteins; turbidimetric urine and serum proteins are often falsely positive or elevated in tests using sulfosalicylic acid or trichloroacetic acid. Nafcillin may cause transient reductions in RBC, WBC, and platelet counts. Abnormal urinalysis results may indicate drug-induced interstitial nephritis.

CONTRAINDICATIONS
Contraindicated in patients with hypersensitivity to the drug or other penicillins.

NURSING CONSIDERATIONS
● Use cautiously in patients with other drug allergies, especially to cephalosporins (possible cross-sensitivity), or in those with GI distress.
● Before giving, ask the patient about any allergic reactions to penicillin. However, a negative history of penicillin

---

allergy is no guarantee against a future
allergic reaction.

● Obtain specimen for culture and sensitivity tests before first dose. Therapy may begin pending results.

● Give 1 to 2 hours before or 2 to 3 hours after meals. When given orally, drug may cause GI disturbances. Food may interfere with absorption.

● **I.V. use:** Reconstitute piggyback containers according to manufacturer's instructions. Reconstitute 500-mg, 1-g, or 2-g vials with sterile water for injection, D₅W, or 0.9% sodium chloride for injection. Add 1.7 ml for each 500 mg of drug. Reconstituted drug may be given I.M. Alternatively, dilute with 15 to 30 ml of sterile water for injection or 0.45% or 0.9% sodium chloride for injection, and give by direct injection into a vein or into the tubing of a free-flowing I.V. solution over 5 to 10 minutes. Or dilute drug to a concentration of 2 to 40 mg/ml, and give by intermittent I.V. infusion over 30 to 60 minutes.

● Avoid continuous I.V. infusions to prevent vein irritation. Change site every 48 hours.

● Give nafcillin at least 1 hour before bacteriostatic antibiotics.

● Observe closely. With large doses and prolonged therapy, bacterial or fungal superinfection may occur, especially in elderly, debilitated, or immunosuppressed patients.

☑ **PATIENT TEACHING**
● Tell the patient to take entire quantity of medication exactly as prescribed, even after he feels better.
● Instruct the patient to take oral form of drug on an empty stomach.
● Tell the patient to call the doctor if rash, fever, or chills develop. A rash is the most common allergic reaction.

---

oxacillin sodium
Bactocill, Prostaphlin

Pregnancy Risk Category: B

HOW SUPPLIED
Capsules: 250 mg, 500 mg
Oral solution: 250 mg/5 ml (after reconstitution)
Injection: 250 mg, 500 mg, 1 g, 2 g, 4 g
I.V. infusion: 1 g, 2 g, 4 g
Pharmacy bulk package: 4 g, 10 g

ACTION
A penicillinase-resistant penicillin that inhibits cell-wall synthesis during microorganism multiplication; bacteria resist penicillins by producing penicillinases—enzymes that convert penicillins to inactive penicillic acid. Oxacillin resists these enzymes.

ONSET, PEAK, DURATION
Onset immediate after I.V. administration, unknown after I.M. injection. Peak serum levels occur immediately after I.V. administration, within ½ to 2 hours of oral dose, within ½ hour of an I.M. dose. Duration unknown.

INDICATIONS & DOSAGE
Systemic infections caused by penicillinase-producing staphylococci—
Adults and children over 40 kg: 500 mg to 1 g P.O. q 4 to 6 hours; or 2 to 12 g I.M. or I.V. daily, in divided doses q 4 to 6 hours.
Children 40 kg or less: 50 to 100 mg/kg P.O. daily, in divided doses q 6 hours; or 50 to 200 mg/kg I.M. or I.V. daily, in divided doses q 4 to 6 hours, depending on severity.

ADVERSE REACTIONS
CNS: neuropathy, neuromuscular irritability, *seizures,* lethargy, hallucinations, anxiety, confusion, agitation, depression, dizziness, fatigue.
GI: oral lesions, nausea, vomiting, diarrhea, enterocolitis, pseudomembranous colitis.
GU: interstitial nephritis, nephropathy.
Hematologic: *thrombocytopenia,* eosinophilia, *hemolytic anemia,* neutropenia, anemia, *agranulocytosis.*
Other: hypersensitivity reactions (fever,

chills, rash, urticaria, ***anaphylaxis***), overgrowth of nonsusceptible organisms, elevated liver enzymes, ***thrombophlebitis***.

INTERACTIONS

Aminoglycosides: possible synergistic effect; monitor closely. Chemical and physical incompatibility; do not mix together in the same I.V. solution.

Oral contraceptives: efficacy of oral contraceptives may be decreased. Additional form of contraception recommended during penicillin therapy.

Probenecid: increased blood levels of oxacillin and other penicillins. Probenecid may be used for this purpose.

Rifampin: possible antagonism. Monitor closely.

EFFECTS ON DIAGNOSTIC TESTS

Oxacillin alters tests for urine and serum proteins; turbidimetric urine and serum proteins are often falsely positive or elevated in tests using sulfosalicylic acid or trichloroacetic acid. Oxacillin may cause transient reductions in RBC, WBC, and platelet counts. Elevations in liver function tests may indicate drug-induced hepatitis or cholestasis. Abnormal urinalysis results may indicate drug-induced interstitial nephritis. Oxacillin may falsely decrease serum aminoglycoside concentrations.

CONTRAINDICATIONS

Contraindicated in patients with hypersensitivity to the drug or other penicillins.

NURSING CONSIDERATIONS

● Use cautiously in patients with other drug allergies, especially to cephalosporins (possible cross-sensitivity); in neonates; and in infants.

● Before giving, ask the patient about any allergic reactions to penicillin. However, a negative history of penicillin allergy is no guarantee against a future allergic reaction.

● Obtain specimen for culture and sensitivity tests before first dose. Therapy may begin pending results.

● **I.V. use:** For direct I.V. injection, reconstitute vials with sterile water for injection or 0.9% sodium chloride for injection. Use 5 ml of diluent for a 250- or 500-mg vial, 10 ml of diluent for a 1-g vial, 20 ml of diluent for a 2-g vial, or 40 ml of diluent for a 4-g vial. When the solution is clear, withdraw the ordered dose and inject over 10 minutes. When giving by piggyback injection, reconstitute the 1-g piggyback vial with 20 to 100 ml of diluent; reconstitute the 2-g vial with 19 to 99 ml of diluent. For intermittent infusion, further dilute the drug to a concentration of 5 to 40 mg/ml.

● To prevent vein irritation, avoid continuous infusions. Change site every 48 hours.

● Give the drug I.M. or I.V. only if ordered and the infection is severe or if the patient can't take oral dose.

● Give 1 to 2 hours before or 2 to 3 hours after meals. When given orally, drug may cause GI disturbances. Food may interfere with absorption.

● Give oxacillin at least 1 hour before bacteriostatic antibiotics.

● Monitor periodic liver function studies; watch for elevated AST and ALT levels.

● Observe closely. With large doses and prolonged therapy, bacterial or fungal superinfection may occur, especially in elderly, debilitated, or immunosuppressed patients.

☑ PATIENT TEACHING

● Tell the patient to take entire quantity of medication exactly as prescribed, even after he feels better.

● Instruct the patient to take drug on an empty stomach.

● Tell the patient to call the doctor if rash, fever, or chills develop. A rash is the most common allergic reaction.

---

penicillin G benzathine
(benzylpenicillin benzathine)
Bicillin L-A, Permapen

Pregnancy Risk Category: B

HOW SUPPLIED
Injection: 300,000 units/ml, 600,000 units/ml

ACTION
A natural penicillin that inhibits cell-wall synthesis during microorganism multiplication; bacteria resist penicillins by producing penicillinases—enzymes that convert penicillins to inactive penicillic acid.

ONSET, PEAK, DURATION
Onset unknown. Serum levels peak 13 to 24 hours after I.M. injection. Detectable in serum 1 to 4 weeks after I.M. injection.

INDICATIONS & DOSAGE
Congenital syphilis—
Children under 2 years: 50,000 units/kg I.M. as a single dose.
Group A streptococcal upper respiratory infections—
Adults: 1.2 million units I.M. as a single injection.
Children over 27 kg: 900,000 units I.M. as a single injection.
Children under 27 kg: 300,000 to 600,000 units I.M. as a single injection.
Prophylaxis of poststreptococcal rheumatic fever—
Adults and children: 1.2 million units I.M. once monthly or 600,000 units twice monthly.
Syphilis of less than 1 year's duration—
Adults: 2.4 million units I.M. as a single dose.
Syphilis of more than 1 year's duration—
Adults: 2.4 million units I.M. weekly for 3 successive weeks.

ADVERSE REACTIONS
CNS: neuropathy, *seizures* (with high doses), lethargy, hallucinations, anxiety, confusion, agitation, depression, dizziness, fatigue.
GI: nausea, vomiting, enterocolitis, pseudomembranous colitis.
GU: interstitial nephritis, nephropathy.
Hematologic: eosinophilia, hemolytic anemia, *thrombocytopenia,* leukopenia, anemia, *agranulocytosis*.
Other: hypersensitivity reactions (maculopapular and *exfoliative dermatitis,* chills, fever, edema, *anaphylaxis*), pain and sterile abscess at injection site.

INTERACTIONS
Aminoglycosides: physical and chemical incompatibility. Administer separately.
Colestipol: decreased serum concentrations of penicillin G benzathine. Administer penicillin G benzathine 1 hour before or 4 hours after colestipol.
Oral contraceptives: efficacy of oral contraceptives may be decreased. Additional form of contraception recommended during penicillin therapy.
Probenecid: increased blood levels of penicillin. Probenecid may be used for this purpose.

EFFECTS ON DIAGNOSTIC TESTS
Penicillin G alters test results for urine and serum protein levels; it interferes with turbidimetric methods using sulfosalicylic acid, trichloracetic acid, acetic acid, and nitric acid. Penicillin G does not interfere with tests using bromphenol blue (Albustix, Albutest, Multistix). Penicillin G alters urine glucose testing using cupric sulfate (Benedict's reagent); use Clinistix or Tes-Tape instead. Penicillin G may cause falsely elevated results of urine specific gravity tests in patients with low urine output and dehydration and falsely elevated Norymberski and Zimmerman tests results for 17-ketogenic steroids; it causes false-positive CSF protein test results (Folin-Ciocalteau method) and may

---

cause positive Coombs' test results. The drug may falsely decrease serum aminoglycoside concentrations. Adding betalactamase to the sample inactivates the penicillin, rendering the assay more accurate. Alternatively, the sample can be spun down and frozen immediately after collection.

CONTRAINDICATIONS

Contraindicated in patients with hypersensitivity to the drug or other penicillins.

NURSING CONSIDERATIONS

● Use cautiously in patients with other drug allergies, especially to cephalosporins (possible cross-sensitivity).
● Before giving, ask the patient about any allergic reactions to penicillin. However, a negative history of penicillin allergy is no guarantee against a future allergic reaction.
● Obtain specimen for culture and sensitivity tests before first dose. Therapy may begin pending results.
● Shake medication well before injection.
Alert: Never give I.V.—inadvertent I.V. administration has caused cardiac arrest and death.
● Inject deeply into upper outer quadrant of buttocks in adults; in midlateral thigh in infants and small children. Avoid injection into or near major nerves or blood vessels to prevent permanent neurovascular damage.
● Give penicillin G benzathine at least 1 hour before bacteriostatic antibiotics.
● Know that drug's extremely slow absorption time makes allergic reactions difficult to treat.
● Observe closely. With large doses and prolonged therapy, bacterial or fungal superinfection may occur, especially in elderly, debilitated, or immunosuppressed patients.

☑ **PATIENT TEACHING**
● Tell the patient to report adverse reactions promptly. Fever and eosino-

philia are the most common reactions.
● Warn the patient that I.M. injection may be painful but that ice applied to the site may ease discomfort.

---

penicillin G potassium (benzylpenicillin potassium)
Megacillin†, Pfizerpen

Pregnancy Risk Category: B

HOW SUPPLIED
Tablets: 500,000 units†
Oral suspension: 250,000 units†, 500,000 units†
Injection: 1 million units, 5 million units, 10 million units, 20 million units

ACTION
A natural penicillin that inhibits cell-wall synthesis during microorganism multiplication; bacteria resist penicillins by producing penicillinases—enzymes that convert penicillins to inactive penicillic acid.

ONSET, PEAK, DURATION
Onset immediate after I.V. infusion, unknown after oral dose and I.M. injection. Peak serum levels occur immediately after I.V. infusion, within 15 to 30 minutes of I.M. injection, within ½ to 1 hour of oral dose. Duration unknown.

INDICATIONS & DOSAGE
Moderate to severe systemic infection—
Adults and children age 12 and over: highly individualized; 1.6 to 3.2 million units P.O. daily in divided doses q 6 hours; 1.2 to 24 million units I.M. or I.V. daily in divided doses q 4 hours.
Children under age 12: 25,000 to 100,000 units/kg P.O. daily in divided doses q 6 hours; or 25,000 to 400,000 units/kg I.M. or I.V. daily in divided doses q 4 hours.

ADVERSE REACTIONS
CNS: neuropathy, *seizures* (with high doses), lethargy, hallucinations, anxiety,

---

Reactions may be *common,* uncommon, *life-threatening,* or COMMON AND LIFE-THREATENING.

confusion, agitation, depression, dizziness, fatigue.

GI: nausea, vomiting, enterocolitis, pseudomembranous colitis.

GU: interstitial nephritis, nephropathy.

Hematologic: *hemolytic anemia,* leukopenia, *thrombocytopenia,* anemia, eosinophilia, *agranulocytosis.*

Other: hypersensitivity reactions (rash, urticaria, maculopapular eruptions, *exfoliative dermatitis,* chills, fever, edema, *anaphylaxis*), overgrowth of nonsusceptible organisms, possible severe potassium poisoning with high doses (hyperreflexia, *seizures, coma*), thrombophlebitis, pain at injection site.

INTERACTIONS

Aminoglycosides: physical and chemical incompatibility. Administer separately.

Colestipol: decreased serum concentrations of penicillin G potassium. Administer penicillin G potassium 1 hour before or 4 hours after colestipol.

Oral contraceptives: efficacy of oral contraceptives may be decreased. Additional form of contraception recommended during penicillin therapy.

Potassium-sparing diuretics: possible increased risk of hyperkalemia. Do not use together.

Probenecid: increased blood levels of penicillin. Probenecid may be used for this purpose.

EFFECTS ON DIAGNOSTIC TESTS

Penicillin G alters test results for urine and serum protein levels; it interferes with turbidimetric methods using sulfosalicylic acid, trichloracetic acid, acetic acid, and nitric acid. Penicillin G does not interfere with tests using bromphenol blue (Albustix, Albutest, Multistix). Penicillin G alters urine glucose testing using cupric sulfate (Benedict's reagent); use Clinistix or Tes-Tape instead. Penicillin G may cause falsely elevated results of urine specific gravity tests in patients with low urine output and dehydration, and falsely elevated

Norymberski and Zimmerman tests results for 17-ketogenic steroids; it causes false-positive CSF protein test results (Folin-Ciocalteau method) and may cause positive Coombs' test results. The drug may falsely decrease serum aminoglycoside concentrations. Adding beta-lactamase to the sample inactivates the penicillin, rendering the assay more accurate. Alternatively, the sample can be spun down and frozen immediately after collection.

CONTRAINDICATIONS

Contraindicated in patients with hypersensitivity to the drug or other penicillins.

NURSING CONSIDERATIONS

● Use cautiously in patients with other drug allergies, especially to cephalosporins (possible cross-sensitivity).

● Before giving, ask the patient about any allergic reactions to penicillin. However, a negative history of penicillin allergy is no guarantee against a future allergic reaction.

● Obtain specimen for culture and sensitivity tests before first dose. Therapy may begin pending results.

● **I.V. use:** Reconstitute vials with sterile water for injection, D_5W, or 0.9% sodium chloride for injection. Volume of diluent varies with manufacturer.

● Give a continuous I.V. infusion when large doses are required (10 million units or more). Otherwise, give via intermittent I.V. infusion over 1 to 2 hours.

● For I.M. injection, administer deeply into large muscle; may be extremely painful.

● Give 1 to 2 hours before or 2 to 3 hours after meals. When given orally, drug may cause GI disturbances. Food may interfere with absorption.

● Give penicillin G potassium at least 1 hour before bacteriostatic antibiotics.

● Monitor renal function closely. Patients with poor renal function are predisposed to high blood levels of this

drug.
- Monitor serum potassium and sodium levels closely in patients receiving more than 10 million units I.V. daily.
- Observe closely. With large doses and prolonged therapy, bacterial or fungal superinfection may occur, especially in elderly, debilitated, or immunosuppressed patients.

Alert: Institute seizure precautions. Patients with high blood levels of this drug may develop seizures.

☑ **PATIENT TEACHING**
- Tell the patient taking oral form to take entire amount exactly as prescribed, even after he feels better.
- Instruct patient to take oral drug on empty stomach.
- Tell the patient to call the doctor if rash, fever, or chills develop. A rash is the most common allergic reaction.
- Warn patient that I.M. injection may be painful but that ice applied to the site may help alleviate discomfort.

---

penicillin G procaine (benzylpenicillin procaine)
Ayercillin†, Crysticillin 300 A.S., Wycillin

Pregnancy Risk Category: B

HOW SUPPLIED
Injection: 300,000 units/ml, 500,000 units/ml, 600,000 units/ml

ACTION
A natural penicillin that inhibits cell-wall synthesis during microorganism multiplication; bacteria resist penicillins by producing penicillinases—enzymes that convert penicillins to inactive penicillic acid.

ONSET, PEAK, DURATION
Onset unknown. Serum levels peak 1 to 4 hours after I.M. dose. Drug persists in serum for 1 to 2 days; after high doses, for 5 days.

INDICATIONS & DOSAGE
Moderate to severe systemic infection—
Adults: 600,000 to 1.2 million units I.M. daily in a single dose.
Children over 1 month: 25,000 to 50,000 units/kg I.M. daily in a single dose.
Uncomplicated gonorrhea—
Adults and children over 12 years: 1 g probenecid P.O.; after 30 minutes, 4.8 million units of penicillin G procaine I.M., divided between two injection sites.
Pneumococcal pneumonia—
Adults and children over 12 years: 600,000 units to 1.2 million units I.M. daily for 7 to 10 days.

ADVERSE REACTIONS
CNS: *seizures,* lethargy, hallucinations, anxiety, confusion, agitation, depression, dizziness, fatigue.
GI: nausea, vomiting, enterocolitis, pseudomembranous colitis.
GU: interstitial nephritis, nephropathy.
Hematologic: *thrombocytopenia, hemolytic anemia,* leukopenia, anemia, eosinophilia, *agranulocytosis.*
Other: arthralgia, hypersensitivity reactions (rash, urticaria, chills, fever, edema, prostration, *anaphylaxis*), overgrowth of nonsusceptible organisms.

INTERACTIONS
Aminoglycosides: physical and chemical incompatibility. Administer separately.
Colestipol: decreased serum concentrations of penicillin G procaine. Administer penicillin G procaine 1 hour before or 4 hours after colestipol.
Oral contraceptives: efficacy of oral contraceptives may be decreased. Additional form of contraception recommended during penicillin therapy.
Probenecid: increased blood levels of penicillin. Probenecid may be used for this purpose.

EFFECTS ON DIAGNOSTIC TESTS
Penicillin G alters test results for urine

Reactions may be *common,* uncommon, *life-threatening,* or COMMON AND LIFE-THREATENING.

and serum protein levels. It interferes with turbidimetric methods using sulfosalicylic acid, trichloracetic acid, acetic acid, and nitric acid. Penicillin G does not interfere with tests using bromphenol blue (Albustix, Albutest, Multistix). Penicillin G alters urine glucose testing using cupric sulfate (Benedict's reagent); use Clinistix or Tes-Tape instead. Penicillin G may cause falsely elevated results of urine specific gravity tests in patients with low urine output and dehydration, and falsely elevated Norymberski and Zimmerman tests results for 17-ketogenic steroids; it causes false-positive CSF protein test results (Folin-Ciocalteau method) and may cause positive Coombs' test results. The drug may falsely decrease serum aminoglycoside concentrations. Adding betalactamase to the sample inactivates the penicillin, rendering the assay more accurate. Alternatively, the sample can be spun down and frozen immediately after collection.

CONTRAINDICATIONS
Contraindicated in patients with hypersensitivity to the drug or other penicillins.

NURSING CONSIDERATIONS
● Use cautiously in patients with other drug allergies, especially to cephalosporins (possible cross-sensitivity). Some formulations contain sulfites, which may cause allergic reactions in sensitive persons.
● Before giving, ask the patient about any allergic reactions to penicillin. However, a negative history of penicillin allergy is no guarantee against a future allergic reaction.
● Obtain specimen for culture and sensitivity tests before first dose. Therapy may begin pending results.
● Give deep I.M. in upper outer quadrant of buttocks in adults; in midlateral thigh in small children. Do not give subcutaneously. Don't massage injection site. Avoid injection near major nerves

or blood vessels to prevent permanent neurovascular damage.
Alert: Never give I.V.—inadvertent I.V. administration has caused death due to CNS toxicity caused by procaine.
● Give penicillin G procaine at least 1 hour before bacteriostatic antibiotics.
● Know that because of drug's slow absorption rate, allergic reactions are hard to treat.
● Monitor renal and hematopoietic function periodically, as ordered.
● Observe closely. With large doses and prolonged therapy, bacterial or fungal superinfection may occur, especially in elderly, debilitated, or immunosuppressed patients.

☑ PATIENT TEACHING
● Tell the patient to report adverse reactions promptly. A rash is the most common allergic reaction.
● Warn the patient that I.M. injection may be painful but that ice applied to the site may help alleviate discomfort.

---

penicillin G sodium (benzylpenicillin sodium)
Crystapen†

Pregnancy Risk Category: B

HOW SUPPLIED
Injection: 5 million-units vial

ACTION
A natural penicillin that inhibits cell-wall synthesis during active multiplication; bacteria resist penicillins by producing penicillinases—enzymes that convert penicillins to inactive penicillic acid.

ONSET, PEAK, DURATION
Onset immediate after I.V. administration, unknown after I.M. injection. Peak serum levels occur 15 to 30 minutes after I.M. injection, immediately after I.V. administration. Duration unknown.

INDICATIONS & DOSAGE
Moderate to severe systemic infection—
Adults and children age 12 and over:
1.2 to 24 million units daily I.M. or I.V.
in divided doses q 4 to 6 hours.
Children under age 12: 25,000 to
400,000 units/kg daily I.M. or I.V. in divided doses q 4 to 6 hours.
*Endocarditis prophylaxis for dental
surgery—*
Adults and children over 27 kg: 2 million units I.V. or I.M. 30 to 60 minutes
before procedure; then 1 million units 6
hours later.

ADVERSE REACTIONS
CNS: neuropathy, *seizures,* lethargy,
hallucinations, anxiety, confusion, agitation, depression, dizziness, fatigue.
CV: *CHF* (with high doses).
GI: nausea, vomiting, enterocolitis,
pseudomembranous colitis.
GU: interstitial colitis, nephropathy.
Hematologic: hemolytic anemia,
leukopenia, *thrombocytopenia,* agranulocytosis, anemia, eosinophilia.
Other: arthralgia, hypersensitivity reactions (*exfoliative dermatitis,* urticaria,
anaphylaxis), overgrowth of nonsusceptible organisms, vein irritation, pain at
injection site, thrombophlebitis.

INTERACTIONS
Aminoglycosides: physical and chemical incompatibility. Administer separately.
Colestipol: decreased serum concentrations of penicillin G sodium. Administer
penicillin G sodium 1 hour before or 4
hours after colestipol.
Oral contraceptives: efficacy of oral
contraceptives may be decreased. Additional form of contraception recommended during penicillin therapy.
Probenecid: increased blood levels of
penicillin. Probenecid may be used for
this purpose.

EFFECTS ON DIAGNOSTIC TESTS
Penicillin G alters test results for urine
and serum protein levels; it interferes

with turbidimetric methods using sulfosalicylic acid, trichloracetic acid,
acetic acid, and nitric acid. Penicillin G
does not interfere with tests using
bromphenol blue (Albustix, Albutest,
Multistix). Penicillin G alters urine glucose testing using cupric sulfate (Benedict's reagent); use Clinistix or Tes-Tape
instead. Penicillin G may cause falsely
elevated results of urine specific gravity
tests in patients with low urine output
and dehydration, and falsely elevated
Norymberski and Zimmerman tests results for 17-ketogenic steroids; it causes
false-positive CSF protein test results
(Folin-Ciocalteau method) and may
cause positive Coombs' test results. The
drug may falsely decrease serum aminoglycoside concentrations. Adding beta-
lactamase to the sample inactivates the
penicillin, rendering the assay more accurate. Alternatively, the sample can be
spun down and frozen immediately after
collection.

CONTRAINDICATIONS
Contraindicated in patients with hypersensitivity to the drug or other penicillins and in patients on sodium-restricted diets.

NURSING CONSIDERATIONS
● Use cautiously in patients with other
drug allergies, especially to cephalosporins (possible cross-allergenicity).
● Before giving, ask the patient about
any allergic reactions to penicillin.
However, a negative history of penicillin
allergy is no guarantee against a future
allergic reaction.
● Obtain specimen for culture and sensitivity tests before first dose. Therapy
may begin pending results.
● **I.V. use:** Reconstitute vials with sterile water for injection, 0.9% sodium
chloride for injection, or D$_5$W. Check
manufacturer's instructions for volume
of diluent necessary to produce desired
drug concentration.
● For patients receiving 10 million units
of drug or more daily, dilute in 1 to 2

liters of compatible solution, and administer over 24 hours. Otherwise, give by intermittent I.V. infusion: Dilute drug in 50 to 100 ml, and give over 1 to 2 hours q 4 to 6 hours.
● In neonates and children, give divided doses over 15 to 30 minutes.
● Give penicillin G sodium at least 1 hour before bacteriostatic antibiotics.
● Observe closely. With large doses and prolonged therapy, bacterial or fungal superinfection may occur, especially in elderly, debilitated, or immunosuppressed patients.
Alert: Institute seizure precautions. Patients with high blood levels of this drug may develop seizures.

☑ **PATIENT TEACHING**
● Tell patient to report adverse reactions promptly.
● Instruct patient to alert nurse if discomfort occurs at I.V. site.
● Warn patient receiving I.M. injection that the injection may be painful but that ice applied to site may help alleviate discomfort.

---

penicillin V
(phenoxymethylpenicillin)

penicillin V potassium
(phenoxymethylpenicillin
potassium)
Abbocillin VK‡, Apo-Pen-VK†, Beepen-VK, Betapen-VK, Cilicane VK‡, Ledercillin VK, Nadopen-V-200†, Nadopen-V-400†, Nadopen-VK†, NovoPen-VK†, Nu-Pen VK†, Pen Vee, Pen Vee K, PVF K†, PVK‡, Robicillin VK, V-Cillin K, Veetids**

Pregnancy Risk Category: B

HOW SUPPLIED
penicillin V
Tablets: 250 mg, 500 mg
Oral suspension: 125 mg/5 ml, 250 mg/5 ml (after reconstitution)
penicillin V potassium

Tablets: 125 mg, 250 mg, 500 mg
Tablets (film-coated): 250 mg, 500 mg
Capsules: 250 mg‡
Oral suspension: 125 mg/5 ml, 250 mg/5 ml (after reconstitution)

ACTION
A natural penicillin that inhibits cell-wall synthesis during microorganism multiplication; bacteria resist penicillins by producing penicillinases—enzymes that convert penicillins to inactive penicillic acid.

ONSET, PEAK, DURATION
Onset and duration unknown. Serum levels peak within 30 to 60 minutes.

INDICATIONS & DOSAGE
Mild to moderate systemic infections—
Adults and children age 12 and over: 250 to 500 mg (400,000 to 800,000 units) P.O. q 6 hours.
Children under age 12: 15 to 62.5 mg/kg (25,000 to 100,000 units/kg) P.O. daily, in divided doses q 6 to 8 hours.
Endocarditis prophylaxis for dental surgery—
Adults: 2 g P.O. 30 to 60 minutes before procedure; then 1 g 6 hours after.
Children under 30 kg: half of the adult dose.

ADVERSE REACTIONS
CNS: neuropathy.
GI: *epigastric distress,* vomiting, diarrhea, *nausea,* black "hairy" tongue.
GU: nephropathy.
Hematologic: eosinophilia, hemolytic anemia, leukopenia, ***thrombocytopenia.***
Other: hypersensitivity reactions (rash, urticaria, fever, laryngeal edema, ***anaphylaxis***), overgrowth of nonsusceptible organisms.

INTERACTIONS
Oral contraceptives: efficacy of oral contraceptives may be decreased. Additional form of contraception recommended during penicillin therapy.
Probenecid: increased blood levels of

penicillin. Probenecid may be used for this purpose.

EFFECTS ON DIAGNOSTIC TESTS
Penicillin V alters test results for urine and serum protein levels; it interferes with turbidimetric methods using sulfosalicylic acid, trichloroacetic acid, acetic acid, and nitric acid. Penicillin V does not interfere with tests using bromphenol blue (Albustix, Albutest, Multistix). Penicillin V may falsely decrease serum aminoglycoside concentrations.

CONTRAINDICATIONS
Contraindicated in patients with hypersensitivity to the drug or other penicillins.

NURSING CONSIDERATIONS
● Use cautiously in patients with other drug allergies, especially to cephalosporins (possible cross-sensitivity), or in those with GI disturbances.
● Before giving, ask the patient about any allergic reactions to penicillins. However, a negative history of penicillin allergy is no guarantee against a future allergic reaction.
● Obtain specimen for culture and sensitivity tests before first dose. Therapy may begin pending results.
● Give penicillin V at least 1 hour before bacteriostatic antibiotics.
● As ordered, periodically assess renal and hematopoietic function in patients receiving long-term therapy.
● Observe closely. With large doses and prolonged therapy, bacterial or fungal superinfection may occur, especially in elderly, debilitated, or immunosuppressed patients.
● Be aware that The American Heart Association considers amoxicillin the preferred agent for endocarditis prophylaxis because GI absorption is better and serum levels are sustained longer. Penicillin V is considered an alternative agent.

☑ **PATIENT TEACHING**
● Tell the patient to take entire quantity of medication exactly as prescribed, even after he feels better.
● Tell the patient to take drug with food if stomach upset occurs.
● Tell the patient to call the doctor if rash, fever, or chills develop. A rash is the most common allergic reaction.

piperacillin sodium
Pipracil, Pipril‡

Pregnancy Risk Category: B

HOW SUPPLIED
Injection: 2 g, 3 g, 4 g
Pharmacy bulk package: 40 g

ACTION
Extended-spectrum penicillin that inhibits cell-wall synthesis during microorganism multiplication; bacteria resist penicillins by producing penicillinases—enzymes that convert penicillins to inactive penicillic acid.

ONSET, PEAK, DURATION
Onset immediate after I.V. administration, unknown after I.M. injection. Peak serum levels occur immediately after I.V. administration, within 30 to 50 minutes of I.M. dose. Duration unknown.

INDICATIONS & DOSAGE
Systemic infections caused by susceptible strains of gram-positive and especially gram-negative organisms (including Proteus *and* Pseudomonas aeruginosa)—
Adults and children over 12 years:
100 to 300 mg/kg I.V. or I.M. daily in divided doses q 4 to 6 hours, not to exceed 24 g daily.
Prophylaxis of surgical infections—
Adults: 2 g I.V., given 30 to 60 minutes before surgery. Dose may be repeated during surgery and once or twice more after surgery.

ADVERSE REACTIONS
CNS: *seizures,* headache, dizziness, fatigue.
GI: nausea, diarrhea, vomiting, pseudomembranous colitis.
GU: interstitial nephritis.
Hematologic: *bleeding* (with high doses), neutropenia, eosinophilia, leukopenia, *thrombocytopenia.*
Other: *hypokalemia,* hypersensitivity reactions (edema, fever, chills, rash, pruritus, urticaria, *anaphylaxis*), overgrowth of nonsusceptible organisms, pain at injection site, vein irritation, phlebitis, prolonged muscle relaxation.

INTERACTIONS
Aminoglycoside antibiotics (such as gentamicin and tobramycin): chemically incompatible. Don't mix in the same I.V. container.
Oral contraceptives: efficacy of oral contraceptives may be decreased. Additional form of contraception recommended during penicillin therapy.
Probenecid: increased blood levels of piperacillin. Probenecid may be used for this purpose.

EFFECTS ON DIAGNOSTIC TESTS
Piperacillin may falsely decrease serum aminoglycoside concentrations.
Piperacillin may cause hypokalemia and hypernatremia and may prolong PT times; it may also cause transient elevations in liver function study results and transient reductions in RBC, WBC, and platelet counts. Drug may cause positive Coombs' tests.

CONTRAINDICATIONS
Contraindicated in patients with hypersensitivity to the drug or other penicillins.

NURSING CONSIDERATIONS
• Use cautiously in patients with other drug allergies, especially to cephalosporins (possible cross-sensitivity), or in those with bleeding tendencies, uremia, and hypokalemia.

• Before giving, ask the patient about any allergic reactions to penicillin. However, a negative history of penicillin allergy is no guarantee against a future allergic reaction.
• Obtain specimen for culture and sensitivity tests before first dose. Therapy may begin pending results.
• **I.V. use:** Reconstitute each gram of drug with 5 ml of diluent, such as sterile or bacteriostatic water for injection, 0.9% sodium chloride for injection (with or without preservative), D_5W, or dextrose 5% in 0.9% sodium chloride for injection. Shake until dissolved. Inject reconstituted solution directly into a vein or into the tubing of a free-flowing I.V. solution over 3 to 5 minutes. Alternatively, dilute with at least 50 ml of a compatible I.V. solution, and give by intermittent infusion over 30 minutes.
• Avoid continuous infusions to prevent vein irritation. Change site every 48 hours.
• For I.M. injection, reconstitute with sterile or bacteriostatic water for injection, 0.9% sodium chloride for injection (with or without preservative), or 0.5% to 1% lidocaine hydrochloride. Add 2 ml of diluent for each gram of drug. Final solution will contain 1 g/2.5 ml.
• Give piperacillin at least 1 hour before bacteriostatic antibiotics.
• Check CBC and platelet counts frequently, as ordered. Drug may cause thrombocytopenia.
• Monitor serum potassium level.
Alert: Institute seizure precautions. Patients with high serum levels of this drug may have seizures.
• Observe closely. With large doses and prolonged therapy, bacterial or fungal superinfection may occur, especially in elderly, debilitated, or immunosuppressed patients.
• Know that dosage should be altered in patients with impaired renal function.
• Be aware that patients with cystic fibrosis tend to be most susceptible to fever or rash.
• Be aware that drug may be better suit-

ed for patients on sodium-free diets than ticarcillin (piperacillin contains 1.85 mEq of sodium/g).

• Keep in mind that piperacillin is typically used with another antibiotic, such as gentamicin.

☑ **PATIENT TEACHING**
• Tell patient to report adverse reactions promptly.
• Instruct patient receiving drug I.V. to report discomfort at I.V. site.
• Advise patient to limit salt intake during drug therapy because drug contains 1.85 mEq of sodium/g.

---

piperacillin sodium and tazobactam sodium
Zosyn

Pregnancy Risk Category: B

HOW SUPPLIED
Powder for injection: 2 g piperacillin and 0.25 g tazobactam per vial, 3 g piperacillin and 0.375 g tazobactam per vial, 4 g piperacillin and 0.5 g tazobactam per vial
Pharmacy bulk package: 40.5 g

ACTION
Piperacillin is an extended-spectrum penicillin that inhibits cell-wall synthesis during microorganism multiplication; tazobactam increases piperacillin's effectiveness by inactivating beta lactamases, which destroy penicillins.

ONSET, PEAK, DURATION
Onset immediate after I.V. infusion. Plasma levels peak immediately after I.V. infusion. Duration unknown.

INDICATIONS & DOSAGE
Appendicitis (complicated by rupture or abscess) and peritonitis caused by Escherichia coli, Bacteroides fragilis, B. ovatus, B. thetaiotaomicron, *or* B. vulgatus; *skin and skin-structure infections caused by* Staphylococcus aureus; *postpartum endometritis or pelvic inflammatory disease caused by* E. coli; *moderately severe community-acquired pneumonia caused by* Haemophilus influenzae—

Adults: 3 g piperacillin and 0.375 g tazobactam I.V. q 6 hours.
In patients with renal impairment—
Adults: if creatinine clearance is 20 to 40 ml/minute, 2 g piperacillin and 0.25 g tazobactam I.V. q 6 hours. If creatinine clearance is below 20 ml/minute, 2 g piperacillin and 0.25 g tazobactam I.V. q 8 hours.

✱ *New indication: Moderate to severe nosocomial pneumonia (moderate to severe) caused by piperacillin-resistant, beta-lactamase-producing strains of* S. aureus—
Adults: initially, 3.375 g I.V. over 30 minutes q 4 hours. Administer with an aminoglycoside.

ADVERSE REACTIONS
CNS: *headache, insomnia,* agitation, dizziness, anxiety.
CV: hypertension, tachycardia, chest pain, edema.
EENT: rhinitis.
GI: *diarrhea, nausea, constipation,* vomiting, dyspepsia, stool changes, abdominal pain.
GU: interstitial nephritis.
Hematologic: leukopenia, anemia, eosinophilia, ***thrombocytopenia.***
Respiratory: dyspnea.
Skin: rash (including maculopapular, bullous, urticarial, and eczematoid), pruritus.
Other: fever; pain; moniliasis; inflammation, phlebitis at I.V. site; ***anaphylaxis.***

INTERACTIONS
Aminoglycoside antibiotics (such as amikacin, gentamicin and tobramycin): chemically incompatible. Don't mix in the same I.V. container.
Oral contraceptives: efficacy of oral contraceptives may be decreased. Additional form of contraception recom-

---

mended during penicillin therapy.
Probenecid: increased blood levels of
piperacillin. Probenecid may be used for
this purpose.
Veruronium: prolongation of neuromuscular blockade. Monitor closely.

EFFECTS ON DIAGNOSTIC TESTS
As with other penicillins, piperacillin/
tazobactam may result in a false-positive reaction for urine glucose using a
copper reduction method, such as Clinitest. Glucose tests based on enzymatic
glucose oxidase reactions (such as Diastix or Tes-Tape) are recommended.

CONTRAINDICATIONS
Contraindicated in patients with hypersensitivity to the drug or other penicillins.

NURSING CONSIDERATIONS
● Use cautiously in patients with other
drug allergies, especially to cephalosporins (possible cross-sensitivity), or in
those with bleeding tendencies, uremia,
and hypokalemia.
● Obtain specimen for culture and sensitivity tests before first dose. Therapy
may begin pending results.
● **I.V. use:** Reconstitute each gram of
piperacillin with 5 ml of diluent, such as
sterile or bacteriostatic water for injection, 0.9% sodium chloride for injection, bacteriostatic 0.9% sodium chloride for injection, D_5W, dextrose 5% in
0.9% sodium chloride for injection, or
dextran 6% in 0.9% sodium chloride for
injection. Don't use lactated Ringer's
injection. Shake until dissolved. Further
dilute to a final volume of 50 ml before
infusion.
● Infuse over at least 30 minutes. Discontinue any primary infusion during
administration if possible. Don't mix
with other drugs.
● Use drug immediately after reconstitution. Discard unused drug after 24
hours if stored at room temperature; 48
hours if refrigerated. Once diluted, drug
is stable in I.V. bags for 24 hours at

room temperature or 1 week if refrigerated.
● Change I.V. site every 48 hours.
● Because hemodialysis removes 6% of
the piperacillin dose and 21% of the
tazobactam dose, be aware that supplemental doses may be needed after hemodialysis.
● Observe closely. With large doses and
prolonged therapy, bacterial and fungal
superinfection may occur, especially in
elderly, debilitated, or immunosuppressed patients.

☑ **PATIENT TEACHING**
● Tell patient to report adverse reactions
promptly.
● Instruct patient to alert nurse if discomfort occurs at I.V. site.

---

ticarcillin disodium
Ticar, Ticillin‡

Pregnancy Risk Category: B

HOW SUPPLIED
Injection: 1 g, 3 g, 6 g
I.V. infusion: 3 g
Pharmacy bulk package: 20 g, 30 g

ACTION
An extended-spectrum penicillin that inhibits cell-wall synthesis during microorganism multiplication; bacteria resist penicillins by producing penicillinases—enzymes that convert penicillins
to inactive penicillic acid.

ONSET, PEAK, DURATION
Onset immediate after I.V. administration, unknown after I.M. injection. Peak
serum levels occur immediately after
I.V. administration, within 30 to 75 minutes of I.M. injection. Duration unknown.

INDICATIONS & DOSAGE
*Severe systemic infections caused by
susceptible strains of gram-positive and
especially gram-negative organisms (in-*

---

cluding Pseudomonas *and* Proteus)—
Adults: 18 g I.V. or I.M. daily, in divided doses q 4 to 6 hours.
Children: 50 to 300 mg/kg I.V. or I.M. daily, in divided doses q 4 to 6 hours.

ADVERSE REACTIONS
CNS: *seizures,* neuromuscular excitability.
GI: nausea, diarrhea, vomiting, pseudomembranous colitis.
Hematologic: leukopenia, neutropenia, eosinophilia, *thrombocytopenia,* hemolytic anemia.
Other: hypersensitivity reactions (rash, pruritus, urticaria, chills, fever, edema, *anaphylaxis*), overgrowth of nonsusceptible organisms, hypokalemia, pain at injection site, vein irritation, phlebitis.

INTERACTIONS
Aminoglycoside antibiotics (such as amikacin, gentamicin, and tobramycin): chemically incompatible. Don't mix in the same I.V. container.
Lithium: altered renal elimination of lithium. Monitor serum lithium levels closely.
Oral contraceptives: efficacy of oral contraceptives may be decreased. Additional form of contraception recommended during penicillin therapy.
Probenecid: increased blood levels of ticarcillin and other penicillins. Probenecid may be used for this purpose.

EFFECTS ON DIAGNOSTIC TESTS
Ticarcillin alters tests for urine or serum proteins; it interferes with turbidimetric methods that use sulfosalicylic acid, trichloroacetic acid, acetic acid, or nitric acid. Ticarcillin does not interfere with tests using bromphenol blue (Albustix, Albutest, Multistix). Ticarcillin may falsely decrease serum aminoglycoside concentrations. Systemic effects of ticarcillin may cause positive Coombs' test, hypokalemia and hypernatremia, and may prolong PT; it may also cause transient elevations in liver function studies and transient reductions in

RBC, WBC, and platelet counts.

CONTRAINDICATIONS
Contraindicated in patients with hypersensitivity to the drug or other penicillins.

NURSING CONSIDERATIONS
● Use cautiously in patients with other drug allergies, especially to cephalosporins (possible cross-sensitivity), or in those with impaired renal function, hemorrhagic conditions, hypokalemia, or sodium restrictions (contains 5.2 to 6.5 mEq sodium/g).
● Before giving, ask the patient about any allergic reactions to penicillin. However, a negative history of penicillin allergy is no guarantee against a future allergic reaction.
● Obtain specimen for culture and sensitivity tests before first dose. Therapy may begin pending results.
● **I.V. use:** Reconstitute vials using D_5W, 0.9% sodium chloride injection, sterile water for injection, or other compatible solution. Add 4 ml of diluent for each gram of drug. Further dilute to a maximum concentration of 50 mg/ml, and inject slowly directly into a vein or into the tubing of a free-flowing I.V. solution. Alternatively, dilute to a concentration of 10 to 100 mg/ml, and give by intermittent infusion over 30 to 120 minutes in adults or 10 to 20 minutes in neonates.
● Avoid continuous infusion to prevent vein irritation. Change site every 48 hours.
● For I.M. injection, reconstitute vials using sterile water for injection, 0.9% sodium chloride for injection, or lidocaine 1% (without epinephrine). Use 2 ml diluent for each gram of drug. Give deep I.M. into large muscle. Don't exceed 2 g per injection.
● Give ticarcillin at least 1 hour before bacteriostatic antibiotics.
● Monitor serum potassium.
● Check CBC and platelet counts frequently, as ordered. Drug may cause

thrombocytopenia.

Alert: Institute seizure precautions. Patients with high blood levels of ticarcillin may develop seizures.

● Be aware that ticarcillin is typically used with another antibiotic, such as gentamicin.

● Observe closely. With large doses and prolonged therapy, bacterial or fungal superinfection may occur, especially in elderly, debilitated, or immunosuppressed patients.

● Know that dosage should be decreased in patients with impaired renal function.

☑ PATIENT TEACHING
● Tell patient to report adverse reactions promptly.

● Instruct patient to alert nurse if discomfort occurs at I.V. insertion site.

ticarcillin disodium/clavulanate potassium
Timentin

Pregnancy Risk Category: B

HOW SUPPLIED
Injection: 3 g ticarcillin and 100 mg clavulanic acid
Pharmacy bulk package: 31 g

ACTION
Ticarcillin is an extended-spectrum penicillin that inhibits cell-wall synthesis during microorganism replication; clavulanic acid increases ticarcillin's effectiveness by inactivating beta lactamases, which destroy ticarcillin.

ONSET, PEAK, DURATION
Onset immediate after I.V. infusion. Peak serum levels occur immediately after I.V. infusion. Duration unknown.

INDICATIONS & DOSAGE
Lower respiratory tract, urinary tract, bone and joint, and skin and skin-structure infections and septicemia when caused by beta-lactamase-producing strains of bacteria or by ticarcillin-susceptible organisms—
Adults: 3.1 g (3 g ticarcillin and 100 mg clavulanic acid) administered by I.V. infusion q 4 to 6 hours.

ADVERSE REACTIONS
CNS: *seizures,* neuromuscular excitability, headache, giddiness.
GI: nausea, diarrhea, stomatitis, vomiting, epigastric pain, flatulence, pseudomembranous colitis, taste and smell disturbances.
Hematologic: leukopenia, neutropenia, eosinophilia, *thrombocytopenia,* hemolytic anemia, anemia.
Other: hypersensitivity reactions (rash, pruritus, urticaria, chills, fever, edema, *anaphylaxis*), overgrowth of nonsusceptible organisms, hypokalemia, pain at injection site, vein irritation, phlebitis.

INTERACTIONS
Aminoglycoside antibiotics (such as amikacin, gentamicin, and tobramycin): chemically incompatible. Don't mix in the same I.V. container.
Oral contraceptives: efficacy of oral contraceptives may be decreased. Additional form of contraception recommended during penicillin therapy.
Probenecid: increased blood levels of ticarcillin. Probenecid may be used for this purpose.

EFFECTS ON DIAGNOSTIC TESTS
Ticarcillin/clavulanate potassium alters tests for urine or serum proteins; it interferes with turbidimetric methods that use sulfosalicylic acid, trichloroacetic acid, acetic acid, or nitric acid. The drug does not interfere with tests using bromphenol blue (Albustix, Albutest, Multistix). Drug may falsely decrease serum aminoglycoside concentrations. Systemic effects of the drug may cause positive Coombs' test, hypokalemia and hypernatremia, and may prolong PT; it may also cause transient elevations in liver function studies and transient re-

ductions in RBC, WBC, and platelet counts.

CONTRAINDICATIONS
Contraindicated in patients with hypersensitivity to the drug or other penicillins.

NURSING CONSIDERATIONS
• Use cautiously in patients with other drug allergies, especially to cephalosporins (possible cross-sensitivity), and in those with impaired renal function, hemorrhagic conditions, hypokalemia, or sodium restrictions (contains 4.5 mEq sodium/g).
• Before giving, ask the patient about any allergic reactions to penicillin. However, a negative history of penicillin allergy is no guarantee against a future allergic reaction.
• Obtain specimen for culture and sensitivity tests before first dose. Therapy may begin pending results.
• I.V. use: Reconstitute drug with 13 ml of sterile water for injection or 0.9% sodium chloride for injection. Further dilute to a maximum of 10 to 100 mg/ml (based on ticarcillin component), and administer by I.V. infusion over 30 minutes. In fluid-restricted patients, dilute to a maximum of 48 mg/ml if using D₅W, 43 mg/ml if using 0.9% sodium chloride for injection, or 86 mg/ml if using sterile water for injection.
• Give drug at least 1 hour before bacteriostatic antibiotics.
• Check CBC and platelet counts frequently, as ordered. Drug may cause thrombocytopenia.
• Observe closely. With large doses and prolonged therapy, bacterial or fungal superinfection may occur, especially in elderly, debilitated, or immunosuppressed patients.
• Know that dosage should be decreased in patients with impaired renal function.

☑ PATIENT TEACHING
• Tell patient to report adverse reactions promptly.
• Instruct patient to alert nurse if discomfort occurs at I.V. site.
• Advise patient to limit salt intake during drug therapy because of high sodium content.

cefaclor
cefadroxil monohydrate
cefazolin sodium
cefepime hydrochloride
cefixime
cefmetazole sodium
cefonicid sodium
cefoperazone sodium
cefotaxime sodium
cefotetan disodium
cefoxitin sodium
cefpodoxime proxetil
cefprozil
ceftazidime
ceftibuten
ceftizoxime sodium
ceftriaxone sodium
cefuroxime axetil
cefuroxime sodium
cephalexin hydrochloride
cephalexin monohydrate
cephapirin sodium
cephradine
loracarbef

COMBINATION PRODUCTS
None.

cefaclor
Ceclor

Pregnancy Risk Category: B

HOW SUPPLIED
Capsules: 250 mg, 500 mg
Oral suspension: 125 mg/5 ml, 250 mg/5 ml, 187 mg/5 ml, 375 mg/5 ml

ACTION
A second-generation cephalosporin that inhibits cell-wall synthesis, promoting osmotic instability; usually bactericidal.

ONSET, PEAK, DURATION
Onset and duration unknown. Peak levels occur within 30 to 60 minutes.

INDICATIONS & DOSAGE
Respiratory or urinary tract, skin, and soft-tissue infections and otitis media caused by Haemophilus influenzae, Streptococcus pneumoniae, S. pyogenes, Escherichia coli, Proteus mirabilis, Klebsiella *species, and* staphylococci—
Adults: 250 to 500 mg P.O. q 8 hours. For pharyngitis or otitis media, daily dosage may be given in two equally divided doses q 12 hours.
Children: 20 mg/kg daily P.O. in divided doses q 8 hours. For pharyngitis or otitis media, daily dosage may be given in two equally divided doses q 12 hours. In more serious infections, 40 mg/kg daily are recommended, not to exceed 1 g daily.

ADVERSE REACTIONS
CNS: dizziness, headache, somnolence, malaise.
GI: *nausea,* vomiting, *diarrhea,* anorexia, dyspepsia, abdominal cramps, pseudomembranous colitis, oral candidiasis.
GU: vaginal moniliasis, vaginitis.
Hematologic: transient leukopenia, anemia, eosinophilia, ***thrombocytopenia,*** lymphocytosis.
Skin: *maculopapular rash,* dermatitis, pruritus.
Other: hypersensitivity reactions (serum sickness, ***anaphylaxis***), fever, transient increases in liver enzymes.

INTERACTIONS
Chloramphenicol: antagonistic effect. Do not use together.
Probenecid: may inhibit excretion and increase blood levels of cefaclor.

---

*Liquid contains alcohol.   **May contain tartrazine.   †Canada only.   ‡Australia only.   ◇OTC.

EFFECTS ON DIAGNOSTIC TESTS
Cefaclor may cause false-positive Coombs' test results. Cefaclor also causes false-positive results in urine glucose tests utilizing cupric sulfate (Benedict's reagent or Clinitest); use glucose oxidase tests (Clinistix or Tes-Tape) instead. Drug causes false elevations in serum or urine creatinine levels in tests using Jaffé's reaction.

CONTRAINDICATIONS
Contraindicated in patients with hypersensitivity to other cephalosporins.

NURSING CONSIDERATIONS
● Use cautiously in patients with impaired renal function or a history of sensitivity to penicillin and in breastfeeding women.
● Obtain specimen for culture and sensitivity tests before first dose. Therapy may begin pending results.
● With large doses or prolonged therapy, monitor for superinfection, especially in high-risk patients.
● Store reconstituted suspension in refrigerator. Stable for 14 days if refrigerated. Shake well before using.

☑ **PATIENT TEACHING**
● Tell the patient to take entire amount of medication exactly as prescribed, even after he feels better.
● Tell the patient that drug may be taken with meals. If suspension is used, instruct the patient to shake container well before measuring dose and to keep the drug refrigerated.
● Tell the patient to call the doctor if rash develops.

cefadroxil monohydrate
Duricef, Ultracef

Pregnancy Risk Category: B

HOW SUPPLIED
Tablets: 1 g
Capsules: 500 mg

Oral suspension: 125 mg/5 ml, 250 mg/5 ml, 500 mg/5 ml

ACTION
A first-generation cephalosporin that inhibits cell-wall synthesis, promoting osmotic instability; usually bactericidal.

ONSET, PEAK, DURATION
Onset and duration unknown. Serum levels peak within 1 to 2 hours after an oral dose.

INDICATIONS & DOSAGE
Urinary tract infections caused by Escherichia coli, Proteus mirabilis, *and* Klebsiella *species; skin and soft-tissue infections caused by staphylococci and streptococci; and pharyngitis or tonsillitis caused by group A beta-hemolytic streptococci—*
Adults: 1 to 2 g P.O. daily, depending on infection being treated. Usually given once daily or b.i.d.
Children: 30 mg/kg P.O. daily in two divided doses q 12 hours.

ADVERSE REACTIONS
CNS: *seizures.*
GI: pseudomembranous colitis, *nausea, vomiting, diarrhea,* glossitis, abdominal cramps, oral candidiasis.
GU: genital pruritus, moniliasis, vaginitis, renal dysfunction.
Hematologic: transient neutropenia, eosinophilia, leukopenia, anemia, *agranulocytosis, thrombocytopenia.*
Skin: *maculopapular and erythematous rashes,* urticaria.
Other: hypersensitivity reactions (serum sickness, *anaphylaxis,* angioedema), transient increases in liver enzymes, dyspnea, fever.

INTERACTIONS
Probenecid: may inhibit excretion and increase blood levels of cefadroxil.

EFFECTS ON DIAGNOSTIC TESTS
Cefadroxil causes false-positive results in urine glucose tests using cupric sul-

fate (Benedict's reagent or Clinitest); use glucose oxidase test (Clinistix or Tes-Tape) instead. Cefadroxil causes false elevations in serum or urine creatinine levels in tests using Jaffé's reaction. Positive Coombs' test results occur in about 3% of patients taking cephalosporins.

CONTRAINDICATIONS

Contraindicated in patients with hypersensitivity to the drug or other cephalosporins.

NURSING CONSIDERATIONS

● Use cautiously in patients with a history of sensitivity to penicillin or in breast-feeding women. Also use cautiously in patients with impaired renal function; dosage adjustments may be necessary.
● Obtain specimen for culture and sensitivity tests before first dose. Therapy may begin pending results.
● Be aware that if creatinine clearance is below 50 ml/minute, dosage interval should be lengthened so drug doesn't accumulate.
● With large doses or prolonged therapy, monitor for superinfection, especially in high-risk patients.

☑ PATIENT TEACHING

● Tell patient to take drug with food or milk to lessen GI discomfort.
● Tell the patient to take entire amount of medication exactly as prescribed, even after he feels better.
● Advise the patient to call the doctor if rash develops.

---

cefazolin sodium
Ancef, Kefzol, Zolicef

Pregnancy Risk Category: B

HOW SUPPLIED

Injection (parenteral): 500 mg, 1 g
Infusion: 500 mg/50-ml vial, 500 mg/100-ml vial

Pharmacy bulk package: 5 g, 10 g, 20 g

ACTION

A first-generation cephalosporin that inhibits cell-wall synthesis, promoting osmotic instability; usually bactericidal.

ONSET, PEAK, DURATION

Onset immediate after I.V. administration, unknown after I.M. injection. Plasma levels peak within 1 to 2 hours after I.M. injection, immediately after I.V. administration. Duration unknown.

INDICATIONS & DOSAGE

Perioperative prophylaxis in contaminated surgery—
Adults: 1 g I.M. or I.V. 30 to 60 minutes before surgery; then 0.5 to 1 g I.M. or I.V. q 6 to 8 hours for 24 hours. In long operations (over 2 hours), another 0.5- to 1-g I.M. dose may be administered intraoperatively.
 Note: In cases where infection would be devastating, prophylaxis may be continued for 3 to 5 days.
Serious infections of respiratory, biliary, and GU tracts; skin, soft-tissue, bone, and joint infections; septicemia; and endocarditis caused by Escherichia coli, *Enterobacteriaceae, gonococci,* Haemophilus influenzae, Klebsiella, Proteus mirabilis, Staphylococcus aureus, Streptococcus pneumoniae, *and group A beta-hemolytic streptococci—*
Adults: 250 mg I.M. or I.V. q 8 hours to 1.5 g P.O. q 6 hours. Maximum 12 g/day in life-threatening situations.
Children over 1 month: 25 to 50 mg/kg or 1.25 g/m² daily I.M. or I.V. in three or four divided doses. In severe infections, dosage may be increased to 100 mg/kg/day.

ADVERSE REACTIONS

GI: pseudomembranous colitis, nausea, anorexia, vomiting, *diarrhea,* glossitis, dyspepsia, abdominal cramps, anal pruritus, oral candidiasis.
GU: genital pruritus and moniliasis,

---

vaginitis.
Hematologic: neutropenia, leukopenia, eosinophilia, ***thrombocytopenia.***
Skin: *maculopapular and erythematous rashes, urticaria, pruritus.*
Other: hypersensitivity reactions (serum sickness, ***anaphylaxis***); transient increases in liver enzymes; ***Stevens-Johnson syndrome;*** at injection site— *pain, induration, sterile abscesses, tissue sloughing;* with I.V. injection— *phlebitis, thrombophlebitis.*

INTERACTIONS
Probenecid: may inhibit excretion and increase blood levels of cefazolin.

EFFECTS ON DIAGNOSTIC TESTS
Cephalosporins cause false-positive results in urine glucose tests using cupric sulfate (Benedict's reagent or Clinitest); use glucose oxidase tests (Clinistix or Tes-Tape) instead. It causes false elevations in serum or urine creatinine levels in tests using Jaffé's reaction. It also causes positive Coombs' test results and may elevate liver function test results.

CONTRAINDICATIONS
Contraindicated in patients with hypersensitivity to other cephalosporins.

NURSING CONSIDERATIONS
● Use cautiously in patients with a history of sensitivity to penicillin and in breast-feeding women. Also use cautiously and with dosage adjustments in patients with renal failure.
● Obtain specimen for culture and sensitivity tests before first dose. Therapy may begin pending results.
● Be aware that dose and dosing interval will be adjusted if creatinine clearance is below 55 ml/minute.
● **I.V. use:** Reconstitute with sterile water, bacteriostatic water, or 0.9% sodium chloride solution as follows: 2 ml to 500-mg vial; 2.5 ml to 1-g vial. Shake well until dissolved. Resultant concentration: 225 mg/ml or 330 mg/ml, respectively.

● Know that reconstituted cefazolin is stable for 24 hours at room temperature or 96 hours under refrigeration.
● For direct injection, further dilute Ancef with 5 ml, or Kefzol with 10 ml, of sterile water for injection. Inject into a large vein or into the tubing of a free-flowing I.V. solution over 3 to 5 minutes. For intermittent infusion, add reconstituted drug to 50 to 100 ml of compatible solution or use premixed solution. Commercially available frozen solutions of cefazolin in D_5W should be given only by intermittent or continuous I.V. infusion.
● Alternate injection sites if I.V. therapy lasts longer than 3 days. Use of small I.V. needles in larger available veins may be preferable.
● After reconstitution, inject I.M. drug without further dilution (this drug is not as painful as other cephalosporins). Injection should be given deeply into a large muscle mass, such as the gluteus maximus or lateral aspect of the thigh.
● With large doses or prolonged therapy, monitor for superinfection, especially in high-risk patients.

☑ **PATIENT TEACHING**
● Instruct patient to report adverse reactions promptly.
● Tell patient to alert nurse if discomfort occurs at I.V. injection site.

---

cefepime hydrochloride
Maxipime

Pregnancy Risk Category: B

HOW SUPPLIED
Injection: 500 mg/15 ml vial, 1 g/100 ml piggyback bottle, 1 g/ADD-Vantage vial, 1 g/15 ml vial, 2 g/100 ml piggyback bottle, 2 g/20 ml vial

ACTION
A fourth-generation cephalosporin that inhibits bacterial cell-wall synthesis, promotes osmotic instability, and de-

stroys bacteria.

ONSET, PEAK, DURATION
Onset occurs within 30 minutes. Peak levels occur in 1 to 2 hours. Duration is unknown.

INDICATIONS & DOSAGE
Mild to moderate urinary tract infections caused by Escherichia coli, Klebsiella pneumoniae, *or* Proteus mirabilis, *including cases associated with concurrent bacteremia with these microorganisms—*
Adults and children 12 years and older: 0.5 to 1 g I.M. (I.M. route used only for infections caused by *E. coli*) or I.V. infused over 30 minutes q 12 hours for 7 to 10 days.
Severe urinary tract infections, including pyelonephritis, caused by E. coli *or* K. pneumoniae—
Adults and children 12 years and older: 2 g I.V. infused over 30 minutes q 12 hours for 10 days.
Moderate to severe pneumonia caused by Streptococcus pneumoniae, Pseudomonas aeruginosa, K. pneumoniae, *or* Enterobacter *species—*
Adults and children 12 years and older: 1 to 2 g I.V. infused over 30 minutes q 12 hours for 10 days.
Moderate to severe skin infections, uncomplicated skin infections, and skin-structure infections caused by Staphylococcus aureus *(methicillin-susceptible strains only) or* Streptococcus pyogenes—
Adults and children 12 years and older: 2 g I.V. infused over 30 minutes q 12 hours for 10 days.

ADVERSE REACTIONS
CNS: headache.
GI: colitis, diarrhea, nausea, vomiting, oral moniliasis.
GU: vaginitis.
Skin: rash, pruritus, urticaria.
Other: phlebitis, pain, inflammation, fever.

INTERACTIONS
Aminoglycosides: may increase risk of nephrotoxicity and ototoxicity. Monitor renal and hearing functions closely.
Potent diuretics such as furosemide: may increase risk of nephrotoxicity. Monitor renal function closely.

EFFECTS ON DIAGNOSTIC TESTS
Cefepime may cause a false-positive reaction for glucose in the urine when using Clinitest tablets. Glucose tests based on enzymatic glucose oxidase reactions (such as Clinistix or Tes-Tape) should be used instead. A positive direct Coombs' test may occur during treatment with the drug.

CONTRAINDICATIONS
Contraindicated in patients with hypersensitivity to the drug, other cephalosporins, penicillins, or other beta-lactam antibiotics.

NURSING CONSIDERATIONS
● Use cautiously in patients with renal impairment, poor nutrition, or history of gastrointestinal disease (particularly colitis); in those receiving a protracted course of antimicrobial therapy; and in breast-feeding women.
● Safety of drug in children under age 12 has not been established.
● Obtain culture and sensitivity tests before first dose, if appropriate. Therapy may begin pending results.
● Dosage adjustment is necessary in patients with impaired renal function.
● I.V. use: Follow manufacturer's guidelines closely when reconstituting drug. Variations occur in constituting drug for administration, depending on concentration of drug ordered and how drug is packaged (piggyback vial, ADD-Vantage vial, or regular vial). Also be aware that the type of diluent used for constitution varies, depending on the product used. Use only solutions recommended by the manufacturer. The resulting solution should be administered over about 30 minutes.

---

*Liquid contains alcohol.   **May contain tartrazine.   †Canada only.   ‡Australia only.   ◇OTC.

• Intermittent I.V. infusion with a Y-type administration set can be accomplished with compatible solutions. However, during infusion of a solution containing cefepime, discontinuing the other solution is recommended.

• For I.M. administration, constitute the drug using sterile water for injection, 0.9% sodium chloride for injection, 5% dextrose injection, 0.5% or 1% lidocaine hydrochloride, or bacteriostatic water for injection with parabens or benzyl alcohol. Follow the manufacturer's guidelines for quantity of diluent to use.

• Inspect solution for particulate matter before administration. The powder and its solutions tend to darken, depending on storage conditions. Product potency is not adversely affected when stored as recommended.

• Monitor the patient for superinfection. Drug may cause overgrowth of nonsusceptible bacteria or fungi.

• Be aware that many cephalosporins can reduce prothrombin activity. Patients at risk include those with renal or hepatic impairment or poor nutrition and those receiving prolonged cefepime therapy. Monitor PT in these patients as ordered. Administer exogenous vitamin K as indicated and ordered.

☑ PATIENT TEACHING
• Warn patient receiving drug I.M. that pain may occur at injection site.
• Instruct patient to report adverse reactions promptly.

---

cefixime
Suprax

Pregnancy Risk Category: B

HOW SUPPLIED
Tablets: 200 mg, 400 mg
Oral suspension: 100 mg/5 ml (after reconstitution)

ACTION
A third-generation cephalosporin that inhibits cell-wall synthesis, promoting osmotic instability; usually bactericidal.

ONSET, PEAK, DURATION
Onset and duration unknown. Serum levels peak within 3.1 to 4.4 hours after an oral dose. Peak serum concentrations are approximately 15% to 50% higher when administered as oral suspension rather than tablets.

INDICATIONS & DOSAGE
Uncomplicated urinary tract infections caused by Escherichia coli *and* Proteus mirabilis; *otitis media caused by* Haemophilus influenzae *(beta-lactamase positive and negative strains),* Moraxella (Branhamella) catarrhalis, *and* Streptococcus pyogenes; *pharyngitis and tonsillitis caused by* S. pyogenes; *acute bronchitis and acute exacerbations of chronic bronchitis caused by* S. pneumoniae *and* H. influenzae *(beta-lactamase positive and negative strains)—*
Adults and children over 12 years or weighing over 50 kg: 400 mg/day P.O. as a single 400-mg tablet or 200 mg q 12 hours.
Children 12 years and younger or weighing 50 kg or less: 8 mg/kg/day suspension P.O. as a single daily dose or 4 mg/kg q 12 hours.
Uncomplicated gonorrhea caused by Neisseria gonorrhoeae—
Adults: 400 mg P.O. as a single dose.

ADVERSE REACTIONS
CNS: headache, dizziness.
GI: *diarrhea,* loose stools, abdominal pain, nausea, vomiting, dyspepsia, flatulence, pseudomembranous colitis.
GU: genital pruritus, vaginitis, genital candidiasis, transient increases in BUN and serum creatinine levels.
Hematologic: *thrombocytopenia,* leukopenia, eosinophilia.
Skin: pruritus, rash, urticaria, *erythema multiforme, Stevens-Johnson syn-*

Reactions may be *common,* uncommon, *life-threatening*, or COMMON AND LIFE-THREATENING.

drome.
Other: drug fever, transient increases in liver enzymes, hypersensitivity reactions (serum sickness, *anaphylaxis*).

INTERACTIONS
Probenecid: may inhibit excretion and increase blood levels of cefixime. Use together cautiously.
Salicylates: may displace cefixime from plasma protein-binding sites. Clinical significance is unknown.

EFFECTS ON DIAGNOSTIC TESTS
Cefixime may cause false-positive results in urine glucose tests using cupric sulfate (Benedict's reagent or Clinitest); use glucose oxidase tests (Clinistix or Tes-Tape) instead. It may cause false-positive results in tests for urine ketones that utilize nitroprusside (but not nitroferricyanide). Positive direct Coombs' test results have been seen with other cephalosporins.

CONTRAINDICATIONS
Contraindicated in patients with hypersensitivity to the drug or other cephalosporins.

NURSING CONSIDERATIONS
Alert: Use cautiously and with reduced dosage in patients with renal dysfunction; reduced dosage is necessary in patients with creatinine clearance below 60 ml/minute.
● Also use cautiously in patients with a history of sensitivity to penicillin and in breast-feeding women.
● Obtain specimen for culture and sensitivity tests before first dose. Therapy may begin pending results.
● To prepare oral suspension: add required amount of water to powder in two portions. Shake well after each addition. After mixing, suspension is stable for 14 days. No need to refrigerate, but keep tightly closed. Shake well before using.
● With large doses or prolonged therapy, monitor for superinfection, especial-

ly in high-risk patients.

☑ PATIENT TEACHING
● Tell the patient to take all of the medication prescribed, even after he feels better.
● Instruct the patient using oral suspension to shake container before measuring dose. Tell him suspension does not need to be refrigerated.
● Tell the patient to call the doctor if rash develops.

---

cefmetazole sodium (cefmetazone)
Zefazone

Pregnancy Risk Category: B

HOW SUPPLIED
Injection: 1 g, 2 g

ACTION
A semisynthetic cephamycin antibiotic pharmacologically similar to second-generation cephalosporins that inhibits cell-wall synthesis, promoting osmotic instability; usually bactericidal.

ONSET, PEAK, DURATION
Onset and duration unknown. Plasma levels peak immediately after I.V. administration.

INDICATIONS & DOSAGE
Lower respiratory tract infections caused by Streptococcus pneumoniae, Staphylococcus aureus *(penicillinase- and non-penicillinase-producing strains),* Escherichia coli, *and* Haemophilus influenzae *(non-penicillinase-producing strains); intra-abdominal infections caused by* E. coli *or* Bacteroides fragilis; *skin and skin-structure infections caused by* S. aureus *(penicillinase- and non-penicillinase-producing strains),* S. epidermidis, Streptococcus pyogenes, Streptococcus agalactiae, E. coli, Proteus mirabilis, Klebsiella pneumoniae, *and* B. fragilis—

---

*Liquid contains alcohol.   **May contain tartrazine.   †Canada only.   ‡Australia only.   ◇OTC.

Adults: 2 g I.V. q 6 to 12 hours for 5 to 14 days.
Urinary tract infections caused by E. coli—
Adults: 2 g I.V. q 12 hours.
Prophylaxis in patients undergoing vaginal hysterectomy—
Adults: 2 g I.V. 30 to 90 minutes before surgery as a single dose; or 1 g I.V. 30 to 90 minutes before surgery, repeated in 8 and 16 hours.
Prophylaxis in patients undergoing abdominal hysterectomy—
Adults: 1 g I.V. 30 to 90 minutes before surgery, repeated in 8 and 16 hours.
Prophylaxis in patients undergoing cesarean section—
Adults: 2 g I.V. as a single dose after clamping cord; or 1 g I.V. after clamping cord, repeated in 8 and 16 hours.
Prophylaxis in patients undergoing colorectal surgery—
Adults: 2 g I.V. as a single dose 30 to 90 minutes before surgery. Some clinicians follow with additional 2-g doses in 8 and 16 hours.
Prophylaxis in high-risk patients undergoing cholecystectomy—
Adults: 1 g I.V. 30 to 90 minutes before surgery, repeated in 8 and 16 hours.

ADVERSE REACTIONS
CNS: headache, hot flashes.
CV: *shock,* hypotension.
EENT: epistaxis.
GI: nausea, vomiting, *diarrhea,* epigastric pain, pseudomembranous colitis, candidiasis, bleeding.
GU: vaginitis.
Respiratory: pleural effusion, dyspnea, respiratory distress.
Skin: rash, pruritus, generalized erythema.
Other: fever, bacterial or fungal superinfection, hypersensitivity reactions (serum sickness, *anaphylaxis*), altered color perception, pain at injection site, phlebitis, thrombophlebitis, joint pain and inflammation.

INTERACTIONS
Aminoglycosides: potential increased risk of nephrotoxicity. Monitor closely.
Ethanol: possible disulfiram-like reaction. Should be avoided for 24 hours before and after administration of cefmetazole.
Probenecid: may inhibit excretion and increase blood levels of cefmetazole. Sometimes used for this effect.

EFFECTS ON DIAGNOSTIC TESTS
Cefmetazole causes false-positive results of urine glucose tests that use cupric sulfate (Benedict's reagent or Clinitest); use glucose oxidase tests (Clinistix or Tes-Tape) instead. It may cause positive Coombs' test results and may elevate liver function test results.

CONTRAINDICATIONS
Contraindicated in patients with hypersensitivity to the drug or other cephalosporins.

NURSING CONSIDERATIONS
● Use cautiously in patients with a history of sensitivity to penicillin and in breast-feeding women.
● Obtain specimen for culture and sensitivity tests before first dose. Therapy may begin pending results.
● **I.V. use:** Reconstitute with bacteriostatic water for injection, sterile water for injection, or 0.9% sodium chloride for injection. After reconstitution, drug may be further diluted to concentrations ranging from 1 to 20 mg/ml by adding it to 0.9% sodium chloride injection, D_5W, or lactated Ringer's injection. Reconstituted or dilute solutions are stable for 24 hours at room temperature (77° F [25° C]) or 1 week if refrigerated at 46° F (8° C).
● Monitor patient for bacterial and fungal superinfections. Prolonged use may result in overgrowth of nonsusceptible organisms.
● Monitor PT in patients at risk (from renal or hepatic impairment, malnutrition, or prolonged therapy), as ordered.

Reactions may be *common*, uncommon, *life-threatening*, or COMMON AND LIFE-THREATENING.

The chemical structure of this drug includes the methylthiotetrazole side chain that has been associated with bleeding disorders. However, such bleeding has not been reported with this drug.

☑ **PATIENT TEACHING**
● Tell patient to report adverse reactions promptly.
● Instruct patient to alert nurse if discomfort occurs at I.V. insertion site.

cefonicid sodium
Monocid

Pregnancy Risk Category: B

HOW SUPPLIED
Injection: 500 mg, 1 g
Infusion: 1 g/100 ml
Pharmacy bulk package: 10 g

ACTION
A second-generation cephalosporin that inhibits cell-wall synthesis, promoting osmotic instability; usually bactericidal.

ONSET, PEAK, DURATION
Onset immediate after I.V. administration, unknown after I.M. injection. Plasma levels peak within 1 to 2 hours after I.M. injection, immediately after I.V. administration. Duration unknown.

INDICATIONS & DOSAGE
Perioperative prophylaxis in contaminated surgery—
Adults: 1 g I.M. or I.V. 30 to 60 minutes before surgery; then 1 g I.M. or I.V. daily for 2 days after surgery. If used for prophylaxis in cesarean section, 1 g I.M. or I.V. after umbilical cord is clamped.
Serious infections of the lower respiratory and urinary tracts, skin and skin-structure infections, septicemia, bone and joint infections, and preoperative prophylaxis. Susceptible microorganisms include Streptococcus pneumoniae,

Klebsiella pneumoniae, Escherichia coli, Haemophilus influenzae, Proteus mirabilis, Staphylococcus aureus, S. epidermidis, *and* Streptococcus pyogenes—
Adults: usual dosage is 1 g I.V. or I.M. q 24 hours; in life-threatening infections, 2 g q 24 hours.

ADVERSE REACTIONS
CNS: dizziness, headache, malaise, paresthesia.
GI: pseudomembranous colitis, diarrhea.
GU: *acute renal failure,* interstitial nephritis.
Hematologic: neutropenia, leukopenia, eosinophilia, anemia, thrombocytosis, *thrombocytopenia.*
Skin: *maculopapular and erythematous rashes, urticaria.*
Other: hypersensitivity reactions (serum sickness, *anaphylaxis*); at injection site—*pain, induration, sterile abscesses, tissue sloughing;* with I.V. injection—*phlebitis, thrombophlebitis,* fever, myalgia.

INTERACTIONS
Probenecid: may inhibit excretion and increase blood levels of cefonicid. Use together cautiously.

EFFECTS ON DIAGNOSTIC TESTS
Cefonicid causes positive Coombs' test results and may elevate liver function test results or PT. It also causes false-positive results in urine glucose tests utilizing cupric sulfate (Benedict's reagent or Clinitest); use glucose oxidase tests (Clinistix or Tes-Tape) instead. Cefonicid causes false elevations in serum or urine creatinine levels in tests using Jaffé's reaction.

CONTRAINDICATIONS
Contraindicated in patients with hypersensitivity to the drug or other cephalosporins.

NURSING CONSIDERATIONS
● Use cautiously in patients with a history of sensitivity to penicillin and in breast-feeding women. Also use cautiously and with dosage adjustments in patients with renal failure.
● Obtain specimen for culture and sensitivity tests before first dose. Therapy may begin pending results.
● Be aware that dosing interval will be adjusted for patients with renal impairment.
● **I.V. use:** Reconstitute 500-mg vial with 2 ml of sterile water for injection (yields a concentration of 220 mg/ml) and 1-g vial with 2.5 ml of sterile water for injection (yields a concentration of 325 mg/ml). Shake well. Reconstitute piggyback vials with 50 to 100 ml of sterile water for injection, bacteriostatic water for injection, or 0.9% sodium chloride solution.
● For I.M. use, when administering 2-g I.M. doses once daily, divide the dose equally and inject deeply into large muscle masses, such as the gluteus maximus or the lateral aspect of the thigh.
● With large doses or prolonged therapy, monitor for superinfection, especially in high-risk patients.
● Be aware that the chemical structure of this drug includes the methylthiotetrazole side chain that has been associated with bleeding disorders. However, such bleeding has not been reported with this drug.

☑ PATIENT TEACHING
● Tell patient to report adverse reactions promptly.
● Instruct patient to alert nurse if discomfort is felt at I.V. insertion site.

---

cefoperazone sodium
Cefobid

Pregnancy Risk Category: B

HOW SUPPLIED
Infusion: 1 g, 2 g piggyback
Parenteral: 1 g, 2 g
Pharmacy bulk package: 10-g vial

ACTION
A third-generation cephalosporin that inhibits cell-wall synthesis, promoting osmotic instability; usually bactericidal.

ONSET, PEAK, DURATION
Onset immediate after I.V. administration, unknown after I.M. injection. Serum levels peak 1 to 2 hours after I.M. injection, immediately after I.V. administration. Duration unknown.

INDICATIONS & DOSAGE
Serious infections of the respiratory tract; intra-abdominal, gynecologic, and skin infections; bacteremia; and septicemia. Susceptible microorganisms include Streptococcus pneumoniae *and* S. pyogenes; Staphylococcus aureus *(penicillinase- and non-penicillinase-producing) and* Staphylococcus epidermidis; *enterococci;* Escherichia coli; Klebsiella; Haemophilus influenzae; Enterobacter; Citrobacter; Proteus; *some* Pseudomonas, *including* P. aeruginosa; *and* Bacteroides fragilis—
Adults: usual dosage is 1 to 2 g q 12 hours I.M. or I.V. In severe infections or in infections caused by less sensitive organisms, the total daily dosage or frequency may be increased up to 16 g/day in certain situations.

ADVERSE REACTIONS
GI: pseudomembranous colitis, nausea, vomiting, *diarrhea.*
Hematologic: transient neutropenia, *eosinophilia,* anemia, hypoprothrombinemia, bleeding.
Skin: *maculopapular and erythematous rashes, urticaria.*
Other: mildly elevated liver enzymes; hypersensitivity reactions (serum sickness, **anaphylaxis**); at injection site— *pain, induration, sterile abscesses, temperature elevation, tissue sloughing;*

Reactions may be *common*, uncommon, *life-threatening*, or COMMON AND LIFE-THREATENING.

with I.V. injection—*phlebitis, thrombophlebitis,* drug fever.

INTERACTIONS
Ethanol: possible disulfiram-like reaction. Warn patients not to drink alcohol for several days after discontinuing cefoperazone.
Probenecid: may inhibit excretion and increase blood levels of cefoperazone. Use together cautiously.

EFFECTS ON DIAGNOSTIC TESTS
Cephalosporins cause false-positive results in urine glucose tests utilizing cupric sulfate (Benedict's reagent or Clinitest); use glucose oxidase (Clinistix or Tes-Tape) instead. Cefoperazone may cause positive Coombs' test results and elevated liver function test results and PT.

CONTRAINDICATIONS
Contraindicated in patients with hypersensitivity to the drug or other cephalosporins.

NURSING CONSIDERATIONS
● Use cautiously in patients with impaired renal function or with a history of sensitivity to penicillin. Also use cautiously in breast-feeding women.
● Doses of 4 g/day should be given cautiously to patients with hepatic disease or biliary obstruction. Higher dosages require monitoring of serum levels.
● Obtain specimen for culture and sensitivity tests before first dose. Therapy may begin pending results.
● **I.V. use:** Reconstitute 1- or 2-g vial with a minimum of 2.8 ml of compatible I.V. solution; the manufacturer recommends using 5 ml/g. Give by direct injection into a large vein or into the tubing of a free-flowing I.V. solution over 3 to 5 minutes. When giving by intermittent infusion, add reconstituted drug to 20 to 40 ml of a compatible I.V. solution and infuse over 15 to 30 minutes.
● To prepare drug for I.M. injection: us-

ing the 1-g vial, dissolve drug with 2 ml of sterile water for injection; then add 0.6 ml of 2% lidocaine hydrochloride for a final concentration of 333 mg/ml. Alternatively, dissolve drug with 2.8 ml of sterile water for injection; then add 1 ml of 2% lidocaine hydrochloride for a final concentration of 250 mg/ml. When using the 2-g vial, dissolve drug with 3.8 ml of sterile water for injection; then add 1.2 ml of 2% lidocaine hydrochloride for a final concentration of 333 mg/ml. Alternatively, dissolve drug with 5.4 ml of sterile water for injection; then add 1.8 ml of 2% lidocaine hydrochloride for a final concentration of 250 mg/ml.
● For I.M. administration, inject deeply into a large muscle mass, such as the gluteus maximus or the lateral aspect of the thigh.
● With large doses or prolonged therapy, monitor for superinfection, especially in high-risk patients.
● Monitor PT regularly. The chemical structure of this drug includes the methylthiotetrazole side chain that has been associated with bleeding disorders. Vitamin K promptly reverses bleeding if it occurs.

☑ PATIENT TEACHING
● Tell patient to report adverse reactions promptly.
● Instruct patient to alert nurse if discomfort occurs at I.V. insertion site.

---

cefotaxime sodium
Claforan

Pregnancy Risk Category: B

HOW SUPPLIED
Injection: 500 mg, 1 g, 2 g
Infusion: 1 g, 2 g
Pharmacy bulk package: 10-g vial

ACTION
A third-generation cephalosporin that inhibits cell-wall synthesis, promoting

---

osmotic instability; usually bactericidal.

ONSET, PEAK, DURATION
Onset immediate after I.V. administration, unknown after I.M. injection. Serum levels peak 30 minutes after I.M. injection, immediately after I.V. administration. Duration unknown.

INDICATIONS & DOSAGE
Perioperative prophylaxis in contaminated surgery—
Adults: 1 g I.M. or I.V. 30 to 60 minutes before surgery. Patients undergoing bowel surgery should receive preoperative mechanical bowel cleansing and a nonabsorbable anti-infective agent such as neomycin. Patients undergoing cesarean section should receive 1 g I.M. or I.V. as soon as the umbilical cord is clamped, then 1 g I.M. or I.V. 6 and 12 hours later.
Uncomplicated gonorrhea caused by penicillinase-producing strains of Neiseria gonorrhoeae *or non-penicillinase-producing strains of the organism—*
Adults and adolescents: 500 mg I.M. as a single dose.
Serious infections of the lower respiratory and urinary tracts, CNS, skin, bone, and joints; gynecologic and intra-abdominal infections; bacteremia; and septicemia. Susceptible microorganisms include streptococci, including Streptococcus pneumoniae *and* S. pyogenes; Staphylococcus aureus *(penicillinase- and non-penicillinase-producing) and* Staphylococcus epidermidis; Escherichia coli; Klebsiella; Haemophilus influenzae; Serratia marcescens; Pseudomonas *species, including* P. aeruginosa; Enterobacter; Proteus; *and* Peptostreptococcus—
Adults: usual dose is 1 g I.V. or I.M. q 6 to 8 hours. Up to 12 g daily can be given in life-threatening infections.
Children weighing 50 kg or more: the usual adult dose, but dosage should not exceed 12 g daily.
Children 1 month to 12 years weighing less than 50 kg: 50 to 180 mg/

kg/day I.M. or I.V. in four to six divided doses.
Neonates to 1 week: 50 mg/kg I.V. q 12 hours.
Neonates 1 to 4 weeks: 50 mg/kg I.V. q 8 hours.

ADVERSE REACTIONS
CNS: headache.
GI: pseudomembranous colitis, nausea, vomiting, *diarrhea.*
GU: vaginitis, moniliasis, interstitial nephritis.
Hematologic: transient neutropenia, eosinophilia, hemolytic anemia, *thrombocytopenia, agranulocytosis.*
Skin: *maculopapular and erythematous rashes, urticaria.*
Other: hypersensitivity reactions (serum sickness, *anaphylaxis*); transient increases in liver enzymes; elevated temperature; at injection site—*pain, induration, sterile abscesses, temperature elevation, tissue sloughing;* with I.V. injection—*phlebitis, thrombophlebitis.*

INTERACTIONS
Aminoglycosides: may increase risk of nephrotoxicity. Monitor closely.
Probenecid: may inhibit excretion and increase blood levels of cefotaxime. Use together cautiously.

EFFECTS ON DIAGNOSTIC TESTS
Cefotaxime may cause positive Coombs' tests results and elevations of liver function test results.

CONTRAINDICATIONS
Contraindicated in patients with hypersensitivity to the drug or other cephalosporins.

NURSING CONSIDERATIONS
● Use cautiously in patients with a history of sensitivity to penicillin and in breast-feeding women. Also use cautiously and with dosage adjustments in patients with renal failure.
● Obtain specimen for culture and sensitivity tests before first dose. Therapy

may begin pending results.
- **I.V. use:** For direct injection, reconstitute 500-mg, 1-g, or 2-g vials with 10 ml of sterile water for injection. Solutions containing 1 g/14 ml are isotonic. Inject drug into a large vein or into the tubing of a free-flowing I.V. solution over 3 to 5 minutes.
- For I.V. infusion, reconstitute infusion vials with 50 to 100 ml of D_5W or 0.9% sodium chloride solution. Infuse drug over 20 to 30 minutes. Interrupt flow of primary I.V. solution during infusion.
- For I.M. administration, inject deeply into a large muscle mass, such as the gluteus maximus or the lateral aspect of the thigh.
- With large doses or prolonged therapy, monitor for superinfection, especially in high-risk patients.

☑ PATIENT TEACHING
- Tell patient to report adverse reactions promptly.
- Instruct patient to alert nurse if discomfort occurs at I.V. insertion site.

---

cefotetan disodium
Cefotan

Pregnancy Risk Category: B

HOW SUPPLIED
Injection: 1 g, 2 g
Infusion: 1 g, 2 g piggyback
Pharmacy bulk package: 10-g vial

ACTION
A semisynthetic cephamycin antibiotic that is pharmacologically similar to the second-generation cephalosporins. Inhibits cell-wall synthesis, promoting osmotic instability; usually bactericidal.

ONSET, PEAK, DURATION
Onset immediate after I.V. administration, unknown after I.M. injection. Peak serum levels occur 1½ to 3 hours after I.M. injection, immediately after I.V. administration. Duration unknown.

INDICATIONS & DOSAGE
Serious urinary tract and lower respiratory tract infections and gynecologic, skin and skin-structure, intra-abdominal, and bone and joint infections caused by susceptible streptococci, Staphylococcus aureus *(penicillinase- and non-penicillinase-producing) and* S. epidermidis, Escherichia coli, Klebsiella, Enterobacter, Proteus, Haemophilus influenzae, Neisseria gonorrhoeae, *and* Bacteroides, *including* B. fragilis—
Adults: 1 to 2 g I.V. or I.M. q 12 hours for 5 to 10 days. Up to 6 g daily in life-threatening infections.
Perioperative prophylaxis—
Adults: 1 to 2 g I.V. given once 30 to 60 minutes before surgery. In cesarean section, dose should be administered as soon as umbilical cord is clamped.

ADVERSE REACTIONS
GI: pseudomembranous colitis, nausea, *diarrhea.*
GU: nephrotoxicity.
Hematologic: transient neutropenia, eosinophilia, hemolytic anemia, hypoprothrombinemia, bleeding, thrombocytosis, *agranulocytosis, thrombocytopenia.*
Skin: *maculopapular and erythematous rashes, urticaria.*
Other: hypersensitivity reactions (serum sickness, *anaphylaxis*); transient increases in liver enzymes; elevated temperature; at injection site—*pain, induration, sterile abscesses, tissue sloughing;* with I.V. injection—*phlebitis, thrombophlebitis.*

INTERACTIONS
Aminoglycosides: possible synergistic effect and possible increased risk of nephrotoxicity. Use with caution.
Ethanol: possible disulfiram-like reaction. Warn patients not to drink alcohol for several days after discontinuing cefotetan.
Probenecid: may inhibit excretion and increase blood levels of cefotetan.

Sometimes used for this effect.

EFFECTS ON DIAGNOSTIC TESTS
Cefotetan causes false-positive results in urine glucose tests utilizing cupric sulfate (Benedict's reagent or Clinitest) use glucose oxidase tests (Clinistix or Tes-Tape) instead. It causes false elevations in serum or urine creatinine levels in tests using Jaffé's reaction. It may cause positive Coombs' test results and may elevate liver function test results and PT.

CONTRAINDICATIONS
Contraindicated in patients with hypersensitivity to the drug or other cephalosporins.

NURSING CONSIDERATIONS
● Use cautiously in patients with a history of sensitivity to penicillin and in breast-feeding women. Also use cautiously and with dosage adjustments in patients with renal failure.
● Obtain specimen for culture and sensitivity tests before first dose. Therapy may begin pending results.
● I.V. use: Reconstitute with sterile water for injection. Then may be mixed with 50 to 100 ml of D_5W or 0.9% sodium chloride solution. Interrupt flow of primary I.V. solution during cefotetan infusion.
● Reconstitute I.M. injection with sterile water or bacteriostatic water for injection, 0.9% sodium chloride for injection, or 0.5% or 1% lidocaine hydrochloride. Shake to dissolve and let stand until clear.
● Know that reconstituted solution is stable for 24 hours at room temperature or 96 hours if refrigerated.
● With large doses or prolonged therapy, monitor for superinfection, especially in high-risk patients.
● Know that chemical structure of drug includes the methylthiotetrazole side chain that has been associated with bleeding disorders. However, such bleeding has not been reported with this drug.

☑ PATIENT TEACHING
● Tell patient to report adverse reactions promptly.
● Instruct patient to alert nurse if discomfort occurs at I.V. site.

---

cefoxitin sodium
Mefoxin

Pregnancy Risk Category: B

HOW SUPPLIED
Injection: 1 g, 2 g
Infusion: 1 g, 2 g in 50-ml or 100-ml container
Pharmacy bulk package: 10 g

ACTION
A semisynthetic cephamycin antibiotic that is pharmacologically similar to the second-generation cephalosporins. Inhibits cell-wall synthesis, promoting osmotic instability; usually bactericidal.

ONSET, PEAK, DURATION
Onset immediate after I.V. administration, unknown after I.M. injection. Serum levels peak occur within 20 to 30 minutes after I.M. injection, immediately after I.V. administration. Duration unknown.

INDICATIONS & DOSAGE
Serious infections of respiratory and GU tracts, skin, soft-tissue, bone, and joint infections, and bloodstream and intra-abdominal infections caused by susceptible Escherichia coli *and other coliform bacteria,* Staphylococcus aureus *(penicillinase- and non-penicillinase-producing) and* S. epidermidis, *streptococci,* Klebsiella, Haemophilus influenzae, *and* Bacteroides, *including* B. fragilis; *and perioperative prophylaxis*—
Adults: 1 to 2 g q 6 to 8 hours for uncomplicated infections. Up to 12 g daily in life-threatening infections.

Children over 3 months: 80 to 160 mg/kg daily given in four to six equally divided doses. Maximum daily dose is 12 g.

Prophylactic use in surgery—
Adults: 2 g I.M. or I.V. 30 to 60 minutes before surgery, then 2 g I.M. or I.V. q 6 hours for 24 hours (72 hours after prosthetic arthroplasty).

Children 3 months or older: 30 to 40 mg/kg I.M. or I.V. 30 to 60 minutes before surgery, then 30 to 40 mg/kg q 6 hours for 24 hours (72 hours after prosthetic arthroplasty).

ADVERSE REACTIONS
CV: hypotension.
GI: pseudomembranous colitis, nausea, vomiting, *diarrhea.*
GU: *acute renal failure.*
Hematologic: transient neutropenia, eosinophilia, *hemolytic anemia,* anemia, *thrombocytopenia.*
Skin: *maculopapular and erythematous rashes, urticaria, exfoliative dermatitis.*
Other: hypersensitivity reactions (serum sickness, *anaphylaxis*); transient increases in liver enzymes; elevated temperature; at injection site—*pain, induration, sterile abscesses, tissue sloughing;* with I.V. injection—*phlebitis, thrombophlebitis,* dyspnea.

INTERACTIONS
Nephrotoxic agents: possible increased risk of nephrotoxicity. Monitor closely.
Probenecid: may inhibit excretion and increase blood levels of cefoxitin. Sometimes used for this effect.

EFFECTS ON DIAGNOSTIC TESTS
Cefoxitin causes false-positive results in urine glucose tests utilizing cupric sulfate (Benedict's reagent or Clinitest); use glucose oxidase tests (Clinistix or Tes-Tape) instead. It also causes false elevations in serum or urine creatinine levels in tests using Jaffé's reaction. Cefoxitin may elevate liver function test results and may cause positive Coombs' test results.

CONTRAINDICATIONS
Contraindicated in patients with hypersensitivity to the drug or other cephalosporins.

NURSING CONSIDERATIONS
● Use cautiously in patients with a history of sensitivity to penicillin and in breast-feeding women. Also use cautiously and with dosage adjustments in patients with renal failure.
● Obtain specimen for culture and sensitivity tests before first dose. Therapy may begin pending results.
● **I.V. use:** Reconstitute 1 g with at least 10 ml of sterile water for injection and 2 g with 10 to 20 ml of sterile water for injection. Solutions of dextrose 5% and 0.9% sodium chloride for injection can also be used. For direct injection, inject drug into a large vein or into the tubing of a free-flowing I.V. solution over 3 to 5 minutes. For intermittent infusion, add reconstituted drug to 50 or 100 ml of dextrose 5% or 10% in water or 0.9% sodium chloride injection. Interrupt flow of primary I.V. solution during infusion.
● Reconstitute I.M. injection with 0.5% or 1% lidocaine hydrochloride (without epinephrine) to minimize pain. Inject deeply into a large muscle mass, such as the gluteus maximus or the lateral aspect of the thigh.
● After reconstitution, store for 24 hours at room temperature or 1 week under refrigeration.
● Assess I.V. site frequently. Such use has been linked to development of thrombophlebitis.
● With large doses or prolonged therapy, monitor for superinfection, especially in high-risk patients.

☑ **PATIENT TEACHING**
● Tell patient to report adverse reactions promptly.
● Instruct patient to alert nurse if discomfort is felt at I.V. site.

---

*Liquid contains alcohol.　　**May contain tartrazine.　　†Canada only.　　‡Australia only.　　◇OTC.

cefpodoxime proxetil
Vantin

Pregnancy Risk Category: B

HOW SUPPLIED
Tablets (film-coated): 100 mg, 200 mg
Oral suspension: 50 mg/5 ml, 100 mg/ 5 ml in 100-ml bottles

ACTION
A second-generation cephalosporin that inhibits cell-wall synthesis, promoting osmotic instability; usually bactericidal.

ONSET, PEAK, DURATION
Onset and duration unknown. Serum levels peak in 2 to 3 hours after an oral dose.

INDICATIONS & DOSAGE
Acute, community-acquired pneumonia caused by non-beta-lactamase-producing strains of Haemophilus influenzae *or* Streptococcus pneumoniae—
Adults and children 13 years and older: 200 mg P.O. q 12 hours for 14 days.
Acute bacterial exacerbation of chronic bronchitis caused by S. pneumoniae, H. influenzae *(non-beta-lactamase-producing strains only), or* Moraxella (Branhamella) catarrhalis—
Adults and children 13 years and older: 200 mg P.O. q 12 hours for 10 days.
Uncomplicated gonorrhea in men and women; rectal gonococcal infections in women—
Adults and children 13 years and older: 200 mg P.O. as a single dose. Follow with doxycycline 100 mg P.O. b.i.d. for 7 days.
Uncomplicated skin and skin-structure infections caused by Staphylococcus aureus *or* Streptococcus pyogenes—
Adults and children 13 years and older: 400 mg P.O. q 12 hours for 7 to 14 days.
Acute otitis media caused by S. pneumoniae, H. influenzae, *or* M. catar-

rhalis—
Children 6 months and over: 5 mg/ kg (not to exceed 200 mg) P.O. q 12 hours for 10 days.
Pharyngitis or tonsillitis caused by S. pyogenes—
Adults: 100 mg P.O. q 12 hours for 10 days.
Children 6 months and over: 5 mg/ kg (not to exceed 100 mg) P.O. q 12 hours for 10 days.
Uncomplicated urinary tract infections caused by Escherichia coli, Klebsiella pneumoniae, Proteus mirabilis, *or* Staphylococcus saprophyticus—
Adults: 100 mg P.O. q 12 hours for 7 days.
  In patients with renal failure: Know that when creatinine clearance is below 30 ml/minute, dosage interval should be increased to q 24 hours. Patients receiving dialysis should get the drug three times weekly after dialysis.

ADVERSE REACTIONS
CNS: headache.
GI: *diarrhea,* nausea, vomiting, abdominal pain.
GU: vaginal fungal infections.
Skin: rash.
Other: hypersensitivity reactions *(anaphylaxis).*

INTERACTIONS
Antacids, H₂ antagonists: decreased absorption of cefpodoxime. Avoid concomitant use.
Probenecid: decreased excretion of cefpodoxime. Monitor for toxicity.

EFFECTS ON DIAGNOSTIC TESTS
Cefpodoxime proxetil may induce a positive direct Coombs' test.

CONTRAINDICATIONS
Contraindicated in patients with hypersensitivity to the drug or other cephalosporins. Safety and efficacy in children under age 6 months have not been established.

Reactions may be *common,* uncommon, *life-threatening,* or COMMON AND LIFE-THREATENING.

NURSING CONSIDERATIONS

• Use cautiously in patients with a history of penicillin hypersensitivity because of the risk of cross-sensitivity and in patients receiving nephrotoxic drugs because other cephalosporins have been shown to have nephrotoxic potential. Because drug is excreted in human breast milk, also use cautiously in breast-feeding women.

• Obtain specimen for culture and sensitivity tests before first dose. Therapy may begin pending results.

• Administer drug with food to enhance absorption. Shake suspension well before using.

• Store suspension in the refrigerator (36° to 46° F [2° to 8° C]). Discard unused portion after 14 days.

• Monitor for superinfection. Drug may cause overgrowth of nonsusceptible bacteria or fungi.

• Keep in mind that urine glucose determinations may be false-positive with copper sulfate tests (Clinitest); glucose enzymatic tests (Clinistix, Tes-Tape) are not affected.

☑ PATIENT TEACHING

• Tell the patient to take all of the medication prescribed, even after he feels better.

• Instruct the patient to take drug with food. If the patient is using suspension, tell him to shake container before measuring dose and to keep it refrigerated.

• Tell the patient to call doctor if rash develops.

---

cefprozil
Cefzil

Pregnancy Risk Category: B

HOW SUPPLIED
Tablets: 250 mg, 500 mg
Oral suspension: 125 mg/5 ml, 250 mg/ 5 ml

ACTION

A second-generation cephalosporin that interferes with cell-wall synthesis during microorganism replication, leading to osmotic instability and cell lysis (bactericidal).

ONSET, PEAK, DURATION

Onset and duration unknown. Serum levels peak within 1½ hours after an oral dose.

INDICATIONS & DOSAGE

Pharyngitis or tonsillitis caused by Streptococcus pyogenes—
Adults and children 13 years and older: 500 mg P.O. daily for at least 10 days.
Otitis media caused by S. pneumoniae, Haemophilus influenzae, *and* Moraxella (Branhamella) catarrhalis—
Infants and children 6 months to 12 years: 15 mg/kg P.O. q 12 hours for 10 days.
Secondary bacterial infections of acute bronchitis and acute bacterial exacerbation of chronic bronchitis caused by S. pneumoniae, H. influenzae, *and* M. catarrhalis—
Adults and children 13 years and older: 500 mg P.O. q 12 hours for 10 days.
Uncomplicated skin and skin-structure infections caused by Staphylococcus aureus *and* S. pyogenes—
Adults and children 13 years and older: 250 mg P.O. b.i.d., or 500 mg daily to b.i.d.
**✱*New indication:* *Acute sinusitis caused by* S. pneumoniae, H. influenzae *(beta-lactamase positive and negative strains), and* M. catarrhalis *(including beta-lactamase-producing strains)*—
Adults and children 13 years and older: 250 mg P.O. q 12 hours for 10 days; for moderate to severe infection, 500 mg P.O. q 12 hours for 10 days.
Children 6 months to 12 years: 7.5 mg/kg P.O. q 12 hours for 10 days; for moderate to severe infections, 15 mg/kg P.O. q 12 hours for 10 days.

---

*Liquid contains alcohol.   **May contain tartrazine.   †Canada only.   ‡Australia only.   ◇ OTC.

ADVERSE REACTIONS
CNS: dizziness, hyperactivity, headache, nervousness, insomnia, confusion, somnolence.
GI: *diarrhea, nausea,* vomiting, abdominal pain.
GU: elevated BUN level, elevated serum creatinine level, genital pruritus, vaginitis.
Hematologic: decreased leukocyte count, eosinophilia.
Hepatic: elevated liver enzymes, cholestatic jaundice (rare).
Skin: rash, urticaria, diaper rash.
Other: superinfection, hypersensitivity reactions (serum sickness, ***anaphylaxis***).

INTERACTIONS
Aminoglycosides: potential increased risk of nephrotoxicity. Monitor closely.
Probenecid: may inhibit excretion and increase blood levels of cefprozil. Use together cautiously.

EFFECTS ON DIAGNOSTIC TESTS
Cephalosporins may produce a false-positive result for urine glucose tests that use copper reduction method (Benedict's reagent, Fehling's solution, or Clinitest tablets); use enzymatic glucose oxidase methods (such as TesTape) instead. A false-negative reaction may occur in the ferricyanide test for blood glucose.

CONTRAINDICATIONS
Contraindicated in patients with hypersensitivity to the drug or other cephalosporins.

NURSING CONSIDERATIONS
• Use cautiously in patients with a history of sensitivity to penicillin and in breast-feeding women. Also use cautiously in patients with impaired hepatic or renal function.
Alert: Know that patients with creatinine clearance less than 30 ml/minute should receive 50% of usual dose.
• Obtain specimen for culture and sensitivity tests before first dose. Therapy may begin pending results.
• Administer after hemodialysis treatment is completed; drug is removed by hemodialysis.
• Monitor for superinfection. May cause overgrowth of nonsusceptible bacteria or fungi.

☑ PATIENT TEACHING
• Tell the patient to take all of the medication as prescribed, even after he feels better.
• Tell the patient to shake suspension well before measuring dose.
• Tell the patient that oral suspensions contain the drug in a bubble-gum-flavored form to improve palatability and promote compliance in children. Tell him to refrigerate reconstituted suspension and to discard unused drug after 14 days.
• Tell the patient to notify doctor if rash occurs.

---

ceftazidime
Ceptaz, Fortaz, Tazicef, Tazidime

Pregnancy Risk Category: B

HOW SUPPLIED
Injection (with sodium carbonate): 500 mg, 1 g, 2 g; 6 g (pharmacy bulk package)
Injection (with arginine): 1 g, 2 g; 6 g, 10 g (pharmacy bulk package)
Infusion: 1 g, 2 g in 50-ml and 100-ml vials (premixed)

ACTION
A third-generation cephalosporin that inhibits cell-wall synthesis, promoting osmotic instability; usually bactericidal.

ONSET, PEAK, DURATION
Onset immediate after I.V. administration, unknown after I.M. injection. Peak serum levels occur within 1 hour after I.M. injection, immediately after I.V. administration. In women, peak serum

concentrations may be lower after I.M. injection into the gluteus maximus than into the vastus lateralis. Duration unknown.

INDICATIONS & DOSAGE
Serious infections of the lower respiratory and urinary tracts; gynecologic, intra-abdominal, CNS, and skin infections; bacteremia; and septicemia.
Among susceptible microorganisms are streptococci, including Streptococcus pneumoniae *and* S. pyogenes; Staphylococcus aureus *(penicillinase- and non-penicillinase-producing);* Escherichia coli; Klebsiella; Proteus; Enterobacter; Haemophilus influenzae; Pseudomonas; *and some strains of* Bacteroides—
Adults and children 12 years and older: 1 g I.V. or I.M. q 8 to 12 hours; up to 6 g daily in life-threatening infections.
Children 1 month to 12 years: 25 to 50 mg/kg I.V. q 8 hours (sodium carbonate formulation).
Neonates 0 to 4 weeks: 30 mg/kg I.V. q 12 hours (sodium carbonate formulation).

ADVERSE REACTIONS
CNS: headache, dizziness, paresthesia, *seizures.*
GI: pseudomembranous colitis, nausea, vomiting, diarrhea, candidiasis, abdominal cramps.
GU: vaginitis.
Hematologic: eosinophilia; thrombocytosis, leukopenia, hemolytic anemia, *agranulocytosis, thrombocytopenia.*
Skin: *maculopapular and erythematous rashes, urticaria.*
Other: hypersensitivity reactions (serum sickness, *anaphylaxis*); transient elevation in liver enzymes; at injection site—*pain, induration, sterile abscesses, tissue sloughing;* with I.V. injection—*phlebitis, thrombophlebitis.*

INTERACTIONS
Aminoglycosides: additive or synergistic effect against some strains of *Pseudo-*

monas aeruginosa and Enterobacteriaceae.
Chloramphenicol: antagonistic effect. Avoid concomitant use.

EFFECTS ON DIAGNOSTIC TESTS
Ceftazidime causes false-positive results in urine glucose tests utilizing cupric sulfate (Benedict's reagent or Clinitest); use glucose oxidase (Clinistix or tesTape) instead. Ceftazidime may cause positive Coombs' test results and elevated liver function test results.

CONTRAINDICATIONS
Contraindicated in patients with hypersensitivity to the drug or other cephalosporins.

NURSING CONSIDERATIONS
● Use cautiously in patients with a history of sensitivity to penicillin and in breast-feeding women. Also use cautiously and with dosage adjustments in patients with renal failure.
● Obtain specimen for culture and sensitivity tests before first dose. Therapy may begin pending results.
● **I.V. use:** Reconstitute sodium carbonate-containing solutions with sterile water for injection. Add 5 ml to a 500-mg vial; 10 ml to a 1-g or 2-g vial. Shake well to dissolve drug. Carbon dioxide is released during dissolution, and positive pressure will develop in the vial. Reconstitute arginine-containing solutions with 10 ml of sterile water for injection. This formulation won't release gas bubbles. Each brand of ceftazidime includes specific instructions for reconstitution. Read and follow these instructions carefully.
● For I.M. administration, inject deeply into a large muscle mass, such as the gluteus maximus or the lateral aspect of the thigh.
● With large doses or prolonged therapy, monitor for superinfection, especially in high-risk patients.
Alert: Keep in mind that commercially available preparations contain either

---

*Liquid contains alcohol.   **May contain tartrazine.   †Canada only.   ‡Australia only.   ◊OTC.

sodium carbonate (Fortaz, Magnacef, Tazicef, Tazidime) or arginine (Ceptaz, Pentacef) to facilitate dissolution of drug. Safety and efficacy of arginine-containing solutions in children 12 years and under have not been established.

● Know that ceftazidime is removed by hemodialysis; a supplemental dose of the drug is indicated after each dialysis period, as ordered.

☑ **PATIENT TEACHING**
● Tell patient to report adverse reactions promptly.
● Instruct patient to alert nurse if discomfort is felt at I.V. insertion site.

▼ *NEW DRUG*

ceftibuten
Cedax

Pregnancy Risk Category: B

HOW SUPPLIED
Capsules: 400 mg
Oral suspension: 90 mg/5 ml, 180 mg/5 ml

ACTION
Ceftibuten exerts its bacterial action by binding to essential target proteins of the bacterial cell wall, which leads to inhibition of cell-wall synthesis.

ONSET, PEAK, DURATION
Onset and duration unknown. Maximum concentrations occur 2 to 4 hours after administration.

INDICATIONS & DOSAGE
Acute bacterial exacerbation of chronic bronchitis due to Haemophilus influenzae, Moraxella catarrhalis, *or penicillin-susceptible strains of* Streptococcus pneumoniae—
Adults and children age 12 and over: 400 mg P.O. daily for 10 days.
Pharyngitis and tonsillitis due to Streptococcus pyogenes; *acute bacterial oti-*

tis media due to H. influenzae, M. catarrhalis, *or* S. pyogenes—
Adults and children age 12 and over: 400 mg P.O. daily for 10 days.
Children under age 12: 9 mg/kg P.O. daily for 10 days.
Children weighing more than 45 kg (99 lb): should receive maximum dose of 400 mg P.O. daily for 10 days.
Adults with renal impairment: if creatinine clearance is 30 to 49 ml/min, 4.5 mg/kg or 200 mg P.O. is given q 24 hours. If creatinine clearance is 5 to 29 ml/min, 2.25 mg/kg or 100 mg P.O. is given q 24 hours. In patients undergoing hemodialysis two or three times a week, a single dose of 400 mg (capsule) or 9 mg/kg (suspension) P.O. is given after each hemodialysis session. Maximum dose is 400 mg.

ADVERSE REACTIONS
CNS: headache, dizziness, aphasia, psychosis.
GI: nausea, vomiting, diarrhea, dyspepsia, abdominal pain, loose stools, pseudomembranous colitis.
Hepatic: hepatic cholestasis, elevated liver enzymes and bilirubin.
Hematologic: elevated levels of eosinophils, decreased hemoglobin levels, altered platelet count, aplastic anemia, hemolytic anemia, *hemorrhage, neutropenia, agranulocytosis, pancytopenia.*
Skin: *Stevens-Johnson syndrome.*
Other: elevated levels of BUN, toxic nephropathy, renal dysfunction, allergic reaction, *anaphylaxis*, drug fever.

INTERACTIONS
Food: decreased bioavailability of the drug, which slows its absorption. Administer drug 2 hours before or 1 hour after a meal.

EFFECTS ON DIAGNOSTIC TESTS
Although ceftibuten has not been known to affect the direct Coombs' test to date, other cephalosporins have caused a false-positive direct Coombs' test. Some

cephalosporins may cause a false-positive test for urinary glucose.

CONTRAINDICATIONS
Contraindicated in patients with hypersensitivity to cephalosporin drugs.

NURSING CONSIDERATIONS
● Use cautiously if administering to patients with history of hypersensitivity to penicillin.
● Use cautiously in patients with impaired renal failure or GI disease, especially colitis.
● Use cautiously when administering to elderly patient.
● Safety and effectiveness in infants under age 6 months have not been established.
● Drug should be used in pregancy only if clearly needed. It is unknown if drug is excreted in breast milk; use cautiously in breast-feeding women.
Alert: If allergic reaction is suspected, drug should be discontinued. Emergency treatment may be required.
● Pseudomembranous colitis has been reported with nearly all antibacterial agents. Consider this diagnosis in patients who develop diarrhea secondary to therapy. Obtain specimens for *Clostridium difficile,* as ordered.
● Obtain specimen for culture and sensitivity tests before giving first dose. Therapy may begin pending test results.
● When preparing oral suspension, first tap the bottle to loosen powder. Follow chart supplied by manufacturer for amount of water to add to powder when mixing oral suspension form. Add water in two portions; shake well after each step. After mixing, suspension is stable for 14 days when refrigerated.
● Shake oral suspension well before administering.
● Drug may cause overgrowth of nonsusceptible bacteria or fungi. Monitor patient for superinfection.

☑ **PATIENT TEACHING**
● Instruct patient to take all of the medication prescribed, even if he feels better.
● Instruct patient using oral suspension to take it at least 2 hours before or 1 hour after a meal.
● Instruct patient using oral suspension to shake bottle well before measuring.
● Instruct patient to store oral suspension in the refrigerator, with lid tightly closed, and to discard any unused drug after 14 days.
● Caution breast-feeding woman that it is unknown whether ceftibuten is excreted in breast milk.
● Tell diabetic patient that the suspension contains 1 gram sucrose/tsp.

ceftizoxime sodium
Cefizox

Pregnancy Risk Category: B

HOW SUPPLIED
Injection: 500 mg, 1 g, 2 g
Infusion: 1 g, 2 g in 100-mg vials or in 50 ml of D_5W
Pharmacy bulk package: 10 g

ACTION
A third-generation cephalosporin that inhibits cell-wall synthesis, promoting osmotic instability; usually bactericidal.

ONSET, PEAK, DURATION
Onset immediate after I.V. administration, unknown after I.M. injection. Serum levels peak ½ to 1½ hours after I.M. injection, immediately after I.V. administration. Duration unknown.

INDICATIONS & DOSAGE
Serious infections of the lower respiratory and urinary tracts, gynecologic infections, bacteremia, septicemia, meningitis, intra-abdominal infections, bone and joint infections, and skin infections. Among susceptible microorganisms are streptococci, including Streptococcus pneumoniae *and* S. pyogenes; *Staphylococcus aureus and* Staphylococcus epidermidis; *Escherichia coli; Klebsiella;*

Haemophilus influenzae; Enterobacter; Proteus; *some* Pseudomonas; *and* Peptostreptococcus—
Adults: usual dosage is 1 to 2 g I.V. or I.M. q 8 to 12 hours. In life-threatening infections, up to 2 g q 4 hours.
Children over 6 months: 33 to 50 mg/kg I.V. q 6 to 8 hours. Serious infections: up to 200 mg/kg/day in divided doses may be used. Don't exceed 12 g/day.

ADVERSE REACTIONS
GI: pseudomembranous colitis, nausea, anorexia, vomiting, *diarrhea.*
GU: vaginitis.
Hematologic: transient neutropenia, eosinophilia, hemolytic anemia, thrombocytosis, anemia, ***thrombocytopenia.***
Skin: *maculopapular and erythematous rashes, urticaria.*
Other: hypersensitivity reactions (serum sickness, ***anaphylaxis***); dyspnea; elevated temperature; at injection site—*pain, induration, sterile abscesses, tissue sloughing;* with I.V. injection—*phlebitis, thrombophlebitis,* transient elevation in liver enzymes.

INTERACTIONS
Probenecid: may inhibit excretion and increase blood levels of ceftizoxime. Sometimes used for this effect.

EFFECTS ON DIAGNOSTIC TESTS
Ceftizoxime causes false-positive results in urine glucose tests utilizing cupric sulfate (Benedict's reagent or Clinitest); use glucose oxidase (Clinistix or Tes-Tape) instead. It also causes false elevations in urine creatinine levels using Jaffé's reaction. Ceftizoxime may cause positive Coombs' test results and elevated liver function test results.

CONTRAINDICATIONS
Contraindicated in patients with hypersensitivity to the drug or other cephalosporins.

NURSING CONSIDERATIONS
● Use cautiously in patients with a history of sensitivity to penicillin and in breast-feeding women. Also use cautiously and with dosage adjustments in patients with renal failure.
● Obtain specimen for culture and sensitivity tests before first dose. Therapy may begin pending results.
● **I.V. use:** To reconstitute powder, add 5 ml of sterile water to a 500-mg vial, 10 ml to a 1-g vial, or 20 ml to a 2-g vial. Reconstitute piggyback vials with 50 to 100 ml of 0.9% sodium chloride solution or D_5W. Shake well.
● For I.M. administration, inject deeply into a large muscle mass, such as the gluteus maximus or the lateral aspect of the thigh. Larger doses (2 g) should be divided and administered at two separate sites.
● With large doses or prolonged therapy, monitor for superinfection, especially in high-risk patients.

☑ PATIENT TEACHING
● Tell patient to report adverse reactions promptly.
● Instruct patient to alert nurse if discomfort is felt at I.V. site.

---

ceftriaxone sodium
Rocephin

Pregnancy Risk Category: B

HOW SUPPLIED
Injection: 250 mg, 500 mg, 1 g, 2 g
Infusion: 1 g, 2 g
Pharmacy bulk package: 10 g

ACTION
A third-generation cephalosporin that inhibits cell-wall synthesis, promoting osmotic instability; usually bactericidal.

ONSET, PEAK, DURATION
Onset immediate after I.V. administra-

Reactions may be *common,* uncommon, ***life-threatening***, or COMMON AND LIFE-THREATENING.

tion, unknown after I.M. injection. Peak serum levels occur 1½ to 4 hours after I.M. injection, immediately after I.V. administration. Duration unknown.

INDICATIONS & DOSAGE
Most infections caused by susceptible organisms—
Adults: 1 to 2 g I.M. or I.V. daily or b.i.d. depending on type and severity of infection.
Uncomplicated gonococcal vulvovaginitis—
Adults: 250 mg I.M. as a single dose, followed with 100 mg of doxycycline P.O. q 12 hours for 10 to 14 days.
Serious infections of the lower respiratory and urinary tracts; gynecologic, bone and joint, intra-abdominal, and skin infections; bacteremia; septicemia; and Lyme disease caused by such susceptible microorganisms as streptococci, including Streptococcus pneumoniae *and* S. pyogenes; Staphylococcus aureus *(penicillinase- and non-penicillinase-producing) and* Staphylococcus epidermidis; Escherichia coli; Klebsiella; Haemophilus influenzae; Neisseria meningitidis; N. gonorrhoeae; Enterobacter; Proteus; Peptostreptococcus, Pseudomonas; *and* Serratia marcescens—
Adults and children over 12 years: 1 to 2 g I.M. or I.V. daily or in equally divided doses b.i.d. Total daily dosage should not exceed 4 g.
Children 12 years and under: 50 to 75 mg/kg I.M. or I.V., not to exceed 2 g/day, given in divided doses q 12 hours.
Meningitis—
Adults and children: initially, 100 mg/kg I.M. or I.V. (not to exceed 4 g); thereafter, 100 mg/kg I.M. or I.V., given once daily or in divided doses q 12 hours, not to exceed 4 g, for 7 to 14 days.
Perioperative prophylaxis—
Adults: 1 g I.V. as a single dose ½ to 2 hours before surgery.

ADVERSE REACTIONS
CNS: headache, dizziness.
GI: pseudomembranous colitis, nausea, vomiting, diarrhea.
GU: genital pruritus, moniliasis, elevated BUN levels.
Hematologic: eosinophilia, thrombocytosis, leukopenia.
Skin: pain, induration, tenderness at injection site; phlebitis; *rash;* pruritus.
Other: hypersensitivity reactions (serum sickness, ***anaphylaxis***), elevated temperature, chills.

INTERACTIONS
Aminoglycosides: additive or synergistic effect against some strains of *Pseudomonas aeruginosa* and Enterobacteriaceae.
Probenecid: high doses (1 or 2 g/day) may enhance hepatic clearance of ceftriaxone and shorten its half-life. Avoid concomitant use.

EFFECTS ON DIAGNOSTIC TESTS
Ceftriaxone causes false-positive results in urine glucose tests utilizing cupric sulfate (Benedict's reagent or Clinitest); instead use glucose oxidase (Clinistix or Tes-Tape). It also causes false elevations in urine creatinine levels in tests using Jaffé's reaction. Ceftriaxone may cause positive Coombs' test results and elevations in liver function test results.

CONTRAINDICATIONS
Contraindicated in patients with hypersensitivity to the drug or other cephalosporins.

NURSING CONSIDERATIONS
● Use cautiously in patients with a history of sensitivity to penicillin and in breast-feeding women.
● Obtain specimen for culture and sensitivity tests before first dose. Therapy may begin pending results.
● **I.V. use:** Reconstitute with sterile water for injection, 0.9% sodium chloride injection, dextrose 5% or 10% injection, or a combination of sodium chloride and dextrose injection and other compatible solutions. Reconstitute by adding 2.4 ml

---

of diluent to the 250-mg vial, 4.8 ml to the 500-mg vial, 9.6 ml to the 1-g vial, and 19.2 ml to the 2-g vial. All reconstituted solutions yield a concentration that averages 100 mg/ml. After reconstitution, dilute further for intermittent infusion to desired concentration. I.V. dilutions are stable for 24 hours at room temperature.
• For I.M. administration, inject deeply into a large muscle mass, such as the gluteus maximus or the lateral aspect of the thigh.
• With large doses or prolonged therapy, monitor for superinfection, especially in high-risk patients.
• Be aware that drug is commonly used in home antibiotic programs for outpatient treatment of serious infections, such as osteomyelitis.

☑ PATIENT TEACHING
• Tell patient to report adverse reactions promptly.
• Instruct patient to alert nurse if discomfort occurs at I.V. insertion site.
• Teach home care patient and family how to prepare and administer drug.
• If home care patient is a diabetic who is testing his urine for glucose, tell him drug may affect results of cupric sulfate tests; instead he should use an enzymatic test.

---

cefuroxime axetil
Ceftin

cefuroxime sodium
Kefurox, Zinacef

Pregnancy Risk Category: B

HOW SUPPLIED
cefuroxime axetil
Tablets: 125 mg, 250 mg, 500 mg
Suspension: 125 mg/5 ml
cefuroxime sodium
Injection: 750 mg, 1.5 g
Infusion: 750 mg, 1.5 g premixed, frozen solution

Pharmacy bulk package: 7.5 g

ACTION
A second-generation cephalosporin that inhibits cell-wall synthesis, promoting osmotic instability; usually bactericidal.

ONSET, PEAK, DURATION
Onset is immediate after I.V. administration, unknown after oral and I.M. administration. Peak serum levels occur within 2 hours after oral administration, 15 to 60 minutes after I.M. injection, immediately after I.V. administration. Duration unknown.

INDICATIONS & DOSAGE
Injectable form is for serious infections of the lower respiratory and urinary tracts; skin and skin-structure infections; bone and joint infections; septicemia; meningitis; and gonorrhea; and for perioperative prophylaxis; oral form is used to treat otitis media, pharyngitis, tonsillitis, infections of the urinary and lower respiratory tracts, and skin and skin-structure infections. Among susceptible organisms are Streptococcus pneumoniae *and* S. pyogenes, Haemophilus influenzae, Klebsiella, Staphylococcus aureus, Escherichia coli, Moraxella (Branhamella) catarrhalis *(including beta-lactamase-producing strains),* Enterobacter, Neisseria gonorrhoeae—
Adults and children 12 years and older: usual dosage of cefuroxime sodium is 750 mg to 1.5 g I.M. or I.V. q 8 hours for 5 to 10 days. For life-threatening infections and infections caused by less susceptible organisms, 1.5 g I.M. or I.V. q 6 hours; for bacterial meningitis, up to 3 g I.V. q 8 hour
Alternatively, administer 250 mg of cefuroxime axetil P.O. q 12 hours. For severe infections, dosage may be increased to 500 mg q 12 hours.
Children and infants over 3 months: 50 to 100 mg/kg/day of cefuroxime sodium I.M. or I.V. in equally divided doses q 6 to 8 hours. Higher doses are

---

Reactions may be *common*, uncommon, *life-threatening*, or COMMON AND LIFE-THREATENING.

administered when treating meningitis. Alternatively, 125 mg of cefuroxime axetil P.O. q 12 hours; for bacterial meningitis, 200 to 240 mg/kg I.V. in divided doses q 6 to 8 hours.

Uncomplicated urinary tract infections—
Adults: 125 to 250 mg P.O. q 12 hours.

Otitis media—
Children under 2 years: 125 mg P.O. q 12 hours.

Children 2 years and over: 250 mg P.O. q 12 hours.

Perioperative prophylaxis—
Adults: 1.5 g I.V. 30 to 60 minutes before surgery; in lengthy operations, 750 mg I.V. or I.M. q 8 hours. For open-heart surgery, 1.5 g I.V. at induction of anesthesia and then q 12 hours for a total dosage of 6 g.

✳ New indication: *Early Lyme disease (erythema migrans) caused by* Borrelia burgdorferi—
Adults and children 13 years and older: 500 mg P.O. b.i.d. for 20 days.

ADVERSE REACTIONS
GI: pseudomembranous colitis, nausea, anorexia, vomiting, *diarrhea.*
Hematologic: transient neutropenia, eosinophilia, **hemolytic anemia, thrombocytopenia,** decreased hemoglobin and hematocrit levels.
Skin: *maculopapular and erythematous rashes, urticaria.*
Other: transient increases in liver enzymes; hypersensitivity reactions (serum sickness, **anaphylaxis**); at injection site—*pain, induration, sterile abscesses, temperature elevation, tissue sloughing;* with I.V. injection—*phlebitis, thrombophlebitis.*

INTERACTIONS
Diuretics: increased risk of adverse renal reactions. Monitor closely.
Probenecid: may inhibit excretion and increase blood levels of cefuroxime. Sometimes used for this effect.

EFFECTS ON DIAGNOSTIC TESTS
Cefuroxime causes false-positive results in urine glucose tests utilizing cupric sulfate (Benedict's reagent or Clinitest); use glucose oxidase tests (Clinistix or Tes-Tape) instead. It also causes false elevations in serum or urine creatinine levels in tests using Jaffé's reaction. Cefuroxime may elevate liver function test results and may cause positive Coombs' test results.

CONTRAINDICATIONS
Contraindicated in patients with hypersensitivity to the drug or other cephalosporins.

NURSING CONSIDERATIONS
● Use cautiously in patients with history of sensitivity to penicillin and in breast-feeding women. Also use cautiously and with reduced dosage in patients with impaired renal function.
● Obtain specimen for culture and sensitivity tests before first dose. Therapy may begin pending results.
● **I.V. use:** For each 750-mg vial of Kefurox, reconstitute with 9 ml of sterile water for injection. Withdraw 8 ml from the vial for the proper dose. For each 1.5-g vial of Kefurox, reconstitute with 16 ml of sterile water for injection; withdraw entire contents of vial for a dose. For each 750-mg vial of Zinacef, reconstitute with 8 ml of sterile water for injection; for each 1.5-g vial, reconstitute with 16 ml. In each case, withdraw entire contents of vial for a dose.
● To give by direct injection, inject into a large vein or into the tubing of a free-flowing I.V. solution over 3 to 5 minutes.
● For intermittent infusion, add reconstituted drug to 100 ml D_5W, 0.9% sodium chloride for injection, or other compatible I.V. solution. Infuse over 15 to 60 minutes.
● For I.M. administration, inject deeply into a large muscle mass, such as the gluteus maximus or the lateral aspect of the thigh.

---

*Liquid contains alcohol.   **May contain tartrazine.   †Canada only.   ‡Australia only.   ◇OTC.

• Know that absorption of cefuroxime axetil is enhanced by food.
• Keep in mind that cefuroxime axetil is available only in tablet form, which may be crushed for patients who cannot swallow tablets. Tablets may be allowed to dissolve in small amounts of apple, orange, or grape juice or chocolate milk. However, the drug has a bitter taste that is difficult to mask, even with food.
• Be aware that cefuroxime axetil film-coated tablet form and the oral suspension are not bioequivalent and are not substitutable on a mg/mg basis.
• With large doses or prolonged therapy, monitor for superinfection, especially in high-risk patients.

☑ **PATIENT TEACHING**
• Tell the patient to take all of the medication as prescribed, even after he feels better.
• Instruct the patient to take oral form with food. If patient has difficulty swallowing tablets, tell him how to dissolve or crush tablets but warn him that the bitter taste that results is hard to mask, even with food. If suspension is being used, tell patient to shake container well before measuring dose.
• Tell the patient to notify doctor if rash occurs.
• Instruct the patient receiving drug I.V. to alert nurse if discomfort occurs at I.V. insertion site.

---

cephalexin hydrochloride
Keftab

cephalexin monohydrate
Apo-Cephalex†, Bio-cef, Cefanex, Ceporex†‡, C-Lexin, Keflex, Novo-Lexin†, Nu-Cephalex†‡

Pregnancy Risk Category: B

HOW SUPPLIED
cephalexin hydrochloride
Tablets: 250 mg, 500 mg
cephalexin monohydrate
Tablets: 250 mg, 500 mg, 1 g
Capsules: 250 mg, 500 mg
Oral suspension: 100 mg/5 ml, 125 mg/5 ml, 250 mg/5 ml

ACTION
A first-generation cephalosporin that inhibits cell-wall synthesis, promoting osmotic instability; usually bactericidal.

ONSET, PEAK, DURATION
Onset unknown. Serum levels peak within 1 hour. Duration unknown.

INDICATIONS & DOSAGE
Respiratory tract, GI tract, skin, soft-tissue, bone, and joint infections and otitis media caused by Escherichia coli *and other coliform bacteria, group A beta-hemolytic streptococci,* Klebsiella, Proteus mirabilis, Streptococcus pneumoniae, *and staphylococci—*
Adults: 250 mg to 1 g P.O. q 6 hours.
Children: 6 to 12 mg/kg P.O. q 6 hours (monohydrate only). Maximum 25 mg/kg q 6 hours.

ADVERSE REACTIONS
CNS: dizziness, headache, fatigue, agitation, confusion, hallucinations.
GI: pseudomembranous colitis, *nausea, anorexia,* vomiting, *diarrhea,* gastritis, glossitis, dyspepsia, abdominal pain, anal pruritus, tenesmus, oral candidiasis.
GU: genital pruritus and moniliasis, vaginitis, interstitial nephritis.
Hematologic: neutropenia, eosinophilia, anemia, ***thrombocytopenia.***
Skin: *maculopapular and erythematous rashes,* urticaria.
Other: transient increases in liver enzymes, hypersensitivity reactions (serum sickness, ***anaphylaxis***), arthritis, arthralgia, joint pain.

INTERACTIONS
Probenecid: may increase blood levels of cephalosporins. Sometimes used for this effect.

Reactions may be *common,* uncommon, *life-threatening,* or COMMON AND LIFE-THREATENING.

EFFECTS ON DIAGNOSTIC TESTS
Cephalexin causes false-positive results in urine glucose tests utilizing cupric sulfate (Benedict's reagent or Clinitest); use glucose oxidase tests (Clinistix or Tes-Tape) instead. It also causes false elevations in serum or urine creatinine levels in tests using Jaffé's reaction. Positive Coombs' test results occur in about 3% of patients taking cephalexin.

CONTRAINDICATIONS
Contraindicated in patients with hypersensitivity to cephalosporins.

NURSING CONSIDERATIONS
● Use cautiously in breast-feeding women and in patients with impaired renal function or history of sensitivity to penicillin.
● Ask the patient if he's had any reaction to cephalosporin or penicillin therapy before giving first dose.
● Obtain specimen for culture and sensitivity tests before first dose. Therapy may begin pending results.
● To prepare oral suspension: Add required amount of water to powder in two portions. Shake well after each addition. After mixing, store in refrigerator. The mixture will remain stable for 14 days without significant loss of potency. Keep tightly closed and shake well before using.
● With large doses or prolonged therapy, monitor for superinfection, especially in high-risk patients.
● Know that group A beta-hemolytic streptococcal infections should be treated for a minimum of 10 days.

☑ PATIENT TEACHING
● Tell the patient to take all of the medication exactly as prescribed, even after he feels better.
● Tell the patient to take drug with food or milk to lessen GI discomfort. If patient is taking suspension form, instruct him to shake container well before measuring dose and to store in refrigerator.
● Instruct the patient to call the doctor if rash develops.

---

cephapirin sodium
Cefadyl

Pregnancy Risk Category: B

HOW SUPPLIED
Injection: 500-mg, 1-g, 2-g vials; 1-g, 2-g, 4-g piggyback vials
Pharmacy bulk package: 20 g

ACTION
Synthetic first-generation cephalosporin that inhibits cell-wall synthesis, promoting osmotic instability; usually bactericidal.

ONSET, PEAK, DURATION
Onset immediate after I.V. administration, unknown after I.M. injection. Serum levels peak within 30 minutes of I.M. injection, immediately after I.V. administration. Duration unknown.

INDICATIONS & DOSAGE
Perioperative prophylaxis in contaminated or potentially contaminated surgery—
Adults: 1 to 2 g I.M. or I.V. 30 to 60 minutes before surgery; then 1 to 2 g I.M. or I.V. q 6 hours for 24 hours. In procedures longer than 2 hours, additional doses may be given during surgery. In cases where infection would be devastating, prophylaxis may be continued for 3 to 5 days.
Serious infections of respiratory, GU, or GI tract; skin and soft-tissue infections; bone and joint infections (including osteomyelitis); septicemia; and endocarditis caused by Streptococcus pneumoniae, Escherichia coli, *group A beta-hemolytic streptococci,* Klebsiella, Proteus mirabilis, Staphylococcus aureus, *and* Streptococcus viridans—
Adults: 500 mg to 1 g I.M. or I.V. q 4 to 6 hours. In life-threatening infections, up to 12 g/day may be used.
Children over 3 months: 10 to 20

---

mg/kg I.V. or I.M. q 6 hours; dose depends on age, weight, and severity of infection.

Patients with reduced renal function may be treated adequately with a lower dose (7.5 to 15 mg/kg q 12 hours), depending on causative organism and severity of dysfunction. Patients with severely reduced renal function who are scheduled for dialysis should receive same dose just before dialysis and q 12 hours thereafter.

ADVERSE REACTIONS
CNS: dizziness, headache, malaise, paresthesia.
GI: pseudomembranous colitis, nausea, anorexia, vomiting, *diarrhea,* abdominal cramps, oral candidiasis.
GU: genital pruritus and moniliasis, vaginitis.
Hematologic: transient neutropenia, eosinophilia, anemia, ***thrombocytopenia.***
Skin: *maculopapular and erythematous rashes, urticaria.*
Other: transient increases in liver enzymes; hypersensitivity reactions (serum sickness, ***anaphylaxis***); at injection site—*pain, induration, sterile abscesses, tissue sloughing;* with I.V. injection—*phlebitis, thrombophlebitis.*

INTERACTIONS
Probenecid: may increase blood levels of cephalosporins. Sometimes used for this effect.

EFFECTS ON DIAGNOSTIC TESTS
Cephapirin causes false-positive results in urine glucose tests utilizing cupric sulfate (Benedict's reagent or Clinitest); use glucose oxidase tests (Clinistix or Tes-Tape) instead. It also causes false elevations in serum or urine creatinine levels in tests using Jaffé's reaction. Cephapirin may cause positive Coombs' test results and may elevate liver function test results.

CONTRAINDICATIONS
Contraindicated in patients with hypersensitivity to the drug or other cephalosporins.

NURSING CONSIDERATIONS
● Use cautiously in patients with a history of sensitivity to penicillin and in breast-feeding women.
● Obtain specimen for culture and sensitivity tests before first dose. Therapy may begin pending results.
● **I.V. use:** Prepare I.V. infusion using dextrose for injection, sodium chloride for injection, or bacteriostatic water for injection as diluent: 20 ml yields 1 g/10 ml; 50 ml yields 1 g/25 ml; 100 ml yields 1 g/50 ml.
● When using I.V. infusion with Y-tubing, dilute 4-g vial with 40 ml of diluent. During infusion of cephapirin solution, stop the flow of the other solution. Check volume of cephapirin solution carefully so that calculated dose is infused.
● When giving this drug I.V., check frequently for vein irritation and phlebitis. Alternate injection sites if I.V. therapy lasts longer than 3 days. Use of small I.V. needles in the larger available veins may be preferable.
● For I.M. use, reconstitute 1-g vial with 2 ml of sterile water for injection or bacteriostatic water for injection so that 1.2 ml contains 500 mg of cephapirin. Prepare patient for painful I.M. injection. Inject deeply into a large muscle mass, such as the gluteus maximus or the lateral aspect of the thigh.
● Store reconstituted cephapirin for 10 days under refrigeration and for 24 hours at room temperature.
● With large doses or prolonged therapy, monitor for superinfection, especially in high-risk patients.

☑ PATIENT TEACHING
● Tell patient to report adverse reactions promptly.
● Instruct patient to alert nurse if discomfort occurs at I.V. insertion site.

• Warn patient receiving drug I.M. that injection is painful but that application of ice to site may help relieve discomfort.

cephradine
Velosef**

Pregnancy Risk Category: B

HOW SUPPLIED
Capsules: 250 mg, 500 mg
Oral suspension: 125 mg/5 ml, 250 mg/5 ml

ACTION
First-generation cephalosporin that inhibits cell-wall synthesis, promoting osmotic instability; usually bactericidal.

ONSET, PEAK, DURATION
Onset and duration unknown. Serum levels peak within 1 hour after oral dose.

INDICATIONS & DOSAGE
Serious infections of respiratory, GU, or GI tract; skin and soft-tissue infections; bone and joint infections; septicemia; endocarditis; and otitis media caused by such susceptible organisms as Escherichia coli *and other coliform bacteria,* group A beta-hemolytic streptococci, Klebsiella, Proteus mirabilis, Staphylococcus aureus, Streptococcus pneumoniae, Streptococcus viridans, *and staphylococci; and perioperative prophylaxis—*
Adults: 250 to 500 mg P.O. q 6 hours.
Children over 9 months: 25 to 50 mg/kg P.O. daily in divided doses.
Otitis media—
Children: 75 to 100 mg/kg P.O. daily. Don't exceed 4 g daily.

All patients, regardless of age and weight, may be given larger doses (up to 1 g q.i.d.) for severe or chronic infections.

ADVERSE REACTIONS
CNS: dizziness, headache, malaise, paresthesia.
GI: pseudomembranous colitis, *nausea, anorexia,* vomiting, heartburn, abdominal cramps, *diarrhea,* oral candidiasis.
GU: genital pruritus and moniliasis, vaginitis.
Hematologic: transient neutropenia, eosinophilia, ***thrombocytopenia.***
Skin: *maculopapular and erythematous rashes, urticaria.*
Other: transient increases in liver enzymes, hypersensitivity reactions (serum sickness, ***anaphylaxis***).

INTERACTIONS
Probenecid: may increase blood levels of cephalosporins. Sometimes used for this effect.

EFFECTS ON DIAGNOSTIC TESTS
Cephradine causes false-positive results in urine glucose tests utilizing cupric sulfate (Benedict's reagent or Clinitest); instead use glucose oxidase tests (Clinistix or Tes-Tape). It also causes false elevations in serum or urine creatinine levels in tests using Jaffé's reaction. Cephradine may cause positive Coombs' test results or elevate liver function test results.

CONTRAINDICATIONS
Contraindicated in patients with hypersensitivity to the drug and to other cephalosporins.

NURSING CONSIDERATIONS
• Use cautiously in patients with impaired renal function or with a history of sensitivity to penicillin. Also use cautiously in breast-feeding women.
• Obtain specimen for culture and sensitivity tests before first dose. Therapy may begin pending results.
• Know that group A beta-hemolytic streptococcal infections should be treated for a minimum of 10 days.
• With large doses or prolonged therapy, monitor for superinfection, especial-

ly in high-risk patients.

☑ **PATIENT TEACHING**
● Tell the patient to take all of the medication as prescribed, even after he feels better.
● Tell the patient to take drug with food or milk to lessen GI discomfort. If patient is taking suspension form, tell him to shake it well before measuring dose.
● Tell the patient to notify doctor if rash occurs.

loracarbef
Lorabid

Pregnancy Risk Category: B

HOW SUPPLIED
Pulvules: 200 mg, 400 mg
Powder for oral suspension: 100 mg/5 ml, 200 mg/5 ml in 50-ml and 100-ml bottles

ACTION
A synthetic beta-lactam antibiotic of the carbacephem class with actions similar to the second-generation cephalosporins. Inhibits cell-wall synthesis, promoting osmotic instability; usually bactericidal.

ONSET, PEAK, DURATION
Onset and duration unknown. Serum levels peak ½ to 1 hour after an oral dose.

INDICATIONS & DOSAGE
Secondary bacterial infections of acute bronchitis—
Adults: 200 to 400 mg P.O. q 12 hours for 7 days.
Acute bacterial exacerbations of chronic bronchitis—
Adults: 400 mg P.O. q 12 hours for 7 days.
Pneumonia—
Adults: 400 mg P.O. q 12 hours for 14 days.
Pharyngitis, sinusitis, or tonsillitis—

Adults: 200 to 400 mg P.O. q 12 hours for 10 days.
Children: 15 mg/kg P.O. daily in divided doses q 12 hours for 10 days.
Acute otitis media—
Children: 30 mg/kg (oral suspension) P.O. daily in divided doses q 12 hours for 10 days.
Uncomplicated skin and skin-structure infections—
Adults: 200 mg P.O. q 12 hours for 7 days.
Impetigo—
Children: 15 mg/kg P.O. daily in divided doses q 12 hours for 7 days.
Uncomplicated cystitis—
Adults: 200 mg P.O. daily for 7 days.
Uncomplicated pyelonephritis—
Adults: 400 mg P.O. q 12 hours for 14 days.

Patients with a creatinine clearance greater than or equal to 50 ml/minute don't require dose and interval changes. Patients with a creatinine clearance of 10 to 49 ml/minute should receive half of the usual dose at the same interval; with a creatinine clearance below 10 ml/minute, the usual dose q 3 to 5 days. Hemodialysis patients require another dose after dialysis.

ADVERSE REACTIONS
CNS: headache, somnolence, nervousness, insomnia, dizziness.
CV: vasodilation.
GI: diarrhea, nausea, vomiting, abdominal pain, anorexia, pseudomembranous colitis.
GU: vaginal candidiasis or moniliasis, transient increases in BUN and creatinine levels.
Hematologic: *transient thrombocytopenia,* leukopenia, eosinophilia.
Skin: rash, urticaria, pruritus, *erythema multiforme.*
Other: hypersensitivity reactions, including *anaphylaxis;* transient elevations in AST, ALT, and alkaline phosphatase levels.

Reactions may be *common,* uncommon, *life-threatening,* or COMMON AND LIFE-THREATENING.

INTERACTIONS
Probenecid: decreased excretion of loracarbef, causing increased plasma levels. Monitor for toxicity.

EFFECTS ON DIAGNOSTIC TESTS
Loracarbef can cause increased PT, positive direct Coombs' test result, elevated lactate dehydrogenase level, pancytopenia, and neutropenia.

CONTRAINDICATIONS
Contraindicated in patients with hypersensitivity to the drug or other cephalosporins and in patients with diarrhea caused by pseudomembranous colitis.

NURSING CONSIDERATIONS
● Use cautiously in pregnant or breastfeeding women. Safety and efficacy of drug have not been established in infants under 6 months.
● Obtain specimen for culture and sensitivity tests before first dose. Therapy may begin pending results.
● To reconstitute powder for oral suspension, add 30 ml of water in two portions to the 50-ml bottle or 60 ml of water in two portions to the 100-ml bottle; shake after each addition.
● After reconstitution, store oral suspension for 14 days at room temperature (59° to 86° F [15° to 30° C]).
● Monitor for superinfection. May cause overgrowth of nonsusceptible bacteria or fungi.
Alert: Monitor the patient for seizures. Beta-lactam antibiotics may trigger seizures in susceptible patients, especially when given without dosage modification to those with renal impairment. If seizures occur, discontinue drug and notify the doctor. Administer anticonvulsants as ordered.
● For otitis media, remember that the more rapidly absorbed oral suspension produces higher peak plasma levels than do the capsules.

☑ PATIENT TEACHING
● Tell the patient to take all of the medication prescribed, even after he feels better.
● Tell the patient to take drug on an empty stomach, at least 1 hour before or 2 hours after meals. Tell him to shake container of suspension well before measuring dose.
● Instruct the patient to discard unused portion after 14 days.
● Instruct the patient to notify doctor if rash appears.

14

Tetracyclines

**demeclocycline hydrochloride
doxycycline calcium
doxycycline hyclate
doxycycline hydrochloride
doxycycline monohydrate
minocycline hydrochloride
oxytetracycline hydrochloride
tetracycline hydrochloride**

COMBINATION PRODUCTS
UROBIOTIC-250: oxytetracycline hydrochloride 250 mg, sulfamethizole 250 mg, and phenazopyridine hydrochloride 50 mg.

---

demeclocycline hydrochloride
Declomycin, Ledermycin‡

Pregnancy Risk Category: D

HOW SUPPLIED
Film coated tablets: 150 mg, 300 mg
Capsules: 150 mg

ACTION
Unknown. Thought to exert bacteriostatic effect by binding to the 30S and possibly 50S ribosomal subunits of microorganisms, thus inhibiting protein synthesis. May also alter the cytoplasmic membrane of susceptible microorganisms.

ONSET, PEAK, DURATION
Onset and duration unknown. Serum levels peak within 3 to 4 hours after oral dose. Half-life is 10 to 17 hours.

INDICATIONS & DOSAGE
Infections caused by susceptible gram-positive and gram-negative organisms (including Haemophilus ducreyi, Yersinia pestis, *and* Campylobacter fetus) Rickettsiae, Mycoplasma pneumo-
niae, Chlamydia trachomatis; *psittacosis; granuloma inguinale—*
Adults: 150 mg P.O. q 6 hours or 300 mg P.O. q 12 hours.
Children over 8 years: 6 to 12 mg/kg P.O. daily, in divided doses q 6 to 12 hours.
Gonorrhea—
Adults: initially, 600 mg P.O.; then 300 mg P.O. q 12 hours for 4 days (for a total of 3 g).

ADVERSE REACTIONS
CNS: *intracranial hypertension (pseudotumor cerebri),* dizziness.
CV: pericarditis.
EENT: dysphagia, glossitis, tinnitus, visual disturbances.
GI: anorexia, *nausea, vomiting, diarrhea,* enterocolitis, anogenital inflammation, pancreatitis.
Hematologic: neutropenia, eosinophilia, *thrombocytopenia, hemolytic anemia.*
Skin: *maculopapular and erythematous rashes, photosensitivity, increased pigmentation, urticaria.*
Other: hypersensitivity reactions *(anaphylaxis),* elevated liver enzymes, *increased BUN level,* diabetes insipidus syndrome (polyuria, polydipsia, weakness), permanent tooth discoloration or bone growth retardation if used in children under 9 years.

INTERACTIONS
Antacids (including sodium bicarbonate) and laxatives containing aluminum, magnesium, or calcium; antidiarrheals; food, milk, or other dairy products: decreased antibiotic absorption. Give antibiotic 1 hour before or 2 hours after any of the above.
Ferrous sulfate and other iron products, zinc: decreased antibiotic absorption. Give antibiotic 3 hours after or 2 hours

---

Reactions may be *common,* uncommon, *life-threatening*, or COMMON AND LIFE-THREATENING.

before iron administration.
Methoxyflurane: may cause nephrotoxicity with tetracyclines. Monitor carefully.
Oral anticoagulants: increased anticoagulant effect. Monitor PT and International Normalized Ratio (INR), and adjust dosage as ordered.
Oral contraceptives: decreased contraceptive effectiveness and increased risk of breakthrough bleeding. Use a nonhormonal birth control method.
Penicillins: may interfere with bactericidal action of penicillins. Avoid using together.

EFFECTS ON DIAGNOSTIC TESTS
Demeclocycline causes false-negative results in urine glucose tests using glucose oxidase reagent (Clinistix or Tes-Tape). It also causes false elevations in fluorometric tests for urine catecholamines. Demeclocycline may elevate serum BUN levels in patients with decreased renal function.

CONTRAINDICATIONS
Contraindicated in patients with hypersensitivity to the drug or other tetracyclines.

NURSING CONSIDERATIONS
● Use cautiously in patients with impaired renal or hepatic function. Use of these drugs during last half of pregnancy and in children under 9 years may cause permanent discoloration of teeth, enamel defects, and bone growth retardation.
● Obtain specimen for culture and sensitivity tests before first dose. Therapy may begin pending test results.
Alert: Check expiration date. Outdated or deteriorated tetracyclines have been associated with reversible nephrotoxicity (Fanconi's syndrome).
● Don't expose these drugs to light or heat; store in tightly capped container.
● With large doses or prolonged therapy, monitor for superinfection, especially in high-risk patients.

● Check the patient's tongue for signs of candidal infection. Stress good oral hygiene.

☑ **PATIENT TEACHING**
● Instruct the patient to take entire amount of medication, exactly as prescribed, even after he feels better.
● Explain to the patient that drug's effectiveness is reduced when taken with milk or other dairy products, food, antacids, or iron products. Tell him to take each dose with a full glass of water on an empty stomach, at least 1 hour before or 2 hours after meals. Also tell him to take drug at least 1 hour before bedtime to prevent esophageal irritation or ulceration.
● Warn the patient to avoid direct sunlight and ultraviolet light, wear protective clothing, and use sunscreen. Photosensitivity reactions may occur within a few minutes to several hours after sun exposure. Photosensitivity persists for some time after discontinuation of drug.

doxycycline calcium
Vibramycin

doxycycline hyclate
Apo-Doxy†, Doryx, Doxy-Caps, Doxy 100, Doxy 200, Doxycin†, Monodox, Novo-Doxylin†, Vibramycin, Vibra-Tabs

doxycycline hydrochloride
Cyclidox‡, Doryx‡, Doxylin‡, Vibramycin‡, Vibra-Tabs 50‡

doxycycline monohydrate
Monodox, Vibramycin

Pregnancy Risk Category: D

HOW SUPPLIED
doxycycline calcium
Oral suspension: 50 mg/5ml
doxycycline hyclate
Tablets (film-coated): 100 mg
Capsules: 50 mg, 100 mg

Capsules (enteric-coated pellets): 100 mg
Injection: 100 mg, 200 mg
doxycycline hydrochloride
Tablets: 50 mg‡, 100 mg‡
Capsules: 50 mg‡, 100 mg‡, 250 mg‡
Injection: 100 mg‡
doxycycline monohydrate
Capsules: 50 mg, 100 mg
Oral suspension: 25 mg/5ml

ACTION

Unknown. Thought to exert bacteriostatic effect by binding to the 30S and possibly 50S ribosomal subunits of microorganisms, thus inhibiting protein synthesis. May also alter the cytoplasmic membrane of susceptible microorganisms.

ONSET, PEAK, DURATION

Onset immediate after I.V. administration, unknown after oral administration. Serum levels peak within 1½ to 4 hours after oral dose; not clearly defined for I.V. use. Duration unknown.

INDICATIONS & DOSAGE

Infections caused by susceptible gram-positive and gram-negative organisms (including Haemophilus ducreyi, Yersinia pestis, *and* Campylobacter fetus), Rickettsiae, Mycoplasma pneumoniae, Chlamydia trachomatis, *and* Borrelia burgdoferi (*Lyme disease*); psittacosis; granuloma inguinale—
Adults and children over 8 years weighing 45 kg and over: 100 mg P.O. q 12 hours on first day, then 100 mg P.O. daily; or 200 mg I.V. on first day in one or two infusions, then 100 to 200 mg I.V. daily.
Children over 8 years weighing under 45 kg: 4.4 mg/kg P.O. or I.V. daily, in divided doses q 12 hours on first day; then 2.2 to 4.4 mg/kg daily in one or two divided doses.
   Give I.V. infusion slowly (minimum 1 hour). Infusion must be completed within 12 hours (within 6 hours in lactated Ringer's solution or dextrose 5% in lactated Ringer's solution).
Gonorrhea in patients allergic to penicillin—
Adults: 100 mg P.O. b.i.d. for 7 days (10 days for epididymitis).
Primary or secondary syphilis in patients allergic to penicillin—
Adults: 300 mg P.O. daily in divided doses for at least 10 days.
Uncomplicated urethral, endocervical, or rectal infections caused by Chlamydia trachomatis *or* Ureaplasma urealyticum—
Adults: 100 mg P.O. b.i.d. for at least 7 days (10 days for epididymitis).
Prophylaxis of malaria—
Adults: 100 mg P.O. daily.
Children over 8 years: 2 mg/kg P.O. once daily. Dosage should not exceed adult dose.
   Note: Prophylaxis should begin 1 to 2 days before travel to endemic area and be continued during travel and for 4 weeks afterward.
Pelvic inflammatory disease—
Adults: 100 mg I.V. q 12 hours combined with cefoxitin or cefotetan and continued for at least 2 days after symptomatic improvement; thereafter, 100 mg P.O. q 12 hours for a total course of 14 days.

ADVERSE REACTIONS

CNS: *intracranial hypertension (pseudotumor cerebri)*.
CV: pericarditis.
EENT: glossitis, dysphagia.
GI: anorexia, *epigastric distress, nausea, vomiting, diarrhea,* oral candidiasis, enterocolitis, anogenital inflammation.
Hematologic: neutropenia, eosinophilia, *thrombocytopenia,* hemolytic anemia.
Skin: *maculopapular and erythematous rashes, photosensitivity, increased pigmentation, urticaria.*
Other: hypersensitivity reactions *(anaphylaxis)*; elevated liver enzymes; permanent discoloration of teeth, enamel defects, and bone growth retardation if

used in children under 9 years; superinfection; thrombophlebitis.

INTERACTIONS
Antacids (including sodium bicarbonate) and laxatives containing aluminum, magnesium, or calcium; antidiarrheals: decreased antibiotic absorption. Give antibiotic 1 hour before or 2 hours after any of the above.

Ferrous sulfate and other iron products, zinc: decreased antibiotic absorption. Give drug 3 hours after or 2 hours before iron administration.

Methoxyflurane: may cause nephrotoxicity with tetracyclines. Monitor carefully.

Oral anticoagulants: increased anticoagulant effect. Monitor PT and International Normalized Ratio (INR), and adjust dosage as ordered.

Oral contraceptives: decreased contraceptive effectiveness and increased risk of breakthrough bleeding. Use a nonhormonal form of birth control.

Penicillins: may interfere with bactericidal action of penicillins. Avoid using together.

Phenobarbital, carbamazepine, alcohol: decreased antibiotic effect. Avoid if possible.

EFFECTS ON DIAGNOSTIC TESTS
Doxycycline causes false-negative results in urine glucose tests using glucose oxidase reagent (Clinistix or Tes-Tape). Parenteral dosage form may cause false-positive Clinitest results. Drug also causes false elevations in fluorometric tests for urine catecholamines.

CONTRAINDICATIONS
Contraindicated in patients with hypersensitivity to the drug or other tetracyclines.

NURSING CONSIDERATIONS
● Use cautiously in patients with impaired renal or hepatic function. Use of these drugs during last half of pregnancy and in children under 9 years may cause permanent discoloration of teeth, enamel defects, and bone growth retardation.

● Obtain specimen for culture and sensitivity tests before first dose. Therapy may begin pending test results.

Alert: Check expiration date. Outdated or deteriorated tetracyclines have been associated with reversible nephrotoxicity (Fanconi's syndrome).

● Administer with milk or food if adverse GI reactions develop.

● **I.V. use:** Reconstitute powder for injection with sterile water for injection. Use 10 ml in 100-mg vial and 20 ml in 200-mg vial. Dilute solution to 100 to 1,000 ml for I.V. infusion. Avoid extravasation. Don't infuse solutions that are more concentrated than 1 mg/ml. Infusion time varies with dose, but usually ranges from 1 to 4 hours. Monitor I.V. infusion site for signs of thrombophlebitis, which may occur with I.V. administration.

● Don't expose drug to light or heat. Protect it from sunlight during infusion.

● Know that reconstituted injectable solution is stable for 72 hours if refrigerated.

● With large doses or prolonged therapy, monitor for superinfection, especially in high-risk patients.

● Check the patient's tongue for signs of fungal infection. Stress good oral hygiene.

● Know that drug is not indicated for the treatment of neurosyphilis.

☑ PATIENT TEACHING
● Tell the patient to take entire amount of medication exactly as prescribed, even after he feels better.

● Instruct the patient to report adverse reactions promptly. If drug is being administered I.V., tell patient to alert nurse if discomfort occurs at I.V site.

● Tell the patient to take oral form of drug with food or milk if stomach upset occurs. Also advise patient not to take oral tablets or capsules within 1 hour of bedtime because of possible esophageal

---

irritation or ulceration.
● Warn patient to avoid direct sunlight and ultraviolet light, wear protective clothing, and use sunscreen. Photosensitivity reactions may occur within a few minutes to several hours after exposure. Photosensitivity persists for some time after therapy ends.

---

minocycline hydrochloride
Apo-Minocycline†, Dynacin, Minocin*, Minomycin‡, Minomycin IV‡, Syn-Mynocycline†

Pregnancy Risk Category: D

HOW SUPPLIED
Tablets (film-coated): 50 mg, 100 mg
Capsules (pellet-filled): 50 mg, 100 mg
Oral suspension: 50 mg/5 ml
Injection: 100 mg

ACTION
Unknown. Thought to exert bacteriostatic effect by binding to the 30S and possibly 50S ribosomal subunits of microorganisms, thus inhibiting protein synthesis. May also alter the cytoplasmic membrane of susceptible microorganisms.

ONSET, PEAK, DURATION
Onset immediate after I.V. administration, unknown after oral administration. Serum levels peak immediately after I.V. administration, within 1 to 4 hours after oral dose. Duration unknown.

INDICATIONS & DOSAGE
Infections caused by susceptible gram-negative and gram-positive organisms (including Haemophilus ducreyi, Yersinia pestis, *and* Campylobacter fetus) Rickettsiae, Mycoplasma pneumoniae, *and* Chlamydia trachomatis; *psittacosis; granuloma inguinale—*
Adults: initially, 200 mg I.V.; then 100 mg I.V. q 12 hours. Not to exceed 400 mg/day. Alternatively, 200 mg P.O. initially; then 100 mg P.O. q 12 hours.

Some clinicians use 100 or 200 mg P.O. initially, followed by 50 mg q.i.d.
Children over 8 years: initially, 4 mg/kg P.O. or I.V., followed by 2 mg/kg q 12 hours.

Given I.V. in 500- to 1,000-ml solution without calcium and administered over 6 hours.
Gonorrhea in patients allergic to penicillin—
Adults: initially, 200 mg P.O.; then 100 mg q 12 hours for at least 4 days.
Syphilis in patients allergic to penicillin—
Adults: initially, 200 mg P.O.; then 100 mg q 12 hours for 10 to 15 days.
Meningococcal carrier state—
Adults: 100 mg P.O. q 12 hours for 5 days.
Uncomplicated urethral, endocervical, or rectal infection caused by Chlamydia trachomatis *or* Ureaplasma urealyticum—
Adults: 100 mg P.O. b.i.d. for at least 7 days.
Uncomplicated gonococcal urethritis in men—
Adults: 100 mg P.O. b.i.d. for 5 days.

ADVERSE REACTIONS
CNS: headache, *intracranial hypertension (pseudotumor cerebri),* light-headedness, dizziness, vertigo.
CV: pericarditis.
EENT: dysphagia, glossitis.
GI: *anorexia,* epigastric distress, oral candidiasis, *nausea,* vomiting, *diarrhea,* enterocolitis, inflammatory lesions in anogenital region.
Hematologic: neutropenia, eosinophilia, *thrombocytopenia,* hemolytic anemia.
Skin: *maculopapular and erythematous rashes, photosensitivity, increased pigmentation,* urticaria.
Other: hypersensitivity reactions (*anaphylaxis*); elevated liver enzymes; increased BUN level; permanent discoloration of teeth, enamel defects, and bone growth retardation if used in children under 9 years; superinfection;

Reactions may be *common,* uncommon, *life-threatening,* or COMMON AND LIFE-THREATENING.

thrombophlebitis.

INTERACTIONS
Antacids (including sodium bicarbonate) and laxatives containing aluminum, magnesium, or calcium; antidiarrheals: decreased antibiotic absorption. Give antibiotic 1 hour before or 2 hours after any of the above.
Ferrous sulfate and other iron products, zinc: decreased antibiotic absorption. Give drug 3 hours after or 2 hours before iron administration.
Methoxyflurane: may cause nephrotoxicity with tetracyclines. Monitor carefully.
Oral anticoagulants: increased anticoagulant effect. Monitor PT and International Normalized Ratio (INR), and adjust dosage as ordered.
Oral contraceptives: decreased contraceptive effectiveness and increased risk of breakthrough bleeding. Use a nonhormonal form of birth control.
Penicillins: may interfere with bactericidal action of penicillins. Avoid using together.

EFFECTS ON DIAGNOSTIC TESTS
Minocycline causes false-negative results in urine glucose tests using glucose oxidase reagent (Clinistix or Tes-Tape). It also causes false elevations in fluorometric tests for urine catecholamines. Parenteral form may cause false-positive reading of copper sulfate tests (Clinitest).

CONTRAINDICATIONS
Contraindicated in patients with hypersensitivity to the drug or other tetracyclines.

NURSING CONSIDERATIONS
● Use cautiously in patients with impaired renal or hepatic function. Use of these drugs during last half of pregnancy and in children under 9 years may cause permanent discoloration of teeth, enamel defects, and bone growth retardation.

● Obtain specimen for culture and sensitivity tests before first dose. Therapy may begin pending test results.
Alert: Check expiration date. Outdated or deteriorated tetracyclines have been associated with reversible nephrotoxicity (Fanconi's syndrome).
● Don't expose drug to light or heat. Keep cap tightly closed.
● **I.V. use:** Reconstitute 100 mg of powder with 5 ml of sterile water for injection, with further dilution to 500 to 1,000 ml for I.V. infusion. Stable for 24 hours at room temperature.
● Be aware that patient may develop thrombophlebitis with I.V. administration of this drug. Avoid extravasation. Switch to oral therapy as soon as possible.
● With large doses or prolonged therapy, monitor for superinfection, especially in high-risk patients.
● Check the patient's tongue for signs of candidal infection. Stress good oral hygiene.
● Be aware that the drug may cause tooth discoloration in young adults. Observe for brown pigmentation, and inform the doctor if it occurs.
● Know that drug is not indicated for the treatment of neurosyphilis.

☑ **PATIENT TEACHING**
● Tell the patient to take entire amount of medication exactly as prescribed, even after he feels better.
● Tell the patient to take oral form of drug with a full glass of water. Drug may be taken with food. Tell patient not to take within 1 hour of bedtime to avoid esophageal irritation or ulceration.
● Warn the patient to avoid driving or other hazardous tasks due to possible adverse CNS effects.
● Warn the patient to avoid direct sunlight and ultraviolet light, wear protective clothing, and use sunscreen. Photosensitivity reactions may occur within a few minutes to several hours after exposure. Photosensitivity persists for some time after discontinuation of therapy.

oxytetracycline hydrochloride
Terramycin, Uri-Tet

Pregnancy Risk Category: D

HOW SUPPLIED
Capsules: 250 mg
Injection: 50 mg/ml, 125 mg/ml (with lidocaine 2%)

ACTION
Unknown. Thought to exert bacteriostatic effect by binding to the 30S and possibly 50S ribosomal subunits of microorganisms, thus inhibiting protein synthesis. May also alter the cytoplasmic membrane of susceptible microorganisms.

ONSET, PEAK, DURATION
Onset and duration unknown. Serum levels peak within 2 to 4 hours after oral dose, unknown after I.M. injection.

INDICATIONS & DOSAGE
Infections caused by susceptible gram-negative and gram-positive organisms (including Haemophilus ducreyi, Yersinia pestis, Campylobacter fetus), Rickettsiae, Mycoplasma pneumoniae, *and* Chlamydia trachomatis; *psittacosis; granuloma inguinale—*
Adults: 1 to 2 g P.O. in four divided doses, 100 mg I.M. q 8 to 12 hours, or 250 mg I.M. as a single dose.
Children over 8 years: 25 to 50 mg/kg P.O. daily, in divided doses q 6 hours; 15 to 25 mg/kg I.M. daily, in divided doses q 8 to 12 hours.
Brucellosis—
Adults: 500 mg P.O. q.i.d. for 3 weeks combined with 1 g of streptomycin I.M. q 12 hours for first week, once daily for second week.
Syphilis in patients allergic to penicillin—
Adults: 30 to 40 g total dosage P.O., divided equally over 10 to 15 days.
Gonorrhea in patients allergic to peni-
cillin—
Adults: initially, 1.5 g P.O., followed by 0.5 g q.i.d., for a total of 9 g.

ADVERSE REACTIONS
CNS: *intracranial hypertension (pseudotumor cerebri).*
CV: pericarditis.
EENT: dysphagia, glossitis.
GI: *anorexia, nausea,* vomiting, *diarrhea,* oral candidiasis, enterocolitis, stomatitis.
GU: *proctitis, anogenital inflammation,* vaginitis.
Hematologic: neutropenia, eosinophilia.
Skin: *maculopapular and erythematous rashes, urticaria, photosensitivity, increased pigmentation.*
Other: hypersensitivity reactions *(anaphylaxis);* elevated liver enzymes; permanent discoloration of teeth, enamel defects, and bone growth retardation if used in children under 9 years; superinfection; increased BUN levels; *irritation after I.M. injection; thrombophlebitis.*

INTERACTIONS
Antacids (including sodium bicarbonate) and laxatives containing aluminum, magnesium, or calcium; antidiarrheals; food, milk, or other dairy products: decreased antibiotic absorption. Give antibiotic 1 hour before or 2 hours after any of the above.
Ferrous sulfate and other iron products, zinc: decreased antibiotic absorption. Give antibiotic 3 hours after or 2 hours before iron administration.
Methoxyflurane: may cause nephrotoxicity with tetracyclines. Monitor carefully.
Oral anticoagulants: increased anticoagulant effect. Monitor PT and International Normalized Ratio (INR), and adjust dosage as ordered.
Oral contraceptives: decreased contraceptive effectiveness and increased risk of breakthrough bleeding. Use a nonhormonal form of birth control.
Penicillins: may interfere with bacterici-

dal action of penicillins. Avoid using together.

EFFECTS ON DIAGNOSTIC TESTS
Oxytetracycline causes false-negative results in urine glucose tests using glucose oxidase reagent (Clinistix or Tes-Tape); parenteral dosage form may cause false-positive Clinitest results. It also causes false elevations in fluorometric tests for urine catecholamines. It may elevate BUN level in patients with decreased renal function.

CONTRAINDICATIONS
Contraindicated in patients with hypersensitivity to the drug or other tetracyclines.

NURSING CONSIDERATIONS
● Use cautiously in patients with impaired renal or hepatic function. Use of these drugs during last half of pregnancy and in children under 9 years may cause permanent discoloration of teeth, enamel defects, and bone growth retardation.
● Obtain specimen for culture and sensitivity tests before first dose. Therapy may begin pending test results.
Alert: Check expiration date. Outdated or deteriorated oxytetracyclines have been associated with reversible nephrotoxicity (Fanconi's syndrome).
● Don't expose this drug to light or heat.
● For I.M. administration, inject deeply into a large muscle mass. Rotate sites. I.M. preparations contain a local anesthetic; ask the patient about hypersensitivity reactions to local anesthetics. With I.M. administration, serum levels are lower than with oral administration of oxytetracycline.
● With large doses or prolonged therapy, monitor for superinfection, especially in high-risk patients.
● Check the patient's tongue for signs of fungal infection. Stress good oral hygiene.
● Know that drug is not indicated for

the treatment of neurosyphilis.

☑ PATIENT TEACHING
● Tell the patient to take entire amount of medication exactly as prescribed, even after he feels better.
● Explain to the patient that oral drug's effectiveness is reduced when taken with milk or other dairy products, food, antacids, or iron products. Tell him to take each dose with a full glass of water on an empty stomach, at least 1 hour before or 2 hours after meals. Also tell him to take drug at least 1 hour before bedtime to prevent esophageal irritation or ulceration.
● Warn the patient that I.M. injection may be painful.
● Warn the patient to avoid direct sunlight and ultraviolet light, wear protective clothing, and use sunscreen. Photosensitivity reactions may occur within a few minutes to several hours after sun exposure. Photosensitivity persists for considerable time after discontinuation of drug.

---

tetracycline hydrochloride
Achromycin V, Ala-Tet, Apo-Tetra†, Austramycin V‡, Hostacicline P‡, Nor-Tet, Novo-Tetra†, Nu-Tetra†, Panmycin**, Panmycin P‡, Robitet, Sumycin, Teline, Tetracap, Tetracyn, Tetralan, Tetram

Pregnancy Risk Category: D

HOW SUPPLIED
Tablets: 250 mg, 500 mg
Capsules: 100 mg, 250 mg, 500 mg
Oral suspension: 125 mg/5 ml

ACTION
Unknown. Thought to exert bacteriostatic effect by binding to the 30S and possibly 50S ribosomal subunits of microorganisms, thus inhibiting protein synthesis. May also alter the cytoplasmic membrane of susceptible microorganisms.

ONSET, PEAK, DURATION
Onset and duration unknown. Serum levels peak within 2 to 4 hours.

INDICATIONS & DOSAGE
Infections caused by susceptible gram-negative and gram-positive organisms (including Haemophilus ducreyi, Yersinia pestis, *and* Campylobacter fetus), Rickettsia, Mycoplasma pneumoniae, *and* Chlamydia trachomatis; *psittacosis; granuloma inguinale—*
Adults: 250 to 500 mg P.O. q 6 hours.
Children over 8 years: 25 to 50 mg/kg P.O. daily, in divided doses q 6 hours.
Uncomplicated urethral, endocervical, or rectal infections caused by Chlamydia trachomatis—
Adults: 500 mg P.O. q.i.d. for at least 7 days, 10 days for epididymitis, and 21 days for lymphogranuloma venereum.
Brucellosis—
Adults: 500 mg P.O. q 6 hours for 3 weeks combined with 1 g of streptomycin I.M. q 12 hours for first week; once daily, for second week.
Gonorrhea in patients allergic to penicillin—
Adults: initially, 1.5 g P.O.; then 500 mg q 6 hours for a total dose of 9 g; for epididymitis, 500 mg P.O. q 6 hours for 7 days.
Syphilis in patients allergic to penicillin—
Adults: total of 30 to 40 g P.O. in equally divided doses over 10 to 15 days.
Acne—
Adults and adolescents: initially, 250 mg P.O. q 6 hours; then 125 to 500 mg daily or q.o.d.
Helicobacter pylori *infection—*
Adults: 500 mg P.O. q 6 hours for 10 to 14 days in combination with other agents, such as metronidazole, bismuth subsalicylate, amoxicillin, or omeprazole.
Cholera—
Adults: 500 mg P.O. q 6 hours for 48 to 72 hours.

Malaria caused by Plasmodium falciparum—
Adults: 250 to 500 mg P.O. daily for 7 days with quinine sulfate 650 mg P.O. q 8 hours for 3 to 7 days.

ADVERSE REACTIONS
CNS: dizziness, headache, ***intracranial hypertension (pseudotumor cerebri).***
CV: pericarditis.
EENT: sore throat, glossitis, dysphagia.
GI: anorexia, *epigastric distress, nausea,* vomiting, *diarrhea,* esophagitis, oral candidiasis, stomatitis, enterocolitis, inflammatory lesions in anogenital region.
Hematologic: neutropenia, eosinophilia, thrombocytopenia.
Skin: *candidal superinfection, maculopapular and erythematous rashes, urticaria, photosensitivity, increased pigmentation.*
Other: hypersensitivity reactions, elevated liver enzymes, *increased BUN levels, permanent discoloration of teeth, enamel defects, and bone growth retardation if used in children under 9 years.*

INTERACTIONS
Antacids (including sodium bicarbonate) and laxatives containing aluminum, magnesium, or calcium; antidiarrheals containing kaolin, pectin, or bismuth subsalicylate; food, milk, or other dairy products: decreased antibiotic absorption. Give antibiotic 1 hour before or 2 hours after any of the above.
Ferrous sulfate and other iron products, zinc: decreased antibiotic absorption. Give tetracyclines 3 hours after or 2 hours before iron administration.
Lithium carbonate: may alter serum lithium levels.
Methoxyflurane: may cause severe nephrotoxicity with tetracyclines. Monitor carefully.
Oral anticoagulants: potentiated anticoagulant effects. Monitor PT and International Normalized Ratio (INR), and adjust anticoagulant dosage as ordered.
Oral contraceptives: decreased contra-

ceptive effectiveness and increased risk of breakthrough bleeding. Use a non-hormonal form of birth control.

Penicillins: may interfere with bactericidal action of penicillins. Avoid using together.

EFFECTS ON DIAGNOSTIC TESTS
Tetracycline causes false-negative results in urine glucose tests using glucose oxidase reagent (Clinistix or Tes-Tape), and false elevations in fluorometric tests for urine catecholamines. It may elevate BUN levels in patients with decreased renal function.

CONTRAINDICATIONS
Contraindicated in patients with hypersensitivity to tetracyclines.

NURSING CONSIDERATIONS
● Use with extreme caution in patients with impaired renal or hepatic function. Also use with extreme caution (if at all) during last half of pregnancy and in children under 9 years because drug may cause permanent discoloration of teeth, enamel defects, and bone growth retardation.
● Obtain specimen for culture and sensitivity tests before giving first dose. Therapy may begin pending test results.
Alert: Check expiration date. Outdated or deteriorated tetracyclines have been associated with reversible nephrotoxicity (Fanconi's syndrome).
● Don't expose drug to light or heat.
● With large doses or prolonged therapy, monitor for superinfection, especially in high-risk patients.
● Check the patient's tongue for signs of candidal infection. Stress good oral hygiene.
● Know that drug is not indicated for the treatment of neurosyphilis.

☑ **PATIENT TEACHING**
● Tell the patient to take drug exactly as prescribed, even after he feels better, and to take entire amount prescribed.
● Explain to the patient that effective-

ness is reduced when taken with milk or other dairy products, food, antacids, or iron products. Tell him to take each dose with a full glass of water on an empty stomach, at least 1 hour before or 2 hours after meals. Also tell him to take it at least 1 hour before bedtime to prevent esophageal irritation or ulceration.
● Warn the patient to avoid direct sunlight and ultraviolet light, wear protective clothing, and use sunscreen. Photosensitivity reactions may occur within a few minutes to several hours after sun exposure. Photosensitivity persists after discontinuation of drug.

co-trimoxazole
sulfadiazine
sulfamethoxazole
sulfisoxazole
sulfisoxazole acetyl

COMBINATION PRODUCTS

AZO GANTANOL, AZO SULFAMETHOXA-ZOLE†, URO GANTANOL† tablets (film-coated): sulfamethoxazole 500 mg and phenazopyridine hydrochloride 100 mg.
AZO GANTRISIN, AZO SULFISOXAZOLE tablets (film-coated): sulfisoxazole 500 mg and phenazopyridine hydrochloride 50 mg.
ERYZOLE, PEDIAZOLE, SULFINEYCIN suspension: sulfisoxazole 600 mg and erythromycin ethylsuccinate 200 mg/5 ml.

---

co-trimoxazole (sulfamethoxazole-trimethoprim)

Apo-Sulfatrim†, Apo-Sulfatrim DS†, Bactrim*, Bactrim DS, Bactrim I.V. Infusion, Cotrim, Cotrim D.S., Novo-Trimel†, Novotrimel DS†, Nu-Cotrimox†, Protrin†, Pro-Trin, Protrin DF†, Resprim‡, Roubac†, Roubac DS†, Septra*, Septra DS, Septra I.V. Infusion, Septrin‡, SMZ-TMP, Sulfatrim, Uroplus DS, Uroplus SS

Pregnancy Risk Category: C (contraindicated at term)

HOW SUPPLIED

Tablets: (single-strength) trimethoprim 80 mg and sulfamethoxazole 400 mg; *(double-strength)* trimethoprim 160 mg and sulfamethoxazole 800 mg
Oral suspension: trimethoprim 40 mg and sulfamethoxazole 200 mg/5 ml
Injection: trimethoprim 16 mg and sulfamethoxazole 80 mg/ml in 5-, 10-, 20-, 30-, and 50-ml vials

ACTION

Sulfamethoxazole inhibits formation of dihydrofolic acid from PABA; trimethoprim inhibits dihydrofolate reductase. Both decrease bacterial folic acid synthesis.

ONSET, PEAK, DURATION

Onset immediate after I.V. administration, unknown after oral administration. Serum levels peak 1 to 4 hours after an oral dose or immediately after an I.V. infusion. Duration unknown.

INDICATIONS & DOSAGE

Shigellosis or urinary tract infections (UTIs) caused by susceptible strains of E. coli, Proteus *(indole positive or negative),* Klebsiella, *or* Enterobacter—
Adults: 160 mg trimethoprim/800 mg sulfamethoxazole (double-strength tablet) P.O. q 12 hours for 10 to 14 days in UTIs and for 5 days in shigellosis. For uncomplicated cystitis or acute urethral syndrome, one double-strength tablet q 12 hours for 3 days. If indicated, I.V. infusion is given: 8 to 10 mg/kg/day (based on trimethoprim component) in two to four divided doses q 6, 8, or 12 hours for up to 14 days for severe UTIs. Maximum daily dose is 960 mg trimethoprim.
Children 2 months and over: 8 mg/kg/day (based on trimethoprim component) P.O., in two divided doses q 12 hours (10 days for UTIs; 5 days for shigellosis). If indicated, I.V. infusion is given: 8 to 10 mg/kg/day (based on trimethoprim component) in two to four divided doses q 6, 8, or 12 hours. Adult dose should not be exceeded.
Otitis media in patients with penicillin allergy or penicillin-resistant infections—
Children 2 months and over: 8 mg/kg/day (based on trimethoprim com-

ponent) P.O., in two divided doses q 12 hours for 10 to 14 days.

Chronic bronchitis and upper respiratory tract infections—
Adults: 160 mg trimethoprim/800 mg sulfamethoxazole P.O. q 12 hours for 10 to 14 days.

Traveler's diarrhea—
Adults: 160 mg trimethoprim/800 mg sulfamethoxazole P.O. b.i.d. for 3 to 5 days. Some patients may require 2 days of therapy or less.

UTIs in men with prostatitis—
Adults: 160 mg trimethoprim/800 mg sulfamethoxazole P.O. b.i.d. for 3 to 6 months.

Prophylaxis for chronic UTIs—
Adults: 40 mg trimethoprim/200 mg sulfamethoxazole (½ tablet) or 80 mg trimethoprim/400 mg sulfamethoxazole P.O. daily or three times a week for 3 to 6 months.

ADVERSE REACTIONS
CNS: headache, mental depression, aseptic meningitis, tinnitus, apathy, *seizures,* hallucinations, ataxia, nervousness, fatigue, muscle weakness, vertigo, insomnia.
GI: *nausea, vomiting, diarrhea,* abdominal pain, anorexia, stomatitis, pancreatitis, pseudomembranous colitis.
GU: *toxic nephrosis with oliguria and anuria,* crystalluria, hematuria, interstitial nephritis, increased BUN and serum creatinine concentrations.
Hematologic: *agranulocytosis, aplastic anemia,* megaloblastic anemia, *thrombocytopenia,* leukopenia, *hemolytic anemia.*
Hepatic: jaundice, *hepatic necrosis.*
Respiratory: pulmonary infiltrates.
Skin: *erythema multiforme (Stevens-Johnson syndrome), generalized skin eruption, epidermal necrolysis, exfoliative dermatitis,* photosensitivity, urticaria, pruritus.
Other: hypersensitivity reactions (*serum sickness, drug fever, anaphylaxis*), thrombophlebitis, arthralgia, myalgia.

INTERACTIONS
Cyclosporine: may decrease cyclosporine levels and increase nephrotoxicity risk.
Oral anticoagulants: increased anticoagulant effect. Monitor for bleeding.
Oral antidiabetic agents: increased hypoglycemic effect. Monitor blood glucose levels.
Oral contraceptives: decreased contraceptive effectiveness and increased risk of breakthrough bleeding. Suggest a nonhormonal contraceptive.
Phenytoin: may inhibit hepatic metabolism of phenytoin. Monitor closely.

EFFECTS ON DIAGNOSTIC TESTS
Trimethoprim can interfere with serum methotrexate assay as determined by the competitive binding protein technique. No interference occurs if radioimmunoassay is used. Co-trimoxazole may elevate liver function test results; it may decrease serum concentration levels of erythrocytes, platelets, or leukocytes.

CONTRAINDICATIONS
Contraindicated in patients with hypersensitivity to trimethoprim or sulfonamides, severe renal impairment (creatinine clearance less than 15 ml/minute), and porphyria; in megaloblastic anemia caused by folate deficiency; in pregnant women at term; in breast-feeding women; and in children under 2 months.

NURSING CONSIDERATIONS
● Use cautiously and in reduced dosages in patients with impaired hepatic or renal function (creatinine clearance of 15 to 30 ml/minute), severe allergy or bronchial asthma, G6PD deficiency, and blood dyscrasia.
● Obtain specimen for culture and sensitivity tests before first dose. Therapy may begin pending results.
● Note that the "DS" or "DF" product means "double strength."
● **I.V. use:** Dilute I.V. infusion in D₅W before administration. Don't mix with other drugs or solutions. Infuse slowly

---

over 60 to 90 minutes. Don't give by rapid infusion or bolus injection. Don't refrigerate, and use within 6 hours.
• Never administer I.M.
• Promptly report complaints of rash, sore throat, fever, or mouth sores—early signs and symptoms of blood dyscrasia.
• Watch for superinfection (fever or other signs of new infection).
Alert: Be aware that adverse reactions, especially hypersensitivity reactions, rash, and fever, occur much more frequently in AIDS patients.

☑ **PATIENT TEACHING**
• Tell the patient to take drug as prescribed, even if he feels better.
• Encourage adequate fluid intake.
• Tell the patient to report adverse reactions promptly.
• Instruct patient receiving drug I.V. to alert nurse if discomfort occurs at I.V. insertion site.
• Advise patient to avoid prolonged sun exposure, wear protective clothing, and use sunscreen.
• Instruct patient to take oral medication with 8 oz (240 ml) of water on an empty stomach.

---

sulfadiazine
Coptin†, Microsulfon

Pregnancy Risk Category: C (contraindicated at term)

HOW SUPPLIED
Tablets: 500 mg

ACTION
Inhibits formation of dihydrofolic acid from PABA, decreasing bacterial folic acid synthesis.

ONSET, PEAK, DURATION
Onset and duration unknown. Serum levels peak within 4 to 6 hours of oral dose.

INDICATIONS & DOSAGE
Asymptomatic meningococcal carriers—
Adults: 1 g P.O. q 12 hours for 2 days.
Children 1 to 12 years: 500 mg P.O. q 12 hours for 2 days.
Children 2 to 12 months: 500 mg P.O. daily for 2 days.
Rheumatic fever prophylaxis, as an alternative to penicillin—
Children over 66 lb (30 kg): 1 g P.O. daily.
Children under 66 lb: 500 mg P.O. daily.
Adjunct treatment in toxoplasmosis—
Adults: 2 to 8 g P.O. daily divided q 6 hours for 6 to 8 weeks or until improvement occurs. Usually given with pyrimethamine.
Children: 100 to 200 mg/kg P.O. daily divided q 6 hours (maximum 6 g daily) for 6 to 8 weeks or until improvement occurs. Usually given with pyrimethamine.
Malaria, treatment of chloroquine-resistant Plasmodium falciparum—
Adults: 500 mg P.O. q.i.d. for 5 days with quinine sulfate and pyrimethamine.
Children: 25 to 50 mg/kg P.O. q.i.d. (maximum 2 g daily) for 5 days with quinine sulfate and pyrimethamine.
Nocardiosis—
Adults: 4 to 8 g P.O daily given in divided doses for a minimum of 6 weeks.

ADVERSE REACTIONS
CNS: headache, mental depression, *seizures,* hallucinations.
GI: *nausea, vomiting, diarrhea,* abdominal pain, anorexia, stomatitis.
GU: *toxic nephrosis* with oliguria and anuria, crystalluria, hematuria.
Hematologic: *agranulocytosis, aplastic anemia,* megaloblastic anemia, *thrombocytopenia,* leukopenia, *hemolytic anemia.*
Skin: *erythema multiforme (Stevens-Johnson syndrome),* generalized skin eruption, *epidermal necrolysis, exfoliative dermatitis,* photosensitivity, urticaria, pruritus.

Reactions may be *common,* uncommon, *life-threatening,* or COMMON AND LIFE-THREATENING.

Other: hypersensitivity reactions (*serum sickness, drug fever,* **anaphylaxis**), jaundice, local irritation, extravasation.

INTERACTIONS
Oral anticoagulants: increased anticoagulant effect. Monitor for bleeding.
Oral antidiabetic agents: increased hypoglycemic effect. Monitor blood glucose levels.
Oral contraceptives: decreased contraceptive effectiveness and increased risk of breakthrough bleeding. Suggest a nonhormonal contraceptive.
PABA-containing drugs: inhibited antibacterial action. Don't use together.

EFFECTS ON DIAGNOSTIC TESTS
Sulfadiazine alters urine glucose tests utilizing cupric sulfate (Benedict's reagent or Clinitest). The drug may elevate liver function test results; it may decrease serum levels of erythrocytes, platelets, or leukocytes. It may also elevate serum creatinine.

CONTRAINDICATIONS
Contraindicated in patients with hypersensitivity to sulfonamides, in those with porphyria, in infants under age 2 months (except in congenital toxoplasmosis), in pregnant women at term, and during breast-feeding.

NURSING CONSIDERATIONS
● Use cautiously and in reduced doses in patients with impaired hepatic or renal function, bronchial asthma, history of multiple allergies, G6PD deficiency, and blood dyscrasia.
● Give drug on schedule to maintain constant blood level.
● Monitor for signs of blood dyscrasia (purpura, ecchymoses, sore throat, fever, and pallor). Report them immediately.
● Monitor urine cultures, CBCs, and urinalyses before and during therapy, as ordered.
● Watch for superinfection (fever or

other signs of new infection).
● Be aware that folic or folinic acid may be used during rest periods in toxoplasmosis therapy to reverse hematopoietic depression or anemia associated with pyrimethamine and sulfadiazine.
● Monitor fluid intake and output. Intake should be sufficient to produce output of 1,500 ml daily (between 3,000 and 4,000 ml daily for adults). If fluid intake is not adequate enough to prevent crystalluria, sodium bicarbonate may be administered to alkalinize urine, as ordered. Monitor urine pH daily.

☑ PATIENT TEACHING
● Tell the patient to take drug as prescribed, even if he feels better.
● Tell him to drink a glass of water with each dose and plenty of water each day to prevent crystalluria.
● Instruct the patient to report adverse reactions promptly.
● Warn the patient to avoid prolonged exposure to sunlight, wear protective clothing, and use sunscreen.

sulfamethoxazole (sulphamethoxazole)
Apo-Sulfamethoxazole†, Gantanol

Pregnancy Risk Category: C (contraindicated at term)

HOW SUPPLIED
Tablets: 500 mg
Oral suspension: 500 mg/5 ml

ACTION
Inhibits formation of dihydrofolic acid from PABA, decreasing bacterial folic acid synthesis.

ONSET, PEAK, DURATION
Onset and duration unknown. Serum levels peak within 2 hours of oral dose.

INDICATIONS & DOSAGE
Urinary tract and systemic infections—
Adults: initially, 2 g P.O., then 1 g P.O.

b.i.d. up to t.i.d. for severe infections.
Chlamydia trachomatis *(lymphogranu-loma venereum)*—
Adults: 1 g P.O. b.i.d. for 21 days.
Children and infants over 2 months:
initially, 50 to 60 mg/kg P.O., then 25 to
30 mg/kg b.i.d. Maximum dosage
should not exceed 75 mg/kg daily.

ADVERSE REACTIONS
CNS: headache, mental depression,
seizures, hallucinations, aseptic meningitis, tinnitus, apathy.
GI: *nausea, vomiting, diarrhea,* abdominal pain, anorexia, stomatitis, pancreatitis, pseudomembranous colitis.
GU: *toxic nephrosis with oliguria and
anuria,* crystalluria, hematuria, interstitial nephritis.
Hematologic: *agranulocytosis, aplastic
anemia,* megaloblastic anemia, thrombocytopenia, leukopenia, *hemolytic
anemia.*
Skin: *erythema multiforme (Stevens-
Johnson syndrome),* generalized skin
eruption, *epidermal necrolysis, exfoliative dermatitis,* photosensitivity, urticaria, pruritus.
Other: hypersensitivity reactions
(*serum sickness, drug fever, anaphylaxis*), *jaundice.*

INTERACTIONS
Oral anticoagulants: increased anticoagulant effect. Monitor for bleeding.
Oral antidiabetic agents: increased hypoglycemic effect. Monitor blood glucose levels.
Oral contraceptives: decreased contraceptive effectiveness and increased risk
of breakthrough bleeding. Suggest a
nonhormonal contraceptive.
Phenytoin: may increase phenytoin effect. Monitor closely.

EFFECTS ON DIAGNOSTIC TESTS
Sulfamethoxazole alters results of urine
glucose tests utilizing cupric sulfate
(Benedict's reagent or Clinitest). The
drug may elevate liver function test results; it may decrease serum levels of

erythrocytes, platelets, or leukocytes.

CONTRAINDICATIONS
Contraindicated in patients with hypersensitivity to sulfonamides; in those
with porphyria, in infants under 2
months (except in congenital toxoplasmosis), in pregnant women at term, and
during breast-feeding.

NURSING CONSIDERATIONS
● Use cautiously and in reduced
dosages in patients with impaired hepatic or renal function, severe allergy or
bronchial asthma, G6PD deficiency, and
blood dyscrasia.
● Obtain specimen for culture and sensitivity tests before first dose. Therapy
may begin pending results.
● Monitor urine cultures, CBCs, and
urinalyses before and during therapy, as
ordered.
● Watch for superinfection (fever or
other signs of new infection).
● Monitor fluid intake and output. Intake should be sufficient to produce output of 1,500 ml daily (between 3,000
and 4,000 ml daily for adults). If fluid
intake is not adequate enough to prevent
crystalluria, sodium bicarbonate may be
administered to alkalinize urine, as ordered. Monitor urine pH daily.

☑ **PATIENT TEACHING**
● Tell the patient to take drug as prescribed, even if he feels better.
● Tell him to drink a glass of water with
each dose and plenty of water each day
to prevent crystalluria.
Alert: Tell the patient to report early
signs of blood dyscrasia (sore throat,
fever, and pallor) to the doctor.
● Warn the patient to avoid prolonged
exposure to sunlight, to wear protective
clothing, and to use sunscreen.

---

sulfisoxazole (sulfafurazole, sulphafurazole)
Azo-Sulfisoxazole†‡, Gantrisin,
Novo-Soxazole†

sulfisoxazole acetyl
Gantrisin Pediatric

Pregnancy Risk Category: C (contraindicated at term)

HOW SUPPLIED
sulfisoxazole
Tablets: 500 mg
sulfisoxazole acetyl
Liquid: 500 mg/5 ml

ACTION
Inhibits formation of dihydrofolic acid from PABA, decreasing bacterial folic acid synthesis.

ONSET, PEAK, DURATION
Onset and duration unknown. Serum levels peak in 1 to 4 hours.

INDICATIONS & DOSAGE
Urinary tract and systemic infections—
Adults: initially, 2 to 4 g P.O., then 4 to 8 g daily divided in four to six doses.
Children over 2 months: initially, 75 mg/kg P.O. daily or 2 g/m² P.O., then 150 mg/kg or 4 g/m² P.O. daily in divided doses q 6 hours. Total daily dose should not exceed 6 g.
Chlamydia trachomatis *(lymphogranuloma venereum)—*
Adults: 500 mg P.O. one to four times daily for 21 days.
Uncomplicated urethral, endocervical, or rectal infections caused by Chlamydia trachomatis—
Adults: 500 mg P.O. q.i.d. for 10 days.

ADVERSE REACTIONS
CNS: headache, mental depression, *seizures,* hallucinations.
CV: tachycardia, palpitations, syncope, cyanosis.
GI: *nausea, vomiting, diarrhea,* abdominal pain, anorexia, stomatitis, *hepatitis,* pseudomembranous colitis.
GU: *toxic nephrosis with oliguria and anuria,* crystalluria, hematuria, *acute renal failure.*

Hematologic: *agranulocytosis, aplastic anemia,* megaloblastic anemia, *thrombocytopenia,* leukopenia, *hemolytic anemia.*
Skin: *erythema multiforme,* generalized skin eruption, *epidermal necrolysis, exfoliative dermatitis,* photosensitivity, urticaria, pruritus.
Other: hypersensitivity reactions (*serum sickness, drug fever, anaphylaxis*), jaundice.

INTERACTIONS
Oral anticoagulants: increased anticoagulant effect. Monitor for bleeding.
Oral antidiabetic agents: increased hypoglycemic effect. Monitor blood glucose levels.
Oral contraceptives: decreased contraceptive effectiveness, increased risk of breakthrough bleeding. Suggest a nonhormonal contraceptive.

EFFECTS ON DIAGNOSTIC TESTS
Sulfisoxazole alters results of urine glucose tests utilizing cupric sulfate (Benedict's reagent or Clinitest). Sulfisoxazole may elevate liver function test results. It may decrease serum levels of erythrocytes, platelets, or leukocytes.

CONTRAINDICATIONS
Contraindicated in patients with hypersensitivity to sulfonamides, in infants under 2 months (except in congenital toxoplasmosis), in pregnant women at term, and during breast-feeding.

NURSING CONSIDERATIONS
● Use cautiously in patients with impaired hepatic or renal function, severe allergy or bronchial asthma, and G6PD deficiency.
● Obtain specimen for culture and sensitivity tests before first dose. Therapy may begin pending results.
● Monitor urine cultures, CBCs, PT, and urinalyses before and during therapy, as ordered.
● When drug is given preoperatively, be aware that the patient should receive a

---

*Liquid contains alcohol.   **May contain tartrazine.   †Canada only.   ‡Australia only.   ◇OTC.

low-residue diet and a minimal number of enemas and cathartics.
● Watch for superinfection (fever or other signs of new infection).
● Monitor fluid intake and output. Maintain intake between 3,000 and 4,000 ml daily for adults to produce output of 1,500 ml daily. If fluid intake is not adequate enough to prevent crystalluria, sodium bicarbonate may be administered to alkalinize urine, as ordered. Monitor urine pH daily.

☑ PATIENT TEACHING
● Tell the patient to take drug as prescribed, even if he feels better.
● Tell him to drink a glass of water with each dose and plenty of water each day to prevent crystalluria.
Alert: Tell the patient to report early signs of blood dyscrasia (sore throat, fever, and pallor) to the doctor.
● Warn the patient to avoid sunlight and to wear protective clothing and use sunscreen.

16

Fluoroquinolones

ciprofloxacin
enoxacin
levofloxacin
lomefloxacin hydrochloride
nalidixic acid
norfloxacin
ofloxacin
sparfloxacin

COMBINATION PRODUCTS
None.

---

ciprofloxacin
Cipro, Cipro I.V., Ciproxin‡

Pregnancy Risk Category: C

HOW SUPPLIED
Tablets (film-coated): 250 mg, 500 mg, 750 mg
Infusion (premixed): 200 mg in 100 ml D_5W, 400 mg in 200 ml D_5W
Injection: 200 mg, 400 mg

ACTION
Inhibits bacterial DNA synthesis, mainly by blocking DNA gyrase; bactericidal.

ONSET, PEAK, DURATION
Onset and duration unknown. Serum levels peak 0.5 to 2.3 hours after oral administration, immediately after I.V. administration.

INDICATIONS & DOSAGE
Mild to moderate urinary tract infection caused by E. coli, K. pneumoniae, E. cloacae, Serratia marcescens, P. mirabilis, Providencia rettgeri, M. morganii, C. diversus, C. freundii, P. aeruginosa, S. epidermidis, *and* Enterococcus faecalis—
Adults: 250 mg P.O. or 200 mg I.V. q 12 hours.

Severe or complicated urinary tract infections; mild to moderate bone and joint infections caused by E. cloacae, P. aeruginosa, *and* Serratia marcescens; *mild to moderate respiratory infections caused by* E. coli, K. pneumoniae, E. cloacae, P. mirabilis, P. aeruginosa, H. influenzae, *and* H. parainfluenzae; *mild to moderate skin and skin-structure infections caused by* E. coli, K. pneumoniae, E. cloacae, P. mirabilis, P. vulgaris, Providencia stuartii, M. morganii, C. freundii, S. pyogenes, P. aeruginosa, S. aureus, *and* S. epidermidis; *infectious diarrhea caused by* E. coli, Campylobacter jejuni, Shigella flexneri, *and* S. sonnei; *typhoid fever*—
Adults: 500 mg P.O. or 400 mg I.V. q 12 hours.
Severe or complicated bone or joint infections; severe respiratory tract infections; severe skin and skin-structure infections—
Adults: 750 mg P.O. q 12 hours.
✳*New indication: Chronic bacterial prostatitis caused by* E. coli *or* P. mirabilis
Adults: 500 mg P.O. q 12 hours for 28 days.
Complicated intra-abdominal infections (used with metronidazole) caused by E. coli, P. aeruginosa, P. mirabilis, K. pneumoniae, *or* Bacteroides fragilis—
Adults: 500 mg P.O., or 400 mg I.V., q 12 hours for 7 to 14 days.

ADVERSE REACTIONS
CNS: headache, restlessness, tremor, dizziness, fatigue, drowsiness, insomnia, depression, light-headedness, confusion, hallucinations, *seizures,* paresthesia.
GI: *nausea, diarrhea,* vomiting, abdominal pain or discomfort, oral candidiasis, pseudomembranous colitis, dyspepsia, flatulence, constipation.

GU: crystalluria, increased serum creatinine and BUN levels, interstitial nephritis.

Musculoskeletal: arthralgia, joint or back pain, joint inflammation, joint stiffness, aching, neck or chest pain.

Skin: *rash,* photosensitivity, ***Stevens-Johnson syndrome, toxic epidermal necrolysis, exfoliative dermatitis.***

Other: elevated liver enzymes; hypersensitivity; with I.V. administration—thrombophlebitis, burning, pruritus, erythema, edema.

INTERACTIONS

Antacids containing magnesium hydroxide or aluminum hydroxide, sucralfate, iron supplements, zinc- or iron-containing multivitamins: decreased ciprofloxacin absorption. Separate administration by at least 2 hours.

Caffeine: increased effect of caffeine. Monitor closely.

Food and dairy products: decreased absorption.

Probenecid: may elevate serum level of ciprofloxacin. Monitor for toxicity.

Theophylline: increased plasma theophylline concentrations and prolonged theophylline half-life. Monitor blood levels of theophylline and observe for adverse effects.

EFFECTS ON DIAGNOSTIC TESTS
None reported.

CONTRAINDICATIONS
Contraindicated in patients sensitive to fluoroquinolone antibiotics.

NURSING CONSIDERATIONS
● Use cautiously in patients with CNS disorders, such as severe cerebral arteriosclerosis or seizure disorders, and in those at increased risk for seizures. May cause CNS stimulation.
● Obtain specimen for culture and sensitivity tests before first dose. Therapy may begin pending results.
● Administer oral form 2 hours after a meal or 2 hours before or after taking antacids, sucralfate, or products that contain iron (such as vitamins with mineral supplements). Food does not affect absorption but may delay peak serum levels.
● **I.V. use:** Dilute drug using D_5W or 0.9% sodium chloride for injection to a final concentration of 1 to 2 mg/ml before use. Infuse slowly (over 1 hour) into a large vein.
● Be aware that dosage adjustments are necessary in patients with renal dysfunction.
● Know that long-term therapy may result in overgrowth of organisms resistant to ciprofloxacin.
● Dosage adjustment is needed for patients with creatinine clearance below 50 ml/minute.
● Safety in children under age 18 has not been established. Erosion of cartilage in immature animals has been reported.

☑ **PATIENT TEACHING**
● Tell the patient to take drug as prescribed, even after he feels better.
● Advise him to drink plenty of fluids to reduce the risk of crystalluria.
● Warn the patient to avoid hazardous tasks that require alertness, such as driving, until CNS effects of the drug are known.
● Advise the patient to avoid caffeine while taking the drug because of potential for cumulative caffeine effects.
● Advise the patient that hypersensitivity reactions may occur even after first dose. If he notices a rash or other allergic reaction, he should stop taking the drug immediately and notify the doctor.
● Tell him to avoid excessive sunlight or artificial ultraviolet light during therapy and to stop drug and call the doctor if phototoxicity occurs.
● Instruct the patient to discontinue breast-feeding during treatment or ask to be treated with another drug. Drug is excreted in breast milk.
● Instruct patient to take drug on an empty stomach.

enoxacin
Penetrex

Pregnancy Risk Category: C

HOW SUPPLIED
Tablets (film-coated): 200 mg, 400 mg

ACTION
Inhibits bacterial DNA synthesis, mainly by blocking DNA gyrase; bactericidal.

ONSET, PEAK, DURATION
Onset and duration unknown. Serum levels peak in 1 to 3 hours.

INDICATIONS & DOSAGE
Uncomplicated urinary tract infections (UTIs) caused by susceptible strains of E. coli, S. epidermis, *and* S. saprophyticus—
Adults age 18 and over: 200 mg P.O. q 12 hours for 7 days.
Severe or complicated UTIs caused by susceptible strains of E. coli, P. mirabilis, P. aeruginosa, S. epidermidis, *and* E. cloacae—
Adults age 18 and over: 400 mg P.O. q 12 hours for 14 days.
Uncomplicated urethral or endocervical gonorrhea—
Adults: 400 mg P.O. as a single dose.
Doxycycline therapy may follow to treat possible coexisting chlamydial infection.
In patients with renal failure: If creatinine clearance is 30 ml/minute or less, therapy is started with usual initial dose. Subsequent doses are decreased by 50%.

ADVERSE REACTIONS
CNS: headache, restlessness, tremor, light-headedness, confusion, hallucinations, *seizures.*
GI: *nausea, diarrhea,* vomiting, abdominal pain or discomfort, oral candidiasis.
GU: crystalluria.

Other: *rash,* photosensitivity, eosinophilia, dyspnea, cough, elevated liver enzymes, pruritus, hypersensitivity.

INTERACTIONS
Aminophylline, cyclosporine, caffeine, theophylline: increased levels of these drugs because of decreased metabolism. Use together cautiously.
Antacids containing magnesium hydroxide or aluminum hydroxide, oral iron supplements, sucralfate: decreased enoxacin absorption. Separate administration times by at least 2 hours.
Bismuth subsalicylate: bioavailability of enoxacin is decreased when given within 60 minutes of bismuth subsalicylate. Avoid concomitant use.
Digoxin: may increase digoxin serum levels. Monitor closely for toxicity.
Oral anticoagulants: increased anticoagulant effect. Use together cautiously.

EFFECTS ON DIAGNOSTIC TESTS
None reported.

CONTRAINDICATIONS
Contraindicated in patients with hypersensitivity to the drug or other fluoroquinolone antibiotics.

NURSING CONSIDERATIONS
● Use cautiously in patients with CNS disorders, such as severe cerebral arteriosclerosis or seizure disorders, and in those at increased risk for seizures. May cause CNS stimulation.
● Use cautiously and with dosage adjustments in patients with impaired renal or hepatic function.
● Obtain specimen for culture and sensitivity tests before first dose. Therapy may begin pending results.
Alert: Patients being treated for gonorrhea should have an initial serologic test for syphilis before therapy starts. Drug has not been effective in treating syphilis and may mask signs and symptoms of infection. Have the serologic test repeated in 1 to 3 months.
● Administer 2 hours after a meal or 2

---

hours before or after antacids containing magnesium hydroxide or aluminum hydroxide, sucralfate, or products that contain iron (such as vitamins with mineral supplements).

• Monitor closely for superinfection.

• Safety in children under age 18 has not been established. Erosion of cartilage in immature animals has been reported.

☑ PATIENT TEACHING

• Tell the patient to take drug as prescribed, even after he feels better.

• Instruct the patient to take drug on an empty stomach.

• Advise him to drink plenty of fluids to reduce risk of crystalluria.

• Warn the patient to avoid hazardous tasks until adverse CNS effects of the drug are known.

• Warn the patient not to drink beverages containing caffeine. Enoxacin inhibits the metabolism of caffeine and can result in toxicity.

• Advise the patient to avoid overexposure to direct sunlight and to use a sunblock and wear protective clothing while outdoors.

▼ NEW DRUG

levofloxacin
Levaquin

Pregnancy Risk Category: C

HOW SUPPLIED
Tablets: 250 mg, 500 mg
Single-use vials: 500 mg
Infusion (premixed): 250 mg in 50 ml D_5W, 500 mg in 100 ml D_5W

ACTION
Inhibits bacterial DNA gyrase and prevents DNA replication, transcription, repair, and recombination in susceptible bacteria.

ONSET, PEAK, DURATION
Onset and duration unknown. Plasma levels peak within 1 to 2 hours.

INDICATIONS & DOSAGE
Indicated for treatment of mild, moderate, and severe infections caused by susceptible microorganisms in adults 18 years and older.

Acute maxillary sinusitis caused by susceptible strains of Streptococcus pneumoniae, Moraxella catarrhalis, *or* Haemophilus influenzae—

Adults: 500 mg P.O. or I.V. daily for 10 to 14 days. (See note below.)

Acute bacterial exacerbation of chronic bronchitis caused by Staphylococcus aureus, S. pneumoniae, M. catarrhalis, H. influenzae, *or* H. parainfluenzae—

Adults: 500 mg P.O. or I.V. daily for 7 days. (See note below.)

Community-acquired pneumonia caused by S. aureus, S. pneumoniae, M. catarrhalis, H. influenzae, H. parainfluenzae, Klebsiella pneumoniae, Chlamydia pneumoniae, Legionella pneumophila, *or* Mycoplasma pneumoniae—

Adults: 500 mg P.O. or I.V. daily for 7 to 14 days. (See note below.)

Mild to moderate skin and skin structure infections caused by S. aureus *or* Streptococcus pyogenes—

Adults: 500 mg P.O. or I.V. daily for 7 to 10 days. (See note below.)

Note: If creatinine clearance is 20 to 49 ml/minute, subsequent dosages are half the initial dose. If creatinine clearance is 10 to 19 ml/minute, subsequent dosages are half the initial dose and the interval is prolonged to q 48 hours.

Urinary tract infections (mild to moderate) caused by Enterococcus faecalis, Enterobacter cloacae, Escherichia coli, K. pneumoniae, Proteus mirabilis, *or* pseudomonas aeruginosa—

Adults: 250 mg P.O. or I.V. daily for 10 days. (See following note.)

Acute pyelonephritis (mild to moderate) caused by E. coli—

Adults: 250 mg P.O. or I.V. daily for 10 days. (See following note.)

Reactions may be *common*, uncommon, *life-threatening*, or COMMON AND LIFE-THREATENING.

Note: If creatinine clearance is 10 to 19 ml/minute, the dosage interval is increased to q 48 hours.

ADVERSE REACTIONS

CNS: headache, insomnia, dizziness, encephalopathy, paresthesia, *seizures*.
CV: chest pain, palpitations, vasodilatation.
GI: nausea, diarrhea, constipation, vomiting, abdominal pain, dyspepsia, flatulence, *pseudomembranous colitis.*
Hematologic: eosinophilia, hemolytic anemia.
Musculoskeletal: back pain, tendon rupture.
Respiratory: allergic pneumonitis.
Skin: rash, photosensitivity, pruritus, erythema multiforme, *Stevens-Johnson syndrome*.
Other: vaginitis, pain, hypersensitivity reactions, *anaphylaxis, multi-system organ failure.*

INTERACTIONS

Antacids containing aluminum or magnesium, iron salts, products containing zinc, sucralfate: may interfere with the GI absorption of levofloxacin. Administer at least 2 hours apart.
Antidiabetic agents: may alter blood glucose levels. Monitor glucose levels closely.
NSAIDs: may increase CNS stimulation. Monitor for seizure activity.
Warfarin and derivatives: increased effect of oral anticoagulant with some fluoroquinolones. Monitor PT and INR.
Theophylline: decreased clearance of theophylline with some fluoroquinolones. Monitor theophylline levels.

EFFECTS ON DIAGNOSTIC TESTS

Levofloxacin may cause abnormal ECG and a decreased glucose level and lymphocyte count.

CONTRAINDICATIONS

Contraindicated in patients with hypersensitivity to drug, its components, or other fluoroquinolones.

NURSING CONSIDERATIONS

● Know that the safety and efficacy of drug in children under age 18 and pregnant and breast-feeding women have not been established.
● Use cautiously in patients with a history of seizure disorders or other CNS diseases, such as cerebral arteriosclerosis. If patient experiences symptoms of excessive CNS stimulation (restlessness, tremor, confusion, hallucinations), discontinue medication and notify doctor. Institute seizure precautions.
● Use cautiously and with dosage adjustment, as ordered, in patients with renal impairment.
● Know that acute hypersensitivity reactions may require treatment with epinephrine, oxygen, I.V. fluids, antihistamines, corticosteroids, pressor amines, and airway management.
● Be aware that most antibacterial agents can cause pseudomembranous colitis. Notify the doctor if diarrhea occurs. Drug may be discontinued.
● **I.V. use:** Know that levofloxacin injection should be administered only by I.V. infusion. Dilute drug in single-use vials according to manufacturer's instructions, with D_5W or 0.9% sodium chloride injection to a final concentration of 5 mg/ml. Reconstituted solution should be clear, slightly yellow, and free of particulate matter. Reconstituted drug is stable for 72 hours at room temperature, for 14 days when refrigerated in plastic containers, and for 6 months when frozen. Thaw at room temperature or in refrigerator only. Do not mix drug with other medications. Infuse over 60 minutes.
● Obtain specimen for culture and sensitivity before starting therapy and as needed to determine if bacterial resistance has occurred.
● Monitor blood glucose and renal, hepatic, and hematopoietic blood studies as ordered.

☑ PATIENT TEACHING

● Tell patient to take drug as prescribed,

even if symptoms disappear.

• Advise patient to take drug with plenty of fluids and to avoid antacids, sucralfate, and products containing iron or zinc for at least 2 hours before and after each dose.

• Warn patient to avoid hazardous tasks until adverse CNS effects of drug are known.

• Advise patient to use sunblock and wear protective clothing when exposed to excessive sunlight.

• Tell patient to stop drug and notify the doctor if rash or other signs of hypersensitivity develop.

• Tell patient to notify the doctor of pain or inflammation; tendon rupture can occur with drug.

• Know that diabetic patients should monitor blood glucose levels and notify the doctor if a hypoglycemic reaction occurs.

---

lomefloxacin hydrochloride
Maxaquin

Pregnancy Risk Category: C

HOW SUPPLIED
Tablets (film-coated): 400 mg

ACTION
Inhibits bacterial DNA gyrase, an enzyme necessary for bacterial replication (bactericidal).

ONSET, PEAK, DURATION
Onset and duration unknown. Plasma levels peak 1½ hours after oral dose.

INDICATIONS & DOSAGE
Acute bacterial exacerbations of chronic bronchitis caused by Haemophilus influenzae *or* Moraxella (Branhamella) catarrhalis—
Adults: 400 mg P.O. daily for 10 days.
Uncomplicated urinary tract infections (cystitis) caused by Escherichia coli, Klebsiella pneumoniae, Proteus mirabilis, *or* Staphylococcus sapro-

phyticus—
Adults: 400 mg P.O. daily for 10 days.
Complicated urinary tract infections caused by E. coli, K. pneumoniae, P. mirabilis, *or* Pseudomonas aeruginosa; *possibly effective against infections caused by* Citrobacter diversus *or* Enterobacter cloacae—
Adults: 400 mg P.O. daily for 14 days.
Prophylaxis of infections after transurethral surgical procedures—
Adults: 400 mg P.O. as a single dose 2 to 6 hours before surgery.

Patients with a creatinine clearance of 10 to 40 ml/minute should receive a loading dose of 400 mg P.O. on the first day, followed by 200 mg daily for the duration of therapy. Hemodialysis removes negligible amounts of drug.
✳ *New indication: Prophylaxis of urinary tract infections after transrectal prostate biopsy—*
Adults: 400 mg P.O. as a single dose 1 to 6 hours before procedure.

ADVERSE REACTIONS
CNS: *dizziness, headache,* abnormal dreams, fatigue, malaise, asthenia, agitation, anorexia, anxiety, confusion, depersonalization, depression, increased appetite, insomnia, nervousness, somnolence, *seizures, coma,* hyperkinesis, tremor, vertigo, paresthesia, arthralgia, myalgia.
CV: flushing, hypotension, hypertension, edema, syncope, arrhythmia, tachycardia, bradycardia, extrasystoles, cyanosis, angina pectoris, *MI, cardiac failure, pulmonary embolism,* cerebrovascular disorder, cardiomyopathy, phlebitis.
EENT: epistaxis, abnormal vision, conjunctivitis, eye pain, earache, tinnitus, tongue discoloration, taste perversion.
GI: *diarrhea, nausea,* dry mouth, pseudomembranous colitis, abdominal pain, dyspepsia, vomiting, flatulence, constipation, inflammation, dysphagia, bleeding.
GU: dysuria, hematuria, anuria, epididymitis, orchitis, vaginitis, vaginal

---

Reactions may be *common,* uncommon, *life-threatening,* or COMMON AND LIFE-THREATENING.

moniliasis, intermenstrual bleeding, perineal pain.

Hematologic: thrombocythemia, *thrombocytopenia,* lymphadenopathy.

Respiratory: dyspnea, *bronchospasm,* respiratory disorder or infection, increased sputum, stridor.

Skin: pruritus, skin disorder, skin exfoliation, eczema, rash, urticaria, *photosensitivity.*

Other: *anaphylaxis,* increased diaphoresis, leg cramps, thirst, chest or back pain, chills, allergic reaction, facial edema, flulike symptoms, decreased heat tolerance, hypoglycemia, elevated liver enzymes, gout.

INTERACTIONS
Antacids, sucralfate: impaired absorption after binding with lomefloxacin in GI tract. Give no less than 4 hours before or 2 hours after a dose.
Cimetidine: increased half-life of other fluoroquinolones when administered to patients taking cimetidine; lomefloxacin has not been tested. Monitor for toxicity.
Probenecid: decreased excretion of lomefloxacin. Monitor for toxicity.
Warfarin, cyclosporine: increased effects or serum levels when combined with other fluoroquinolones; lomefloxacin has not been tested. Monitor for toxicity.

EFFECTS ON DIAGNOSTIC TESTS
None reported.

CONTRAINDICATIONS
Contraindicated in patients with hypersensitivity to lomefloxacin or other fluoroquinolones.

NURSING CONSIDERATIONS
• Use cautiously in patients with known or suspected CNS disorders, such as seizure disorder or cerebral arteriosclerosis, that may predispose the patient to seizures.
• Obtain culture and sensitivity tests before first dose. Therapy may begin

pending results.
• Be aware that although most fluoroquinolones exhibit photosensitizing effects, early studies suggest that photosensitization and phototoxicity are more common with lomefloxacin.
• Keep in mind that prolonged use may result in overgrowth of organisms resistant to lomefloxacin.
• Safety in children under age 18 has not been established. Erosion of cartilage in immature animals has been reported.

☑ PATIENT TEACHING
• Tell the patient to take drug as prescribed, even after he feels better.
• Advise the patient that hypersensitivity reactions may occur even after first dose. If rash or other allergic reaction occurs, the patient should stop taking the drug and notify the doctor.
• Warn the patient to avoid hazardous tasks until CNS effects of drug are known.
• Advise the patient to wear protective clothing, use a sunscreen, and avoid prolonged exposure to sunlight during treatment and for a few days after therapy ends. If sunburn occurs, the patient should call the doctor as soon as possible.
• Tell patient the drug may be taken with or without food.

nalidixic acid
NegGram

Pregnancy Risk Category: B (safe use in first trimester not known)

HOW SUPPLIED
Caplets: 250 mg, 500 mg, 1 g
Oral suspension: 250 mg/5 ml

ACTION
Inhibits microbial DNA synthesis.

ONSET, PEAK, DURATION
Onset and duration unknown. Serum

levels peak 1 to 2 hours after an oral dose. Urine levels peak 3 to 4 hours after a dose.

INDICATIONS & DOSAGE
Acute and chronic urinary tract infections caused by susceptible gram-negative organisms (Proteus, Klebsiella, Enterobacter, *and* Escherichia coli)—
Adults: 1 g P.O. q.i.d. for 7 to 14 days; 2 g daily for long-term use.
Children over 3 months: 55 mg/kg P.O. daily divided q.i.d. for 7 to 14 days; 33 mg/kg daily for long-term use.

ADVERSE REACTIONS
CNS: drowsiness, weakness, headache, dizziness, vertigo, *seizures,* malaise, confusion, hallucinations, psychosis.
EENT: sensitivity to light, change in color perception, diplopia, blurred vision.
GI: *abdominal pain, nausea, vomiting,* diarrhea.
Hematologic: eosinophilia, *leukopenia, thrombocytopenia,* hemolytic anemia.
Skin: pruritus, photosensitivity, urticaria, rash.
Other: angioedema, *increased intracranial pressure and bulging fontanelles in infants and children,* arthralgia, joint stiffness, anaphylactoid reaction.

INTERACTIONS
Oral anticoagulants: increased anticoagulant effect. Monitor for bleeding.

EFFECTS ON DIAGNOSTIC TESTS
Nalidixic acid may cause false-positive results in urine glucose tests using cupric sulfate (such as Benedict's reagent, Fehling's solution, and Clinitest). Urine 17-ketosteroid and urine 17-ketogenic steroid levels may be falsely elevated because nalidixic acid interacts with *M*-dinitrobenzene, used to measure these urine metabolites. Urine vanillylmandelic acid levels may also be falsely elevated. Drug may cause transient decreases in circulating RBC, WBC, and platelet counts during therapy.

CONTRAINDICATIONS
Contraindicated in patients with hypersensitivity to the drug, in those with seizure disorders, and in infants under age 3 months.

NURSING CONSIDERATIONS
● Use with extreme caution in prepubertal children; erosion of cartilage in immature animals has been reported.
● Use cautiously in patients with impaired hepatic or renal function or with severe cerebral arteriosclerosis.
● Obtain specimen for culture and sensitivity tests before starting therapy and repeat p.r.n. Therapy may begin pending results.
● Monitor CBC, renal, and liver function studies during long-term therapy, as ordered.
● Be aware that resistant bacteria may emerge in the first 48 hours of therapy.

☑ PATIENT TEACHING
● Tell the patient to take drug as prescribed, even after he feels better.
● Instruct the patient to take drug with food to prevent GI upset.
● Tell the patient to avoid exposure to sunlight, to wear protective clothing, and to use sunscreen.
● Tell the patient to report visual disturbances or CNS symptoms immediately.

norfloxacin
Noroxin

Pregnancy Risk Category: C

HOW SUPPLIED
Film-coated tablets: 400 mg

ACTION
Inhibits bacterial DNA synthesis, mainly by blocking DNA gyrase; bactericidal.

ONSET, PEAK, DURATION
Onset and duration unknown. Plasma levels peak 1 to 2 hours after oral dose.

INDICATIONS & DOSAGE
Complicated or uncomplicated urinary tract infections caused by susceptible strains of Enterococcus faecalis, Escherichia coli, Klebsiella pneumoniae, Enterobacter aerogenes, E. cloacae, Proteus mirabilis, P. vulgaris, Pseudomonas aeruginosa, Citrobacter freundii, Staphylococcus agalactiae, S. aureus, S. epidermidis, S. saprophyticus, *and* Serratia marcescens—
Adults: for uncomplicated infections, 400 mg P.O. q 12 hours for 7 to 10 days. For complicated infections, 400 mg P.O. q 12 hours for 10 to 21 days.
Cystitis caused by E. coli, K. pneumoniae, *or* P. mirabilis—
Adults: 400 mg P.O. q 12 hours for 3 days.
Acute, uncomplicated urethral and cervical gonorrhea—
Adults: 800 mg P.O. as a single dose, followed by doxycycline therapy to treat any coexisting chlamydial infection.
Note: Adults with creatinine clearance 30 ml/minute or less should receive 400 mg once daily for above indications.

ADVERSE REACTIONS
CNS: fatigue, somnolence, headache, dizziness, *seizures,* depression, insomnia.
GI: nausea, constipation, flatulence, heartburn, dry mouth, abdominal pain, diarrhea, vomiting, anorexia.
GU: increased serum creatinine and BUN levels, crystalluria.
Hematologic: eosinophilia.
Musculoskeletal: back pain.
Skin: rash, photosensitivity.
Other: hypersensitivity reactions (rash, *anaphylactoid reaction*), transient elevations of AST and ALT, fever, hyperhidrosis.

INTERACTIONS
Antacids, iron products, sucralfate: may hinder absorption. Separate administration times by 2 hours.
Cyclosporine: increased serum concentrations of cyclosporine. Monitor serum levels.
Oral anticoagulants: increased anticoagulant effect. Monitor closely.
Probenecid: may increase serum levels of norfloxacin by decreasing its excretion. Monitor for toxicity.
Theophylline: possibly impaired theophylline metabolism, resulting in increased plasma levels and risk of toxicity. Monitor closely.

EFFECTS ON DIAGNOSTIC TESTS
BUN, serum creatinine, ALT, AST, and alkaline phosphatase levels may increase; hematocrit may decrease; and eosinophilia and neutropenia may occur during norfloxacin therapy.

CONTRAINDICATIONS
Contraindicated in patients with hypersensitivity to fluoroquinolones.

NURSING CONSIDERATIONS
● Use cautiously in patients with conditions that may predispose them to seizure disorders, such as cerebral arteriosclerosis. Also use cautiously in those with renal impairment.
● Safety in children under age 18 has not been established. Erosion of cartilage in immature animals has been reported.

☑ PATIENT TEACHING
● Tell the patient to take drug as prescribed, even after he feels better.
● Advise the patient to take the drug 1 hour before or 2 hours after meals because food, antacids, iron products, and sucralfate may hinder absorption.
● Warn the patient not to exceed the recommended dosages and to drink several glasses of water throughout the day to maintain hydration and adequate urine output.
● Warn the patient to avoid hazardous tasks that require alertness until CNS

effects of the drug are known.
● Instruct patient to avoid exposure to sunlight, to wear protective clothing, and to use sunscreen.

---

ofloxacin
Floxin, Floxin I.V.

Pregnancy Risk Category: C

HOW SUPPLIED
Tablets (film-coated): 200 mg, 300 mg, 400 mg
Injection: 20 mg/ml, 40 mg/ml; 4 mg/ml premixed in D_5W

ACTION
Inhibits bacterial DNA synthesis by blocking DNA gyrase; bactericidal.

ONSET, PEAK, DURATION
Onset and duration unknown. Plasma levels peak immediately after an I.V. infusion, within 1 to 2 hours after an oral dose.

INDICATIONS & DOSAGE
Lower respiratory tract infections caused by susceptible strains of Haemophilus influenzae *or* Streptococcus pneumoniae—
Adults: 400 mg I.V. or P.O. q 12 hours for 10 days.
Cervicitis or urethritis caused by Chlamydia trachomatis *or* Neisseria gonorrhoeae—
Adults: 300 mg I.V. or P.O. q 12 hours for 7 days.
Acute, uncomplicated gonorrhea—
Adults: 400 mg I.V. or P.O. as a single dose with doxycycline.
Mild to moderate skin and skin-structure infections caused by susceptible strains of Staphylococcus aureus, Streptococcus pyogenes, *or* Proteus mirabilis—
Adults: 400 mg I.V. or P.O. q 12 hours for 10 days.
Cystitis caused by Escherichia coli *or* Klebsiella pneumoniae—
Adults: 200 mg I.V. or P.O. q 12 hours for 3 days.
Urinary tract infections caused by susceptible strains of Citrobacter diversus, Enterobacter aerogenes, E. coli, P. mirabilis, *or* Pseudomonas aeruginosa—
Adults: 200 mg I.V. or P.O. q 12 hours for 7 days. Complicated infections may require therapy for 10 days.
Prostatitis caused by E. coli—
Adults: 300 mg I.V. or P.O. q 12 hours for 6 weeks.
Epididymitis—
Adults: 300 mg P.O. q 12 hours for 10 days.
Pelvic inflammatory disease (outpatient)—
Adults: 400 mg P.O. q 12 hours for 14 days in combination with clindamycin or metronidazole.

If creatinine clearance is 10 to 50 ml/minute, dosage interval is decreased to once q 24 hours. If creatinine clearance is less than 10 ml/minute, half the recommended dose is given q 24 hours.

ADVERSE REACTIONS
CNS: headache, dizziness, fatigue, lethargy, malaise, drowsiness, sleep disorders, nervousness, insomnia, visual disturbances, *seizures*.
CV: chest pain.
GI: *nausea,* anorexia, abdominal pain or discomfort, diarrhea, vomiting, constipation, dry mouth, flatulence, dysgeusia.
GU: vaginitis, vaginal discharge, genital pruritus.
Musculoskeletal: trunk pain.
Skin: rash, pruritus, photosensitivity.
Other: hypersensitivity reactions *(anaphylactoid reaction)*, elevated liver enzymes, fever, phlebitis.

INTERACTIONS
Antacids containing aluminum or magnesium hydroxide, iron salts, sucralfate, products containing zinc: may interfere with the GI absorption of ofloxacin.

Reactions may be *common*, uncommon, *life-threatening*, or COMMON AND LIFE-THREATENING.

Separate administration by at least 2 hours.

Antidiabetic agents: may cause alterations in blood glucose levels. Monitor concentrations closely.

Antineoplastic agents: may lower serum levels of fluoroquinolones. Monitor for lack of effect.

Oral anticoagulants: increased effect. Monitor for bleeding and altered PT.

Theophylline: decreased clearance of theophylline with some fluoroquinolones. Monitor theophylline levels.

EFFECTS ON DIAGNOSTIC TESTS
Drug may increase blood glucose levels.

CONTRAINDICATIONS
Contraindicated in patients with hypersensitivity to the drug or other fluoroquinolones.

NURSING CONSIDERATIONS
● Use cautiously in patients with a history of seizure disorders or other CNS diseases, such as cerebral arteriosclerosis.

● Use cautiously and with dosage adjustment in patients with renal failure, as prescribed, because the drug is mainly eliminated by renal excretion.

● **I.V. use:** Dilute concentrate for injection before use. Single-use vials containing 20 or 40 mg/ml must be diluted to a maximum concentration of 4 mg/ml with a compatible I.V. solution, such as D₅W, 0.9% sodium chloride for injection, D₅W in 0.9% sodium chloride for injection, or sterile water for injection. Infuse over not less than 60 minutes.

● Because compatibility with other drugs is not known, don't mix ofloxacin with other drugs. If giving infusion at a Y-site, discontinue the flow of the other solution.

● Monitor regular blood studies and hepatic and renal function tests during prolonged therapy, as ordered.

Alert: Know that patients treated for gonorrhea should have a serologic test for syphilis. Drug is not effective against syphilis, and treatment of gonorrhea may mask or delay symptoms of syphilis.

● Safety in children under age 18 is unknown. Erosion of cartilage in immature animals has been reported.

☑ **PATIENT TEACHING**
● Tell the patient to take drug as prescribed, even after he feels better.

● Advise the patient to take the drug with plenty of fluids, but not with meals, and to avoid antacids, sucralfate, and products containing iron or zinc for at least 2 hours before and after each dose.

● Warn the patient to avoid hazardous tasks until adverse CNS effects of drug are known.

● Advise the patient to use sunscreen and wear protective clothing.

● Tell the patient to stop drug and notify the doctor if a rash or other signs of hypersensitivity develop.

▼ *NEW DRUG*

sparfloxacin
Zagam

Pregnancy Risk Category: C

HOW SUPPLIED
Tablets: 200 mg

ACTION
Inhibits bacterial DNA gyrase and prevents DNA replication, transcription, repair, and deactivation in susceptible bacteria.

ONSET, PEAK, DURATION
Onset and duration unknown. Plasma levels peak within 3 to 6 hours.

INDICATIONS & DOSAGE
Acute bacterial exacerbation of chronic bronchitis caused by Staphylococcus aureus, Streptococcus pneumoniae, Chlamydia pneumoniae, Enterobacter

cloacae, Klebsiella pneumoniae, Moraxella catarrhalis, Haemophilus influenzae, *or* H. parainfluenzae—

Adults over 18 years: 400 mg P.O. on the first day as a loading dose, then 200 mg daily for a total of 10 days of therapy.

Community-acquired pneumonia caused by S. pneumoniae, M. catarrhalis, H. influenzae, H. parainfluenzae, C. pneumoniae, *or* Mycoplasma pneumoniae—

Adults over 18 years: 400 mg P.O. on the first day as a loading dose, then 200 mg daily for a total of 10 days of therapy.

In patients with renal impairment, if creatinine clearance is below 50 ml/minute, a loading dose of 400 mg P.O. is given; thereafter, 200 mg P.O. q 48 hours is given for a total of 9 days of therapy.

ADVERSE REACTIONS
CNS: headache, dizziness, insomnia, taste perversion, asthenia, somnolence, *seizures.*
CV: QT interval prolongation, vasodilatation.
EENT: dry mouth.
GI: nausea, diarrhea, vomiting, abdominal pain, dyspepsia, flatulence, *pseudomembranous colitis.*
GU: vaginal moniliasis.
Musculoskeletal: tendon rupture.
Skin: rash, photosensitivity, pruritus.
Other: elevated ALT and AST levels and white blood cell counts, hypersensitivity reactions, *anaphylaxis.*

INTERACTIONS
Antacids containing aluminum or magnesium, iron salts, zinc, sucralfate: may interfere with GI absorption of levofloxacin. Administer at least 4 hours apart.
Drugs that prolong the QT interval or cause torsades de pointes (including bepridil, terfenadine, disopyramide, amiodarone, class Ia antiarrythmics such as quinidine and procainamide, and class III drugs such as sotalol): may

cause torsades de pointes. Sparfloxacin is contraindicated in these patients.

EFFECTS ON DIAGNOSTIC TESTS
Sparfloxacin may produce false-negative culture results for *Mycobacterium tuberculosis* and elevations in ALT and AST levels and WBC count.

CONTRAINDICATIONS
Contraindicated in patients with a history of hypersensitivity or photosensitivity reactions to drug and those who cannot stay out of the sun. Avoid concomitant administration with drugs known to prolong the QT interval or cause torsades de pointes. Sparfloxacin is not recommended for patients with heart conditions that predispose them to arrhythmias.

NURSING CONSIDERATIONS
● Know that the safety and efficacy of levofloxacin in pregnant and breast-feeding women and patients under age 18 have not been established.
● Use cautiously in patients with a history of seizure disorder or other CNS diseases, such as cerebral arteriosclerosis. If patient experiences symptoms of excessive CNS stimulation (restlessness, tremor, confusion, hallucinations), discontinue medication and notify the doctor. Then institute seizure precautions.
● Use cautiously and with dosage adjustment in patients with renal impairment.
● Know that acute hypersensitivity reactions may require treatment with epinephrine, oxygen, I.V. fluids, antihistamines, corticosteroids, pressor amines, and airway management.
● Obtain specimen for culture and sensitivity before starting therapy and as needed and ordered to determine if bacterial resistance has occurred.

☑ PATIENT TEACHING
● Drug may be taken with food, milk, or products that contain caffeine.
● Tell patient to take drug as prescribed,

Reactions may be *common*, uncommon, *life-threatening*, or COMMON AND LIFE-THREATENING.

even if symptoms disappear.
● Advise patient to take drug with plenty of fluids and to avoid antacids, sucralfate, and products containing iron or zinc for at least 4 hours after each dose.
● Warn patient to avoid hazardous tasks until adverse CNS effects of drug are known.
Alert: Advise patient to avoid direct, indirect, and artificial ultraviolet light, even with sunscreen on, during treatment and for 5 days after treatment. Patient should stop taking drug and notify the doctor if signs or symptoms of phototoxicity (skin burning, redness, swelling, blisters, rash, itching) occur.
● Tell patient to stop drug and notify the doctor if a rash or other signs of hypersensitivity develop.
● Tell patient to discontinue drug and notify the doctor of pain or inflammation; tendon rupture can occur with drug. The patient should rest and refrain from exercise until a diagnosis is made.

17

Antivirals

acyclovir sodium
amantadine hydrochloride
cidofovir
didanosine
famciclovir
foscarnet sodium
ganciclovir
indinavir sulfate
lamivudine
nevirapine
ribavirin
rimantadine hydrochloride
ritonavir
saquinavir mesylate
stavudine
valacyclovir hydrochloride
zalcitabine
zidovudine

COMBINATION PRODUCTS
None.

---

acyclovir sodium
Avirax†, Zovirax

Pregnancy Risk Category: C

HOW SUPPLIED
Capsules: 200 mg
Tablets: 400 mg, 800 mg
Suspension: 200 mg/5 ml
Injection: 500 mg/vial, 1 g/vial

ACTION
Interferes with DNA synthesis and inhibits viral multiplication.

ONSET, PEAK, DURATION
Onset immediate after I.V. infusion, unknown after oral administration. Serum levels peak immediately after I.V. infusion, within 1.5 to 2.5 hours of oral dose. Duration unknown.

INDICATIONS & DOSAGE
Initial and recurrent episodes of mucocutaneous herpes simplex virus (HSV-1 and HSV-2) infections in immunocompromised patients; severe initial episodes of genital herpes in patients who are not immunocompromised—
Adults and children 12 years and over: 5 mg/kg, given at a constant rate over a period of 1 hour by I.V. q 8 hours for 7 to 14 days (5 to 7 days for severe initial episode of genital herpes).
Children under 12 years: 250 mg/m², given at a constant rate over a period of 1 hour by I.V. q 8 hours for 7 days.
Initial genital herpes—
Adults: 200 mg P.O. q 4 hours while awake (a total of 5 capsules daily); or 400 mg P.O. q 8 hours. Treatment should continue for 7 to 10 days for treatment of initial genital herpes episodes.
Intermittent therapy for recurrent genital herpes—
Adults: 200 mg P.O. q 4 hours while awake (a total of 5 capsules daily). Treatment should continue for 5 days. Initiate therapy at the first sign of recurrence.
Chronic suppressive therapy for recurrent genital herpes—
Adults: 400 mg P.O. b.i.d. for up to 12 months. Alternatively, 200 mg P.O. three to five times daily for up to 12 months.
Treatment of varicella (chickenpox) infections in immunocompromised patients—
Adults and children 12 years and over: 10 mg/kg I.V. infused at a constant rate over 1 hour q 8 hours for 7 days. Dosage for obese patients based on ideal body weight.
Children under 12 years: 500 mg/m² I.V. infused at a constant rate over 1 hour q 8 hours for 7 to 10 days.

Reactions may be *common*, uncommon, **life-threatening**, or COMMON AND LIFE-THREATENING.

Varicella infection in immunocompetent patients—

Adults and children 2 years and over: 20 mg/kg (maximum 800 mg/dose) P.O. q.i.d. for 5 days. Start therapy as soon as symptoms appear to achieve maximum efficacy. Alternatively, adults and children who weigh more than 40 kg: 800 mg P.O. q.i.d. for 5 days. Children 2 years and older who weigh 40 kg or less: 20 mg/kg P.O. q.i.d. for 5 days.

Acute herpes zoster infection in immunocompetent patients—

Adults and children 12 years and over: 800 mg P.O. q 4 hours five times daily for 5 to 10 days.

Herpes simplex encephalitis—

Adults and children over 6 months: 10 mg/kg I.V. infused at a constant rate over 1 hour q 8 hours for 10 days. Alternatively, in children 6 months to 12 years: 500 mg/m^2 I.V. infused at a constant rate over 1 hour q 8 hours for 10 days.

ADVERSE REACTIONS

CNS: *malaise, headache, encephalopathic changes (lethargy, obtundation, tremor, confusion, hallucinations, agitation, **seizures, coma**).*

GI: *nausea, vomiting,* diarrhea.

GU: *transient elevations of serum creatinine and BUN levels,* hematuria, acute renal failure.

Skin: rash, itching, urticaria.

Other: *inflammation and phlebitis at injection site.*

INTERACTIONS

Probenecid: increased acyclovir blood levels. Monitor for possible toxicity.
Zidovudine: may cause drowsiness or lethargy. Use together cautiously.

EFFECTS ON DIAGNOSTIC TESTS

Serum creatinine and BUN levels may increase during acyclovir therapy.

CONTRAINDICATIONS

Contraindicated in patients with hypersensitivity to the drug.

NURSING CONSIDERATIONS

● Use cautiously in patients with underlying neurologic problems, renal disease, or dehydration and in those receiving other nephrotoxic drugs.

● Be aware that it is recommended that acyclovir be administered in a reduced dosage to patients with impaired renal function.

● **I.V. use:** Administer I.V. infusion over at least 1 hour to prevent renal tubular damage. Bolus injection, dehydration (decreased urine output), preexisting renal disease, and the concomitant use of other nephrotoxic drugs increase the risk of renal toxicity.

Alert: Don't give by bolus injection or administer I.M. or S.C.

● Be alert that concentrated solutions (7 mg/ml or more) may be associated with a higher incidence of phlebitis.

● Encourage fluid intake because the patient must be adequately hydrated during acyclovir infusion.

● Know that encephalopathic changes are more likely in patients with neurologic disorders or in those who have had neurologic reactions to cytotoxic drugs.

● Keep in mind that Glaxo-Wellcome, the manufacturer of Zovirax, maintains an ongoing registry of women exposed to the drug during pregnancy. Follow-up studies to date have not shown an increased risk for birth defects for infants born to patients exposed to the drug during pregnancy. Health care providers are encouraged to report such exposures to the registrar at 1-800-722-9292, ext. 58465.

☑ PATIENT TEACHING

● Tell the patient to take drug as prescribed, even after he feels better.

● Instruct the patient that drug is effective in managing herpes infection but does not eliminate or cure it. Warn the patient that acyclovir will not prevent spread of infection to others.

● Urge the patient to recognize early symptoms of herpes infection (such as tingling, itching, or pain). He can then

---

notify his doctor and get a prescription for acyclovir before the infection fully develops.

---

amantadine hydrochloride
Antadine‡, Symadine, Symmetrel

Pregnancy Risk Category: C

HOW SUPPLIED
Capsules: 100 mg
Syrup: 50 mg/5 ml

ACTION
Unknown. Possibly inhibits the uncoating of the virus.

ONSET, PEAK, DURATION
Onset unknown for antiviral activity. Peak plasma levels occur 1 to 4 hours after an oral dose. Duration unknown.

INDICATIONS & DOSAGE
Prophylaxis or symptomatic treatment of influenza type A virus, respiratory tract illnesses—
Adults up to 65 years with normal renal function and children 9 years and over who weigh more than 45 kg: 200 mg P.O. daily in a single dose.
Children 1 to 9 years or weighing less than 45 kg: 4.4 to 8.8 mg/kg P.O. daily, as a single dose or divided b.i.d. Maximum dose is 150 mg daily.
Adults over 65 years with normal renal function: 100 mg P.O. once daily.

Treatment should begin within 24 to 48 hours after symptoms appear and should continue for 24 to 48 hours after symptoms disappear (usually 2 to 7 days of therapy). Prophylaxis should start as soon as possible after initial exposure and continue for at least 10 days after exposure. May continue prophylactic treatment up to 90 days for repeated or suspected exposures if influenza vaccine unavailable. If used with influenza vaccine, dose is continued for 2 to 3 weeks until antibody response to vaccine has developed.

ADVERSE REACTIONS
CNS: depression, fatigue, confusion, *dizziness,* hallucinations, anxiety, *irritability,* ataxia, *insomnia,* headache, *light-headedness.*
CV: peripheral edema, orthostatic hypotension, CHF.
GI: anorexia, *nausea,* constipation, vomiting, dry mouth.
Skin: *livedo reticularis* (with prolonged use).

INTERACTIONS
Anticholinergics: additive adverse anticholinergic effects. Use together cautiously. Dosage of anticholinergic agent may be reduced prior to initiation of amantadine by some doctors.
CNS stimulants: additive CNS stimulation. Use together cautiously.

EFFECTS ON DIAGNOSTIC TESTS
None reported.

CONTRAINDICATIONS
Contraindicated in patients with hypersensitivity to the drug.

NURSING CONSIDERATIONS
● Use cautiously in those with seizure disorders, CHF, peripheral edema, hepatic disease, mental illness, eczematoid rash, renal impairment, orthostatic hypotension, and CV disease and in elderly patients.
Alert: Be aware that elderly patients are more susceptible to adverse neurologic effects.

☑ PATIENT TEACHING
● If insomnia occurs, tell the patient to take the drug several hours before bedtime.
● If orthostatic hypotension occurs, instruct the patient not to stand or change positions too quickly.
● Instruct the patient to report adverse reactions to the doctor, especially dizziness, depression, anxiety, nausea, and urine retention.

Reactions may be *common*, uncommon, *life-threatening*, or COMMON AND LIFE-THREATENING.

▼ NEW DRUG

cidofovir
Vistide

Pregnancy Risk Category: C

HOW SUPPLIED
Injection: 75 mg/ml in 5-ml vial

ACTION
Suppresses CMV replication by selective inhibition of viral DNA synthesis.

ONSET, PEAK, DURATION
Unknown.

INDICATIONS & DOSAGE
CMV retinitis in patients with AIDS—
Adults: initially, 5 mg/kg I.V. infused over 1 hour once weekly for 2 consecutive weeks, followed by a maintenance dosage of 5 mg/kg I.V. infused over 1 hour q 2 weeks. Probenecid and prehydration with 0.9% sodium chloride solution I.V. must be administered concomitantly and may reduce potential for nephrotoxicity.

Dosages may need adjustment in patients with renal impairment.

ADVERSE REACTIONS
CNS: *asthenia, headache,* amnesia, anxiety, confusion, *seizure,* depression, dizziness, abnormal gait, hallucinations, insomnia, neuropathy, paresthesia, somnolence.
CV: hypotension, postural hypotension, pallor, syncope, tachycardia, vasodilation.
EENT: amblyopia, conjunctivitis, eye disorders, *ocular hypotony,* iritis, retinal detachment, uveitis, abnormal vision, taste perversion.
GI: *nausea and vomiting, diarrhea, anorexia, abdominal pain,* dry mouth, colitis, constipation, tongue discoloration, dyspepsia, dysphagia, flatulence, gastritis, melena, oral candidiasis, rectal disorders, stomatitis, aphthous stomatitis, mouth ulcerations.

GU: *elevated creatinine levels, nephrotoxicity, proteinuria,* decreased creatinine clearance levels, glycosuria, hematuria, urinary incontinence, urinary tract infection.
Hematologic: NEUTROPENIA, *anemia, thrombocytopenia.*
Hepatic: hepatomegaly, abnormal liver function tests, increased alkaline phosphatase levels.
Metabolic: fluid imbalance, hyperglycemia, hyperlipemia, hypocalcemia, hypokalemia, weight loss, decreased serum bicarbonate level.
Musculoskeletal: arthralgia, myasthenia, myalgia.
Respiratory: asthma, bronchitis, coughing, *dyspnea,* hiccups, increased sputum, lung disorders, pharyngitis, pneumonia, rhinitis, sinusitis.
Skin: *rash, alopecia,* acne, skin discoloration, dry skin, herpes simplex, pruritis, sweating, urticaria.
Other: *fever, infections, chills,* allergic reactions, facial edema, malaise, *sarcoma, sepsis,* pain in back, chest, or neck.

INTERACTIONS
Nephrotoxic agents, such as amphotericin B, aminoglycosides, foscarnet, I.V. pentamidine: may increase nephrotoxicity. Avoid concomitant use.
Probenecid: known to interact with the metabolism or renal tubular excretion of many drugs. Monitor closely.

EFFECTS ON DIAGNOSTIC TESTS
None reported.

CONTRAINDICATIONS
Contraindicated in patients with hypersensitivity to drug or history of clinically severe hypersensitivity to probenecid or other sulfur-containing medication. Do not administer as a direct intraocular injection (may be associated with significant decreases in intraocular pressure and vision impairment). Do not administer to breast-feeding women.

---

*Liquid contains alcohol. **May contain tartrazine. †Canada only. ‡Australia only. ◊ OTC.

NURSING CONSIDERATIONS

- Use cautiously in patients with impaired renal function.
- Administer 1 L 0.9% sodium chloride as ordered, usually over 1- to 2-hour period immediately before each cidofovir infusion.
- Administer probenecid, as ordered, with cidofovir.
- Because of the potential for increased nephrotoxicity, do not exceed recommended doses or frequency or rate of administration.
- To prepare cidofovir for infusion, extract the appropriate amount of cidofovir from the vial using a syringe and transfer the dose to an infusion bag containing 100 ml of 0.9% sodium chloride solution. Infuse the entire volume I.V. at a constant rate over a 1-hour period. Use a standard infusion pump for administration.
- Be aware that because of the mutagenic properties of cidofovir, drug should be prepared in a class II laminar flow biological safety cabinet. Personnel preparing drug should wear surgical gloves and a closed front surgical gown with knit cuffs.
- If drug contacts the skin, wash membranes and flush thoroughly with water. Excess drug and all other materials used in the admixture preparation and administration should be placed in a leakproof, puncture-proof container. Recommended method of disposal is high temperature incineration.
- Know that cidofovir infusion admixtures should be administered within 24 hours of preparation; refrigerator or freezer storage should not be used to extend this 24-hour period. If admixtures are not used immediately, they may be refrigerated at 36° to 46° F (2° to 8° C) for no more than 24 hours. Allow cidofovir to reach room temperature prior to use.
- Know that no other drugs or supplements should be added to admixture for concurrent administration.
- Be aware that compatibility with Ringer's solution, lactated Ringer's solution, or bacteriostatic infusion fluids has not been evaluated.
- Monitor WBC counts with differential before each dose.
- Know that renal function (serum creatinine and urine protein) should be monitored before each dose and the dosage modified by a doctor for changes in renal function.
- Be aware that drug should not be used in patients with baseline serum creatinine exceeding 1.5 mg/dl or calculated creatinine clearance of 55 ml/minute or below unless potential benefits outweigh potential risks.
- Know that Fanconi's syndrome and decreased serum bicarbonate levels associated with renal tubular damage have been reported in patients receiving cidofovir. Monitor patient closely.
- Be aware that granulocytopenia has been observed in association with drug treatment. Monitor neutrophil counts during therapy.
- Be aware that intraocular pressure, visual acuity, and ocular symptoms should be monitored periodically.
- Know that cidofovir is indicated only for the treatment of CMV retinitis in patients with AIDS. Safety and efficacy of drug have not been established for treating other CMV infections, congenital or neonatal CMV disease, or CMV disease in patients not infected with HIV.
- Know that in animal studies, cidofovir was carcinogenic and teratogenic and caused hypospermia.
- Discontinue zidovudine therapy or reduce dosage by 50%, as ordered, on the days cidofovir is administered; probenecid reduces metabolic clearance of zidovudine.
- Know that dosage adjustment may be necessary in elderly patients with renal impairment.
- Be aware that safety and effectiveness in children have not been established.
- Be aware that it is unknown whether cidofovir is excreted in breast milk.

☑ **PATIENT TEACHING**
● Inform patient that drug is not a cure for CMV retinitis and that regular ophthalmologic follow-up examinations are necessary.
● Alert patients on zidovudine therapy that they'll need to obtain dosage guidelines on days cidofovir is administered.
● Tell patient that close monitoring of renal function will be needed and that abnormalities may require a change in cidofovir therapy.
● Stress importance of completing a full course of probenecid with each cidofovir dose. Tell patient to take probenecid after a meal to decrease nausea.
● Advise women of childbearing age to use effective contraception during and for 1 month following treatment with cidofovir.
● Advise men to practice barrier contraception during and for 3 months after treatment with the drug.
● Advise breast-feeding women that it is unknown whether cidofovir is excreted in breast milk.

---

didanosine (ddI)
Videx

Pregnancy Risk Category: B

HOW SUPPLIED
Tablets (buffered, chewable): 25 mg, 50 mg, 100 mg, 150 mg
Powder for oral solution (buffered): 100 mg/packet, 167 mg/packet, 250 mg/packet, 375 mg/packet
Powder for oral solution (pediatric): 10 mg/ml in 2- and 4-g bottles

ACTION
Inhibits the enzyme HIV-RNA-dependent DNA polymerase (reverse transcriptase) and terminates DNA chain growth.

ONSET, PEAK, DURATION
Onset and duration unknown. Peak levels occur in $\frac{1}{2}$ to 1 hour.

INDICATIONS & DOSAGE
Treatment of HIV infection when antiretroviral therapy is warranted—
Adults 60 kg and over: 200 mg (tablets) P.O. q 12 hours; or 250 mg buffered powder P.O. q 12 hours.
Adults less than 60 kg: 125 mg (tablets) P.O. q 12 hours; or 167 mg buffered powder P.O. q 12 hours.
Children: 120 mg/m^2 P.O. q 12 hours.

ADVERSE REACTIONS
CNS: *headache, seizures,* confusion, anxiety, nervousness, abnormal thinking, twitching, depression, *peripheral neuropathy.*
GI: *diarrhea, nausea, vomiting, abdominal pain, pancreatitis,* dry mouth, anorexia.
Hematologic: *leukopenia,* granulocytosis, *thrombocytopenia,* anemia.
Hepatic: *hepatic failure,* elevated liver enzymes.
Skin: rash, pruritus.
Other: asthenia, pain, pneumonia, infection, sarcoma, dyspnea, allergic reactions, myopathy, increased serum uric acid levels, *chills, fever.*

INTERACTIONS
Antacids containing magnesium or aluminum hydroxides: enhanced adverse effects of the antacid component (including diarrhea or constipation) when administered with didanosine tablets or pediatric suspension. Avoid concomitant use.
Dapsone, ketoconazole, drugs that require gastric acid for adequate absorption: decreased absorption from buffering action. Administer these drugs 2 hours before didanosine.
Fluoroquinolones, tetracyclines: decreased absorption from buffering agents in didanosine tablets or antacids in pediatric suspension.
Itraconazole: decreased serum concentrations of itraconazole. Avoid concomitant use.

EFFECTS ON DIAGNOSTIC TESTS
None reported.

CONTRAINDICATIONS
Contraindicated in patients with a history of hypersensitivity to any component of the formulation.

NURSING CONSIDERATIONS
● Use cautiously in patients with a history of pancreatitis; fatalities have occurred. Also use cautiously in patients with peripheral neuropathy, renal or hepatic impairment, or hyperuricemia.
● Administer didanosine on an empty stomach, regardless of the dosage form used; administering the drug with meals can decrease absorption by 50%.
● To administer single-dose packets containing buffered powder for oral solution, pour contents into 4 oz (120 ml) of water. Do not use fruit juice or other beverages that may be acidic. Stir for 2 or 3 minutes until the powder dissolves completely. Administer immediately.
● Keep in mind that in early clinical trials, the powder for oral solution was associated with a high incidence of diarrhea. The manufacturer suggests switching to the tablet formulation if diarrhea is a problem.
Alert: Know that the pediatric powder for oral solution must be prepared by a pharmacist before dispensing. It must be constituted with purified USP water and then diluted with an antacid (either Mylanta Double Strength Liquid or Maalox TC Suspension) to a final concentration of 10 mg/ml. The admixture is stable for 30 days if refrigerated (at 36° to 46° F [2° to 8° C]). Shake the solution well before measuring the dose.

☑ **PATIENT TEACHING**
● Instruct the patient to take drug on an empty stomach.
● Because the tablets contain buffers that raise stomach pH to levels that prevent degradation of the active drug, instruct the patient to chew tablets thoroughly before swallowing and drink at least 1

oz (30 ml) of water with each dose. Teach the patient how to prepare crushed tablets or buffered powder form for ingestion, if appropriate.
● Inform the patient receiving a sodium-restricted diet that each two-tablet dose of didanosine contains 529 mg of sodium; each single packet of buffered powder for oral solution contains 1.38 g of sodium.

___

famciclovir
Famvir

Pregnancy Risk Category: B

HOW SUPPLIED
Tablets: 125 mg, 250 mg, 500 mg

ACTION
A guanosine nucleoside that is converted to penciclovir, which enters viral cells and inhibits DNA polymerase and viral DNA synthesis.

ONSET, PEAK, DURATION
Onset and duration unknown. Serum levels peak within 1 hour.

INDICATIONS & DOSAGE
Acute herpes zoster infection (shingles)—
Adults: 500 mg P.O. q 8 hours for 7 days.

  In patients with reduced renal function: if creatinine clearance is greater than or equal to 60 ml/minute, give 500 mg P.O. q 8 hours; if 40 to 59 ml/minute, 500 mg P.O. q 12 hours; if 20 to 39 ml/minute, 500 mg P.O. q 24 hours; if less than 20 ml/minute, 250 mg P.O. q 48 hours.

  Hemodialysis patients: 250 mg P.O. after each hemodialysis session.
✷New indication: *Recurrent episodes of genital herpes—*
Adults: 125 mg P.O. b.i.d. for 5 days. Therapy begins as soon as symptoms occur.

  In patients with reduced renal func-

___

tion: If creatinine clearance is greater than 40 ml/minute, give 125 mg P.O. q 12 hours; if 20 to 39 ml/minute, 125 mg P.O. q 24 hours; if less than 20 ml/minute, 125 mg P.O. q 48 hours.

Hemodialysis patients: 125 mg P.O. after each hemodialysis session.

ADVERSE REACTIONS
CNS: *headache,* fatigue, dizziness, paresthesia, somnolence.
GI: diarrhea, *nausea,* vomiting, constipation, anorexia, abdominal pain.
Musculoskeletal: back pain, arthralgia.
Respiratory: pharyngitis, sinusitis.
Skin: pruritus; zoster-related signs, symptoms, and complications.

INTERACTIONS
Probenecid: may increase plasma concentrations of famciclovir. Monitor patient for increased adverse effects.

EFFECTS ON DIAGNOSTIC TESTS
None known.

CONTRAINDICATIONS
Contraindicated in patients with hypersensitivity to the drug.

NURSING CONSIDERATIONS
● Use cautiously in patients with renal or hepatic impairment. Know that dosage adjustment may be needed.
● Famciclovir may be taken without regard to meals.

☑ PATIENT TEACHING
● Inform the patient that famciclovir is not a cure for genital herpes but can decrease the length and severity of symptoms.
● Teach the patient how to prevent spread of infection to others.
● Urge the patient to recognize the early symptoms of herpes infection, such as tingling, itching, or pain, and to report them. Treatment is more effective if therapy is started within 48 hours of rash onset.

foscarnet sodium (phosphonoformic acid)
Foscavir

Pregnancy Risk Category: C

HOW SUPPLIED
Injection: 24 mg/ml in 250- and 500-ml bottles

ACTION
Inhibits all known herpesviruses in vitro by blocking the pyrophosphate binding site on DNA polymerases and reverse transcriptases.

ONSET, PEAK, DURATION
Onset and duration are unknown. Peak levels occur immediately after I.V. infusion.

INDICATIONS & DOSAGE
CMV retinitis in patients with AIDS—
Adults: initially, 60 mg/kg I.V. as an induction treatment in patients with normal renal function. Administer I.V. over 1 hour q 8 hours for 2 to 3 weeks, depending on clinical response. Followed with a maintenance infusion of 90 to 120 mg/kg daily, administered over 2 hours. Dosage must be adjusted when creatinine clearance is less than 1.5 ml/minute/kg.

ADVERSE REACTIONS
CNS: *headache,* **seizures,** *fatigue, malaise, asthenia, paresthesia, dizziness, hypoesthesia, neuropathy,* tremor, ataxia, generalized spasms, dementia, stupor, sensory disturbances, meningitis, aphasia, abnormal coordination, EEG abnormalities, depression, confusion, anxiety, insomnia, somnolence, nervousness, amnesia, agitation, aggressive reaction, hallucinations.
CV: *hypertension, palpitations, ECG abnormalities, sinus tachycardia,* cerebrovascular disorder, *first-degree AV block, hypotension, flushing,* edema.
EENT: *visual disturbances,* taste perversion, eye pain, conjunctivitis.

GI: *nausea, diarrhea, vomiting, abdominal pain, anorexia,* constipation, dysphagia, rectal hemorrhage, dry mouth, dyspepsia, melena, flatulence, ulcerative stomatitis, *pancreatitis.*

GU: *abnormal renal function, decreased creatinine clearance and increased serum creatinine levels, albuminuria, dysuria, polyuria, urethral disorder, urine retention, urinary tract infections, acute renal failure,* candidiasis.

Hematologic: *anemia, granulocytopenia, leukopenia, bone marrow suppression, thrombocytopenia,* platelet abnormalities, thrombocytosis, WBC count abnormalities, lymphadenopathy.

Respiratory: *cough, dyspnea,* pneumonitis, sinusitis, pharyngitis, rhinitis, respiratory insufficiency, pulmonary infiltration, stridor, pneumothorax, *bronchospasm,* hemoptysis, flulike symptoms.

Skin: *rash, diaphoresis,* pruritus, skin ulceration, erythematous rash, seborrhea, skin discoloration, facial edema.

Other: *death, fever,* pain, sepsis, hypokalemia, hypomagnesemia, hypophosphatemia or hyperphosphatemia, hypocalcemia, hyponatremia, leg cramps, rigors, inflammation and pain at infusion site, lymphoma-like disorder, sarcoma, back or chest pain, abnormal hepatic function, bacterial or fungal infections, abscess, increased liver enzymes, arthralgia, myalgia.

INTERACTIONS
Nephrotoxic drugs such as amphotericin B, aminoglycosides: increased risk of nephrotoxicity. Avoid concomitant use.
Pentamidine: increased risk of nephrotoxicity; severe hypocalcemia has also been reported. Avoid concomitant use.
Zidovudine: possible increased incidence or severity of anemia. Monitor blood counts.

EFFECTS ON DIAGNOSTIC TESTS
Drug may increase serum bilirubin, alkaline phosphatase, ALT, and AST levels. It may also alter serum creatinine, calcium, phosphate, magnesium, and potassium levels.

CONTRAINDICATIONS
Contraindicated in patients with hypersensitivity to the drug.

NURSING CONSIDERATIONS
• Use cautiously and with reduced dosage in patients with abnormal renal function as ordered. Because foscarnet is nephrotoxic, it has the potential to worsen renal impairment. Some degree of nephrotoxicity occurs in most patients treated with the drug.
• Because the drug is highly toxic and toxicity is probably dose-related, keep in mind that the lowest effective maintenance dose should be used throughout therapy.
• **I.V. use:** Use an infusion pump to administer foscarnet. To minimize renal toxicity, make sure the patient is adequately hydrated before and during the infusion.
Alert: Do not exceed the recommended dosage, infusion rate, or frequency of administration. All doses must be individualized according to the patient's renal function.
• Monitor creatinine clearance frequently during therapy because of the drug's adverse effects on renal function. A baseline 24-hour creatinine clearance is recommended, followed by regular determinations two to three times weekly during induction and at least once every 1 to 2 weeks during maintenance. If creatinine clearance falls below 0.4 ml/minute/kg, drug should be discontinued.
• Because the drug can alter serum electrolytes, monitor levels using a schedule similar to that established for creatinine clearance. Assess the patient for tetany and seizures associated with abnormal electrolyte levels.
• Monitor the patient's hemoglobin and hematocrit levels. Anemia is common (in up to 33% of patients treated with the drug). It may be severe enough to

require transfusions.
• Keep in mind that administration of the drug is associated with a dose-related transient decrease in ionized serum calcium, which may not always be reflected in the patient's laboratory values.

☑ **PATIENT TEACHING**
• Explain to the patient the importance of adequate hydration throughout therapy.
• Advise the patient to report perioral tingling, numbness in the extremities, and paresthesia.
• Instruct the patient to alert the nurse if discomfort occurs at I.V. insertion site.

---

ganciclovir
Cytovene

Pregnancy Risk Category: C

HOW SUPPLIED
Capsules: 250 mg
Injection: 500 mg/vial

ACTION
Inhibits binding of deoxyguanosine triphosphate to DNA polymerase, resulting in inhibition of DNA synthesis.

ONSET, PEAK, DURATION
Onset and duration unknown. Peak serum levels occur immediately after I.V. infusion.

INDICATIONS & DOSAGE
CMV retinitis in immunocompromised individuals, including patients with AIDS and normal renal function—
Adults: induction treatment—5 mg/kg I.V. q 12 hours for 14 to 21 days; maintenance treatment—5 mg/kg I.V. daily for 7 days each week, or 6 mg/kg daily for 5 days each week. Alternatively, 1,000 mg P.O. t.i.d. with food.
Dosage is adjusted for patients with impaired renal function and is based on creatinine clearance levels.

✳*New indication: Prevention of CMV disease in patients with advanced HIV infection and normal renal function—*
Adults: 1,000 mg P.O. t.i.d. with food.
Prevention of CMV disease in transplant recipients with normal renal function—
Adults: 5 mg/kg I.V. (given at a constant rate over 1 hour) q 12 hours for 7 to 14 days, then 5 mg/kg daily for 7 days each week, or 6 mg/kg daily for 5 days each week. Duration of therapy depends on degree of immunosuppression.

ADVERSE REACTIONS
CNS: altered dreams, confusion, ataxia, headache, *seizures, coma,* dizziness, somnolence, tremor, abnormal thinking, agitation, amnesia, anxiety, neuropathy, paresthesia, asthenia.
CV: phlebitis.
GI: *nausea, vomiting, diarrhea, anorexia, abdominal pain,* flatulence, dyspepsia, dry mouth.
GU: *increased serum creatinine levels.*
Hematologic: *agranulocytosis, thrombocytopenia, leukopenia, anemia.*
Other: retinal detachment in CMV retinitis patients; abnormal liver function tests results; *fever;* infection; chills; sepsis; *rash; sweating;* pruritus; pneumonia; at injection site—inflammation, pain, phlebitis.

INTERACTIONS
Cytotoxic agents: increased toxic effects, especially hematologic effects and stomatitis. Monitor closely.
Imipenem/cilastatin: heightened seizure activity with concomitant use. Monitor closely.
Immunosuppressants such as azathioprine, cyclosporine, corticosteroids: enhanced immune and bone marrow suppression. Use together cautiously.
Probenecid: increased ganciclovir blood levels. Monitor closely.
Zidovudine: increased incidence of agranulocytosis with concurrent use. Monitor closely.

EFFECTS ON DIAGNOSTIC TESTS
None reported.

CONTRAINDICATIONS
Contraindicated in patients with hypersensitivity to the drug or acyclovir and in those with an absolute neutrophil count below 500/mm^3 or a platelet count below 25,000/mm^3.

NURSING CONSIDERATIONS
• Use cautiously and in reduced dosage in patients with renal dysfunction.
• Dosage adjustment is necessary in patients with creatinine clearance less than 70 ml/minute.
• **I.V. use:** Administer infusion over at least 1 hour. Too-rapid infusions will result in increased toxicity. Use an infusion pump. Do not administer as an I.V. bolus.
• Use caution when preparing ganciclovir solution, which is alkaline.
Alert: Do not administer S.C. or I.M.
• Because of the frequency of agranulocytosis and thrombocytopenia, obtain neutrophil and platelet counts every 2 days during twice-daily ganciclovir dosing and at least weekly thereafter.

☑ **PATIENT TEACHING**
• Explain to patient the importance of adequate hydration during therapy.
• Instruct patient to report adverse reactions promptly.
• Tell patient to alert the nurse if discomfort occurs at I.V. insertion site.

▼ *NEW DRUG*

---

indinavir sulfate
Crixivan

Pregnancy Risk Category: C

HOW SUPPLIED
Capsules: 200 mg, 400 mg

ACTION
Inhibits HIV protease, enzyme required for the proteolytic cleavage of viral polyprotein precursors into individual functional proteins found in infectious HIV. Indinavir binds to the protease active site and inhibits activity of the enzyme, preventing cleavage of the viral polyproteins and resulting in the formation of immature noninfectious viral particles.

ONSET, PEAK, DURATION
Indinavir plasma concentrations peak in less than 1 hour. Average half-life is 1.8 hours.

INDICATIONS & DOSAGE
Treatment of patients with HIV infection when antiretroviral therapy is warranted—
Adults: 800 mg P.O. q 8 hours. Dosage should be reduced to 600 mg P.O. q 8 hours in mild to moderate hepatic insufficiency due to cirrhosis.

ADVERSE REACTIONS
CNS: headache, insomnia, dizziness, somnolence, asthenia, fatigue.
GI: abdominal pain, *nausea,* diarrhea, vomiting, acid regurgitation, anorexia, dry mouth.
GU: nephrolithiasis.
Hematologic: decreased hemoglobin or neutrophil count.
Other: *hyperbilirubinemia,* flank pain, malaise, back pain, taste perversion, elevation in ALT, AST, and serum amylase levels.

INTERACTIONS
Didanosine: possible degradation of didanosine, formulated with buffering agents to increase pH. If administered concomitantly with indinavir, administer at least 1 hour apart on an empty stomach. Normal gastric pH (acidic) may be necessary for optimum absorption of indinavir but rapidly degrades didanosine
Food: substantially decreased absorption of oral indinavir.
Ketoconazole: increased plasma concentration of indinavir. Dosage reduc-

tion of indinavir to 600 mg P.O. q 8 hours should be considered when they are administered together.

Rifabutin: increased plasma concentrations. Reduce dosage of rifabutin by 50% if administered concomitantly with indinavir.

Rifampin: markedly diminished plasma concentrations of indinavir. Concomitant administration of indinavir and rifampin is not recommended.

Terfenadine, astemizole, cisapride, triazolam, or midazolam: possible inhibition of the metabolism of these drugs as a result of competition for CYP3A4 by indinavir, creating potential for serious or life-threatening events, such as cardiac arrhythmias or prolonged sedation. Do not administer concurrently.

EFFECTS ON DIAGNOSTIC TESTS
None reported.

CONTRAINDICATIONS
Contraindicated in patients with hypersensitivity to any component of the drug.

NURSING CONSIDERATIONS
● Use cautiously in patients with hepatic insufficiency due to cirrhosis.
● Know that drug must be taken at 8-hour intervals.
● Know that drug may cause nephrolithiasis. If signs and symptoms of nephrolithiasis occur, doctor may stop drug for 1 to 3 days during acute phases.
● Be aware that to prevent nephrolithiasis, patient should maintain adequate hydration (at least 48 oz or 1½ L of fluids q 24 hours while on indinavir).
● Know that safety and effectiveness in children have not been established.

☑ **PATIENT TEACHING**
● Tell patient that indinavir is not a cure for HIV infection and that he may continue to develop opportunistic infections and other complications associated with HIV disease. Drug has not been shown to reduce the risk of HIV transmission.

● Instruct patient on use of barrier protection during sexual activity.
● Caution patient not to adjust dosage or discontinue indinavir therapy without first consulting his doctor.
● Advise patient that if a dose of indinavir is missed, he should take the next dose at the regular, scheduled time and should not double the dose.
● Instruct patient to take drug on an empty stomach with water 1 hour before or 2 hours after a meal. Alternatively, he may take it with other liquids (such as skim milk, juice, coffee, or tea) or a light meal.
● Inform patient that a meal high in fat, calories, and protein reduces absorption of drug.
● Instruct patient to store and use capsules in the original container and to keep desiccant in the bottle; capsules are sensitive to moisture.
● Instruct patient to drink at least 48 oz (1.5 L) of fluid daily.
● Advise female patient to avoid breastfeeding because indinavir may be excreted in breast milk. In addition, an HIV-positive woman should not breastfeed to prevent transmitting the virus to the infant.

---

lamivudine
Epivir

Pregnancy Risk Category: C

HOW SUPPLIED
Tablets: 150 mg
Oral solution: 10 mg/ml

ACTION
A synthetic nucleoside analogue that inhibits HIV reverse transcription via viral DNA chain termination. RNA- and DNA-dependent DNA polymerase activities are also inhibited.

ONSET, PEAK, DURATION
Unknown.

INDICATIONS & DOSAGE

Treatment of HIV infection concomitantly with zidovudine—
Adults weighing 50 kg (110 lbs) or more and children 12 years and older: 150 mg P.O. b.i.d.
Adults weighing less than 50 kg (110 lbs): 2 mg/kg P.O. b.i.d.
Children 3 months to 12 years: 4 mg/kg P.O. b.i.d. Maximum dosage is 150 mg b.i.d.

ADVERSE REACTIONS

NOTE: Adverse reactions pertain to the combination therapy of lamivudine and zidovudine.
CNS: *headache, fatigue, neuropathy, dizziness, insomnia and other sleep disorders,* depressive disorders.
GI: *nausea, diarrhea, vomiting, anorexia,* abdominal pain, abdominal cramps, dyspepsia, pancreatitis (in children 3 months to 12 years).
EENT: *nasal symptoms.*
Hematologic: neutropenia, anemia, *thrombocytopenia.*
Respiratory: *cough.*
Skin: rash.
Other: *malaise, fever, chills, musculoskeletal pain,* myalgia, arthralgia, elevated liver enzymes and bilirubin.

INTERACTIONS

Trimethoprim/sulfamethoxazole: may cause increased blood level of lamivudine because of decreased clearance of lamivudine. Monitor patient closely.
Zidovudine: Increased serum zidovudine concentration. Monitor patient closely.

EFFECTS ON DIAGNOSTIC TESTS

None reported.

CONTRAINDICATIONS

Contraindicated in patients with hypersensitivity to the drug.

NURSING CONSIDERATIONS

Alert: Know that this drug should be used with extreme caution, if at all, in pediatric patients with a history of pancreatitis or other significant risk factors for development of pancreatitis. Treatment with lamivudine should be stopped immediately and the doctor notified if clinical signs, symptoms, or laboratory abnormalities suggest pancreatitis.

● Use cautiously in patients with renal impairment. Know that dosage reduction is necessary.
● Breast-feeding should be discontinued if lamivudine is prescribed.
● Drug must be administered concomitantly with zidovudine. It is not currently indicated for use alone.
● Monitor the patient's CBC, platelet count, and liver function studies, as ordered. Report abnormalities.
● Be aware that an Antiretroviral Pregnancy Registry has been established to monitor maternal-fetal outcomes of pregnant women exposed to lamivudine. To register a pregnant patient, the doctor can call 1-800-722-9292, ext. 58465.

☑ PATIENT TEACHING

● Inform the patient that long-term effects of lamivudine are unknown.
● Stress the importance of taking lamivudine exactly as prescribed.
● For a pediatric patient, teach parents the signs and symptoms of pancreatitis, and tell them to report such occurrences immediately.

▼ *NEW DRUG*

nevirapine
Viramune

Pregnancy Risk Category: C

HOW SUPPLIED

Tablets: 200 mg

ACTION

Binds directly to reverse transcriptase and blocks RNA-dependent and DNA-dependent DNA polymerase activities by causing a disruption of the enzyme's catalytic site.

ONSET, PEAK, DURATION
Onset and duration unknown. Peak plasma concentrations occur 4 hours following a single 200-mg dose.

INDICATIONS & DOSAGE
Adjunct treatment in patients with HIV-1 infection who have experienced clinical or immunologic deterioration—
Adults: 200 mg P.O. daily for the first 14 days, followed by 200 mg P.O. b.i.d. Used in combination with nucleoside analog antiretroviral agents.

ADVERSE REACTIONS
CNS: headache, paresthesia.
GI: *nausea,* diarrhea, abdominal pain, ulcerative stomatitis.
Hematologic: *decreased neutrophil count,* decreased hemoglobin.
Hepatic: hepatitis, increased ALT, AST, gamma-glutamyl transpeptidase (GGT), and total bilirubin levels.
Skin: *rash, blistering, Stevens-Johnson syndrome.*
Other: *fever,* myalgia

INTERACTIONS
Drugs extensively metabolized by P450 CYP3A: may lower plasma concentration of these drugs, requiring dosage adjustment.
Protease inhibitors, oral contraceptives, other hormonal contraceptives: may decrease plasma concentrations of these drugs; do not administer concomitantly.
Rifabutin, rifampin: more data needed to assess whether dosage adjustments are necessary. When administering concurrently with nevirapine, monitor closely.

EFFECTS ON DIAGNOSTIC TESTS
None reported.

CONTRAINDICATIONS
Contraindicated in patients with hypersensitivity to drug.

NURSING CONSIDERATIONS
● Use cautiously in patients with impaired renal and hepatic function; pharmacokinetics have not been evaluated in those patients.
● Know that clinical chemistry tests, including liver function tests, should be performed before initiating and regularly throughout therapy.
● Know that drug should be used in conjunction with at least one additional antiretroviral agent.
Alert: Monitor patient for blistering, oral lesions, conjunctivitis, muscle or joint aches, or general malaise. Be especially alert for a severe rash or rash accompanied by fever. Report such signs and symptoms to doctor. Patients who experience a rash during the initial 14 days of therapy should not have the dosage increased until the rash has resolved. Most rashes occur within the first 6 weeks of therapy.
● Know that moderate and severe liver function test abnormalities may warrant temporary discontinuance of therapy; drug may be restarted at half the previous dose level as ordered.
● Know that patients who have nevirapine therapy interrupted for more than 7 days should restart therapy as if receiving drug for the first time.
● Know that antiretroviral therapy may be changed if disease progression occurs while a patient is receiving nevirapine.
● Know that safety and effectiveness in children have not been established.
● Be aware that nevirapine is excreted in breast milk.

☑ PATIENT TEACHING
● Inform the patient that nevirapine is not a cure for HIV and that illnesses associated with advanced HIV-1 infection may still occur. Explain that drug does not reduce risk of HIV-1 transmission.
● Instruct patient to report rash immediately and to discontinue drug until told to resume.
● Stress importance of taking drug ex-

actly as prescribed. If a dose is missed, tell patient to take the next dose as soon as possible. If a dose is skipped, patient should not double next dose.

● Tell patient not to use other medications unless approved by a doctor.

● Advise women of childbearing age that oral contraceptives and other hormonal methods of birth control should not be used with nevirapine.

● Advise women to avoid breast-feeding while taking drug to reduce risk of postnatal HIV transmission.

---

ribavirin
Virazole

Pregnancy Risk Category: X

HOW SUPPLIED
Powder to be reconstituted for inhalation: 6 g in 100-ml glass vial

ACTION
Inhibits viral activity by an unknown mechanism, possibly by inhibiting RNA and DNA synthesis by depleting intracellular nucleotide pools.

ONSET, PEAK, DURATION
Onset, peak, and duration are unknown.

INDICATIONS & DOSAGE
Hospitalized infants and young children infected by respiratory syncytial virus (RSV)—

Infants and young children: solution in concentration of 20 mg/ml delivered via the Viratek Small Particle Aerosol Generator (SPAG-2) and mechanical ventilator or oxygen hood, face mask, or oxygen tent at a rate of about 12.5 liters of mist per minute. Treatment is carried out for 12 to 18 hours/day for at least 3 days, and no more than 7 days.

ADVERSE REACTIONS
CV: *cardiac arrest*, hypotension.
EENT: conjunctivitis.
Hematologic: reticulocytosis.

Respiratory: worsening respiratory state, apnea, bacterial pneumonia, pneumothorax.
Other: rash or erythema of eyelids.

INTERACTIONS
None significant.

EFFECTS ON DIAGNOSTIC TESTS
None reported.

CONTRAINDICATIONS
Contraindicated in patients with hypersensitivity to the drug. Know that although the drug is used in children, manufacturer states that it's also contraindicated in women who are or may become pregnant during treatment.

NURSING CONSIDERATIONS
● Administer ribavirin aerosol by the Viratek Small Particle Aerosol Generator (SPAG-2) only. Don't use any other aerosol-generating device.

● Use sterile USP water for injection, *not* bacteriostatic water. Water used to reconstitute this drug must not contain any antimicrobial agent.

● Discard solutions placed in the SPAG-2 unit at least every 24 hours before adding newly reconstituted solution.

● The most frequent adverse effects reported in health care personnel exposed to aerosolized ribavirin include eye irritation and headache.

Alert: Monitor ventilator function frequently. Ribavirin may precipitate in ventilator apparatus, causing equipment malfunction with serious consequences.

● Store reconstituted solutions at room temperature for 24 hours.

● Keep in mind that ribavirin aerosol is indicated only for severe lower respiratory tract infection caused by RSV. Although treatment may begin while awaiting diagnostic test results, existence of RSV infection must eventually be documented.

● Be aware that most infants and children with RSV infection don't require treatment because the disease is com-

---

Reactions may be *common*, uncommon, *life-threatening*, or COMMON AND LIFE-THREATENING.

monly mild and self-limiting. Infants with underlying conditions, such as prematurity or cardiopulmonary disease, get RSV in its severest form and benefit most from treatment with ribavirin aerosol.

☑ PATIENT TEACHING
● Inform parents of need for drug and answer any questions.
● Encourage parents to report any subtle change in child immediately to nurse.

---

rimantadine hydrochloride
Flumadine

Pregnancy Risk Category: C

HOW SUPPLIED
Tablets (film-coated): 100 mg
Syrup: 50 mg/5 ml

ACTION
Unknown. Appears to prevent viral uncoating, an early step in virus reproductive cycle.

ONSET, PEAK, DURATION
Onset and duration unknown. Peak plasma levels occur in 1 to 4 hours.

INDICATIONS & DOSAGE
Prophylaxis of influenza A—
Adults and children 10 years and over: 100 mg P.O. b.i.d.
Children under 10 years: 5 mg/kg (not to exceed 150 mg) P.O. once a day.
Elderly patients, patients with severe hepatic or renal dysfunction, or those experiencing adverse effects with normal dosage: 100 mg P.O. daily.

Prophylaxis should begin as soon as possible after initial exposure and should be continued through course of influenza A outbreak. Safety of prolonged therapy over 6 months has not been established. Can be used for prophylaxis in children up to 6 weeks after first dose of influenza vaccine or until 2 weeks after second dose of vaccine.

Treatment of influenza A—
Adults: 100 mg P.O. b.i.d. initiated within 24 to 48 hours after onset of symptoms and continued for 48 hours after symptoms disappear (usually 7-day total course).

ADVERSE REACTIONS
CNS: insomnia, headache, dizziness, nervousness, fatigue, asthenia.
GI: nausea, vomiting, anorexia, dry mouth, abdominal pain.

INTERACTIONS
Acetaminophen, aspirin: reduced concentration of rimantadine. Monitor for decreased effectiveness of rimantadine.
Cimetidine: may decrease clearance of rimantadine. Monitor for adverse reactions.

EFFECTS ON DIAGNOSTIC TESTS
None reported.

CONTRAINDICATIONS
Contraindicated in patients with hypersensitivity to the drug or amantadine.

NURSING CONSIDERATIONS
● Use cautiously in patients with renal or hepatic impairment and in patients with a history of seizures. Pregnant patients should consider the risks compared to the benefits before taking this drug.
● Consider the risk to contacts of treated patients who may be subject to morbidity from influenza A. Influenza A-resistant strains can emerge during therapy. Patients taking the drug may still be able to spread the disease.

☑ PATIENT TEACHING
● Instruct the patient to take drug several hours before bedtime to prevent insomnia.
● Inform the patient that he may still be able to infect others with influenza A and to take infection-control precautions.

---

*Liquid contains alcohol.   **May contain tartrazine.   †Canada only.   ‡Australia only.   ◇ OTC.

▼ *NEW DRUG*

ritonavir
Norvir

Pregnancy Risk Category: B

HOW SUPPLIED
Capsules: 100 mg
Oral solution: 80 mg/ml

ACTION
An HIV protease inhibitor with activity against HIV-1 and HIV-2 proteases. HIV protease is an enzyme required for the proteolytic cleavage of viral polyprotein precursors into the individual functional proteins in infectious HIV. Ritonavir binds to the protease active site and inhibits activity of the enzyme, preventing cleavage of the viral polyproteins and resulting in the formation of immature noninfectious viral particles.

ONSET, PEAK, DURATION
Ritonavir is well absorbed following oral administration, Onset is unknown, but drug peaks within 2 to 4 hours. Plasma half-life averages 3 to 5 hours.

INDICATIONS & DOSAGE
Treatment of HIV infection in combination with nucleoside analogues or as monotherapy when antiretroviral therapy is warranted—
Adults: 600 mg P.O. b.i.d with meals. If nausea occurs, increased dosage may provide some relief: 300 mg b.i.d. for 1 day, 400 mg b.i.d. for 2 days, 500 mg b.i.d. for 1 day, and then 600 mg b.i.d. thereafter.

ADVERSE REACTIONS
CNS: *asthenia,* headache, malaise, circumoral paresthesia, dizziness, insomnia, paresthesia, peripheral paresthesia, somnolence, thinking abnormality, *taste perversion,* migraine headache.
CV: vasodilation.
GI: abdominal pain, anorexia, constipa-tion, *diarrhea, nausea, vomiting,* dyspepsia, flatulence.
Musculoskeletal: myalgia.
Respiratory: pharyngitis.
Skin: rash, sweating.
Other: fever, local throat irritation, increased CK level, hyperlipidemia.

INTERACTIONS
Agents that increase CYP3A activity (for example, phenobarbital, carbamazepine, dexamethasone, phenytoin, rifampin, rifabutin): may increase clearance of ritonavir, resulting in decreased ritonavir plasma concentrations. Monitor patient closely.
Alprazolam, clorazepate, diazepam, estazolam, flurazepam, midazolam, triazolam, and zolpidem: significantly increased levels of these drugs. Because of the potential for extreme sedation and respiratory depression, these agents should not be administered concurrently with ritonavir.
Amiodarone, astemizole, bepridil, bupropion, cisapride, clozapine, encainide, flecainide, meperidine, piroxicam, propafenone, propoxyphene, quinidine, rifabutin,terfenadine: significantly increased plasma concentrations of these drugs, which increases patient's risk of arrhythmias, hematologic abnormalities, seizures, or other potentially serious adverse effects. Do not administer drug concurrently.
Clarithromycin: reduced creatinine clearance. Patients with impaired renal function receiving drug concomitantly with ritonavir require a 50% reduction in clarithromycin dose if creatinine clearance is 30 to 60 ml/minute and a 75% reduction if it is below 30 ml/minute.
Desipramine: increased overall serum concentrations of desipramine. Concomitant administration may require a dosage adjustment when administered with ritonavir. Monitor patient.
Directly glucuronidated agents: ritonavir may increase activity of glucoronosyl transferases with loss of therapeutic effects from these agents; may signify

---

Reactions may be *common,* uncommon, ***life-threatening***, or COMMON AND LIFE-THREATENING.

need for dosage alteration of these agents. Concomitant use should be accompanied by therapeutic drug concentration monitoring and increased monitoring of therapeutic and adverse effects, especially for agents with narrow therapeutic margins, such as oral anticoagulants and immunosuppressants. Dosage reduction greater than 50% may be required for agents extensively metabolized by CYP3A.

Disulfiram or other drugs that produce disulfiram-like reactions such as metronidazole: increased risk of disulfiram-like reactions. Ritonavir formulations contain alcohol that can produce reactions when co-administered. Monitor patient.

Oral contraceptives containing ethinyl estradiol: decreased overall serum concentrations of the contraceptive. Advise patient that concomitant therapy may require a dosage increase in the oral contraceptive or use of other contraceptive measures.

Saquinivir: inhibited metabolism of saquinivir, resulting in greatly increased plasma levels. The safety of this combination has not been established.

Theophylline: decreased overall serum concentrations of theophylline. Increased dosage may be required when coadministered with ritonavir. Monitor level.

Tobacco: decreased overall serum concentrations of ritonavir. Advise against tobacco use.

EFFECTS ON DIAGNOSTIC TESTS
Ritonavir may alter triglyceride, AST, ALT, gamma-glutamytransferase (GGT), CK, and uric acid levels, as well as alkaine phosphatase, total bilirubin, glucose, potassium, hemoglobin, and hematocrit levels; RBC and WBC counts; neutrophil and eosinophil levels; and PT.

CONTRAINDICATIONS
Contraindicated in patients with hypersensitivity to any component of drug.

NURSING CONSIDERATIONS
● Use cautiously in patients with hepatic insufficiency.
● Know that drug may be administered alone or in combination with nucleoside analogs.
● Know that patients beginning combination regimens with ritonavir and nucleosides may improve GI tolerance by starting ritonavir alone and subsequently adding nucleosides before completing 2 weeks of ritonavir.
● Be aware that safety and effectiveness in children under 12 years have not been established.
● Be aware that it is not known whether ritonavir is excreted in breast milk

☑ PATIENT TEACHING
● Inform patient that drug is not a cure for HIV infection. Patient may continue to develop opportunistic infections and other complications associated with HIV infection. Drug has not been shown to reduce the risk of transmitting HIV to others through sexual contact or blood contamination.
● Caution patient to take drug as prescribed and not to adjust dosage or discontinue therapy without first consulting the doctor.
● Tell patient he may improve the taste of ritonavir oral solution by mixing it with chocolate milk, Ensure, or Advera within 1 hour of the scheduled dose.
● Instruct patient to take drug with a meal to improve absorption.
● Tell patient that if a dose is missed, he should take the next dose as soon as possible. If a dose is skipped, he should not double the next dose.
● Advise patient to report use of other medications, including nonprescription drugs; ritonavir interacts with some drugs when taken together.
● Advise breast-feeding women not to breast-feed, to prevent transmission of infection.

saquinavir mesylate
Invirase

Pregnancy Risk Category: B

HOW SUPPLIED
Capsules: 200 mg

ACTION
Inhibits the activity of HIV protease and prevents the cleavage of HIV polyproteins, which are essential for HIV maturation.

ONSET, PEAK, DURATION
Unknown.

INDICATIONS & DOSAGE
Adjunct treatment of advanced HIV infection in selected patients—
Adults: 600 mg P.O. t.i.d. taken within 2 hours after a full meal and in combination with a nucleoside analogue, such as zalcitabine at a dosage of 0.75 mg P.O. t.i.d. or zidovudine at a dosage of 200 mg P.O. t.i.d.

ADVERSE REACTIONS
CNS: paresthesia, headache.
GI: diarrhea, ulcerated buccal mucosa, abdominal pain, nausea.
Other: asthenia, rash, musculoskeletal pain.

INTERACTIONS
Astemizole, terfenadine: increased serum levels of these drugs and increased risk of arrhythmias and sudden death. Avoid concomitant use.
Ketoconazole, ritonavir: increased serum saquinavir concentrations. Monitor patient closely.
Phenobarbital, phenytoin, rifabutin, rifampin: reduces the steady state concentration of saquinavir. Use together cautiously.

EFFECTS ON DIAGNOSTIC TESTS
None reported.

CONTRAINDICATIONS
Contraindicated in patients with hypersensitivity to the drug or to any component contained in the capsule.

NURSING CONSIDERATIONS
● Safety of drug is not established in pregnant or breast-feeding women or in children under 16 years.
● CBC, platelets, electrolytes, uric acid, liver enzymes, and bilirubin should be evaluated before therapy begins and at appropriate intervals throughout therapy, as ordered.
● Be aware that if serious toxicity occurs during treatment, saquinavir should be discontinued until the etiology of the event is identified or the toxicity resolves. When drug is resumed, it may be done with no dosage modifications.
● Monitor patient's hydration if adverse GI reactions occur.
● Notify doctor if adverse reactions occur. Obtain an order for a mild analgesic if drug causes headache, an antiemetic if drug causes nausea, or an antidiarrheal agent if drug causes diarrhea.
● Be alert for adverse reactions associated with adjunct therapy (zidovudine or zalcitabine).

☑ PATIENT TEACHING
● Advise the patient to take drug within 2 hours after a full meal.
● Inform the patient that drug is usually administered with other AIDS-related antiviral agents.
● Instruct the patient to take the drug around the clock, not missing any doses, to decrease the risk of developing HIV resistance.

stavudine (2,3 didehydro-3-deoxythymidine, d4T)
Zerit

Pregnancy Risk Category: C

HOW SUPPLIED
Capsules: 15 mg, 20 mg, 30 mg, 40 mg

Reactions may be *common*, uncommon, *life-threatening*, or COMMON AND LIFE-THREATENING.

ACTION
A primidine nucleoside analogue that prevents replication of retroviruses, including HIV, by inhibiting the enzyme reverse transcriptase and causing termination of DNA chain growth.

ONSET, PEAK, DURATION
Onset and duration unknown. Serum levels peak within 1 hour.

INDICATIONS & DOSAGE
✳ *New indication: Treatment of HIV-infected patients who have received prolonged prior zidovudine therapy—*
Adults weighing 60 kg or more: 40 mg P.O. q 12 hours.
Adults weighing less than 60 kg: 30 mg P.O. q 12 hours.
Children: 2 mg/kg/day P.O. in divided doses q 12 hours for children weighing under 30 kg; adult dose should be used for children weighing 30 kg or more.

ADVERSE REACTIONS
CNS: *peripheral neuropathy, headache, malaise, insomnia, anxiety, depression, nervousness,* dizziness.
CV: chest pain.
GI: *abdominal pain, diarrhea, nausea, vomiting, anorexia,* dyspepsia, constipation, weight loss.
Hematologic: *neutropenia, **thrombocytopenia,*** anemia.
Skin: *rash, diaphoresis, pruritus,* maculopapular rash.
Other: *myalgia, hepatotoxicity, chills, fever, asthenia, back pain, arthralgia, dyspnea,* conjunctivitis.

INTERACTIONS
Myelosuppressants: additive myelosuppression. Avoid concurrent use.

EFFECTS ON DIAGNOSTIC TESTS
Stavudine may cause a mild to moderate increase in AST and ALT levels.

CONTRAINDICATIONS
Contraindicated in patients with hypersensitivity to the drug.

NURSING CONSIDERATIONS
● Use cautiously in patients with renal impairment or history of peripheral neuropathy. Dosage adjustment is necessary for creatinine clearance less than 50 ml/minute; dosage adjustment or discontinuation is necessary in onset of peripheral neuropathy. Also use cautiously in pregnant women.
Alert: Know that peripheral neuropathy appears to be the major dose-limiting adverse effect of stavudine. It may or may not resolve after drug is discontinued.
● Monitor CBC and serum levels of creatinine, AST, ALT, and alkaline phosphatase, as ordered.

☑ PATIENT TEACHING
● Tell the patient that the drug may be taken without regard to meals.
● Warn the patient not to take any other drugs for HIV or AIDS unless the doctor has approved them.
● Teach the patient signs and symptoms of peripheral neuropathy—pain, burning, aching, weakness, or pins and needles in the extremities—and tell him to report these immediately.

valacyclovir hydrochloride
Valtrex

Pregnancy Risk Category: B

HOW SUPPLIED
Tablets: 500 mg

ACTION
Rapidly converts to acyclovir, which in turn becomes incorporated into viral DNA thereby terminating growth of the DNA chain and inhibits viral DNA polymerase, causing inhibition of viral replication.

ONSET, PEAK, DURATION
Onset occurs about 30 minutes after oral administration. Peak and duration are unknown.

INDICATIONS & DOSAGE

Herpes zoster infection (shingles)—
Adults: 1 g P.O. t.i.d. for 7 days. Dosage is adjusted for patients with impaired renal function based on creatinine clearance level. For creatinine clearance greater than 50 ml/minute, use regular dose; for 30 to 49 ml/minute, use 1 g P.O. q 12 hours; for 10 to 29 ml/minute, use 1 g P.O. q 24 hours; for less than 10 ml/minute, use 500 mg P.O. q 24 hours.
Hemodialysis patients: 1 g P.O. after hemodialysis.
✳ *New indications: For initial episode of genital herpes—*
Adults: 1 g P.O. b.i.d. for 10 days. For patients with creatinine clearance of 30 ml/minute or greater, dosage is 1 g P.O. q 12 hours; for 10 to 29 ml/minute, 1 g P.O. q 24 hours; for below 10 ml/minute, 500 mg P.O. q 24 hours.
Hemodialysis patients: 1 g P.O. after hemodialysis.
Recurrent genital herpes—
Adults: 500 mg P.O. b.i.d. for 5 days, given at the first sign or symptom of an episode. For patients with creatinine clearance of 30 ml/minute or greater, dosage is 500 mg P.O. q 12 hours; for 29 ml/minute or less, 500 mg P.O. q 24 hours.
Hemodialysis patients: 500 mg P.O. after hemodialysis.

ADVERSE REACTIONS

CNS: *headache,* dizziness.
GI: *nausea,* vomiting, diarrhea, constipation, abdominal pain, anorexia.
Other: asthenia.

INTERACTIONS

Cimetidine, probenecid: reduces the rate but not the extent of conversion of valacyclovir to acyclovir and reduces the renal clearance of acyclovir, thus increasing acyclovir blood levels. Monitor for possible toxicity.

EFFECTS ON DIAGNOSTIC TESTS

None reported.

CONTRAINDICATIONS

Contraindicated in patients with hypersensitivity or intolerance to valacyclovir, acyclovir, or any component of the formulation.

NURSING CONSIDERATIONS

● Know that valacyclovir is not recommended for use in patients with HIV or bone marrow or organ transplant recipients. Thrombotic thrombocytopenic purpura and hemolytic uremic syndrome have occurred, resulting in death in some patients with advanced HIV disease and in bone marrow transplant and renal transplant recipients participating in clinical trials of valacyclovir.
● Use cautiously in patients with renal impairment, the elderly, and those receiving other nephrotoxic drugs.
● Safety and efficacy in children have not been established.
● Glaxo-Wellcome, the manufacturer, maintains an ongoing registry of women exposed to the drug during pregnancy. Use during pregnancy should only be considered if the benefits outweigh the risks. Health care providers are encouraged to report such exposures to the registrar at 1-800-722-9292, ext 58465.
● Alert the doctor if the patient is breast-feeding; the drug may need to be discontinued.
● Although there have been no reports of overdosage, precipitation of acyclovir in renal tubules may occur when solubility (2.5 mg/ml) is exceeded in the intratubular fluid. With acute renal failure and anuria, the patient may benefit from hemodialysis until renal function is restored.

☑ PATIENT TEACHING

● Inform the patient that valacyclovir may be taken without regard to meals.
● Teach the patient the signs and symptoms of herpes infection (rash, tingling, itching, and pain), and advise him to notify the doctor immediately if they occur. Treatment should be initiated as soon as possible after symptoms appear,

---

Reactions may be *common*, uncommon, *life-threatening*, or COMMON AND LIFE-THREATENING.

preferably within 48 hours of the onset of zoster rash.
● Inform patient that valacyclovir is not a cure for herpes but may decrease the length and severity of symptoms.

---

zalcitabine (dideoxycytidine, ddC)
Hivid

Pregnancy Risk Category: C

HOW SUPPLIED
Tablets: 0.375 mg, 0.75 mg

ACTION
Inhibits replication of HIV by blocking viral DNA synthesis.

ONSET, PEAK, DURATION
Onset and duration unknown. Peak plasma levels occur 1 to 2 hours after an oral dose.

INDICATIONS & DOSAGE
Monotherapy for treatment of advanced HIV disease in patients who either cannot tolerate zidovudine or who have disease progression while receiving zidovudine—
Adults and children 13 years or older: 0.75 mg P.O. q 8 hours.
Combination therapy with zidovudine for treatment of advanced HIV disease (CD4$^+$ cell count equal to or less than 300 cells /mm^3)—
Adults and children 13 years or older: 0.75 mg P.O. q 8 hours administered concomitantly with zidovudine 200 mg P.O. q 8 hours.

ADVERSE REACTIONS
CNS: *peripheral neuropathy, headache, fatigue,* dizziness, confusion, ***seizures,*** impaired concentration, amnesia, insomnia, mental depression, tremor, hypertonia, anxiety.
EENT: pharyngitis, cough, ocular pain, abnormal vision, ototoxicity, nasal discharge.

GI: nausea, vomiting, diarrhea, abdominal pain, anorexia, constipation, stomatitis, esophageal ulcer, glossitis, ***pancreatitis.***
Hematologic: anemia, neutropenia, leukopenia, ***thrombocytopenia.***
Skin: pruritus; night sweats; *erythematous, maculopapular, or follicular rash;* urticaria.
Other: myalgia, arthralgia, *fever,* hypoglycemia, increased liver enzymes.

INTERACTIONS
Aminoglycosides, amphotericin B, foscarnet, and other drugs that may impair renal function: increased risk of nephrotoxicity. Avoid concomitant use when possible.
Chloramphenicol, cisplatin, dapsone, didanosine, disulfiram, ethionamide, glutethimide, gold salts, hydralazine, iodoquinol, isoniazid, metronidazole, nitrofurantoin, phenytoin, ribavirin, and vincristine as well as other drugs that can cause peripheral neuropathy: increased risk of peripheral neuropathy. Avoid concomitant use.
Pentamidine: increased risk of pancreatitis. Avoid concomitant use when possible.
Cimetidine, probenecid: increased serum zalcitabine levels. Monitor the patient carefully.

EFFECTS ON DIAGNOSTIC TESTS
Toxic effects of the drug may cause abnormalities in several laboratory tests, including CBC; hemoglobin; leukocyte, reticulocyte, granulocyte, and platelet counts; and AST, ALT, and alkaline phosphatase levels.

CONTRAINDICATIONS
Contraindicated in patients with hypersensitivity to the drug or any component of the formulation.

NURSING CONSIDERATIONS
● Use with extreme caution in patients with preexisting peripheral neuropathy.
● Use cautiously in patients with renal

---

*Liquid contains alcohol.   **May contain tartrazine.   †Canada only.   ‡Australia only.   ◊ OTC.

impairment (creatinine clearance below 40 ml/minute) because they may be at increased risk for toxicity to the drug. Dosage adjustments are necessary. Also use cautiously in patients with hepatic failure, history of pancreatitis, baseline cardiomyopathy, or history of CHF.

● Do not administer the drug with food because it decreases the rate and extent of absorption.

● Assess for signs of peripheral neuropathy, characterized by numbness and burning in the extremities, which are the major toxic effects of the drug. If drug isn't withdrawn, peripheral neuropathy can progress to sharp shooting pain or severe continuous burning pain requiring opioid analgesics. It may or may not be reversible.

● If the patient experiences symptoms that resemble peripheral neuropathy, prepare to withdraw the drug, as ordered. It should be discontinued if symptoms are bilateral and persist beyond 72 hours. If symptoms persist or worsen beyond 1 week, drug should be permanently discontinued. However, if all findings relevant to peripheral neuropathy have resolved to minor symptoms, the drug may be reintroduced at 0.375 mg P.O. q 8 hours.

☑ **PATIENT TEACHING**
● Instruct the patient to take drug on an empty stomach.

● Make sure the patient understands that the drug doesn't cure HIV infection and that opportunistic infections may still occur despite continued use. Review safe sex practices with the patient.

● Inform the patient that peripheral neuropathy is the major toxicity associated with this drug and that pancreatitis is the major life-threatening toxic reaction. Review the signs and symptoms of these adverse reactions, and instruct the patient to call the doctor promptly if any appear.

● Instruct the patient of childbearing age to use an effective contraceptive while taking this drug.

zidovudine
(azidothymidine, AZT)
Apo-Zidovudine†, Novo-AZT†, Retrovir

Pregnancy Risk Category: C

HOW SUPPLIED
Capsules: 100 mg
Tablets: 300 mg
Syrup: 50 mg/5 ml
Injection: 10 mg/ml

ACTION
Inhibits replication of HIV by blocking DNA synthesis.

ONSET, PEAK, DURATION
Onset unknown after oral administration. Peak plasma levels occur in $\frac{1}{2}$ to $1\frac{1}{2}$ hours. Duration unknown.

INDICATIONS & DOSAGE
Symptomatic HIV infection, including AIDS—
Adults and children 12 years and over: 100 mg P.O. q 4 hours around the clock or 300 mg (1 tablet) P.O. q 12 hours.
Children 3 months to 12 years: 180 mg/m^2 P.O. q 6 hours (720 mg/m^2/ day), not to exceed 200 mg q 6 hours.
Asymptomatic HIV infection—
Adults and children 12 years and over: 100 mg P.O. q 4 hours while awake (500 mg daily).
Children 3 months to 12 years: 180 mg/m^2 P.O. q 6 hours (720 mg/m^2/ day), not to exceed 200 mg q 6 hours.
To reduce risk of transmission of HIV from infected mother with a baseline CD4$^+$ lymphocyte count greater than 200 cells/mm^3 to the newborn—
Adults: 100 mg P.O. 5 times daily given initially between 14 and 34 weeks' gestation and continued throughout pregnancy. During labor, administer loading dose of 2 mg/kg I.V. over 1 hour followed by continuous I.V. infusion of 1 mg/kg/hour until umbilical cord is

clamped.

Neonates: 2 mg/kg P.O. (syrup) q 6 hours for 6 weeks, beginning within 12 hours after birth. Or, 1.5 mg/kg I.V. q 6 hours.

Combination therapy with zalcitabine or other antiretroviral agents for treatment of advanced HIV disease—

Adults and children 13 years or older: 200 mg P.O. q 8 hours or 300 mg (1 tablet) P.O. q 12 hours administered concomitantly with zalcitabine 0.75 mg P.O. q 8 hours or other antiretroviral agents.

ADVERSE REACTIONS
CNS: *headache,* **seizures,** *paresthesia, malaise,* insomnia, *dizziness,* somnolence.
GI: *nausea, anorexia, abdominal pain, vomiting,* constipation, *diarrhea,* dyspepsia.
Hematologic: *severe bone marrow suppression (resulting in anemia), agranulocytosis, thrombocytopenia.*
Skin: *rash.*
Other: myalgia, diaphoresis, *fever, asthenia,* taste perversion.

INTERACTIONS
Acetaminophen, aspirin, co-trimoxazole, indomethacin: may impair hepatic metabolism of zidovudine, increasing the drug's toxicity. Monitor closely.
Acyclovir: possible seizures, lethargy, and fatigue. Use together cautiously.
Amphotericin B, dapsone, flucytosine, pentamidine: increased risk of nephrotoxicity and bone marrow suppression. Monitor closely.
Ganciclovir: increased risk of hematologic toxicity. Monitor closely.
Other cytotoxic drugs: additive adverse effects on the bone marrow. Avoid concomitant use.
Probenecid: may decrease the renal clearance of zidovudine. Avoid concomitant use.
Ribavirin: antagonizes the antiviral activity of zidovudine against HIV. Avoid concomitant use.

EFFECTS ON DIAGNOSTIC TESTS
Zidovudine may cause depression of formed elements (erythrocytes, leukocytes, and platelets) in peripheral blood.

CONTRAINDICATIONS
Contraindicated in patients with hypersensitivity to the drug.

NURSING CONSIDERATIONS
● Use cautiously and with close monitoring in patients with advanced symptomatic HIV infection and in patients with severe bone marrow depression.
● Use with caution in any patient with hepatomegaly, hepatitis, or other known risk factors for liver disease and in patients with renal insufficiency. Dosage must be adjusted in end-stage renal disease.
● **I.V. use:** Dilute before administration. Remove the calculated dose from the vial; add to D_5W to achieve a concentration that does not exceed 4 mg/ml. Infuse drug over 1 hour at a constant rate. Avoid rapid infusion or bolus injection. Adding mixture to biological or colloidal fluids (for example, blood products, protein solutions) is not recommended. After drug is diluted, the solution is physically and chemically stable for 24 hours at room temperature and for 48 hours if refrigerated at 35.6° to 46.4°F (2° to 8° C) to minimize the risk of microbial contamination. Store undiluted vials at 59° to 77° F (15° to 25° C) and protect them from light.
● Monitor blood studies every 2 weeks, as ordered, to detect anemia or agranulocytosis. Patients may require dosage reduction or temporary discontinuation of the drug.
● Be aware that zidovudine may temporarily decrease morbidity and mortality in certain patients with AIDS.

☑ PATIENT TEACHING
● Tell patient to take drug exactly as directed and not to share it with others.
● Instruct patient to take drug on an empty stomach. To avoid esophageal ir-

---

*Liquid contains alcohol.   **May contain tartrazine.   †Canada only.   ‡Australia only.   ◇OTC.

ritation, tell patient to take drug while sitting upright and with adequate amount of fluids.

● Remind patient that he *must* comply with the dosage schedule. Suggest ways to avoid missing doses, perhaps by using an alarm clock.

● Advise patient that blood transfusions may be needed during treatment. Zidovudine frequently causes a low RBC count.

● Warn patient not to take any other drugs for AIDS unless the doctor has approved them.

● Advise pregnant, HIV-infected patient that zidovudine therapy only *reduces* the risk of HIV transmission to her newborn. Long-term risks to infants are unknown.

● Advise health care workers who consider zidovudine prophylaxis after occupational exposure (following needlestick injury, for example) that animal and human studies have not yet proved the drug's safety or efficacy.

18

Macrolide anti-infectives

azithromycin
clarithromycin
dirithromycin
erythromycin base
erythromycin estolate
erythromycin ethylsuccinate
erythromycin lactobionate
erythromycin stearate

COMBINATION PRODUCTS
None.

---

azithromycin
Zithromax

Pregnancy Risk Category: B

HOW SUPPLIED
Capsules: 250 mg; Z-pak (contains 5
days of therapy)
Oral suspension: 100 mg/5ml, 200
mg/5ml
Single-dose powder for oral suspension:
1 g
Tablets: 250 mg, 600 mg

ACTION
Binds to the 50S subunit of bacterial ribosomes, blocking protein synthesis;
bacteriostatic or bactericidal, depending
on concentration.

ONSET, PEAK, DURATION
Onset and duration unknown. Serum
levels peak in young patients in 2.5 to
3.2 hours, in elderly patients in 3.8 to
4.4 hours.

INDICATIONS & DOSAGE
*Acute bacterial exacerbations of COPD
caused by* Haemophilus influenzae,
Moraxella (Branhamella) catarrhalis, *or*
Streptococcus pneumoniae; *mild com-
munity-acquired pneumonia caused by*
H. influenzae *or* S. pneumoniae; *un-*

*complicated skin and skin-structure in-
fections caused by* Staphylococcus aureus, Streptococcus pyogenes, *or* S.
agalactiae; *second-line therapy of
pharyngitis or tonsillitis caused by* S.
pyogenes—
**Adults and adolescents 16 years and
over:** 500 mg P.O. as a single dose on
day 1, followed by 250 mg daily on
days 2 through 5. Total dose is 1.5 g.
*Nongonococcal urethritis or cervicitis
caused by* Chlamydia trachomatis—
**Adults and adolescents 16 years and
over:** 1 g P.O. as a single dose.
✴*New indication: Prevention of disseminated* Mycobacterium avium *complex (MAC) disease in patients with
advanced HIV infection—*
Adults: 1,200 mg P.O. once weekly, as
indicated.
Urethritis and cervicitis due to Neisseria gonorrhoeae—
Adults: 2 g P.O. as a single dose.
Genital ulcer disease in men due to
Haemophilus ducreyi *(chancroid)—*
Adults: 1 g P.O. as a single dose.

ADVERSE REACTIONS
CNS: dizziness, vertigo, headache, fa-
tigue, somnolence.
CV: palpitations, chest pain.
GI: *nausea, vomiting, diarrhea, abdom-
inal pain,* dyspepsia, flatulence, melena,
cholestatic jaundice, pseudomembra-
nous colitis.
GU: candidiasis, vaginitis, nephritis.
Skin: rash, photosensitivity.
Other: angioedema.

INTERACTIONS
*Aluminum- and magnesium-containing
antacids:* lowered peak plasma levels of
azithromycin. Separate administration
times by at least 2 hours.
Astemizole, terfenadine: prolongation of
QT interval and ventricular tachycardia

---

have been associated with other macrolide anti-infectives. Monitor patient closely.

Digoxin: may cause elevated digoxin levels. Monitor closely.

Food: decreases absorption. take drug on an empty stomach.

Theophylline: may increase plasma theophylline levels with other macrolides; effect of azithromycin is unknown. Monitor theophylline levels carefully.

Warfarin: may increase PT with other macrolides; effect of azithromycin is unknown. Monitor PT carefully.

EFFECTS ON DIAGNOSTIC TESTS
None reported.

CONTRAINDICATIONS
Contraindicated in patients with hypersensitivity to erythromycin or other macrolides.

NURSING CONSIDERATIONS
● Use cautiously in patients with impaired hepatic function.
● Obtain specimen for culture and sensitivity tests before first dose. Therapy may begin pending results.
● Administer capsules 1 hour before or 2 hours after meals; do not administer with antacids. Oral suspension can be taken with or without food.
● Monitor for superinfection. May cause overgrowth of nonsusceptible bacteria or fungi.
● Single-dose 1-g packets for suspension should be reconstituted with 2 oz (60 ml) water, mixed, and administered to patient. Patient should rinse glass with additional 2 oz of water and drink to ensure he has consumed entire dose.

☑ PATIENT TEACHING
● Tell the patient to take drug as prescribed, even after he feels better.

clarithromycin
Biaxin

Pregnancy Risk Category: C

HOW SUPPLIED
Tablets (film-coated): 250 mg, 500 mg
Suspension: 125 mg/5 ml, 250 mg/5 ml

ACTION
Binds to the 50S subunit of bacterial ribosomes, blocking protein synthesis; bacteriostatic or bactericidal, depending on concentration.

ONSET, PEAK, DURATION
Onset and duration unknown. Serum levels peak in 2 to 4 hours.

INDICATIONS & DOSAGE
Pharyngitis or tonsillitis caused by Streptococcus pyogenes—
Adults: 250 mg P.O. q 12 hours for 10 days.
Children: 15 mg/kg/day P.O. in divided doses q 12 hours for 10 days.
Acute maxillary sinusitis caused by S. pneumoniae, Haemophilus influenzae, or Moraxella (Branhamella) catarrhalis—
Adults: 500 mg P.O. q 12 hours for 14 days.
Children: 15 mg/kg/day P.O. in divided doses q 12 hours for 10 days.
Acute exacerbations of chronic bronchitis caused by M. catarrhalis *or* S. pneumoniae; *pneumonia caused by* S. pneumoniae *or* Mycoplasma pneumoniae—
Adults: 250 mg P.O. q 12 hours for 7 to 14 days.
Acute exacerbations of chronic bronchitis caused by H. influenzae—
Adults: 500 mg P.O. q 12 hours for 7 to 14 days.
Uncomplicated skin and skin-structure infections caused by Staphylococcus aureus *or* S. pyogenes—
Adults: 250 mg P.O. q 12 hours for 7 to 14 days.
Children: 15 mg/kg/day P.O. in divided

doses q 12 hours for 10 days.
Acute otitis media caused by H. influenzae, M. catarrhalis, *or* S. pneumoniae—
Children: 7.5 mg/kg P.O. q 12 hours
for 10 days.
Mycobacterium avium *complex (MAC)*
disease in patients with HIV infection—
Adults: 500 mg P.O. q 12 hours, in
combination with other antimycobacterial drugs, for life.
Children: 7.5 mg/kg P.O. (maximum of
500 mg) q 12 hours, in combination
with other antimycobacterial drugs, for
life.
Prophylaxis against MAC disease in pa-
tients with advanced HIV infection—
Adults: 500 mg P.O. q 12 hours.
Children: 7.5 mg/kg P.O. (maximum of
500 mg) q 12 hours.
Helicobacter pylori *infection*—
Adults: 500 mg P.O. q 8 hours for 14
days with omeprazole 40 mg P.O. each
morning. Omeprazole therapy should
continue at a dose of 20 mg P.O. each
morning for a total of 28 days.

ADVERSE REACTIONS
CNS: headache.
GI: *diarrhea, nausea, abnormal taste,*
dyspepsia, abdominal pain or discomfort.

INTERACTIONS
Carbamazepine: may increase serum
levels of carbamazepine. Monitor blood
levels.
Digoxin: may increase serum digoxin
levels. Monitor for digitalis toxicity.
Terfenadine: altered metabolism of terfenadine, with prolongation of QT interval and ventricular tachycardia. Avoid
concurrent use.
Theophylline: increased plasma theophylline levels possible with other
macrolides; effect of clarithromycin is
unknown. Monitor theophylline levels
carefully.
Warfarin: increased PT possible with
other macrolides; effect of clarithromycin is unknown. Monitor PT carefully.

Zidovudine: decreased zidovudine levels. Monitor effectiveness of zidovudine
closely.

EFFECTS ON DIAGNOSTIC TESTS
None reported.

CONTRAINDICATIONS
Contraindicated in patients with hypersensitivity to erythromycin or other
macrolides.

NURSING CONSIDERATIONS
● Use cautiously in patients with hepatic or renal impairment.
● Obtain specimen for culture and sensitivity tests before first dose. Therapy
may begin pending results.
● Monitor the patient for superinfection.
Drug may cause overgrowth of nonsusceptible bacteria or fungi.

☑ PATIENT TEACHING
● Tell the patient to take drug as prescribed, even after he feels better.
● Instruct the patient to report persistent
adverse reactions.
● Inform the patient the drug may be
taken with or without food. He should
not refrigerate the suspension form.

---

dirithromycin
Dynabac

Pregnancy Risk Category: C

HOW SUPPLIED
Tablets (enteric-coated): 250 mg

ACTION
Inhibits bacterial RNA-dependent protein synthesis by binding to the 50S
subunit of the ribosome.

ONSET, PEAK, DURATION
Onset and duration are unknown. Peak
serum levels occur in about 4 hours.

INDICATIONS & DOSAGE
Acute bacterial exacerbations of chron-

---

*Liquid contains alcohol.   **May contain tartrazine.   †Canada only.   ‡Australia only.   ◇OTC.

ic bronchitis due to Moraxella catarrhalis *or* Streptococcus pneumoniae; *secondary bacterial infection of acute bronchitis due to* M. catarrhalis *or* S. pneumoniae; *uncomplicated skin and skin-structure infections due to* Staphylococcus aureus *(methicillin-susceptible strains)—*

Adults and children 12 years and older: 500 mg P.O. daily with food (or within 1 hour after eating) for 7 days.
Community-acquired pneumonia due to Legionella pneumophila, Mycoplasma pneumoniae, *or* S. pneumoniae—

Adults and children 12 years and older: 500 mg P.O. daily with food (or within 1 hour after eating) for 14 days.
Pharyngitis or tonsillitis due to Streptococcus pyogenes—

Adults and children 12 years and older: 500 mg P.O. daily with food (or within 1 hour after eating) for 10 days.

ADVERSE REACTIONS
CNS: headache, dizziness, vertigo, insomnia.
GI: abdominal pain, nausea, diarrhea, vomiting, dyspepsia, flatulence.
Hematologic: increased platelet, eosinophil, and neutrophil counts.
Respiratory: increased cough, dyspnea.
Skin: rash, pruritus, urticaria.
Other: pain (nonspecific), asthenia, hyperkalemia, decreased bicarbonate levels, increased CK and liver enzyme levels.

INTERACTIONS
Antacids, histamine$_2$ antagonists: may slightly increase the absorption of dirithromycin when it is administered immediately after these drugs.
Terfenadine: may decrease terfenadine metabolism, leading to increased levels of terfenadine and to cardiotoxicity. Concomitant use should be avoided if possible until further recommendations are available.
Theophylline: may alter steady-state plasma concentration of theophylline. Monitor theophylline plasma concentra-

tions. Dosage adjustments may be needed.

Note: Alfentanil, oral anticoagulants, astemizole, bromocriptine, carbamazepine, cyclosporine, digoxin, disopyramide, ergotamine, hexobarbital, lovastatin, phenytoin, triazolam, and valproate have been reported to interact with erythromycin products. It's unknown whether these same drugs interact with dirithromycin. Until further data are available, use caution during coadministration.

EFFECTS ON DIAGNOSTIC TESTS
None reported.

CONTRAINDICATIONS
Contraindicated in patients with hypersensitivity to the drug, erythromycin, or any other macrolide antibiotic.

NURSING CONSIDERATIONS
● Use cautiously in patients with hepatic insufficiency and in breast-feeding women.
● Safety of the drug in children under age 12 has not been established.
● Obtain culture and sensitivity results to ensure organism is sensitive to dirithromycin. This drug is not recommended for empiric use.
● Be aware that drug should not be used in patients with known, suspected, or potential bacteremias because serum levels are inadequate to provide antibacterial coverage of organisms within the bloodstream.
● Administer drug with food or within 1 hour of food intake.
● Monitor the patient for superinfection. Drug may cause overgrowth of nonsusceptible bacteria or fungi.

☑ PATIENT TEACHING
● Tell patient to take drug as prescribed, even after he feels better.
● Tell patient to take drug with food or within 1 hour after eating and not to cut, chew, or crush the tablet.

Reactions may be *common,* uncommon, *life-threatening,* or COMMON AND LIFE-THREATENING.

erythromycin base
Apo-Erythro†, EMU-V‡, E-Mycin, Er-amycin, Erybid†, ERYC, Erythromid†, Erythromycin Base Filmtab, Erythromycin Delayed-Release, Novo-rythro†, PCE Dispertab, Robimycin

erythromycin estolate
Ilosone, Ilosone pulvules, Novo-rythro†

erythromycin ethylsuccinate
Apo-Erythro-ES†, EEG Dulcets‡, E.E.S., EES-400‡, EES granules‡, EryPed, EryPed 200, EryPed 400

erythromycin lactobionate
Erythrocin, Erythromycin Lactobionate

erythromycin stearate
Apo-Erythro-S†, Erythrocin Stearate, Novo-rythro†

Pregnancy Risk Category: B

HOW SUPPLIED
erythromycin base
Tablets (enteric-coated): 250 mg, 333 mg, 500 mg
Tablets (filmtabs): 250 mg, 500 mg
Capsules (enteric-coated): 250 mg
erythromycin estolate
Tablets: 500 mg
Capsules: 250 mg
Oral suspension: 125 mg/5 ml, 250 mg/5 ml
erythromycin ethylsuccinate
Tablets (film-coated): 400 mg
Tablets (chewable): 200 mg
Oral suspension: 200 mg/5 ml, 400 mg/5 ml, 100 mg/2.5 ml
erythromycin lactobionate
Injection: 500-mg, 1-g vials
erythromycin stearate
Tablets (film-coated): 250 mg, 500 mg

ACTION
Inhibits bacterial protein synthesis by binding to the 50S subunit of the ribo-some. Bacteriostatic or bactericidal, depending on concentration.

ONSET, PEAK, DURATION
Onset and duration unknown. Peak serum levels occur 1 to 4 hours after an oral dose or immediately after I.V. infusion.

INDICATIONS & DOSAGE
Acute pelvic inflammatory disease caused by Neisseria gonorrhoeae—
Adults: 500 mg I.V. (lactobionate) q 6 hours for 3 days, then 250 mg (base, estolate, stearate) or 400 mg (ethylsuccinate) P.O. q 6 hours for 7 days.
Endocarditis prophylaxis for dental procedures in patients allergic to penicillin—
Adults: initially, 1,600 mg (ethylsuccinate) or 1 g (base, estolate, stearate) P.O. 1½ to 2 hours before procedure; then 800 mg (ethylsuccinate) or 500 mg (base, estolate, stearate) P.O. 6 hours later.
Children: initially, 20 mg/kg (base, ethylsuccinate, stearate) P.O. 1½ to 2 hours before procedure; then half the initial dose 6 hours later.
Intestinal amebiasis due to Entamoeba histolytica—
Adults: 250 mg P.O. (base, estolate, stearate) four times daily for 10 to 14 days. I.V. therapy not effective.
Children: 30 to 50 mg/kg (oral salts) P.O. daily, in divided doses, for 10 to 14 days. I.V. therapy not effective.
Erythrasma—
Adults: 250 mg P.O. (base, estolate, stearate) t.i.d. for 21 days.
Rheumatic fever prophylaxis—
Adults: 250 mg (base, estolate, stearate) P.O. q 12 hours.
Mild to moderately severe respiratory tract, skin, and soft-tissue infections caused by sensitive group A beta-hemolytic streptococci, Streptococcus pneumoniae, Mycoplasma pneumoniae, Corynebacterium diphtheriae, Bordetella pertussis—
Adults: 250 to 500 mg (base, estolate,

stearate) P.O. q 6 hours; or 400 to 800 mg (ethylsuccinate) P.O. q 6 hours; or 15 to 20 mg/kg I.V. daily, as continuous infusion or in divided doses q 6 hours for 10 days (3 weeks for *Mycoplasma* infection).

Children: 30 to 50 mg/kg (oral erythromycin salts) P.O. daily, in divided doses q 6 hours; or 15 to 20 mg/kg I.V. daily, in divided doses q 4 to 6 hours for 10 days (3 weeks for *Mycoplasma* infection).

Listeria monocytogenes infection—
Adults: 250 mg (base, estolate, stearate) P.O. q 6 hours or 500 mg P.O. q 12 hours.

Nongonococcal urethritis due to Ureaplasma urealyticum—
Adults: 500 mg (base, estolate, stearate) P.O. q 6 hours for at least 7 days.

Syphilis in patients allergic to penicillin—
Adults: 500 mg (base, estolate, stearate) P.O. q.i.d. for 10 days.

Legionnaire's disease—
Adults: 500 mg to 1 g I.V. or P.O. (base, estolate, stearate) or 800 to 1,600 mg (ethylsuccinate) q 6 hours for 21 days.

Uncomplicated urethral, endocervical, or rectal infections due to Chlamydia trachomatis *when tetracyclines are contraindicated—*
Adults: 500 mg (base, estolate, stearate) or 800 mg (ethylsuccinate) P.O. q.i.d. for 14 days.

Urogenital Chlamydia trachomatis *infections during pregnancy—*
Adults: 500 mg (base, estolate, stearate) P.O. q.i.d. for at least 7 days or 250 mg (base, estolate, stearate) or 400 mg (ethylsuccinate) P.O. q.i.d. for at least 14 days.

Conjunctivitis caused by C. trachomatis *in neonates—*
Neonates: 50 mg/kg (base, estolate, stearate) P.O. daily in four divided doses for 14 days.

Pneumonia in infants caused by C. trachomatis—

Infants: 50 mg/kg/day (base, estolate, lactiobionate, stearate) P.O. or I.V. in four divided doses for 10 to 14 days.

ADVERSE REACTIONS
EENT: hearing loss with high I.V. doses.
GI: *abdominal pain and cramping, nausea, vomiting, diarrhea.*
Hepatic: cholestatic jaundice (with erythromycin estolate).
Skin: urticaria, rash, eczema.
Other: overgrowth of nonsusceptible bacteria or fungi; *anaphylaxis;* fever; *vein irritation, thrombophlebitis after I.V. injection.*

INTERACTIONS
Astemizole, terfenadine: decreased metabolism, leading to increased levels of these antihistamines and cardiotoxicity. Avoid concomitant use.
Carbamazepine: increased carbamazepine blood levels and increased risk of toxicity. Monitor closely.
Clindamycin, lincomycin: may be antagonistic. Don't use together.
Cyclosporine: increased concentrations of cyclosporine. Monitor closely.
Digoxin: increased serum digoxin levels. Monitor for digoxin toxicity.
Disopyramide: increased disopyramide plasma levels resulting, in some cases, in arrhythmias and increased QT intervals. Monitor ECG.
Midazolam, triazolam: increased effects of these drugs. Monitor closely.
Oral anticoagulants: increased anticoagulant effect. Monitor PT and INR closely.
Theophylline: decreased erythromycin blood level and increased theophylline toxicity. Use together cautiously.

EFFECTS ON DIAGNOSTIC TESTS
Erythromycin may interfere with fluorometric determination of urine catecholamines. Liver function test results may become abnormal during erythromycin therapy (rare).

Reactions may be *common,* uncommon, *life-threatening,* or COMMON AND LIFE-THREATENING.

CONTRAINDICATIONS

Contraindicated in patients with hypersensitivity to the drug or other macrolides. Erythromycin estolate is contraindicated in patients with hepatic disease.

NURSING CONSIDERATIONS

• Use erythromycin salts cautiously in patients with impaired hepatic function.
• Be aware that erythromycin estolate is not recommended during pregnancy because of the potential adverse effects on the mother and the fetus.
• Obtain urine specimen for culture and sensitivity tests before first dose. Therapy may begin pending results.
• When administering suspension, be sure to note the concentration.
• **I.V. use:** Reconstitute according to manufacturer's directions and dilute each 250 mg in at least 100 ml of 0.9% sodium chloride solution. Infuse over 1 hour.
Alert: Do not administer erythromycin lactobionate with other drugs.
• Monitor the patient for superinfection. May cause overgrowth of nonsusceptible bacteria or fungi.
• Monitor hepatic function (increased serum levels of alkaline phosphatase, ALT, AST, and bilirubin may occur). Erythromycin estolate may cause serious hepatotoxicity in adults (reversible cholestatic jaundice). Other erythromycin salts cause hepatotoxicity to a lesser degree.
• Keep in mind that the drug may falsely elevate concentrations of urinary 17-hydroxycorticosteroids and 17-ketosteroids.
• Be aware that drug may interfere with colorimetric assays, resulting in falsely elevated AST and ALT levels.
• Keep in mind that coated tablets or encapsulated pellets have caused fewer instances of GI upset; they may be better tolerated by patients who cannot tolerate erythromycin.
• Know that drug is not indicated for the treatment of neurosyphilis.

☑ PATIENT TEACHING

• Tell the patient to take drug as prescribed, even after he feels better.
• For best absorption, instruct the patient to take oral form of drug with full glass of water 1 hour before or 2 hours after meals. May be taken with food if GI upset occurs. Coated tablets may be taken with meals. Tell the patient not to drink fruit juice with drug. Chewable erythromycin tablets should not be swallowed whole.
• Instruct the patient to report adverse reactions, especially nausea, abdominal pain, and fever.

---

*Liquid contains alcohol.   **May contain tartrazine.   †Canada only.   ‡Australia only.   ◇ OTC.

19

Miscellaneous anti-infectives

aztreonam
bacitracin
chloramphenicol
chloramphenicol palmitate
chloramphenicol sodium
    succinate
clindamycin hydrochloride
clindamycin palmitate
    hydrochloride
clindamycin phosphate
fosfomycin tromethamine
imipenem/cilastatin sodium
meropenem
methenamine hippurate
methenamine mandelate
nitrofurantoin macrocrystals
nitrofurantoin microcrystals
polymyxin B sulfate
spectinomycin hydrochloride
trimethoprim
trimetrexate glucuronate
vancomycin hydrochloride

COMBINATION PRODUCTS
CYSTEX: methenamine 165 mg, sodium salicylate 162.5 mg, and benzoic acid 32 mg.
ATROSEPT, DOLSED, UAA, URIDON MODIFIED, URINARY ASEPTIC NO. 2, URISED, URITIN: methenamine 40.8 mg, phenylsalicylate 18.1 mg, atropine sulfate 0.03 mg, hyoscyamine 0.03 mg, benzoic acid 4.5 mg, and methylene blue 5.4 mg.
MACROBID: nitrofurantoin macrocrystals 25 mg and nitrofurantoin monohydrate 75 mg.
PROSED/DS: methenamine 81.6 mg, phenylsalicylate 36.2 mg, methylene blue 10.8 mg, benzoic acid 9 mg, atropine sulfate 0.06 mg, hyoscyamine sulfate 0.06 mg.
TRAC TABS 2X: methenamine 120 mg, methylene blue 6 mg, phenyl salicylate 30 mg, atropine sulfate 0.06 mg, hyoscyamine sulfate 0.03 mg, and ben-

zoic acid 7.5 mg.
URIMAR-T, UROGESIC BLUE: methenamine 81.6 mg, sodium biphosphate 40.8 mg, phenylsalicylate 36.2 mg, methylene blue 10.8 mg, hyoscyamine sulfate 0.12 mg.
URISEDAMINE: methenamine mandelate 500 mg and hyoscyamine 0.15 mg.
URO PHOSPHATE: methenamine 300 mg and sodium acid phosphate 434.78 mg. Sugar coated.
UROQUID-ACID NO. 2: methenamine mandelate 500 mg and sodium acid phosphate 500 mg.

---

aztreonam
Azactam

Pregnancy Risk Category: B

HOW SUPPLIED
Injection: 500-mg, 1-g, 2-g vials

ACTION
Inhibits bacterial cell-wall synthesis, ultimately causing cell-wall destruction; bactericidal.

ONSET, PEAK, DURATION
Onset and duration unknown. Serum levels peak in 0.6 to 1.3 hours after I.M. injection, immediately after I.V. infusion.

INDICATIONS & DOSAGE
Urinary tract infections, lower respiratory tract infections, septicemia, skin and skin-structure infections, intra-abdominal infections, surgical infections, and gynecologic infections caused by susceptible strains of the following gram-negative aerobic organisms: E. coli, Klebsiella pneumoniae, Proteus mirabilis, Pseudomonas aeruginosa, Enterobacter cloacae, Klebsiella oxytoca,

Citrobacter *species,* Serratia marcescens. *Also respiratory infections caused by* Haemophilus influenzae—
Adults: 500 mg to 2 g I.V. or I.M. q 8 to 12 hours. For severe systemic or life-threatening infections, 2 g q 6 to 8 hours may be given. Maximum dosage is 8 g daily.

ADVERSE REACTIONS
CNS: *seizures,* headache, insomnia, confusion.
CV: hypotension.
GI: diarrhea, nausea, vomiting.
Hematologic: neutropenia, anemia, pancytopenia, ***thrombocytopenia,*** leukocytosis, thrombocytosis.
Other: hypersensitivity reactions (rash, ***anaphylaxis***), transient elevation of ALT and AST, thrombophlebitis at I.V. site, discomfort and swelling at I.M. injection site.

INTERACTIONS
Aminoglycosides, beta-lactam antibiotics and other anti-infectives: synergistic effectiveness.
Cefoxitin, imipenem: possible antagonistic effect. Do not use together.
Probenecid: increased serum aztreonam levels. Avoid concomitant use.

EFFECTS ON DIAGNOSTIC TESTS
Aztreonam therapy alters urine glucose determinations using cupric sulfate (Clinitest or Benedict's reagent). Coombs' test results may become positive during therapy. Drug may prolong PT and PTT, and may transiently increase ALT, AST, lactate dehydrogenase, and serum creatinine concentrations.

CONTRAINDICATIONS
Contraindicated in patients with hypersensitivity to the drug.

NURSING CONSIDERATIONS
● Use cautiously in elderly patients and in those with impaired renal function. Dosage adjustment may be necessary.

● Obtain culture and sensitivity tests before first dose. Therapy may begin pending results.
● **I.V. use:** To administer a bolus of aztreonam, inject drug slowly (over 3 to 5 minutes) directly into a vein or I.V. tubing. Give infusions over 20 minutes to 1 hour.
● Administer I.M. injections deep into a large muscle mass, such as the upper outer quadrant of the gluteus maximus or the lateral aspect of the thigh. Know that doses greater than 1 g should be given I.V.
● Observe the patient for signs of super-infection.
● Because aztreonam is ineffective against gram-positive and anaerobic organisms, anticipate using it with other antibiotics for immediate treatment of life-threatening illnesses. Aztreonam is a narrow-spectrum antibiotic, effective only against gram-negative organisms.
● Be aware that patients who are allergic to penicillins or cephalosporins may not be allergic to aztreonam. However, close monitoring of those who have had an immediate hypersensitivity reaction to these antibiotics is recommended.

☑ **PATIENT TEACHING**
● Warn patient receiving I.M. drug that pain and swelling at the injection site may occur.
● Tell patient to alert nurse if discomfort occurs at I.V. insertion site.
● Instruct patient to report adverse reactions promptly.

---

bacitracin
Baciguent, Baci-IM, Bacitin†

Pregnancy Risk Category: C

HOW SUPPLIED
Injection: 10,000-unit, 50,000-unit vials

ACTION
Hinders bacterial cell-wall synthesis, damaging the bacterial plasma mem-

brane and making the cell more vulnerable to osmotic pressure.

ONSET, PEAK, DURATION
Onset and duration unknown. Plasma levels peak within 1 to 2 hours of an I.M. injection.

INDICATIONS & DOSAGE
Pneumonia or empyema caused by susceptible staphylococci—
Infants over 2.5 kg: 1,000 units/kg I.M. daily, divided q 8 to 12 hours.
Infants under 2.5 kg: 900 units/kg I.M. daily, divided q 8 to 12 hours.

ADVERSE REACTIONS
EENT: ototoxicity.
GI: nausea, vomiting.
GU: *nephrotoxicity (albuminuria,* cylindruria, oliguria, anuria, increased BUN, *tubular and glomerular necrosis*).
Skin: urticaria, rash.
Other: pain at injection site.

INTERACTIONS
Nephrotoxic drugs (such as aminoglycosides): increased nephrotoxicity. Use together cautiously.
Neuromuscular blockers, inhalation anesthetics: prolonged muscle weakness. Monitor the patient for excessive muscle weakness or respiratory distress.

EFFECTS ON DIAGNOSTIC TESTS
Urinary sediment tests may show increased protein and cast excretion. Serum creatinine and BUN levels may increase during bacitracin therapy.

CONTRAINDICATIONS
Contraindicated in patients with hypersensitivity to the drug or impaired renal function. Due to significant risk of neurotoxicity, limit I.M. use to infants with staphylococcal pneumonia.

NURSING CONSIDERATIONS
• Use cautiously in those with myasthenia gravis and neuromuscular disease.

• Obtain culture and sensitivity tests before first dose.
• Assess baseline renal function studies before and during therapy.
• Administer by deep I.M. injection only.
• Know that concentration of bacitracin should be between 5,000 and 10,000 units/ml. Reconstitute 50,000-unit vial with 9.8 ml of diluent. Store in refrigerator. Drug is inactivated if stored at room temperature.
• Maintain adequate fluid intake, and monitor urine output closely.
• Provide measures to keep urine pH above 6.0 to reduce the risk of nephrotoxicity.
• Be aware that prolonged therapy may result in overgrowth of nonsusceptible organisms, especially *Candida albicans.*

☑ **PATIENT TEACHING**
• Warn the patient that injection may be painful.
• Instruct the patient to report adverse reactions promptly.

---

chloramphenicol
AK-Chlor, Chloromycetin, Chloromycetin Kapseals, Chloroptic, Diochloram†, Novochlorocap†, Sopamycetin†

chloramphenicol palmitate
Chloromycetin Palmitate

chloramphenicol sodium succinate
Chloromycetin Sodium Succinate, Pentamycetin†

Pregnancy Risk Category: C

HOW SUPPLIED
chloramphenicol
Capsules: 250 mg
chloramphenicol palmitate
Oral suspension: 150 mg/5 ml
chloramphenicol sodium succinate
Injection: 1-g vial

ACTION
Inhibits bacterial protein synthesis by binding to the 50S subunit of the ribosome; bacteriostatic.

ONSET, PEAK, DURATION
Onset and duration unknown. Serum levels peak immediately after I.V. administration, 1 to 3 hours after oral dose.

INDICATIONS & DOSAGE
Haemophilus influenzae *meningitis, acute* Salmonella typhi *infection, and meningitis, bacteremia, or other severe infections caused by sensitive* Salmonella *species,* Rickettsia, *lymphogranuloma, psittacosis, or various sensitive gram-negative organisms*—
Adults: 50 to 100 mg/kg P.O. or I.V. daily, divided q 6 hours. Maximum dosage is 100 mg/kg daily.
Full-term infants older than 2 weeks with normal metabolic processes: up to 50 mg/kg P.O. or I.V. daily, divided q 6 hours.
Premature infants, neonates 2 weeks or younger, and children and infants with immature metabolic processes: 25 mg/kg P.O. or I.V. once daily. I.V. route must be used to treat meningitis.

ADVERSE REACTIONS
CNS: headache, mild depression, confusion, delirium, peripheral neuropathy with prolonged therapy.
EENT: optic neuritis (in patients with cystic fibrosis), glossitis, decreased visual acuity.
GI: nausea, vomiting, stomatitis, diarrhea, enterocolitis.
Hematologic: *aplastic anemia, hypoplastic anemia, granulocytopenia, thrombocytopenia.*
Other: hypersensitivity reactions (fever, rash, urticaria, *anaphylaxis*), jaundice, *gray syndrome in neonates (abdominal distention, gray cyanosis, vasomotor collapse, respiratory distress, death within a few hours of onset of symptoms).*

INTERACTIONS
Anticoagulants, barbiturates, hydantoins, iron salts, sulfonylureas: increased blood levels of these agents possible. Monitor for toxicity.
Penicillins: synergistic effects may develop in the treatment of certain microorganisms, but antagonism may also occur. Monitor effectiveness closely.
Rifampin: may reduce chloramphenicol levels. Monitor for changes in effectiveness.
Vitamin B$_{12}$: may decrease response of vitamin B in patients with pernicious anemia. Monitor closely.

EFFECTS ON DIAGNOSTIC TESTS
False elevation of urine PABA levels will result if chloramphenicol is administered during a bentiromide test for pancreatic function. Treatment with chloramphenicol will cause false-positive results on tests for urine glucose using cupric sulfate (Clinitest). Erythrocyte, platelet, and leukocyte counts in the blood and possibly the bone marrow may decrease during chloramphenicol therapy (from reversible or irreversible bone marrow depression). Hemoglobinuria or lactic acidosis may also occur.

CONTRAINDICATIONS
Contraindicated in patients with hypersensitivity to the drug.

NURSING CONSIDERATIONS
● Use cautiously in patients with impaired hepatic or renal function, acute intermittent porphyria, and G6PD deficiency and with other drugs that cause bone marrow suppression or blood disorders.
● Obtain specimen for culture and sensitivity tests before first dose. Therapy may begin pending results.
● **I.V. use:** Give I.V. slowly over at least 1 minute. Check injection site daily for phlebitis and irritation.
● Reconstitute 1-g vial of powder for injection with 10 ml of sterile water for injection. Concentration will be 100

mg/ml. Stable for 30 days at room temperature, but refrigeration recommended. Do not use cloudy solutions.

● Obtain plasma concentration levels. Therapeutic plasma concentrations are as follows: peak, 10 to 20 mcg/ml; trough, 5 to 10 mcg/ml.

● Monitor CBC, platelets, serum iron, and reticulocytes before and every 2 days during therapy, as ordered. Stop drug immediately if anemia, reticulocytopenia, leukopenia, or thrombocytopenia develops, and notify doctor.

● Monitor for evidence of superinfection.

☑ **PATIENT TEACHING**
● Tell the patient to take medication for as long as prescribed, exactly as directed, even after he feels better.

● Instruct the patient to report adverse reactions to the doctor, especially nausea, vomiting, diarrhea, fever, confusion, sore throat, or mouth sores.

● Tell the patient receiving drug I.V. to alert nurse if discomfort occurs at I.V. insertion site.

---

clindamycin hydrochloride
Cleocin HCl, Dalacin C†‡

clindamycin palmitate hydrochloride
Cleocin Pediatric, Dalacin C Palmitate†‡

clindamycin phosphate
Cleocin Phosphate, Cleocin T, Dalacin C†‡, Dalacin C Phosphate

Pregnancy Risk Category: B

HOW SUPPLIED
clindamycin hydrochloride
Capsules: 75 mg, 150 mg, 300 mg
clindamycin palmitate hydrochloride
Granules for oral solution: 75 mg/5 ml
clindamycin phosphate
Injection: 150 mg base/ml, 300 mg base/2ml, 600 mg base/4ml, 900 mg base/6 ml, 9,000 mg base/60 ml
Injectable infusion (in 5% dextrose): 300 mg (50 ml), 600 mg (50 ml), 900 mg (50 ml)

ACTION
Inhibits bacterial protein synthesis by binding to the 50S subunit of the ribosome.

ONSET, PEAK, DURATION
Onset and duration unknown. Serum levels peak immediately after I.V. administration, 3 hours after an I.M. injection, or within 45 minutes to 1 hour after an oral dose.

INDICATIONS & DOSAGE
Infections caused by sensitive staphylococci, streptococci, pneumococci, Bacteroides, Fusobacterium, Clostridium perfringens, *and other sensitive aerobic and anaerobic organisms—*
Adults: 150 to 450 mg P.O. q 6 hours; or 300 to 600 mg I.M. or I.V. q 6, 8, or 12 hours.
Children over 1 month: 8 to 20 mg/kg P.O. daily, in divided doses q 6 to 8 hours; or 20 to 40 mg/kg I.M. or I.V. daily, in divided doses q 6 or 8 hours.
Endocarditis prophylaxis for dental procedures in patients allergic to penicillin—
Adults: initially, 300 mg P.O. 1 hour before procedure; then 150 mg 6 hours later.
Children: initially, 10 mg/kg P.O. 1 hour before procedure; then half the initial dose 6 hours later.
Pelvic inflammatory disease—
Adults: 900 mg I.V. q 8 hours with gentamicin. Continue at least 48 hours after improvement in symptoms, then switch to oral clindamycin 450 mg 5 times daily for a total course of 10 to 14 days or doxycycline 100 mg P.O. q 12 hours for a total of 10 to 14 days.
Pneumocystis carinii pneumonia—
Adults: 600 mg I.V. q 6 hours or 300 to 450 mg P.O. q 6 hours with primaquine.

ADVERSE REACTIONS
GI: *nausea,* vomiting, abdominal pain, ***diarrhea, pseudomembranous colitis.***
Hematologic: transient leukopenia, eosinophilia, ***thrombocytopenia.***
Skin: maculopapular rash, urticaria.
Other: ***anaphylaxis,*** jaundice, abnormal liver function tests.

INTERACTIONS
Erythromycin: may block access of clindamycin to its site of action. Don't use together.
Kaolin: decreased absorption of oral clindamycin. Separate administration times.
Neuromuscular blockers: potentiated neuromuscular blockade possible. Monitor closely.

EFFECTS ON DIAGNOSTIC TESTS
Liver function test results may become abnormal in some patients during clindamycin therapy.

CONTRAINDICATIONS
Contraindicated in patients with hypersensitivity to this drug or lincomycin.

NURSING CONSIDERATIONS
• Use cautiously in neonates and patients with renal or hepatic disease, asthma, history of GI disease, or significant allergies.
• Know that drug does not penetrate blood-brain barrier.
• Obtain culture and sensitivity tests before first dose. Therapy may begin pending results.
• **I.V. use:** When giving I.V., check site daily for phlebitis and irritation. For I.V. infusion, dilute each 300 mg in 50 ml solution, and give no faster than 30 mg/minute (over 10 to 60 minutes). Never give undiluted as a bolus.
• For I.M. administration, inject deeply. Rotate sites. Doses greater than 600 mg per injection are not recommended.
• Be aware that I.M. injection may raise CK in response to muscle irritation.
• Don't refrigerate reconstituted oral so-

lution because it will thicken. Drug is stable for 2 weeks at room temperature.
• Monitor renal, hepatic, and hematopoietic functions during prolonged therapy, as ordered.
• Observe the patient for signs of superinfection.
Alert: Don't give opioid antidiarrheals to treat drug-induced diarrhea. They may prolong and worsen diarrhea.

☑ **PATIENT TEACHING**
• Advise the patient taking the capsule form to take it with a full glass of water to prevent esophageal irritation.
• Warn the patient that I.M. injection may be painful.
• Tell the patient to alert nurse if discomfort occurs at I.V. insertion site.
• Instruct the patient to report adverse reactions, especially diarrhea, to the doctor. Warn the patient not to treat such diarrhea himself.

▼ *NEW DRUG*

fosfomycin tromethamine
Monurol

Pregnancy Risk Category: B

HOW SUPPLIED
Single-dose sachet: 3 g

ACTION
Bactericidal; inhibits bacterial cell wall synthesis. It is effective in the urinary tract because it reduces adherence of bacteria to uroepithelial cells.

ONSET, PEAK, DURATION
Onset and duration unknown. Rapidly absorbed after oral administration. Plasma levels peak within 2 hours.

INDICATIONS & DOSAGE
Uncomplicated urinary tract infections (acute cystitis) in women caused by susceptible strains of Escherichia coli *and* Enterococcus faecalis—

Women over 18 years: 1 sachet P.O. mixed with cold water just before ingestion.

ADVERSE REACTIONS
CNS: headache, dizziness, asthenia.
GI: diarrhea, nausea, dyspepsia.
GU: vaginitis.

INTERACTIONS
Metoclopramide: lowers serum concentration of fosfomycin. Avoid concomitant use.

EFFECTS ON DIAGNOSTIC TESTS
None reported.

CONTRAINDICATIONS
Contraindicated in patients with known hypersensitivity to the drug.

NURSING CONSIDERATIONS
• Use cautiously in patients with renal impairment.
• Know that fosfomycin should not be used during pregnancy unless clearly needed. Breast-feeding women should not take the drug.
• Know that safety and effectiveness in children age 12 and under have not been established.
• Obtain urine specimens for culture and sensitivity before and after therapy has been completed.
• Know that using more than one single-dose sachet to treat a single episode of acute cystitis will not improve clinical success and may cause adverse reactions.

☑ **PATIENT TEACHING**
• Instruct patient about the proper way to take fosfomycin. Drug should not be taken in its dry form. The entire contents of a single-dose sachet should be mixed with 3 to 4 oz (½ cup) cold water. Stir to dissolve, and drink immediately.
• Tell patient to notify the doctor if symptoms have not improved in 2 to 3 days.

imipenem/cilastatin sodium
Primaxin IM, Primaxin IV

Pregnancy Risk Category: C

HOW SUPPLIED
Powder for injection: 250 mg, 500 mg

ACTION
Imipenem is bactericidal and inhibits bacterial cell-wall synthesis. Cilastatin inhibits the enzymatic breakdown of imipenem in the kidneys, thereby preventing formation of a renally toxic metabolite.

ONSET, PEAK, DURATION
Onset unknown. Serum levels peak immediately after I.V. infusion, within 1 hour for cilastatin and within 2 hours for imipenem after I.M. administration. Duration is 4 to 6 hours.

INDICATIONS & DOSAGE
Serious infections of the lower respiratory and urinary tracts, intra-abdominal and gynecologic infections, bacterial septicemia, bone and joint infections, skin and soft-tissue infections, and endocarditis. Most known microorganisms are susceptible: Acinetobacter, Enterococcus, Staphylococcus, Streptococcus, Escherichia coli, Haemophilus, Klebsiella, Morganella, Proteus, Enterobacter, Pseudomonas aeruginosa, *and* Bacteroides, *including* B. fragilis—
Adults and children weighing over 40 kg: 250 mg to 1 g by I.V. infusion q 6 to 8 hours. Maximum daily dosage is 50 mg/kg/day or 4 g/day, whichever is less. Alternatively, 500 to 750 mg I.M. q 12 hours. Maximum daily dosage is 1,500 mg/day.
Children weighing less than 40 kg: 60 mg/kg I.V. daily in divided doses.
Premature infants less than 36 weeks gestational age: 20 mg/kg I.V. q 12 hours.

Reactions may be *common*, uncommon, *life-threatening*, or COMMON AND LIFE-THREATENING.

ADVERSE REACTIONS
CNS: *seizures,* dizziness, somnolence.
CV: hypotension.
GI: nausea, vomiting, diarrhea, *pseudo-membranous colitis.*
Skin: rash, urticaria, pruritus.
Other: *hypersensitivity reactions (anaphylaxis);* thrombophlebitis, pain at injection site; fever; transient increases in liver enzymes.

INTERACTIONS
Beta-lactam antibiotics: possible in vitro antagonism. Avoid concomitant use.
Ganciclovir: may cause seizures. Avoid concomitant use.
Probenicid: increased serum concentrations of cilastatin. Avoid concomitant use.

EFFECTS ON DIAGNOSTIC TESTS
Serum levels of AST, ALT, alkaline phosphatase, lactate dehydrogenase, and bilirubin may be elevated, and erythrocyte, platelet, and leukocyte counts reduced during drug therapy.

CONTRAINDICATIONS
Contraindicated in patients with hypersensitivity to the drug.

NURSING CONSIDERATIONS
● Use cautiously in patients allergic to penicillins or cephalosporins because this drug has similar properties.
● Also use cautiously in patients who have a history of seizure disorders, especially if they also have compromised renal function.
● Use with caution in children under age 3 months.
● Obtain culture and sensitivity tests before first dose. Therapy may begin pending results.
● Adjust dosage for patients with a creatinine clearance less than 70 ml/minute.
● **I.V. use:** Don't administer by direct I.V. bolus injection. Each 250- or 500-mg dose should be given by I.V. infusion over 20 to 30 minutes. Each 1-g dose should be infused over 40 to 60

minutes. If nausea occurs, the infusion may be slowed.
● When reconstituting powder, shake until the solution is clear. Solutions may range from colorless to yellow, and variations of color within this range do not affect the drug's potency. After reconstitution, solution is stable for 10 hours at room temperature and for 48 hours when refrigerated.
Alert: If seizures develop and persist, despite anticonvulsant therapy, notify the doctor. The drug should then be discontinued.
● Monitor patients for bacterial or fungal superinfections and resistant infections during and after therapy.

☑ **PATIENT TEACHING**
● Instruct patient to report adverse reactions promptly.
● Tell patient to alert nurse if discomfort occurs at I.V. insertion site.

▼ *NEW DRUG*

meropenem
Merrem I.V.

Pregnancy Risk Category: B

HOW SUPPLIED
Powder for injection: 500 mg/15 ml, 500 mg/20 ml, 500 mg/100 ml, 1g/15 ml, 1 g/30 ml, 1 g/100 ml

ACTION
Meropenem inhibits cell wall synthesis in bacteria. It readily penetrates cell wall of most gram-positive and gram-negative bacteria to reach penicillin-binding-protein targets.

ONSET, PEAK, DURATION
Onset unknown. After a single dose, peak concentrations have been found usually 1 hour after the start of the infusion. Elimination half-life in adults with normal renal function and children 2 years and older is about 1 hour and is 1½

hours in children 3 months to 2 years.

INDICATIONS & DOSAGE
Complicated appendicitis and peritonitis caused by viridans group streptococci, Escherichia coli, Klebsiella pneumoniae, Pseudomonas aeruginosa, Bacteroides fragilis, B. thetaiotaomicron, *and* Peptostreptococcus species; bacterial meningitis *(pediatric patients only) caused by* Streptococcus pneumoniae, Haemophilus influenzae, *and* Neisseria meningitidis—

Adults: 1 g I.V. q 8 hours over 15 to 30 minutes as I.V. infusion or over about 3 to 5 minutes as I.V. bolus injection (5 to 20 ml).

Children 3 months and older: 20 mg/kg (intra-abdominal infection) or 40 mg/kg (bacterial meningitis) q 8 hours over 15 to 30 minutes as I.V. infusion or over about 3 to 5 minutes as I.V. bolus injection (5 to 20 ml). Maximum dosage is 2 g I.V. q 8 hours.

Children weighing more than 50 kg (110 lb): 1 g I.V. q 8 hours for intra-abdominal infections and 2 g I.V. q 8 hours for meningitis.

Note: Dosages need to be adjusted for patients with renal insufficiency or renal failure or with creatinine clearance below 51 ml/min.

ADVERSE REACTIONS
CNS: *seizures,* headache.
GI: diarrhea, nausea, vomiting, constipation, oral moniliasis, glossitis.
GU: increased creatinine or BUN levels, presence of RBCs in urine.
Hematologic: increased or decreased platelet count, increased eosinophil count, prolonged or shortened PT or PTT, positive direct or indirect Coombs' test, decreased hemoglobin or hematocrit, decreased WBC count.
Hepatic: increased levels of ALT, AST, alkaline phosphatase, LDH, and bilirubin.
Respiratory: *apnea.*
Skin: rash, pruritus.
Other: *hypersensitivity, anaphylactic reaction;* inflammation, phlebitis, or thrombophlebitis at the injection site.

INTERACTIONS
Probenecid: inhibited renal excretion of meropenem. Drug competes with meropenem for active tubular secretion, which significantly increases elimination half-life of drug and the extent of systemic exposure. Concomitant administration of probenecid with meropenem is not recommended.

EFFECTS ON DIAGNOSTIC TESTS
Meropenem may increase creatinine, BUN, eosinophil, ALT, AST, alkaline phosphatase, LDH, bilirubin, and platelet count levels. It may also lead to RBCs in the urine, a postitive direct or indirect Coombs' test, or altered PT or PTT. Drug may decrease hemoglobin or hematocrit levels or WBC count.

CONTRAINDICATIONS
Contraindicated in patients with hypersensitivity to a component of drug or other drugs in the same class and in those who have demonstrated anaphylactic reactions to beta-lactams.

NURSING CONSIDERATIONS
● Use cautiously in the elderly and in patients with history of seizure disorders or impaired renal function.
● Know that safety and effectiveness of drug have not been established for patients under 3 months.
● Be aware that it is not known whether meropenem is excreted in breast milk. Use drug cautiously in breast-feeding women.
● Know that meropenem is not used to treat methicillin-resistant staphylococci.
● Obtain specimen for culture and sensitivity test before first dose. Therapy may begin pending test results.
● For I.V. bolus administration, add 10 ml of sterile water for injection to 500 mg/20-ml vial size or 20 ml to 1 g/30-ml vial size. Shake to dissolve, and let stand until clear.

Reactions may be *common*, uncommon, *life-threatening*, or COMMON AND LIFE-THREATENING.

• For I.V. infusion, infusion vials (500 mg/100 ml and 1 g/100 ml) may be directly reconstituted with a compatible infusion fluid. Alternatively, an injection vial may be reconstituted, then the resulting solution added to an I.V. container and further diluted with an appropriate infusion fluid. Do not use ADD-Vantage vials for this purpose. For ADD-Vantage vials, constitute only with 0.45% sodium chloride injection, 0.9% sodium chloride injection, or 5% dextrose injection in 50-, 100-, or 250-ml Abbott ADD-Vantage flexible diluent containers. Follow manufacturer's guidelines closely when using ADD-Vantage vials.

• Do not mix or add meropenem to solutions containing other drugs.

• Use freshly prepared solutions of drug immediately whenever possible. Stability of drug varies with type of drug used (injection vial, infusion vial, or ADD-Vantage container). Consult manufacturer's literature for details.

Alert: Know that serious and occasionally fatal hypersensitivity reactions have been reported in patients receiving therapy with beta-lactams. Before therapy is initiated, determine whether previous hypersensitivity reactions to penicillins, cephalosporins, or other beta-lactams or to other allergens have occurred.

• Discontinue drug and notify doctor if an allergic reaction occurs. Serious anaphylactic reactions require immediate, emergency treatment.

• Know that seizures and other CNS adverse reactions associated with meropenem therapy can occur in patients with CNS disorders, bacterial meningitis, and compromised renal function.

• If seizures occur during meropenem therapy, discontinue infusion and notify the doctor. Dosage adjustment may be ordered.

• Monitor patient for signs and symptoms of superinfection. Drug may cause overgrowth of nonsusceptible bacteria or fungi.

• Be aware that periodic assessment of organ system functions—including renal, hepatic, and hematopoietic function—is recommended during prolonged therapy.

☑ **PATIENT TEACHING**
• Advise breast-feeding patients of the risk of transmitting drug to baby through breast milk.
• Instruct patient to report adverse reactions.

---

methenamine hippurate
Hiprex**, Hip-Rex†, Urex

methenamine mandelate
Mandelamine, Sterinet†

Pregnancy Risk Category: C

HOW SUPPLIED
methenamine hippurate
Tablets: 1 g
methenamine mandelate
Tablets: 500 mg, 1 g
Tablets (enteric-coated): 500 mg, 1 g
Tablets (film-coated): 500 mg, 1 g
Suspension: 500 mg/5 ml

ACTION
Hydrolyzed to ammonia and to formaldehyde in urine, causing antibacterial action against gram-positive and gram-negative organisms. Mandelic and hippuric acids, with which methenamines are combined, are also antibacterial by unknown mechanisms.

ONSET, PEAK, DURATION
Onset and duration unknown. Plasma levels peak within 1 hour of administration. Urine levels of formaldehyde peak within 2 hours of administration of a film-coated tablet, or 3 to 8 hours after an enteric-coated tablet.

INDICATIONS & DOSAGE
Long-term prophylaxis or suppression of chronic urinary tract infections (UTIs)—

Note: Use only after eradication of acute infection with other appropriate antibiotic therapy.

Adults and children over 12 years: 1 g (hippurate) P.O. q 12 hours; or 1 g (mandelate) P.O. q.i.d. after meals and h.s.

Children 6 to 12 years: 500 mg to 1 g (hippurate) P.O. q 12 hours; or 500 mg (mandelate) P.O. q.i.d. after meals and h.s.

Children under 6 years: 50 mg/kg (mandelate) P.O. divided in four doses after meals and h.s.

ADVERSE REACTIONS
GI: nausea, vomiting, abdominal cramps, anorexia.
GU: with high doses, urinary tract irritation, dysuria, frequency, hematuria.
Skin: rash, pruritus.
Other: elevated liver enzymes, headache, dyspnea.

INTERACTIONS
Acetazolamide: antagonize methenamine effect. Use together cautiously.
Sulfamethizole: forms an insoluble precipitate in acid urine. Do not administer together.
Urine alkalinizing agents: inhibits methenamine action. Don't use together.

EFFECTS ON DIAGNOSTIC TESTS
Formaldehyde formation from methenamine may cause false elevations in catecholamine and 17-hydroxycorticosteroid levels and false decreases in 5-hydroxyindoleacetic acid and estriol levels in urine. Liver function test results may become abnormal during methenamine therapy.

CONTRAINDICATIONS
Contraindicated in patients with renal insufficiency, severe hepatic disease, or severe dehydration.

NURSING CONSIDERATIONS
● Administer cautiously to elderly or debilitated patients because aspiration

could cause lipid pneumonia. Oral suspension contains vegetable oil.
● Obtain a clean-catch urine specimen for culture and sensitivity tests before starting therapy, and repeat as needed.
● Administer after meals to minimize GI upset.
● Monitor fluid intake and output. Fluid intake should be at least 1,500 to 2,000 ml daily.
● For best results, maintain urine pH at 5.5 or below. Use Nitrazine paper to check pH. Large doses of ascorbic acid (12 g/day) may be necessary to effectively acidify urine.
● Monitor liver function studies periodically during long-term therapy.
Alert: If rash appears, withhold dose and contact the doctor.

☑ **PATIENT TEACHING**
● Instruct the patient to take medication for as long as prescribed, exactly as directed, even after he feels better.
● Tell the patient to take drug after meals.
● Instruct the patient to limit intake of alkaline foods, such as vegetables, milk, and peanuts. Patient may drink cranberry, plum, and prune juices. These juices or ascorbic acid may be used to acidify urine.
● Warn the patient not to take antacids, including Alka-Seltzer and sodium bicarbonate.

---

nitrofurantoin macrocrystals
Macrobid, Macrodantin

nitrofurantoin microcrystals
Apo-Nitrofurantoin†, Furadantin, Furalan, Furan, Furanite, Macrodantin, Nephronex†, Novo-Furan†

Pregnancy Risk Category: B

HOW SUPPLIED
nitrofurantoin macrocrystals
Capsules: 25 mg, 50 mg, 100 mg
nitrofurantoin microcrystals

Reactions may be *common*, uncommon, *life-threatening*, or COMMON AND LIFE-THREATENING.

Oral suspension: 25 mg/5 ml

ACTION
Unknown. Appears to interfere with bacterial enzyme systems and possibly with bacterial cell-wall formation.

ONSET, PEAK, DURATION
Unknown.

INDICATIONS & DOSAGE
Urinary tract infections caused by susceptible Escherichia coli, Staphylococcus aureus, *enterococci; or certain strains of* Klebsiella *and* Enterobacter—
Adults and children over 12 years: 50 to 100 mg P.O. q.i.d. with meals and h.s.
Children 1 month to 12 years: 5 to 7 mg/kg P.O. daily, divided q.i.d.
Long-term suppression therapy—
Adults: 50 to 100 mg P.O. daily h.s.
Children: 1 to 2 mg/kg P.O. daily in a single dose h.s. or divided into two doses given q 12 hours.

ADVERSE REACTIONS
CNS: *peripheral neuropathy,* headache, dizziness, drowsiness, *ascending polyneuropathy with high doses or renal impairment.*
GI: *anorexia, nausea, vomiting,* abdominal pain, *diarrhea.*
Hematologic: *hemolysis in patients with G6PD deficiency* (reversed after stopping drug), *agranulocytosis, thrombocytopenia.*
Hepatic: *hepatitis, hepatic necrosis.*
Respiratory: *pulmonary sensitivity reactions* (cough, chest pain, fever, chills, dyspnea, pulmonary infiltration with consolidation or pleural effusion), *asthmatic attacks in patients with history of asthma.*
Skin: maculopapular, erythematous, or eczematous eruption; pruritus; urticaria; *exfoliative dermatitis; Stevens-Johnson syndrome.*
Other: hypersensitivity reactions *(anaphylaxis),* transient alopecia, drug fever, overgrowth of nonsusceptible organisms in the urinary tract.

INTERACTIONS
Magnesium-containing antacids: decreased nitrofurantoin absorption. Separate administration times by 1 hour.
Probenecid, sulfinpyrazone: increased blood levels and decreased urine levels. May result in increased toxicity and lack of therapeutic effect. Don't use together.

EFFECTS ON DIAGNOSTIC TESTS
Nitrofurantoin may cause false-positive results in urine glucose tests using cupric sulfate (such as Benedict's reagent, Fehling's solution, or Clinitest) because it reacts with these agents. Serum glucose may be decreased; bilirubin and alkaline phosphatase may be elevated.

CONTRAINDICATIONS
Contraindicated in children 1 month and under and in patients with moderate to severe renal impairment, anuria, oliguria, or creatinine clearance under 60 ml/minute. Contraindicated in pregnancy at term.

NURSING CONSIDERATIONS
● Use cautiously in patients with renal impairment, anemia, diabetes mellitus, electrolyte abnormalities, vitamin B deficiency, debilitating disease, and G6PD deficiency.
● Obtain urine specimen for culture and sensitivity tests before starting therapy and repeat p.r.n. Therapy may begin pending results.
● Give with food or milk to minimize GI distress and improve absorption.
● Monitor fluid intake and output carefully. May turn urine brown or darker.
● Monitor CBC and pulmonary status regularly.
● Monitor the patient for signs of superinfection. Use of nitrofurantoin may result in growth of nonsusceptible organisms, especially *Pseudomonas.*
Alert: Know that hypersensitivity may develop when used for long-term therapy.

• Be aware that some patients may experience fewer adverse GI effects with nitrofurantoin macrocrystals.

• Know that dual-release capsules (25 mg nitrofurantoin macrocrystals combined with 75 mg nitrofurantoin monohydrate) enable patients to take drug only twice daily.

• Continue treatment for 3 days after sterile urine specimens have been obtained.

• Store drug in amber container. Keep away from metals other than stainless steel or aluminum to avoid precipitate formation.

☑ **PATIENT TEACHING**

• Instruct patient to take medication for as long as prescribed, exactly as directed, even after he feels better.

• Tell patient to take drug with food or milk to minimize stomach upset.

• Instruct patient to report adverse reactions.

• Alert patient that drug may turn urine a harmless dark yellow or brown color.

• Warn patient not to store drug in container made of metal other than stainless steel or aluminum.

---

polymyxin B sulfate
Aerosporin

Pregnancy Risk Category: B

HOW SUPPLIED
Powder for injection: 500,000-unit vials

ACTION
Hinders bacterial cell-wall synthesis, damaging the bacterial plasma membrane and making the cell more vulnerable to osmotic pressure (bactericidal).

ONSET, PEAK, DURATION
Onset and duration unknown. Peak serum levels occur immediately after I.V. infusion, within 2 hours of an I.M. injection.

INDICATIONS & DOSAGE
Meningitis caused by sensitive P. aeruginosa *or* Haemophilus influenzae *when other antibiotics are ineffective or contraindicated—*

Adults and children over 2 years: 50,000 units intrathecally once daily for 3 to 4 days, then 50,000 units every other day for at least 2 weeks after CSF tests are negative and CSF glucose level is normal.

Children under 2 years: 20,000 units intrathecally once daily for 3 to 4 days, then 25,000 units q.o.d. for at least 2 weeks after CSF tests are negative and CSF glucose level is normal.

ADVERSE REACTIONS
CNS: *neurotoxicity,* irritability, drowsiness, facial flushing, weakness, ataxia, *respiratory paralysis,* headache and meningeal irritation with intrathecal administration, peripheral and perioral paresthesias.
EENT: blurred vision.
GU: *nephrotoxicity* (albuminuria, cylindruria, hematuria, proteinuria, decreased urine output, increased BUN level).
Skin: urticaria.
Other: drug fever, pain or thrombophlebitis at injection site.

INTERACTIONS
Aminoglycosides, amphotericin B, cisplatin, vancomycin, zidovudine: increased risk of nephrotoxicity. Avoid concomitant use.
Neuromuscular blockers: may potentiate neuromuscular blockade. Monitor closely.

EFFECTS ON DIAGNOSTIC TESTS
BUN and serum creatinine levels may increase during polymyxin B therapy. CSF protein and leukocyte levels may increase during intrathecal polymyxin B therapy.

CONTRAINDICATIONS
Contraindicated in patients with hypersensitivity to the drug.

Reactions may be *common,* uncommon, *life-threatening,* or COMMON AND LIFE-THREATENING.

NURSING CONSIDERATIONS
● Use cautiously in those with impaired renal function or myasthenia gravis.
● Give only to hospitalized patient under constant supervision.
● Obtain culture and sensitivity tests before first dose. Therapy may begin pending results.
● Know that for meningitis, the drug is given intrathecally to achieve adequate CSF levels.
● Don't give solution containing local anesthetics.
● Drug is extremely nephrotoxic. Monitor renal function (BUN, serum creatinine, creatinine clearance, urine output) before and during therapy, as ordered. Fluid intake should be sufficient to maintain output at 1,500 ml/day (between 3,000 and 4,000 ml/day for adults).
● Notify the doctor immediately if the patient develops fever, adverse CNS effects, rash, or symptoms of nephrotoxicity.
● If the patient is scheduled for surgery, tell the anesthesiologist about preoperative treatment with this drug because it may prolong neuromuscular blockade.

☑ PATIENT TEACHING
● Instruct patient to drink at least 3,000 to 4,000 ml/day of fluid to maintain adequate output, if not contraindicated.
● Tell patient to report adverse reactions promptly.

---

spectinomycin hydrochloride
Trobicin

Pregnancy Risk Category: B

HOW SUPPLIED
Powder for injection: 2 g, 4 g

ACTION
Inhibits protein synthesis by binding to the 30S subunit of the ribosome.

ONSET, PEAK, DURATION
Onset and duration unknown. Serum levels peak 1 hour after a single 2-g I.M. dose, 2 hours after a single 4-g I.M. dose.

INDICATIONS & DOSAGE
Acute gonococcal urethritis and proctitis in men and cervicitis and proctitis in women. Alternative therapy for patient allergic to beta-lactam antibiotics—
Adults: 2 to 4 g I.M. single dose injected deeply into the upper outer quadrant of the buttock.

ADVERSE REACTIONS
CNS: insomnia, dizziness.
GI: nausea.
GU: decreased urine output and creatinine clearance, increased BUN.
Hematologic: decreased hemoglobin and hematocrit levels.
Skin: urticaria.
Other: fever, chills (may mask or delay symptoms of incubating syphilis), transient increases in liver enzymes, pain at injection site.

INTERACTIONS
None significant.

EFFECTS ON DIAGNOSTIC TESTS
BUN, AST, and serum alkaline phosphatase levels increase, and hemoglobin, hematocrit, and creatinine clearance levels decrease during spectinomycin therapy.

CONTRAINDICATIONS
Contraindicated in patients with hypersensitivity to the drug.

NURSING CONSIDERATIONS
● Spectinomycin isn't effective for pharyngeal gonorrhea.
● Shake vial vigorously after reconstitution and before withdrawing dose. Store at room temperature after reconstitution and use within 24 hours.
● Use 20G needle to administer drug. Divide the 4-g dose (10 ml) into two 5-

---

ml injections—give one in each buttock.

☑ **PATIENT TEACHING**
● Inform patient that drug is not effective in the treatment of syphilis. Tell him that serologic test for syphilis should be done before therapy begins and for 3 months afterward.
● Tell patient to report adverse reactions promptly.

---

trimethoprim
Proloprim, Trimpex, Triprim‡

Pregnancy Risk Category: C

HOW SUPPLIED
Tablets: 100 mg, 200 mg

ACTION
Interferes with the action of dihydrofolate reductase, inhibiting bacterial synthesis of folic acid.

ONSET, PEAK, DURATION
Onset and duration unknown. Plasma levels peak 1 to 4 hours after an oral dose.

INDICATIONS & DOSAGE
Uncomplicated urinary tract infections caused by susceptible strains of Escherichia coli, Proteus mirabilis, Klebsiella pneumoniae, Enterobacter *species, and* coagulase-negative Staphylococcus, *including* S. saprophyticus—
Adults: 200 mg P.O. daily as a single dose or in divided doses q 12 hours for 10 days.

Not recommended for children under age 12.

ADVERSE REACTIONS
GI: *epigastric distress, nausea, vomiting,* glossitis.
Hematologic: *thrombocytopenia,* leukopenia, megaloblastic anemia, methemoglobinemia.
Skin: *rash, pruritus, exfoliative dermatitis.*

Other: fever.

INTERACTIONS
Phenytoin: may decrease phenytoin metabolism and increase its serum levels. Monitor for toxicity.

EFFECTS ON DIAGNOSTIC TESTS
Liver enzyme levels and renal function indices (BUN and serum creatinine levels) may increase during trimethoprim therapy.

CONTRAINDICATIONS
Contraindicated in patients with hypersensitivity to the drug and in those with documented megaloblastic anemia caused by folate deficiency.

NURSING CONSIDERATIONS
● Use cautiously in patients with impaired hepatic or renal function. Dosage should be decreased in patients with severely impaired renal function. Be aware that the drug is not recommended for use in patients with creatinine clearance less than 15 ml/minute. Dosage should be adjusted for patients with creatinine clearance of 15 to 30 ml/minute. Also use cautiously in patients with possible folate deficiency.
● Obtain urine specimen for culture and sensitivity tests before first dose. Therapy may begin pending results.
● Monitor CBC routinely. Clinical signs such as sore throat, fever, pallor, or purpura may be early indications of serious blood disorders.
Alert: Prolonged use of trimethoprim at high doses may cause bone marrow suppression.
● Keep in mind that because resistance to trimethoprim develops rapidly when administered alone, it is usually given in combination with other drugs.

☑ **PATIENT TEACHING**
● Instruct the patient to take entire amount of the drug, as prescribed, even after he feels better.
● Tell the patient to report adverse reac-

tions promptly, especially signs of infection or unusual bruising.

---

trimetrexate glucuronate
Neutrexin

Pregnancy Risk Category: D

HOW SUPPLIED
Injection: 25-mg vials, parenteral kit with leucovorin calcium, 50-mg vial

ACTION
Prevents reduction of folic acid to tetrahydrofolate by binding to dihydrofolate reductase.

ONSET, PEAK, DURATION
Unknown.

INDICATIONS & DOSAGE
Alternative treatment of moderate to severe Pneumocystis carinii *pneumonia in immunocompromised patients, including HIV-infected patients who are intolerant or refractory to trimethoprim-sulfamethoxazole*—
Adults: 45 mg/m^2 I.V. infusion over 60 to 90 minutes daily for 21 days, administered with 20 mg/m^2 of leucovorin I.V. or P.O. q 6 hours for 24 days.

ADVERSE REACTIONS
GI: nausea, vomiting, stomatitis.
Hematologic: *neutropenia, thrombocytopenia, anemia.*
Hepatic: hepatotoxicity.
Skin: rash.

INTERACTIONS
Acetaminophen, cimetidine, clotrimazole, erythromycin, fluconazole, ketoconazole, miconazole, rifampin, rifabutin: may interfere with trimetrexate metabolism and lead to toxicity. Monitor closely.
Chloride-containing solutions, leucovorin: precipitate will form if mixed with trimetrexate. Administer separately.

Hepatotoxic, myelosuppressive, or nephrotoxic drugs: enhanced toxicity. Use together cautiously and monitor closely.

EFFECTS ON DIAGNOSTIC TESTS
Information not available.

CONTRAINDICATIONS
Contraindicated in patients with hypersensitivity to trimetrexate, methotrexate, or leucovorin.

NURSING CONSIDERATIONS
● Use cautiously in patients with impaired hematologic, renal, or hepatic function and in women of childbearing age because the drug may cause fetal harm. Avoid using during pregnancy.
● Follow institutional policy when administering parenteral form of this drug because parenteral form is associated with carcinogenic, mutagenic, and teratogenic risks for personnel.
● **I.V. use:** Reconstitute 25-mg vial with 2 ml of D$_5$W or sterile water for injection to yield a solution of 12.5 mg/ml. Complete dissolution usually occurs within 30 seconds. Further dilute reconstituted solution with D$_5$W to yield a final concentration of 0.25 to 2 mg/ml. Infuse over 60 minutes. After reconstitution, the drug is stable at room temperature or refrigerated for 24 hours.
● Use only D$_5$W for I.V. infusion. Drug is incompatible with chloride-containing solutions (including 0.9% sodium chloride solution) and leucovorin.
● Flush the I.V. line with at least 10 ml of D$_5$W immediately before and after the trimetrexate infusion.
● Administer leucovorin either before or after trimetrexate. When giving I.V., be sure to flush the I.V. line with D$_5$W because the two drugs are incompatible. Leucovorin calcium may be infused over 5 to 10 minutes.
Alert: Know that leucovorin therapy must accompany trimetrexate treatments to avoid potentially life-threatening toxicity. Leucovorin therapy must extend

---

for 3 days after trimetrexate therapy.
• When calculating the oral dose of leucovorin, round dosage up to the next increment of 25 mg.
• Monitor patients closely. Many adverse effects may be decreased by adjusting the dosage of leucovorin.
• Avoid I.M. injections in patients with thrombocytopenia.

☑ **PATIENT TEACHING**
• Instruct patient to alert nurse if discomfort occurs at I.V. site.
• Warn patient to watch for signs and symptoms of infection (fever, sore throat, fatigue) and bleeding (easy bruising, epistaxis, bleeding gums, melena) and instruct how to take infection control and bleeding precautions. Tell patients to take temperature daily.
• Advise women of childbearing age to avoid becoming pregnant during therapy. Also recommend consulting doctor before becoming pregnant.

---

vancomycin hydrochloride
Lyphocin, Vancocin, Vancoled

Pregnancy Risk Category: C

HOW SUPPLIED
Capsules: 125 mg, 250 mg
Powder for oral solution: 1-g, 10-g bottles
Powder for injection: 500-mg, 1-g vials
Pharmacy bulk package: 5 g, 10 g
I.V. infusion (frozen): 500 mg in 100 ml 5% dextrose

ACTION
Hinders bacterial cell-wall synthesis, damaging the bacterial plasma membrane and making the cell more vulnerable to osmotic pressure. Also interferes with RNA synthesis.

ONSET, PEAK, DURATION
Onset and duration unknown. Serum levels peak immediately after I.V. infusion.

INDICATIONS & DOSAGE
Serious or severe infections when other antibiotics are ineffective or contraindicated, including those caused by methicillin-resistant Staphyloccus aureus, S. epidermidis, *and diphtheroid organisms—*
Adults: 1 to 1.5 g I.V. q 12 hours (dose based on weight and renal function; longer dosing intervals necessary in renal dysfunction).
Children: 10 mg/kg I.V. q 6 hours.
Neonates and young infants: 15 mg/kg I.V. loading dose, followed by 10 mg/kg I.V. q 12 hours if less than 1 week of age or 10 mg/kg I.V. q 8 hours if older than 1 week but less than 1 month.
Antibiotic-associated pseudomembranous (Clostridium difficile) *and staphylococcal enterocolitis—*
Adults: 125 to 500 mg P.O. q 6 hours for 7 to 10 days.
Children: 40 mg/kg P.O. daily, in divided doses q 6 hours for 7 to 10 days. Maximum daily dosage is 2 g.
Endocarditis prophylaxis for dental procedures—
Adults: 1 g I.V. slowly over 1 hour, starting 1 hour before procedure.
Children: 20 mg/kg I.V. over 1 hour, starting 1 hour before procedure.

ADVERSE REACTIONS
EENT: tinnitus, ototoxicity.
GI: nausea.
GU: nephrotoxicity.
Hematologic: neutropenia.
Skin: "red-neck" syndrome with rapid I.V. infusion (maculopapular rash on face, neck, trunk, and extremities; pruritus and hypotension associated with histamine release).
Other: chills, fever, *anaphylaxis,* superinfection, pain or thrombophlebitis at injection site, hypotension, wheezing, dyspnea.

INTERACTIONS
Aminoglycosides, amphotericin B, cisplatin, pentamidine: increased risk of nephrotoxicity and ototoxicity. Monitor

---

Reactions may be *common,* uncommon, *life-threatening,* or COMMON AND LIFE-THREATENING.

closely.

EFFECTS ON DIAGNOSTIC TESTS
BUN and serum creatinine levels may increase, and neutropenia and eosinophilia may occur during vancomycin therapy.

CONTRAINDICATIONS
Contraindicated in patients with hypersensitivity to the drug.

NURSING CONSIDERATIONS
● Use cautiously in patients receiving other neurotoxic, nephrotoxic, or ototoxic drugs; in patients over 60 years, and in those with impaired hepatic or renal function, preexisting hearing loss, or allergies to other antibiotics. Patients with renal dysfunction require dosage adjustment. Serum levels should be monitored to adjust I.V. dosage. Normal therapeutic levels of vancomycin are as follows: peak, 30 to 40 mg/L (drawn 1 hour after infusion ends); trough, 5 to 10 mg/L (drawn just before next dose is given).
● Obtain culture and sensitivity tests before first dose. Therapy may begin pending results.
● Obtain hearing evaluation and renal function studies before therapy.
● **I.V. use:** For I.V. infusion, dilute in 200 ml 0.9% sodium chloride injection or D_5W, and infuse over 60 to 90 minutes. Check site daily for phlebitis and irritation. Report pain at infusion site. Avoid extravasation. Severe irritation and necrosis can result.
● Monitor the patient carefully for "redneck" syndrome, which can occur if drug is infused too rapidly. If this reaction occurs, stop infusion and report to the doctor.
● Oral administration is ineffective for systemic infections, and I.V. administration is ineffective for pseudomembranous (*Clostridium difficile*) diarrhea.
● Refrigerate I.V. solution after reconstitution and use within 96 hours.
● Do not give drug I.M..

● Know that the oral preparation is stable for 2 weeks if refrigerated.
● Monitor renal function (BUN, serum creatinine, urinalysis, creatinine clearance, and urine output) during therapy. Also monitor for signs of superinfection.
● Have the patient's hearing evaluated during prolonged therapy.
● Be aware that when using the drug to treat staphylococcal endocarditis, it will be given for at least 4 weeks.

☑ **PATIENT TEACHING**
● Tell the patient to take entire amount of medication exactly as directed, even after he feels better.
● Instruct the patient receiving drug I.V. to alert nurse if discomfort occurs at I.V. insertion site.

20

Inotropics

amrinone lactate
digoxin
milrinone lactate

COMBINATION PRODUCTS
None.

---

amrinone lactate
Inocor

Pregnancy Risk Category: C

HOW SUPPLIED
Injection: 5 mg/ml in 20-ml ampules

ACTION
Unknown. Thought to produce inotropic action by increasing cellular levels of cAMP. Produces vasodilation through a direct relaxant effect on vascular smooth muscle.

ONSET, PEAK, DURATION
Onset begins within 2 to 5 minutes. Serum levels peak in 10 minutes. Effects persist ½ to 2 hours after dose.

INDICATIONS & DOSAGE
Short-term management of CHF—
Adults: initially, 0.75 mg/kg I.V. bolus over 2 to 3 minutes. Then begin maintenance infusion of 5 to 10 mcg/kg/minute. Additional bolus of 0.75 mg/kg may be given 30 minutes after start of therapy. Total daily dosage should not exceed 10 mg/kg.

ADVERSE REACTIONS
CV: *arrhythmias,* hypotension.
GI: nausea, vomiting, anorexia, abdominal pain.
Hematologic: *thrombocytopenia* (depends on dose and duration of therapy).
Hepatic: elevated enzymes, hepatotoxicity (rare).

Other: burning at injection site, *hypersensitivity reactions* (pericarditis, ascites, myositis vasculitis, pleuritis), fever, chest pain.

INTERACTIONS
Digitalis glycosides: enhanced inotropic effect. Beneficial drug interaction.

EFFECTS ON DIAGNOSTIC TESTS
The physiologic effects of amrinone may decrease serum potassium or increase serum hepatic enzymes.

CONTRAINDICATIONS
Contraindicated in patients with hypersensitivity to amrinone or bisulfites.

NURSING CONSIDERATIONS
● Know that amrinone should not be used in patients with severe aortic or pulmonic valvular disease in place of surgical correction of the obstruction or during acute phase of MI.
● Use cautiously in patients with hypertrophic cardiomyopathy.
● Be aware that amrinone is primarily prescribed for patients who have not responded to digitalis glycosides, diuretics, and vasodilators.
● Dosage depends on clinical response, including assessment of pulmonary artery wedge pressure and cardiac output.
● Anticipate that amrinone may be added to digitalis glycoside therapy in patients with atrial fibrillation and flutter because it slightly enhances AV conduction and increases ventricular response rate.
● **I.V. use:** Administer amrinone with an infusion pump and use as supplied, or dilute in 0.45% or 0.9% sodium chloride solution to a concentration of 1 to 3 mg/ml. Use diluted solution within 24 hours.

Reactions may be *common,* uncommon, *life-threatening,* or COMMON AND LIFE-THREATENING.

• Don't dilute with solutions containing dextrose because a slow chemical reaction occurs over 24 hours. Amrinone can be injected into free-flowing dextrose infusions through a Y-connector or directly into tubing.

Alert: Don't administer furosemide and amrinone through the same I.V. line because precipitation occurs.

• Monitor blood pressure and heart rate throughout the infusion. If the patient's blood pressure falls, slow or stop infusion and notify the doctor.

• Monitor platelet count. If it falls below 150,000/mm³, decrease dosage as ordered.

• Patients with end-stage cardiac disease may receive home treatment with an amrinone drip while awaiting heart transplantation.

☑ **PATIENT TEACHING**
• Warn patient that burning may occur at the site of injection.
• Instruct home care patient and family on administration; tell them to report adverse reactions promptly.

---

digoxin
Digoxin, Lanoxicaps, Lanoxin*, Novodigoxin†

Pregnancy Risk Category: C

HOW SUPPLIED
Tablets: 0.125 mg, 0.25 mg, 0.5 mg
Capsules: 0.05 mg, 0.1 mg, 0.2 mg
Elixir: 0.05 mg/ml
Injection: 0.05 mg/ml†, 0.1 mg/ml (pediatric), 0.25 mg/ml

ACTION
Inhibits sodium-potassium activated adenosine triphosphatase, thereby promoting movement of calcium from extracellular to intracellular cytoplasm and strengthening myocardial contraction. Also acts on CNS to enhance vagal tone, slowing conduction through the SA and AV nodes and providing an an-

tiarrhythmic effect.

ONSET, PEAK, DURATION
Onset occurs ½ to 2 hours after oral dose or 5 to 30 minutes after I.V. administration. Serum levels peak 2 to 6 hours after oral dose or 1 to 4 hours after I.V. administration. Effects persist 3 to 4 days after last dose.

INDICATIONS & DOSAGE
CHF, paroxysmal supraventricular tachycardia, atrial fibrillation and flutter—
Adults: loading dose is 0.5 to 1 mg I.V. or P.O. in divided doses over 24 hours; maintenance dosage is 0.125 to 0.5 mg I.V. or P.O. daily (average is 0.25 mg). Depending on response, larger doses may be needed for arrhythmias. Smaller loading and maintenance doses are given to patients with impaired renal function.
Adults over 65 years: 0.125 mg P.O. daily as maintenance dose. Frail or underweight elderly patients may require only 0.0625 mg daily or 0.125 mg every other day.
Premature neonates: loading dose is 0.015 to 0.025 mg/kg I.V. in three divided doses over 24 hours; maintenance dosage is 0.01 mg/kg daily, divided q 12 hours.
Neonates: loading dose is 0.025 to 0.035 mg/kg P.O., divided q 8 hours over 24 hours; I.V. loading dose is 0.02 to 0.03 mg/kg; maintenance dosage is 0.01 mg/kg P.O. daily, divided q 12 hours.
Children 1 month to 2 years: loading dose is 0.035 to 0.06 mg/kg P.O. in three divided doses over 24 hours; I.V. loading dose is 0.03 to 0.05 mg/kg; maintenance dosage is 0.01 to 0.02 mg/kg P.O. daily, divided q 12 hours.
Children over 2 years: loading dose is 0.02 to 0.04 mg/kg P.O. daily, divided q 8 hours over 24 hours; I.V. loading dose is 0.015 to 0.035 mg/kg; maintenance dosage is 0.012 mg/kg P.O. daily, divided q 12 hours.

---

*Liquid contains alcohol.   **May contain tartrazine.   †Canada only.   ‡Australia only.   ◇OTC.

ADVERSE REACTIONS

The following signs of toxicity may occur with all digitalis glycosides:

CNS: *fatigue, generalized muscle weakness, agitation, hallucinations,* headache, malaise, dizziness, vertigo, stupor, paresthesia.

CV: *arrhythmias* (most commonly, conduction disturbances with or without AV block, PVCs, and supraventricular arrhythmias); arrhythmias may lead to increased severity of CHF and hypotension. *Toxic effects on the heart may be life-threatening and require immediate attention.*

EENT: *yellow-green halos around visual images, blurred vision,* light flashes, photophobia, diplopia.

GI: *anorexia, nausea,* vomiting, diarrhea.

INTERACTIONS

Amiloride: inhibited digoxin effect and increased digoxin excretion. Monitor for altered digoxin effect.

Amiodarone, diltiazem, nifedipine, quinidine, verapamil: increased digoxin blood levels. Monitor for toxicity.

Amphotericin B, carbenicillin, corticosteroids, diuretics (including loop diuretics, chlorthalidone, metolazone, and thiazides), ticarcillin: hypokalemia, predisposing patient to digitalis toxicity. Monitor serum potassium levels.

Antacids, kaolin-pectin: decreased absorption of oral digoxin. Schedule doses as far as possible from oral digoxin administration.

Anticholinergics: may increase digoxin absorption of oral digoxin tablets. Monitor blood levels and observe for toxicity.

Cholestyramine, colestipol, metoclopramide: decreased absorption of oral digoxin. Monitor for decreased digitoxin effect and low blood levels. Increase dosage as ordered.

Parenteral calcium, thiazides: hypercalcemia and hypomagnesemia, predisposing patient to digitalis toxicity. Monitor serum calcium and serum magnesium

levels.

EFFECTS ON DIAGNOSTIC TESTS

None reported.

CONTRAINDICATIONS

Contraindicated in patients with hypersensitivity to the drug; any digitalis-induced toxicity; ventricular fibrillation; or ventricular tachycardia unless caused by CHF.

NURSING CONSIDERATIONS

● Use with extreme caution in elderly patients and in those with acute MI, incomplete AV block, sinus bradycardia, PVCs, chronic constrictive pericarditis, hypertrophic cardiomyopathy, renal insufficiency, severe pulmonary disease, or hypothyroidism. Reduce dosage in patients with renal impairment.

● Be aware that hypothyroid patients are extremely sensitive to digitalis glycosides; hyperthyroid patients may need larger doses.

● Before administering the loading dose, obtain baseline data (heart rate and rhythm, blood pressure, and electrolytes) and question the patient about use of digitalis glycosides within the previous 2 to 3 weeks.

● Be aware that the loading dose is divided over the first 24 hours unless the situation indicates otherwise.

● Before giving, take apical-radial pulse for a full minute. Record and report to the doctor significant changes (sudden increase or decrease in pulse rate, pulse deficit, irregular beats and, particularly, regularization of a previously irregular rhythm). If any occurs, check blood pressure and obtain a 12-lead ECG.

● **I.V. use:** Infuse drug slowly over at least 5 minutes.

● Absorption of digoxin from liquid-filled capsules is superior to absorption from tablets or elixir. Expect dosage reduction of 20% to 25% when changing from tablets or elixir to liquid-filled capsules or parenteral therapy.

● Monitor serum digoxin levels. Therapeutic levels range from 0.5 to 2.0 ng/ml. Obtain blood for digoxin levels 8 hours after last oral dose.

Alert: Excessive slowing of the pulse rate (60 beats/minute or less) may be a sign of digitalis toxicity. Withhold drug and notify the doctor.

● Monitor serum potassium levels carefully. Take corrective action before hypokalemia occurs.

● Withhold drug for 1 to 2 days before elective cardioversion. Adjust dose after cardioversion.

☑ **PATIENT TEACHING**

● Instruct the patient and a responsible family member about drug action, dosage regimen, how to take pulse, reportable signs, and follow-up care.

● Encourage the patient to eat potassium-rich foods.

● Tell the patient not to substitute one brand of digoxin for another.

---

milrinone lactate
Primacor

Pregnancy Risk Category: C

HOW SUPPLIED
Injection: 1 mg/ml

ACTION
Produces inotropic action by increasing cellular levels of cAMP. Produces vasodilation by directly relaxing vascular smooth muscle.

ONSET, PEAK, DURATION
Onset occurs within 5 to 15 minutes. Serum levels peak within 1 to 2 hours. Duration is 3 to 6 hours.

INDICATIONS & DOSAGE
Short-term treatment of CHF—
Adults: initial loading dose is 50 mcg/kg I.V., administered slowly over 10 minutes, followed by continuous I.V. infusion of 0.375 to 0.75 mcg/kg/minute. Adjust infusion dose

according to clinical and hemodynamic responses, as ordered.

In patients with renal failure: if creatinine clearance is 50 ml/minute or less, dosage is titrated to maximum clinical effect and not to exceed 1.13 mg/kg/day.

ADVERSE REACTIONS
CNS: headache.
CV: VENTRICULAR ARRHYTHMIAS, *ventricular ectopic activity,* nonsustained ventricular tachycardia, *sustained ventricular tachycardia, ventricular fibrillation.*

INTERACTIONS
None significant.

EFFECTS ON DIAGNOSTIC TESTS
None reported.

CONTRAINDICATIONS
Contraindicated in patients with hypersensitivity to the drug.

NURSING CONSIDERATIONS
● Know that milrinone should not be used in patients with severe aortic or pulmonic valvular disease in place of surgical correction of the obstruction or during acute phase of MI.

● Use cautiously in patients with atrial flutter or fibrillation because drug slightly shortens AV node conduction time and may increase ventricular response rate. Administer a digitalis glycoside, if ordered, before beginning milrinone therapy.

● Be aware that milrinone is typically given with digoxin and diuretics.

● Be aware that inotropic agents may aggravate outflow tract obstruction in hypertrophic subaortic stenosis.

● **I.V. use:** Prepare I.V. infusion solution using 0.45% or 0.9% sodium chloride or D_5W. Prepare the 100-mcg/ml solution by adding 180 ml of diluent per 20-mg (20-ml) vial, the 150-mcg/ml solution by adding 113 ml of diluent per 20-mg (20-ml) vial, and the 200-mcg/ml solu-

---

*Liquid contains alcohol.   **May contain tartrazine.   †Canada only.   ‡Australia only.   ◇OTC.

tion by adding 80 ml of diluent per 20-mg (20-ml) vial.

● Be aware that improved cardiac output may enhance urine output. Expect dosage reduction in patient's diuretic therapy as CHF improves. Potassium loss may predispose patient to digitalis toxicity.

● Monitor fluid and electrolyte status, blood pressure, heart rate, and renal function during therapy. Excessive decrease in blood pressure requires discontinuing or slowing rate of infusion. *Alert:* Do not administer furosemide and amrinone through the same I.V. line because precipitation will occur.

☑ **PATIENT TEACHING**
● Instruct patient to report adverse reactions promptly.
● Tell patient to alert the nurse if discomfort is felt at I.V. insertion site.

21

Antiarrhythmics

adenosine
amiodarone hydrochloride
atropine sulfate
bretylium tosylate
diltiazem hydrochloride
(See Chapter 22, antianginals.)
disopyramide
disopyramide phosphate
esmolol hydrochloride
flecainide acetate
ibutilide fumarate
lidocaine hydrochloride
mexiletine hydrochloride
moricizine hydrochloride
phenytoin
(See Chapter 30, anticonvulsants.)
phenytoin sodium
(See Chapter 30, anticonvulsants.)
procainamide hydrochloride
propafenone hydrochloride
propranolol hydrochloride
(See Chapter 22, antianginals.)
quinidine bisulfate
quinidine gluconate
quinidine polygalacturonate
quinidine sulfate
sotalol
tocainide hydrochloride
verapamil hydrochloride
(See Chapter 22, antianginals.)

COMBINATION PRODUCTS
None.

---

adenosine
Adenocard

Pregnancy Risk Category: C

HOW SUPPLIED
Injection: 3 mg/ml in 2-ml and 5-ml
vials

ACTION
A naturally occurring nucleoside that
acts on the AV node to slow conduction
and inhibit reentry pathways. Adenosine
is also useful in treating paroxysmal
supraventricular tachycardia (PSVT) associated with accessory bypass tracts
(Wolff-Parkinson-White syndrome).

ONSET, PEAK, DURATION
Onset and peak serum levels occur immediately. Duration is extremely short;
the exact time is unknown. However,
half-life is estimated to be under 10 seconds.

INDICATIONS & DOSAGE
Conversion of PSVT to sinus rhythm—
Adults: 6 mg I.V. by rapid bolus injection over 1 to 2 seconds. If PSVT is not
eliminated in 1 to 2 minutes, 12 mg by
rapid I.V. push may be given and repeated (if necessary). Single doses over 12
mg are not recommended.

ADVERSE REACTIONS
CNS: apprehension, back pain, blurred
vision, burning sensation, dizziness,
heaviness in arms, light-headedness,
neck pain, numbness, tingling in arms.
CV: chest pain, *facial flushing,*
headache, hypotension, palpitations, diaphoresis.
GI: metallic taste, nausea.
Respiratory: chest pressure, *dyspnea,
shortness of breath,* hyperventilation.
Other: *throat tightness, groin pressure.*

INTERACTIONS
Carbamazepine: higher degrees of heart
block may occur.
Dipyridamole: may potentiate adenosine's effects. Smaller doses may be
necessary.
Methylxanthines: antagonism of adenosine's effects. Patients receiving theophylline or caffeine may require higher
doses or may not respond to adenosine

---

therapy.

EFFECTS ON DIAGNOSTIC TESTS
None reported.

CONTRAINDICATIONS
Contraindicated in patients with hyper-sensitivity to the drug and also in those with second- or third-degree heart block or sick sinus syndrome, unless an artificial pacemaker is present, because adenosine decreases conduction through the AV node and may produce first-, second-, or third-degree heart block. Patients who develop significant heart block after a dose of adenosine should not receive additional doses.

NURSING CONSIDERATIONS
• Use cautiously in patients with asthma because bronchoconstriction may occur.
• Crystals may form if solution is cold. If crystals are visible, gently warm solution to room temperature. Don't use solutions that aren't clear.
• Because adenosine contains no preservatives, discard any unused drug.
• **I.V. use:** Rapid I.V. injection is necessary to ensure drug action. Administer directly into a vein if possible; when giving through an I.V. line, use the port closest to the patient, and flush immediately and rapidly with 0.9% sodium chloride solution to ensure that the drug reaches the systemic circulation quickly.
• Monitor patient's ECG for arrhythmias. In clinical trials, more than half the patients exhibited new arrhythmias, including sinus bradycardia or tachycardia, premature atrial contractions, various degrees of AV block, PVCs, and skipped beats, when adenosine was used to convert to normal sinus rhythm. Such arrhythmias are usually transient.

☑ **PATIENT TEACHING**
• Instruct patient to report adverse reactions promptly.
• Tell patient to alert nurse if discomfort occurs at I.V. site.

amiodarone hydrochloride
Aratac‡, Cordarone, Cordarone X‡

Pregnancy Risk Category: D

HOW SUPPLIED
Tablets: 100 mg†‡, 200 mg
Injection: 50 mg/ml

ACTION
Unknown. Thought to prolong the refractory period and action potential duration.

ONSET, PEAK, DURATION
Onset may occur in 2 to 3 days despite more rapid peak concentration, but more commonly takes 1 to 3 weeks, even with loading doses. Serum levels peak 3 to 7 hours after oral administration. With I.V. use, electrophysiologic effects (prolonged QTc) can be seen within hours. Duration of antiarrhythmic effects may last for weeks or months but rate variable and unpredictable.

INDICATIONS & DOSAGE
Recurrent ventricular fibrillation and recurrent hemodynamically unstable ventricular tachycardia refractory to other antiarrhythmics—
Adults: give loading dose of 800 to 1,600 mg P.O. daily for 1 to 3 weeks until initial therapeutic response occurs, then 600 to 800 mg/day P.O. for 1 month, and then, for maintenance, 200 to 600 mg P.O. daily.
Or, give loading dose of 150 mg I.V. over 10 minutes (15 mg/minute); then 360 mg I.V. over the next 6 hours (1 mg/minute); then 540 mg I.V. over the next 18 hours (0.5 mg/minute). After the first 24 hours, a maintenance I.V. infusion of 720 mg/24 hours (0.5 mg/minute) should be continued.

ADVERSE REACTIONS
CNS: peripheral neuropathy, ataxia, paresthesia, tremor, insomnia, sleep dis-

turbances, headache, *malaise, fatigue*.
CV: bradycardia, hypotension, ***arrhythmias, CHF, heart block, sinus arrest***.
EENT: *corneal microdeposits,* visual disturbances.
GI: *nausea, vomiting,* constipation, abdominal pain.
Hepatic: *altered liver enzymes,* hepatic dysfunction, ***hepatic failure***.
Respiratory: severe pulmonary toxicity (pneumonitis, alveolitis).
Skin: *photosensitivity,* blue-gray skin pigmentation, solar dermatitis.
Other: hypothyroidism, hyperthyroidism, edema, coagulation abnormalities.

INTERACTIONS
Antiarrhythmics: amiodarone may reduce the hepatic or renal clearance of certain antiarrhythmics (especially flecainide, procainamide, or quinidine); concomitant use of amiodarone with other antiarrhythmics (especially mexiletine, propafenone, quinidine, disopyramide, or procainamide) may induce torsades de pointes.
Antihypertensives: increased hypotensive effect. Use together cautiously.
Beta blockers, calcium channel blockers: increased cardiac depressant effects; may potentiate slowing of SA node and AV conduction. Use together cautiously.
Digitalis glycosides: increased serum digoxin levels (average of 70% to 100%). Monitor digoxin levels closely and adjust dosage as ordered.
Phenytoin: may decrease phenytoin metabolism. Monitor serum phenytoin levels and adjust dosage as ordered.
Theophylline: increased theophylline levels with toxicity may occur. Monitor serum theophylline levels.
Warfarin: increased PT (average of 100% within 1 to 4 weeks of therapy). Decrease warfarin dosage 33% to 50% when amiodarone is initiated. Monitor patient closely.

EFFECTS ON DIAGNOSTIC TESTS
Amiodarone alters thyroid function test results, causing increased serum thyroxine (T_4) and decreased triiodothyronine (T_3) levels. (However, most patients maintain normal thyroid function during therapy.)

CONTRAINDICATIONS
Contraindicated in patients with hypersensitivity to the drug and in those with severe SA node disease resulting in preexisting bradycardia. Unless an artificial pacemaker is present, drug is also contraindicated in patients with cardiogenic shock or second- or third-degree AV block and in those in whom bradycardia has caused syncope.

NURSING CONSIDERATIONS
● Use with extreme caution in those receiving other antiarrhythmics.
● Use cautiously in patients with pulmonary or thyroid disease.
● Be aware that although amiodarone is often effective for treatment of arrhythmias resistant to other drug therapy, the high incidence of adverse reactions limits its use.
● Obtain baseline pulmonary, liver, and thyroid function tests.
● Administer loading doses in a hospital setting and with continuous ECG monitoring because of the slow onset of antiarrhythmic effect and risk of life-threatening arrhythmias.
● Divide oral loading dose into three equal doses and give with meals to decrease GI intolerance. Maintenance dosage may be given once daily, but may be divided into two doses taken with meals if GI intolerance occurs.
● **I.V. use:** Know that amiodarone may be given I.V. where facilities for close monitoring of cardiac function and resuscitation are available. Initial dosage of 150 mg should be mixed in 100 ml of dextrose 5% solution. Repeat doses should be administered through a central venous catheter.
● Continuously monitor cardiac status of patient receiving drug I.V.
● Monitor blood pressure and heart rate

and rhythm frequently. Perform continuous ECG monitoring during initiation and alteration of dosage. Notify doctor of significant change.

Alert: Monitor carefully for pulmonary toxicity, which can be fatal. Incidence increases in patients receiving more than 400 mg/day.

● Monitor for symptoms of pneumonitis—exertional dyspnea, nonproductive cough, and pleuritic chest pain. Monitor pulmonary function tests and chest X-ray.

● Monitor liver and thyroid function tests and serum electrolytes, particularly potassium and magnesium levels.

● Instillation of methylcellulose ophthalmic solution is recommended during amiodarone therapy to minimize corneal microdeposits. Within 1 to 4 months after beginning amiodarone therapy, most patients show corneal microdeposits upon slit-lamp ophthalmic examination. However, only 2% to 3% have actual vision disturbances.

☑ **PATIENT TEACHING**
● Advise the patient to use a sunscreen or protective clothing to prevent photosensitivity reaction. Monitor for burning or tingling skin followed by erythema and possible skin blistering. A blue-gray discoloration of the exposed skin may occur.

● Tell the patient to take oral drug with food if GI reactions occur.

● Inform the patient that amiodarone's adverse effects are more prevalent at high doses but are generally reversible when drug therapy is stopped. Resolution of adverse reactions may take up to 4 months.

---

atropine sulfate

Pregnancy Risk Category: C

HOW SUPPLIED
Tablets: 0.4 mg, 0.6 mg
Injection: 0.05 mg/ml, 0.1 mg/ml, 0.3 mg/ml, 0.4 mg/ml, 0.5 mg/ml, 0.6 mg/ml, 0.8 mg/ml, 1 mg/ml, 1.2 mg/ml

ACTION
An anticholinergic that inhibits acetylcholine at the parasympathetic neuroeffector junction, blocking vagal effects on the SA and AV nodes; this enhances conduction through the AV node and speeds heart rate.

ONSET, PEAK, DURATION
Onset occurs 30 minutes to 1 hour after oral administration, 30 minutes after I.M. administration, and immediately after I.V. administration. Serum levels peak 2 hours after oral administration, 1 to 1.6 hours after I.M. administration, and 2 to 4 minutes after I.V. administration. Duration is about 4 hours.

INDICATIONS & DOSAGE
Symptomatic bradycardia, brady-arrhythmia (junctional or escape rhythm)—
Adults: usually 0.5 to 1 mg I.V. push; repeated q 3 to 5 minutes to maximum of 2 mg as needed. Lower doses (less than 0.5 mg) can cause bradycardia.
Children: 0.01 mg/kg I.V.; may repeat q 4 to 6 hours; maximum dose is 0.4 mg or 0.3 mg/m^2.
Antidote for anticholinesterase insecticide poisoning—
Adults: 2 to 3 mg I.V. repeated q 5 to 10 minutes until muscarinic symptoms disappear or signs of atropine toxicity appear. Severe poisoning may require up to 6 mg q hour.
Children: 0.05 mg/kg I.M. or I.V. repeated q 10 to 30 minutes until muscarinic signs and symptoms subside (may be repeated if they appear) or until atropine toxicity occurs.
Preoperatively to diminish secretions and block cardiac vagal reflexes—
Adults and children weighing 20 kg or more: 0.4 to 0.6 mg I.M. or S.C. 30 to 60 minutes before anesthesia.
Children weighing less than 20 kg: 0.01 mg/kg I.M. or S.C. up to maximum

---

dose of 0.4 mg 30 to 60 minutes before anesthesia.

Adjunct treatment of peptic ulcer disease; treatment of functional GI disorders such as irritable bowel syndrome—

Adults: 0.4 to 0.6 mg P.O. q 4 to 6 hours.

Children: 0.01 mg/kg or 0.3 mg/m^2 (not to exceed 0.4 mg) q 4 to 6 hours.

ADVERSE REACTIONS

CNS: *headache, restlessness,* ataxia, disorientation, hallucinations, delirium, *insomnia, dizziness,* excitement, agitation, confusion (especially in elderly patients).

CV: palpitations and bradycardia following low dose of atropine, tachycardia after higher doses.

EENT: photophobia, *blurred vision, mydriasis,* cycloplegia, increased intraocular pressure.

GI: *dry mouth,* thirst, *constipation,* nausea, vomiting.

GU: urine retention, impotence.

Hematologic: leukocytosis.

Other: severe allergic reactions, including ***anaphylaxis*** and urticaria.

INTERACTIONS

Antacids: decreased absorption of anticholinergics. Separate administration times by at least 1 hour.

Anticholinergics or drugs with anticholinergic effects, such as amantadine, glutethimide, meperidine, antiarrhythmics, antiparkinsonian agents, phenothiazines, and tricyclic antidepressants: additive anticholinergic effects. Use together cautiously.

Ketoconazole, levodopa: decreased absorption. Avoid concomitant use.

Methotrimeprazine: may produce extrapyramidal symptoms. Monitor patient carefully.

Potassium chloride wax-matrix tablets: increased risk of mucosal lesions. Use cautiously.

EFFECTS ON DIAGNOSTIC TESTS
None reported.

CONTRAINDICATIONS

Contraindicated in patients with hypersensitivity to drug, acute angle-closure glaucoma, obstructive uropathy, obstructive disease of GI tract, paralytic ileus, toxic megacolon, intestinal atony, unstable CV status in acute hemorrhage, tachycardia, myocardial ischemia, asthma, and myasthenia gravis.

NURSING CONSIDERATIONS

● Use cautiously in patients with Down syndrome because they may be more sensitive to the drug.

● **I.V. use:** Administer via direct I.V. into a large vein or I.V. tubing over at least 1 minute.

● Be aware that many adverse reactions (such as dry mouth and constipation) vary with the dose.

● Monitor patients for paradoxical initial bradycardia, especially those receiving small doses (0.4 to 0.6 mg). This usually disappears within 2 minutes.

Alert: Watch for tachycardia in cardiac patients because it may precipitate ventricular fibrillation.

● Monitor fluid intake and urine output. Drug causes urine retention and urinary hesitancy.

☑ PATIENT TEACHING

● Teach patient receiving oral form of drug how to handle distressing anticholinergic effects.

● Instruct patient to report serious or persistent adverse reactions promptly.

---

bretylium tosylate
Bretylate†‡, Bretylol, Critifib‡

Pregnancy Risk Category: C

HOW SUPPLIED

Injection: 50 mg/ml in 10-ml ampules, vials, and syringes and in 20-ml vials

---

ACTION
Unknown but considered a class III antiarrhythmic that initially exerts transient adrenergic stimulation through release of norepinephrine. Subsequent depletion of norepinephrine causes adrenergic blocking actions to predominate, prolonging repolarization and increasing the duration of action potential and an effective refractory period.

ONSET, PEAK, DURATION
Onset occurs within a few minutes but suppression of ventricular tachycardia and ventricular fibrillation may not occur for 20 minutes to 6 hours. Peak serum levels occur at the end of an I.V. bolus or 1 hour following I.M. administration. Effects may persist 6 to 24 hours.

INDICATIONS & DOSAGE
Ventricular fibrillation or hemodynamically unstable ventricular tachycardia unresponsive to other antiarrhythmics—
Adults: 5 mg/kg by I.V. push over 1 minute. If necessary, dose increased to 10 mg/kg and repeated q 15 to 30 minutes until 30 to 35 mg/kg have been given. For continuous suppression, diluted solution administered at 1 to 2 mg/minute continuously or 5 to 10 mg/kg diluted over more than 8 minutes q 6 hours.

ADVERSE REACTIONS
CNS: *vertigo, dizziness, light-headedness, syncope* (usually secondary to hypotension).
CV: SEVERE HYPOTENSION (especially orthostatic), bradycardia, anginal pain, transient arrhythmias, transient hypertension, increased PVCs.
GI: severe nausea, vomiting (with rapid infusion).

INTERACTIONS
All antihypertensives: may potentiate hypotension. Monitor blood pressure.
Other antiarrhythmics: additive or an-tagonistic antiarrhythmic effects. Monitor for additive toxicity.
Sympathomimetics: bretylium may potentiate effects of drugs given to correct hypotension.

EFFECTS ON DIAGNOSTIC TESTS
None reported.

CONTRAINDICATIONS
Contraindicated in digitalized patients unless the arrhythmia is life-threatening, not caused by digitalis, and unresponsive to other antiarrhythmics.

NURSING CONSIDERATIONS
● Use with extreme caution in patients with fixed cardiac output (aortic stenosis and pulmonary hypertension) to avoid severe and sudden drop in blood pressure.
● Bretylium is used with other cardiac life-support measures, such as cardiopulmonary resuscitation, countershock, epinephrine, sodium bicarbonate, and lidocaine.
● **I.V. use:** When used for maintenance therapy, dilute using dextrose or sodium chloride for injection before administration. Follow manufacturer's guidelines for specific dilution guidelines (varies according to dosage). When administering as direct I.V. injection, use a 20G to 22G needle and inject over 1 minute into a vein or I.V. line containing a free-flowing, compatible solution.
● To prevent nausea and vomiting, follow dosage directions carefully.
● Keep the patient supine until tolerance to hypotension develops.
● Monitor the patient closely. The initial release of norepinephrine caused by bretylium may induce transient hypertension and arrhythmias.
● Monitor blood pressure and heart rate and rhythm continuously. Notify doctor immediately of any significant change. If supine systolic blood pressure falls below 75 mm Hg, the doctor may order norepinephrine, dopamine, or volume expanders.

Reactions may be *common*, uncommon, *life-threatening*, or COMMON AND LIFE-THREATENING.

• Observe for increased anginal pain in susceptible patients.

☑ **PATIENT TEACHING**
• Instruct the patient to report adverse reactions immediately.
• Tell the patient to alert nurse if discomfort occurs at I.V. insertion site.
• Tell the patient to avoid sudden postural changes.

disopyramide
Rythmodan†

disopyramide phosphate
Norpace, Norpace CR, Rythmodan LA†

Pregnancy Risk Category: C

HOW SUPPLIED
disopyramide
Capsules: 100 mg†, 150 mg†
disopyramide phosphate
Tablets (sustained-release): 250 mg†
Capsules: 100 mg, 150 mg
Capsules (controlled-release): 100 mg, 150 mg
Injection: 10 mg/ml‡

ACTION
Unknown, but the drug is considered a class Ia antiarrhythmic that depresses phase O and prolongs the action potential. All class I drugs have membrane-stabilizing effects.

ONSET, PEAK, DURATION
Onset occurs within ½ to 3½ hours after an oral dose. Plasma levels peak within 2 to 2½ hours after an oral dose. Effects persist for 1½ to 8½ hours after last dose.

INDICATIONS & DOSAGE
Ventricular tachycardia and ventricular arrhythmias believed to be life-threatening—
Adults weighing more than 50 kg: 150 mg q 6 hours with conventional cap-

sules or 300 mg q 12 hours with extended-release preparations.
Adults weighing 50 kg or less: highly individualized.
Children under 1 year: 10 to 30 mg/kg P.O. daily.
Children 1 to 4 years: 10 to 20 mg/kg P.O. daily.
Children 4 to 12 years: 10 to 15 mg/kg P.O. daily.
Children 12 to 18 years: 6 to 15 mg/kg P.O. daily.
For pediatric dosages, divide into equal amounts and give q 6 hours.
Recommended dosages in advanced renal insufficiency: If creatinine clearance is 30 to 40 ml/minute, 100 mg q 8 hours; if 15 to 30 ml/minute, 100 mg q 12 hours; if less than 15 ml/minute, 100 mg q 24 hours.
For parenteral use in adults, initially give 2 mg/kg I.V. slowly (over not less than 15 minutes). Administer until arrhythmia is eliminated or patient has received 150 mg. Repeat dosage if conversion is successful but arrhythmia returns. Total I.V. dosage should not exceed 300 mg in the first hour. Follow with an I.V. infusion of 0.4 mg/kg/hour (usually 20 to 30 mg/hour) to a maximum of 800 mg/day.

ADVERSE REACTIONS
CNS: dizziness, agitation, depression, fatigue, headache, acute psychosis.
CV: *hypotension, CHF, heart block,* edema, weight gain, *arrhythmias,* syncope, shortness of breath, chest pain.
EENT: *blurred vision, dry eyes or nose.*
GI: nausea, vomiting, anorexia, bloating, abdominal pain, diarrhea.
Hepatic: cholestatic jaundice.
Skin: rash, pruritus, dermatosis.
Other: aches, pain, muscle weakness, hypoglycemia (rare).

INTERACTIONS
Antiarrhythmics: possible additive or antagonized antiarrhythmic effects.
Phenytoin: increased metabolism of disopyramide. Monitor for decreased

antiarrhythmic effect.
Rifampin: may decrease disopyramide levels. Monitor closely.

EFFECTS ON DIAGNOSTIC TESTS
The physiologic effects of disopyramide may cause a decrease in blood glucose concentrations.

CONTRAINDICATIONS
Contraindicated in patients with hypersensitivity to the drug, sick sinus syndrome, cardiogenic shock, or second- or third-degree heart block in the absence of an artificial pacemaker.

NURSING CONSIDERATIONS
● Use with extreme caution and avoid, if possible, in patients with CHF. Use cautiously in patients with underlying conduction abnormalities, urinary tract diseases (especially prostatic hyperplasia), hepatic or renal impairment, myasthenia gravis, or acute angle-closure glaucoma.
● Correct electrolyte abnormalities before therapy begins, as ordered.
● Check apical pulse before administering drug. Notify the doctor if pulse rate is slower than 60 beats/minute or faster than 120 beats/minute.
● Know that sustained or controlled-release preparations should not be used for rapid control of ventricular arrhythmias, when therapeutic blood levels must be rapidly attained, in patients with cardiomyopathy or possible cardiac decompensation, or in those with severe renal impairment.
● For administration to young children, pharmacist may prepare disopyramide suspension, using 100-mg capsules and cherry syrup. Suspension should be dispensed in amber glass bottles and protected from light.
● **I.V. use:** Add 200 mg to 200 to 500 ml of a compatible solution, such as 0.9% sodium chloride or D₅W. Do not mix with other drugs; switch to oral therapy as soon as possible.
● Watch for recurrence of arrhythmias

and check for adverse reactions; notify the doctor if any occur.
● Discontinue drug if heart block develops, if QRS complex widens by more than 25%, or if QT interval lengthens by more than 25% above baseline; also notify the doctor.
● When transferring the patient from immediate-release to sustained-release capsules, advise him to take the first sustained-release capsule 6 hours after taking the last immediate-release capsule.

☑ PATIENT TEACHING
● Teach the patient the importance of taking drug on time and exactly as prescribed. This may require use of an alarm clock for overnight doses.
● Advise the patient to chew gum or hard candy to relieve dry mouth and to increase fiber and fluid intake to relieve constipation, if not contraindicated.

esmolol hydrochloride
Brevibloc

Pregnancy Risk Category: C

HOW SUPPLIED
Injection: 10 mg/ml in 10-ml vials, 250 mg/ml in 10-ml ampules

ACTION
A class II antiarrhythmic and ultra-short-acting selective beta₁-adrenergic blocker that decreases heart rate, contractility, and blood pressure.

ONSET, PEAK, DURATION
Onset occurs almost immediately. Peak serum levels vary with infusion rate but typically occur in 30 minutes. Effects subside within 30 minutes after infusion ends.

INDICATIONS & DOSAGE
Supraventricular tachycardia; to control ventricular rate in patients with atrial fibrillation or flutter in periopera-

---

Reactions may be *common*, uncommon, *life-threatening*, or COMMON AND LIFE-THREATENING.

tive, postoperative, or other emergent circumstances; noncompensatory sinus tachycardia when heart rate requires specific interventions—
Adults: loading dose is 500 mcg/kg/minute by I.V. infusion over 1 minute, followed by 4-minute maintenance infusion of 50 mcg/kg/minute. If adequate response does not occur within 5 minutes, loading dose is repeated and followed by maintenance infusion of 100 mcg/kg/minute for 4 minutes. Loading dose is repeated and maintenance infusion is increased by 50-mcg/kg/minute increments. Maximum maintenance infusion for tachycardia is 200 mcg/kg/minute.
Perioperative and postoperative tachycardia or hypertension—
Adults: for perioperative treatment of tachycardia or hypertension, 80 mg (approximately 1 mg/kg) I.V. bolus over 30 seconds, followed by 150 mcg/kg/minute I.V. infusion, if needed. Adjust the infusion rate as needed up to a maximum of 300 mcg/kg/minute; dosage for postoperative treatment of tachycardia and hypertension is the same as for supraventricular tachycardia.

ADVERSE REACTIONS
CNS: dizziness, somnolence, headache, agitation, fatigue, confusion.
CV: HYPOTENSION (sometimes with diaphoresis), peripheral ischemia.
GI: *nausea,* vomiting.
Respiratory: *bronchospasm,* wheezing, dyspnea, nasal congestion.
Other: inflammation and induration at infusion site.

INTERACTIONS
Digoxin: serum digoxin levels may be increased by 10% to 20%. Monitor serum digoxin levels.
Morphine: may increase esmolol blood levels. Titrate esmolol carefully.
Reserpine (and other catecholamine-depleting drugs): may cause additive bradycardia and hypotension. Titrate es-

molol carefully.
Succinylcholine: esmolol may prolong neuromuscular blockade.

EFFECTS ON DIAGNOSTIC TESTS
None reported.

CONTRAINDICATIONS
Contraindicated in patients with sinus bradycardia, heart block greater than first-degree, cardiogenic shock, or overt heart failure.

NURSING CONSIDERATIONS
● Use cautiously in patients with impaired renal function, diabetes, or bronchospasm.
● **I.V. use:** Don't give esmolol by I.V. push; use an infusion control device. The 10-mg/ml single-dose vials may be used without diluting, but the injection concentrate (250 mg/ml) must be diluted to a maximum concentration of 10 mg/ml before infusion. Remove 20 ml from 500 ml of D_5W, lactated Ringer's solution, or 0.45% or 0.9% sodium chloride solution and add two ampules of esmolol (final concentration 10 mg/ml).
● Remember that esmolol solutions are incompatible with diazepam, furosemide, sodium bicarbonate, and thiopental sodium.
*Alert:*Monitor ECG and blood pressure continuously during infusion. Up to 50% of all patients treated with esmolol develop hypotension. Monitor closely, especially if patient's pretreatment blood pressure was low.
● Hypotension can usually be reversed within 30 minutes by decreasing the dose or, if necessary, by stopping the infusion. Notify doctor if this becomes necessary.
● If a local reaction develops at the infusion site, change to another site. Avoid using butterfly needles.
● Be aware that esmolol is recommended only for short-term use, for no longer than 48 hours.
● When the patient's heart rate becomes

stable, esmolol will be replaced by alternative (longer-acting) antiarrhythmics, such as propranolol, digoxin, or verapamil. A half hour after the first dose of the alternative agent is administered, reduce infusion rate by 50%. Monitor patient response and, if heart rate is controlled for 1 hour after administration of the second dose of the alternative drug, discontinue esmolol infusion.

☑ **PATIENT TEACHING**
● Instruct patient to report adverse reactions promptly.
● Tell patient to alert nurse if discomfort occurs at I.V. site.

---

flecainide acetate
Tambocor

Pregnancy Risk Category: C

HOW SUPPLIED
Tablets: 50 mg, 100 mg, 150 mg
Injection: 10 mg/ml‡

ACTION
A class Ic antiarrhythmic that decreases excitability, conduction velocity, and automaticity as a result of slowed atrial, AV node, His-Purkinje system, and intraventricular conduction and causes a slight but significant prolongation of refractory periods in these tissues.

ONSET, PEAK, DURATION
Onset immediate with I.V. administration, unknown with oral administration. Serum levels peak immediately after I.V. infusion, 2 to 3 hours after oral administration. Duration unknown.

INDICATIONS & DOSAGE
Paroxysmal supraventricular tachycardia, paroxysmal atrial fibrillation or flutter in patients without structural heart disease; life-threatening ventricular arrhythmias, such as sustained ventricular tachycardia—
Adults: for paroxysmal supraventricular tachycardia, 50 mg P.O. q 12 hours. Increased in increments of 50 mg b.i.d. q 4 days. Maximum dosage is 300 mg/day.

In patients with renal impairment (creatinine clearance of 35 ml/minute or less), initial dosage is 100 mg once daily or 50 mg b.i.d.

For life-threatening ventricular arrhythmias, 100 mg P.O. q 12 hours. Increase in increments of 50 mg b.i.d. q 4 days until efficacy is achieved. Maximum dosage is 400 mg daily for most patients.

Initial dosage for patients with CHF is 50 mg P.O. q 12 hours.

Where available, flecainide may be given by I.V. injection‡—
Adults: 2 mg/kg I.V. push over not less than 10 minutes to a maximum dose of 150 mg; or dilute the dose and administer as an infusion.

ADVERSE REACTIONS
CNS: *dizziness, headache,* fatigue, tremor, anxiety, insomnia, depression, malaise, paresthesia, ataxia, vertigo, *light-headedness, syncope,* asthenia.
CV: ***new or worsened arrhythmias,*** chest pain, ***CHF, cardiac arrest,*** palpitations.
EENT: *blurred vision and other visual disturbances.*
GI: nausea, constipation, abdominal pain, dyspepsia, vomiting, diarrhea, anorexia.
Other: *dyspnea,* edema, skin rash, flushing, fever.

INTERACTIONS
Amiodarone, cimetidine: altered pharmacokinetics. Monitor for toxicity.
Digitalis glycosides: flecainide may increase plasma digoxin levels by 15% to 25%. Monitor serum digoxin levels.
Propranolol, other beta blockers: both flecainide and propranolol plasma levels increase by 20% to 30%. Monitor for propranolol and flecainide toxicity.
Urine acidifying and alkalinizing

Reactions may be *common*, uncommon, *life-threatening*, or COMMON AND LIFE-THREATENING.

agents: extremes of urine pH may substantially alter excretion of flecainide. Monitor for flecainide toxicity or decreased effectiveness.

Disopyramide, verapamil: negative inotropic properties may be additive with flecainide; avoid concurrent adminstration.

EFFECTS ON DIAGNOSTIC TESTS
None reported.

CONTRAINDICATIONS
Contraindicated in patients with hypersensitivity to the drug; preexisting second- or third-degree AV block or right bundle-branch block when associated with a left hemiblock (in the absence of an artificial pacemaker); recent MI; and cardiogenic shock.

NURSING CONSIDERATIONS
• Use cautiously in patients with preexisting CHF, cardiomyopathy, severe renal or hepatic disease, prolonged QT interval, sick sinus syndrome, or blood dyscrasia.
• Know that when used to prevent ventricular arrhythmias, flecainide should be reserved for patients with documented life-threatening arrhythmias.
• Check that pacing threshold was determined 1 week before and after initiating therapy in patients with pacemakers because flecainide can alter endocardial pacing thresholds.
• Correct hypokalemia or hyperkalemia as ordered before giving flecainide because these electrolyte disturbances may alter its effect.
• Know that most patients can be adequately maintained on an every-12-hour dosing schedule, but that some need to receive flecainide every 8 hours.
• **I.V. use:** When administering by I.V. push, give over at least 10 minutes. For I.V. infusion, mix only with D_5W.
• Be aware that dosage adjustments should be made only once every 3 to 4 days.
• Because of flecainide's long half-life,

its full therapeutic effect may take 3 to 5 days. Administer concomitant I.V. lidocaine as ordered for the first several days.
• Monitor serum flecainide levels, especially in patients with renal failure or CHF. Therapeutic serum levels of flecainide range from 0.2 to 1 mcg/ml. Incidence of adverse effects increases when trough blood levels exceed 1 mcg/ml.

☑ **PATIENT TEACHING**
• Stress importance of taking drug exactly as prescribed.
• Instruct patient to report adverse reactions promptly and to limit fluid and sodium intake to minimize fluid retention.
• Tell patient receiving drug I.V. to alert nurse if discomfort occurs at the insertion site.

---

ibutilide fumarate
Corvert

Pregnancy Risk Category: C

HOW SUPPLIED
Injection: 0.1 mg/ml in 10-ml vials

ACTION
Prolongs action potential in isolated cardiac myocyte and increases atrial and ventricular refractoriness, namely class III electrophysiologic effects.

ONSET, PEAK, DURATION
Unknown. May convert arrhythmia 30 to 90 minutes after infusion starts, with most patients in normal sinus rhythm 24 hours later.

INDICATIONS & DOSAGE
Rapid conversion of atrial fibrillation or atrial flutter of recent onset to sinus rhythm—
Adults weighing 60 kg (132 lb) or more: 1 mg I.V. over 10 minutes.
Adults weighing less than 60 kg:

0.01 mg/kg I.V. over 10 minutes.

Alert: Infusion should be stopped if arrhythmia is terminated or patient develops ventricular tachycardia (VT) or marked prolongation of QT or QTc. If arrhythmia is not terminated 10 minutes after infusion ends, a second 10-minute infusion of equal strength may be given.

ADVERSE REACTIONS
CNS: headache.
CV: ventricular extrasystoles, nonsustained VT, hypotension, bundle branch block, *sustained polymorphic VT,* AV block, hypertension, QT segment prolongation, bradycardia, palpitation, tachycardia.
GI: nausea.

INTERACTIONS
Class Ia antiarrhythmics (disopyramide, quinidine, procainamide) and other class III drugs (amiodarone, sotalol): increased potential for prolonged refractoriness. Don't give these drugs for at least 5 half-lives before and 4 hours after ibutilide dose.
Digoxin: supraventricular arrhythmias may mask cardiotoxicity associated with excessive digoxin levels. Use cautiously.
Phenothiazines, tricyclic antidepressants, tetracyclic antidepressants, H_1-receptor antagonist antihistamines, and other drugs that prolong QT interval: increased risk for proarrhythmia. Monitor closely.

EFFECTS ON DIAGNOSTIC TESTS
None reported.

CONTRAINDICATIONS
Contraindicated in patients with hypersensitivity to drug or its components.

NURSING CONSIDERATIONS
● Drug is not recommended for patients with a history of polymorphic VT and in breast-feeding women.
● Use cautiously in patients with hepatic or renal dysfunction.

● Safety of drug has not been established in children.
● Drug should be given only by skilled personnel. Cardiac monitor, intracardiac pacing, cardioverter or defibrillator, and medication for sustained VT must be available.
● Before therapy, hypokalemia and hypomagnesemia should be corrected to reduce the potential for proarrhythmia. Patients with atrial fibrillation of more than 2 to 3 days' duration must be adequately anticoagulated, generally for at least 2 weeks.
● **I.V. use:** Drug may be given undiluted or diluted in 50 ml of diluent; may be added to 0.9% sodium chloride injection or 5% dextrose injection before infusion. Contents of 10-ml vial (0.1 mg/ml) may be added to 50-ml infusion bag to form admixture of about 0.017 mg/ml ibutilide fumarate. Use aseptic technique. Drug can be used with polyvinyl chloride plastic bags or polyolefin bags.
● Admixtures with approved diluents are stable for 24 hours at room temperature; 48 hours if refrigerated.
● Inspect parenteral products for particulate and discoloration before administration.
● Monitor ECG continuously during administration and for at least 4 hours afterward or until QTc returns to baseline; drug can induce or worsen ventricular arrhythmias. Longer monitoring is required if ECG shows arrhythmia.

☑ PATIENT TEACHING
● Tell patient to report adverse reactions promptly.
● Instruct patient to alert nurse of discomfort at injection site.

---

lidocaine hydrochloride (lignocaine hydrochloride)
LidoPen Auto-Injector, Xylocaine, Xylocard†‡

Pregnancy Risk Category: B

Reactions may be *common,* uncommon, *life-threatening,* or COMMON AND LIFE-THREATENING.

HOW SUPPLIED
Injection (for I.M. use): 300 mg/3 ml automatic injection device
Injection (for direct I.V. use): 1% (10 mg/ml), 2% (20 mg/ml)
Injection (for I.V. admixtures): 4% (40 mg/ml), 10% (100 mg/ml), 20% (200 mg/ml)
Infusion (premixed): 0.2% (2 mg/ ml), 0.4% (4 mg/ml), 0.8% (8 mg/ml)

ACTION
Lidocaine, a class 1b antiarrhythmic, decreases the depolarization, automaticity, and excitability in the ventricles during the diastolic phase by direct action on the tissues, especially the Purkinje network.

ONSET, PEAK, DURATION
Onset is immediate (45 to 90 seconds) with I.V. bolus administration, 5 to 15 minutes with I.M. administration. After an I.M. injection, plasma levels peak in about 10 minutes. Effects of an I.V. bolus dose last for 10 to 20 minutes; effective blood levels persist for up to 2 hours after an I.M. injection.

INDICATIONS & DOSAGE
Ventricular arrhythmias resulting from MI, cardiac manipulation, or digitalis glycosides—
Adults: 50 to 100 mg (1 to 1.5 mg/kg) by I.V. bolus at 25 to 50 mg/minute. Half this amount is given to elderly patients or patients under 50 kg and to those with CHF or hepatic disease. Bolus dose is repeated q 3 to 5 minutes until arrhythmias subside or adverse reactions develop. Don't exceed 300-mg total bolus during a 1-hour period. Simultaneously, constant infusion of 20 to 50 mcg/kg/minute (1 to 4 mg/minute) is begun. If single bolus has been given, smaller bolus dose may be repeated 15 to 20 minutes after start of infusion to maintain therapeutic serum level. Alter-

natively, 200 to 300 mg I.M., followed by second I.M. dose 60 to 90 minutes later, if needed.
Children: 0.5 to 1 mg/kg by I.V. bolus, followed by infusion of 10 to 50 mcg/kg/minute.

ADVERSE REACTIONS
CNS: *confusion, tremor,* lethargy, somnolence, *stupor, restlessness,* anxiety, hallucinations, nervousness, *light-headedness,* paresthesia, muscle twitching, *seizures.*
CV: *hypotension,* bradycardia, ***new or worsened arrhythmias, cardiac arrest.***
EENT: *tinnitus, blurred or double vision.*
Other: ***anaphylaxis, respiratory depression and arrest,*** soreness at injection site, sensation of cold, vomiting.

INTERACTIONS
Beta blockers, cimetidine: decreased metabolism of lidocaine. Monitor for toxicity.
Phenytoin, procainamide, propranolol, quinidine: additive cardiac depressant effects. Monitor carefully.
Tocainide, mexiletine: additive pharmacologic effects; avoid concomitant use.

EFFECTS ON DIAGNOSTIC TESTS
Because I.M. lidocaine therapy may increase CK levels, isoenzyme tests should be performed for differential diagnosis of acute MI.

CONTRAINDICATIONS
Contraindicated in patients with hypersensitivity to the amide-type local anesthetics; Adams-Stokes syndrome; Wolff-Parkinson-White syndrome; and severe degrees of SA, AV, or intraventricular block in absence of artificial pacemaker.

NURSING CONSIDERATIONS
● Use cautiously in patients with complete or second-degree heart block or sinus bradycardia, in elderly patients, in those with CHF or renal or hepatic disease, and in those who weigh under 50

kg. Reduced dosage in these patients is required.

● **I.V. use:** Patients receiving infusions must be on a cardiac monitor and must be attended *at all times*. Use an infusion control device for administering infusion precisely. Do not exceed rate of 4 mg/minute; faster rate greatly increases risk of toxicity.

● Give I.M. injections in the deltoid muscle only.

● Monitor isoenzymes when using I.M. drug for suspected MI. A patient who has received I.M. lidocaine will show a seven-fold increase in serum CK level. Such an increase originates in the skeletal muscle, not the heart.

● Monitor serum levels as ordered. Therapeutic levels are 2 to 5 mcg/ml. *Alert:* Monitor patient for toxicity. In many severely ill patients, seizures may be the first clinical sign of toxicity. However, severe reactions usually are preceded by somnolence, confusion, and paresthesia.

● If signs of toxicity (such as dizziness) occur, stop drug at once and notify the doctor. Continuing could lead to seizures and coma. Give oxygen via nasal cannula if not contraindicated. Keep oxygen and cardiopulmonary resuscitation equipment available.

● Monitor the patient's response, especially blood pressure and serum electrolytes, BUN, and creatinine levels, as ordered. Notify the doctor promptly if abnormalities develop.

● Discontinue infusion and notify the doctor if arrhythmias worsen or ECG changes, such as widening QRS complex or substantially prolonged PR interval, are evident.

☑ **PATIENT TEACHING**
● Inform patient receiving drug I.M. that drug may cause soreness at injection site. Instruct patient receiving drug I.V. to alert nurse if discomfort occurs at the insertion site.

● Tell patient to report adverse reactions promptly as toxicity can occur.

mexiletine hydrochloride
Mexitil

Pregnancy Risk Category: C

HOW SUPPLIED
Capsules: 50 mg‡, 100 mg†, 150 mg, 200 mg, 250 mg
Injection: 250 mg/10 ml‡

ACTION
A class Ib antiarrhythmic that blocks the fast sodium channel in cardiac tissues, especially the Purkinje network, without involving the autonomic nervous system. Reduces the rate of rise and amplitude of the action potential and decreases automaticity in the Purkinje fibers. Shortens the duration of the action potential and, to a lesser extent, decreases the effective refractory period in the Purkinje fibers.

ONSET, PEAK, DURATION
Onset occurs ½ to 2 hours after oral administration, immediately after I.V. administration. Serum levels peak 2 to 3 hours after oral administration, immediately after I.V. administration. Duration unknown.

INDICATIONS & DOSAGE
Refractory life-threatening ventricular arrhythmias, including ventricular tachycardia and PVCs—
Adults: 200 to 400 mg P.O. followed by 200 mg q 8 hours. Dose increased every 2 to 3 days to 400 mg q 8 hours if satisfactory control is not obtained. Patients who respond well to an every-12-hour schedule may be given up to 450 mg q 12 hours.
Where available, mexiletine may be given I.V.‡—
Adults: loading dose is 100 to 250 mg I.V. at a rate of 25 mg/minute. Then prepare an infusion solution of 250 mg mexiletine in 500 ml of D_5W, and administer the first 120 ml (60 mg) over 1 hour. If clinical response is inadequate,

give another bolus of 200 mg over 10 to 20 minutes. Maintenance dosage is 0.5 mg/minute (1 ml/minute of prepared solution).

ADVERSE REACTIONS
CNS: *tremor, dizziness,* blurred vision, diplopia, confusion, *light-headedness, incoordination,* changes in sleep habits, paresthesia, weakness, fatigue, speech difficulties, tinnitus, depression, *nervousness,* headache.
CV: *new or worsened arrhythmias,* palpitations, chest pain, nonspecific edema, angina.
GI: *nausea, vomiting, upper GI distress, heartburn,* diarrhea, constipation, dry mouth, changes in appetite, abdominal pain.
Skin: rash.

INTERACTIONS
Antacids, atropine, narcotics: slowed mexiletine absorption. Monitor patient.
Cimetidine: increased or decreased mexiletine blood levels. Monitor carefully.
Methylxanthines, such as caffeine or theophylline: reduced clearance of methylxanthines, possibly resulting in toxicity. Monitor carefully.
Metoclopramide: mexiletine absorption may be accelerated. Monitor for toxicity.
Phenobarbital, phenytoin, rifampin, urine acidifiers: decreased mexiletine blood levels. Monitor carefully.
Urine alkalinizers: increased mexiletine blood levels. Monitor carefully.

EFFECTS ON DIAGNOSTIC TESTS
Liver function test results may be transiently altered during mexiletine therapy.

CONTRAINDICATIONS
Contraindicated in patients with cardiogenic shock or preexisting second- or third-degree AV block in the absence of an artificial pacemaker.

NURSING CONSIDERATIONS
• Use cautiously in patients with preex-

isting first-degree heart block, a ventricular pacemaker, preexisting sinus node dysfunction, intraventricular conduction disturbances, hypotension, severe CHF, or seizure disorder.
• When changing from lidocaine to mexiletine, stop the lidocaine infusion when the first mexiletine dose is given. Keep the infusion line open, however, until the arrhythmia appears to be satisfactorily controlled.
• **I.V. use:** Mexiletine injection is compatible with 0.9% sodium chloride, D_5W, 5% sodium bicarbonate, 1/6 M sodium lactate, and 10% fructose (levulose) solutions.
• To lessen GI distress, administer oral dose with meals or antacids.
• If you feel the patient is a good candidate for every-12-hour therapy, notify the doctor. Twice-daily dosage enhances compliance.
• Monitor therapeutic levels, as ordered. Levels range from 0.5 to 2 mcg/ml.
• Monitor patient for toxicity. An early sign of mexiletine toxicity is tremor, usually a fine tremor of the hands. This progresses to dizziness and later to ataxia and nystagmus as the drug's blood level increases. Question patients about these symptoms.
• Monitor blood pressure and heart rate and rhythm frequently. Notify the doctor of any significant change.

☑ PATIENT TEACHING
• Tell patient to take drug exactly as prescribed and to take with food or antacids if GI reactions occur.
• Instruct patient to report adverse reactions promptly.
• Tell patient receiving drug I.V. to report discomfort at the insertion site.

---

moricizine hydrochloride
Ethmozine

Pregnancy Risk Category: B

HOW SUPPLIED
Tablets: 200 mg, 250 mg, 300 mg

ACTION
A class I antiarrhythmic that reduces the fast inward current carried by sodium ions across myocardial cell membranes. Has potent local anesthetic activity and membrane-stabilizing effect.

ONSET, PEAK, DURATION
Onset occurs in 2 hours. Serum levels peak in $1/2$ to 2 hours; effects peak in 10 to 14 hours. Effects persist 10 to 24 hours after last dose.

INDICATIONS & DOSAGE
Life-threatening ventricular arrhythmias—
Adults: individualized dosage is based on clinical response and patient tolerance. Therapy should begin in the hospital. Most patients respond to 600 to 900 mg P.O. daily in divided doses q 8 hours. Daily dosage increased q 3 days by 150 mg until the desired clinical effect is seen.

In patients with hepatic or renal impairment, 600 mg or less P.O. daily.

ADVERSE REACTIONS
CNS: *dizziness, headache, fatigue,* hyperesthesias, anxiety, asthenia, nervousness, paresthesia, sleep disorders.
CV: *proarrhythmic events (ventricular tachycardia, PVCs, supraventricular arrhythmias), ECG abnormalities (including conduction defects, sinus pause, junctional rhythm, or AV block), CHF,* palpitations, chest pain, **cardiac death,** hypotension, hypertension, vasodilation, cerebrovascular events.
EENT: blurred vision.
GI: *nausea, vomiting, abdominal pain, dyspepsia, diarrhea, dry mouth.*
GU: urine retention, urinary frequency, dysuria.
Respiratory: dyspnea.
Skin: rash.
Other: drug-induced fever, diaphoresis, musculoskeletal pain, thrombophlebitis.

INTERACTIONS
Cimetidine: increased plasma levels and decreased clearance of moricizine. Begin moricizine therapy at low dosage (not more than 600 mg daily), and monitor plasma levels and therapeutic effect closely.
Digoxin, propranolol: additive prolongation of PR interval. Monitor closely.
Theophylline: increased clearance and reduced plasma levels of theophylline. Monitor plasma levels and therapeutic response; adjust theophylline dosage as needed.

EFFECTS ON DIAGNOSTIC TESTS
Drug may elevate liver function test results.

CONTRAINDICATIONS
Contraindicated in patients with hypersensitivity to the drug; preexisting second- or third-degree AV block or right bundle branch block when associated with left hemiblock (bifascicular block) unless an artificial pacemaker is present; and cardiogenic shock.

NURSING CONSIDERATIONS
● Know that because drug has been detected in breast milk, a decision should be made to discontinue breast-feeding or discontinue the drug, depending on drug's potential benefit to the mother.
● Use with extreme caution in patients with sick sinus syndrome because drug may cause sinus bradycardia or sinus arrest. Also use with extreme caution in patients with coronary artery disease and left ventricular dysfunction because these patients may be at risk for sudden death when treated with the drug.
● Administer cautiously to patients with liver impairment.
● Patients with hepatic or renal dysfunction will have decreased moricizine clearance. Administer cautiously and

---

Reactions may be *common,* uncommon, *life-threatening,* or COMMON AND LIFE-THREATENING.

monitor effects closely.

● Know that when substituting moricizine for another antiarrhythmic, previous drug should be withdrawn for one to two of the drug's half-lives before moricizine is started. Patients who have shown a tendency to develop life-threatening arrhythmias after withdrawal of previous antiarrhythmic drug therapy should be hospitalized during withdrawal and adjustment to moricizine. Guidelines doctors use for when to start moricizine therapy are as follows:

—disopyramide, 6 to 12 hours after the last dose.

—flecainide, 12 to 24 hours after last dose.

—mexiletine, 8 to 12 hours after the last dose.

—procainamide, 3 to 6 hours after the last dose.

—propafenone, 8 to 12 hours after the last dose.

—quinidine, 6 to 12 hours after the last dose.

—tocainide, 8 to 12 hours after the last dose.

● Determine electrolyte status and correct imbalances before therapy as ordered. Hypokalemia, hyperkalemia, and hypomagnesemia may alter the effects of the drug.

☑ **PATIENT TEACHING**
● Instruct patient to take drug exactly as prescribed.
● Tell patient to avoid hazardous activities if adverse CNS reactions or blurred vision occurs.
● Instruct patient to report persistent or serious adverse reactions promptly.

---

procainamide hydrochloride
Procainamide Durules‡, Procanbid, Procan SR, Promine, Pronestyl**, Pronestyl-SR

Pregnancy Risk Category: C

HOW SUPPLIED
Tablets: 250 mg, 375 mg, 500 mg
Tablets (sustained-release): 250 mg, 500 mg, 750 mg, 1,000 mg
Capsules: 250 mg, 375 mg, 500 mg
Injection: 100 mg/ml, 500 mg/ml

ACTION
A class Ia antiarrhythmic that decreases excitability, conduction velocity, automaticity, and membrane responsiveness with prolonged refractory period. Larger than usual doses may induce AV block.

ONSET, PEAK, DURATION
Onset occurs immediately with I.V. injection, 10 to 30 minutes after I.M. injection, and 2 hours after oral dose. Peak serum levels occur immediately after I.V. infusion, 15 to 60 minutes after I.M. injection, and 1 to 1½ hours after oral dose. Duration unknown.

INDICATIONS & DOSAGE
Life-threatening ventricular arrhythmias—
Adults: 100 mg by slow I.V. push q 5 minutes, no faster than 25 to 50 mg/minute until arrhythmias disappear, adverse reactions develop, or 1 g has been given. Usual effective dose is 500 to 600 mg. When arrhythmias disappear, give continuous infusion of 1 to 6 mg/minute. If arrhythmias recur, repeat bolus as above and increase infusion rate. Alternatively, give 0.5 to 1 g I.M. q 4 to 8 hours until oral therapy begins.

For oral therapy, give 50 mg/kg daily in divided doses q 3 hours (average is 250 to 500 mg q 3 hours); for sustained-release tablets, give 50 mg/kg daily in divided doses q 6 hours.

In patients with renal or hepatic dysfunction, decreased dosages or longer dosing intervals may be needed.

ADVERSE REACTIONS
CNS: hallucinations, confusion, *seizures,* depression, dizziness.
CV: *hypotension,* bradycardia, AV

block, *ventricular fibrillation* (after parenteral use), *ventricular asystole.*
GI: nausea, vomiting, anorexia, diarrhea, bitter taste.
Hematologic: *thrombocytopenia, neutropenia, agranulocytosis, hemolytic anemia.*
Skin: *maculopapular rash, urticaria, pruritus, flushing, angioneurotic edema.*
Other: *fever, lupuslike syndrome* (especially after prolonged administration).

INTERACTIONS
Amiodarone: increased procainamide levels and toxicity; additive effects on QT interval and QRS complex. Avoid concomitant use.
Anticholinergics: additive anticholinergic effects. Monitor closely.
Anticholinesterase agents: May decrease effect of anticholinesterase agents. Anticholinesterase dosage may need to be increased.
Cimetidine, ranitidine, trimethoprim: may increase procainamide blood levels. Monitor for toxicity.
Neuromuscular blockers: increased skeletal muscle relaxant effects. Monitor the patient closely.

EFFECTS ON DIAGNOSTIC TESTS
Procainamide will invalidate bentiromide test results; discontinue at least 3 days before bentiromide test. Procainamide may alter edrophonium test results; positive antinuclear antibody (ANA) titers, positive direct antiglobulin (Coombs) tests, and ECG changes may be seen. The physiologic effects of the drug may result in decreased leukocytes and platelets and increased bilirubin, lactate dehydrogenase, alkaline phosphatase, ALT, and AST.

CONTRAINDICATIONS
Contraindicated in patients with hypersensitivity to procaine and related drugs; in those with complete, second-, or third-degree heart block in the absence of an artificial pacemaker; and in patients with myasthenia gravis or sys-

temic lupus erythematosus. Also contraindicated in patients with atypical ventricular tachycardia (torsades de pointes) because procainamide may aggravate this condition.

NURSING CONSIDERATIONS
● Use with extreme caution when treating patients with ventricular tachycardia during coronary occlusion.
● Use cautiously in patients with CHF or other conduction disturbances, such as bundle-branch heart block, sinus bradycardia, or digitalis glycoside intoxication, or with hepatic or renal insufficiency. Also use cautiously in those with preexisting blood dyscrasias or bone marrow suppression.
● **I.V. use:** Patients receiving infusions must be attended *at all times.* Use an infusion control device to administer the infusion precisely.
● Note that the vials for I.V. injection contain 1 g of drug: 100 mg/ml (10 ml) or 500 mg/ml (2 ml).
● Keep patients in the supine position during I.V. administration. If drug is given too rapidly, hypotension can occur. Watch closely for adverse reactions during infusion, and notify the doctor if they occur.
● If procainamide solution becomes discolored, check with pharmacy and expect to discard.
Alert: Monitor blood pressure and ECG continuously during I.V. administration. Watch for prolonged QT intervals and QRS complexes, heart block, or increased arrhythmias. If these occur, withhold drug, obtain rhythm strip, and notify the doctor immediately.
● Monitor plasma levels of procainamide and its active metabolite NAPA. To suppress ventricular arrhythmias, therapeutic serum concentrations of procainamide are 4 to 8 mcg/ml; therapeutic levels of NAPA are 10 to 30 mcg/ml.
● Monitor QT interval closely in patients with renal failure.
● Hypokalemia predisposes patients to

arrhythmias; therefore, monitor serum electrolytes, especially potassium level.
● Elderly patients may be more likely to develop hypotension. Monitor blood pressure carefully.
● Monitor CBC frequently during first 3 months of therapy.
● Be aware that positive ANA titer is common in about 60% of patients who don't have symptoms of lupuslike syndrome. This response seems to be related to prolonged use, not dosage. May progress to systemic lupus erythematosus if drug is not discontinued.

☑ **PATIENT TEACHING**
● Stress to the patient the importance of taking the drug exactly as prescribed. This may require use of an alarm clock for nighttime doses.
● Instruct the patient to report fever, rash, muscle pain, diarrhea, bleeding, bruises, or pleuritic chest pain.
● Reassure the patient who is taking the extended-release form that a wax-matrix "ghost" from the tablet may be passed in stools. The drug is completely absorbed before this occurs.

---

propafenone hydrochloride
Rythmol

Pregnancy Risk Category: C

HOW SUPPLIED
Tablets: 150 mg, 225 mg, 300 mg

ACTION
A class Ic antiarrhythmic that reduces inward sodium current in Purkinje and myocardial cells. Decreases excitability, conduction velocity, and automaticity in AV nodal, His-Purkinje, and intraventricular tissue; causes slight but significant prolongation of refractory period in AV nodal tissue.

ONSET, PEAK, DURATION
Onset and duration unknown. Plasma levels peak within 3½ hours.

INDICATIONS & DOSAGE
Suppression of life-threatening ventricular arrhythmias, such as sustained ventricular tachycardia—
Adults: initially, 150 mg P.O. q 8 hours. Dosage may be increased at 3- to 4-day intervals to 225 mg q 8 hours, if necessary, increase dosage to 300 mg q 8 hours. Maximum daily dosage is 900 mg.

ADVERSE REACTIONS
CNS: anxiety, ataxia, *dizziness,* drowsiness, fatigue, headache, insomnia, syncope, tremor.
CV: atrial fibrillation, bradycardia, bundle branch block, *CHF,* angina, chest pain, edema, first-degree AV block, hypotension, increased QRS duration, intraventricular conduction delay, palpitations, *proarrhythmic events (ventricular tachycardia, PVCs, ventricular fibrillation).*
EENT: blurred vision.
GI: abdominal pain or cramps, constipation, diarrhea, dyspepsia, anorexia, flatulence, *nausea, vomiting,* dry mouth, unusual taste.
Respiratory: dyspnea.
Skin: rash.
Other: diaphoresis, joint pain.

INTERACTIONS
Antiarrhythmics: increased risk of CHF. Monitor closely.
Cimetidine: decreased metabolism of propafenone. Monitor closely.
Digitalis glycosides, oral anticoagulants, cyclosporine: propafenone may increase serum levels of these agents by about 35% to 85%, resulting in toxicity. Monitor closely.
Local anesthetics: increased risk of CNS toxicity. Monitor closely.
Metoprolol, propranolol: propafenone slows the metabolism of these agents. Adjust dosage as ordered.
Quinidine: slowed metabolism of propafenone. Avoid concomitant use.
Rifampin: increased clearance of propafenone. Monitor closely.

EFFECTS ON DIAGNOSTIC TESTS
Although the drug may slow conduction and increase PR interval and QRS duration, ECG changes alone cannot be used to predict plasma concentration or drug efficacy.

Increased liver enzymes have been rarely reported (less than 0.2% of patients). Hematologic abnormalities have also been rarely reported (positive antinuclear antibody titer, decreased CBC, and altered electrolyte levels).

CONTRAINDICATIONS
Contraindicated in patients with hypersensitivity to the drug and in those with severe or uncontrolled CHF; cardiogenic shock; SA, AV, or intraventricular disorders of impulse conduction in the absence of a pacemaker; bradycardia; marked hypotension; bronchospastic disorders; and electrolyte imbalance.

NURSING CONSIDERATIONS
● Use cautiously in patients with CHF because propafenone can exert a negative inotropic effect on the heart. Also use cautiously in patients taking other cardiac depressant drugs and in those with hepatic or renal failure.
● To minimize adverse GI reactions, administer drug with food.
● Continuous cardiac monitoring is recommended during initiation of therapy and during dosage adjustments. If PR interval or QRS complex increases by more than 25%, a reduction in dosage may be necessary.
● During concomitant use with digoxin, frequently monitor ECG and serum digoxin levels.

☑ PATIENT TEACHING
● Stress importance of taking drug exactly as prescribed.
● Tell patient to report adverse reactions promptly.

quinidine bisulfate
(66.4% quinidine base)
Biquin Durules†, Kinidin Durules‡

quinidine gluconate
(62% quinidine base)
Quinaglute Dura-Tabs, Quinalan, Quinate†

quinidine polygalacturonate
(60.5% quinidine base)
Cardioquin

quinidine sulfate
(83% quinidine base) Apo-Quinidine†, Cin-Quin, Novoquinidin†, Quinidex Extentabs, Quinora

Pregnancy Risk Category: C

HOW SUPPLIED
quinidine bisulfate
Tablets (extended-release): 250 mg†‡
quinidine gluconate
Tablets (extended-release): 324 mg, 325 mg†, 330 mg
Injection: 80 mg/ml
quinidine polygalacturonate
Tablets: 275 mg
quinidine sulfate
Tablets: 200 mg, 300 mg
Tablets (extended-release): 300 mg
Capsules: 200 mg, 300 mg
Injection: 200 mg/ml†

ACTION
A class Ia antiarrhythmic, quinidine has both direct and indirect (anticholinergic) effects on cardiac tissue. Automaticity, conduction velocity, and membrane responsiveness are decreased. The effective refractory period is prolonged. The anticholinergic action reduces vagal tone.

ONSET, PEAK, DURATION
Onset is immediate after I.V. administration, 30 to 90 minutes after I.M. administration, and 1 to 3 hours after oral administration. Peak plasma levels oc-

cur immediately after I.V. injection; for oral form, depends on the salt used: sulfate, 1 to 3 hours; gluconate, 3 to 5 hours; and polygalacturonate, about 6 hours. The extended-release sulfate peaks at 3 to 5 hours. Effects persist 6 to 8 hours after oral dose.

INDICATIONS & DOSAGE
Atrial flutter or fibrillation—
Adults: 200 mg quinidine sulfate or equivalent base P.O. q 2 to 3 hours for five to eight doses, with subsequent daily increases until sinus rhythm is restored or toxic effects develop. Quinidine is administered only after AV node has been blocked with a beta blocker, digoxin, or a calcium channel blocker to avoid increasing AV conduction. Maximum dosage is 3 to 4 g daily.
Paroxysmal supraventricular tachycardia—
Adults: 400 to 600 mg I.M. or P.O. gluconate q 2 to 3 hours until toxic adverse reactions develop or arrhythmia subsides.
Premature atrial and ventricular contractions; paroxysmal AV junctional rhythm; paroxysmal atrial tachycardia; paroxysmal ventricular tachycardia; maintenance after cardioversion of atrial fibrillation or flutter—
Adults: test dose is 200 mg P.O. or I.M. Quinidine sulfate or equivalent base 200 to 400 mg P.O. q 4 to 6 hours; or initially, quinidine gluconate 600 mg I.M., then up to 400 mg q 2 hours, p.r.n.; or quinidine gluconate 800 mg (10 ml of the commercially available solution) added to 40 ml of D_5W, infused I.V. at 16 mg (1 ml)/minute.
Children: 30 mg/kg/24 hours or 900 mg/m^2/24 hours P.O. in five divided doses.
Severe Plasmodium falciparum *malaria—*
Adults: 10 mg/kg gluconate I.V. diluted in 250 ml of 0.9% sodium chloride solution and infused over 1 to 2 hours, followed by a continuous maintenance infusion of 0.02 mg/kg/minute for 72

hours or until parasitemia is reduced to less than 1%.
Patients with impaired hepatic function and those with CHF require a reduced dosage.

ADVERSE REACTIONS
CNS: *vertigo, headache, light-headedness,* confusion, ataxia, depression, dementia.
CV: *PVCs; ventricular tachycardia; atypical ventricular tachycardia (torsades de pointes); hypotension; complete AV block,* tachycardia; *aggravated CHF; ECG changes (particularly widening of QRS complex, widened QT and PR intervals).*
EENT: *tinnitus,* excessive salivation, blurred vision, diplopia, photophobia.
GI: *diarrhea, nausea, vomiting,* anorexia, abdominal pain.
Hematologic: *hemolytic anemia, thrombocytopenia, agranulocytosis.*
Hepatic: *hepatotoxicity.*
Respiratory: acute asthmatic attack, *respiratory arrest.*
Skin: rash, petechial hemorrhage of buccal mucosa, pruritus, urticaria, lupus erythematosus, photosensitivity.
Other: angioedema, *fever, cinchonism.*

INTERACTIONS
Acetazolamide, antacids, sodium bicarbonate, thiazide diuretics: may increase quinidine blood levels because of alkaline urine. Monitor for increased effect.
Amiodarone, cimetidine: increased serum quinidine levels. Monitor for increased effect.
Barbiturates, phenytoin, rifampin: may lower blood levels of quinidine. Monitor for decreased effect.
Digoxin: increased serum digoxin levels after initiating quinidine therapy. Monitor closely.
Nifedipine: may decrease quinidine blood levels. Monitor carefully.
Other antiarrhythmics, such as lidocaine, phenytoin, procainamide, and propranolol: increased risk of toxicity. Use together cautiously.

---

*Liquid contains alcohol.   **May contain tartrazine.   †Canada only.   ‡Australia only.   ◇ OTC.

Verapamil: may result in hypotension, bradycardia, or AV block. Monitor blood pressure and heart rate.

Warfarin: increased anticoagulant effect. Monitor closely.

Tricyclic antidepressants: increased blood levels with increased effect.

EFFECTS ON DIAGNOSTIC TESTS
None reported.

CONTRAINDICATIONS
Contraindicated in patients with idiosyncrasy or hypersensitivity to quinidine or related cinchona derivatives, myasthenia gravis, intraventricular conduction defects, digitalis toxicity when AV conduction is grossly impaired, and abnormal rhythms due to escape mechanisms.

NURSING CONSIDERATIONS
● Use cautiously in patients with asthma, muscle weakness, or infection accompanied by fever because hypersensitivity reactions to the drug may be masked.
● Also use cautiously in patients with hepatic or renal impairment because systemic accumulation may occur.
● Check apical pulse rate and blood pressure before therapy. If you detect extremes in pulse rate, withhold drug and notify the doctor at once.
● Know that anticoagulant therapy is commonly advised before quinidine therapy in long-standing atrial fibrillation because restoration of normal sinus rhythm may result in thromboembolism caused by dislodgment of thrombi from atrial wall.
● When changing route of administration or oral salt form, be aware that dosage needs to be altered to compensate for variations in quinidine base content.
● Never use discolored (brownish) quinidine solution.
● Do not crush extended-release tablets.
Alert: When used to treat severe malaria, patients should be hospitalized in an intensive-care setting. Continuous monitoring is necessary. Decrease infusion rate if plasma quinidine level exceeds 6 mcg/ml, uncorrected QT interval exceeds 0.6 second, or QRS complex widening exceeds 25% of baseline.
● Monitor liver function tests during the first 4 to 8 weeks of therapy.
● Monitor serum quinidine levels as ordered. Therapeutic plasma levels for antiarrhythmic effects are 2 to 5 mcg/ml.
● Monitor patient response carefully. Adverse GI reactions, especially diarrhea, are signs of toxicity. Notify the doctor. Check quinidine blood levels, which are toxic when greater than 8 mcg/ml. GI symptoms may be decreased by giving drug with meals.
● Store drug away from heat and direct light.

☑ **PATIENT TEACHING**
● Stress importance of taking drug exactly as prescribed and to take it with food if adverse GI reactions occur.
● Tell patient to report persistent or serious adverse reactions promptly, especially signs and symptoms of quinidine toxicity.

---

sotalol
Betapace, Sotacor†‡

Pregnancy Risk Category: B

HOW SUPPLIED
Tablets: 80 mg, 120 mg, 160 mg, 240 mg

ACTION
A nonselective beta-adrenergic blocker that depresses sinus heart rate, slows AV conduction, decreases cardiac output, and lowers systolic and diastolic blood pressure.

ONSET, PEAK, DURATION
Onset and duration not clearly defined. Peak plasma levels occur within $2\frac{1}{2}$ to

---

4 hours.

INDICATIONS & DOSAGE
Documented, life-threatening ventricular arrhythmias—
Adults: initially, 80 mg P.O. b.i.d. Dosage is increased q 2 to 3 days as needed and tolerated; most patients respond to daily dosage of 160 to 320 mg. A few patients with refractory arrhythmias have received as much as 640 mg daily.

In patients with renal failure: If creatinine clearance is greater than 60 ml/minute, no adjustment in dosage interval is necessary. If creatinine clearance is 30 to 60 ml/minute, dosage interval is increased to q 24 hours; 10 to 30 ml/minute, q 36 to 48 hours; less than 10 ml/minute, dosage must be individualized.

Hypertension—
Adults: 80 mg P.O. b.i.d. Dosage is increased at weekly intervals in 80-mg increments b.i.d. as needed and tolerated. Most patients respond to daily dosage of 160 to 320 mg; patients taking 320 mg or less daily may take drug as a single morning dose.

Angina—
Adults: 80 mg P.O. b.i.d. Dosage is increased at weekly intervals in 80-mg increments b.i.d. as needed and tolerated. Most patients respond to doses of 160 mg b.i.d.; maximum daily dosage is 480 mg.

ADVERSE REACTIONS
CNS: *asthenia, headache, dizziness, weakness, fatigue,* sleep problems, *light-headedness.*
CV: *bradycardia, arrhythmias, CHF, AV block, proarrhythmic events (polymorphic ventricular tachycardia, PVCs, ventricular fibrillation),* edema, *palpitations, chest pain,* ECG abnormalities, hypotension.
GI: *nausea, vomiting,* diarrhea, dyspepsia.
Respiratory: *dyspnea, bronchospasm.*

INTERACTIONS
Antiarrhythmics: additive effects. Avoid concomitant use.
Antihypertensives, catecholamine-depleting drugs (such as reserpine and guanethidine): enhanced hypotensive effects. Monitor closely.
Calcium channel blockers: enhanced myocardial depression. Avoid concomitant use.
Clonidine: beta blockers may enhance rebound effect after withdrawal of clonidine. Discontinue sotalol several days before withdrawing clonidine.
General anesthetics: may cause additional myocardial depression. Monitor closely.
Insulin, oral hypoglycemics: may cause hyperglycemia; adjust dosage. May mask symptoms of hypoglycemia.

EFFECTS ON DIAGNOSTIC TESTS
Sotalol may increase blood glucose and liver enzyme levels.

CONTRAINDICATIONS
Contraindicated in patients with hypersensitivity to the drug, severe sinus node dysfunction, sinus bradycardia, second- and third-degree AV block in the absence of an artificial pacemaker, congenital or acquired long QT syndrome, cardiogenic shock, uncontrolled CHF, and bronchial asthma.

NURSING CONSIDERATIONS
• Use cautiously in patients with renal impairment or diabetes mellitus. Beta blockers may mask signs and symptoms of hypoglycemia.
• Because proarrhythmic events may occur at start of therapy and during dosage adjustments, patient should be hospitalized. Facilities and personnel should be available for cardiac rhythm monitoring and interpretation of ECG.
• Note that although patients receiving I.V. lidocaine have started sotalol therapy without ill effect, other antiarrhythmic drugs should be withdrawn before therapy with sotalol. Sotalol therapy

---

typically is delayed until two or three half-lives of the withdrawn drug have elapsed. After withdrawal of amiodarone, sotalol shouldn't be administered until the QT interval normalizes.

• Be aware that dosage should be adjusted slowly, allowing 2 to 3 days between dosage increments for adequate monitoring of QT intervals and for plasma levels of drug to reach a steady-state level.

• Monitor serum electrolytes regularly, especially if patient is receiving diuretics. Electrolyte imbalances, such as hypokalemia or hypomagnesemia, may enhance QT-interval prolongation and increase the risk of serious arrhythmias, such as torsades de pointes.

☑ **PATIENT TEACHING**
• Explain to the patient the importance of taking this drug as prescribed, even when he is feeling well. Caution him not to discontinue drug suddenly.

• Because food can interfere with absorption, tell the patient to take this drug on an empty stomach, 1 hour before or 2 hours after meals.

---

tocainide hydrochloride
Tonocard

Pregnancy Risk Category: C

HOW SUPPLIED
Tablets: 400 mg, 600 mg

ACTION
A class Ib antiarrhythmic that blocks the fast sodium channel in cardiac tissues, especially the Purkinje network, without involvement of the autonomic nervous system. It reduces the rate of rise and amplitude of the action potential and decreases automaticity in the Purkinje fibers. It shortens the duration of action potential and, to a lesser extent, decreases the effective refractory period in the Purkinje fibers.

ONSET, PEAK, DURATION
Onset unknown. Plasma levels peak in ½ to 2 hours. Duration is 8 hours.

INDICATIONS & DOSAGE
Suppression of symptomatic life-threatening ventricular arrhythmias—
Adults: initially, 400 mg P.O. q 8 hours. Usual dosage is between 1,200 and 1,800 mg daily in three divided doses. Patients with renal or hepatic impairment may be adequately treated with dosages less than 1,200 mg daily.

ADVERSE REACTIONS
CNS: *light-headedness, tremor,* paresthesia, *dizziness, vertigo,* drowsiness, fatigue, confusion, headache.
CV: hypotension, *new or worsened arrhythmias, CHF,* bradycardia, palpitations.
EENT: blurred vision, tinnitus.
GI: *nausea, vomiting,* diarrhea, anorexia.
Hematologic: *blood dyscrasias.*
Hepatic: hepatitis.
Respiratory: *respiratory arrest, pulmonary fibrosis, pneumonitis, pulmonary edema.*
Skin: rash, diaphoresis.

INTERACTIONS
Beta blockers: decreased myocardial contractility; increased CNS toxicity. Monitor closely.
Cimetidine: may decrease tocainide peak concentration. Monitor closely.
Rifampin: increased clearance of tocainide. Monitor efficacy of tocainide.
Lidocaine, mexiletine: additive pharmacologic effect and CNS toxicity.

EFFECTS ON DIAGNOSTIC TESTS
Drug may cause abnormal liver function tests, especially during early stages of therapy.

CONTRAINDICATIONS
Contraindicated in patients with hypersensitivity to lidocaine or other amidetype local anesthetics and in those with

---

second- or third-degree AV block in the absence of an artificial pacemaker.

NURSING CONSIDERATIONS

• Use cautiously in patients with CHF or diminished cardiac reserve and in those with hepatic or renal impairment. These patients often may be treated effectively with a lower dose.

• Be aware that drug may ease transition from I.V. lidocaine to oral antiarrhythmic. Monitor patient carefully.

• Correct potassium deficits, as ordered; drug may be ineffective in hypokalemia.

• Monitor the patient for tremor, which may indicate that the maximum dosage has been reached.

• Monitor blood levels as ordered. Therapeutic range is 4 to 10 mcg/ml.

☑ PATIENT TEACHING

• Tell the patient to report immediately any unusual bruising or bleeding or signs of infection. Agranulocytosis and bone marrow suppression have been reported in patients taking usual doses of the drug, typically within the first 12 weeks of therapy.

• Tell the patient to report sudden onset of any pulmonary symptoms, such as coughing, wheezing, or exertional dyspnea. Drug has been associated with serious pulmonary toxicity.

• Tell the patient to take safety precautions, especially if he is elderly because dizziness and falling are more likely to occur in such patients.

22
Antianginals

amlodipine besylate
amyl nitrite
bepridil hydrochloride
diltiazem hydrochloride
isosorbide dinitrate
isosorbide mononitrate
nadolol
nicardipine
nifedipine
nitroglycerin
propranolol hydrochloride
verapamil
verapamil hydrochloride

COMBINATION PRODUCTS
NITROTYM-PLUS: nitroglycerin 2.5 mg
and butabarbital sodium 48 mg.

---

amlodipine besylate
Norvasc

Pregnancy Risk Category: C

HOW SUPPLIED
Tablets: 2.5 mg, 5 mg, 10 mg

ACTION
Inhibits calcium ion influx across cardiac and smooth-muscle cells, thus decreasing myocardial contractility and
oxygen demand. Also dilates coronary
arteries and arterioles.

ONSET, PEAK, DURATION
Onset unknown. Serum levels peak in 6
to 12 hours. Effects persist for 24 hours.

INDICATIONS & DOSAGE
*Chronic stable angina; vasospastic
angina (Prinzmetal's [variant]
angina)—*
Adults: initially, 5 to 10 mg P.O. daily.
Small, frail, or elderly patients or patients with hepatic insufficiency should
begin therapy at 5 mg daily. Most patients require 10 mg daily.
Hypertension—
Adults: initially, 2.5 to 5 mg P.O. daily.
Small, frail, or elderly patients; patients
currently receiving other antihypertensives; or patients with hepatic insufficiency should begin therapy at 2.5 mg
daily. Dosage adjusted according to patient response and tolerance. Maximum
daily dosage is 10 mg.

ADVERSE REACTIONS
CNS: *headache,* somnolence, fatigue,
dizziness, light-headedness, paresthesia.
CV: *edema,* flushing, palpitations.
GI: nausea, abdominal pain.
Other: dyspnea, muscle pain, rash, pru-
ritus.

INTERACTIONS
None significant.

EFFECTS ON DIAGNOSTIC TESTS
None reported.

CONTRAINDICATIONS
Contraindicated in patients with hypersensitivity to the drug.

NURSING CONSIDERATIONS
• Use cautiously in patients receiving
other peripheral vasodilators, especially
those with severe aortic stenosis, and in
those with CHF. Because drug is metabolized by the liver, use cautiously and in
reduced dosage in patients with severe
hepatic disease.
Alert: Monitor the patient carefully.
Some patients, especially those with severe obstructive coronary artery disease,
have developed increased frequency, duration, or severity of angina or even
acute MI after initiation of calcium
channel blocker therapy or at time of
dosage increase.
• Monitor blood pressure frequently

Reactions may be *common*, uncommon, *life-threatening*, or COMMON AND LIFE-THREATENING.

during initiation of therapy. Because drug-induced vasodilation has a gradual onset, acute hypotension is rare.
• Notify the doctor if signs of CHF occur, such as swelling of hands and feet or shortness of breath.

☑ **PATIENT TEACHING**
• Caution patient to continue taking the drug, even when feeling better.
• Tell patient sublingual nitroglycerin may be taken as needed when anginal symptoms are acute. If the patient continues nitrate therapy during titration of amlodipine dosage, urge continued compliance.

---

amyl nitrite

Pregnancy Risk Category: X

HOW SUPPLIED
Ampules (crushable): 0.3 ml

ACTION
Antianginal action unknown. Thought to be the result of dilation of both arterial and venous beds. The net effect is a reduction in myocardial oxygen demand, improving perfusion to the ischemic myocardium. Converts hemoglobin to methemoglobin (which binds cyanide) to treat cyanide poisoning.

ONSET, PEAK, DURATION
Onset occurs in 30 seconds. Peak unknown. Effects persist 3 to 5 minutes.

INDICATIONS & DOSAGE
Relief of angina pectoris—
Adults and children: 0.3 ml by inhalation (one glass ampule) p.r.n.
Antidote for cyanide poisoning—
0.3 ml by inhalation for 15 to 60 seconds q 5 minutes until conscious.

ADVERSE REACTIONS
CNS: *headache, sometimes with throbbing;* dizziness; weakness.
CV: *orthostatic hypotension, tachycar-*
dia, flushing, palpitations, syncope.
GI: nausea, vomiting.
Hematologic: methemoglobinemia.
Skin: cutaneous vasodilation, rash.
Other: hypersensitivity reactions.

INTERACTIONS
Alcohol: severe hypotension and CV collapse may occur.
Calcium channel blockers: increased risk of symptomatic orthostatic hypotension.

EFFECTS ON DIAGNOSTIC TESTS
Amyl nitrite alters the Zlatkis-Zak color reaction, causing a false decrease in serum cholesterol levels.

CONTRAINDICATIONS
Contraindicated in patients with hypersensitivity to nitrates, severe anemia, angle-closure glaucoma, postural hypotension, early MI, increased intracranial pressure and in pregnant patients.

NURSING CONSIDERATIONS
• Use cautiously in patients with glaucoma (except angle-closure type which is a contraindication), volume depletion, or hypotension.
• Extinguish all cigarettes before use, or ampule may ignite.
• Wrap ampule in cloth and crush. Hold near the patient's nose and mouth so vapor is inhaled.
• Watch for orthostatic hypotension.
• Store away from light.
• Be aware that drug is often abused (claimed to have aphrodisiac benefits). Street name is "Amy."

☑ **PATIENT TEACHING**
• Instruct patient how to administer drug. Stress importance of extinguishing all cigarettes before use.
• Tell patient to sit and avoid any position changes while inhaling drug to prevent orthostatic hypotension.
• Instruct patient to take a mild analgesic for drug-induced headache.

bepridil hydrochloride
Bepadin‡, Vascor

Pregnancy Risk Category: C

HOW SUPPLIED
Tablets: 200 mg, 300 mg, 400 mg

ACTION
A calcium channel blocker that inhibits calcium ion influx across cardiac and smooth-muscle cells. This action dilates coronary arteries as well as peripheral arteries and arterioles; it may reduce heart rate, decrease myocardial contractility, and slow AV node conduction.

ONSET, PEAK, DURATION
Onset of action after oral administration is 60 minutes. Plasma levels peak within 2 to 3 hours. Effects persist for 24 hours.

INDICATIONS & DOSAGE
Chronic stable angina in patients who cannot tolerate or who fail to respond to other agents—
Adults: initially, 200 mg P.O. daily. After 10 days, dosage increased based on response. Maintenance dosage in most patients is 300 mg/day. Maximum daily dosage is 400 mg.

ADVERSE REACTIONS
CNS: *dizziness,* drowsiness, *nervousness, headache,* insomnia, paresthesia, *asthenia,* tremor.
CV: edema, flushing, palpitations, tachycardia, ***ventricular arrhythmias, including torsades de pointes, ventricular tachycardia, ventricular fibrillation.***
EENT: tinnitus.
GI: *nausea, diarrhea,* constipation, abdominal discomfort, dry mouth, anorexia.
Respiratory: dyspnea, shortness of breath.
Skin: rash.
Other: flu syndrome.

INTERACTIONS
Antiarrhythmics, digitalis glycosides, drugs that increase QT interval: may exaggerate prolongation of the QT interval or depression of AV node with bepridil.
Digoxin: serum digoxin levels may be increased; monitor combined use.
Fentanyl anesthesia: severe hypotension has been reported with concomitant use of a beta blocker and a calcium channel blocker. Inform anesthesiologist that the patient is taking a calcium channel blocker.

EFFECTS ON DIAGNOSTIC TESTS
Increased ALT levels and abnormal liver function test results have been observed.

CONTRAINDICATIONS
Contraindicated in patients with hypersensitivity to the drug; uncompensated cardiac insufficiency, sick sinus syndrome or second- or third-degree AV block unless pacemaker is present; hypotension (below 90 mm Hg systolic); congenital QT interval prolongation; or history of serious ventricular arrhythmias. Also contraindicated in those receiving other drugs that prolong the QT interval.

NURSING CONSIDERATIONS
● Use cautiously in patients with left bundle branch block, sinus bradycardia, impaired renal or hepatic function, or CHF.
● Monitor patient for adverse reactions. Bepridil has been associated with severe ventricular arrhythmias, including torsades de pointes.
● Know that dosage should not be adjusted more frequently than every 10 to 14 days because of bepridil's long half-life and time it takes to reach steady-state blood levels.

☑ PATIENT TEACHING
● Instruct patient to take drug exactly as directed.

Reactions may be *common*, uncommon, *life-threatening*, or COMMON AND LIFE-THREATENING.

diltiazem hydrochloride
Apo-Diltiaz†, Cardizem, Cardizem
CD, Cardizem SR, Dilacor XR, Vaso-
cardol SR‡

Pregnancy Risk Category: C

HOW SUPPLIED
Tablets: 30 mg, 60 mg, 90 mg, 120 mg
*Capsules (extended-release; Cardizem
CD, Dilacor XR):* 120 mg, 180 mg, 240
mg, 300 mg
*Capsules (sustained-release; Cardizem
SR, Vasocardol SR‡):* 60 mg, 90 mg,
120 mg, 180 mg, 240 mg
Injection: 5 mg/ml

ACTION
A calcium channel blocker that inhibits
calcium ion influx across cardiac and
smooth-muscle cells, decreasing myocardial contractility and oxygen demand. Also dilates coronary arteries and
arterioles.

ONSET, PEAK, DURATION
Onset is about 3 minutes after I.V. bolus
injection, 30 to 60 minutes after oral administration of regular tablets, 2 to 3
hours after extended- or sustained-release preparations. Peak plasma levels
occur immediately after I.V. injection, 2
to 3 hours after regular tablet, 6 to 11
hours after sustained-release capsule, or
10 to 14 hours after extended-release
capsule. Effects persist 1 to 3 hours after I.V. bolus, up to 10 hours after I.V.
infusion, 6 to 8 hours after regular
tablet, about 12 hours after sustained-release capsule, about 24 hours after extended-release capsule.

INDICATIONS & DOSAGE
*Vasospastic angina (Prinzmetal's [vari-
ant] angina) and classic chronic stable
angina pectoris—*
Adults: 30 mg P.O. t.i.d. or q.i.d. before
meals and h.s. Dosage increased gradually to maximum of 360 mg/day in divided doses. Alternatively, 120 or 180

mg (extended-release capsule). Titrated
as needed and tolerated to a maximum
of 480 mg daily.
Hypertension—
Adults: 60 to 120 mg P.O. b.i.d. (sustained-release). Titrated to effect. Maximum recommended dosage is 360
mg/day. Alternatively, 180 to 240 mg
daily (extended-release) initially.
Dosage adjusted as necessary.
*Atrial fibrillation or flutter; paroxysmal
supraventricular tachycardia—*
Adults: 0.25 mg/kg as an I.V. bolus injection over 2 minutes. If response is inadequate, 0.35 mg/kg I.V. after 15 minutes followed with a continuous infusion of 10 mg/hour. Some patients
respond well to rates of 5 mg/hour; the
maximum dose is 15 mg/hour.

ADVERSE REACTIONS
CNS: *headache,* dizziness, asthenia,
somnolence.
CV: *edema, arrhythmias,* flushing,
bradycardia, hypotension, conduction
abnormalities, *CHF,* AV block, abnormal ECG.
GI: *nausea, constipation,* abdominal
discomfort.
Hepatic: acute hepatic injury.
Skin: *rash.*

INTERACTIONS
Anesthetics: effects may be potentiated.
Cimetidine: may inhibit diltiazem metabolism. Monitor for toxicity.
Cyclosporine: diltiazem may increase
serum cyclosporine levels, possibly by
decreasing its metabolism, leading to increased risk of cyclosporine toxicity. If
used concurrently, monitor cyclosporine
levels.
Digoxin: diltiazem may increase serum
levels of digoxin. Monitor for toxicity.
Furosemide: forms a precipitate when
mixed with diltiazem injection. Administer through separate I.V. lines.
Propranolol, other beta blockers: may
precipitate CHF or prolong conduction
time. Use together cautiously.

EFFECTS ON DIAGNOSTIC TESTS
None reported.

CONTRAINDICATIONS
Contraindicated in patients with sick sinus syndrome or second- or third-degree AV block in the absence of an artificial pacemaker, systolic blood pressure below 90 mm Hg, hypersensitivity to the drug, acute MI, and pulmonary congestion (documented by X-ray).

NURSING CONSIDERATIONS
● Use cautiously in elderly patients and in those with CHF or impaired hepatic or renal function.
● **I.V. use:** Infusions lasting longer than 24 hours are not recommended.
● Monitor blood pressure and heart rate during initiation of therapy and dosage adjustments.
● If systolic blood pressure is below 90 mm Hg or heart rate is below 60 beats/minute, withhold dose and notify the doctor.

☑ **PATIENT TEACHING**
● Advise patient to avoid hazardous activities during initiation of therapy.
● If nitrate therapy is prescribed during titration of diltiazem dosage, urge patient compliance. Tell patient that sublingual nitroglycerin, especially, may be taken concomitantly as needed when anginal symptoms are acute.
● Tell patient to swallow Dilacor XR whole, not to open, crush, or chew it.

isosorbide dinitrate
Apo-ISDN†, Cedocard-SR†, Coradur†, Coronex†, Dilatrate-SR, Isonate, Isorbid, Isordil, Isordil Tembids, Isordil Titradose, Isotrate, Nitro-Spray‡, Novosorbide†, Sorbitrate

isosorbide mononitrate
Imdur, ISMO, Monoket

Pregnancy Risk Category: C

HOW SUPPLIED
isosorbide dinitrate
Tablets: 5 mg, 10 mg, 20 mg, 30 mg, 40 mg
Tablets (chewable): 5 mg, 10 mg
Tablets (sublingual): 2.5 mg, 5 mg, 10 mg
Tablets (sustained-release): 40 mg
Capsules: 40 mg
Capsules (sustained-release): 40 mg
Topical spray: 10%‡, 12.5 mg metered spray‡
isosorbide mononitrate
Tablets: 10 mg, 20 mg
Tablets (extended-release): 30 mg, 60 mg, 120 mg

ACTION
Not completely known. Thought to reduce cardiac oxygen demand by decreasing preload and afterload. Drug also may increase blood flow through the collateral coronary vessels.

ONSET, PEAK, DURATION
Onset and peak levels occur as follows: isosorbide dinitrate—2 to 5 minutes after administration of S.L. or chewable form, 15 to 40 minutes after oral form, 30 minutes to 4 hours after extended-release form. Isosorbide mononitrate—30 to 60 minutes. Duration is as follows: isosorbide dinitrate—effective for 1 to 1½ hours after administration of S.L. form, 2 to 2½ hours after chewable form, 4 to 6 hours after oral form, 12 hours after extended-release form. Isosorbide mononitrate—not determined.

INDICATIONS & DOSAGE
Acute anginal attacks (S.L. and chewable tablets of isosorbide dinitrate only), prophylaxis in situations likely to cause anginal attacks—
Adults: *S.L. form*—2.5 to 5 mg under the tongue for prompt relief of anginal pain, repeated q 5 to 10 minutes (maximum of three doses for each 30-minute period). For prophylaxis, 2.5 to 10 mg q 2 to 3 hours.

Chewable form—5 to 10 mg p.r.n. for acute attack or q 2 to 3 hours for prophylaxis, but only after initial test dose of 5 mg to determine risk of severe hypotension.

Oral form (isosorbide dinitrate)—5 to 30 mg P.O. t.i.d. or q.i.d. for prophylaxis only (use smallest effective dose); 20 to 40 mg P.O. (sustained-release form) q 6 to 12 hours.

Oral form (isosorbide mononitrate using Imdur)—30 to 60 mg P.O. once daily upon arising; increased to 120 mg once daily after several days, if needed.

Oral form (isosorbide mononitrate using ISMO or Monoket)—20 mg b.i.d. with the two doses given 7 hours apart.

Topical form‡ (where available)—initially, 2 sprays to chest in morning from about 8″ (20 cm). Rub solution in. Increase dosage gradually as needed to 2 to 5 sprays, daily or b.i.d. (in morning and h.s.).

ADVERSE REACTIONS

CNS: *headache* (sometimes with throbbing); dizziness; weakness.
CV: *orthostatic hypotension, tachycardia, palpitations, ankle edema,* fainting.
GI: nausea, vomiting.
Skin: cutaneous vasodilation, *flushing,* rash.
Other: hypersensitivity reactions, sublingual burning.

INTERACTIONS

Antihypertensives: may increase hypotensive effects. Monitor closely during initial therapy.
Ethanol: may increase hypotension. Avoid concomitant use.

EFFECTS ON DIAGNOSTIC TESTS

May interfere with serum cholesterol determination tests using the Zlatkis-Zak color reaction, causing a falsely decreased value.

CONTRAINDICATIONS

Contraindicated in patients with hypersensitivity or idiosyncrasy to nitrates, severe hypotension, angle-closure glaucoma, increased intracranial pressure, shock, or acute MI with low left ventricular filling pressure.

NURSING CONSIDERATIONS

• Use cautiously in patients with blood volume depletion (such as from diuretic therapy) or mild hypotension.
• To prevent development of tolerance, a nitrate-free interval of 8 to 12 hours per day has been recommended. The regimen for isosorbide mononitrate (one tablet upon awakening with the second dose in 7 hours, or one extended-release tablet daily) is intended to minimize nitrate tolerance by providing a substantial nitrate-free interval.
• Monitor blood pressure and intensity and duration of drug response.
• May cause headaches, especially at beginning of therapy. Dosage may be reduced temporarily, but tolerance usually develops. Treat headache with aspirin or acetaminophen.

☑ PATIENT TEACHING

• Caution the patient to take medication regularly, as prescribed, and to keep it accessible at all times.
Alert: Advise the patient that abrupt discontinuation of drug may cause coronary vasospasm with increased anginal symptoms and potential risk of MI.
• Tell patient to take S.L. tablet at first sign of attack. The tablet should be wet with saliva and placed under the tongue until absorbed, and the patient should sit down and rest. Dose may be repeated every 10 to 15 minutes for a maximum of three doses. If drug doesn't provide relief, medical help should be obtained promptly.
• Advise patient who complains of tingling sensation with S.L. drug to try holding tablet in buccal pouch.
• Warn the patient not to confuse S.L. with oral form.

● Teach the patient taking oral form of isosorbide dinitrate to take oral tablet on an empty stomach, either ½ before or 1 to 2 hours after meals; to swallow oral tablets whole; and to chew chewable tablets thoroughly before swallowing.
● Tell the patient to minimize orthostatic hypotension by changing to upright position slowly. Advise him to go up and down stairs carefully and to lie down at the first sign of dizziness.
● Tell the patient to store drug in a cool place, in a tightly closed container, away from light.

---

nadolol
Corgard

Pregnancy Risk Category: C

HOW SUPPLIED
Tablets: 20 mg, 40 mg, 80 mg, 120 mg, 160 mg

ACTION
A beta-adrenergic blocker that reduces cardiac oxygen demand by blocking catecholamine-induced increases in heart rate, blood pressure, and force of myocardial contraction. Depresses renin secretion.

ONSET, PEAK, DURATION
Onset and duration unknown. Plasma levels peak within 2 to 4 hours.

INDICATIONS & DOSAGE
Angina pectoris—
Adults: 40 mg P.O. once daily. Dosage increased in 40- to 80-mg increments until optimum response occurs. Usual maintenance dosage is 40 to 80 mg once daily; up to 240 mg once daily may be needed.
Hypertension—
Adults: 40 mg P.O. once daily. Dosage increased in 40- to 80-mg increments until optimum response occurs. Usual maintenance dosage is 40 to 80 mg once daily. Doses of 320 mg may be needed.

ADVERSE REACTIONS
CNS: fatigue, dizziness.
CV: *bradycardia, hypotension, CHF,* peripheral vascular disease, rhythm and conduction disturbances.
GI: nausea, vomiting, diarrhea, abdominal pain, constipation, anorexia.
Respiratory: *increased airway resistance.*
Skin: rash.
Other: fever.

INTERACTIONS
Antihypertensives: enhanced antihypertensive effect.
Digitalis glycosides: excessive bradycardia and additive effects on AV conduction. Use together cautiously.
Epinephrine: severe vasoconstriction and reflex bradycardia. Monitor blood pressure carefully.
Insulin, oral antidiabetic agents: can alter dosage requirements in previously stabilized diabetic patients. Observe the patient carefully.
NSAIDs: decreased antihypertensive effect. Monitor blood pressure and adjust dosage.

EFFECTS ON DIAGNOSTIC TESTS
None reported.

CONTRAINDICATIONS
Contraindicated in patients with bronchial asthma, sinus bradycardia and greater than first-degree heart block, and cardiogenic shock.

NURSING CONSIDERATIONS
● Use cautiously in patients with heart failure, chronic bronchitis, emphysema, or renal or hepatic impairment and in patients undergoing major surgery involving general anesthesia. Also use cautiously in diabetic patients because beta-adrenergic blockers may mask certain signs and symptoms of hypoglycemia.
● Check apical pulse before giving drug. If slower than 60 beats/minute, withhold drug and call doctor.

Reactions may be *common*, uncommon, *life-threatening*, or COMMON AND LIFE-THREATENING.

• Monitor blood pressure frequently. If the patient develops severe hypotension, administer a vasopressor, as prescribed.
Alert: Know that abrupt discontinuation can exacerbate angina and precipitate MI. Dosage should be reduced gradually over 1 to 2 weeks.
• Be aware that nadolol masks signs of shock and hyperthyroidism.

☑ **PATIENT TEACHING**
• Explain to the patient the importance of taking the drug as prescribed, even when he's feeling well.
• Teach the patient how to check pulse rate and to do so before each dose. If pulse rate is below 60 beats/minute, tell the patient to notify the doctor.
• Caution the patient not to discontinue the drug suddenly.

---

nicardipine
Cardene, Cardene IV, Cardene SR

Pregnancy Risk Category: C

HOW SUPPLIED
Capsules (immediate-release): 20 mg, 30 mg
Capsules (sustained-release): 30 mg, 45 mg, 60 mg
Injection: 2.5 mg/ml

ACTION
A calcium channel blocker that inhibits calcium ion influx across cardiac and smooth-muscle cells, decreasing myocardial contractility and oxygen demand. Also dilates coronary arteries and arterioles.

ONSET, PEAK, DURATION
Onset is immediate after I.V. administration, within 20 minutes for both oral formulations. Serum levels peak within minutes after I.V. injection, within ½ to 2 hours after immediate-release capsules, 1 to 4 hours after sustained-release capsule. Effects of immediate-release product persist for 6 to 8 hours, of sustained-release preparation, up to 12 hours; rapid decline after cessation of I.V. infusion.

INDICATIONS & DOSAGE
Chronic stable angina (used alone or in combination with other antianginal agents)—
Adults: initially, 20 mg P.O. t.i.d. (immediate-release only). Dosage titrated according to patient response q 3 days. Usual dosage range is 20 to 40 mg t.i.d.
Hypertension—
Adults: initially, 20 mg P.O. t.i.d. (immediate-release); range, 20 to 40 mg t.i.d. Or, 30 mg b.i.d. (sustained-release); range, 30 to 60 mg b.i.d. Dosage increased according to patient response. Alternatively, for patients unable to take oral nicardipine, 50 ml/hour (5 mg/hour) I.V. infusion initially; then increased by 25 ml/hour (2.5 mg/hour) every 15 minutes up to a maximum of 150 ml/hour (15 mg/hour).

ADVERSE REACTIONS
CNS: *dizziness, light-headedness, headache, asthenia.*
CV: *peripheral edema, palpitations,* angina, tachycardia.
GI: nausea, abdominal discomfort, dry mouth.
Skin: rash, *flushing.*

INTERACTIONS
Antihypertensives: enhanced antihypertensive effect. Monitor closely.
Beta blockers: may increase cardiac depressant effects. Monitor closely.
Cimetidine: may decrease metabolism of calcium channel blockers. Monitor for increased pharmacologic effect.
Cyclosporine: nicardipine may increase plasma levels of cyclosporine. Monitor for toxicity.
Theophylline: pharmacologic effects of theophylline may be enhanced. Monitor for toxicity.

EFFECTS ON DIAGNOSTIC TESTS
None reported.

---

*Liquid contains alcohol. **May contain tartrazine. †Canada only. ‡Australia only. ◇OTC.

CONTRAINDICATIONS
Contraindicated in patients with hypersensitivity to the drug and in those with advanced aortic stenosis.

NURSING CONSIDERATIONS
• Use cautiously in patients with hypotension, CHF, and impaired hepatic and renal function.
• **I.V. use:** When switching to oral therapy other than nicardipine, initiate therapy upon discontinuation of the infusion. If oral nicardipine is to be used, administer first dose of t.i.d. regimen 1 hour prior to discontinuation of infusion.
• Adjust infusion rate if hypotension or tachycardia occurs, as ordered.
• Measure blood pressure frequently during initial therapy. Maximum blood pressure response occurs about 1 hour after dosing with the immediate-release form and 2 to 4 hours with the sustained-release form. Check for potential orthostatic hypotension. Because large swings in blood pressure may occur based on blood level of drug, assess adequacy of antihypertensive effect 8 hours after dosing.

☑ PATIENT TEACHING
• Tell the patient to take oral form of drug exactly as prescribed.
• Advise the patient to report chest pain immediately. Some patients may experience increased frequency, severity, or duration of chest pain at beginning of therapy or during dosage adjustments.

nifedipine
Adalat, Adalat CC, Adalat FT†, Adalat P.A.†, Anpine‡, Apo-Nifed†, Novonifedin†, Nu-Nifed†, Procardia, Procardia XL

Pregnancy Risk Category: C

HOW SUPPLIED
Tablets (extended-release): 30 mg, 60 mg, 90 mg

Capsules: 10 mg, 20 mg

ACTION
Unknown. Thought to inhibit calcium ion influx across cardiac and smooth-muscle cells, decreasing contractility and oxygen demand. Also may dilate coronary arteries and arterioles.

ONSET, PEAK, DURATION
Onset occurs in 20 minutes. Serum levels peak in about 30 to 60 minutes for capsules, 6 hours for tablets. Effects persist for 4 to 8 hours for capsules; 24 hours for extended-release formulations.

INDICATIONS & DOSAGE
Vasospastic angina (also called Prinzmetal's [variant] angina) and classic chronic stable angina pectoris—
Adults: starting dose is 10 mg P.O. t.i.d. Usual effective dose range is 10 to 20 mg t.i.d. Some patients may require up to 30 mg q.i.d. Maximum daily dosage is 180 mg.
Hypertension—
Adults: 30 or 60 mg P.O. (extended-release form) once daily. Titrated over 7 to 14 days. Doses larger than 90 mg (for Adalat CC) and 120 mg (for Procardia XL) are not recommended.

ADVERSE REACTIONS
CNS: *dizziness, light-headedness, flushing, headache, weakness,* syncope, nervousness.
CV: *peripheral edema,* hypotension, palpitations, CHF, ***MI,*** pulmonary edema.
EENT: nasal congestion.
GI: *nausea,* diarrhea, constipation, abdominal discomfort.
Respiratory: dyspnea, cough.
Skin: rash, pruritus.
Other: muscle cramps, hypokalemia.

INTERACTIONS
Cimetidine, ranitidine: decreased nifedipine metabolism.
Propranolol, other beta blockers: may cause hypotension and heart failure. Use

together cautiously.

EFFECTS ON DIAGNOSTIC TESTS
Mild to moderate increase in serum concentrations of alkaline phosphate, lactate dehydrogenase, AST, and ALT have been noted.

CONTRAINDICATIONS
Contraindicated in patients with hypersensitivity to the drug.

NURSING CONSIDERATIONS
● Use cautiously in patients with CHF or hypotension and in elderly patients. Use extended-release tablets cautiously in patients with severe GI narrowing.
● When a rapid response to the drug is desired, have the patient bite and swallow the capsule. If he can't chew capsules, the liquid can be withdrawn by puncturing the capsule with a needle and squeezing the contents into the mouth. When these methods are used, continuous blood pressure and ECG monitoring is recommended.
● Despite widespread S.L. use of nifedipine capsules, this route of administration should be avoided. Peak serum levels are lower and take longer to occur than when capsules are bitten and swallowed.
● Monitor blood pressure regularly, especially in patients who are taking beta blockers or antihypertensives.
● Be aware that although rebound effect hasn't been observed when drug is stopped, dosage should be reduced slowly under doctor's supervision.

☑ **PATIENT TEACHING**
● If the patient is kept on nitrate therapy while nifedipine dosage is being titrated, urge continued compliance. S.L. nitroglycerin, especially, may be taken as needed when anginal symptoms are acute.
● Patient may briefly develop anginal exacerbation when beginning drug therapy or when dosage is increased.
● Instruct the patient to swallow extend-ed-release tablets without breaking, crushing, or chewing.
● Reassure the patient who is taking the extended-release form that a wax-matrix "ghost" from the tablet may be passed in the stools. Drug is completely absorbed before this occurs.
● Warn the patient not to switch brands. Procardia XL and Adalat CC are not therapeutically equivalent because of major differences in their pharmacokinetics.
● Tell the patient to protect capsules from direct light and moisture and to store at room temperature.

nitroglycerin (glyceryl trinitrate)
Anginine‡, Coro-Nitra, Deponit, GTN-Pohl‡, Minitran, Nitradisc‡, Nitro-Bid, Nitro-Bid I.V., Nitrocine, Nitrodisc, Nitro-Dur, Nitrogard, Nitrogard-SR†, Nitroglyn, Nitroject, Nitrol, Nitrolate‡, Nitrolingual, Nitrong, Nitrostat, Nitro-Time, NTS, Transdermal-NTG, Transderm-Nitro, Transiderm-Nitro‡, Tridil

Pregnancy Risk Category: C

HOW SUPPLIED
Tablets (buccal): 1 mg, 2 mg, 3 mg
Tablets (sublingual): 0.15 mg ($^1/_{400}$ gr), 0.3 mg ($^1/_{200}$ gr), 0.4 mg ($^1/_{150}$ gr), 0.6 mg ($^1/_{100}$ gr)
Tablets (sustained-release): 2.6 mg, 6.5 mg, 9 mg, 13 mg
Capsules (sustained-release): 2.5 mg, 6.5 mg, 9 mg, 13 mg
Aerosol (translingual): 0.4 mg metered spray
Topical: 2% ointment
Transdermal: 0.1 mg, 0.2 mg, 0.3 mg, 0.4 mg, 0.6 mg, 0.8 mg per hour release rate
Injection: 0.5 mg/ml, 5 mg/ml

ACTION
A nitrate that reduces cardiac oxygen demand by decreasing left ventricular end-diastolic pressure (preload) and, to

---

*Liquid contains alcohol.   **May contain tartrazine.   †Canada only.   ‡Australia only.   ◇OTC.

a lesser extent, systemic vascular resistance (afterload). Also increases blood flow through the collateral coronary vessels.

ONSET, PEAK, DURATION
Onset and peak immediate after I.V. form, 1 to 3 minutes after S.L. form, 2 to 4 minutes after translingual form, 3 minutes after buccal form, 20 to 45 minutes after oral form, 30 minutes after topical ointment, 30 minutes after transdermal system. With I.V. form, effects last 3 to 5 minutes; with S.L. form, 30 to 60 minutes; with translingual form, 30 to 60 minutes; with buccal form, 3 to 5 hours; with oral form, 3 to 8 hours; with topical ointment, 2 to 12 hours; with transdermal system, up to 24 hours with system in place (otherwise, effects last several hours after removal).

INDICATIONS & DOSAGE
Prophylaxis against chronic anginal attacks—
Adults: 2.5 mg or 2.6 mg sustained-release capsule q 8 to 12 hours, titrated upward to an effective dose in 2.5- or 2.6-mg increments 2 to 4 times daily. Or, use of 2% ointment: Dosage started with ½″ ointment, increasing by ½″ increments until desired results are achieved. Range of dosage with ointment is ½″ to 5″. Usual dose is 1″ to 2″. Alternatively, transdermal disc or pad (Nitrodisc, Nitro-Dur, or Transderm-Nitro) 0.2 to 0.4 mg/hour once daily.
Acute angina pectoris, prophylaxis to prevent or minimize anginal attacks before stressful events—
Adults: 1 S.L. tablet (gr ¹/₄₀₀, ¹/₂₀₀, ¹/₁₅₀, ¹/₁₀₀) dissolved under the tongue or in the buccal pouch as soon as angina begins. Repeat q 5 minutes, if needed, for 15 minutes. Or, using Nitrolingual spray, one or two sprays into mouth, preferably onto or under the tongue. Repeat q 3 to 5 minutes, if needed, to a maximum of three doses within a 15-minute period. Or, 1 to 3 mg transmucosally q 3 to 5 hours during waking hours.

Hypertension associated with surgery; CHF associated with MI; angina pectoris in acute situations; to produce controlled hypotension during surgery (by I.V. infusion)—
Adults: initial infusion rate is 5 mcg/minute, increased as needed by 5 mcg/minute q 3 to 5 minutes until a response is noted. If a 20 mcg/minute rate doesn't produce a response, dosage is increased by as much as 20 mcg/minute q 3 to 5 minutes. Up to 100 mcg/minute may be needed.

ADVERSE REACTIONS
CNS: *headache, sometimes with throbbing; dizziness;* weakness.
CV: *orthostatic hypotension, tachycardia, flushing, palpitations,* fainting.
GI: nausea, vomiting.
Skin: cutaneous vasodilation, contact dermatitis (patch), rash.
Other: hypersensitivity reactions, sublingual burning.

INTERACTIONS
Antihypertensives: possible enhanced hypotensive effect. Monitor closely.
Ethanol: possible increased hypotension. Advise patient to avoid ethanol.
Heparin: I.V. nitroglycerin interferes with anticoagulant effect of heparin in some patients.

EFFECTS ON DIAGNOSTIC TESTS
Nitroglycerin may interfere with serum cholesterol determination tests using the Zlatkis-Zak color reaction, resulting in falsely decreased values.

CONTRAINDICATIONS
Contraindicated in patients with hypersensitivity to nitrates and in those with early MI (sublingual nitroglycerin), severe anemia, increased intracranial pressure, angle-closure glaucoma, postural hypotension, and allergy to adhesives (transdermal). I.V. nitroglycerin is contraindicated in patients with hypersensitivity to I.V. form, cardiac tamponade,

---

restrictive cardiomyopathy, or constrictive pericarditis.

NURSING CONSIDERATIONS
● Use cautiously in patients with hypotension or volume depletion.
● **I.V. use:** Dilute with D_5W or 0.9% sodium chloride for injection. Concentration should not exceed 400 mcg/ml. Always administer with an infusion control device and titrate to desired response. Also, always mix in glass bottles and avoid use of I.V. filters because drug binds to plastic. Regular polyvinyl chloride (PVC) tubing can bind up to 80% of the drug, making it necessary to infuse higher dosages. A special nonabsorbent (non-PVC) tubing is available from the manufacturer; patients receive more drug when these infusion sets are used. Always use the same type of infusion set when changing I.V. lines.
● When changing the concentration of infusion, flush the I.V. administration set with 15 to 20 ml of the new concentration before use. This will clear the line of the old drug solution.
● Closely monitor vital signs during infusion. Be particularly aware of blood pressure, especially in a patient with an MI. Excessive hypotension may worsen the MI.
● To apply ointment, measure the prescribed amount on the application paper; then place the paper on any nonhairy area. Do not rub in. Cover with plastic film to aid absorption and to protect clothing. If using Tape-Surrounded Appli-Ruler (TSAR) system, keep the TSAR on skin to protect patient's clothing and to ensure that ointment remains in place. Remove all excess ointment from previous site before applying the next dose. Avoid getting ointment on fingers.
● Know that transdermal dosage forms can be applied to any nonhairy part of the skin except distal parts of the arms or legs (absorption will not be maximal at distal sites).
● Remove transdermal patch before defibrillation. Because of its aluminum backing, the electric current may cause arcing that can result in damage to paddles and burns to the patient.
● When stopping transdermal treatment of angina, gradually reduce the dose and frequency of application over 4 to 6 weeks, as ordered.
● Monitor blood pressure and intensity and duration of drug response.
● May cause headaches, especially at beginning of therapy. Dosage may be reduced temporarily, but tolerance usually develops. Treat headache with aspirin or acetaminophen.
● Tolerance to the drug can be minimized with a 10- to 12-hour nitrate-free interval. To achieve this, remove the transdermal system in the early evening and apply a new system the next morning or omit the last daily dose of a buccal, sustained-release, or ointment form. Check with the doctor for alterations in dosage regimen if tolerance is suspected.

☑ PATIENT TEACHING
● Caution the patient to take nitroglycerin regularly, as prescribed, and to have it accessible at all times.
Alert: Advise the patient that abrupt discontinuation of drug causes coronary vasospasms.
● Teach the patient how to administer the prescribed form of nitroglycerin.
● Tell patient to take S.L. tablet at first sign of attack. The tablet should be wet with saliva and placed under the tongue until absorbed, and the patient should sit down and rest. Dose may be repeated every 10 to 15 minutes for a maximum of three doses. If drug doesn't provide relief, medical help should be obtained promptly.
● Advise patient who complains of a tingling sensation with S.L. drug to try holding tablet in buccal pouch.
● Tell the patient to take oral tablets on an empty stomach, either 30 minutes before or 1 to 2 hours after meals; to swallow oral tablets whole; and not to

---

chew tablets.
• Remind the patient using translingual aerosol form that he should *not* inhale the spray, but should release it onto or under the tongue. Also tell him to wait about 10 seconds or so before swallowing.
• Tell the patient to place the buccal tablet between the lip and gum above the incisors or between the cheek and gum. Tablets should not be swallowed or chewed.
• Tell him to take an additional dose before anticipated stress or at bedtime if angina is nocturnal.
• Instruct the patient to use caution when wearing transdermal patch near microwave oven. Leaking radiation may heat patch's metallic backing and cause burns.
• Advise him to avoid alcohol.
• To minimize orthostatic hypotension, tell the patient to change to upright position slowly. Advise him to go up and down stairs carefully and to lie down at the first sign of dizziness.
• Tell the patient to store drug in cool, dark place in a tightly closed container. Remove cotton from container because it absorbs the drug.
• Tell the patient to store S.L. tablets in original container or other container specifically approved for this use and to carry the container in a jacket pocket or purse, not in a pocket close to the body.

propranolol hydrochloride
Apo-Propranolol†, Betachron E-R, Deralin‡, Detensol†, Inderal, Inderal LA, Novopranol†, pms Propranolol†

Pregnancy Risk Category: C

HOW SUPPLIED
Tablets: 10 mg, 20 mg, 40 mg, 60 mg, 80 mg, 90 mg
Capsules (extended-release): 60 mg, 80 mg, 120 mg, 160 mg
Oral solution: 4 mg/ml, 8 mg/ml, 80 mg/ml (concentrate)

Injection: 1 mg/ml

ACTION
Reduces cardiac oxygen demand by blocking catecholamine-induced increases in heart rate, blood pressure, and force of myocardial contraction. Depresses renin secretion and prevents vasodilation of cerebral arteries.

ONSET, PEAK, DURATION
Onset occurs within 1 minute after I.V. injection, 30 minutes after oral administration. Peak plasma levels occur 60 to 90 minutes after oral administration or immediately after I.V. injection. Effects persist for about 12 hours after oral administration. Drug undetectable in the plasma 5 minutes after I.V. bolus administration.

INDICATIONS & DOSAGE
Angina pectoris—
Adults: Total daily doses of 80 to 320 mg P.O. when given b.i.d., t.i.d., or q.i.d. Or one 80-mg extended-release capsule daily. Dosage increased at 7- to 10-day intervals.
Mortality reduction after MI—
Adults: 180 to 240 mg P.O. daily in divided doses beginning 5 to 21 days after MI has occurred. Usually administered t.i.d. or q.i.d.
Supraventricular, ventricular, and atrial arrhythmias; tachyarrhythmias caused by excessive catecholamine action during anesthesia, hyperthyroidism, or pheochromocytoma—
Adults: 0.5 to 3 mg by slow I.V. push, not to exceed 1 mg/minute. After 3 mg have been given, another dose may be given in 2 minutes; subsequent doses, no sooner than q 4 hours. May be diluted and infused slowly. Usual maintenance dosage is 10 to 30 mg P.O. t.i.d. or q.i.d.
Hypertension—
Adults: initially, 80 mg P.O. daily in two to four divided doses or the extended-release form once daily. Increased at 3- to 7-day intervals to maximum daily

dosage of 640 mg. Usual maintenance dosage is 160 to 480 mg daily.
Prevention of frequent, severe, uncontrollable, or disabling migraine or vascular headache—
Adults: initially, 80 mg P.O. daily in divided doses or 1 extended-release capsule daily. Usual maintenance dosage is 160 to 240 mg daily, t.i.d. or q.i.d.
Essential tremor—
Adults: 40 mg (tablets, oral solution) P.O. b.i.d. Usual maintenance dosage is 120 to 320 mg daily in three divided doses.
Hypertrophic subaortic stenosis—
Adults: 20 to 40 mg P.O. t.i.d. or q.i.d., or 80 to 160 mg extended-release capsules once daily.
Adjunct therapy in pheochromocytoma—
Adults: 60 mg P.O. daily in divided doses with an alpha-adrenergic blocker 3 days before surgery.

ADVERSE REACTIONS
CNS: *fatigue, lethargy,* vivid dreams, hallucinations, mental depression, lightheadedness, insomnia.
CV: *bradycardia, hypotension, CHF,* intermittent claudication, intensification of AV block.
GI: nausea, vomiting, diarrhea, abdominal cramping.
Respiratory: bronchospasm.
Skin: rash.
Other: fever, *agranulocytosis.*

INTERACTIONS
Aminophylline: antagonized beta-blocking effects of propranolol. Use together cautiously.
Cimetidine: inhibits propranolol's metabolism. Monitor for increased beta-blocking effect.
Digitalis glycosides, diltiazem, verapamil: hypotension, bradycardia, and increased depressant effect on myocardium. Use together cautiously.
Epinephrine: severe vasoconstriction. Monitor blood pressure and observe the patient carefully.

Glucagon, isoproterenol: antagonized propranolol effect. May be used therapeutically and in emergencies.
Insulin, oral antidiabetic agents: can alter requirements for these drugs in previously stabilized diabetics. Monitor for hypoglycemia.

EFFECTS ON DIAGNOSTIC TESTS
Propranolol may elevate serum transaminase, alkaline phosphatase, and lactate dehydrogenase levels, and may elevate BUN levels in patients with severe heart disease.

CONTRAINDICATIONS
Contraindicated in patients with bronchial asthma, sinus bradycardia and heart block greater than first-degree, cardiogenic shock, and CHF (unless failure is secondary to a tachyarrhythmia that can be treated with propranolol).

NURSING CONSIDERATIONS
● Use cautiously in patients with renal impairment, nonallergic bronchospastic diseases, or hepatic disease and in those taking other antihypertensives. Because drug blocks some symptoms of hypoglycemia, use with caution in patients with diabetes mellitus. Also use cautiously in patients with thyrotoxicosis because drug may mask some signs of that disorder. Elderly patients may experience enhanced adverse reactions and may need dosage adjustment.
● Always check patient's apical pulse before giving drug. If you detect extremes in pulse rates, withhold drug and call the doctor immediately.
● Double-check dose and route. I.V. doses are much smaller than oral doses.
● **I.V. use:** Give by direct injection into a large vessel or into the tubing of a free-flowing, compatible I.V. solution; continuous I.V. infusion generally is not recommended. Alternatively, dilute drug with 0.9% sodium chloride and give by intermittent infusion over 10 to 15 minutes in 0.1- to 0.2-mg increments. Drug

is compatible with D_5W and 0.45% and 0.9% sodium chloride and lactated Ringer's solutions.

• Give consistently with meals. Food may increase absorption of propranolol.

• Monitor blood pressure, ECG, and heart rate and rhythm frequently, especially during I.V. administration. If the patient develops severe hypotension, notify the doctor; a vasopressor may be prescribed.

• Be aware that drug masks common signs of shock and hypoglycemia.

• *Don't discontinue drug before surgery for pheochromocytoma.* Before any surgical procedure, tell the anesthesiologist that the patient is receiving propranolol.

• For overdose, give I.V. isoproterenol, I.V. atropine, or glucagon; refractory cases may require a pacemaker.

• Compliance may be improved by administering drug twice daily or as extended-release capsule. Check with the doctor.

☑ **PATIENT TEACHING**
• Caution the patient to continue taking this drug as prescribed, even when he is feeling well.

• Instruct the patient to take drug with food.

Alert: Tell the patient not to discontinue the drug suddenly because this can exacerbate angina and precipitate MI.

---

verapamil
Apo-Verap†, Calan, Isoptin, Novo-Veramil†, Nu-Verap†

verapamil hydrochloride
Anpec‡, Calan, Calan SR, Cordilox‡,Cordilox SR‡, Isoptin, Isoptin SR, Novoveramil†, Veracaps SR‡, Verelan

Pregnancy Risk Category: C

HOW SUPPLIED
verapamil
Tablets: 40 mg, 80 mg, 120 mg

verapamil hydrochloride
Tablets: 40 mg, 80 mg, 120 mg, 160 mg‡
Tablets (extended-release): 120 mg, 180 mg, 240 mg, 360 mg
Capsules (extended-release): 120 mg, 160 mg‡, 180 mg, 240 mg
Injection: 2.5 mg/ml

ACTION
Not clearly defined. Verapamil is a calcium channel blocker that inhibits calcium ion influx across cardiac and smooth-muscle cells, thus decreasing myocardial contractility and oxygen demand; it also dilates coronary arteries and arterioles.

ONSET, PEAK, DURATION
Onset occurs within 30 minutes with oral administration, within 1 to 5 minutes with I.V. administration. Serum levels peak within 1 to 2 hours (tablets), 7 to 9 hours (extended-release capsules), 5 to 7 hours (extended-release tablets), and immediately after I.V. administration. Effects persist 1 to 6 hours with I.V. form, about 8 to 10 hours with tablets, and about 24 hours with extended-release oral forms.

INDICATIONS & DOSAGE
Vasospastic angina (also called Prinzmetal's [variant] angina) and classic chronic, stable angina pectoris; chronic atrial fibrillation—
Adults: starting dose is 80 to 120 mg P.O. t.i.d. Dosage increased at weekly intervals as needed. Some patients may require up to 480 mg daily.
Supraventricular arrhythmias—
Adults: 0.075 to 0.15 mg/kg (5 to 10 mg) by I.V. push over 2 minutes with ECG and blood pressure monitoring. Repeat dose in 30 minutes if no response occurs.
Children under 1 year: 0.1 to 0.2 mg/kg as I.V. bolus over 2 minutes with continuous ECG monitoring. Repeat dose in 30 minutes if no response occurs.

Reactions may be *common*, uncommon, *life-threatening*, or COMMON AND LIFE-THREATENING.

Children 1 to 15 years: 0.1 to 0.3 mg/kg as I.V. bolus over 2 minutes.
Hypertension—
Adults: 240 mg extended-release tablet P.O. once daily in the morning. If response is not adequate, give an additional ½ tablet in the evening or one tablet q 12 hours or an 80 mg immediate-release tablet t.i.d.

ADVERSE REACTIONS
CNS: dizziness, headache, asthenia.
CV: *transient hypotension, CHF,* pulmonary edema, bradycardia, AV block, ***ventricular asystole, ventricular fibrillation,*** peripheral edema.
GI: *constipation,* nausea.
Hepatic: elevated liver enzymes.
Skin: rash.

INTERACTIONS
Antihypertensives, quinidine: may result in hypotension. Monitor blood pressure.
Carbamazepine, digitalis glycosides: may increase serum levels of these drugs. Monitor for toxicity.
Cyclosporine: may increase cyclosporine serum levels. Monitor cyclosporine levels.
Disopyramide, flecainide, propranolol (and other beta blockers, including ophthalmic timolol): may cause heart failure. Use together cautiously.
Lithium: may decrease or increase serum lithium levels. Monitor closely.
Rifampin: may decrease oral bioavailability of verapamil. Monitor the patient for lack of effect.

EFFECTS ON DIAGNOSTIC TESTS
None reported.

CONTRAINDICATIONS
Contraindicated in patients with hypersensitivity to the drug; severe left ventricular dysfunction; cardiogenic shock; second- or third-degree AV block or sick sinus syndrome except in presence of functioning pacemaker; atrial flutter or fibrillation and accessory bypass tract syndrome; severe CHF (unless secondary to verapamil therapy); and severe hypotension. In addition, I.V. verapamil is contraindicated in patients receiving I.V. beta-adrenergic blocking agents and in those with ventricular tachycardia.

NURSING CONSIDERATIONS
● Use cautiously in elderly patients; in patients with increased intracranial pressure; and in patients with hepatic or renal disease.
● Although the drug should be taken with food, be aware that taking extended-release tablets with food may decrease rate and extent of absorption but allows smaller fluctuations of peak and trough blood levels.
● Patients with severely compromised cardiac function or those receiving beta blockers should receive lower doses of verapamil. Monitor these patients closely.
● **I.V. use:** Give by direct injection into a vein or into the tubing of a free-flowing, compatible I.V. solution. Compatible solutions include D_5W and 0.45%, 0.9% sodium chloride, Ringer's, and lactated Ringer's solutions. Administer I.V. doses over at least 3 minutes to minimize the risk of adverse reactions.
● All patients receiving I.V. verapamil should be on a cardiac monitor. Monitor the R-R interval.
● Be aware that if verapamil is being used to terminate supraventricular tachycardia, the doctor may have the patient perform vagal maneuvers after receiving drug.
● Monitor blood pressure at the start of therapy and during dosage adjustments. Assist the patient with ambulation because dizziness may occur.
● Notify the doctor if signs of CHF, such as swelling of hands and feet or shortness of breath, occur.
● Monitor liver function during prolonged treatment, as ordered.

☑ **PATIENT TEACHING**
● Instruct the patient to take oral form

---

of drug exactly as prescribed.
- Tell the patient to take drug with food.
- If the patient is kept on nitrate therapy during titration of oral verapamil dosage, urge continued compliance. Sublingual nitroglycerin, especially, may be taken as needed when anginal symptoms are acute.
- Encourage the patient to increase fluid and fiber intake to combat constipation. Administer a stool softener as ordered.

23 Antihypertensives

acebutolol
acebutolol hydrochloride
amlodipine besylate
(See Chapter 22, antianginals.)
atenolol
benazepril hydrochloride
betaxolol hydrochloride
bisoprolol fumarate
captopril
carteolol
clonidine
clonidine hydrochloride
diazoxide
diltiazem hydrochloride
(See Chapter 22, antianginals.)
doxazosin mesylate
enalaprilat
enalapril maleate
felodipine
fosinopril sodium
guanabenz acetate
guanadrel sulfate
guanethidine monosulfate
guanfacine hydrochloride
hydralazine hydrochloride
isradipine
labetalol hydrochloride
lisinopril
losartan potassium
methyldopa
methyldopate hydrochloride
metoprolol succinate
metoprolol tartrate
minoxidil
moexipril hydrochloride
nadolol
(See Chapter 22, antianginals.)
nicardipine
(See Chapter 22, antianginals.)
nifedipine
(See Chapter 22, antianginals.)
nisoldipine
nitroprusside sodium
penbutolol sulfate
phentolamine mesylate
pindolol
prazosin hydrochloride
propranolol hydrochloride
(See Chapter 22, antianginals.)
quinapril hydrochloride
ramipril
reserpine
terazosin hydrochloride
timolol maleate
trandolapril
valsartan
verapamil hydrochloride
(See Chapter 22, antianginals.)

COMBINATION PRODUCTS

ALDOCLOR-150: chlorothiazide 150 mg and methyldopa 250 mg.
ALDOCLOR-250: chlorothiazide 250 mg and methyldopa 250 mg.
ALDORIL-15: hydrochlorothiazide 15 mg and methyldopa 250 mg.
ALDORIL-25: hydrochlorothiazide 25 mg and methyldopa 250 mg.
ALDORIL D30: hydrochlorothiazide 30 mg and methyldopa 500 mg.
ALDORIL D50: hydrochlorothiazide 50 mg and methyldopa 500 mg.
APRESAZIDE 25/25: hydrochlorothiazide 25 mg and hydralazine hydrochloride 25 mg.
APRESAZIDE 50/50: hydrochlorothiazide 50 mg and hydralazine hydrochloride 50 mg.
APRESAZIDE 100/50: hydrochlorothiazide 50 mg and hydralazine hydrochloride 100 mg.
APRESODEX: hydrochlorothiazide 15 mg and hydralazine hydrochloride 25 mg.
APRESOLINE-ESIDRIX: hydrochlorothiazide 15 mg and hydralazine hydrochloride 25 mg.
CAM-AP-ES: hydrochlorothiazide 15 mg, hydralazine hydrochloride 25 mg, and reserpine 0.1 mg.
CAPOZIDE 25/15: hydrochlorothiazide 15 mg and captopril 25 mg.
CAPOZIDE 25/25: hydrochlorothiazide

*Liquid contains alcohol. **May contain tartrazine. †Canada only. ‡Australia only. ◇ OTC.

25 mg and captopril 25 mg.

CAPOZIDE 50/15: hydrochlorothiazide 15 mg and captopril 50 mg.

CAPOZIDE 50/25: hydrochlorothiazide 25 mg and captopril 50 mg.

CHERAPAS: hydrochlorothiazide 15 mg, hydralazine hydrochloride 25 mg, and reserpine 0.1 mg.

COMBIPRES 0.1: chlorthalidone 15 mg and clonidine hydrochloride 0.1 mg.

COMBIPRES 0.2: chlorthalidone 15 mg and clonidine hydrochloride 0.2 mg.

CORZIDE: nadolol 40 mg or 80 mg and bendroflumethiazide 5 mg.

DEMI-REGROTON: chlorthalidone 25 mg and reserpine 0.125 mg.

DIUPRES-250: chlorothiazide 250 mg and reserpine 0.125 mg.

DIUPRES-500: chlorothiazide 500 mg and reserpine 0.125 mg.

DIURESE-R: trichlormethiazide 4 mg and reserpine 0.1 mg.

DIURIGEN WITH RESERPINE: chlorothiazide 250 mg and reserpine 0.125 mg.

DIUTENSEN-R: methyclothiazide 2.5 mg and reserpine 0.1 mg.

ESIMIL: hydrochlorothiazide 25 mg and guanethidine monosulfate 10 mg.

EXNA-R TABLETS: benzthiazide 50 mg and reserpine 0.125 mg.

H.H.R.: hydrochlorothiazide 15 mg, hydralazine hydrochloride 25 mg, and reserpine 0.1 mg.

HYDROMOX-R: quinethazone 50 mg and reserpine 0.125 mg.

HYDROPINE: hydroflumethiazide 25 mg and reserpine 0.125 mg.

HYDROPINE HP: hydroflumethiazide 50 mg and reserpine 0.125 mg.

HYDROPRES-25: hydrochlorothiazide 25 mg and reserpine 0.125 mg.

HYDRO-RESERP: hydrochlorothiazide 25 or 50 mg and reserpine 0.125 mg.

HYDRO-SERP: hydrochlorothiazide 25 or 50 mg and reserpine 0.125 mg.

HYDROSERPINE: hydrochlorothiazide 25 or 50 mg and reserpine 0.125 mg.

HYDROTENSIN-25 Tablets: hydrochlorothiazide 25 mg and reserpine 0.125 mg.

HYZAAR: losartan 50 mg and hydrochlorothiazide 12.5 mg.

INDERIDE 40/25: propranolol hydrochloride 40 mg and hydrochlorothiazide 25 mg.

INDERIDE 80/25: propranolol hydrochloride 80 mg and hydrochlorothiazide 25 mg.

INDERIDE LA 80/50: propranolol hydrochloride 80 mg and hydrochlorothiazide 50 mg.

INDERIDE LA 120/50: propranolol hydrochloride 120 mg and hydrochlorothiazide 50 mg.

INDERIDE LA 160/50: propranolol hydrochloride 160 mg and hydrochlorothiazide 50 mg.

LOPRESSOR HCT 50/25: metoprolol tartrate 50 mg and hydrochlorothiazide 25 mg.

LOPRESSOR HCT 100/25: metoprolol tartrate 100 mg and hydrochlorothiazide 25 mg.

LOPRESSOR HCT 100/50: metoprolol tartrate 100 mg and hydrochlorothiazide 50 mg.

MAXZIDE: triamterene 75 mg and hydrochlorothiazide 50 mg.

METATENSIN TABLETS #2 or #4: trichlormethiazide 2 or 4 mg and reserpine 0.1 mg.

MINIZIDE 1: polythiazide 0.5 mg and prazosin hydrochloride 1 mg.

MINIZIDE 2: polythiazide 0.5 mg and prazosin hydrochloride 2 mg.

MINIZIDE 5: polythiazide 0.5 mg and prazosin hydrochloride 5 mg.

NAQUIVAL: trichlormethiazide 4 mg and reserpine 0.1 mg.

NORMOZIDE 100/25: labetalol hydrochloride 100 mg and hydrochlorothiazide 25 mg.

NORMOZIDE 200/25: labetalol hydrochloride 200 mg and hydrochlorothiazide 25 mg.

NORMOZIDE 300/25: labetalol hydrochloride 300 mg and hydrochlorothiazide 25 mg.

PRINZIDE 10-12.5: lisinopril 10 mg and hydrochlorothiazide 12.5 mg.

PRINZIDE 20-12.5: lisinopril 20 mg and hydrochlorothiazide 12.5 mg.

Reactions may be *common*, uncommon, *life-threatening*, or COMMON AND LIFE-THREATENING.

PRINZIDE 20-25: lisinopril 20 mg and hydrochlorothiazide 25 mg.

RAUZIDE**: bendroflumethiazide 4 mg and powdered rauwolfia serpentina 50 mg.

REGROTON: chlorthalidone 50 mg and reserpine 0.25 mg.

RENESE-R: polythiazide 2 mg and reserpine 0.25 mg.

REZIDE: hydrochlorothiazide 15 mg, hydralazine hydrochloride 25 mg, and reserpine 0.1 mg.

R-HCTZ-H: hydrochlorothiazide 15 mg, hydralazine hydrochloride 25 mg, and reserpine 0.1 mg.

SALUTENSIN: hydroflumethiazide 50 mg and reserpine 0.125 mg.

SALUTENSIN DEMI: hydroflumethiazide 25 mg and reserpine 0.125 mg.

SER-A-GEN: hydrochlorothiazide 15 mg, hydralazine hydrochloride 25 mg, and reserpine 0.1 mg.

SERALAZIDE: hydrochlorothiazide 15 mg, hydralazine hydrochloride 25 mg, and reserpine 0.1 mg.

SER-AP-ES: hydrochlorothiazide 15 mg, reserpine 0.1 mg, and hydralazine hydrochloride 25 mg.

SERPASIL-APRESOLINE #1**: reserpine 0.1 mg and hydralazine hydrochloride 25 mg.

SERPASIL-APRESOLINE #2: reserpine 0.2 mg and hydralazine hydrochloride 50 mg.

SERPASIL-ESIDRIX #1: hydrochlorothiazide 25 mg and reserpine 0.1 mg (Serpasil-Esidrix 25 in Canada).

SERPASIL ESIDRIX #2: hydrochlorothiazide 50 mg and reserpine 0.1 mg.

SERPAZIDE: hydrochlorothiazide 15 mg, hydralazine hydrochloride 25 mg, and reserpine 0.1 mg.

TENORETIC 50: atenolol 50 mg and chlorthalidone 25 mg.

TENORETIC 100: atenolol 100 mg and chlorthalidone 25 mg.

TIMOLIDE 10/25: timolol maleate 10 mg and hydrochlorothiazide 25 mg.

TRI-HYDROSERPINE: hydrochlorothiazide 15 mg, hydralazine hydrochloride 25 mg, and reserpine 0.1 mg.

UNIPRES: hydrochlorothiazide 15 mg, reserpine 0.1 mg, and hydralazine hydrochloride 25 mg.

VASERETIC: enalapril maleate 10 mg and hydrochlorothiazide 25 mg.

ZESTORETIC 20-12.5: lisinopril 20 mg and hydrochlorothiazide 12.5 mg

ZESTORETIC 20-25: lisinopril and hydrochlorothiazide 25 mg

ZIAC: bisoprolol fumarate 2.5 mg, 5 mg, or 10 mg and hydrochlorothiazide 6.5 mg.

---

acebutolol
Monitan†, Sectral

acebutolol hydrochloride

Pregnancy Risk Category: B

HOW SUPPLIED
Capsules: 200 mg, 400 mg

ACTION
Antihypertensive action is unknown. Possible mechanisms include reduced cardiac output, decreased sympathetic outflow to peripheral vasculature, and inhibition of renin release. Drug decreases myocardial contractility and decreases heart rate. Drug has mild intrinsic sympathomimetic activity.

ONSET, PEAK, DURATION
Onset occurs within 1 to 1½ hours. Plasma levels of parent drug peak by 2½ hours; 3½ hours for active metabolite. Effects persist up to 24 hours.

INDICATIONS & DOSAGE
Hypertension—
Adults: 400 mg P.O. either as a single daily dose or in divided doses b.i.d. Patients may receive as much as 1,200 mg daily.
Ventricular arrhythmias—
Adults: 400 mg P.O. daily divided b.i.d. Dosage increased to provide an adequate clinical response. Usual dosage is 600 to 1,200 mg daily. In patients with

impaired renal function, dosage is reduced. Elderly patients may require lower dosage; dosage should not exceed 800 mg daily.

ADVERSE REACTIONS
CNS: *fatigue,* headache, dizziness, insomnia, depression.
CV: chest pain, edema, bradycardia, *CHF,* hypotension.
GI: nausea, constipation, diarrhea, dyspepsia, flatulence.
Respiratory: dyspnea, *bronchospasm,* cough.
Skin: rash.
Other: arthralgia, myalgia.

INTERACTIONS
Catecholamine-depleting drugs (such as reserpine): effects may be additive. Monitor closely.
Digitalis glycosides, diltiazem, verapamil: excessive bradycardia and increased depressant effect on myocardium. Use together cautiously.
Diuretics, other antihypertensive agents: increased hypotensive effect. Use together cautiously.
Insulin, oral antidiabetic agents: can alter dosage requirements in previously stabilized diabetic patients. Observe the patient carefully.
NSAIDs: decreased antihypertensive effect. Monitor blood pressure and adjust dosage.
Sympathomimetic agents: effects antagonized by acebutolol. Greater than usual dosages of beta-adrenergic agonist bronchodilators may be required.

EFFECTS ON DIAGNOSTIC TESTS
Acebutolol may cause positive antinuclear antibody titers.

CONTRAINDICATIONS
Contraindicated in patients with persistent severe bradycardia, second- and third-degree heart block, overt cardiac failure, and cardiogenic shock.

NURSING CONSIDERATIONS
● Use cautiously in those with cardiac failure, peripheral vascular disease, bronchospastic disease, and diabetes.
● Check apical pulse before giving drug; if slower than 60 beats/minute, withhold drug and call the doctor. Also monitor blood pressure.
● Before surgery, tell the anesthesiologist that the patient is taking this drug.
● Be aware that acebutolol may mask signs of hyperthyroidism.

☑ PATIENT TEACHING
● Instruct patient to take drug exactly as prescribed.
● Warn patient not to discontinue drug suddenly, but to notify the doctor of unpleasant adverse reactions.
● Teach patient how to take his pulse and instruct him to withhold the dose and notify doctor if pulse rate is below 60 beats/minute.

atenolol
Apo-Atenolol†, Noten‡, Nu-Atenol†, Tenormin

Pregnancy Risk Category: D

HOW SUPPLIED
Tablets: 25 mg, 50 mg, 100 mg
Injection: 5 mg/10 ml

ACTION
A beta-adrenergic blocker that selectively blocks beta$_1$-adrenergic receptors; decreases cardiac output, peripheral resistance, and cardiac oxygen consumption; and depresses renin secretion.

ONSET, PEAK, DURATION
Onset occurs 5 minutes after I.V. injection, 1 hour after oral administration. Peak effects occur 2 to 4 hours after oral dose or 5 minutes after direct I.V. injection. Effects persist less than 12 hours after I.V. dose or 24 hours after oral dose.

INDICATIONS & DOSAGE
Hypertension—
Adults: initially, 50 mg P.O. daily as a single dose, increased to 100 mg once daily after 7 to 14 days. Dosages over 100 mg are unlikely to produce further benefit. Adjust dosage in patients with creatinine clearance below 35 ml/minute.
Angina pectoris—
Adults: 50 mg P.O. once daily, increased as needed to 100 mg daily after 7 days for optimal effect. Maximum dosage is 200 mg daily.
To reduce cardiovascular mortality and risk of reinfarction in patients with acute MI—
Adults: 5 mg I.V. over 5 minutes, followed by another 5 mg 10 minutes later. After an additional 10 minutes, 50 mg P.O., followed by 50 mg P.O. in 12 hours. Thereafter, 100 mg P.O. daily (as a single dose or 50 mg b.i.d.) for at least 7 days.

In patients with renal insufficiency: If creatinine clearance is 15 to 35 ml/minute, a maximum of 50 mg daily; if creatinine clearance is less than 15 ml/minute, maximum dosage is 25 mg daily. Hemodialysis patients require 25 to 50 mg after each dialysis session, but supervise closely because of the risk of hypotension.

ADVERSE REACTIONS
CNS: *fatigue,* lethargy, vertigo, drowsiness, *dizziness*.
CV: *bradycardia, hypotension, CHF,* intermittent claudication.
GI: nausea, diarrhea.
Respiratory: dyspnea, *bronchospasm*.
Skin: rash.
Other: fever, leg pain.

INTERACTIONS
Antihypertensives: enhanced hypotensive effect. Use together cautiously.
Digitalis glycosides, diltiazem, verapamil: excessive bradycardia and increased depressant effect on myocardium. Use together cautiously.

Insulin, oral antidiabetic agents: can alter dosage requirements in previously stabilized diabetic patients. Observe the patient carefully.

EFFECTS ON DIAGNOSTIC TESTS
Atenolol may increase or decrease serum glucose levels in diabetic patients; it does not potentiate insulin-induced hypoglycemia or delay recovery of serum glucose to normal levels.

Atenolol also may cause changes in exercise tolerance and ECG; it has reportedly elevated platelet count as well as serum levels of potassium, uric acid, transaminase, alkaline phosphatase, lactate dehydrogenase, creatinine, and BUN.

CONTRAINDICATIONS
Contraindicated in patients with sinus bradycardia, greater than first-degree heart block, overt cardiac failure, or cardiogenic shock.

NURSING CONSIDERATIONS
• Use cautiously in patients at risk for CHF and in patients with bronchospastic disease, diabetes, and hyperthyroidism.
• Check apical pulse before giving drug; if slower than 60 beats/minute, withhold drug and call the doctor.
• **I.V. use:** Give by slow I.V. injection, not exceeding 1 mg/minute. I.V. doses may be mixed with D_5W, 0.9% sodium chloride, or dextrose and sodium chloride solutions. Solution is stable for 48 hours after mixing.
• Monitor blood pressure.
Alert: Know that drug should be withdrawn gradually over 2 weeks to avoid serious adverse reactions.

☑ PATIENT TEACHING
• Instruct patient to take drug exactly as prescribed, at the same time every day.
• Caution patient not to stop drug suddenly, but to call the doctor if unpleasant adverse reactions occur.
• Teach patient how to take his pulse.

*Liquid contains alcohol.   **May contain tartrazine.   †Canada only.   ‡Australia only.   ◇OTC.

Tell him to withhold drug and call doctor if pulse rate is below 60 beats/minute.

• Tell female patient to notify doctor if pregnancy occurs. Drug will need to be discontinued.

---

benazepril hydrochloride
Lotensin

Pregnancy Risk Category: C (D in 2nd and 3rd trimesters)

HOW SUPPLIED
Tablets: 5 mg, 10 mg, 20 mg, 40 mg

ACTION
Benazepril and its active metabolite, benazeprilat, inhibit ACE, preventing conversion of angiotensin I to angiotensin II, a potent vasoconstrictor. Reduced formation of angiotensin II decreases peripheral arterial resistance, thus decreasing aldosterone secretion. This reduces sodium and water retention and lowers blood pressure. Benazepril also has antihypertensive activity in patients with low-renin hypertension.

ONSET, PEAK, DURATION
Onset occurs within 1 hour. Peak effects occur within 2 to 4 hours. Effects persist for 24 hours.

INDICATIONS & DOSAGE
Hypertension—
Adults: In a patient not receiving a diuretic, 10 mg P.O. daily initially. Dosage titrated as needed and tolerated; most patients take 20 to 40 mg daily in one or two doses; a patient receiving a diuretic, 5 mg P.O. daily.

ADVERSE REACTIONS
CNS: headache, dizziness, anxiety, fatigue, insomnia, nervousness, paresthesia.
CV: symptomatic hypotension, palpitations.
EENT: dysphagia, increased salivation.

GI: nausea, vomiting, abdominal pain, constipation.
Respiratory: dry, persistent, nonproductive cough; dyspnea.
Skin: hypersensitivity reactions (rash, pruritus).
Other: *angioedema,* arthralgia, arthritis, impotence, increased diaphoresis, myalgia, hyperkalemia.

INTERACTIONS
Diuretics, other antihypertensives: risk of excessive hypotension. Discontinue diuretic or lower dose of benazepril as needed.
Lithium: increased serum lithium levels and lithium toxicity. Coadminister with caution; monitor serum lithium levels.
Potassium-sparing diuretics, potassium supplements, sodium substitutes containing potassium: risk of hyperkalemia. Monitor closely.

EFFECTS ON DIAGNOSTIC TESTS
ACE inhibitors may cause agranulocytosis and bone marrow depression; however, available data are insufficient to show that benazepril does not affect the CBC in the same way. Benazepril may increase serum creatinine and BUN levels. Elevations of liver enzymes, serum bilirubin, uric acid, and blood glucose have been reported, along with scattered incidents of hyponatremia, ECG changes, leukopenia, eosinophilia, and proteinuria.

CONTRAINDICATIONS
Contraindicated in patients with hypersensitivity to ACE inhibitors.

NURSING CONSIDERATIONS
• Use cautiously in patients with impaired hepatic or renal function.
• Monitor for hypotension. Excessive hypotension can occur when drug is given with diuretics. If possible, diuretic therapy should be discontinued 2 to 3 days before starting benazepril to decrease potential for excessive hypotensive response. If benazepril does not ad-

---

Reactions may be *common,* uncommon, *life-threatening,* or COMMON AND LIFE-THREATENING.

equately control blood pressure, diuretic may be reinstituted with care.

• Measure blood pressure when drug levels are at peak (2 to 6 hours after administration) and at trough (just before a dose) to verify adequate blood pressure control.

• Assess renal and hepatic function before and periodically throughout therapy. Monitor serum potassium levels, as ordered.

• Know that other ACE inhibitors have been associated with agranulocytosis and neutropenia. Monitor CBC with differential counts before therapy and periodically thereafter.

☑ **PATIENT TEACHING**
• Tell patient to avoid sodium substitutes; these products may contain potassium, which can cause hyperkalemia in patients taking this drug.

• Light-headedness can occur, especially during the first few days of therapy. Tell patient to rise slowly to minimize this effect and to report symptoms to doctor. Patients who experience syncope should stop taking the drug and call the doctor immediately.

• Tell patient to use caution in hot weather and during exercise. Inadequate fluid intake, vomiting, diarrhea, and excessive perspiration can lead to light-headedness and syncope.

• Advise patient to report signs of infection, such as fever and sore throat. Tell him to call the doctor if the following signs or symptoms occur: easy bruising or bleeding; swelling of tongue, lips, face, eyes, mucous membranes, or extremities; difficulty swallowing or breathing; and hoarseness.

• Tell female patient to notify doctor if pregnancy occurs. Drug will need to be discontinued.

---

betaxolol hydrochloride
Kerlone

Pregnancy Risk Category: C

HOW SUPPLIED
Tablets: 10 mg, 20 mg

ACTION
Unknown. A selective beta$_1$-adrenergic blocker that decreases blood pressure, possibly by slowing heart rate and decreasing cardiac output.

ONSET, PEAK, DURATION
Onset occurs within 3 hours. Serum levels peak within 2 to 4 hours after a dose. Peak antihypertensive effects occur after 7 to 14 days of therapy. Effects persist for 24 to 48 hours.

INDICATIONS & DOSAGE
Hypertension (used alone or with other antihypertensives)—
Adults: initially, 10 mg P.O. once daily; if necessary, 20 mg P.O. once daily if desired response is not achieved in 7 to 14 days.

ADVERSE REACTIONS
CNS: dizziness, fatigue, headache, insomnia, lethargy, anxiety.
CV: bradycardia, chest pain, *CHF,* edema.
GI: nausea, diarrhea, dyspepsia.
Respiratory: dyspnea, pharyngitis, *bronchospasm.*
Skin: rash.
Other: impotence, arthralgia.

INTERACTIONS
Calcium channel blockers: increased risk of hypotension, left ventricular failure, and AV conduction disturbances. Use I.V. calcium channel blockers with caution.
Catecholamine-depleting drugs, reserpine: may have an additive effect. Monitor closely.
General anesthetics: increased hypotensive effects. Observe carefully for excessive hypotension or bradycardia or orthostatic hypotension.
Lidocaine: may increase lidocaine's effects.

EFFECTS ON DIAGNOSTIC TESTS
Oral beta blockers have been reported to decrease serum glucose levels from blockage of normal glycogen release after hypoglycemia. Oral beta blockers may alter the results of glucose tolerance tests.

CONTRAINDICATIONS
Contraindicated in patients with hypersensitivity to the drug, severe bradycardia, greater than first-degree heart block, cardiogenic shock, or uncontrolled CHF.

NURSING CONSIDERATIONS
• Use cautiously in patients with CHF controlled by digitalis glycosides and diuretics because these patients may exhibit signs of cardiac decompensation with beta-blocker therapy.
• Monitor blood pressure closely.
• Monitor blood glucose levels regularly in patients with diabetes. Beta blockade may inhibit glycogenolysis as well as the signs and symptoms of hypoglycemia (such as tachycardia and blood pressure changes).
• Know that withdrawal of beta-blocker therapy before surgery is controversial. Some clinicians advocate withdrawal to prevent any impairment of cardiac responsiveness to reflex stimuli and decreased responsiveness to administration of catecholamines. Advise the anesthesiologist that the patient is receiving a beta blocker so that isoproterenol or dobutamine is made readily available for reversal of drug's cardiac effects.
• Beta blockers may mask tachycardia associated with hyperthyroidism. In patients with suspected thyrotoxicosis, withdraw beta blocker gradually, as ordered, to avoid thyroid storm.

☑ **PATIENT TEACHING**
• Instruct patient to take drug exactly as prescribed.
Alert: Advise patient that abrupt discontinuation may precipitate angina pectoris in patients with unrecognized coronary artery disease.

• Emphasize the importance of promptly reporting signs of CHF, including shortness of breath or difficulty breathing, unusually fast heartbeat, cough, or fatigue with exertion.

---

bisoprolol fumarate
Zebeta

Pregnancy Risk Category: C

HOW SUPPLIED
Tablets: 5 mg, 10 mg

ACTION
Not completely defined. Bisoprolol is a beta₁-selective blocker that decreases myocardial contractility, heart rate, and cardiac output; lowers blood pressure; and reduces myocardial oxygen consumption.

ONSET, PEAK, DURATION
Onset unknown. Peak effects occur within 1 to 4 hours. Effects last about 24 hours.

INDICATIONS & DOSAGE
Hypertension (used alone or in combination with other antihypertensives)—
Adults: initially, 5 mg P.O. once daily. If response is inadequate, increase to 10 mg once daily or to 20 mg P.O. daily if needed. Maximum recommended dosage is 20 mg daily.
For patients with renal or hepatic impairment, 2.5 mg P.O. daily initially. Subsequent dosage titration is done cautiously.

ADVERSE REACTIONS
CNS: asthenia, fatigue, dizziness, *headache,* hypoesthesia, vivid dreams, depression, insomnia.
CV: bradycardia, peripheral edema, chest pain, *CHF.*
EENT: pharyngitis, rhinitis, sinusitis.
GI: nausea, vomiting, diarrhea, dry mouth.
Respiratory: cough, dyspnea.

Other: arthralgia.

INTERACTIONS
NSAIDs: decreased antihypertensive effect. Monitor blood pressure and adjust dosage.

EFFECTS ON DIAGNOSTIC TESTS
May produce hypoglycemia and interfere with glucose or insulin tolerance tests.

CONTRAINDICATIONS
Contraindicated in patients with hypersensitivity to the drug and in those with cardiogenic shock, overt cardiac failure, marked sinus bradycardia, or second- or third-degree AV block.

NURSING CONSIDERATIONS
• Use cautiously in patients with bronchospastic disease. In general, these patients should avoid beta-adrenergic blockers because blockade of pulmonary beta$_2$-receptors may result in worsening of symptoms. For patients who cannot tolerate or do not respond to other antihypertensives, bisoprolol is given in low doses, starting with 2.5 mg P.O. daily. Know that bisoprolol blocks beta$_2$-receptors in higher doses (20 mg daily or more).
• Also use cautiously in patients with diabetes, peripheral vascular disease, or thyroid disease and in those with a history of heart failure.
• Monitor blood pressure frequently.
• Monitor blood glucose levels in diabetic patients closely. Beta blockers may mask some manifestations of hypoglycemia, such as tachycardia. Nonselective beta blockers can potentiate insulin-induced hypoglycemia and delay recovery of serum glucose levels. Because bisoprolol is a selective agent, this problem is minimal.
• Know that drug must be withdrawn gradually over 1 to 2 weeks.

☑ PATIENT TEACHING
• Explain the importance of taking drug as prescribed, even when he's feeling well.
• Tell the patient not to stop drug suddenly but to call the doctor if unpleasant adverse reactions occur.
• Tell the patient to check with the doctor or pharmacist before taking OTC medications.

---

captopril
Apo-Capto†, Capoten, Novo-Captopril†, Syn-Captopril†

Pregnancy Risk Category: C (D in 2nd and 3rd trimesters)

HOW SUPPLIED
Tablets: 12.5 mg, 25 mg, 50 mg, 100 mg

ACTION
Not clearly defined. Thought to inhibit ACE, preventing conversion of angiotensin I to angiotensin II, a potent vasoconstrictor. Reduced formation of angiotensin II decreases peripheral arterial resistance, thus decreasing aldosterone secretion. This reduces sodium and water retention and lowers blood pressure.

ONSET, PEAK, DURATION
Onset occurs in 15 to 60 minutes; peak effects, in 60 to 90 minutes. Effects are dose-related but typically persist for 6 to 12 hours.

INDICATIONS & DOSAGE
Hypertension—
Adults: 25 mg P.O. b.i.d. or t.i.d. initially. If blood pressure isn't satisfactorily controlled in 1 to 2 weeks, dosage increased to 50 mg b.i.d. or t.i.d. If not satisfactorily controlled after another 1 to 2 weeks, expect a diuretic to be added. If further blood pressure reduction is necessary, dosage may be raised to 150 mg t.i.d. while continuing the diuretic. Maximum dosage is 450 mg daily.
CHF; to reduce risk of death and to slow

---

*Liquid contains alcohol.   **May contain tartrazine.   †Canada only.   ‡Australia only.   ◇OTC.

development of heart failure after MI—
Adults: 6.25 to 12.5 mg P.O. t.i.d. initially. Gradually increased to 50 mg t.i.d. as needed. Maximum daily dosage is 450 mg.
Diabetic nephropathy—
Adults: 25 mg P.O. t.i.d.

ADVERSE REACTIONS
CNS: dizziness, fainting, headache, malaise, fatigue.
CV: *tachycardia, hypotension,* angina pectoris.
GI: anorexia, *dysgeusia,* nausea, vomiting, abdominal pain, constipation, dry mouth.
Hematologic: *leukopenia, agranulocytosis, pancytopenia,* anemia, *thrombocytopenia.*
Hepatic: transient increase in hepatic enzymes.
Respiratory: *dry, persistent, nonproductive cough,* dyspnea.
Skin: *urticarial rash, maculopapular rash,* pruritus, alopecia.
Other: fever, *angioedema of face and extremities,* hyperkalemia.

INTERACTIONS
Antacids: decreased captopril effect. Separate administration times.
Digitalis glycosides: may increase serum digoxin concentration by 15% to 30%.
Diuretics, other antihypertensives: risk of excessive hypotension. Diuretic may need to be discontinued or captopril dosage lowered.
Insulin, oral antidiabetic agents: risk of hypoglycemia when captopril therapy is initiated. Monitor closely.
Lithium: increased lithium levels and symptoms of toxicity may occur. Monitor patient closely.
NSAIDs: may reduce antihypertensive effect. Monitor blood pressure.
Potassium supplements, potassium-sparing diuretics: increased risk of hyperkalemia. Avoid these agents unless hypokalemic blood levels are confirmed.

EFFECTS ON DIAGNOSTIC TESTS
Captopril may cause false-positive results for urinary acetone; it also may cause hyperkalemia and may transiently elevate liver enzyme levels.

CONTRAINDICATIONS
Contraindicated in patients with hypersensitivity to the drug or any other ACE inhibitor.

NURSING CONSIDERATIONS
● Use cautiously in patients with impaired renal function or serious autoimmune disease (particularly systemic lupus erythematosus) or in patients who have been exposed to other drugs known to affect WBC counts or immune response.
● Monitor the patient's blood pressure and pulse rate frequently.
Alert: Be aware that elderly patients may be more sensitive to the drug's hypotensive effects.
● In patients with impaired renal function or collagen vascular disease, monitor WBC and differential counts before starting treatment, every 2 weeks for the first 3 months of therapy, and periodically thereafter, as ordered.

☑ **PATIENT TEACHING**
● Instruct patient to take this medication 1 hour before meals; food in the GI tract may reduce absorption.
● Inform patient that light-headedness can occur, especially during the first few days of therapy. Tell patient to rise slowly to minimize this effect and to report symptoms to the doctor. If he experiences syncope, he should stop taking the drug and call the doctor immediately.
● Tell patient to use caution in hot weather and during exercise. Inadequate fluid intake, vomiting, diarrhea, and excessive perspiration can lead to light-headedness and syncope.
● Advise patient to report signs of infection, such as fever and sore throat.
● Tell female patient to notify doctor if

Reactions may be *common,* uncommon, *life-threatening,* or COMMON AND LIFE-THREATENING.

pregnancy occurs. Drug will need to be discontinued.

---

carteolol
Cartrol

Pregnancy Risk Category: C

HOW SUPPLIED
Tablets: 2.5 mg, 5 mg

ACTION
Unknown. Carteolol is a nonselective beta-adrenergic blocker with intrinsic sympathomimetic activity. Its antihypertensive effects are probably caused by decreased sympathetic outflow from the brain and decreased cardiac output. Carteolol does not have a consistent effect on renin output.

ONSET, PEAK, DURATION
Onset and duration unknown. Serum levels peak within 1 to 3 hours. Effects persist for at least 24 hours.

INDICATIONS & DOSAGE
Hypertension—
Adults: initially, 2.5 mg P.O. as a single daily dose; gradually increased to 5 or 10 mg as a single daily dose as needed. Dosages that exceed 10 mg daily do not produce a greater response and may actually decrease it.

In patients with substantial renal failure: If creatinine clearance is more than 60 ml/minute, give drug at 24-hour intervals; if 20 to 60 ml/minute, at 48-hour intervals; if less than 20 ml/minute, at 72-hour intervals.

ADVERSE REACTIONS
CNS: lassitude, fatigue, somnolence, *asthenia,* paresthesia.
CV: conduction disturbances, bradycardia.
GI: diarrhea, nausea, abdominal pain.
Other: *muscle cramps,* arthralgia, rash.

INTERACTIONS
Calcium channel blockers: increased risk of hypotension, left ventricular failure, and AV conduction disturbances. Use I.V. calcium antagonists with caution.
Catecholamine-depleting drugs, reserpine: may have an additive effect. Monitor closely.
Digitalis glycosides: may produce additive effects on slowing AV node conduction. Avoid concomitant use.
General anesthetics: increased hypotensive effects. Observe carefully for excessive hypotension or bradycardia or orthostatic hypotension.
Insulin, oral antidiabetic agents: may alter hypoglycemic response. Adjust dosage as necessary.

EFFECTS ON DIAGNOSTIC TESTS
None reported.

CONTRAINDICATIONS
Contraindicated in patients with bronchial asthma, severe bradycardia, greater than first-degree heart block, cardiogenic shock, or uncontrolled CHF.

NURSING CONSIDERATIONS
● Use cautiously in patients with CHF controlled by digitalis glycosides and diuretics because these patients may exhibit signs of cardiac decompensation with beta-blocker therapy.
● Monitor blood pressure frequently.
● Know that beta blockade may inhibit glycogenolysis and the signs and symptoms of hypoglycemia (such as tachycardia and blood pressure changes). It may also attenuate insulin release. Monitor blood glucose levels frequently.
● Know that withdrawal of beta-blocker therapy before surgery is controversial. Some clinicians advocate withdrawal to prevent any impairment of cardiac responsiveness to reflex stimuli and decreased responsiveness to administration of catecholamines. However, the beta-blocking effects of carteolol may

---

persist for weeks, and discontinuing drug before surgery may be impractical. Advise the anesthesiologist that the patient is receiving a beta blocker so that isoproterenol or dobutamine is made readily available for reversal of the drug's cardiac effects.

• Beta blockers may mask tachycardia associated with hyperthyroidism. In patients with suspected thyrotoxicosis, gradually withdraw beta blocker therapy, as ordered, to avoid thyroid storm. *Alert:* Be aware that patients with unrecognized coronary artery disease may exhibit signs of angina pectoris on withdrawal of drug. Monitor closely.

☑ **PATIENT TEACHING**
• Instruct patient to take drug exactly as prescribed.
• Tell patient not to stop drug suddenly but to call doctor and discuss unpleasant adverse reactions.
• Emphasize the importance of reporting signs of CHF, including shortness of breath or difficulty breathing, unusually fast heartbeat, cough, or fatigue with exertion.

---

clonidine
Catapres-TTS

clonidine hydrochloride
Catapres, Dixarit††‡

Pregnancy Risk Category: C

HOW SUPPLIED
clonidine
Transdermal: TTS-1 (releases 0.1 mg/24 hours), TTS-2 (releases 0.2 mg/24 hours), TTS-3 (releases 0.3 mg/24 hours)
clonidine hydrochloride
Tablets: 0.025 mg††‡, 0.1 mg, 0.2 mg, 0.3 mg

ACTION
Unknown. Thought to stimulate alpha$_2$-adrenergic receptors centrally and inhib-

it the central vasomotor centers, thereby decreasing sympathetic outflow to the heart, kidneys, and peripheral vasculature; this results in decreased peripheral vascular resistance, decreased systolic and diastolic blood pressure, and decreased heart rate.

ONSET, PEAK, DURATION
Onset occurs within 30 to 60 minutes after oral administration, 2 to 3 days after transdermal application. Peak effects occur within 2 to 4 hours after oral dose, about 2 to 3 days after transdermal application. Effects persist for 12 to 24 hours after an oral dose and decline over several days after transdermal system removal.

INDICATIONS & DOSAGE
Essential and renal hypertension—
Adults: initially, 0.1 mg P.O. b.i.d. Then increased by 0.1 to 0.2 mg daily on a weekly basis. Usual dosage range is 0.2 to 0.8 mg daily in divided doses; infrequently, dosages as high as 2.4 mg daily are used.

Or, a transdermal patch is applied to a nonhairy area of intact skin on the upper arm or torso once every 7 days, starting with 0.1-mg system and titrated with another 0.1-mg system or larger system.

ADVERSE REACTIONS
CNS: *drowsiness, dizziness,* fatigue, *sedation, weakness,* malaise, agitation, depression.
CV: orthostatic hypotension, bradycardia, ***severe rebound hypertension.***
GI: *constipation, dry mouth,* nausea, vomiting, anorexia.
GU: urine retention, impotence, loss of libido.
Skin: *pruritus, dermatitis* (with transdermal patch), rash.
Other: weight gain.

INTERACTIONS
CNS depressants: enhanced CNS depression. Use together cautiously.

Reactions may be *common,* uncommon, *life-threatening,* or COMMON AND LIFE-THREATENING.

Diuretics, other antihypertensive agents: increased hypotensive effect. Monitor closely.
MAO inhibitors, tricyclic antidepressants: may decrease antihypertensive effect. Use together cautiously.
Propranolol, other beta blockers: paradoxical hypertensive response. Monitor carefully.

EFFECTS ON DIAGNOSTIC TESTS
Clonidine may decrease urinary excretion of vanillylmandelic acid and catecholamines; it may slightly increase blood or serum glucose levels and may cause a weakly positive Coombs' test.

CONTRAINDICATIONS
Contraindicated in patients with hypersensitivity to the drug. Transdermal form is contraindicated in patients with hypersensitivity to any component of the adhesive layer of the transdermal system.

NURSING CONSIDERATIONS
● Use cautiously in patients with severe coronary insufficiency, recent MI, cerebrovascular disease, chronic renal failure, or impaired liver function.
● Know that clonidine may be given to rapidly lower blood pressure in some hypertensive emergencies.
● Monitor blood pressure and pulse rate frequently. Dosage is usually adjusted to patient's blood pressure and tolerance.
● Elderly patients may be more sensitive to drug's hypotensive effects.
● Observe for patient tolerance to drug's therapeutic effects, which may require increased dosage.
● Antihypertensive effects of transdermal clonidine may take 2 to 3 days to become apparent. Oral antihypertensive therapy may have to be continued in the interim.
Alert: Remove transdermal patch before defibrillation to prevent arcing.
● When stopping therapy in patients receiving both clonidine and a beta blocker, gradually withdraw the beta blocker

first to minimize adverse reactions, as ordered.
● Be aware that discontinuation for surgery is not recommended.

☑ **PATIENT TEACHING**
● Instruct the patient to take drug exactly as prescribed.
● Advise the patient that abrupt discontinuation of drug may cause severe rebound hypertension. Tell him dosage must be reduced gradually over 2 to 4 days as instructed by doctor.
● Tell the patient to take the last dose immediately before retiring.
● Reassure the patient that the transdermal patch usually adheres despite showering and other routine daily activities. Instruct him on the use of the adhesive "overlay" to provide additional skin adherence if necessary. Also tell the patient to place the patch at a different site each week.
● Caution the patient that drug may cause drowsiness but that this adverse effect will usually diminish over 4 to 6 weeks.
● Inform the patient that orthostatic hypotension can be minimized by rising slowly and avoiding sudden position changes.

diazoxide
Hyperstat IV

Pregnancy Risk Category: C

HOW SUPPLIED
Injection: 300 mg/20 ml, 15 mg/ml

ACTION
Exact antihypertensive action unknown. Directly relaxes arteriolar smooth muscle and decreases peripheral vascular resistance.

ONSET, PEAK, DURATION
Onset occurs within 1 minute after I.V. bolus. Peak effects occur within 2 to 5 minutes after I.V. bolus. Effects persist

2 to 12 hours.

INDICATIONS & DOSAGE

Hypertensive crisis—

Adults and children: 1 to 3 mg/kg by
I.V. bolus (up to a maximum of 150 mg)
q 5 to 15 minutes until adequate response is seen. Repeat at 4- to 24-hour
intervals as needed.

ADVERSE REACTIONS

CNS: *headache,* dizziness, light-headedness, weakness, ***seizures, paralysis,***
euphoria, ***cerebral ischemia.***
CV: *sodium and water retention,* orthostatic hypotension, diaphoresis, flushing, warmth, angina, myocardial ischemia, ***arrhythmias,*** ECG changes,
shock, MI.
GI: *nausea, vomiting,* abdominal discomfort, dry mouth, constipation, diarrhea.
Other: inflammation and pain resulting
from extravasation, *hyperglycemia,* hyperuricemia, optic nerve infarction.

INTERACTIONS

Antihypertensives, such as hydralazine:
may cause severe hypotension. Use together cautiously.
Thiazide diuretics: may increase diazoxide's effects. Use together cautiously.

EFFECTS ON DIAGNOSTIC TESTS

Diazoxide inhibits glucose-stimulated
insulin release and may cause false-negative insulin response to glucagon. Prolonged use of oral diazoxide may decrease hemoglobin and hematocrit levels.

CONTRAINDICATIONS

Contraindicated in patients with hypersensitivity to the drug, other thiazides,
or other sulfonamide-derived drugs.
Also contraindicated in the treatment of
compensatory hypertension (such as
that associated with coarctation of the
aorta or arteriovenous shunt).

NURSING CONSIDERATIONS

● Use cautiously in patients with impaired cerebral or cardiac function or
uremia.
● **I.V. use:** Monitor blood pressure and
ECG continuously. Place the patient in
the supine position or in Trendelen-
burg's position during and for 1 hour after infusion. Notify the doctor immediately if severe hypotension develops.
Keep norepinephrine available.
● Protect I.V. solutions from light.
Darkened I.V. solutions of diazoxide are
subpotent and should not be used.
● Take care to avoid extravasation.
● Check the patient's standing blood
pressure before discontinuing close
monitoring for hypotension.
● Monitor the patient's fluid intake and
output carefully. If fluid or sodium retention develops, the doctor may order
diuretics.
● Weigh the patient daily and notify the
doctor of any weight increase.
● Diazoxide may alter requirements for
insulin, diet, or oral antidiabetic agents
in previously controlled diabetic patients. Monitor blood glucose daily;
watch for signs of severe hyperglycemia
or hyperosmolar nonketotic syndrome.
Insulin may be needed.
● Check uric acid levels frequently and
report abnormalities to the doctor.

☑ **PATIENT TEACHING**
● Inform the patient that orthostatic hypotension can be minimized by rising
slowly and avoiding sudden position
changes. Instruct the patient to remain
in the supine position for 60 minutes after injection.
● Tell the patient to alert nurse if discomfort occurs at I.V. insertion site.

doxazosin mesylate
Cardura

Pregnancy Risk Category: C

HOW SUPPLIED
Tablets: 1 mg, 2 mg, 4 mg, 8 mg

ACTION
An alpha$_1$-adrenergic blocker that acts on the peripheral vasculature to reduce peripheral vascular resistance and produce vasodilation.

ONSET, PEAK, DURATION
Onset occurs in 1 to 2 hours. Peak antihypertensive effect occurs in 2 to 6 hours. Effects persist about 24 hours.

INDICATIONS & DOSAGE
Essential hypertension—
Adults: initially, 1 mg P.O. daily and determine effect on standing and supine blood pressure at 2 to 6 hours and 24 hours after dosing. If necessary, dose is increased to 2 mg daily. To minimize adverse reactions, dosage is titrated slowly (dosage typically increased only q 2 weeks). If necessary, dose increased to 4 mg daily, then 8 mg. Maximum daily dosage is 16 mg, but dosage that exceeds 4 mg daily is associated with a greater incidence of adverse reactions.
Benign prostatic hyperplasia—
Adults: initially, 1 mg P.O. once daily in the morning or evening; may be increased to 2 mg and, thereafter, 4 mg and 8 mg once daily, as needed. The recommended titration interval is 1 to 2 weeks.

ADVERSE REACTIONS
CNS: *dizziness,* vertigo, somnolence, drowsiness, *asthenia, headache.*
CV: *orthostatic hypotension,* hypotension, edema, palpitations, ***arrhythmias,*** tachycardia.
GI: nausea, vomiting, diarrhea, constipation.
Skin: rash, pruritus.
Other: rhinitis, arthralgia, myalgia, pain, dyspnea, pharyngitis, abnormal vision.

INTERACTIONS
None significant.

EFFECTS ON DIAGNOSTIC TESTS
Mean WBC and neutrophil counts may be decreased.

CONTRAINDICATIONS
Contraindicated in patients with hypersensitivity to the drug and quinazoline derivatives (including prazosin and terazosin).

NURSING CONSIDERATIONS
● Use cautiously in patients with impaired hepatic function.
● Monitor blood pressure closely.
● If syncope occurs, place the patient in a recumbent position and treat supportively. A transient hypotensive response is not considered a contraindication to continued therapy.

☑ **PATIENT TEACHING**
● Instruct patient to take drug exactly as prescribed.
Alert: Advise patient that he is susceptible to a "first-dose" effect similar to that produced by other alpha-adrenergic blockers—marked orthostatic hypotension accompanied by dizziness or syncope. Orthostatic hypotension is most common after first dose but also can occur during dosage adjustment or interruption of therapy. Warn patient that dizziness or fainting may occur. Advise him to avoid driving and other hazardous activities until drug's CNS effects are known.

---

enalaprilat
Vasotec I.V.

enalapril maleate
Amprace‡, Renitec‡, Vasotec

Pregnancy Risk Category: C (D in 2nd and 3rd trimesters)

HOW SUPPLIED
enalaprilat
Injection: 1.25 mg/ml
enalapril maleate

Tablets: 2.5 mg, 5 mg, 10 mg, 20 mg

ACTION

Unknown, but does inhibit ACE, preventing conversion of angiotensin I to angiotensin II, a potent vasoconstrictor. Reduced formation of angiotensin II decreases peripheral arterial resistance, thus decreasing aldosterone secretion.

ONSET, PEAK, DURATION

Onset occurs 15 minutes after I.V. injection, 1 hour after oral dose. Peak effects occur 1 to 4 hours after I.V. injection or 4 to 6 hours after oral dose. Effects persist about 6 hours after I.V. injection or 24 hours after oral dose.

INDICATIONS & DOSAGE

Hypertension—
Adults: for patient not receiving diuretics, initially 5 mg P.O. once daily, then adjusted according to response. Usual dosage range is 10 to 40 mg daily as a single dose or two divided doses. Alternatively, 1.25 mg I.V. infusion q 6 hours over 5 minutes. For patient on diuretics, initially 2.5 mg P.O. once daily. Alternatively, 0.625 mg I.V. over 5 minutes, repeated in 1 hour if needed, then followed by 1.25 mg I.V. q 6 hours.
To convert from I.V. therapy to oral therapy—
Adults: initially, 5 mg P.O. once daily; if patient was receiving 0.625 mg I.V. q 6 hours, then 2.5 mg P.O. once daily. Dosage is adjusted to response.
To convert from oral therapy to I.V. therapy—
Adults: 1.25 mg I.V. over 5 minutes q 6 hours. Higher doses have not demonstrated greater efficacy.
Renal impairment or hyponatremia—
If serum creatinine is above 1.6 mg/dl or serum sodium is below 130 mEq/L, dosage is initiated at 2.5 mg P.O. daily and titrated slowly.

ADVERSE REACTIONS

CNS: *headache, dizziness, fatigue,* vertigo, asthenia, syncope.
CV: *hypotension,* chest pain.
GI: diarrhea, nausea, abdominal pain, vomiting.
GU: decreased renal function (in patients with bilateral renal artery stenosis or CHF).
Hematologic: *neutropenia, thrombocytopenia, agranulocytosis.*
Respiratory: *dry, persistent, tickling, nonproductive cough,* dyspnea.
Skin: rash.
Other: *angioedema.*

INTERACTIONS

Insulin, oral antidiabetic agents: risk of hypoglycemia, especially at initiation of enalapril therapy. Monitor closely.
Lithium: lithium toxicity can occur. Monitor lithium levels.
NSAIDs: may reduce antihypertensive effect. Monitor blood pressure.
Potassium supplements, potassium-sparing diuretics: increased risk of hyperkalemia. Avoid these drugs unless hypokalemic blood levels are confirmed.
Diuretics: excessive reduction of blood pressure.

EFFECTS ON DIAGNOSTIC TESTS

Enalapril may elevate BUN and serum creatinine levels and, less commonly, liver enzyme and bilirubin levels; it may slightly decrease hemoglobin and hematocrit levels. Rare cases of neutropenia, thrombocytopenia, and bone marrow depression have been reported.

CONTRAINDICATIONS

Contraindicated in patients with hypersensitivity to the drug or history of angioedema related to previous treatment with an ACE inhibitor.

NURSING CONSIDERATIONS

● Use cautiously in patients with renal impairment.
● **I.V. use:** Inject drug slowly over at least 5 minutes, or dilute in 50 ml of a compatible solution and infuse over 15 minutes. Compatible solutions include

D_5W, 0.9% sodium chloride injection, dextrose 5% in lactated Ringer's injection, and dextrose 5% in 0.9% sodium chloride injection.
• Monitor blood pressure response to drug closely.
• Monitor CBC with differential counts before and during therapy.
• Diabetic patients, those with impaired renal function or CHF, and those receiving drugs that can increase serum potassium may develop hyperkalemia. Monitor potassium intake and serum potassium level.

☑ **PATIENT TEACHING**
• Advise the patient to report breathing difficulty or swelling of face, eyes, lips, or tongue. Angioedema (including laryngeal edema) may occur, especially after the first dose.
• Advise him to report signs of infection, such as fever and sore throat.
• Advise the patient that light-headedness can occur, especially during the first few days of therapy. Tell the patient to rise slowly to minimize this effect and to report symptoms to the doctor. Patients who experience syncope should stop taking drug and call the doctor immediately.
• Tell the patient to use caution in hot weather and during exercise. Inadequate fluid intake, vomiting, diarrhea, and excessive perspiration can lead to light-headedness and syncope.
• Advise him to avoid salt substitutes; these products may contain potassium, which can cause hyperkalemia in patients taking this drug.
• Tell the female patient to notify doctor if pregnancy occurs. Drug will need to be discontinued.

felodipine
Agon‡, Agon SR‡, Plendil, Plendil ER‡, Renedil†

Pregnancy Risk Category: C

HOW SUPPLIED
Tablets: 5 mg‡
Tablets (extended-release): 2.5 mg, 5 mg, 10 mg

ACTION
Unknown. A dihydropyridine-derivative calcium channel blocker that prevents the entry of calcium ions into vascular smooth-muscle and cardiac cells; shows some selectivity for smooth muscle as compared with cardiac muscle.

ONSET, PEAK, DURATION
Onset occurs within 2 to 5 hours. Plasma levels peak within 2½ to 5 hours. Effects persist for 24 hours.

INDICATIONS & DOSAGE
Hypertension—
Adults: initially, 5 mg P.O. daily. Dosage is adjusted according to patient response, generally at intervals not less than 2 weeks. Usual dose is 5 to 10 mg daily; maximum recommended dosage is 20 mg daily.
   In elderly patients and patients with impaired hepatic function, 5 mg P.O. is given daily; dosage is adjusted as for adults. Maximum recommended dosage is 10 mg daily.

ADVERSE REACTIONS
CNS: *headache,* dizziness, paresthesia, asthenia.
CV: *peripheral edema,* chest pain, palpitations.
EENT: rhinorrhea, pharyngitis.
GI: abdominal pain, nausea, constipation, diarrhea.
Respiratory: upper respiratory infection, cough.
Skin: rash, *flushing.*
Other: muscle cramps, back pain, gingival hyperplasia.

INTERACTIONS
Anticonvulsants: decreased plasma concentration of felodipine. Avoid concomitant use.
Cimetidine: decreased clearance of

felodipine. Use lower doses of felodipine.

Metoprolol: may alter pharmacokinetics of metoprolol. No dosage adjustment appears necessary; monitor for adverse effects.

Theophylline: may slightly decrease theophylline levels. Monitor patient's response closely.

Grapefruit juice: increased bioavailability and effect when taken together.

EFFECTS ON DIAGNOSTIC TESTS
None reported.

CONTRAINDICATIONS
Contraindicated in patients with hypersensitivity to the drug.

NURSING CONSIDERATIONS
• Use cautiously in patients with heart failure, particularly those receiving beta-adrenergic blockers, and in patients with impaired hepatic function.
• Monitor blood pressure for response.
• Monitor patient for peripheral edema. Peripheral edema appears to be both dose- and age-dependent: it's more common in patients taking higher doses, especially those over age 60.

☑ **PATIENT TEACHING**
• Tell the patient to swallow tablets whole and not to crush or chew them.
• Teach the patient to continue taking the drug even when he feels better; to watch his diet; and to check with the doctor or pharmacist before taking any other medications, including OTC drugs.
• Advise the patient to observe good oral hygiene and to see a dentist regularly; use of drug has been associated with mild gingival hyperplasia.

fosinopril sodium
Monopril

Pregnancy Risk Category: C (D in 2nd and 3rd trimesters)

HOW SUPPLIED
Tablets: 10 mg, 20 mg

ACTION
Antihypertensive action not clearly defined. Inhibits ACE, preventing conversion of angiotensin I to angiotensin II, a potent vasoconstrictor. Reduced formation of angiotensin II decreases peripheral arterial resistance, thus decreasing aldosterone secretion.

ONSET, PEAK, DURATION
Onset occurs within 1 hour. Serum levels peak in approximately 3 hours. Effects peak at 2 to 6 hours and persist about 24 hours.

INDICATIONS & DOSAGE
Hypertension—
Adults: initially, 10 mg P.O. daily. Dosage is adjusted based on blood pressure response at peak and trough levels. Usual dosage is 20 to 40 mg, up to 80 mg daily. Dosage is divided if needed.
Heart failure—
Adults: initially, 10 mg P.O. once daily. Dosage increased over several weeks to a maximum dosage of 40 mg P.O. daily, if needed. For patients with moderate to severe renal failure or vigorous diuresis, initially, 5 mg P.O. once daily.

ADVERSE REACTIONS
CNS: headache, dizziness, fatigue, syncope, paresthesia, sleep disturbance, *CVA.*
CV: chest pain, angina, *MI,* rhythm disturbances, palpitations, hypotension, orthostatic hypotension.
EENT: tinnitus, sinusitis.
GI: nausea, vomiting, diarrhea, pancreatitis, hepatitis, dry mouth, abdominal distention, abdominal pain, constipation.
GU: sexual dysfunction, decreased libido, renal insufficiency.
Respiratory: *dry, persistent, tickling,*

nonproductive cough; **bronchospasm.**
Skin: urticaria, rash, photosensitivity, pruritus.
Other: *angioedema,* arthralgia, musculoskeletal pain, myalgia, gout, hyperkalemia.

INTERACTIONS
Antacids: may impair absorption. Separate administration times by at least 2 hours.
Diuretics, other antihypertensives: risk of excessive hypotension. Diuretic may need to be discontinued or fosinopril dosage lowered.
Lithium: increased serum lithium levels and lithium toxicity. Monitor serum lithium levels.
Potassium-sparing diuretics, potassium supplements, salt substitutes containing potassium: risk of hyperkalemia. Monitor closely during concomitant use.

EFFECTS ON DIAGNOSTIC TESTS
False low measurements of digoxin levels may result with the DIGI TAB radioimmunoassay kit for digoxin; other kits may be used. Transient elevations of BUN and serum creatinine levels and liver function tests and decreases in hematocrit or hemoglobin may also occur.

CONTRAINDICATIONS
Contraindicated in patients with hypersensitivity to this drug or other ACE inhibitors and in breast-feeding patients.

NURSING CONSIDERATIONS
● Use cautiously in patients with impaired renal or hepatic function.
● Monitor blood pressure for effect.
● Monitor potassium intake and serum potassium level. Diabetic patients, those with impaired renal function, and those receiving drugs that can increase serum potassium may develop hyperkalemia.
● Other ACE inhibitors have been associated with agranulocytosis and neutropenia. Monitor CBC with differential counts, as ordered, before therapy and periodically thereafter.

● Assess renal and hepatic function before and periodically throughout therapy.

✓ PATIENT TEACHING
● Tell the patient to avoid salt substitutes; these products may contain potassium, which can cause hyperkalemia in patients taking this drug.
● Advise the patient to report any signs of infection, such as fever and sore throat.
● Also tell the patient to call the doctor if any of the following signs or symptoms occur: easy bruising or bleeding; swelling of tongue, lips, face, eyes, mucous membranes, or extremities; difficulty swallowing or breathing; and hoarseness.
● Tell the patient to use caution in hot weather and during exercise. Inadequate fluid intake, vomiting, diarrhea, and excessive perspiration can lead to lightheadedness and syncope.
● Tell the female patient to notify doctor if pregnancy occurs. Drug will need to be discontinued.

---

guanabenz acetate
Wytensin

Pregnancy Risk Category: C

HOW SUPPLIED
Tablets: 4 mg, 8 mg

ACTION
Unknown. A centrally acting antihypertensive, its action is thought to be due to central alpha-adrenergic stimulation, which results in decreased sympathetic outflow to the heart, kidneys, and peripheral vasculature.

ONSET, PEAK, DURATION
Onset occurs within 1 hour. Peak effects occur within 2 to 5 hours. Effects for persist about 12 hours.

INDICATIONS & DOSAGE
Hypertension—
Adults: initially, 4 mg P.O. b.i.d. Dosage increased in increments of 4 to 8 mg/day q 1 to 2 weeks. Maximum daily dosage is 32 mg b.i.d. To ensure adequate overnight blood pressure control, give last dose h.s.

ADVERSE REACTIONS
CNS: *drowsiness, sedation, dizziness, weakness,* headache.
CV: *rebound hypertension.*
GI: *dry mouth.*

INTERACTIONS
CNS depressants: may cause increased sedation. Use together cautiously.
Diuretics, other antihypertensive agents: increased risk of excessive hypotension.
Tricyclic antidepressants, MAO inhibitors: may decrease antihypertensive effect.

EFFECTS ON DIAGNOSTIC TESTS
Guanabenz may reduce serum cholesterol and total triglyceride levels slightly, but it does not alter high-density lipoprotein fraction; drug may cause nonprogressive elevations in liver enzyme levels.

Chronic use of guanabenz decreases plasma norepinephrine, dopamine, beta-hydroxylase, and plasma renin activity.

CONTRAINDICATIONS
Contraindicated in patients with hypersensitivity to the drug.

NURSING CONSIDERATIONS
• Use cautiously in patients with severe coronary insufficiency, recent MI, cerebrovascular disease, or severe hepatic or renal failure. Also use cautiously in elderly patients.
• Monitor blood pressure for effects. Elderly patients may be more sensitive to drug's hypotensive effects.

☑ **PATIENT TEACHING**
• Caution the patient that abrupt discontinuation of drug may cause rebound hypertension.
• Advise him to avoid hazardous tasks that require alertness until drug's CNS effects are known.
• Inform the patient that orthostatic hypotension can be minimized by rising slowly and avoiding sudden position changes. Dry mouth can be relieved with chewing gum, sour hard candy, or ice chips.
• Warn the patient that tolerance to alcohol or other CNS depressants may be diminished.

---

guanadrel sulfate
Hylorel

Pregnancy Risk Category: B

HOW SUPPLIED
Tablets: 10 mg, 25 mg

ACTION
Acts peripherally, inhibiting norepinephrine release and depleting norepinephrine stores in adrenergic nerve endings.

ONSET, PEAK, DURATION
Onset occurs in 2 hours. Peak effects occur within 4 to 6 hours. Effects persist for 4 to 14 hours.

INDICATIONS & DOSAGE
Hypertension—
Adults: initially, 5 mg P.O. b.i.d. Dosage adjusted until blood pressure is controlled. Most patients require dosages of 20 to 75 mg/day, usually given b.i.d.; however, tolerance to hypotensive effect may necessitate upward titration to 100 to 400 mg daily in three to four divided doses.

In patients with renal impairment, dosage is reduced to 5 mg P.O. once daily if creatinine clearance is 30 to 60 ml/minute; if creatinine clearance is less than 30 ml/minute, increase dosage interval to 48 hours. Dosage is adjusted every 7 to 14 days.

ADVERSE REACTIONS
CNS: *fatigue, drowsiness, faintness, headache, confusion, paresthesia.*
CV: *palpitations, chest pain, peripheral edema, orthostatic hypotension.*
GI: *diarrhea,* dry mouth, *indigestion, constipation, anorexia,* nausea, vomiting, abdominal pain.
GU: impotence, *ejaculation disturbances, nocturia, urination frequency.*
Respiratory: *shortness of breath, cough.*
Other: *weight gain, aching limbs, leg cramps, visual disturbances,* glossitis.

INTERACTIONS
Amphetamines, ephedrine, methylphenidate, norepinephrine, phenothiazines, tricyclic antidepressants: may inhibit guanadrel's antihypertensive effect. Adjust dose accordingly.
Diuretics, other antihypertensives: hypotensive effect of guanadrel increased. Monitor blood pressure closely.
MAO inhibitors: antagonized hypotensive effects of guanadrel. Don't give guanadrel concurrently or within 1 week of MAO inhibitor therapy.

EFFECTS ON DIAGNOSTIC TESTS
None reported.

CONTRAINDICATIONS
Contraindicated in patients with hypersensitivity to the drug, known or suspected pheochromocytoma, and frank CHF. Avoid concurrent use with or within 1 week of MAO inhibitor therapy.

NURSING CONSIDERATIONS
● Use cautiously in patients with regional vascular disease, bronchial asthma, or history of peptic ulcer disease.
● Monitor both supine and standing blood pressure, especially during dosage adjustment periods.

● Be aware that elderly patients may be more sensitive to drug's hypotensive effects.
● Know that guanadrel should be discontinued 48 to 72 hours before surgery to minimize risk of vascular collapse during anesthesia.

☑ **PATIENT TEACHING**
● Inform the patient that orthostatic hypotension can be minimized by rising slowly from a supine position and by avoiding sudden position changes. Dry mouth can be relieved with chewing gum, sour hard candy, or ice chips.
● Warn the patient to avoid strenuous exercise and hot showers; these may cause a hypotensive reaction. An ambient temperature that is too hot also may potentiate the hypotensive effects of guanadrel as can alcohol ingestion.

guanethidine monosulfate
Apo-Guanethidine†, Ismelin

Pregnancy Risk Category: C

HOW SUPPLIED
Tablets: 10 mg, 25 mg

ACTION
An adrenergic neuron blocker that acts peripherally, inhibiting norepinephrine release and depleting norepinephrine stores in adrenergic nerve endings. This reduces arteriolar vasoconstriction.

ONSET, PEAK, DURATION
Onset unknown. Serum levels peak within 8 hours after single dose. Effects persist for 3 to 4 days; blood pressure returns to pretreatment levels in 1 to 3 weeks.

INDICATIONS & DOSAGE
Moderate to severe hypertension and renal hypertension—
Adults: initially, 10 mg P.O. daily. Increase by 10 mg at weekly to monthly intervals, p.r.n. Usual dosage is 25 to 50

mg daily. Some patients may require up to 300 mg daily.

ADVERSE REACTIONS

CNS: *syncope, fatigue, headache, drowsiness, paresthesia, confusion.*
CV: *palpitations, chest pain, orthostatic hypotension, peripheral edema, bradycardia,* CHF.
EENT: *visual disturbances,* glossitis.
GI: *diarrhea, indigestion, constipation, anorexia,* nausea, vomiting.
GU: *nocturia, urination frequency, ejaculation disturbances,* impotence.
Respiratory: shortness of breath, cough.
Other: *weight gain, aching limbs, leg cramps.*

INTERACTIONS

Amphetamines, ephedrine, MAO inhibitors, methylphenidate, norepinephrine, phenothiazines, tricyclic antidepressants: may inhibit guanethidine's antihypertensive effect. Adjust dose accordingly. Discontinue MAO inhibitor therapy 1 week before starting guanethidine.
Ethanol, levodopa: may increase hypotensive effect of guanethidine. Use together cautiously.
Digoxin: may note increased slowing of heart rate.

EFFECTS ON DIAGNOSTIC TESTS

None reported.

CONTRAINDICATIONS

Contraindicated in patients with pheochromocytoma, frank CHF, or hypersensitivity to drug and in those receiving MAO inhibitor therapy.

NURSING CONSIDERATIONS

● Use cautiously in patients with severe cardiac disease, recent MI, cerebrovascular disease, peptic ulceration, impaired renal function, or bronchial asthma and in those taking other antihypertensives.
● Monitor blood pressure for effects, especially after dosage adjustments.
● Elderly patients may be more sensitive to drug's hypotensive effects.
● Know that drug should be discontinued 2 to 3 weeks before elective surgery to reduce the possibility of vascular collapse and cardiac arrest during anesthesia.
● Know that if the patient develops diarrhea, the doctor may prescribe atropine or paregoric.

☑ **PATIENT TEACHING**
● Inform the patient that orthostatic hypotension can be minimized by rising slowly and avoiding sudden position changes. Dry mouth can be relieved with chewing gum, sour hard candy, or ice chips.
● Patients should receive instruction on a low-salt diet. Monitor for possible weight gain and edema.
● Warn the patient to avoid strenuous exercise and hot showers; these may cause a hypotensive reaction. An ambient temperature that is too hot also may potentiate the hypotensive effects of guanethidine.

guanfacine hydrochloride
Tenex

Pregnancy Risk Category: B

HOW SUPPLIED
Tablets: 1 mg, 2 mg

ACTION
Unknown. Thought to be due to inhibition of the central vasomotor center, thereby decreasing sympathetic outflow to the heart, kidneys, and peripheral vasculature. This decreases blood pressure.

ONSET, PEAK, DURATION
Onset unknown. Serum levels peak in 1 to 4 hours. Effects persist for 24 hours.

INDICATIONS & DOSAGE

Hypertension—
Adults: initially, 1 mg P.O. daily h.s.
Dosage may be increased to 2 mg P.O.
h.s. after 3 to 4 weeks, as needed.
Dosage may be further increased to 3
mg P.O. h.s. after an additional 3 to 4
weeks, as needed. Average dosage is 1
to 3 mg daily.

ADVERSE REACTIONS

CNS: *dizziness,* fatigue, headache, insomnia, *somnolence,* asthenia.
CV: bradycardia.
GI: *constipation,* diarrhea, nausea, *dry mouth.*
Skin: dermatitis, pruritus.

INTERACTIONS

CNS depressants: may potentially increase sedation.

EFFECTS ON DIAGNOSTIC TESTS

Drug alters urinary catecholamine concentrations and urinary vanillylmandelic acid (VMA) excretion (may be decreased during therapy but may increase on abrupt withdrawal). Plasma growth hormone levels may be increased after a single dose; chronic elevation does not follow long-term use.

CONTRAINDICATIONS

Contraindicated in patients with hypersensitivity to the drug.

NURSING CONSIDERATIONS

● Use cautiously in patients with severe coronary insufficiency, recent MI, cerebrovascular disease, or chronic renal or hepatic insufficiency.
● Monitor blood pressure frequently.
● Be aware that the incidence and severity of adverse reactions increase with higher dosages.
● Know that guanfacine may be used alone or with a diuretic.

☑ **PATIENT TEACHING**
● Tell patient not to discontinue therapy abruptly. Rebound hypertension is less

common than with similar drugs but may occur.
● Because guanfacine causes drowsiness, advise the patient to avoid activities that require alertness until response to drug is established.

---

hydralazine hydrochloride

Alphapress‡, Apresoline**, Novo-Hylazin†, Supres‡

Pregnancy Risk Category: C

HOW SUPPLIED

Tablets: 10 mg, 25 mg, 50 mg, 100 mg
Injection: 20 mg/ml

ACTION

Unknown. A direct-acting vasodilator, its predominant effect relaxes arteriolar smooth muscle.

ONSET, PEAK, DURATION

Onset occurs within 10 to 20 minutes of I.V. injection, 20 to 30 minutes of oral dose, unknown after I.M. administration. Peak effects occur 15 to 30 minutes after I.V. administration or 1 to 2 hours after oral dose. Unknown after I.M. administration. Effects persist for 3 to 8 hours.

INDICATIONS & DOSAGE

Essential hypertension (orally, alone or in combination with other antihypertensives); severe essential hypertension (parenterally, to lower blood pressure quickly)—
Adults: *oral*—initially, 10 mg P.O.
q.i.d.; gradually increased to 50 mg
q.i.d. as needed. Maximum recommended dosage is 200 mg daily, but some patients may require 300 to 400 mg daily.
I.V.—20 to 40 mg given slowly and repeated as necessary, switching to oral antihypertensives as soon as possible.
I.M.—10 to 50 mg, repeated as necessary, switching to oral form as soon as possible.
Children: *oral*—initially, 0.75

mg/kg/day P.O. divided into 4 doses; gradually increased over 3 to 4 weeks to a maximum of 7.5 mg/kg or 200 mg daily.
I.V.—0.1 to 0.2 mg/kg I.V. every 4 to 6 hours as needed.

ADVERSE REACTIONS
CNS: peripheral neuritis, *headache, dizziness.*
CV: orthostatic hypotension, *tachycardia,* edema, *angina, palpitations.*
GI: *nausea, vomiting, diarrhea, anorexia,* constipation.
Hematologic: neutropenia, leukopenia, *agranulocytopenia.*
Skin: rash.
Other: *lupuslike syndrome* (especially with high doses).

INTERACTIONS
Diazoxide, MAO inhibitors: may cause severe hypotension. Use together cautiously.
Indomethacin: may decrease effects of hydralazine. Monitor blood pressure.

EFFECTS ON DIAGNOSTIC TESTS
Hydralazine may cause positive antinuclear antibody titer; positive lupus erythematosus cell preparation; blood dyscrasias, including leukopenia, agranulocytosis, and purpura; and hematologic abnormalities, including decreased hemoglobin and RBC count.

CONTRAINDICATIONS
Contraindicated in patients with hypersensitivity to the drug, coronary artery disease, or mitral valvular rheumatic heart disease.

NURSING CONSIDERATIONS
● Use cautiously in patients with suspected cardiac disease, CVA, or severe renal impairment and in those taking other antihypertensives.
● **I.V. use:** Give slowly and repeat as necessary, generally every 4 to 6 hours. Hydralazine will undergo color changes in most infusion solutions; these color

changes do not indicate loss of potency. Compatible with 0.9% sodium chloride, Ringer's, and lactated Ringer's solutions, and several other common I.V. solutions. Drug may undergo a reaction with dextrose. The manufacturer does not recommend mixing the drug in infusion solutions. Check with the pharmacist for additional compatibility information.
● Monitor the patient's blood pressure, pulse rate, and body weight frequently. Some clinicians combine hydralazine therapy with diuretics and beta-adrenergic blockers to decrease sodium retention and tachycardia and to prevent anginal attacks.
● Be aware that elderly patients may be more sensitive to drug's hypotensive effects.
● Monitor CBC, lupus erythematosus cell preparation, and antinuclear antibody titer determination before therapy and periodically during long-term therapy, as ordered.
Alert: Watch the patient closely for signs of lupuslike syndrome (sore throat, fever, muscle and joint aches, and rash). Call the doctor immediately if any of these develop.
● Compliance may be improved by administering drug b.i.d. Check with the doctor.

☑ **PATIENT TEACHING**
● Instruct the patient to take oral form with meals to increase absorption.
● Inform the patient that orthostatic hypotension can be minimized by rising slowly and avoiding sudden position changes.

isradipine
DynaCirc

Pregnancy Risk Category: C

HOW SUPPLIED
Capsules: 2.5 mg, 5 mg

ACTION
Unknown. A calcium channel blocker that inhibits calcium ion influx across cardiac and smooth-muscle cells and is thought to decrease arteriolar resistance and blood pressure.

ONSET, PEAK, DURATION
Onset occurs within 2 hours. Serum levels peak within 1½ hours. Effects persist more than 12 hours.

INDICATIONS & DOSAGE
Essential hypertension—
Adults: initially, 1.25 to 2.5 mg P.O. b.i.d., alone or with a thiazide diuretic. Dosage increased by gradual titration. If response is inadequate after first 2 to 4 weeks, dosage increased to 5 mg b.i.d., then increased at 5-mg daily intervals q 2 to 4 weeks to a maximum of 20 mg daily.

ADVERSE REACTIONS
CNS: dizziness, *headache,* fatigue.
CV: edema, flushing, syncope, angina, tachycardia.
GI: nausea, diarrhea, abdominal discomfort, vomiting.
Respiratory: dyspnea.
Skin: rash.

INTERACTIONS
Fentanyl anesthesia: severe hypotension has been reported with concomitant use of a beta blocker and a calcium channel blocker.
Cimetidine: increases levels of isradipine; monitor for increased effects.

EFFECTS ON DIAGNOSTIC TESTS
None reported.

CONTRAINDICATIONS
Contraindicated in patients with hypersensitivity to the drug.

NURSING CONSIDERATIONS
● Use cautiously in patients with CHF, especially if combined with a beta blocker.

● Monitor patient for adverse reactions. Like other calcium channel blockers, isradipine is known to cause symptomatic hypotension. Most adverse reactions are mild and transient and related to vasodilation (dizziness, edema, flushing, palpitations, and tachycardia).
● Monitor blood pressure closely.
● Before surgery, inform the anesthesiologist that the patient is taking a calcium channel blocker.

☑ PATIENT TEACHING
● Tell patient that isradipine has some diuretic activity. He may note an increased need to void.
● Advise him to avoid hazardous tasks if adverse CNS reactions occur.

---

labetalol hydrochloride
Normodyne, Presolol‡, Trandate

Pregnancy Risk Category: C

HOW SUPPLIED
Tablets: 100 mg, 200 mg, 300 mg
Injection: 5 mg/ml

ACTION
Unknown. May be related to reduced peripheral vascular resistance mainly as a result of beta-adrenergic blockade.

ONSET, PEAK, DURATION
Onset occurs 2 to 5 minutes after I.V. administration, within 20 minutes after oral dose. Peak effects occur within 5 minutes of I.V. administration, 2 to 4 hours of oral dose. Effects persist for 2 to 4 hours after I.V. dose and 8 to 12 hours after oral dose.

INDICATIONS & DOSAGE
Hypertension—
Adults: 100 mg P.O. b.i.d. with or without a diuretic. If needed, dosage is increased to 200 mg b.i.d. after 2 days. Further increases may be made q 2 to 3 days until optimum response is reached. Usual maintenance dosage is 200 to 400

mg b.i.d.
Severe hypertension and hypertensive emergencies—
Adults: 200 mg diluted in 160 ml of D_5W, infused at 2 mg/minute until satisfactory response is obtained; then infusion is stopped. May be repeated q 6 to 12 hours.

Alternatively, administered by repeated I.V. injection: initially, 20 mg I.V. slowly over 2 minutes. Then repeat injections of 40 to 80 mg q 10 minutes until maximum dosage of 300 mg is reached, as needed.

ADVERSE REACTIONS
CNS: vivid dreams, fatigue, headache, paresthesia, syncope, transient scalp tingling.
CV: *orthostatic hypotension, dizziness, ventricular arrhythmias.*
EENT: nasal stuffiness.
GI: nausea, vomiting.
GU: sexual dysfunction, urine retention.
Respiratory: dyspnea, bronchospasm.
Skin: rash.

INTERACTIONS
Beta-adrenergic agonists: may blunt bronchodilator effect of these drugs in patients with bronchospasm; therefore, greater than normal dose of these agents may be required.
Cimetidine: may enhance labetalol's effect. Give together cautiously.
Halothane: additive hypotensive effect. Monitor blood pressure closely.
Insulin, oral antidiabetic agents: can alter dosage requirements in previously stabilized diabetic patients. Observe the patient carefully.

EFFECTS ON DIAGNOSTIC TESTS
Labetalol therapy may cause a false-positive increase of urine free and total catecholamine levels when measured by a nonspecific trihydroxindole fluorometric method.

CONTRAINDICATIONS
Contraindicated in patients with bronchial asthma, overt cardiac failure, greater than first-degree heart block, cardiogenic shock, severe bradycardia, other conditions associated with severe and prolonged hypotension, and hypersensitivity to the drug.

NURSING CONSIDERATIONS
● Use cautiously in patients with CHF, hepatic failure, chronic bronchitis, emphysema, preexisting peripheral vascular disease, and pheochromocytoma.
● **I.V. use:** Administer labetalol injection with an infusion control device. Monitor blood pressure closely: every 5 minutes for 30 minutes, then every 30 minutes for 2 hours, then hourly for 6 hours. The patient should remain in a supine position for 3 hours after infusion.
Alert: Be aware that sodium bicarbonate injection is incompatible with I.V. labetalol.
● Monitor blood pressure frequently. Know that drug masks common signs of shock.
● Be aware that when administered I.V. for hypertensive emergencies, labetalol produces a rapid, predictable fall in blood pressure within 5 to 10 minutes.
● If dizziness occurs, ask doctor if patient may take a dose at bedtime or take smaller doses t.i.d. to help minimize this adverse reaction.
● Monitor blood glucose levels in diabetic patients closely because beta blockers may mask certain signs and symptoms of hypoglycemia.

☑ PATIENT TEACHING
● Tell the patient that abrupt discontinuation of therapy can exacerbate angina and precipitate MI.
● Dizziness is the most troublesome adverse reaction and tends to occur in early stages of treatment, in patients also receiving diuretics, and in those receiving higher dosages. Inform the patient that this can be minimized by rising slowly and avoiding sudden position changes.

• Warn the patient that transient scalp tingling may occur, especially at beginning of therapy, but is harmless.

lisinopril
Prinivil, Zestril

Pregnancy Risk Category: C (D in 2nd and 3rd trimesters)

HOW SUPPLIED
Tablets: 2.5 mg, 5 mg, 10 mg, 20 mg, 40 mg

ACTION
Unknown. Thought to result primarily from suppression of the renin-angiotensin-aldosterone system.

ONSET, PEAK, DURATION
Onset occurs within 1 hour. Plasma levels peak within 7 hours. Effects persist for 24 hours.

INDICATIONS & DOSAGE
Hypertension—
Adults: initially, 10 mg P.O. daily for the patient not receiving a diuretic; 5 mg P.O. daily for the patient receiving a diuretic. Most patients are well controlled on 20 to 40 mg daily as a single dose.
Treatment adjunct in heart failure (with diuretics and digitalis glycosides)—
Adults: initially, 5 mg P.O. daily; increased as needed to a maximum of 20 mg P.O. daily.
✳*New indication:* *Treatment of hemodynamically stable patients within 24 hours of acute MI to improve survival—*
Adults: initially 5 mg P.O., followed by 5 mg after 24 hours, 10 mg after 48 hours, and then 10 mg once daily for 6 weeks.
   In patients with low systolic blood pressure (120 mm Hg or less) when treatment is started or during the first 3 days after an infarct, dose should be decreased to 2.5 mg P.O. If hypotension occurs (systolic blood pressure 100

mm Hg or less), daily maintenance dose of 5 mg may be reduced to 2.5 mg if needed. If prolonged hypotension occurs (systolic blood pressure below 90 mm Hg for over 1 hour), drug should be withdrawn.

ADVERSE REACTIONS
CNS: *dizziness, headache, fatigue, paresthesia.*
CV: hypotension, *orthostatic hypotension,* chest pain.
EENT: *nasal congestion.*
GI: *diarrhea,* nausea, dyspepsia.
GU: impotence.
Hematologic: neutropenia, *agranulocytopenia.*
Respiratory: dry, persistent, tickling, nonproductive cough, dyspnea.
Skin: rash.
Other: *angioedema,* hyperkalemia.

INTERACTIONS
Diuretics, thiazide diuretics: excessive hypotension with diuretics. Monitor closely. Thiazide diuretics cause attenuation of potassium loss; combined use may lead to increases in serum potassium.
Indomethacin: attenuated hypotensive effect. Monitor closely.
Insulin, oral antidiabetic agents: risk of hypoglycemia, especially at initiation of lisinopril therapy. Monitor closely.
Potassium-sparing diuretics, potassium supplements, potassium-containing sodium substitutes: possible hyperkalemia. Monitor closely.

EFFECTS ON DIAGNOSTIC TESTS
Drug's physiologic effects may lead to elevations in serum potassium, serum creatinine, BUN, and serum bilirubin levels; minor reductions of hemoglobin and hematocrit; and changes in liver enzymes.

CONTRAINDICATIONS
Contraindicated in patients with hypersensitivity to ACE inhibitors or history of angioedema related to previous treat-

ment with ACE inhibitor.

NURSING CONSIDERATIONS
● Use cautiously in patients with impaired renal function; dosage adjustment is required. Also use cautiously in patients at risk for hyperkalemia.
● When used in acute MI, patient should receive, as appropriate, the standard recommended treatment, such as thrombolytics, aspirin, and beta blockers.
● Monitor blood pressure often. Know that if drug does not adequately control blood pressure, diuretics may be added.
● Monitor WBC with differential counts before therapy, every 2 weeks for the first 3 months of therapy, and periodically thereafter.

☑ PATIENT TEACHING
Alert: Angioedema (including laryngeal edema) may occur, especially after first dose. Advise the patient to report signs or symptoms, such as swelling of face, eyes, lips, or tongue or breathing difficulty.
● Light-headedness can occur, especially during the first few days of therapy. Tell the patient to rise slowly to minimize this effect and to report symptoms to the doctor. Patients who experience syncope should stop taking drug and call the doctor immediately.
● Tell the patient not to discontinue drug suddenly, but to call the doctor, if unpleasant adverse reactions occur.
● Advise him to report signs of infection, such as fever and sore throat.
● Tell the female patient to notify doctor if pregnancy occurs. Drug will need to be discontinued.
● Instruct the patient not to use salt substitutes that contain potassium without first consulting the doctor.

---

losartan potassium
Cozaar

Pregnancy Risk Category: C (D in 2nd and 3rd trimesters)

HOW SUPPLIED
Tablets: 25 mg, 50 mg

ACTION
An angiotensin II receptor antagonist that inhibits the vasoconstricting and aldosterone-secreting effects of angiotensin II by selectively blocking the binding of angiotensin II to its receptor sites that are found in many tissues, including vascular smooth muscle and adrenal glands.

ONSET, PEAK, DURATION
Onset and duration unknown. Serum levels peak in 1 hour for losartan and in 3 to 4 hours for its active metabolite. Although the effect of losartan is substantially present within 1 week, some studies have shown that maximal effect occurs within 3 to 6 weeks.

INDICATIONS & DOSAGE
Hypertension—
Adults: initially, 25 to 50 mg P.O. daily. Maximum daily dosage is 100 mg in one or two divided doses.

ADVERSE REACTIONS
CNS: dizziness, insomnia.
GI: diarrhea, dyspepsia.
Musculoskeletal: muscle cramps, myalgia, back or leg pain.
Respiratory: nasal congestion, cough, upper respiratory tract infection, sinusitis.

INTERACTIONS
None significant.

EFFECTS ON DIAGNOSTIC TESTS
None reported.

CONTRAINDICATIONS
Contraindicated in patients with hypersensitivity to the drug.

NURSING CONSIDERATIONS
● Know that breast-feeding is not recommended during losartan therapy.
● Use cautiously in patients with im-

paired renal or hepatic function.
• Know that drugs that act directly on the renin-angiotensin system (such as losartan) can cause fetal and neonatal morbidity and death when administered to pregnant women. These problems have not been detected when exposure has been limited to the first trimester. If pregnancy is suspected, notify doctor because drug should probably be discontinued.
• Know that the lowest dosage (25 mg) should be used initially in patients with impaired hepatic function and in those who are intravascularly volume-depleted (such as those receiving diuretics).
• Be aware that losartan can be used alone or with other antihypertensives.
• Be aware that if the antihypertensive effect measured by the serum trough level of the drug, using once-daily dosing, is inadequate, a twice-daily regimen using the same total daily dosage or an increase in dosage may give a more satisfactory response.
• Monitor the patient's blood pressure closely to evaluate effectiveness of therapy. Know that when losartan is used alone, the effect on blood pressure is notably less in black patients than in patients of other races.
• Monitor patients who also are taking diuretics for symptomatic hypotension.
• Regularly assess the patient's renal function (via serum creatinine and BUN levels), as ordered.
• Be aware that patients with severe CHF whose renal function depends on the angiotensin-aldosterone system have experienced acute renal failure during ACE inhibitor therapy. Manufacturer of losartan states that drug would be expected to do the same. Closely monitor patient, especially during the first few weeks of therapy.

☑ **PATIENT TEACHING**
• Tell the patient to avoid sodium substitutes; these products may contain potassium, which can cause hyperkalemia in patients taking losartan.

• Inform the female patient of childbearing age about the consequences of second- and third-trimester exposure to losartan, and instruct her to notify the doctor immediately if she suspects that she is pregnant.

---

methyldopa
Aldomet, Aldomet M‡, Apo-Methyldopa†, Dopamet†, Hydopa‡, Novomedopa†, Nu-Medopa†

methyldopate hydrochloride
Aldomet, Aldomet Ester Injection‡

Pregnancy Risk Category: B

HOW SUPPLIED
methyldopa
Tablets: 125 mg, 250 mg, 500 mg
Oral suspension: 250 mg/5 ml
methyldopate hydrochloride
Injection: 250 mg/5 ml

ACTION
Unknown. Thought to involve inhibition of the central vasomotor centers, thereby decreasing sympathetic outflow to the heart, kidneys, and peripheral vasculature.

ONSET, PEAK, DURATION
Onset unknown. Serum levels peak within 4 to 6 hours after I.V. or oral administration. Effects persist for 12 to 24 hours after single oral dose, 24 to 48 hours after multiple oral doses, and 10 to 16 hours after I.V. administration.

INDICATIONS & DOSAGE
Hypertension, hypertensive crisis—
Adults: *oral—*initially, 250 mg P.O. b.i.d. to t.i.d. in first 48 hours. Then increased as needed q 2 days. May give entire daily dosage in the evening or h.s. Adjust dosages as needed if other antihypertensives are added to or deleted from therapy. Maintenance dosage is 500 mg to 2 g daily in two to four divided doses. Maximum recommended dai-

ly dosage is 3 g.

I.V.—250 to 500 mg q 6 hours, diluted in D₅W and administered over 30 to 60 minutes. Maximum dosage is 1 g q 6 hours. Switch to oral antihypertensives as soon as possible.

Children: initially, 10 mg/kg P.O. daily in two to four divided doses; or 20 to 40 mg/kg I.V. daily in four divided doses. Increase dose daily until desired response occurs. Maximum daily dosage is 65 mg/kg or 3 g, whichever is least.

ADVERSE REACTIONS

CNS: *sedation,* headache, weakness, dizziness, *decreased mental acuity,* paresthesia, parkinsonism, involuntary choreoathetoid movements, psychic disturbances, depression, nightmares.

CV: bradycardia, *orthostatic hypotension,* aggravated angina, ***myocarditis,*** edema.

EENT: *nasal congestion.*

GI: nausea, vomiting, diarrhea, pancreatitis, *dry mouth,* constipation.

Hematologic: ***hemolytic anemia, thrombocytopenia,*** leukopenia, bone marrow depression.

Hepatic: ***hepatic necrosis,*** abnormal liver function tests, hepatitis.

Skin: rash.

Other: gynecomastia, galactorrhea, drug-induced fever.

INTERACTIONS

Amphetamines, norepinephrine, phenothiazines, tricyclic antidepressants: possible hypertensive effects. Monitor carefully.

Anesthetics: may require lower doses of anesthetics while on methyldopa therapy.

Haloperidol: adverse mental symptoms and increased sedation when used concomitantly with methyldopa.

Levodopa: additive hypotensive effects may increase adverse CNS reactions. Monitor closely.

Lithium: may increase lithium levels. Monitor for increased lithium levels.

EFFECTS ON DIAGNOSTIC TESTS

Methyldopa alters urinary uric acid, serum creatinine, and AST levels; it may also cause falsely high levels of urinary catecholamines, interfering with the diagnosis of pheochromocytoma. A positive direct antiglobulin (Coombs') test may also occur.

CONTRAINDICATIONS

Contraindicated in patients with hypersensitivity to the drug or active hepatic disease (such as acute hepatitis) and active cirrhosis. Also contraindicated if previous methyldopa therapy has been associated with liver disorders.

NURSING CONSIDERATIONS

• Use cautiously in patients with history of impaired hepatic function and in breast-feeding patients.

• **I.V. use:** Observe for and report any involuntary choreoathetoid movements. The doctor may decide to discontinue drug if this occurs.

• Monitor patient's blood pressure regularly. Be aware that elderly patients are more likely to experience hypotension and sedation.

• After dialysis, monitor the patient for hypertension and notify doctor if necessary. The patient may need an extra dose of methyldopa.

• Monitor CBC with differential counts before therapy and periodically thereafter.

• Patients who require blood transfusions should have direct and indirect Coombs' tests to prevent crossmatching problems.

• Monitor patient's Coombs' test results. In patients who have received this drug for several months, positive reaction to direct Coombs' test indicates hemolytic anemia.

☑ **PATIENT TEACHING**

• Tell the patient not to suddenly stop taking drug, but to contact the doctor, if unpleasant adverse reactions occur.

• Tell him to report signs of infection.

Reactions may be *common,* uncommon, *life-threatening,* or COMMON AND LIFE-THREATENING.

• Tell the patient to check his weight daily and to notify the doctor of weight gain over 5 lb (about 2 kg). Sodium and water retention may occur but can be relieved with diuretics.

• Warn the patient that drug may impair ability to perform tasks that require mental alertness, particularly at start of therapy. A once-daily dosage at bedtime will minimize daytime drowsiness.

• Inform the patient that orthostatic hypotension can be minimized by rising slowly and avoiding sudden position changes. Dry mouth can be relieved with chewing gum, sour hard candy, or ice chips.

• Tell him that urine may turn dark if left standing in toilet bowls or in toilet bowls treated with bleach.

---

metoprolol succinate
Toprol XL

metoprolol tartrate
Apo-Metoprolol†, Apo-Metoprolol (Type L)†, Betaloc†‡, Betaloc Durules†, Lopresor†, Lopresor SR†, Lopressor, Minax‡, Novometoprol†, Nu-Metop†

Pregnancy Risk Category: C

HOW SUPPLIED
metoprolol succinate
Tablets (extended-release): 50 mg, 100 mg, 200 mg
metoprolol tartrate
Tablets: 50 mg, 100 mg
Tablets (extended-release): 100 mg†, 200 mg†
Injection: 1 mg/ml in 5-ml ampules

ACTION
Unknown for antihypertensive action. A beta$_1$-selective blocking agent that decreases myocardial contractility, heart rate, cardiac output, and blood pressure and reduces myocardial oxygen use. Also depresses renin secretion.

ONSET, PEAK, DURATION
Onset occurs within 5 minutes of I.V. dose, 15 minutes of oral dose. Peak effects occur within 20 minutes of I.V. dose, 1 hour after regular-release tablet, or 6 to 12 hours after extended-release dosage forms. Effects persist for 5 to 8 hours after I.V. dose, 6 to 12 hours after regular-release oral tablets, up to 24 hours after extended-release forms.

INDICATIONS & DOSAGE
Hypertension—
Adults: initially, 50 mg P.O. b.i.d. or 100 mg P.O. once daily, then up to 100 to 450 mg daily in two or three divided doses. Alternatively, 50 to 100 mg of extended-release tablets (tartrate equivalent) once daily. Dosage is adjusted as needed and tolerated at intervals of not less than 1 week to a maximum of 400 mg daily.
Early intervention in acute MI (metoprolol tartrate)—
Adults: three 5-mg I.V. boluses q 2 minutes. Then, beginning 15 minutes after last dose, 25 to 50 mg P.O. q 6 hours for 48 hours. Maintenance dosage is 100 mg P.O. b.i.d. for 3 months to 3 years.
Angina pectoris—
Adults: initially, 100 mg P.O. daily as a single dose or in two equally divided doses; increased at weekly intervals until an adequate response or a pronounced decrease in heart rate is seen. Daily dosage beyond 400 mg has not been studied. Alternatively, give 100 mg of extended-release tablets (tartrate equivalent) once daily. Dosage adjusted as needed and tolerated at intervals of not less than 1 week to a maximum of 400 mg daily.

ADVERSE REACTIONS
CNS: *fatigue, dizziness,* depression.
CV: *bradycardia, hypotension,* **CHF, AV block.**
GI: nausea, diarrhea.
Respiratory: dyspnea, **bronchospasm.**
Skin: rash.

INTERACTIONS

Barbiturates, rifampin: increased metabolism of metoprolol. Monitor for decreased effect.

Catecholamine-depleting drugs (such as reserpine): may have additive effect when given with beta blockers. Monitor for hypotension and bradycardia.

Chlorpromazine, cimetidine, verapamil: decreased hepatic clearance. Monitor for greater beta-blocking effect.

Digitalis glycosides, diltiazem, verapamil: excessive bradycardia and increased depressant effect on myocardium. Use together cautiously.

Indomethacin: decreased antihypertensive effect. Monitor blood pressure and adjust dosage.

Insulin, oral antidiabetic agents: can alter dosage requirements in previously stabilized diabetic patients. Observe the patient carefully.

EFFECTS ON DIAGNOSTIC TESTS

May elevate serum transaminase, alkaline phosphatase, lactate dehydrogenase, and uric acid levels.

CONTRAINDICATIONS

Contraindicated in patients with hypersensitivity to the drug or other beta blockers. Also contraindicated in patients with sinus bradycardia, heart block greater than first-degree, cardiogenic shock, or overt cardiac failure when used to treat hypertension or angina. When used to treat MI, drug also is contraindicated in patients with heart rate less than 45 beats/minute, second- or third-degree heart block, PR interval of 0.24 seconds or longer with first-degree heart block, systolic blood pressure less than 100 mm Hg, or moderate to severe cardiac failure.

NURSING CONSIDERATIONS

● Use cautiously in patients with heart failure, diabetes, or respiratory or hepatic disease.
● Always check the patient's apical pulse rate before giving drug. If it's slower than 60 beats/minute, withhold drug and call the doctor immediately.
● **I.V. use:** Give undiluted by direct injection. Although mixing with other drugs should be avoided, studies have shown that metoprolol is compatible when mixed with meperidine hydrochloride or morphine sulfate or when administered with alteplase infusion at a Y-site connection.
● Food may increase drug absorption. Give consistently with meals.
● Monitor blood glucose levels closely in diabetic patients because drug masks common signs of hypoglycemia.
● Monitor blood pressure frequently. Know that metoprolol masks common signs of shock.
● Store drug at room temperature and protect from light. Discard solution if it's discolored or contains particles.

☑ PATIENT TEACHING

● Instruct the patient to take drug exactly as prescribed and to take it with meals.
● Tell the patient not to stop drug suddenly but to notify the doctor about unpleasant adverse reactions. Inform him that drug must be withdrawn gradually over 1 to 2 weeks.

---

minoxidil
Loniten, Minodyl

Pregnancy Risk Category: C

HOW SUPPLIED
Tablets: 2.5 mg, 10 mg, 25 mg‡

ACTION
Unknown. Predominant effect produces direct arteriolar vasodilation.

ONSET, PEAK, DURATION
Onset occurs in about 30 minutes. Peak effects occur within 2 to 3 hours. Effects persist for 2 to 5 days.

INDICATIONS & DOSAGE

Severe hypertension—
Adults: initially, 5 mg P.O. as a single dose. Effective dosage range is usually 10 to 40 mg daily. Maximum dosage is 100 mg daily.
Children under 12 years: 0.2 mg/kg P.O. (maximum 5 mg) as a single daily dose. Effective dosage range usually is 0.25 to 1 mg/kg daily. Maximum dosage is 50 mg.

ADVERSE REACTIONS

CV: *edema, tachycardia, pericardial effusion and tamponade,* **CHF,** ECG changes, rebound hypertension.
GI: nausea, vomiting.
Skin: rash, *Stevens-Johnson syndrome*.
Other: *hypertrichosis* (elongation, thickening, and enhanced pigmentation of fine body hair), breast tenderness, weight gain.

INTERACTIONS

Guanethidine: severe orthostatic hypotension. Advise the patient to stand up slowly.

EFFECTS ON DIAGNOSTIC TESTS

May elevate serum alkaline phosphatase, serum creatinine, and BUN levels, as well as antinuclear antibody titers; drug may transiently decrease hemoglobin and hematocrit levels. Minoxidil may also alter direction and magnitude of T waves on ECG.

CONTRAINDICATIONS

Contraindicated in patients with pheochromocytoma or hypersensitivity to the drug.

NURSING CONSIDERATIONS

• Use cautiously in those with impaired renal function and after acute MI.
• Closely monitor blood pressure and pulse at beginning of therapy.
• Know that elderly patients may be more sensitive to drug's hypotensive effects.
• Minoxidil is removed by hemodialy-

sis. Be sure to administer dose after dialysis.
• Monitor fluid intake and urine output. Check for weight gain and edema.

☑ PATIENT TEACHING

• Make sure the patient receives and reads the manufacturer's package insert that describes in layman's terms the drug and its adverse reactions. Also provide an oral explanation.
• Tell the patient not to suddenly stop taking the drug, but to call the doctor, if unpleasant adverse effects occur.
• Make sure the patient understands the importance of compliance with total treatment regimen. Minoxidil usually is prescribed with a beta blocker to control tachycardia and a diuretic to counteract fluid retention.
• Teach the patient how to take his own pulse and to report increases greater than 20 beats/minute to the doctor.
• Tell the patient to weigh himself at least weekly and to report weight gain of over 5 lb (about 2 kg).
• About 8 out of 10 patients will experience hypertrichosis within 3 to 6 weeks of beginning treatment. Unwanted hair can be controlled with a depilatory or shaving. Assure the patient that extra hair will disappear within 1 to 6 months of stopping minoxidil. Advise the patient, however, not to discontinue drug without the doctor's approval.

---

moexipril hydrochloride
Univasc

Pregnancy Risk Category: C (first trimester), D (second and third trimester)

HOW SUPPLIED

Tablets: 7.5 mg, 15 mg

ACTION

Unknown. Thought to result primarily from suppression of renin-angiotensin-aldosterone system.

ONSET, PEAK, DURATION
Onset occurs in about 1 hour. Plasma levels peak in about 1½ hours and antihypertensive effects between 3 and 6 hours. Effects persist for 24 hours.

INDICATIONS & DOSAGE
Hypertension—
Adults: initially, 7.5 mg (3.75 mg if patient is receiving a diuretic) P.O. once daily 1 hour before meal. If control is inadequate, dose may be increased or divided. Recommended maintenance dosage is 7.5 mg to 30 mg daily, in one or two divided doses 1 hour before meal. Subsequent dosage depends on response.

ADVERSE REACTIONS
CNS: *dizziness,* headache, fatigue.
CV: peripheral edema, hypotension, orthostatic hypotension, chest pain, flushing.
EENT: pharyngitis, rhinitis, sinusitis.
GI: diarrhea, dyspepsia, nausea.
GU: urinary frequency.
Hematologic: neutropenia.
Respiratory: *persistent, nonproductive cough,* upper respiratory infection.
Skin: rash.
Other: myalgia, ***anaphylactoid reactions, angioedema,*** hyperkalemia, flu syndrome, pain.

INTERACTIONS
Diuretics: risk of excessive hypotension. Expect diuretic to be discontinued or moexipril dose lowered.
Lithium: increased serum lithium level and lithium toxicity. Use together cautiously and monitor serum lithium levels frequently.
Potassium-sparing diuretics, potassium supplements, salt substitutes containing potassium: risk of hyperkalemia. Monitor serum potassium level closely.

EFFECTS ON DIAGNOSTIC TESTS
May cause minor elevations in creatinine and BUN levels. Elevations of liver enzymes and uric acid may also occur.

CONTRAINDICATIONS
Contraindicated in patients with hypersensitivity to drug or history of angioedema related to treatment with ACE inhibitor.

NURSING CONSIDERATIONS
● Safety of drug is not established in children.
● Use cautiously in patients with impaired renal function, CHF, or renal artery stenosis and in breast-feeding women.
● Monitor for excessive hypotension.
● Measure blood pressure at trough (just before dose) to verify blood pressure control.
● Assess renal function before and during therapy. Monitor serum potassium level, as ordered.
● Know that other ACE inhibitors have been associated with agranulocytosis and neutropenia. Monitor CBC with differential before therapy, especially in patients who have collagen-vascular disease with impaired renal function.
● Because angioedema associated with the tongue, glottis, or larynx can cause a fatal airway obstruction, be prepared with appropriate therapy, such as S.C. epinephrine 1:1,000 (0.3 to 0.5 ml), and equipment to ensure a patent airway.

☑ **PATIENT TEACHING**
● Tell patient to take this drug on an empty stomach; meals can impair absorption.
● Advise patient to avoid salt substitutes with potassium, which can cause hyperkalemia in patients taking this drug.
● Tell patient to use caution in hot weather and during exercise. Inadequate fluid intake, vomiting, diarrhea, and excessive perspiration can lead to lightheadedness and syncope.
● Urge patient to rise slowly to minimize light-headedness. Tell him to stop taking drug and to call the doctor immediately if syncope occurs.
● Advise patient to report fever; sore throat; easy bruising or bleeding;

swelling of tongue, lips, face, eyes, mucous membranes, or extremities; difficulty swallowing or breathing; or hoarseness.
● Tell female patient to notify doctor if pregnancy occurs. Drug must be discontinued.

---

nisoldipine
Sular

Pregnancy Risk Category: C

HOW SUPPLIED
Extended-release tablets: 10 mg, 20 mg, 30 mg, 40 mg

ACTION
Prevents calcium ions from entering vascular smooth muscle cells, thereby causing dilation of arterioles, which in turn decreases peripheral vascular resistance.

ONSET, PEAK, DURATION
Onset unknown. Peak plasma levels occur in 6 to 12 hours. Duration is up to 24 hours for the extended-release tablet.

INDICATIONS & DOSAGE
Hypertension—
Adults: initially, 20 mg (10 mg if patient is over 65 or has liver dysfunction) P.O. once daily; increased by 10 mg/week or at longer intervals, as needed. Usual maintenance dosage is 20 to 40 mg/day. Dosages greater than 60 mg/day are not recommended.

ADVERSE REACTIONS
CNS: *headache,* dizziness.
CV: vasodilation, palpitation, chest pain.
EENT: sinusitis.
GI: nausea.
Respiratory: pharyngitis.
Skin: rash.
Other: *peripheral edema.*

INTERACTIONS
Cimetidine: increased bioavailability and peak concentration of nisoldipine.
Quinidine: decreased bioavailability of nisoldipine.
High-fat meal: increased peak drug concentration.
Grapefruit juice: increased bioavailability and concentration of drug.

EFFECTS ON DIAGNOSTIC TESTS
None reported.

CONTRAINDICATIONS
Contraindicated in patients with hypersensitivity to dihydropyridine calcium channel blockers.

NURSING CONSIDERATIONS
● Use cautiously in patients with CHF or compromised ventricular function, particularly in those receiving beta blockers and in patients with severe hepatic dysfunction.
● Know that drug should not be used in breast-feeding women.
● Monitor patient carefully. Some patients, especially those with severe obstructive coronary artery disease, have developed increased frequency, duration, or severity of angina or even acute MI after starting calcium channel blocker therapy or at time of dosage increase.
● Monitor blood pressure regularly, especially during the initial administration and titration of drug.

☑ PATIENT TEACHING
● Tell the patient to take drug as prescribed, even if he feels better.
● Advise patient to swallow tablet whole and not to chew, divide, or crush it.
● Remind patient not to take drug with a high-fat meal or with grapefruit products. Both may increase the amount of drug in the body over the intended amount.

---

nitroprusside sodium
Nitropress

Pregnancy Risk Category: C

HOW SUPPLIED
Injection: 50 mg/vial in 2-ml, 5-ml vials

ACTION
Relaxes both arteriolar and venous smooth muscle.

ONSET, PEAK, DURATION
Onset occurs within 1 to 2 minutes. Peak effects are evident almost immediately. Effects dissipate within 10 minutes after infusion.

INDICATIONS & DOSAGE
To lower blood pressure quickly in hypertensive emergencies; to produce controlled hypotension during anesthesia; to reduce preload and afterload in cardiac pump failure or cardiogenic shock (may be used with or without dopamine)—
Adults: 50 mg vial diluted with 2 to 3 ml of D_5W and then added to 250, 500, or 1,000 ml of D_5W; infused at 0.3 to 10 mcg/kg/minute. Average dose is 3 mcg/kg/minute. Maximum infusion rate is 10 mcg/kg/minute.
Patients taking other antihypertensives along with nitroprusside are extremely sensitive to nitroprusside. Dosage is adjusted accordingly.

ADVERSE REACTIONS
CNS: *headache, dizziness,* loss of consciousness, apprehension, *restlessness, muscle twitching, diaphoresis.*
CV: bradycardia, hypotension, tachycardia, palpitations, ECG changes.
GI: *nausea, abdominal pain,* ileus.
Skin: pink color, flushing, rash.
Other: acidosis, *thiocyanate toxicity, methemoglobinemia, cyanide toxicity,*

venous streaking, irritation at infusion site, *increased intracranial pressure,* hypothyroidism.

INTERACTIONS
Antihypertensives: may cause sensitivity to nitroprusside. Adjust dosage as ordered.
Ganglionic blocking agents, general anesthetics, negative inotropic agents, other antihypertensives: additive effects. Monitor blood pressure closely.

EFFECTS ON DIAGNOSTIC TESTS
An increase in serum creatinine concentration may occur during therapy.

CONTRAINDICATIONS
Contraindicated in patients with hypersensitivity to the drug, compensatory hypertension (such as in arteriovenous shunt or coarctation of the aorta), inadequate cerebral circulation, acute CHF associated with reduced peripheral vascular resistance, congenital optic atrophy, or tobacco-induced amblyopia.

NURSING CONSIDERATIONS
● Use with extreme caution in patients with increased intracranial pressure. Use cautiously in patients with hypothyroidism, hepatic or renal disease, hyponatremia, or low vitamin B_{12} concentration.
● Obtain baseline vital signs before giving drug, and find out what parameters the doctor wants to achieve.
● Keep the patient in the supine position when initiating or titrating nitroprusside therapy.
● **I.V. use:** Don't use bacteriostatic water for injection or sterile sodium chloride solution for reconstitution.
● Because the drug is sensitive to light, wrap I.V. solution in foil; it's not necessary to wrap the tubing. Fresh solution should have faint brownish tint. Discard after 24 hours.
● Infuse with an infusion pump. Drug is

Reactions may be *common,* uncommon, *life-threatening,* or COMMON AND LIFE-THREATENING.

best given via piggyback through a peripheral line with no other medication. Don't adjust rate of main I.V. line while drug is being infused. Even a small bolus of nitroprusside can cause severe hypotension.

• Check blood pressure every 5 minutes at start of infusion and every 15 minutes thereafter. If severe hypotension occurs, discontinue nitroprusside infusion—effects of drug quickly reverse. Notify the doctor. If possible, start an arterial pressure line. Regulate drug flow to specified level.

Alert: Excessive doses or rapid infusion greater than 10 mcg/kg/minute can cause cyanide toxicity; therefore, check serum thiocyanate levels every 72 hours. Levels above 100 mcg/ml are associated with toxicity. Watch for profound hypotension, metabolic acidosis, dyspnea, headache, loss of consciousness, ataxia, and vomiting. If these occur, discontinue drug immediately and notify the doctor.

☑ **PATIENT TEACHING**
• Instruct patient to report adverse reactions promptly.
• Tell patient to alert nurse if discomfort occurs at I.V. insertion site.

---

penbutolol sulfate
Levatol, Lobeta‡

Pregnancy Risk Category: C

HOW SUPPLIED
Tablets: 20 mg

ACTION
Unknown.

ONSET, PEAK, DURATION
Onset occurs within 1 hour. Peak effects occur within 1½ to 3 hours. Effects persist up to 24 hours.

INDICATIONS & DOSAGE
Mild to moderate hypertension—

Adults: 20 mg P.O. once daily. Usually given with other antihypertensives, such as thiazide diuretics.

ADVERSE REACTIONS
CNS: *dizziness,* headache, fatigue, insomnia, asthenia.
CV: chest pain, *CHF.*
GI: nausea, diarrhea, dyspepsia.
GU: impotence.
Respiratory: cough, dyspnea.
Skin: excessive diaphoresis.

INTERACTIONS
Clonidine: may cause paradoxical hypertension. Also, beta blockers may enhance rebound hypertension when clonidine is withdrawn.
Digoxin, diltiazem, verapamil: may produce additive depressant effects on AV node conduction. Monitor closely.
Insulin, oral antidiabetic agents: hypoglycemic response to these drugs may be altered. Monitor patient closely.
NSAIDs: may decrease antihypertensive effects.
Prazosin, terazosin: "first-dose" orthostatic hypotension seen with these drugs may be enhanced.
Sympathomimetics, including isoproterenol, dopamine, dobutamine, or norepinephrine: decreased hypotensive response.
Theophylline: may decrease bronchodilator effect.

EFFECTS ON DIAGNOSTIC TESTS
Drug may interfere with glucose or insulin tolerance tests.

CONTRAINDICATIONS
Contraindicated in patients with hypersensitivity to the drug or other beta blockers and in those with sinus bradycardia, cardiogenic shock, overt cardiac failure, greater than first-degree heart block, or bronchial asthma.

NURSING CONSIDERATIONS
• Use cautiously in patients with CHF controlled by drug therapy and in those

with a history of bronchospastic disease. Also use cautiously in diabetic patients because beta-adrenergic blockers may mask certain signs and symptoms of hypoglycemia.

● Always check the patient's apical pulse before giving drug. If you detect extremes in pulse rates, withhold drug and call the doctor immediately.

● Monitor blood pressure, ECG, and heart rate and rhythm frequently.

☑ **PATIENT TEACHING**

● Instruct the patient to take drug exactly as prescribed.

● Tell the patient not to stop drug suddenly but to notify the doctor about unpleasant adverse reactions.

● Teach the patient the signs and symptoms of CHF (edema and pulmonary congestion). Advise him to contact the doctor if these occur.

---

phentolamine mesylate
Regitine, Rogitine†

Pregnancy Risk Category: C

HOW SUPPLIED
Injection: 5 mg/ml in 1-ml vials, 10 mg/ml‡

ACTION
An alpha-adrenergic blocker that competitively blocks the effects of catecholamines on alpha-adrenergic receptors.

ONSET, PEAK, DURATION
Unknown.

INDICATIONS & DOSAGE
To aid in diagnosis of pheochromocytoma; to control or prevent hypertension before or during pheochromocytomectomy—
Adults: I.V. diagnostic dose is 2.5 mg with close monitoring of blood pressure. Before surgical removal of tumor, 5 mg I.M. or I.V. During surgery, the patient

may need 5 mg I.V.
Children: I.V. diagnostic dose is 1 mg with close monitoring of blood pressure. Before surgical removal of tumor, 1 mg I.V. or I.M. During surgery, the patient may need 1 mg I.V.
Dermal necrosis and sloughing after I.V. extravasation of norepinephrine—
Adults and children: infiltrate area with 5 to 10 mg phentolamine in 10 ml of 0.9% sodium chloride solution, or give half the dosage through the infiltrated I.V. and the other half around the site. Must be done within 12 hours.

ADVERSE REACTIONS
CNS: *dizziness, weakness, flushing, cerebrovascular occlusion,* cerebrovascular spasm.
CV: *hypotension, shock, arrhythmias, tachycardia, MI.*
EENT: *nasal congestion.*
GI: *diarrhea, nausea, vomiting.*

INTERACTIONS
Epinephrine: excessive hypotension. Don't use together.
Narcotics, sedatives, rauwolfia alkaloids: false-positive test results for pheochromocytoma. Don't give 24 hours before phentolamine is given as a diagnostic test. Withdraw rauwolfia alkaloids at least 4 weeks before such testing.

EFFECTS ON DIAGNOSTIC TESTS
None reported.

CONTRAINDICATIONS
Contraindicated in patients with angina, coronary artery disease, MI or history of MI, or hypersensitivity to the drug.

NURSING CONSIDERATIONS
● Use cautiously in patients with gastritis or peptic ulcer.

● When drug is given as a diagnostic test for pheochromocytoma, take the patient's blood pressure first; also monitor blood pressure frequently during administration.

Reactions may be *common*, uncommon, *life-threatening*, or COMMON AND LIFE-THREATENING.

● Know that test is positive for pheochromocytoma if I.V. test dose causes severe hypotension.

Alert: Don't administer epinephrine to treat phentolamine-induced hypotension because it may cause additional fall in blood pressure ("epinephrine reversal"). Use norepinephrine instead, as ordered.

☑ **PATIENT TEACHING**
● Explain to patient why and how drug is administered.
● Tell patient to report adverse reactions promptly.

---

pindolol
Apo-Pindol†, Barbloc‡, Novo-Pindol†, Syn-Pindolol†, Visken

Pregnancy Risk Category: B

HOW SUPPLIED
Tablets: 5 mg, 10 mg, 15 mg‡

ACTION
Unknown. A nonselective beta-adrenergic blocker that has intrinsic sympathomimetic activity. Possible mechanisms include reduced cardiac output, decreased sympathetic outflow to peripheral vasculature, and inhibition of renin release by the kidneys.

ONSET, PEAK, DURATION
Onset unknown. Peak effects occur in 1 to 2 hours. Effects persist for 24 hours.

INDICATIONS & DOSAGE
Hypertension—
Adults: initially, 5 mg P.O. b.i.d. Dosage increased as needed and tolerated to a maximum of 60 mg daily.

ADVERSE REACTIONS
CNS: *insomnia, fatigue, dizziness, nervousness,* vivid dreams, weakness, paresthesia.
CV: *edema,* bradycardia, *CHF,* chest pain.
GI: *nausea,* abdominal discomfort.

Respiratory: *increased airway resistance,* dyspnea.
Skin: rash, pruritus.
Other: *muscle pain, joint pain.*

INTERACTIONS
Catecholamine-depleting drugs (such as reserpine): may have additive effects. Monitor for hypotension and bradycardia.
Digitalis glycosides, diltiazem, verapamil: excessive bradycardia and additive depression of AV node. Use together cautiously.
Epinephrine: severe vasoconstriction. Monitor blood pressure and observe the patient carefully.
Indomethacin: decreased antihypertensive effect. Monitor blood pressure and adjust dosage.
Insulin, oral antidiabetic agents: can alter requirements for these drugs in previously stabilized diabetic patients. Monitor the patient for hypoglycemia.

EFFECTS ON DIAGNOSTIC TESTS
Pindolol may elevate serum transaminase, alkaline phosphatase, lactate dehydrogenase, and uric acid levels.

CONTRAINDICATIONS
Contraindicated in patients with hypersensitivity to the drug, bronchial asthma, severe bradycardia, heart block greater than first degree, cardiogenic shock, or overt cardiac failure.

NURSING CONSIDERATIONS
● Use cautiously in patients with CHF, nonallergic bronchospastic disease, diabetes, hyperthyroidism, and impaired renal or hepatic function.
● Always check the patient's apical pulse rate before giving this drug. If you detect extremes in pulse rates, withhold medication and call the doctor immediately.
● Monitor blood pressure frequently and notify the doctor if severe hypotension occurs. A vasopressor may be required.
● Withdraw drug over 1 to 2 weeks after

---

long-term therapy, as ordered.
● Monitor blood glucose levels in diabetic patients closely because drug masks certain signs and symptoms of hypoglycemia.

☑ PATIENT TEACHING
● Tell the patient to take drug exactly as prescribed.
● Tell the patient not to stop drug suddenly but to call doctor to discuss unpleasant adverse drug reactions.

---

prazosin hydrochloride
Minipress

Pregnancy Risk Category: C

HOW SUPPLIED
Capsules: 1 mg, 2 mg, 5 mg

ACTION
Unknown. Its alpha-adrenergic blocking activity is thought to account primarily for its effects.

ONSET, PEAK, DURATION
Onset occurs in 30 to 90 minutes. Peak effects occur in 2 to 4 hours, but maximal antihypertensive effect may not occur for 3 to 4 weeks. Effects persist about 7 to 10 hours.

INDICATIONS & DOSAGE
Mild to moderate hypertension, alone or in combination with a diuretic or other antihypertensive—
Adults: P.O. test dose is 1 mg h.s. to prevent "first-dose syncope." Initial dose is 1 mg P.O. b.i.d. or t.i.d. Dosage increased slowly. Maximum daily dosage is 20 mg. Maintenance dosage is 6 to 15 mg daily in three divided doses. Some patients need dosages larger than this (up to 40 mg daily). If other antihypertensives or diuretics are added to this drug, prazosin is decreased to 1 to 2 mg t.i.d. and retitrated.

ADVERSE REACTIONS
CNS: *dizziness,* headache, drowsiness, nervousness, paresthesia, weakness, *"first-dose syncope,"* depression.
CV: orthostatic hypotension, *palpitations.*
EENT: blurred vision, tinnitus, conjunctivitis.
GI: vomiting, diarrhea, abdominal cramps, *nausea.*
GU: priapism, impotence, urinary frequency, incontinence.
Respiratory: dyspnea, nasal congestion, epistaxis.
Other: arthralgia, myalgia, pruritus, edema, fever.

INTERACTIONS
Propranolol and other beta blockers: increased frequency of syncope with loss of consciousness. Advise the patient to sit or lie down if dizziness occurs.

EFFECTS ON DIAGNOSTIC TESTS
Prazosin alters results of screening tests for pheochromocytoma and causes increases in levels of the urinary metabolite of norepinephrine and vanillylmandelic acid; it may cause positive antinuclear antibody titer and liver function test abnormalities. A transient fall in leukocyte count and increased serum uric acid and BUN levels may also occur.

CONTRAINDICATIONS
None known.

NURSING CONSIDERATIONS
● Use cautiously in patients receiving other antihypertensives.
● Monitor the patient's blood pressure and pulse rate frequently.
● Know that elderly patients may be more sensitive to drug's hypotensive effects.
● Compliance *might* be improved with twice-daily dosing. Suggest this dosing change with the doctor if you suspect compliance problems.

Alert: Be aware that if initial dose is greater than 1 mg, severe syncope with loss of consciousness may occur ("first-dose syncope").

☑ **PATIENT TEACHING**
● Warn the patient that dizziness may occur with first dose. If he experiences dizziness, tell him to sit or lie down. Reassure him that this effect disappears with continued dosing.
● Tell the patient not to suddenly stop taking this drug but to call the doctor if unpleasant adverse reactions occur.
● Advise the patient to minimize orthostatic hypotension by rising slowly and avoiding sudden position changes. Dry mouth can be relieved with chewing gum, sour hard candy, or ice chips.

---

quinapril hydrochloride
Accupril, Asig‡

Pregnancy Risk Category: C (D in 2nd and 3rd trimesters)

HOW SUPPLIED
Tablets: 5 mg, 10 mg, 20 mg, 40 mg

ACTION
Unknown, but thought to be related to inhibition of angiotensin I to angiotensin II, a potent vasoconstrictor. Reduced formation of angiotensin II decreases peripheral arterial resistance, thus decreasing aldosterone secretion.

ONSET, PEAK, DURATION
Onset occurs within 1 hour. Peak serum levels of quinapril are seen in 1 hour; quinaprilat, in 2 hours. Peak effects occur within 2 to 4 hours. Effects persist about 24 hours.

INDICATIONS & DOSAGE
Hypertension—
Adults: initially, 10 mg daily. Dosage adjusted based on patient response at intervals of about 2 weeks. Most patients are controlled at 20, 40, or 80 mg daily

as a single dose or in two divided doses. If patient is taking a diuretic, initiate therapy with 5 mg daily.
Heart failure—
Adults: initially, 5 mg P.O. b.i.d. if patient is receiving a diuretic and 10 mg P.O. b.i.d. if patient not receiving a diuretic. Dosage increased at weekly intervals. Usual effective dose is 20 to 40 mg b.i.d. in equally divided doses.

ADVERSE REACTIONS
CNS: somnolence, vertigo, nervousness, headache, dizziness, fatigue, depression.
CV: palpitations, tachycardia, angina, hypertensive crisis, orthostatic hypotension, rhythm disturbances.
GI: dry mouth, abdominal pain, constipation, vomiting, nausea, hemorrhage.
Hepatic: elevated liver enzymes.
Respiratory: *dry, persistent, tickling, nonproductive cough.*
Skin: pruritus, *exfoliative dermatitis,* photosensitivity, diaphoresis.
Other: *angioedema,* hyperkalemia.

INTERACTIONS
Diuretics, other antihypertensives: risk of excessive hypotension. Discontinue diuretic or lower dose of quinapril as needed.
Lithium: increased serum lithium levels and lithium toxicity. Monitor serum lithium levels.
Potassium-sparing diuretics, potassium supplements, salt substitutes containing potassium: risk of hyperkalemia. Monitor closely during concomitant use.
Tetracycline: absorption decreased with administration of quinapril.

EFFECTS ON DIAGNOSTIC TESTS
In clinical trials, up to 2% of patients exhibited elevated serum potassium levels.

CONTRAINDICATIONS
Contraindicated in patients with hypersensitivity to ACE inhibitors or with a history of angioedema related to treat-

---

ment with an ACE inhibitor.

NURSING CONSIDERATIONS

• Use cautiously in patients with impaired renal function.
• Assess renal and hepatic function before and periodically throughout therapy. Know that dosage adjustment is necessary for patients with renal impairment.
• Monitor blood pressure for effectiveness of therapy.
• Monitor serum potassium levels as ordered. Be aware that risk factors for the development of hyperkalemia include renal insufficiency, diabetes, and concomitant use of drugs that raise potassium level.
• Other ACE inhibitors have been associated with agranulocytosis and neutropenia. Monitor CBC with differential counts before therapy and periodically thereafter, as ordered.

☑ PATIENT TEACHING

• Advise the patient to report any signs of infection, such as fever and sore throat.
Alert: Angioedema (including laryngeal edema) may occur, especially after the first dose. Advise the patient to report any signs or symptoms, such as swelling of face, eyes, lips, or tongue or breathing difficulty.
• Light-headedness can occur, especially during the first few days of therapy. Tell the patient to rise slowly to minimize effect and to report symptoms to the doctor. Patients who experience syncope should stop taking drug and call the doctor immediately.
• Inadequate fluid intake, vomiting, diarrhea, and excessive perspiration can lead to light-headedness and syncope. Tell the patient to use caution in hot weather and during exercise.
• Tell the patient to avoid salt substitutes; these products may contain potassium, which can cause hyperkalemia in patients taking quinapril.
• Tell the female patient to notify doctor

if pregnancy occurs. Drug will need to be discontinued.

ramipril
Altace, Ramace‡, Tritace‡

Pregnancy Risk Category: C (D in 2nd and 3rd trimesters)

HOW SUPPLIED
Capsules: 1.25 mg, 2.5 mg, 5 mg, 10 mg

ACTION
Unknown, but thought to be related to inhibition of angiotensin I to angiotensin II, a potent vasoconstrictor. Reduced formation of angiotensin II decreases peripheral arterial resistance, thus decreasing aldosterone secretion.

ONSET, PEAK, DURATION
Onset occurs within 1 to 2 hours. Peak serum levels of ramipril occur within 1 hour; of ramiprilat, in 3 hours. Peak effects occur in 3 to 6 hours. Effects persist about 24 hours.

INDICATIONS & DOSAGE
Hypertension—
Adults: initially, 2.5 mg P.O. once daily for patients not receiving a diuretic, and 1.25 mg P.O. once daily for patients receiving a diuretic. Dosage increased as necessary based on patient response. Maintenance dosage is 2.5 to 20 mg daily as a single dose or in divided doses.
   In patients with renal insufficiency: If creatinine clearance is less than 40 ml/minute, 1.25 mg P.O. daily. Dosage is titrated gradually according to response. Maximum daily dosage is 5 mg.
Heart failure—
Adults: initially, 2.5 mg P.O. b.i.d. If hypotension occurs, dosage should be decreased to 1.25 mg P.O. b.i.d. Dosage may be gradually increased to a maximum of 5 mg P.O. b.i.d. as needed.
   In patients with renal insufficiency: If creatinine clearance is less than 40

ml/minute, 1.25 mg P.O. daily. Dosage is titrated gradually according to response. Maximum daily dosage is 2.5 mg b.i.d.

ADVERSE REACTIONS
CNS: headache, dizziness, fatigue, asthenia, malaise, light-headedness, anxiety, amnesia, *seizures,* depression, insomnia, nervousness, neuralgia, neuropathy, paresthesia, somnolence, tremor, vertigo.
CV: orthostatic hypotension, syncope, angina, *arrhythmias,* chest pain, palpitations, *MI.*
EENT: epistaxis, tinnitus.
GI: nausea, vomiting, abdominal pain, anorexia, constipation, diarrhea, dyspepsia, dry mouth, gastroenteritis.
GU: impotence.
Respiratory: *dry, persistent, tickling, nonproductive cough;* dyspnea.
Skin: hypersensitivity reactions, rash, dermatitis, pruritus, photosensitivity.
Other: *angioedema,* edema, hyperkalemia, increased diaphoresis, weight gain, arthralgia, arthritis, myalgia.

INTERACTIONS
Diuretics: excessive hypotension, especially at the start of therapy. Discontinue diuretic at least 3 days before therapy begins, increase sodium intake, or reduce starting dose of ramipril.
Insulin, oral antidiabetic agents: risk of hypoglycemia, especially at initiation of ramipril therapy. Monitor closely.
Lithium: increased serum lithium levels. Use together cautiously and monitor serum lithium levels.
Potassium-sparing diuretics, potassium supplements, sodium substitutes containing potassium: increased risk of hyperkalemia because ramipril attenuates potassium loss. Monitor plasma potassium levels closely.

EFFECTS ON DIAGNOSTIC TESTS
Transient increases in BUN and creatinine levels, decreases in hemoglobin and hematocrit, and elevations of liver enzymes, serum bilirubin, uric acid, and blood glucose levels have been reported.

CONTRAINDICATIONS
Contraindicated in patients with hypersensitivity to ACE inhibitors or a history of angioedema related to treatment with an ACE inhibitor.

NURSING CONSIDERATIONS
● Use cautiously in patients with renal impairment.
● Monitor blood pressure regularly for drug effectiveness.
● Closely assess renal function in patients during first few weeks of therapy. Regular assessment of renal function (serum creatinine and BUN levels) is advisable. Patients with severe CHF whose renal function depends on the angiotensin-aldosterone system have experienced acute renal failure during ACE inhibitor therapy. Hypertensive patients with renal artery stenosis also may show signs of worsening renal function at start of therapy.
● Monitor CBC with differential counts before therapy and periodically thereafter. These effects may occur especially in patients with impaired renal function or collagen vascular diseases (systemic lupus erythematosus or scleroderma).
● Monitor serum potassium levels. Risk factors for the development of hyperkalemia include renal insufficiency, diabetes, and concomitant use of agents that raise potassium levels.

☑ PATIENT TEACHING
● Tell the patient to avoid abrupt discontinuation of therapy but to call doctor to discuss any unpleasant adverse reactions.
Alert: Angioedema (including laryngeal edema) may occur, especially after the first dose. Advise the patient to report any signs or symptoms, such as swelling of face, eyes, lips, or tongue or breathing difficulty.
● Light-headedness can occur, especial-

ly during the first few days of therapy. Tell the patient to rise slowly to minimize this effect and to report symptoms to the doctor. Patients who experience syncope should stop taking drug and call the doctor immediately.

● Advise him to report signs of infection, such as fever and sore throat.

● Tell the patient to avoid sodium substitutes; these products may contain potassium, which can cause hyperkalemia in patients taking ramipril.

● Tell the female patient to notify doctor if pregnancy occurs. Drug will need to be discontinued.

reserpine
Novoreserpine†, Sandril, Serpalan, Serpasil*

Pregnancy Risk Category: C

HOW SUPPLIED
Tablets: 0.1 mg, 0.25 mg

ACTION
Unknown. Thought to be due to reduced cardiac output and possibly decreased peripheral resistance.

ONSET, PEAK, DURATION
Onset occurs in several days to 3 weeks. Peak effect occurs in 3 to 6 weeks. Effects persist for 1 to 6 weeks.

INDICATIONS & DOSAGE
Mild to moderate essential hypertension—
Adults: initially, 0.5 mg daily for 1 to 2 weeks, then maintenance dose of 0.1 to 0.25 mg P.O. daily.
Children: 5 to 20 mcg/kg P.O. daily.

ADVERSE REACTIONS
CNS: *drowsiness, sedation, nervousness, paradoxical anxiety,* dizziness, *nightmares, depression,* extrapyramidal symptoms.
CV: angina, arrhythmias, *bradycardia,* syncope.

EENT: *nasal congestion,* glaucoma, epistaxis.
GI: *hyperacidity, nausea, vomiting, dry mouth,* bleeding, anorexia, diarrhea.
GU: *impotence.*
Skin: pruritus, rash.
Other: *weight gain,* **thrombocytopenic purpura,** dyspnea.

INTERACTIONS
Digitalis glycosides, quinidine: arrhythmias may occur. Monitor patient closely.
Diuretics and other antihypertensives: increased risk of hypotension. Monitor blood pressure closely.
MAO inhibitors: may cause excitability and hypertension. Use together cautiously.

EFFECTS ON DIAGNOSTIC TESTS
Reserpine therapy alters the detection of urinary corticosteroids by colorimetric assay and may interfere with excretion of urinary catecholamines and vanillylmandelic acid.

CONTRAINDICATIONS
Contraindicated in patients with hypersensitivity to the drug, mental depression, ulcerative colitis or peptic ulcer disease and in those receiving electroconvulsive therapy.

NURSING CONSIDERATIONS
● Use cautiously in patients with history of peptic ulcer, ulcerative colitis, or gallstones.
● Monitor blood pressure and pulse rate frequently.

☑ PATIENT TEACHING
● Tell the patient that drug should be taken with meals.
● Tell the patient not to discontinue drug suddenly, but to call the doctor, if unpleasant adverse reactions occur.
● Warn the patient not to perform hazardous tasks that require alertness and coordination until drug's CNS effects are known.

Reactions may be *common,* uncommon, *life-threatening,* or COMMON AND LIFE-THREATENING.

• Advise the patient to minimize orthostatic hypotension by rising slowly and
avoiding sudden position changes. Dry
mouth can be relieved with chewing
gum, sour hard candy, or ice chips. Tell
him to contact the doctor if he needs relief for nasal congestion.
• Tell the patient to weigh himself daily
and to notify the doctor of any weight
gain over 5 lb (about 2 kg).
• Advise the patient to have periodic
eye examinations.
• Tell caregivers to watch the patient
closely for signs of mental depression.
Warn the patient to notify the doctor
promptly if nightmares occur.

terazosin hydrochloride
Hytrin

Pregnancy Risk Category: C

HOW SUPPLIED
Tablets: 1 mg, 2 mg, 5 mg, 10 mg
Capsules: 1 mg, 2 mg, 5 mg, 10 mg

ACTION
Decreases blood pressure by vasodilation produced in response to blockade
of alpha$_1$-adrenergic receptors. Improves urine flow in patients with benign prostatic hyperplasia (BPH) by
blocking alpha$_1$-adrenergic receptors in
the smooth muscle of the bladder neck
and prostate, thus relieving urethral
pressure and reestablishing urine flow.

ONSET, PEAK, DURATION
Onset occurs within 15 minutes. Peak
effects occur within 2 to 3 hours. Effects persist for 24 hours.

INDICATIONS & DOSAGE
Hypertension—
Adults: initially, 1 mg P.O. h.s. Dosage
increased gradually according to patient
response. Usual dosage range is 1 to 5
mg daily. Maximum recommended
dosage is 20 mg/day.
Symptomatic BPH—

Adults: initially, 1 mg P.O. h.s. Dosage
increased in a stepwise fashion to 2, 5,
or 10 mg once daily to achieve optimal
response. Most patients require 10 mg
daily for optimal response.

ADVERSE REACTIONS
CNS: *asthenia, dizziness, headache,*
nervousness, paresthesia, somnolence.
CV: *palpitations,* postural hypotension,
tachycardia, *peripheral edema.*
EENT: *nasal congestion,* sinusitis,
blurred vision.
GI: *nausea.*
GU: impotence.
Respiratory: dyspnea.
Other: back pain, muscle pain.

INTERACTIONS
Antihypertensives: excessive hypotension. Use together cautiously.

EFFECTS ON DIAGNOSTIC TESTS
Terazosin therapy causes small but significant decreases in hematocrit, hemoglobin, WBCs, total protein, and albumin; the magnitude of these decreases
has not been shown to worsen with
time, suggesting the possibility of he-
modilution.

CONTRAINDICATIONS
Contraindicated in patients with hypersensitivity to the drug.

NURSING CONSIDERATIONS
• Monitor blood pressure frequently.
Alert: Know that if terazosin is discontinued for several days, the patient will
need to be retitrated using initial dosing
regimen (1 mg P.O. h.s.).

☑ PATIENT TEACHING
• Tell the patient not to discontinue
drug suddenly, but to call the doctor, if
adverse reactions occur.
• Warn the patient to avoid hazardous
activities that require mental alertness,
such as driving or operating heavy machinery, for 12 hours after the first dose.

timolol maleate
Apo-Timol†, Blocadren

Pregnancy Risk Category: C

HOW SUPPLIED
Tablets: 5 mg, 10 mg, 20 mg

ACTION
Mechanism of antihypertensive action unknown. In MI, may decrease myocardial oxygen requirements. Prevents arterial dilation through beta blockade for migraine headache prophylaxis.

ONSET, PEAK, DURATION
Onset occurs in 15 to 30 minutes. Peak effects occur in 1 to 2 hours. Effects persist for 6 to 12 hours.

INDICATIONS & DOSAGE
Hypertension—
Adults: initially, 10 mg P.O. b.i.d. Usual daily maintenance dosage is 20 to 40 mg. Maximum daily dosage is 60 mg. Allow at least 7 days to elapse between increases in dosage.
MI (long-term prophylaxis in patients who have survived acute phase)—
Adults: 10 mg P.O. b.i.d.
Migraine headache prophylaxis—
Adults: initially, 20 mg P.O. daily as a single dose or in divided doses b.i.d. Increase dosage as needed and tolerated to maximum of 30 mg daily. Discontinue treatment if no response occurs after 6 to 8 weeks of therapy at maximum dosage.

ADVERSE REACTIONS
CNS: fatigue, lethargy, dizziness.
CV: *bradycardia, hypotension, CHF,* peripheral vascular disease, arrhythmias, pulmonary edema.
GI: nausea, vomiting, diarrhea.
Respiratory: dyspnea, *bronchospasm, increased airway resistance.*
Skin: pruritus.

INTERACTIONS
Catecholamine-depleting drugs (such as reserpine): may have additive effect when given with beta blockers. Monitor for hypotension and bradycardia.
Digitalis glycosides, diltiazem, verapamil: excessive bradycardia and increased depressant effect on myocardium. Use together cautiously.
Indomethacin: decreased antihypertensive effect. Monitor blood pressure and adjust dosage.
Insulin, oral antidiabetic agents: can alter requirements for these drugs in previously stabilized diabetic patients. Monitor the patient for hypoglycemia.

EFFECTS ON DIAGNOSTIC TESTS
May slightly increase BUN, serum potassium, uric acid, and blood glucose levels and may slightly decrease hemoglobin and hematocrit levels.

CONTRAINDICATIONS
Contraindicated in patients with bronchial asthma, severe COPD, sinus bradycardia and heart block greater than first-degree, cardiogenic shock, overt CHF, or hypersensitivity to the drug.

NURSING CONSIDERATIONS
● Use cautiously in patients with compensated CHF; hepatic, renal, or respiratory disease; diabetes; and hyperthyroidism.
● Check the patient's apical pulse rate before giving drug. If you detect extremes in pulse rates, withhold drug and call the doctor immediately.
● Monitor blood pressure frequently.
● Monitor blood glucose levels in diabetic patients; drug can mask signs and symptoms of hypoglycemia.

☑ PATIENT TEACHING
● Tell the patient to take drug exactly as prescribed.
● Instruct the patient not to discontinue drug suddenly but to call doctor to discuss any unpleasant adverse reactions. Tell him dosage should be reduced

---

Reactions may be *common*, uncommon, *life-threatening*, or COMMON AND LIFE-THREATENING.

gradually over 1 to 2 weeks.

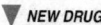 **NEW DRUG**

trandolapril
Mavik

Pregnancy Risk Category: C (D, in 2nd and 3rd trimesters)

HOW SUPPLIED
Tablets: 1 mg, 2 mg, 4 mg

ACTION
Unknown. Thought to result primarily from the inhibition of circulating and tissue ACE activity, thereby reducing angiotensin II formation, decreasing vasoconstriction, decreasing aldosterone secretion, and increasing plasma renin. Decreased aldosterone secretion leads to diuresis, natriuresis, and a small increase in serum potassium. Trandolapril is converted in the liver to the prodrug, trandolaprilat.

ONSET, PEAK, DURATION
Onset unknown. Peak levels of trandolapril occur in 1 hour; 4 and 10 hours for trandolaprilat. Elimination half-lives of trandolapril and trandolaprilat are about 6 and 10 hours, respectively. Like other ACE inhibitors, drug has a prolonged terminal elimination phase.

INDICATIONS & DOSAGE
Hypertension—
Adults: for patient not receiving a diuretic, initially 1 mg for a nonblack patient and 2 mg for a black patient P.O. once daily. If control is not adequate, dosage can be increased at intervals of at least 1 week. Maintenance dosages range from 2 to 4 mg daily for most patients. Some patients receiving oncedaily doses of 4 mg may need b.i.d. doses. For a patient receiving a concurrent diuretic, the initial dose of trandolapril should be 0.5 mg P.O. once daily. Subsequent dosage adjustment is made according to blood pressure response.

ADVERSE REACTIONS
CNS: dizziness, headache, fatigue, drowsiness, insomnia, paresthesia, vertigo, anxiety.
CV: chest pain, first-degree AV block, bradycardia, edema, flushing, hypotension, palpitations.
EENT: epistaxis, throat irritation, upper respiratory tract infection.
GI: diarrhea, dyspepsia, abdominal distention, abdominal pain or cramps, constipation, vomiting, pancreatitis.
GU: urinary frequency, impotence, decreased libido.
Hematologic: neutropenia, leukopenia.
Respiratory: persistent, nonproductive cough; dyspnea.
Skin: rash, pruritus, pemphigus.
Other: *anaphylactic reactions, angioedema,* hyperkalemia, hyponatremia.

INTERACTIONS
Diuretics: increased risk of excessive hypotension. Diuretic may be discontinued or treatment initiated with a lower dose of trandolapril, as ordered.
Lithium: increased serum lithium levels and lithium toxicity. Avoid concomitant use. Monitor serum lithium levels.
Potassium-sparing diuretics, potassium supplements, salt substitutes containing potassium: increased risk of hyperkalemia. Monitor serum potassium closely.

EFFECTS ON DIAGNOSTIC TESTS
Trandolapril may cause minor elevations in creatinine and BUN levels. Elevations of liver enzyme and potassium levels may also occur. Sodium levels and WBC and neutrophil counts may decrease.

CONTRAINDICATIONS
Contraindicated in patients with hypersensitivity to drug and history of angioedema related to previous treatment with an ACE inhibitor. Drug is not recommended for use in pregnant women.

NURSING CONSIDERATIONS

● Use cautiously in patients with impaired renal function, CHF, or renal artery stenosis.

● Monitor serum potassium levels closely.

● Monitor for hypotension. Excessive hypotension can occur when drug is given with diuretics. If possible, diuretic therapy should be discontinued 2 to 3 days before starting trandolapril to decrease potential for excessive hypotension response. If trandolapril does not adequately control blood pressure, diuretic therapy may be reinstituted cautiously, as ordered.

● Assess patient's renal function before and periodically throughout therapy.

● Know that other ACE inhibitors have been associated with agranulocytosis and neutropenia. Monitor CBC with differential before therapy, especially in patients with collagen vascular disease with impaired renal function.

Alert: Be aware that angioedema associated with involvement of the tongue, glottis, or larynx may be fatal because of airway obstruction. Appropriate therapy should be ordered, including epinephrine 1:1,000 (0.3 to 0.5 ml) S.C., and resuscitation equipment for maintaining a patent airway should be readily available.

● If patient develops jaundice, discontinue drug under doctor's advice because, although rare, ACE inhibitors have been associated with a syndrome of cholestatic jaundice, fulminant hepatic necrosis, and death.

● Safety and effectiveness in children have not been established.

● Be aware that it is unknown whether trandolapril is excreted in breast milk. Drug should not be given to breast-feeding women.

☑ PATIENT TEACHING

● Instruct patient to report jaundice.

● Advise patient to report signs of infection, such as fever and sore throat, and any of the following signs or symptoms:

easy bruising or bleeding; swelling of the tongue, lips, face, eyes, mucous membranes, or extremities; difficulty swallowing or breathing; hoarseness; and nonproductive, persistent cough.

● Tell patient to avoid salt substitutes; these products may contain potassium, which can cause hyperkalemia in those taking this drug.

● Tell patient that light-headedness can occur, especially during the first few days of therapy. The patient should rise slowly to minimize this effect and report it immediately.

● Tell patient to use caution in hot weather and during exercise. Inadequate fluid intake, vomiting, diarrhea, and excessive perspiration can lead to light-headedness and syncope.

● Tell female patient to report suspected pregnancy immediately. Drug will need to be discontinued.

● Advise a patient planning to undergo surgery or anesthesia to inform the doctor that he is taking this drug.

▼ *NEW DRUG*

valsartan
Diovan

Pregnancy Risk Category: C (D in 2nd and 3rd trimesters)

HOW SUPPLIED
Capsules: 80 mg, 160 mg

ACTION
Blocks the binding of angiotensin II to receptor sites in vascular smooth muscle and the adrenal gland, which inhibits the pressor effects of the renin-angiotensin system.

ONSET, PEAK, DURATION
Onset occurs within 2 hours. Plasma levels peak within 2 to 4 hours, and effects persist for 24 hours.

INDICATIONS & DOSAGE
Hypertension, used alone or in combi-

nation with other antihypertensives—
Adults: initially, 80 mg P.O. once daily.
Expect to see a reduction in blood pressure in 2 to 4 weeks. If additional antihypertensive effect is needed, dosage may be increased to 160 or 320 mg daily, or a diuretic may be added. (Addition of a diuretic has a greater effect than dosage increases beyond 80 mg.) Usual dosage range is 80 to 320 mg daily.

ADVERSE REACTIONS
CNS: headache, dizziness.
CV: hyperkalemia, edema.
GI: abdominal pain, diarrhea, nausea.
Hematologic: neutropenia.
Musculoskeletal: arthralgia.
Respiratory: upper respiratory infection, cough, rhinitis, sinusitis, pharyngitis.
Other: viral infection, fatigue.

INTERACTIONS
Diuretics: risk of excessive hypotension. Assess fluid status before starting concomitant therapy. Monitor closely.

EFFECTS ON DIAGNOSTIC TESTS
None reported.

CONTRAINDICATIONS
Contraindicated in patients with known hypersensitivity to drug.

NURSING CONSIDERATIONS
● Use cautiously in patients with renal or hepatic disease.
● Know that valsartan can cause fetal or neonatal morbidity and death if administered to a pregnant woman in the second or third trimester. Breast-feeding women should not take drug.
● Be aware that safety and effectiveness in children have not been established.
● Monitor for hypotension. Excessive hypotension can occur when drug is given with high doses of diuretics. Correct volume and salt depletions as ordered before starting drug.

☑ PATIENT TEACHING
● Tell female patient to notify doctor if pregnancy occurs; drug will need to be discontinued.
● Tell patient drug may be taken with or without food.

Antilipemics

atorvastatin calcium
cholestyramine
colestipol hydrochloride
fluvastatin sodium
gemfibrozil
lovastatin
niacin
   (See Chapter 90, vitamins and
   minerals.)
pravastatin sodium
simvastatin

COMBINATION PRODUCTS
None.

▼ NEW DRUG

atorvastatin calcium
Lipitor

Pregnancy Risk Category: X

HOW SUPPLIED
Tablets: 10 mg, 20 mg, 40 mg

ACTION
Inhibits 3-hydroxy-3-methylglutaryl-
coenzyme A reductase, an early (and
rate-limiting) step in cholesterol biosynthesis.

ONSET, PEAK, DURATION
Rapidly absorbed. Plasma levels peak
within 1 to 2 hours. Therapeutic response can be seen within 2 weeks;
peaks within 4 weeks.

INDICATIONS & DOSAGE
*Adjunct to diet to reduce low-density
lipoprotein (LDL), total cholesterol,
apo B, and triglyceride levels in patients with primary hypercholesterolemia and mixed dyslipidemia—*
Adults: initially, 10 mg P.O. once daily.
Dosage increased as needed to a maximum of 80 mg daily as a single dose.

Dosage based on blood lipid levels
drawn within 2 to 4 weeks after starting
therapy.
*Alone or as an adjunct to lipid-lowering
treatments such as LDL apheresis in patients with homozygous familial hypercholesterolemia—*
Adults: 10 to 80 mg P.O. once daily.

ADVERSE REACTIONS
CNS: *headache,* asthenia.
GI: abdominal pain, constipation, diar-
rhea, dyspepsia, flatulence.
Musculoskeletal: back pain, arthralgia,
myalgia.
Respiratory: sinusitis, pharyngitis.
Skin: rash.
Other: *infection,* accidental injury, flu-
like syndrome, allergic reaction.

INTERACTIONS
*Azole antifungals, cyclosporine, ery-
thromycin, fibric acid derivatives,
niacin:* possible risk of rhabdomyolysis.
Avoid concomitant use.
Digoxin: may increase plasma digoxin
levels. Monitor serum digoxin levels.
Erythromycin: will increase plasma
concentration of drug. Monitor patient.
Oral contraceptives: increased levels of
hormones. Consider when selecting an
oral contraceptive.

EFFECTS ON DIAGNOSTIC TESTS
Drug may increase liver function test results.

CONTRAINDICATIONS
Contraindicated in patients hypersensitive to the drug or with active liver disease or conditions associated with unexplained persistent elevations of serum
transaminase levels; in pregnant and
breast-feeding women; and in women of
childbearing age (except in women not
at risk for becoming pregnant).

NURSING CONSIDERATIONS
• Use cautiously in patients with a history of liver disease or heavy alcohol use.
• Know that drug should be withheld or discontinued in patients with serious, acute conditions that suggest myopathy or those at risk for renal failure secondary to rhabdomyolysis as a result of trauma; major surgery; severe metabolic, endocrine, and electrolyte disorders; severe acute infection; hypotension; or uncontrolled seizures.
• Know that experience in pediatric patients has been limited to patients with homozygous familial hypercholesterolemia over 9 years.
• Atorvastatin therapy should be initiated only after diet and other nonpharmacologic treatments prove ineffective. Patient should follow a standard low-cholesterol diet before and during therapy.
• Before initiating treatment, secondary causes for hypercholesterolemia should be excluded and a baseline lipid profile done. Periodic liver function tests and lipid levels should be done, as ordered, before starting treatment, at 6 and 12 weeks after initiation or after an increase in dosage and periodically thereafter.
• Know that drug may be given as a single dose at any time of day, with or without food.
• Watch for signs of myositis.

☑ PATIENT TEACHING
• Teach patient about proper dietary management, weight control, and exercise. Explain their importance in controlling elevated serum lipid levels.
• Warn patient to avoid alcohol.
• Tell patient to inform the doctor of adverse reactions, such as muscle pain, malaise, and fever.
Alert: Inform female patient that drug is contraindicated during pregnancy due to the potential of danger to the fetus. Advise her to notify doctor immediately if pregnancy occurs.

cholestyramine
Cholybar, Prevalite, Questran**, Questran Light, Questran Lite‡

Pregnancy Risk Category: NR

HOW SUPPLIED
Powder: 378-g cans, 9-g single-dose packets. Each scoop of powder or single-dose packet contains 4 g of cholestyramine resin.
Tablets: 1 g

ACTION
A bile-acid sequestrant that combines with bile acid to form an insoluble compound that is excreted. The liver must synthesize new bile acid from cholesterol, which reduces low-density-lipoprotein cholesterol levels.

ONSET, PEAK, DURATION
Fall in low-density lipoprotein concentration occurs in 4 to 7 days. Reduction of plasma cholesterol concentrations generally within 1 month of therapy. After withdrawal of drug, cholesterol concentrations return to baseline in about 2 to 4 weeks.

INDICATIONS & DOSAGE
Primary hyperlipidemia or pruritus caused by partial bile obstruction; adjunct for reduction of elevated serum cholesterol in patients with primary hypercholesterolemia—
Adults: 4 g once or twice daily. Maintenance dosage is 8 to 16 g daily divided into two doses. Maximum daily dosage is 24 g.

ADVERSE REACTIONS
CNS: headache, anxiety, vertigo, dizziness, insomnia, fatigue, syncope, tinnitus.
GI: *constipation, fecal impaction,* hemorrhoids, *abdominal discomfort,* flatulence, *nausea,* vomiting, steatorrhea, GI bleeding, diarrhea, anorexia.
GU: hematuria, dysuria.

*Liquid contains alcohol.　**May contain tartrazine.　†Canada only.　‡Australia only.　◇OTC.

Skin: *rash;* irritation of skin, tongue, and perianal area.
Other: *vitamin A, D, E, and K deficiencies from decreased absorption,* hyperchloremic acidosis with long-term use or very high dosage, anemia, ecchymoses, backache, muscle and joint pains, bleeding tendencies, osteoporosis.

INTERACTIONS
Acetaminophen, beta-adrenergic blockers, corticosteroids, digitalis glycosides, fat-soluble vitamins (A, D, E, and K), iron preparations, thiazide diuretics, thyroid hormones, warfarin and other coumarin derivatives: absorption may be substantially decreased by cholestyramine. Administer other drugs 1 hour before or 4 to 6 hours after cholestyramine resin.

EFFECTS ON DIAGNOSTIC TESTS
Drug therapy alters serum concentrations of alkaline phosphatase, AST, chloride, phosphorous, potassium, calcium, and sodium. Impaired calcium absorption may lead to osteoporosis. Cholecystography using iopanoic acid is also bound by cholestyramine.

CONTRAINDICATIONS
Contraindicated in patients with hypersensitivity to bile-acid sequestering resins and in those with complete biliary obstruction.

NURSING CONSIDERATIONS
● Use cautiously in patients predisposed to constipation and in those with conditions aggravated by constipation, such as severe, symptomatic coronary artery disease.
● Monitor serum cholesterol and triglyceride levels regularly during therapy.
● Monitor serum levels of digitalis glycosides in patients receiving digitalis glycosides and cholestyramine concurrently. If cholestyramine therapy is discontinued, adjust dosage of digitalis glycosides as ordered to avoid toxicity.
● Monitor bowel habits. Encourage a diet high in fiber and fluids. If severe constipation develops, decrease dosage, add a stool softener, or discontinue drug, as ordered.
● Be aware that long-term use may be associated with deficiencies of vitamins A, D, E, and K and folic acid.

☑ PATIENT TEACHING
Alert: Tell the patient never to take drug in its dry form; esophageal irritation or severe constipation may result.
● Instruct the patient to mix powder as follows: Using a large glass, the patient should sprinkle the powder on the surface of preferred beverage; let the mixture stand a few minutes; then stir thoroughly. The best diluents are water, milk, and juice (especially pulpy fruit juice). Mixing with carbonated beverages may result in excessive foaming. After drinking this preparation, the patient should swirl a small additional amount of liquid in the same glass and then drink it to ensure ingestion of the entire dose.
● Advise the patient to take all other drugs at least 1 hour before or 4 to 6 hours after cholestyramine to avoid blocking their absorption.
● Teach the patient about proper dietary management of serum lipids. When appropriate, recommend weight-control, exercise, and smoking-cessation programs.

colestipol hydrochloride
Colestid

Pregnancy Risk Category: NR

HOW SUPPLIED
Granules: 300-g and 500-g bottles, 5-g packets
Tablets: 1 g

ACTION
Combines with bile acid to form an in-

soluble compound that is excreted in feces. The liver must synthesize new bile acid from cholesterol; this leads to reduced low-density-lipoprotein cholesterol levels.

ONSET, PEAK, DURATION
Antilipemic effects evident at about 1 month of therapy. Lipid levels return to pretreatment values within 1 month of discontinuing treatment.

INDICATIONS & DOSAGE
Primary hypercholesterolemia—
Adults: granules: 5 to 30 g P.O. once daily or in divided doses; tablets: 2 to 16 g/day given once or in divided doses.

ADVERSE REACTIONS
CNS: headache, dizziness, anxiety, vertigo, insomnia, fatigue, syncope, tinnitus.
CNS: *constipation, fecal impaction,* hemorrhoids, abdominal discomfort, flatulence, nausea, vomiting, steatorrhea, GI bleeding, diarrhea, anorexia.
GU: dysuria, hematuria.
Skin: rash; irritation of tongue and perianal area.
Other: vitamin A, D, E, and K deficiencies from decreased absorption; hyperchloremic acidosis with long-term use or high dosage, anemia, ecchymoses, bleeding tendencies, backache, muscle and joint pain, osteoporosis.

INTERACTIONS
Oral antidiabetic agents: may antagonize response to colestipol. Monitor serum lipids.
Orally administered drugs: colestipol may decrease absorption. Separate administration times; give other drugs at least 1 hour before or 4 hours after colestipol.

EFFECTS ON DIAGNOSTIC TESTS
Colestipol alters serum levels of alkaline phosphatase, ALT, AST, chloride, phosphorous, potassium, and sodium.

CONTRAINDICATIONS
Contraindicated in patients with hypersensitivity reactions to bile-acid sequestering resins.

NURSING CONSIDERATIONS
● Use cautiously in patients predisposed to constipation and in those with conditions aggravated by constipation, such as severe, symptomatic coronary artery disease.
● Monitor serum cholesterol and triglyceride levels regularly during therapy.
● Monitor bowel habits; if severe constipation develops, decrease dosage or add stool softener as ordered. Encourage a diet high in fiber and fluids.
● Monitor serum levels of digitalis glycosides in patients receiving digitalis glycosides and colestipol concurrently. If colestipol therapy is discontinued, adjust dosage of digitalis glycosides to avoid toxicity, as ordered.

☑ PATIENT TEACHING
Alert: Tell the patient never to take drug in its dry form; esophageal irritation or severe constipation may result.
● To prepare, instruct the patient to use a large glass containing water, milk, or juice (especially pulpy fruit juice). The patient should sprinkle the powder on the surface of the preferred beverage; let the mixture stand a few minutes; then stir thoroughly to obtain a uniform suspension. After drinking this preparation, the patient should swirl a small additional amount of liquid in the same glass and then drink it to ensure ingestion of the entire dose.
● To enhance palatability, tell the patient to mix and refrigerate the next daily dose the previous evening.
● Instruct the patient taking tablet form to swallow tablets whole and not to crush, cut, or chew them.
● Advise the patient to take all other drugs at least 1 hour before or 4 to 6 hours after colestipol to avoid blocking their absorption.

---

*Liquid contains alcohol. **May contain tartrazine. †Canada only. ‡Australia only. ◇OTC.

• Teach the patient about proper dietary management of serum lipids. When appropriate, recommend weight-control, exercise, and smoking-cessation programs.

• Inform the patient that long-term use may be associated with deficiencies of vitamins A, D, E, and K and folic acid. Instruct patient to report any unusual signs and symptoms.

---

fluvastatin sodium
Lescol

Pregnancy Risk Category: X

HOW SUPPLIED
Capsules: 20 mg, 40 mg

ACTION
Inhibits 3-hydroxy-3-methylglutaryl coenzyme A reductase. This enzyme is an early (and rate-limiting) step in the synthetic pathway of cholesterol.

ONSET, PEAK, DURATION
Onset and duration is unknown. Peak plasma levels occur about 1 hour after oral administration; maximal lipid-lowering effect occurs within 4 weeks.

INDICATIONS & DOSAGE
Reduction of low-density lipoprotein and total cholesterol levels in patients with primary hypercholesterolemia (types IIa and IIb)—
Adults: initially, 20 mg P.O. h.s. Increase dosage as needed to a maximum of 40 mg daily.

ADVERSE REACTIONS
CNS: headache, fatigue, dizziness, insomnia.
GI: dyspepsia, diarrhea, nausea, vomiting, abdominal pain, constipation, flatulence, tooth disorder.
Hematologic: *thrombocytopenia, hemolytic anemia, leukopenia.*
Respiratory: sinusitis, *upper respiratory infection,* rhinitis, cough, pharyngitis,

bronchitis.
Other: arthropathy, muscle pain, hypersensitivity reactions (rash, pruritus), increased liver enzyme levels.

INTERACTIONS
Cholestyramine, colestipol: may bind with fluvastatin in the GI tract and decrease absorption. Separate administration times by at least 4 hours.
Cimetidine, omeprazole, ranitidine: decreased fluvastatin metabolism. Monitor for enhanced effects.
Cyclosporine and other immunosuppressants, erythromycin, gemfibrozil, niacin: possible increased risk of polymyositis and rhabdomyolysis. Avoid concomitant use.
Digoxin: may alter digoxin pharmacokinetics. Monitor serum digoxin levels carefully.
Ethanol: increased risk of hepatotoxicity. Avoid concomitant use.
Rifampin: enhanced fluvastatin metabolism and decreased plasma levels. Monitor for lack of effect.
Warfarin: increased anticoagulant effect with bleeding. Monitor patient.

EFFECTS ON DIAGNOSTIC TESTS
May elevate serum ALT, AST, CK, alkaline phosphatase, and bilirubin levels. Thyroid function test abnormalities also can occur.

CONTRAINDICATIONS
Contraindicated in patients with hypersensitivity to the drug; in those with active liver disease or conditions associated with unexplained persistent elevations of serum transaminase levels; in pregnant and breast-feeding women; and in women of childbearing age unless there is no risk of pregnancy.

NURSING CONSIDERATIONS
• Use cautiously in patients with severe renal impairment and history of liver disease or heavy alcohol use.
• Know that fluvastatin should be initiated only after diet and other nonphar-

---

Reactions may be *common*, uncommon, *life-threatening*, or COMMON AND LIFE-THREATENING.

macologic therapies prove ineffective. The patient should be on a standard low-cholesterol diet during therapy.
● Be aware that liver function tests should be performed at the start of therapy and periodically thereafter.
● Watch for signs of myositis.

☑ **PATIENT TEACHING**
● Tell the patient that drug may be taken without regard to meals; however, efficacy is enhanced if the drug is taken in the evening.
● Teach the patient about proper dietary management, weight control, and exercise. Explain their importance in controlling elevated serum lipids levels.
● Warn the patient to avoid alcohol.
● Tell the patient to inform the doctor of any adverse reactions, particularly muscle aches and pains.
Alert: Inform the female patient that drug is contraindicated during pregnancy. Advise her to notify doctor immediately if pregnancy occurs.

---

gemfibrozil
Lopid

Pregnancy Risk Category: C

HOW SUPPLIED
Tablets: 600 mg
Capsules: 300 mg

ACTION
Inhibits peripheral lipolysis and also reduces triglyceride synthesis in the liver. Lowers serum triglyceride levels and increases high-density-lipoprotein cholesterol levels.

ONSET, PEAK, DURATION
Onset occurs in 2 to 5 days. Peak effect occurs after 4 weeks of treatment. Duration unknown.

INDICATIONS & DOSAGE
Types IV and V hyperlipidemia unresponsive to diet and other drugs; reduc-tion of risk of coronary heart disease in patients with type IIb hyperlipidemia who cannot tolerate or who are refractory to treatment with bile acid sequestrants or niacin—
Adults: 1,200 mg P.O. daily in two divided doses, 30 minutes before morning and evening meals.

ADVERSE REACTIONS
CNS: headache, fatigue, vertigo.
CV: atrial fibrillation.
GI: *abdominal and epigastric pain, diarrhea, nausea,* vomiting, *dyspepsia,* constipation, acute appendicitis.
Hematologic: *anemia, leukopenia,* eosinophilia, *thrombocytopenia.*
Hepatic: bile duct obstruction, elevated liver enzymes.
Skin: rash, dermatitis, pruritus, eczema.

INTERACTIONS
Lovastatin: myopathy with rhabdomyolysis has been reported. Don't use together.
Oral anticoagulants: gemfibrozil may enhance the clinical effects of oral anticoagulants. Monitor closely.

EFFECTS ON DIAGNOSTIC TESTS
Gemfibrozil therapy may elevate serum levels of creatinine phosphokinase, ALT, AST, alkaline phosphatase, and lactate dehydrogenase; it may also decrease serum potassium, hematocrit, hemoglobin, and leukocyte counts.

CONTRAINDICATIONS
Contraindicated in patients with hypersensitivity to the drug, or hepatic or severe renal dysfunction (including primary biliary cirrhosis), and preexisting gallbladder disease.

NURSING CONSIDERATIONS
● Know that periodic CBCs and liver function tests should be performed during the first 12 months of therapy.
● If the drug has no beneficial effects after 3 months of therapy, expect the doctor to discontinue the drug.

---

*Liquid contains alcohol.   **May contain tartrazine.   †Canada only.   ‡Australia only.   ◇OTC.

☑ **PATIENT TEACHING**
● Instruct the patient to take drug ½ hour before breakfast and dinner.
● Teach the patient about proper dietary management of serum lipids. When appropriate, recommend weight-control, exercise, and smoking-cessation programs.
● Because of possible dizziness and blurred vision, advise the patient to avoid driving or other potentially hazardous activities until drug's CNS effects are known.
● Tell the patient to observe bowel movements and to report any evidence of steatorrhea or other signs of bile duct obstruction.

lovastatin (mevinolin)
Mevacor

Pregnancy Risk Category: X

HOW SUPPLIED
Tablets: 10 mg, 20 mg, 40 mg

ACTION
Inhibits 3-hydroxy-3-methylglutaryl coenzyme A reductase. This enzyme is an early (and rate-limiting) step in the synthetic pathway of cholesterol.

ONSET, PEAK, DURATION
Plasma levels peak within 2 hours after a dose. After withdrawal of continuous therapy, effects persist for 4 to 6 weeks. Maximal therapeutic effect occurs within 4 to 6 weeks.

INDICATIONS & DOSAGE
Reduction of low-density lipoprotein and total cholesterol levels in patients with primary hypercholesterolemia (types IIa and IIb)—
Adults: initially, 20 mg P.O. once daily with evening meal. For patients with severely elevated cholesterol levels (for example, over 300 mg/dl), initial dose is 40 mg. Recommended daily dosage range is 10 to 80 mg in single or divided

doses.

ADVERSE REACTIONS
CNS: headache, dizziness, peripheral neuropathy, insomnia.
EENT: blurred vision.
GI: constipation, diarrhea, dyspepsia, flatulence, abdominal pain or cramps, heartburn, nausea, vomiting.
Skin: rash, pruritus, alopecia.
Other: muscle cramps, myalgia, myositis, *rhabdomyolysis*, abnormal liver test results, chest pain.

INTERACTIONS
Cyclosporine or other immunosuppressants, erythromycin, gemfibrozil, niacin: possible increased risk of polymyositis and rhabdomyolysis (maximum recommended lovastatin dosage is 20 mg daily); monitor the patient closely.
Ethanol: increased risk of hepatotoxicity. Avoid concomitant use.
Oral anticoagulants: lovastatin may enhance the clinical effects of oral anticoagulants. Monitor the patient closely.

EFFECTS ON DIAGNOSTIC TESTS
May elevate serum CK or serum transaminase levels.

CONTRAINDICATIONS
Contraindicated in patients with hypersensitivity to the drug; in those with active liver disease or conditions associated with unexplained persistent elevations of serum transaminase levels; in pregnant and breast-feeding patients; and in women of childbearing age unless there is no risk of pregnancy.

NURSING CONSIDERATIONS
● Use cautiously in patients who consume substantial quantities of alcohol or have a past history of liver disease.
● Know that lovastatin should be initiated only after diet and other nonpharmacologic therapies prove ineffective. The patient should be on a standard low-cholesterol diet during therapy.
● Be aware that liver function tests

Reactions may be *common,* uncommon, *life-threatening,* or COMMON AND LIFE-THREATENING.

should be performed at the start of therapy and periodically thereafter.

☑ PATIENT TEACHING
● Instruct the patient to take lovastatin with the evening meal, when absorption is enhanced and cholesterol biosynthesis is greater.
● Teach the patient about proper dietary management of serum lipids. When appropriate, recommend weight-control, exercise, and smoking-cessation programs.
● Advise him to have periodic eye examinations; related compounds have caused cataracts in laboratory animals.
● Tell him to store tablets at room temperature in a light-resistant container.
Alert: Inform the female patient that drug is contraindicated during pregnancy. Advise her to notify doctor immediately if pregnancy occurs.

---

pravastatin sodium (eptastatin)
Pravachol

Pregnancy Risk Category: X

HOW SUPPLIED
Tablets: 10 mg, 20 mg, 40 mg

ACTION
Inhibits 3-hydroxy-3-methylglutaryl coenzyme A reductase. This enzyme is an early (and rate-limiting) step in the synthetic pathway of cholesterol.

ONSET, PEAK, DURATION
Onset and duration are unknown. Plasma levels peak within 1 to 1½ hours.

INDICATIONS & DOSAGE
Reduction of low-density lipoprotein and total cholesterol levels in patients with primary hypercholesterolemia (types IIa and IIb)—
Adults: initially, 10 or 20 mg P.O. daily h.s. Dosage adjusted q 4 weeks based on patient tolerance and response; maxi-

mum daily dosage is 40 mg. Most elderly patients respond to a daily dosage of 20 mg or less.

ADVERSE REACTIONS
CNS: headache, dizziness, fatigue.
CV: chest pain.
EENT: rhinitis.
GI: vomiting, diarrhea, heartburn, abdominal pain, constipation, flatulence, nausea.
GU: renal failure secondary to myoglobinuria, urinary abnormality.
Respiratory: cough, influenza, common cold.
Skin: rash.
Other: flulike symptoms, myositis, myopathy, *localized muscle pain,* myalgia, ***rhabdomyolysis.***

INTERACTIONS
Cholestyramine, colestipol: concomitant administration decreases plasma levels of pravastatin. Administer pravastatin 1 hour before or 4 hours after these drugs.
Drugs that decrease levels or activity of endogenous steroids (such as cimetidine, ketoconazole, spironolactone): may increase risk of developing endocrine dysfunction. No intervention appears necessary; take complete drug history in patients who develop endocrine dysfunction.
Erythromycin, fibric acid derivatives (such as clofibrate or gemfibrozil), immunosuppressants (such as cyclosporine), high doses (1 g or more daily) of niacin (nicotinic acid): may increase the risk of rhabdomyolysis. Monitor the patient closely if concomitant use cannot be avoided.
Ethanol, hepatotoxic drugs: increased risk of hepatotoxicity. Avoid concomitant use.
Gemfibrozil: decreases protein-binding and urinary clearance of pravastatin. Avoid concomitant use.

EFFECTS ON DIAGNOSTIC TESTS
Serum ALT, AST, CK, alkaline phos-

---

phatase, and bilirubin levels are increased; thyroid function test is abnormal.

CONTRAINDICATIONS
Contraindicated in patients with hypersensitivity to the drug; in those with active liver disease or conditions that cause unexplained, persistent elevations of serum transaminase levels; in pregnant and breast-feeding patients; and in women of childbearing age unless there is no risk of pregnancy.

NURSING CONSIDERATIONS
● Use cautiously in patients who consume large quantities of alcohol or have history of liver disease.
● Know that pravastatin should be initiated only after diet and other nonpharmacologic therapies prove ineffective. Patients should be on a standard low-cholesterol diet during therapy.
● Know that liver function tests should be performed at the start of therapy and periodically thereafter. A liver biopsy may be performed if liver enzyme elevations persist.

☑ **PATIENT TEACHING**
● Instruct the patient to take the recommended dosage in the evening, preferably at bedtime.
● Teach the patient about proper dietary management of serum lipids. When appropriate, recommend weight-control, exercise, and smoking-cessation programs.
Alert: Inform the female patient that drug is contraindicated during pregnancy. Advise her to notify doctor immediately if pregnancy occurs.

---

simvastatin (syvinolin)
Lipex‡, Zocor

Pregnancy Risk Category: X

HOW SUPPLIED
Tablets: 5 mg, 10 mg, 20 mg, 40 mg

ACTION
Inhibits 3-hydroxy-3-methylglutaryl coenzyme A reductase. This enzyme is an early (and rate-limiting) step in the synthetic pathway of cholesterol.

ONSET, PEAK, DURATION
Onset and duration unknown. Peak plasma levels occur in 1.3 to 2.4 hours.

INDICATIONS & DOSAGE
Reduction of low-density lipoprotein (LDL) and total cholesterol levels in patients with primary hypercholesterolemia (types IIa and IIb)—
Adults: initially, 5 to 10 mg P.O. daily in the evening. Dosage adjusted q 4 weeks based on patient tolerance and response; maximum daily dosage is 40 mg.

ADVERSE REACTIONS
CNS: headache, asthenia.
GI: abdominal pain, constipation, diarrhea, dyspepsia, flatulence, nausea, vomiting.
Hepatic: elevated liver enzymes.
Respiratory: upper respiratory tract infection.

INTERACTIONS
Digoxin: simvastatin may elevate digoxin levels slightly. Closely monitor plasma digoxin levels at initiation of simvastatin therapy.
Drugs that decrease levels or activity of endogenous steroids (such as cimetidine, ketoconazole, spironolactone): may increase risk of developing endocrine dysfunction. No intervention appears necessary; take complete drug history in patients who develop endocrine dysfunction.
Erythromycin, fibric acid derivatives (such as clofibrate or gemfibrozil), immunosuppressants (such as cyclosporine), high doses (1 g or more daily) of niacin (nicotinic acid): may increase risk of rhabdomyolysis. Monitor the patient closely if concomitant use cannot be avoided. Limit daily dosage of sim-

---

vastatin to 10 mg if the patient must take cyclosporine.

Ethanol, hepatotoxic drugs: increased risk of hepatotoxicity. Avoid concomitant use.

Warfarin: anticoagulant effect may be slightly enhanced. Monitor the patient's PT at start of therapy and during dosage adjustments.

EFFECTS ON DIAGNOSTIC TESTS
As expected, simvastatin will reduce total plasma cholesterol, very-low-density lipoprotein (VLDL), and LDL, and may variably increase high-density lipoprotein (HDL). The ratios of total cholesterol to HDL, total cholesterol to LDL, and LDL to HDL are reduced. Modest decreases in triglycerides may also occur.

Toxic effects of the drug may be evident by marked, persistent elevations of serum transaminases. During clinical trials, about 5% of patients had asymptomatic marked elevations in the noncardiac fraction of CK.

CONTRAINDICATIONS
Contraindicated in patients with hypersensitivity to the drug and in those with active liver disease or conditions that cause unexplained persistent elevations of serum transaminase; in pregnant and breast-feeding patients; and in women of childbearing age unless there is no risk of pregnancy.

NURSING CONSIDERATIONS
● Use cautiously in patients who consume substantial quantities of alcohol or have a history of liver disease.
● Know that simvastatin is initiated only after diet and other nonpharmacologic therapies prove ineffective. The patient should be on a standard low-cholesterol diet during therapy.
● Know that liver function tests should be performed at the start of therapy and periodically thereafter. A liver biopsy may be performed if enzyme elevations persist.

☑ **PATIENT TEACHING**
● Instruct the patient to take simvastatin with the evening meal; absorption is enhanced and cholesterol biosynthesis is greater.
● Teach the patient about proper dietary management of serum lipids. When appropriate, recommend weight-control, exercise, and smoking-cessation programs.
● Tell the patient to inform the doctor of any adverse reactions, particularly muscle aches and pains.
Alert: Inform the female patient that drug is contraindicated during pregnancy. Advise her to notify the doctor immediately if pregnancy occurs.

alprostadil
dipyridamole
isoxsuprine hydrochloride
midodrine hydrochloride
papaverine hydrochloride
pentoxifylline
ticlopidine hydrochloride
tolazoline hydrochloride

COMBINATION PRODUCTS
None.

---

alprostadil
Prostin VR Pediatric

Pregnancy Risk Category: NR

HOW SUPPLIED
Injection: 500 mcg/ml

ACTION
A prostaglandin derivative that relaxes the smooth muscle of the ductus arteriosus.

ONSET, PEAK, DURATION
Onset occurs within 20 minutes. Peak levels occur within 1 to 2 hours. Effects persist for length of infusion.

INDICATIONS & DOSAGE
Palliative therapy for temporary maintenance of patency of ductus arteriosus until surgery can be performed—
Infants: 0.05 to 0.1 mcg/kg/minute by I.V. infusion. When therapeutic response is achieved, infusion rate reduced to lowest dosage that will maintain response. Maximum dosage is 0.4 mcg/kg/minute. Or, drug can be administered through umbilical artery catheter placed at ductal opening.

ADVERSE REACTIONS
CNS: *seizures.*

CV: bradycardia, hypotension, tachycardia, ***cardiac arrest,*** edema.
GI: diarrhea.
Hematologic: ***disseminated intravascular coagulation.***
Other: **apnea,** *flushing, fever, sepsis,* hypokalemia.

INTERACTIONS
None significant.

EFFECTS ON DIAGNOSTIC TESTS
None reported.

CONTRAINDICATIONS
None known.

NURSING CONSIDERATIONS
● Know that a differential diagnosis should be made between respiratory distress syndrome and cyanotic heart disease before drug is administered. Drug should not be used in neonates with respiratory distress syndrome.
● Use cautiously in neonates with bleeding tendencies because drug inhibits platelet aggregation.
● Dilute drug before administering. Prepare fresh solution daily; discard solution after 24 hours.
● Do not use diluents that contain benzyl alcohol. Fatal toxic syndrome may occur.
● **I.V. use:** Know that this drug is not recommended for direct injection or intermittent infusion. Administer by continuous infusion using a constant-rate pump. Infuse through a large peripheral or central vein or through an umbilical artery catheter placed at the level of the ductus arteriosus. If flushing occurs from peripheral vasodilation, reposition catheter.
● Reduce infusion rate if fever or significant hypotension occurs.
● Keep respiratory support available.

Reactions may be *common,* uncommon, ***life-threatening,*** or COMMON AND LIFE-THREATENING.

• In infants with restricted pulmonary blood flow, measure drug's effectiveness by monitoring blood oxygenation. In infants with restricted systemic blood flow, measure drug's effectiveness by monitoring systemic blood pressure and blood pH.
• Monitor arterial pressure by umbilical artery catheter, auscultation, or Doppler transducer. Slow rate of infusion if arterial pressure falls significantly.
Alert: If apnea and bradycardia (may reflect drug overdose) occur, stop infusion immediately.
• Keep in mind that CV and CNS adverse reactions are more frequent in infants weighing less than 2 kg and in those receiving infusions for longer than 48 hours.

☑ **PATIENT TEACHING**
• Inform parents of the need for alprostadil and explain its use.
• Encourage parents to ask questions and express concerns.

dipyridamole
Apo-Dipyridamole†, Dipridacot, I.V. Persantine, Novodipiradol†, Persantin‡, Persantin 100‡, Persantine**

Pregnancy Risk Category: B

HOW SUPPLIED
Tablets: 25 mg, 50 mg, 75 mg
Injection: 10 mg/2 ml

ACTION
Unknown but may involve its ability to increase adenosine, which is a coronary vasodilator and platelet aggregation inhibitor.

ONSET, PEAK, DURATION
Onset and duration are unknown. Plasma levels peak about 75 minutes after oral dose; within 2 minutes after I.V. administration.

INDICATIONS & DOSAGE
Inhibition of platelet adhesion in prosthetic heart valves (in combination with warfarin or aspirin)—
Adults: 75 to 100 mg P.O. q.i.d.
Alternative to exercise in evaluation of coronary artery disease during thallium (^{201}Tl) myocardial perfusion scintigraphy—
Adults: 0.57 mg/kg as an I.V. infusion at a constant rate over 4 minutes (0.142 mg/kg/minute).
Acute coronary insufficiency—
Adults: 10 mg I.V. or I.M.

ADVERSE REACTIONS
CNS: *headache, dizziness.*
CV: flushing, syncope, hypotension; angina, chest pain, *ECG abnormalities,* blood pressure lability, hypertension (with I.V. infusion).
GI: *nausea,* vomiting, diarrhea, abdominal distress.
Skin: rash, irritation (with undiluted injection), pruritus.

INTERACTIONS
Heparin: may increase risk of bleeding. Monitor closely.
Theophylline: may prevent the coronary vasodilation by I.V. dipyridamole.

EFFECTS ON DIAGNOSTIC TESTS
Drug's physiologic effects on platelet aggregation will cause an increase in bleeding time.

CONTRAINDICATIONS
Contraindicated in patients with hypersensitivity to dipyridamole.

NURSING CONSIDERATIONS
• Use cautiously in patients with hypotension.
• If the patient develops GI distress, administer 1 hour before meals or with meals.
• **I.V. use:** If administering as a diagnostic agent, dilute in 0.45% or 0.9% sodium chloride solution or D_5W in at least a 1:2 ratio for a total volume of

20 to 50 ml. Inject ^{201}Tl within 5 minutes after completing the 4-minute dipyridamole infusion.

● Observe for adverse reactions, especially with large doses. Monitor blood pressure.

● Observe for signs of bleeding; note prolonged bleeding time (especially with large doses or long-term therapy).

● Know that dipyridamole's value as part of an antithrombotic regimen is controversial; using it may not provide significantly better results than using aspirin alone.

☑ **PATIENT TEACHING**
● Instruct the patient to take drug exactly as prescribed.
● Tell patient to report adverse reactions promptly.
● Tell patient receiving drug I.V. to alert nurse if discomfort occurs at insertion site.

---

isoxsuprine hydrochloride
Duvadilan‡, Vasodilan

Pregnancy Risk Category: NR

HOW SUPPLIED
Tablets: 10 mg, 20 mg

ACTION
Produces peripheral vasodilation by a direct effect on vascular smooth muscle.

ONSET, PEAK, DURATION
Onset and duration unknown. Serum levels peak in 1 hour after oral administration.

INDICATIONS & DOSAGE
Adjunct for relief of symptoms associated with cerebrovascular insufficiency, peripheral vascular diseases (such as arteriosclerosis obliterans, thromboangiitis obliterans, Raynaud's disease)—
Adults: 10 to 20 mg P.O. t.i.d. or q.i.d.

ADVERSE REACTIONS
CNS: trembling, weakness, dizziness.
CV: tachycardia, hypotension, chest pain.
GI: vomiting, abdominal distress, nausea.
Skin: severe rash.

INTERACTIONS
None significant.

EFFECTS ON DIAGNOSTIC TESTS
No information available.

CONTRAINDICATIONS
Contraindicated in immediate postpartum period and in patients with arterial bleeding.

NURSING CONSIDERATIONS
● Use cautiously in patients with cardiovascular or cerebrovascular disease.
● Know that safe use during pregnancy and lactation has not been established.
● Discontinue drug if rash develops.

☑ **PATIENT TEACHING**
● Instruct the patient to take drug exactly as prescribed.
● To minimize the risk of orthostasis, instruct the patient to avoid sudden position changes.
● Drug may cause palpitations; tell the patient to notify doctor if they become a problem.

▼ *NEW DRUG*

---

midodrine hydrochloride
ProAmatine

Pregnancy Risk Category: C

HOW SUPPLIED
Tablets: 2.5 mg, 5 mg

ACTION
Midodrine forms an active metabolite, desglymidodrine, which is an alpha-$_1$ agonist. It increases blood pressure by

---

Reactions may be *common*, uncommon, *life-threatening*, or COMMON AND LIFE-THREATENING.

activating alpha-adrenergic receptors in arteriolar and venous vasculature.

ONSET, PEAK, DURATION
Onset and duration unknown. Plasma levels peak within 1 to 2 hours. Effects may persist up to 3 hours.

INDICATIONS & DOSAGE
Treatment of symptomatic orthostatic hypotension unresponsive to standard clinical care—
Adults: 10 mg P.O. t.i.d. Suggested dosing schedule: Dose 1 shortly before or upon arising in the morning; dose 2 at midday; and dose 3 in late afternoon but no later than 6 p.m. Use cautiously in patients with abnormal renal function; initially, 2.5-mg doses are recommended.

ADVERSE REACTIONS
CNS: *paresthesia,* headache, confusion, anxiety.
CV: *supine hypertension, vasodilation.*
GU: urine retention, frequency, and urgency; *dysuria.*
Skin: *piloerection (goosebumps), pruritus,* rash.
Other: pain, chills, dry mouth.

INTERACTIONS
Alpha-adrenergics: enhanced vasopressor effects. Monitor blood pressure closely.
Alpha-adrenergic blockers: may antagonize drug effects. Avoid concomitant use.
Digitalis glycosides, psychopharmacologic agents, beta blockers: may enhance or cause bradycardia, AV block, or arrhythmia. Avoid concomitant use.
Fludrocortisone acetate: may increase risk of supine hypertension. Monitor closely.

EFFECTS ON DIAGNOSTIC TESTS
None reported.

CONTRAINDICATIONS
Contraindicated in patients with severe organic heart disease, persistent and excessive supine hypertension, acute renal disease, urine retention, pheochromocytoma, or thyrotoxicosis.

NURSING CONSIDERATIONS
● Use cautiously in patients with a history of urine retention, visual problems, diabetes, or renal or hepatic impairment and in breast-feeding women.
● Know that drug should be used in pregnancy only if the benefit justifies the potential risk to the fetus.
● Know that safety and effectiveness in children have not been established.
● Monitor supine and sitting blood pressures closely, and notify doctor if supine blood pressure increases excessively.
● Know that drug should be taken during the day when patient can be upright and performing activities of daily living. Space doses at least 3 hours apart. Midodrine should not be given after the evening meal or within 4 hours before bedtime, to reduce potential for supine hypertension during sleep.
● Know that midodrine should be continued only if patient attains symptomatic improvement during initial therapy.
● Renal and hepatic tests should be done before and during drug therapy as ordered.

☑ PATIENT TEACHING
● Instruct patient about proper dosing intervals and to take last dose of the day 4 hours before bedtime.
● Tell patient to report symptoms of supine hypertension (cardiac awareness, pounding in ears, headache, blurred vision) immediately to the doctor and to stop drug.
● Tell patient to consult the doctor before taking OTC medications.

---

*Liquid contains alcohol.   **May contain tartrazine.   †Canada only.   ‡Australia only.   ◇ OTC.

papaverine hydrochloride
Cerespan, Genabid, Pavabid,
Pavabid HP, Pavabid Plateau,
Pavacels, Pavagen, Pavarine,
Pavased, Pavasule, Pavatine, Pa-
vatym, Paverolan Lanacaps

Pregnancy Risk Category: C

HOW SUPPLIED
Tablets: 30 mg, 60 mg, 100 mg, 150
mg, 200 mg, 300 mg
Tablets (timed-release): 200 mg
Capsules (timed-release): 150 mg
Injection: 30 mg/ml, 32.5 mg/ml†

ACTION
Has a direct, nonspecific relaxant effect on vascular, cardiac, and other
smooth muscle.

ONSET, PEAK, DURATION
Onset is fairly rapid. Peak unknown.
Persists for 12 hours after administration of timed-release form. Unknown
for other forms of the drug.

INDICATIONS & DOSAGE
*Relief from vascular spasm associated
with acute MI (coronary occlusion),
angina pectoris, peripheral and pulmonary embolism, peripheral vascular
disease in which there is a vasospastic
element or certain cerebral angiostatic
states; and visceral spasm, as in
ureteral, biliary, or gastrointestinal
colic—*
Adults: 75 to 300 mg P.O. three to five
times daily, or 150- to 300-mg timed-
release preparations q 8 to 12 hours;
30 to 120 mg I.M. or I.V. slowly over 1
to 2 minutes q 3 hours, as indicated.

ADVERSE REACTIONS
CNS: *headache,* vertigo, drowsiness,
sedation, malaise.
CV: *increased heart rate, increased
blood pressure* (with parenteral use),
depressed AV and intraventricular conduction, *arrhythmias.*

GI: constipation, *nausea,* anorexia, abdominal pain, diarrhea.
Hepatic: *hepatitis* (jaundice,
eosinophilia, abnormal liver function
tests), *cirrhosis.*
Respiratory: increased depth and rate
of respiration.
Skin: *diaphoresis, flushing,* skin rash.

INTERACTIONS
Lactated Ringer's solution: precipitate
forms when mixed with papaverine.
Don't mix together.
Levodopa: papaverine may interfere
with levodopa's therapeutic effects in
patients with Parkinson's disease.
Monitor for decreased effectiveness.

EFFECTS ON DIAGNOSTIC TESTS
Drug therapy alters serum concentrations of eosinophils, ALT, alkaline
phosphatase, and bilirubin. Elevated
serum bilirubin levels signal hepatic
hypersensitivity to papaverine.

CONTRAINDICATIONS
I.V. use is contraindicated in patients
with Parkinson's disease or complete
AV block.

NURSING CONSIDERATIONS
● Use cautiously in patients with glaucoma.
● **I.V. use:** Give by direct injection
over 1 to 2 minutes. Slow administration minimizes the risk of serious adverse reactions. Do not add to lactated
Ringer's injection because precipitation occurs.
● Be aware that drug is most effective
when given early in the course of a
disorder.
● Know that the FDA has declared that
this drug may not be effective for the
disease states indicated.
● Monitor blood pressure and heart
rate and rhythm, especially in patients
with cardiac disease. Withhold dose
and notify the doctor immediately if
changes occur.

Alert: Monitor for adverse hepatic reactions in patients receiving long-term therapy.

☑ **PATIENT TEACHING**
● Tell the patient to take medication regularly; long-term therapy is required.
● Advise the patient to avoid tasks that require mental alertness, such as driving or operating heavy machinery, until drug's CNS effects are known.
● To minimize the risk of orthostatic hypotension, instruct the patient to avoid sudden posture changes.

---

pentoxifylline
Trental

Pregnancy Risk Category: C

HOW SUPPLIED
Tablets (extended-release): 400 mg

ACTION
Unknown. Improves capillary blood flow probably by increasing RBC flexibility and lowering blood viscosity.

ONSET, PEAK, DURATION
Onset and duration unknown. Serum levels peak within 1 hour but are not related to drug effect.

INDICATIONS & DOSAGE
Intermittent claudication caused by chronic occlusive vascular disease—
Adults: 400 mg P.O. t.i.d. with meals. May decrease to 400 mg b.i.d. if GI and CNS adverse effects occur.

ADVERSE REACTIONS
CNS: headache, dizziness.
GI: dyspepsia, nausea, vomiting.

INTERACTIONS
Anticoagulants: increased anticoagulant effect. Adjust anticoagulant dosage as ordered.

Antihypertensives: increased hypotensive effect. Dosage adjustments may be necessary.
Nicotine: vasoconstriction. Advise patient to avoid smoking; it may worsen his condition.

EFFECTS ON DIAGNOSTIC TESTS
None reported.

CONTRAINDICATIONS
Contraindicated in patients who are intolerant to methylxanthines, such as caffeine, theophylline, and theobromine, and in patients with recent cerebral or retinal hemorrhage.

NURSING CONSIDERATIONS
● Know that drug is useful in patients who are not good surgical candidates.
● Be aware that elderly patients may be more sensitive to drug's effects.

☑ **PATIENT TEACHING**
● Advise the patient to take with meals to minimize GI upset.
● Instruct the patient to swallow medication whole, without breaking, crushing, or chewing.
● Tell the patient to report any GI or CNS adverse reactions; the doctor may reduce the dosage.
● Tell the patient not to discontinue drug during the first 8 weeks of therapy unless directed by the doctor.

---

ticlopidine hydrochloride
Ticlid

Pregnancy Risk Category: B

HOW SUPPLIED
Tablets: 250 mg

ACTION
Unknown. An antiplatelet agent that probably blocks adenosine diphosphate-induced platelet-to-fibrinogen and platelet-to-platelet binding.

---

*Liquid contains alcohol. **May contain tartrazine. †Canada only. ‡Australia only. ◊ OTC.

ONSET, PEAK, DURATION
Onset occurs within 4 days. Serum levels peak in about 2 hours, although time to peak effect takes 8 to 11 days. Effects persist for 1 to 2 weeks.

INDICATIONS & DOSAGE
To reduce risk of thrombotic stroke in patients with history of stroke or who have experienced stroke precursors—
Adults: 250 mg P.O. b.i.d. with meals.

ADVERSE REACTIONS
CNS: dizziness, *intracerebral bleeding*, peripheral neuropathy.
CV: vasculitis.
EENT: epistaxis, conjunctival hemorrhage.
GI: *diarrhea, nausea, dyspepsia, abdominal pain,* anorexia, vomiting, flatulence, bleeding.
GU: hematuria, *nephrotic syndrome,* dark-colored urine.
Hematologic: *neutropenia, pancytopenia, agranulocytosis, immune thrombocytopenia.*
Hepatic: hepatitis, cholestatic jaundice, abnormal liver function tests.
Respiratory: *allergic pneumonitis.*
Skin: *rash,* pruritus, ecchymoses, maculopapular rash, urticaria, *thrombocytopenic purpura.*
Other: hypersensitivity reactions, postoperative bleeding, systemic lupus erythematosus, *serum sickness,* arthropathy, myositis, *hyponatremia.*

INTERACTIONS
Antacids: decreased plasma ticlopidine levels. Separate administration times by at least 2 hours.
Aspirin: effects of aspirin on platelets potentiated. Avoid concomitant use.
Cimetidine: decreased clearance of ticlopidine and increased risk of toxicity. Avoid concomitant use.
Digoxin: slight decrease in serum digoxin levels. Monitor serum digoxin levels.
Theophylline: decreased theophylline clearance and risk of toxicity. Monitor

closely and adjust theophylline dosage as ordered.

EFFECTS ON DIAGNOSTIC TESTS
Pharmacologic effects of drug result in prolonged bleeding time. Toxic effects are evident in a decreased neutrophil or platelet count and elevated liver function tests. A positive antinuclear antibody titer has been reported rarely.

CONTRAINDICATIONS
Contraindicated in patients hypersensitive to drug; in patients with hematopoietic disorders, active pathologic bleeding from peptic ulceration or active intracranial bleeding, and in those with severe hepatic impairment.

NURSING CONSIDERATIONS
● Use cautiously and with close monitoring of CBC and WBC differentials. Moderate to severe neutropenia and agranulocytosis have occurred in patients taking ticlopidine.
● Monitor baseline liver function tests prior to therapy.
● Determine CBC and WBC differentials at the 2nd week of therapy and repeat every 2 weeks until the end of the 3rd month, as ordered.
● Monitor liver function tests and repeat if dysfunction is suspected.
● Know that thrombocytopenia has occurred rarely. Drug should be discontinued in patients having a platelet count of 80,000/mm^3 or less. If necessary, give methylprednisolone 20 mg I.V. to normalize bleeding time within 2 hours, as ordered.
● Know that when used preoperatively, ticlopidine may decrease incidence of graft occlusion in patients receiving coronary artery bypass grafts and reduce severity of drop in platelet count in patients receiving extracorporeal hemoperfusion during open heart surgery.

☑ **PATIENT TEACHING**
● Tell patient to take drug with meals.

Reactions may be *common,* uncommon, *life-threatening,* or COMMON AND LIFE-THREATENING.

• Tell patient to avoid aspirin and aspirin-containing products and to check with the doctor or pharmacist before taking OTC medications.

• Explain that drug will prolong bleeding time and that unusual or prolonged bleeding should be reported. Advise patient to tell dentists and other doctors that he is taking ticlopidine.

• Stress importance of regular blood tests. Because neutropenia can result from increased risk of infection, tell patient to immediately report signs of infection, such as fever, chills, or sore throat.

• If ticlopidine is being substituted for a fibrinolytic or anticoagulant, tell patient to discontinue those drugs before starting ticlopidine therapy as ordered.

• Advise patient to discontinue drug 10 to 14 days before undergoing elective surgery, as ordered. Also tell patient to immediately report yellow skin or sclera, severe or persistent diarrhea, rashes, subcutaneous bleeding, light-colored stools, or dark urine.

---

tolazoline hydrochloride
Priscoline

Pregnancy Risk Category: C

HOW SUPPLIED
Injection: 25 mg/ml in 4-ml ampules

ACTION
Direct-acting vasodilator. May have some alpha-receptor blocking effects.

ONSET, PEAK, DURATION
Onset occurs within 30 minutes. Peak and duration unknown.

INDICATIONS & DOSAGE
Persistent pulmonary hypertension in neonates—
Neonates: initially, 1 to 2 mg/kg I.V. over 10 minutes, followed by infusion of 1 to 2 mg/kg/hour.

ADVERSE REACTIONS
CV: *arrhythmias,* pain, *hypertension, flushing,* tachycardia, *hypotension.*
GI: nausea, vomiting, diarrhea, *GI hemorrhage.*
GU: edema, oliguria, hematuria.
Hematologic: leukopenia, *thrombocytopenia.*
Respiratory: *pulmonary hemorrhage.*
Skin: increased pilomotor activity with tingling and chilliness, rash.

INTERACTIONS
Vasopressors (epinephrine, norepinephrine): may cause paradoxical fall in blood pressure.

EFFECTS ON DIAGNOSTIC TESTS
None reported.

CONTRAINDICATIONS
Contraindicated in neonates with hypersensitivity to the drug.

NURSING CONSIDERATIONS
• Use cautiously in patients with known or suspected mitral stenosis.
• **I.V. use:** Know that response should be evident within 30 minutes. Little information exists regarding infusions lasting longer than 48 hours.
• Place the patient in the supine position during infusion.
• Keep patient warm during parenteral administration.
Alert: Appearance of flushing usually indicates maximum tolerable dose.
• Monitor vital signs for blood pressure changes and arrhythmias.

☑ PATIENT TEACHING
• Inform parents of need for drug and explain its use.
• Encourage parents to ask questions and express concerns.

---

*Liquid contains alcohol. **May contain tartrazine. †Canada only. ‡Australia only. ◇OTC.

acetaminophen
aspirin
choline magnesium trisalicylate
choline salicylate
diflunisal
magnesium salicylate
salsalate

COMBINATION PRODUCTS

ALLEREST NO DROWSINESS TABLETS ◊, COLDRINE ◊, ORNEX NO DROWSINESS CAPLETS ◊, SINUS RELIEF TABLETS, SINUTAB WITHOUT DROWSINESS ◊: acetaminophen 325 mg and pseudoephedrine hydrochloride 30 mg.

AMAPHEN, ANOQUAN, BUTACE, ENDOLOR, ESGIC, FEMCET, FIORICET, ISOPAP, MEDIGESIC, REPAN, TENCET, TRIAD, TWO-DYNE: acetaminophen 325 mg, caffeine 40 mg, and butalbital 50 mg.

ASCRIPTIN, MAGNAPRIN: aspirin 325 mg, magnesium hydroxide 50 mg, aluminum hydroxide 50 mg, and calcium carbonate 50 mg. ◊

ASCRIPTIN A/D, MAGNAPRIN ARTHRITIS STRENGTH: aspirin 325 mg, magnesium hydroxide 75 mg, aluminum hydroxide 75 mg, and calcium carbonate 75 mg. ◊

AXOTAL: aspirin 650 mg and butalbital 50 mg.

CAMA ARTHRITIS PAIN RELIEVER: aspirin 500 mg, magnesium oxide 150 mg, and aluminum hydroxide 150 mg.

COPE: aspirin 421 mg, caffeine 32 mg, magnesium hydroxide 50 mg, and aluminum hydroxide 25 mg.

DOAN'S P.M. EXTRA STRENGTH ◊, magnesium salicylate 500 mg and diphenhydramine 25 mg.

EXCEDRIN EXTRA STRENGTH ◊: aspirin 250 mg, acetaminophen 250 mg, and caffeine 65 mg.

EXCEDRIN P.M., BUFFERIN AF NITE TIME ◊: acetaminophen 500 mg and diphenhydramine citrate 38 mg.

FIORINAL, FIORGEN PF, ISOLLYL IM-PROVED, LANORINAL, MARNEL: aspirin 325 mg, caffeine 40 mg, and butalbital 50 mg.

MIDRIN: isometheptene mucate 65 mg, dichloralphenazone 100 mg, and acetaminophen 325 mg.

P-A-C TABLETS ◊: aspirin 400 mg and caffeine 32 mg.

PHRENILIN: acetaminophen 325 mg and butalbital 50 mg.

PHRENILIN FORTE: acetaminophen 650 mg and butalbital 50 mg.

SINUS EXCEDRIN EXTRA STRENGTH ◊: acetaminophen 500 mg and pseudophedrine hydrochloride 30 mg.

SINUTAB ◊: acetaminophen 325 mg, chlorpheniramine 2 mg, and pseudoephedrine hydrochloride 30 mg.

SINUTAB MAXIMUM STRENGTH ◊: acetaminophen 500 mg, pseudoephedrine hydrochloride 30 mg, and chlorpheniramine maleate, 2 mg.

TECNAL†: aspirin 330 mg, caffeine 40 mg, and butalbital 50 mg.

VANQUISH ◊: aspirin 227 mg, acetaminophen 194 mg, caffeine 33 mg, aluminum hydroxide 25 mg, and magnesium hydroxide 50 mg.

---

acetaminophen
(APAP, paracetamol)

Abenol† ◊; Aceta Elixir* ◊; Acetaminophen Uniserts ◊; Aceta Tablets ◊; Actamin ◊; Actamin Extra ◊; Actimol† ◊; Aminofen ◊; Aminofen Max ◊; Anacin-3 ◊; Anacin-3 Children's Elixir* ◊; Anacin-3 Children's Tablets ◊; Anacin-3 Extra Strength ◊; Anacin-3 Infants' ◊; Anacin-3 Maximum Strength Caplets ◊; Apacet Capsules ◊; Apacet Elixir* ◊; Apacet Extra Strength Caplets ◊; Apacet Extra Strength Tablets ◊; Apacet Infants' ◊; Apacet Regular Strength Tablets ◊;

Apo-Acetaminophen† ◊ ; Arthritis Pain Formula Aspirin Free ◊ ; Atasol Caplets† ◊ ; Atasol Drops† ◊ ; Atasol Elixir*† ◊ ; Atasol Forte Caplets† ◊ ; Atasol Forte Tablets† ◊ ; Atasol Tablets† ◊ ; Banesin ◊ ; Dapa ◊ ; Dapa X-S ◊ ; Datril Extra-Strength; Dolanex* ◊ ; Dorcol Children's Fever and Pain Reducer ◊ ; Dymadon‡ ◊ ; Dymadon P‡ ◊ ; Exdol† ◊ ; Exdol Strong† ◊ ; Feverall, Children's‡; Feverall Junior Strength‡; Feverall Sprinkle Caps, Children's‡; Feverall Sprinkle Caps, Junior Strength‡; Genapap Children's Elixir ◊ ; Genapap Children's Tablets ◊ ; Genapap Extra Strength Caplets ◊ ; Genapap Extra Strength Tablets ◊ ; Genapap, Infants' ◊ ; Genapap Regular Strength Tablets ◊ ; Genebs Extra Strength Caplets ◊ ; Genebs Regular Strength Tablets ◊ ; Genebs X-Tra ◊ ; Halenol Children's* ◊ ; Liquiprin Infants' Drops ◊ ; Meda Cap ◊ ; Myapap Elixir* ◊ ; Myapap, Infants' ◊ ; Neopap ◊ ; Oraphen-PD ◊ ; Panadol ◊ ; Panadol, Children's ◊ ; Panadol Extra Strength ◊ ; Panadol, Infants' ◊ ; Panadol Junior Strength Caplets ◊ ; Panadol Maximum Strength Caplets ◊ ; Panadol Maximum Strength Tablets ◊ ; Panamax‡ ◊ ; Panex ◊ ; Panex-500 ◊ ; Paralgin‡ ◊ ; Paraspen‡ ◊ ; Redutemp ◊ ; Ridenol Caplets ◊ ; Robigesic† ◊ ; Rounox† ◊ ; Setamol-500‡ ◊ ; Snaplets-FR ◊ ; Stanback AF Extra Strength Powder; St. Joseph Aspirin-Free Fever Reducer for Children ◊ ; Suppap-120 ◊ ; Suppap-325 ◊ ; Suppap-650 ◊ ; Tapanol Extra Strength Caplets ◊ ; Tapanol Extra Strength Tablets ◊ ; Tempra ◊ ; Tempra Caplets ◊ ; Tempra Chewable Tablets ◊ ; Tempra Drops ◊ ; Tempra D.S. ◊ ; Tempra, Infants' ◊ ; Tempra Syrup ◊ ; Tenol ◊ ; Tylenol Caplets ◊ ; Tylenol Chewable Tablets ◊ ; Tylenol Children's Elixir ◊ ; Tylenol Children's Tablets ◊ ; Tylenol Drops ◊ ; Tylenol Elixir* ◊ ; Tylenol Extended Relief ◊ ; Tylenol Extra Strength Adult Liquid Pain Reliever ◊ ; Tylenol Extra Strength Caplets ◊ ; Tylenol Extra Strength Gelcaps ◊ ; Tylenol Extra Strength Tablets ◊ ; Tylenol Infants' ◊ ; Tylenol Junior Strength Caplets ◊ ; Tylenol Junior Strength Tablets ◊ ; Tylenol Regular Strength Caplets ◊ ; Tylenol Regular Strength Tablets ◊ ; Tylenol Tablets ◊ ; Ty-Pap ◊ ; Ty-Pap, Infants' ◊ ; Ty-Pap Syrup ◊ ; Ty-Tab Caplets ◊ ; Ty-Tab Capsules ◊ ; Ty-Tab, Children's ◊ ; Ty-Tab Tablets ◊ ; Valorin ◊ ; Valorin Extra ◊

Pregnancy Risk Category: NR

HOW SUPPLIED
Tablets: 160 mg ◊ , 325 mg ◊ , 500 mg ◊ , 650 mg ◊
Tablets (chewable): 80 mg ◊ , 160 mg ◊
Caplets (extended-release): 650 mg
Capsules: 500 mg ◊
Oral liquid: 160 mg/5 ml ◊ , 500 mg/15 ml ◊
Oral solution: 48 mg/ml ◊ , 100 mg/ml ◊
Oral suspension: 120 mg/5 ml‡, 100 mg/ml ◊ , 160 mg/5 ml ◊
Elixir: 120 mg/5 ml, 130 mg/5 ml* ◊ , 160 mg/5 ml* ◊ , 325 mg/5 ml* ◊
Granules: 80 mg/packet ◊ , 325 mg/dosage measure ◊
Powder for solution: 1 g/packet
Sprinkles: 80 mg/capsule, 160 mg/capsule
Suppositories: 80 mg ◊ , 120 mg ◊ , 125 mg ◊ , 300 mg ◊ , 325 mg ◊ , 650 mg ◊

ACTION
Unknown. Thought to produce analgesia by blocking generation of pain impulses, probably by inhibiting prostaglandin synthesis in the CNS or the synthesis or action of other substances that sensitize pain receptors to mechanical or chemical stimulation. It is thought to relieve fever by central action in the hypothalamic heat-regulating center.

---

*Liquid contains alcohol.   **May contain tartrazine.   †Canada only.   ‡Australia only.   ◊OTC.

ONSET, PEAK, DURATION
Onset unknown. Peak effects vary; average peak blood levels occur in 1 to 3 hours. Effects persist about 3 to 4 hours.

INDICATIONS & DOSAGE
Mild pain or fever—
Adults and children over 11 years: 325 to 650 mg P.O. q 4 to 6 hours; or 1 g P.O. t.i.d. or q.i.d., p.r.n. Alternatively, 2 extended-release caplets P.O. q 8 hours. Maximum dosage should not exceed 4 g daily. Dosage for long-term therapy should not exceed 2.6 g daily.
Children 11 years: 480 mg P.O. or rectally q 4 to 6 hours.
Children 9 to 10 years: 400 mg P.O. or rectally q 4 to 6 hours.
Children 6 to 8 years: 320 mg P.O. or rectally q 4 to 6 hours.
Children 4 to 5 years: 240 mg P.O. or rectally q 4 to 6 hours.
Children 2 to 3 years: 160 mg P.O. or rectally q 4 to 6 hours.
Children 12 to 23 months: 120 mg P.O. q 4 to 6 hours.
Children 4 to 11 months: 80 mg P.O. q 4 to 6 hours.
Children up to 3 months: 40 mg P.O. q 4 to 6 hours.

ADVERSE REACTIONS
Hematologic: hemolytic anemia, neutropenia, leukopenia, *pancytopenia, thrombocytopenia* (rare).
Hepatic: *severe liver damage* (with toxic doses), jaundice.
Skin: rash, urticaria.
Other: hypoglycemia.

INTERACTIONS
Barbiturates, carbamazepine, hydantoins, rifampin, sulfinpyrazone: high doses or long-term use of these drugs may reduce the therapeutic effects and enhance the hepatotoxic effects of acetaminophen. Avoid concomitant use.
Caffeine: may enhance analgesic effects of acetaminophen.
Ethanol: increased risk of hepatic damage. Avoid concomitant use.

Warfarin: may increase hypoprothrombinemic effects with long-term use with high doses of acetaminophen. Monitor PTs closely.
Zidovudine: may increase the incidence of bone marrow suppression because of impaired zidovudine metabolism. Monitor patient closely.

EFFECTS ON DIAGNOSTIC TESTS
May cause a false-positive test result for urinary 5-hydroxyindoleacetic acid (5-HIAA).

CONTRAINDICATIONS
Contraindicated in patients with hypersensitivity to acetaminophen.

NURSING CONSIDERATIONS
● Use cautiously in patients with history of chronic alcohol use because hepatotoxicity has occurred after therapeutic doses.
● Many OTC products contain acetaminophen; be aware of this when calculating total daily dosage.
● Liquid form is recommended for children and for all patients who have difficulty swallowing.
● Know that acetaminophen may produce false-positive decreases in blood glucose levels in home monitoring systems.

☑ PATIENT TEACHING
● Tell parents to consult a doctor before giving this drug to child under 2 years.
● Tell patient this drug is only for short-term use. Tell patient to consult a doctor if administering to child for more than 5 days or adults for more than 10 days.
● Tell patient not to use for self-medication of marked fever (over 103.1° F [39.5° C]), fever persisting longer than 3 days, or recurrent fever unless directed by doctor.
Alert: Warn patient that high doses or unsupervised long-term use can cause hepatic damage. Excessive ingestion of alcoholic beverages may increase the risk of hepatotoxicity.

Reactions may be *common*, uncommon, *life-threatening*, or COMMON AND LIFE-THREATENING.

• Tell breast-feeding patient that acetaminophen is found in breast milk in low concentrations (less than 1% of dose). Such patients may use it safely if therapy is short-term and does not exceed recommended doses.

---

aspirin (acetylsalicylic acid)

Ancasal†◊, Arthrinol†◊, Artria S.R.◊, ASA◊, ASA Enseals◊, Aspergum◊, Aspro‡, Astrin†◊, Bayer Aspirin◊, Bex‡, Coryphen†◊, Easprin◊, Ecotrin◊, Empirin◊, Entrophen†◊, Halfprin, Measurin◊, Norwich Aspirin Extra Strength◊, Novasent†◊, Riphen-10†◊, Sal-Adult†◊, Sal-Infant†◊, Solprin‡, Supasat†◊, Triaphen-10†◊, Vincent's Powders‡, Winsprin Capsules‡, ZORprin◊

Pregnancy Risk Category: C (D in 3rd trimester)

HOW SUPPLIED
Tablets◊: 325 mg, 500 mg, 650 mg
Tablets (chewable): 81 mg◊
Tablets (enteric-coated): 81 mg, 162 mg, 165 mg, 325 mg◊, 500 mg◊, 650 mg◊, 975 mg
Tablets (extended-release): 650 mg, 800 mg
Tablets (timed-release): 650 mg◊
Chewing gum: 227.5 mg◊
Suppositories◊: 60 mg, 120 mg, 125 mg, 130 mg, 195 mg, 200 mg, 300 mg, 325 mg, 600 mg, 650 mg, 1.2 g

ACTION
Produces analgesia by blocking prostaglandin synthesis (peripheral action). Aspirin and other salicylates may prevent the lowering of the pain threshold that occurs when prostaglandins sensitize pain receptors to mechanical and chemical stimulation. Exerts its anti-inflammatory effect by inhibiting prostaglandin synthesis; also may inhibit the synthesis or action of other mediators of the inflammatory response. Relieves fever by acting on the hypothalamic heat-regulating center to cause peripheral vasodilation. This increases peripheral blood supply and promotes sweating, which leads to heat loss and to cooling by evaporation. In low doses, aspirin also appears to impede clotting by blocking prostaglandin synthesis, which prevents formation of the platelet-aggregating substance thromboxane A_2.

ONSET, PEAK, DURATION
Onset occurs 5 to 30 minutes after an oral, rapidly absorbed dose. With oral solution, serum aspirin levels peak in 15 to 40 minutes; peak serum levels of salicylate, its active metabolite, in ½ to 1 hour. With regular tablets, peak serum aspirin levels in 25 to 40 minutes; peak serum salicylate levels, in 1 to 2 hours. With buffered tablets, peak serum aspirin and salicylate levels occur in 1 to 2 hours. With extended-release tablets, peak aspirin levels occur in 1 to 2 hours; peak salicylate levels, in 3 to 4 hours. With enteric-coated tablets, peak aspirin and salicylate levels occur in 4 to 8 hours. With suppositories, peak aspirin and salicylate levels occur in 3 to 4 hours. Effects persist for 1 to 4 hours.

INDICATIONS & DOSAGE
Rheumatoid arthritis, osteoarthritis, or other polyarthritic or inflammatory conditions—
Adults: initially, 2.4 to 3.6 g P.O. daily in divided doses. Maintenance dosage is 3.2 to 6 g P.O. daily in divided doses.
Juvenile rheumatoid arthritis—
Children: weighing 25 kg or less, 60 to 90 mg/kg P.O. daily in divided doses; weighing more than 25 kg, 2.4 to 3.6 g P.O. daily in divided doses.
Mild pain or fever—
Adults and children over 11 years: 325 to 650 mg P.O. or P.R. q 4 hours, p.r.n.
Children 2 to 11 years: 1.5 g/m^2 or 65 mg/kg P.O. or P.R. daily in 4 to 6 divided doses.

Prevention of thrombosis—
Adults: 1.3 g P.O. daily in 2 to 4 divided doses.
Reduction of risk of heart attack in patients with previous MI or unstable angina—
Adults: 160 to 325 mg P.O. daily.
Kawasaki syndrome (mucocutaneous lymph node syndrome)—
Adults: 80 to 100 mg/kg P.O. daily in 4 divided doses during the febrile phase. Some patients may need up to 120 mg/kg. When fever subsides, dosage decreased to 3 to 8 mg/kg once daily, adjusted according to serum salicylate concentration.

ADVERSE REACTIONS
EENT: *tinnitus and hearing loss.*
GI: *nausea, GI distress, occult bleeding, dyspepsia, **GI bleeding.***
Hematologic: leukopenia, ***thrombocytopenia,*** *prolonged bleeding time.*
Hepatic: abnormal liver function studies, hepatitis.
Skin: *rash,* bruising, urticaria, angioedema.
Other: hypersensitivity reactions, (***ana-phylaxis,*** asthma), ***Reye's syndrome.***

INTERACTIONS
Ammonium chloride and other urine acidifiers: increased blood levels of aspirin products. Monitor for aspirin toxicity.
Angiotensin-converting enzyme inhibitors: may decrease antihypertensive effects. Monitor blood pressure closely.
Antacids in high doses (and other urine alkalinizers): decreased levels of aspirin products. Monitor for decreased aspirin effect.
Anticoagulants: increased risk of bleeding. Avoid using together if possible.
Beta blockers: decreased antihypertensive effect. Avoid long-term aspirin use if patient is taking antihypertensives.
Corticosteroids: enhanced salicylate elimination. Monitor for decreased salicylate effect.
Ethanol, NSAIDs, steroids: increased

risk of GI bleeding. Avoid concomitant use.
Methotrexate: increased risk of methotrexate toxicity. Avoid concomitant use.
Nizatidine: may increase risk of salicylate toxicity in patients receiving high doses of aspirin. Monitor closely.
NSAIDs, including diflunisal, fenoprofen, ibuprofen, indomethacin, piroxicam, meclofenamate, naproxen: altered pharmacokinetics of these agents, leading to lowered serum levels and decreased effectiveness. Avoid concomitant use.
Oral antidiabetic agents: increased hypoglycemic effect. Monitor closely.
Probenecid, sulfinpyrazone: decreased uricosuric effect. Avoid aspirin during therapy with these agents.
Valproic acid: may increase serum valproic acid concentrations. Avoid concomitant use.

EFFECTS ON DIAGNOSTIC TESTS
Aspirin will cause an increased bleeding time. It interferes with urinary glucose analysis performed with Clinistix, Tes-Tape, Clinitest, and Benedict's solution, and with urinary 5-hydroxyindoleacetic acid (5-HIAA) and vanillylmandelic acid tests. Serum uric acid levels may be falsely increased. Aspirin may also interfere with the Gerhardt test for urine acetoacetic acid.

CONTRAINDICATIONS
Contraindicated in patients with hypersensitivity to the drug, G6PD deficiency, bleeding disorders such as hemophilia, von Willebrand's disease, or telangiectasia. Also contraindicated in patients with NSAID-induced sensitivity reactions.

NURSING CONSIDERATIONS
● Use cautiously in patients with GI lesions, impaired renal function, hypoprothrombinemia, vitamin K deficiency, thrombocytopenia, thrombotic thrombocytopenic purpura, or severe hepatic im-

pairment.

Alert: Because of epidemiologic association with Reye's syndrome, the Centers for Disease Control and Prevention recommends not giving salicylates to children or teenagers with chickenpox or influenza-like illness.

● Be aware that for inflammatory conditions, rheumatic fever, and thrombosis, aspirin is administered on a scheduled, rather than p.r.n., basis.

● Know that because enteric-coated and sustained-release tablets are slowly absorbed, they are not suitable for rapid relief of acute pain, fever, or inflammation. They do cause less GI bleeding and may be more suited for long-term therapy, such as for the treatment of arthritis.

● For patient with swallowing difficulties, crush non-enteric-coated aspirin and dissolve in soft food or liquid. Administer liquid immediately after mixing because drug will break down rapidly.

● For patients who cannot tolerate oral medications, ask doctor about the possibility of using aspirin rectal suppositories. Watch for rectal mucosal irritation or bleeding.

● Be aware that febrile, dehydrated children can develop toxicity rapidly.

● Monitor elderly patients closely because they may be more susceptible to aspirin's toxic effects.

● Monitor blood salicylate levels as indicated and ordered. Therapeutic blood salicylate level in arthritis is 10 to 30 mg/100 ml. Tinnitus may occur at plasma levels of 30 mg/100 ml and above, but this is not a reliable indicator of toxicity, especially in very young patients and those over age 60. With chronic therapy, mild toxicity may occur at plasma levels of 20 mg/100 ml.

● During prolonged therapy, hematocrit, hemoglobin level, PT, and renal function should be assessed periodically as ordered.

● Know that aspirin irreversibly inhibits platelet aggregation. It should be discontinued 5 to 7 days before elective surgery as ordered to allow time for the production and release of new platelets.

☑ PATIENT TEACHING
● Advise patient allergic to tartrazine dye not to take aspirin.

● To reduce adverse GI reactions, advise patient to take with food, milk, antacid, or large glass of water.

● Tell patient that sustained-release or enteric-coated preparations should not be crushed or chewed but swallowed whole.

● Tell patient that aspirin tablets with a strong vinegar-like odor should be discarded.

● Tell patient to consult a doctor if administering to child for more than 5 days or adult for more than 10 days.

● Advise patient receiving prolonged treatment with large doses of aspirin to watch for petechiae, bleeding gums, and signs of GI bleeding, and to maintain adequate fluid intake. Encourage the use of a soft-bristled toothbrush.

● Because of the many possible drug interactions involving aspirin, warn patient taking prescription drugs to check with a doctor or pharmacist before taking aspirin or OTC combination products containing aspirin.

● Inform female patient that she should not take aspirin during last trimester of pregnancy unless specifically directed to do so by a doctor.

● Caution parents to keep out of reach of children—aspirin is one of the leading causes of poisoning in children. Encourage the use of child-resistant containers.

choline magnesium trisalicylate (choline salicylate and magnesium salicylate)
Tricosal, Trilisate

Pregnancy Risk Category: C

HOW SUPPLIED
Tablets: 500 mg, 750 mg, 1,000 mg of salicylate
Solution: 500 mg of salicylate/5 ml

ACTION
Produces analgesia by blocking prostaglandin synthesis (peripheral action). Salicylates may prevent the lowering of the pain threshold that occurs when prostaglandins sensitize pain receptors to mechanical and chemical stimulation. Exerts its anti-inflammatory effect by inhibiting prostaglandin synthesis. Relieves fever by acting on the hypothalamic heat-regulating center to produce peripheral vasodilation. This increases peripheral blood supply and promotes sweating, which leads to heat loss and to cooling by evaporation.

ONSET, PEAK, DURATION
Onset and duration unknown. Serum levels peak within 1 to 2 hours.

INDICATIONS & DOSAGE
Rheumatoid arthritis and osteoarthritis or other polyarthritic or inflammatory conditions—
Adults: initially, 1.5 to 2.5 g P.O. daily as a single dose or in 2 or 3 divided doses. Dosage is adjusted according to patient response. Maintenace dosage range is 1 to 4.5 g daily.
Juvenile rheumatoid arthritis—
Children: 60 to 110 mg/kg/day P.O. in divided doses (q 6 to 8 hours).
Mild to moderate pain and fever—
Adults: 2 to 3 g P.O. daily in divided doses q 4 to 6 hours.
Children: for children weighing 37 kg or less, 50 mg/kg/day P.O. in divided doses b.i.d.; for those weighing over 37 kg, 2,250 mg/day.

ADVERSE REACTIONS
EENT: tinnitus and hearing loss.
GI: GI distress, nausea, vomiting.
Skin: rash.
Other: hypersensitivity reactions *(anaphylaxis), Reye's syndrome.*

INTERACTIONS
ACE inhibitors, beta blockers, diuretics: effects of these agents may be decreased.
Ammonium chloride and other urine acidifiers: increased blood levels of salicylates. Monitor for salicylate toxicity.
Antacids in high doses (and other urine alkalinizers): decreased levels of salicylates. Monitor for decreased salicylate effect.
Corticosteroids: enhanced salicylate elimination. Monitor for decreased salicylate effect.
Ethanol, steroids, and other NSAIDs: enhanced risk of adverse GI effects. Avoid concomitant use.
Methotrexate: increased risk of methotrexate toxicity. Avoid concomitant use.
Oral anticoagulants: increased risk of bleeding. Use together cautiously.
Uricosuric agents: decreased uricosuric effect. Avoid concomitant use.

EFFECTS ON DIAGNOSTIC TESTS
Choline salicylates may interfere with urinary glucose analysis performed via Clinistix, Tes-Tape, Clinitest, and Benedict's solution. These drugs also interfere with urinary 5-hydroxyindoleacetic acid (5-HIAA) and vanillylmandelic acid.

CONTRAINDICATIONS
Contraindicated in patients hypersensitive to the drug. Also contraindicated in patients with hemophilia, bleeding ulcers, and hemorrhagic states.

NURSING CONSIDERATIONS
● Use cautiously in patients with renal insufficiency, hepatic impairment, peptic ulcer disease, and gastritis.
Alert: Because of epidemiologic association with Reye's syndrome, the Centers for Disease Control and Prevention recommends not giving salicylates to children or teenagers with chickenpox or influenza-like illness.
● Be aware that febrile, dehydrated chil-

dren can develop toxicity rapidly.
• Monitor serum salicylate levels in long-term therapy. Therapeutic blood salicylate level in arthritis is 10 to 30 mg/100 ml. Tinnitus may occur at plasma levels of 30 mg/100 ml and above, but this is not a reliable indicator of toxicity, especially in the very young and those over age 60. In chronic therapy, mild toxicity may occur at plasma levels of 20 mg/100 ml.
• Periodically monitor hemoglobin level and PT in patients receiving long-term treatment with large doses.
• Know that this drug causes less GI distress than aspirin. If an antacid is needed, give it 2 hours after meals and choline magnesium trisalicylate before meals.

☑ **PATIENT TEACHING**
• Tell patient to take tablets with food or a full glass of water. Solution may be mixed with fruit juice, but not antacids.
• Warn patient not to take drug longer than prescribed or to increase dosage without consulting doctor.

---

choline salicylate
Arthropan, Teejel†*

Pregnancy Risk Category: NR

HOW SUPPLIED
Liquid: 870 mg/5 ml ◊
Gel: 87 mg/g†*

ACTION
Produces analgesia by blocking prostaglandin synthesis (peripheral action). Salicylates may prevent the lowering of the pain threshold that occurs when prostaglandins sensitize pain receptors to mechanical and chemical stimulation. Exerts its anti-inflammatory effect by inhibiting prostaglandin synthesis. Relieves fever by acting on the hypothalamic heat-regulating center to produce peripheral vasodilation. This increases peripheral blood supply and

promotes sweating, which leads to heat loss and to cooling by evaporation.

ONSET, PEAK, DURATION
Unknown.

INDICATIONS & DOSAGE
Rheumatoid arthritis, osteoarthritis, mild to moderate pain or fever—
Adults and children over 12 years: ½ to 1 tsp (435 to 870 mg of choline salicylate) P.O. q 4 hours, p.r.n. If tolerated and needed, dosage may be increased to 2 tsp. Not to exceed 8 tsp daily.
Relief of pain from inflamed gums—
Adults and children over 2 years: apply 1 cm of gel to affected area q 3 to 4 hours and h.s., p.r.n.

ADVERSE REACTIONS
EENT: *tinnitus,* hearing loss.
GI: nausea, vomiting, GI distress.
Skin: rash.
Other: hypersensitivity reactions *(anaphylaxis), Reye's syndrome.*

INTERACTIONS
ACE inhibitors, beta blockers, diuretics: effects of these drugs may be decreased.
Ammonium chloride and other urine acidifiers: increased blood levels of salicylates. Monitor for salicylate toxicity.
Antacids in high doses and other urine alkalinizers: decreased levels of salicylates. Monitor for decreased salicylate effect.
Corticosteroids: enhanced salicylate elimination. Monitor for decreased salicylate effect.
Ethanol, other NSAIDs, steroids: enhanced risk of adverse GI reactions. Avoid concomitant use.
Methotrexate: increased risk of methotrexate toxicity. Avoid concomitant use.

EFFECTS ON DIAGNOSTIC TESTS
Choline salicylates may interfere with urinary glucose analysis performed via Clinistix, Tes-Tape, Clinitest, and Benedict's solution. These drugs also inter-

---

fere with urinary 5-hydroxyindoleacetic acid and vanillylmandelic acid.

CONTRAINDICATIONS
Contraindicated in patients with hypersensitivity to the drug, hemophilia, bleeding ulcers, and hemorrhagic states.

NURSING CONSIDERATIONS
• Use cautiously in impaired hepatic or renal function, hypoprothrombinemia, vitamin K deficiency, peptic ulcer disease, and gastritis, and in a known allergy to salicylates.
Alert: Because of epidemiologic association with Reye's syndrome, the Centers for Disease Control and Prevention recommends not giving salicylates to children or teenagers with chickenpox or influenza-like illness.
• Know that febrile, dehydrated children can develop toxicity rapidly.
• Monitor serum salicylate levels in prolonged therapy. Therapeutic blood salicylate level in arthritis is 10 to 30 mg/100 ml. Tinnitus may occur at plasma levels of 30 mg/100 ml and above, but this is not a reliable indicator of toxicity, especially in the very young and those over age 60. With chronic therapy, mild toxicity may occur at plasma levels of 20 mg/100 ml.
• Periodically monitor hemoglobin level and PT in patients receiving long-term treatment with large doses.

☑ PATIENT TEACHING
• Tell patient that drug should be mixed with water, fruit juice, or carbonated drinks, but not antacids.
• Inform patient that drug causes less GI distress than aspirin. If an antacid is needed, he should take it 2 hours after meals and drug before meals.

---

diflunisal
Dolobid

Pregnancy Risk Category: C

HOW SUPPLIED
Tablets: 250 mg, 500 mg

ACTION
Unknown. Probably related to inhibition of prostaglandin synthesis.

ONSET, PEAK, DURATION
Onset in 1 hour for pain relief; unknown for anti-inflammatory action. Peak plasma levels and analgesic effects in 2 to 3 hours. Effects persist for pain relief 8 to 12 hours; unknown for anti-inflammatory effects.

INDICATIONS & DOSAGE
Mild to moderate pain, osteoarthritis, and rheumatoid arthritis—
Adults: 500 to 1,000 mg P.O. daily in two divided doses, usually q 12 hours. Maximum dosage is 1,500 mg daily.
Adults over 65 years: one-half the usual adult dose.

ADVERSE REACTIONS
CNS: *dizziness,* somnolence, insomnia, *headache,* fatigue.
EENT: *tinnitus,* visual disturbances (rare).
GI: *nausea, dyspepsia, GI pain, diarrhea,* vomiting, constipation, flatulence.
GU: renal impairment, hematuria, *interstitial nephritis.*
Skin: rash, pruritus, sweating, stomatitis, erythema multiforme, *Stevens-Johnson syndrome.*

INTERACTIONS
Acetaminophen, hydrochlorothiazide, indomethacin: diflunisal may substantially increase blood levels, increasing the risk of toxicity. Avoid concomitant use.
Antacids, aspirin: decreased diflunisal blood levels. Monitor for possible decreased therapeutic effect.
Anticoagulants, thrombolytic agents: diflunisal may enhance pharmacologic effects of these agents. Use together cautiously.

Reactions may be *common,* uncommon, *life-threatening,* or COMMON AND LIFE-THREATENING.

Cyclosporine: diflunisal may enhance the nephrotoxicity of cyclosporine. Avoid concomitant use.
Methotrexate: diflunisal may enhance the toxicity of methotrexate. Avoid concomitant use.
Sulindac: diflunisal decreases blood levels of sulindac's active metabolite. Monitor for reduced effect.

EFFECTS ON DIAGNOSTIC TESTS
Physiologic effects of the drug may prolong bleeding time; increase serum BUN, creatinine, and potassium levels; decrease serum uric acid; and increase liver function tests.

CONTRAINDICATIONS
Contraindicated in patients with hypersensitivity to the drug, or for whom acute asthmatic attacks, urticaria, or rhinitis are precipitated by aspirin or other NSAIDs.

NURSING CONSIDERATIONS
● Use cautiously in GI bleeding, history of peptic ulcer disease, renal impairment, and compromised cardiac function, hypertension, or other conditions predisposing patient to fluid retention.
Alert: Because of the epidemiologic association with Reye's syndrome, the Centers for Disease Control and Prevention recommends not giving salicylates to children and teenagers with chickenpox or influenza-like illness.

☑ PATIENT TEACHING
● Advise the patient to take with water, milk, or meals.
● Tell patient that tablets must be swallowed whole.
● Tell him to avoid aspirin or acetaminophen while using diflunisal unless ordered.
● Inform breast-feeding patients that drug is excreted in breast milk and that a decision should be made to discontinue either nursing or the drug.

magnesium salicylate
Doan's, Extra-Strength Doan's
P.M.◊, Magan◊, Mobidin◊

Pregnancy Risk Category: NR

HOW SUPPLIED
Tablets: 545 mg, 600 mg
Caplets: 325 mg◊, 500 mg◊

ACTION
Produces analgesia by blocking prostaglandin synthesis (peripheral action). Salicylates may prevent the lowering of the pain threshold that occurs when prostaglandins sensitize pain receptors to mechanical and chemical stimulation. Exerts its anti-inflammatory effect by inhibiting prostaglandin synthesis. Relieves fever by acting on the hypothalamic heat-regulating center to produce peripheral vasodilation. This increases peripheral blood supply and promotes sweating, which leads to heat loss and to cooling by evaporation.

ONSET, PEAK, DURATION
Onset and duration unknown. Blood levels peak within 1½ to 2 hours of a dose.

INDICATIONS & DOSAGE
Arthritis—
Adults: 545 mg to 1.2 g P.O. t.i.d. or q.i.d.
Mild pain or fever—
Adults and children over 11 years: 300 to 600 mg P.O. q 4 hours, not to exceed 3.5 g/day.

ADVERSE REACTIONS
EENT: *tinnitus and hearing loss.*
GI: *nausea, vomiting, GI distress.*
Hepatic: abnormal liver function studies, hepatitis.
Skin: *rash,* bruising.
Other: hypersensitivity reactions (***anaphylaxis,*** asthma), ***Reye's syndrome.***

INTERACTIONS

ACE inhibitors, beta blockers, diuretics, uricosuric agents: effects of these drugs may be decreased.

Ammonium chloride and other urine acidifiers: increased blood levels of salicylates. Monitor for salicylate toxicity.

Antacids in high doses and other urine alkalinizers: decreased levels of salicylates. Monitor for decreased salicylate effect.

Anticoagulants: increased risk of bleeding. Avoid using together.

Corticosteroids: enhanced salicylate elimination. Monitor for decreased salicylate effect.

Ethanol, other NSAIDs, steroids: increased risk of GI bleeding. Avoid concomitant use.

Methotrexate: increased risk of methotrexate toxicity. Avoid concomitant use.

EFFECTS ON DIAGNOSTIC TESTS

In high doses, drug may cause false-positive urine glucose test results using copper sulfate method; it may cause false-negative urine glucose test results using glucose enzymatic method. False increases or decreases have been seen in urine vanillylmandelic acid tests; false increases in serum uric acid have been seen. Magnesium salicylate may interfere with the Gerhardt test for urine acetoacetic acid. Magnesium salicylate may increase serum levels of AST, ALT, alkaline phosphatase, and bilirubin.

CONTRAINDICATIONS

Contraindicated in patients with hypersensitivity to the drug, or severe chronic renal insufficiency because of risk of magnesium toxicity. Also contraindicated in patients with bleeding disorders, or aspirin hypersensitivity.

NURSING CONSIDERATIONS

● Use cautiously in hypoprothrombinemia and vitamin K deficiency.

Alert: Because of epidemiologic association with Reye's syndrome, the Centers for Disease Control and Prevention rec-

ommends not giving salicylates to children or teenagers with chickenpox or influenza-like illness.

● Know that febrile, dehydrated children can develop toxicity rapidly.

● Monitor serum salicylate levels when drug used long term, as ordered. Therapeutic blood salicylate level in arthritis is 10 to 30 mg/100 ml. Tinnitus may occur at plasma levels of 30 mg/100 ml and above, but this is not a reliable indicator of toxicity, especially in very young patients and those over age 60. With chronic therapy, mild toxicity may occur at plasma levels of 20 mg/100 ml.

● Monitor hemoglobin level and PT in long-term treatment with large doses.

☑ **PATIENT TEACHING**
● Tell patient to take drug with food, milk, antacid, or large glass of water.
● Tell patient that tablets or caplets must be swallowed whole.

---

salsalate (disalicylic acid, salicylsalicylic acid)

Amigesic, Argesic-SA, Arthra-G, Disalcid, Mono-Gesic, Salflex, Salgesic, Salsitab

Pregnancy Risk Category: C

HOW SUPPLIED

Tablets: 500 mg, 750 mg
Caplets: 750 mg
Capsules: 500 mg

ACTION

Each molecule of salsalate is hydrolyzed to two molecules of salicylate in vivo. Produces analgesia by blocking prostaglandin synthesis (peripheral action). Salicylates prevent the lowering of the pain threshold that occurs when prostaglandins sensitize pain receptors to mechanical and chemical stimulation. Drug also has an ill-defined effect on the hypothalamus. Exact mechanism of its anti-inflammatory action is unknown.

Reactions may be *common*, uncommon, *life-threatening*, or COMMON AND LIFE-THREATENING.

ONSET, PEAK, DURATION
Onset and duration unknown. Plasma levels of salsalate peak within 1½ hours of oral dose; of salicylate, 2 to 4 hours.

INDICATIONS & DOSAGE
Arthritis—
Adults: 3 g P.O. daily in divided doses b.i.d. or t.i.d.

ADVERSE REACTIONS
EENT: *tinnitus and hearing loss.*
GI: *nausea, vomiting, GI distress,* occult bleeding (rare).
Hepatic: abnormal liver function studies, hepatitis.
Skin: *rash,* bruising.
Other: hypersensitivity reactions (*anaphylaxis,* asthma), *Reye's syndrome.*

INTERACTIONS
Ammonium chloride and other urine acidifiers: increased blood levels of salicylates. Monitor for salicylate toxicity.
Antacids in high doses and other urine alkalinizers: decreased levels of salicylates. Monitor for decreased effect.
Corticosteroids: enhanced salicylate excretion. Monitor for decreased salicylate effect.
Ethanol, NSAIDs, steroids: increased risk of GI bleeding. Avoid concomitant use.
Methotrexate: increased risk of methotrexate toxicity. Avoid concomitant use.
Oral anticoagulants: possible increased risk of bleeding. Avoid using together.
Uricosuric agents: decreased uricosuric effect. Avoid concomitant use.

EFFECTS ON DIAGNOSTIC TESTS
Doses of 1 to 8 g/day or more may cause false-positive copper sulfate uric test results or false-negative enzymatic uric sugar test results. False elevations of serum uric acid tests may result. Salsalate may interfere with the Gerhardt test for uric acetoacetic acid. Increases or decreases or urine vanillylmandelic acid may occur. Physiologic effects of the drug may increase serum AST, prothrombin time, and T_3 resin uptake; the drug may decrease uric phenolsulfonphthalein concentrations, serum T_3 and T_4 concentrations, serum potassium levels, and serum cholesterol levels. Increases or decreases in serum uric acid levels may be seen.

CONTRAINDICATIONS
Contraindicated in patients with salsalate hypersensitivity.

NURSING CONSIDERATIONS
• Use cautiously in bleeding disorders, peptic ulcer disease, renal insufficiency, hypoprothrombinemia, vitamin K deficiency, thrombocytopenia, thrombotic thrombocytopenic purpura, or severe hepatic impairment.
Alert: Because of epidemiologic association with Reye's syndrome, the Centers for Disease Control and Prevention recommends not giving salicylates to children or teenagers with chickenpox or influenza-like illness.
• Monitor serum salicylate level as ordered. Therapeutic blood salicylate level in arthritis is 10 to 30 mg/100 ml. Tinnitus may occur at plasma levels of 30 mg/100 ml and above, but this is not a reliable indicator of toxicity, especially in very young patients and those over age 60. With long-term therapy, mild toxicity may occur at plasma levels of 20 mg/100 ml.
• In long-term therapy, obtain hemoglobin and PT tests periodically.

☑ PATIENT TEACHING
• Tell patient to take drug with food, milk, antacid, or large glass of water.
• Advise patient receiving long-term treatment with large doses to watch for petechiae, bleeding gums, and signs of GI bleeding, and to maintain adequate fluid intake. Encourage the use of a soft-bristled toothbrush.

---

diclofenac sodium
diclofenac potassium
etodolac
fenoprofen calcium
flurbiprofen
ibuprofen
indomethacin
indomethacin sodium trihydrate
ketoprofen
ketorolac tromethamine
meclofenamate
mefenamic acid
nabumetone
naproxen
naproxen sodium
oxaprozin
piroxicam
sulindac
tolmetin sodium

COMBINATION PRODUCTS

ADVIL COLD AND SINUS ◊ , DIMETAPP
SINUS, DRISTAN SINUS CAPLETS ◊ ,
MOTRIN IB SINUS, SINE-AID IB: pseudoephedrine hydrochloride 30 mg and
ibuprofen 200 mg.

---

diclofenac sodium
Fenac‡, Voltaren, Voltaren SR†

diclofenac potassium
Cataflam

Pregnancy Risk Category: B

HOW SUPPLIED
Tablets: 50 mg
Tablets (enteric-coated): 25 mg, 50 mg,
75 mg
Tablets (slow-release): 100 mg
Suppositories: 50 mg†, 100 mg†

ACTION
Unknown. Produces anti-inflammatory,
analgesic, and antipyretic effects, possibly by inhibiting prostaglandin synthesis.

ONSET, PEAK, DURATION
Onset occurs in 30 minutes. Plasma levels peak within 2 to 3 hours of oral administration of enteric-coated tablets;
unknown for regular tablets. Analgesic
effects persist for up to 8 hours.

INDICATIONS & DOSAGE
Ankylosing spondylitis—
Adults: 25 mg P.O. q.i.d. (and h.s.,
p.r.n.)
Osteoarthritis—
Adults: 50 mg P.O. b.i.d. or t.i.d., or 75
mg P.O. b.i.d. (diclofenac sodium only).
Rheumatoid arthritis—
Adults: 50 mg P.O. t.i.d. or q.i.d. Alternatively, 75 mg P.O. b.i.d. (diclofenac
sodium only) or 50 to 100 mg P.R.
(where available) h.s. as a substitute for
the last oral dose of the day. Not to exceed 225 mg daily.
Analgesia and primary dysmenorrhea—
Adults: 50 mg P.O. t.i.d. (diclofenac
potassium only).

ADVERSE REACTIONS
CNS: anxiety, depression, dizziness,
drowsiness, insomnia, irritability,
headache.
CV: *CHF,* hypertension, edema, fluid
retention.
EENT: *tinnitus,* laryngeal edema,
swelling of the lips and tongue, blurred
vision, eye pain, night blindness, epistaxis, taste disorder, reversible hearing
loss.
GI: *abdominal pain or cramps, constipation, diarrhea, indigestion, nausea,*
abdominal distention, flatulence, peptic
ulceration, *bleeding,* melena, bloody diarrhea, appetite change, colitis.
GU: proteinuria, *acute renal failure,*
oliguria, interstitial nephritis, papillary

Reactions may be *common,* uncommon, *life-threatening*, or COMMON AND LIFE-THREATENING.

necrosis, *nephrotic syndrome, fluid retention.*
Hepatic: elevated liver enzymes, jaundice, hepatitis, *hepatotoxicity.*
Respiratory: asthma.
Skin: rash, pruritus, urticaria, eczema, dermatitis, alopecia, photosensitivity, bullous eruption, *Stevens-Johnson syndrome* (rare), allergic purpura.
Other: *anaphylaxis; anaphylactoid reactions;* angioedema; back, leg, or joint pain; hypoglycemia; hyperglycemia.

INTERACTIONS

Anticoagulants (including warfarin): possible increased incidence of bleeding. Monitor patient closely.
Aspirin: may decrease effectiveness of diclofenac. Concomitant use not recommended by manufacturer.
Cyclosporine, digoxin, lithium, methotrexate: diclofenac may reduce renal clearance of these drugs and increase risk of toxicity. Monitor patient closely.
Diuretics: decreased effectiveness of diuretics. Avoid concomitant use.
Insulin, oral antidiabetic agents: diclofenac may alter requirements for antidiabetic agents. Monitor patient closely.
Phenytoin: increased serum levels. Monitor for toxicity.
Potassium-sparing diuretics: enhanced potassium retention and increased serum potassium levels. Monitor serum potassium level.

EFFECTS ON DIAGNOSTIC TESTS

Diclofenac increases plasma aggregation time but does not alter bleeding time, plasma thrombin clotting time, plasma fibrinogen, or Factors V and VII to XII.

CONTRAINDICATIONS

Contraindicated in patients with hypersensitivity to this drug, hepatic porphyria and in patients with a history of asthma, urticaria, or other allergic reactions after taking aspirin or other NSAIDs. Not recommended for use during late pregnancy or while breast-feeding.

NURSING CONSIDERATIONS

● Use cautiously in patients with a history of peptic ulcer disease, hepatic dysfunction, cardiac disease, hypertension, conditions associated with fluid retention, or impaired renal function.
● Because NSAIDs impair the synthesis of renal prostaglandins, they can decrease renal blood flow and lead to reversible renal impairment, especially in patients with preexisting renal failure, liver dysfunction, or heart failure; in elderly patients; and in those taking diuretics. Monitor these patients closely.
● Elevations of liver tests may occur during therapy. Monitor serum transaminase, especially ALT levels, periodically in patients undergoing long-term therapy as ordered. Know that the first serum transaminase measurement should be no later than 8 weeks after initiation of therapy.
● Be aware that because of their antipyretic and anti-inflammatory actions, NSAIDs may mask the signs and symptoms of infection.

☑ PATIENT TEACHING

● To minimize GI distress, tell patient to take diclofenac with milk or meals.
● Instruct patient not to crush, break, or chew enteric-coated tablets.
● Serious GI toxicity, including peptic ulceration and bleeding, can occur in patients taking NSAIDs despite the absence of GI symptoms. Teach patient the signs and symptoms of GI bleeding, and tell him to contact the doctor immediately if any of these occurs.
● Teach patient the signs and symptoms of hepatotoxicity, including nausea, fatigue, lethargy, pruritus, jaundice, right upper quadrant tenderness, and flulike symptoms. Tell him to contact doctor immediately if these symptoms appear.
● Advise patient to avoid consumption of alcoholic beverages or asprin while taking diclofenac.
● Tell patient to wear sunscreen or protective clothing because drug may cause photosensitivity reactions.

---

*Liquid contains alcohol.   **May contain tartrazine.   †Canada only.   ‡Australia only.   ◇OTC.

- Warn patient to avoid hazardous activities that require alertness until adverse CNS effects of drug are known.
- Tell patient that use during last trimester of pregnancy should be avoided.

---

etodolac (ultradol)
Lodine

Pregnancy Risk Category: C

HOW SUPPLIED
Capsules: 200 mg, 300 mg
Tablets: 400 mg

ACTION
Unknown, but believed related to inhibition of prostaglandin biosynthesis.

ONSET, PEAK, DURATION
Onset occurs within 30 minutes. Plasma levels peak within 1 to 2 hours. Analgesic effects persist 4 to 12 hours.

INDICATIONS & DOSAGE
Acute and chronic management of osteoarthritis and pain—
Adults: 200 to 400 mg P.O. q 6 to 8 hours, p.r.n., not to exceed 1,200 mg daily. For patients weighing 60 kg or less, total daily dose should not exceed 20 mg/kg.

ADVERSE REACTIONS
CNS: *asthenia, malaise, dizziness,* depression, drowsiness, nervousness, insomnia.
CV: hypertension, *CHF,* syncope, flushing, palpitations, edema, fluid retention.
EENT: blurred vision, tinnitus, photophobia, dry mouth.
GI: *dyspepsia*, flatulence, abdominal pain, diarrhea, nausea, constipation, gastritis, melena, vomiting, anorexia, peptic ulceration with or without *GI bleeding* or perforation, ulcerative stomatitis, thirst.
GU: dysuria, urinary frequency, *renal failure.*

Hematologic: anemia (rare), leukopenia, *thrombocytopenia,* hemolytic anemia, *agranulocytosis.*
Hepatic: hepatitis.
Respiratory: asthma.
Skin: pruritus, rash, *Stevens-Johnson syndrome.*
Other: chills, fever, weight gain.

INTERACTIONS
Antacids: may decrease peak levels of the drug. Monitor for decreased effect of etodolac.
Aspirin: reduced protein-binding of etodolac without altering its clearance. Clinical significance unknown. Recommend avoiding concomitant use.
Cyclosporine: impaired elimination and increased risk of nephrotoxicity. Avoid concomitant use.
Digoxin, lithium, methotrexate: etodolac may impair elimination of these drugs, resulting in increased levels and risk of toxicity. Monitor blood levels.
Phenytoin: increased serum levels of phenytoin. Monitor for toxicity.
Warfarin: etodolac decreases the protein-binding of warfarin but does not change its clearance. Although no dosage adjustment is necessary, monitor PT closely and watch for bleeding.

EFFECTS ON DIAGNOSTIC TESTS
A false-positive test for urinary bilirubin may be caused by phenolic metabolites. Decreased serum uric acid levels and borderline elevations of one or more liver test results may occur.

CONTRAINDICATIONS
Contraindicated in patients with hypersensitivity to the drug and in those with a history of aspirin- or NSAID-induced asthma, rhinitis, urticaria, or other allergic reactions.

NURSING CONSIDERATIONS
- Use cautiously in patients with a history of GI bleeding, ulceration, and perforation and renal or hepatic impairment.

Reactions may be *common*, uncommon, *life-threatening*, or COMMON AND LIFE-THREATENING.

• Because NSAIDs impair the synthesis of renal prostaglandins, they can decrease renal blood flow and lead to reversible renal impairment, especially in patients with preexisting renal failure, liver dysfunction, or heart failure; in elderly patients; and in those taking diuretics. Monitor these patients closely during therapy.

Alert: Know that etodolac appears to cause fewer GI problems than most NSAIDs. Minimal GI blood loss has been reported at dosages up to 1,200 mg daily.

☑ **PATIENT TEACHING**
• To minimize GI discomfort, tell patient to take etodolac with milk or meals.
• Serious GI toxicity, including peptic ulceration and bleeding, can occur in patient taking NSAIDs despite the absence of GI symptoms. Teach patient the signs and symptoms of GI bleeding, and tell him to contact the doctor immediately if any of these occurs.
• Advise patient to avoid consumption of alcoholic beverages or aspirin while taking drug.
• Warn patient to avoid hazardous activities that require alertness until adverse CNS effects of drug are known.
• This drug has been associated with photosensitivity reactions. Advise patient to use a sunblock, wear protective clothing, and avoid prolonged exposure to sunlight.
• Tell patient that use during last trimester of pregnancy should be avoided.

---

fenoprofen calcium
Nalfon, Nalfon 200

Pregnancy Risk Category: NR

HOW SUPPLIED
Tablets: 600 mg
Capsules: 200 mg, 300 mg

ACTION
Unknown. Produces anti-inflammatory, analgesic, and antipyretic effects, possibly by inhibiting prostaglandin synthesis.

ONSET, PEAK, DURATION
Onset occurs within 15 to 30 minutes. Plasma levels peak in about 2 hours. Analgesic effects persist 4 to 6 hours.

INDICATIONS & DOSAGE
Rheumatoid arthritis and osteoarthritis—
Adults: 300 to 600 mg P.O. t.i.d. or q.i.d. Maximum dosage is 3.2 g daily.
Mild to moderate pain—
Adults: 200 mg P.O. q 4 to 6 hours, p.r.n.

ADVERSE REACTIONS
CNS: *headache,* dizziness, *somnolence,* fatigue, nervousness, asthenia, tremor, confusion.
CV: peripheral edema, palpitations.
EENT: tinnitus, blurred vision, decreased hearing.
GI: *epigastric distress, nausea, GI bleeding,* vomiting, occult blood loss, peptic ulceration, constipation, anorexia, *dyspepsia,* flatulence.
GU: oliguria, interstitial nephritis, proteinuria, *reversible renal failure, papillary necrosis,* cystitis, hematuria.
Hematologic: prolonged bleeding time, anemia, *aplastic anemia, agranulocytosis, thrombocytopenia, hemorrhage,* bruising, hemolytic anemia.
Hepatic: elevated enzymes, hepatitis.
Respiratory: dyspnea, upper respiratory tract infections, nasopharyngitis.
Skin: *pruritus,* rash, urticaria, *anaphylaxis,* increased diaphoresis.
Other: angioedema.

INTERACTIONS
Aspirin: decreased fenoprofen half-life; may increase GI toxicity. Avoid concomitant use.
Diuretics: decreased diuretic effectiveness. Monitor patient closely.

---

*Liquid contains alcohol.   **May contain tartrazine.   †Canada only.   ‡Australia only.   ◇OTC.

Ethanol, corticosteroids: increased risk of adverse GI reactions. Avoid concomitant use.
Oral anticoagulants, sulfonylureas: fenoprofen enhances pharmacologic effects of these drugs. Use together cautiously.
Phenobarbital: enhanced metabolism of fenoprofen. Monitor for lack of fenoprofen effectiveness.

EFFECTS ON DIAGNOSTIC TESTS
Physiologic effects of the drug may increase bleeding time, BUN, serum creatinine, potassium, alkaline phosphatase, lactate dehydrogenase, and transaminase concentrations. Drug may also cause false elevations in both free and total serum triiodothyronine (T_3), but thyroid-stimulating hormone and thyroxine are unaffected.

CONTRAINDICATIONS
Contraindicated in patients with hypersensitivity to this drug, significantly impaired renal function, or history of aspirin- or NSAID-induced asthma, rhinitis, or urticaria. Also contraindicated in pregnancy.

NURSING CONSIDERATIONS
● Use cautiously in elderly patients; in patients with history of serious GI events or peptic ulcer disease, compromised cardiac function or hypertension.
● Be aware that safety has not been established for pregnancy. Administration to pregnant patients is not recommended.
● Because NSAIDs impair the synthesis of renal prostaglandins, they can decrease renal blood flow and lead to reversible renal impairment, especially in patients with preexisting renal failure, liver dysfunction, or heart failure; in elderly patients; and in those taking diuretics. Monitor these patients closely during therapy.
● Know that because of their antipyretic and anti-inflammatory actions, NSAIDs may mask the signs and symptoms of infection.
● Be aware that renal, hepatic, ocular, and auditory function should be checked periodically in long-term therapy. Drug should be stopped if abnormalities occur.
● Fenoprofen or its metabolite may cross-react with the antibody used in the Amerlex-M assay. Limited data suggest that drug may alter free and total T_3 concentrations determined by the Corning method.
● Know that fenoprofen is not recommended for use in children.

☑ PATIENT TEACHING
● Tell patient that full therapeutic effect for arthritis may be delayed for 2 to 4 weeks.
● Tell patient to take this drug 30 minutes before or 2 hours after meals. If adverse GI reactions occur, drug may be taken with milk or meals.
● Serious GI toxicity, including peptic ulceration and bleeding, can occur in patients taking NSAIDs despite the absence of GI symptoms. Teach patient the signs and symptoms of GI bleeding, and tell him to contact the doctor immediately if any occurs.
● Advise patient to avoid consumption of alcoholic beverages or aspirin while taking drug.
● Warn patient to avoid hazardous activities that require alertness until adverse CNS effects of the drug are known.

flurbiprofen
Ansaid, Apo-Flurbiprofen†, Froben†, Froben SR†

Pregnancy Risk Category: B

HOW SUPPLIED
Tablets: 50 mg, 100 mg
Capsules (extended-release)†: 200 mg

ACTION
Unknown. Possibly inhibits prostaglandin synthesis.

ONSET, PEAK, DURATION
Onset and duration unknown. Serum levels peak about 1½ hours after a dose.

INDICATIONS & DOSAGE
Rheumatoid arthritis and osteoarthritis—
Adults: 200 to 300 mg P.O. daily, divided b.i.d. to q.i.d. Where available, patients maintained on 200 mg daily may switch to one 200-mg extended-release capsule P.O. daily, taken in the evening after food.

ADVERSE REACTIONS
CNS: *headache,* anxiety, insomnia, dizziness, increased reflexes, tremors, amnesia, asthenia, drowsiness, malaise, depression.
CV: *edema, CHF,* hypertension, vasodilation.
EENT: rhinitis, tinnitus, visual changes, epistaxis.
GI: *dyspepsia, diarrhea, abdominal pain, nausea,* constipation, *bleeding,* flatulence, vomiting.
GU: *symptoms suggesting urinary tract infection,* hematuria, interstitial nephritis, *renal failure.*
Hematologic: *thrombocytopenia,* neutropenia, anemia, *aplastic anemia.*
Hepatic: elevated liver enzymes, jaundice.
Respiratory: asthma.
Skin: rash, photosensitivity, urticaria, angioedema.
Other: weight changes.

INTERACTIONS
Anticoagulants: increased risk of bleeding. Monitor patient closely.
Aspirin: decreased flurbiprofen levels. Concomitant use is not recommended.
Beta-adrenergic blockers: antihypertensive effect of beta blockers may be impaired. Monitor blood pressure.
Cyclosporine: increased risk of nephrotoxicity.
Diuretics: possible decreased diuretic effect. Monitor patient closely.
Lithium: serum lithium levels may be increased.
Methotrexate: increased risk of methotrexate toxicity. Monitor patient closely.

EFFECTS ON DIAGNOSTIC TESTS
None reported.

CONTRAINDICATIONS
Contraindicated in patients with hypersensitivity to the drug, or history of aspirin- or NSAID-induced asthma, urticaria, or other allergic-type reactions.

NURSING CONSIDERATIONS
● Use cautiously in patients with a history of peptic ulcer disease, hepatic dysfunction, cardiac disease, or other conditions associated with fluid retention or impaired renal function.
● Safety and effectiveness of drug use in children have not been established.
● Know that use during pregnancy is not recommended in last trimester.
● Be aware that elderly or debilitated patients and those patients with hepatic or renal dysfunction should be closely monitored and probably should receive lower doses. These patients may be at risk for renal toxicity, jaundice, or toxic hepatitis. Periodically monitor renal and hepatic function as ordered.
● Because NSAIDs impair the synthesis of renal prostaglandins, they can decrease renal blood flow and lead to reversible renal impairment, especially in patients with preexisting renal failure, liver dysfunction, or heart failure; in elderly patients; and in those taking diuretics. Monitor these patients closely during therapy.
● Know that patients receiving long-term therapy should have periodic liver function studies, eye examinations, and hematocrit determinations.

☑ PATIENT TEACHING
● Tell patient to take drug with food, milk, or antacid if GI upset occurs.
● Tell patient taking extended-release capsules to swallow them whole; do not crush, chew, or break open the capsules.

*Liquid contains alcohol. **May contain tartrazine. †Canada only. ‡Australia only. ◇OTC.

• Serious GI toxicity, including peptic ulceration and bleeding, can occur in patients taking NSAIDs despite the absence of GI symptoms. Teach patient the signs and symptoms of GI bleeding, and tell him to contact the doctor immediately if they occur.

• Advise patients to avoid consumption of alcoholic beverages or aspirin while taking drug.

• Warn patient to avoid hazardous activities that require mental alertness until CNS effects are known.

ibuprofen

Aches-N-Pain◇, ACT-3‡, Advil◇, Amersol†, Apo-Ibuprofen†, Bayer Select Pain Relief, Brufen‡, Children's Advil, Children's Motrin◇, Excedrin IB, Caplets◇, Excedrin IB Tablets◇, Genpril Caplets◇, Genpril Tablets◇, Haltran◇, Ibu-Cream‡, Ibuprin◇, Ibuprohm Caplets◇, Ibuprohm Tablets◇, Ibu-Tab◇, Inflam‡, Medipren Caplets◇, Medipren Tablets◇, Menadol, Midol IB, Midol-200◇, Motrin, Motrin IB Caplets◇, Motrin IB Tablets◇, Novo-Profen†, Nuprin Caplets◇, Nuprin Tablets◇, Nurofen‡, Pamprin-IB, PediaProfen, Rafen‡, Rufen, Saleto-200, Saleto-400, Saleto-600, Saleto-800, Trendar◇

Pregnancy Risk Category: NR

HOW SUPPLIED
Tablets: 100 mg, 200 mg◇, 300 mg, 400 mg, 600 mg, 800 mg
Tablets (chewable): 50 mg, 100 mg
Caplets: 200 mg◇
Oral suspension: 100 mg/5 ml

ACTION
Unknown. Produces anti-inflammatory, analgesic, and antipyretic effects, possibly by inhibiting prostaglandin synthesis.

ONSET, PEAK, DURATION
Analgesic and antipyretic effects occur within 30 minutes. Plasma levels peak 1 to 2 hours after oral dose and last 4 to 6 hours. Onset of antirheumatic action occurs within 7 days and peaks at 1 to 2 weeks.

INDICATIONS & DOSAGE
Rheumatoid arthritis, osteoarthritis, arthritis—
Adults: 300 to 800 mg P.O. t.i.d. or q.i.d. not to exceed 3.2 g/day.
Mild to moderate pain, dysmenorrhea—
Adults: 400 mg P.O. q 4 to 6 hours p.r.n.
Fever—
Adults: 200 to 400 mg P.O. q 4 to 6 hours. Do not exceed 1.2 g daily or give longer than 3 days.
Children 6 months to 12 years: if fever is below 102.5° F (39.2° C), the recommended dose is 5 mg/kg P.O. q 6 to 8 hours. Treat higher fevers with 10 mg/kg q 6 to 8 hours. Do not exceed 40 mg/kg daily.
External treatment of joint pain; swelling of tissues adjacent to joints†—
Adults: apply a 4- to 10-cm strip of cream to the skin and massage briskly. Apply t.i.d.
Juvenile arthritis—
Children: 30 to 70 mg/kg/day in three or four divided doses.

ADVERSE REACTIONS
CNS: *headache, dizziness,* nervousness, aseptic meningitis.
CV: *peripheral edema,* fluid retention, edema.
EENT: *tinnitus.*
GI: *epigastric distress, nausea, occult blood loss, peptic ulceration,* diarrhea, constipation, dyspepsia, flatulence, heartburn, decreased appetite.
GU: *acute renal failure,* azotemia, cystitis, hematuria.
Hematologic: prolonged bleeding time, anemia, neutropenia, pancytopenia, ***thrombocytopenia, aplastic anemia,*** leukopenia, ***agranulocytosis.***

Reactions may be *common,* uncommon, *life-threatening,* or COMMON AND LIFE-THREATENING.

Hepatic: elevated enzymes.
Respiratory: *bronchospasm.*
Skin: pruritus, *rash,* urticaria, *Stevens-Johnson syndrome.*

INTERACTIONS

Antihypertensives, furosemide, thiazide diuretics: ibuprofen may decrease the effectiveness of diuretics or antihypertensives. Monitor patient closely.
Aspirin: may decrease serum levels of ibuprofen. Avoid concomitant use.
Aspirin, corticosteroids, ethanol: increased risk of adverse GI reactions. Avoid concomitant use.
Cyclosporine: nephrotoxicity of both agents may be increased.
Digoxin, lithium, oral anticoagulants: ibuprofen may increase plasma levels or effects of these drugs. Monitor for toxicity.
Methotrexate: decreased methotrexate clearance and increased toxicity. Use together cautiously.

EFFECTS ON DIAGNOSTIC TESTS

Physiologic effects of drug may prolong bleeding time; decrease blood glucose concentrations (note that each ml of suspension contains 0.3 g sucrose); increase BUN and serum creatinine and potassium levels; decrease serum uric acid, hemoglobin, and hematocrit levels; increase PT; and increase serum alkaline phosphatase, lactate dehydrogenase, and transaminase levels.

CONTRAINDICATIONS

Contraindicated in patients with hypersensitivity to this drug, or who have the syndrome of nasal polyps, angioedema, and bronchospastic reaction to aspirin or other NSAIDs.

NURSING CONSIDERATIONS

● Use cautiously in patients with GI disorders, history of peptic ulcer disease, hepatic or renal disease, cardiac decompensation, hypertension, known intrinsic coagulation defects.
● Know that use during pregnancy is not recommended.
● Check renal and hepatic function periodically in patients on long-term therapy. Stop drug if abnormalities occur and notify doctor.
● Be aware that because of their antipyretic and anti-inflammatory actions, NSAIDs may mask the signs and symptoms of infection.
● Know that blurred or diminished vision and changes in color vision have occurred.

☑ PATIENT TEACHING

● To reduce adverse GI reactions, tell patient to take with meals or milk.
Alert: Drug is available OTC in several brands (200 mg). Instruct patient not to exceed 1.2 g daily, give to children under 12 years, or self-medicate for extended periods without consulting the doctor.
● Tell patient that full therapeutic effect for arthritis may be delayed for 2 to 4 weeks. Although analgesic effect occurs at low dosage levels, anti-inflammatory effect does not occur at dosages below 400 mg q.i.d.
● Caution patient that concomitant use with aspirin, alcohol, or corticosteroids may increase the risk of GI adverse reactions.
● Serious GI toxicity, including peptic ulceration and bleeding, can occur in patients taking NSAIDs despite the absence of GI symptoms. Teach patients the signs and symptoms of GI bleeding, and tell them to contact the doctor immediately if they occur.
● Warn patient to avoid hazardous activities that require mental alertness until CNS effects are known.
● Drug may cause photosensitivity reaction; advise the patient to wear sunscreen.

---

indomethacin

Apo-Indomethacin†, Arthrexin‡, Indochron E-R, Indocid†‡, Indocid

---

SR†, Indocin, Indocin SR, Novo-Methacin†, Rheumacin‡

indomethacin sodium trihydrate

Apo-Indomethacin†, Indocid PDA†, Indocin I.V., Novomethacin†

Pregnancy Risk Category: NR

HOW SUPPLIED
indomethacin
Capsules: 25 mg, 50 mg
Capsules (sustained-release): 75 mg
Oral suspension: 25 mg/5 ml
Suppositories: 50 mg
indomethacin sodium trihydrate
Injection: 1-mg vials

ACTION
Unknown. Produces anti-inflammatory, analgesic, and antipyretic effects, possibly by inhibiting prostaglandin synthesis.

ONSET, PEAK, DURATION
Onset occurs within 30 minutes. Serum levels peak within 1 to 2 hours after a dose of immediate-release capsules or oral suspension, within 2 to 4 hours of a sustained-release capsule, or immediately following an I.V. injection. Peak antirheumatic effects occur after 1 to 2 weeks of therapy. Analgesic effects persist 4 to 6 hours.

INDICATIONS & DOSAGE
Moderate to severe rheumatoid arthritis or osteoarthritis, ankylosing spondylitis—
Adults: 25 mg P.O. or P.R. b.i.d. or t.i.d. with food or antacids; increase daily dosage by 25 or 50 mg q 7 days, up to 200 mg daily. Or, sustained-release capsules (75 mg): 75 mg P.O. to start, in the morning or h.s., followed, if necessary, by 75 mg b.i.d.
Acute gouty arthritis—
Adults: 50 mg P.O. t.i.d. Dose reduced as soon as possible; then discontinued. Sustained-release capsules shouldn't be used for this condition.
Acute painful shoulders (bursitis or tendinitis)—
Adults: 75 to 150 mg P.O. daily in divided doses t.i.d. or q.i.d. for 7 to 14 days.
To close a hemodynamically significant patent ductus arteriosus in premature infants (I.V. form only)—
Neonates under 48 hours: 0.2 mg/kg I.V. followed by two doses of 0.1 mg/kg at 12- to 24-hour intervals.
Neonates 2 to 7 days: 0.2 mg/kg I.V. followed by two doses of 0.2 mg/kg at 12- to 24-hour intervals.
Neonates over 7 days: 0.2 mg/kg I.V. followed by two doses of 0.25 mg/kg at 12- to 24-hour intervals.

ADVERSE REACTIONS
Oral and rectal forms:
CNS: *headache, dizziness,* depression, drowsiness, confusion, somnolence, fatigue, peripheral neuropathy, *seizures, vertigo,* psychic disturbances, syncope, *vertigo.*
CV: hypertension, *edema, CHF.*
EENT: blurred vision, corneal and retinal damage, hearing loss, tinnitus.
GI: *nausea,* anorexia, *diarrhea, peptic ulceration, GI bleeding,* constipation, dyspepsia, pancreatitis.
GU: hematuria, *acute renal failure.*
Hematologic: *hemolytic anemia, aplastic anemia, agranulocytosis,* leukopenia, *thrombocytopenic purpura,* iron deficiency anemia.
Skin: pruritus, urticaria, *Stevens-Johnson syndrome.*
Other: hypersensitivity (rash, respiratory distress, **anaphylaxis, angioedema**), hyperkalemia.
I.V. form:
GU: *renal failure,* hematuria, proteinuria, interstitial nephritis.

INTERACTIONS
Aminoglycosides, cyclosporine, methotrexate: indomethacin may enhance the toxicity of these agents. Avoid concomitant use.
Anticoagulants: increased risk of bleed-

ing. Monitor patient closely.
Antihypertensives: reduced antihypertensive effect. Monitor patient closely.
Aspirin: decreased blood levels of indomethacin. Avoid concomitant use.
Corticosteroids, ethanol: increased risk of GI toxicity. Don't use together.
Diflunisal, probenecid: decreased indomethacin excretion; watch for increased incidence of indomethacin adverse reactions.
Digoxin: indomethacin may prolong the half-life of digoxin. Use together cautiously.
Dipyridamole: enhanced fluid retention. Avoid concomitant use.
Furosemide, thiazide diuretics: impaired response to both drugs. Avoid using together if possible.
Lithium: increased plasma lithium levels. Monitor for toxicity.
Phenytoin: increased serum phenytoin levels may occur.
Triamterene: possible nephrotoxicity. Monitor patient closely.

EFFECTS ON DIAGNOSTIC TESTS
Drug may interfere with results of the dexamethasone suppression test. It may also interfere with urinary 5-hydroxyindoleacetic acid determinations.

CONTRAINDICATIONS
Contraindicated in patients with hypersensitivity to this drug, or history of aspirin- or NSAID-induced asthma, rhinitis, or urticaria; in pregnancy or while breast-feeding. Also contraindicated in infants with untreated infection, active bleeding, coagulation defects or thrombocytopenia, congenital heart disease in whom patency of the ductus arteriosus is necessary, necrotizing enterocolitis, or impaired renal function. Suppositories are contraindicated in patients with a history of proctitis or recent rectal bleeding.

NURSING CONSIDERATIONS
• Use cautiously in patients with epilepsy, parkinsonism, hepatic or renal disease, cardiovascular disease, infection, and mental illness or depression. Also use cautiously in elderly patients and patients with history of GI disease.
• Be aware that because of its high incidence of adverse effects during chronic use, indomethacin should not be used routinely as an analgesic or antipyretic.
• Know that use during pregnancy is not recommended.
• Administer oral dosage with food, milk, or antacid if GI upset occurs.
• **I.V. use:** Reconstitute powder for injection with sterile water or 0.9% sodium chloride for injection or 0.9% sodium chloride. For each 1-mg vial, add 1 ml of diluent for a solution containing 1 mg/ml.
Alert: Use only preservative-free sterile sodium chloride or sterile water to prepare I.V. injection. Never use diluents containing benzyl alcohol because this has been associated with toxicity in newborns. Because the injection contains no preservatives, reconstitute immediately before administration, and discard any unused solution.
• Don't administer second or third scheduled I.V. dose if anuria or marked oliguria is evident; instead, notify doctor.
• Be aware that if ductus arteriosus reopens, a second course of one to three doses may be given. If ineffective, surgery may be necessary.
• Monitor carefully for bleeding and for reduced urine output with I.V. administration.
• Monitor for bleeding in patients receiving anticoagulants, patients with coagulation defects, and neonates.
• Because NSAIDs impair the synthesis of renal prostaglandins, they can decrease renal blood flow and lead to reversible renal impairment, especially in patients with preexisting renal failure, liver dysfunction, or heart failure; in elderly patients; and in those taking diuretics. Monitor these patients closely during therapy.
• Causes sodium retention; monitor for

weight gain (especially in elderly patients) and increased blood pressure in patients with hypertension.

• Know that because of their antipyretic and anti-inflammatory actions, NSAIDs may mask the signs and symptoms of infection.

☑ **PATIENT TEACHING**
• Tell patient to take oral form of this drug with food, milk, or antacid if GI upset occurs.
• Alert patient that concomitant use of oral form with aspirin, alcohol, or corticosteroids may increase the risk of adverse GI reactions.
• Serious GI toxicity, including peptic ulceration and bleeding, can occur in patient taking oral NSAIDs despite the absence of GI symptoms. Teach patient the signs and symptoms of GI bleeding, and tell him to contact the doctor immediately if they occur.
• Warn patient to avoid hazardous activities that require mental alertness until CNS effects are known.
• Tell patient to notify the doctor immediately if any visual or hearing changes occurs. Patient on long-term oral therapy should have regular eye examinations, hearing tests, CBC, and renal function tests to monitor for toxicity.

ketoprofen
Actron, Apo-Keto†, Apo-Keto-E†, Novo-Keto-EC†, Orudis, Orudis-E†, Orudis KT, Orudis-SR†‡, Oruvail, Rhodist†, Rhodis-E†, Rhodis-EC†

Pregnancy Risk Category: B

HOW SUPPLIED
Tablets: 12.5 mg ◊
Tablets (extended-release): 100 mg, 150 mg, 200 mg†
Tablets (enteric-coated): 50 mg†, 100 mg†
Capsules (extended-release): 100 mg, 150 mg, 200 mg
Capsules: 25 mg, 50 mg, 75 mg

Suppositories: 100 mg†

ACTION
Unknown. Produces anti-inflammatory, analgesic, and antipyretic effects, possibly by inhibiting prostaglandin synthesis.

ONSET, PEAK, DURATION
Analgesic onset occurs in 1 to 2 hours; unknown for arthritis. Serum levels peak ½ to 2 hours. Effects persist for 3 to 4 hours when used for analgesia; unknown for arthritis.

INDICATIONS & DOSAGE
Rheumatoid arthritis and osteoarthritis—
Adults: 75 mg t.i.d. or 50 mg q.i.d. or 200 mg as an extended-release tablet once daily. Maximum dosage is 300 mg/day. Reduce initial dose to one-half to one-third in elderly patients or in those with impaired renal function.
Alternatively, where suppository is available, 100 mg P.R. b.i.d.; or 1 suppository h.s. (in conjunction with oral ketoprofen during the day).
Mild to moderate pain; dysmenorrhea—
Adults: 25 to 50 mg P.O. q 6 to 8 hours p.r.n.
Minor aches and pain or fever—
Adults: 12.5 mg q 4 to 6 hours. Do not exceed 25 mg in a 4- to 6-hour period or 75 mg in 24 hours.

ADVERSE REACTIONS
CNS: *headache,* dizziness, *CNS excitation* or depression.
EENT: tinnitus, visual disturbances.
GI: *nausea, abdominal pain, diarrhea, constipation, flatulence, **peptic ulceration,** dyspepsia,* anorexia, vomiting, stomatitis.
GU: *nephrotoxicity, elevated BUN.*
Hematologic: prolonged bleeding time, **thrombocytopenia, agranulocytosis.**
Hepatic: elevated liver enzymes.
Respiratory: dyspnea, **bronchospasm, laryngeal edema.**
Skin: rash, photosensitivity, *exfoliative*

dermatitis.
Other: peripheral edema.

INTERACTIONS
Antihypertensives: reduced antihypertensive effect.
Aspirin, corticosteroids, ethanol: increased risk of adverse GI reactions. Avoid concomitant use.
Aspirin, probenecid: increased plasma levels of ketoprofen. Avoid concomitant use.
Cyclosporine: increased nephrotoxicity.
Hydrochlorothiazide, other diuretics: decreased diuretic effectiveness. Monitor for lack of effect.
Lithium, methotrexate, phenytoin: increased levels of these drugs, leading to toxicity. Monitor patient closely.
Warfarin: increased risk of bleeding. Monitor patient closely.

EFFECTS ON DIAGNOSTIC TESTS
In vitro interactions with glucose determinations have been reported with glucose oxidase and peroxidase methods.

Drug may interfere with serum iron determinations (false increases or decreases depending on method used) and produce false increases in serum bilirubin levels. These interactions were reported with drug concentrations above those seen clinically (60 mg/ml).

CONTRAINDICATIONS
Contraindicated in patients with hypersensitivity to this drug, or history of aspirin- or NSAID-induced asthma, urticaria, or other allergic-type reactions.

NURSING CONSIDERATIONS
● Use cautiously in patients with history of peptic ulcer disease, renal dysfunction, hypertension, heart failure, or fluid retention.
● Know that use during last trimester of pregnancy should be avoided.
● Know that the sustained-release dosage form is not recommended for patients in acute pain.
● Because NSAIDs impair the synthesis of renal prostaglandins, they can decrease renal blood flow and lead to reversible renal impairment, especially in patients with preexisting renal failure, liver dysfunction, or heart failure; in elderly patients; and in those taking diuretics. Monitor these patients closely during therapy.
● Check renal and hepatic function every 6 months or as indicated.
● Be aware that NSAIDs may mask the signs and symptoms of infection because of their antipyretic and anti-inflammatory actions.
● Know that drug is not recommended for use in pediatric patients.

☑ PATIENT TEACHING
Alert: Drug is available OTC. Instruct the patient not to exceed dosage of 75 mg/day.
● Tell patient to take drug 30 minutes before or 2 hours after meals. If adverse GI reactions occur, patient may take the drug with milk or meals.
● Tell patient that full therapeutic effect may be delayed for 2 to 4 weeks.
● Serious GI toxicity, including peptic ulceration and bleeding, can occur in patient taking NSAIDs despite the absence of GI symptoms. Teach patient the signs and symptoms of GI bleeding, and tell him to contact the doctor immediately if they occur.
● Alert patient that concomitant use with aspirin, alcohol, or corticosteroids may increase the risk of adverse GI reactions.
● Warn patient to avoid hazardous activities that require mental alertness until CNS effects are known.
● This drug has been associated with photosensitivity reactions. Advise patient to use a sunblock, wear protective clothing, and avoid prolonged exposure to sunlight.
● Tell patient to report visual or auditory adverse reactions immediately.

---

*Liquid contains alcohol.   **May contain tartrazine.   †Canada only.   ‡Australia only.   ◇ OTC.

ketorolac tromethamine
Toradol

Pregnancy Risk Category: C

HOW SUPPLIED
Tablets: 10 mg
Injection: 15 mg, 30 mg, 60 mg

ACTION
Unknown. Thought to inhibit prostaglandin synthesis.

ONSET, PEAK, DURATION
Onset immediate with I.V. administration; within 10 minutes of an I.M. injection; 30 to 60 minutes after oral dose. Plasma levels peak in ½ to 1 hour after either oral or I.M. administration, immediately after I.V. injection. Analgesic effects persist up to 8 hours.

INDICATIONS & DOSAGE
Short-term management of moderately severe, acute pain for single-dose treatment—
Adults under 65 years: 60 mg I.M. or 30 mg I.V.
Adults 65 years or older, renally impaired patients, or patients weighing less than 50 kg: 30 mg I.M. or 15 mg I.V.
Short-term management of moderately severe, acute pain for multiple-dose treatment—
Adults under 65 years: 30 mg I.M. or I.V. q 6 hours. Maximum daily dose should not exceed 120 mg.
Adults 65 years or older, renally impaired patients, or patients weighing less than 50 kg: 15 mg I.M. or I.V. q 6 hours. Maximum daily dose should not exceed 60 mg.
Short-term management of moderately severe, acute pain when switching from parenteral to oral administration (oral therapy is indicated only as continuation of parenterally administered drug and should never be given without the patient first having received parenteral therapy)—
Adults under 65 years: 20 mg P.O. as single dose followed by 10 mg P.O. q 4 to 6 hours, not to exceed 40 mg/day.
Adults 65 years or older, renally impaired patients, or patients weighing less than 50 kg: 10 mg P.O. as single dose followed by 10 mg P.O. q 4 to 6 hours, not to exceed 40 mg/day.

ADVERSE REACTIONS
CNS: *drowsiness, sedation,* dizziness, headache.
CV: edema, hypertension, palpitations, arrhythmias.
GI: *nausea, dyspepsia, GI pain,* diarrhea, *peptic ulceration,* vomiting, constipation, flatulence, stomatitis.
GU: *acute renal failure.*
Hematologic: decreased platelet adhesion, purpura, *thrombocytopenia.*
Other: pain at injection site, pruritus, rash, diaphoresis, *bronchospasm.*

INTERACTIONS
ACE inhibitors: may increase risk of renal impairment, particularly in volume-depleted patients. Do not use together in volume-depleted patients.
Antihypertensives, diuretics: decreased effectiveness. Monitor patient closely.
Lithium: increased lithium levels. Monitor patient closely.
Methotrexate: decreased methotrexate clearance and increased toxicity. Don't use together.
Salicylates, anticoagulants: ketorolac may increase the levels of free (unbound) salicylates or anticoagulants in the blood. Use with extreme caution and monitor patient closely.

EFFECTS ON DIAGNOSTIC TESTS
Like other NSAIDs, ketorolac has been associated with borderline elevations of one or more liver function test results. Meaningful elevations of AST or ALT—three times the upper limit—occur in less than 1% of the patients. Because this drug inhibits platelet aggregation, it can prolong bleeding time.

Reactions may be *common*, uncommon, *life-threatening*, or COMMON AND LIFE-THREATENING.

CONTRAINDICATIONS

Contraindicated in patients with hypersensitivity to this drug and in patients with active peptic ulcer disease, recent GI bleeding or perforation, advanced renal impairment, risk for renal impairment due to volume depletion, suspected or confirmed cerebrovascular bleeding, hemorrhagic diathesis, incomplete hemostasis, or high risk of bleeding.

Drug is also contraindicated in patients with a history of peptic ulcer disease or GI bleeding, past allergic manifestations to aspirin or other NSAIDs, and during labor and delivery or breastfeeding. In addition, drug is contraindicated as prophylactic analgesic before major surgery or intraoperatively when hemostasis is critical; and in patients currently receiving aspirin, an NSAID, or probenecid. Drug should not be administered epidurally or intrathecally because of alcohol content.

NURSING CONSIDERATIONS

● Use of ketorolac is not recommended in pediatric patients.
● Use cautiously in patients with hepatic or renal impairment.
Alert: The maximum combined duration of therapy (parenteral and oral) must be limited to 5 days.
● I.M. administration may cause pain at the injection site. Holding pressure over the site for 15 to 30 seconds after the injection may minimize local effects.
● Do not mix with morphine sulfate, meperidine hydrochloride, promethazine hydrochloride, or hydroxyzine hydrochloride. Toradol will precipitate out in solution.
● Carefully observe patients with coagulopathies and those who are taking anticoagulants. Ketorolac inhibits platelet aggregation and can prolong bleeding time. This effect will disappear within 48 hours of discontinuing the drug. It will not alter platelet count, PTT, or PT.
● Be aware that NSAIDs may mask the signs and symptoms of infection because of their antipyretic and anti-inflammatory actions.

☑ PATIENT TEACHING
● Warn patient receiving drug I.M. that pain may occur at injection site.
● Serious GI toxicity, including peptic ulceration and bleeding, can occur in patient taking NSAIDs despite the absence of GI symptoms. Teach patient the signs and symptoms of GI bleeding, and tell him to notify the doctor immediately if they occur.

meclofenamate
Meclomen

Pregnancy Risk Category: NR

HOW SUPPLIED
Capsules: 50 mg, 100 mg

ACTION
Unknown. Produces anti-inflammatory, analgesic, and antipyretic effects, possibly by inhibiting prostaglandin synthesis.

ONSET, PEAK, DURATION
Onset occurs within 30 minutes for analgesic effects; antirheumatic effects, within a few days of therapy. Plasma levels peak in $\frac{1}{2}$ to 1 hour; peak antirheumatic activity occurs after 2 to 3 weeks of therapy. Duration unknown.

INDICATIONS & DOSAGE
Rheumatoid arthritis and osteoarthritis—
Adults: 200 to 400 mg/day P.O. in three or four equally divided doses.
Mild to moderate pain—
Adults: 50 to 100 mg P.O. q 4 to 6 hours. Maximum dosage is 400 mg/day.
Dysmenorrhea or menorrhagia—
Adults: 100 mg P.O. t.i.d. for up to 6 days, starting on first day of menstrual flow.

ADVERSE REACTIONS
CNS: *dizziness, headache.*

CV: edema.
EENT: tinnitus.
GI: *abdominal pain, flatulence, peptic ulceration,* constipation, anorexia, stomatitis, *GI bleeding.*
GU: *acute renal failure, hyperkalemia, hematuria.*
Hematologic: leukopenia, *thrombocytopenia, agranulocytosis, hemolytic anemia.*
Hepatic: *renal failure,* alterations in liver function tests.
Skin: rash, urticaria.

INTERACTIONS
Antihypertensives, diuretics: decreased effectiveness. Monitor patient closely.
Aspirin: decreased plasma levels of meclofenamate. Avoid concomitant use.
Corticosteroids, ethanol, other NSAIDs: increased risk of GI adverse reactions. Avoid concomitant use.
Cyclosporine, methotrexate: toxicity may be increased.
Lithium, phenytoin: increased serum levels. Monitor patient.
Oral anticoagulants: enhanced anticoagulant effect. Monitor for toxicity.

EFFECTS ON DIAGNOSTIC TESTS
False-positive test results for urine bilirubin by the Di-Azo tablet test have been reported.

CONTRAINDICATIONS
Contraindicated in patients with hypersensitivity to the drug or with a history of aspirin- or NSAID-induced bronchospasm, urticaria, or rhinitis.

NURSING CONSIDERATIONS
● Use cautiously in patients with hepatic or renal disease, cardiovascular disease, blood dyscrasia, and in those with a history of peptic ulcer disease; and in elderly patients, who are more likely to experience adverse reactions.
● Know that use during pregnancy is not recommended, especially during 1st and 3rd trimesters.
● Because NSAIDs impair the synthesis

of renal prostaglandins, they can decrease renal blood flow and lead to reversible renal impairment, especially in patients with preexisting renal failure, liver dysfunction, or heart failure; in elderly patients; and in those taking diuretics. Monitor these patients closely during therapy.
● Know that NSAIDs may mask the signs and symptoms of infection because of their anti-inflammatory and antipyretic actions.
● Be aware that CBC and renal and hepatic function should be assessed every 6 months or as indicated in patients receiving long-term therapy.

☑ **PATIENT TEACHING**
● Tell patient to take this drug with food to minimize adverse GI reactions.
● Tell patient to stop drug and contact the doctor immediately if rash, visual disturbances, or diarrhea develops.
● Caution patient that concomitant use with other NSAIDs, alcohol, or corticosteroids may increase the risk of GI adverse reactions.
● Serious GI toxicity, including peptic ulceration and bleeding, can occur in patient taking NSAIDs despite the absence of GI symptoms. Teach patient the signs and symptoms of GI bleeding, and tell him to contact the doctor immediately if they occur.
● Advise patient to avoid hazardous activities that require mental alertness until CNS effects are known.

---

mefenamic acid
Mefic‡, Ponstan†, Ponstel

Pregnancy Risk Category: C

HOW SUPPLIED
Capsules: 250 mg

ACTION
Produces anti-inflammatory, analgesic, and antipyretic effects, possibly by inhibiting prostaglandin synthesis.

ONSET, PEAK, DURATION

Onset and duration unknown. Serum levels peak 2 to 4 hours after a dose.

INDICATIONS & DOSAGE

Mild to moderate pain, dysmenorrhea—
Adults and children over 14 years: initially, 500 mg P.O.; then 250 mg q 6 hours, p.r.n. Maximum therapy is 1 week for pain.

ADVERSE REACTIONS

CNS: drowsiness, dizziness, nervousness, headache, insomnia.
EENT: blurred vision.
GI: nausea, *diarrhea, peptic ulceration, GI bleeding,* anorexia, flatulence, constipation.
GU: dysuria, hematuria, *renal failure.*
Hematologic: leukopenia, *thrombocytopenia, agranulocytosis, hemolytic anemia.*
Hepatic: *hepatotoxicity.*
Skin: rash, urticaria.

INTERACTIONS

Antihypertensives, diuretics: decreased effect. Monitor patient closely.
Aspirin, corticosteroids, ethanol: increased risk of GI adverse reactions. Avoid concomitant use.
Oral anticoagulants, sulfonylureas, and other highly protein-bound drugs: increased risk of toxicity. Monitor patient closely.

EFFECTS ON DIAGNOSTIC TESTS

False-positive results for urine bilirubin by the Di-Azo tablet test have been reported. Serum BUN, transaminase, and potassium levels may be increased by the drug; hematocrit may be decreased. Mefenamic acid may also increase PT.

CONTRAINDICATIONS

Contraindicated in patients with hypersensitivity to the drug; history of aspirin- or NSAID-induced bronchospasm, allergic rhinitis, or urticaria; GI ulceration or inflammation; or renal disease.

NURSING CONSIDERATIONS

● Use cautiously in patients with hepatic disease, cardiovascular disease, and in those with a history of peptic ulcer disease.
● Know that use during third trimester of pregnancy is not recommended.
Alert: Be aware that mefenamic acid should not be administered for more than 1 week at a time because of increased risk of toxicity.
● Severe hemolytic anemia may occur with prolonged use. Monitor CBC every 4 to 6 months as ordered or as indicated.
● Because NSAIDs impair the synthesis of renal prostaglandins, they can decrease renal blood flow and lead to reversible renal impairment, especially in patients with preexisting renal failure, liver dysfunction, or heart failure; in elderly patients; and in those taking diuretics. Monitor these patients closely during therapy.
● Know that NSAIDs may mask the signs and symptoms of infection because of their anti-inflammatory and antipyretic actions.

☑ PATIENT TEACHING

● Tell patient to take this drug with food to minimize adverse GI reactions.
● Tell patient to stop drug and contact the doctor immediately if rash, visual disturbances, or diarrhea develops.
● Caution patient that concomitant use with aspirin, alcohol, or corticosteroids may increase the risk of GI adverse reactions.
● Serious GI toxicity, including peptic ulceration and bleeding, can occur in patient taking NSAIDs despite the absence of GI symptoms. Teach patient the signs and symptoms of GI bleeding, and tell him to contact the doctor immediately if they occur.
● Warn patient against hazardous activities that require alertness until CNS effects are known.

---

*Liquid contains alcohol.   **May contain tartrazine.   †Canada only.   ‡Australia only.   ◇OTC.

nabumetone
Relafen

Pregnancy Risk Category: C

HOW SUPPLIED
Tablets: 500 mg, 750 mg

ACTION
Unknown. Probably acts by inhibiting prostaglandin synthesis.

ONSET, PEAK, DURATION
Onset and duration unknown. Plasma levels peak 2 to 4 hours after a dose.

INDICATIONS & DOSAGE
Rheumatoid arthritis or osteoarthritis—
Adults: initially, 1,000 mg P.O. daily as a single dose or in divided doses b.i.d. Maximum daily dosage is 2,000 mg.

ADVERSE REACTIONS
CNS: *dizziness, headache,* fatigue, insomnia, nervousness, somnolence.
CV: vasculitis, edema.
EENT: *tinnitus.*
GI: *diarrhea, dyspepsia, abdominal pain, constipation, flatulence, nausea,* dry mouth, gastritis, stomatitis, anorexia, vomiting, ***bleeding,*** ulceration.
Respiratory: dyspnea, pneumonitis.
Skin: *pruritus, rash,* increased diaphoresis.

INTERACTIONS
Diuretics: NSAIDs may decrease diuretic effectiveness. Monitor patients closely during therapy.
Ethanol: associated with an increased risk of additive GI toxicity. Concomitant use should be avoided.
Warfarin and other highly protein-bound drugs: increased risk of adverse effects from displacement of drugs by nabumetone. Use cautiously.

EFFECTS ON DIAGNOSTIC TESTS
None reported.

CONTRAINDICATIONS
Contraindicated in patients with hypersensitivity reactions, or history of aspirin- or NSAID-induced asthma, urticaria, or other allergic-type reactions.

NURSING CONSIDERATIONS
• Use cautiously in patients with renal or hepatic impairment; CHF, hypertension, or other conditions that may predispose the patient to fluid retention; and in patients with a history of peptic ulcer disease.
• Know that use during 3rd trimester of pregnancy is not recommended.
• Because NSAIDs impair the synthesis of renal prostaglandins, they can decrease renal blood flow and lead to reversible renal impairment, especially in patients with preexisting renal failure, liver dysfunction, or heart failure; in elderly patients; and in those taking diuretics. Monitor these patients closely during therapy.
• During long-term therapy, periodically monitor renal and liver function, CBC, and hematocrit as ordered; assess these patients for signs and symptoms of GI bleeding.
• Know that drug is not recommended for use in children.

☑ PATIENT TEACHING
• Instruct patient to take this drug with food, milk, or antacids. Nabumetone is absorbed more rapidly when administered with food or milk.
• Advise patient to limit alcohol intake because of additive GI toxicity risk.
• Serious GI toxicity, including peptic ulceration and bleeding, can occur in patient taking NSAIDs despite the absence of GI symptoms. Teach patient the signs and symptoms of GI bleeding and tell him to contact the doctor immediately if they occur.
• Warn patient against hazardous activities that require mental alertness until CNS effects are known.

naproxen
Apo-Naproxen†, EC-Naprosyn, Inza-250‡, Inza-500‡, Naprosyn, Naprosyn-E†, Naprosyn SR†‡, Naxen†‡, Novo-Naprox†, Nu-Naprox†

naproxen sodium
Aleve ◊, Anaprox, Anaprox DS, Apo-Napro-Na†, Naprelan, Naprogesic‡, Novo-Naprox Sodium†, Synflex†

Pregnancy Risk Category: B

HOW SUPPLIED
naproxen
Tablets: 250 mg, 375 mg, 500 mg
Tablets (delayed-release): 375 mg, 500 mg
Tablets (extended-release)†: 750 mg, 1,000 mg
Oral suspension: 125 mg/5 ml
Suppositories: 500 mg‡
naproxen sodium
Tablets (controlled-release): 421.5 mg, 550 mg
Tablets (film-coated): 220 mg ◊, 275 mg, 550 mg
Note: 275 mg of naproxen sodium contains 250 mg of naproxen

ACTION
Unknown. Produces anti-inflammatory, analgesic, and antipyretic effects, possibly by inhibiting prostaglandin synthesis.

ONSET, PEAK, DURATION
Onset of analgesic effect within 1 hour, antirheumatic effect within 14 days. Peak serum levels after administration of naproxen sodium occur within 1 to 2 hours; peak levels after naproxen (base) occur in 2 to 4 hours. Analgesic effects persist about 7 hours.

INDICATIONS & DOSAGE
Rheumatoid arthritis, osteoarthritis, ankylosing spondylitis, pain, dysmenorrhea, tendinitis, bursitis—
Adults: 250 to 500 mg (naproxen) b.i.d.; maximum is 1.5 g/day for a limited time. Or, 375 to 500 mg delayed-release (EC-Naprosyn) b.i.d.; or 750 to 1,000 mg controlled-release (Naprelan) b.i.d.; or 275 to 550 mg naproxen sodium b.i.d.
Juvenile arthritis—
Children: 10 mg/kg P.O. in two divided doses.
Acute gout—
Adults: 750 mg (naproxen) P.O., followed by 250 mg q 8 hours until attack subsides. Or, 825 mg naproxen sodium, followed by 275 mg q 8 hours until attack subsides; or 1,000 to 1,500 mg/day controlled-release (Naprelan) on first day, followed by 1,000 mg daily until attack subsides.
Mild to moderate pain, primary dysmenorrhea—
Adults: 500 mg (naproxen) P.O., followed by 250 mg q 6 to 8 hours up to 1.25 g/day. Or, 550 mg naproxen sodium, followed by 275 mg q 6 to 8 hours up to 1.375 g/day; or 1,000 mg controlled-release (Naprelan) once daily.

ADVERSE REACTIONS
CNS: *headache, drowsiness, dizziness,* vertigo.
CV: *edema,* palpitations.
EENT: visual disturbances, *tinnitus,* auditory disturbances.
GI: *epigastric distress, occult blood loss, nausea, **peptic ulceration,*** constipation, dyspepsia, heartburn, diarrhea, stomatitis, thirst.
GU: nephrotoxicity, ***acute renal failure.***
Hematologic: ***thrombocytopenia,*** eosinophilia, ***agranulocytosis,*** neutropenia.
Hepatic: elevated liver enzyme levels.
Respiratory: dyspnea.
Skin: *pruritus, rash,* urticaria, ecchymosis, diaphoresis, purpura.

INTERACTIONS
ACE inhibitors: may increase risk of renal impairment. Use together cautiously.
Antihypertensives, diuretics: decreased

---

effect of these drugs. Monitor patient closely.

Aspirin, corticosteroids, ethanol: increased risk of adverse GI reactions. Avoid concomitant use.

Methotrexate: increased risk of toxicity. Monitor patient closely.

Oral anticoagulants, sulfonylureas, and other highly protein-bound drugs: increased risk of toxicity. Monitor patient closely.

Probenecid: decreased elimination of naproxen. Monitor for toxicity.

EFFECTS ON DIAGNOSTIC TESTS
Naproxen and its metabolite may interfere with urinary 5-hydroxyindoleacetic acid (5-HIAA) and 17-hydroxycorticosteroid determinations. The physiologic effects of naproxen may lead to an increase in bleeding time (may persist for 4 days after withdrawal of drug); serum creatinine and potassium, BUN, and serum transaminase levels may also increase.

CONTRAINDICATIONS
Contraindicated in patients with hypersensitivity to this drug or with the syndrome of asthma, rhinitis, and nasal polyps.

NURSING CONSIDERATIONS
● Use cautiously in elderly patients and in patients with renal disease, cardiovascular disease, GI disorders, hepatic disease, or a history of peptic ulcer disease.
● Know that use during last trimester of pregnancy should be avoided.
● Because NSAIDs impair the synthesis of renal prostaglandins, they can decrease renal blood flow and lead to reversible renal impairment, especially in patients with preexisting renal failure, liver dysfunction, or heart failure; in elderly patients; and in those taking diuretics. Monitor these patients closely during therapy.
● Monitor CBC and renal and hepatic function every 4 to 6 months or as indicated and ordered during long-term

therapy.
● Be aware that because of their antipyretic and anti-inflammatory actions, NSAIDs may mask the signs and symptoms of infection.

☑ **PATIENT TEACHING**
Alert: Drug is available OTC (naproxen sodium, 200 mg). Instruct the patient not to exceed 600 mg in 24 hours. Patient over 65 years should not exceed 400 mg/day.
● Advise patient to take drug with food or milk to minimize GI upset. A full glass of water or other liquid should be taken with each dose.
● Tell patient taking prescription doses of naproxen for arthritis that full therapeutic effect may be delayed 2 to 4 weeks.
● Warn patient against taking both naproxen and naproxen sodium at the same time because both circulate in the blood as the naproxen anion.
● Serious GI toxicity, including peptic ulceration and bleeding, can occur in patient taking NSAIDs despite the absence of GI symptoms. Teach patient the signs and symptoms of GI bleeding and tell him to contact the doctor immediately if they occur.
● Caution patient that concomitant use with aspirin, alcohol, or corticosteroids may increase the risk of adverse GI reactions.
● Warn patient against hazardous activities that require mental alertness until CNS effects are known.

---

oxaprozin
Daypro

Pregnancy Risk Category: C

HOW SUPPLIED
Caplets: 600 mg

ACTION
Unknown. Produces anti-inflammatory, analgesic, and antipyretic effects, possi-

bly by inhibiting prostaglandin synthesis.

ONSET, PEAK, DURATION
Onset and duration unknown. Serum levels peak 3 to 5 hours after a dose.

INDICATIONS & DOSAGE
Osteoarthritis or rheumatoid arthritis—
Adults: initially, 1,200 mg P.O. daily. Then, individualized to the smallest effective dosage to minimize adverse reactions. Smaller patients or those with mild symptoms may require only 600 mg daily. Maximum is 1,800 mg or 26 mg/kg, whichever is lower, in divided doses.

ADVERSE REACTIONS
CNS: depression, sedation, somnolence, confusion, sleep disturbances.
EENT: tinnitus, blurred vision.
GI: *nausea, dyspepsia, diarrhea, constipation,* abdominal pain or distress, anorexia, flatulence, vomiting, ***hemorrhage,*** stomatitis.
GU: dysuria, urinary frequency.
Hepatic: elevated liver function test results (with chronic use); severe hepatic dysfunction (rare).
Skin: *rash,* photosensitivity.

INTERACTIONS
Antihypertensives, diuretics: decreased effect. Monitor patient closely and adjust dosage, as ordered.
Aspirin: oxaprozin displaces salicylates from plasma protein-binding sites, increasing risk of salicylate toxicity. Avoid concomitant use.
Aspirin, corticosteroids, ethanol: increased risk of adverse GI reactions. Avoid concomitant use.
Cyclosporine: nephrotoxicity may be increased.
Methotrexate: increased risk of methotrexate toxicity. Avoid concomitant use.
Oral anticoagulants: although problems haven't been reported, there is an increased risk of bleeding. Use together

cautiously.
Phenytoin, lithium: serum levels of these drugs may be increased.

EFFECTS ON DIAGNOSTIC TESTS
Drug can alter platelet aggregation and prolong bleeding time. It also may decrease hemoglobin levels, causing anemia, and elevate liver function studies.

CONTRAINDICATIONS
Contraindicated in patients with hypersensitivity to this drug or with the syndrome of nasal polyps, angioedema, and bronchospastic reaction to aspirin or other NSAIDs.

NURSING CONSIDERATIONS
● Use cautiously in patients with a history of peptic ulcer disease, hepatic or renal dysfunction, hypertension, cardiovascular disease, or conditions predisposing patient to fluid retention.
● Because renal prostaglandins play a role in the maintenance of renal perfusion, patients with preexisting conditions leading to a reduction in renal blood flow may experience renal toxicity with NSAID therapy. Those at greatest risk are elderly patients, patients taking diuretics, and those with impaired renal, hepatic, or cardiac function. Closely monitor renal function in these patients, and discontinue NSAID therapy if problems develop.
● Elevations of liver function tests can occur after chronic use. These abnormal findings may persist, worsen, or resolve with continued therapy. Rarely, patients may progress to severe hepatic dysfunction. Periodically monitor liver function tests in patients receiving long-term therapy, and closely monitor patients with abnormal test results.
● Be aware that because of their antipyretic and anti-inflammatory actions, NSAIDs may mask the signs and symptoms of infection.

☑ PATIENT TEACHING
● Tell patient to take this drug 30 min-

---

*Liquid contains alcohol.   **May contain tartrazine.   †Canada only.   ‡Australia only.   ◇OTC.

utes before or 2 hours after meals. If adverse GI reactions occur, drug may be taken with milk or meals.
• Tell patient that full therapeutic effects may be delayed for 2 to 4 weeks.
• Serious GI toxicity, including peptic ulceration and bleeding, can occur in patient taking NSAIDs despite the absence of GI symptoms. Teach patient the signs and symptoms of GI bleeding and tell him to contact the doctor immediately if they occur.
• Tell patient to report adverse visual or auditory reactions immediately.
• Warn patient against hazardous activities that require mental alertness until CNS effects are known.
• This drug has been associated with photosensitivity reactions. Advise patient to use a sunblock, wear protective clothing, and avoid prolonged exposure to sunlight.

---

piroxicam
Apo-Piroxicam†, Feldene, Novo-Pirocam†

Pregnancy Risk Category: NR

HOW SUPPLIED
Capsules: 10 mg, 20 mg

ACTION
Unknown. Produces anti-inflammatory, analgesic, and antipyretic effects, possibly by inhibiting prostaglandin synthesis.

ONSET, PEAK, DURATION
Onset occurs within 1 hour for analgesia; antirheumatic action, 7 to 12 days. Serum levels peak in 3 to 5 hours; peak rheumatic action occurs after 2 to 3 weeks of therapy. Analgesic effects persist for 48 to 72 hours.

INDICATIONS & DOSAGE
Osteoarthritis and rheumatoid arthritis—
Adults: 20 mg P.O. daily. If desired, the

dosage may be divided b.i.d.

ADVERSE REACTIONS
CNS: headache, drowsiness, dizziness, somnolence, vertigo.
CV: peripheral edema.
EENT: auditory disturbances.
GI: *epigastric distress, nausea, occult blood loss,* **peptic ulceration, severe GI bleeding,** diarrhea, constipation, abdominal pain, dyspepsia, flatulence, anorexia, stomatitis.
GU: *nephrotoxicity,* elevated BUN level.
Hematologic: prolonged bleeding time, anemia, leukopenia, *aplastic anemia, agranulocytosis,* eosinophilia, *thrombocytopenia.*
Hepatic: elevated liver enzymes.
Respiratory: *bronchospasm.*
Skin: pruritus, rash, urticaria, *photosensitivity.*

INTERACTIONS
Antihypertensives, diuretics: decreased effects.
Aspirin, corticosteroids, ethanol: increased risk of GI toxicity. Decreased plasma levels of piroxicam. Avoid concomitant use.
Lithium: increased plasma lithium levels. Monitor for toxicity.
Methotrexate, cyclosporine: increased toxicity. Monitor patient closely.
Oral anticoagulants and other highly protein-bound drugs: enhanced risk of bleeding. Monitor patient closely.
Oral antidiabetic agents: enhanced antidiabetic effects. Monitor patient closely.

EFFECTS ON DIAGNOSTIC TESTS
Physiologic effects of the drug may prolong bleeding time (may persist for 2 weeks after discontinuing drug); increase BUN, creatinine, and potassium levels or PT; decrease serum glucose (in diabetic patients), hemoglobin, hematocrit, or uric acid levels; and increase liver function test results (alkaline phosphatase, lactate dehydrogenase, or transaminase levels).

Reactions may be *common*, uncommon, *life-threatening*, or COMMON AND LIFE-THREATENING.

CONTRAINDICATIONS
Contraindicated in patients with hypersensitivity to this drug or with bronchospasm or angioedema precipitated by aspirin or NSAIDs and during pregnancy or while breast-feeding.

NURSING CONSIDERATIONS
● Use cautiously in elderly patients and in patients with GI disorders, history of renal or peptic ulcer disease, cardiac disease, hypertension, or conditions predisposing to fluid retention.
● Because NSAIDs impair the synthesis of renal prostaglandins, they can decrease renal blood flow and lead to reversible renal impairment, especially in patients with preexisting renal failure, liver dysfunction, or heart failure; in elderly patients; and in those taking diuretics. Monitor these patients closely.
● Check renal, hepatic, and auditory function and CBC periodically during prolonged therapy. Discontinue drug if abnormalities occur and notify doctor.
● Be aware that NSAIDs may mask the signs and symptoms of infection because of their antipyretic and anti-inflammatory actions.

☑ PATIENT TEACHING
● Tell patient to take this drug with milk, antacids, or meals if GI adverse reactions occur.
● Tell patient that full therapeutic effects may be delayed for 2 to 4 weeks.
● Serious GI toxicity, including peptic ulceration and bleeding, can occur in patient taking NSAIDs despite the absence of GI symptoms. Teach patient what signs and symptoms of GI bleeding to look for and when to report them.
● Warn patient against hazardous activities that require mental alertness until CNS effects are known.
● Advise patient to use a sunblock, wear protective clothing, and avoid prolonged exposure to sunlight. Causes adverse skin reactions more often than other drugs in its class. Photosensitivity reactions are the most common.

sulindac
Aclin‡, Apo-Sulin†, Clinoril, Novo-Sundac†

Pregnancy Risk Category: NR

HOW SUPPLIED
Tablets: 100 mg‡, 150 mg, 200 mg

ACTION
Produces anti-inflammatory, analgesic, and antipyretic effects, possibly by inhibiting prostaglandin synthesis.

ONSET, PEAK, DURATION
Onset and duration unknown. Plasma levels peak 2 to 4 hours after a dose; peak antirheumatic effects occur in 2 to 3 weeks.

INDICATIONS & DOSAGE
Osteoarthritis, rheumatoid arthritis, ankylosing spondylitis—
Adults: initially, 150 mg P.O. b.i.d.; increased to 200 mg b.i.d., p.r.n.
Acute subacromial bursitis or supraspinatus tendinitis, acute gouty arthritis—
Adults: 200 mg P.O. b.i.d. for 7 to 14 days. Dose reduced as symptoms subside.

ADVERSE REACTIONS
CNS: dizziness, headache, nervousness, psychosis.
CV: hypertension, CHF, palpitations.
EENT: tinnitus, transient visual disturbances.
GI: *epigastric distress,* **peptic ulceration, pancreatitis,** occult blood loss, nausea, constipation, dyspepsia, flatulence, anorexia, *GI bleeding.*
GU: interstitial nephritis, *nephrotic syndrome, renal failure.*
Hematologic: prolonged bleeding time, *aplastic anemia, thrombocytopenia,* neutropenia, *agranulocytosis,* hemolytic anemia.
Skin: *rash,* pruritus.
Other: edema, drug fever, *anaphylaxis,*

---

*Liquid contains alcohol.   **May contain tartrazine.   †Canada only.   ‡Australia only.   ◇OTC.

angioedema, *hypersensitivity syndrome.*

INTERACTIONS
Anticoagulants: increased risk of bleeding. Monitor PT closely.
Aspirin: decreased sulindac plasma concentration and increased risk of GI adverse reactions. Concomitant use not recommended.
Cyclosporine: increased nephrotoxicity of cyclosporine. Avoid concomitant use.
Diflunisal, dimethyl sulfoxide: decreased metabolism of sulindac to its active metabolite, reducing its effectiveness. Don't use together.
Methotrexate: increased methotrexate toxicity. Avoid concomitant use.
Probenecid: increased plasma levels of sulindac and its active metabolite. Monitor for toxicity.
Sulfonamides, sulfonylureas, other highly protein-bound drugs: possible displacement of these drugs from plasma protein-binding sites, leading to increased toxicity. Monitor closely.

EFFECTS ON DIAGNOSTIC TESTS
Physiologic effects of the drug may result in in creased bleeding time; increased BUN and serum creatinine and potassium levels; and increased serum alkaline phosphatase and transaminase concentrations.

CONTRAINDICATIONS
Contraindicated in patients with hypersensitivity to this drug or in whom acute asthmatic attacks, urticaria, or rhinitis is precipitated by aspirin or NSAIDs.

NURSING CONSIDERATIONS
● Use cautiously in patients with a history of ulcers and GI bleeding, renal dysfunction, compromised cardiac function, hypertension, or conditions predisposing to fluid retention.
● Know that use during pregnancy is not recommended.
● Periodically monitor hepatic and renal function and CBC in patients receiving long-term therapy as ordered.

● Be aware that NSAIDs may mask the signs and symptoms of infection.

☑ PATIENT TEACHING
● Tell patient to take this drug with food, milk, or antacids.
● Serious GI toxicity, including peptic ulceration and bleeding, can occur in patient taking NSAIDs despite the absence of GI symptoms. Teach patient the signs and symptoms of GI bleeding and tell him to contact the doctor immediately if they occur.
Alert: Tell patient to notify the doctor immediately if easy bruising or prolonged bleeding occurs.
● Advise patient to avoid hazardous activities that require mental alertness until CNS effects are known.
● Instruct patient to report edema and have blood pressure checked monthly. Drug causes sodium retention but is thought to have less effect on the kidneys than other NSAIDs.
● Patient should notify the doctor and have complete eye examinations if any visual disturbances occur.

---

tolmetin sodium
Tolectin 200, Tolectin 400, Tolectin 600, Tolectin DS

Pregnancy Risk Category: C

HOW SUPPLIED
Tablets: 200 mg, 600 mg
Capsules: 400 mg

ACTION
Produces anti-inflammatory, analgesic, and antipyretic effects, possibly by inhibiting prostaglandin synthesis.

ONSET, PEAK, DURATION
Onset and duration unknown. Serum levels peak in ½ to 1 hour; peak effect occurs after 1 to 2 weeks.

INDICATIONS & DOSAGE
Rheumatoid arthritis, osteoarthritis, ju-

venile rheumatoid arthritis—
Adults: 400 mg P.O. t.i.d. Maximum daily dosage is 1.8 g.
Children 2 years or over: initially, 20 mg/kg/day P.O. in divided doses (t.i.d. or q.i.d.), followed by maintenance dosage of 15 to 30 mg/kg P.O. daily in divided doses (t.i.d. or q.i.d.).

ADVERSE REACTIONS
CNS: *headache,* dizziness, drowsiness, asthenia, depression.
CV: chest pain, hypertension, edema.
EENT: tinnitus, visual disturbances.
GI: *epigastric distress,* **peptic ulceration,** occult blood loss, *nausea,* vomiting, diarrhea, constipation, dyspepsia, flatulence, anorexia, ***GI bleeding.***
GU: hematuria, proteinuria, dysuria, ***renal failure.***
Hematologic: prolonged bleeding time, granulocytopenia, ***thrombocytopenia, agranulocytosis,*** hemolytic anemia.
Skin: rash, urticaria, pruritus.
Other: ***anaphylaxis,*** *weight gain,* weight loss.

INTERACTIONS
Anticoagulants: increased risk of bleeding. Monitor patient closely.
Aspirin: increased tolmetin levels. Avoid concurrent use.
Ethanol: increased risk of GI toxicity. Avoid concomitant use.
Methotrexate: increased risk of methotrexate toxicity. Monitor closely.

EFFECTS ON DIAGNOSTIC TESTS
Tolmetin falsely elevates results of urinary protein assays (pseudoproteinuria) in tests using sulfosalicylic acid (not reagent strips like Albustix or Unistix). The physiologic effects may result in an increased bleeding time; increased BUN, serum potassium, and serum transaminase levels; and decreased hemoglobin and hematocrit levels.

CONTRAINDICATIONS
Contraindicated in patients with hypersensitivity to this drug or in whom acute asthmatic attacks, urticaria, or rhinitis is precipitated by aspirin or NSAIDs as well as in lactation.

NURSING CONSIDERATIONS
● Use cautiously in patients with cardiac or renal disease, GI bleeding, history of peptic ulcer disease, hypertension, or conditions predisposing to fluid retention.
● NSAIDs can decrease renal blood flow and lead to reversible renal impairment, especially in patients with preexisting renal failure, liver dysfunction, or heart failure; in elderly patients; and in those taking diuretics. Monitor closely.
● Know that NSAIDs may mask the signs and symptoms of infection because of their antipyretic and anti-inflammatory actions.

☑ **PATIENT TEACHING**
● Tell patient to take this drug with food, milk, or antacids to reduce adverse GI reactions.
● Tell patient that therapeutic effect begins within 1 week, but full effect may be delayed 2 to 4 weeks.
● Serious GI toxicity, including peptic ulceration and bleeding, can occur in patient taking NSAIDs despite the absence of GI symptoms. Teach patient the signs and symptoms of GI bleeding and tell him to contact the doctor immediately if they occur.
● Tell patient to notify the doctor immediately if any visual or hearing change occurs. During prolonged therapy, patient should have regular eye examinations, hearing tests, CBCs, and renal function tests.
● Advise patient to avoid hazardous activities that require alertness until the CNS effects of the drug are known.
● Advise patient to wear sunblock and protective clothing when in the sun.

28

Narcotic and opioid analgesics

alfentanil hydrochloride
buprenorphine hydrochloride
butorphanol tartrate
codeine phosphate
codeine sulfate
fentanyl citrate
fentanyl transdermal system
fentanyl transmucosal
hydromorphone hydrochloride
meperidine hydrochloride
methadone hydrochloride
morphine hydrochloride
morphine sulfate
morphine tartrate
nalbuphine hydrochloride
oxycodone hydrochloride
oxycodone pectinate
oxymorphone hydrochloride
pentazocine hydrochloride
pentazocine hydrochloride and
**   naloxone hydrochloride**
pentazocine lactate
propoxyphene hydrochloride
propoxyphene napsylate
sufentanil citrate
tramadol hydrochloride

COMBINATION PRODUCTS

222†: aspirin 375 mg, codeine phosphate 8 mg, and caffeine citrate 30 mg.
222 FORTE†: aspirin 500 mg, codeine phosphate 8 mg, and caffeine citrate 30 mg.
282†: aspirin 375 mg, codeine phosphate 15 mg, and caffeine citrate 30 mg.
292†: aspirin 375 mg, codeine phosphate 30 mg, and caffeine citrate 30 mg.
293†: aspirin 375 mg, codeine phosphate 30 mg, codeine phosphate (slow-release) 30 mg, and caffeine citrate 30 mg.
692†: aspirin 375 mg, propoxyphene hydrochloride 65 mg, and caffeine 30 mg.
A.C. & C.†: aspirin 375 mg, codeine phosphate 8 mg, and caffeine 30 mg.

ACETA WITH CODEINE, EMPRACET-30†, EMTEC-30†: acetaminophen 300 mg and codeine phosphate 30 mg.
ANACIN WITH CODEINE†: aspirin 325 mg, codeine phosphate 8 mg, and caffeine 32 mg.
ANCASAL 8†, C2 WITH CODEINE†: aspirin 375 mg, codeine phosphate 8 mg, and caffeine 15 mg.
ANCASAL 15†: aspirin 375 mg, codeine phosphate 15 mg, and caffeine 15 mg.
ANCASAL 30†: aspirin 375 mg, codeine phosphate 30 mg, and caffeine 15 mg.
ANEXIA 5/500: hydrocodone bitartrate 5 mg, acetaminophen 500 mg
BUFF-A-COMP NO. 3: aspirin 325 mg, codeine phosphate 30 mg, caffeine 40 mg, and butalbital 50 mg.
CAPITAL WITH CODEINE, MAPAP WITH CODEINE*, TYLENOL WITH CODEINE ELIXIR*, TY-PAP WITH CODEINE ELIXIR*: acetaminophen 120 mg and codeine phosphate 12 mg/5 ml.
DARVOCET-N 50: acetaminophen 325 mg and propoxyphene napsylate 50 mg.
DARVOCET-N 100, DOXAPAP-N, propacet 100: acetaminophen 650 mg and propoxyphene napsylate 100 mg.
DARVON COMPOUND†: aspirin 325 mg, propoxyphene hydrochloride 32 mg, and caffeine 32.4 mg.
DARVON COMPOUND-65†: aspirin 389 mg, propoxyphene hydrochloride 65 mg, and caffeine 32.4 mg.
DARVON NC-COMPOUND†: aspirin 375 mg, propoxyphene napsylate 100 mg, and caffeine 30 mg.
DARVON COMPOUND WITH A.S.A.†: aspirin 325 mg and propoxyphene napsylate 100 mg.
DARVON COMPOUND WITH A.S.A.†: aspirin 325 mg and propoxyphene hydrochloride 65 mg.
DOLENE-AP-65, D-REX-65, E-L, GENAGESIC, PRO POX WITH APAP, WY-GESIC: acetaminophen 650 mg and

propoxyphene hydrochloride 65 mg.
EMPIRIN WITH CODEINE NO. 2: aspirin
325 mg and codeine phosphate 15 mg.
EMPIRIN WITH CODEINE NO. 3: aspirin
325 mg and codeine phosphate 30 mg.
EMPIRIN WITH CODEINE NO. 4: aspirin
325 mg and codeine phosphate 60 mg.
EMPRACET-60†: acetaminophen 300 mg
and codeine phosphate 60 mg.
ENDOCAN†, OXYCODAN†, PERCODAN†:
aspirin 325 mg and oxycodone hydrochloride 5 mg.
ENDOCET†, OXYCOCET†, PERCOCET,
ROXICET: acetaminophen 325 mg and
oxycodone hydrochloride 5 mg.
FIORICET WITH CODEINE: acetaminophen
325 mg, butalbital 50 mg, caffeine 40
mg, and codeine phosphate 30 mg.
FIORINAL WITH CODEINE: aspirin 325
mg, butalbital 50 mg, caffeine 40 mg,
and codeine 30 mg.
INNOVAR INJECTION: droperidol 2.5 mg
and fentanyl citrate 0.05 mg/ml.
LENOLTEC WITH CODEINE NO. 1†,
NOVOGESIC C8†: acetaminophen 300
mg, codeine phosphate 8 mg, and caffeine 15 mg.
LORCET 10/650: acetaminophen 650 mg
and hydrocodone bitartrate 10mg.
LORCET PLUS: acetaminophen 650 mg,
hydrocodone bitartrate 7.5 mg
LORTAB 2.5/500: acetaminophen 500 mg
and hydrocodone bitartrate 2.5 mg.
LORTAB 5/500: acetaminophen 500 mg
and hydrocodone bitartrate 5 mg.
LORTAB 7.5/500: acetaminophen 500 mg
and hydrocodone bitartrate 7.5 mg.
PERCODAN-DEMI: aspirin 325 mg, oxycodone hydrochloride 2.25 mg, and
oxycodone terephthalate 0.19 mg.
PERCODAN-DEMI:†: aspirin 325 mg and
oxycodone hydrochloride 2.5 mg.
PERCODAN-ROXIPRIN: aspirin 325 mg,
oxycodone hydrochloride 4.5 mg, and
oxycodone terephthalate 0.38 mg.
PHENAPHEN-650 WITH CODEINE: acetaminophen 650 mg and codeine phosphate 30 mg.
ROUNOX AND CODEINE 15†: acetaminophen 325 mg and codeine phosphate 15 mg.

ROUNOX AND CODEINE 30†: acetaminophen 325 mg and codeine phosphate 30 mg.
ROUNOX AND CODEINE 60†: acetaminophen 325 mg and codeine phosphate 60 mg.
ROXICET 5/500, TYLOX: acetaminophen
500 mg and oxycodone hydrochloride 5
mg.
ROXICET ORAL SOLUTION*: acetaminophen 325 mg and oxycodone hydrochloride 5 mg/5 ml.
TALACEN: acetaminophen 650 mg and
pentazocine hydrochloride 25 mg.
TALWIN COMPOUND: aspirin 325 mg and
pentazocine hydrochloride 12.5 mg.
TYLENOL WITH CODEINE NO. 1: acetaminophen 300 mg and codeine phosphate 7.5 mg.
TYLENOL WITH CODEINE NO. 2: acetaminophen 300 mg and codeine phosphate 15 mg.
TYLENOL WITH CODEINE NO. 3: acetaminophen 300 mg and codeine phosphate 30 mg.
TYLENOL WITH CODEINE NO. 4: acetaminophen 300 mg and codeine phosphate 60 mg.
VICODIN: acetaminophen 500 mg and
hydrocodone bitartrate 5 mg.
VICODIN ES: acetaminophen 750 mg
and hydrocodone bitartrate 7.5 mg.

alfentanil hydrochloride
Alfenta

Controlled Substance Schedule II
Pregnancy Risk Category: C

HOW SUPPLIED
Injection: 500 mcg/ml

ACTION
Binds with opiate receptors in the CNS,
altering both perception of and emotional response to pain through an unknown
mechanism.

ONSET, PEAK, DURATION
Onset within 1 minute. Serum levels

peak within 1½ to 2 minutes. Effects persist 5 to 10 minutes.

INDICATIONS & DOSAGE
Adjunct to general anesthetic—
Adults: initially, 8 to 50 mcg/kg I.V.; then increments of 3 to 15 mcg/kg I.V. q 5 to 20 minutes.
As a primary anesthetic—
Adults: initially, 130 to 245 mcg/kg I.V.; then 0.5 to 1.5 mcg/kg/minute I.V.

In elderly and debilitated patients, dosage should be reduced. In obese patients, dosage is based on lean body weight.

ADVERSE REACTIONS
CNS: anxiety, headache, confusion, sleepiness, sedation.
EENT: blurred vision.
CV: *hypotension, hypertension, bradycardia, tachycardia,* **arrhythmias, asystole hypercarbia.**
GI: *nausea, vomiting.*
Respiratory: *chest wall rigidity,* **bronchospasm, respiratory depression,** hypercapnia, **respiratory arrest,** laryngospasm.
Skin: pruritus, urticaria.

INTERACTIONS
Cimetidine: CNS toxicity.
CNS depressants, ethanol: additive effects. Use together cautiously.
Diazepam: CV depression and decreased blood pressure with high doses of alfentanil.

EFFECTS ON DIAGNOSTIC TESTS
May increase biliary tract pressure with resultant increases in amylase and lipase plasma levels.

CONTRAINDICATIONS
Contraindicated in patients with hypersensitivity to this drug.

NURSING CONSIDERATIONS
• Use cautiously in patients with head injury, pulmonary disease, decreased respiratory reserve, or hepatic or renal impairment.
• Be aware drug should be administered only by persons specifically trained in the use of I.V. anesthetics.
• **I.V. use:** Compatible with D_5W, D_5W in lactated Ringer's solution, and 0.9% sodium chloride solution. Most clinicians use infusions containing 25 to 80 mcg/ml.
• Discontinue infusion at least 10 to 15 minutes before the end of surgery.
Alert: To administer small volumes of alfentanil accurately, use a tuberculin syringe.
• Keep narcotic antagonist (naloxone) and resuscitation equipment available when giving drug I.V.
• Accidental skin contact should be treated by rinsing the area with water.
• Periodically monitor postoperative vital signs and bladder function. Because drug decreases both rate and depth of respirations, monitoring of arterial oxygen saturation may aid in assessing respiratory depression.

☑ **PATIENT TEACHING**
• Explain the anesthetic effect of alfentanil as well as preoperative and postoperative care measures.
• Inform the patient that another analgesic will be available to relieve pain after effects of alfentanil have worn off.

---

buprenorphine hydrochloride
Buprenex, Temgesic Injection‡

Controlled Substance Schedule V
Pregnancy Risk Category: C

HOW SUPPLIED
Injection: 0.324 mg (equivalent to 0.3 mg base/ml)

ACTION
Binds with opiate receptors in the CNS, altering both perception of and emotional response to pain through an unknown mechanism.

ONSET, PEAK, DURATION
Onset occurs within 15 minutes after
I.M. administration; more rapid after
I.V. administration. Analgesic effects
peak in 2 to 5 minutes after I.M. administration, 2 minutes after I.V. administration. Effects persist about 6 hours.

INDICATIONS & DOSAGE
Moderate to severe pain—
**Adults and children 13 years and
over:** 0.3 mg I.M. or slow I.V. q 6
hours, p.r.n. or around the clock; dosage
repeated (up to 0.3 mg) if required, 30
to 60 minutes after initial dose.
Children 2 to 12 years: 2 to 6 mcg/kg
I.M. or I.V. q 4 to 6 hours.
    Reduce dose by one-half in high-risk
patients, such as debilitated or elderly
patients.

ADVERSE REACTIONS
CNS: *dizziness, sedation, headache,*
confusion, nervousness, euphoria, *verti-
go,* increased intracranial pressure.
CV: *hypotension,* bradycardia, tachycar-
dia, hypertension.
EENT: *miosis,* blurred vision.
GI: *nausea,* vomiting, constipation, dry
mouth.
GU: urine retention.
Respiratory: *respiratory depression,*
hypoventilation, dyspnea.
Skin: pruritus, *diaphoresis.*

INTERACTIONS
*CNS depressants, ethanol, MAO in-
hibitors:* additive effects. Use together
cautiously.

EFFECTS ON DIAGNOSTIC TESTS
None reported.

CONTRAINDICATIONS
Contraindicated in patients with hypersensitivity to this drug.

NURSING CONSIDERATIONS
● Use cautiously in elderly or debilitated patients or patients with head injury,
intracranial lesions, and increased in-

tracranial pressure; severe respiratory,
liver, or kidney impairment; CNS depression or coma; thyroid irregularities;
adrenal insufficiency; and prostatic hyperplasia, urethral stricture, acute alcoholism, delirium tremens, or kyphoscol-
iosis.
● **I.V. use:** Give by direct I.V. injection,
slowly into a vein or through the tubing
of a free-flowing, compatible I.V. solution over not less than 2 minutes.
● S.C. administration is not recommended.
● Be aware that buprenorphine 0.3 mg
is equal to 10 mg of morphine and 75
mg of meperidine in analgesic potency.
It has longer duration of action than
morphine or meperidine.
Alert: Know that naloxone will not completely reverse the respiratory depression caused by buprenorphine overdose;
an overdose may necessitate mechanical
ventilation. Larger than customary doses of naloxone (more than 0.4 mg) and
doxapram also may be ordered.
● Accidental skin exposure should be
treated by removing exposed clothing
and rinsing skin with water.
● Be aware that drug's narcotic antagonist properties may precipitate withdrawal syndrome in narcotic-dependent
patients.
● Know that if dependence occurs,
withdrawal symptoms may appear up to
14 days after drug is stopped.

☑ **PATIENT TEACHING**
● Caution ambulatory patient about getting out of bed or walking.
● When drug is used postoperatively,
encourage patient to turn, cough, and
deep breathe to prevent atelectasis.

---

butorphanol tartrate
Stadol, Stadol NS

Pregnancy Risk Category: C

HOW SUPPLIED
Injection: 1 mg/ml, 2 mg/ml

Nasal spray: 10 mg/ml

ACTION
Binds with opiate receptors in the CNS, altering both perception of and emotional response to pain through an unknown mechanism.

ONSET, PEAK, DURATION
Onset occurs within 2 to 3 minutes after an I.V. injection; within 10 to 30 minutes after I.M. injection; within 15 minutes of nasal use. Analgesic effects peak within ½ to 1 hour of I.M. or I.V. use, within 1 to 2 hours of nasal use. Analgesic effects persist 3 to 4 hours after I.M. use, 2 to 4 hours after I.V. use, or 4 to 5 hours after nasal administration.

INDICATIONS & DOSAGE
Moderate to severe pain—
Adults: 1 to 4 mg I.M. q 3 to 4 hours, p.r.n. or around the clock; or 0.5 to 2 mg I.V. q 3 to 4 hours, p.r.n. or around the clock. Not to exceed 4 mg per dose. Alternatively, 1 mg by nasal spray q 3 to 4 hours (1 spray in one nostril); repeated in 60 to 90 minutes if pain relief is inadequate.
Labor for patients at full term and in early labor—
Adults: 1 to 2 mg I.V. or I.M., repeated after 4 hours as needed.
Preoperative anesthesia or preanesthesia—
Adults: 2 mg. I.M. 60 to 90 minutes before surgery.
Adjunct to balanced anesthesia—
Adults: 2 mg I.V. shortly before induction or 0.5 to 1.0 mg I.V. in increments during anesthesia.

In patients with renal or hepatic impairment: Increase dosage interval to 6 to 8 hours. In elderly patients, use one-half of the usual dose at twice the interval for I.V. use; for nasal use, allow 1½ to 2 hours to elapse before repeating dose.

ADVERSE REACTIONS
CNS: *confusion,* nervousness, lethargy, headache, *somnolence, dizziness, insomnia,* anxiety, paresthesia, euphoria, hallucinations, flushing, increased intracranial pressure.
CV: palpitations, vasodilation, hypotension.
EENT: blurred vision, *nasal congestion* (with nasal spray), tinnitus, unpleasant taste.
GI: *nausea, vomiting, constipation,* anorexia.
Respiratory: *respiratory depression.*
Skin: rash, hives, *clamminess, excessive diaporesis.*
Other: sensation of heat.

INTERACTIONS
CNS depressants, ethanol: additive effects. Use together cautiously.

EFFECTS ON DIAGNOSTIC TESTS
None reported.

CONTRAINDICATIONS
Contraindicated in patients with narcotic addiction; may precipitate withdrawal syndrome. Also contraindicated in patient with hypersensitivity to the drug or to the preservative, benzethonium chloride.

NURSING CONSIDERATIONS
● Use cautiously in patients with head injury, increased intracranial pressure, acute MI, ventricular dysfunction, coronary insufficiency, respiratory disease or depression, and renal or hepatic dysfunction. Also administer cautiously to patients who have recently received repeated doses of narcotic analgesic medication.
● **I.V. use:** Give by direct injection into a vein or into the tubing of a free-flowing I.V. solution. Compatible solutions include D_5W and 0.9% sodium chloride.
● S.C. route is not recommended.
● Know that respiratory depression apparently does not increase with larger dosage.
● Be aware that psychological and physical addiction may occur.

Reactions may be *common,* uncommon, *life-threatening,* or COMMON AND LIFE-THREATENING.

• Periodically monitor postoperative vital signs and bladder function. Because drug decreases both rate and depth of respirations, monitoring of arterial oxygen saturation may aid in assessing respiratory depression.

☑ **PATIENT TEACHING**
• Caution ambulatory patient about getting out of bed or walking. Warn outpatient to avoid driving and other potentially hazardous activities that require mental alertness until drug's CNS effects are known.
• Instruct patient about administration technique for and storage of nasal spray, if applicable.

---

codeine phosphate
Paveral†

codeine sulfate
Controlled Substance Schedule II
Pregnancy Risk Category: C

HOW SUPPLIED
codeine phosphate
Oral solution: 15 mg/5 ml, 10 mg/ml†
Injection: 30 mg/ml, 60 mg/ml
Soluble tablets: 30 mg, 60 mg
codeine sulfate
Tablets: 15 mg, 30 mg, 60 mg

ACTION
Binds with opiate receptors in the CNS, altering both perception of and emotional response to pain through an unknown mechanism. Also suppresses the cough reflex by direct action on the cough center in the medulla.

ONSET, PEAK, DURATION
Onset occurs immediately with I.V. administration, 10 to 30 minutes after I.M. or S.C. injection, 30 to 45 minutes after oral use. Peak effects occur immediately after I.V. administration, within ½ to 1 hour after I.M. injection, unknown after S.C. administration, and 1 to 2 hours after oral administration. Effects persist 4

to 6 hours.

INDICATIONS & DOSAGE
Mild to moderate pain—
Adults: 15 to 60 mg P.O. or 15 to 60 mg (phosphate) S.C., I.M., or I.V. q 4 to 6 hours, p.r.n.
Children over 1 year: 0.5 mg/kg P.O., S.C., or I.M. q 4 hours, p.r.n.
Nonproductive cough—
Adults: 10 to 20 mg P.O. q 4 to 6 hours. Maximum dosage is 120 mg/day.
Children 6 to 12 years: 5 to 10 mg P.O. q 4 to 6 hours. Maximum dosage is 60 mg/day.
Children 2 to 6 years: 2.5 to 5 mg P.O. q 4 to 6 hours. Do not exceed 30 mg/day.

ADVERSE REACTIONS
CNS: *sedation, clouded sensorium, euphoria, dizziness, light-headedness.*
CV: *hypotension,* bradycardia.
GI: *nausea, vomiting, constipation, dry mouth,* ileus.
GU: *urine retention.*
Respiratory: *respiratory depression.*
Skin: pruritus, flushing, *diaphoresis.*
Other: physical dependence.

INTERACTIONS
CNS depressants, ethanol, general anesthetics, hypnotics, MAO inhibitors, other narcotic analgesics, sedatives, tranquilizers, tricyclic antidepressants: additive effects. Use together with extreme caution. Monitor patient response.

EFFECTS ON DIAGNOSTIC TESTS
Codeine may increase plasma amylase and lipase levels, delay gastric emptying, increase biliary tract pressure resulting from contraction of the sphincter of Oddi, and may interfere with hepatobiliary imaging studies.

CONTRAINDICATIONS
Contraindicated in patients with hypersensitivity to this drug.

---

*Liquid contains alcohol.   **May contain tartrazine.   †Canada only.   ‡Australia only.   ◊OTC.

NURSING CONSIDERATIONS

• Use with extreme caution in patients with head injury, increased intracranial pressure, increased CSF pressure, hepatic or renal disease, hypothyroidism, Addison's disease, acute alcoholism, seizures, severe CNS depression, bronchial asthma, COPD, respiratory depression, and shock. Also use with extreme caution in elderly or debilitated patients.

• **I.V. use:** Give by direct injection into a large vein. Administer very slowly. *Alert:* Don't mix with other solutions because codeine phosphate is incompatible with many drugs.

• Don't administer discolored injection solution.

• Know that codeine and aspirin or acetaminophen are often prescribed together to provide enhanced pain relief.

• For full analgesic effect, administer drug before patient has intense pain.

• Be aware that drug is an antitussive and should not be used when cough is a valuable diagnostic sign or is beneficial (as after thoracic surgery).

• Monitor cough type and frequency.

• Monitor respiratory and circulatory status.

• Opiates may cause constipation. Assess bowel function and need for stool softeners or laxatives.

☑ **PATIENT TEACHING**

• To minimize GI distress caused by oral administration, advise patient to take this drug with milk or meals.

• Instruct patient to ask for or to take drug before pain is intense.

• Caution ambulatory patient about getting out of bed or walking. Warn outpatient to avoid driving and other potentially hazardous activities that require mental alertness until drug's CNS effects are known.

---

fentanyl citrate
Sublimaze

fentanyl transdermal system
Duragesic-25, Duragesic-50, Duragesic-75, Duragesic-100

fentanyl transmucosal
Fentanyl Oralet

Controlled Substance Schedule II
Pregnancy Risk Category: C

HOW SUPPLIED
Injection: 50 mcg/ml
Transdermal system: patches designed to release 25 mcg, 50 mcg, 75 mcg, or 100 mcg of fentanyl per hour
Transmucosal: 200 mcg, 300 mcg, 400 mcg

ACTION
Unknown. Binds with opiate receptors in the CNS, altering both perception of and emotional response to pain through an unknown mechanism.

ONSET, PEAK, DURATION
Onset within 1 to 2 minutes with I.V. administration; within 7 to 15 minutes of I.M. injection; within 5 to 15 minutes of transmucosal use; onset after transdermal use may take 12 to 24 hours. Peak effects after I.V. use occur in 3 to 5 minutes; after I.M. or transmucosal use, 20 to 30 minutes; after transdermal use, 1 to 3 days. Effects persist ½ to 1 hour after I.V. use or 1 to 2 hours after I.M. use; variable with transdermal system; not clearly defined with transmucosal use.

INDICATIONS & DOSAGE
Adjunct to general anesthetic—
Adults: for low-dose therapy, 2 mcg/kg I.V. For moderate-dose therapy, 2 to 20 mcg/kg I.V.; then 25 to 100 mcg I.V. p.r.n. For high-dose therapy, 20 to 50 mcg/kg I.V.; then 25 mcg to one-half the initial loading dose I.V. p.r.n.
Adjunct to regional anesthesia—
Adults: 50 to 100 mcg I.M. or slowly I.V. over 1 to 2 minutes, p.r.n.

Reactions may be *common,* uncommon, *life-threatening,* or COMMON AND LIFE-THREATENING.

Induction and maintenance of anesthesia—
Children 2 to 12 years: 2 to 3 mcg/kg I.V.
Postoperatively—
Adults: 50 to 100 mcg I.M. q 1 to 2 hours p.r.n.
Preoperatively—
Adults: 50 to 100 mcg I.M. 30 to 60 minutes before surgery. Alternatively, 5 mcg/kg dispensed as oralet unit, 20 to 40 minutes prior to need of desired effects.
Management of chronic pain—
Adults: one transdermal system applied to a portion of the upper torso on an area of skin that is not irritated and has not been irradiated. Therapy initiated with the 25-mcg/hour system; dosage adjusted as needed and tolerated. Each system may be worn for 72 hours although a small number of patients may require systems to be applied q 48 hours.

ADVERSE REACTIONS
CNS: *sedation, somnolence, clouded sensorium, euphoria,* dizziness, headache, *confusion, asthenia,* nervousness, hallucinations, anxiety, depression, **seizures.**
CV: *hypotension,* hypertension, arrhythmias, chest pain.
GI: *nausea, vomiting, constipation,* ileus, abdominal pain, *dry mouth,* anorexia, diarrhea, dyspepsia.
GU: *urine retention.*
Respiratory: *respiratory depression,* hypoventilation, dyspnea, apnea.
Skin: reaction at application site (erythema, papules, edema), *pruritus, diaphoresis.*
Other: physical dependence.

INTERACTIONS
CNS depressants, ethanol, general anesthetics, hypnotics, MAO inhibitors, other narcotic analgesics, sedatives, tricyclic antidepressants: additive effects. Use together with extreme caution. Fentanyl dose should be reduced by one-quarter to one-third. Also give above drugs in reduced dosages.
Diazepam: CV depression when given with high doses of fentanyl.
Droperidol: hypotension and decreased pulmonary arterial pressure.

EFFECTS ON DIAGNOSTIC TESTS
Fentanyl increases plasma amylase and lipase levels.

CONTRAINDICATIONS
Contraindicated in patients with known intolerance of the drug.

NURSING CONSIDERATIONS
● Use with caution in patients with head injury, increased CSF pressure, COPD, decreased respiratory reserve, potentially compromised respirations, hepatic or renal disease, and cardiac bradyarrhythmias. Also use with caution in elderly or debilitated patients.
● Keep narcotic antagonist (naloxone) and resuscitation equipment available when giving drug I.V.
● For better analgesic effect, administer drug before patient has intense pain.
Alert: Be aware that high doses can produce muscle rigidity, which can be reversed with neuromuscular blockers; however, patient must be artificially ventilated.
● Monitor circulatory and respiratory status and urinary function carefully. Drug may cause respiratory depression, hypotension, urine retention, nausea, vomiting, ileus, or altered level of consciousness without regard to route of administration.
● Periodically monitor postoperative vital signs and bladder function. Because drug decreases both rate and depth of respirations, monitoring of arterial oxygen saturation (SaO_2) may help assess respiratory depression. Immediately report respiratory rate below 12 breaths/minute, decreased respiratory volume, or decreased SaO_2.
I.V. form:
● Know that only staff trained in admin-

istration of I.V. anesthetics and management of their potential adverse effects should administer I.V. fentanyl.

● Be aware that drug is often used I.V. with droperidol to produce neuroleptanalgesia.

Transmucosal form:

● Remove foil overwrap of fentanyl oralet just prior to administration.

● Have patient place the fentanyl oralet in mouth and suck (not chew or swallow) it.

● Remove fentanyl oralet unit using the handle after it has been consumed, patient shows adequate effect, or patient shows signs of respiratory depression. Place any remaining portion in the plastic overwrap provided, and dispose accordingly for Schedule II drugs, or flush down the toilet.

Transdermal form:

● Know that transdermal fentanyl is not recommended for postoperative pain.

● Dosage equivalent charts are available to calculate the fentanyl transdermal dose based on the daily morphine intake—for example, for every 90 mg of oral morphine or 15 mg of I.M. morphine per 24 hours, 25 mcg/hour of transdermal fentanyl is required. Some patients will require alternative means of opiate administration when the dosage exceeds 300 mcg/hour.

● Be aware that dosage adjustments in patients using the transdermal system should be made gradually. Reaching steady-state levels of a new dosage may take up to 6 days; delay dosage adjustment until after at least two applications.

● Monitor patients who develop adverse reactions to the transdermal system for at least 12 hours after removal. Serum levels of fentanyl drop gradually and may take as long as 17 hours to decline by 50%.

● Most patients experience good control of pain for 3 days while wearing the transdermal system, but a few may need a new application after 48 hours. Because serum fentanyl concentration rises

for the first 24 hours after application, analgesic effect cannot be evaluated on the first day. Be sure the patient has adequate supplemental analgesic to prevent breakthrough pain.

● When reducing opiate therapy or switching to a different analgesic, know the transdermal system should be withdrawn gradually. Because fentanyl's serum level drops gradually after removal, give half of the equianalgesic dose of the new analgesic 12 to 18 hours after removal as ordered.

☑ PATIENT TEACHING

● When used for pain control, instruct patient to ask for drug before pain becomes intense.

● When drug is used postoperatively, encourage patient turning, coughing, and deep breathing to prevent atelectasis.

● Instruct patient to avoid performing hazardous activities until CNS effects subside.

● Tell home care patient to avoid drinking alcohol or taking other CNS-type drugs while receiving fentanyl because additive effects can occur.

● Teach patient about the proper application of the prescribed transdermal patch. Tell patient to clip hair at the application site, but not to use a razor, which may irritate the skin. Wash area with clear water if necessary, but not with soaps, oils, lotions, alcohol, or other substances that may irritate the skin or prevent adhesion. Dry the area completely before application.

● Tell patient to remove the transdermal system from the package just before applying. Hold in place for 30 seconds, and be sure the edges of the patch adhere to the skin.

● Teach patient to dispose of the transdermal patch by folding so the adhesive side adheres to itself and then flushing it down the toilet.

● Tell patient if another patch is needed after 48 to 72 hours, apply to a new site.

● Inform patient that heat from fever or

Reactions may be *common,* uncommon, *life-threatening*, or COMMON AND LIFE-THREATENING.

environment, such as from heating pads, electric blankets, heat lamps, hot tubs, or water beds, may increase transdermal delivery and cause toxicity requiring dosage adjustment. Instruct patient to notify doctor if fever occurs or if he'll be spending time in a hot climate.

hydromorphone hydrochloride (dihydromorphinone hydrochloride)
Dilaudid, Dilaudid-HP

Controlled Substance Schedule II
Pregnancy Risk Category: C

HOW SUPPLIED
Tablets: 1 mg, 2 mg, 3 mg, 4 mg
Injection: 1 mg/ml, 2 mg/ml, 3 mg/ml, 4 mg/ml, 10 mg/ml
Suppositories: 3 mg
Syrup: 1 mg/5 ml

ACTION
Binds with opiate receptors in the CNS, altering both perception of and emotional response to pain through an unknown mechanism. Also suppresses the cough reflex by direct action on the cough center in the medulla.

ONSET, PEAK, DURATION
Onset occurs 10 to 15 minutes after I.V. injection, about 15 minutes after S.C. or I.M. administration, about 30 minutes after oral dose. Peak effects occur 15 to 30 minutes after I.V. injection, 30 to 60 minutes after I.M. injection, 30 to 90 minutes after S.C. administration, 1 1/2 to 2 hours after oral administration. Effects persist about 2 to 3 hours after I.V. injection, 4 to 5 hours after I.M. injection, 4 hours after S.C. or oral administration.

INDICATIONS & DOSAGE
Moderate to severe pain—
Adults: 2 to 4 mg P.O. q 4 to 6 hours, p.r.n.; or 1 to 4 mg I.M., S.C., or I.V. (slowly over at least 2 to 3 minutes) q 4

to 6 hours p.r.n.; or 3 mg rectal suppository q 6 to 8 hours p.r.n.
Cough—
Adults and children over 12 years: 1 teaspoon (5 ml) P.O. q 3 to 4 hours p.r.n.

ADVERSE REACTIONS
CNS: *sedation, somnolence, clouded sensorium, dizziness, euphoria.*
CV: *hypotension,* bradycardia.
EENT: blurred vision, diplopia, nystagmus.
GI: *nausea, vomiting, constipation,* ileus.
GU: *urine retention.*
Respiratory: *respiratory depression, bronchospasm.*
Other: induration with repeated S.C. injections, physical dependence.

INTERACTIONS
CNS depressants, ethanol, general anesthetics, hypnotics, MAO inhibitors, other narcotic analgesics, sedatives, tranquilizers, tricyclic antidepressants: additive effects. Use together with extreme caution. Reduce hydromorphone dose and monitor patient response.

EFFECTS ON DIAGNOSTIC TESTS
Hydromorphone increases plasma amylase and lipase levels. Hydromorphone may delay gastric emptying; increased biliary tract pressure resulting from contraction of the sphincter of Oddi may interfere with hepatobiliary imaging studies.

CONTRAINDICATIONS
Contraindicated in patients with hypersensitivity to this drug, intracranial lesions associated with increased intracranial pressure, and whenever ventilator function is depressed such as in status asthmaticus, COPD, cor pulmonale, emphysema, and kryphoscoliosis.

NURSING CONSIDERATIONS
● Use with extreme caution in patients with hepatic or renal disease, hypothy-

roidism, Addison's disease, prostatic hyperplasia, or urethral stricture. Also use with caution in elderly or debilitated patients.

● For better analgesic effect, give this drug before patient has intense pain.

● Dilaudid-HP, a highly concentrated form (10 mg/ml), may be administered in smaller volumes to prevent the discomfort associated with large-volume I.M. or S.C. injections. Check dosage carefully.

● Rotate injection sites to avoid induration with S.C. injection.

● **I.V. use:** Give by direct injection over no less than 2 minutes. For infusion, drug may be mixed in D_5W, 0.9% sodium chloride, dextrose 5% in 0.9% sodium chloride, dextrose 5% in 0.45% sodium chloride, or Ringer's or lactated Ringer's solutions.

● Respiratory depression and hypotension can occur with I.V. administration. Give very slowly and monitor constantly. Keep resuscitation equipment available.

● Monitor respiratory and circulatory status and bowel function.

● Keep narcotic antagonist (naloxone) available.

● Be aware that drug may worsen or mask gallbladder pain.

● Be aware that drug is a commonly abused narcotic.

☑ **PATIENT TEACHING**

● Instruct patient to ask for or take drug before pain becomes intense.

● Tell patient to store suppositories in refrigerator.

● Tell patient to take drug with food if GI upset occurs.

● When drug is used postoperatively, encourage patient to turn, cough, and deep breathe to avoid atelectasis.

● Caution ambulatory patient about getting out of bed or walking. Warn outpatient to avoid hazardous activities that require mental alertness until drug's CNS effects are known.

meperidine hydrochloride (pethidine hydrochloride)
Demerol

Controlled Substance Schedule II
Pregnancy Risk Category: B

HOW SUPPLIED
Tablets: 50 mg, 100 mg
Syrup: 50 mg/5 ml
Injection: 10 mg/ml, 25 mg/ml, 50 mg/ml, 75 mg/ml, 100 mg/ml

ACTION
Binds with opiate receptors in the CNS, altering both perception of and emotional response to pain through an unknown mechanism.

ONSET, PEAK, DURATION
Onset occurs about 1 minute following I.V. administration, 10 to 15 minutes after S.C. or I.M. injection, about 15 minutes after oral administration. Peak effects occur within 5 to 7 minutes after I.V. injection, 30 to 50 minutes after I.M. or S.C. injection, and 60 to 90 minutes after oral administration. Effects persist 2 to 4 hours for all routes of administration.

INDICATIONS & DOSAGE
Moderate to severe pain—
Adults: 50 to 150 mg P.O., I.M., or S.C. q 3 to 4 hours, p.r.n.; or 15 to 35 mg/hour by continuous I.V. infusion.
Children: 1.1 to 1.8 mg/kg P.O., I.M., or S.C. q 3 to 4 hours. Maximum dosage is 100 mg q 4 hours, p.r.n.
Preoperatively—
Adults: 50 to 100 mg I.M. or S.C. 30 to 90 minutes before surgery.
Children: 1 to 2.2 mg/kg I.M. or S.C. up to the adult dose 30 to 90 minutes before surgery.
Adjunct to anesthesia—
Adults: Repeated slow I.V. injections of fractional doses (10 mg/ml); alternatively, continuous I.V. infusion of a more dilute solution (1 mg/ml) titrated to pa-

---

Reactions may be *common*, uncommon, *life-threatening*, or COMMON AND LIFE-THREATENING.

NARCOTIC AND OPIOID ANALGESICS

tient's needs.
Obstetric analgesia—
Adults: 50 to 100 mg I.M. or S.C. when pain becomes regular, repeated at 1- to 3-hour intervals.

ADVERSE REACTIONS
CNS: *sedation, somnolence, clouded sensorium, euphoria,* paradoxical excitement, tremor, *dizziness,* **seizures** (with large doses), headache, hallucinations, syncope, *light-headedness.*
CV: *hypotension,* bradycardia, tachycardia, **cardiac arrest, shock.**
GI: *constipation,* ileus, dry mouth, *nausea, vomiting,* biliary tract spasms.
GU: *urine retention.*
Respiratory: *respiratory depression,* respiratory arrest.
Skin: pruritus, urticaria, *diaphoresis.*
Other: physical dependence, muscle twitching, phlebitis after I.V. delivery, pain at injection site, local tissue irritation and induration after S.C. injection.

INTERACTIONS
Aminophylline, barbiturates, heparin, methicillin, morphine sulfate, phenytoin, sodium bicarbonate, sulfonamides: incompatible when mixed in the same I.V. container.
CNS depressants, ethanol, general anesthetics, hypnotics, other narcotic analgesics, phenothiazines, sedatives, tricyclic antidepressants: possible respiratory depression, hypotension, profound sedation, or coma. Use together with extreme caution. Reduce meperidine dosage.
MAO inhibitors: increased CNS excitation or depression that can be severe or fatal. Don't use together.
Phenytoin: decreased blood levels of meperidine. Monitor for decreased analgesia.

EFFECTS ON DIAGNOSTIC TESTS
Meperidine increases plasma amylase and lipase levels through increased biliary tract pressure; levels may be unreliable for 24 hours after meperidine ad-

ministration.

CONTRAINDICATIONS
Contraindicated in patients with hypersensitivity to this drug and in patients who have received MAO inhibitors within past 14 days.

NURSING CONSIDERATIONS
● Use with extreme caution in patients with increased intracranial pressure, head injury, asthma, and other respiratory conditions; in supraventricular tachycardias, seizures, acute abdominal conditions, hepatic or renal disease, hypothyroidism, Addison's disease, urethral stricture, and prostatic hyperplasia; and in elderly or debilitated patients.
● May be used in some patients allergic to morphine.
● **I.V. use:** Give slowly by direct I.V. injection. Meperidine also may be given by slow continuous I.V. infusion. Drug is compatible with most I.V. solutions, including D_5W, 0.9% sodium chloride, and Ringer's or lactated Ringer's solutions.
● Keep narcotic antagonist (naloxone) available when giving this drug I.V.
● S.C. injection is not recommended because it is very painful.
Alert: Oral dose is less than half as effective as parenteral dose. Give I.M. if possible. When changing from parenteral to oral route, know that dosage should be increased.
● Syrup has local anesthetic effect. Give with full glass of water.
● Meperidine and its active metabolite normeperidine accumulate in the body. Monitor for increased toxic effect, especially in patients with impaired renal function.
● Because meperidine toxicity often appears after several days of treatment, this drug is not recommended for treatment of chronic pain.
● Monitor respirations of neonates exposed to drug during labor. Have resuscitation equipment and naloxone avail-

---

*Liquid contains alcohol.   **May contain tartrazine.   †Canada only.   ‡Australia only.   ◇OTC.

able.
● Monitor respiratory and cardiovascular status carefully. Don't give if respirations are below 12 breaths/minute, if respiratory rate or depth is decreased, or if change in pupils is noted.
● Watch for withdrawal symptoms if drug is discontinued abruptly after long-term use.
● Monitor bladder function in postoperative patients.
● Monitor bowel function. Patient may need a laxative or stool softener.

☑ PATIENT TEACHING
● When drug is used postoperatively, encourage patient to turn, cough, and deep breathe and to use an incentive spirometer to prevent atelectasis.
● Caution ambulatory patient about getting out of bed or walking. Warn outpatient to avoid driving and other potentially hazardous activities that require mental alertness until drug's CNS effects are known.

---

methadone hydrochloride
Dolophine, Methadose, Physeptone‡

Controlled Substance Schedule II
Pregnancy Risk Category: NR

HOW SUPPLIED
Tablets: 5 mg, 10 mg
Dispersible tablets (for methadone maintenance therapy): 40 mg
Oral solution: 5 mg/5 ml, 10 mg/10 ml, 10 mg/ml (concentrate)
Injection: 10 mg/ml

ACTION
Binds with opiate receptors at many sites in the CNS (brain, brain stem, and spinal cord), altering both perception of and emotional response to pain through an unknown mechanism.

ONSET, PEAK, DURATION
Onset occurs immediately after I.V. administration, 10 to 20 minutes after I.M.

injection, 30 to 60 minutes after oral administration. Peak effects occur within 15 to 30 minutes after I.V injection, 1 to 2 hours after I.M. injection, 1 ½ to 2 hours after oral administration. Effects persist 3 to 4 hours after I.V. use, 4 to 5 hours after I.M. use, 4 to 6 hours after oral use.

INDICATIONS & DOSAGE
Severe pain—
Adults: 2.5 to 10 mg P.O., I.M., or S.C. q 3 to 4 hours, p.r.n.
Narcotic withdrawal syndrome—
Adults: 15 to 40 mg P.O. daily (highly individualized). Maintenance dosage is 20 to 120 mg P.O. daily. Dosage adjusted as needed. Daily dosages greater than 120 mg require special state and federal approval.

ADVERSE REACTIONS
CNS: *sedation, somnolence, clouded sensorium, euphoria, dizziness,* choreic movements, *seizures* (with large doses), headache, insomnia, agitation, *lightheadedness,* syncope.
CV: *hypotension,* bradycardia, *shock, cardiac arrest,* palpitations.
EENT: visual disturbances.
GI: *nausea, vomiting, constipation,* ileus, dry mouth, anorexia, biliary tract spasm.
GU: *urine retention,* decreased libido.
Respiratory: *respiratory depression, respiratory arrest.*
Skin: *diaphoresis,* pruritus, urticaria, edema.
Other: physical dependence; pain at injection site; tissue irritation, induration (following S.C. injection).

INTERACTIONS
Ammonium chloride and other urine acidifiers, phenytoin: may reduce methadone effect. Monitor for decreased pain control.
CNS depressants, ethanol, general anesthetics, hypnotics, MAO inhibitors, sedatives, tranquilizers, tricyclic antidepressants: possible respiratory depres-

---

Reactions may be *common*, uncommon, *life-threatening*, or COMMON AND LIFE-THREATENING.

sion, hypotension, profound sedation, or coma. Use together with extreme caution. Monitor patient response.
Rifampin: withdrawal symptoms; reduced blood levels of methadone. Use together cautiously.

EFFECTS ON DIAGNOSTIC TESTS
Methadone increases plasma amylase levels.

CONTRAINDICATIONS
Contraindicated in patients with hypersensitivity to this drug.

NURSING CONSIDERATIONS
● Use with extreme caution in patients with acute abdominal conditions, severe hepatic or renal impairment, hypothyroidism, Addison's disease, prostatic hyperplasia, urethral stricture, head injury, increased intracranial pressure, asthma, and other respiratory conditions. Also use with caution in elderly or debilitated patients.
● Oral liquid form legally required in maintenance programs. Completely dissolve tablets in 120 ml of orange juice or powdered citrus drink.
● For parenteral use, I.M. injection is preferred. Rotate injection sites.
● **I.V. use:** Dilute to a maximum concentration of 10 mg/ml using 0.9% sodium chloride. Give slowly by direct injection. Alternatively, dilute to 1 mg/ml and give as a slow I.V. infusion (15 to 35 mg/hour).
● Know that oral dose is half as potent as injected dose.
● Know that an around-the-clock regimen is necessary to manage severe, chronic pain.
● Be aware that patient treated for narcotic withdrawal syndrome usually will require an additional analgesic if pain control is necessary.
● Monitor patient closely; has cumulative effect; marked sedation can occur after repeated doses.
● Monitor circulatory and respiratory status and bladder and bowel function.

Patient may need a laxative.
● Be aware that when used as an adjunct in the treatment of narcotic addiction (maintenance), withdrawal usually will be delayed and mild.

☑ **PATIENT TEACHING**
● Caution ambulatory patient about getting out of bed or walking. Warn outpatient to avoid hazardous activities that require mental alertness until drug's CNS effects are known.
● Instruct patient to increase fluid and fiber in diet, if not contraindicated, to combat constipation.

morphine hydrochloride
Morphitec†, M.O.S.†, M.O.S.-S.R.†

morphine sulfate
Astramorph PF, Duramorph, Duramorph PF, Epimorph†, Infumorph 200, Infumorph 500, Morphine H.P.†, MS Contin, MSIR, MS/L, OMS Concentrate, Oramorph SR, RMS Uniserts, Roxanol, Roxanol 100, Roxanol Rescudose, Roxanol SR, Roxanol UD, Statex

morphine tartrate†
Controlled Substance Schedule II
Pregnancy Risk Category: C

HOW SUPPLIED
morphine hydrochloride
Tablets: 10 mg†, 20 mg†, 40 mg†, 60 mg†
Tablets (extended-release): 30 mg†, 60 mg†
Oral solution†: 1 mg/ml, 5 mg/ml, 10 mg/ml, 20 mg/ml, 50 mg/ml
Syrup: 1 mg/ml†, 5 mg/ml†, 10 mg/ml†, 20 mg/ml†, 50 mg/ml†
Suppositories: 10 mg†, 20 mg†, 30 mg†
morphine sulfate
Tablets: 15 mg, 30 mg
Tablets (extended-release): 15 mg, 30 mg, 60 mg, 100 mg, 200 mg
Soluble tablets: 10 mg, 15 mg, 30 mg
Oral solution: 10 mg/5 ml, 20 mg/5 ml,

20 mg/ml (concentrate)
Syrup: 1 mg/ml, 5 mg/ml
Injection (with preservative): 0.5 mg/ml, 1 mg/ml, 2 mg/ml, 3 mg/ml, 4 mg/ml, 5 mg/ml, 8 mg/ml, 10 mg/ml, 15 mg/ml, 25 mg/ml, 50 mg/ml
Injection (without preservative): 0.5 mg/ml, 1 mg/ml, 10 mg/ml, 25 mg/ml
Suppositories: 5 mg, 10 mg, 20 mg, 30 mg

morphine tartrate
Injection: 80 mg/ml‡

ACTION
Binds with opiate receptors in the CNS, altering both perception of and emotional response to pain through an unknown mechanism.

ONSET, PEAK, DURATION
Onset occurs within 1 hour after oral dose, 20 to 60 minutes after rectal dose, 10 to 30 minutes after S.C. or I.M. dose, less than 5 minutes after I.V. dose, 15 to 60 minutes after epidural or intrathecal dose. Peak analgesic effect is 1 to 2 hours after oral dose, 20 to 60 minutes after rectal dose, 50 to 90 minutes after S.C. dose, 30 to 60 minutes after I.M. dose, 20 minutes after direct I.V. injection, 15 to 60 minutes after epidural injection. Effects persist 4 to 5 hours after immediate-release oral forms, 8 to 12 hours after extended-release oral forms, 4 to 5 hours after rectal, S.C., I.M., or I.V. dose, up to 24 hours after intrathecal or epidural dose.

INDICATIONS & DOSAGE
Severe pain—
Adults: 5 to 20 mg S.C. or I.M. or 2.5 to 15 mg I.V. q 4 hours p.r.n.; or 10 to 30 mg P.O. or 10 to 20 mg rectally q 4 hours, p.r.n. When given by continuous I.V. infusion, a loading dose of 15 mg I.V. may be followed by a continuous infusion of 0.8 to 10 mg/hour. 15 to 30 mg controlled-release tablets P.O. q 8 to 12 hours may also be administered. As an epidural injection, 5 mg by epidural catheter; then, if adequate pain relief not

obtained within 1 hour, additional doses of 1 to 2 mg given at intervals sufficient to assess efficacy. Maximum total epidural dose should not exceed 10 mg/24 hours.
Children: 0.1 to 0.2 mg/kg S.C. or I.M. q 4 hours. Maximum single dose is 15 mg.

ADVERSE REACTIONS
CNS: *sedation, somnolence, clouded sensorium, euphoria, **seizures** (with large doses), dizziness, nightmares (with long-acting oral forms), light-headedness,* hallucinations, nervousness, depression, syncope.
CV: *hypotension,* bradycardia, ***shock, cardiac arrest,*** tachycardia, hypertension.
GI: *nausea, vomiting, constipation,* ileus, dry mouth, biliary tract spasms, anorexia.
GU: *urine retention,* decreased libido.
Hematologic: ***thrombocytopenia.***
Respiratory: ***respiratory depression, apnea, respiratory arrest.***
Skin: pruritus and skin flushing (with epidural administration), *diaphoresis,* edema.
Other: *physical dependence.*

INTERACTIONS
CNS depressants, ethanol, general anesthetics, hypnotics, MAO inhibitors, other narcotic analgesics, sedatives, tranquilizers, tricyclic antidepressants: possible respiratory depression, hypotension, profound sedation, or coma. Use together with extreme caution. Reduce morphine dosage and monitor patient response.

EFFECTS ON DIAGNOSTIC TESTS
Morpine increases plasma amylase levels.

CONTRAINDICATIONS
Contraindicated in patients with hypersensitivity to this drug or conditions that would preclude administration of opioids by I.V. route (acute bronchial asth-

ma or upper airway obstruction).

NURSING CONSIDERATIONS
• Use with extreme caution in patients with head injury, increased intracranial pressure, seizures, chronic pulmonary disease, prostatic hyperplasia, severe hepatic or renal disease, acute abdominal conditions, hypothyroidism, Addison's disease, and urethral stricture. Also use with extreme caution in elderly or debilitated patients.
• Keep narcotic antagonist (naloxone) and resuscitation equipment available.
• **I.V. use:** When given by direct injection, 2.5 to 15 mg may be diluted in 4 or 5 ml of sterile water for injection and given over 4 to 5 minutes. Alternatively, the drug may be mixed with D_5W to a concentration of 0.1 to 1 mg/ml and administered by a continuous infusion device. Morphine sulfate is compatible with most common I.V. solutions.
• Oral solutions of various concentrations are available as well as an intensified oral solution (20 mg/ml). Carefully note the strength administered.
• Do not crush, break, or chew extended-release tablets.
• Oral capsules may be carefully opened and the entire beaded contents poured into cool, soft foods, such as water, orange juice, applesauce, or pudding; mixture should be consumed immediately.
• S.L. administration may be ordered. Measure oral solution with tuberculin syringe. Administer dose a few drops at a time to allow maximal S.L. absorption and minimize swallowing.
• Refrigeration of rectal suppository is not necessary. In some patients, rectal and oral absorption may not be equivalent.
• Preservative-free preparations are available for epidural and intrathecal administration.
• When given epidurally, monitor closely for respiratory depression up to 24 hours after the injection. Check respiratory rate and depth every 30 to 60 min-

utes for 24 hours.
• Know that morphine is the drug of choice in relieving pain of MI. May cause transient decrease in blood pressure.
• Be aware that an around-the-clock regimen best manages severe, chronic pain.
• Be aware morphine may worsen or mask gallbladder pain.
• Monitor circulatory, respiratory, bladder, and bowel functions carefully. Drug may cause respiratory depression, hypotension, urine retention, nausea, vomiting, ileus, or altered level of consciousness regardless of the route used. Withhold dose and notify doctor if respirations are below 12 breaths/minute.
• Constipation is often severe with maintenance dosage. Ensure that stool softener or other laxative is ordered.

☑ PATIENT TEACHING
• When drug is used postoperatively, encourage patient to turn, cough, and deep breathe and to use incentive spirometer to prevent atelectasis.
• Caution ambulatory patient about getting out of bed or walking. Warn outpatient to avoid driving and other potentially hazardous activities that require mental alertness until drug's adverse CNS effects are known.

---

nalbuphine hydrochloride
Nubain

Pregnancy Risk Category: NR

HOW SUPPLIED
Injection: 10 mg/ml, 20 mg/ml

ACTION
Binds with opiate receptors in the CNS, altering both perception of and emotional response to pain through an unknown mechanism.

ONSET, PEAK, DURATION
Onset occurs 2 to 3 minutes after I.V.

---

administration, within 15 minutes of S.C. or I.M. injection. Peak effects occur within 30 minutes of I.V. administration, 60 minutes of I.M. injection. Effects persist 3 to 4 hours after I.V. use, 3 to 6 hours after S.C. or I.M. injection.

INDICATIONS & DOSAGE
Moderate to severe pain—
Adults: For an average (70 kg) person, give 10 to 20 mg S.C., I.M., or I.V. q 3 to 6 hours, p.r.n. Maximum daily dosage is 160 mg.
Adjunct to balanced anesthesia—
Adults: 0.3 mg/kg to 3.0 mg/kg I.V. over 10 to 15 minutes followed by maintenance doses of 0.25 to 0.50 mg/kg in single I.V. dose, p.r.n.

ADVERSE REACTIONS
CNS: *headache, sedation, dizziness, vertigo,* nervousness, depression, restlessness, crying, euphoria, hostility, unusual dreams, confusion, hallucinations, speech difficulty, delusions.
CV: hypertension, hypotension, tachycardia, bradycardia.
EENT: blurred vision, *dry mouth.*
GI: cramps, dyspepsia, bitter taste, *nausea, vomiting,* constipation, biliary tract spasms.
GU: urinary urgency.
Respiratory: *respiratory depression,* dyspnea, asthma, *pulmonary edema.*
Skin: pruritus, burning, urticaria, *clamminess.*

INTERACTIONS
CNS depressants, ethanol, general anesthetics, hypnotics, MAO inhibitors, sedatives, tranquilizers, tricyclic antidepressants: possible respiratory depression, hypertension, profound sedation, or coma. Use together with extreme caution. Monitor patient response.
Narcotic analgesics: possible decreased analgesic effect. Avoid concomitant use.

EFFECTS ON DIAGNOSTIC TESTS
None reported.

CONTRAINDICATIONS
Contraindicated in patients with hypersensitivity to the drug.

NURSING CONSIDERATIONS
• Use cautiously in patients with history of drug abuse or in patients with emotional instability, head injury, increased intracranial pressure, impaired ventilation, MI accompanied by nausea and vomiting, upcoming biliary surgery, and hepatic or renal disease.
• Respiratory depression can be reversed with naloxone. Keep resuscitation equipment available, particularly when administering I.V.
• Acts as a narcotic antagonist; may precipitate withdrawal syndrome. For patients who have chronically received opiates, administer 25% of the usual dose initially as ordered. Observe for signs of withdrawal.
• **I.V. use:** Inject slowly over at least 2 to 3 minutes into a vein or into an I.V. line containing a compatible, free-flowing I.V. solution, such as D_5W, 0.9% sodium chloride, or lactated Ringer's solution.
Alert: Causes respiratory depression, which at 10 mg is equal to the respiratory depression produced by 10 mg of morphine.
• Monitor circulatory and respiratory status and bladder and bowel function. Withhold dose and notify doctor if respirations are shallow or rate is below 12 breaths/minute.
• Constipation is often severe with maintenance therapy. Make sure stool softener or other laxative is ordered.
• Know that psychological and physical dependence may occur with prolonged use.

☑ **PATIENT TEACHING**
• Caution ambulatory patient about getting out of bed or walking. Warn outpatient to avoid driving and other potentially hazardous activities that require mental alertness until drug's CNS effects are known.

Reactions may be *common,* uncommon, *life-threatening,* or COMMON AND LIFE-THREATENING.

NARCOTIC AND OPIOID ANALGESICS 383

• Instruct patient on how to manage troublesome adverse effects such as constipation.

---

oxycodone hydrochloride
Endone‡, Roxicodone, Roxicodone Intensol, Supeudol†

oxycodone pectinate
Proladone‡

Controlled Substance Schedule II
Pregnancy Risk Category: NR

HOW SUPPLIED
oxycodone hydrochloride
Capsules: 5 mg
Tablets: 5 mg
Tablets (controlled-release): 10 mg, 20 mg, 40 mg
Oral solution: 5 mg/5 ml, 20 mg/ml (concentrate)
Suppositories: 10 mg, 20 mg
oxycodone pectinate
Suppositories: 30 mg‡

ACTION
Binds with opiate receptors in the CNS, altering both perception of and emotional response to pain through an unknown mechanism.

ONSET, PEAK, DURATION
Onset occurs in 10 to 15 minutes. Peak effects occur within 1 hour. Effects persist 3 to 6 hours.

INDICATIONS & DOSAGE
Moderate to severe pain—
Adults: 5 mg P.O. q 6 hours, p.r.n. Alternatively, 1 to 3 suppositories P.R. daily, p.r.n.

ADVERSE REACTIONS
CNS: *sedation, somnolence, clouded sensorium, euphoria, dizziness, lightheadedness.*
CV: *hypotension,* bradycardia.
GI: *nausea, vomiting, constipation,* ileus.

GU: *urine retention.*
Respiratory: ***respiratory depression.***
Skin: *diaphoresis,* pruritus.
Other: physical dependence.

INTERACTIONS
Anticoagulants: oxycodone hydrochloride products containing aspirin may increase anticoagulant effect. Monitor clotting times. Use together cautiously.
CNS depressants, ethanol, general anesthetics, hypnotics, MAO inhibitors, other narcotic analgesics, sedatives, tranquilizers, tricyclic antidepressants: additive effects. Use together with extreme caution. Reduce oxycodone dose and monitor patient response.

EFFECTS ON DIAGNOSTIC TESTS
Oxycodone increases plasma amylase and lipase and liver enzyme levels.

CONTRAINDICATIONS
Contraindicated in patients with hypersensitivity to this drug.

NURSING CONSIDERATIONS
• Use with extreme caution in patients with head injury, increased intracranial pressure, seizures, asthma, COPD, prostatic hyperplasia, severe hepatic or renal disease, acute abdominal conditions, urethral stricture, hypothyroidism, Addison's disease, and arrhythmias. Also use with extreme caution in elderly or debilitated patients.
• For full analgesic effect, administer drug before patient has intense pain.
• To minimize GI upset, administer drug after meals or with milk.
• Be aware that single-agent oxycodone solution or tablets are especially good for patients who shouldn't take aspirin or acetaminophen.
• Monitor circulatory and respiratory status. Withhold dose and notify doctor if respirations are shallow or if respiratory rate falls below 12 breaths/minute.
• Monitor patient's bladder and bowel patterns. Patient may require a laxative because drug has a constipating effect.

---

*Liquid contains alcohol.   **May contain tartrazine.   †Canada only.   ‡Australia only.   ◊ OTC.

☑ **PATIENT TEACHING**
● Instruct patient to ask for drug before pain is intense.
● Tell patient to take drug with milk or after eating.
● Caution ambulatory patient about getting out of bed or walking. Warn outpatient to avoid driving and other potentially hazardous activities that require mental alertness until drug's CNS effects are known.

oxymorphone hydrochloride
Numorphan, Numorphan H.P.

Controlled Substance Schedule II
Pregnancy Risk Category: NR

HOW SUPPLIED
Injection: 1 mg/ml, 1.5 mg/ml
Suppositories: 5 mg

ACTION
Binds with opiate receptors in the CNS, altering both perception of and emotional response to pain through an unknown mechanism.

ONSET, PEAK, DURATION
Onset occurs within 5 to 10 minutes after I.V. use, 10 to 15 minutes after I.M. use, 10 to 20 minutes after S.C. use, 15 to 30 minutes after rectal use. Peak effects occur within 15 to 30 minutes after I.V. use, 30 to 90 minutes after I.M. use, 60 to 90 minutes after S.C. use, 2 hours after rectal use. Effects persist 3 to 4 hours after I.V. use; 3 to 6 hours after I.M., S.C., or rectal use.

INDICATIONS & DOSAGE
Moderate to severe pain—
Adults: 1 to 1.5 mg I.M. or S.C. q 4 to 6 hours, p.r.n.; or 0.5 mg I.V. q 4 to 6 hours, p.r.n.; or 5 mg P.R. q 4 to 6 hours, p.r.n.
Analgesia during labor—
Adults: 0.5 to 1 mg I.M.

ADVERSE REACTIONS
CNS: *sedation, somnolence, clouded sensorium, euphoria,* dizziness, *seizures* (with large doses), light-headedness, headache.
CV: *hypotension,* bradycardia.
GI: *nausea, vomiting, constipation,* ileus.
GU: *urine retention.*
Respiratory: *respiratory depression.*
Skin: pruritus.
Other: physical dependence.

INTERACTIONS
CNS depressants, ethanol, general anesthetics, MAO inhibitors, tricyclic antidepressants: additive effects. Use together with extreme caution.

EFFECTS ON DIAGNOSTIC TESTS
Oxymorphone increases plasma amylase levels.

CONTRAINDICATIONS
Contraindicated in patients with hypersensitivity to this drug.

NURSING CONSIDERATIONS
● Use with extreme caution in patients with head injury, increased intracranial pressure, seizures, asthma, COPD, acute abdominal conditions, prostatic hyperplasia, severe hepatic or renal disease, urethral stricture, respiratory depression, hypothyroidism, Addison's disease, and arrhythmias. Also use with extreme caution in elderly or debilitated patients.
● Keep narcotic antagonist (naloxone) and resuscitation equipment available.
● Drug is not for mild to moderate pain. May worsen gallbladder pain.
● For better effect, administer drug before patient has intense pain.
● **I.V. use:** Give by direct I.V. injection. If necessary, drug may be diluted in 0.9% sodium chloride solution.
● Monitor cardiovascular and respiratory status. Withhold dose and notify doctor if respirations decrease or rate is below 12 breaths/minute.

Reactions may be *common,* uncommon, *life-threatening,* or COMMON AND LIFE-THREATENING.

• Monitor patient's bladder and bowel function. Patient may need laxative.

☑ PATIENT TEACHING
• Instruct patient to ask for drug before pain is intense.
• When drug is used postoperatively, encourage patient to turn, cough, and deep breathe and to use incentive spirometer to avoid atelectasis.
• Caution ambulatory patient about getting out of bed or walking. Warn outpatient to avoid driving and other potentially hazardous activities that require mental alertness until drug's CNS effects are known.
• Instruct patient to store suppositories in refrigerator.

---

pentazocine hydrochloride
Fortral†‡, Talwin†

pentazocine hydrochloride and naloxone hydrochloride
Talwin-Nx

pentazocine lactate
Fortral‡, Talwin

Controlled Substance Schedule IV
Pregnancy Risk Category: C

HOW SUPPLIED
pentazocine hydrochloride
Tablets: 25 mg‡, 50 mg†‡
pentazocine hydrochloride and naloxone hydrochloride
Tablets: 50 mg pentazocine hydrochloride and 500 mcg naloxone hydrochloride
pentazocine lactate
Injection: 30 mg/ml

ACTION
Binds with opiate receptors at many sites in the CNS, altering both perception of and emotional response to pain through an unknown mechanism.

ONSET, PEAK, DURATION
Onset occurs within 2 to 3 minutes after I.V. use, 15 to 20 minutes after I.M. or S.C. use, 15 to 30 minutes after oral use. Peak effects occur within 15 to 30 minutes after I.V. use, 30 to 60 minutes after I.M. or S.C. use, 60 to 180 minutes after oral use. Effects persist 2 to 3 hours after parenteral use, 2 to 3 hours after oral use.

INDICATIONS & DOSAGE
Moderate to severe pain—
Adults: 50 to 100 mg P.O. q 3 to 4 hours, p.r.n. Maximum oral dosage is 600 mg/day. Alternatively, 30 mg I.M., I.V., or S.C. q 3 to 4 hours, p.r.n. Maximum parenteral dosage is 360 mg/day. Single doses above 30 mg I.V. or 60 mg I.M. or S.C. are not recommended.
Labor—
Adults: 30 mg I.M. or 20 mg I.V. q 2 to 3 hours when contractions become regular.

ADVERSE REACTIONS
CNS: *sedation,* visual disturbances, hallucinations, drowsiness, *dizziness, lightheadedness,* confusion, *euphoria,* headache, psychotomimetic effects.
CV: circulatory depression, *shock,* hypertension.
EENT: dry mouth.
GI: *nausea, vomiting,* constipation.
GU: urine retention.
Respiratory: *respiratory depression,* dyspnea, *apnea.*
Skin: induration, nodules, sloughing, and sclerosis of injection site; diaphoresis; pruritus.
Other: hypersensitivity reactions *(anaphylaxis),* physical and psychological dependence.

INTERACTIONS
CNS depressants, ethanol: additive effects. Use together cautiously.
Narcotic analgesics: possible decreased analgesic effect. Avoid concomitant use.

---

*Liquid contains alcohol.   **May contain tartrazine.   †Canada only.   ‡Australia only.   ◊OTC.

EFFECTS ON DIAGNOSTIC TESTS
None reported.

CONTRAINDICATIONS
Contraindicated in patients with hypersensitivity to the drug or any product component. Not recommended for children under 12 years.

NURSING CONSIDERATIONS
• Use cautiously in patients with hepatic or renal disease, acute MI, head injury, increased intracranial pressure, and respiratory depression.
• Have naloxone readily available. Respiratory depression can be reversed with naloxone.
• **I.V. use:** Give by direct I.V. injection slowly. Do not mix in syringe with aminophylline, barbiturates, or other alkaline substances.
Alert: When giving by S.C. or I.M. injection, rotate injection sites to minimize tissue irritation. If possible, avoid giving by S.C.route.
• Know that drug possesses narcotic antagonist properties. May precipitate withdrawal syndrome in narcotic-dependent patients.
• Psychological and physical dependence may occur with prolonged use.
• Know that Talwin-Nx, the oral pentazocine available in the U.S., contains the narcotic antagonist naloxone. This prevents illicit I.V. use.
• Know that pentazocine may interfere with certain laboratory tests for urinary 17-hydroxycorticosteroids.

☑ **PATIENT TEACHING**
• Instruct patient to ask for drug before pain is intense.
• Caution ambulatory patient about getting out of bed or walking. Warn outpatient to avoid driving and other potentially hazardous activities that require mental alertness until drug's CNS effects are known.

propoxyphene hydrochloride (dextropropoxyphene hydrochloride)
Darvon, Dolene, Novopropoxyn†, 642†

propoxyphene napsylate (dextropropoxyphene napsylate)
Darvon-N, Doloxene‡, Doloxene Co‡

Controlled Substance Schedule IV
Pregnancy Risk Category: C

HOW SUPPLIED
propoxyphene hydrochloride
Capsules: 32 mg, 65 mg
propoxyphene napsylate
Tablets: 100 mg
Oral suspension: 10 mg/ml

ACTION
Binds with opiate receptors in the CNS, altering both perception of and emotional response to pain through an unknown mechanism.

ONSET, PEAK, DURATION
Onset occurs within 15 to 60 minutes. Plasma levels peak in 2 to 2½ hours. Effects persist 4 to 6 hours.

INDICATIONS & DOSAGE
Mild to moderate pain—
Adults: 65 mg (hydrochloride) P.O. q 4 hours p.r.n. Maximum dosage is 390 mg/day.
Mild to moderate pain—
Adults: 100 mg (napsylate) P.O. q 4 hours p.r.n. Maximum dosage is 600 mg/day.

ADVERSE REACTIONS
CNS: *dizziness,* headache, *sedation,* euphoria, light-headedness, weakness, hallucinations.
GI: *nausea, vomiting,* constipation, abdominal pain.
Respiratory: *respiratory depression.*
Other: psychological and physical de-

pendence, abnormal liver function tests.

INTERACTIONS
Carbamazepine: may increase carbamazepine levels. Monitor closely.
CNS depressants, ethanol: additive effects. Use together cautiously.
Warfarin: may increase anticoagulant effect. Monitor PT.
Cigarette smoking: increased metabolism of propoxyphene.

EFFECTS ON DIAGNOSTIC TESTS
Propoxyphene may cause false decreases in tests for urinary steroid excretion.

CONTRAINDICATIONS
Contraindicated in patients with hypersensitivity to this drug.

NURSING CONSIDERATIONS
• Use cautiously in hepatic or renal disease, emotional instability, or history of drug or alcohol abuse.
• Remember that 65 mg of propoxyphene hydrochloride equals 100 mg of propoxyphene napsylate.
• Drug is considered a mild narcotic analgesic, but pain relief is equivalent to that provided by aspirin. Tolerance and physical dependence may occur. Used with aspirin or acetaminophen to maximize analgesia.
• Know that smokers may need increased dosage because smoking may induce liver enzymes responsible for the metabolism of the drug thereby decreasing its efficacy.

☑ PATIENT TEACHING
• To minimize GI upset, advise patient to take drug with food or milk.
• Warn patient not to exceed recommended dosage. Respiratory depression, hypotension, profound sedation, and coma may result if used in excessive doses or with other CNS depressants. Advise patient to avoid alcohol intake or use of other CNS-type drugs when taking propoxyphene.
• Caution ambulatory patient about get-

ting out of bed or walking. Warn outpatient to avoid driving and other hazardous activities that require mental alertness until drug's CNS effects are known.

---

sufentanil citrate
Sufenta

Controlled Substance Schedule II
Pregnancy Risk Category: C

HOW SUPPLIED
Injection: 50 mcg/ml

ACTION
Binds with opiate receptors in the CNS, altering both perception of and emotional response to pain through an unknown mechanism.

ONSET, PEAK, DURATION
Onset and peak for analgesic effects occur within 1 minute . Time to loss of consciousness depends on rate of administration, generally within 1 to 2 minutes. Analgesic effects persist for 5 minutes. Time to awakening is 0.7 to 2.9 hours after average dose.

INDICATIONS & DOSAGE
Adjunct to general anesthetic—
Adults: 1 to 8 mcg/kg I.V. administered with nitrous oxide and oxygen; additional 10 to 25 mcg I.V. may be administered, p.r.n., when movement or changes in vital signs indicate surgical stress or lightening of analgesia.
As a primary anesthetic—
Adults: 8 to 30 mcg/kg I.V. administered with 100% oxygen and a muscle relaxant; additional 10 to 50 mcg I.V. may be administered p.r.n., when movement or changes in vital signs indicate surgical stress or lightening of analgesia.
Children under 12 years undergoing CV surgery: 10 to 25 mcg/kg I.V. administered with 100% oxygen and a muscle relaxant. Additional doses up to

50 mcg may be given p.r.n.

ADVERSE REACTIONS
CNS: chills, somnolence.
CV: *hypotension,* hypertension, arrhythmias, *bradycardia,* tachycardia.
GI: nausea, vomiting.
Respiratory: ***chest wall rigidity, apnea, bronchospasm.***
Skin: *pruritus,* erythema.
Other: intraoperative muscle movement.

INTERACTIONS
CNS depressants, ethanol: additive effects. Use together cautiously.

EFFECTS ON DIAGNOSTIC TESTS
Sufentanil may increase plasma amylase and lipase and serum prolactin levels.

CONTRAINDICATIONS
Contraindicated in patients with hypersensitivity to this drug.

NURSING CONSIDERATIONS
● Use with extreme caution in head injury; in pulmonary, hepatic, or renal disease; in decreased respiratory reserve; and in elderly or debilitated patients.
● Should be administered only by persons trained in the use of I.V. anesthetics.
● Reduced dosage is required for elderly and debilitated patients.
● For obese patients who exceed 20% of their ideal body weight, dosage calculations should be based upon an estimate of ideal weight.
● When used at doses over 8 mcg/kg, postoperative mechanical ventilation and observation are essential because of prolonged respiratory depression.
● Keep narcotic antagonist (naloxone) and resuscitation equipment available.
● **I.V. use:** Give by direct I.V. injection. Drug has been given by intermittent I.V. infusion, but drug compatibility and stability in I.V. solutions have not been fully investigated.

● Because drug decreases both rate and depth of respirations, monitoring of arterial oxygen saturation may aid in assessing respiratory depression. Notify the doctor if respirations decrease or rate falls below 12 breaths/minute.
● Monitor respirations of neonates exposed to the drug during labor.
Alert: Know that high doses can produce muscle rigidity reversible by neuromuscular blockers; however, patient must be artificially ventilated.
● Monitor postoperative vital signs frequently, including circulatory and respiratory status and urinary function. Drug may cause respiratory depression, hypotension, urine retention, nausea, vomiting, ileus, or altered level of consciousness.

☑ PATIENT TEACHING
● Inform patient and family of need for drug and answer any questions.
● Encourage turning, coughing, and deep breathing postoperatively to prevent atelectasis.

tramadol hydrochloride
Ultram

Pregnancy Risk Category: C

HOW SUPPLIED
Tablets: 50 mg

ACTION
Unknown. A centrally acting synthetic analgesic compound not chemically related to opiates. Thought to bind to opioid receptors and inhibit reuptake of norepinephrine and serotonin.

ONSET, PEAK, DURATION
Onset and duration unknown. Serum levels peak in about 2 hours.

INDICATIONS & DOSAGE
Moderate to moderately severe pain—
Adults: 50 to 100 mg P.O. q 4 to 6 hours, p.r.n. Maximum dosage is 400

mg daily. In patients over 75 years, maximum dosage is 300 mg/day in divided doses.

ADVERSE REACTIONS
CNS: *dizziness, vertigo, headache, somnolence, CNS stimulation, asthenia,* anxiety, confusion, coordination disturbance, euphoria, nervousness, sleep disorder, *seizures.*
CV: vasodilation.
EENT: visual disturbances.
GI: *nausea, constipation, vomiting,* dyspepsia, dry mouth, diarrhea, abdominal pain, anorexia, flatulence.
GU: urine retention, urinary frequency, menopausal symptoms.
Respiratory: *respiratory depression.*
Skin: *pruritus,* diaphoresis, rash.
Other: malaise, hypertonia.

INTERACTIONS
Carbamazepine: increased tramadol metabolism. Patients receiving chronic carbamazepine therapy at a dosage of up to 800 mg daily may require up to twice the recommended dose of tramadol.
CNS depressants: additive effects. Use together with caution. Dosage of tramadol may need to be reduced.
MAO inhibitors, neuroleptics: increased risk of seizures. Monitor patient closely.

EFFECTS ON DIAGNOSTIC TESTS
Tramadol may increase creatinine clearance and liver enzyme levels, decrease hemoglobin levels, and cause proteinuria.

CONTRAINDICATIONS
Contraindicated in patients with hypersensitivity to drug or with acute intoxication from alcohol, hypnotics, centrally acting analgesics, opioids, or psychotropic drugs.

NURSING CONSIDERATIONS
● Use cautiously in risk for seizures or respiratory depression; in increased intracranial pressure or head injury, acute abdominal conditions, or renal or hepatic impairment; and in physical dependence on opioids.
● Monitor CV and respiratory status. Withhold dose and notify doctor if respirations decrease or rate is below 12 breaths/minute.
● Monitor bowel and bladder function. Anticipate the need for a laxative.
● For better analgesic effect, give drug before onset of intense pain.
● Monitor patients at risk for seizures. Drug may reduce seizure threshold.
● Monitor patient for drug dependence. It can produce dependence similar to that of codeine or dextropropoxyphene and thus has potential for abuse.

☑ PATIENT TEACHING
● Tell patient to take drug as prescribed and not to increase dosage or dosage interval unless ordered by doctor.
● Caution ambulatory patient to be careful when rising and walking. Warn outpatient to avoid driving and other potentially hazardous activities that require mental alertness until drug's CNS effects are known.
● Advise patient to check with doctor before taking OTC medications; drug interactions can occur.

butabarbital sodium
chloral hydrate
estazolam
ethchlorvynol
flurazepam hydrochloride
pentobarbital
pentobarbital sodium
phenobarbital sodium
  (See Chapter 30, ANTICONVULSANTS.)
quazepam
secobarbital sodium
temazepam
triazolam
zolpidem tartrate

COMBINATION PRODUCTS
TRI-BARBS CAPSULES: phenobarbital 32 mg, butabarbital sodium 32 mg, and secobarbital sodium 32 mg.
TUINAL 50 MG PULVULES: amobarbital sodium 25 mg and secobarbital sodium 25 mg.
TUINAL 100 MG PULVULES: amobarbital sodium 50 mg and secobarbital sodium 50 mg.
TUINAL 200 MG PULVULES: amobarbital sodium 100 mg and secobarbital sodium 100 mg.

---

butabarbital sodium
(butabarbitone sodium)
Butalan*, Butisol* **, Sanery‡, Sarisol No. 2* **

Controlled Substance Schedule III
Pregnancy Risk Category: D

HOW SUPPLIED
Tablets: 15 mg, 30 mg, 50 mg, 100 mg
Elixir: 30 mg/5 ml, 33.3 mg/5 ml

ACTION
Unknown. A barbiturate that probably interferes with transmission of impulses from the thalamus to the cortex of the brain.

ONSET, PEAK, DURATION
Onset occurs in 45 to 60 minutes. Peak levels occur within 3 hours. Effects persist 6 to 8 hours.

INDICATIONS & DOSAGE
Sedation—
Adults: 15 to 30 mg P.O. t.i.d. or q.i.d.
Children: 6 mg/kg or 180 mg/m² P.O. divided t.i.d. Dosage range is 7.5 to 30 mg P.O. t.i.d.
Preoperatively—
Adults: 50 to 100 mg P.O. 60 to 90 minutes before surgery.
Children: 2 to 6 mg/kg P.O. (not to exceed 100 mg) 60 to 90 minutes before surgery.
Insomnia—
Adults: 50 to 100 mg P.O. h.s.

ADVERSE REACTIONS
CNS: *drowsiness, lethargy, hangover,* paradoxical excitement in elderly patients, somnolence.
GI: nausea, vomiting.
Hematologic: exacerbation of porphyria.
Respiratory: *respiratory depression, apnea.*
Skin: rash, urticaria, *Stevens-Johnson syndrome.*
Other: *angioedema,* physical and psychological dependence.

INTERACTIONS
Chloramphenicol, MAO inhibitors, valproic acid: inhibited metabolism of barbiturates; may cause prolonged CNS depression. Reduce barbiturate dosage.
Corticosteroids, digitoxin, doxycycline, estrogens and oral contraceptives, oral anticoagulants, tricyclic antidepressants: barbiturates may enhance the metabolism of these drugs. Monitor for de-

---

Reactions may be *common*, uncommon, *life-threatening*, or COMMON AND LIFE-THREATENING.

creased effectiveness.

Ethanol or other CNS depressants, including narcotic analgesics: excessive CNS and respiratory depression. Use together cautiously.

Griseofulvin: decreased absorption of griseofulvin. Monitor effectiveness of griseofulvin.

Rifampin: may decrease barbiturate levels. Monitor for decreased effect.

EFFECTS ON DIAGNOSTIC TESTS
Butabarbital may cause a false-positive phentolamine test. The physiologic effects of the drug may impair the absorption of cyanocobalamin ^{57}Co; it may decrease serum bilirubin concentrations in neonates, epileptic patients, and patients with congenital nonhemolytic unconjugated hyperbilirubinemia. EEG patterns are altered, with a change in low-voltage, fast activity; changes persist for a time after discontinuation of therapy. Barbiturates may increase sulfobromophthalein retention.

CONTRAINDICATIONS
Contraindicated in patients with bronchopneumonia, or other severe pulmonary insufficiency, hypersensitivity to barbiturates, or porphyria.

NURSING CONSIDERATIONS
• Use cautiously in patients with acute or chronic pain, depression, suicidal tendencies, history of drug abuse, or hepatic or renal impairment.
• Elderly patients are more sensitive to drug's adverse CNS reactions. Assess mental status before and after initiating therapy.
• Take precautions to prevent hoarding or self-overdosing by patients who are depressed, suicidal, or drug-dependent or who have a history of drug abuse.
• Watch for signs of barbiturate toxicity: coma, pupillary constriction, cyanosis, clammy skin, and hypotension. Overdose can be fatal.
• Discontinue drug when skin reactions occur because skin eruptions may pre-

cede potentially fatal reactions to barbiturate therapy. In some patients, high fever, stomatitis, headache, or rhinitis may precede skin reactions.
• Long-term use is not recommended; drug loses its efficacy in promoting sleep after 14 days. A drug-free interval of at least 1 week is advised if continued treatment is appropriate. Long-term high dosage may cause drug dependence, and patients may experience withdrawal symptoms if drug is suddenly stopped. Withdraw barbiturates gradually.

☑ **PATIENT TEACHING**
• Tell patient that morning "hangover" common after hypnotic dose. Hypnotic doses suppress REM sleep. Patients may experience increased dreaming after drug is discontinued.
• Tell patient to avoid alcohol use while taking drug.
• Caution patient about performing activities that require mental alertness or physical coordination.
• Tell patient who uses oral contraceptives that she should consider alternate birth control methods because drug may enhance contraceptive hormone metabolism and decrease its effect.

---

chloral hydrate
Aquachloral Supprettes, Dormel‡, Noctec, Novo-Chlorhydrate†

Controlled Substance Schedule IV
Pregnancy Risk Category: C

HOW SUPPLIED
Capsules: 250 mg, 500 mg
Syrup: 250 mg/5 ml, 500 mg/5 ml
Suppositories: 324 mg, 500 mg, 648 mg

ACTION
Unknown. Sedative effects may be caused by its primary metabolite, trichloroethanol.

---

*Liquid contains alcohol.   **May contain tartrazine.   †Canada only.   ‡Australia only.   ◇OTC.

ONSET, PEAK, DURATION
Onset occurs within 30 minutes. Peak unknown. Effects persist 4 to 8 hours.

INDICATIONS & DOSAGE
Sedation—
Adults: 250 mg P.O. or P.R. t.i.d. after meals.
Children: 8.3 mg/kg or 250 mg/m² P.O. or P.R. t.i.d. Maximum daily dosage is 500 mg t.i.d.
Insomnia—
Adults: 500 mg to 1 g P.O. or P.R. 15 to 30 minutes before bedtime.
Children: 50 mg/kg or 1.5 g/m² P.O. or P.R. 15 to 30 minutes before bedtime. Maximum single dose is 1 g.
Preoperatively—
Adults: 500 mg to 1 g P.O. or P.R. 30 minutes before surgery.
Premedication for EEG—
Children: 20 to 25 mg/kg P.O. or P.R.
Management of alcohol withdrawal symptoms—
Adults: 500 mg to 1 g P.O. or P.R. q 6 hours p.r.n., not to exceed 2 g daily.

ADVERSE REACTIONS
CNS: drowsiness, nightmares, dizziness, ataxia, paradoxical excitement, hangover, somnolence, disorientation, delirium, light-headedness, hallucinations, confusion, vertigo, malaise.
GI: *nausea, vomiting, diarrhea,* flatulence.
Hematologic: eosinophilia, leukopenia.
Skin: hypersensitivity reactions (rash, urticaria).
Other: physical and psychological dependence.

INTERACTIONS
Alkaline solutions: incompatible with aqueous solutions of chloral hydrate. Don't mix together.
Ethanol or other CNS depressants, including narcotic analgesics: excessive CNS depression or vasodilation reaction. Use together cautiously.
Furosemide I.V.: causes sweating, flushes, variable blood pressure, nausea, and uneasiness. Use together cautiously or use a different hypnotic drug.
Oral anticoagulants: increased risk of bleeding. Monitor patient closely.
Phenytoin: decreased phenytoin levels. Monitor closely.

EFFECTS ON DIAGNOSTIC TESTS
Chloral hydrate therapy may produce false-positive results for urine glucose with tests using cupric sulfate, such as Benedict's reagent and possibly Clinitest. It does not interfere with Clinistix or Tes-Tape results. It will interfere with fluorometric tests for urine catecholamines; do not use drug for 48 hours before the test. Drug may interfere with Reddy-Jenkins-Thorn test for urinary 17-hydroxycorticosteroids. May also cause a false-positive phentolamine test.

CONTRAINDICATIONS
Contraindicated in patients with hepatic or renal impairment, severe cardiac disease, or in those with hypersensitivity to chloral hydrate. Oral administration contraindicated in patients with gastric disorders.

NURSING CONSIDERATIONS
● Use with extreme caution in patients with severe cardiac disease. Use cautiously in patients with mental depression, suicidal tendencies, or history of drug abuse.
Alert: Note two strengths of oral liquid form. Double-check dose, especially when administering to children. Fatal overdoses have occurred.
● To minimize unpleasant taste and stomach irritation, dilute or administer with liquid. Drug should be taken after meals.
● Take precautions to prevent hoarding or self-overdosing by patients who are depressed, suicidal, or drug-dependent or who have a history of drug abuse.
● Be aware that long-term use is not recommended; drug loses its efficacy in promoting sleep after 14 days of continued use. Long-term use may cause drug

---

Reactions may be *common,* uncommon, *life-threatening,* or COMMON AND LIFE-THREATENING.

dependence, and patient may experience withdrawal symptoms if drug is suddenly stopped.

• Do not administer drug for 48 hours before fluorometric test, as ordered.

• Monitor BUN levels as ordered. Large dosage may raise BUN levels.

☑ **PATIENT TEACHING**

• Instruct patient to take capsules with a full glass of water or juice and to swallow the capsule whole.

• Tell patient to avoid alcohol use while taking drug.

• Caution patients about performing activities that require mental alertness or physical coordination.

• Tell patient to store drug in dark container; store suppositories in refrigerator.

---

estazolam
ProSom

Controlled Substance Schedule IV
Pregnancy Risk Category: X

HOW SUPPLIED
Tablets: 1 mg, 2 mg

ACTION
Unknown. Thought to act on the limbic system and thalamus of the CNS by binding to specific benzodiazepine receptors.

ONSET, PEAK, DURATION
Onset and duration unknown. Serum levels peak in 1 to 3 hours.

INDICATIONS & DOSAGE
Insomnia—
Adults: 1 mg P.O. h.s. Some patients may require 2 mg.
Elderly patients: 1 mg P.O. h.s. Use higher doses with extreme care. Frail elderly or debilitated patients may take 0.5 mg, but this low dose may be only marginally effective.

ADVERSE REACTIONS
CNS: fatigue, dizziness, *daytime drowsiness, somnolence, asthenia, hypokinesia,* abnormal thinking.
GI: dyspepsia, abdominal pain.
Other: back pain, stiffness.

INTERACTIONS
Cigarette smoking, rifampin: may increase metabolism and clearance and decrease plasma half-life. Monitor for decreased effectiveness.
Cimetidine, disulfiram, isoniazid, oral contraceptives: may impair the metabolism and clearance of benzodiazepines and prolong their plasma half-life. Monitor for increased CNS depression.
CNS depressants, including antihistamines, opiate analgesics, and other benzodiazepines; ethanol: increased CNS depression. Avoid concomitant use.
Theophylline: pharmacologic antagonism. Monitor for decreased effectiveness.

EFFECTS ON DIAGNOSTIC TESTS
AST levels may be increased.

CONTRAINDICATIONS
Contraindicated in pregnant patients or patients with hypersensitivity to drug.

NURSING CONSIDERATIONS
• Use cautiously in patients with hepatic, renal, or pulmonary disease; depression, or suicidal tendencies.
• Liver and renal function and CBC should be checked before and periodically during long-term therapy as ordered.
• Take precautions to prevent hoarding by depressed, suicidal, or drug-dependent patients or those who have a history of drug abuse.
• Be aware that patients who receive prolonged treatment with benzodiazepines may experience withdrawal symptoms if the drug is suddenly discontinued (possibly after 6 weeks of continuous therapy).

---

*Liquid contains alcohol.   **May contain tartrazine.   †Canada only.   ‡Australia only.   ◊OTC.

☑ **PATIENT TEACHING**

● Tell patient not to increase dosage of the drug but to inform the doctor if he thinks that the drug is no longer effective.

● Caution patient about performing activities that require mental alertness or physical coordination.

● Warn patient that additive depressant effects can occur if alcohol is consumed while taking this drug or within 24 hours after taking drug.

● Tell patient who uses oral contraceptives that she should consider alternate birth control methods when taking this drug because drug may enhance contraceptive hormone metabolism and decrease its effect.

ethchlorvynol
Placidyl**

*Controlled Substance Schedule IV
Pregnancy Risk Category: C*

HOW SUPPLIED
Capsules: 200 mg, 500 mg, 750 mg**

ACTION
Unknown; pharmacologic effects are similar to those produced by barbiturates.

ONSET, PEAK, DURATION
Onset occurs within 30 minutes to 1 hour. Plasma levels peak within 1 to 2 hours. Effects persist about 5 hours.

INDICATIONS & DOSAGE
Insomnia—
Adults: 500 mg to 1 g P.O. h.s. An additional 200 mg dose P.O. if awakened in early morning after a 500 mg or 750 mg bedtime dose.

ADVERSE REACTIONS
CNS: facial numbness, dizziness, hangover, ataxia, transient giddiness, syncope, hysteria, muscular weakness.
CV: hypotension.

EENT: unpleasant aftertaste, blurred vision.
GI: nausea, vomiting, gastric upset.
Hematologic: *thrombocytopenia,* exacerbation of porphyria.
Skin: rashes, urticaria.
Other: physical and psychological dependence, cholestatic jaundice.

INTERACTIONS
Ethanol or other CNS depressants, including MAO inhibitors, narcotic analgesics, and tricyclic antidepressants: excessive CNS depression. Use together cautiously.
Oral anticoagulants: ethchlorvynol may enhance the metabolism of coumarin derivatives, decreasing their effectiveness. Monitor patient closely.

EFFECTS ON DIAGNOSTIC TESTS
Ethchlorvynol may cause a false-positive phentolamine test.

CONTRAINDICATIONS
Contraindicated in patients with hypersensitivity to this drug and in those with porphyria.

NURSING CONSIDERATIONS
● Use cautiously in patients with hepatic or renal impairment, in elderly or debilitated patients, mental depression, and in those with suicidal tendencies.
● Minimize transient dizziness or ataxia, which is caused by rapid absorption, by giving this drug with milk or food.
● Take precautions to prevent hoarding or self-overdosing by patients who are depressed, suicidal, or drug-dependent or who have a history of drug abuse. Overdose is difficult to treat and is associated with high mortality.
● Monitor patient for allergic reactions. The 750-mg strength contains tartrazine dye, which may cause allergic reactions in susceptible patients.
● Watch for signs of toxicity, such as poor muscle coordination, confusion, hypothermia, speech or vision disturbances, tremor, and weakness.

Reactions may be *common,* uncommon, *life-threatening,* or COMMON AND LIFE-THREATENING.

• Be aware that drug is effective for short-term use only; treatment period should not exceed 1 week.

☑ **PATIENT TEACHING**
• Tell patient to take drug with milk or food if dizziness or ataxia occurs.
• Tell patient to avoid alcohol use while taking drug.
• Caution patient about performing activities that require mental alertness or physical coordination.

flurazepam hydrochloride
Apo-Flurazepam†, Dalmane, Novoflu-pam†

Controlled Substance Schedule IV
Pregnancy Risk Category: NR

HOW SUPPLIED
Capsules: 15 mg, 30 mg

ACTION
Unknown. A benzodiazepine that is thought to act on the limbic system, thalamus, and hypothalamus of the CNS to produce hypnotic effects.

ONSET, PEAK, DURATION
Onset and duration unknown. Peak effects occur in ½ to 1 hour.

INDICATIONS & DOSAGE
Insomnia—
Adults: 15 to 30 mg P.O. h.s. Dose repeated once, p.r.n.

ADVERSE REACTIONS
CNS: *daytime sedation, dizziness, drowsiness, disturbed coordination,* lethargy, confusion, *headache,* light-headedness, nervousness, hallucinations, staggering, ataxia, disorientation, ***coma.***
GI: nausea, vomiting, heartburn, diarrhea, abdominal pain.
Hepatic: elevated liver enzymes.
Other: physical or psychological dependence.

INTERACTIONS
Cigarette smoking, rifampin: enhanced metabolism of benzodiazepines. Monitor for decreased effectiveness.
Cimetidine: increased sedation. Monitor carefully.
Disulfiram, isoniazid, oral contraceptives: decreased metabolism of benzodiazepines, leading to toxicity. Monitor closely.
Ethanol or other CNS depressants, including narcotic analgesics: excessive CNS depression. Use together cautiously.
Phenytoin: increased phenytoin levels. Monitor for toxicity.

EFFECTS ON DIAGNOSTIC TESTS
Flurazepam therapy may elevate liver function test results. Minor changes in EEG patterns, usually low-voltage, fast activity, may occur during and after flurazepam therapy.

CONTRAINDICATIONS
Contraindicated in patients with hypersensitivity to the drug and during pregnancy.

NURSING CONSIDERATIONS
• Use cautiously in patients with impaired hepatic or renal function, chronic pulmonary insufficiency, mental depression, suicidal tendencies, or history of drug abuse.
• Check hepatic and renal function and CBC before and periodically during long-term therapy. May cause elevations in certain liver function tests (AST, ALT, total and direct bilirubin, and alkaline phosphatase).
• Assess mental status before initiating therapy. Elderly patients are more sensitive to the drug's adverse CNS reactions.
• Take precautions to prevent hoarding or self-overdosing by patients who are depressed, suicidal, or drug-dependent or who have a history of drug abuse.
• Be aware that physical and psychological dependence is possible with long-term use.

☑ **PATIENT TEACHING**
● Advise patient that this drug is more effective on second, third, and fourth nights because active metabolite accumulates. Encourage him to continue drug even if it doesn't relieve insomnia the first night.
● Tell patient to avoid alcohol use while taking this drug.
● Caution patient about performing activities that require mental alertness or physical coordination.
● Tell patient who uses oral contraceptives that she should consider alternate birth control methods when taking this drug.

---

pentobarbital
(pentobarbitone)
Nembutal*,**

pentobarbital sodium
Carbrital‡, Nembutal Sodium*, Nova Rectal†, Novopentobarb†

Controlled Substance Schedule II (suppositories: III)
Pregnancy Risk Category: D (suppositories: C)

HOW SUPPLIED
pentobarbital
Elixir: 18.2 mg/5 ml
pentobarbital sodium
Capsules: 50 mg, 100 mg
Injection: 50 mg/ml
Suppositories: 30 mg, 60 mg, 120 mg, 200 mg

ACTION
Unknown. Probably interferes with transmission of impulses from the thalamus to the cortex of the brain. A barbiturate.

ONSET, PEAK, DURATION
Onset occurs immediately after I.V. administration, within 10 to 25 minutes after I.M. administration, within 15 minutes after oral or rectal administration.

Serum levels peak immediately after I.V. administration, 30 to 60 minutes with oral dose, unknown for I.M. or rectal routes. Effects persist 1 to 4 hours following oral or rectal administration, 15 minutes following I.V. administration, unknown for I.M. administration.

INDICATIONS & DOSAGE
Sedation—
Adults: 20 to 40 mg P.O. b.i.d., t.i.d., or q.i.d.
Children: 2 to 6 mg/kg daily P.O. in 3 divided doses. Maximum daily dosage is 100 mg.
Insomnia—
Adults: 100 to 200 mg P.O. h.s. or 150 to 200 mg deep I.M.; 100 mg initially I.V., then additional doses up to 500 mg; 120 or 200 mg P.R.
Children: 2 to 6 mg/kg or 125 mg/m² I.M. Maximum dosage is 100 mg. P.R. dose for child 2 months to 1 year is 30 mg; 1 to 4 years, 30 or 60 mg; 5 to 11 years, 60 mg; 12 to 14 years, 60 or 120 mg.
Preoperative sedation—
Adults: 150 to 200 mg I.M.
Children: 5 mg/kg P.O. or I.M. if 10 years or older; 5 mg/kg I.M. or P.R. if younger than 10 years.

ADVERSE REACTIONS
CNS: *drowsiness, lethargy, hangover,* paradoxical excitement in elderly patients, somnolence.
GI: nausea, vomiting.
Hematologic: exacerbation of porphyria.
Respiratory: *respiratory depression.*
Skin: rash, urticaria, *Stevens-Johnson syndrome.*
Other: *angioedema,* physical and psychological dependence.

INTERACTIONS
Corticosteroids, doxycycline, estrogens and oral contraceptives, oral anticoagulants: pentobarbital may enhance the metabolism of these drugs. Monitor for decreased effect.

Reactions may be *common,* uncommon, *life-threatening,* or COMMON AND LIFE-THREATENING.

Ethanol or other CNS depressants, including narcotic analgesics: excessive CNS and respiratory depression. Use together cautiously.

Griseofulvin: decreased absorption of griseofulvin. Monitor effectiveness of griseofulvin.

MAO inhibitors: inhibited metabolism of barbiturates; may cause prolonged CNS depression. Reduce barbiturate dosage.

Rifampin: may decrease barbiturate levels. Monitor for decreased effect.

EFFECTS ON DIAGNOSTIC TESTS

Pentobarbital may cause a false-positive phentolamine test. The physiologic effects of the drug may impair the absorption of cyanocobalamin ^{57}Co; it may decrease serum bilirubin concentrations in neonates, epileptic patients, and patients with congenital nonhemolytic unconjugated hyperbilirubinemia. EEG patterns show a change in low-voltage, fast activity; changes persist for a time after discontinuation of therapy.

CONTRAINDICATIONS

Contraindicated in patients with hypersensitivity to barbiturates, or porphyria.

NURSING CONSIDERATIONS

● Use cautiously in patients with acute or chronic pain, mental depression, suicidal tendencies, history of drug abuse, or hepatic impairment. Also administer cautiously to elderly or debilitated patients.

● Assess mental status before initiating therapy and use reduced doses as ordered. Elderly patients are more sensitive to the drug's adverse CNS effects.

● **I.V. use:** I.V. administration of barbiturates may cause severe respiratory depression, laryngospasm, or hypotension. Have emergency resuscitation equipment available.

● To minimize deterioration, use I.V injection solution within 30 minutes after opening container. Don't use cloudy solution.

● Reserve I.V. injection for emergency treatment, which should be given under close supervision. Administer slowly at a rate not exceeding 50 mg/minute.

● Parenteral solution is alkaline. Local tissue reactions and injection site pain have followed I.V. use. Avoid extravasation. Assess patency of I.V. site before and during administration.

● Do not mix in syringe or in I.V. solutions or lines with other drugs.

Alert: Administer I.M. injection deeply. Superficial injection may cause pain, sterile abscess, and sloughing.

● To ensure accurate dosage, don't divide suppositories.

● Take precautions to prevent hoarding or self-overdosing by patients who are depressed, suicidal, or drug-dependent or who have a history of drug abuse.

● Watch for signs of barbiturate toxicity: coma, pupillary constriction, cyanosis, clammy skin, and hypotension. Overdose can be fatal.

● Inspect patient's skin. Skin eruptions may precede potentially fatal reactions to barbiturate therapy. Discontinue drug when skin reactions occur and call doctor. In some patients, high fever, stomatitis, headache, or rhinitis may precede skin reactions.

● Know that pentobarbital has no analgesic effect and may cause restlessness or delirium in patients with pain.

● Be aware that long-term use is not recommended; drug loses its efficacy in promoting sleep after 14 days of continued use. Long-term high dosage may cause drug dependence, and patient may experience withdrawal symptoms if drug is suddenly discontinued. Withdraw barbiturates gradually.

☑ PATIENT TEACHING

● Inform patient that morning "hangover" is common after hypnotic dose, which suppresses REM sleep. Patient may experience increased dreaming after drug is discontinued.

● Caution patient about performing activities that require mental alertness or physical coordination.

• Tell patient to avoid alcohol use while taking drug.

• Tell patient who uses oral contraceptives that she should consider alternate birth control methods because drug may enhance contraceptive hormone metabolism and decrease its effect.

quazepam
Doral

Controlled Substance Schedule IV
Pregnancy Risk Category: X

HOW SUPPLIED
Tablets: 7.5 mg, 15 mg

ACTION
Unknown, although drug acts on the limbic system and thalamus of the CNS by binding to specific benzodiazepine receptors.

ONSET, PEAK, DURATION
Onset and duration unknown. Plasma levels peak in about 2 hours.

INDICATIONS & DOSAGE
Insomnia—
Adults: 15 mg P.O. h.s. Some patients may respond to lower dosages. Dosage decreased in elderly patients after 2 days of therapy if possible.

ADVERSE REACTIONS
CNS: *fatigue, dizziness, daytime drowsiness, headache.*
GI: dry mouth, dyspepsia.
Other: physical and psychological dependence.

INTERACTIONS
Anticonvulsants, antihistamines, ethanol, psychotropic drugs, and other drugs that produce CNS depression: additive CNS depressant effects. Avoid concomitant use.

EFFECTS ON DIAGNOSTIC TESTS
None reported.

CONTRAINDICATIONS
Contraindicated in patients with hypersensitivity to this drug or other benzodiazepines, in pregnant patients, and in patients with suspected or established sleep apnea.

NURSING CONSIDERATIONS
• Use cautiously in patients with hepatic, renal, or respiratory disease, depression, and in elderly patients.
• Take precautions to prevent hoarding or self-overdosing by patients who are depressed, suicidal, or drug-dependent or who have a history of drug abuse.
• Be aware that patients on long-term therapy with benzodiazepines may experience withdrawal symptoms if the drug is suddenly withdrawn (possibly after 6 weeks of continuous therapy).

☑ PATIENT TEACHING
• Warn patient not to increase the drug dosage but to inform the doctor if he thinks that drug is not effective.
• Caution patient about performing activities that require mental alertness or physical coordination.
• Warn patient about the possible additive depressant effects that can occur if alcohol is consumed within 24 hours of quazepam.

secobarbital sodium
Novosecobarb†, Seconal Sodium

Controlled Substance Schedule II
Pregnancy Risk Category: D

HOW SUPPLIED
Capsules: 50 mg, 100 mg
Injection: 50 mg/ml

ACTION
Unknown. Probably interferes with transmission of impulses from the thalamus to the cortex of the brain. A barbiturate.

ONSET, PEAK, DURATION
Onset occurs within 15 minutes with oral dose, almost immediate with I.V. dose, unknown for I.M. administration. Serum levels peak 1 to 3 minutes with I.V. administration, 7 to 10 minutes with I.M. administration, and 15 to 30 minutes with oral dose. Effects persist for 1 to 4 hours for oral dose, 15 minutes for I.V. dose, unknown for I.M. dose.

INDICATIONS & DOSAGE
Preoperative sedation—
Adults: 200 to 300 mg P.O. 1 to 2 hours before surgery.
Children: 2 to 6 mg/kg P.O. Maximum single dose is 100 mg.
Insomnia—
Adults: 100 to 200 mg P.O. or I.M.
Children: 3 to 5 mg/kg I.M. or 125 mg/m², not to exceed 100 mg, with no more than 5 ml injected in any one site.
Acute tetanus seizure—
Adults and children: 5.5 mg/kg I.M. or slow I.V., repeated q 3 to 4 hours, if needed; I.V. injection rate not to exceed 50 mg/15 seconds.
Status epilepticus—
Children: 15 to 20 mg/kg I.V. over 15 minutes.

ADVERSE REACTIONS
CNS: *drowsiness, lethargy, hangover,* paradoxical excitement in elderly patients, somnolence.
CV: hypotension (with I.V. use).
GI: nausea, vomiting.
Hematologic: exacerbation of porphyria.
Respiratory: *respiratory depression.*
Skin: rash, urticaria, *Stevens-Johnson syndrome,* tissue reactions and injection-site pain.
Other: *angioedema,* physical and psychological dependence.

INTERACTIONS
Chloramphenicol, MAO inhibitors, valproic acid: inhibited metabolism of barbiturates; may cause prolonged CNS depression. Reduce barbiturate dosage.

Corticosteroids, digitoxin, doxycycline, estrogens and oral contraceptives, oral anticoagulants, tricyclic antidepressants: secobarbital may enhance the metabolism of these drugs. Monitor for decreased effect.
Ethanol or other CNS depressants, including narcotic analgesics: excessive CNS and respiratory depression. Use together cautiously.
Griseofulvin: decreased absorption of griseofulvin. Monitor effectiveness of griseofulvin.
Lactated Ringer's solution, acidic solutions: incompatible with I.V. form of drug. Don't mix.
Rifampin: may decrease barbiturate levels. Monitor for decreased effect.

EFFECTS ON DIAGNOSTIC TESTS
Secobarbital may cause a false-positive phentolamine test. The physiologic effects of the drug may impair the absorption of cyanocobalamin ^{57}Co; it may decrease serum bilirubin concentrations in neonates, epileptic patients, and patients with congenital nonhemolytic unconjugated hyperbilirubinemia. EEG patterns are altered, with a change in low-voltage, fast activity; changes persist for a time after discontinuation of therapy.

CONTRAINDICATIONS
Contraindicated in patients with marked liver impairment, respiratory disease in which dyspnea or obstruction is evident, hypersensitivity to barbiturates, or porphyria.

NURSING CONSIDERATIONS
● Use cautiously in patients with acute or chronic pain, depression, suicidal tendencies, history of drug abuse, or hepatic impairment.
● Assess mental status before initiating therapy. Elderly patients are more sensitive to the drug's adverse CNS effects.
● **I.V. use:** Know that I.V. injection is reserved for emergency treatment and given under close supervision by direct injection and administered slowly at a

rate not exceeding 50 mg/15 seconds. May be administered as supplied or diluted.

● Local tissue reactions and injection-site pain have been noted with I.V. use. Assess patency of I.V. site before and during administration.

● I.V. administration of barbiturates may cause severe respiratory depression, laryngospasm, or hypotension. Have emergency resuscitation equipment readily available.

● Know that secobarbital sodium injection is not compatible with lactated Ringer's solution, but is compatible with Ringer's solution, sterile water for injection, and 0.9% sodium chloride. Don't mix with acidic solutions.

● Use injection solution within 30 minutes after opening container to minimize deterioration. Don't use cloudy solution.
Alert: Give I.M. injection deeply. Superficial injection may cause pain, sterile abscess, and sloughing.

● Take precautions to prevent hoarding or self-overdosing by patients who are depressed, suicidal, or drug-dependent or who have a history of drug abuse.

● Watch for signs of barbiturate toxicity: coma, pupillary constriction, cyanosis, clammy skin, and hypotension. Overdose can be fatal.

● Inspect patient's skin. Skin eruptions may precede potentially fatal reactions to barbiturate therapy. Discontinue drug when skin reactions occur and notify doctor. In some patients, high fever, stomatitis, headache, or rhinitis may precede skin reactions.

● Be aware that long-term use is not recommended; drug loses its efficacy in promoting sleep after 14 days of continued use.

☑ PATIENT TEACHING
● Tell patient that morning "hangover" is common after hypnotic dose, which suppresses REM sleep. Patient may experience increased dreaming after drug is discontinued.

● Tell patient to avoid alcohol use while taking drug.

● Caution patient about performing activities that require mental alertness or physical coordination.

● Tell patient who uses oral contraceptives that she should consider alternate birth control methods.

---

temazepam
Euhypnos 10‡, Euhypnos 20‡, Normison‡, Restoril, Temaze‡

Controlled Substance Schedule IV
Pregnancy Risk Category: X

HOW SUPPLIED
Capsules: 10 mg‡, 15 mg, 20 mg‡, 30 mg

ACTION
Unknown. A benzodiazepine that probably acts on the limbic system, thalamus, and hypothalamus of the CNS to produce hypnotic effects.

ONSET, PEAK, DURATION
Onset and duration unknown. Serum levels peak in 1 to 2 hours.

INDICATIONS & DOSAGE
Insomnia—
Adults: 7.5 to 30 mg P.O. h.s.
Adults over 65 years: 7.5 mg P.O. h.s.

ADVERSE REACTIONS
CNS: *drowsiness, dizziness, lethargy,* disturbed coordination, daytime sedation, confusion, nightmares, vertigo, euphoria, weakness, headache, fatigue, nervousness, anxiety, depression.
EENT: blurred vision.
GI: diarrhea, nausea, dry mouth.
Other: physical and psychological dependence.

INTERACTIONS
Ethanol or other CNS depressants: increased CNS depression. Use together cautiously.

Reactions may be *common,* uncommon, *life-threatening,* or COMMON AND LIFE-THREATENING.

EFFECTS ON DIAGNOSTIC TESTS
Temazepam therapy may increase liver function test results. Minor changes in EEG patterns, usually low-voltage, fast activity, may occur during and after temazepam therapy.

CONTRAINDICATIONS
Contraindicated in patients with hypersensitivity to this drug or other benzodiazepines and during pregnancy.

NURSING CONSIDERATIONS
• Use cautiously in patients with chronic pulmonary insufficiency, impaired hepatic or renal function, severe or latent mental depression, suicidal tendencies, and history of drug abuse.
• Assess mental status before initiating therapy. Elderly patients are more sensitive to the drug's adverse CNS effects.
• Take precautions to prevent hoarding or self-overdosing by patients who are depressed, suicidal, or drug-dependent or who have a history of drug abuse.

☑ PATIENT TEACHING
• Tell patient to avoid alcohol use while taking drug.
• Caution patient about performing activities that require mental alertness or physical coordination.
• Tell patient that onset of the drug's effects may take as long as 2 to 2½ hours.

---

triazolam
Apo-Triazo†, Halcion, Novo-Triolam†, Nu-Triazo†

Controlled Substance Schedule IV
Pregnancy Risk Category: X

HOW SUPPLIED
Tablets: 0.125 mg, 0.25 mg

ACTION
Unknown. A benzodiazepine that probably acts on the limbic system, thalamus, and hypothalamus of the CNS to produce hypnotic effects.

ONSET, PEAK, DURATION
Onset and duration unknown. Serum levels peak in 1 to 2 hours.

INDICATIONS & DOSAGE
Insomnia—
Adults: 0.125 to 0.5 mg P.O. h.s.
Adults over 65: 0.125 mg P.O. h.s.; increased, as needed, to 0.25 mg P.O. h.s.

ADVERSE REACTIONS
CNS: *drowsiness, dizziness, headache,* rebound insomnia, amnesia, lack of coordination, mental confusion, depression, nervousness, ataxia.
GI: nausea, vomiting.
Other: physical or psychological dependence.

INTERACTIONS
Cimetidine, erythromycin: may cause prolonged triazolam blood levels. Monitor for increased sedation.
Ethanol or other CNS depressants: excessive CNS depression. Use together cautiously.

EFFECTS ON DIAGNOSTIC TESTS
Triazolam therapy may increase liver function test results. Minor changes in EEG patterns, usually low-voltage, fast activity, may occur during and after triazolam therapy.

CONTRAINDICATIONS
Contraindicated in patients with hypersensitivity to benzodiazepines and during pregnancy.

NURSING CONSIDERATIONS
• Use cautiously in nursing mothers and patients with impaired hepatic or renal function, chronic pulmonary insufficiency, sleep apnea, mental depression, suicidal tendencies, or history of drug abuse.
• Assess mental status before initiating therapy. Elderly patients are more sensitive to the drug's CNS effects.
• Take precautions to prevent hoarding or self-overdosing by patients who are

---

depressed, suicidal, or drug-dependent or who have a history of drug abuse.

☑ PATIENT TEACHING
● Warn patient not to take more than the prescribed amount; overdose can occur at a total daily dose of 2 mg (or four times highest recommended amount).
● Tell patient to avoid alcohol while taking drug.
● Caution patient about performing activities that require mental alertness or physical coordination.
● Inform patient that drug tends not to cause morning drowsiness.
● Tell patient that rebound insomnia may develop for one or two nights after stopping therapy.

---

zolpidem tartrate
Ambien

Controlled Substance Schedule IV
Pregnancy Risk Category: B

HOW SUPPLIED
Tablets: 5 mg, 10 mg

ACTION
Although zolpidem interacts with one of three identified gamma-aminobutyric acid-benzodiazepine receptor complexes, it's not a benzodiazepine. It exhibits hypnotic activity, but no muscle relaxant or anticonvulsant properties.

ONSET, PEAK, DURATION
Onset rapid. Serum levels peak within ½ to 2 hours. Duration unknown.

INDICATIONS & DOSAGE
Short-term management of insomnia—
Adults: 10 mg P.O. immediately before bedtime.
    In elderly or debilitated patients and in patients with hepatic insufficiency, 5 mg P.O. immediately before bedtime. Maximum daily dosage is 10 mg.

ADVERSE REACTIONS
CNS: daytime drowsiness, light-headedness, abnormal dreams, amnesia, dizziness, *headache,* hangover, sleep disorder, lethargy, depression.
CV: palpitations.
EENT: sinusitis, pharyngitis, dry mouth.
GI: nausea, vomiting, diarrhea, dyspepsia, constipation, abdominal pain.
Skin: rash.
Other: back or chest pain, flulike-symptoms, hypersensitivity reactions, myalgia, arthralgia.

INTERACTIONS
Ethanol or other CNS depressants: enhanced CNS depression. Avoid concomitant use.

EFFECTS ON DIAGNOSTIC TESTS
None reported.

CONTRAINDICATIONS
None known.

NURSING CONSIDERATIONS
● Use cautiously in patients with compromised respiratory status.
● Be aware that hypnotics should be used only for short-term management of insomnia, usually 7 to 10 days.
● Know that the smallest effective dose should be used in all patients.
● Take precautions to prevent hoarding or self-overdosing by patients who are depressed, suicidal, or drug-dependent or who have a history of drug abuse.

☑ PATIENT TEACHING
● For faster sleep onset, instruct patient not to take drug with or immediately after meals.
● Tell patient to avoid alcohol.
● Caution patient about performing activities that require mental alertness or physical coordination.

Anticonvulsants

acetazolamide sodium
(See Chapter 62, DIURETICS.)
carbamazepine
clonazepam
clorazepate dipotassium
(See Chapter 32, ANTIANXIETY
DRUGS.)
diazepam
(See Chapter 32, ANTIANXIETY
DRUGS.)
ethosuximide
fosphenytoin sodium
gabapentin
lamotrigine
magnesium sulfate
mephobarbital
phenobarbital
phenobarbital sodium
phensuximide
phenytoin
phenytoin sodium
phenytoin sodium (extended)
primidone
valproate sodium
valproic acid
divalproex sodium

COMBINATION PRODUCTS
DILANTIN WITH PHENOBARBITAL
KAPSEALS: phenytoin sodium 100 mg
and phenobarbital 16 mg; phenytoin
sodium 100 mg and phenobarbital 32
mg.

---

carbamazepine
Apo-Carbamazepine†, Epitol,
Mazepine†, Novocarbamaz†, PMS-
Carbamazepine†, Tegretol, Tegretol
Chewable Tablets, Tegretol CR†, Ter-
il‡

Pregnancy Risk Category: C

HOW SUPPLIED
Tablets: 200 mg

Tablets (chewable): 100 mg
Tablets (extended-release)†: 200 mg,
400 mg
Oral suspension: 100 mg/5 ml

ACTION
Unknown. Thought to stabilize neuronal
membranes and limit seizure activity by
either increasing efflux or decreasing influx of sodium ions across cell membranes in the motor cortex during generation of nerve impulses.

ONSET, PEAK, DURATION
For trigeminal neuralgia, onset occurs in
8 to 72 hours; for anticonvulsant effect,
in hours to days. Serum levels peak in
1½ hours after oral suspension, 4 to 12
hours after tablets. Duration unknown.

INDICATIONS & DOSAGE
*Generalized tonic-clonic and complex
partial seizures, mixed seizure
patterns—*
Adults and children over 12 years:
initially, 200 mg P.O. b.i.d. for tablets or
1 tsp of suspension P.O. q.i.d. May be
increased at weekly intervals by 200 mg
P.O. daily, in divided doses at 6- to 8-
hour intervals. Adjusted to minimum effective level. Maximum daily dosage is
1 g/day in children ages 12 to 15, or 1.2
g/day in patients over age 15.
Children 6 to 12 years: initially, 100
mg P.O. b.i.d. or ½ tsp of suspension
P.O. q.i.d. Increased at weekly intervals
by 100 mg P.O. daily. Maximum daily
dosage is 1 g/day.
Trigeminal neuralgia—
Adults: initially, 100 mg P.O. b.i.d. or ½
tsp of suspension q.i.d. with meals. Increased by 100 mg q 12 hours for
tablets or ½ tsp of suspension q.i.d. until
pain is relieved. Maximum daily dosage
is 1.2 g/day. Maintenance dosage is 200
to 400 mg P.O. b.i.d.

---

*Liquid contains alcohol. **May contain tartrazine. †Canada only. ‡Australia only. ◇OTC.

ADVERSE REACTIONS

CNS: *dizziness, vertigo, drowsiness*, fatigue, *ataxia*, **worsening of seizures** (usually in patients with mixed seizure disorders, including atypical absence seizures), confusion, headache, syncope.

CV: *CHF*, hypertension, hypotension, aggravation of coronary artery disease, arrhythmias, AV block.

EENT: conjunctivitis, dry mouth and pharynx, blurred vision, diplopia, nystagmus.

GI: *nausea, vomiting*, abdominal pain, diarrhea, anorexia, stomatitis, glossitis.

GU: urinary frequency, urine retention, impotence, albuminuria, glycosuria, elevated BUN.

Hematologic: *aplastic anemia, agranulocytosis,* eosinophilia, leukocytosis, *thrombocytopenia.*

Hepatic: abnormal liver function test results, *hepatitis.*

Respiratory: pulmonary hypersensitivity.

Skin: rash, urticaria, erythema multiforme, *Stevens-Johnson syndrome.*

Other: excessive diaphoresis, fever, chills, SIADH.

INTERACTIONS

Cimetidine, danazol, diltiazem, fluoxetine, flouoxamine, macrolides (such as erythromycin), isoniazid, propoxyphene, terfenadine, valproic acid, verapamil: may increase carbamazepine blood levels. Use cautiously.

Lithium: increased CNS toxicity of lithium. Avoid concomitant use.

MAO inhibitors: increased depressant and anticholinergic effects. Don't use together.

Oral contraceptives, doxycycline, felbamate, haloperidol, phenytoin, theophylline, warfarin: carbamazepine may decrease blood levels of these drugs. Monitor for decreased effect.

Phenobarbital, phenytoin, primidone: may decrease carbamazepine levels. Monitor for decreased effect.

EFFECTS ON DIAGNOSTIC TESTS

Carbamazepine may elevate liver enzyme levels; it also may decrease values of thyroid function tests.

CONTRAINDICATIONS

Contraindicated in patients with history of previous bone marrow suppression or hypersensitivity to carbamazepine or tricyclic antidepressants and in patients who have taken an MAO inhibitor within 14 days of therapy.

NURSING CONSIDERATIONS

● Use cautiously in patients with mixed seizure disorders because they may experience an increased incidence of seizures.

● Obtain baseline determinations of urinalysis, BUN level, liver function, CBC, platelet and reticulocyte counts, and serum iron level as ordered. Monitor periodically thereafter.

● Shake oral suspension well before measuring dose.

● When administering by nasogastric tube, mix dose with an equal volume of water, 0.9% sodium chloride solution, or D_5W. Flush tube with 100 ml of diluent after administering dose.

● Never discontinue suddenly when treating seizures. Notify doctor immediately if adverse reactions occur.

● Adverse reactions may be minimized by increasing dosage gradually.

● Therapeutic carbamazepine blood level is 4 to 12 mcg/ml. Monitor blood levels and effects closely. Ask the patient when last dose of medication was taken to better evaluate blood levels.

● When managing seizures, institute appropriate precautions.

Alert: Observe for signs of anorexia or subtle appetite changes, which may indicate excessive blood levels.

☑ PATIENT TEACHING

● Tell patient to take carbamazepine with food to minimize GI distress. Tell patient who takes suspension form to shake container well before measuring

---

dose.
- Tell patient to keep tablets in the original container, tightly closed, and away from moisture. Some formulations may harden when exposed to excessive moisture, resulting in decreased bioavailability and loss of seizure control.
- Inform patient that when used for trigeminal neuralgia, an attempt to decrease dosage or withdraw drug is usually done every 3 months.
- Tell patient to notify the doctor immediately if fever, sore throat, mouth ulcers, or easy bruising or bleeding occurs.
- Tell patient that drug may cause mild to moderate dizziness and drowsiness when first taken. Advise him to avoid hazardous activities until effects disappear. Effect usually disappears within 3 to 4 days.
- Advise patient that periodic eye examinations are recommended.

---

clonazepam
Klonopin

Controlled Substance Schedule IV
Pregnancy Risk Category: NR

HOW SUPPLIED
Tablets: 0.5 mg, 1 mg, 2 mg
Drops: 2.5 mg/ml‡
Injection: 1 mg/ml‡

ACTION
Unknown. A benzodiazepine that probably acts by facilitating the effects of the inhibitory neurotransmitter gamma-aminobutyric acid.

ONSET, PEAK, DURATION
Onset and duration unknown. Serum levels peak in 1 to 2 hours, although peak concentrations may not be achieved for 4 to 8 hours.

INDICATIONS & DOSAGE
Lennox-Gastaut syndrome; atypical ab-

sence seizures; akinetic and myoclonic seizures—
Adults: initially, not to exceed 1.5 mg P.O. daily in three divided doses. May be increased by 0.5 to 1 mg q 3 days until seizures are controlled. If given in unequal doses, the largest dose given h.s. Maximum recommended daily dosage is 20 mg.
Children up to 10 years or 30 kg: initially, 0.01 to 0.03 mg/kg P.O. daily (not to exceed 0.05 mg/kg daily), in 2 or 3 divided doses. Increased by 0.25 to 0.5 mg q third day to a maximum maintenance dosage of 0.1 to 0.2 mg/kg daily as needed.
Status epilepticus (where parenteral form is available)—
Adults: 1 mg by slow I.V. infusion.
Children: 0.5 mg by slow I.V. infusion.

ADVERSE REACTIONS
CNS: *drowsiness, ataxia, behavioral disturbances* (especially in children), slurred speech, tremor, confusion, psychosis, agitation.
CV: palpitations.
EENT: nystagmus, abnormal eye movements, sore gums.
GI: constipation, gastritis, change in appetite, nausea, anorexia, diarrhea.
GU: dysuria, enuresis, nocturia, urine retention.
Hematologic: leukopenia, *thrombocytopenia,* eosinophilia.
Respiratory: *respiratory depression,* chest congestion, shortness of breath.
Skin: rash.

INTERACTIONS
Ethanol or other CNS depressants: increased CNS depression. Monitor patient closely.
Phenytoin: levels of phenytoin may be increased.

EFFECTS ON DIAGNOSTIC TESTS
Clonazepam may elevate phenytoin levels and liver function test results.

---

*Liquid contains alcohol.   **May contain tartrazine.   †Canada only.   ‡Australia only.   ◊OTC.

CONTRAINDICATIONS

Contraindicated in patients with significant hepatic disease; in those with sensitivity to benzodiazepines; or in patients with acute angle-closure glaucoma.

NURSING CONSIDERATIONS

• Use cautiously in patients with mixed type of seizure because drug may precipitate generalized tonic-clonic seizures. Also use cautiously in children and in patients with chronic respiratory disease, or open-angle glaucoma.

• **I.V. use‡:** Give slowly by direct injection or by slow I.V. infusion. Drug may be diluted with D_5W, dextrose 2.5% in water, or 0.9% sodium chloride or 0.45% sodium chloride solution.

• Mix solutions in glass bottles because the drug binds to polyvinyl chloride (PVC) plastic. If PVC infusion bags are used, administer immediately and infuse at a rate of 60 ml/hour or faster.

• Never withdraw suddenly because seizures may worsen. Call the doctor at once if adverse reactions develop.

• Monitor blood levels. Therapeutic blood level is 20 to 80 ng/ml.

• Assess elderly patient's response closely. Elderly patients are more sensitive to the drug's CNS effects.

• Monitor patient for oversedation.

• Monitor CBCs and liver function tests as ordered.

• Know that withdrawal symptoms are similar to those of barbiturates.

☑ PATIENT TEACHING

• Advise patient to avoid driving and other potentially hazardous activities that require mental alertness until drug's CNS effects are known.

• Instruct parent to monitor child's school performance because clonazepam may interfere with attentiveness in school.

• Instruct patient and parents never to stop drug abruptly because seizures may occur.

ethosuximide
Zarontin

Pregnancy Risk Category: NR

HOW SUPPLIED

Capsules: 250 mg
Syrup: 250 mg/5 ml

ACTION

Not clearly defined. A succinimide derivative that probably increases seizure threshold. Reduces the paroxysmal spike-and-wave pattern of absence seizures by depressing nerve transmission in the motor cortex.

ONSET, PEAK, DURATION

Onset and duration unknown. Peak effect occurs in 3 to 7 hours.

INDICATIONS & DOSAGE

Absence seizures—

Adults and children 6 years and older: 500 mg P.O. daily. Optimal dose is 20 mg/kg/day.

Children 3 to 6 years: 250 mg P.O. daily. Adjust dosage until control is achieved. Optimal dose is 20 mg/kg/day.

Alert: Dosages exceeding 1.5 g daily require administration under the doctor's strict supervision.

ADVERSE REACTIONS

CNS: *drowsiness, headache, fatigue, dizziness, ataxia, irritability, hiccups, euphoria, lethargy, depression, psychosis.*

EENT: myopia, tongue swelling, gingival hyperplasia.

GI: *nausea, vomiting, diarrhea, weight loss, cramps, anorexia, epigastric and abdominal pain.*

GU: vaginal bleeding, urinary frequency.

Hematologic: leukopenia, eosinophilia, ***agranulocytosis,*** pancytopenia.

Skin: urticaria, pruritic and erythematous rashes, hirsutism.

Reactions may be *common*, uncommon, *life-threatening*, or COMMON AND LIFE-THREATENING.

INTERACTIONS
Phenytoin: serum phenytoin levels may be increased.
Valproic acid: may increase or decrease serum levels of ethosuximide.

EFFECTS ON DIAGNOSTIC TESTS
Ethosuximide may elevate liver enzyme levels and may cause false-positive Coombs' test results. It may also cause abnormal results of renal function tests.

CONTRAINDICATIONS
Contraindicated in patients with hypersensitivity to succinimide derivatives.

NURSING CONSIDERATIONS
• Use with extreme caution in patients with hepatic or renal disease.
• Be aware that ethosuximide is currently the drug of choice for treating absence seizures.
• Never withdraw drug suddenly. Call doctor immediately if adverse reactions develop.
• Monitor blood levels. Therapeutic blood levels are 40 to 100 mcg/ml.
• Obtain CBC every 3 to 6 months as ordered.
• Know that drug may increase frequency of generalized tonic-clonic seizures when used alone in patients who have mixed types of seizures.
• Know that drug may cause positive direct Coombs' test.

☑ PATIENT TEACHING
• Advise patient to take ethosuximide with food to minimize GI distress.
• Advise patient to avoid hazardous activities that require mental alertness until drug's CNS effects are known.
• Warn patient and parents not to stop drug abruptly.

▼ *NEW DRUG*

fosphenytoin sodium
Cerebyx

Pregnancy Risk Category: D

HOW SUPPLIED
Injection: 2 ml (150 mg fosphenytoin sodium equivalent to 100 mg phenytoin sodium), 10 ml (750 mg fosphenytoin sodium equivalent to 500 mg phenytoin sodium)

ACTION
Fosphenytoin is a prodrug of phenytoin, so its anticonvulsant action is that of phenytoin. Phenytoin is thought to stabilize neuronal membranes and limit seizure activity by modulation of voltage-dependent sodium channels of neurons, inhibition of calcium flux across neuronal membranes, modulation of voltage-dependent calcium channels of neurons, and enhancement of sodium-potassium ATPase activity of neurons and glial cells.

ONSET, PEAK, DURATION
Onset is unknown. Peak plasma concentrations of fosphenytoin occur about 30 minutes after I.M. administration or at the end of an I.V. infusion. Conversion half-life of fosphenytoin to phenytoin is about 15 minutes.

INDICATIONS & DOSAGE
Status epilepticus—
Adults: 15 to 20 mg phenytoin sodium equivalent (PE)/kg I.V. at 100 to 150 mg PE/ minute as loading dose; then 4 to 6 mg PE/kg/day I.V. as maintenance dose. (Phenytoin may be used instead of fosphenytoin as maintenance, using the appropriate dose.)
Prevention and treatment of seizures during neurosurgery (nonemergent loading or maintenance dosing)—
Adults: loading dose of 10 to 20 mg PE/kg I.M. or I.V. at infusion rate not exceeding 150 mg PE/minute. Maintenance dose is 4 to 6 mg PE/kg/day I.V. or I.M.
Short-term substitution for oral phenytoin therapy—
Adult: same total daily dosage equivalent as oral phenytoin sodium therapy given as a single daily dose I.M. or I.V.

at infusion rate not exceeding 150 mg PE/minute. Some patients may require more frequent dosing.

ADVERSE REACTIONS
CNS: increased or decreased reflexes, speech disorders, dysarthria, asthenia, intracranial hypertension, thinking abnormalities, nervousness, hypesthesia, extrapyramidal syndrome, brain edema, headache, *nystagmus, dizziness, somnolence, ataxia,* stupor, incoordination, paresthesia, tremor, agitation, vertigo.
CV: hypertension, vasodilation, tachycardia, hypotension.
GI: constipation, taste perversion.
Hematologic: *thrombocytopenia,* leukopenia, agranulocytosis, granulocytopenia, pancytopenia.
Respiratory: pneumonia.
Skin: rash, ecchymosis, *pruritus.*
Other: lymphadenopathy, hypokalemia, hyperglycemia, pelvic pain, back pain, accidental injury, myasthenia, injection site reaction and pain, infection, chills.

INTERACTIONS
Most significant drug interactions expected to occur are those that are commonly seen with phenytoin.
Acute alcohol intake, amiodarone, chloramphenicol, chlordiazepoxide, cimetidine, diazepam, dicumarol, disulfuram, estrogens, ethosuximide, fluoxetine, H_2 antagonists, halothane, isoniazid, methylphenidate, phenothiazines, phenylbutazone, salicylates, succinimides, sulfonamides, tolbutamide, trazodone: may increase plasma phenytoin concentrations and thus its therapeutic effects. Use together cautiously.
Carbamazepine, chronic alcohol abuse, reserpine: may decrease plasma phenytoin levels. Monitor patient.
Phenobarbital, valproic acid, sodium valproate: may increase or decrease plasma phenytoin levels. Similarly, the effects of phenytoin on the concentrations of these drugs is unpredictable. Monitor patient.
Coumarin, digitoxin, doxycycline, estro-gens, furosemide, oral contraceptives, rifampin, quinidine, theophylline, vitamin D: efficacy may be decreased by phenytoin due to increased hepatic metabolism. Monitor closely.
Tricyclic antidepressants: may lower seizure threshold and require adjustments in phenytoin dosage. Use cautiously.

EFFECTS ON DIAGNOSTIC TESTS
Fosphenytoin may decrease serum concentrations of T_4. It may also produce artificially low results in dexamethasone or metyrapone tests. Phenytoin may cause increased serum concentrations of glucose, alkaline phosphatase, and gamma glutamyl transpeptidase. Can lower serum folate levels.

CONTRAINDICATIONS
Contraindicated in patients with hypersensitivity to drug or its components, phenytoin, or other hydantoins. Also contraindicated in patients with sinus bradycardia, SA block, second- or third-degree AV block, and Adams-Stokes syndrome.

NURSING CONSIDERATIONS
● Use cautiously in patients with porphyria and those with history of hypersensitivity to similarly structured drugs, such as barbiturates, oxazolidinediones, and succinimides.
Alert: Know that fosphenytoin should always be prescribed and dispensed in phenytoin sodium equivalent units (PE). Do not make any adjustments in the recommended doses when substituting fosphenytoin for phenytoin, and vice versa.
● Before I.V. infusion, dilute fosphenytoin in 5% dextrose or 0.9% sodium chloride solution for injection to a concentration ranging from 1.5 to 25 mg PE/ml. Do not administer at a rate exceeding 150 mg PE/minute.
● Administer the dose of I.V. fosphenytoin used to treat status epilepticus at a maximum rate of 150 mg PE/minute. The typical infusion to a 50 kg patient

---

Reactions may be *common,* uncommon, **life-threatening**, or COMMON AND LIFE-THREATENING.

takes 5 to 7 minutes. (An infusion of an identical molar dose of phenytoin cannot be accomplished in less than 15 to 20 minutes because of adverse CV effects that accompany direct I.V. administration of phenytoin at rates above 50 mg/minute.) Do not use fosphenytoin I.M. for status epilepticus because therapeutic phenytoin concentrations may not be reached as rapidly as with I.V. administration.

● Know that if rapid phenytoin loading is a primary goal, I.V. administration of drug is preferred because it takes longer to achieve therapeutic plasma phenytoin concentrations after I.M. injection than after I.V. infusion.

● Monitor patient's ECG, blood pressure, and respiration continuously throughout the period during which maximal serum phenytoin concentrations occur—about 10 to 20 minutes after the end of fosphenytoin infusions. Severe CV complications are most commonly encountered in elderly or gravely ill patients. Reducing the rate of administration or discontinuing the drug may be necessary.

● Know that patients receiving 20 mg PE/kg of drug infused at a rate of 150 mg PE/minute are expected to experience sensory discomfort, most often in the groin. Occurrence and intensity of the discomfort can be lessened by slowing or temporarily stopping the infusion.

● Be aware that the phosphate load provided by fosphenytoin (0.0037 mmol phosphate/mg PE fosphenytoin) must be taken into consideration when treating patients who require phosphate restriction, such as those with severe renal impairment. Monitor labaratory values.

● Discontinue fosphenytoin if a rash appears, and notify the doctor. If the rash is exfoliative, purpuric, or bullous or if lupus erythematosus, Stevens-Johnson syndrome, or epidermal necrolysis is suspected, know that the drug should be discontinued and alternative therapy considered. If the rash is mild (measle-like or scarlatiniform), therapy may be resumed after the rash has disappeared. If rash recurs on reinstitution of therapy, further fosphenytoin or phenytoin administration is contraindicated. Document that the patient is allergic to drug.

● Know that in patients with acute hepatoxicity, drug should be discontinued.

● Know that I.M. administration generates systemic phenytoin concentrations similar enough to oral phenytoin sodium to allow essentially interchangeable use when ordered.

● Keep in mind that following fosphenytoin administration, phenytoin concentrations should not be monitored until conversion to phenytoin is essentially complete—about 2 hours after the end of an I.V. infusion or 4 hours after I.M. administration.

● Interpret total phenytoin plasma concentration levels cautiously in patients with renal or hepatic disease or with hypoalbuminemia due to an increased fraction in unbound phenytoin. Unbound phenytoin concentrations may be more useful in these patients. When administering drug I.V., monitor patients with renal and hepatic disease because they're at an increased risk for more frequent and severe adverse reactions.

● Know that abrupt withdrawal of drug may precipitate status epilepticus.

● Be aware that safety and effectiveness in children have not been established.

● Be aware that it is not known if fosphenytoin is excreted in breast milk.

☑ **PATIENT TEACHING**
● Warn patient that sensory disturbances may occur with I.V. administration.

● Instruct patient to immediately report adverse reactions, especially a rash.

● Warn patient to never stop drug abruptly or adjust dosage without discussing with his doctor.

● Inform women that breast-feeding is not recommended.

gabapentin
Neurontin

Pregnancy Risk Category: C

HOW SUPPLIED
Capsules: 100 mg, 300 mg, 400 mg

ACTION
Unknown. Although structurally related to gamma-amino butyric acid (GABA), the drug doesn't interact with GABA receptors and isn't converted metabolically into GABA or a GABA agonist.

ONSET, PEAK, DURATION
Unknown.

INDICATIONS & DOSAGE
Adjunctive treatment of partial seizures with and without secondary generalization in adults with epilepsy—
Adults: initially 300 mg P.O. h.s. on day 1; 300 mg P.O. b.i.d. on day 2; then 300 mg P.O. t.i.d. on day 3. Dosage increased as needed and tolerated to 1,800 mg daily in divided doses. Dosages up to 3,600 mg daily have been well tolerated.

Patients with renal failure: if creatinine clearance is over 60 ml/minute, 400 mg P.O. t.i.d.; if creatinine clearance is 30 to 60 ml/minute, 300 mg P.O. b.i.d.; if creatinine clearance is 15 to 30 ml/minute, 300 mg P.O. daily; if creatinine clearance is under 15 ml/minute, 300 mg P.O. every other day. Patients on dialysis should receive a loading dose of 300 to 400 mg P.O.; then 200 to 300 mg P.O. following every 4 hours of hemodialysis.

ADVERSE REACTIONS
CNS: *fatigue, somnolence, dizziness, ataxia, nystagmus, tremor,* nervousness, dysarthria, amnesia, depression, abnormal thinking, twitching, incoordination.
CV: peripheral edema, vasodilation.
EENT: *diplopia, rhinitis,* pharyngitis, dry throat, coughing, *amblyopia.*

GI: nausea, vomiting, dyspepsia, dry mouth, constipation.
GU: impotence.
Hematologic: leukopenia, decreased WBC count.
Skin: pruritus, abrasion.
Other: dental abnormalities, increased appetite, weight gain, back pain, myalgia, fractures.

INTERACTIONS
Antacids: decreased absorption of gabapentin. Separate administration times by at least 2 hours.

EFFECTS ON DIAGNOSTIC TESTS
Gabapentin causes false-positive results with the Ames-N-Multistix SG dipstick test for urinary protein when added to other antiepileptic drugs. The more specific sulfosalicylic acid precipitation procedure is recommended to determine the presence of urine protein.

CONTRAINDICATIONS
Contraindicated in patients hypersensitive to the drug.

NURSING CONSIDERATIONS
● Know that first dose should be given at bedtime to minimize drowsiness, dizziness, fatigue, and ataxia.
● If gabapentin therapy is discontinued or alternative medication is substituted, do so gradually over at least 1 week, as ordered, to minimize risk of precipitating seizures.
Alert: Do not suddenly withdraw other anticonvulsants in patients starting gabapentin therapy.
● Know that routine monitoring of plasma levels of gabapentin is not necessary. The drug does not appear to alter plasma levels of other anticonvulsants.
● Know that it may cause false-positive tests for urine protein when the Ames-N-Multistix SG dipstick test is used.

☑ PATIENT TEACHING
● Instruct patient to take first dose at bedtime to minimize adverse reactions.

Reactions may be *common*, uncommon, *life-threatening*, or COMMON AND LIFE-THREATENING.

• Warn patient to avoid driving and operating heavy machinery until drug's CNS effects are known.

lamotrigine
Lamictal

Pregnancy Risk Category: C

HOW SUPPLIED
Tablets: 25 mg, 100 mg, 150 mg, 200 mg

ACTION
Unknown. May cause inhibited release of glutamate and aspartate (excitatory neurotransmitters), in the brain. This may occur by way of an action at voltage-sensitive sodium channels.

ONSET, PEAK, DURATION
Onset and duration unknown. Serum levels peak in 1.4 to 4.8 hours.

INDICATIONS & DOSAGE
Adjunct therapy in treatment of partial seizures caused by epilepsy—
Adults: 50 mg P.O. daily for 2 weeks, followed by 100 mg daily in two divided doses for 2 weeks. Thereafter, usual maintenance dosage is 300 to 500 mg P.O. daily in two divided doses. For patients also taking valproic acid, 25 mg P.O. every other day for 2 weeks, followed by 25 mg P.O. daily for 2 weeks. Thereafter, no more than 150 mg P.O. daily in two divided doses.

ADVERSE REACTIONS
CNS: *dizziness, headache, ataxia, somnolence,* incoordination, insomnia, tremor, depression, anxiety, seizures, irritability, speech disorder, decreased memory, aggravated reaction, concentration disturbance, sleep disorder, emotional lability, vertigo, mind racing.
EENT: *diplopia, blurred vision,* vision abnormality, nystagmus.
GI: *nausea, vomiting,* diarrhea, dyspepsia, abdominal pain, constipation, tooth disorder, anorexia, dry mouth.
Respiratory: *rhinitis,* pharyngitis, cough, dyspnea.
Skin: *rash,* **Stevens-Johnson syndrome, toxic epidermal necrolysis,** pruritus, hot flashes, alopecia, acne.
Other: palpitations, dysarthria, muscle spasm, flulike syndrome, fever, infection, neck pain, malaise, chills, dysmenorrhea, vaginitis, amenorrhea.

INTERACTIONS
Carbamazepine, phenobarbital, phenytoin, primidone: decreased lamotrigine's steady-state concentrations. Monitor patient closely.
Folate inhibitors (such as cotrimoxazole, methotrexate): lamotrigine inhibits dihydrofolate reductase, an enzyme involved in folic acid synthesis. May have an additive effect. Monitor patient.
Valproic acid: decreased clearance of lamotrigine, which increases the drug's steady-state concentrations. Monitor patient closely for toxicity.

EFFECTS ON DIAGNOSTIC TESTS
None reported.

CONTRAINDICATIONS
Contraindicated in patients with hypersensitivity to the drug and children under 16 years of age.

NURSING CONSIDERATIONS
• Use cautiously in patients with renal, hepatic, or cardiac impairment.
• Know that drug should not be discontinued abruptly because of the possibility of increased seizure frequency. Instead, drug should be tapered over at least 2 weeks.
Alert: Know that drug should be stopped at first sign of rash unless it is not drug-related.
• Be aware that lamotrigine dose should be lowered if drug is added to a multidrug regimen that includes valproate.
• Know that a lowered maintenance dosage should be used in a patient with severe renal impairment.

• Be aware that patients should be evaluated for changes in seizure activity. Adjunct anticonvulsant's serum levels should be checked, as ordered.

☑ **PATIENT TEACHING**
• Inform patient that lamotrigine may cause a rash. Combination therapy of valproic acid and lamotrigine may be more likely to cause a serious rash. Tell patient to report rash or any signs or symptoms of hypersensitivity promptly to the doctor because they may warrant drug discontinuation.
• Warn patient not to engage in hazardous activity until drug's CNS effects are known.

---

magnesium sulfate

Pregnancy Risk Category: A

HOW SUPPLIED
Injection: 4%, 8%, 10%, 12.5%, 25%, 50%
Injection solution: 1% in 5% dextrose, 2% in 5% dextrose

ACTION
May decrease acetylcholine released by nerve impulses, but its anticonvulsant mechanism is unknown.

ONSET, PEAK, DURATION
Onset occurs 1 to 2 minutes after I.V. use; 1 hour after I.M. injection. Serum levels peak almost immediately after I.V. administration, unknown after I.M. administration. Effects persist about 30 minutes after I.V. administration, 3 to 4 hours after I.M. injection.

INDICATIONS & DOSAGE
Prevention or control of seizures in preeclampsia or eclampsia—
Women: initially, 4 g I.V. in 250 ml D₅W and 4 to 5 g deep I.M. each buttock; then 4 to 5 g deep I.M. into alternate buttock q 4 hours, p.r.n. Alternatively, 4 g I.V. loading dose, followed by 1 to 2 g hourly as I.V. infusion. Total dosage should not exceed 30 to 40 g daily.
Hypomagnesemia—
Adults: 1 g I.M. q 6 hours for four doses for mild deficiency; for severe deficiency, 5 g in 1,000 ml of D₅W or normal saline solution infused over 3 hours.
Seizures, hypertension, and encephalopathy associated with acute nephritis in children—
Children: 0.2 ml/kg of 50% solution I.M. q 4 to 6 hours, p.r.n. For severe symptoms, 100 to 200 mg/kg I.V. slowly over 1 hour with one-half of the dose administered in first 15 to 20 minutes. Dosage titrated according to blood magnesium levels and seizure response.
Management of paroxysmal atrial tachycardia—
Adults: 3 to 4 g I.V. over 30 seconds.
Management of life-threatening ventricular arrhythmias, such as sustained ventricular tachycardia or torsades de pointes—
Adults: 2 to 6 g I.V. over several minutes, followed by a continuous I.V. infusion of 3 to 20 mg/minute for 5 to 48 hours. Dosage and duration of therapy depend on patient response and serum magnesium levels.

ADVERSE REACTIONS
CNS: drowsiness, *depressed reflexes, flaccid paralysis, hypothermia.*
CV: *hypotension, flushing, **circulatory collapse,** depressed cardiac function.*
Other: diaphoresis, ***respiratory paralysis,*** hypocalcemia.

INTERACTIONS
Anesthetics, CNS depressants: may cause additive CNS depression. Use cautiously.
Digitalis glycosides: concomitant use may exacerbate arrhythmias. Use together cautiously.
Neuromuscular blockers: may cause increased neuromuscular blockade. Use cautiously.

EFFECTS ON DIAGNOSTIC TESTS
None reported.

CONTRAINDICATIONS
Parenteral administration of drug contraindicated in patients with heart block or myocardial damage.

NURSING CONSIDERATIONS
• Use cautiously in patients with impaired renal function. Also use cautiously in women who are in labor.
• If used to treat seizures, institute appropriate seizure precautions.
• **I.V. use:** If necessary, dilute to a maximum concentration of 20%. Infuse no faster than 150 mg/minute (1.5 ml/minute of a 10% solution or 0.75 ml/minute of a 20% solution). Drug is compatible with D_5W.
• Maximum infusion rate is 150 mg/minute. Too-rapid infusion will induce uncomfortable feeling of heat.
• Monitor vital signs every 15 minutes when giving drug I.V.
Alert: Watch for respiratory depression and signs of heart block.
• Keep I.V. calcium gluconate available to reverse magnesium intoxication; however, use cautiously in patients undergoing digitalization because of danger of arrhythmias.
• Check blood magnesium levels after repeated doses. Disappearance of knee-jerk and patellar reflexes is a sign of impending magnesium toxicity.
• Signs of hypermagnesemia begin to appear at blood levels of 4 mEq/liter.
• Monitor fluid intake and output. Urine output should be 100 ml or more in 4-hour period before each dose.
• Observe neonates for signs of magnesium toxicity, including neuromuscular or respiratory depression, when giving I.V. form of drug to toxemic mothers within 24 hours before delivery.

☑ PATIENT TEACHING
• Inform patient of short-term need for drug, and answer any questions and address concerns.

• Review adverse reactions associated with drug and tell patient to report adverse reactions promptly. Reassure patient that although drug may cause adverse reactions, vital signs, reflexes, and blood levels will be checked frequently to ensure his safety.

---

mephobarbital
Mebaral

Controlled Substance Schedule IV
Pregnancy Risk Category: D

HOW SUPPLIED
Tablets: 32 mg, 50 mg, 100 mg

ACTION
Unknown. A barbiturate that probably depresses monosynaptic and polysynaptic transmission in the CNS and increases the threshold for seizure activity in the motor cortex. Some activity comes from phenobarbital, an active metabolite.

ONSET, PEAK, DURATION
Onset occurs in 60 minutes or longer. Peak unknown. Effects persist for 10 to 12 hours.

INDICATIONS & DOSAGE
Generalized tonic-clonic or absence seizures—
Adults: 400 to 600 mg P.O. once daily or in divided doses.
Children under 5 years: 16 to 32 mg P.O. t.i.d. or q.i.d.
Children 5 years and over: 32 to 64 mg P.O. t.i.d. or q.i.d.
Relief of anxiety, tension, and apprehension—
Adults: 32 to 100 mg P.O. t.i.d. or q.i.d.
Children: 16 to 32 mg P.O. t.i.d. or q.i.d.

ADVERSE REACTIONS
CNS: headache, *hangover,* confusion, paradoxical excitation, drowsiness, somnolence, agitation, ataxia, nervous-

---

ness, hallucinations, insomnia, anxiety, dizziness, nightmares, syncope.
CV: hypotension, bradycardia.
GI: nausea, vomiting, constipation.
Respiratory: *respiratory depression,* apnea.
Other: allergic reactions (facial edema, rashes, exfoliative dermatitis), physical and psychological dependence.

INTERACTIONS
Chloramphenicol, MAO inhibitors, valproic acid: potentiated barbiturate effect. Monitor patient for increased CNS and respiratory depression.
Corticosteroids, digitoxin, doxycycline, estrogens and oral contraceptives, oral anticoagulants, tricyclic antidepressants: mephobarbital may enhance the metabolism of these drugs. Monitor for decreased effect.
Ethanol or other CNS depressants, including narcotic analgesics: excessive CNS depression. Use cautiously.
Griseofulvin: decreased absorption of griseofulvin. Monitor effectiveness of griseofulvin.
Rifampin: may decrease barbiturate levels. Monitor for decreased effect.

EFFECTS ON DIAGNOSTIC TESTS
Mephobarbital may elevate liver function test results.

CONTRAINDICATIONS
Contraindicated in patients with barbiturate hypersensitivity or porphyria.

NURSING CONSIDERATIONS
● Use cautiously in patients with acute or chronic pain, depression, suicidal tendencies, or history of drug abuse; hepatic, renal, cardiac, or respiratory function impairment; myasthenia gravis; or myxedema. Also use cautiously in elderly or debilitated patients.
● Know that dosage should be reduced in elderly or debilitated patients because these patients may be more sensitive to barbiturates. Dosage also should be reduced for patients with impaired renal

or hepatic disease.
● Never withdraw drug suddenly because seizures may worsen. Call the doctor at once if adverse reactions develop.
● Monitor phenobarbital blood levels. Therapeutic blood levels of phenobarbital are 15 to 40 mcg/ml.
● Periodically monitor CBC and BUN and creatinine levels.

☑ PATIENT TEACHING
● Advise patient to avoid driving and other potentially hazardous activities that require mental alertness until drug's CNS effects are known.
● Advise adults with nighttime seizures to take total or largest dose at night after checking with doctor.
● Warn patient and parents never to stop drug abruptly.
● Instruct patient to store in light-resistant container.
● Inform patient who uses oral contraceptives that she should consider another birth-control method because drug may enhance contraceptive hormone metabolism and decrease its effectiveness.
● Tell patient that drug suppresses REM sleep. When drug is discontinued, patient may experience increased dreaming.

---

phenobarbital (phenobarbitone)
Ancalixir†, Barbita, Solfoton

phenobarbital sodium (phenobarbitone sodium)
Luminal Sodium

Controlled Substance Schedule IV
Pregnancy Risk Category: D

HOW SUPPLIED
Tablets: 15 mg, 16 mg, 30 mg, 32 mg, 60 mg, 65 mg, 100 mg
Capsules: 16 mg
Elixir*: 15 mg/5 ml, 20 mg/5 ml
Injection: 30 mg/ml, 60 mg/ml, 65

mg/ml, 130 mg/ml

ACTION
Unknown. A barbiturate that probably depresses monosynaptic and polysynaptic transmission in the CNS and increases the threshold for seizure activity in the motor cortex. As a sedative, probably interferes with transmission of impulses from the thalamus to the cortex of the brain.

ONSET, PEAK, DURATION
Onset occurs in 60 minutes or longer. Peak concentration levels are reached in 8 to 12 hours. Effects persist for as long as 10 to 12 hours.

INDICATIONS & DOSAGE
All forms of epilepsy, febrile seizures—
Adults: 60 to 200 mg P.O. daily in divided dose t.i.d. or as single dose h.s.
Children: 3 to 6 mg/kg P.O. daily, usually divided q 12 hours. It can be administered once daily, usually h.s.
Status epilepticus—
Adults: 200 to 600 mg I.V.
Children: 100 to 400 mg I.V. Do not exceed 50 mg/minute.
Sedation—
Adults: 30 to 120 mg P.O. daily in two or three divided doses.
Children: 3 to 5 mg/kg P.O. daily in divided doses t.i.d.
Insomnia—
Adults: 100 to 200 mg P.O. or I.M. h.s.
Preoperative sedation—
Adults: 100 to 200 mg I.M. 60 to 90 minutes before surgery.
Children: 16 to 100 mg I.M. or 1 to 3 mg/kg I.V., I.M., or P.O. 60 to 90 minutes before surgery.

ADVERSE REACTIONS
CNS: *drowsiness, lethargy, hangover,* paradoxical excitement in elderly patients, somnolence.
CV: bradycardia, hypotension.
GI: nausea, vomiting.
Hematologic: exacerbation of porphyria.

Respiratory: *respiratory depression,* apnea.
Skin: rash, *erythema multiforme, Stevens-Johnson syndrome,* urticaria; pain, swelling, thrombophlebitis, necrosis, nerve injury at injection site.
Other: *angioedema,* physical and psychological dependence.

INTERACTIONS
Chloramphenicol, MAO inhibitors, valproic acid: potentiated barbiturate effect. Monitor patient for increased CNS and respiratory depression.
Corticosteroids, digitoxin, doxycycline, estrogens and oral contraceptives, oral anticoagulants, tricyclic antidepressants: phenobarbital may enhance the metabolism of these drugs. Monitor for decreased effect.
Diazepam: increased effects of both drugs. Use together cautiously.
Ethanol or other CNS depressants, including narcotic analgesics: excessive CNS depression. Alcohol should not be consumed while taking phenobarbital.
Griseofulvin: decreased absorption of griseofulvin. Monitor effectiveness of griseofulvin.
Mephobarbital, primidone: excessive phenobarbital blood levels; monitor closely.
Rifampin: may decrease barbiturate levels. Monitor for decreased effect.
Valproic acid: increased phenobarbital levels. Monitor for toxicity.

EFFECTS ON DIAGNOSTIC TESTS
Phenobarbital may cause a false-positive phentolamine test. The physiologic effects of the drug may impair the absorption of cyanocobalamin ^{57}Co. It may decrease serum bilirubin concentrations in neonates, epileptics, and in patients with congenital nonhemolytic unconjugated hyperbilirubinemia. Barbiturates may increase sulfobromophthalein retention. EEG patterns show a change in low-voltage, fast activity. Changes persist for a time after discontinuation of therapy.

---

*Liquid contains alcohol.   **May contain tartrazine.   †Canada only.   ‡Australia only.   ◊OTC.

CONTRAINDICATIONS
Contraindicated in patients with barbiturate hypersensitivity, history of manifest or latent porphyria, hepatic dysfunction, respiratory disease with dyspnea or obstruction, and nephritis.

NURSING CONSIDERATIONS
● Use cautiously in patients with acute or chronic pain, depression, suicidal tendencies, history of drug abuse, blood pressure alterations, cardiovascular disease, shock, uremia, and in elderly or debilitated patients.
● **I.V. use:** Know that I.V. injection is reserved for emergency treatment. Give slowly under close supervision. Monitor respirations closely. When administering, do not give more than 60 mg/minute. Have resuscitation equipment available.
● Do not mix parenteral form with acidic solutions; precipitation may result.
● Do not use injectable solution if it contains a precipitate.
● Give I.M. injection deeply. Superficial injection may cause pain, sterile abscess, and tissue sloughing.
● Know that elderly patients are more sensitive to the drug's effects.
Alert: Watch for signs of barbiturate toxicity: coma, asthmatic breathing, cyanosis, clammy skin, and hypotension. Overdose can be fatal.
● Therapeutic blood levels are 15 to 40 mcg/ml.
● Don't stop drug abruptly because seizures may worsen. Call the doctor immediately if adverse reactions develop.

☑ **PATIENT TEACHING**
● Make sure that patient is aware that phenobarbital is available in different milligram strengths and sizes. Advise him to check prescription and refills closely.
● Inform patient that full therapeutic effects are not seen for 2 to 3 weeks, except when loading dose is used.

● Advise patient to avoid driving and other potentially hazardous activities that require mental alertness until drug's CNS effects are known.
● Warn patient and parents not to discontinue drug abruptly.
● Tell patient who uses oral contraceptives that she should consider another birth-control method because drug may enhance contraceptive hormone metabolism and decrease its effect.

---

phensuximide
Milontin

Pregnancy Risk Category: NR

HOW SUPPLIED
Capsules: 500 mg

ACTION
Unknown. A succinimide that probably increases seizure threshold. Reduces the paroxysmal spike-and-wave pattern of absence seizures by depressing nerve transmission in the motor cortex. A succinimide derivative.

ONSET, PEAK, DURATION
Onset and duration unknown. Serum levels peak in 1 to 4 hours.

INDICATIONS & DOSAGE
Absence seizures—
Adults and children: 500 mg to 1 g P.O. b.i.d. or t.i.d.

ADVERSE REACTIONS
CNS: muscular weakness, *drowsiness,* dizziness, ataxia, headache, lethargy.
GI: *nausea, vomiting,* anorexia.
GU: urinary frequency, renal damage, hematuria.
Hematologic: transient leukopenia, *pancytopenia, fatal blood dyscrasias.*
Skin: pruritus, eruptions, erythema, Stevens-Johnson syndrome, alopecia.
Other: lupuslike syndrome.

Reactions may be *common,* uncommon, *life-threatening,* or COMMON AND LIFE-THREATENING.

INTERACTIONS
May interact with other antiepileptic drugs. Monitor serum levels.

EFFECTS ON DIAGNOSTIC TESTS
None reported.

CONTRAINDICATIONS
Contraindicated in patients with hypersensitivity to succinimide derivatives.

NURSING CONSIDERATIONS
● Use with extreme caution in patients with hepatic or renal disease.
● Monitor blood levels, as ordered. Therapeutic blood level is 40 to 80 mcg/ml.
● Check CBC every 3 to 4 months; urinalysis and liver function tests every 6 months, as ordered.
● Never withdraw drug suddenly. Abrupt withdrawal may precipitate absence seizures. Call the doctor immediately if adverse reactions develop.

☑ PATIENT TEACHING
● Advise patient to avoid driving and other potentially hazardous activities that require mental alertness until drug's CNS effects are known.
● Warn patient and parents not to stop drug therapy suddenly.
● Tell patient to report lupuslike symptoms immediately.
● Caution patient that this drug may color urine pink, red, or reddish brown.

---

phenytoin (diphenylhydantoin)
Dilantin, Dilantin-30 Pediatric, Dilantin-125, Dilantin Infatabs,

phenytoin sodium
Dilantin, Phenytex

phenytoin sodium (extended)
Dilantin Kapseals

Pregnancy Risk Category: NR

HOW SUPPLIED
phenytoin
Tablets (chewable): 50 mg
Oral suspension: 30 mg/5 ml, 125 mg/5 ml
phenytoin sodium
Capsules: 30 mg (27.6-mg base), 100 mg (92-mg base)
Injection: 50 mg/ml (46-mg base)
phenytoin sodium (extended)
Capsules: 30 mg (27.6-mg base), 100 mg (92-mg base)

ACTION
Unknown. A hydantoin derivative that probably stabilizes neuronal membranes and limits seizure activity by either increasing efflux or decreasing influx of sodium ions across cell membranes in the motor cortex during generation of nerve impulses.

ONSET, PEAK, DURATION
Onset immediate with I.V. administration, unknown for other routes. Peak levels occur 1 to 2 hours after I.V. injection, 1½ to 3 hours after tablets or oral solution, 4 to 12 hours after extended-release capsules. Duration unknown.

INDICATIONS & DOSAGE
Control of tonic-clonic (grand mal) and complex partial (temporal lobe) seizures—
Adults: highly individualized. Initially, 100 mg P.O. t.i.d., increased in increments of 100 mg P.O. every 2 to 4 weeks until desired response is obtained. Usual range is 300 to 600 mg daily. If patient stabilized with extended-release capsules, once-daily dosing with 300 mg extended-release capsules possible as an alternative.
Children: 5 mg/kg or 250 mg/m² P.O. divided b.i.d. or t.i.d. Maximum daily dosage is 300 mg.
For patient requiring a loading dose—
Adults: initially, 1 g P.O. daily divided into 3 doses and administered at 2-hour intervals. Alternatively, 10 to 15 mg/kg I.V. at a rate not exceeding 50

---

*Liquid contains alcohol. **May contain tartrazine. †Canada only. ‡Australia only. ◇OTC.

mg/minute. Normal maintenance dosage instituted 24 hours later.

Children: 5 mg/kg/day P.O. in 2 or 3 equally divided doses with subsequent dosage individualized to a maximum of 300 mg daily.

Prevention and treatment of seizures occurring during neurosurgery—

Adults: 100 to 200 mg I.M. q 4 hours during surgery and continued during the postoperative period.

Status epilepticus—

Adults: loading dose of 10 to 15 mg/kg I.V. (1 to 1.5 g may be needed) at a rate not exceeding 50 mg/minute, followed by maintenance doses of 100 mg P.O. or I.V. q 6 to 8 hours.

Children: loading dose of 15 to 20 mg/kg I.V., at a rate not exceeding 1 to 3 mg/kg/minute, followed by highly individualized maintenance dosages.

ADVERSE REACTIONS

CNS: *ataxia, slurred speech,* dizziness, insomnia, nervousness, twitching, headache, *mental confusion, decreased coordination.*

CV: periarteritis nodosa.

EENT: *nystagmus, diplopia,* blurred vision, *gingival hyperplasia* (especially in children).

GI: *nausea, vomiting,* constipation.

Hematologic: ***thrombocytopenia, leukopenia, agranulocytosis, pancytopenia,*** macrocythemia, megaloblastic anemia.

Hepatic: ***toxic hepatitis.***

Skin: scarlatiniform or morbilliform rash; bullous, ***exfoliative,*** or purpuric dermatitis; ***Stevens-Johnson syndrome;*** lupus erythematosus; *hirsutism;* ***toxic epidermal necrolysis;*** photosensitivity; pain, necrosis, and inflammation at injection site; discoloration of skin ("purple-glove syndrome") if given by I.V. push in back of hand.

Other: lymphadenopathy, hyperglycemia, osteomalacia, hypertrichosis.

INTERACTIONS

Amiodarone, antihistamines, chloramphenicol, cimetidine, cycloserine, diazepam, disulfiram, influenza vaccine, isoniazid, phenylbutazone, salicylates, sulfamethizole, valproate: may increase phenytoin activity and toxicity.

Barbiturates, carbamazepine, dexamethasone, diazoxide, ethanol (with chronic use), folic acid, rifampin: decreased phenytoin activity. Inform patient that heavy alcohol use may diminish drug's benefits.

Carbamazepine, digitalis glycosides, oral contraceptives, quinidine, theophylline, valproic acid: effects may be decreased by phenytoin.

Oral tube feedings with Osmolite or Isocal: may interfere with absorption of oral phenytoin.

EFFECTS ON DIAGNOSTIC TESTS

Phenytoin may raise blood glucose levels by inhibiting pancreatic insulin release; it may decrease serum levels of protein-bound iodine and may interfere with the 1-mg dexamethasone suppression test.

CONTRAINDICATIONS

Contraindicated in patients with hydantoin hypersensitivity, sinus bradycardia, SA block, second- or third-degree AV block, or Adams-Stokes syndrome.

NURSING CONSIDERATIONS

● Use cautiously in patients with hepatic dysfunction, hypotension, myocardial insufficiency, diabetes, and respiratory depression; in elderly or debilitated patients; and in patients receiving other hydantoin derivatives.

● Be aware that elderly patients tend to metabolize phenytoin slowly and may require lower dosages.

● Know that phenytoin requirements usually increase during pregnancy.

● Suspension available as 30 mg/5 ml or 125 mg/5 ml. Read label carefully. Shake suspension well before each dose.

● Use only clear solution for injection. A slight yellow color is acceptable.

Don't refrigerate.

● **I.V. use:** Administer slowly (50 mg/minute) as I.V. bolus. If giving as an infusion, don't mix drug with D_5W because it will precipitate. Clear I.V. tubing first with 0.9% sodium chloride solution. Never use cloudy solution. May mix with 0.9% sodium chloride solution if necessary and give as an infusion over $\frac{1}{2}$ to 1 hour, when possible. Infusion must begin within 1 hour after preparation and should run through an in-line filter. Discard 4 hours after preparation. *Alert:* Check patency of I.V. catheter before administering. Extravasation has caused severe local tissue damage.

● Avoid administering phenytoin by I.V. push into veins on the back of the hand to avoid discoloration known as purple-glove syndrome. Inject into larger veins or central venous catheter if available.

● Check vital signs, blood pressure, and ECG during I.V. administration.

● Do not give I.M. unless dosage adjustments are made. Drug may precipitate at injection site, cause pain, and be absorbed erratically.

● Divided doses given with or after meals may decrease adverse GI reactions.

● Be aware that drug should be discontinued if rash appears. If rash is scarlatiniform or morbilliform, drug may be resumed after rash clears. If rash reappears, therapy should be discontinued. If rash is exfoliative, purpuric, or bullous, drug will not be resumed.

● Don't withdraw drug suddenly because seizures may worsen. Call the doctor at once if adverse reactions develop.

● Monitor blood levels as ordered. Therapeutic phenytoin blood level is 10 to 20 mcg/ml.

● Monitor CBC and serum calcium level every 6 months, and periodically monitor hepatic function as ordered. If megaloblastic anemia is evident, the doctor may order folic acid and vitamin B_{12}.

● If using to treat seizures, take appropriate safety precautions.

● Mononucleosis may decrease phenytoin levels. Monitor for increased seizure activity.

● Know that therapy with phenytoin may cause altered laboratory test results, including reduced serum protein-bound iodine and free thyroxine levels without clinical signs of hypothyroidism; a slight decrease in urinary 17-hydroxysteroid and 17-ketosteroid levels; increased urine 6-β hydroxycortisol excretion and serum levels of alkaline phosphatase or gamma-glutamyltransferase; and decreased values for dexamethasone suppression or metyrapone tests.

☑ **PATIENT TEACHING**
● Advise patient to avoid driving and other potentially hazardous activities that require mental alertness until drug's CNS effects are known.

● Advise patient not to change brands or dosage forms once he's stabilized on therapy.

● Dilantin capsules are the only oral form that can be given once daily. Toxic levels may result if any other brand or form is given once daily. Dilantin brand tablets and oral suspension should never be taken once daily.

● Warn patient and parents not to stop drug abruptly.

● Stress importance of good oral hygiene and regular dental examinations. Gingivectomy may be necessary periodically if dental hygiene is poor.

● Caution patient that this drug may color urine pink, red, or reddish brown.

---

primidone
Apo-Primidone†, Mysoline, PMS Primidone†, Sertan†

Pregnancy Risk Category: NR

HOW SUPPLIED
Tablets: 50 mg, 250 mg
Oral suspension: 250 mg/5 ml

ACTION
Unknown, but some activity may be caused by phenylethylmalonamide and phenobarbital, which are active metabolites.

ONSET, PEAK, DURATION
Onset and duration unknown. Serum levels peak in 3 to 4 hours.

INDICATIONS & DOSAGE
Tonic-clonic, complex partial, and simple partial seizures—
Adults and children 8 years and over: initially, 100 to 125 mg P.O. h.s. on days 1 to 3; then 100 to 125 mg P.O. b.i.d. on days 4 to 6; then 100 to 125 mg P.O. t.i.d. on days 7 to 9; followed by maintenance dosage of 250 mg P.O. t.i.d. Maintenance dosage increased to 250 mg q.i.d., if needed. Dosage may be increased to a maximum of 2 g daily in divided doses.
Children under 8 years: initially, 50 mg P.O. h.s. for 3 days, then 50 mg P.O. b.i.d. for days 4 to 6, then 100 mg P.O. b.i.d. for days 7 to 9, followed by maintenance dosage of 125 to 250 mg P.O. t.i.d.

ADVERSE REACTIONS
CNS: *drowsiness, ataxia,* emotional disturbances, vertigo, hyperirritability, fatigue, paranoia.
EENT: *diplopia,* nystagmus.
GI: anorexia, *nausea, vomiting.*
GU: impotence, polyuria.
Hematologic: megaloblastic anemia, ***thrombocytopenia.***
Skin: morbilliform rash.

INTERACTIONS
Acetazolamide, succinimide: may decrease primidone concentrations.
Carbamazepine: increased carbamazepine levels and decreased primidone and phenobarbital levels. Observe for toxicity.
Isoniazid: increased primidone concentration.
Phenytoin: stimulated conversion of primidone to phenobarbital. Observe for increased phenobarbital effect.

EFFECTS ON DIAGNOSTIC TESTS
Primidone may cause abnormalities in liver function test results.

CONTRAINDICATIONS
Contraindicated in patients with phenobarbital hypersensitivity or porphyria.

NURSING CONSIDERATIONS
● Shake liquid suspension well.
● Don't withdraw drug suddenly because seizures may worsen. Call the doctor immediately if adverse reactions develop.
● Therapeutic blood level of primidone is 5 to 12 mcg/ml. Therapeutic blood level of phenobarbital is 15 to 40 mcg/ml.
● Monitor CBC and routine blood chemistry every 6 months.

☑ PATIENT TEACHING
● Advise patient to avoid driving and other potentially hazardous activities that require mental alertness until drug's CNS effects are known.
● Warn patient and parents not to stop drug therapy suddenly.
● Tell patient that full therapeutic response may take 2 weeks or more.

---

valproate sodium
Depakene Syrup, Epilim‡, Myproic Acid Syrup

valproic acid
Depakene, Myproic Acid

divalproex sodium
Depakote, Depakote Sprinkle, Epival†, Valcote‡

Pregnancy Risk Category: D

HOW SUPPLIED
valproate sodium
Syrup: 250 mg/ml

---

valproic acid
Tablets (enteric-coated): 200 mg‡, 500 mg‡
Crushable tablets: 100 mg‡
Capsules: 250 mg
Syrup: 200 mg/5 ml‡
divalproex sodium
Capsules (delayed-release): 125 mg
Tablets (enteric-coated): 125 mg, 250 mg, 500 mg

ACTION
Unknown. Probably increases brain levels of gamma-aminobutyric acid, which transmits inhibitory nerve impulses in the CNS.

ONSET, PEAK, DURATION
Onset and duration unknown. Serum levels peak within 1 to 4 hours after capsules or syrup; 3 to 4 hours after tablets and delayed-release capsules.

INDICATIONS & DOSAGE
Simple and complex absence seizures, mixed seizure types (including absence seizures)—
Adults and children: initially, 15 mg/kg P.O. daily; then increased by 5 to 10 mg/kg daily at weekly intervals up to maximum of 60 mg/kg daily.
Mania (delayed-release capsules)—
Adults and children: initially, 750 mg daily in divided doses. Adjust dosage according to patient's response; maximum dosage is 60 mg/kg/day.
Migraine—
✳*New indication: Prophylaxis for migraine headache (Depakote only)—*
Adults: initially, 250 mg P.O. b.i.d. Some patients may require up to 1,000 mg/day.

ADVERSE REACTIONS
Because drug usually is used in combination with other anticonvulsants, adverse reactions reported may not be caused by valproic acid alone.
CNS: *sedation,* emotional upset, depression, psychosis, aggressiveness, hyperactivity, behavioral deterioration, muscle weakness, tremor, ataxia, headache, dizziness, incoordination.
EENT: nystagmus, diplopia.
GI: *nausea, vomiting, indigestion,* diarrhea, abdominal cramps, constipation, increased appetite and weight gain, anorexia, *pancreatitis.* (*Note:* lower incidence of GI effects occur with divalproex sodium.)
Hematologic: *thrombocytopenia,* increased bleeding time, petechiae, bruising, eosinophilia, hemorrhage, leukopenia, bone marrow suppression.
Hepatic: *elevated liver enzymes, toxic hepatitis.*
Skin: rash, alopecia, pruritus, photosensitivity, erythema multiforme.

INTERACTIONS
Aspirin, chlorpromazine, cimetidine, felbamate: May cause valproic acid toxicity. Use together cautiously and monitor blood levels. Monitor patient closely.
Ethanol: excessive CNS depression. Avoid concomitant use.
Lamotrogine: increased lamotrogine levels.
Phenobarbital: increased phenobarbital levels. Monitor patient closely.
Phenytoin: increased or decreased phenytoin levels. Monitor patient closely.
Rifampin: may decrease valproate levels.
Warfarin: valproic acid may displace warfarin from binding sites.

EFFECTS ON DIAGNOSTIC TESTS
Drug may produce false-positive results for urine ketones; it may also cause abnormalities in liver function test results. Valproic acid reportedly alters thyroid function tests but clinical importance of this is not known.

CONTRAINDICATIONS
Should not be administered to patients with hepatic disease or significant hepatic dysfunction. Contraindicated in patients with hypersensitivity.

NURSING CONSIDERATIONS

● Monitor liver function studies, platelet counts, and PT before starting drug and periodically thereafter as ordered.

● Don't administer syrup to patients who need sodium restriction. Check with the doctor.

● Never withdraw the drug suddenly because sudden withdrawal may worsen seizures. Call the doctor at once if adverse reactions develop.

Alert: Be aware serious or fatal hepatotoxicity may follow nonspecific symptoms, such as malaise, fever, and lethargy. Notify doctor at once as drug will need to be discontinued in the presence of suspected or apparent substantial hepatic dysfunction.

● Know that patients at high risk for hepatotoxicity include those with congenital metabolic disorders, mental retardation or presence of organic brain disease; those taking multiple anticonvulsants; and children under age 2.

● Notify doctor if tremors occur (a dosage reduction may be necessary).

● Monitor blood levels, as ordered. Therapeutic blood level is 50 to 100 mcg/ml.

● Know that drug may produce false-positive test results for ketones in urine.

☑ PATIENT TEACHING

● To reduce adverse GI effects, tell patient this drug may be taken with food or milk.

● Advise patient not to chew capsules; irritation of mouth and throat may result.

● Tell patient and parents that syrup shouldn't be mixed with carbonated beverages; may be irritating to mouth and throat.

● Tell patient and parents to keep drug out of children's reach.

● Warn patient and parents not to stop drug therapy abruptly.

● Advise patient to avoid driving and other potentially hazardous activities that require mental alertness until drug's CNS effects are known.

Reactions may be *common*, uncommon, *life-threatening*, or COMMON AND LIFE-THREATENING.

amitriptyline hydrochloride
amitriptyline pamoate
amoxapine
bupropion hydrochloride
clomipramine hydrochloride
desipramine hydrochloride
doxepin hydrochloride
fluoxetine hydrochloride
imipramine hydrochloride
imipramine pamoate
maprotiline hydrochloride
mirtazapine
nefazodone hydrochloride
nortriptyline hydrochloride
paroxetine hydrochloride
phenelzine sulfate
protriptyline hydrochloride
sertraline hydrochloride
tranylcypromine sulfate
trazodone hydrochloride
trimipramine maleate
venlafaxine hydrochloride

COMBINATION PRODUCTS
ETRAFON: perphenazine 2 mg and
amitriptyline hydrochloride 25 mg.
ETRAFON 2-10: perphenazine 2 mg and
amitriptyline hydrochloride 10 mg.
ETRAFON-A: perphenazine 4 mg and
amitriptyline hydrochloride 10 mg.
ETRAFON-FORTE: perphenazine 4 mg
and amitriptyline hydrochloride 25 mg.
LIMBITROL DS: chlordiazepoxide 10 mg
and amitriptyline hydrochloride 25 mg.
TRIAVIL 2-10, TRIAVIL 4-10, TRIAVIL 2-
25, TRIAVIL 4-25 are products identical
to the Etrafon products listed above. Triavil is also available as TRIAVIL 4-50
(perphenazine 4 mg and amitriptyline
hydrochloride 50 mg).

---

amitriptyline hydrochloride
Apo-Amitriptyline†, Elavil, Emitrip,
Endep, Enovil, Levate†, Novotriptyn†,
PMS-Amitriptyline, Tryptanol‡

amitriptyline pamoate
Elavil†

Pregnancy Risk Category: NR

HOW SUPPLIED
amitriptyline hydrochloride
Tablets: 10 mg, 25 mg, 50 mg, 75 mg,
100 mg, 150 mg
Injection: 10 mg/ml
amitriptyline pamoate
Syrup: 10 mg/5 ml

ACTION
Unknown, but a tricyclic antidepressant
(TCA) that increases the amount of nor-
epinephrine, serotonin, or both in the
CNS by blocking their reuptake by the
presynaptic neurons.

ONSET, PEAK, DURATION
Onset unknown although thought to
take several weeks. Serum levels peak
in 2 to 12 hours. Duration unknown.

INDICATIONS & DOSAGE
Depression—
Adults: initially, 50 to 100 mg P.O. h.s.,
increasing to 150 mg daily; maximum
dosage is 300 mg daily, if needed.
Maintenance dose: 50 to 100 mg/day.
Or 20 to 30 mg I.M. q.i.d.
Elderly patients and adolescents: 10
mg P.O. t.i.d. and 20 mg h.s. daily.

ADVERSE REACTIONS
CNS: *coma, seizures,* hallucinations,
delusions, disorientation, ataxia, tremor,
peripheral neuropathy, anxiety, insomnia, restlessness, drowsiness, dizziness,
weakness, fatigue, headache, extrapyramidal reactions.
CV: *MI, stroke, arrhythmias,* heart
block, *orthostatic hypotension, tachycardia, ECG changes,* hypertension.
EENT: *blurred vision,* tinnitus, mydria-

---

sis, increased intraocular pressure.
GI: *dry mouth,* nausea, vomiting, anorexia, epigastric distress, diarrhea, constipation, paralytic ileus.
GU: urine retention.
Hematologic: *agranulocytosis, thrombocytopenia,* leukopenia, eosinophilia.
Skin: rash, urticaria, photosensitivity.
Other: *diaphoresis,* hypersensitivity reaction, edema.
After abrupt withdrawal of long-term therapy: nausea, headache, malaise (does not indicate addiction).

INTERACTIONS
Barbiturates, CNS depressants, ethanol: enhanced CNS depression. Avoid concomitant use.
Cimetidine, methylphenidate, oral contraceptives: increased TCA blood levels. Monitor for enhanced antidepressant effect.
Clonidine: may cause hypertensive crisis. Avoid coadministration.
Epinephrine, norepinephrine: increased hypertensive effect. Use with caution.
MAO inhibitors: may cause severe excitation, hyperpyrexia, or seizures, usually with high dosage. Use with caution.

EFFECTS ON DIAGNOSTIC TESTS
Drug may prolong conduction time (elongation of QT and PR intervals, flattened T waves on ECG); it also may elevate liver function test results, decrease WBC counts, and decrease or increase serum glucose levels.

CONTRAINDICATIONS
Contraindicated during acute recovery phase of MI, in patients with hypersensitivity, and in patients who have received an MAO inhibitor within the past 14 days.

NURSING CONSIDERATIONS
● Use cautiously in patients with history of seizures, urine retention, angle-closure glaucoma, or increased intraocular pressure; in those with hyperthyroidism, CV disease, diabetes, or impaired liver function; and in those receiving thyroid medications.
Alert: Know that parenteral form of drug is for I.M. administration only. Drug should not be given I.V.
● Amitriptyline has strong anticholinergic effects and is one of the most sedating TCAs. Be aware that anticholinergic effects have a rapid onset even though therapeutic effect is delayed for weeks.
● If signs of psychosis occur or increase, expect doctor to reduce dosage. Record mood changes. Monitor patients for suicidal tendencies, and allow them only a minimum supply of the drug.
● Because hypertensive episodes have occurred during surgery in patients receiving TCAs, be aware drug should be gradually discontinued several days before surgery.
● Do not withdraw drug abruptly.

☑ **PATIENT TEACHING**
● Advise patient to take full dose at bedtime, but warn him of possible morning orthostatic hypotension.
● Tell patient to avoid alcohol while taking this drug.
● Tell patient to consult his doctor before taking other medications.
● Warn patient to avoid activities that require alertness and good psychomotor coordination until CNS effects of drug are known. Drowsiness and dizziness usually subside after a few weeks.
● Tell patient that dry mouth may be relieved with sugarless hard candy or gum. Saliva substitutes may be needed.
● To prevent photosensitivity reactions, advise patient to use a sunblock, wear protective clothing, and avoid prolonged exposure to strong sunlight.
● Warn patient not to stop drug therapy abruptly.

amoxapine
Asendin

Pregnancy Risk Category: C

HOW SUPPLIED
Tablets: 25 mg, 50 mg, 100 mg, 150 mg

ACTION
Unknown, but a tricyclic antidepressant (TCA) that increases the amount of norepinephrine, serotonin, or both in the CNS by blocking their reuptake by the presynaptic neurons.

ONSET, PEAK, DURATION
Onset thought to occur in 2 to 4 weeks. Serum levels peak in about 90 minutes. Duration unknown.

INDICATIONS & DOSAGE
Depression—
Adults: initially, 50 mg P.O. b.i.d. or t.i.d. Increased to 100 mg b.i.d. or t.i.d. by the end of the first week of therapy if tolerated. Increases above 300 mg daily are made only if 300 mg daily has been ineffective during a trial period of at least 2 weeks. Maximum recommended dosage for outpatients is 400 mg daily. When effective dosage is established, entire dosage (not to exceed 300 mg) may be given h.s.
Elderly patients: initially, 25 mg b.i.d. or t.i.d. If tolerated by end of first week, increase to 50 mg b.i.d. or t.i.d. Carefully increase up to 300 mg daily.

ADVERSE REACTIONS
CNS: *drowsiness, dizziness,* excitation, tremor, weakness, confusion, anxiety, insomnia, restlessness, nightmares, ataxia, fatigue, headache, nervousness, *tardive dyskinesia, EEG changes, seizures,* extrapyramidal reactions (rare), **neuroleptic malignant syndrome** (high fever, tachycardia, tachypnea, profuse diaphoresis).
CV: *orthostatic hypotension, tachycardia,* hypertension, palpitations.
EENT: *blurred vision.*
GI: *dry mouth, constipation,* nausea, excessive appetite.
GU: *urine retention, acute renal failure* (with overdose).
Skin: rash, edema, *diaphoresis.*

After abrupt withdrawal of long-term therapy: nausea, headache, malaise (does not indicate addiction).

INTERACTIONS
Barbiturates: decreased TCA blood levels. Monitor for decreased antidepressant effect.
Cimetidine, methylphenidate, oral contraceptives: may increase amoxapine serum levels. Monitor for increased adverse effects.
Clonidine, epinephrine, norepinephrine: increased hypertensive effect. Use with caution.
CNS depressants, ethanol: enhanced CNS depression. Avoid concomitant use.
MAO inhibitors: may cause severe excitation, hyperpyrexia, or seizures, usually with high dosage.

EFFECTS ON DIAGNOSTIC TESTS
Drug may prolong conduction time (elongation of QT and PR intervals, flattened T waves on ECG); it also may elevate liver function tests, decrease WBC counts, and decrease or increase serum glucose levels.

CONTRAINDICATIONS
Contraindicated in patients with hypersensitivity, during acute recovery phase of MI, and in patients who have received an MAO inhibitor within the past 14 days.

NURSING CONSIDERATIONS
• Use cautiously in patients with history of urine retention, angle-closure glaucoma, or increased intraocular pressure, as well as patients with CV disease. Use with extreme caution in patients with history of seizure disorders.
• Be aware that dosage should be reduced in elderly or debilitated persons and adolescents.
• Know that safe use of drug in children under 16 years has not been determined.
• Do not withdraw drug abruptly.
• Because hypertensive episodes have

---

*Liquid contains alcohol.   **May contain tartrazine.   †Canada only.   ‡Australia only.   ◊ OTC.

occurred during surgery in patients receiving TCAs, be aware that drug should be gradually discontinued several days before surgery.
• Expect delay of 2 weeks or more before noticeable effect. Full effect may take 4 weeks or more. However, know that adverse anticholinergic effects can occur rapidly.
• If signs of psychosis occur or increase, expect doctor to reduce dosage. Record mood changes. Monitor patients for suicidal tendencies, and allow them only a minimum supply of the drug.
• Monitor for signs and symptoms of tardive dyskinesia, especially in elderly women.
• Amoxapine therapy has been associated with neuroleptic malignant syndrome, a rare but life-threatening syndrome usually seen with phenothiazines. Discontinue drug immediately and institute appropriate therapy if symptoms occur.
• Relieve dry mouth with sugarless hard candy or gum. Saliva substitutes may be necessary.

☑ **PATIENT TEACHING**
• Whenever possible, tell patient to take full dose at bedtime.
• Warn patient not to stop drug therapy abruptly.
• Warn patient to avoid activities that require alertness and good psychomotor coordination until CNS effects of the drug are known. Drowsiness and dizziness usually subside after first few weeks.
• Some patients may experience photosensitivity reactions. Advise patient to use a sunblock, wear protective clothing, and avoid prolonged exposure to strong sunlight.

---

bupropion hydrochloride
Wellbutrin

Pregnancy Risk Category: B

HOW SUPPLIED
Tablets: 75 mg, 100 mg

ACTION
Unknown. Bupropion is not a tricyclic antidepressant (TCA), does not inhibit MAO, and is a weak inhibitor of norepinephrine, dopamine, and serotonin reuptake.

ONSET, PEAK, DURATION
Onset occurs in 1 to 3 weeks. Serum levels peak within 2 hours. Duration unknown.

INDICATIONS & DOSAGE
Depression—
Adults: initially, 100 mg P.O. b.i.d., increased after 3 days to 100 mg P.O. t.i.d. if needed. If no response occurs after several weeks of therapy, dosage increased to 150 mg t.i.d. No single dose should exceed 150 mg.

ADVERSE REACTIONS
CNS: *headache,* **seizures,** anxiety, *confusion,* delusions, euphoria, hostility, impaired sleep quality, *insomnia, sedation, tremor,* akinesia, akathisia, *agitation, dizziness,* fatigue.
CV: *arrhythmias,* hypertension, hypotension, palpitations, syncope, *tachycardia.*
EENT: *auditory disturbances,* blurred vision.
GI: *dry mouth,* taste disturbance, increased appetite, *constipation,* dyspepsia, *nausea, vomiting, weight loss, anorexia, weight gain,* diarrhea.
GU: impotence, menstrual complaints, urinary frequency, decreased libido, urine retention.
Skin: pruritus, rash, cutaneous temperature disturbance, *excessive diaphoresis.*
Other: arthritis, fever and chills.

INTERACTIONS
Ethanol, levodopa, phenothiazines, MAO inhibitors, or TCAs; recent and rapid withdrawal of benzodiazepines: increased risk of adverse reactions, in-

---

Reactions may be *common,* uncommon, *life-threatening,* or COMMON AND LIFE-THREATENING.

cluding seizures. Monitor patient closely.

EFFECTS ON DIAGNOSTIC TESTS
None reported.

CONTRAINDICATIONS
Contraindicated in patients who are hypersensitive to the drug, who have taken MAO inhibitors within the previous 14 days, and in patients with seizure disorders. Also contraindicated in patients with a history of bulimia or anorexia nervosa because of a higher incidence of seizures.

NURSING CONSIDERATIONS
● Use cautiously in patients with recent history of MI or unstable heart disease, as well as impaired renal or hepatic impairment.
● Know that many patients experience a period of increased restlessness, especially at initiation of therapy. This may include agitation, insomnia, and anxiety.
Alert: Risk of seizure may be minimized by not exceeding 450 mg/day and by administering daily dosage in three to four equally divided doses. Be aware that patients who experience seizures often have predisposing factors, including history of head trauma, prior seizures, or CNS tumors, or they may be taking a drug that lowers the seizure threshold.
● Monitor patients with history of bipolar disorders closely. Antidepressants can cause manic episodes during the depressed phase of bipolar disorder.
● From 28% to 30% of patients taking this drug may experience a weight loss of 5 lb (2.3 kg) or more. Consider this if weight loss is a major factor in the patient's depressive illness.

☑ **PATIENT TEACHING**
● Advise patient to take the drug as scheduled and to take each day's dosage in three divided doses to minimize the risk of seizures.
● Advise patient to consult his doctor before taking other prescription or OTC medications.
● Tell patient to avoid alcohol while taking this drug because it may contribute to the development of seizures.
● Advise patient to avoid hazardous activities that require alertness and good psychomotor coordination until CNS effects of the drug are known.

---

clomipramine hydrochloride
Anafranil

Pregnancy Risk Category: C

HOW SUPPLIED
Capsules: 25 mg, 50 mg, 75 mg

ACTION
Unknown, but a tricyclic antidepressant (TCA) that selectively inhibits reuptake of serotonin.

ONSET, PEAK, DURATION
Unknown, although onset is thought to take 2 weeks or longer.

INDICATIONS & DOSAGE
Obsessive-compulsive disorder—
Adults: initially, 25 mg P.O. daily with meals, gradually increased to 100 mg daily in divided doses during first 2 weeks. Thereafter, increased to maximum dosage of 250 mg daily in divided doses with meals as needed. After titration, total daily dosage may be given h.s.
Children and adolescents: initially, 25 mg P.O. daily with meals, gradually increased over first 2 weeks to daily maximum of 3 mg/kg or 100 mg P.O. in divided doses, whichever is smaller. Maximum daily dosage is 3 mg/kg or 200 mg, whichever is smaller; may be given h.s. after titration. Periodic reassessment and adjustment necessary.

ADVERSE REACTIONS

CNS: *somnolence, tremor, dizziness, headache, insomnia, nervousness, myoclonus, fatigue,* EEG changes, ***seizures.***

CV: *postural hypotension,* palpitations, tachycardia.

EENT: *pharyngitis, rhinitis, visual changes.*

GI: *dry mouth, constipation, nausea, dyspepsia, increased appetite,* diarrhea, anorexia, abdominal pain.

GU: *urinary hesitancy,* urinary tract infection, *dysmenorrhea, ejaculation failure, impotence.*

Hematologic: *purpura.*

Skin: *diaphoresis,* rash, pruritus, dry skin.

Other: *myalgia, weight gain, altered libido.*

INTERACTIONS

Barbiturates: decreased TCA blood levels. Monitor for decreased antidepressant effect.

Cimetidine, methylphenidate, oral contraceptives: increased TCA blood levels. Monitor for enhanced antidepressant effect.

Clonidine, epinephrine, norepinephrine: increased hypertensive effect. Use with caution.

CNS depressants, ethanol: enhanced CNS depression. Avoid concomitant use.

MAO inhibitors: may cause hyperpyretic crisis, seizures, coma, or death. Don't use together.

EFFECTS ON DIAGNOSTIC TESTS
None reported.

CONTRAINDICATIONS
Contraindicated in patients with hypersensitivity to drug or other TCAs, who have taken MAO inhibitors within the previous 14 days, and in patients during acute recovery period after MI.

NURSING CONSIDERATIONS
● Use cautiously in patients with history of seizure disorders or with brain damage of varying etiology; in patients receiving other seizure threshold-lowering drugs; in patients at risk for suicide; in patients with history of urine retention or angle-closure glaucoma, increased intraocular pressure, CV disease, impaired hepatic or renal function, or hyperthyroidism; in patients with tumors of the adrenal medulla; in patients receiving thyroid medication or electroconvulsive therapy; and in those undergoing elective surgery.

● Know that total daily dose may be taken at bedtime after titration. During titration, dosage may be divided.

● Do not withdraw drug abruptly.

● Because hypertensive episodes have occurred during surgery in patients receiving TCAs, know that drug should be gradually discontinued several days before surgery.

● Be aware that adverse anticholinergic effects can occur rapidly.

● Relieve dry mouth with sugarless candy or gum. Saliva substitutes may be necessary.

☑ PATIENT TEACHING
● Warn patient to avoid hazardous activities requiring alertness and good psychomotor coordination, especially during titration. Daytime sedation and dizziness may occur.

● Tell patient to avoid alcohol while taking this drug.

● Warn patient not to withdraw drug suddenly.

● To prevent photosensitivity reactions, advise patient to use sunblock, wear protective clothing, and avoid prolonged exposure to strong sunlight.

---

desipramine hydrochloride
Norpramin**, Pertofran‡, Pertofrane

Pregnancy Risk Category: NR

HOW SUPPLIED
Tablets: 10 mg, 25 mg, 50 mg, 75 mg,

100 mg, 150 mg
Capsules: 25 mg, 50 mg

ACTION
Unknown, but a tricyclic antidepressant (TCA) that increases the amount of norepinephrine, serotonin, or both in the CNS by blocking their reuptake by the presynaptic neurons.

ONSET, PEAK, DURATION
Onset unknown but thought to occur in 2 to 4 weeks or longer. Serum levels peak within 4 to 6 hours. Duration unknown.

INDICATIONS & DOSAGE
Depression—
Adults: 100 to 200 mg P.O. daily in divided doses, increased to maximum of 300 mg daily. Or entire dosage can be given at h.s.
Elderly patients and adolescents: 25 to 100 mg P.O. daily in divided doses, increased gradually to maximum of 150 mg daily if needed.

ADVERSE REACTIONS
CNS: *drowsiness, dizziness,* excitation, tremor, weakness, confusion, anxiety, restlessness, agitation, headache, nervousness, EEG changes, *seizures,* extrapyramidal reactions.
CV: orthostatic hypotension, *tachycardia, ECG changes,* hypertension.
EENT: *blurred vision,* tinnitus, mydriasis.
GI: *dry mouth, constipation,* nausea, vomiting, anorexia, paralytic ileus.
GU: *urine retention.*
Skin: rash, urticaria, photosensitivity.
Other: *diaphoresis,* hypersensitivity reaction, *sudden death* (in children).
After abrupt withdrawal of long-term therapy: nausea, headache, malaise (does not indicate addiction).

INTERACTIONS
Barbiturates, CNS depressants, ethanol: enhanced CNS depression. Avoid concomitant use.

Cimetidine, methylphenidate, oral contraceptives: may increase serum desipramine levels. Monitor for adverse reactions.
Clonidine, epinephrine, norepinephrine: increased hypertensive effect. Use with caution.
MAO inhibitors: may cause severe excitation, hyperpyrexia, or seizures, usually with high dosage. Use with caution.

EFFECTS ON DIAGNOSTIC TESTS
Drug may prolong conduction time (elongation of QT and PR intervals, flattened T waves on ECG); it also may elevate liver function test results, decrease WBC counts, and decrease or increase serum glucose levels.

CONTRAINDICATIONS
Contraindicated in patients with hypersensitivity to drug, who have taken MAO inhibitors within the previous 14 days, and in patients during acute recovery phase of MI.

NURSING CONSIDERATIONS
• Use with extreme caution in patients with CV disease, history of urine retention, or glaucoma, thyroid disease, or those taking thyroid medication, and in patients with history of seizure disorders.
• Do not withdraw drug abruptly.
• Because hypertensive episodes have occurred during surgery in patients receiving TCAs, know that drug should be gradually discontinued several days before surgery.
• If signs of psychosis occur or increase, expect the doctor to reduce dosage. Record mood changes. Monitor patients for suicidal tendencies, and allow them only a minimum supply of the drug.
• Know that because desipramine produces fewer anticholinergic effects than other TCAs, it is often prescribed for cardiac patients.
• Be aware that adverse anticholinergic effects can occur rapidly.

• Relieve dry mouth with sugarless hard candy or gum. Saliva substitutes may be necessary.

☑ **PATIENT TEACHING**
• Advise patient to take full dose at bedtime.
• Warn patient to avoid hazardous activities that require alertness and good psychomotor coordination until CNS effects of the drug are known. Drowsiness and dizziness usually subside after a few weeks.
• Tell patient to avoid alcohol while taking this drug because it may antagonize effects of desipramine.
• Tell patient to consult his doctor before taking other prescription or OTC medications.
• Warn patient not to stop drug therapy suddenly.
• To prevent photosensitivity reactions, advise patient to use sunblock, wear protective clothing, and avoid prolonged exposure to strong sunlight.

---

doxepin hydrochloride
Deptran‡, Novo-Doxepin†, Sinequan, Triadapin†

Pregnancy Risk Category: NR

HOW SUPPLIED
Capsules: 10 mg, 25 mg, 50 mg, 75 mg, 100 mg, 150 mg
Oral concentrate: 10 mg/ml

ACTION
Unknown, but a tricyclic antidepressant (TCA) that increases the amount of norepinephrine, serotonin, or both in the CNS by blocking their reuptake by the presynaptic neurons.

ONSET, PEAK, DURATION
Onset unknown but thought to take 2 to 4 weeks or longer. Serum levels peak within 2 hours. Duration unknown.

INDICATIONS & DOSAGE
Depression or anxiety—
Adults: initially, 25 to 75 mg P.O. daily in divided doses to maximum of 300 mg daily. Alternatively, entire maintenance dosage may be given once daily with a maximum dose of 150 mg P.O.

ADVERSE REACTIONS
CNS: *drowsiness, dizziness,* confusion, numbness, hallucinations, paresthesia, ataxia, weakness, headache, *seizures,* extrapyramidal reactions.
CV: *orthostatic hypotension, tachycardia.*
EENT: *blurred vision,* tinnitus.
GI: *dry mouth, constipation,* nausea, vomiting, anorexia.
GU: urine retention.
Skin: rash, urticaria, photosensitivity, *diaphoresis.*
Other: hypersensitivity reaction.
After abrupt withdrawal of long-term therapy: nausea, headache, malaise (does not indicate addiction).

INTERACTIONS
Barbiturates, CNS depressants, ethanol: enhanced CNS depression. Avoid concomitant use.
Cimetidine, methylphenidate: may increase serum doxepin levels. Monitor for increased adverse reactions.
Clonidine, epinephrine, norepinephrine: increased hypertensive effect.
MAO inhibitors: may cause severe excitation, hyperpyrexia, or seizures, usually with high dosage. Avoid concomitant use.

EFFECTS ON DIAGNOSTIC TESTS
Drug may prolong conduction time (elongation of QT and PR intervals, flattened T waves on ECG); it also may elevate liver function test results, decrease WBC counts, and decrease or increase serum glucose levels.

CONTRAINDICATIONS
Contraindicated in patients with hypersensitivity to drugs, glaucoma, or ten-

dency to urine retention and in those who have received an MAO inhibitor within the past 14 days or during acute recovery phase of an MI.

NURSING CONSIDERATIONS
● Be aware that dosage should be reduced in elderly or debilitated patients, adolescents, and those receiving other medications.
● Drug is not recommended for use in children under 12 years.
● Do not withdraw drug abruptly.
● Because hypertensive episodes have occurred during surgery in patients receiving TCAs, be aware that drug should be gradually discontinued several days before surgery.
● If signs of psychosis occur or increase, expect doctor to reduce dosage. Record mood changes. Monitor patients for suicidal tendencies, and allow them only a minimum supply of the drug.
● Doxepin has strong anticholinergic effects; it is one of the most sedating TCAs. Adverse anticholinergic effects can occur rapidly.
● Relieve dry mouth with sugarless hard candy or gum. Saliva substitutes may be necessary.

☑ PATIENT TEACHING
● Tell patient to dilute oral concentrate with 120 ml (4 oz) of water, milk, or juice (orange, grapefruit, tomato, prune, or pineapple, but not grape juice); preparation is incompatible with carbonated beverages.
● Advise patient to take full dose at bedtime but warn him of possible morning orthostatic hypotension.
● Advise patient to consult his doctor before taking other prescription or OTC medications.
● Warn patient to avoid hazardous activities that require alertness and good psychomotor coordination until CNS effects of the drug are known. Drowsiness and dizziness usually subside after a few weeks.
● Tell patient to avoid alcohol while tak-

ing this drug.
● Warn patient not to stop drug therapy suddenly.
● To prevent photosensitivity reactions, advise patient to use sunblock, wear protective clothing, and avoid prolonged exposure to strong sunlight.

fluoxetine hydrochloride
Prozac, Prozac-20‡

Pregnancy Risk Category: B

HOW SUPPLIED
Pulvules: 10 mg, 20 mg
Oral solution: 20 mg/5 ml

ACTION
Unknown, but presumed to be linked to its inhibition of CNS neuronal uptake of serotonin.

ONSET, PEAK, DURATION
Onset occurs in 1 to 4 weeks. Serum levels peak in 6 to 8 hours. Duration unknown.

INDICATIONS & DOSAGE
Depression, obsessive-compulsive disorder—
Adults: initially, 20 mg P.O. in the morning; dosage increased according to patient response. May be given b.i.d. in the morning and at noon. Maximum dosage is 80 mg/day.
✱*New indication: Treatment of binge-eating and vomiting behavior in patients with moderate to severe bulimia nervosa—*
Adults: 60 mg/day P.O. in the morning.

ADVERSE REACTIONS
CNS: *nervousness, anxiety, insomnia, headache, drowsiness,* fatigue, tremor, dizziness, asthenia.
CV: palpitations, hot flashes.
EENT: nasal congestion, pharyngitis, cough, sinusitis.
GI: *nausea, diarrhea, dry mouth, anorexia,* dyspepsia, constipation, ab-

dominal pain, vomiting, flatulence, increased appetite.
GU: sexual dysfunction.
Respiratory: upper respiratory infection, respiratory distress.
Skin: rash, pruritus, diaphoresis.
Other: flulike syndrome, muscle pain, weight loss, fever.

INTERACTIONS
Flecainide, carbamazepine, vinblastine: increased serum levels of these drugs. Monitor serum levels and the patient for adverse effects.
Insulin, oral antidiabetic agents: altered blood glucose levels and possible altered requirements for antidiabetic medication. Adjust dosage, as ordered.
Lithium, tricyclic antidepressants: risk of increased adverse CNS effects. Avoid concomitant use.
Phenytoin: increased plasma phenytoin levels and risk of toxicity. Monitor serum phenytoin levels and adjust dosage, as ordered.
Tryptophan: increased toxic reaction exhibited by agitation, GI distress, and restlessness. Do not use together.
Warfarin, other highly protein-bound agents: may increase plasma levels of fluoxetine or other highly protein-bound drugs. Monitor patient closely.

EFFECTS ON DIAGNOSTIC TESTS
None reported.

CONTRAINDICATIONS
Contraindicated in patients hypersensitive to the drug and in patients taking MAO inhibitors within 14 days of starting therapy.

NURSING CONSIDERATIONS
● Use cautiously in patients at high risk for suicide and in patients with history of hepatic, renal, or CV disease; diabetes mellitus; or history of seizures.
● Be aware that elderly or debilitated patients and patients with renal or hepatic dysfunction may require lower dosages or less frequent dosing.

● Use antihistamines or topical corticosteroids as ordered to treat rashes or pruritus.

☑ PATIENT TEACHING
● Tell patient to avoid taking drug in the afternoon because fluoxetine commonly causes nervousness and insomnia.
● Drug may cause dizziness or drowsiness in some patients. Warn patient to avoid driving and other hazardous activities that require alertness and good psychomotor coordination until CNS effects of the drug are known.
● Tell patient to consult his doctor before taking other prescription or OTC medications.
● Warn patient to avoid food high in tryptophan, including meats, poultry, fish, liver, kidney, eggs, nuts, peanut butter, broad beans, and wheat germ.

---

imipramine hydrochloride
Apo-Imipramine†, Imiprin‡, Impril†, Janimine**, Melipramine‡, Norfranil, Novopramine†, Tipramine, Tofranil**

imipramine pamoate
Tofranil-PM**

Pregnancy Risk Category: NR

HOW SUPPLIED
imipramine hydrochloride
Tablets: 10 mg, 25 mg, 50 mg
Injection: 12.5 mg/ml
imipramine pamoate
Capsules: 75 mg, 100 mg, 125 mg, 150 mg

ACTION
Unknown, but a tricyclic antidepressant (TCA) that increases the amount of norepinephrine, serotonin, or both in the CNS by blocking their reuptake by the presynaptic neurons.

ONSET, PEAK, DURATION
Onset unknown but thought to take 2 to 4 weeks or longer. Peak plasma concen-

---

trations occur within 1 to 2 hours after oral administration and 30 minutes after I.M. administration. Duration unknown.

INDICATIONS & DOSAGE
Depression—
Adults: 75 to 100 mg P.O. or I.M. daily in divided doses, increased in 25- to 50-mg increments. Maximum dosage for outpatients is 200 mg daily; 300 mg daily may be used for hospitalized patients. Entire dosage may be given h.s.
Elderly and adolescent patients: initially, 30 to 40 mg daily; usually not necessary to exceed 100 mg daily.
Childhood enuresis—
Children 6 years and over:
25 mg P.O. 1 hour before bedtime. If no response within 1 week, increased to 50 mg if child is under 12 years; increased to 75 mg for children 12 years and over. In either case, maximum dosage is 2.5 mg/kg/day.

ADVERSE REACTIONS
CNS: *drowsiness, dizziness,* excitation, tremor, confusion, hallucinations, anxiety, ataxia, paresthesia, nervousness, EEG changes, *seizures,* extrapyramidal reactions.
CV: *orthostatic hypotension, tachycardia, ECG changes,* hypertension, *MI, stroke,* arrhythmias, heart block, precipitation of CHF.
EENT: *blurred vision,* tinnitus, mydriasis.
GI: *dry mouth, constipation,* nausea, vomiting, anorexia, paralytic ileus, abdominal cramps.
GU: *urine retention.*
Skin: rash, urticaria, photosensitivity, pruritus.
Other: *diaphoresis,* hypersensitivity reaction.
After abrupt withdrawal of long-term therapy: nausea, headache, malaise (does not indicate addiction).

INTERACTIONS
Barbiturates, CNS depressants, ethanol: enhanced CNS depression. Avoid con-

comitant use.
Cimetidine, methylphenidate: may increase serum imipramine levels. Monitor for adverse reactions.
Clonidine, epinephrine, norepinephrine: increased hypertensive effect.
MAO inhibitors: may cause hyperpyretic crisis, severe seizures, and death. Avoid concomitant use.

EFFECTS ON DIAGNOSTIC TESTS
Drug may prolong conduction time (elongation of QT and PR intervals, flattened T waves on ECG); it also may elevate liver function test results, decrease WBC counts, and decrease or increase serum glucose levels.

CONTRAINDICATIONS
Contraindicated during acute recovery phase of MI, in patients with hypersensitivity to drug, and in those receiving MAO inhibitors.

NURSING CONSIDERATIONS
● Use with extreme caution in patients at risk for suicide; in patients with history of urine retention or angle-closure glaucoma, increased intraocular pressure, CV disease, impaired hepatic function; or hyperthyroidism, history of seizure disorders, impaired renal function; and in patients receiving thyroid medications. Injectable form contains sulfites, which may cause allergic reactions in hypersensitive patients.
● Be aware that reduced dosage in elderly or debilitated persons, adolescents, and patients with aggravated psychotic symptoms is necessary.
● Do not withdraw drug abruptly.
● Because of hypertensive episodes during surgery in patients receiving TCAs, be aware that drug should be gradually discontinued several days before surgery.
● If signs of psychosis occur or increase, expect doctor to reduce dosage. Record mood changes. Monitor patients for suicidal tendencies, and allow them only a minimum supply of the drug.

• To prevent relapse in children receiving the drug for enuresis, be aware that drug should be withdrawn gradually.
• Relieve dry mouth with sugarless hard candy or gum. Saliva substitutes may be necessary.

☑ **PATIENT TEACHING**
• Advise patient to take full dose at bedtime but warn him of possible morning orthostatic hypotension.
• If the child is an "early night" bedwetter, tell parents it may be more effective to divide dosage and administer the first dose earlier in the day.
• Tell patient to avoid alcohol while taking this drug.
• Advise patient to consult his doctor before taking other prescription or OTC medications.
• Warn patient to avoid hazardous activities that require alertness and good psychomotor coordination until CNS effects of the drug are known. Drowsiness and dizziness usually subside after a few weeks.
• Warn patient not to stop drug suddenly.
• To prevent photosensitivity reactions, advise patient to use sunblock, wear protective clothing, and avoid prolonged exposure to strong sunlight.

---

maprotiline hydrochloride
Ludiomil

Pregnancy Risk Category: B

HOW SUPPLIED
Tablets: 25 mg, 50 mg, 75 mg

ACTION
Unknown. A tetracyclic antidepressant similar to tricyclic derivatives. Probably increases the amount of norepinephrine, serotonin, or both in the CNS by blocking their reuptake by the presynaptic neurons.

ONSET, PEAK, DURATION
Onset usually occurs in 2 to 3 weeks, although sometimes it occurs within 7 days. Serum levels peak in 12 hours. Duration unknown.

INDICATIONS & DOSAGE
Depression—
Adults: initially, 25 to 75 mg P.O. daily for patients with mild to moderate depression, increased gradually in increments of 25 mg to 150 mg daily, if needed. Maximum dosage is 225 mg daily.

ADVERSE REACTIONS
CNS: *drowsiness, dizziness, seizures,* tremor, confusion, headache, nervousness, extrapyramidal reactions, anxiety, insomnia, agitation, numbness, weakness.
CV: *orthostatic hypotension, tachycardia, ECG changes,* hypertension, arrhythmias, heart block, syncope.
EENT: *blurred vision,* tinnitus, mydriasis.
GI: *dry mouth, constipation,* nausea, diarrhea, vomiting.
GU: urine retention.
Skin: rash, urticaria, photosensitivity.
Other: *diaphoresis,* hypersensitivity reaction.
After abrupt withdrawal of long-term therapy: nausea, headache, malaise (does not indicate addiction).

INTERACTIONS
Barbiturates: decreased blood maprotiline levels. Monitor for decreased antidepressant effect.
Cimetidine, methylphenidate: may increase serum maprotiline levels. Monitor for adverse reactions.
Clonidine, epinephrine, norepinephrine: increased hypertensive effect. Use with caution.
CNS depressants, ethanol: enhanced CNS depression. Avoid concomitant use.
MAO inhibitors: may cause severe excitation, hyperpyrexia, or seizures, usually

---

Reactions may be *common*, uncommon, *life-threatening*, or COMMON AND LIFE-THREATENING.

with high dosage. Use with caution. *Tricyclic antidepressants:* drug shares toxic potentials with tricyclic antidepressants and may cause hypertensive episodes during surgery. Gradually withdraw drug several days before surgery.

EFFECTS ON DIAGNOSTIC TESTS
Drug may prolong conduction time (elongation of QT and PR intervals, flattened T waves on ECG); it also may elevate liver function test results, decrease WBC counts, and decrease or increase serum glucose levels.

CONTRAINDICATIONS
Contraindicated during acute recovery phase of MI and in patients with hypersensitivity to drug, seizure disorders, or within 14 days of MAO inhibitor therapy.

NURSING CONSIDERATIONS
• Use with extreme caution in patients with history of MI or CV disease. Use cautiously in patients with suicidal tendency, increased intraocular pressure, or history of urine retention or angle-closure glaucoma.
• Know that dosage needs to be reduced in elderly or debilitated patients and adolescents.
• Do not withdraw drug abruptly.
• If signs of psychosis occur or increase, expect doctor to reduce dosage. Record mood changes. Monitor patients for suicidal tendencies, and allow them only a minimum supply of the drug.
• Relieve dry mouth with sugarless hard candy or gum. Saliva substitutes may be necessary.

☑ **PATIENT TEACHING**
• Warn patient to avoid activities that require alertness and good psychomotor coordination until CNS effects of the drug are known. Drowsiness and dizziness usually subside after a few weeks.
• Advise patient to take full dose at bedtime, but warn him of possible morning orthostatic hypotension.
• Tell patient to avoid alcohol while taking this drug.
• Advise patient to consult his doctor before taking other prescription or OTC medications.
• Warn patient not to withdraw drug suddenly.
• To prevent photosensitivity reactions, advise patient to use sunblock, wear protective clothing, and avoid prolonged exposure to strong sunlight.

▼ *NEW DRUG*

mirtazapine
Remeron

Pregnancy Risk Category: C

HOW SUPPLIED
Tablets: 15 mg, 30 mg

ACTION
Antidepressant action is thought to be due to enhancement of central noradrenergic and serotonergic activity.

ONSET, PEAK, DURATION
Onset unknown. Peak plasma concentrations reached within about 2 hours of administration. Half-life is 20 to 40 hours.

INDICATIONS & DOSAGE
Depression—
Adults: initially, 15 mg P.O. h.s. Maintenance dosage ranges from 15 to 45 mg daily. Dosage adjustments should be made at intervals of at least 1 to 2 weeks.

ADVERSE REACTIONS
CNS: *somnolence,* dizziness, asthenia, abnormal dreams, abnormal thinking, tremors, confusion.
GI: nausea, *increased appetite, dry mouth, constipation.*
GU: urinary frequency.
Hematologic: *agranulocytosis* (rare).

Respiratory: dyspnea.
Other: *weight gain,* back pain, flu syndrome, edema, peripheral edema, myalgia.

INTERACTIONS
Alcohol, diazepam, other CNS depressants: possible additive CNS effects. Avoid concomitant use.
MAO inhibitor: sometimes fatal reactions. Drug should not be used with MAO inhibitor or within 14 days of initiating or discontinuing therapy with MAO inhibitor. At least 14 days should elapse after stopping mirtazapine before starting an MAO inhibitor.

EFFECTS ON DIAGNOSTIC TESTS
Drug may increase cholesterol, triglyceride, and ALT levels.

CONTRAINDICATIONS
Contraindicated in patients with hypersensitivity to drug.

NURSING CONSIDERATIONS
● Use cautiously in patients with CV or cerebrovascular disease, seizure disorders, suicidal ideations, impaired hepatic or renal function, or history of mania or hypomania.
● Use cautiously in patients with conditions that predispose them to hypotension, such as dehydration, hypovolemia, or treatment with antihypertensive medication.
● Know that although incidence of agranulocytosis is rare, discontinue drug and monitor patient closely if he develops a sore throat, fever, stomatitis, or other signs of infection together with a low WBC count.
● Monitor patient closely for signs of dependence; it is not known whether mirtazapine causes physical or psychological dependence.
● Administer drug cautiously to elderly patients; pharmacokinetic studies reveal decreased clearance in the elderly.
● Safety and effectiveness in children have not been established.

● Be aware that it is not known whether drug is excreted in breast milk; use cautiously when administering drug to breast-feeding women.

☑ **PATIENT TEACHING**
● Caution patient not to perform hazardous activities if somnolence occurs.
● Tell patient to report signs and symptoms of infection, such as fever, chills, sore throat, mucous membrane ulceration, or flulike symptoms.
● Instruct patient not to use alcohol or other CNS depressants while taking drug.
● Stress importance of compliance with therapy.
● Instruct patient not to take concomitant medications without a doctor's approval.
● Tell women of childbearing age to report suspected pregnancy immediately and to notify doctor if they are breastfeeding.

---

nefazodone hydrochloride
Serzone

Pregnancy Risk Category: C

HOW SUPPLIED
Tablets: 100 mg, 150 mg, 200 mg, 250 mg

ACTION
Not precisely defined. Nefazodone inhibits neuronal uptake of serotonin (5-HT-2) and norepinephrine; it also occupies serotonin and alpha$_1$-adrenergic receptors in the CNS.

ONSET, PEAK, DURATION
Onset and duration unknown. Serum levels peak in about 1 hour.

INDICATIONS & DOSAGE
Depression—
Adults: initially, 200 mg/day P.O. in two divided doses. Dosage increased in increments of 100 to 200 mg/day at intervals of no less than 1 week, p.r.n.

Usual dosage range is 300 to 600 mg/day.
Elderly or debilitated patients: initially, 100 mg/day P.O. b.i.d.

ADVERSE REACTIONS
CNS: *headache, somnolence, dizziness, asthenia,* insomnia, *light-headedness, confusion,* memory impairment, paresthesia, vasodilation, abnormal dreams, decreased concentration, ataxia, incoordination, taste perversion, psychomotor retardation, tremor, hypertonia.
CV: postural hypotension, hypotension, peripheral edema.
EENT: *blurred vision, abnormal vision,* tinnitus, visual field defect.
GI: *dry mouth, nausea, constipation,* dyspepsia, diarrhea, increased appetite, vomiting.
GU: urinary frequency, urinary tract infection, urine retention, vaginitis.
Respiratory: pharyngitis, cough.
Skin: pruritus, rash.
Other: infection, flulike syndrome, chills, fever, neck rigidity, breast pain, thirst, arthralgia.

INTERACTIONS
Alprazolam, triazolam: coadministration with nefazodone potentiates the effects of these drugs. Do not administer concurrently. However, if necessary, dosage of alprazolam and triazolam may need to be reduced greatly.
Astemizole, terfenadine: may cause decreased metabolism, leading to increased levels of these antihistamines and cardiotoxicity. Avoid concomitant use.
CNS drugs: may alter CNS activity. Use together cautiously.
Digoxin: may increase digoxin level. Use together cautiously and monitor digoxin levels.
MAO inhibitors: may cause severe excitation, hyperpyrexia, seizures, delirium, or coma. Avoid concomitant use.
Other highly protein-bound drugs: may increase incidence and severity of adverse reactions. Monitor patient closely.

EFFECTS ON DIAGNOSTIC TESTS
None reported.

CONTRAINDICATIONS
Contraindicated in patients with hypersensitivity to the drug or to other phenylpiperazine antidepressants. Also contraindicated within 14 days of MAO inhibitor therapy and in coadministration with terfenadine or astemizole.

NURSING CONSIDERATIONS
● Use cautiously in patients with CV or cerebrovascular disease that could be exacerbated by hypotension (such as history of MI, angina, or CVA) and conditions that would predispose patients to hypotension (such as dehydration, hypovolemia, and treatment with antihypertensives). Also use cautiously in patients with a history of mania.
● Know that at least 1 week should elapse between stopping nefazodone and starting MAO inhibitor therapy, and that at least 14 days should elapse before a patient begins taking nefazodone after MAO inhibitor therapy has been discontinued.
● Record mood changes. Monitor patients for suicidal tendencies, and allow them only a minimum supply of the drug.

☑ PATIENT TEACHING
● Warn patient not to engage in hazardous activity until drug's CNS effects are known.
Alert: Instruct men who experience prolonged or inappropriate erections to stop drug immediately and notify doctor.
● Instruct women to notify doctor if they become pregnant or intend to become pregnant during therapy.
● Tell patient who develops a rash, hives, or a related allergic reaction to notify doctor.
● Instruct patient to avoid alcoholic beverages while on therapy.
● Tell patient to notify doctor before

taking any OTC drugs.
● Inform patient that several weeks of therapy may be required to obtain the full antidepressant effect. Once improvement occurs, advise patient not to discontinue drug until directed by doctor.

---

nortriptyline hydrochloride
Allegron‡, Aventyl*, Nortab‡, Pamelor*

Pregnancy Risk Category: NR

HOW SUPPLIED
Tablets: 10 mg‡, 25 mg‡
Capsules: 10 mg, 25 mg, 50 mg, 75 mg
Oral solution: 10 mg/5 ml (4% alcohol)

ACTION
Unknown, but a tricyclic antidepressant (TCA) that increases the amount of norepinephrine, serotonin, or both in the CNS by blocking their reuptake by the presynaptic neurons.

ONSET, PEAK, DURATION
Onset unknown but thought to take at least 2 to 4 weeks or longer. Peak plasma concentrations occur within 7 to 8.5 hours. Duration unknown.

INDICATIONS & DOSAGE
Depression—
Adults: 25 mg P.O. t.i.d. or q.i.d., gradually increased to maximum of 150 mg daily. Entire dosage may be given h.s. Monitor plasma levels when doses above 100 mg/day are given.
Elderly and adolescent patients: 30 to 50 mg daily given once or in divided doses.

ADVERSE REACTIONS
CNS: *drowsiness, dizziness, seizures,* tremor, weakness, confusion, headache, nervousness, EEG changes, extrapyramidal reactions, insomnia, nightmares, hallucinations, paresthesia, ataxia, agitation.

CV: *tachycardia,* hypertension, hypotension, *MI,* heart block, *stroke.*
EENT: *blurred vision,* tinnitus, mydriasis.
GI: dry mouth, *constipation,* nausea, vomiting, anorexia, paralytic ileus.
GU: *urine retention.*
Hematologic: bone marrow depression, *agranulocytosis,* eosinophilia, *thrombocytopenia.*
Skin: rash, urticaria, photosensitivity.
Other: *diaphoresis,* hypersensitivity reaction.
After abrupt withdrawal of long-term therapy: nausea, headache, malaise (does not indicate addiction).

INTERACTIONS
Barbiturates, CNS depressants, ethanol: enhanced CNS depression. Avoid concomitant use.
Cimetidine, methylphenidate: may increase nortriptyline serum levels. Monitor for adverse reactions.
Clonidine, epinephrine, norepinephrine: increased hypertensive effect. Use with caution.
MAO inhibitors: may cause severe excitation, hyperpyrexia, or seizures, usually with high dosage. Use with caution.

EFFECTS ON DIAGNOSTIC TESTS
Drug may prolong conduction time (elongation of QT and PR intervals, flattened T waves on ECG); it also may elevate liver function test results, decrease WBC counts, and decrease or increase serum glucose levels.

CONTRAINDICATIONS
Contraindicated during acute recovery phase of MI and in patients with hypersensitivity to drug or MAO therapy within past 14 days.

NURSING CONSIDERATIONS
● Use with extreme caution in patients with glaucoma, suicidal tendency, history of urine retention or seizures, CV disease, or hyperthyroidism and in those receiving thyroid medication.

Reactions may be *common,* uncommon, *life-threatening,* or COMMON AND LIFE-THREATENING.

• Know that dosage should be reduced in elderly or debilitated patients and adolescents.

• Do not withdraw drug abruptly.

• Because hypertensive episodes have occurred during surgery in patients receiving TCAs, know that dosage should be gradually discontinued several days before surgery.

• If signs of psychosis occur or increase, expect doctor to reduce dosage. Record mood changes. Monitor patients for suicidal tendencies, and allow them only a minimum supply of the drug.

• Be aware that adverse anticholinergic effects can occur rapidly. Drug has anticholinergic effects similar to other TCAs.

• Relieve dry mouth with sugarless hard candy or gum. Saliva substitutes may be necessary.

☑ **PATIENT TEACHING**
• Whenever possible, advise patient to take full dose at bedtime to reduce the risk of orthostatic hypotension.

• Warn patient to avoid activities that require alertness and good psychomotor coordination until CNS effects of the drug are known. Drowsiness and dizziness usually subside after a few weeks.

• Tell patient to consult his doctor before taking other prescription or OTC drugs.

• Warn patient not to stop drug suddenly.

• To prevent photosensitivity reactions, advise patient to use sunblock, wear protective clothing, and avoid prolonged exposure to strong sunlight.

---

paroxetine hydrochloride
Paxil

Pregnancy Risk Category: B

HOW SUPPLIED
Tablets: 20 mg, 30 mg

ACTION
Unknown, but presumed to be linked to its inhibition of CNS neuronal uptake of serotonin.

ONSET, PEAK, DURATION
Onset usually occurs within 1 to 4 weeks. Serum levels peak in 2 to 8 hours. Duration unknown.

INDICATIONS & DOSAGE
Depression—
Adults: initially, 20 mg P.O. daily, preferably in the morning as indicated. If patient does not respond after full antidepressant effect has occurred, dosage may be increased in 10-mg/day increments at weekly intervals, to a maximum of 50 mg daily.
Elderly or debilitated patients; patients with severe hepatic or renal disease: initially, 10 mg P.O. daily, preferably in the morning as indicated. If patient does not respond after full antidepressant effect has occurred, dosage may be increased in 10-mg/day increments at weekly intervals, to a maximum of 40 mg daily.
Panic disorder—
Adults: initially, 10 mg/day. Dosage may be increased in 10-mg/week increments and at weekly intervals. Maximum dosage should not exceed 60 mg/day.

ADVERSE REACTIONS
CNS: *somnolence, dizziness, insomnia, tremor, nervousness,* anxiety, paresthesia, confusion, *headache,* agitation.
CV: palpitations, vasodilation, postural hypotension.
EENT: lump or tightness in throat, dysgeusia.
GI: *dry mouth, nausea, constipation, diarrhea,* flatulence, vomiting, dyspepsia, increased appetite, abdominal pain.
GU: ejaculatory disturbances, male genital disorders (including anorgasmy, erectile difficulties, delayed ejaculation or orgasm, impotence, and sexual dysfunction), urinary frequency, other uri-

---

*Liquid contains alcohol.   **May contain tartrazine.   †Canada only.   ‡Australia only.   ◇OTC.

nary disorders, female genital disorders (including anorgasmy, difficulty with orgasm).
Skin: rash, pruritus.
Other: *asthenia, diaphoresis,* myopathy, myalgia, myasthenia, decreased libido, yawning.

INTERACTIONS
Cimetidine: decreased hepatic metabolism of paroxetine, leading to risk of toxicity. Dosage adjustments may be necessary.
Digoxin: may decrease digoxin levels. Monitor closely.
MAO inhibitors: may increase risk of serious, sometimes fatal, adverse reactions. Avoid concomitant use.
Phenobarbital, phenytoin: may alter pharmacokinetics of both drugs. Dosage adjustments may be necessary.
Procyclidine: may increase procyclidine levels. Monitor for excessive anticholinergic effects.
Tryptophan: may increase incidence of adverse reactions, such as diaphoresis, headache, nausea, and dizziness. Avoid concomitant use.
Warfarin: increased risk of bleeding. Use concomitantly with caution.

EFFECTS ON DIAGNOSTIC TESTS
None reported.

CONTRAINDICATIONS
Contraindicated in patients taking MAO inhibitors or within 14 days of discontinuing MAO inhibitor therapy and in those hypersensitive to the drug.

NURSING CONSIDERATIONS
● Use cautiously in patients with a history of seizure disorders or mania and in those with severe, concomitant systemic illness.
● Use cautiously in patients at risk for volume depletion, and monitor appropriately.
● If signs of psychosis occur or increase, expect doctor to reduce dosage. Record mood changes. Monitor patients for suicidal tendencies, and allow them only a minimum supply of the drug.

☑ PATIENT TEACHING
● Warn patient to avoid activities that require alertness and good psychomotor coordination until CNS effects of the drug are known.
● Tell patient to avoid alcohol and to consult his doctor before taking other prescription or OTC drugs.

phenelzine sulfate
Nardil

Pregnancy Risk Category: C

HOW SUPPLIED
Tablets: 15 mg

ACTION
Unknown. An MAO inhibitor that probably promotes accumulation of neurotransmitters by inhibiting their metabolism.

ONSET, PEAK, DURATION
Onset occurs in 7 to 10 days, although up to 4 to 8 weeks may be needed to achieve full therapeutic effect. Peak levels occur in 2 to 4 hours. Effects persist for up to 10 days after therapy is stopped.

INDICATIONS & DOSAGE
Depression—
Adults: 15 mg P.O. t.i.d., increased rapidly to 60 mg daily. Maximum dosage is 90 mg daily. Then dosage can usually be reduced to 15 mg daily.

ADVERSE REACTIONS
CNS: *dizziness,* vertigo, headache, hyperreflexia, tremor, muscle twitching, *insomnia,* drowsiness, weakness, fatigue.
CV: postural hypotension, edema.
GI: dry mouth, *anorexia,* nausea, constipation.
Other: diaphoresis, weight gain.

INTERACTIONS
Amphetamines, antihistamines, buspiron, ephedrine, levodopa, meperidine, metaraminol, methylphenidate, phenylephrine, phenylpropanolamine, sympathomimetics: enhanced pressor effects. Avoid concomitant use.

Antihypertensives containing thiazide diuretics, spinal anesthetics, barbiturates, dextromethorphan, ethanol, methotrimeprazine, narcotics, other sedatives, serotonin reuptake inhibitors, tricyclic antidepressants: unpredictable interaction. Use these agents with caution and in reduced dosage.

Insulin, oral antidiabetic agents: increased risk of hypoglycemia. Use with caution and in reduced dosages.

Foods high in tryptophan, tyramine, caffeine: may precipitate hypertensive crisis. Avoid concomitant use.

EFFECTS ON DIAGNOSTIC TESTS
Phenelzine therapy elevates liver function test results and urinary catecholamine levels and may elevate WBC count.

CONTRAINDICATIONS
Contraindicated in patients with hypersensitivity to drug, CHF, pheochromocytoma, hypertension, significant renal impairment, cerebrovascular defect, liver disease, and CV disease. Also contraindicated during therapy with other MAO inhibitors (isocarboxazid, tranylcypromine) or within 10 days of such therapy or within 10 days of elective surgery requiring general anesthesia, cocaine use, or local anesthesia containing sympathomimetic vasoconstrictors.

NURSING CONSIDERATIONS
● Use cautiously with antihypertensives containing thiazide diuretics, with spinal anesthetics, and in patients at risk for suicide, diabetes, or seizure disorders.
● Obtain baseline blood pressure, heart rate, CBC, and liver function test results before therapy, and continue to monitor

throughout treatment.
● Be aware dosage usually is reduced to maintenance level as soon as possible.
● In most patients, discontinue MAO inhibitors 14 days before elective surgery as ordered to avoid drug interactions that may occur during anesthesia.
● Monitor patients closely for suicidal tendencies, and allow them only a minimum supply of the drug.
● If patients develop symptoms of overdose (severe hypotension, palpitations, or frequent headaches), withhold dose and notify the doctor.
Alert: Have phentolamine available to combat severe hypertension.
● Continue precautions 14 days after stopping drug because it has long-lasting effects.

☑ **PATIENT TEACHING**
● Severe adverse effects can occur if MAO inhibitors are taken with OTC cold, hay-fever, or diet preparations.
● Advise patient to avoid alcohol and to consult doctor before taking any other prescription or OTC medications.
● Warn patient about the probability of orthostatic hypotension. Supervise walking. Tell patient to get out of bed slowly, sitting up first for 1 minute.
● Because MAO inhibitors may suppress chest pain in patient with angina, warn such a patient to engage in moderate activities and to avoid overexertion.

---

protriptyline hydrochloride
Triptil†, Vivactil

Pregnancy Risk Category: NR

HOW SUPPLIED
Tablets: 5 mg, 10 mg

ACTION
Unknown, but a tricyclic antidepressant (TCA) that increases the amount of norepinephrine, serotonin, or both in the CNS by blocking their reuptake by the presynaptic neurons.

ONSET, PEAK, DURATION
Onset unknown, although therapeutic effect thought to take 2 to 4 weeks or longer. Serum levels peak in 24 to 30 hours. Duration unknown.

INDICATIONS & DOSAGE
Depression—
Adults: 15 to 40 mg P.O. daily in divided doses, increasing gradually to maximum of 60 mg daily.
Elderly and adolescent patients: initially, 5 mg t.i.d., increasing dosage gradually. In elderly patients receiving doses over 20 mg/day, monitor CV status closely.

ADVERSE REACTIONS
CNS: *seizures,* tremor, hallucinations, disorientation, anxiety, restlessness, insomnia, ataxia, paresthesia, dizziness, weakness, confusion, headache, nervousness, EEG changes, extrapyramidal reactions.
CV: *tachycardia,* orthostatic hypotension, hypertension, *MI, stroke,* heart block, arrhythmias.
EENT: *blurred vision,* tinnitus, mydriasis.
GI: *dry mouth, constipation,* nausea, vomiting, anorexia, paralytic ileus.
GU: *urine retention.*
Skin: rash, urticaria, photosensitivity.
Other: *diaphoresis,* hypersensitivity reaction.
After abrupt withdrawal of long-term therapy: nausea, headache, malaise (does not indicate addiction).

INTERACTIONS
Barbiturates: decreased TCA blood levels. Monitor for decreased antidepressant effect.
Cimetidine, methylphenidate: may increase serum protriptyline levels. Monitor for adverse reactions.
Clonidine, epinephrine, norepinephrine: increased hypertensive effect.
CNS depressants, ethanol: enhanced CNS depression. Avoid concomitant use.

MAO inhibitors: may cause severe excitation, hyperpyrexia, seizures, or death, usually with high dosage.

EFFECTS ON DIAGNOSTIC TESTS
Drug may prolong conduction time (elongation of QT and PR intervals, flattened T waves on ECG); it also may elevate liver enzyme levels, decrease WBC counts, and decrease or increase serum glucose levels.

CONTRAINDICATIONS
Contraindicated during acute recovery phase of MI, in patients with hypersensitivity to the drug, and within 14 days of MAO inhibitor therapy.

NURSING CONSIDERATIONS
● Use cautiously in elderly patients; in patients with history of seizures, suicidal tendencies, history of urine retention, increased intraocular pressure, CV disorders, hyperthyroidism, and in those receiving thyroid medications.
● Do not withdraw drug abruptly.
● Because hypertensive episodes have occurred during surgery in patients receiving TCAs, know that drug should be gradually discontinued several days before surgery.
● If signs of psychosis occur or increase, expect doctor to reduce dosage. Record mood changes. Monitor patients for suicidal tendencies, and allow them only a minimum supply of the drug. To prevent insomnia, avoid late-day dosing.
● Know that protriptyline has strong anticholinergic effects.
● Relieve dry mouth with sugarless hard candy or gum. Saliva substitutes may be necessary.

☑ **PATIENT TEACHING**
● Tell patient to avoid alcohol while taking this drug.
● Advise patient to consult doctor before taking other prescription or OTC drugs.
● Warn patient not to withdraw drug suddenly.

Reactions may be *common*, uncommon, *life-threatening*, or COMMON AND LIFE-THREATENING.

• To prevent photosensitivity reactions, advise patient to use sunblock, wear protective clothing, and avoid prolonged exposure to strong sunlight.

---

sertraline hydrochloride
Zoloft

Pregnancy Risk Category: B

HOW SUPPLIED
Tablets: 50 mg, 100 mg

ACTION
Unknown, but presumed to be linked to its inhibition of neuronal uptake of serotonin in the CNS.

ONSET, PEAK, DURATION
Onset occurs in 2 to 4 weeks. Serum levels peak 4½ to 8½ hours after dose. Duration unknown.

INDICATIONS & DOSAGE
Depression—
Adults: 50 mg P.O. daily. Dosage adjusted as tolerated and needed; clinical trials involved dosage of 50 to 200 mg daily. Dosage adjustments should be made at intervals of no less than 1 week.
✷ **New indication:** *Obsessive-compulsive disorder—*
Adults: 50 mg P.O. once daily. If no response, dose may be increased to maximum of 200 mg/day. Dosage adjustments should be made at intervals of no less than 1 week.

ADVERSE REACTIONS
CNS: *headache, tremor, dizziness, insomnia, somnolence,* paresthesia, hypoesthesia, *fatigue,* nervousness, anxiety, agitation, hypertonia, twitching, confusion.
CV: palpitations, chest pain, hot flashes.
GI: *dry mouth, nausea, diarrhea, loose stools, dyspepsia,* vomiting, constipation, thirst, flatulence, anorexia, abdominal pain, increased appetite.
GU: *male sexual dysfunction.*

Skin: rash, pruritus.
Other: *diaphoresis,* myalgia.

INTERACTIONS
Diazepam, tolbutamide: decreased clearance of these drugs. Clinical significance unknown; however, monitor patients for increased drug effects.
MAO inhibitors: may cause serious, sometimes fatal, reactions including myoclonus rigidity, mental status changes, hyperthermia, autonomic nervous system instability, rapid fluctuations of vital signs, delirium, coma, and death. Avoid concomitant use.
Warfarin, other highly protein-bound drugs: may increase plasma levels of sertraline or other highly bound drug. Small (8%) increases in PT have been seen with concomitant use of warfarin. Monitor closely.

EFFECTS ON DIAGNOSTIC TESTS
Minor changes in several laboratory values have occurred. Elevated serum AST and ALT levels have occurred, usually within the first 9 weeks of therapy; values returned to normal after discontinuing drug. Minor increases in serum cholesterol and triglycerides and minor decreases in uric acid have also been seen. Clinical significance is unknown.

CONTRAINDICATIONS
Contraindicated in patients taking MAO inhibitors or within 14 days of discontinuing MAO inhibitor therapy.

NURSING CONSIDERATIONS
• Use cautiously in patients at risk for suicide, and in those with seizure disorder, major affective disorder, or diseases or conditions that affect metabolism or hemodynamic responses.
• Administer sertraline once daily, either in the morning or evening. May be given with or without food.
• Record mood changes. Monitor patients for suicidal tendencies, and allow them only a minimum supply of the drug.

---

*Liquid contains alcohol.   **May contain tartrazine.   †Canada only.   ‡Australia only.   ◇OTC.

☑ PATIENT TEACHING
● Advise patient to use caution when performing hazardous tasks that require alertness.
● Tell patient to avoid alcohol and to notify his doctor before taking any OTC drugs.

---

tranylcypromine sulfate
Parnate

Pregnancy Risk Category: NR

HOW SUPPLIED
Tablets: 10 mg

ACTION
Unknown. An MAO inhibitor that probably promotes accumulation of neurotransmitters by inhibiting MAO.

ONSET, PEAK, DURATION
Onset in 48 hours to 3 weeks may be needed to achieve full therapeutic effect. Peak levels occur in 1 to 3.5 hours. Effects persist for up to 10 days after therapy is stopped.

INDICATIONS & DOSAGE
Depression—
Adults: 10 mg P.O. t.i.d. Increased by 10 mg P.O. daily at 1- to 3-week intervals to maximum of 60 mg daily, if necessary, after 2 weeks of therapy.

ADVERSE REACTIONS
CNS: *dizziness,* headache, anxiety, agitation, paresthesia, drowsiness, weakness, numbness, tremor, jitters, confusion.
CV: *orthostatic hypotension, tachycardia,* paradoxical hypertension, palpitations.
EENT: blurred vision, tinnitus.
GI: dry mouth, *anorexia,* nausea, diarrhea, constipation, abdominal pain.
GU: impotence, SIADH, urine retention, impaired ejaculation.
Hematologic: anemia, leukopenia, ***agranulocytosis, thrombocytopenia.***

Skin: rash.
Other: edema, hepatitis, muscle spasm, myoclonic jerks, chills.

INTERACTIONS
Amphetamines, antihistamines, antihypertensives, diuretics, ephedrine, levodopa, meperidine, metaraminol, methylphenidate, phenylephrine, phenylpropanolamine, sympathomimetics: enhanced pressor effects of these drugs. Avoid concomitant use.
Antiparkinsonian drugs, barbiturates, dextromethorphan, ethanol, methotrimeprazine, narcotics, other sedatives, selective serotonin reuptake inhibitors, spinal anesthetics, tricyclic antidepressants: enhanced adverse CNS effects. Avoid concomitant use. If necessary, use with caution and in reduced dosage.
Buspirone: may elevate blood pressure. Monitor patient closely.
Insulin, oral antidiabetic agents: increased risk of hypoglycemia. Use with caution and in reduced dosages.
Foods high in tryptophan, tyramine, caffeine: may cause hypertensive crisis. Avoid concomitant use.

EFFECTS ON DIAGNOSTIC TESTS
Drug therapy elevates liver function tests and urinary catecholamine levels.

CONTRAINDICATIONS
● Contraindicated in patients receiving MAO inhibitors or dibenzazepine derivatives; sympathomimetics (including amphetamines); some CNS depressants (including narcotics and alcohol); antihypertensive, diuretic, antihistaminic, sedative or anesthetic drugs; bupropion hydrochloride, buspirone hydrochloride, dextromethorphan, meperidine; cheese or other foods with a high tyramine or tryptophan content; or excessive quantities of caffeine.
● Also contraindicated in patients with a confirmed or suspected cerebrovascular defect, hypersensitivity to the drug, pheochromocytoma, CHF, CV disease,

---

hypertension, hepatic disease, significant renal impairment, or history of headache and in those undergoing elective surgery.

NURSING CONSIDERATIONS
● Use cautiously in patients with renal disease, diabetes, seizure disorder, Parkinson's disease, or hyperthyroidism; and in patients at risk for suicide.
● Obtain baseline blood pressure, heart rate, CBC, and liver function test results before beginning therapy, and continue to monitor throughout treatment.
● Know that dosage usually is reduced to maintenance level as soon as possible.
● Do not withdraw drug abruptly.
● In most patients, discontinue MAO inhibitors 14 days before elective surgery as ordered to avoid drug interactions that may occur during anesthesia.
● Monitor patients for suicidal tendencies, and allow them only a minimum supply of the drug.
● If patients develop symptoms of overdose (palpitations, severe hypotension, or frequent headaches), withhold dose and notify the doctor.
Alert: Have phentolamine available to combat severe hypertension.
● Continue precautions for 10 days after stopping drug because it has long-lasting effects.

☑ **PATIENT TEACHING**
● Warn patient to avoid foods high in tyramine or tryptophan and large amounts of caffeine. Tranylcypromine is the MAO inhibitor most often reported to cause hypertensive crisis with ingestion of tyramine-rich foods, including aged cheese, Chianti wine, beer, avocados, chicken livers, chocolate, bananas, soy sauce, meat tenderizers, salami, and bologna.
● Tell patient to avoid alcohol and to consult his doctor before taking other prescription or OTC drugs.
● To prevent dizziness resulting from

orthostatic hypotension, tell patient to get out of bed slowly, sitting up for 1 minute first.
● Because MAO inhibitors may suppress anginal pain, warn patient to moderate activities and to avoid overexertion.
● Warn patient not to stop drug suddenly.

---

trazodone hydrochloride
Desyrel, Trazon, Trialodine

Pregnancy Risk Category: C

HOW SUPPLIED
Tablets: 50 mg, 100 mg, 150 mg, 300 mg

ACTION
Unknown, although it inhibits serotonin uptake in the brain. Not a tricyclic derivative.

ONSET, PEAK, DURATION
Onset occurs in 2 to 4 weeks or longer. Plasma levels peak after 1 hour if taken on an empty stomach, 2 hours if taken with food. Duration unknown.

INDICATIONS & DOSAGE
Depression—
Adults: initial dosage, 150 mg P.O. daily in divided doses; increased by 50 mg daily q 3 to 4 days, p.r.n. Average dosage ranges from 150 mg to 400 mg daily. Maximum daily dosage is 600 mg for inpatients and 400 mg for outpatients.

ADVERSE REACTIONS
CNS: *drowsiness, dizziness,* nervousness, fatigue, confusion, tremor, weakness, hostility, anger, nightmares, vivid dreams, headache, insomnia.
CV: orthostatic hypotension, tachycardia, hypertension, syncope, shortness of breath.
EENT: blurred vision, tinnitus, nasal congestion.

GI: dry mouth, dysgeusia, constipation, nausea, vomiting, anorexia.
GU: urine retention; priapism, possibly leading to impotence; decreased libido; hematuria.
Hematologic: anemia.
Skin: rash, urticaria.
Other: diaphoresis.

INTERACTIONS
Antihypertensives: increased hypotensive effect of trazodone. Antihypertensive dosage may have to be decreased.
Clonidine, CNS depressants, ethanol: enhanced CNS depression. Avoid concomitant use.
Digoxin, phenytoin: may increase serum levels of these drugs. Monitor for toxicity.
MAO inhibitors: effects unknown. Use together with extreme caution.

EFFECTS ON DIAGNOSTIC TESTS
Trazodone may prolong conduction time (elongation of QT and PR intervals, flattened T waves on ECG); it also may elevate liver function tests, decrease WBC counts, and alter serum glucose levels.

CONTRAINDICATIONS
Contraindicated during initial recovery phase of MI or in patients with hypersensitivity to drug.

NURSING CONSIDERATIONS
● Use cautiously in patients with cardiac disease and in patients at risk for suicide.
● Administer after meals or a light snack for optimal absorption and to decrease incidence of dizziness.
● Record mood changes. Monitor patients for suicidal tendencies, and allow them only minimum supply of the drug.

☑ PATIENT TEACHING
Alert: Inform male patient that priapism is a potential problem in men taking trazodone and to report its presence immediately; it may require surgical intervention.
● Warn patient to avoid activities that require alertness and good psychomotor coordination until CNS effects of the drug are known. Drowsiness and dizziness usually subside after the first few weeks.
● Teach caregivers how to recognize signs of suicidal tendency or suicidal ideation.

---

trimipramine maleate
Apo-Trimip†, Novo-Tripramine†, Rhotrimine†, Surmontil

Pregnancy Risk Category: C

HOW SUPPLIED
Tablets: 25 mg‡
Capsules: 25 mg, 50 mg, 100 mg

ACTION
Unknown, but a tricyclic antidepressant (TCA) that increases the amount of norepinephrine, serotonin, or both in the CNS by blocking their reuptake by the presynaptic neurons.

ONSET, PEAK, DURATION
Onset unknown, although thought to occur in 2 to 4 weeks or longer. Plasma concentrations peak in 2 hours. Duration unknown.

INDICATIONS & DOSAGE
Depression—
Adults: 75 to 100 mg P.O. daily in divided doses, increased to 200 to 300 mg daily. Dosages over 300 mg daily not recommended in hospitalized patients; not over 200 mg in outpatients. Total dosage requirement may be given h.s.
Elderly and adolescent patients: initially, 50 mg/day, gradually increased to 100 mg/day.

ADVERSE REACTIONS
CNS: *drowsiness, dizziness,* paresthesia, ataxia, hallucinations, delusions, anxiety, agitation, insomnia, tremor,

---

weakness, confusion, headache, EEG changes, *seizures,* extrapyramidal reactions.
CV: *orthostatic hypotension, tachycardia,* hypertension, arrhythmias, heart block, *MI, stroke.*
EENT: *blurred vision,* tinnitus, mydriasis.
GI: *dry mouth, constipation,* nausea, vomiting, anorexia, paralytic ileus.
GU: *urine retention.*
Skin: rash, urticaria, photosensitivity.
Other: *diaphoresis,* hypersensitivity reaction.
After abrupt withdrawal of long-term therapy: nausea, headache, malaise (does not indicate addiction).

INTERACTIONS
Barbiturates: decreased TCA blood levels. Monitor for decreased antidepressant effect.
Cimetidine, methylphenidate: may increase serum trimipramine levels. Monitor for increased adverse reactions.
Clonidine, epinephrine, norepinephrine: increased hypertensive effect. Use with caution.
CNS depressants, ethanol: enhanced CNS depression. Avoid concomitant use.
MAO inhibitors: may cause severe excitation, hyperpyrexia, or seizures, usually with high dosage. Use with caution.

EFFECTS ON DIAGNOSTIC TESTS
Drug may prolong conduction time (elongation of QT and PR intervals, flattened T waves of ECG); it also may elevate liver function test levels, decrease WBC counts, and alter serum glucose levels. Trimipramine may alter prothrombin time.

CONTRAINDICATIONS
Contraindicated during acute recovery phase of MI and in patients with hypersensitivity to drug or receiving MAO inhibitor therapy within 14 days.

NURSING CONSIDERATIONS
● Use with extreme caution in patients with CV disease, history of urine retention or angle-closure glaucoma, increased intraocular pressure, hyperthyroidism, impaired hepatic function, or history of seizures and in those receiving thyroid medications, guanethidine, or similar agents.
● Do not withdraw drug abruptly.
● Because hypertensive episodes have occurred during surgery in patients receiving TCAs, be aware that dosage should be gradually discontinued several days before surgery.
● If signs of psychosis occur or increase, expect doctor to reduce dosage. Record mood changes. Monitor patients for suicidal tendencies, and allow them only a minimum supply of the drug.
● Relieve dry mouth with sugarless hard candy or gum. Saliva substitutes may be necessary.

☑ PATIENT TEACHING
● To reduce daytime sedation, tell patient to take full dose at bedtime. Warn him about possible morning orthostatic hypotension.
● Tell patient to avoid alcohol and to consult his doctor before taking other prescription or OTC drugs.
● Warn patient to avoid hazardous activities that require alertness and good psychomotor coordination until CNS effects of the drug are known. Drowsiness and dizziness usually subside after a few weeks.
● Warn patient not to stop drug suddenly.
● To prevent photosensitivity reactions, advise patient to use sunblock, wear protective clothing, and avoid prolonged exposure to strong sunlight.

---

venlafaxine hydrochloride
Effexor

Pregnancy Risk Category: C

HOW SUPPLIED
Tablets: 25 mg, 37.5 mg, 50 mg, 75 mg,

100 mg

ACTION
Blocks reuptake of norepinephrine and serotonin into neurons in the CNS.

ONSET, PEAK, DURATION
Onset unknown but thought to take several weeks. Peak and duration unknown.

INDICATIONS & DOSAGE
Depression—
Adults: initially, 75 mg P.O. daily, in two or three divided doses with food. Dosage increased as tolerated and needed in increments of 75 mg/day at intervals of no less than 4 days. For moderately depressed outpatients, usual maximum dosage is 225 mg/day; in certain severely depressed patients, dosage may be as high as 375 mg/day.

ADVERSE REACTIONS
CNS: *headache, somnolence, dizziness, nervousness, insomnia,* anxiety, tremor, abnormal dreams, paresthesia, agitation.
CV: hypertension.
EENT: blurred vision.
GI: *nausea, constipation,* vomiting, *dry mouth, anorexia,* diarrhea, dyspepsia, flatulence.
GU: *abnormal ejaculation,* impotence, urinary frequency, impaired urination.
Other: *diaphoresis, asthenia,* weight loss, rash, yawning, chills, infection.

INTERACTIONS
MAO inhibitors: may precipitate a syndrome similar to neuroleptic malignant syndrome (myoclonus, hyperthermia, seizures, and death). Do not start venlafaxine within 14 days of discontinuing therapy with an MAO inhibitor, and don't start MAO inhibitor therapy within 7 days of stopping venlafaxine.

EFFECTS ON DIAGNOSTIC TESTS
None reported.

CONTRAINDICATIONS
Contraindicated in patients hypersensi-

tive to the drug. Also contraindicated for use within 14 days of MAO inhibitor therapy.

NURSING CONSIDERATIONS
● Use cautiously in patients with renal impairment, diseases or conditions that could affect hemodynamic responses or metabolism, and in those with history of mania or seizures.
● Know that total daily dosage should be reduced by 50% in patients with hepatic impairment. In patients with moderate renal impairment (glomerular filtration rate of 10 to 70 ml/minute), total daily dosage should be reduced by 25%. In patients undergoing hemodialysis, know that dose should be withheld until dialysis session is completed and daily dosage is reduced by 50%.
● Carefully monitor blood pressure. Venlafaxine therapy is associated with sustained, dose-dependent increases in blood pressure. Greatest increases (averaging about 7 mm Hg above baseline) occur in patients taking 375 mg daily.

☑ PATIENT TEACHING
● Inform patient who has received drug for 6 weeks or more that drug should be gradually discontinued by tapering dosage over a 2-week period as instructed by doctor.
● Warn patient to avoid hazardous activities that require alertness and good psychomotor coordination until CNS effects of the drug are known.

32

Antianxiety drugs

alprazolam
buspirone hydrochloride
chlordiazepoxide
chlordiazepoxide hydrochloride
clorazepate dipotassium
diazepam
doxepin hydrochloride
   (See Chapter 31, ANTIDEPRESSANTS.)
hydroxyzine embonate
hydroxyzine hydrochloride
hydroxyzine pamoate
lorazepam
meprobamate
midazolam hydrochloride
oxazepam

COMBINATION PRODUCTS
EQUAGESIC: meprobamate 200 mg and aspirin 325 mg.
LIBRAX: chlordiazepoxide hydrochloride 5 mg and clidinium bromide 2.5 mg.
LIMBITROL DS: chlordiazepoxide 10 mg and amitriptyline hydrochloride 25 mg.

---

alprazolam
Apo-Alpraz†, Novo-Alprazol†, Nu-Alpraz†, Xanax

Controlled Substance Schedule IV
Pregnancy Risk Category: D

HOW SUPPLIED
Tablets: 0.25 mg, 0.5 mg, 1 mg, 2 mg
Oral solution: 0.5 mg/5 ml, 1 mg/ml (concentrate)

ACTION
Unknown. A benzodiazepine that probably potentiates the effects of gamma-aminobutyric acid, an inhibitory neurotransmitter, and depresses the CNS at the limbic and subcortical levels of the brain.

ONSET, PEAK, DURATION
Onset and duration unknown. Serum levels peak within 1 to 2 hours.

INDICATIONS & DOSAGE
Anxiety—
Adults: usual initial dose, 0.25 to 0.5 mg P.O. t.i.d. Maximum dosage is 4 mg daily in divided doses.
Elderly or debilitated patients or those with advanced liver disease: usual initial dose, 0.25 mg P.O. b.i.d. or t.i.d. Maximum dosage is 4 mg daily in divided doses.
Panic disorders—
Adults: 0.5 mg P.O. t.i.d., increased at intervals of 3 to 4 days in increments of no more than 1 mg. Maximum dosage is 10 mg daily in divided doses.

ADVERSE REACTIONS
CNS: *drowsiness, light-headedness,* headache, confusion, tremor, dizziness, syncope, *depression,* insomnia, nervousness.
CV: hypotension, tachycardia.
EENT: blurred vision, nasal congestion.
GI: *dry mouth,* nausea, vomiting, *diarrhea,* constipation.
Skin: dermatitis.
Other: muscle rigidity, weight gain or loss.

INTERACTIONS
Cimetidine: increased sedation. Monitor patient carefully.
Digoxin: may increase serum digoxin levels, increasing toxicity. Monitor patient closely.
Ethanol, other CNS depressants: increased CNS depression. Avoid concomitant use.
Smoking: increased clearance of benzodiazepines. Monitor for lack of effect.

---

*Liquid contains alcohol.   **May contain tartrazine.   †Canada only.   ‡Australia only.   ◇OTC.

Tricyclic antidepressants (TCAs): increased plasma levels of TCAs. Monitor for toxicity.

EFFECTS ON DIAGNOSTIC TESTS
Drug therapy may elevate liver function test results. Minor changes in EEG patterns, usually low-voltage, fast activity, may occur during and after alprazolam therapy.

CONTRAINDICATIONS
Contraindicated in patients with hypersensitivity to drug or other benzodiazepines or acute angle-closure glaucoma.

NURSING CONSIDERATIONS
• Use cautiously in patients with hepatic, renal, or pulmonary disease.
• Also know that drug should not be prescribed for everyday stress or for long-term use (more than 4 months).
• Know that drug should not be withdrawn abruptly after long-term use; withdrawal symptoms may occur. Abuse or addiction is possible.
• Monitor liver, renal, and hematopoietic function studies periodically in patients receiving repeated or prolonged therapy, as ordered.

☑ **PATIENT TEACHING**
• Warn patient to avoid hazardous activities that require alertness and good psychomotor coordination until CNS effects of the drug are known.
• Tell patient to avoid alcohol while taking this drug.

---

buspirone hydrochloride
BuSpar

Pregnancy Risk Category: B

HOW SUPPLIED
Tablets: 5 mg, 10 mg

ACTION
Unknown. May inhibit neuronal firing and reduce serotonin turnover in cortical, amygdaloid, and septohippocampal tissue.

ONSET, PEAK, DURATION
Onset unknown but for therapeutic effect, possibly 1 to 2 weeks; optimal results, possibly 3 to 4 weeks. Serum levels peak within 40 to 90 minutes. Duration unknown.

INDICATIONS & DOSAGE
Anxiety disorders; short-term relief of anxiety—
Adults: initially, 5 mg P.O. t.i.d. Dosage increased at 3-day intervals in 5-mg increments. Usual maintenance dosage is 20 to 30 mg daily in divided doses. Do not exceed 60 mg daily.

ADVERSE REACTIONS
CNS: *dizziness, drowsiness,* nervousness, insomnia, headache, light-headedness, fatigue, numbness.
GI: dry mouth, nausea, diarrhea, abdominal distress.
Other: blurred vision.

INTERACTIONS
Ethanol, other CNS depressants: increased CNS depression. Avoid concomitant use.
MAO inhibitors: may elevate blood pressure. Avoid concomitant use.

EFFECTS ON DIAGNOSTIC TESTS
None reported.

CONTRAINDICATIONS
Contraindicated in patients hypersensitive to the drug or within 14 days of therapy with an MAO inhibitor.

NURSING CONSIDERATIONS
• Use cautiously in patients with hepatic or renal failure.
• Monitor patient closely for adverse CNS reactions. Buspirone is less sedating than other antianxiety agents. How-

---

ever, CNS effects in individual patients may be unpredictable.

• Be aware that drug has shown no potential for abuse and has not been classified as a controlled substance. However, it is not recommended for relief of everyday stress.

☑ PATIENT TEACHING
Alert: Before initiating buspirone therapy in patient already being treated with benzodiazepines, warn him against stopping the benzodiazepine abruptly; withdrawal reaction may occur.

• Warn patient to avoid hazardous activities that require alertness and good psychomotor coordination until CNS effects of the drug are known.

• Tell patient to avoid alcohol during drug therapy.

---

chlordiazepoxide
Libritabs

chlordiazepoxide hydrochloride
Apo-Chlordiazepoxide†, Librium, Novopoxide†, Sereen, Solium†

Controlled Substance Schedule IV
Pregnancy Risk Category: NR

HOW SUPPLIED
chlordiazepoxide
Tablets: 5 mg, 10 mg, 25 mg
chlordiazepoxide hydrochloride
Capsules: 5 mg, 10 mg, 25 mg
Powder for injection: 100-mg ampule

ACTION
Unknown. Thought to depress the CNS at the limbic and subcortical levels of the brain.

ONSET, PEAK, DURATION
Onset and duration unknown. Plasma levels peak in 30 minutes to 4 hours.

INDICATIONS & DOSAGE
Mild to moderate anxiety—
Adults: 5 to 10 mg P.O. t.i.d. or q.i.d.
Children over 6 years: 5 mg P.O. b.i.d. to q.i.d. Maximum dosage is 10 mg P.O. b.i.d. or t.i.d.
Severe anxiety—
Adults: 20 to 25 mg P.O. t.i.d. or q.i.d. In geriatric patients, 5 mg b.i.d. to q.i.d.
Withdrawal symptoms of acute alcoholism—
Adults: 50 to 100 mg P.O., I.M., or I.V. Repeated in 2 to 4 hours, p.r.n. Maximum dosage is 300 mg daily.
Preoperative apprehension and anxiety—
Adults: 5 to 10 mg P.O. t.i.d. or q.i.d. on day preceding surgery; or 50 to 100 mg I.M. 1 hour before surgery.
Note: Parenteral form not recommended in children under 12 years.

ADVERSE REACTIONS
CNS: *drowsiness, lethargy,* ataxia, confusion, extrapyramidal symptoms, EEG changes.
GI: nausea, constipation.
GU: increased or decreased libido, menstrual irregularities.
Hematologic: *agranulocytosis.*
Hepatic: jaundice.
Skin: *swelling, pain at injection site,* skin eruptions, edema.

INTERACTIONS
Cimetidine: increased sedation. Monitor patient carefully.
Digoxin: increased serum digoxin levels and risk of toxicity. Monitor patient closely.
Ethanol, other CNS depressants: increased CNS depression. Avoid concomitant use.
Smoking: increased clearance of benzodiazepines. Monitor for lack of effect.

EFFECTS ON DIAGNOSTIC TESTS
Drug therapy may elevate results of liver function tests. Minor changes in

EEG patterns, usually low-voltage, fast activity, may occur during and after therapy. Drug may cause a false-positive pregnancy test, depending on method used. It may also alter urinary 17-ketosteroids (Zimmerman reaction), urine alkaloid determination (Frings thin layer chromatography method), and urinary glucose determinations (with Clinistix and Diastix, but not Tes-Tape).

CONTRAINDICATIONS
Contraindicated in patients hypersensitive to the drug.

NURSING CONSIDERATIONS
• Use cautiously in patients with mental depression, porphyria, or hepatic or renal disease.
• Know that drug should be avoided during pregnancy, especially during first trimester.
• Know that dosage should be reduced in elderly or debilitated patients.
• Also know that drug should not be prescribed regularly for everyday stress.
• Injectable form (as hydrochloride) comes in two types of ampules—as diluent and as powdered drug. Read directions carefully.
• Keep powder away from light and refrigerate; mix just before use and discard remainder.
• For I.M. use, add 2 ml of diluent to powder and agitate gently until clear. Use immediately. I.M. form may be absorbed erratically.
Alert: Recommended for I.M. use only, but may be given I.V.
• **I.V. use:** Use 5 ml of 0.9% sodium chloride solution or sterile water for injection as diluent; do not give packaged diluent I.V. Administer over 1 minute.
• When giving drug I.V., be sure equipment and personnel needed for emergency airway management are available. Monitor respirations every 5 to 15 minutes and before each repeated I.V. dose.
• Monitor liver, renal, and hematopoiet-

ic function studies periodically in patients receiving repeated or prolonged therapy, as ordered.
• Possibility of abuse and addiction exists. Drug should not be withdrawn abruptly after long-term administration; withdrawal symptoms may occur.

☑ **PATIENT TEACHING**
• Warn patient to avoid hazardous activities that require alertness and good psychomotor coordination until CNS effects of the drug are known.
• Tell patient to avoid alcohol while taking this drug.

clorazepate dipotassium
Apo-Clorazepate†, Gen-XENE, Novoclopate†, Tranxene, Tranxene-SD, Tranxene-T-Tab

Controlled Substance Schedule IV
Pregnancy Risk Category: D

HOW SUPPLIED
Tablets: 3.75 mg, 7.5 mg, 11.25 mg, 15 mg, 22.5 mg
Capsules: 3.75 mg, 7.5 mg, 15 mg

ACTION
Unknown. A benzodiazepine that probably facilitates the action of the inhibitory neurotransmitter gamma-aminobutyric acid. Depresses the CNS at the limbic and subcortical levels of the brain and suppresses the spread of seizure activity produced by epileptogenic foci in the cortex, thalamus, and limbic structures.

ONSET, PEAK, DURATION
Onset and duration unknown. Plasma levels peak within ½ to 2 hours.

INDICATIONS & DOSAGE
Acute alcohol withdrawal—
Adults: day 1—30 mg P.O. initially, followed by 30 to 60 mg P.O. in divided doses; day 2—45 to 90 mg P.O. in divided doses; day 3—22.5 to 45 mg

P.O. in divided doses; day 4—15 to 30 mg P.O. in divided doses; then gradually reduce dosage to 7.5 to 15 mg daily. Maximum recommended daily dosage is 90 mg.

Anxiety—
Adults: 15 to 60 mg P.O. daily.
Elderly or debilitated patients: initially, 7.5 to 15 mg daily in divided doses or as a single dose h.s.

Adjunct in partial seizure disorder—
Adults and children over 12 years: Maximum recommended initial dosage is 7.5 mg P.O. t.i.d. Dosage increases should be no greater than 7.5 mg/week. Maximum dosage should not exceed 90 mg daily.

Children 9 and 12 years: Maximum recommended initial dosage is 7.5 mg P.O. b.i.d. Dosage increases should be no greater than 7.5 mg/week. Maximum dosage should not exceed 60 mg daily.

ADVERSE REACTIONS
CNS: *drowsiness,* dizziness, nervousness, confusion, headache, insomnia, depression, irritability, tremor.
CV: hypotension.
EENT: blurred vision, diplopia.
GI: nausea, vomiting, abdominal discomfort, dry mouth
GU: urine retention, incontinence.
Skin: rashes.

INTERACTIONS
Cimetidine: increased sedation. Monitor patient carefully.
Digoxin: may increase serum digoxin levels and risk of toxicity. Monitor patient closely.
Ethanol, other CNS depressants: increased CNS depression. Avoid concomitant use.
Smoking: increased clearance of benzodiazepines. Monitor for lack of effect.

EFFECTS ON DIAGNOSTIC TESTS
Clorazepate therapy may elevate liver function test results. Minor changes in

EEG patterns, usually low-voltage, fast activity, may occur during and after drug therapy.

CONTRAINDICATIONS
Contraindicated in patients with hypersensitivity to the drug and acute angle-closure glaucoma.

NURSING CONSIDERATIONS
● Know that drug should be avoided during pregnancy, especially the first trimester.
● Use cautiously in patients with suicidal tendencies, renal or hepatic impairment, or history of drug abuse.
● Know that dosage should be reduced in elderly or debilitated patients.
● Monitor liver, renal, and hematopoietic function studies periodically in patients receiving repeated or prolonged therapy as ordered.
● Possibility of abuse and addiction exists. Do not withdraw drug abruptly after prolonged use; withdrawal symptoms may occur.
● Drug is not recommended for use in children under 9 years.

☑ PATIENT TEACHING
● Warn patient to avoid activities that require alertness and good psychomotor coordination until CNS effects of the drug are known.
● Tell patient to avoid alcohol while taking this drug.
● Tell patient that sugarless chewing gum or hard candy can relieve dry mouth.

---

diazepam
Apo-Diazepam†, Atenex‡, Diazemuls†‡, Diazepam Intensol, Ducene‡, Novodipam†, PMS- Diazepam†, T-Quil, Valium, Valrelease, Vazepam, Vivol†, Zetran

Controlled Substance Schedule IV
Pregnancy Risk Category: D

HOW SUPPLIED
Tablets: 2 mg, 5 mg, 10 mg
Capsules (extended-release): 15 mg
Oral solution: 5 mg/5 ml, 5 mg/ml
Injection: 5 mg/ml
Sterile emulsion for injection: 5 mg/ml†

ACTION
Unknown. A benzodiazepine that probably depresses the CNS at the limbic and subcortical levels of the brain. Suppresses spread of seizure activity produced by epileptogenic foci in the cortex, thalamus, and limbic structures.

ONSET, PEAK, DURATION
Onset occurs 30 minutes after oral dose, 1 to 5 minutes after I.V. injection. Plasma levels peak « to 2 hours after oral dose, immediately after I.V. injection; peak levels after administration of injectable emulsion occur 15 minutes after I.V. injection, 2 hours after I.M. injection. Effects persist for 3 to 8 hours after oral dose, 15 minutes to 1 hour after I.V. injection.

INDICATIONS & DOSAGE
Anxiety—
Adults: depending on severity, 2 to 10 mg P.O. 2 to 4 times daily or 15 to 30 mg extended-release capsules P.O. once daily. Alternatively, 2 to 10 mg I.M. or I.V. q 3 to 4 hours, p.r.n.
Elderly patients: initially, 2 to 2.5 mg once or twice daily; increased gradually.
Children 6 months and older: 1 to 2.5 mg P.O. 3 to 4 times daily, increased gradually, as needed and tolerated.
Acute alcohol withdrawal—
Adults: 10 mg P.O. 3 or 4 times first 24 hours, reduced to 5 mg P.O. three or four times daily, p.r.n. Alternatively, initially, 10 mg I.M. or I.V., then 5 to 10 mg I.M. or I.V. q 3 to 4 hours, p.r.n.
Before endoscopic procedures—

Adults: I.V. dose titrated to desired sedative response (up to 20 mg). Alternatively, 5 to 10 mg I.M. 30 minutes before procedure.
Muscle spasm—
Adults: 2 to 10 mg P.O. two to four times daily or 15 to 30 mg extended-release capsules once daily. Alternatively, 5 to 10 mg I.M. or I.V. initially, then 5 to 10 mg I.M. or I.V. q 3 to 4 hours, p.r.n. For tetanus, larger doses may be required.
Children over 30 days to 5 years: 1 to 2 mg I.M. or I.V. slowly, repeated q 3 to 4 hours, p.r.n.
Children 5 years or older: 5 to 10 mg I.M. or I.V. q 3 to 4 hours, p.r.n.
Preoperative sedation—
Adults: 10 mg I.M. (preferred) or I.V. before surgery.
Cardioversion—
Adults: 5 to 15 mg I.V. within 5 to 10 minutes prior to procedure
Adjunct in seizure disorders—
Adults: 2 to 10 mg P.O. two to four times daily.
Children 6 months and older: 1 to 2.5 mg P.O. three or four times daily initially; increased as tolerated and needed.
Status epilepticus and severe recurrent seizures—
Adults: 5 to 10 mg I.V. (preferred) or I.M. initially. Repeated q 10 to 15 minutes, p.r.n., up to a maximum dose of 30 mg. Repeated q 2 to 4 hours, if necessary.
Children over 30 days to 5 years: 0.2 to 0.5 mg I.V. slowly q 2 to 5 minutes up to a maximum of 5 mg. Repeated q 2 to 4 hours, if necessary.
Children 5 years and older: 1 mg I.V. q 2 to 5 minutes up to maximum of 10 mg. Repeated q 2 to 4 hours, if necessary.

ADVERSE REACTIONS
CNS: *drowsiness,* slurred speech, tremor, transient amnesia, fatigue, ataxia, headache, insomnia, paradoxical anxiety, hallucinations.

Reactions may be *common,* uncommon, *life-threatening,* or COMMON AND LIFE-THREATENING.

CV: hypotension, *cardiovascular collapse,* bradycardia.
EENT: diplopia, blurred vision, nystagmus.
GI: nausea, constipation.
GU: incontinence, urine retention, altered libido.
Respiratory: respiratory depression.
Skin: rash.
Other: physical or psychological dependence, *acute withdrawal syndrome* after sudden discontinuation in physically dependent persons, *pain, phlebitis at injection site, dysarthria, jaundice, neutropenia.*

INTERACTIONS
Cimetidine: increased sedation. Monitor patient carefully.
Digoxin: may increase serum digoxin levels and risk of toxicity. Monitor patient closely.
Ethanol, other CNS depressants: increased CNS depression. Avoid concomitant use.
Phenobarbital: increased effects of both drugs. Use together cautiously.
Smoking: increased clearance of benzodiazepines. Monitor for lack of effect.

EFFECTS ON DIAGNOSTIC TESTS
Drug may elevate liver function test results. Minor changes in EEG patterns, usually low-voltage, fast activity, may occur during and after drug therapy.

CONTRAINDICATIONS
Contraindicated in patients with hypersensitivity or angle-closure glaucoma; in patients experiencing shock, coma, or acute alcohol intoxication (parenteral form); and in children under 6 months (oral form).

NURSING CONSIDERATIONS
● Know that drug should be avoided during pregnancy, especially the first trimester.
● Use cautiously in patients with liver or renal impairment, depression, or chronic open-angle glaucoma; and in elderly and debilitated patients.
● Do not mix injectable diazepam with other drugs; also, do not store parenteral solution in plastic syringes.
● Be aware dosage should be reduced in elderly or debilitated patients, who may be more susceptible to the adverse CNS effects of the drug.
● When oral concentrate solution is used, dilute the dose just before administering.
● I.V. route is the most reliable parenteral route; I.M. administration is not recommended because absorption is variable and injection is painful.
● I.V. use: Give at rate not exceeding 5 mg/minute. When injecting, administer directly into the vein. If this is impossible, inject slowly through the infusion tubing as near to the vein insertion site as possible. Watch daily for phlebitis at injection site.
● Avoid extravasation. Do not inject into small veins.
Alert: Monitor respirations every 5 to 15 minutes and before each repeated I.V. dose. Have emergency resuscitation equipment and oxygen at bedside.
● Parenteral emulsion—a stabilized oil-in-water emulsion—should appear milky white and uniform. Avoid mixing with any other drugs or solutions, and avoid infusion sets or containers made from polyvinyl chloride. If dilution is necessary, drug may be mixed with I.V. fat emulsion. Use the admixture within 6 hours.
● Monitor periodic liver, renal, and hematopoietic function studies in patients receiving repeated or prolonged therapy, as ordered.
● Possibility of abuse and addiction exists. Do not withdraw drug abruptly after long-term use; withdrawal symptoms may occur.

☑ **PATIENT TEACHING**
● Warn patient to avoid activities that require alertness and good psychomotor coordination until CNS effects of the

drug are known.
• Tell patient to avoid alcohol while taking this drug.

hydroxyzine embonate‡
Atarax

hydroxyzine hydrochloride
Anxanil, Apo-Hydroxyzine†, Atarax*, Atozine, Durrax, E-Vista, Hydroxacen, Hyzine-50, Multipax†, Novohydroxyzin†, Quiess, Vistacon-50, Vistaject-25, Vistaject-50, Vistaquel, Vistaril, Vistazine 50

hydroxyzine pamoate
Hy-Pam, Vamate, Vistaril

Pregnancy Risk Category: NR

HOW SUPPLIED
hydroxyzine embonate‡
Capsules: 25 mg, 50 mg
hydroxyzine hydrochloride
Tablets: 10 mg, 25 mg, 50 mg, 100 mg
Capsules: 10 mg†‡, 25 mg†‡, 50 mg†‡
Syrup: 10 mg/5 ml
Injection: 25 mg/ml, 50 mg/ml
hydroxyzine pamoate
Capsules: 25 mg, 50 mg, 100 mg
Oral suspension: 25 mg/5 ml

ACTION
Unknown. A piperazine antihistamine whose action may be due to a suppression of activity in certain key regions of the subcortical area of the CNS.

ONSET, PEAK, DURATION
Onset occurs in 15 to 30 minutes with oral administration, unknown after I.M. administration. Serum levels peak about 2 hours after oral dose, unknown after I.M. administration. Effects persist for 4 to 6 hours.

INDICATIONS & DOSAGE
Anxiety—
Adults: 50 to 100 mg P.O. q.i.d.

Children under 6 years: 50 mg P.O. daily in divided doses.
Children 6 years and over: 50 to 100 mg P.O. daily in divided doses.
Preoperative and postoperative adjunctive therapy—
Adults: 25 to 100 mg I.M. q 4 to 6 hours.
Children: 1.1 mg/kg I.M. q 4 to 6 hours.
Pruritus due to allergies—
Adults: 25 mg P.O. t.i.d. or q.i.d.
Children under 6 years: 50 mg P.O. daily in divided doses.
Children 6 years and over: 50 to 100 mg P.O. daily in divided doses.
Psychiatric and emotional emergencies, including acute alcoholism—
Adults: 50 to 100 mg I.M. q 4 to 6 hours, p.r.n.
Nausea and vomiting (excluding nausea and vomiting of pregnancy)—
Adults: 25 to 100 mg I.M.
Children: 1.1 mg/kg I.M.
Prepartum and postpartum adjunctive therapy—
Adults: 25 to 100 mg I.M.

ADVERSE REACTIONS
CNS: *drowsiness,* involuntary motor activity.
GI: *dry mouth.*
Other: marked discomfort at I.M. injection site, hypersensitivity reactions (wheezing, dyspnea, chest tightness).

INTERACTIONS
Ethanol, other CNS depressants: increased CNS depression. Avoid concomitant use.

EFFECTS ON DIAGNOSTIC TESTS
Drug therapy causes falsely elevated urinary 17-hydroxycorticosteroid levels. It also may cause false-negative skin allergen tests by attenuating or inhibiting the cutaneous response to histamine.

Reactions may be *common,* uncommon, *life-threatening,* or COMMON AND LIFE-THREATENING.

CONTRAINDICATIONS

Contraindicated in patients hypersensitive to the drug, during early pregnancy, and in breast-feeding women.

NURSING CONSIDERATIONS

● Know that dosage should be reduced in elderly or debilitated patients.
● Parenteral form (hydroxyzine hydrochloride) for I.M. use only; never administer I.V. The Z-track injection method is preferred.
● Aspirate I.M. injection carefully to prevent inadvertent intravascular injection. Inject deeply into a large muscle mass.
● If the patient is taking other CNS drugs, observe for oversedation.
● Be aware that drug may cause false elevations of urine 17-hydroxycorticosteroids, depending on test method used.

☑ **PATIENT TEACHING**
● Warn patient to avoid hazardous activities that require alertness and good psychomotor coordination until CNS effects of the drug are known.
● Tell patient to avoid alcohol while taking this drug.
● To relieve dry mouth, suggest sugarless hard candy or gum.

---

lorazepam

Alzapam, Apo-Lorazepam†, Ativan, Lorazepam Intensol, Novo-Lorazem†, Nu-Loraz†

Controlled Substance Schedule IV
Pregnancy Risk Category: D

HOW SUPPLIED

Tablets: 0.5 mg, 1 mg, 2 mg
Tablets (sublingual): 0.5 mg†, 1 mg†, 2 mg†
Oral solution (concentrated): 2 mg/ml
Injection: 2 mg/ml, 4 mg/ml

ACTION

Unknown. Probably stimulates gamma-aminobutyric receptors in the ascending reticular activating system.

ONSET, PEAK, DURATION

Onset occurs within 5 minutes after I.V. administration, 15 to 30 minutes after I.M. injection, about 1 hour after oral administration. Plasma levels peak within 1 to 1½ hours after I.V. or I.M. injection, 2 hours after oral dose. Effects persist for 12 to 24 hours after oral dose, 6 to 8 hours after I.M. or I.V. dose.

INDICATIONS & DOSAGE

Anxiety—
Adults: 2 to 6 mg P.O. daily in divided doses. Maximum dosage is 10 mg daily.
Geriatric patients: initially, 1 to 2 mg/day.
Insomnia due to anxiety—
Adults: 2 to 4 mg P.O. h.s.
Preoperative sedation—
Adults: 0.05 mg/kg I.M. 2 hours before procedure. Total dosage should not exceed 4 mg. Alternatively, 2 mg I.V. total or 0.044 mg/kg I.V., whichever is smaller. Larger doses up to 0.05 mg/kg I.V., up to a total of 4 mg, may be required.

ADVERSE REACTIONS

CNS: *drowsiness,* amnesia, insomnia, agitation, *sedation,* dizziness, weakness, unsteadiness, disorientation, depression, headache.
EENT: visual disturbances.
GI: abdominal discomfort, nausea, change in appetite.
Other: *acute withdrawal syndrome* (following sudden discontinuation in physically dependent persons).

INTERACTIONS

Digoxin: may increase serum digoxin levels and risk of toxicity. Monitor patient closely.

Ethanol, other CNS depressants: increased CNS depression. Avoid concomitant use.
Smoking: increased clearance of benzodiazepines. Monitor for lack of effect.

EFFECTS ON DIAGNOSTIC TESTS
Lorazepam therapy may increase the results of liver function tests.

CONTRAINDICATIONS
Contraindicated in patients with acute angle-closure glaucoma or hypersensitivity to drug, other benzodiazepines or its vehicle (used in parenteral dosage form).

NURSING CONSIDERATIONS
● Know that drug should be avoided during pregnancy, especially the first trimester.
● Use cautiously in patients with pulmonary, renal, or hepatic impairment. Also use cautiously in elderly, acutely ill, or debilitated patients.
● Know that dosage should be reduced in elderly or debilitated patients. Preoperative I.V. dose should not exceed 2 mg in patients over age 50.
● For I.M. administration, inject deeply into a muscle mass. Don't dilute.
● **I.V. use:** Give slowly, at rate not exceeding 2 mg/minute. Dilute with an equal volume of sterile water for injection, 0.9% sodium chloride for injection, or dextrose 5% injection.
Alert: Monitor respirations every 5 to 15 minutes and before each repeated I.V. dose. Have emergency resuscitation equipment and oxygen available.
● Refrigerate parenteral form to prolong shelf life.
● Monitor liver, renal, and hematopoietic function studies periodically in patients receiving repeated or prolonged therapy, as ordered.
● Possibility of abuse and addiction exists. Do not withdraw drug abruptly after long-term use; withdrawal symptoms may occur.

☑ **PATIENT TEACHING**
● Warn patient to avoid hazardous activities that require alertness or good psychomotor coordination until CNS effects of the drug are known.
● Tell patient to avoid alcohol while taking this drug.
● As a premedication before surgery, lorazepam provides substantial preoperative amnesia. Patient teaching requires extra care to ensure adequate recall. Provide written materials or inform a family member, if possible.

---

meprobamate
Apo-Meprobamate†, Equanil**, Meprospan 200, Meprospan-400, Miltown-200, Miltown-400, Miltown-600, Probate, Trancot

Controlled Substance Schedule IV
Pregnancy Risk Category: NR

HOW SUPPLIED
Tablets: 200 mg, 400 mg, 600 mg
Capsules (sustained-release): 200 mg, 400 mg

ACTION
Unknown. It appears to act at multiple sites in the CNS.

ONSET, PEAK, DURATION
Unknown.

INDICATIONS & DOSAGE
Anxiety—
Adults: 1.2 to 1.6 g P.O. daily in three or four equally divided doses. Maximum dosage is 2.4 g daily. Alternatively, 400 to 800 mg sustained-release capsule P.O. b.i.d.
Children 6 to 12 years: 200 to 600 mg P.O. in two or three divided doses. Or, 200 mg sustained-release capsule P.O. b.i.d. Not recommended for children under 6 years.

ADVERSE REACTIONS
CNS: *drowsiness,* ataxia, dizziness, slurred speech, headache, vertigo, *seizures.*
CV: palpitations, tachycardia, hypotension, arrhythmias, syncope.
GI: nausea, vomiting, diarrhea.
Hematologic: *aplastic anemia, thrombocytopenia, agranulocytosis.*
Skin: pruritus, urticaria, erythematous maculopapular rash, *hypersensitivity reactions.*
Alert: After abrupt withdrawal of long-term therapy, severe generalized tonic-clonic seizures may occur.

INTERACTIONS
Ethanol, other CNS depressants: increased CNS depression. Avoid concomitant use.

EFFECTS ON DIAGNOSTIC TESTS
Drug therapy may falsely elevate urinary 17-ketosteroids, 17-ketogenic steroids (as determined by the Zimmerman reaction), and 17-hydroxycorticosteroid levels (as determined by the Glenn-Nelson technique).

CONTRAINDICATIONS
Contraindicated in patients hypersensitive to meprobamate or related compounds (such as carisoprodol, mebutamate, tybamate, and carbromal) and in patients with porphyria.

NURSING CONSIDERATIONS
● Know that drug should be avoided during pregnancy, especially the first trimester.
● Use cautiously in patients with impaired hepatic or renal function, seizure disorders, or suicidal tendencies.
● Be aware that dosage should be reduced in elderly or debilitated patients.
● Know that Miltown-600 is not recommended for use in children.
● Give drug with meals to reduce GI distress.
● Possibility of abuse and addiction exists with long-term use. Withdraw drug

gradually over 2 weeks to avoid withdrawal symptoms.
● Periodically monitor CBC and renal and liver function tests in patients receiving high doses, as ordered.

☑ **PATIENT TEACHING**
● Advise patient to take drug with meals and not to crush or chew sustained-release capsules but to swallow them whole.
● Warn patient to avoid hazardous activities that require alertness and good psychomotor coordination until CNS effects of the drug are known.
● Tell patient to avoid alcohol while taking this drug.
● Tell patient to report any unusual bruising or bleeding, fever, or sore throat. These symptoms may indicate serious hematologic toxicity.

---

midazolam hydrochloride
Hypnovel‡, Versed

Controlled Substance Schedule IV
Pregnancy Risk Category: D

HOW SUPPLIED
Injection: 1 mg/ml, 5 mg/ml

ACTION
Unknown. Thought to depress CNS at the limbic and subcortical levels of the brain by potentiating the effects of gamma-aminobutyric acid.

ONSET, PEAK, DURATION
Onset occurs 1½ to 5 minutes after I.V. injection, within 15 minutes of I.M. injection. Peak effect occurs rapidly after I.V. administration, within 15 to 60 minutes after I.M. injection. Effects typically persist about 2 hours, but may last up to 6 hours.

INDICATIONS & DOSAGE
Preoperative sedation (to induce sleepiness or drowsiness and relieve apprehension)—

Adults: 0.07 mg to 0.08 mg/kg I.M. approximately 1 hour before surgery.
Conscious sedation before short diagnostic or endoscopic procedures—
Adults under 60 years: initially, small dose not to exceed 2.5 mg I.V. administered slowly; repeated in 2 minutes, if needed, in small increments of initial dose over at least 2 minutes to achieve desired effect. Total dose of up to 5 mg may be used. For maintenance, additional doses to maintain desired level of sedation may be given by slow titration in increments of 25% of the dose used to first reach the sedative endpoint.
Adults 60 years and over: 1.5 mg or less over at least 2 minutes. If additional titration is needed, give at rate not exceeding 1 mg over 2 minutes. Total doses exceeding 3.5 mg are not usually necessary.
Induction of general anesthesia—
Unpremedicated adults under 55 years: 0.3 to 0.35 mg/kg I.V. over 20 to 30 seconds if patient has not received any preanesthesia medication, or 0.2 to 0.25 mg/kg I.V. over 20 to 30 seconds if patient has received preanesthesia medication. Additional increments of 25% of the initial dose may be needed to complete induction.
Unpremedicated adults 55 years and over: initially, 0.3 mg/kg. For debilitated patients, initial dose is 0.2 to 0.25 mg/kg.
Premedicated patients: 0.15 mg/kg may be sufficient.

ADVERSE REACTIONS
CNS: headache, oversedation, drowsiness, amnesia.
CV: variations in blood pressure and pulse rate.
GI: *nausea,* vomiting, *hiccups.*
Respiratory: *decreased respiratory rate,* APNEA.
Other: *pain at injection site.*

INTERACTIONS
Ethanol or other CNS depressants: may increase the risk of apnea. Avoid concomitant use. Prepare to adjust dosage of midazolam if used with opiates or other CNS depressants.

EFFECTS ON DIAGNOSTIC TESTS
None reported.

CONTRAINDICATIONS
Contraindicated in patients with hypersensitivity to drug, acute angle-closure glaucoma, shock, coma, or acute alcohol intoxication.

NURSING CONSIDERATIONS
● Use cautiously in patients with uncompensated acute illness and in elderly or debilitated patients.
Alert: Before administering, have oxygen and resuscitation equipment available in case of severe respiratory depression. Excessive dosage or rapid infusion has been associated with respiratory arrest.
● May be mixed in the same syringe with morphine sulfate, meperidine, atropine sulfate, or scopolamine.
● When injecting I.M., give deep into a large muscle mass.
● **I.V. use:** Administer slowly over at least 2 minutes, and wait at least 2 minutes when titrating doses to effect.
● When administering I.V., take care to avoid extravasation.
● Monitor blood pressure, heart rate and rhythm, respirations, airway integrity, and arterial oxygen saturation during procedure.

☑ **PATIENT TEACHING**
● Midazolam's beneficial amnestic effect diminishes a patient's recall of perioperative events. This effect requires extra caution when teaching patients. Written information, family member instruction, and follow-up contact may be required to ensure that the patient has adequate information.
● Warn patient to avoid hazardous activ-

Reactions may be *common,* uncommon, *life-threatening,* or COMMON AND LIFE-THREATENING.

ities that require alertness or good psychomotor coordination until CNS effects of the drug are known.

---

oxazepam
Alepam‡, Apo-Oxazepam†, Murelax‡, Novoxapam†, Ox-Pam†, Serax**, Serepax‡, Zapex†

Controlled Substance Schedule IV
Pregnancy Risk Category: NR

HOW SUPPLIED
Tablets: 10 mg, 15 mg, 30 mg
Capsules: 10 mg, 15 mg, 30 mg

ACTION
Unknown. Believed to stimulate gamma-aminobutyric acid receptors in the ascending reticular activating system.

ONSET, PEAK, DURATION
Onset and duration unknown. Serum levels peak in about 3 hours.

INDICATIONS & DOSAGE
Alcohol withdrawal, severe anxiety—
Adults: 15 to 30 mg P.O. t.i.d. or q.i.d.
Mild to moderate anxiety—
Adults: 10 to 15 mg P.O. t.i.d. or q.i.d.
Geriatric patients: initially 10 mg t.i.d., increased to 15 mg t.i.d. to q.i.d. p.r.n.

ADVERSE REACTIONS
CNS: *drowsiness, lethargy,* dizziness, vertigo, headache, syncope, tremor, slurred speech.
CV: edema.
GI: nausea.
Hematologic: *leukopenia* (rare).
Hepatic: *hepatic dysfunction.*
Skin: rash.
Other: altered libido.

INTERACTIONS
Digoxin: may increase serum digoxin levels and risk of toxicity. Monitor patient closely.

Ethanol, cimetidine, other CNS depressants: increased CNS depression. Avoid concomitant use.
Smoking: increased clearance of benzodiazepines. Monitor for lack of effect.

EFFECTS ON DIAGNOSTIC TESTS
Drug therapy may increase liver function test results. Changes in EEG patterns, usually low-voltage, fast activity, may occur during and after drug therapy.

CONTRAINDICATIONS
Contraindicated in patients with psychoses or hypersensitivity to drug.

NURSING CONSIDERATIONS
• Know that drug should be avoided during pregnancy, especially the first trimester.
• Use cautiously in elderly patients and in patients with a history of drug abuse or in whom a drop in blood pressure might lead to cardiac problems.
• Know that dosage should be reduced in elderly or debilitated patients.
• Monitor liver, renal, and hematopoietic function studies periodically in patients receiving repeated or prolonged therapy as ordered.
• Possibility of abuse and addiction exists. Do not stop drug abruptly; withdrawal symptoms may occur.

☑ PATIENT TEACHING
• Warn patient to avoid hazardous activities that require alertness or good psychomotor coordination until CNS effects of the drug are known.
• Tell patient to avoid alcohol while taking this drug.

---

chlorpromazine hydrochloride
clozapine
fluphenazine decanoate
fluphenazine enanthate
fluphenazine hydrochloride
haloperidol
haloperidol decanoate
haloperidol lactate
loxapine hydrochloride
loxapine succinate
mesoridazine besylate
molindone hydrochloride
olanzapine
perphenazine
pimozide
prochlorperazine
(See Chapter 51, ANTIEMETICS.)
promazine hydrochloride
risperidone
thioridazine hydrochloride
thiothixene
thiothixene hydrochloride
trifluoperazine hydrochloride

COMBINATION PRODUCTS
ETRAFON 2-10: perphenazine 2 mg and amitriptyline hydrochloride 10 mg.
ETRAFON-A: perphenazine 2 mg and amitriptyline hydrochloride 25 mg.
ETRAFON-FORTE: perphenazine 4 mg and amitriptyline hydrochloride 25 mg.
TRIAVIL 2-10, TRIAVIL 4-10, TRIAVIL 2-25 are identical to Etrafon products above. Triavil also is available as TRI-AVIL 4-25 (perphenazine 4 mg and amitriptyline hydrochloride 25 mg) and TRIAVIL 4-50 (perphenazine 4 mg and amitriptyline hydrochloride 50 mg).

---

chlorpromazine hydrochloride
Chlorpromanyl-5†, Chlorpromanyl-20†, Chlorpromanyl-40†, Largactil†‡, Novo-Chlorpromazine†, Ormazine, Thorazine, Thor-Prom

Pregnancy Risk Category: NR

HOW SUPPLIED
Tablets: 10 mg, 25 mg, 50 mg, 100 mg, 200 mg
Capsules (controlled-release): 30 mg, 75 mg, 150 mg, 200 mg, 300 mg
Oral concentrate: 30 mg/ml, 100 mg/ml
Syrup: 10 mg/5 ml
Injection: 25 mg/ml
Suppositories: 25 mg, 100 mg

ACTION
Unknown. An aliphatic phenothiazine that probably blocks postsynaptic dopamine receptors in the brain and inhibits the medullary chemoreceptor trigger zone.

ONSET, PEAK, DURATION
Onset for full antipsychotic effects, 6 weeks or longer. Onset for other effects, peak, and duration vary.

INDICATIONS & DOSAGE
Psychosis—
Adults: 25 to 75 mg P.O. daily in two to four divided doses. Dosage increased by 20 to 50 mg twice weekly until symptoms are controlled. Up to 800 mg daily may be required in some patients. Or, 25 to 50 mg I.M. q 1 to 4 hours, p.r.n. Subsequent I.M. doses should be gradually increased over several days to a maximum of 400 mg q 4 to 6 hours. Should progress to oral therapy as soon as possible.
Children 6 months and older: 0.55 mg/kg P.O. q 4 to 6 hours or I.M. q 6 to 8 hours; or 1.1 mg/kg P.R. q 6 to 8 hours. Maximum I.M. dose in children under 5 years or weighing less than

22.7 kg is 40 mg. Maximum I.M. dose in children 5 to 12 years or weighing 22.7 to 45.5 kg is 75 mg.

Nausea and vomiting—
Adults: 10 to 25 mg P.O. q 4 to 6 hours, p.r.n.; or 50 to 100 mg P.R. q 6 to 8 hours, p.r.n., or 25 mg I.M. (if no hypotension occurs), 25 to 50 mg I.M. q 3 to 4 hours, p.r.n., until vomiting stops.
Children 6 months and older: 0.55 mg/kg P.O. q 4 to 6 hours or I.M. q 6 to 8 hours; or 1.1 mg/kg P.R. q 6 to 8 hours. Maximum I.M. dose in children under 5 years or weighing less than 22.7 kg is 40 mg. Maximum I.M. dose in children 5 to 12 years or weighing 22.7 to 45.5 kg is 75 mg.

Intractable hiccups, acute intermittent porphyria—
Adults: 25 to 50 mg P.O. t.i.d. or q.i.d. If symptoms persist for 2 to 3 days, 25 to 50 mg I.M. For hiccups, if symptoms still persist 25 to 50 mg diluted in 500 to 1,000 ml of 0.9% sodium chloride solution and infused slowly with patient in supine position.

Tetanus—
Adults: 25 to 50 mg I.V. or I.M. t.i.d. or q.i.d.
Children 6 months or older: 0.55 mg/kg I.M. or I.V. q 6 to 8 hours. Maximum parenteral dosage in children weighing less than 22.7 kg. is 40 mg daily; for children weighing 22.7 to 45.5 kg is 75 mg, except in severe cases.

Surgery—
Adults: preoperatively, 25 to 50 mg P.O. 2 to 3 hours before surgery or 12.5 to 25 mg I.M. 1 to 2 hours before surgery; during surgery, 12.5 mg I.M., repeated in 30 minutes if needed, or fractional 2-mg doses I.V. at 2-minute intervals up to a maximum dose of 25 mg; postoperatively, 10 to 25 mg P.O. q 4 to 6 hours or 12.5 to 25 mg I.M., repeated in 1 hour, if needed.
Children 6 months and older: preoperatively, 0.55 mg/kg P.O. 2 to 3 hours before surgery or I.M. 1 to 2 hours be-

fore surgery; during surgery, 0.275 mg/kg I.M., repeated in 30 minutes if needed, or fractional 1 mg doses I.V. at 2-minute intervals up to a total of 0.275 mg/kg; may repeat fractional I.V. regimen in 30 minutes if needed; postoperatively, 0.55 mg/kg P.O. or I.M. q 4 to 6 hours (oral dose) or 1 hour (I.M. dose), if needed, and hypotension does not occur.

ADVERSE REACTIONS
CNS: *extrapyramidal reactions,* drowsiness, *sedation, seizures, tardive dyskinesia,* pseudoparkinsonism, dizziness.
CV: *orthostatic hypotension,* tachycardia, ECG changes.
EENT: ocular changes, blurred vision, nasal congestion.
GI: *dry mouth, constipation,* nausea.
GU: *urine retention,* menstrual irregularities, gynecomastia, inhibited ejaculation, priapism.
Hematologic: leukopenia, *agranulocytosis,* eosinophilia, hemolytic anemia, *aplastic anemia, thrombocytopenia.*
Hepatic: jaundice, abnormal liver function test results.
Skin: *mild photosensitivity,* allergic reactions, *I.M. injection site pain,* sterile abscess, skin pigmentation.
Other: *neuroleptic malignant syndrome.*
After abrupt withdrawal of long-term therapy: gastritis, nausea, vomiting, dizziness, tremor.

INTERACTIONS
Antacids: inhibited absorption of oral phenothiazines. Separate antacid and phenothiazine doses by at least 2 hours.
Anticholinergics (including antidepressants and antiparkinsonian agents): increased anticholinergic activity, aggravated parkinsonian symptoms. Use with caution.
Anticonvulsants: may lower seizure threshold.

Barbiturates, lithium: may decrease phenothiazine effect. Observe patient.
Centrally acting antihypertensives: decreased antihypertensive effect. Monitor blood pressure.
Ethanol, other CNS depressants: increased CNS depression. Avoid concomitant use.
Insulin, electroconvulsive therapy: may precipitate severe reactions.
Propranolol: increased levels of both propranolol and chlorpromazine. Monitor patient closely.
Warfarin: decreased effect of oral anticoagulants. Monitor PT.

EFFECTS ON DIAGNOSTIC TESTS
Drug causes false-positive test results for urinary porphyrins, urobilinogen, amylase, and 5-hydroxyindoleacetic acid (5-HIAA) because of darkening of urine by metabolites; it also causes false-positive results in urine pregnancy tests using human chorionic gonadotropin. Chlorpromazine elevates tests for liver function and protein-bound iodine and causes quinidine-like ECG effects.

CONTRAINDICATIONS
Contraindicated in patients with hypersensitivity or in patients experiencing CNS depression, bone marrow suppression, subcortical damage, and coma.

NURSING CONSIDERATIONS
● Use cautiously in elderly or debilitated patients and in patients with hepatic or renal disease; severe CV disease (may cause sudden drop in blood pressure); exposure to extreme heat or cold (including antipyretic therapy), to organophosphate insecticides; respiratory disorders; hypocalcemia; glaucoma; or prostatic hyperplasia.
● Use cautiously in acutely ill or dehydrated children.
● Obtain baseline measures of blood pressure before starting therapy and monitor regularly. Watch for orthostat-

ic hypotension, especially with parenteral administration. Monitor blood pressure before and after I.M. administration. Keep patient supine for 1 hour afterward and have him get up slowly.
● **I.V. use:** For direct injection, drug may be diluted with 0.9% sodium chloride for injection and administered into a large vein or through the tubing of a free-flowing I.V. solution. Do not exceed 1 mg/minute for adults or 0.5 mg/minute for children. Drug also may be given as an intermittent I.V. infusion; dilute with 50 or 100 ml of a compatible solution and infuse over 30 minutes. Chlorpromazine is compatible with most common I.V. solutions, including D_5W, Ringer's injection, lactated Ringer's injection, and 0.9% sodium chloride for injection.
● Slight yellowing of injection or concentrate is common and does not affect potency. Discard markedly discolored solutions.
● Give deep I.M. only in upper outer quadrant of buttocks. Massage slowly afterward to prevent sterile abscess. Injection stings.
● Wear gloves when preparing solutions, and prevent any contact with skin and clothing. Oral liquid and parenteral forms can cause contact dermatitis.
● Protect liquid concentrate from light. Dilute with fruit juice, milk, or semisolid food just before administration.
● Monitor patient for tardive dyskinesia, which may occur after prolonged use. It may not appear until months or years later and may disappear spontaneously or persist for life, despite discontinuation of drug.
● Watch for symptoms of neuroleptic malignant syndrome. It is rare, but frequently fatal. It is not necessarily related to length of drug use or type of neuroleptic, but over 60% of affected patients are men.
● Monitor therapy with weekly bilirubin tests during first month; periodic blood tests (CBC and liver function);

Reactions may be *common,* uncommon, *life-threatening,* or COMMON AND LIFE-THREATENING.

and ophthalmic tests (long-term use) as ordered.
● Do not withdraw drug abruptly unless required by severe adverse reactions.
● Withhold dose and notify doctor if patient develops jaundice, symptoms of blood dyscrasia (fever, sore throat, infection, cellulitis, weakness), persistent extrapyramidal reactions (longer than a few hours), or any such reaction in pregnancy or in children.
● Know that acute dystonic reactions may be treated with diphenhydramine.

☑ **PATIENT TEACHING**
● Warn patient to avoid activities that require alertness or good psychomotor coordination until CNS effects of the drug are known. Drowsiness and dizziness usually subside after first few weeks.
● Tell patient to avoid alcohol while taking this drug.
● Have patient report urine retention or constipation.
● Tell patient to use sunblock and to wear protective clothing to avoid photosensitivity reactions. Chlorpromazine causes higher incidence of photosensitivity than any other drug in its class.
● Tell patient to relieve dry mouth with sugarless gum or hard candy.

clozapine
Clozaril

Pregnancy Risk Category: B

HOW SUPPLIED
Tablets: 25 mg, 100 mg

ACTION
Unknown. Binds to dopaminergic receptors (both D-1 and D-2) within the limbic system of the CNS and may interfere with adrenergic, cholinergic, histaminergic, and serotoninergic receptors.

ONSET, PEAK, DURATION
Onset unknown. Serum levels peak in about 2½ hours. Effects persist for 4 to 12 hours.

INDICATIONS & DOSAGE
Schizophrenia in severely ill patients unresponsive to other therapies—
Adults: initially, 12.5 mg P.O. once daily or b.i.d., titrated upward at 25 to 50 mg daily (if tolerated) to 300 to 450 mg daily by the end of 2 weeks. Individual dosage is based on clinical response, patient tolerance, and adverse reactions. Subsequent dosage should not be increased more than once or twice weekly, and should not exceed 100 mg. Many patients respond to dosages of 300 to 600 mg daily, but some may require as much as 900 mg daily. Do not exceed 900 mg daily.

ADVERSE REACTIONS
CNS: *drowsiness, sedation, seizures, dizziness,* syncope, vertigo, headache, tremor, disturbed sleep or nightmares, restlessness, hypokinesia or akinesia, agitation, rigidity, hakathisia, confusion, fatigue, insomnia, hyperkinesia, weakness, lethargy, ataxia, slurred speech, depression, myoclonus, anxiety.
CV: *tachycardia, hypotension,* hypertension, chest pain, ECG changes, orthostatic hypotension.
GI: *dry mouth, constipation,* nausea, vomiting, *excessive salivation,* heartburn, constipation, diarrhea.
GU: urinary abnormalities (urinary frequency or urgency, urine retention), incontinence, abnormal ejaculation.
Hematologic: *leukopenia, agranulocytosis.*
Skin: rash.
Other: fever, muscle pain or spasm, muscle weakness, weight gain, visual disturbances, diaphoresis.
After abrupt withdrawal of long-term therapy: possible abrupt recurrence of psychotic symptoms. Monitor closely.

---

*Liquid contains alcohol.   **May contain tartrazine.   †Canada only.   ‡Australia only.   ◊OTC.

INTERACTIONS

Anticholinergics: may potentiate anticholinergic effects of clozapine. Avoid concomitant use. Monitor blood pressure.

Antihypertensives: may potentiate hypotensive effects. Monitor blood pressure.

Bone marrow suppressants: may increase bone marrow toxicity. Don't use together.

Psychoactive drugs: may produce additive effects. Use together cautiously.

Warfarin, digoxin, and other highly protein-bound drugs: may increase serum levels of these drugs. Monitor closely for adverse reactions.

EFFECTS ON DIAGNOSTIC TESTS

Toxic effects of the drug may be evidenced by depressed blood counts.

CONTRAINDICATIONS

Contraindicated in patients with uncontrolled epilepsy, a history of clozapine-induced agranulocytosis; in patients with a WBC count below 3,500/mm^3; in patients with severe CNS depression or coma; in patients taking other drugs that suppress bone marrow function; and in those with myelosuppressive disorders.

NURSING CONSIDERATIONS

● Use cautiously in patients with prostatic hyperplasia or angle-closure glaucoma because clozapine has potent anticholinergic effects and also in patients with hepatic, renal, or cardiac disease or those receiving general anesthesia.

Alert: Clozapine carries significant risk of agranulocytosis. If possible, patients should receive at least two trials of drug therapy with a standard antipsychotic before clozapine therapy is initiated. Baseline WBC and differential counts are required before therapy. Monitor WBC counts weekly for at least 4 weeks after clozapine therapy is discontinued, as ordered.

● When administering clozapine, ensure that WBC counts and blood tests are performed weekly. Also ensure that no more than a 1-week supply of drug is dispensed.

● If WBC count drops below 3,500/mm^3 after therapy is initiated or if it exhibits a substantial drop from baseline, monitor patient closely for signs of infection. If WBC count is 3,000 to 3,500/mm^3 and granulocyte count is above 1,500/mm^3, perform WBC and differential count twice weekly. If WBC count drops below 3,000/mm^3 and granulocyte count drops below 1,500/mm^3, interrupt therapy, notify doctor, and monitor the patient for signs of infection. Be aware that therapy may be restarted cautiously if WBC count returns to above 3,000/mm^3 and granulocyte count returns above 1,500/mm^3. Continue monitoring of WBC and differential counts twice weekly until WBC count exceeds 3,500/mm^3, as ordered.

● If the WBC count drops below 2,000/mm^3 and granulocyte count drops below 1,000/mm^3, the patient may require protective isolation. If the patient develops infection, prepare cultures according to institutional policy and administer antibiotics, as ordered. Some clinicians may perform bone marrow aspiration to assess bone marrow function. Know that future clozapine therapy is contraindicated in such patients.

● Be aware that seizures may occur, especially in patients receiving high doses.

● Some patients experience transient fevers (temperature over 100.4° F [38° C]), especially in the first 3 weeks of therapy. Monitor patients closely.

● If clozapine therapy must be discontinued, the drug usually is withdrawn gradually (over a 1- to 2-week period). However, changes in the patient's medical condition (including the development of leukopenia) may require abrupt discontinuation of the drug.

Monitor closely for the recurrence of psychotic symptoms.

• If therapy is reinstated in patients withdrawn from the drug, follow usual guidelines for dosage increase. However, reexposure of the patient to this drug may increase the severity and risk of adverse reactions. If therapy was terminated because WBC counts were below 2,000/mm^3 or granulocyte counts below 1,000/mm^3, do not expect the drug to be continued.

☑ PATIENT TEACHING
• Warn patient about the risk of agranulocytosis. Tell patient that the drug is available only through a special monitoring program that requires weekly blood tests to monitor for agranulocytosis. Advise him to report flulike symptoms, fever, sore throat, lethargy, malaise, or other signs of infection.
• Warn patient to avoid hazardous activities that require alertness and good psychomotor coordination while taking this drug.
• Tell patient to check with the doctor before taking OTC drugs or alcohol.
• Tell patient to rise slowly to avoid orthostatic hypotension.
• Recommend ice chips or sugarless candy or gum to help relieve dry mouth.

---

fluphenazine decanoate
Modecate†‡, Modecate Concentrate†, Prolixin Decanoate

fluphenazine enanthate
Moditen Enanthate†, Prolixin Enanthate

fluphenazine hydrochloride
Anatensol‡*, Apo-Fluphenazine†, Moditen HCl†, Moditen HCl-H.P.†, Permitil* **, Permitil Concentrate, Prolixin* **, Prolixin Concentrate

Pregnancy Risk Category: NR

HOW SUPPLIED
fluphenazine decanoate
Depot injection: 25 mg/ml
fluphenazine enanthate
Depot injection: 25 mg/ml
fluphenazine hydrochloride
Tablets: 1 mg, 2.5 mg, 5 mg, 10 mg
Oral concentrate: 5 mg/ml (contains 1% alcohol)
Elixir: 2.5 mg/5 ml (with 14% alcohol)
I.M. injection: 2.5 mg/ml

ACTION
Unknown. A piperazine phenothiazine that probably blocks postsynaptic dopamine receptors in the brain.

ONSET, PEAK, DURATION
Following administration of fluphenazine hydrochloride, onset occurs within 1 hour although full therapeutic effect may take up to several weeks. Serum levels peak within 1½ to 2 hours after I.M. administration; ½ hour after oral administration. Effects persist for 6 to 8 hours. Following I.M. administration of fluphenazine decanoate or enanthate, onset of action occurs within 24 to 72 hours and duration of action is 1 to 6 weeks.

INDICATIONS & DOSAGE
Psychotic disorders—
Adults: initially, 2.5 to 10 mg hydrochloride P.O. daily in divided doses q 6 to 8 hours; may increase cautiously to 20 mg. Higher doses (50 to 100 mg) have been given. Maintenance dosage is 1 to 5 mg P.O. daily. I.M. doses are one-third to one-half of oral doses. Usual I.M. dose is 1.25 mg. Use dosages above 10 mg/day with caution. Use lower dosages for elderly patients (1 to 2.5 mg daily).

Alternatively, 12.5 to 25 mg of long-acting esters (decanoate or enanthate) I.M. or S.C. q 1 to 6 weeks; maintenance dosage is 25 to 100 mg, p.r.n.

ADVERSE REACTIONS

CNS: *extrapyramidal reactions, tardive dyskinesia,* sedation, pseudoparkinsonism, EEG changes, drowsiness, *seizures,* dizziness.

CV: *orthostatic hypotension,* tachycardia, ECG changes.

EENT: ocular changes, *blurred vision,* nasal congestion.

GI: *dry mouth, constipation.*

GU: *urine retention,* dark urine, menstrual irregularities, gynecomastia, inhibited ejaculation.

Hematologic: leukopenia, *agranulocytosis,* eosinophilia, hemolytic anemia, *aplastic anemia, thrombocytopenia.*

Hepatic: cholestatic jaundice, abnormal liver function test results.

Skin: *mild photosensitivity,* allergic reactions.

Other: weight gain; increased appetite; rarely, *neuroleptic malignant syndrome.*

After abrupt withdrawal of long-term therapy: gastritis, nausea, vomiting, dizziness, tremor, feeling of warmth or cold, diaphoresis, tachycardia, headache, insomnia.

INTERACTIONS

Antacids: inhibited absorption of oral phenothiazines. Separate antacid and phenothiazine doses by at least 2 hours.

Anticholinergics: increased anticholinergic effects. Avoid concomitant use.

Barbiturates, lithium: may decrease phenothiazine effect. Observe patient.

Centrally acting antihypertensives: decreased antihypertensive effect. Monitor blood pressure.

Ethanol, other CNS depressants: increased CNS depression. Avoid concomitant use.

EFFECTS ON DIAGNOSTIC TESTS

Drug causes false-positive test results for urinary porphyrins, urobilinogen, amylase, and 5-hydroxyindoleacetic acid (5-HIAA) because of darkening of urine by metabolites; it also causes false-positive urine pregnancy test results using human chorionic gonadotropin. Fluphenazine elevates test results for liver enzymes and protein-bound iodine and causes quinidine-like ECG effects.

CONTRAINDICATIONS

Contraindicated in patients with hypersensitivity or in patients experiencing coma, CNS depression, bone marrow suppression or other blood dyscrasia, subcortical damage, or liver damage.

NURSING CONSIDERATIONS

● Use cautiously in elderly or debilitated patients and in those with pheochromocytoma; severe CV disease (may cause sudden drop in blood pressure); peptic ulcer; exposure to extreme heat or cold (including antipyretic therapy) or phosphorus insecticides; respiratory disorder; hypocalcemia; seizure disorder (may lower seizure threshold); severe reactions to insulin or electroconvulsive therapy; mitral insufficiency; glaucoma; or prostatic hyperplasia. Use parenteral form cautiously in asthmatic patients and patients allergic to sulfites.

● Prolixin Concentrate and Permitil Concentrate are 10 times more concentrated than Prolixin elixir (5 mg/ml versus 0.5 mg/ml). Check dosage order carefully.

● Dilute liquid concentrate with water, fruit juice, milk, or semisolid food just before administration.

● For long-acting forms (decanoate and enanthate), which are oil preparations, use a dry needle of at least 21G. Allow 24 to 96 hours for onset of action. Note and report adverse reactions in patients taking these drug forms.

● Oral liquid and parenteral forms can cause contact dermatitis. Wear gloves when preparing solutions, and prevent contact with skin and clothing.

● Protect medication from light. Slight yellowing of injection or concentrate is

---

common and does not affect potency. Discard markedly discolored solutions.

• Monitor patient for tardive dyskinesia, which may occur after prolonged use. It may not appear until months or years later and disappear spontaneously or persist for life, despite discontinuation of drug.

• Watch patient for neuroleptic malignant syndrome. It is rare, but frequently fatal. It is not necessarily related to length of drug use or type of neuroleptic, but over 60% of affected patients are men.

• Monitor therapy with weekly bilirubin tests during first month; periodic blood tests (CBC and liver function); and periodic renal function and ophthalmic tests (long-term use) as ordered.

• Do not withdraw drug abruptly unless serious adverse reactions occur.

• Withhold dose and notify doctor if patient develops symptoms of blood dyscrasia (fever, sore throat, infection, cellulitis, weakness), persistent extrapyramidal reactions (longer than a few hours) especially in pregnant patients or in children.

• Acute dystonic reactions may be treated with diphenhydramine.

☑ **PATIENT TEACHING**
• Warn patient to avoid activities that require alertness and good psychomotor coordination until CNS effects of the drug are known. Drowsiness and dizziness usually subside after first few weeks.

• Tell patient to avoid alcohol while taking this drug.

• Tell patient to relieve dry mouth with sugarless gum or hard candy.

• Have patient report urine retention or constipation.

• Tell patient to use sunblock and to wear protective clothing to avoid photosensitivity reactions.

• Tell patient that drug may discolor urine.

haloperidol
Apo-Haloperidol†, Haldol**, Novo-Peridol†, Peridol†, Serenace‡

haloperidol decanoate
Haldol Decanoate, Haldol LA†

haloperidol lactate
Haldol

Pregnancy Risk Category: C

HOW SUPPLIED
haloperidol
Tablets: 0.5 mg, 1 mg, 2 mg, 5 mg, 10 mg, 20 mg
haloperidol decanoate
Injection: 50 mg/ml, 100 mg/ml
haloperidol lactate
Oral concentrate: 2 mg/ml
Injection: 5 mg/ml

ACTION
Unknown. A butyrophenone that probably blocks postsynaptic dopamine receptors in the brain.

ONSET, PEAK, DURATION
Onset unknown. Serum levels peak in 3 to 6 hours with oral dose, 10 to 20 minutes with I.M. injection (lactate), or 3 to 9 days with long-acting I.M. injection (decanoate). Duration unknown.

INDICATIONS & DOSAGE
Psychotic disorders—
Adults and children 12 and older: dosage varies for each patient. Initial range, 0.5 to 5 mg P.O. b.i.d. or t.i.d.; or 2 to 5 mg I.M. q 4 to 8 hours although hourly administration may be needed until control obtained. Maximum dosage is 100 mg P.O. daily.
Children 3 to 12 years: 0.05 mg/kg to 0.15 mg/kg P.O. daily. Severely disturbed children may require higher doses.
Chronic psychotic patients who require prolonged therapy—

Adults: 50 to 100 mg I.M. haloperidol decanoate q 4 weeks.
Nonpsychotic behavior disorders—
Children 3 to 12 years: 0.05 mg/kg P.O. daily. Maximum daily dosage is 6 mg.
Tourette syndrome—
Adults: 0.5 to 5 mg P.O. b.i.d. or t.i.d. or p.r.n.
Children 3 to 12 years: 0.05 to 0.075 mg/kg P.O. daily in two or three divided doses.

ADVERSE REACTIONS
CNS: *severe extrapyramidal reactions, tardive dyskinesia,* sedation, drowsiness, lethargy, headache, insomnia, confusion, vertigo, *seizures.*
CV: tachycardia, hypotension, hypertension, ECG changes.
EENT: *blurred vision.*
GI: dry mouth, anorexia, constipation, diarrhea, nausea, vomiting, dyspepsia.
GU: urine retention, menstrual irregularities, gynecomastia, priapism.
Hematologic: leukopenia and leukocytosis.
Skin: rash and other skin reactions, diaphoresis.
Other: rarely, *neuroleptic malignant syndrome, altered liver function tests, jaundice.*

INTERACTIONS
Ethanol, other CNS depressants: increased CNS depression. Avoid concomitant use.
Lithium: lethargy and confusion after high doses. Monitor the patient.
Methyldopa: may cause symptoms of dementia or psychosis. Monitor the patient.

EFFECTS ON DIAGNOSTIC TESTS
None reported.

CONTRAINDICATIONS
Contraindicated in patients with hypersensitivity or in patients experiencing parkinsonism, coma, or CNS depression.

NURSING CONSIDERATIONS
● Use cautiously in elderly and debilitated patients; in patients with history of seizures or EEG abnormalities, severe CV disorders, allergies, glaucoma, or urine retention; and in conjunction with anticonvulsant, anticoagulant, antiparkinsonian, or lithium medications.
● Know that elderly patients usually require lower initial doses and a more gradual dosage titration.
Alert: Do not administer the decanoate form I.V.
● When changing from tablets to decanoate injection, know that patient should be given 10 to 15 times the oral dose once a month (maximum 100 mg).
● Protect medication from light. Slight yellowing of injection or concentrate is common and does not affect potency. Discard markedly discolored solutions.
● Do not withdraw drug abruptly unless required by severe adverse reactions.
● Monitor patient for tardive dyskinesia, which may occur after prolonged use. It may not appear until months or years later and disappear spontaneously or persist for life, despite discontinuation of drug.
● Watch patient for neuroleptic malignant syndrome. It is rare, but frequently fatal. It is not necessarily related to length of drug use or type of neuroleptic, but over 60% of affected patients are men.
● Know that acute dystonic reactions may be treated with diphenhydramine.

☑ PATIENT TEACHING
● Drug is the least sedating of the antipsychotics, but warn the patient to avoid activities that require alertness and good psychomotor coordination until CNS effects of the drug are known. Drowsiness and dizziness usually subside after a few weeks.
● Tell the patient to avoid alcohol while taking this drug.

Reactions may be *common,* uncommon, *life-threatening,* or COMMON AND LIFE-THREATENING.

• Tell the patient to relieve dry mouth with sugarless gum or hard candy.

---

loxapine hydrochloride
Loxapac†, Loxitane C, Loxitane IM

loxapine succinate
Loxapac†, Loxitane

Pregnancy Risk Category: NR

HOW SUPPLIED
loxapine hydrochloride
Oral concentrate: 25 mg/ml
Injection: 50 mg/ml
loxapine succinate
Capsules: 5 mg, 10 mg, 25 mg, 50 mg
Tablets: 5 mg†, 10 mg†, 25 mg†, 50 mg†

ACTION
Unknown. A dibenzoxazepine that probably blocks postsynaptic dopamine receptors in the brain.

ONSET, PEAK, DURATION
Onset of action occurs in 30 minutes. Serum levels peak in 1.5 to 3 hours. Effects persist up to 12 hours.

INDICATIONS & DOSAGE
Psychotic disorders—
Adults: 10 mg P.O. b.i.d. to q.i.d., rapidly increasing to 60 to 100 mg P.O. daily for most patients; dosage varies from patient to patient. If patient is unable to take oral dose, 12.5 to 50 mg I.M. q 4 to 6 hours or longer, both dose and interval depending on patient response. Dosages greater than 250 mg/day are not recommended.

ADVERSE REACTIONS
CNS: *extrapyramidal reactions, sedation,* drowsiness, **seizures,** numbness, confusion, syncope, *tardive dyskinesia,* pseudoparkinsonism, EEG changes, dizziness.
CV: *orthostatic hypotension,* tachycardia, ECG changes, hypertension.

EENT: *blurred vision,* nasal congestion.
GI: *dry mouth, constipation,* nausea, vomiting, paralytic ileus.
GU: *urine retention,* menstrual irregularities, gynecomastia.
Hematologic: leukopenia, *agranulocytosis, thrombocytopenia.*
Skin: *mild photosensitivity,* allergic reactions, rash, pruritus.
Other: weight gain, *neuroleptic malignant syndrome,* jaundice.

INTERACTIONS
Ethanol, other CNS depressants: increased CNS depression. Avoid concomitant use.

EFFECTS ON DIAGNOSTIC TESTS
Loxapine causes false-positive test results for urinary porphyrins, urobilinogen, amylase. and 5-hydroxyindoleacetic acid (5-HIAA) because of darkening of urine by metabolites; it also causes false-positive urine pregnancy test results using human chorionic gonadotropin.

Drug elevates test results for liver enzymes and protein-bound iodine and causes quinidine-like effects on the ECG.

CONTRAINDICATIONS
Contraindicated in patients with hypersensitivity to dibenzoxazepines and in patients experiencing coma, severe CNS depression, or drug-induced depressed states.

NURSING CONSIDERATIONS
• Use with extreme caution in patients with seizure disorder, CV disorder, glaucoma, and history of urine retention.
• Obtain baseline measures of blood pressure before starting therapy and monitor regularly.
• Dilute liquid concentrate with orange or grapefruit juice just before giving.

---

*Liquid contains alcohol.   **May contain tartrazine.   †Canada only.   ‡Australia only.   ◇OTC.

• Monitor patient for tardive dyskinesia, which may occur after prolonged use. It may not appear until months or years later and disappear spontaneously or persist for life, despite discontinuation of drug.
• Monitor patient for neuroleptic malignant syndrome. It is rare, but frequently fatal. It is not necessarily related to length of drug use or type of neuroleptic, but over 60% of affected patients are men.
• Know that acute dystonic reactions may be treated with diphenhydramine.

☑ **PATIENT TEACHING**
• Warn patient to avoid activities that require alertness and good psychomotor coordination until CNS effects of the drug are known. Drowsiness and dizziness usually subside after first few weeks.
• Tell patient to avoid alcohol while taking this drug.
• Advise patient to get up slowly to avoid orthostatic hypotension.
• Tell patient to relieve dry mouth with sugarless gum or hard candy.
• Tell patient that periodic eye examinations are recommended.

---

mesoridazine besylate
Serentil* **, Serentil Concentrate

Pregnancy Risk Category: NR

HOW SUPPLIED
Tablets: 10 mg, 25 mg, 50 mg, 100 mg
Oral concentrate: 25 mg/ml (0.6% alcohol)
Injection: 25 mg/ml

ACTION
Unknown. A piperidine phenothiazine and the major sulfoxide metabolite of thioridazine that probably blocks postsynaptic dopamine receptors in the brain.

ONSET, PEAK, DURATION
Onset of antipsychotic effect is gradual (up to several weeks) and varies among patients. Peak and duration not clearly defined.

INDICATIONS & DOSAGE
Alcoholism—
Adults and children over 12 years: 25 mg P.O. b.i.d. up to maximum of 200 mg daily.
Behavioral problems associated with chronic organic mental syndrome—
Adults and children over 12 years: 25 mg P.O. t.i.d. up to maximum of 300 mg daily.
Psychoneurotic manifestations (anxiety)—
Adults and children over 12 years: 10 mg P.O. t.i.d. up to maximum of 150 mg daily.
Schizophrenia—
Adults and children over 12 years: initially, 50 mg P.O. t.i.d. or 25 mg I.M. repeated in 30 to 60 minutes, p.r.n. Maximum oral dosage is 400 mg daily; maximum I.M. dosage is 200 mg.

ADVERSE REACTIONS
CNS: extrapyramidal reactions, *tardive dyskinesia, sedation,* drowsiness, tremor, rigidity, weakness, EEG changes, dizziness.
CV: *hypotension,* tachycardia, ECG changes.
EENT: *ocular changes, blurred vision,* retinitis pigmentosa, nasal congestion.
GI: *dry mouth, constipation,* nausea, vomiting.
GU: *urine retention,* menstrual irregularities, gynecomastia, inhibited ejaculation.
Hematologic: leukopenia, *agranulocytosis, aplastic anemia,* eosinophilia, *thrombocytopenia.*
Hepatic: jaundice, abnormal liver function test results.

Reactions may be *common,* uncommon, *life-threatening,* or COMMON AND LIFE-THREATENING.

Skin: *mild photosensitivity,* allergic reactions, pain at I.M. injection site, sterile abscess, rash.

Other: weight gain, *neuroleptic malignant syndrome.*

After abrupt withdrawal of long-term therapy: gastritis, nausea, vomiting, dizziness, tremor, feeling of warmth or cold, diaphoresis, tachycardia, headache, insomnia.

INTERACTIONS

Antacids: inhibited absorption of oral phenothiazines. Separate antacid and phenothiazine doses by at least 2 hours.

Anticholinergics: may increase anticholinergic effects. Use together cautiously.

Barbiturates: may decrease phenothiazine effect. Observe patient.

Ethanol: increased CNS depression. Avoid concomitant use.

Other CNS depressants: increased CNS depression. Use together cautiously.

EFFECTS ON DIAGNOSTIC TESTS

Drug causes false-positive test results for urinary porphyrins, urobilinogen, amylase, and 5-hydroxyindoleacetic acid (5-HIAA) because of darkening of urine by metabolites; it also causes false-positive urine pregnancy test results using human chorionic gonadotropin.

Mesoridazine elevates tests for liver function and protein-bound iodine and causes quinidine-like effects on the ECG.

CONTRAINDICATIONS

Contraindicated in patients with hypersensitivity to the drug or experiencing severe CNS depression or comatose states.

NURSING CONSIDERATIONS

● Obtain baseline measures of blood pressure before starting therapy and monitor regularly. Watch for orthostat-ic hypotension, especially with parenteral administration.

● Oral liquid and parenteral forms may cause contact dermatitis. Wear gloves when preparing solutions, and prevent contact with skin and clothing.

● Give deep I.M. only in upper outer quadrant of buttocks. Massage slowly afterward to prevent sterile abscess. Injection may sting.

● Protect medication from light. Slight yellowing of injection or concentrate is common and does not affect potency. Discard markedly discolored solutions.

● Monitor patient for tardive dyskinesia, which may occur after prolonged use. It may not appear until months or years later and disappear spontaneously or persist for life, despite discontinuation of drug.

● Assess patient for neuroleptic malignant syndrome. It is rare, but frequently fatal. It is not necessarily related to length of drug use or type of neuroleptic, but over 60% of affected patients are men.

● Withhold dose and notify the doctor if patient develops jaundice, symptoms of blood dyscrasia (fever, sore throat, infection, cellulitis, weakness), persistent extrapyramidal reactions (longer than a few hours), especially in pregnant patients or in children.

● Monitor therapy with weekly bilirubin tests during first month; periodic blood tests (CBC and liver function); and ophthalmic tests (long-term use), as ordered.

● Know that acute dystonic reactions may be treated with diphenhydramine.

● Do not withdraw drug abruptly unless required by severe adverse reactions.

☑ PATIENT TEACHING

● Warn patient to avoid activities that require alertness and good psychomotor coordination until CNS effects of the drug are known. Drowsiness and dizziness usually subside after a few weeks.

---

*Liquid contains alcohol.   **May contain tartrazine.   †Canada only.   ‡Australia only.   ◇ OTC.

• Advise patient to change position slowly.

• Tell patient to avoid alcohol while taking this drug.

• Have patient report urine retention or constipation.

• Tell patient that drug may discolor urine.

• Instruct patient to relieve dry mouth with sugarless gum or hard candy.

• Tell patient to use sunblock and to wear protective clothing to avoid photosensitivity reactions.

---

molindone hydrochloride
Moban

Pregnancy Risk Category: NR

HOW SUPPLIED
Tablets: 5 mg, 10 mg, 25 mg, 50 mg, 100 mg
Oral solution: 20 mg/ml

ACTION
Unknown. A dihydroindolone that probably blocks postsynaptic dopamine receptors in the brain.

ONSET, PEAK, DURATION
Onset unknown but thought to take several weeks. Serum levels peak in 1.5 hours. Effects persist for 24 to 36 hours.

INDICATIONS & DOSAGE
Psychotic disorders—
Adults: initially, 50 to 75 mg P.O. daily, then increased to 100 to 225 mg/day in 3 or 4 days. Maintenance dosage as follows: mild severity—5 to 15 mg P.O. t.i.d. to q.i.d.; moderate severity—10 to 25 mg P.O. t.i.d. or q.i.d.; or severe severity—225 mg/day P.O.

ADVERSE REACTIONS
CNS: *extrapyramidal reactions, tardive dyskinesia, sedation,* drowsiness, depression, euphoria, pseudoparkinsonism, EEG changes, dizziness.
CV: *orthostatic hypotension,* tachycardia, ECG changes.
EENT: *blurred vision.*
GI: *dry mouth, constipation,* nausea.
GU: *urine retention,* menstrual irregularities, gynecomastia, inhibited ejaculation.
Hematologic: leukopenia, leukocytosis.
Hepatic: jaundice, abnormal liver function test results.
Skin: *mild photosensitivity,* allergic reactions.
Other: rarely, ***neuroleptic malignant syndrome.***

INTERACTIONS
Ethanol, other CNS depressants: increased CNS depression. Avoid concomitant use.

EFFECTS ON DIAGNOSTIC TESTS
Drug causes false-positive results in urine pregnancy tests using human chorionic gonadotropin and additive potential for causing convulsions with metrizamide myelography.

Molindone elevates levels of liver enzymes (AST, ALT), free fatty acids, and BUN; drug may alter WBC counts and may increase or decrease serum glucose levels.

CONTRAINDICATIONS
Contraindicated in patients with hypersensitivity to drug or experiencing coma or severe CNS depression.

NURSING CONSIDERATIONS
• Use cautiously when increased physical activity would be harmful because this agent increases activity and in patients subject to seizures (may lower seizure threshold).

• Monitor patient for tardive dyskinesia, which may occur after prolonged use. It may not appear until months or years later and may disappear sponta-

---

neously or persist for life, despite discontinuation of drug.
● Assess patient for neuroleptic malignant syndrome. It is rare, but frequently fatal. It is not necessarily related to length of drug use or type of neuroleptic, but over 60% of affected patients are men.
● Know that acute dystonic reactions may be treated with diphenhydramine.

☑ **PATIENT TEACHING**
● Warn patient to avoid activities that require alertness or good psychomotor coordination until CNS effects of the drug are known. Drowsiness and dizziness usually subside after first few weeks.
● Tell patient to avoid alcohol while taking this drug.
● Tell patient to relieve dry mouth with sugarless gum or hard candy.

▼ *NEW DRUG*

olanzapine
Zyprexa

Pregnancy Risk Category: C

HOW SUPPLIED
Tablets: 5 mg, 7.5 mg, 10 mg

ACTION
Unknown. Binds to dopamine and serotonin receptors; may interfere with adrenergic, cholinergic, and histaminergic receptors.

ONSET, PEAK, DURATION
Onset and duration unknown. Plasma levels peak in 6 hours. May take up to 1 week to obtain steady-state concentrations.

INDICATIONS & DOSAGE
Psychotic disorders—
Adults: initially, 5 to 10 mg P.O. once daily. Dosage adjustments in 5-mg daily increments should occur at intervals of not less than 1 week. Most pa-

tients respond to dosages of 10 mg/day. Do not exceed 20 mg/day. Patients who are debilitated, predisposed to hypotension, or have an alteration in metabolism due to smoking status, gender, or age or who are pharmacologically sensitive to drug should be given 5 mg initially.

ADVERSE REACTIONS
CNS: *somnolence, agitation, insomnia, headache, nervousness, hostility, parkinsonism, dizziness,* anxiety, personality disorder, *akathesia,* hypertonia, tremor, amnesia, articulation impairment, euphoria, stuttering, tardive dyskinesia.
CV: orthostatic hypotension, tachycardia, chest pain, hypotension, edema.
EENT: amblyopia, blepharitis, corneal lesion.
GI: constipation, dry mouth, abdominal pain, increased appetite, increased salivation, nausea, vomiting, thirst.
GU: premenstrual syndrome, hematuria, metrorrhagia, urinary incontinence, UTI.
Musculoskeletal: joint pain, extremity pain, back pain, neck rigidity, twitching.
Respiratory: *rhinitis,* increased cough, pharyngitis, dyspnea.
Skin: vesiculobullous rash.
Other: weight gain or loss, fever, intentional injury.

INTERACTIONS
Alcohol, antihypertensives, diazepam: may potentiate hypotensive effects. Monitor BP closely.
Carbamazepine, omeprazole, rifampin: increased clearance of olanzapine. Monitor patient.
Levodopa, dopamine agonists: antagonized activity of these agents. Monitor patient.

EFFECTS ON DIAGNOSTIC TESTS
Olanzapine may cause asymptomatic increases in AST, ALT, GGT, serum prolactin, eosinophil count, and CK.

---

*Liquid contains alcohol.   **May contain tartrazine.   †Canada only.   ‡Australia only.   ◇OTC.

CONTRAINDICATIONS
Contraindicated in patients with known hypersensitivity to drug.

NURSING CONSIDERATIONS
● Use cautiously in patients with heart disease, cerebrovascular disease, conditions that predispose patient to hypotension, history of seizures or conditions that might lower the seizure threshold, and hepatic impairment. Also use cautiously in elderly patients, those with a history of paralytic ileus, and those at risk for aspiration pneumonia, prostatic hypertrophy, or narrow-angle glaucoma.
● Know that drug should be used in pregnancy only if the benefit justifies the potential risk to the fetus. Women taking drug should not breast-feed.
● Know that safety and effectiveness in patients under 18 years have not been established.
● Monitor patient for signs of neuroleptic malignant syndrome (hyperpyrexia, muscle rigidity, altered mental status, autonomic instability)—a rare, but frequently fatal adverse reaction that can occur with the administration of antipsychotic drugs. Drug should be stopped immediately and patient monitored and treated as required.
● Monitor patient for tardive dyskinesia, which may occur after prolonged use. It may not appear until months or years later and may disappear spontaneously or persist for life, despite discontinuation of drug.
● Obtain baseline and periodic liver function tests, as ordered.

☑ **PATIENT TEACHING**
● Warn patient to avoid hazardous tasks until adverse CNS effects of drug are known.
● Warn patient against exposure to extreme heat; drug may impair the body's ability to reduce core temperature.
● Tell patient to avoid alcohol.
● Tell patient to rise slowly to avoid orthostatic hypotension.
● Recommend ice chips or sugarless candy or gum to relieve dry mouth.
● Tell patient to notify the doctor if she becomes pregnant or intends to become pregnant during drug therapy. Advise her not to breast-feed during therapy.

---

perphenazine
Apo-Perphenazine†, PMS Perphenazine†, Trilafon, Trilafon Concentrate

Pregnancy Risk Category: NR

HOW SUPPLIED
Tablets: 2 mg, 4 mg, 8 mg, 16 mg
Oral concentrate: 16 mg/5 ml
Syrup: 2 mg/5 ml†
Injection: 5 mg/ml

ACTION
Unknown. Probably blocks postsynaptic dopamine receptors in the brain and inhibits the medullary chemoreceptor trigger zone.

ONSET, PEAK, DURATION
Onset of antipsychotic effect is gradual (up to several weeks) and varies among patients. Peak and duration not clearly defined.

INDICATIONS & DOSAGE
Psychosis in nonhospitalized patients—
Adults: initially, 4 to 8 mg P.O. t.i.d., reduced as soon as possible to minimum effective dosage.
Children over 12 years: lowest adult dose.
Psychosis in hospitalized patients—
Adults: initially, 8 to 16 mg P.O. b.i.d., t.i.d., or q.i.d., increased to 64 mg daily, p.r.n. Alternatively, 5 to 10 mg I.M. q 6 hours, p.r.n. Maximum dosage is 30 mg.

Children over 12 years: lowest limit of adult dosage.

Severe nausea and vomiting—

Adults: 8 to 16 mg P.O. daily in divided doses up to maximum of 24 mg. Alternatively, 5 to 10 mg I.M., p.r.n. May be given I.V., diluted to 0.5 mg/ml with saline solution. Dose should not exceed 5 mg.

ADVERSE REACTIONS

CNS: *extrapyramidal reactions, tardive dyskinesia,* sedation, pseudoparkinsonism, EEG changes, dizziness, *seizures,* drowsiness.
CV: *orthostatic hypotension,* tachycardia, ECG changes.
EENT: ocular changes, *blurred vision,* nasal congestion.
GI: *dry mouth, constipation,* nausea, vomiting, diarrhea.
GU: *urine retention,* dark urine, menstrual irregularities, gynecomastia, inhibited ejaculation.
Hematologic: leukopenia, *agranulocytosis,* eosinophilia, *hemolytic anemia, thrombocytopenia.*
Hepatic: jaundice.
Skin: *mild photosensitivity,* allergic reactions, pain at I.M. injection site, sterile abscess.
Other: weight gain, *neuroleptic malignant syndrome.*
After abrupt withdrawal of long-term therapy: gastritis, nausea, vomiting, dizziness, tremor, feeling of warmth or cold, diaphoresis, tachycardia, headache, insomnia.

INTERACTIONS

Antacids: inhibited absorption of oral phenothiazines. Separate antacid and phenothiazine doses by at least 2 hours.
Barbiturates: may decrease phenothiazine effect. Observe patient.
Ethanol, other CNS depressants: increased CNS depression. Avoid concomitant use.

EFFECTS ON DIAGNOSTIC TESTS

Drug causes false-positive test results for urinary porphyrins, urobilinogen, amylase, and 5-hydroxyindoleacetic acid (5-HIAA) because of darkening of urine by metabolites; it also causes false-positive urine pregnancy test results using human chorionic gonadotropin. Drug elevates test results for liver enzymes and protein-bound iodine and causes quinidine-like effects on the ECG.

CONTRAINDICATIONS

Contraindicated in patients with hypersensitivity to the drug; in patients experiencing coma; in those with CNS depression, blood dyscrasia, bone marrow depression, liver damage, or subcortical damage; and in those receiving large doses of CNS depressants.

NURSING CONSIDERATIONS

● Use cautiously with other CNS depressants or anticholinergics, and in elderly or debilitated patients.
● Also use cautiously in patients with alcohol withdrawal, psychic depression, suicidal tendency, severe adverse reactions to other phenothiazines, impaired renal function, and respiratory disorders.
● Obtain baseline measures of blood pressure before starting therapy and monitor regularly. Watch for orthostatic hypotension, especially with parenteral administration. Keep patient supine for 1 hour afterward; tell him to change positions slowly.
● Prevent contact dermatitis by keeping drug away from skin and clothes. Wear gloves when preparing liquid forms.
● Dilute liquid concentrate with fruit juice, milk, carbonated beverage, or semisolid food just before giving. Exceptions: Oral concentrate causes turbidity or precipitation in colas, black coffee, grape or apple juice, or tea. Do not mix with these liquids.

---

*Liquid contains alcohol.   **May contain tartrazine.   †Canada only.   ‡Australia only.   ◊ OTC.

• Protect drug from light. Slight yellowing of injection or concentrate is common and does not affect potency. Discard markedly discolored solutions.
• Give deep I.M. only in upper outer quadrant of buttocks. Massage slowly afterward to prevent sterile abscess. Injection may sting.
• Monitor patient for tardive dyskinesia, which may occur after prolonged use. It may not appear until months or years later and disappear spontaneously or persist for life, despite discontinuation of drug.
• Assess patient for neuroleptic malignant syndrome. It is rare, but frequently fatal. It is not necessarily related to length of drug use or type of neuroleptic, but over 60% of affected patients are men.
• Know that acute dystonic reactions may be treated with diphenhydramine.
• Monitor therapy with weekly bilirubin tests during first month; periodic blood tests (CBC and liver function); and ophthalmic tests (long-term use), as ordered.
• Do not withdraw drug abruptly unless required by severe adverse reactions.
• Withhold dose and notify doctor if patient develops jaundice, symptoms of blood dyscrasia (fever, sore throat, infection, cellulitis, weakness), or persistent extrapyramidal reactions (longer than a few hours).

☑ **PATIENT TEACHING**
• Instruct patient what beverages to use to dilute oral concentrate.
• Warn patient to avoid activities that require alertness or good psychomotor coordination until CNS effects of the drug are known. Drowsiness and dizziness usually subside after a few weeks.
• Tell patient to avoid alcohol while taking this drug.
• Advise patient to report urine retention or constipation.

• Tell patient to use sunblock and to wear protective clothing to avoid photosensitivity reactions.
• Tell patient to relieve dry mouth with sugarless gum or hard candy.

---

pimozide
Orap

Pregnancy Risk Category: C

HOW SUPPLIED
Tablets: 2 mg, 4 mg†, 10 mg†

ACTION
Unknown. Although thought to block dopamine nonselectively at both the presynaptic and postsynaptic receptors on neurons in the CNS.

ONSET, PEAK, DURATION
Onset and duration unknown. Serum levels peak within 4 to 12 hours.

INDICATIONS & DOSAGE
Suppression of motor and phonic tics in patients with Tourette syndrome refractory to first-line therapy—
Adults and children over 12 years: initially, 1 to 2 mg P.O. daily in divided doses, then increased every other day, p.r.n. Maintenance dose: under 0.2 mg/kg/day or 10 mg/day, whichever is less. Maximum dosage is 10 mg daily.

ADVERSE REACTIONS
CNS: *parkinsonian-like symptoms,* drowsiness, headache, insomnia, other extrapyramidal symptoms (dystonia, akathisia, hyperreflexia, opisthotonos, oculogyric crisis), *tardive dyskinesia, sedation.*
CV: *ECG changes (prolonged QT interval),* hypotension, hypertension, tachycardia.
EENT: visual disturbances.
GI: *dry mouth, constipation.*
GU: impotence, urinary frequency.
Skin: rash, diaphoresis.

Reactions may be *common,* uncommon, *life-threatening,* or COMMON AND LIFE-THREATENING.

Other: *neuroleptic malignant syndrome,* muscle rigidity.

INTERACTIONS
Ethanol, other CNS depressants: increased CNS depression. Avoid concomitant use.
Phenothiazines, tricyclic antidepressants, antiarrhythmics: increased incidence of ECG abnormalities. Monitor patient closely.

EFFECTS ON DIAGNOSTIC TESTS
Drug causes quinidine-like ECG effects (including prolongation of QT interval and flattened T waves).

CONTRAINDICATIONS
Contraindicated in patients with hypersensitivity to drug, in the treatment of simple tics or tics other than those associated with Tourette syndrome, concurrent drug therapy known to cause motor and phonic tics, congenital long QT syndrome or history of arrhythmias, patients with severe toxic CNS depression, and patients experiencing coma.

NURSING CONSIDERATIONS
● Use cautiously in patients with hepatic or renal dysfunction, glaucoma, prostatic hyperplasia, seizure disorder, or EEG abnormalities.
Alert: Perform an ECG before treatment begins and periodically thereafter as ordered. Monitor for prolonged QT interval.
● Know that concurrent administration of other drugs that prolong the QT interval, such as antiarrhythmics, should be avoided.
● Monitor patient for tardive dyskinesia, which may occur after prolonged use. It may not appear until months or years later and may disappear spontaneously or persist for life, despite discontinuation of drug.
● Assess patient for neuroleptic malignant syndrome. It is rare, but frequently fatal. It is not necessarily related to

length of drug use or type of neuroleptic, but over 60% of affected patients are men.
● Know that acute dystonic reactions may be treated with diphenhydramine.
● Monitor patients who also are taking anticonvulsants for increased seizure activity. Pimozide may lower the seizure threshold.

☑ PATIENT TEACHING
● Warn patient not to stop taking drug abruptly and not to exceed prescribed dosage.
● Tell patient to avoid alcohol while taking this drug.
● Tell patient to use sugarless hard candy, gum, and liquids to relieve dry mouth.

---

promazine hydrochloride
Primazine, Prozine-50, Sparine**

Pregnancy Risk Category: NR

HOW SUPPLIED
Tablets: 25 mg, 50 mg, 100 mg
Injection: 25 mg/ml, 50 mg/ml

ACTION
Unknown. An aliphatic phenothiazine that probably blocks postsynaptic dopamine receptors in the brain.

ONSET, PEAK, DURATION
Onset of antipsychotic effect is gradual (up to several weeks) and varies among patients. Peak and duration unknown.

INDICATIONS & DOSAGE
Psychosis—
Adults: 10 to 200 mg P.O. or I.M. q 4 to 6 hours, up to 1 g daily, p.r.n. For acutely agitated patients, initial dose is 50 to 150 mg I.M.; repeat within 30 minutes, if necessary, up to a total of 300 mg.
Children over 12 years: 10 to 25 mg P.O. or I.M. q 4 to 6 hours.

ADVERSE REACTIONS

CNS: extrapyramidal reactions, tardive dyskinesia, drowsiness, *seizures, sedation,* pseudoparkinsonism, EEG changes, dizziness.
CV: *orthostatic hypotension,* tachycardia, ECG changes.
EENT: ocular changes, blurred vision.
GI: *dry mouth, constipation.*
GU: *urine retention,* menstrual irregularities, gynecomastia, inhibited ejaculation.
Hematologic: leukopenia, *hemolytic anemia, thrombocytopenia,* eosinophilia, *agranulocytosis.*
Hepatic: jaundice.
Skin: *mild photosensitivity,* allergic reactions, pain at I.M. injection site, sterile abscess.
Other: weight gain, *neuroleptic malignant syndrome.*
After abrupt withdrawal of long-term therapy: gastritis, nausea, vomiting, dizziness, tremor, feeling of warmth or cold, diaphoresis, tachycardia, headache, insomnia.

INTERACTIONS

Antacids: inhibited absorption of oral phenothiazines. Use together cautiously. Separate antacid and phenothiazine doses by at least 2 hours.
Anticholinergics (including antidepressants and antiparkinsonian agents): increased anticholinergic activity, aggravated parkinsonian symptoms. Use together cautiously.
Barbiturates, lithium: may decrease phenothiazine effect. Observe patient.
Centrally acting antihypertensives: decreased antihypertensive effect. Monitor blood pressure.
Ethanol: increased CNS depression. Avoid concomitant use.
Other CNS depressants: increased CNS depression. Use together cautiously.

EFFECTS ON DIAGNOSTIC TESTS

Drug causes false-positive test results for urinary porphyrins, urobilinogen, amylase, and 5-hydroxyindoleacetic acid (5-HIAA) because of darkening of urine by metabolites; it also causes false-positive urine pregnancy test results in tests using human chorionic gonadotropin.

Promazine elevates test results for liver enzymes and protein-bound iodine and causes quinidine-like effects on the ECG.

CONTRAINDICATIONS

Contraindicated in patients with hypersensitivity to the drug or in patients experiencing coma or CNS depression, bone marrow suppression, or subcortical damage.

NURSING CONSIDERATIONS

● Use cautiously in elderly or debilitated patients and in patients with hepatic or renal disease, severe CV disease (may cause sudden drop in blood pressure); exposure to extreme heat or cold (including antipyretic therapy) or to organophosphate insecticides; respiratory disorder; hypocalcemia; seizure disorder (may lower seizure threshold); severe reactions to insulin or electroconvulsive therapy; glaucoma; or prostatic hyperplasia.
● Monitor blood pressure with patient lying and standing before therapy and routinely throughout treatment.
● Keep drug away from skin and clothes. Wear gloves when preparing liquid forms.
● Protect drug from light. Slight yellowing of injection or concentrate does not affect potency. Discard markedly discolored solutions.
● Give deeply I.M. only in upper outer quadrant of buttocks. Massage slowly afterward to prevent sterile abscess. Injection may sting.
● Watch for orthostatic hypotension, especially with parenteral administration. Keep the patient supine for 1 hour afterward and have patient change positions slowly.

Reactions may be *common,* uncommon, *life-threatening,* or COMMON AND LIFE-THREATENING.

• Monitor patient for tardive dyskinesia, which may occur after prolonged use. It may not appear until months or years later and disappear spontaneously or persist for life, despite discontinuation of drug.

• Assess patient for neuroleptic malignant syndrome. It is rare, but frequently fatal. It is not necessarily related to length of drug use or type of neuroleptic, but over 60% of affected patients are men.

• Monitor therapy with weekly bilirubin tests during first month; periodic blood tests (CBC and liver function); and ophthalmic tests (long-term use).

• Do not withdraw abruptly unless required by severe adverse reactions.

• Withhold dose and notify doctor if patient develops jaundice, blood dyscrasia (fever, sore throat, infection, cellulitis, weakness), or persistent extrapyramidal reactions, especially in pregnant patients or in children.

• Acute dystonic reactions may be treated with diphenhydramine.

☑ PATIENT TEACHING
• Warn patient to avoid activities that require alertness until CNS effects of the drug are known.

• Tell patient to avoid alcohol.

• Have patient report urine retention or constipation.

• Tell patient to use sunblock and to wear protective clothing outdoors.

• Tell patient to relieve dry mouth with sugarless gum or hard candy.

risperidone
Risperdal

Pregnancy Risk Category: C

HOW SUPPLIED
Tablets: 1 mg, 2 mg, 3 mg, 4 mg

ACTION
Blocks dopamine and serotonin receptors; also blocks alpha$_1$, alpha$_2$, and histamine$_1$ receptors in the CNS.

ONSET, PEAK, DURATION
Onset and duration unknown. Plasma levels peak in about 1 hour.

INDICATIONS & DOSAGE
Psychosis—
Adults: initially, 1 mg P.O. b.i.d. Increased in increments of 1 mg b.i.d. on days 2 and 3 of treatment to a target dose of 3 mg b.i.d. At least 1 week must pass before dosage is adjusted further. Safety of dosages exceeding 16 mg/day has not been evaluated.
Elderly or debilitated patients, hypotensive patients, or patients with severe renal or hepatic impairment: initially, 0.5 mg P.O. b.i.d. Increased in increments of 0.5 mg b.i.d. on days 2 and 3 of treatment to a target dosage of 1.5 mg P.O. b.i.d. At least 1 week must pass before dosage increased further.

ADVERSE REACTIONS
CNS: *somnolence, extrapyramidal symptoms, headache, insomnia, agitation, anxiety,* tardive dyskinesia, aggressiveness.
CV: tachycardia, chest pain, orthostatic hypotension, prolonged QT interval.
EENT: *rhinitis,* coughing, upper respiratory infection, sinusitis, pharyngitis, abnormal vision.
GI: *constipation, nausea, vomiting, dyspepsia.*
Skin: rash, dry skin, photosensitivity.
Other: arthralgia; back pain; fever; rarely, ***neuroleptic malignant syndrome.***

INTERACTIONS
Carbamazepine: increased clearance of risperidone, leading to decreased effectiveness. Monitor patient closely.
Clozapine: decreased clearance of risperidone, increasing toxicity. Monitor patient closely.

---

*Liquid contains alcohol.   **May contain tartrazine.   †Canada only.   ‡Australia only.   ◊ OTC.

Ethanol, CNS depressants: additive CNS depression. Avoid concomitant use.

Levodopa: antagonized effects. Don't use together.

EFFECTS ON DIAGNOSTIC TESTS
Drug may increase serum prolactin levels.

CONTRAINDICATIONS
Contraindicated in patients hypersensitive to the drug. Also contraindicated in breast-feeding patients.

NURSING CONSIDERATIONS
● Use cautiously in patients with prolonged QT interval, CV disease, cerebrovascular disease, dehydration, hypovolemia, history of seizures, exposure to extreme heat, or conditions that could affect metabolism or hemodynamic responses.
Alert: Obtain baseline measures of blood pressure before starting therapy and monitor regularly. Watch for orthostatic hypotension, especially during initial dosage titration.
● Monitor patient for tardive dyskinesia, which may occur after prolonged use. It may not appear until months or years later and disappear spontaneously or persist for life, despite discontinuation of drug.
● Assess for neuroleptic malignant syndrome. It is rare, but frequently fatal. It is not necessarily related to length of drug use or type of neuroleptic, but over 60% of patients are men.

☑ **PATIENT TEACHING**
● Warn patient to avoid activities that require alertness until CNS effects of the drug are known.
● Warn patient to rise slowly, avoid hot showers, and use extra caution during the first few days of therapy to avoid fainting.
● Advise patient to use caution in hot weather to prevent heatstroke.
● Tell patient to avoid alcohol.

● Tell patient to use sunblock and to wear protective clothing outdoors.
● Tell female patient to notify her doctor if she is or plans to become pregnant during therapy.

---

thioridazine hydrochloride
Aldazine‡, Apo-Thioridazine†, Mellaril*, Mellaril Concentrate, Novo-Ridazine†, PMS Thioridazine†

Pregnancy Risk Category: NR

HOW SUPPLIED
Tablets: 10 mg, 15 mg, 25 mg, 50 mg, 100 mg, 150 mg, 200 mg
Oral suspension: 25 mg/5 ml, 100 mg/5 ml
Oral concentrate: 30 mg/ml, 100 mg/ml (3% to 4.2% alcohol)

ACTION
Unknown. A piperidine phenothiazine that probably blocks postsynaptic dopamine receptors in the brain.

ONSET, PEAK, DURATION
Onset of antipsychotic effect is gradual (up to several weeks) and variable between patients. Peak and duration unknown.

INDICATIONS & DOSAGE
Psychosis—
Adults: initially, 50 to 100 mg P.O. t.i.d., with gradual increments up to 800 mg daily in divided doses, if needed. Dosage varies.
Short term treatment of moderate to marked depression with variable degrees of anxiety, treatment of multiple symptoms, such as agitation, anxiety, depressed mood, tension, sleep disturbances, and fears in geriatric patients—
Adults: initially, 25 mg P.O. t.i.d. Maximum daily dosage is 200 mg.
Children 2 to 12 years: 0.5 to 3 mg/kg P.O. daily in divided doses.

Reactions may be *common,* uncommon, *life-threatening,* or COMMON AND LIFE-THREATENING.

ADVERSE REACTIONS
CNS: extrapyramidal reactions (low incidence), *tardive dyskinesia, sedation* (high incidence), EEG changes, dizziness.
CV: *orthostatic hypotension,* tachycardia, ECG changes.
EENT: *ocular changes, blurred vision,* retinitis pigmentosa.
GI: *dry mouth, constipation.*
GU: *urine retention,* dark urine, menstrual irregularities, gynecomastia, inhibited ejaculation.
Hematologic: transient leukopenia, *agranulocytosis,* hyperprolactinemia.
Hepatic: cholestatic jaundice.
Skin: *mild photosensitivity,* allergic reactions.
Other: weight gain; increased appetite; rarely, *neuroleptic malignant syndrome.*
After abrupt withdrawal of long-term therapy: gastritis, nausea, vomiting, dizziness, tremor, feeling of warmth or cold, diaphoresis, tachycardia, headache, insomnia.

INTERACTIONS
Antacids: inhibited absorption of oral phenothiazines. Separate antacid and phenothiazine doses by at least 2 hours.
Barbiturates, lithium: may decrease phenothiazine effect. Observe patient.
Centrally acting antihypertensives: decreased antihypertensive effect. Monitor blood pressure.
Ethanol: increased CNS depression. Avoid concomitant use.
Other CNS depressants: increased CNS depression. Use together cautiously.

EFFECTS ON DIAGNOSTIC TESTS
Drug causes false-positive test results for urinary porphyrins, urobilinogen, amylase, 5-hydroxyindoleacetic acid (5-HIAA) because of darkening of urine by metabolites; it also causes false-positive urine pregnancy results in tests using human chorionic gonadotropin as the indicator.

Drug elevates test results for liver enzymes and protein-bound iodine and causes quinidine-like effects on the ECG.

CONTRAINDICATIONS
Contraindicated in patients with hypersensitivity to the drug or in patients experiencing coma or CNS depression, or severe hypertensive or hypotensive cardiac disease.

NURSING CONSIDERATIONS
● Use cautiously in elderly or debilitated patients and in patients with hepatic disease; CV disease; exposure to extreme heat or cold (including antipyretic therapy) or to organophosphate insecticides; respiratory disorder; hypocalcemia; seizure disorder; or severe reactions to insulin or electroconvulsive therapy.
Alert: Remember that different liquid formulations have different concentrations. Check dosage carefully.
● Prevent contact dermatitis by keeping drug away from skin and clothes. Wear gloves when preparing liquid forms.
● Dilute liquid concentrate with water or fruit juice just before giving.
● Shake suspension well before using.
● Monitor patient for tardive dyskinesia, which may occur after prolonged use. It may not appear until months or years later and disappear spontaneously or persist for life, despite discontinuation of drug.
● Assess for neuroleptic malignant syndrome. It is rare, but frequently fatal. Not necessarily related to length of drug use or type of neuroleptic, but over 60% of patients are men.
● Monitor therapy with weekly bilirubin tests during first month; periodic blood tests (CBC and liver function); and ophthalmic tests (long-term use).
● Do not stop drug abruptly unless required by severe adverse reactions.

● Withhold dose and notify doctor if patient develops jaundice, blood dyscrasia (fever, sore throat, infection, cellulitis, weakness), or persistent extrapyramidal reactions, especially in pregnant patients or in children.
● Acute dystonic reactions may be treated with diphenhydramine.

☑ **PATIENT TEACHING**
● Tell patient to shake suspension.
● Warn patient to avoid activities that require alertness until CNS effects of the drug are known.
● Tell patient to watch for orthostatic hypotension, especially with parenteral administration. Advise patient to change positions slowly.
● Tell patient to avoid alcohol.
● Have patient report urine retention, constipation, or blurred vision.
● Tell patient that drug may discolor the urine.
● Advise patient to relieve dry mouth with sugarless gum or hard candy.
● Tell patient to use sunblock and to wear protective clothing outdoors.

---

thiothixene
Navane

thiothixene hydrochloride
Navane*

Pregnancy Risk Category: NR

HOW SUPPLIED
thiothixene
Capsules: 1 mg, 2 mg, 5 mg, 10 mg, 20 mg
thiothixene hydrochloride
Oral concentrate: 5 mg/ml (7% alcohol)
Injection: 2 mg/ml, 5 mg/ml

ACTION
Unknown. A thioxanthene that probably blocks postsynaptic dopamine receptors in the brain.

ONSET, PEAK, DURATION
Onset of antipsychotic effect is gradual (up to several weeks). Peak and duration unknown.

INDICATIONS & DOSAGE
Mild to moderate psychosis—
Adults: initially, 2 mg P.O. t.i.d. Increased gradually to 15 mg daily, p.r.n.
Severe psychosis—
Adults: initially, 5 mg P.O. b.i.d. Increased gradually to 20 to 30 mg daily, p.r.n. Maximum recommended dosage is 60 mg daily. Alternatively, 4 mg I.M. b.i.d. or q.i.d. Maximum dosage is 30 mg I.M. daily. An oral form should replace the injectable form as soon as possible.

ADVERSE REACTIONS
CNS: *extrapyramidal reactions,* drowsiness, restlessness, agitation, insomnia, *tardive dyskinesia,* sedation, pseudoparkinsonism, EEG changes, dizziness.
CV: *hypotension,* tachycardia, ECG changes.
EENT: ocular changes, *blurred vision,* nasal congestion.
GI: *dry mouth, constipation.*
GU: *urine retention,* menstrual irregularities, gynecomastia, inhibited ejaculation.
Hematologic: transient leukopenia, leukocytosis, ***agranulocytosis.***
Hepatic: jaundice.
Skin: *mild photosensitivity,* allergic reactions, pain at I.M. injection site, sterile abscess.
Other: weight gain, ***neuroleptic malignant syndrome.***
After abrupt withdrawal of long-term therapy: gastritis, nausea, vomiting, dizziness, tremor, feeling of warmth or cold, diaphoresis, tachycardia, headache, insomnia.

INTERACTIONS
Ethanol, other CNS depressants: increased CNS depression. Avoid concomitant use.

EFFECTS ON DIAGNOSTIC TESTS
Drug causes false-positive test results for urinary porphyrins, urobilinogen, amylase, 5-hydroxyindoleacetic acid (5-HIAA) because of darkening of urine by metabolites; it also causes false-positive urine pregnancy results in tests using human chorionic gonadotropin as the indicator.

Thiothixene elevates test results for liver enzymes and protein-bound iodine and causes quinidine-like effects on the ECG.

CONTRAINDICATIONS
Contraindicated in patients with hypersensitivity to the drug or in patients experiencing circulatory collapse, coma, CNS depression, or blood dyscrasia.

NURSING CONSIDERATIONS
● Use with extreme caution in patients with history of seizure disorder or in a state of alcohol withdrawal.
● Use cautiously in elderly or debilitated patients and in those with CV disease (may cause sudden drop in blood pressure), heat exposure, glaucoma, or prostatic hyperplasia.
● Prevent contact dermatitis by keeping drug off skin and clothes. Wear gloves when preparing liquid forms.
● Dilute liquid concentrate with fruit juice, milk, or semisolid food just before administering.
● Slight yellowing of injection or concentrate is common and does not affect potency. Discard markedly discolored solutions.
● Give I.M. only in upper outer quadrant of buttocks or midlateral thigh. Massage slowly afterward to prevent sterile abscess. Injection may sting.
● Monitor patient for tardive dyskinesia, which may occur after prolonged use; it may not appear until months or years later and disappear spontaneously or persist for life, despite discontinuation of drug.
● Assess for neuroleptic malignant syndrome. It is rare, but frequently fa-

tal. Not necessarily related to length of drug use or type of neuroleptic, but over 60% of patients are men.
● Do not withdraw abruptly unless required by severe adverse reactions.
● Withhold dose and notify doctor if patient develops jaundice, blood dyscrasia (fever, sore throat, infection, cellulitis, weakness), or persistent extrapyramidal reactions, especially in pregnant patients.
● Monitor therapy with weekly bilirubin tests during first month; periodic blood tests (CBC and liver function); and ophthalmic tests (long-term use).
● Acute dystonic reactions may be treated with diphenhydramine.
● Watch for orthostatic hypotension, especially with parenteral administration. Keep the patient in supine position for 1 hour afterward and tell him to change positions slowly.

☑ **PATIENT TEACHING**
● Warn patient to avoid activities that require alertness until CNS effects of the drug are known.
● Tell patient to watch for orthostatic hypotension. Advise him to change positions slowly.
● Tell patient to avoid alcohol.
● Have him report urine retention, constipation, or blurred vision.
● Tell patient to use sunblock and to wear protective clothing outdoors.

---

trifluoperazine hydrochloride
Apo-Trifluoperazine†, Calmazine‡, Novo-Flurazine†, PMS Trifluoperazine†, Solazine†, Stelazine, Stelazine Concentrate, Terfluzine†, Terfluzine Concentrate†

Pregnancy Risk Category: NR

HOW SUPPLIED
Tablets (regular and film-coated): 1 mg, 2 mg, 5 mg, 10 mg
Oral concentrate: 10 mg/ml
Injection: 2 mg/ml

---

*Liquid contains alcohol.   **May contain tartrazine.   †Canada only.   ‡Australia only.   ◇OTC.

ACTION
Unknown. A piperazine phenothiazine that probably blocks postsynaptic dopamine receptors in the brain.

ONSET, PEAK, DURATION
Onset of antipsychotic effect is gradual (up to several weeks) and variable between patients. Peak and duration unknown.

INDICATIONS & DOSAGE
Anxiety states—
Adults: 1 to 2 mg P.O. b.i.d. Maximum dosage is 6 mg/day and drug should not be used longer than 12 weeks for this indication.
Schizophrenia and other psychotic disorders—
Adults: 2 to 5 mg P.O. b.i.d., gradually increased until therapeutic response. Or 1 to 2 mg deep I.M. q 4 to 6 hours, p.r.n. Most patients respond to 15 to 20 mg P.O. daily, although some may require dosages of 40 mg/day or more. More than 6 mg I.M. in 24 hours is rarely required.
Children 6 to 12 years (hospitalized or under close supervision): 1 mg P.O. daily or b.i.d.; may increase gradually to 15 mg daily, if needed.

ADVERSE REACTIONS
CNS: *extrapyramidal reactions, tardive dyskinesia,* pseudoparkinsonism, dizziness, drowsiness, insomnia, fatigue, headache.
CV: *orthostatic hypotension,* tachycardia, ECG changes.
EENT: ocular changes, *blurred vision.*
GI: *dry mouth, constipation,* nausea.
GU: *urine retention.*
Hematologic: transient leukopenia, *agranulocytosis.*
Hepatic: cholestatic jaundice.
Skin: *photosensitivity,* allergic reactions, pain at I.M. injection site, sterile abscess, rash.
Other: weight gain; rarely, *neuroleptic malignant syndrome* (fever, tachycardia, tachypnea, profuse diaphore-

sis), menstrual irregularities, gynecomastia, inhibited lactation.
After abrupt withdrawal of long-term therapy: gastritis, nausea, vomiting, dizziness, tremor, feeling of warmth or cold, diaphoresis, tachycardia, headache, insomnia, anorexia, muscle rigidity, altered mental status and evidence of autonomic instability.

INTERACTIONS
Antacids: inhibited absorption of oral phenothiazines. Separate antacid and phenothiazine doses by at least 2 hours.
Barbiturates, lithium: may decrease phenothiazine effect. Monitor patient.
Centrally acting antihypertensives: decreased antihypertensive effect. Monitor blood pressure.
Ethanol: increased CNS depression. Avoid concomitant use.
Other CNS depressants: increased CNS depression. Use together cautiously.
Propranolol: increased levels of both propranolol and trifluoperazine. Monitor closely.
Warfarin: decreased effect of oral anticoagulants. Monitor PT.

EFFECTS ON DIAGNOSTIC TESTS
Drug causes false-positive test results for urinary porphyrins, urobilinogen, amylase, 5-hydroxyindoleacetic acid (5-HIAA) because of darkening of urine by metabolites; it also causes false-positive urine pregnancy results in tests using human chorionic gonadotropin as the indicator.

Trifluoperazine elevates test results for liver enzymes and protein-bound iodine and causes quinidine-like effects on the ECG.

CONTRAINDICATIONS
Contraindicated in patients with hypersensitivity to phenothiazines or in patients experiencing coma, CNS depression, bone marrow suppression, or liver damage.

Reactions may be *common,* uncommon, *life-threatening,* or COMMON AND LIFE-THREATENING.

NURSING CONSIDERATIONS

● Use cautiously in elderly or debilitated patients and in patients with CV disease (may cause drop in blood pressure), exposure to extreme heat, seizure disorder, glaucoma, or prostatic hyperplasia.

● Wear gloves when preparing liquid forms.

● Dilute liquid concentrate with 60 ml of tomato or fruit juice, carbonated beverages, coffee, tea, milk, water, or semisolid food just before giving.

● Protect drug from light. Slight yellowing of injection or concentrate is common and does not affect potency. Discard markedly discolored solutions.

● Give deeply I.M. only in upper outer quadrant of buttocks. Massage slowly afterward to prevent sterile abscess. Injection may sting.

● Watch for orthostatic hypotension, especially with parenteral administration. Keep patient supine for 1 hour, and tell him to change positions slowly.

● Monitor patient for tardive dyskinesia, which may occur after prolonged use. It may not appear until months or years later and disappear spontaneously or persist for life, despite discontinuation of drug.

● Assess for neuroleptic malignant syndrome. It is rare, but frequently fatal. It is not necessarily related to length of drug use or type of neuroleptic, but over 60% of patients are men.

● Do not withdraw drug abruptly unless severe adverse reactions occur.

● Withhold dose and notify doctor if patient develops jaundice, symptoms of blood dyscrasia (fever, sore throat, infection, cellulitis, weakness), persistent extrapyramidal reactions (longer than a few hours), especially in pregnant patients or in children.

● Monitor therapy with weekly bilirubin tests during first month; periodic blood tests (CBC and liver function); and ophthalmic tests (long-term use).

● Acute dystonic reactions may be treated with diphenhydramine.

☑ PATIENT TEACHING

● Warn patient to avoid activities that require alertness until CNS effects of the drug are known.

● Tell patient to avoid alcohol.

● Have him report urine retention or constipation.

● Tell him to use sunblock and to wear protective clothing outdoors.

● Tell patient to relieve dry mouth with sugarless gum or hard candy.

amphetamine sulfate
benzphetamine hydrochloride
caffeine
dexfenfluramine hydrochloride
dextroamphetamine sulfate
diethylpropion hydrochloride
doxapram hydrochloride
fenfluramine hydrochloride
**methamphetamine
    hydrochloride**
methylphenidate hydrochloride
pemoline
phentermine hydrochloride

COMBINATION PRODUCTS
None.

---

amphetamine sulfate

Controlled Substance Schedule II
Pregnancy Risk Category: C

HOW SUPPLIED
Tablets: 5 mg, 10 mg

ACTION
Unknown. Probably promotes nerve impulse transmission by releasing stored norepinephrine from nerve terminals in the brain. Main sites of activity appear to be the cerebral cortex and the reticular activating system.

ONSET, PEAK, DURATION
Unknown.

INDICATIONS & DOSAGE
Attention deficit disorder with hyperactivity—
Children 3 to 5 years: 2.5 mg P.O. daily, with 2.5-mg increments weekly, p.r.n.
Children 6 years and older: 5 mg P.O. daily to b.i.d., with 5-mg increments weekly, p.r.n. Give first dose on awak-

ening; additional doses (one or two) at intervals of 4 to 6 hours. Dosage rarely exceeds 40 mg/day.
Narcolepsy—
Adults and children 12 years and older: 10 mg P.O. daily. Dosage increased in 10-mg increments weekly, p.r.n. Daily dosage may be divided with first dose given on awakening, additional doses at intervals of 4 to 6 hours.
Children 6 to 12 years: 5 mg P.O. daily. Dosage increased in 5-mg increments weekly, p.r.n. Daily dosage may be divided with first dose given on awakening, additional doses at intervals of 4 to 6 hours.
Short-term adjunct in exogenous obesity—
Adults: 5 to 30 mg P.O. daily in divided doses 30 to 60 minutes before meals.

ADVERSE REACTIONS
CNS: *restlessness,* tremor, *hyperactivity, talkativeness, insomnia,* irritability, dizziness, headache, chills, dysphoria, euphoria.
CV: *tachycardia, palpitations,* hypertension, arrhythmias.
GI: dry mouth, metallic taste, diarrhea, constipation, anorexia, weight loss.
GU: impotence.
Skin: urticaria.
Other: altered libido.

INTERACTIONS
Ammonium chloride, ascorbic acid: decreased serum levels and increased renal excretion of amphetamine. Monitor for decreased amphetamine effect.
Antacids, sodium bicarbonate, acetazolamide: increased renal reabsorption. Monitor for enhanced effect.
Antihypertensives: reversal of antihypertensive action. Monitor blood pressure.
Caffeine: may increase amphetamine

---

and related amine effects. Avoid concomitant use.

Haloperidol, phenothiazines, tricyclic antidepressants: altered CNS effect. Avoid concomitant use.

Insulin, oral antidiabetic agents: may decrease antidiabetic agent requirements. Monitor blood glucose level.

MAO inhibitors: may cause severe hypertension, possibly hypertensive crisis. Don't use together or within 14 days after an MAO inhibitor has been discontinued.

EFFECTS ON DIAGNOSTIC TESTS
Amphetamines may elevate plasma corticosteroid levels and also may interfere with urinary steroid determinations.

CONTRAINDICATIONS
Contraindicated in patients with hypersensitivity or idiosyncrasy to the sympathomimetic amines, symptomatic CV disease, hyperthyroidism, moderate to severe hypertension, glaucoma, advanced arteriosclerosis, or history of drug abuse; within 14 days of MAO inhibitor therapy; and in agitated patients.

NURSING CONSIDERATIONS
● Use cautiously in elderly, debilitated, or hyperexcitable patients; or those with psychopathic personalities or history of suicidal or homicidal tendencies.
● Know that drug is not recommended for first-line treatment of obesity or for treatment of obesity in children under 12 years. Use as an anorexigenic agent is prohibited in some states.
● Be aware that drug should not be used to combat fatigue.
● Make sure obese patient is on a weight-reduction program. Give drug 30 to 60 minutes before meals. Monitor dietary intake and count calories, if necessary.
● If tolerance to anorexigenic effect develops, know that drug should be discontinued. Notify doctor.

☑ **PATIENT TEACHING**
● To avoid sleep interference, tell the patient to take drug at least 6 hours before bedtime.
● Warn the patient to avoid activities that require alertness or good psychomotor coordination until CNS effects of the drug are known.
● Tell the patient to avoid drinks containing caffeine, which increases the effects of amphetamines and related amines.
● Tell the patient to report signs of excessive stimulation.
● Inform patient that fatigue may result as drug effects wear off. The patient will need more rest.

benzphetamine hydrochloride
Didrex**

Controlled Substance Schedule III
Pregnancy Risk Category: X

HOW SUPPLIED
Tablets: 25 mg, 50 mg

ACTION
Unknown. Probably promotes nerve impulse transmission by releasing stored norepinephrine from nerve terminals in the brain. Main sites of activity appear to be the cerebral cortex and the reticular activating system.

ONSET, PEAK, DURATION
Onset and peak unknown. Effects persist for about 4 hours.

INDICATIONS & DOSAGE
Short-term adjunct in exogenous obesity—
Adults: 25 to 50 mg P.O. daily, b.i.d. or t.i.d. Increased as needed in dosage or interval.

ADVERSE REACTIONS
CNS: *restlessness,* tremor, *hyperactivity, talkativeness, insomnia,* irritability,

dizziness, headache, chills, dysphoria, euphoria.
CV: *tachycardia, palpitations,* hypertension.
GI: dry mouth, metallic taste, diarrhea, constipation, anorexia, weight loss.
GU: impotence.
Skin: urticaria.
Other: altered libido.

INTERACTIONS
Ammonium chloride, ascorbic acid: decreased serum levels and increased renal excretion of benzphetamine. Monitor for decreased amphetamine effects.
Antacids, sodium bicarbonate, acetazolamide: increased renal reabsorption. Monitor for enhanced effects.
Caffeine: may increase amphetamine and related amine effects. Avoid concomitant use.
Insulin, oral antidiabetic agents: may decrease antidiabetic agent requirement. Monitor blood glucose levels.
MAO inhibitors: may cause severe hypertension, possibly hypertensive crisis. Don't use together or within 14 days after MAO inhibitor has been discontinued.
Phenothiazines, haloperidol, tricyclic antidepressants: increased CNS effects. Avoid concomitant use.

EFFECTS ON DIAGNOSTIC TESTS
Benzphetamine may elevate plasma corticosteroid levels and may also interfere with urinary steroid determinations.

CONTRAINDICATIONS
Contraindicated in patients with hypersensitivity or idiosyncrasy to sympathomimetic amines; within 14 days of MAO inhibitor therapy; in those with symptomatic CV disease, hyperthyroidism, moderate to severe hypertension, glaucoma, advanced arteriosclerosis, or history of drug abuse; and in agitated patients.

NURSING CONSIDERATIONS
• Use cautiously in patients with dia-
betes mellitus and mild hypertension.
• Use in conjunction with a weight-reduction program. Monitor dietary intake and count calories, if necessary. Give 30 to 60 minutes before meals.
• Give a single daily dose in midmorning or midafternoon, according to patient's eating habits.
• If tolerance to anorexigenic effect develops, know that drug should be discontinued. Notify doctor.

☑ PATIENT TEACHING
• Instruct the patient when to take drug.
• To avoid sleep interference, tell the patient to take drug at least 6 hours before bedtime.
• Warn the patient to avoid activities that require alertness or good psychomotor coordination until CNS effects of the drug are known.
• Tell the patient to avoid drinks containing caffeine, which increases the effects of amphetamines and related amines.
• Tell the patient to report signs of excessive stimulation.
• Inform the patient that fatigue may result as drug effects wear off. The patient will need more rest.

caffeine
Caffedrine Caplets ◇, Dexitac ◇, NoDoz ◇, Quick Pep ◇, Vivarin ◇

Pregnancy Risk Category: C

HOW SUPPLIED
Tablets: 100 mg ◇, 150 mg ◇, 200 mg ◇
Tablets (timed-release): 200 mg ◇
Capsules (timed-release): 200 mg ◇
Injection: caffeine (250 mg/ml) with sodium benzoate (250 mg/ml)

ACTION
Inhibits phosphodiesterase, the enzyme that degrades cAMP.

ONSET, PEAK, DURATION
Onset and duration unknown. Serum levels peak within 50 to 75 minutes after oral administration.

INDICATIONS & DOSAGE
CNS stimulant—
Adults: 100 to 200 mg anhydrous caffeine P.O. q 3 to 4 hours, p.r.n. Alternatively, 500 mg to 1 g I.M. (or slowly I.V.). Total daily dosage should seldom exceed 2.5 g.

ADVERSE REACTIONS
CNS: *insomnia,* restlessness, nervousness, headache, excitement, agitation, muscle tremor, twitching.
CV: *tachycardia, palpitations,* extrasystoles.
GI: nausea, vomiting, diarrhea, stomach pain.
GU: *diuresis.*
Other: abrupt withdrawal symptoms (headache, irritability), tinnitus.

INTERACTIONS
Beta-adrenergic agonists, cimetidine, fluoroquinolones, oral contraceptives, phenylpropanolamine, theophylline: excessive CNS stimulation. Avoid concomitant use.

EFFECTS ON DIAGNOSTIC TESTS
Caffeine may increase blood glucose levels and cause false-positive urate levels; it may also cause false-positive test results for pheochromocytoma or neuroblastoma by increasing certain urinary catecholamines.

CONTRAINDICATIONS
Contraindicated in patients with hypersensitivity to the drug.

NURSING CONSIDERATIONS
• Use cautiously in patients with history of peptic ulcer, symptomatic arrhythmias, or palpitations, and during the first several days to weeks after an acute MI.
• Know that caffeine does not reverse alcohol intoxication or CNS depressant

effects of alcohol. Overvigorous therapy with caffeine may aggravate depression in an already depressed patient.
Alert: Be aware single dose should not exceed 1 g.
• Restrict caffeine-containing beverages in patients who experience palpitations. Caffeine content: cola beverages, 17 to 55 mg/180 ml; tea, 40 to 100 mg/180 ml; instant coffee, 60 to 180 mg/180 ml; brewed coffee, 100 to 150 mg/180 ml; decaffeinated coffee, 1 to 6 mg/180 ml.
• Be alert for signs of overdose: GI pain, mild delirium, insomnia, diuresis, dehydration, and fever. Treat with short-acting barbiturates, gastric emesis, or lavage as ordered.
• Monitor patient for tolerance or psychological dependence.
• Be aware that sudden discontinuation of caffeine may cause headache and irritability.

☑ **PATIENT TEACHING**
• Stress to patient the importance of not exceeding recommended dosage.
• Tell patient to stop taking caffeine if increased or abnormal heart rate, dizziness, or palpitations occur.
• Inform patient that caffeine is not intended for use as a substitute for sleep.

▼ *NEW DRUG*

dexfenfluramine hydrochloride
Redux

Controlled Substance Schedule IV
Pregnancy Risk Category: C

HOW SUPPLIED
Capsules: 15 mg

ACTION
Enhances serotoninergic transmission in feeding center of the brain (located in the ventromedial nucleus of the hypothalamus), leading to decreased caloric intake associated with increased serotonin levels.

ONSET, PEAK, DURATION
Onset and duration after oral administration unknown. Peak plasma levels occur from 1½ to 8 hours after oral dose.

INDICATIONS & DOSAGE
*Management of obesity and mainte-
nance of weight loss in patients on a re-
duced-calorie diet—*
Adults: 15 mg P.O. b.i.d. with meals.
Maximum daily dosage is 30 mg.

ADVERSE REACTIONS
CNS: *insomnia, headache, asthenia,*
somnolence, dizziness, depression, vertigo, emotional lability, abnormal
dreams, abnormal thinking, nervousness, anxiety, increased libido, hypertonia, paresthesia.
CV: Hypertension, angina pectoris, palpitations, vasodilatation.
GI: *diarrhea, dry mouth,* abdominal
pain, vomiting, constipation, nausea,
dyspepsia, gastritis, gastroenteritis, flatulence, rectal disorder.
GU: urinary frequency, polyuria, menstrual disorders, UTI.
Musculoskeletal: *arthralgia, myalgia,
arthritis, back pain.*
Respiratory: *pulmonary hypertension,*
pharyngitis, increased cough, bronchitis,
rhinitis, sinusitis.
Skin: rash, sweating, alopecia, urticaria,
pruritus.
Other: chills, fever, thirst, accidental
injury, infection, flulike syndrome, pain,
allergic reaction, taste perversion, amblyopia.

INTERACTIONS
*Alcohol and other drugs with CNS ac-
tion:* sedative effects may be potentiated
with drug. Use cautiously.
MAO inhibitors: possible severe, fatal
reactions. Do not use concomitantly or
within 14 days after an MAO inhibitor
has been discontinued.
*Serotonin reuptake inhibitors, agents for
migraine therapy (sumatriptan succinate or Imitrex, dihydroergotamine):*
may cause "serotonin syndrome," re-

quiring immediate medical attention.
Monitor for symptoms such as excitement, loss of consciousness, hyperreflexia, and tachycardia.
Serotoninergic agents: unknown. Appropriate interval between administra-
tions has not been established. Do not
give concomitantly.

EFFECTS ON DIAGNOSTIC TESTS
False-positive urine drug test for amphetamines by ELISA method for up to
24 hours after a 30-mg dose.

CONTRAINDICATIONS
Contraindicated in patients with known
hypersensitivity to the drug, fenfluramine, or related compounds; in patients with pulmonary hypertension; and
in patients receiving MAO inhibitors.

NURSING CONSIDERATIONS
● Use cautiously in the elderly and in
patients with glaucoma.
● Dexfenfluramine is not recommended
for pregnant or breast-feeding women.
● Know that safety and effectiveness in
pediatric patients have not been established.
● Be aware that before therapy begins,
organic causes of obesity should be excluded.
● Know that drug is recommended for
obese patients with an initial body mass
index (BMI) of at least 30 kg/m^2 or at
least 27 kg/m^2 in the presence of other
risk factors such as hypertension, diabetes, or hyperlipidemia. BMI is calculated by dividing the patient's weight in
kilograms by his height in meters, and
then squaring the results.
● Because weight loss can reduce hyperglycemia in diabetics, reduce blood
pressure in hypertensive patients and
improve the lipid profile, these conditions should be monitored and drug
therapy adjusted as needed.
● Make sure patient is involved in a
weight-reduction program.
● Know that if patient has not lost at
least 4 pounds in the first 4 weeks of

treatment, therapy should be reevaluated.

☑ **PATIENT TEACHING**
● Warn patient to avoid hazardous tasks until adverse CNS effects of the drug are known.
● Tell patient to avoid alcohol and to report symptoms of intolerance, such as nausea or vomiting.
● Tell patient that because drug therapy involves an associated risk of developing primary pulmonary hypertension, he should report signs and symptoms of dyspnea, angina, syncope, and lower extremity edema immediately.
● Tell patient not to discontinue drug abruptly; doing so may precipitate an acute depressive reaction.
● Tell patient the drug may cause a false-positive urine test for amphetamines.

---

dextroamphetamine sulfate
Dexedrine* **, Dexedrine Spansule, Oxydess II, Robese, Spancap #1

Controlled Substance Schedule II
Pregnancy Risk Category: C

HOW SUPPLIED
Tablets: 5 mg, 10 mg
Capsules (sustained-release): 5 mg, 10 mg, 15 mg

ACTION
Unknown. Probably promotes nerve impulse transmission by releasing stored norepinephrine from nerve terminals in the brain. Main sites of activity appear to be the cerebral cortex and the reticular activating system. In children with hyperkinesis, amphetamines have a paradoxical calming effect.

ONSET, PEAK, DURATION
Unknown.

INDICATIONS & DOSAGE
Narcolepsy—

Adults: 5 to 60 mg P.O. daily in divided doses.
Children 6 to 12 years: 5 mg P.O. daily, with 5-mg increments weekly, p.r.n.
Children 12 years and older: 10 mg P.O. daily, with 10-mg increments weekly, p.r.n. Give first dose on awakening; additional doses (one or two) at intervals of 4 to 6 hours.
Short-term adjunct in exogenous obesity—
Adults and children 12 years and older: 5 to 30 mg P.O. daily 30 to 60 minutes before meals in divided doses of 5 to 10 mg. Alternatively, one 10- or 15-mg sustained-release capsule daily as a single dose in the morning.
Attention deficit disorder with hyperactivity—
Children 3 to 5 years: 2.5 mg P.O. daily, with 2.5-mg increments weekly, p.r.n.
Children 6 years and older: 5 mg P.O. once daily or b.i.d., with 5-mg increments weekly, p.r.n. Only in rare cases will it be necessary to exceed a total dosage of 40 mg/day.

ADVERSE REACTIONS
CNS: *restlessness,* tremor, *insomnia,* dizziness, headache, chills, overstimulation, dysphoria, euphoria.
CV: *tachycardia, palpitations,* hypertension, arrhythmias.
GI: dry mouth, unpleasant taste, diarrhea, constipation, anorexia, weight loss and other GI disturbances.
GU: impotence.
Skin: urticaria.
Other: altered libido.

INTERACTIONS
Acidifying agents, ammonium chloride, ascorbic acid: decreased blood levels and increased renal clearance of dextroamphetamine. Monitor for decreased amphetamine effects.
Adrenergic blockers: adrenergic blockers inhibited by amphetamines. Avoid concomitant use.
Alkalizing agents, antacids, sodium bicarbonate, acetazolamide: increased re-

---

*Liquid contains alcohol.   **May contain tartrazine.   †Canada only.   ‡Australia only.   ◇OTC.

nal reabsorption. Monitor for enhanced amphetamine effects.

Antihistamines: amphetamines may counteract the sedative effects of antihistamines.

Caffeine: may increase amphetamine and related amine effects.

Chlorpromazine: inhibits the central stimulant effects of amphetamines. Can be used to treat amphetamine poisoning.

Insulin, oral antidiabetic agents: may decrease antidiabetic agent requirements. Monitor blood glucose levels.

Lithium carbonate: may inhibit antiobesity and stimulating effects of amphetamines. Monitor patient closely.

MAO inhibitors: may cause severe hypertension, possibly hypertensive crisis. Don't use together or within 14 days after MAO inhibitor has been discontinued.

Meperidine: amphetamines potentiate analgesic effect. Use together cautiously.

Methenamine therapy: increased urinary excretion of amphetamines and efficacy reduced. Monitor effects.

Norepinephrine: amphetamines enhance the adrenergic effect of norepinephrine.

Phenobarbital, phenytoin: amphetamines may delay absorption. Monitor patient closely.

Phenothiazines, haloperidol, tricyclic antidepressants: increased CNS effects. Avoid concomitant use.

Propoxyphene: in cases of propoxyphene overdose, amphetamine CNS stimulation is potentiated, and fatal seizures can occur.

Veratrum alkaloids: amphetamines inhibit hypotensive effect of veratrum alkaloids. Monitor blood pressure closely.

EFFECTS ON DIAGNOSTIC TESTS
Dextroamphetamine may elevate plasma corticosteroid levels and may also interfere with urinary steroid determinations.

CONTRAINDICATIONS
Contraindicated in patients with hypersensitivity or idiosyncrasy to the sympa-

thomimetic amines; within 14 days of MAO inhibitor therapy; and in those with hyperthyroidism, moderate to severe hypertension, symptomatic CV disease, glaucoma, advanced arteriosclerosis, and history of drug abuse.

NURSING CONSIDERATIONS
● Use cautiously in patients with motor and phonic tics, Tourette syndrome, and in agitated states.
● Be aware drug not recommended for first-line treatment of obesity. Use as an anorexigenic agent is prohibited in some states.
● Be aware drug is not to be used to prevent fatigue.
● Make sure the obese patient is on a weight-reduction program.
● If tolerance to anorexigenic effect develops, know that drug should be discontinued. Notify doctor.

☑ **PATIENT TEACHING**
● Tell the patient to take drug 30 to 60 minutes before meals if used for weight reduction and at least 6 hours before bedtime to avoid sleep interference.
● Warn the patient to avoid activities that require alertness or good psychomotor coordination until CNS effects of the drug are known.
● Tell the patient to avoid drinks containing caffeine, which increases the effects of amphetamines and related amines.
● Tell the patient that fatigue may result as drug effects wear off. The patient will need more rest.
● Have the patient report signs of excessive stimulation.

---

diethylpropion hydrochloride
M-Orexic, Nobesine†, Nobesine-75†, Propion†, Tenuate, Tenuate Dospan, Tepanil, Tepanil Ten-Tab

Controlled Substance Schedule IV
Pregnancy Risk Category: B

HOW SUPPLIED
Tablets: 25 mg
Tablets (extended-release): 75 mg
Capsules (extended-release): 75 mg†

ACTION
Unknown. Probably promotes nerve impulse transmission by releasing stored norepinephrine from nerve terminals in the brain. Main sites of activity appear to be the cerebral cortex and the reticular activating system.

ONSET, PEAK, DURATION
Onset and peak unknown. Effects of regular-release tablets persist for 4 hours; effects of extended-release tablets and capsules, for 12 hours.

INDICATIONS & DOSAGE
Short-term adjunct in exogenous obesity—
Adults: 25 mg P.O. before meals t.i.d.; or 75 mg extended-release tablet or capsule P.O. in midmorning.

ADVERSE REACTIONS
CNS: headache, *nervousness,* insomnia, fatigue, anxiety, drowsiness.
CV: *tachycardia, palpitations,* elevated blood pressure, **pulmonary hypertension,** ECG changes, arrhythmias.
EENT: blurred vision, mydriasis.
GI: dry mouth, nausea, abdominal cramps, diarrhea, constipation, unpleasant taste, vomiting.
GU: impotence.
Hematologic: decreased blood glucose levels.
Skin: urticaria, rash.
Other: altered libido, changes in menstruation.

INTERACTIONS
Caffeine: may increase amphetamine and related amine effects. Avoid concomitant use.
Guanethidine: decrease antihypertensive effect. Monitor blood pressure.
Insulin, oral antidiabetic agents: may decrease antidiabetic agent requirements. Monitor blood glucose levels.
MAO inhibitors: may cause hypertension, possibly hypertensive crisis. Don't use together or within 14 days after MAO inhibitor has been discontinued.

EFFECTS ON DIAGNOSTIC TESTS
None reported.

CONTRAINDICATIONS
Contraindicated in patients with hypersensitivity or idiosyncrasy to sympathomimetic amines; within 14 days of MAO inhibitor therapy; in those with hyperthyroidism, severe hypertension, advanced arteriosclerosis, glaucoma, or history of drug abuse; and in agitated patients.

NURSING CONSIDERATIONS
● Use cautiously in patients with mild to moderate hypertension, symptomatic CV disease (including arrhythmias), or seizure disorders.
● Be sure the patient also is on a weight-reduction program.
● Monitor patient for habituation or psychic dependence.
● If tolerance to anorexigenic effect develops, notify doctor because drug will need to be discontinued.

☑ PATIENT TEACHING
● Tell the patient to take drug at least 6 hours before bedtime to avoid sleep interference, although it seldom causes insomnia.
● Tell the patient to avoid drinks containing caffeine, which increases the effects of diethylpropion and related amines.
● Tell the patient to report signs of excessive stimulation.
● Tell the patient that fatigue may result as drug effects wear off.

doxapram hydrochloride
Dopram

Pregnancy Risk Category: B

HOW SUPPLIED
Injection: 20 mg/ml (benzyl alcohol 0.9%)

ACTION
Not clearly defined. Acts either directly on the central respiratory centers in the medulla or indirectly on chemoreceptors.

ONSET, PEAK, DURATION
Onset occurs in 20 to 40 seconds. Levels peak in 1 to 2 minutes. Effects persist for 5 to 12 minutes.

INDICATIONS & DOSAGE
Postanesthesia respiratory stimulation—
Adults: 0.5 to 1 mg/kg as a single I.V. injection (not to exceed 1.5 mg/kg) or as multiple injections q 5 minutes, not to exceed 2 mg/kg total dosage. Alternatively, 250 mg in 250 ml of 0.9% sodium chloride solution or D_5W infused at an initial rate of 5 mg/minute I.V. until a satisfactory response is achieved. Maintain at 1 to 3 mg/minute. Recommended total dosage for infusion should not exceed 4 mg/kg.
Drug-induced CNS depression—
Adults: for injection, priming dose of 2 mg/kg I.V., repeated in 5 minutes and again q 1 to 2 hours until patient awakens (and if relapse occurs). Maximum daily dosage is 3 g.
 For infusion, priming dose of 2 mg/kg I.V., repeated in 5 minutes and again in 1 to 2 hours if needed. If response occurs, give I.V. infusion (1 mg/ml) at 1 to 3 mg/minute until patient awakens. Do not infuse for longer than 2 hours or administer more than 3 g/day. May resume I.V. infusion after a rest period of 30 minutes to 2 hours, if needed.
Chronic pulmonary disease associated with acute hypercapnia—
Adults: 1 to 2 mg/minute by I.V. infusion (using 2 mg/ml solution). Maximum dosage is 3 mg/minute for a maximum duration of 2 hours.

ADVERSE REACTIONS
CNS: *seizures,* headache, dizziness, apprehension, disorientation, hyperactivity, bilateral Babinski's signs, paresthesia.
CV: *chest pain and tightness, variations in heart rate, hypertension,* arrhythmias.
EENT: sneezing, *laryngospasm.*
GI: nausea, vomiting, diarrhea.
GU: urine retention, bladder stimulation with incontinence.
Respiratory: cough, *bronchospasm, dyspnea.*
Skin: pruritus.
Other: hiccups, rebound hypoventilation, muscle spasms, diaphoresis, flushing.

INTERACTIONS
MAO inhibitors, sympathomimetics: potentiate adverse CV effects. Use together cautiously.

EFFECTS ON DIAGNOSTIC TESTS
Doxapram may cause T-wave depression on ECG, decreased erythrocyte and leukocyte counts, reduced hemoglobin and hematocrit levels, increased BUN levels, and albuminuria.

CONTRAINDICATIONS
Contraindicated in patients with seizure disorders; head injury; CV disorders; frank, uncompensated heart failure; severe hypertension; CVA; respiratory failure or incompetence secondary to neuromuscular disorders, muscle paresis, flail chest, obstructed airway, pulmonary embolism, pneumothorax, restrictive respiratory disease, acute bronchial asthma, or extreme dyspnea; or hypoxia not associated with hypercapnia.

NURSING CONSIDERATIONS
● Use cautiously in patients with bronchial asthma, severe tachycardia or arrhythmias, cerebral edema or increased CSF pressure, hyperthyroidism, pheochromocytoma, or metabolic disorders.

Reactions may be *common,* uncommon, *life-threatening,* or COMMON AND LIFE-THREATENING.

• Be aware that drug is used only in surgical or emergency department situations.

Alert: Establish an adequate airway before administering drug. Prevent patients from aspirating vomitus by placing them on their side.

• **I.V. use:** Administer slowly; rapid infusion may cause hemolysis. Doxapram is physically incompatible with strongly alkaline drugs, such as thiopental sodium, aminophylline, and sodium bicarbonate.

• Avoid extravasation, which may lead to thrombophlebitis and local skin irritation.

• Monitor blood pressure, heart rate, deep tendon reflexes, and arterial blood gases before giving drug and every 30 minutes afterward.

• Be alert for signs of overdosage: hypertension, tachycardia, arrhythmias, skeletal muscle hyperactivity, and dyspnea. Discontinue drug and notify doctor if patients show signs of increased arterial carbon dioxide or oxygen tension, or if mechanical ventilation is necessary.

☑ **PATIENT TEACHING**
• Inform patient, if alert, and family of need for drug.
• Answer the patient's questions and address his concerns.

---

fenfluramine hydrochloride
Ponderal†, Ponderal Pacaps†, Ponderax‡, Ponderax Pacaps‡, Pondimin, Pondimin Extentabs

Controlled Substance Schedule IV
Pregnancy Risk Category: C

HOW SUPPLIED
Tablets: 20 mg
Capsules (sustained-release): 60 mg†‡

ACTION
Unknown. Stimulates ventromedian nucleus of the hypothalamus. Also may affect serotonin metabolism.

ONSET, PEAK, DURATION
Onset occurs in 1 to 2 hours. Peak unknown. Effects persist for 4 to 6 hours.

INDICATIONS & DOSAGE
Short-term adjunct in exogenous obesity—
Adults: initially, 20 mg P.O. t.i.d. before meals. May increase by 20 mg/day at weekly intervals. Dosage adjusted according to patient response. Maximum dosage is 40 mg t.i.d.

ADVERSE REACTIONS
CNS: *drowsiness,* incoordination, headache, euphoria or depression, anxiety, *insomnia,* weakness, fatigue, agitation.
CV: *palpitations,* hypotension, hypertension, chest pain.
EENT: eye irritation, blurred vision.
GI: dry mouth, *diarrhea,* nausea, vomiting, abdominal pain, constipation.
GU: dysuria, increased urinary frequency, impotence.
Skin: rash, urticaria, burning sensation.
Other: diaphoresis, chills, fever, increased libido.

INTERACTIONS
Centrally acting antihypertensives: decreased antihypertensive effect. Monitor blood pressure.
Ethanol, CNS depressants: enhanced CNS depression. Don't use together.
Insulin, oral antidiabetic agents: may decrease antidiabetic agent requirements. Monitor blood glucose levels.
MAO inhibitors: may cause severe hypertension, possibly hypertensive crisis. Don't use together or within 14 days after an MAO inhibitor has been discontinued.

EFFECTS ON DIAGNOSTIC TESTS
None reported.

---

*Liquid contains alcohol.   **May contain tartrazine.   †Canada only.   ‡Australia only.   ◊OTC.

CONTRAINDICATIONS
Contraindicated in patients with psychotic disorders, severe hypertension, glaucoma, hypersensitivity to sympathomimetic amines, symptomatic CV disease (including arrhythmias), alcoholism, or history of drug abuse.

NURSING CONSIDERATIONS
• Use cautiously in patients with mild to moderate hypertension and history of mental depression.
• Make sure patient is on a weight-reduction program.
• Monitor patient for tolerance or physical or psychological dependence.
• Monitor blood pressure.

☑ PATIENT TEACHING
• Have the patient report signs of excessive sedation, depression, or excessive stimulation.
• Tell patient to avoid alcohol while taking this drug.
• Tell patient not to discontinue abruptly; may precipitate an acute depressive reaction.

---

methamphetamine hydrochloride
Desoxyn, Desoxyn Gradumet

Controlled Substance Schedule II
Pregnancy Risk Category: C

HOW SUPPLIED
Tablets: 5 mg
Tablets (long-acting): 5 mg, 10 mg, 15 mg**

ACTION
Unknown. Probably promotes nerve impulse transmission by releasing stored norepinephrine from nerve terminals in the brain. Main sites of activity appear to be the cerebral cortex and the reticular activating system. In children with hyperkinesis, methamphetamine has a paradoxical calming effect.

ONSET, PEAK, DURATION
Onset and peak unknown. Effects persist up to 24 hours.

INDICATIONS & DOSAGE
Attention deficit disorder with hyperactivity—
Children 6 years and older: 2.5 to 5 mg P.O. once daily or b.i.d., with 5-mg increments weekly, p.r.n. Usual effective dosage is 20 to 25 mg daily.
Short-term adjunct in exogenous obesity—
Adults: 2.5 to 5 mg P.O. b.i.d. to t.i.d., 30 minutes before meals; or 10- to 15-mg long-acting tablet daily before breakfast.

ADVERSE REACTIONS
CNS: *nervousness, insomnia,* irritability, *talkativeness,* dizziness, headache, hyperexcitability, tremor, euphoria.
CV: hypertension, *tachycardia, palpitations,* arrhythmias.
EENT: blurred vision, mydriasis.
GI: dry mouth, metallic taste, diarrhea, constipation, anorexia.
GU: impotence.
Skin: urticaria.
Other: altered libido.

INTERACTIONS
Ammonium chloride, ascorbic acid: decreased serum levels and increased renal excretion of methamphetamine. Monitor for decreased methamphetamine effects.
Antacids, sodium bicarbonate, acetazolamide: increased renal reabsorption. Monitor for enhanced effects.
Caffeine: may increase amphetamine and related amine effects. Avoid concomitant use.
Insulin, oral antidiabetic agents: may decrease antidiabetic agent requirements. Monitor blood glucose levels.
MAO inhibitors: may cause severe hypertension, possibly hypertensive crisis. Don't use together or within 14 days after stopping MAO inhibitor.
Phenothiazines, haloperidol, tricyclic antidepressants: altered CNS effects.

Reactions may be *common*, uncommon, *life-threatening*, or COMMON AND LIFE-THREATENING.

Avoid concomitant use.

EFFECTS ON DIAGNOSTIC TESTS
Methamphetamine may elevate plasma
corticosteroid levels and may also interfere with urinary steroid determinations.

CONTRAINDICATIONS
Contraindicated in moderate to severe
hypertension, hyperthyroidism, symptomatic CV disease, advanced arteriosclerosis, glaucoma, hypersensitivity or
idiosyncrasy to sympathomimetic
amines, history of drug abuse; within 14
days of MAO inhibitor therapy; and in
agitated patients.

NURSING CONSIDERATIONS
● Use cautiously in patients who are elderly, debilitated, asthenic, psychopathic, or who have a history of suicidal or
homicidal tendencies.
● Be aware that drug is not recommended for first-line treatment of obesity.
Use as an anorexigenic agent is prohibited in some states.
● When used for obesity, be sure patient
is on a weight-reduction program.
● If tolerance to anorexigenic effect develops, notify doctor because drug will
need to be discontinued.

☑ **PATIENT TEACHING**
● Tell the patient to take drug at least 6
hours before bedtime to avoid sleep interference.
● Warn the patient of high potential for
abuse. Advise him that drug should not
be used to prevent fatigue.
● Tell the patient never to crush sustained-release tablets.
● Warn the patient to avoid activities
that require alertness or good psychomotor coordination until CNS effects of the drug are known.
● Tell the patient to avoid drinks containing caffeine, which increases the effects of amphetamines and related
amines. Have him report signs of excessive stimulation.

methylphenidate hydrochloride
PMS-Methylphenidate‡, Ritalin, Ritalin-SR

Controlled Substance Schedule II
Pregnancy Risk Category: NR

HOW SUPPLIED
Tablets: 5 mg, 10 mg, 20 mg
Tablets (sustained-release): 20 mg

ACTION
Unknown. Probably promotes nerve impulse transmission by releasing stored
norepinephrine from nerve terminals in
the brain. Main site of activity appears
to be the cerebral cortex and the reticular activating system. In children with
hyperkinesis, methylphenidate has a
paradoxical calming effect.

ONSET, PEAK, DURATION
Onset and duration unknown. Peak levels occur about 2 hours after regular-release tablets, 4 or 5 hours after sustained-release tablets.

INDICATIONS & DOSAGE
Attention deficit disorder with hyperac-
tivity (ADDH)—
Children 6 years and older: initial
dose, 5 to 10 mg P.O. daily before
breakfast and lunch, with 5- to 10-mg
increments weekly p.r.n., up to 60 mg
daily.
Narcolepsy—
Adults: 10 mg P.O. b.i.d. or t.i.d. 30 to
45 minutes before meals. Dosage varies
with patient needs.

ADVERSE REACTIONS
CNS: *nervousness, insomnia,* Tourette
syndrome, dizziness, headache,
akathisia, dyskinesia, *seizures,* drowsiness.
CV: *palpitations,* angina, *tachycardia,*
changes in blood pressure and pulse
rate, arrhythmias.
GI: nausea, abdominal pain, anorexia,

weight loss.
Hematologic: *thrombocytopenia,* thrombocytopenic purpura, leukopenia, anemia.
Skin: rash, urticaria, *exfoliative dermatitis, erythema multiforme.*

INTERACTIONS
Caffeine: may increase amphetamine and related amine effects. Avoid concomitant use.
Centrally acting antihypertensives: decreased antihypertensive effect. Monitor blood pressure.
MAO inhibitors: may cause severe hypertension, possibly hypertensive crisis. Don't use together or within 14 days after an MAO inhibitor has been discontinued.
Tricyclic antidepressants: increased plasma levels of these drugs. Avoid concomitant use.

EFFECTS ON DIAGNOSTIC TESTS
None reported.

CONTRAINDICATIONS
Contraindicated in patients with hypersensitivity to drug, glaucoma, motor tics, family history of or diagnosis of Tourette syndrome, or history of marked anxiety, tension, or agitation.

NURSING CONSIDERATIONS
• Use cautiously in history of drug abuse, hypertension, history of seizures, or EEG abnormalities.
• Pemoline is the drug of choice for ADDH. It is usually stopped after puberty.
• Drug is not used to prevent fatigue.
• May precipitate Tourette syndrome in children. Monitor especially at start of therapy.
• Observe for signs of excessive stimulation. Monitor blood pressure.
• Monitor results of periodic CBC, differential, and platelet counts with long-term use.
• Monitor height and weight in children on long-term therapy. May delay growth

spurt, but children will attain normal height when drug is stopped.
• Monitor patient for tolerance or psychological dependence.

☑ PATIENT TEACHING
• Tell the patient to take drug at least 6 hours before bedtime to prevent insomnia and after meals to reduce appetite-suppressant effects.
• Warn the patient against chewing sustained-release tablets.
• Warn the patient to avoid activities that require alertness or good psychomotor coordination until CNS effects of the drug are known.
• Tell the patient to avoid drinks containing caffeine, which increases the effects of amphetamines and related amines.
• Warn patient with seizure disorder that drug may decrease seizure threshold. Instruct him to notify the doctor if seizure occurs.
• Inform the patient that he will need more rest as drug effects wear off.

---

pemoline
Cylert, Cylert Chewable

Controlled Substance Schedule IV
Pregnancy Risk Category: B

HOW SUPPLIED
Tablets: 18.75 mg, 37.5 mg, 75 mg
Tablets (chewable): 37.5 mg

ACTION
Unknown. Probably promotes nerve impulse transmission by releasing stored norepinephrine from nerve terminals in the brain. Main sites of activity appear to be the cerebral cortex and the reticular activating system.

ONSET, PEAK, DURATION
Onset and duration unknown. Serum levels peak 2 to 4 hours after dose.

INDICATIONS & DOSAGE

Because of the drug's association with life-threatening hepatic failure, it ordinarily should not be considered as first-line therapy for attention deficit disorder with hyperactivity.

Attention deficit disorder with hyperactivity—

Children 6 years and older: initially, 37.5 mg P.O. in the morning with daily dosage raised by 18.75 mg weekly, p.r.n. Effective dosage range is 56.25 to 75 mg daily; maximum dosage is 112.5 mg daily.

ADVERSE REACTIONS

CNS: *insomnia,* dyskinetic movements, irritability, fatigue, mild depression, dizziness, headache, drowsiness, hallucinations, *seizures, Tourette syndrome,* abnormal oculomotor function.
GI: anorexia, abdominal pain, nausea.
Hepatic: *acute hepatic failure,* hepatitis, jaundice, elevated liver enzymes.
Skin: rash, *aplastic anemia.*

INTERACTIONS

Insulin, oral antidiabetic agents: may decrease antidiabetic agent requirements. Monitor blood glucose levels.

EFFECTS ON DIAGNOSTIC TESTS

Pemoline may cause abnormalities in liver function test results.

CONTRAINDICATIONS

Contraindicated in patients with hepatic dysfunction and hypersensitivity or idiosyncrasy to the drug.

NURSING CONSIDERATIONS

Alert: Be aware that drug should be discontinued if significant hepatic dysfunction is observed during its use.
● Be aware that liver function tests should be performed prior to starting, and periodically during, therapy. Liver function tests may not predict the onset of acute liver failure. Treatment should be initiated only in individuals without liver disease and with normal baseline liver function tests.
● Use cautiously in patients with impaired renal function.
● Be aware drug is structurally dissimilar to amphetamines or methylphenidate; however, it may produce similar adverse reactions. Drug has greater potential for abuse and dependence than previously thought.
● May precipitate Tourette syndrome in children. Monitor especially at start of therapy.
● Closely monitor patients on long-term therapy for possible blood or hepatic function abnormalities and for growth suppression.

☑ PATIENT TEACHING

● Tell patient to take drug at least 6 hours before bedtime to avoid sleep interference.
● Tell patient to avoid activities that require alertness or good psychomotor coordination until CNS effects of the drug are known.
● Warn patient with seizure disorder that drug may decrease seizure threshold. Instruct him to notify doctor if seizure occurs.

---

phentermine hydrochloride
Adipex-P, Duromine‡, Fastin, Obe-Mar, Obe-Nix, Obephen, Oby-Trim, Panshape M, Phentercot, Phentride, Phentride Caplets, Phentrol, Phentrol-2, Phentrol-4, Phentrol-5, T-Diet

Controlled Substance Schedule IV
Pregnancy Risk Category: NR

HOW SUPPLIED

Tablets: 8 mg, 30 mg, 37.5 mg
Capsules: 15 mg, 18.75 mg, 30 mg, 37.5 mg
Capsules (resin complex, sustained-release): 15 mg, 30 mg

ACTION

Unknown. Probably promotes nerve impulse transmission by releasing stored norepinephrine from nerve terminals in the brain. Main sites of activity appear to be the cerebral cortex and the reticular activating system.

ONSET, PEAK, DURATION
Onset and peak unknown. Effects persist for 12 to 14 hours.

INDICATIONS & DOSAGE
Short-term adjunct in exogenous obesity—
Adults: 8 mg P.O. t.i.d. ½ hour before meals. Alternatively, 15 to 30 mg (resin complex) or 15 to 37.5 mg (phentermine hydrochloride) P.O. daily as a single dose in the morning.

ADVERSE REACTIONS
CNS: overstimulation, headache, euphoria, dysphoria, dizziness, *insomnia.*
CV: *palpitations, tachycardia,* increased blood pressure.
GI: dry mouth, dysgeusia, constipation, diarrhea, other GI disturbances.
GU: impotence.
Skin: urticaria.
Other: altered libido.

INTERACTIONS
Ammonium chloride, ascorbic acid: decreased plasma levels and increased renal excretion of phentermine. Monitor for decreased phentermine effects.
Antacids, sodium bicarbonate, acetazolamide: increased renal reabsorption. Monitor for enhanced effects.
Caffeine: may increase CNS stimulation.
Insulin, oral antidiabetic agents: may alter antidiabetic agent requirements. Monitor blood glucose levels.
MAO inhibitors: may cause severe hypertension, possibly hypertensive crisis. Don't use together or within 14 days after MAO inhibitor has been discontinued.
Phenothiazines, haloperidol, tricyclic antidepressants: altered CNS effects. Avoid concomitant use.

EFFECTS ON DIAGNOSTIC TESTS
None reported.

CONTRAINDICATIONS
Contraindicated in patients with hyperthyroidism, moderate to severe hypertension, advanced arteriosclerosis, symptomatic CV disease, glaucoma, or hypersensitivity or idiosyncrasy to sympathomimetic amines; within 14 days of MAO inhibitor therapy; and in agitated patients.

NURSING CONSIDERATIONS
● Use cautiously in patients with mild hypertension.
● Use in conjunction with a weight-reduction program.
● Monitor for tolerance or dependence.

☑ PATIENT TEACHING
● Tell the patient to take drug at least 6 hours before bedtime to avoid sleep interference.
● Advise the patient to avoid drinks containing caffeine. Tell him to report signs of excessive stimulation.
● Warn the patient that fatigue may result as drug effects wear off and that the patient will need more rest.

Reactions may be *common,* uncommon, *life-threatening,* or COMMON AND LIFE-THREATENING.

35
Antiparkinsonian drugs

amantadine hydrochloride
(See Chapter 17, ANTIVIRALS.)
benztropine mesylate
biperiden hydrochloride
biperiden lactate
bromocriptine mesylate
carbidopa-levodopa
levodopa
pergolide mesylate
selegiline hydrochloride
trihexyphenidyl hydrochloride

COMBINATION PRODUCTS
MADOPAR‡: levodopa 200 mg and benserazide 50 mg.
MADOPAR HBS‡: levodopa 100 mg and benserazide 25 mg.
MADOPAR Q‡: levodopa 50 mg and benserazide 12.5 mg.
SINEMET 10-100: carbidopa 10 mg and levodopa 100 mg.
SINEMET 25-100: carbidopa 25 mg and levodopa 100 mg.
SINEMET 25-250: carbidopa 25 mg and levodopa 250 mg.
SINEMET CR: carbidopa 50 mg and levodopa 200 mg, in extended-release tablets.

---

benztropine mesylate
Apo-Benztropine†, Bensylate†, Cogentin, PMS Benztropine†

Pregnancy Risk Category: NR

HOW SUPPLIED
Tablets: 0.5 mg, 1 mg, 2 mg
Injection: 1 mg/ml in 2-ml ampules

ACTION
Unknown. Thought to block central cholinergic receptors, helping to balance cholinergic activity in the basal ganglia.

ONSET, PEAK, DURATION
Onset occurs within 15 minutes of parenteral use, or within 1 to 2 hours of oral use. Peak unknown. Effects persist for 24 hours.

INDICATIONS & DOSAGE
Drug-induced extrapyramidal disorders (except tardive dyskinesia)
Adults: 1 to 4 mg P.O. or I.M. once or twice daily.
Acute dystonic reaction—
Adults: 1 to 2 mg I.V. or I.M., followed by 1 to 2 mg P.O. b.i.d. to prevent recurrence.
Parkinsonism—
Adults: 0.5 to 6 mg P.O. or I.M. daily. Initial dose is 0.5 mg to 1 mg., increased by 0.5 mg q 5 to 6 days. Dosage adjusted to meet individual requirements.

ADVERSE REACTIONS
CNS: disorientation, hallucinations, depression, toxic psychosis, confusion, memory impairment, nervousness.
CV: tachycardia.
EENT: dilated pupils, blurred vision.
GI: dry mouth, *constipation,* nausea, vomiting, paralytic ileus.
GU: urine retention, dysuria.
Some adverse reactions may result from atropine-like toxicity and are dose-related.

INTERACTIONS
Amantadine, phenothiazines, tricyclic antidepressants: additive anticholinergic adverse reactions, such as confusion and hallucinations. Reduce dosage before administering.

EFFECTS ON DIAGNOSTIC TESTS
None reported.

---

*Liquid contains alcohol.   **May contain tartrazine.   †Canada only.   ‡Australia only.   ◊OTC.

CONTRAINDICATIONS

Contraindicated in patients with hypersensitivity to drug or its components or narrow-angle glaucoma and in children under age 3.

NURSING CONSIDERATIONS

● Use cautiously in hot weather, in patients with mental disorders, and in children age 3 and older.
● Administer after meals.
● **I.V. use:** Route is seldom used because of small difference in onset when compared with I.M. route.
● Monitor vital signs carefully. Watch closely for adverse reactions, especially in elderly or debilitated patients. Call the doctor promptly.
● Be aware that drug produces atropine-like adverse reactions and may aggravate tardive dyskinesia.
● Watch for intermittent constipation and abdominal distention and pain; may indicate onset of paralytic ileus.
Alert: Never discontinue this drug abruptly. Reduce dosage gradually.

☑ PATIENT TEACHING

● Warn patient to avoid activities that require alertness until CNS effects of the drug are known. If the patient is to receive a single daily dose, tell him to take it at bedtime.
● Advise patient to report signs of urinary hesitancy or urine retention.
● Tell patient to relieve dry mouth with cool drinks, ice chips, sugarless gum, or hard candy.
● Advise limiting activities during hot weather because drug-induced anhydrosis may cause hyperthermia.

---

biperiden hydrochloride
Akineton

biperiden lactate
Akineton Lactate

Pregnancy Risk Category: C

HOW SUPPLIED
biperiden hydrochloride
Tablets: 2 mg
biperiden lactate
Injection: 5 mg/ml in 1-ml ampules

ACTION
Unknown. Blocks central cholinergic receptors, helping to balance cholinergic activity in the basal ganglia.

ONSET, PEAK, DURATION
Onset occurs within 30 minutes of parenteral use, within 1 hour of oral use. Peak unknown. Effects persist for 1 to 8 hours after I.V. use, for 6 to 12 hours after oral use.

INDICATIONS & DOSAGE
Drug-induced extrapyramidal disorders—
Adults: 2 mg P.O. once daily, b.i.d., or t.i.d., depending on severity. Usual dosage is 2 mg daily, or 2 mg I.M. or I.V. q ½ hour, not to exceed four doses or 8 mg daily.
Parkinsonism—
Adults: 2 mg P.O. t.i.d. or q.i.d. Dosage is individualized and titrated to a maximum of 16 mg/24 hours.

ADVERSE REACTIONS
CNS: disorientation, euphoria, drowsiness, agitation.
CV: transient postural hypotension (with parenteral use).
EENT: blurred vision.
GI: dry mouth, *constipation.*
GU: urine retention.
   Adverse reactions are dose-related and may resemble atropine toxicity.

INTERACTIONS
Amantadine, phenothiazines, tricyclic antidepressants: excessive CNS anticholinergic effects. Avoid concomitant use.
Antacids: decreased biperiden absorption. Administer antacids at least 1 hour after biperiden.

Reactions may be *common*, uncommon, *life-threatening*, or COMMON AND LIFE-THREATENING.

EFFECTS ON DIAGNOSTIC TESTS
None reported.

CONTRAINDICATIONS
Contraindicated in patients with hypersensitivity to the drug, narrow-angle glaucoma, bowel obstruction, or megacolon.

NURSING CONSIDERATIONS
• Use cautiously in patients with prostatic hyperplasia, arrhythmias, manifest glaucoma, and seizure disorder.
• To decrease adverse GI effects, give oral doses with or after meals.
• **I.V. use:** Administer very slowly.
• When giving parenterally, keep patient in supine position. Parenteral administration may cause transient postural hypotension and coordination disturbances.
• Monitor vital signs carefully. Watch closely for adverse reactions, especially in elderly or debilitated patients. Call the doctor promptly.
• Monitor patient for tolerance. If it develops, notify doctor because dosage will need to be increased.
• Know that in severe parkinsonism, tremors may increase as spasticity is relieved.

☑ **PATIENT TEACHING**
• Tell the patient to take oral form of drug with or after meals to decrease adverse GI effects.
• Warn the patient to avoid activities that require alertness until CNS effects of the drug are known.
• Because of possible dizziness, help the patient when he gets out of bed.
• Advise the patient to report signs of urinary hesitancy or urine retention.
• Advise the patient to relieve dry mouth with cool drinks, ice chips, sugarless gum, or hard candy.

bromocriptine mesylate
Parlodel

Pregnancy Risk Category: NR

HOW SUPPLIED
Tablets: 2.5 mg
Capsules: 5 mg

ACTION
Inhibits secretion of prolactin and acts as a dopamine-receptor agonist by activating postsynaptic dopamine receptors.

ONSET, PEAK, DURATION
Antiparkinsonian effects occur in 30 to 90 minutes; effects on serum prolactin, within 2 hours. Antiparkinsonian effects peak in 1 to 3 hours. Peak effects on serum prolactin occur within 8 hours. Antiparkinsonian effects persist for 12 to 18 hours; effects on serum prolactin, about 24 hours.

INDICATIONS & DOSAGE
Amenorrhea and galactorrhea associated with hyperprolactinemia; female infertility—
Adults: 1.25 to 2.5 mg P.O. daily, increased by 2.5 mg daily at 3- to 7-day intervals until desired effect is achieved. Therapeutic dosage ranges from 2.5 to 15 mg/day. Safety and efficacy of doses greater than 100 mg daily have not been established.
Parkinson's disease—
Adults: 1.25 mg P.O. b.i.d. with meals. Dosage increased q 14 to 28 days, up to 100 mg daily, p.r.n.
Acromegaly—
Adults: 1.25 to 2.5 mg P.O. with h.s. snack for 3 days. An additional 1.25 to 2.5 mg may be added q 3 to 7 days until patient receives therapeutic benefit. Maximal dosage is 100 mg/day.

ADVERSE REACTIONS
CNS: *dizziness, headache,* fatigue, mania, light-headedness, drowsiness, delusions, nervousness, insomnia, depres-

sion, *seizures.*
CV: *hypotension, stroke, acute MI.*
EENT: nasal congestion, blurred vision.
GI: *nausea,* vomiting, *abdominal cramps, constipation,* diarrhea, anorexia.
GU: urine retention, urinary frequency.
Skin: coolness and pallor of fingers and toes.

INTERACTIONS
Antihypertensives: increased hypotensive effects. Adjust dosage of the antihypertensive.
Haloperidol, loxapine, methyldopa, metoclopramide, MAO inhibitors, phenothiazines, reserpine: interferes with bromocriptine's effects. Bromocriptine dosage may need to be increased.
Levodopa: additive effects. Adjust dosage of levodopa.
Oral contraceptives, estrogens, progestins: interfere with effects of bromocriptine. Concurrent use not recommended.

EFFECTS ON DIAGNOSTIC TESTS
Transient elevation of BUN, ALT, AST, CK, alkaline phosphatase, and uric acid levels may occur.

CONTRAINDICATIONS
Contraindicated in patients with hypersensitivity to ergot derivatives, uncontrolled hypertension, toxemia of pregnancy, severe ischemic heart disease, or peripheral vascular disease.

NURSING CONSIDERATIONS
● Use cautiously in patients with impaired renal or hepatic function and history of MI with residual arrhythmias.
● Be aware that patients with impaired renal function may require dosage adjustments.
● Know that for Parkinson's disease, bromocriptine usually is given in addition to either levodopa or carbidopa-levodopa.
● Give drug with meals.
Alert: Monitor patient for adverse reactions. Incidence of adverse reactions is high (about 68%), particularly at beginning of therapy; however, most are mild to moderate, with nausea being the most common. Minimize adverse reactions by gradually titrating doses to effective levels as ordered. Adverse reactions are more frequent when drug is used for Parkinson's disease.
● Know that baseline and periodic evaluations of cardiac, hepatic, renal, and hematopoietic function are recommended during prolonged therapy.
● May lead to early postpartum conception. Test for pregnancy every 4 weeks or whenever period is missed after menses resumes.

☑ PATIENT TEACHING
● Instruct patient to take drug with meals.
● Advise patient to use contraceptive methods other than oral contraceptives or subdermal implants during treatment.
● Advise patient to avoid dizziness and fainting by rising slowly to an upright position and avoiding sudden position changes.
● Advise patient that it may take 8 weeks or longer for menses to resume and galactorrhea to be suppressed.

---

carbidopa-levodopa
Sinemet, Sinemet CR

Pregnancy Risk Category: NR

HOW SUPPLIED
Tablets: carbidopa 10 mg with levodopa 100 mg (Sinemet 10-100), carbidopa 25 mg with levodopa 100 mg (Sinemet 25-100), carbidopa 25 mg with levodopa 250 mg (Sinemet 25-250)
Tablets (extended-release): carbidopa 50 mg with levodopa 200 mg (Sinemet CR)

ACTION
Unknown for levodopa. Thought to be decarboxylated to dopamine, countering

---

the depletion of striatal dopamine in extrapyramidal centers. Carbidopa inhibits the peripheral decarboxylation of levodopa without affecting levodopa's metabolism within the CNS. Therefore, more levodopa is available to be decarboxylated to dopamine in the brain.

ONSET, PEAK, DURATION
Onset and duration unknown. Peak serum levels occur in about 40 minutes for regular-release tablets, or 2½ hours for extended-release tablets.

INDICATIONS & DOSAGE
Idiopathic Parkinson's disease, postencephalitic parkinsonism, and symptomatic parkinsonism resulting from carbon monoxide or manganese intoxication—
Adults: one tablet of 25 mg carbidopa/100 mg levodopa P.O. t.i.d. followed by an increase of one tablet every day or every other day, p.r.n., to a maximum daily dosage of eight tablets. 25 mg carbidopa/250 mg levodopa or 10 mg carbidopa/100 mg levodopa tablets are substituted as required to obtain maximum response. Optimum daily dosage must be determined by careful titration for each patient.

Patients treated with conventional tablets may receive extended-release tablets; dosage is calculated on current levodopa intake. Initially, the extended-release tablets given should amount to 10% more levodopa per day, increased, as needed and tolerated, to 30% more levodopa per day. Administered in divided doses at intervals of 4 to 8 hours.

ADVERSE REACTIONS
CNS: *choreiform, dystonic, dyskinetic movements; involuntary grimacing, head movements, myoclonic body jerks, ataxia,* tremor, muscle twitching; bradykinetic episodes; psychiatric disturbances, anxiety, disturbing dreams, euphoria, malaise, fatigue; severe depression, suicidal tendencies, dementia, delirium, hallucinations (may necessitate reduction or withdrawal of drug), confusion, insomnia, agitation.
CV: *orthostatic hypotension, cardiac irregularities,* phlebitis.
EENT: blepharospasm, blurred vision, diplopia, mydriasis or miosis, oculogyric crises, excessive salivation.
GI: *dry mouth,* bitter taste, *nausea, vomiting, anorexia,* weight loss may occur at start of therapy; constipation; flatulence; diarrhea; abdominal pain.
GU: urinary frequency, urine retention, urinary incontinence, darkened urine, priapism.
Hematologic: *hemolytic anemia,* thrombocytopenia, leukopenia, *agranulocytosis.*
Hepatic: hepatotoxicity.
Other: dark perspiration, hyperventilation, hiccups.

INTERACTIONS
Antihypertensives: additive hypotensive effects. Use together cautiously.
MAO inhibitors: risk of severe hypertension. Avoid concomitant use.
Papaverine, phenytoin: antagonism of antiparkinsonian actions. Don't use together.
Phenothiazines and other antipsychotics: may antagonize antiparkinsonian actions. Use together cautiously.

EFFECTS ON DIAGNOSTIC TESTS
Levodopa elevates serum and urinary uric acid concentrations when colorimetric test methods are used; it may produce false-positive test results for urinary glucose when cupric sulfate reagent is used and false-negative results in tests using glucose oxidase. False-positive results may occur for urine ketones tests using sodium nitroprusside reagent. Levodopa interferes with urine screening tests for phenyketonuria, falsely elevates urinary catecholamine levels, and may falsely decrease urinary vanillylmandelic acid (VMA) levels.

CONTRAINDICATIONS

Contraindicated in patients with hypersensitivity to drug, narrow-angle glaucoma, melanoma, or undiagnosed skin lesions, and within 14 days of MAO inhibitor therapy.

NURSING CONSIDERATIONS

• Use cautiously in patients with severe CV, renal, hepatic, endocrine, or pulmonary disorders; history of peptic ulcer; psychiatric illness; MI with residual arrhythmias; bronchial asthma; emphysema; and well-controlled, chronic open-angle glaucoma.

• If the patient is being treated with levodopa, the drug should be discontinued at least 8 hours before starting carbidopa-levodopa.

• Know that carbidopa-levodopa typically decreases amount of levodopa needed by 75%, reducing the incidence of adverse reactions.

• Be aware that therapeutic and adverse reactions occur more rapidly with carbidopa-levodopa than with levodopa alone. Observe and monitor vital signs, especially while adjusting dosage. Report significant changes.

• Carefully monitor patients receiving antihypertensives.

Alert: Muscle twitching and blepharospasm may be early signs of drug overdose; report immediately.

• Know that patients receiving long-term therapy should be tested regularly for diabetes and acromegaly and have periodic tests of liver, renal, and hematopoietic function as ordered.

• An accurate measure for urine glucose can be obtained if the paper strip is only partially immersed in the urine sample. Urine will migrate up the strip, as with an ascending chromatographic system. Read only the top of the strip.

☑ PATIENT TEACHING

• Tell patient to take the drug with food to minimize GI upset.

• Warn the patient and his caregivers not to increase dosage without doctor's orders.

• Warn the patient of possible dizziness and orthostatic hypotension, especially at start of therapy. Tell him to change position slowly and dangle legs before getting out of bed. Elastic stockings may control this adverse reaction in some patients.

• Instruct the patient to report adverse reactions and therapeutic effects.

• Inform the patient that pyridoxine (vitamin B_6) does not reverse the beneficial effects of carbidopa-levodopa. Multivitamins can be taken without losing control of symptoms.

---

levodopa
Dopar, Larodopa

Pregnancy Risk Category: NR

HOW SUPPLIED
Tablets: 100 mg, 250 mg, 500 mg
Capsules: 100 mg, 250 mg, 500 mg

ACTION
Unknown. Thought to be decarboxylated to dopamine, countering the depletion of striatal dopamine in extrapyramidal centers, which is thought to produce parkinsonism.

ONSET, PEAK, DURATION
Onset for maximal effects, 3 weeks to 6 months. Plasma levels peak in 1 to 3 hours. Effects vary but usually persist for about 5 hours.

INDICATIONS & DOSAGE
Idiopathic parkinsonism, postencephalitic parkinsonism, and symptomatic parkinsonism after carbon monoxide or manganese intoxication or in association with cerebral arteriosclerosis—
Adults and children over 12 years: initially, 0.5 to 1 g P.O. daily, divided in two or more doses with food; increased by no more than 0.75 g daily q 3 to 7 days until maximum response is

---

achieved. Do not exceed 8 g/day. Dosage adjusted to patient requirements, tolerance, and response. Higher dosage requires close supervision.

ADVERSE REACTIONS
CNS: *aggressive behavior; choreiform, dystonic, and dyskinetic movements; involuntary grimacing, head movements, myoclonic body jerks,* **seizures,** *ataxia, tremor, muscle twitching; bradykinetic episodes; psychiatric disturbances; mood changes, nervousness, anxiety, disturbing dreams, euphoria, malaise, fatigue; severe depression, suicidal tendencies, dementia, delirium, hallucinations* (may require reduction or withdrawal of drug).
CV: *orthostatic hypotension,* cardiac irregularities, phlebitis.
EENT: blepharospasm, blurred vision, diplopia, mydriasis or miosis, activation of latent Horner's syndrome, oculogyric crises, excessive salivation.
GI: dry mouth, bitter taste, *nausea, vomiting, anorexia,* weight loss (at start of therapy), constipation, flatulence, diarrhea, abdominal pain.
GU: urinary frequency, urine retention, incontinence, darkened urine, priapism.
Hematologic: *hemolytic anemia,* leukopenia, *agranulocytosis.*
Hepatic: hepatotoxicity.
Other: dark perspiration, hyperventilation, hiccups.

INTERACTIONS
Antacids: increased absorption of levodopa. Administer antacids 1 hour after levodopa.
Cocaine, sympathomimetic agents, inhalation anesthetics: increased risk of arrhythmias. Monitor closely.
MAO inhibitors, furazolidone, procarbazine: risk of severe hypertension. Avoid concomitant use.
Metoclopramide: accelerated gastric emptying of levodopa. Give metoclopramide 1 hour after levodopa.
Papaverine, phenothiazines and other antipsychotics, phenytoin, rauwolfia al-

kaloids: decreased levodopa effect. Avoid concomitant use, if possible.
Pyridoxine: reversal of antiparkinsonian effects. Check vitamin preparations and nutritional supplements for pyridoxine (vitamin B$_6$) content. Don't give together.
Foods high in protein: decreased absorption of levodopa. Don't give levodopa with high-protein foods.

EFFECTS ON DIAGNOSTIC TESTS
Coombs' test occasionally becomes positive during extended therapy. Colorimetric test for uric acid has shown false elevations. Copper-reduction method has shown false-positive results for urine glucose; glucose oxidase method has shown false-negative results. Levodopa also may interfere with tests for urine ketones.

CONTRAINDICATIONS
Contraindicated in concurrent therapy with MAO inhibitors within 14 days, and in hypersensitivity to the drug, acute angle-closure glaucoma, melanoma, or undiagnosed skin lesions.

NURSING CONSIDERATIONS
● Use cautiously in severe CV, renal, liver, and pulmonary disorders; peptic ulcer; psychiatric illness; MI with residual arrhythmias; bronchial asthma; emphysema; and endocrine disease.
● Patients who must undergo surgery should continue levodopa therapy as long as oral intake is permitted, generally 6 to 24 hours before surgery. Drug should be resumed as soon as patient is able to take oral medication.
● Carbidopa-levodopa typically decreases amount of levodopa needed by 75%, reducing the incidence of adverse reactions.
● Monitor vital signs, especially while adjusting dosage. Report changes.
● Muscle twitching and blepharospasm may be early signs of drug overdose; report immediately.
● Know that alkaline phosphatase, AST,

ALT, lactate dehydrogenase, bilirubin, BUN, and protein-bound iodine show transient elevations in patients receiving levodopa; WBC count, hemoglobin, and hematocrit show occasional reductions.
• Depending on reagent and test method used, expect possible false-positive increases in levels of uric acid, urine ketones, urine catecholamines, and urine vanillylmandelic acid.
• An accurate measure for urine glucose can be obtained if the paper strip is only partially immersed in the urine sample. Urine will migrate up the strip, as with an ascending chromatographic system. Read only the top of the strip.
• Know that patients receiving long-term therapy should be tested regularly for diabetes and acromegaly; periodically monitor renal, liver, and hematopoietic function as ordered.
• A doctor-supervised period of drug discontinuance (called a drug holiday) may reestablish the effectiveness of a lower dosage regimen.

☑ PATIENT TEACHING
• Tell the patient to take the drug with food to minimize GI upset. However, taking the drug with high-protein meals can impair absorption and reduce effectiveness.
• For the patient who has difficulty swallowing pills, tell him and his caregivers to crush tablets and mix with applesauce or baby food fruits.
• Warn the patient and his caregivers not to increase dosage unless ordered. Daily dosage should not exceed 8 g.
• Tell the patient to protect drug from heat, light, and moisture. If preparation darkens, it has lost potency and should be discarded.
• Warn the patient of possible dizziness and orthostatic hypotension, especially at start of therapy. Tell him to change position slowly and dangle legs before rising. Elastic stockings may control this adverse reaction.
• Advise the patient and his caregivers that multivitamin preparations, fortified

cereals, and certain OTC medications may contain pyridoxine (vitamin B_6), which can block the effects of levodopa by enhancing its peripheral metabolism.

---

pergolide mesylate
Permax

Pregnancy Risk Category: B

HOW SUPPLIED
Tablets: 0.05 mg, 0.25 mg, 1 mg

ACTION
A dopamine agonist that directly stimulates dopamine receptors in the nigrostriatal system.

ONSET, PEAK, DURATION
Unknown.

INDICATIONS & DOSAGE
Adjunctive treatment with carbidopa-levodopa in the management of the symptoms in Parkinson's disease—
Adults: initially, 0.05 mg P.O. daily for the first 2 days followed by increased dosage of 0.1 to 0.15 mg every third day over 12 days. Subsequent dosage increased by 0.25 mg every third day, if needed, until optimum response is seen. The drug usually is administered in divided doses t.i.d. Gradual reductions in carbidopa-levodopa dosage could be made during dosage titration.

ADVERSE REACTIONS
CNS: headache, asthenia, *dyskinesia, dizziness, hallucinations, dystonia, confusion, somnolence,* insomnia, anxiety, depression, tremor, abnormal dreams, personality disorder, psychosis, abnormal gait, akathisia, extrapyramidal syndrome, incoordination, akinesia, hypertonia, neuralgia, speech disorder, twitching.
CV: *orthostatic hypotension,* vasodilation, palpitations, hypotension, syncope, hypertension, ***arrhythmias, MI.***
EENT: *rhinitis,* epistaxis, abnormal vi-

---

sion, diplopia, eye disorder.
GI: dry mouth, taste perversion, abdominal pain, *nausea, constipation,* diarrhea, dyspepsia, anorexia, vomiting.
GU: urinary frequency, urinary tract infection, hematuria.
Skin: rash, diaphoresis, paresthesia.
Other: flulike syndrome; chest, neck, and back pain; chills; infection; facial, peripheral, or generalized edema; weight gain; arthralgia; bursitis; myalgia; dyspnea.
Note: The preceding adverse reactions, although not always attributable to the drug, occurred in more than 1% of the study population.

INTERACTIONS
Butyrophenones, metoclopramide, dopamine antagonists, phenothiazines, thioxanthenes: may antagonize effects of pergolide. Avoid concomitant use.

EFFECTS ON DIAGNOSTIC TESTS
None reported.

CONTRAINDICATIONS
Contraindicated in patients hypersensitive to the drug or to ergot alkaloids.

NURSING CONSIDERATIONS
● Use cautiously in patients prone to arrhythmias.
Alert: Monitor BP. Symptomatic orthostatic or sustained hypotension may occur especially at the start of therapy.

☑ **PATIENT TEACHING**
● Inform patient of potential adverse reactions, especially hallucinations and confusion (27% incidence).
● Warn patient to avoid activities that could result in injury from orthostatic hypotension and syncope.

---

selegiline hydrochloride
(L-deprenyl hydrochloride)
Eldepryl

Pregnancy Risk Category: C

HOW SUPPLIED
Tablets: 5 mg

ACTION
Unknown. May selectively inhibit MAO type B (found mostly in the brain). At higher-than-recommended doses, it is a nonselective inhibitor of MAO, including MAO type A (found in the GI tract). Also may directly increase dopaminergic activity by decreasing the reuptake of dopamine into nerve cells. Its active metabolites, amphetamine and methamphetamine, may contribute to this effect.

ONSET, PEAK, DURATION
Onset and duration unknown. Serum levels peak in ½ to 2 hours.

INDICATIONS & DOSAGE
Adjunctive treatment with carbidopa-levodopa in the management of the symptoms in Parkinson's disease—
Adults: 10 mg P.O. daily, taken as 5 mg at breakfast and 5 mg at lunch. After 2 or 3 days, gradual decrease of carbidopa-levodopa dosage.

ADVERSE REACTIONS
CNS: *dizziness,* increased tremor, chorea, loss of balance, restlessness, increased bradykinesia, facial grimacing, stiff neck, dyskinesia, involuntary movements, twitching, increased apraxia, behavioral changes, fatigue, headache, confusion, hallucinations, vivid dreams, anxiety, insomnia, lethargy.
CV: orthostatic hypotension, hypertension, hypotension, *arrhythmias,* palpitations, new or increased anginal pain, tachycardia, peripheral edema, syncope.
EENT: blepharospasm.
GI: dry mouth, *nausea,* vomiting, constipation, weight loss, abdominal pain, anorexia or poor appetite, dysphagia, diarrhea, heartburn.
GU: slow urination, transient nocturia, prostatic hyperplasia, urinary hesitancy, urinary frequency, urine retention, sexual dysfunction.

Skin: rash, hair loss.
Other: malaise, diaphoresis.

INTERACTIONS
Adrenergic agents: possible increased pressor response, particularly in patients who have taken an overdose of selegiline. Use together cautiously.
Meperidine: may cause stupor, muscle rigidity, severe agitation, and elevated temperature. Avoid concomitant use.
Foods high in tyramine: possible hypertensive crisis. Monitor blood pressure.

EFFECTS ON DIAGNOSTIC TESTS
None reported.

CONTRAINDICATIONS
Contraindicated in patients with hypersensitivity to the drug and in patients receiving meperidine.

NURSING CONSIDERATIONS
Alert: Some patients experience increased adverse reactions with levodopa and require a 10% to 30% reduction of carbidopa-levodopa dosage.

☑ PATIENT TEACHING
● Warn patient to move cautiously at the start of therapy because he may experience dizziness.
● Advise patient not to take more than 10 mg daily. A greater amount may increase adverse reactions.

---

trihexyphenidyl hydrochloride
Aparkane†, Apo-Trihex†, Artane*, Artane Sequels, Novohexidyl†, Trihexane, Trihexy-2, Trihexy-5

Pregnancy Risk Category: NR

HOW SUPPLIED
Tablets: 2 mg, 5 mg
Capsules (sustained-release): 5 mg
Elixir: 2 mg/5 ml

ACTION
Unknown. Blocks central cholinergic receptors, helping to balance cholinergic activity in the basal ganglia.

ONSET, PEAK, DURATION
Onset within 1 hour. Peak unknown. Effects persist for 6 to 12 hours.

INDICATIONS & DOSAGE
All forms of parkinsonism, drug-induced parkinsonism, and adjunctive treatment to levodopa in the management of parkinsonism—
Adults: 1 mg P.O. first day, 2 mg second day; then increased in 2-mg increments q 3 to 5 days until total of 6 to 10 mg is given daily. Usually given t.i.d. with meals, sometimes given q.i.d. (last dose h.s.) or switched to extended-release form b.i.d. Postencephalitic parkinsonism may require total daily dosage of 12 to 15 mg.

ADVERSE REACTIONS
CNS: nervousness, dizziness, headache, hallucinations, drowsiness, weakness.
CV: tachycardia.
EENT: blurred vision, mydriasis, increased intraocular pressure.
GI: *dry mouth,* constipation, *nausea,* vomiting.
GU: urinary hesitancy, urine retention.

INTERACTIONS
Amantadine: additive anticholinergic adverse reactions, such as confusion and hallucinations. Reduce dosage of trihexyphenidyl before administering.
Levodopa: increased effect when used concomittantly with levodopa. May require lower doses of both agents.

EFFECTS ON DIAGNOSTIC TESTS
None reported.

CONTRAINDICATIONS
Contraindicated in patients hypersensitive to the drug.

Reactions may be *common,* uncommon, *life-threatening,* or COMMON AND LIFE-THREATENING.

NURSING CONSIDERATIONS
● Use cautiously in glaucoma; cardiac, hepatic, or renal disorders; obstructive disease of the GI and GU tracts; and prostatic hyperplasia.
● Be aware that dosage may need to be gradually increased in patients who develop a tolerance to the drug.
● Monitor patient. Adverse reactions are dose-related and transient.
● Gonioscopic evaluation and monitoring of intraocular pressure are needed, especially in patients over 40 years.

☑ **PATIENT TEACHING**
● Advise the patient that drug may cause nausea if given before meals.
● Tell the patient to avoid activities that require alertness until CNS effects of the drug are known.
● Advise the patient to report signs of urinary hesitancy or urine retention.
● Tell the patient to relieve dry mouth with cool drinks, ice chips, or sugarless gum or hard candy.

donepezil hydrochloride
fluvoxamine maleate
lithium carbonate
lithium citrate
nicotine polacrilex
nicotine transdermal system
sumatriptan succinate
tacrine hydrochloride

COMBINATION PRODUCTS
None.

▼ NEW DRUG

donepezil hydrochloride
Aricept

Pregnancy Risk Category: C

HOW SUPPLIED
Tablets: 5 mg, 10 mg

ACTION
Believed to inhibit the enzyme acetylcholinesterase in the CNS, increasing the concentration of acetylcholine and temporarily improving cognitive function in patients with Alzheimer's disease.

ONSET, PEAK, DURATION
Onset and duration unknown. Plasma levels peak in 3 to 4 hours.

INDICATIONS & DOSAGE
Mild to moderate dementia of the Alzheimer's type—
Adults: initially, 5 mg P.O. daily at bedtime. After 4 to 6 weeks, dosage may be increased to 10 mg daily.

ADVERSE REACTIONS
CNS: *headache, insomnia,* dizziness, depression, abnormal dreams, somnolence, seizures, tremor, irritability, paresthesia, aggression, vertigo, ataxia, increased libido, restlessness, abnormal crying, nervousness, aphasia.
CV: syncope, chest pain, hypertension, vasodilation, atrial fibrillation, hot flashes, hypotension.
EENT: *cataract, blurred vision, eye irritation.*
GI: *nausea, diarrhea,* vomiting, anorexia, fecal incontinence, GI bleeding, bloating, epigastric pain.
GU: frequent urination.
Hematologic: ecchymosis.
Musculoskeletal: muscle cramps, arthritis, toothache, bone fracture.
Respiratory: *dyspnea, sore throat, bronchitis.*
Skin: *pruritus, urticaria, diaphoresis.*
Other: pain, accident, fatigue, weight decrease, influenza, dehydration.

INTERACTIONS
Anticholinergics: drug may interfere with anticholinergic activity. Monitor patient.
Carbamazepine, dexamethasone, rifampin, phenytoin, phenobarbital: may increase rate of elimination of donepezil. Monitor patient.
Cholinomimetics, cholinesterase inhibitors: synergistic effect. Monitor patient closely.
Succinylcholine, bethanechol: Additive effects. Monitor patient closely.

EFFECTS ON DIAGNOSTIC TESTS
None reported.

CONTRAINDICATIONS
Contraindicated in patients with known hypersensitivity to drug or to piperidine derivatives.

NURSING CONSIDERATIONS
● Use cautiously in patients with cardiovascular disease, asthma or obstructive pulmonary disease, urinary outflow im-

pairment, or a history of ulcer disease, and in those patients presently taking nonsteroidal anti-inflammatory drugs (NSAIDs).

• Know that donepezil should be used in pregnancy only if the benefit justifies the risk to the fetus. Women taking the drug should not breast-feed.

• Know that safety and effectiveness in pediatric patients have not been established.

• Monitor for symptoms of active or occult GI bleeding.

☑ **PATIENT TEACHING**
• Patient and caregivers should understand that drug does not alter underlying degenerative disease but can alleviate symptoms. Effects of therapy depend on administration of drug at regular intervals.

• Tell the caregiver to give drug in the evening, just before bedtime.

• Advise patient and caregivers to immediately report significant adverse effects or changes in overall health status and to inform health care team that patient takes drug before he has anesthesia.

---

fluvoxamine maleate
Luvox

Pregnancy Risk Category: C

HOW SUPPLIED
Tablets: 50 mg, 100 mg

ACTION
Unknown. Selectively inhibits the neuronal uptake of serotonin, which is thought to improve obsessive-compulsive disorders.

ONSET, PEAK, DURATION
Onset and duration unknown. Serum levels peak in 3 to 8 hours.

INDICATIONS & DOSAGE
Obsessive-compulsive disorder—

Adults: initially, 50 mg P.O. daily h.s., increased in 50-mg increments q 4 to 7 days until maximum benefit achieved. Maximum daily dosage is 300 mg. Total daily doses of more than 100 mg should be given in two divided doses.

ADVERSE REACTIONS
CNS: *headache, asthenia, somnolence, insomnia, nervousness*, dizziness, tremor, anxiety, hypertonia, *agitation*, depression, CNS stimulation, taste perversion.
CV: palpitations, vasodilation.
EENT: amblyopia.
GI: *nausea, diarrhea, constipation, dyspepsia*, anorexia, *vomiting*, flatulence, tooth disorder, dysphagia, *dry mouth*.
GU: decreased libido, abnormal ejaculation, urinary frequency, impotence, anorgasmia, urine retention.
Respiratory: upper respiratory tract infection, dyspnea, yawning.
Skin: sweating.
Other: flulike syndrome, chills.

INTERACTIONS
Astemizole, terfenadine: may cause decreased metabolism, leading to increased levels of these antihistamines and cardiotoxicity. Avoid concomitant use.
Benzodiazepines, theophylline, warfarin: reduced clearance of these drugs by fluvoxamine. Use together cautiously (except for diazepam, which should not be administered together with fluvoxamine). Dosage adjustments may be necessary.
Carbamazepine, clozapine, methadone, metopranolol, propranolol, tricyclic antidepressants: elevated serum levels of these drugs caused by fluvoxamine. Use together cautiously. Monitor patient closely for adverse reactions. Dosage adjustments may be necessary.
Diltiazem: bradycardia may occur. Monitor heart rate.
Lithium, tryptophan: may enhance effects of fluvoxamine. Use together cautiously.

---

*Liquid contains alcohol.   **May contain tartrazine.   †Canada only.   ‡Australia only.   ◊ OTC.

MAO inhibitors: may cause severe excitation, hyperpyrexia, myoclonus, delirium, and coma. Avoid concomitant use.
Tobacco products: decreased effectiveness of the drug. Advise patient that smoking may decrease effectiveness of the drug.

EFFECTS ON DIAGNOSTIC TESTS
None reported.

CONTRAINDICATIONS
Contraindicated in patients with hypersensitivity to the drug or to other phenylpiperazine antidepressants and within 14 days of MAO inhibitor therapy.

NURSING CONSIDERATIONS
● Use cautiously in patients with hepatic dysfunction, concomitant conditions that may affect hemodynamic responses or metabolism, or history of mania or seizures.
● Know that at least 14 days should elapse after stopping fluvoxamine before patient is started on an MAO inhibitor and that at least 14 days should elapse before a patient is started on fluvoxamine after MAO inhibitor therapy has been discontinued.
● Record mood changes. Monitor patients for suicidal tendencies, and allow them only a minimum supply of the drug.

☑ **PATIENT TEACHING**
● Warn patient not to engage in hazardous activity until drug's CNS effects are known.
● Instruct female patient who becomes pregnant or intends to become pregnant during therapy to notify doctor.
● Tell patient who develops a rash, hives, or a related allergic reaction to notify doctor.
● Inform patient that several weeks of therapy may be required to obtain the full antidepressant effect. Once improvement is seen, advise patient not to discontinue the drug until directed by

doctor.
● Advise patient to check with doctor before taking any OTC medication; drug interactions can occur.

---

lithium carbonate
Carbolith†, Duralith†, Eskalith, Eskalith CR, Lithane**, Lithicarb‡, Lithizine†, Lithobid, Lithonate, Lithotabs, Priadel‡

lithium citrate
Cibalith-S*

Pregnancy Risk Category: NR

HOW SUPPLIED
lithium carbonate
Tablets: 250 mg‡, 300 mg (300 mg equals 8.12 mEq lithium)
Tablets (controlled-release): 300 mg, 400 mg‡, 450 mg
Capsules: 150 mg, 300 mg, 600 mg
lithium citrate
Syrup (sugarless): 8 mEq (of lithium) per 5 ml
   Note: 5 ml of lithium citrate (liquid) contains 8 mEq lithium, equal to 300 mg of lithium carbonate.

ACTION
Unknown. Probably alters chemical transmitters in the CNS, possibly by interfering with ionic pump mechanisms in brain cells, and may compete with or replace sodium ions.

ONSET, PEAK, DURATION
Onset of clinical effects usually within 1 to 3 weeks. Serum levels peak in $1/2$ to 3 hours depending on dosage form used. Duration unknown.

INDICATIONS & DOSAGE
Prevention or control of mania—
Adults: 300 to 600 mg P.O. up to q.i.d. or 900 mg P.O. q 12 hours of controlled-release tablets; increase on the basis of

blood levels to achieve optimal dosage. Recommended therapeutic lithium blood levels: 1.5 mEq/L for acute mania; 0.6 to 1.2 mEq/L for maintenance therapy; and 2 mEq/L as maximum level.

ADVERSE REACTIONS

CNS: tremors, drowsiness, headache, confusion, restlessness, dizziness, psychomotor retardation, lethargy, *coma*, blackouts, *epileptiform seizures*, EEG changes, worsened organic mental syndrome, impaired speech, ataxia, muscle weakness, incoordination.

CV: reversible ECG changes, *arrhythmias*, hypotension, bradycardia, *peripheral vascular collapse* (rare).

EENT: tinnitus, blurred vision.

GI: dry mouth, metallic taste, nausea, vomiting, anorexia, diarrhea, *thirst*, abdominal pain, flatulence, indigestion.

GU: *polyuria*, glycosuria, renal toxicity with long-term use, decreased creatinine clearance, albuminuria.

Hematologic: *leukocytosis with leukocyte count of 14,000 to 18,000/mm³* (reversible).

Skin: pruritus, rash, diminished or absent sensation, drying and thinning of hair, psoriasis, acne, alopecia.

Other: transient hyperglycemia, goiter, hypothyroidism (lowered T_3, T_4, and protein-bound iodine, but elevated ^{131}I uptake), hyponatremia, ankle and wrist edema.

INTERACTIONS

Aminophylline, sodium bicarbonate, urine alkalinizers: increased lithium excretion. Avoid excessive salt and monitor lithium levels.

Carbamazepine, fluoxetine, indomethacin, methyldopa, piroxicam, probenecid: increased effect of lithium. Monitor for lithium toxicity.

Diuretics: increased reabsorption of lithium by kidneys, with possible toxic effect. Use with extreme caution, and monitor lithium and electrolyte levels (especially sodium).

Neuroleptics: may cause encephalopathy. Watch for signs and symptoms (lethargy, tremor, extrapyramidal symptoms), and stop drug if it occurs.

Neuromuscular blockers: may cause prolonged paralysis or weakness. Monitor patient closely.

Thyroid hormones: may induce hypothyroidism. Monitor thyroid function.

EFFECTS ON DIAGNOSTIC TESTS

Lithium causes false-positive test results on thyroid function tests; drug also elevates neutrophil count.

CONTRAINDICATIONS

Contraindicated if therapy cannot be closely monitored.

NURSING CONSIDERATIONS

● Know that drug should not be administered during pregnancy.

● Use with extreme caution in patients receiving neuroleptics, neuromuscular blockers, and diuretics; in elderly or debilitated patients; and in patients with thyroid disease, seizure disorder, renal or CV disease, severe debilitation or dehydration, and sodium depletion.

Alert: Be aware that determination of lithium blood concentration is crucial to the safe use of the drug. Drug should not be used in patients who can't have regular lithium blood level checks. Monitor lithium blood levels 8 to 12 hours after first dose, usually before morning dose, two or three times weekly first month, then weekly to monthly during maintenance therapy.

● Know that when blood levels of lithium are below 1.5 mEq/L, adverse reactions are usually mild.

● Monitor baseline ECG, thyroid and renal studies, as well as electrolyte levels, as ordered.

● Check fluid intake and output, especially when surgery is scheduled.

● Weigh the patient daily; check for signs of edema or sudden weight gain.

● Adjust fluid and salt ingestion to compensate if excessive loss occurs as a result of protracted diaphoresis or diarrhea. Under normal conditions, patients should have fluid intake of 2,500 to 3,000 ml daily and a balanced diet with adequate salt intake.

● Check urine specific gravity and report level below 1.005, which may indicate diabetes insipidus.

● May alter glucose tolerance in diabetics. Monitor blood glucose closely.

● Perform outpatient follow-up of thyroid and renal functions every 6 to 12 months. Palpate thyroid to check for enlargement.

☑ PATIENT TEACHING

● Tell patient to take drug with plenty of water and after meals to minimize GI upset.

● Explain to patient that lithium has a narrow therapeutic margin of safety. A blood level that is even slightly high can be dangerous.

● Warn patient and caregivers to watch for signs of toxicity (diarrhea, vomiting, tremor, drowsiness, muscle weakness, ataxia) and to expect transient nausea, polyuria, thirst, and discomfort during first few days. Patients should withhold one dose and call the doctor if toxic symptoms appear, but not stop drug abruptly.

● Warn ambulatory patient to avoid hazardous activities that require alertness and good psychomotor coordination until CNS effects of the drug are known.

● Tell patient not to switch brands of lithium or take other prescription or OTC drugs without the doctor's guidance.

● Tell patient to carry medical identification at all times.

---

nicotine polacrilex (nicotine-polacrilin resin complex)
Nicorette, Nicorette DS

Pregnancy Risk Category: C

HOW SUPPLIED
Chewing gum: 2 mg/square, 4 mg/square

ACTION
Provides nicotine, which stimulates nicotinic acetylcholine receptors in the CNS, neuromuscular junction, autonomic ganglia, and adrenal medulla.

ONSET, PEAK, DURATION
Onset and duration unknown. Serum levels peak within 15 to 30 minutes after the patient begins to chew the gum.

INDICATIONS & DOSAGE
Relief of nicotine withdrawal symptoms in patients undergoing smoking cessation—
Adults: initially, one 2-mg square; highly dependent patients should start treatment with 4-mg squares. Patients should chew 1 piece of gum slowly and intermittently for 30 minutes whenever the urge to smoke occurs. Most patients require 9 to 12 pieces of gum daily during the first month. For patients using 4-mg squares, maximum dosage is 20 pieces daily. For patients using 2-mg squares, maximum dosage is 30 pieces daily.

ADVERSE REACTIONS
CNS: dizziness, light-headedness, irritability, insomnia, headache.
CV: atrial fibrillation.
EENT: *throat soreness, jaw muscle ache* (from chewing).
GI: nausea, vomiting, indigestion, eructation, anorexia, excessive salivation.
Other: *hiccups.*

INTERACTIONS
Beta blockers, methylxanthines, propoxyphene, propranolol: decreased metabolism of these agents, increasing therapeutic effects. Dosage adjustments of these agents may be needed.
Tobacco products: reduced effectiveness of drug. Warn patient to avoid smoking while taking the drug.

EFFECTS ON DIAGNOSTIC TESTS
None significant.

CONTRAINDICATIONS
Contraindicated in nonsmokers; in patients with recent MI, life-threatening arrhythmias, severe or worsening angina pectoris, or active temporomandibular joint disease; and during pregnancy.

NURSING CONSIDERATIONS
● Use cautiously in patients with hyperthyroidism, pheochromocytoma, insulin-dependent diabetes, peptic ulcer disease, history of esophagitis, oral or pharyngeal inflammation, or dental conditions that might be exacerbated by chewing gum.
● Know that smokers most likely to benefit from nicotine gum are those with high "physical" nicotine dependence—those who smoke more than 15 cigarettes daily, prefer brands of cigarettes with high nicotine levels, usually inhale the smoke, smoke the first cigarette within 30 minutes of rising, find the first morning cigarette the hardest to give up, smoke most frequently during the morning, find it difficult to refrain from smoking in places where it's forbidden, or smoke even when ill and confined to bed during the day.

☑ PATIENT TEACHING
● Instruct patient to chew gum slowly and intermittently (chew several times; then place between cheek and gum) for about 30 minutes to promote slow and even buccal absorption of nicotine. Fast chewing tends to produce more adverse reactions.
● Be sure that patient reads and understands the instruction sheet included in the package.
● Emphasize the importance of withdrawing the gum gradually.
● Tell patient that successful abstainers will begin to gradually withdraw gum usage after 3 months. Use of the gum for longer than 6 months is not recommended. For gradual withdrawal, cut gum in halves or quarters and mix with other sugarless gum.

nicotine transdermal system
Habitrol, Nicoderm, Nicotrol, ProStep

Pregnancy Risk Category: D

HOW SUPPLIED
Transdermal system: designed to release nicotine at a fixed rate
Habitrol—21 mg/day, 14 mg/day, 7 mg/day
Nicoderm—21 mg/day, 14 mg/day, 7 mg/day
Nicotrol—15 mg/16 hours, 10 mg/16 hours, 5 mg/16 hours
ProStep—22 mg/day, 11 mg/day

ACTION
Provides nicotine, which stimulates nicotinic acetylcholine receptors in the CNS, neuromuscular junction, autonomic ganglia, and adrenal medulla.

ONSET, PEAK, DURATION
Users of Habitrol exhibit peak serum levels 5 to 6 hours after application; Nicoderm, 4 hours after application; Nicotrol, 3 to 6 hours; ProStep, 9 hours after application. Duration varies.

INDICATIONS & DOSAGE
Relief of nicotine withdrawal symptoms in patients undergoing smoking cessation—
Adults: initially, one transdermal system, delivering the largest available dosage of nicotine in its dosage series, applied once daily to a nonhairy part of body. For Habitrol, Nicoderm, and ProStep, patch should be kept on for 24 hours, then removed and a new system applied to an alternate skin site. For Nicotrol, the patch should be applied upon awakening and removed at bedtime. After 4 to 12 weeks (depending on the brand used), dosage tapered to next lowest available dosage of nicotine in its dosage series, followed in 2 to 4 weeks

by lowest nicotine dosage system in series being used. Drug is then stopped in 2 to 4 weeks.

ADVERSE REACTIONS

CNS: somnolence, dizziness, *headache, insomnia,* paresthesia, abnormal dreams, nervousness.
EENT: pharyngitis, sinusitis.
GI: abdominal pain, constipation, dyspepsia, nausea, diarrhea, vomiting, dry mouth.
GU: dysmenorrhea.
Respiratory: increased cough, pharyngitis, sinusitis.
Skin: *local or systemic erythema, pruritus, burning at application site,* cutaneous hypersensitivity, rash.
Other: back pain, myalgia, diaphoresis, hypertension.

INTERACTIONS

Acetaminophen, caffeine, imipramine, oxazepam, pentazocine, propranolol, theophylline: may decrease induction of hepatic enzymes that help metabolize certain drugs. Dosage reductions may be necessary.
Adrenergic agonists, such as isoproterenol or phenylephrine: may decrease circulating catecholamines. Dosage increases may be necessary.
Adrenergic antagonists, such as prazosin or labetalol: may decrease circulating catecholamines. Dosage reductions may be necessary.
Insulin: may increase amount of S.C. insulin absorbed. Dosage reduction of insulin may be necessary.

EFFECTS ON DIAGNOSTIC TESTS
None reported.

CONTRAINDICATIONS

Contraindicated in patients with hypersensitivity to nicotine or any component of the transdermal system. Also contraindicated in nonsmokers; in patients with recent MI, life-threatening arrhythmias, and severe or worsening angina pectoris.

NURSING CONSIDERATIONS

● Use cautiously in patients with hyperthyroidism, pheochromocytoma, hypertension, insulin-dependent diabetes, or peptic ulcer disease.
● Health care workers' exposure to nicotine within transdermal systems probably is minimal; however, avoid unnecessary contact with the system. Wash hands with water alone because soap may enhance absorption.

☑ PATIENT TEACHING

● Inform patient that use of the transdermal system for more than 3 months is not recommended. Warn patient that chronic nicotine consumption by any route can be dangerous and habit-forming.
● Patient should also be warned not to smoke. If he continues to smoke while using the system, he may experience serious adverse effects because peak serum nicotine levels will be substantially higher than those achieved by smoking alone.
● Be sure that patient reads and understands the information that's dispensed with the drug.
● Advise patient to apply the patch promptly because the nicotine can evaporate from the transdermal system once it's removed from its protective packaging. Patch should not be altered in any way (folded or cut) before application. Do not store at temperatures above 86° F (30° C).
● Teach patient proper disposal of the transdermal system. After removal, fold the patch in half, bringing the adhesive sides together. If it comes in a protective pouch, place the used patch in the pouch that contained the system. Careful disposal is necessary to prevent accidental poisoning of children or pets.
● Tell patient who experiences persistent or severe local skin reactions or generalized rash to immediately discontinue use of the patch and contact the doctor.
● Inform patient that patients who can-

not stop cigarette smoking during the initial 4 weeks of therapy probably will not benefit from the continued use of the drug. Such patients may benefit from counseling to identify factors that led to treatment failure. Encourage patient to minimize or eliminate factors contributing to treatment failure and to try again, possibly after some time has passed.

---

sumatriptan succinate
Imitrex

Pregnancy Risk Category: C

HOW SUPPLIED
Tablets: 25 mg, 50 mg, 100 mg (base)†
Injection: 6 mg/0.5 ml (12 mg/ml) in 0.5-ml prefilled syringes and vials

ACTION
Unknown. Thought to selectively activate vascular serotonin (5-hydroxytryptamine, 5-HT) receptors. Stimulation of the specific receptor subtype 5-HT_1, present on cranial arteries and the dura mater, causes vasoconstriction of cerebral vessels but has minimal effects on systemic vessels, tissue perfusion, and blood pressure.

ONSET, PEAK, DURATION
Onset occurs within 10 to 20 minutes after S.C. injection, or 30 minutes after oral administration. Serum levels peak about 12 minutes after S.C. injection, within 1½ hours after oral administration. Peak effect occurs within 1 to 2 hours after S.C. administration, within 2 to 4 hours after oral administration. Duration unknown.

INDICATIONS & DOSAGE
Acute migraine attacks (with or without aura)—
Adults: 6 mg S.C. Maximum recommended dosage is two 6-mg injections daily, with at least 1 hour allowed between injections. Alternatively, an initial dose of 25 to 100 mg P.O. and a second dose of up to 100 mg in 2 hours, if needed. Additional doses may be given q 2 hours, p.r.n., up to a maximum oral dosage of 300 mg/day.

ADVERSE REACTIONS
CNS: *dizziness, vertigo,* drowsiness, headache, anxiety, malaise, fatigue.
CV: *atrial fibrillation, ventricular fibrillation, ventricular tachycardia, MI, ECG changes such as ischemic ST-segment elevation* (rare).
EENT: discomfort of throat, nasal cavity or sinus, mouth, jaw, or tongue; altered vision.
GI: abdominal discomfort, dysphagia.
Skin: flushing.
Other: *tingling; warm or hot sensation; burning sensation; heaviness, pressure or tightness;* feeling of strangeness; tight feeling in head; cold sensation; pressure or tightness in chest; myalgia; muscle cramps; diaphoresis; neck pain; *injection site reaction.*

INTERACTIONS
Ergot and ergot derivatives: prolonged vasospastic effects. Don't use these drugs and sumatriptan within the same 24-hour period.
MAO inhibitors: increases sumatriptan's effects. Avoid concomitant use or within 2 weeks of discontinuing MAO inhibitor therapy.

EFFECTS ON DIAGNOSTIC TESTS
None reported.

CONTRAINDICATIONS
Contraindicated in patients with hypersensitivity to the drug; in patients with uncontrolled hypertension or ischemic heart disease (such as angina pectoris, Prinzmetal's angina, history of MI, or documented silent ischemia); in patients with hemiplegic or basilar migraine; in patients taking ergotamine; and within 14 days of MAO therapy.

---

*Liquid contains alcohol.   **May contain tartrazine.   †Canada only.   ‡Australia only.   ◊OTC.

NURSING CONSIDERATIONS
● Use cautiously in patients who are or intend to become pregnant.
● Also use cautiously in patients who may have unrecognized coronary artery disease (CAD), such as postmenopausal women; male patients over age 40; or patients with risk factors such as hypertension, hypercholesterolemia, obesity, diabetes, smoking, or family history of CAD.
● When giving the drug to patients at risk for unrecognized CAD, consider administering the first dose in the doctor's office. Serious adverse cardiac effects can follow S.C. administration of this drug, but such events are rare.
● After S.C. injection, most patients experience relief within 1 to 2 hours.
● Redness or pain at the injection site should subside within 1 hour after the injection.

☑ PATIENT TEACHING
● Tell the patient that the drug is intended only to treat migraine attacks, not to prevent or reduce their occurrence.
● Tell the patient who is pregnant or intends to become pregnant not to use this drug. Advise her to discuss with the doctor the risks and benefits of using the drug during pregnancy.
● Tell the patient that the drug may be given any time during a migraine attack, but should be given as soon as symptoms appear.
● Review information about the drug's injectable form, which is available in a spring-loaded injector system that facilitates self-administration. Be sure the patient understands how to load the injector, administer the injection, and dispose of the used syringes.
Alert: Tell the patient to notify the doctor immediately of persistent or severe chest pain. Tell the patient to stop using the drug and call the doctor if he experiences pain or tightness in the throat, wheezing, heart throbbing, rash, lumps, hives, or swollen eyelids, face, or lips.

tacrine hydrochloride
Cognex

Pregnancy Risk Category: C

HOW SUPPLIED
Capsules: 10 mg, 20 mg, 30 mg, 40 mg

ACTION
Reversibly inhibits the enzyme cholinesterase in the CNS, allowing the buildup of acetylcholine and thereby temporarily improving cognitive function in patients with Alzheimer's disease.

ONSET, PEAK, DURATION
Onset and duration unknown. Serum levels peak in $\frac{1}{2}$ to 3 hours.

INDICATIONS & DOSAGE
Mild to moderate dementia of the Alzheimer's type—
Adults: initially, 10 mg P.O. q.i.d. After 6 weeks and if the patient tolerates treatment and there are no transaminase elevations, dosage increased to 20 mg q.i.d. After 6 weeks, dosage titrated upward to 30 mg q.i.d. If still tolerated, dosage increased to 40 mg q.i.d. after another 6 weeks.

ADVERSE REACTIONS
CNS: agitation, ataxia, insomnia, abnormal thinking, somnolence, depression, anxiety, *headache*, fatigue, *dizziness*, confusion.
GI: *nausea, vomiting, diarrhea*, dyspepsia, loose stools, changes in stool color, anorexia, abdominal pian, flatulence, constipation.
Respiratory: rhinitis, upper respiratory tract infection, cough.
Skin: rash, jaundice, facial flushing.
Other: *elevations in transaminases* (especially ALT), myalgia, chest pain, weight loss.

INTERACTIONS
Anticholinergics: may decrease the ef-

fectiveness of anticholinergics. Monitor patient closely.

Cholinesterase inhibitors, cholinergics (such as bethanechol): additive effects. Monitor for toxicity.

Succinylcholine: enhanced neuromuscular blockade and prolonged duration of action. Monitor patient closely.

Theophylline: increased serum theophylline levels and prolonged theophylline half-life. Carefully monitor theophylline plasma levels, and adjust dosage, as ordered.

Food: decreased absorption of tacrine if taken concomitantly. Give drug 1 hour before meals.

EFFECTS ON DIAGNOSTIC TESTS
Tacrine may cause significant abnormalities in serum transaminase (ALT, AST), bilirubin, and gamma-glutamyl transpeptidase (GGT) levels.

CONTRAINDICATIONS
Contraindicated in patients hypersensitive to the drug or acridine derivatives. Also contraindicated in patients who have previously developed tacrine-related jaundice, which has been confirmed with an elevated total bilirubin level of more than 3 mg/dl.

NURSING CONSIDERATIONS
● Use cautiously in patients with sick sinus syndrome or bradycardia; in patients at risk for peptic ulceration (including patients taking NSAIDs or those with history of peptic ulcer); and in patients with history of hepatic disease. Also use cautiously in patients with renal disease, asthma, prostatic hyperplasia, or other urinary outflow impairment.
● Know that if the drug is discontinued for 4 weeks or more, the full dosage titration and monitoring schedule must be restarted.
● Monitor serum ALT levels weekly during the first 18 weeks of therapy as ordered. If ALT is modestly elevated after the first 18 weeks of monitoring

(twice the upper limit of normal range), continue weekly monitoring. If no problems are detected, frequency of serum determinations is decreased to once every 3 months. On each occasion that dosage is increased, resume weekly monitoring for at least 6 weeks as ordered.

☑ PATIENT TEACHING
● Patient and caregivers should understand that this drug does not alter the underlying degenerative disease, but can alleviate symptoms. Effect of therapy depends upon drug administration at regular intervals.
● Remind caregivers that dosage titration is an integral part of the safe use of this drug. Abrupt discontinuation or a large reduction in daily dosage (80 mg or more per day) may precipitate behavioral disturbances and a decline in cognitive function.
● Tell caregiver to give the patient the drug between meals whenever possible. If GI upset becomes a problem, the drug may be taken with meals, although doing so may reduce plasma levels by 30% to 40%.
● Advise the patient and caregivers to immediately report any significant adverse effects or changes in status.

37

Cholinergics (parasympathomimetics)

ambenonium chloride
bethanechol chloride
edrophonium chloride
neostigmine methylsulfate
physostigmine salicylate
pyridostigmine bromide

COMBINATION PRODUCTS
None.

---

ambenonium chloride
Mytelase Caplets

Pregnancy Risk Category: NR

HOW SUPPLIED
Tablets: 10 mg

ACTION
Inhibits the destruction of acetylcholine
released from the parasympathetic and
somatic efferent nerves. Acetylcholine
accumulates, promoting increased stimulation of the receptors.

ONSET, PEAK, DURATION
Onset ranges from 20 to 30 minutes.
Peak unknown. Effects persist for 4 to 8
hours.

INDICATIONS & DOSAGE
*Symptomatic treatment of myasthenia
gravis in patients who cannot take
neostigmine bromide or pyridostigmine
bromide—*
Adults: dosage individualized for each
patient, but usually ranges from 5 to 25
mg P.O. t.i.d. or q.i.d. Starting dose usually is 5 mg P.O. t.i.d. or q.i.d. Increased
and adjusted at 1- to 2-day intervals to
avoid drug accumulation and overdosage. Usual dosage range is 5 to 25
mg P.O. t.i.d. or q.i.d., but some patients
may require as much as 75 mg b.i.d. to
q.i.d.

ADVERSE REACTIONS
CNS: headache, dizziness, muscle
weakness, *seizures,* mental confusion,
drowsiness.
CV: bradycardia, hypotension, tachycardia, *cardiac arrest,* syncope, AV
block.
EENT: miosis, lacrimation, diplopia.
GI: *nausea, vomiting, diarrhea, abdominal cramps,* increased salivation, dysphagia.
GU: urinary frequency, incontinence.
Respiratory: bronchospasm, *bronchoconstriction,* increased bronchial secretions, *respiratory paralysis,* dyspnea.
Skin: rash, flushing, urticaria.
Other: muscle cramps, diaphoresis.

INTERACTIONS
*Aminoglycosides, anesthetics, atropine,
corticosteroids, magnesium, procainamide, quinidine:* prolonged or enhanced muscle weakness. Monitor
closely.
*Mecamylamine, other ganglionic block-
ers:* increased toxicity. Avoid concomitant use.
Cholinergics: increased effects. Discontinue all other cholinergics, as ordered,
before administering this drug.

EFFECTS ON DIAGNOSTIC TESTS
None reported.

CONTRAINDICATIONS
Contraindicated in patients with hypersensitivity to anticholinesterase agents
and in those with mechanical obstruction of intestine or urinary tract and in
patients receiving ganglionic blockers.

NURSING CONSIDERATIONS
● Use with extreme caution in patients
with bronchial asthma. Use cautiously
in patients with seizure disorders,
bradycardia, recent coronary occlusion,

vagotonia, peptic ulcer, hyperthy-roidism, arrhythmias, postoperative at-electasis, and pneumonia.
• Know that large doses should be avoided in patients with decreased GI motility or megacolon.
• Administer each dose exactly as or-dered, on time. Amount and frequency of dose should vary with the patient's activity level. The doctor probably will order larger doses when the patient is fatigued, for example, in the afternoon and at mealtime.
• Give with milk or food to produce fewer adverse muscarinic reactions.
• Monitor vital signs frequently, espe-cially respirations, and document. Al-ways have atropine injection available and be prepared to give 0.5 to 1 mg S.C. or by slow I.V. push as ordered. Provide respiratory support as needed.
Alert: Watch the patient very closely for adverse reactions, particularly if total dosage is greater than 200 mg daily. When adverse reactions indicate drug toxicity, such as weakness that occurs within 30 to 60 minutes of drug admin-istration, notify the doctor immediately.
• If muscle weakness is severe, know that the doctor must determine if it is caused by drug toxicity or exacerbation of myasthenia gravis. A test dose of edrophonium I.V. will aggravate drug-induced weakness but will temporarily relieve weakness resulting from the dis-ease.
• Seek approval, when indicated, for hospitalized patients to have bedside supply of tablets. Patients with long-standing disease often insist on taking pills themselves.
• Record the patient's variations in mus-cle strength.
• Be aware that patients may develop resistance to drug.

☑ **PATIENT TEACHING**
• Instruct the patient to take drug with milk or food.
• Show the patient how to monitor vari-ations in his muscle strength and to

keep a record of this information.
• When given for myasthenia gravis, explain that this drug will relieve symp-toms of ptosis, double vision, difficulty in chewing and swallowing, and trunk and limb weakness. Stress the impor-tance of taking this drug exactly as or-dered.
• Explain to the patient and his family that ambenonium chloride is a long-term drug. Teach them about the disease and the drug's effect on symptoms.
• Advise the patient to wear medical identification bracelet indicating myas-thenia gravis.

---

bethanechol chloride
Duvoid, Myotonachol, Urabeth, Ure-choline, Urocarb Liquid‡, Urocarb Tablets‡

Pregnancy Risk Category: C

HOW SUPPLIED
Tablets: 5 mg, 10 mg, 25 mg, 50 mg
Injection: 5 mg/ml

ACTION
Directly stimulates cholinergic recep-tors, mimicking the action of acetyl-choline.

ONSET, PEAK, DURATION
Onset occurs within 5 to 15 minutes of S.C. dose, within 30 to 90 minutes of oral dose. Serum levels peak 15 to 30 minutes after S.C. administration, about 1 hour after oral dose. Effects persist for about 2 hours after S.C. administration, up to 6 hours after oral administration, depending on dose.

INDICATIONS & DOSAGE
Acute postoperative and postpartum nonobstructive (functional) urine reten-tion, neurogenic atony of urinary blad-der with urine retention—
Adults: 10 to 50 mg P.O. t.i.d. to q.i.d. Or, 2.5 to 5 mg S.C. Never give I.M. or I.V. When used for urine retention,

526 AUTONOMIC NERVOUS SYSTEM DRUGS

some patients may require 50 to 100 mg P.O. per dose. Use such doses with extreme caution.

Test dose is 2.5 mg S.C., repeated at 15- to 30-minute intervals to total of four doses to determine the minimal effective dose; then minimal effective dose used q 6 to 8 hours. All doses must be adjusted individually.

ADVERSE REACTIONS
CNS: headache, malaise.
CV: hypotension, reflex tachycardia.
EENT: lacrimation, miosis.
GI: *abdominal cramps, diarrhea,* excessive salivation, nausea, belching, borborygmus.
GU: urinary urgency.
Respiratory: *bronchoconstriction,* increased bronchial secretions.
Skin: flushing, diaphoresis.

INTERACTIONS
Atropine, anticholinergic agents, procainamide, quinidine: may reverse cholinergic effects. Observe for lack of drug effect.
Cholinergic agonists, anticholinesterase agents: may cause additive effects, or increase toxicity. Avoid concomitant use.
Ganglionic blockers: may cause hypotension. Avoid concomitant use.

EFFECTS ON DIAGNOSTIC TESTS
Bethanechol increases serum levels of amylase, lipase, bilirubin, and AST, and increases sulfobromophthalein retention time.

CONTRAINDICATIONS
Contraindicated for I.M. or I.V. use and in patients with hypersensitivity to drug or any of its components; in patients with uncertain strength or integrity of bladder wall; when increased muscular activity of GI or urinary tract is harmful; in patients with mechanical obstructions of GI or urinary tract; in patients with hyperthyroidism, peptic ulceration, latent or active bronchial asthma, pro-

nounced bradycardia or hypotension, vasomotor instability, cardiac or coronary artery disease, seizure disorder, Parkinson's disease, spastic GI disturbances, acute inflammatory lesions of the GI tract, peritonitis, or marked vagotonia.

NURSING CONSIDERATIONS
● Use cautiously in pregnant patients.
● Give on empty stomach; otherwise, may cause nausea and vomiting.
Alert: Never give I.M. or I.V.; could cause circulatory collapse, hypotension, severe abdominal cramping, bloody diarrhea, shock, or cardiac arrest.
● Monitor vital signs frequently, especially respirations. Always have atropine injection available and be prepared to give 0.5 mg S.C. or by slow I.V. push as ordered. Provide respiratory support if needed.
● Watch for toxicity, especially with S.C. administration. Edrophonium is not effective against muscle relaxation caused by bethanechol.
● Watch closely for adverse reactions that may indicate drug toxicity.
● Know that oral drug absorption is poor and variable, requiring larger oral doses. Oral and S.C. doses are not interchangeable.

☑ PATIENT TEACHING
● Instruct patient to take oral form on an empty stomach.
● Inform patient that drug is usually effective within 30 to 90 minutes after oral administration and 5 to 15 minutes after S.C. administration.

---

edrophonium chloride
Enlon, Reversol, Tensilon

Pregnancy Risk Category: NR

HOW SUPPLIED
Injection: 10 mg/ml in 1-ml ampules or in 10-ml or 15-ml vials

ACTION
Inhibits the destruction of acetylcholine released from the parasympathetic and somatic efferent nerves. Acetylcholine accumulates, promoting increased stimulation of the receptors.

ONSET, PEAK, DURATION
Onset occurs within 30 to 60 seconds of I.V. administration, within 2 to 10 minutes of I.M. injection. Peak unknown. Effects persist for 5 to 10 minutes after I.V. administration, 5 to 30 minutes after I.M. injection. Duration of action is extremely short.

INDICATIONS & DOSAGE
As a curare antagonist (to reverse nondepolarizing neuromuscular blocking action)—
Adults: 10 mg I.V. given over 30 to 45 seconds. Dose may be repeated as necessary to 40 mg maximum dosage. Larger dosages may potentiate effect of curare.
Diagnostic aid in myasthenia gravis (Tensilon test)—
Adults: 1 to 2 mg I.V. over 15 to 30 seconds, then 8 mg if no response (increase in muscular strength) occurs. Alternatively, 10 mg I.M. If cholinergic reaction occurs, 2 mg I.M. 30 minutes later is given to rule out false-negative response.
Children over 34 kg: 2 mg I.V. If no response within 45 seconds, 1 mg q 45 seconds to maximum of 10 mg.
Children up to 34 kg: 1 mg I.V. If no response within 45 seconds, 1 mg q 45 seconds to maximum of 5 mg.

I.M. route may be used in children because of difficulty with I.V. route: for children under 34 kg, 2 mg I.M.; for children over 34 kg, 5 mg I.M. Expect same reactions as with I.V. test, but these appear after 2- to 10-minute delay.
To differentiate myasthenic crisis from cholinergic crisis—
Adults: 1 mg I.V. If no response in 1 minute, dose repeated once. Increased muscular strength confirms myasthenic crisis; no increase or exaggerated weakness confirms cholinergic crisis.

ADVERSE REACTIONS
CNS: *seizures,* weakness, dysarthria, dysphagia.
CV: hypotension, bradycardia, AV block, *cardiac arrest.*
EENT: excessive lacrimation, diplopia, miosis, conjunctival hyperemia.
GI: nausea, vomiting, *diarrhea, abdominal cramps,* excessive salivation.
GU: urinary frequency, incontinence.
Respiratory: *paralysis of muscles of respiration, central respiratory paralysis, bronchospasm, laryngospasm,* increased bronchial secretions.
Other: muscle cramps, muscle fasciculation, diaphoresis.

INTERACTIONS
Aminoglycosides, anesthetics: prolonged or enhanced muscle weakness. Monitor closely.
Corticosteroids, magnesium, procainamide, quinidine: may antagonize cholinergic effects. Observe for lack of drug effect.
Digitalis glycosides: may increase the heart's sensitivity to edrophonium. Use together cautiously.
Cholinergics: increased effects. Stop all other cholinergics before giving this drug, as ordered.

EFFECTS ON DIAGNOSTIC TESTS
None reported.

CONTRAINDICATIONS
Contraindicated in patients with hypersensitivity to anticholinesterase agents and in those with mechanical obstruction of the intestine or urinary tract.

NURSING CONSIDERATIONS
● Use cautiously in patients with bronchial asthma or cardiac arrhythmias.
● **I.V. use:** For easier parenteral administration, use tuberculin syringe with an I.V. needle. When giving drug to differentiate myasthenic crisis from choliner-

gic crisis, observe patient's muscle
strength closely.
• Monitor vital signs frequently, especially respirations. Always have atropine injection available and be prepared to give 0.5 to 1 mg S.C. or by
slow I.V. push as ordered. Provide respiratory support as needed.
• Watch closely for adverse reactions;
they may indicate toxicity.
• Keep in mind that the drug is effective
against muscle relaxation induced by
decamethonium bromide and succinylcholine chloride.
• Be aware that this cholinergic has the
most rapid onset but shortest duration;
therefore, it is not used to treat myasthenia gravis.

☑ **PATIENT TEACHING**
• Teach patient to report adverse reactions promptly.
• Tell patient to alert nurse if discomfort
occurs at I.V. site.

---

neostigmine methylsulfate
Prostigmin

Pregnancy Risk Category: C

HOW SUPPLIED
Injection: 0.25 mg/ml, 0.5 mg/ml, 1
mg/ml

ACTION
Inhibits the destruction of acetylcholine
released from the parasympathetic and
somatic efferent nerves. Acetylcholine
accumulates, promoting increased stimulation of the receptors.

ONSET, PEAK, DURATION
Onset occurs 4 to 8 minutes after I.V.
administration or 20 to 30 minutes after
I.M. injection. Peak levels occur within
1 to 2 hours, with considerable individual variations. Effects persist for 2 to 4
hours.

INDICATIONS & DOSAGE
Treatment of myasthenia gravis—
Adults: 0.5 to 2 mg S.C., I.M., or I.V. q
1 to 3 hours.
Children: 0.01 to 0.04 mg/kg/dose I.M.
or S.C. q 2 to 3 hours, p.r.n.
   Dosage must be highly individual-
ized, depending on response and toler-
ance of adverse effects. Therapy may be
required day and night.
Diagnosis of myasthenia gravis—
Adults: 0.022 mg/kg I.M. 30 minutes
after 0.011 mg/kg of atropine sulfate
I.M.
Children: 0.025 to 0.04 mg/kg I.M. after 0.011 mg/kg atropine sulfate S.C.
*Postoperative abdominal distention and
bladder atony—*
Adults: 0.5 to 1 mg I.M. or S.C. q 4 to
6 hours (treatment); 0.25 mg S.C. or
I.M. q 4 to 6 hours for 2 to 3 days (prevention).
*Antidote for nondepolarizing neuromus-
cular blocking agents—*
Adults: 0.5 to 2.5 mg I.V. slowly. Repeat p.r.n. to a total of 5 mg. Before antidote dose, 0.6 to 1.2 mg atropine sulfate is given I.V.
   Note: 1:1,000 solution of injectable
solution contains 1 mg/ml; 1:2,000 solution contains 0.5 mg/ml.

ADVERSE REACTIONS
CNS: dizziness, headache, muscle
weakness, loss of consciousness,
drowsiness.
CV: bradycardia, hypotension, tachycardia, AV block, syncope, *cardiac arrest.*
EENT: blurred vision, lacrimation,
miosis.
GI: *nausea, vomiting, diarrhea, abdominal cramps,* excessive salivation, flatulence, increased peristalsis.
GU: urinary frequency.
Respiratory: *bronchospasm,* dyspnea,
respiratory depression, *respiratory arrest,* increased secretions.
Skin: rash, urticaria, diaphoresis, flushing.
Other: *muscle cramps,* muscle fascicu-

lations, arthralgia, hypersensitivity reactions *(anaphylaxis).*

INTERACTIONS
Atropine, anticholinergic agents, corticosteroids, magnesium sulfate, procainamide, aminoglycosides, quinidine: may reverse cholinergic effects. Observe for lack of drug effect. Stop all other cholinergics before giving this drug, as ordered.

Succinylcholine: may worsen blockade produced by succinylcholine when used to reverse the effects of nondepolarizing neuromuscular blockers in patients who have undergone surgery.

EFFECTS ON DIAGNOSTIC TESTS
None reported.

CONTRAINDICATIONS
Contraindicated in patients with hypersensitivity to cholinergics and in those with peritonitis or mechanical obstruction of the intestine or urinary tract.

NURSING CONSIDERATIONS
● Use cautiously in patients with bronchial asthma, bradycardia, seizure disorders, recent coronary occlusion, vagotonia, hyperthyroidism, arrhythmias, and peptic ulcer.
● In myasthenia gravis, schedule doses before periods of fatigue. For example, if the patient has dysphagia, schedule dose 30 minutes before each meal.
● **I.V. use:** Give at a slow, controlled rate, not exceeding 1 mg/minute in adults and 0.5 mg/minute in children.
● Monitor vital signs frequently, especially respirations. Have atropine injection available and be prepared to give as ordered; provide respiratory support, as needed.
● Monitor and document the patient's response after each dose. Optimum dosage is difficult to judge. Observe closely for improvement in strength, vision, and ptosis 45 to 60 minutes after each dose.
● If patient's muscle weakness is severe,

keep in mind that the doctor determines if it is caused by drug-induced toxicity or exacerbation of myasthenia gravis. Test dose of edrophonium I.V. will aggravate drug-induced weakness but will temporarily relieve weakness caused by disease.
● Be aware that I.M. neostigmine may be used instead of edrophonium to diagnose myasthenia gravis. May be preferable to edrophonium when limb weakness is the only symptom.
● When drug is used to prevent abdominal distention and GI distress, be aware that the doctor may order a rectal tube inserted to help passage of gas.
● Know that patients sometimes develop a resistance to neostigmine.
● If appropriate, obtain a doctor's order for a hospitalized patient to have bedside supply of tablets. Patients with long-standing disease often insist on self-administration.

☑ PATIENT TEACHING
● Tell the patient to take the drug with food or milk to reduce adverse GI reactions.
● When using for myasthenia gravis, explain that this drug will relieve ptosis, double vision, difficulty in chewing and swallowing, and trunk and limb weakness. Stress importance of taking drug exactly as ordered. Explain that drug may have to be taken for life.
● Show the patient how to observe and record variations in muscle strength.
● Advise the patient to wear medical identification bracelet indicating myasthenia gravis.

physostigmine salicylate (eserine salicylate)
Antilirium

Pregnancy Risk Category: NR

HOW SUPPLIED
Injection: 1 mg/ml

ACTION

Inhibits the destruction of acetylcholine released from the parasympathetic and somatic efferent nerves. Acetylcholine accumulates, promoting increased stimulation of the receptor.

ONSET, PEAK, DURATION

Onset occurs within 3 to 5 minutes of injection. Peak levels occur within 5 minutes of I.V. injection, 20 to 30 minutes after I.M. injection. Effects persist for 30 to 60 minutes after parenteral use.

INDICATIONS & DOSAGE

To reverse the CNS toxicity associated with clinical or toxic dosages of drugs capable of producing anticholinergic syndrome—
Adults: 0.5 to 2 mg I.M. or I.V. (1 mg/minute I.V.) repeated q 20 minutes as necessary if life-threatening signs recur (coma, seizures, arrhythmias). Additional doses of 1 to 4 mg I.M. or I.V. q 30 to 60 minutes may be given.
Children: reserved for life-threatening situations only. Requires dose of 0.02 mg/kg I.M. or slow I.V., repeated q 5 to 10 minutes until response occurs. Maximum dosage is 2 mg.

ADVERSE REACTIONS

CNS: *seizures,* muscle weakness, *restlessness, excitability.*
CV: bradycardia, hypotension.
EENT: miosis.
GI: nausea, vomiting, epigastric pain, *diarrhea, excessive salivation.*
GU: urinary urgency.
Respiratory: *bronchospasm,* bronchial constriction, dyspnea.
Other: diaphoresis.

INTERACTIONS

Atropine, anticholinergic agents, procainamide, quinidine: may reverse cholinergic effects. Observe for lack of drug effect.
Ganglionic blockers: may decrease blood pressure. Avoid concomitant use.

EFFECTS ON DIAGNOSTIC TESTS

None reported.

CONTRAINDICATIONS

Contraindicated in patients with mechanical obstruction of the intestine or urogenital tract, asthma, gangrene, diabetes, CV disease, or vagotonia and in those receiving choline esters or depolarizing neuromuscular blockers.

NURSING CONSIDERATIONS

● Use cautiously in pregnant patients.
● **I.V. use:** Give I.V. at controlled rate; use direct injection at no more than 1 mg/minute.
● Use only clear solution. Darkening may indicate loss of potency.
● Monitor vital signs frequently, especially respirations. Position the patient to ease breathing. Have atropine injection available and be prepared to give 0.5 mg S.C. or by slow I.V. push as ordered. Provide respiratory support as needed. Best administered in presence of a doctor.
● Watch closely for adverse reactions, particularly CNS disturbances. Raise side rails if the patient becomes restless or hallucinates. Adverse reactions may indicate drug toxicity.
● Know that effectiveness is often immediate and dramatic but may be transient and may require repeated doses.

☑ PATIENT TEACHING

● Inform patient of need for drug, explain its use and adverse reactions, and answer any questions or concerns.
● Tell patient to report adverse reactions promptly.
● Instruct patient to alert nurse if discomfort occurs at I.V. site.

---

pyridostigmine bromide
Mestinon*, Mestinon†, Mestinon Timespans, Regonol

Pregnancy Risk Category: NR

HOW SUPPLIED
Tablets: 60 mg
Tablets (extended-release): 180 mg
Syrup: 60 mg/5 ml
Injection: 5 mg/ml in 2-ml ampules or 5-ml vials

ACTION
Inhibits the destruction of acetylcholine released from the parasympathetic and somatic efferent nerves. Acetylcholine accumulates, promoting increased stimulation of the receptors.

ONSET, PEAK, DURATION
Onset occurs within 2 to 5 minutes of I.V. injection, 15 minutes after I.M. injection, 30 to 45 minutes after oral ingestion of regular-release tablets or syrup, 30 to 60 minutes after ingestion of extended-release tablets. Levels peak within 1 to 2 hours of oral administration. Effects persist for 2 to 4 hours after parenteral use, 3 to 6 hours after regular-release tablets or syrup, 6 to 12 hours after extended-release tablets.

INDICATIONS & DOSAGE
Antidote for nondepolarizing neuromuscular blockers—
Adults: 10 to 20 mg I.V. preceded by atropine sulfate 0.6 to 1.2 mg I.V.
Myasthenia gravis—
Adults: 60 to 120 mg P.O. q 3 or 4 hours. Usual dosage is 600 mg daily but higher dosage may be needed (up to 1,500 mg daily). For I.M. or I.V. use, $\frac{1}{30}$ of oral dosage is given. Dosage must be adjusted for each patient, depending on response and tolerance. Alternatively, 180 to 540 mg extended-release tablets (1 to 3 tablets) P.O. b.i.d., with at least 6 hours between doses.
Children: 7 mg/kg or 200 mg/m² daily in five or six divided doses.
Supportive treatment of neonates born to myasthenic mothers—
Neonates: 0.05 to 0.15 mg/kg I.M. q 4 to 6 hours. Dosage decreased daily until drug can be withdrawn.

ADVERSE REACTIONS
CNS: headache (with high doses), weakness.
CV: bradycardia, hypotension.
EENT: miosis.
GI: abdominal cramps, nausea, vomiting, diarrhea, excessive salivation, increased peristalsis.
Respiratory: *bronchospasm, bronchoconstriction,* increased bronchial secretions.
Skin: rash, diaphoresis.
Other: muscle cramps, muscle fasciculations, thrombophlebitis.

INTERACTIONS
Aminoglycosides, anesthetics: may decrease response to pyridostigmine. Use together cautiously.
Atropine, anticholinergic agents, corticosteroids, magnesium, procainamide, quinidine: may antagonize cholinergic effects. Observe for lack of drug effect.
Ganglionic blockers: increased risk of hypotension. Monitor closely.

EFFECTS ON DIAGNOSTIC TESTS
None reported.

CONTRAINDICATIONS
Contraindicated in patients with hypersensitivity to anticholinesterase agents and in those with mechanical obstruction of the intestine or urinary tract.

NURSING CONSIDERATIONS
● Use cautiously in patients with bronchial asthma, bradycardia, and arrhythmias.
● Stop all other cholinergics before giving this drug, as ordered.
● **I.V. use:** Administer I.V. injection no faster than 1 mg/minute. With too-rapid I.V. infusion, bradycardia and seizures may result. Monitor vital signs frequently, especially respirations. Position patient to ease breathing. Have atropine injection available and be prepared to give as ordered; provide respiratory support as needed.
● Don't crush the extended-release

(Timespans) tablets.

● When using sweet syrup for patients who have difficulty swallowing, give over ice chips if the patient can't tolerate flavor.

● Monitor and document patient's response after each dose. Optimum dosage is difficult to judge.

● If patient's muscle weakness is severe, keep in mind that the doctor determines if it is caused by drug-induced toxicity or exacerbation of myasthenia gravis. Test dose of edrophonium I.V. will aggravate drug-induced weakness, but will temporarily relieve weakness caused by disease.

Alert: In the United States, be aware that Regonol contains benzyl ethanol preservative that may cause toxicity in neonates if administered in high doses. The Canadian formulation of this drug does not contain benzyl ethanol.

● If appropriate, obtain a doctor's order for a hospitalized patient to have bedside supply of tablets. Patients with long-standing disease often insist on self-administration.

☑ **PATIENT TEACHING**

● When using for myasthenia gravis, stress importance of taking drug exactly as ordered, on time, in evenly spaced doses. If the doctor has ordered extended-release tablets, explain that patients must take tablets at the same time each day, at least 6 hours apart. Explain that patients may have to take drug for life.

● Advise patient to wear medical identification indicating he has myasthenia gravis.

38

Anticholinergics

atropine sulfate
  (See Chapter 21, ANTIARRHYTHMICS.)
dicyclomine hydrochloride
glycopyrrolate
hyoscyamine
hyoscyamine sulfate
propantheline bromide
scopolamine
scopolamine butylbromide
scopolamine hydrobromide

COMBINATION PRODUCTS

BARBIDONNA ELIXIR*: atropine sulfate 0.034 mg/5 ml, phenobarbital 21.6 mg/5 ml, hyoscyamine hydrobromide or sulfate 0.174 mg/5 ml, scopolamine hydrobromide 0.01 mg/5 ml, and ethanol 15%.

BARBIDONNA No. 2 TABLETS: atropine sulfate 0.025 mg, scopolamine hydrobromide 0.0074 mg, hyoscyamine hydrobromide or sulfate 0.1286 mg, and phenobarbital 32 mg.

BARBIDONNA TABLETS: atropine sulfate 0.025 mg, scopolamine hydrobromide 0.0074 mg, hyoscyamine hydrobromide or sulfate 0.1286 mg, and phenobarbital 16 mg.

DONNATAL ELIXIR*: atropine sulfate 0.0194 mg/5 ml, scopolamine hydrobromide 0.0065 mg/5 ml, ethanol 23%, hyoscyamine hydrobromide or sulfate 0.1037 mg/5 ml, and phenobarbital 16 mg/5 ml.

DONNATAL EXTENTABS: atropine sulfate 0.0582 mg, scopolamine hydrobromide 0.0195 mg, hyoscyamine sulfate 0.3111 mg, and phenobarbital 48.6 mg.

DONNATAL No. 2 TABLETS: atropine sulfate 0.0194 mg, scopolamine hydrobromide 0.0065 mg, hyoscyamine hydrobromide or sulfate 0.1037 mg, and phenobarbital 32.4 mg.

DONNATAL TABLETS AND CAPSULES: atropine sulfate 0.0194 mg, scopolamine hydrobromide 0.0065 mg, hyoscyamine hydrobromide or sulfate 0.1037 mg, and phenobarbital 16 mg.

KINESED TABLETS: atropine sulfate 0.02 mg, scopolamine hydrobromide 0.007 mg, hyoscyamine hydrobromide or sulfate 0.1 mg, and phenobarbital 16 mg.

---

dicyclomine hydrochloride
Antispas, A-Spas, Bemote, Bentyl, Bentylol†, Byclomine, Dibent, Dilomine, Di-Spaz, Formulex†, Lomine†, Merbentyl‡, Neoquess, Or-Tyl, Spasmoban†, Spasmoject

Pregnancy Risk Category: B

HOW SUPPLIED
Tablets: 10 mg‡, 20 mg
Capsules: 10 mg, 20 mg
Syrup: 5 mg/5 ml‡, 10 mg/5 ml
Injection: 10 mg/ml

ACTION
Unknown. Appears to exert a nonspecific, nondirect spasmolytic action on smooth muscle. Also possesses local anesthetic properties that may be partly responsible for spasmolysis.

ONSET, PEAK, DURATION
Onset and duration unknown. Peak effects occur 1 to 1½ hours after administration.

INDICATIONS & DOSAGE
Irritable bowel syndrome and other functional GI disorders—
Adults: initially, 20 mg P.O. q.i.d., increased to 40 mg q.i.d., or 20 mg I.M. q 4 to 6 hours.

ADVERSE REACTIONS
CNS: *headache; dizziness;* insomnia; light-headedness; drowsiness; nervousness, confusion, excitement (in elderly

patients).

CV: *palpitations,* tachycardia.

EENT: blurred vision, increased intraocular pressure, mydriasis.

GI: nausea, vomiting, *constipation, dry mouth,* abdominal distention, heartburn, paralytic ileus.

GU: *urinary hesitancy, urine retention,* impotence.

Skin: urticaria, decreased sweating or possible anhidrosis, other dermal manifestations, local irritation.

Other: fever, allergic reactions. Dicyclomine is a synthetic tertiary derivative that may have atropine-like adverse reactions.

Note: Overdose may cause curare-like effects, such as respiratory paralysis.

INTERACTIONS

Amantadine, antihistamines, antiparkinsonian agents, disopyramide, glutethimide, meperidine, phenothiazines, procainamide, quinidine, tricyclic antidepressants: additive adverse effects. Avoid concomitant use.

Antacids: decreased absorption of oral anticholinergics. Separate administration times by 2 to 3 hours.

Ketoconazole: anticholinergics may interfere with ketoconazole absorption. Avoid concomitant use.

Methotrimeprazine: anticholinergics may enhance risk of extrapyramidal reactions. Avoid concomitant use.

EFFECTS ON DIAGNOSTIC TESTS
None reported.

CONTRAINDICATIONS
Contraindicated in patients with obstructive uropathy, obstructive disease of the GI tract, reflux esophagitis, severe ulcerative colitis, myasthenia gravis, hypersensitivity to anticholinergics, unstable cardiovascular status in acute hemorrhage, or glaucoma. Also contraindicated in breast-feeding patients and in children under 6 months.

NURSING CONSIDERATIONS
● Use cautiously in patients with autonomic neuropathy, hyperthyroidism, coronary artery disease, arrhythmias, CHF, hypertension, hiatal hernia, hepatic or renal disease, prostatic hyperplasia, and ulcerative colitis.

● Give 30 minutes to 1 hour before meals and h.s. Bedtime dose can be larger; give at least 2 hours after last meal of the day.

Alert: Do not give S.C. or I.V.

● Be prepared to adjust dosage according to patient's needs and response, as ordered. Doses up to 40 mg P.O. q.i.d. have been used in adults, but safety and efficacy for more than 2 weeks has not been established.

● Monitor patient's vital signs and urine output carefully.

☑ **PATIENT TEACHING**

● Instruct the patient when to take drug.

● Advise the patient to avoid driving and other hazardous activities if he is drowsy, dizzy, or has blurred vision; to drink plenty of fluids to help prevent constipation; and to report any rash or other skin eruption.

glycopyrrolate
Robinul, Robinul Forte

Pregnancy Risk Category: B

HOW SUPPLIED
Tablets: 1 mg, 2 mg
Injection: 0.2 mg/ml

ACTION
Inhibits cholinergic (muscarinic) actions of acetylcholine on autonomic effectors innervated by postganglionic cholinergic nerves.

ONSET, PEAK, DURATION
Onset occurs in 1 minute after I.V. administration, 15 to 30 minutes after S.C. or I.M. injection. Serum levels peak in 30 to 45 minutes after I.M. injection.

Vagal blocking effects persist about 3 hours; effect on secretions, up to 7 hours.

INDICATIONS & DOSAGE
Blockade of adverse cholinergic effects caused by anticholinesterase agents used to reverse neuromuscular blockade—
Adults and children: 0.2 mg I.V. for each 1 mg neostigmine or 5 mg of pyridostigmine. May be given I.V. without dilution or may be added to dextrose injection and given by infusion.
Preoperatively to diminish secretions and block cardiac vagal reflexes—
Adults and children 2 years and older: 0.0044 mg/kg of body weight I.M. 30 to 60 minutes before anesthesia.
Children under 2 years: 0.0088 mg/kg I.M. 30 to 60 minutes before anesthesia.
Adjunctive therapy in peptic ulcerations and other GI disorders—
Adults: 1 to 2 mg P.O. t.i.d. or 0.1 to 0.2 mg I.M. or I.V. t.i.d. or q.i.d. Dosage must be individualized. Maximum oral dosage is 8 mg/day.

ADVERSE REACTIONS
CNS: weakness, nervousness, insomnia, drowsiness, dizziness, headache, confusion or excitement (in elderly patients).
CV: palpitations, tachycardia.
EENT: *dilated pupils, blurred vision,* photophobia, increased intraocular pressure.
GI: *constipation, dry mouth,* nausea, loss of taste, abdominal distension, vomiting, epigastric distress.
GU: *urinary hesitancy, urine retention,* impotence.
Skin: urticaria, decreased sweating or anhidrosis, other dermal manifestations.
Other: allergic reactions *(anaphylaxis)*, fever.

INTERACTIONS
Amantadine, antihistamines, antiparkinsonian agents, disopyramide, glutethimide, meperidine, phenothiazines, procainamide, quinidine, tri-
cyclic antidepressants: additive adverse effects. Avoid concomitant use.
Antacids: decreased absorption of oral anticholinergics. Separate administration times by 2 to 3 hours.
Ketoconazole: anticholinergics may interfere with ketoconazole absorption. Avoid concomitant use.
Methotrimeprazine: anticholinergics may enhance risk of extrapyramidal reactions. Avoid concomitant use.

EFFECTS ON DIAGNOSTIC TESTS
None reported.

CONTRAINDICATIONS
Contraindicated in patients with hypersensitivity to drug and in those with glaucoma, obstructive uropathy, obstructive disease of the GI tract, myasthenia gravis, paralytic ileus, intestinal atony, unstable cardiovascular status in acute hemorrhage, severe ulcerative colitis, or toxic megacolon.

NURSING CONSIDERATIONS
● Use cautiously in patients with autonomic neuropathy, hyperthyroidism, coronary artery disease, arrhythmias, CHF, hypertension, hiatal hernia, hepatic or renal disease, and ulcerative colitis. Also use cautiously in patients in hot or humid environment. Drug-induced heatstroke is possible.
● Administer oral form 30 minutes to 1 hour before meals.
● **I.V. use:** Administer by direct injection without dilution. Alternatively, inject into the tubing of a free-flowing I.V. solution.
● Don't mix with I.V. solution containing sodium bicarbonate or alkaline solutions with a pH higher than 6. Alkaline drugs, such as barbiturates, chloramphenicol, dexamethasone, dimenhydrinate, diazepam, methylprednisolone, and pentazocine are incompatible with glycopyrrolate.
Alert: Check all dosages carefully; slight overdose can lead to toxicity.
● Monitor vital signs carefully. Watch

closely for adverse reactions, especially in elderly or debilitated patients. Call the doctor promptly if they occur.
● Be aware that elderly patients typically receive smaller dosages.

☑ **PATIENT TEACHING**
● Instruct patient to take oral drug 30 to 60 minutes before meals.
● Warn patient to avoid activities that require alertness until drug's CNS effects are known.
● Advise patient to report signs of urinary hesitancy or urine retention.

---

hyoscyamine
Cystospaz

hyoscyamine sulfate
Anaspaz, Bellaspaz, Cystospaz, Cystospaz-M, Gastrosed, Levsin*, Levsin Drops, Levsinex Timecaps, Levsin S/L, Neoquess

Pregnancy Risk Category: C

HOW SUPPLIED
hyoscyamine
Tablets: 0.15 mg
hyoscyamine sulfate
Tablets: 0.125 mg, 0.13 mg, 0.15 mg
Capsules (extended-release): 0.375 mg
Elixir: 125 mcg/5 ml
Oral solution: 0.125 mg/ml
Injection: 0.5 mg/ml

ACTION
Competitively blocks acetylcholine, which decreases GI motility and inhibits gastric acid secretion.

ONSET, PEAK, DURATION
Onset occurs within 2 minutes after I.V. injection, 5 to 20 minutes after oral elixir, 20 to 30 minutes after oral tablets. Serum levels peak within 15 to 30 minutes after parenteral use, 30 to 60 minutes after oral use. Effects persist for 4 to 12 hours.

INDICATIONS & DOSAGE
GI tract disorders caused by spasm; to diminish secretions and block cardiac vagal reflexes preoperatively; adjunctive therapy for peptic ulcerations—
Adults and children 12 years or older: 0.125 to 0.25 mg P.O. or S.L. t.i.d. or q.i.d. before meals and h.s.; 0.375-mg extended-release form P.O. q 8 to 12 hours; or 0.25 to 0.5 mg (1 or 2 ml) I.M., I.V., or S.C. b.i.d. to q.i.d. (Oral medication substituted when symptoms are controlled.) Maximum daily dosage is 1.5 mg.
Children under 12 years: dosage individualized according to weight.

ADVERSE REACTIONS
CNS: headache, insomnia, drowsiness, dizziness, *confusion or excitement* (in elderly patients), nervousness, weakness.
CV: *palpitations,* tachycardia.
EENT: *blurred vision,* mydriasis, increased intraocular pressure, cycloplegia, photophobia.
GI: *dry mouth,* dysphagia, *constipation,* heartburn, loss of taste, nausea, vomiting, *paralytic ileus.*
GU: *urinary hesitancy, urine retention,* impotence.
Skin: urticaria, decreased or lack of sweating, other skin conditions.
Other: fever, allergic reactions.
Note: Overdose may cause curare-like effects, such as respiratory paralysis.

INTERACTIONS
Amantadine, antihistamines, antiparkinsonian agents, disopyramide, glutethimide, meperidine, phenothiazines, procainamide, quinidine, tricyclic antidepressants: additive adverse effects. Avoid concomitant use.
Antacids: decreased absorption of oral anticholinergics. Separate administration times by 2 to 3 hours.
Ketoconazole: anticholinergics may interfere with ketoconazole absorption. Avoid concomitant use.
Methotrimeprazine: anticholinergics

Reactions may be *common,* uncommon, *life-threatening,* or COMMON AND LIFE-THREATENING.

may enhance risk of extrapyramidal reactions. Avoid concomitant use.

EFFECTS ON DIAGNOSTIC TESTS
None reported.

CONTRAINDICATIONS
Contraindicated in patients with glaucoma, obstructive uropathy, obstructive disease of the GI tract, severe ulcerative colitis, myasthenia gravis, hypersensitivity to anticholinergics, paralytic ileus, intestinal atony, unstable cardiovascular status in acute hemorrhage, or toxic megacolon.

NURSING CONSIDERATIONS
● Use cautiously in patients with autonomic neuropathy, hyperthyroidism, coronary artery disease, arrhythmias, CHF, hypertension, hiatal hernia associated with reflux esophagitis, hepatic or renal disease, and ulcerative colitis. Also use cautiously in patients in hot or humid environment. Drug-induced heatstroke can develop.
● Give 30 minutes to 1 hour before meals and h.s. Bedtime dose can be larger; give at least 2 hours after the last meal of the day.
● Monitor the patient's vital signs and urine output carefully.
● Be aware that injection contains sodium metabisulfite, which may cause allergic reaction in certain individuals.

☑ **PATIENT TEACHING**
● Instruct the patient when to take drug.
● Advise the patient to avoid driving and other hazardous activities if he is drowsy, dizzy, or has blurred vision; to drink plenty of fluids to help prevent constipation; and to report any rash or other skin eruption.

---

propantheline bromide
Pantheline‡, Pro-Banthine, Propanthel†

Pregnancy Risk Category: C

HOW SUPPLIED
Tablets: 7.5 mg, 15 mg

ACTION
Blocks acetylcholine, which decreases GI motility and inhibits gastric acid secretion.

ONSET, PEAK, DURATION
Onset unknown. Serum levels may peak in 2 hours. Effects persist for 6 hours.

INDICATIONS & DOSAGE
Adjunctive treatment of peptic ulceration—
Adults: 15 mg P.O. t.i.d. before meals and 30 mg h.s.
Elderly patients: 7.5 mg P.O. t.i.d. before meals.

ADVERSE REACTIONS
CNS: headache, insomnia, drowsiness, dizziness, *confusion or excitement in elderly patients,* nervousness, weakness.
CV: *palpitations,* tachycardia.
EENT: *blurred vision,* mydriasis, increased intraocular pressure, cycloplegia, drying of salivary secretions.
GI: *dry mouth,* constipation, loss of taste, nausea, vomiting, paralytic ileus, bloated feeling.
GU: *urinary hesitancy, urine retention,* impotence.
Skin: urticaria, decreased sweating or possible anhidrosis, other dermal manifestations.
Other: allergic reactions *(anaphylaxis).*
Note: Overdose may cause curare-like effects, such as respiratory paralysis.

INTERACTIONS
Amantadine, antihistamines, antiparkinsonian agents, disopyramide, glutethimide, meperidine, phenothiazines, procainamide, quinidine, tricyclic antidepressants: additive adverse effects. Avoid concomitant use.

Antacids: decreased absorption of oral anticholinergics. Separate administration times by 2 to 3 hours.
Digoxin: increased serum digoxin levels. Monitor closely for digitalis toxicity.
Ketoconazole: anticholinergics may interfere with ketoconazole absorption. Avoid concomitant use.
Methotrimeprazine: anticholinergics may enhance risk of extrapyramidal reactions. Avoid concomitant use.

EFFECTS ON DIAGNOSTIC TESTS
None reported.

CONTRAINDICATIONS
Contraindicated in patients with angle-closure glaucoma, obstructive uropathy, obstructive disease of the GI tract, severe ulcerative colitis, myasthenia gravis, hypersensitivity to anticholinergics, paralytic ileus, intestinal atony, unstable cardiovascular status in acute hemorrhage, or toxic megacolon.

NURSING CONSIDERATIONS
● Use cautiously in patients with autonomic neuropathy, hyperthyroidism, coronary artery disease, arrhythmias, CHF, hypertension, hiatal hernia associated with reflux esophagitis, hepatic or renal disease, and ulcerative colitis. Also use cautiously in patients in hot or humid environment. Drug-induced heatstroke can develop.
● Give 30 minutes to 1 hour before meals and h.s. Bedtime doses can be larger; give at least 2 hours after last meal of the day.
● Monitor the patient's vital signs and urine output carefully.

☑ **PATIENT TEACHING**
● Instruct the patient when to take drug.
● Advise the patient to avoid driving and other hazardous activities if he is drowsy, dizzy, or has blurred vision; to drink plenty of fluids to help prevent constipation; and to report any rash or other skin eruption.

scopolamine (hyoscine)
Scop‡, Transderm-Scōp, Transderm-V†

scopolamine butylbromide (hyoscine butylbromide)
Buscospan†‡

scopolamine hydrobromide (hyoscine hydrobromide)

Pregnancy Risk Category: C

HOW SUPPLIED
scopolamine
Transdermal patch: 1.5 mg
scopolamine butylbromide
Capsules: 0.25 mg
Suppositories: 10 mg†
Tablets: 10 mg†
scopolamine hydrobromide
Injection: 0.3 mg, 0.4 mg, 0.5 mg, 0.6 mg, and 1 mg/ml in 1-ml vials and ampules; 0.86 mg/ml in 0.5-ml ampules

ACTION
Inhibits muscarinic actions of acetylcholine on autonomic effectors innervated by postganglionic cholinergic neurons. Also may affect neural pathways originating in the labyrinth (inner ear) to inhibit nausea and vomiting.

ONSET, PEAK, DURATION
Onset occurs within 30 minutes after parenteral administration, 30 to 60 minutes after oral administration, unknown after transdermal patch application. Peak unknown. Effects persist about 4 hours after parenteral administration, 4 to 6 hours after oral administration, and up to 72 hours after applying transdermal patch.

INDICATIONS & DOSAGE
Spastic states—
Adults: 10 to 20 mg P.O. t.i.d. or q.i.d. Dosage adjusted as needed. Or 10 to 20 mg (butylbromide) S.C., I.M., or I.V. t.i.d. or q.i.d.

Delirium, preanesthetic sedation and obstetric amnesia in conjunction with analgesics—
Adults: 0.3 to 0.65 mg I.M., S.C., or I.V. Dilute solution with sterile water for injection before administering I.V.
Children: 0.006 mg/kg I.M., S.C., I.V.; maximum dosage is 0.3 mg. Dilute solution with sterile water for injection before administering I.V.
Prevention of nausea and vomiting associated with motion sickness—
Adults: one Transderm-Scōp or Transderm-V patch (a circular flat unit) programmed to deliver 0.5 mg scopolamine daily over 3 days (72 hours), applied to the skin behind the ear several hours before the antiemetic is required. Or 300 to 600 mcg (hydrobromide) S.C., I.M., or I.V.
Children: 6 mcg/kg or 200 mcg/m^2 of body surface (hydrobromide) S.C., I.M., or I.V.

ADVERSE REACTIONS
CNS: disorientation, restlessness, irritability, dizziness, drowsiness, headache, confusion, hallucinations, delirium.
CV: palpitations, tachycardia, paradoxical bradycardia.
EENT: dilated pupils, blurred vision, photophobia, increased intraocular pressure, difficulty swallowing.
GI: *constipation, dry mouth, nausea, vomiting, epigastric distress.*
GU: urinary hesitancy, urine retention.
Respiratory: bronchial plugging, depressed respirations.
Skin: rash, flushing, dryness, contact dermatitis (with transdermal patch).
Other: fever.
   Adverse reactions may be caused by pending atropine-like toxicity and are dose-related. Individual tolerance varies greatly.
   Many adverse reactions (such as dry mouth, constipation) are an expected extension of the drug's pharmacologic activity.

INTERACTIONS
Centrally acting anticholinergics (tricyclic antidepressants, antihistamines, phenothiazines): increased incidence of adverse CNS reactions. Avoid concomitant use.
Digoxin: increased digoxin levels. Monitor for digitalis toxicity.
Ethanol, CNS depressants: increased incidence of CNS depression. Monitor patient closely.

EFFECTS ON DIAGNOSTIC TESTS
None reported.

CONTRAINDICATIONS
Contraindicated in patients with angle-closure glaucoma, obstructive uropathy, obstructive disease of the GI tract, asthma, chronic pulmonary disease, myasthenia gravis, paralytic ileus, intestinal atony, unstable cardiovascular status in acute hemorrhage, or toxic megacolon.

NURSING CONSIDERATIONS
● Use cautiously in patients with autonomic neuropathy, hyperthyroidism, coronary artery disease, arrhythmias, CHF, hypertension, hiatal hernia associated with reflux esophagitis, hepatic or renal disease, and ulcerative colitis and in children under 6 years. Also use cautiously in patients in hot or humid environment. Drug-induced heatstroke possible.
● **I.V. use:** Keep in mind that intermittent and continuous infusions are not recommended. For direct injection, dilute with sterile water and inject diluted drug at ordered rate through patent I.V. line.
● Protect I.V. solutions from freezing and light, and store at room temperature.
● Raise the bed's side rails as a precaution because some patients become temporarily excited, disoriented, or they develop amnesia or drowsiness. Reorient the patient as needed.
● Be aware that tolerance may develop when given over a long time.

☑ PATIENT TEACHING

• Advise the patient to apply patch the night before a planned trip. Transdermal method releases a controlled therapeutic amount of scopolamine. Transderm-Scōp is effective if applied 2 to 3 hours before experiencing motion, but more effective if applied 12 hours before.

• Advise the patient to wash and dry hands thoroughly before and after applying the transdermal patch on dry skin behind the ear and before touching the eye, as pupil may dilate. After removing the system, discard it. Wash hands and application site thoroughly.

• Tell patient that if patch becomes displaced, he should remove it and apply another patch on a fresh skin site behind the ear.

• Alert the patient to possible withdrawal symptoms (nausea, vomiting, headache, dizziness) when the transdermal system is used longer than 72 hours.

• Warn the patient to avoid activities that require alertness until drug's CNS effects are known.

• Have the patient ask the pharmacist for the brochure that comes with the transdermal product.

• Advise the patient to report signs of urinary hesitancy or urine retention.

39

Adrenergics (sympathomimetics)

dobutamine hydrochloride
dopamine hydrochloride
mephentermine sulfate
metaraminol bitartrate
norepinephrine bitartrate
phenylephrine hydrochloride
pseudoephedrine hydrochloride
pseudoephedrine sulfate

COMBINATION PRODUCTS
ENTEX: phenylephrine hydrochloride 5 mg, phenylpropanolamine hydrochloride 45 mg, and guaifenesin 400 mg.
ENTEX LIQUID: phenylephrine hydrochloride 5 mg/5 ml, phenylpropanolamine hydrochloride 20 mg/5 ml, and guaifenesin 100 mg/5 ml (alcohol 5%).
ENTEX PSE: pseudoephedrine 120 mg and guaifenesin 600 mg.
SEMPREX-D: acrivastine 8 mg and pseudoephedrine hydrochloride 60 mg.

---

dobutamine hydrochloride
Dobutrex

Pregnancy Risk Category: B

HOW SUPPLIED
Injection: 12.5 mg/ml in 20-ml vials (parenteral)

ACTION
Directly stimulates beta$_1$ receptors of the heart to increase myocardial contractility and stroke volume. At therapeutic dosages, decreases peripheral vascular resistance (afterload), reduces ventricular filling pressure (preload), and may facilitate AV node conduction. Net result is increased cardiac output.

ONSET, PEAK, DURATION
Onset occurs in 1 to 2 minutes, up to 10 minutes if I.V. infusion rate is slow. Peak effects usually occur within 10 minutes of starting I.V. infusion. Effects persist for less than 5 minutes after infusion is stopped.

INDICATIONS & DOSAGE
To increase cardiac output in the short-term treatment of cardiac decompensation caused by depressed contractility, such as during refractory heart failure, and as adjunct in cardiac surgery—
Adults: 2.5 to 10 mcg/kg/minute I.V. infusion. Infusion rates up to 40 mcg/kg/minute may be needed (rare).

ADVERSE REACTIONS
CNS: headache.
CV: *increased heart rate, **hypertension, PVCs,*** angina, nonspecific chest pain, palpitations, hypotension.
GI: nausea, vomiting.
Respiratory: shortness of breath, ***asthmatic episodes.***
Other: phlebitis, hypersensitivity reactions *(anaphylaxis).*

INTERACTIONS
Beta blockers: may antagonize dobutamine effects. Don't use together.
General anesthetics: greater incidence of ventricular arrhythmias. Monitor ECG closely.
Bretylium: may potentiate action of vasopressors on adrenergic receptors; arrhythmias may result.
Tricyclic antidepressants: may potentiate pressor response.

EFFECTS ON DIAGNOSTIC TESTS
None reported.

CONTRAINDICATIONS
Contraindicated in patients with hypersensitivity to the drug or any component of the formulation and in those with idiopathic hypertrophic subaortic stenosis.

---

*Liquid contains alcohol.   **May contain tartrazine.   †Canada only.   ‡Australia only.   ◇OTC.

NURSING CONSIDERATIONS
● Use cautiously in patients with a history of hypertension. Drug may precipitate an exaggerated pressor response.
● Before initiating therapy with dobutamine, correct hypovolemia with plasma volume expanders, as ordered.
● Administer a digitalis glycoside before dobutamine as ordered. Because drug increases AV node conduction, patients with atrial fibrillation may develop a rapid ventricular rate.
● Do not mix with sodium bicarbonate injection because the drug is incompatible with alkaline solutions. Infusions for up to 72 hours produce no more adverse effects than shorter infusions.
● **I.V. use:** Administer through a central venous catheter or large peripheral vein. Titrate infusion according to the doctor's orders and the patient's condition. Use an infusion pump.
● Dilute concentrate for injection before administration. Compatible solutions include D_5W, 0.45% sodium chloride or 0.9% sodium chloride for injection and lactated Ringer's injection. The contents of one vial (250 mg) diluted with 1,000 ml of solution yields a concentration of 250 mcg/ml; diluted with 500 ml, a concentration of 500 mcg/ml; diluted with 250 ml, a concentration of 1,000 mcg/ml. Maximum concentration should not exceed 5 mg/ml.
● Avoid extravasation; may cause an inflammatory response. Change I.V. sites regularly to avoid phlebitis.
● Don't administer through the same I.V. line with other drugs. Drug is incompatible with heparin, hydrocortisone sodium succinate, cefazolin, cefamandole, neutral cephalothin, penicillin, and ethacrynate sodium.
● Keep in mind that I.V. solutions remain stable for 24 hours.
● Be aware that oxidation of drug may slightly discolor admixtures containing dobutamine. This does not indicate a significant loss of potency provided drug is used within 24 hours of reconstitution.

● Continuously monitor ECG, blood pressure, pulmonary capillary wedge pressure, cardiac condition, and urine output.
● Monitor serum electrolytes, as ordered. Drug may lower serum potassium levels.

☑ PATIENT TEACHING
● Tell patient to report adverse reactions promptly, especially dyspnea and drug-induced headache.
● Instruct patient to report discomfort at I.V. insertion site.

---

dopamine hydrochloride
Intropin, Revimine†‡

Pregnancy Risk Category: C

HOW SUPPLIED
Injection: 40 mg/ml, 80 mg/ml, 160 mg/ml parenteral concentrate for injection for I.V. infusion; 0.8 mg/ml (200 or 400 mg) in dextrose 5%; 1.6 mg/ml (400 or 800 mg) in dextrose 5%, 3.2 mg/ml (800 mg) in dextrose 5% parenteral injection for I.V. infusion.

ACTION
Stimulates dopaminergic, beta-adrenergic, and alpha-adrenergic receptors of the sympathetic nervous system.

ONSET, PEAK, DURATION
Onset occurs within 5 minutes of starting I.V. infusion. Peak unknown. Effects subside within 10 minutes of discontinuing infusion.

INDICATIONS & DOSAGE
To treat shock and correct hemodynamic imbalances; to improve perfusion to vital organs; to increase cardiac output; to correct hypotension—
Adults: initially, 1 to 5 mcg/kg/minute by I.V. infusion. Dosage titrated to desired hemodynamic or renal response; infusion may be increased by 1 to 4 mcg/kg/minute at 10- to 30-minute in-

tervals.

ADVERSE REACTIONS
CNS: headache.
CV: ectopic beats, tachycardia, anginal pain, palpitations, *hypotension.* Less frequently, bradycardia, widening of QRS complex, conduction disturbances, vasoconstriction, hypertension.
GI: nausea, vomiting.
Other: necrosis and tissue sloughing with extravasation, piloerection, dyspnea, *anaphylactic reactions, asthmatic episodes,* azotemia.

INTERACTIONS
Alpha blockers, beta blockers: may antagonize dopamine's effects. Don't use together.
Ergot alkaloids: extreme elevations in blood pressure. Don't use together.
Inhalation anesthetics: increased risk of arrhythmias or hypertension. Monitor closely.
MAO inhibitors: may cause hypertensive crisis. Avoid if possible.
Phenytoin: may lower blood pressure of dopamine-stabilized patients. Monitor carefully.

EFFECTS ON DIAGNOSTIC TESTS
Dopamine may cause elevated urinary catecholamine levels. Drug may also cause increased serum glucose levels, though level usually doesn't rise above normal limits.

CONTRAINDICATIONS
Contraindicated in patients with uncorrected tachyarrhythmias, pheochromocytoma, or ventricular fibrillation.

NURSING CONSIDERATIONS
• Use cautiously in patients with occlusive vascular disease, cold injuries, diabetic endarteritis, and arterial embolism; in pregnant patients; and in those taking MAO inhibitors.
• Remember that drug is not a substitute for blood or fluid volume deficit. If deficit exists, replace fluid before ad-

ministering vasopressors, as ordered.
• **I.V. use:** Use a central line or large vein, such as in the antecubital fossa, to minimize risk of extravasation. Watch infusion site carefully for signs of extravasation; if it occurs, stop infusion immediately and call doctor. Extravasation may require treatment by infiltration of the area with 5 to 10 mg phentolamine and 10 to 15 ml 0.9% sodium chloride solution. Don't mix with alkaline solutions. Use D_5W, 0.9% sodium chloride solution, or a combination of D_5W and 0.9% sodium chloride solution. Mix just before use.
• Use a continuous infusion pump to regulate flow rate. Keep in mind that patient response depends on dosage and pharmacologic effects. Dosages of 0.5 to 2 mcg/kg/minute predominantly stimulate dopamine receptors and produce vasodilation of the renal vasculature. Dosages of 2 to 10 mcg/kg/minute stimulate beta-adrenergic receptors for a positive inotropic effect. Higher dosages also stimulate alpha-adrenergic receptors, causing vasoconstriction and increased blood pressure. Know that most patients are satisfactorily maintained on dosage less than 20 mcg/kg/minute.
• Don't mix other drugs in I.V. container with dopamine. Don't give alkaline drugs through I.V. line containing dopamine.
• Discard after 24 hours (dopamine solutions deteriorate after 24 hours) or earlier if solution is discolored.
• During infusion, frequently monitor ECG, blood pressure, cardiac output, central venous pressure, pulmonary capillary wedge pressure, pulse rate, urine output, and color and temperature of extremities.
• If a disproportionate rise in diastolic pressure (a marked decrease in pulse pressure) is observed in patients receiving dopamine, decrease infusion rate as ordered and observe carefully for further evidence of predominant vasoconstrictor activity, unless such an effect is desired.

- Observe patients closely for adverse effects. If they develop, the doctor will adjust dosage or discontinue the drug.
- Check urine output often. If urine flow decreases without hypotension, notify doctor because dosage may need to be reduced.

Alert: After drug is stopped, watch closely for sudden drop in blood pressure. Taper dosage slowly to evaluate stability of blood pressure, as ordered.

- Be aware that acidosis decreases effectiveness of dopamine.

☑ **PATIENT TEACHING**
- Tell patient to report adverse reactions promptly.
- Instruct patient to alert nurse if discomfort occurs at I.V. insertion site.

---

mephentermine sulfate
Wyamine

Pregnancy Risk Category: C

HOW SUPPLIED
Injection: 15 mg/ml, 30 mg/ml

ACTION
Unknown. Appears to indirectly stimulate beta- and alpha-adrenergic receptors by releasing norepinephrine.

ONSET, PEAK, DURATION
Onset occurs immediately after I.V. administration, within 5 to 15 minutes after I.M. injection. Peak unknown. Effects persist for 15 to 30 minutes after I.V. administration, 1 to 4 hours after I.M. injection.

INDICATIONS & DOSAGE
Hypotension after spinal anesthesia—
Adults: 30 to 45 mg I.V. as a single injection, then 30 mg I.V. repeated p.r.n. for maintenance of blood pressure, continuous I.V. infusion of 0.1% solution of mephentermine in D₅W.
Children: 0.4 mg/kg I.M. or I.V.
Hypotension after spinal anesthesia

during obstetric procedures—
Adults: initially, 15 mg I.V., then repeated p.r.n.
Prevention of hypotension during spinal anesthesia—
Adults: 30 to 45 mg I.M. 10 to 20 minutes before anesthesia.

ADVERSE REACTIONS
CNS: nervousness, anxiety, headache, dizziness, tremor, weakness.
CV: *arrhythmias, marked elevation of blood pressure* (with large doses), AV block, tachycardia.

INTERACTIONS
Antihypertensives, guanethidine, nitrates phenothiazines, reserpine: decreased effects of these adrenergic blockers. Monitor patient closely.
Beta-adrenergic blockers, rauwolfia alkaloids: mutual inhibition of therapeutic effects. Avoid concomitant use.
CNS stimulants, mazindol, methylphenidate, sympathomimetics: increased CNS stimulation. Monitor patient closely.
Digitalis glycosides, levodopa, inhalation anesthetics: increased risk of arrhythmias. Monitor ECG.
Ergot alkaloids, oxytocin: enhanced vasoconstriction. Use together cautiously.
Inhalation anesthetics: increased risk of hypertension. Monitor closely.
MAO inhibitors: may precipitate hypertension, headache, and related symptoms. Don't use together.
Maprotiline, tricyclic antidepressants: decreased pressure response of mephentermine. Monitor for decreased effectiveness.
Thyroid hormones: enhanced risk of coronary insufficiency. Monitor patient closely.

EFFECTS ON DIAGNOSTIC TESTS
None significant.

CONTRAINDICATIONS
Contraindicated in patients with hyper-

---

sensitivity to the drug and in those with hypotension resulting from hemorrhage, except in emergencies.

NURSING CONSIDERATIONS
● Use cautiously in patients with CV disease, hyperthyroidism, hypertension, and chronic illness.
● Remember that the drug is not a substitute for blood or fluid volume deficit. If deficit exists, replace fluid before administering vasopressors, as ordered.
● Keep in mind that hypercapnia, hypoxia, or acidosis may reduce effectiveness or increase adverse effects. Identify and correct before and during administration, as ordered.
● **I.V. use:** Administer at 1 to 5 mg/minute. Can be given undiluted; I.V. drug is not irritating to tissue and extravasation has no serious effects. To prepare 0.1% I.V. solution, add 16.6 ml of mephentermine (30 mg/ml) to 500 ml of D_5W.
● Don't mix with I.V. hydralazine or epinephrine, which are physically incompatible with drug.
● During infusion, frequently monitor ECG, blood pressure, cardiac output, central venous pressure, pulmonary capillary wedge pressure, pulse rate, urine output, and color and temperature of extremities. Titrate infusion rate according to findings and the doctor's guidelines. Use a continuous infusion pump to regulate flow rate.
Alert: During infusion, check blood pressure every 2 minutes until stabilized; then check every 10 to 15 minutes.
● Know that the I.M. route may be used because drug is not irritating to tissue.
● Monitor blood pressure until stable, even after discontinuing drug.
● Observe patients closely for adverse effects. If they develop, the doctor will adjust dosage or discontinue the drug.
● Be aware that the drug may increase uterine contractions during third trimester of pregnancy.

☑ PATIENT TEACHING
● Tell patient to report adverse reactions promptly.
● Instruct patient to alert nurse if discomfort occurs at I.V. insertion site.

---

metaraminol bitartrate
Aramine

Pregnancy Risk Category: C

HOW SUPPLIED
Injection: 10 mg/ml

ACTION
Stimulates alpha- and beta$_1$-adrenergic receptors within the sympathetic nervous system.

ONSET, PEAK, DURATION
Onset occurs in 1 to 2 minutes after I.V. administration, 10 minutes after I.M. administration, 5 to 20 minutes after S.C. administration. Peak unknown. Effects last 20 minutes after I.V. administration, up to 90 minutes after S.C. or I.M. administration.

INDICATIONS & DOSAGE
Prevention of hypotension associated with spinal anesthesia—
Adults: 2 to 10 mg I.M. or S.C.
Treatment of hypotension associated with spinal anesthesia—
Adults: 0.5 to 5 mg by direct I.V. injection, followed by I.V. infusion titrated to maintain blood pressure.
Children: 0.01 mg/kg as single I.V. injection; 1 mg/25 ml of D_5W as I.V. infusion. Rate adjusted to maintain blood pressure in normal range. Alternatively, 0.1 mg/kg I.M. as single dose, p.r.n. At least 10 minutes should elapse before dosage increased because maximum effect is not immediately apparent.

ADVERSE REACTIONS
CNS: apprehension, dizziness, headache, tremor.
CV: hypertension; hypotension; palpita-

---

tions; *arrhythmias,* including sinus or *ventricular tachycardia; cardiac arrest.*
GI: nausea.
Skin: flushing, diaphoresis.
Other: abscess, necrosis, sloughing upon extravasation.

INTERACTIONS

Beta-adrenergic blockers: mutual inhibition of drug effects, with possible hypertension, bradycardia, and heart block. Avoid concomitant use.
Cocaine, digitalis glycosides, doxapram, ergot alkaloids, general anesthetics, levodopa, maprotiline, other sympathomimetics, thyroid hormones, tricyclic antidepressants: increased risk of adverse cardiac effects. Monitor closely.
Furazolidone, MAO inhibitors, procarbazine: may cause severe hypertension (hypertensive crisis) and increase action of metaraminol. Avoid this combination.
Guanadrel, guanethidine: metaraminol may decrease the hypotensive effect of these drugs; guanadrel and guanethidine may enhance the pressor effect of metaraminol. Avoid concomitant use.

EFFECTS ON DIAGNOSTIC TESTS
None reported.

CONTRAINDICATIONS
Contraindicated in patients with hypersensitivity to the drug and in patients receiving anesthesia with cyclopropane and halogenated hydrocarbon anesthetics.

NURSING CONSIDERATIONS
● Use cautiously in patients with heart disease, hypertension, peripheral vascular disease, thyroid disease, diabetes, cirrhosis, history of malaria, or sulfite sensitivity and in patients receiving digitalis glycosides.
● Know that drug is not a substitute for blood or fluid volume deficit. If deficit exists, replace fluid before administering vasopressors, as ordered.
● Don't mix metaraminol with other drugs.
● **I.V. use:** To prepare an I.V. infusion, mix 15 to 100 mg in 500 ml of 0.9% sodium chloride solution or D_5W. Adjust rate to maintain blood pressure.
● During infusion, check blood pressure every 5 minutes until stabilized; then check every 15 minutes. Frequently monitor ECG, blood pressure, cardiac output, central venous pressure, pulmonary capillary wedge pressure, pulse rate, urine output, and color and temperature of extremities. Titrate infusion rate according to findings and the doctor's guidelines.
● Use a central venous catheter or large vein, such as in the antecubital fossa, to minimize risk of extravasation. Use a continuous infusion pump to regulate infusion flow rate and a piggyback setup so I.V. line remains open if drug is stopped. Watch infusion site carefully for signs of extravasation. If it occurs, stop infusion immediately and call the doctor.
● To treat extravasation, infiltrate site promptly with 10 to 15 ml of 0.9% sodium chloride for injection containing 5 to 10 mg phentolamine. Use a fine needle.
Alert: Keep in mind that blood pressure should be raised to slightly less than the patient's normal level. Be careful to avoid excessive blood pressure response. Headache may be a symptom of hypertension. Rapidly induced hypertensive response can cause acute pulmonary edema, arrhythmias, and cardiac arrest.
● Allow at least 10 minutes between doses. Drug effects are not always immediately apparent.
● Be aware that because of prolonged action, a cumulative effect is possible. With an excessive vasopressor response, elevated blood pressure may persist after drug is stopped.
● Observe patients closely for adverse effects. If they develop, notify the doctor, who will adjust or discontinue dosage.
● Keep emergency drugs on hand to re-

verse effects of metaraminol: atropine for reflex bradycardia; phentolamine to decrease vasopressor, effects; and propranolol for arrhythmias.

• Report persistent decreased urine output. Urine output may decrease initially, then increase as blood pressure returns to normal level.

• Closely monitor patients with diabetes; insulin dosage may need to be adjusted.

• When discontinuing drug, gradually slow infusion rate, as ordered. Continue monitoring vital signs, watching for possible severe drop in blood pressure. Keep equipment nearby to resume drug, if necessary. Do not reinstate vasopressor therapy until the systolic blood pressure falls below 70 to 80 mm Hg, as ordered.

• Keep solution in light-resistant container, away from heat.

☑ PATIENT TEACHING
• Tell patient to report adverse reactions promptly.
• Instruct patient to alert nurse if discomfort occurs at I.V. site.

**norepinephrine bitartrate
(levarterenol bitartrate,
noradrenaline acid tartrate)**
Levophed

Pregnancy Risk Category: C

HOW SUPPLIED
Injection: 1 mg/ml

ACTION
Stimulates alpha- and beta₁-adrenergic receptors within the sympathetic nervous system.

ONSET, PEAK, DURATION
Onset and peak immediately after I.V. infusion begins. Effects persist for 1 to 2 minutes after I.V. infusion ends.

INDICATIONS & DOSAGE
To restore blood pressure in acute hypotensive states—
Adults: initially, 8 to 12 mcg/minute I.V. infusion, then adjusted to maintain normal blood pressure. Average maintenance dosage is 2 to 4 mcg/minute.
Children: 2 mcg/m²/minute I.V. infusion; dosage adjusted based on patient response.
Severe hypotension during cardiac arrest—
Children: initial I.V. infusion rate is 0.1 mcg/kg/minute. Rate adjusted according to patient response.

ADVERSE REACTIONS
CNS: *headache,* anxiety, weakness, dizziness, tremor, restlessness, insomnia.
CV: bradycardia, *severe hypertension, arrhythmias.*
Respiratory: respiratory difficulties, *asthmatic episodes.*
Other: *anaphylaxis,* irritation with extravasation.

INTERACTIONS
Alpha-adrenergic blockers: may antagonize drug effects. Avoid concomitant use.
Antihistamines, ergot alkaloids, guanethidine, methyldopa, tricyclic antidepressants: when given with sympathomimetics, may cause severe hypertension (hypertensive crisis). Don't give together.
Inhalation anesthetics: increased risk of arrhythmias. Monitor closely.
MAO inhibitors: increased risk of hypertensive crisis. Don't use together.

EFFECTS ON DIAGNOSTIC TESTS
None reported.

CONTRAINDICATIONS
Contraindicated in patients with mesenteric or peripheral vascular thrombosis, profound hypoxia, hypercapnia, or hypotension resulting from blood volume deficit and during cyclopropane and

halothane anesthesia.

NURSING CONSIDERATIONS
● Use with extreme caution in patients receiving MAO inhibitors or triptyline- or imipramine-type antidepressants. Use cautiously in patients with sulfite sensitivity.
● Know that drug is not a substitute for blood or fluid volume deficit. If deficit exists, replace fluid before administering vasopressors.
● **I.V. use:** Use a central venous catheter or a large vein, such as in the antecubital fossa, to minimize risk of extravasation. Administer in dextrose 5% in 0.9% sodium chloride for injection; 0.9% sodium chloride for injection alone is not recommended. Use continuous infusion pump to regulate infusion flow rate and a piggyback setup so I.V. line remains open if norepinephrine is stopped.
Alert: Never leave patients unattended during infusion. Also, check blood pressure every 2 minutes until stabilized; then check every 5 minutes. In previously hypertensive patients, blood pressure should be raised no higher than 40 mm Hg below preexisting systolic pressure.
● Also during infusion, frequently monitor ECG, cardiac output, central venous pressure, pulmonary capillary wedge pressure, pulse rate, urine output, and color and temperature of extremities. Titrate infusion rate according to findings and the doctor's guidelines.
● Check site frequently for signs of extravasation. If it occurs, stop infusion immediately and call the doctor. He may counteract effect by infiltrating area with 5 to 10 mg phentolamine and 10 to 15 ml of 0.9% sodium chloride solution. Also check for blanching along course of infused vein; may progress to superficial sloughing.
● If prolonged I.V. therapy is necessary, change injection site frequently.
● Keep emergency drugs on hand to reverse effects of norepinephrine: atropine

for reflex bradycardia; phentolamine for increased vasopressor effects; and propranolol for arrhythmias.
● Report decreased urine output to the doctor immediately.
● When discontinuing drug, gradually slow infusion rate, as ordered. Continue monitoring vital signs, watching for possible severe drop in blood pressure.
● Be aware that norepinephrine solutions deteriorate after 24 hours.
● Protect drug from light. Discard discolored solutions or solutions that contain a precipitate.

☑ PATIENT TEACHING
● Tell patient to report adverse reactions promptly.
● Advise patient to alert nurse if discomfort occurs at I.V. insertion site.

---

phenylephrine hydrochloride
Neo-Synephrine

Pregnancy Risk Category: C

HOW SUPPLIED
Injection: 10 mg/ml

ACTION
Predominantly stimulates alpha-adrenergic receptors in the sympathetic nervous system.

ONSET, PEAK, DURATION
Onset occurs immediately after I.V. administration, within 10 to 15 minutes after S.C. or I.M. injection. Peak unknown. Effects persist for 15 to 20 minutes after I.V. administration, $\frac{1}{2}$ to 2 hours after I.M. injection, 50 minutes to 1 hour after S.C. injection.

INDICATIONS & DOSAGE
Hypotensive emergencies during spinal anesthesia—
Adults: initially, 0.2 mg; subsequent doses should not exceed the preceding dose by more than 0.2 mg. Maximum single dose should not exceed 0.5 mg.

Maintenance of blood pressure during spinal or inhalation anesthesia—
Adults: 2 to 3 mg S.C. or I.M. 3 or 4 minutes before anesthesia.
Children: 0.044 mg to 0.088 mg/kg S.C. or I.M.
Prolongation of spinal anesthesia—
Adults: 2 to 5 mg added to anesthetic solution.
Vasoconstrictor for regional anesthesia—
Adults: 1 mg phenylephrine added to 20 ml local anesthetic.
Mild to moderate hypotension—
Adults: 2 to 5 mg S.C. or I.M.; repeated in 1 to 2 hours as needed and tolerated. Initial dose should not exceed 5 mg. Alternatively, 0.1 to 0.5 mg slow I.V., not to be repeated more often than 10 to 15 minutes.
Children: 0.1 mg/kg I.M. or S.C.; repeated in 1 to 2 hours as needed and tolerated.
Severe hypotension and shock (including drug-induced)—
Adults: 10 mg in 250 to 500 ml of D_5W or 0.9% sodium chloride for injection. I.V. infusion started at 100 to 180 mcg/minute, then decreased to a maintenance infusion of 40 to 60 mcg/minute when blood pressure stabilizes.
Paroxysmal supraventricular tachycardia—
Adults: initially, 0.5 mg rapid I.V.; subsequent doses should not exceed the preceding dose by more than 0.1 to 0.2 mg and should not exceed 1 mg.

ADVERSE REACTIONS
CNS: *headache,* excitability.
CV: bradycardia, *arrhythmias,* hypertension.
Other: tachyphylaxis (may occur with continued use), ***anaphylaxis, asthmatic episodes,*** decreased organ perfusion (with prolonged use), tissue sloughing with extravasation.

INTERACTIONS
Alpha-adrenergic blockers, phenothiazines: decreased vasopressor re-

sponse. Monitor closely.
Beta-adrenergic blockers: blocked cardiostimulatory effects. Monitor closely.
Bretylium, halogenated hydrocarbon anesthetics: may cause serious arrhythmias. Use with extreme caution.
Guanethidine, oxytocics, tricyclic antidepressants: increased pressor response. Observe patient.
MAO inhibitors: may cause severe hypertension (hypertensive crisis). Don't use together.

EFFECTS ON DIAGNOSTIC TESTS
Phenylephrine may lower intraocular pressure in normal eyes or in open-angle glaucoma. The drug also may cause false-normal tonometry readings.

CONTRAINDICATIONS
Contraindicated in patients with hypersensitivity to the drug and in those with severe hypertension or ventricular tachycardia.

NURSING CONSIDERATIONS
● Use with extreme caution in patients with heart disease, hyperthyroidism, severe atherosclerosis, bradycardia, partial heart block, myocardial disease, or sulfite sensitivity and in elderly patients.
● **I.V. use:** For direct injection, dilute 10 mg (1 ml) with 9 ml sterile water for injection to provide a solution containing 1 mg/ml. I.V. infusions are usually prepared by adding 10 mg of drug to 500 ml of D_5W or 0.9% sodium chloride for injection. The initial infusion rate is usually 100 to 180 mcg/minute; the maintenance infusion rate is usually 40 to 60 mcg/minute.
● Use a central venous catheter or a large vein, as in the antecubital fossa, to minimize risk of extravasation. Use a continuous infusion pump to regulate infusion flow rate.
● With prolonged I.V. infusions, avoid abrupt withdrawal. During infusion, frequently monitor ECG, blood pressure, cardiac output, central venous pressure,

pulmonary capillary wedge pressure, pulse rate, urine output, and color and temperature of extremities. Titrate infusion rate according to findings and the doctor's guidelines. Use a continuous infusion pump to regulate flow rate and avoid severe increase. Maintain blood pressure slightly below the patient's normal level, as ordered. In previously normotensive patients, maintain systolic blood pressure at 80 to 100 mm Hg; in previously hypertensive patients, maintain systolic blood pressure at 30 to 40 mm Hg below usual level.

• To treat extravasation, infiltrate site promptly with 10 to 15 ml of 0.9% sodium chloride for injection containing 5 to 10 mg phentolamine, as ordered. Use a fine needle.

• Remember that drug causes little or no CNS stimulation.

• Keep in mind that drug is incompatible with butacaine sulfate, alkalis, ferric salts, and oxidizing agents.

☑ **PATIENT TEACHING**
• Tell patient to report adverse reactions promptly.

• Instruct patient to alert nurse if discomfort occurs at I.V. insertion site.

pseudoephedrine hydrochloride
Afrinol Repetabs ◇, Allerid ◇, Allermed ◇, Cenafed ◇, Children's Congestion Relief ◇, Children's Sudafed Liquid ◇, Congestac N.D. Caplets† ◇, Congestion Relief ◇, Decofed ◇, De-Fed-60 ◇, Dorcol Children's Decongestant Liquid ◇, Drixoral Non-Drowsy Formula ◇, Efidac/24 ◇, Eltor 120† ◇, Genaphed ◇, Halofed ◇, Halofed Adult Strength ◇, Maxenal† ◇, Myfedrine ◇, NeoFed ◇, Novafed ◇, Ornex Cold† ◇, PediaCare Infant's Decongestant ◇, PediaCare Infants' Oral Decongestant Drops ◇, Pseudo ◇, Pseudofrin† ◇, Pseudo-gest ◇, Robidrine ◇, Seudotabs ◇, Sinufed ◇, Sinustat ◇, Si-

nustop Pro ◇, Sudafed ◇, Sudafed 12 Hour ◇, Sudafed-60 ◇, Sudrin ◇, Sufedrin ◇

pseudoephedrine sulfate
Afrin ◇, Drixoral Non-Drowsy Formula ◇, Drixoral‡

Pregnancy Risk Category: C

HOW SUPPLIED
pseudoephedrine hydrochloride
Tablets: 30 mg ◇, 60 mg ◇
Tablets (extended-release): 120 mg ◇, 240 mg ◇
Capsules: 60 mg
Capsules (extended-release): 120 mg
Oral solution: 15 mg/5 ml ◇, 30 mg/5 ml ◇, 7.5 mg/0.8 ml ◇
Syrup: 30 mg/5 ml
pseudoephedrine sulfate
Tablets (extended-release): 120 mg (60 mg immediate-release, 60 mg delayed-release) ◇

ACTION
Stimulates alpha-adrenergic receptors in the respiratory tract, producing vasoconstriction.

ONSET, PEAK, DURATION
Onset occurs in 15 to 30 minutes. Serum levels peak within 30 to 60 minutes. Effects persist for 3 to 4 hours after administration of tablets, oral solution, and syrup, 8 to 12 hours after administration of extended-release capsules and tablets.

INDICATIONS & DOSAGE
Nasal and eustachian tube decongestion—
Adults: 60 mg P.O. q 4 hours. Maximum dosage is 240 mg daily. Or, 120 mg extended-release tablet P.O. q 12 hours or 240 mg extended-release (Efidac/24) once daily.
Children over 12 years: 120 mg P.O. q 12 hours, or 240 mg P.O. (Efidac/24) once daily.
Children 6 to 12 years: 30 mg P.O.

regular-release form q 4 to 6 hours.
Maximum dosage is 120 mg daily.
Children 2 to 6 years: 15 mg P.O. regular-release form q 4 to 6 hours. Maximum dosage is 60 mg/day.
Children 1 to 2 years: 7 drops (0.2 ml)/kg q 4 to 6 hours up to 4 doses/day.
Children 3 to 12 months: 3 drops/kg q 4 to 6 hours up to 4 doses/day.
Relief of nasal congestion—
Adults: 120 mg q 12 hours.

ADVERSE REACTIONS
CNS: *anxiety,* transient stimulation, tremor, dizziness, headache, insomnia, *nervousness.*
CV: arrhythmias, *palpitations,* tachycardia.
GI: anorexia, nausea, vomiting, dry mouth.
GU: difficulty urinating.
Respiratory: respiratory difficulties.
Skin: pallor.

INTERACTIONS
Antihypertensives: may attenuate hypotensive effect. Monitor blood pressure closely.
MAO inhibitors: may cause severe hypertension (hypertensive crisis). Don't use together.

EFFECTS ON DIAGNOSTIC TESTS
None reported.

CONTRAINDICATIONS
Contraindicated in patients with severe hypertension or severe coronary artery disease, in patients receiving MAO inhibitors, and in breast-feeding patients. Extended-release preparations are contraindicated in children under age 12.

NURSING CONSIDERATIONS
● Use cautiously in patients with hypertension, cardiac disease, diabetes, glaucoma, hyperthyroidism, and prostatic hyperplasia.
● Be aware that elderly patients are more sensitive to the drug's effects.

☑ PATIENT TEACHING
● Tell the patient not to crush or break extended-release forms.
● Warn against using OTC products containing other sympathomimetics.
● Tell the patient not to take drug within 2 hours of bedtime because it can cause insomnia.
● Tell the patient to stop drug if he becomes unusually restless and to notify the doctor promptly.

**dihydroergotamine mesylate
ergotamine tartrate
methysergide maleate
propranolol hydrochloride**
(See Chapter 22, antianginals.)

COMBINATION PRODUCTS
BELLERGAL-S**, BEL-PHEN-ERGOT-S, PHENERBEL-S: ergotamine tartrate 0.6 mg, levorotatory belladonna alkaloids 0.2 mg, and phenobarbital 40 mg.
CAFERGOT, ERCAF, WIGRAINE: ergotamine tartrate 1 mg and caffeine 100 mg.
CAFERGOT SUPPOSITORIES, CAFATIN SUPPOSITORIES, CAFETRATE SUPPOSITORIES: ergotamine tartrate 2 mg and caffeine 100 mg.
HYDERGINE: dihydroergocornine mesylate 0.167 mg, dihydroergocristine mesylate 0.167 mg, and dihydroergocryptine mesylate 0.167 mg.
WIGRAINE SUPPOSITORIES: ergotamine tartrate 2 mg and caffeine 100 mg.

---

dihydroergotamine mesylate
D.H.E. 45, Dihydergot‡, Dihydroergotamine-Sandoz†

Pregnancy Risk Category: X

HOW SUPPLIED
Injection: 1 mg/ml

ACTION
Causes peripheral vasoconstriction primarily by stimulating alpha-adrenergic receptors; may abort vascular headaches by direct vasoconstriction of dilated carotid artery bed with a decline in amplitude of pulsations.

ONSET, PEAK, DURATION
Onset occurs within 5 minutes of I.V. administration, within 15 to 30 minutes of I.M. injection. Serum levels peak within 15 minutes of I.V. administration, 30 minutes after I.M. injection, 15 to 45 minutes after S.C. injection. Effects persist for about 8 hours after parenteral use.

INDICATIONS & DOSAGE
To prevent or abort vascular or migraine headache—
Adults: 1 mg I.M. or I.V. Repeated q 1 to 2 hours, p.r.n., up to total of 2 mg I.V. or 3 mg I.M. per attack. Maximum weekly dosage is 6 mg.

ADVERSE REACTIONS
CV: numbness and tingling in fingers and toes, transient tachycardia or bradycardia, precordial distress and pain, increased arterial pressure.
GI: *nausea, vomiting.*
Skin: itching.
Other: weakness in legs, muscle pain in extremities, localized edema.

INTERACTIONS
Erythromycin, other macrolides: may cause symptoms of ergot toxicity. Vasodilators (nitroprusside, nifedipine, or prazosin) may be ordered to treat such an attack. Monitor closely.
Propranolol, other beta blockers: blocked natural pathway for vasodilation in patients receiving ergot alkaloids; may result in excessive vasoconstriction and cold extremities. Watch closely if drugs are used together.

EFFECTS ON DIAGNOSTIC TESTS
None reported.

CONTRAINDICATIONS
Contraindicated in patients with hypersensitivity to the drug, during pregnancy or breast-feeding, and in patients with peripheral and occlusive vascular disease, coronary artery disease, uncon-

trolled hypertension, severe hepatic or renal dysfunction, and sepsis.

NURSING CONSIDERATIONS
● Know that the drug is most effective when used at first sign of migraine or soon after onset.
● **I.V. use:** Directly inject solution into the vein over 3 minutes. Continuous and intermittent infusion are not recommended.
● Avoid prolonged administration; don't exceed recommended dosage, as ordered. Adjust to most effective minimal dosage, as ordered, for best results.
● Be alert for ergotamine rebound, or an increase in frequency and duration of headache, which may occur when drug is stopped.
● Protect ampules from heat and light. Discard if solution is discolored.

☑ **PATIENT TEACHING**
● Instruct patient to lie down and relax in a quiet, low-light environment after administration of drug.
● Tell patient to report any feeling of coldness in extremities or of tingling in fingers and toes. Severe vasoconstriction may result in tissue damage. Keep extremities warm and administer vasodilators as ordered.
● Help patient evaluate underlying causes of stress, which may precipitate attacks.

---

ergotamine tartrate
Ergodryl Mono‡, Ergomar, Ergostat, Gynergen†, Medihaler Ergotamine

Pregnancy Risk Category: X

HOW SUPPLIED
Capsules: 1 mg‡
Tablets: 1 mg†
Tablets (sublingual): 2 mg
Aerosol inhaler: 360 mcg/metered spray

ACTION
Stimulates alpha-adrenergic receptors, causing peripheral vasoconstriction. Also inhibits reuptake of norepinephrine, increasing vasoconstrictor activity.

ONSET, PEAK, DURATION
Onset and duration variable. Serum levels peak in ½ to 3 hours or longer after oral dose, unknown for other routes of administration.

INDICATIONS & DOSAGE
Vascular or migraine headache—
Adults: initially, 2 mg P.O. or S.L., then 1 to 2 mg P.O. q hour or S.L. q ½ hour, to maximum of 6 mg daily and 10 mg weekly. Alternatively, use aerosol inhaler: 1 spray (360 mcg) initially, repeated q 5 minutes p.r.n. to a maximum of 6 sprays (2.16 mg) per 24 hours or 15 sprays (5.4 mg) per week.

ADVERSE REACTIONS
CV: numbness and tingling in fingers and toes, transient tachycardia or bradycardia, precordial distress and pain, increased arterial pressure, angina pectoris, peripheral vasoconstriction.
GI: nausea, vomiting.
Skin: pruritus, localized edema.
Other: weakness in legs, muscle pain in extremities.

INTERACTIONS
Erythromycin, other macrolides: may cause symptoms of ergot toxicity. Vasodilators (nitroprusside, nifedipine, or prazosin) may be ordered to treat such an attack. Monitor closely.
Propranolol, other beta blockers: blocked natural pathway for vasodilation in patients receiving ergot alkaloids; may result in excessive vasoconstriction. Watch closely if drugs are used together.

EFFECTS ON DIAGNOSTIC TESTS
None reported.

CONTRAINDICATIONS
Contraindicated in patients with hypersensitivity to ergot alkaloids, during

---

pregnancy, and in patients with peripheral and occlusive vascular diseases, coronary artery disease, hypertension, hepatic or renal dysfunction, severe pruritus, or sepsis.

NURSING CONSIDERATIONS
• Obtain an accurate dietary history from the patient to determine if a relationship exists between certain foods and onset of headache.
• Be aware that drug is most effective when used during prodromal stage of headache or as soon as possible after onset.
• Avoid prolonged administration; don't exceed recommended dosage.
• Provide a quiet, low-light environment to help patients relax.
• Be alert for ergotamine rebound, or an increase in frequency and duration of headache, which may occur if drug is suddenly discontinued.

☑ **PATIENT TEACHING**
• Tell patient not to eat, drink, or smoke while the tablet is dissolving. S.L. tablet is preferred during early stage of attack because of its rapid absorption.
• Warn patient not to increase dosage without first consulting the doctor.
• Advise patient to avoid prolonged exposure to cold weather whenever possible. Cold may increase many of the adverse reactions to the drug.
• Instruct patient on long-term therapy to check for and report feeling of coldness in extremities or of tingling in fingers and toes. Severe vasoconstriction may result in tissue damage. Keep extremities warm and administer vasodilators as ordered.
• Instruct patient how to use inhaler correctly.
• Help patient evaluate underlying causes of stress, which may precipitate attacks.

---

methysergide maleate
Deseril‡, Sansert**

Pregnancy Risk Category: X

HOW SUPPLIED
Tablets: 1 mg‡, 2 mg

ACTION
Unknown. Specifically blocks serotonin (a neurotransmitter) in the peripheral nervous system. In CNS, drug may act as a serotonin agonist.

ONSET, PEAK, DURATION
Onset occurs within 1 to 2 days after therapy initiated. Peak unknown. Effects persist for 1 to 2 days.

INDICATIONS & DOSAGE
Prevention of frequent, severe, uncontrollable, or disabling migraine or vascular headaches—
Adults: 4 to 8 mg P.O. daily with meals. There must be a drug-free interval of 3 to 4 weeks following every 6-month course of treatment.

ADVERSE REACTIONS
CNS: insomnia, drowsiness, *euphoria, vertigo,* ataxia, *light-headedness,* hyperesthesia, weakness, hallucinations or feelings of dissociation, rapid speech, lethargy.
CV: *fibrotic thickening of cardiac valves and aorta, inferior vena cava, and common iliac branches (retroperitoneal fibrosis);* vasoconstriction, causing chest pain, abdominal pain, vascular insufficiency of lower limbs; cold, numb, painful extremities with or without paresthesia and diminished or absent pulses; postural hypotension; tachycardia; peripheral edema; murmurs; bruits.
GI: nausea, vomiting, diarrhea, constipation, heartburn.
Hematologic: neutropenia, eosinophilia.
Respiratory: *pulmonary fibrosis* (caus-

Reactions may be *common,* uncommon, *life-threatening,* or COMMON AND LIFE-THREATENING.

ing dyspnea, tightness and pain in chest, pleural friction rubs, and effusion). **Skin:** hair loss, flushing, rash. **Other:** arthralgia, myalgia.

INTERACTIONS

Beta blockers: may result in peripheral ischemia by cold extremities and possible gangrene. Monitor closely.

EFFECTS ON DIAGNOSTIC TESTS

None reported.

CONTRAINDICATIONS

Contraindicated in patients with severe hypertension or arteriosclerosis, peripheral vascular insufficiency, renal or hepatic disease, coronary artery disease (CAD), phlebitis or cellulitis of lower limbs, collagen diseases, fibrotic processes, or valvular heart disease; in debilitated patients; and during pregnancy.

NURSING CONSIDERATIONS

• Use cautiously in patients with peptic ulcerations or suspected CAD. ECG and cardiac status evaluation advisable before giving to patients over age 40. Also use cautiously in patients sensitive to aspirin or tartrazine.

Alert: Know that the drug is indicated only for patients who are unresponsive to other drugs and who can be kept under close medical supervision.

• Gradually introduce medication, as ordered, and administer with meals to prevent GI effects.

• Give drug, as ordered, for 3 weeks before evaluating effectiveness.

• Monitor laboratory studies of cardiac and renal function, CBC, and erythrocyte sedimentation rate before and during therapy.

• Know that drug should not be used for treatment of migraine or vascular headache or tension (muscle contraction) headaches.

• Be aware that drug may be withdrawn gradually every 6 months; then restarted after at least 3 weeks.

☑ PATIENT TEACHING

• Instruct patient to take drug with meals.

• Instruct patient to keep daily weight record and report unusually rapid weight gain. Teach patient to check for peripheral edema. Explain and suggest low-salt diet if necessary.

• Tell patient not to stop drug abruptly; may cause rebound headaches. Stop gradually over 2 to 3 weeks.

• Tell patient to promptly report any of the following symptoms to the doctor: cold, numb, or painful hands and feet; leg cramps when walking; and pelvic, chest, or flank pain.

---

*Liquid contains alcohol.   **May contain tartrazine.   †Canada only.   ‡Australia only.   ◇ OTC.

Skeletal muscle relaxants

baclofen
carisoprodol
chlorzoxazone
cyclobenzaprine hydrochloride
dantrolene sodium
methocarbamol
tizanidine hydrochloride

COMBINATION PRODUCTS
NORGESIC: orphenadrine citrate 25 mg, aspirin 385 mg, and caffeine 30 mg.
NORGESIC FORTE: orphenadrine citrate 50 mg, aspirin 770 mg, and caffeine 60 mg.
ROBAXISAL: methocarbamol 400 mg and aspirin 325 mg.
SOMA COMPOUND: carisoprodol 200 mg and aspirin 325 mg.
SOMA COMPOUND WITH CODEINE: carisoprodol 200 mg, aspirin 325 mg, and codeine phosphate 16 mg.

---

baclofen
Clofen‡, Lioresal, Lioresal Intrathecal

Pregnancy Risk Category: C

HOW SUPPLIED
Tablets: 10 mg, 20 mg, 25 mg‡
Intrathecal injection: 500 mcg/ml, 2,000 mcg/ml

ACTION
Unknown. Appears to reduce transmission of impulses from the spinal cord to skeletal muscle.

ONSET, PEAK, DURATION
Onset occurs hours to weeks after oral administration, ½ to 1 hour after intrathecal administration. Serum levels peak 2 to 3 hours after an oral dose; peak effects occur about 4 hours after intrathecal administration. Effects of intrathecal injection persist for about 4 to 8 hours, unknown for oral administration.

INDICATIONS & DOSAGE
Spasticity in multiple sclerosis, spinal cord injury—
Adults: initially, 5 mg P.O. t.i.d. for 3 days, then 10 mg t.i.d. for 3 days, 15 mg t.i.d. for 3 days, 20 mg t.i.d. for 3 days. Increased according to response up to maximum of 80 mg daily.
Management of severe spasticity in patients who do not respond to or cannot tolerate oral baclofen therapy—
Adults: *Screening phase*—After a test dose to check responsiveness, drug is given by an implantable infusion pump. The test dose is 1 ml of a 50-mcg/ml dilution administered into the intrathecal space by barbotage over 1 minute or more. Significantly decreased severity or frequency of muscle spasm or reduced muscle tone should appear within 4 to 8 hours. If the response is inadequate, a second test dose of 75 mcg/1.5 ml is given 24 hours after the first. If response is still inadequate, a final test dose of 100 mcg/2 ml is given 24 hours later. Patients unresponsive to the 100-mcg dose shouldn't be considered candidates for the implantable pump.

Maintenance therapy— Initial dose is titrated based on the screening dose that elicited an adequate response. This effective dose is doubled and administered over 24 hours. However, if the screening dose efficacy was maintained for 12 hours or more, the dose is not doubled. After the first 24 hours, the dose is increased slowly as needed and tolerated by 10% to 30% daily. During prolonged maintenance therapy, daily dose may be increased by 10% to 40% if needed; if the patient experiences adverse effects, dosage may be decreased by 10% to 20%. Maintenance dosages

---

Reactions may be *common,* uncommon, *life-threatening,* or COMMON AND LIFE-THREATENING.

have ranged from 12 mcg to 1,500 mcg daily; however, experience with dosages over 1,000 mcg daily is limited. Most patients need 300 to 800 mcg daily.

ADVERSE REACTIONS
CNS: *drowsiness, dizziness,* headache, *weakness, fatigue,* hypotonia, *confusion,* insomnia, dysarthria, SEIZURES.
CV: hypotension, hypertension.
EENT: blurred vision, nasal congestion, slurred speech.
GI: *nausea,* constipation, *vomiting.*
GU: urinary frequency.
Hepatic: increased AST and alkaline phosphatase levels.
Skin: rash, pruritus.
Other: excessive perspiration, hyperglycemia, weight gain, dyspnea.

INTERACTIONS
Ethanol, CNS depressants: increased CNS depression. Avoid concomitant use.

EFFECTS ON DIAGNOSTIC TESTS
Baclofen therapy increases blood glucose, AST, and alkaline phosphatase levels.

CONTRAINDICATIONS
Contraindicated in patients with hypersensitivity to the drug.

NURSING CONSIDERATIONS
● Use cautiously in patients with impaired renal function or seizure disorder or when spasticity is used to maintain motor function.
● Give oral form with meals or with milk to prevent GI distress.
● Know that orally administered drug should not be used to treat muscle spasm caused by rheumatic disorders, cerebral palsy, Parkinson's disease, or CVA because efficacy hasn't been established. Do not administer intrathecal injection by I.V., I.M., S.C., or epidural route.
● Watch for sensitivity reactions, such as fever, skin eruptions, and respiratory distress.
● Look for increased risk of seizures in patients with seizure disorder.
● Be aware that amount of relief determines if dosage (and drowsiness) can be reduced.
● Do not withdraw drug abruptly after long-term use unless required by severe adverse reactions; may precipitate hallucinations or rebound spasticity.
● Know that experience with long-term intrathecal use suggests that about 10% of patients may develop tolerance to the drug. In some cases, this may be treated by hospitalizing the patient and slowly withdrawing the drug over a 2-week period.

☑ **PATIENT TEACHING**
● Instruct patient to take oral form with meals or milk.
● Tell patients to avoid activities that require alertness until drug's CNS effects are known. Drowsiness usually is transient.
● Tell patients to avoid alcohol while taking this drug.
● Advise the patient to follow the doctor's orders regarding rest and physical therapy.

---

carisoprodol
Rela, Sodol, Soma, Soprodol, Soridol

Pregnancy Risk Category: NR

HOW SUPPLIED
Tablets: 350 mg

ACTION
Unknown. Drug appears to modify central perception of pain without modifying pain reflexes. Blocks interneuronal activity in descending reticular activating system and spinal cord.

ONSET, PEAK, DURATION
Onset occurs within 30 minutes. Serum levels peak within 4 hours. Effects persist for 4 to 6 hours.

INDICATIONS & DOSAGE
As an adjunct in acute, painful musculoskeletal conditions—
Adults: 350 mg P.O. t.i.d. and h.s.

ADVERSE REACTIONS
CNS: *drowsiness, dizziness,* vertigo, ataxia, tremor, agitation, irritability, headache, depressive reactions, insomnia.
CV: *orthostatic hypotension,* tachycardia, facial flushing.
GI: nausea, vomiting, hiccups, epigastric distress.
Hematologic: eosinophilia.
Respiratory: asthmatic episodes.
Skin: rash, *erythema multiforme,* pruritus.
Other: fever, *angioedema, anaphylaxis.*

INTERACTIONS
Ethanol, CNS depressants: increased CNS depression. Avoid concomitant use.

EFFECTS ON DIAGNOSTIC TESTS
None significant.

CONTRAINDICATIONS
Contraindicated in patients with hypersensitivity to related compounds (for example, meprobamate or tybamate) or intermittent porphyria.

NURSING CONSIDERATIONS
● Use cautiously in patients with impaired hepatic or renal function.
Alert: Watch for idiosyncratic reactions after first to fourth dose (weakness, ataxia, visual and speech difficulties, fever, skin eruptions, and mental changes) and for severe reactions, including bronchospasm, hypotension, and anaphylactic shock. Withhold dose and notify the doctor immediately of any unusual reactions.
● Record amount of relief to help the doctor determine whether dosage can be reduced.
● Do not stop drug abruptly; mild withdrawal effects, such as insomnia, headache, nausea, and abdominal cramps, may result.

☑ PATIENT TEACHING
● Warn patient to avoid activities that require alertness until drug's CNS effects are known. Drowsiness is transient.
● Advise patient to avoid combining drug with alcohol or other CNS depressants.
● Advise patient to follow doctor's orders regarding rest and physical therapy.

---

chlorzoxazone
Paraflex, Parafon Forte DSC, Remular-S

Pregnancy Risk Category: NR

HOW SUPPLIED
Tablets: 250 mg, 500 mg
Caplets: 250 mg, 500 mg

ACTION
Unknown. Appears to modify central perception of pain without modifying pain reflexes. Blocks interneuronal activity in descending reticular activating system and in spinal cord.

ONSET, PEAK, DURATION
Onset occurs within 1 hour. Serum levels peak within 1 to 2 hours. Effects persist for 3 to 4 hours.

INDICATIONS & DOSAGE
As an adjunct in acute, painful musculoskeletal conditions—
Adults: 250 to 750 mg P.O. t.i.d. or q.i.d.
Children: 20 mg/kg P.O. or 600 mg/m^2 daily in divided doses t.i.d. or q.i.d.

ADVERSE REACTIONS
CNS: *drowsiness, dizziness, light-headedness,* malaise, headache, overstimulation, tremor.
GI: anorexia, nausea, vomiting, heart-

burn, abdominal distress, constipation, diarrhea.
GU: urine discoloration (orange or purple-red).
Hepatic: hepatic dysfunction.
Skin: urticaria, redness, pruritus, petechiae, bruising, angioneurotic edema, *anaphylaxis.*

INTERACTIONS
Ethanol, CNS depressants: increased CNS depression. Avoid concomitant use.

EFFECTS ON DIAGNOSTIC TESTS
None reported.

CONTRAINDICATIONS
Contraindicated in patients with hypersensitivity to the drug or impaired hepatic function.

NURSING CONSIDERATIONS
● Use cautiously in patients with history of drug allergies.
● Know that the amount of relief determines if dosage (and drowsiness) can be reduced.
● Monitor patient's liver enzyme levels, as ordered. Watch for early signs of hepatic dysfunction or abnormal liver enzyme levels. If they occur, withhold dose and notify the doctor. Serious (including fatal) hepatocellular toxicity has been reported in patients receiving this drug.

☑ **PATIENT TEACHING**
● Tell patient to take drug with meals or milk.
● Warn patient to avoid activities that require alertness until drug's CNS effects are known.
● Instruct patient to report to doctor fever, rash, anorexia, nausea, vomiting, fatigue, right upper quadrant pain, dark urine, or jaundice immediately because these may be signs of hepatocellular toxicity, which warrants immediate discontinuation of drug.
● Warn patient to avoid alcohol or other

CNS depressants; concomitant use with drug may increase risk of hepatocellular toxicity.
● Tell patient that the drug may discolor urine orange or purple-red.
● Advise patient to follow the doctor's orders regarding physical activity.

---

cyclobenzaprine hydrochloride
Flexeril

Pregnancy Risk Category: B

HOW SUPPLIED
Tablets: 10 mg

ACTION
Unknown.

ONSET, PEAK, DURATION
Onset occurs within 1 hour. Serum levels peak in 3 to 8 hours. Effects persist for 12 to 24 hours.

INDICATIONS & DOSAGE
Short-term treatment of muscle spasm—
Adults: 10 mg P.O. t.i.d. Maximum dosage is 60 mg daily; maximum duration of treatment is 2 to 3 weeks.

ADVERSE REACTIONS
CNS: *drowsiness,* headache, insomnia, fatigue, asthenia, nervousness, confusion, paresthesia, *dizziness,* depression, visual disturbances, *seizures.*
CV: tachycardia, syncope, arrhythmias, palpitations, hypotension, vasodilation.
EENT: blurred vision, *dry mouth.*
GI: dyspepsia, abnormal taste, constipation, nausea.
GU: urine retention, urinary frequency.
Skin: rash, urticaria, pruritus.
Other: with high doses, watch for adverse reactions similar to those of other tricyclic antidepressants.

INTERACTIONS
Anticholinergics: additive anticholinergic effects. Avoid concomitant use.

Ethanol, CNS depressants: may cause additive CNS depression. Avoid concomitant use.

MAO inhibitors: may exacerbate CNS depression or anticholinergic effects. Don't give within 14 days after discontinuing MAO inhibitors.

EFFECTS ON DIAGNOSTIC TESTS
None significant.

CONTRAINDICATIONS
Contraindicated in patients who have received MAO inhibitors within 14 days; during acute recovery phase of MI; and in patients with hyperthyroidism, hypersensitivity to the drug, heart block, arrhythmias, conduction disturbances, or CHF.

NURSING CONSIDERATIONS
• Use cautiously in patients with history of urine retention, acute angle-closure glaucoma, and increased intraocular pressure and in elderly or debilitated patients.
• Be alert for nausea, headache, and malaise, which may occur if drug is stopped abruptly after long-term use.
• Watch for symptoms of overdose, including possible cardiac toxicity. Notify the doctor immediately and have physostigmine available.

☑ **PATIENT TEACHING**
• Advise patient to report urinary hesitancy or urine retention. If constipation is a problem, increase fluid intake and suggest a stool softener.
• Warn patient to avoid activities that require alertness until drug's CNS effects are known.
• Warn patient not to combine with alcohol or other CNS depressants.

---

dantrolene sodium
Dantrium, Dantrium Intravenous

Pregnancy Risk Category: NR

HOW SUPPLIED
Capsules: 25 mg, 50 mg, 100 mg
Injection: 20 mg/vial

ACTION
Acts directly on skeletal muscle to interfere with intracellular calcium movement.

ONSET, PEAK, DURATION
Onset and duration unknown. Peak levels occur 5 hours after oral administration.

INDICATIONS & DOSAGE
Spasticity and sequelae secondary to severe chronic disorders (such as multiple sclerosis, cerebral palsy, spinal cord injury, CVA)—
Adults: 25 mg P.O. daily. Increased gradually in 25-mg increments, up to 100 mg b.i.d. to q.i.d., to maximum of 400 mg daily.
Children: initially, 0.5 mg/kg P.O. b.i.d.; increased to t.i.d. then q.i.d. Dosage increased as needed by 0.5 mg/kg daily to 3 mg/kg b.i.d. to q.i.d. Maximum dosage is 100 mg q.i.d.
Management of malignant hyperthermia crisis—
Adults and children: 1 mg/kg I.V. initially; dose repeated as needed up to cumulative dosage of 10 mg/kg.
Prevention or attenuation of malignant hyperthermia crisis in susceptible patients who require surgery—
Adults: 4 to 8 mg/kg P.O. daily in three to four divided doses for 1 to 2 days before procedure. Final dose administered 3 to 4 hours before procedure.
Prevention of recurrence of malignant hyperthermia crisis—
Adults: 4 to 8 mg/kg/day P.O. in four divided doses for up to 3 days after hyperthermic crisis.

ADVERSE REACTIONS
CNS: *muscle weakness, drowsiness, dizziness,* light-headedness, *malaise, fatigue,* headache, confusion, nervousness, insomnia, **seizures.**

Reactions may be *common,* uncommon, *life-threatening,* or COMMON AND LIFE-THREATENING.

CV: tachycardia, blood pressure changes.
EENT: excessive lacrimation, speech disturbance, altered taste, diplopia, visual disturbances.
GI: anorexia, constipation, cramping, dysphagia, metallic taste, severe diarrhea, GI bleeding.
GU: urinary frequency, hematuria, incontinence, nocturia, dysuria, crystalluria, difficult erection, urine retention.
Hepatic: *hepatitis.*
Respiratory: pleural effusion with pericarditis.
Skin: eczematous eruption, pruritus, urticaria.
Other: abnormal hair growth, diaphoresis, myalgia, chills, fever, back pain.

INTERACTIONS

Estrogens: may increase risk of hepatotoxicity. Use together cautiously.
Ethanol, CNS depressants: increased CNS depression. Avoid concomitant use.
I.V. verapamil: may result in cardiovascular collapse. Stop verapamil before administering I.V. dantrolene.

EFFECTS ON DIAGNOSTIC TESTS

Dantrolene therapy alters liver function test results (increased ALT, AST, alkaline phosphatase, and lactate dehydrogenase), BUN levels, and total serum bilirubin.

CONTRAINDICATIONS

Contraindicated in patients when spasticity is used to maintain motor function, in those with upper motor neuron disorders, for spasms in rheumatic disorders, in patients with active hepatic disease, and in breast-feeding patients.

NURSING CONSIDERATIONS

● Use cautiously in patients with severely impaired cardiac or pulmonary function or preexisting hepatic disease, in women, and in patients over age 35.
● Obtain liver function tests at the beginning of therapy.

● Prepare oral suspension for single dose by dissolving capsule contents in juice or other liquid. For multiple doses, use acid vehicle, and refrigerate. Use within several days.
● **I.V. use:** Give as soon as malignant hyperthermia reaction is recognized, as ordered. Reconstitute each vial by adding 60 ml of sterile water for injection and shaking vial until clear. Don't use a diluent that contains a bacteriostatic agent. Protect contents from light, and use within 6 hours. Avoid extravasation.
● Watch for hepatitis (fever and jaundice), severe diarrhea, severe weakness, or sensitivity reactions (fever and skin eruptions). Withhold dose and notify the doctor.
● Know that amount of relief in patient determines if dosage (and drowsiness) can be reduced.

☑ PATIENT TEACHING

● Instruct patient to take drug with meals or milk in four divided doses.
● Tell patient to use caution when eating to avoid choking. Some patients may experience difficulty swallowing during therapy.
● Warn patient to avoid driving and other hazardous activities until drug's CNS effects are known.
● Advise patient to avoid combining drug with alcohol and other CNS depressants.
● Tell patient to avoid photosensitivity reactions by using sunblock and wearing protective clothing, to report abdominal discomfort or GI problems immediately, and to follow the doctor's orders regarding rest and physical therapy.

---

methocarbamol
Delaxin, Marbaxin-750, Robaxin, Robaxin-750, Robomol-500, Robomol-750

Pregnancy Risk Category: NR

HOW SUPPLIED
Tablets: 500 mg, 750 mg
Injection: 100 mg/ml

ACTION
Unknown. Probably modifies central perception of pain without modifying pain reflexes.

ONSET, PEAK, DURATION
Onset is immediate after I.V. administration; within ½ hour after oral administration. Peak levels occur immediately after I.V. administration, or within 2 hours of an oral dose. Duration unknown.

INDICATIONS & DOSAGE
As an adjunct in acute, painful musculoskeletal conditions—
Adults: 1.5 g P.O. q.i.d. for 2 to 3 days, then 1 g P.O. q.i.d., or not more than 500 mg (5 ml) I.M. into each gluteal region. Repeated q 8 hours p.r.n. Or 1 to 3 g daily (10 to 30 ml) I.V. directly into vein at 3 ml/minute, or 10 ml may be added to no more than 250 ml of D$_5$W or 0.9% sodium chloride solution. Maximum dosage is 3 g daily for not more than 3 days.
Supportive therapy in tetanus management—
Adults: 1 to 2 g by direct I.V. or 1 to 3 g as infusion q 6 hours.
Children: 15 mg/kg I.V. q 6 hours.

ADVERSE REACTIONS
CNS: drowsiness, dizziness, light-headedness, headache, syncope, mild muscular incoordination (with I.M. or I.V. use), *seizures* (with I.V. use only), vertigo.
CV: hypotension, bradycardia (with I.M. or I.V. use).
EENT: blurred vision, conjunctivitis, nystagmus, diplopia.
GI: nausea, GI upset, metallic taste.
GU: hematuria (with I.V. use only), discoloration of urine.
Skin: urticaria, pruritus, rash.
Respiratory: thrombophlebitis.
Other: extravasation (with I.V. use

only), fever, flushing, *anaphylactic reactions* (with I.M. or I.V. use).

INTERACTIONS
Ethanol, CNS depressants: increased CNS depression. Avoid concomitant use.

EFFECTS ON DIAGNOSTIC TESTS
Drug therapy alters laboratory test results for urine 5-hydroxyindoleacetic acid (5-HIAA) using quantitative method of Undenfriend (false-positive) and urine vanillylmandelic acid (false-positive when Gitlow screening test used; no problem when quantitative method of Sunderman used).

CONTRAINDICATIONS
Contraindicated in patients with hypersensitivity to the drug, impaired renal function (injectable form), or seizure disorder (injectable form).

NURSING CONSIDERATIONS
● For nasogastric tube administration, prepare liquid by crushing tablets into water or sodium chloride solution.
● In tetanus management, be aware methocarbamol is used with tetanus antitoxin, penicillin; tracheotomy, and aggressive supportive care. Long course of I.V. methocarbamol therapy is required.
● **I.V. use:** Dilute 10 ml of drug in not more than 250 ml of solution. Use D$_5$W or 0.9% sodium chloride for injection. Infuse slowly; maximum rate is 300 mg (3 ml)/minute.
● Know that drug irritates veins; may cause phlebitis, aggravate seizures, and cause fainting if injected rapidly. Make sure the patient remains in a supine position during infusion. Drug is an irritant; avoid extravasation.
● Give I.M. deeply, only into upper outer quadrant of buttocks, with maximum of 5 ml in each buttock.
● Do not give S.C.
● Watch for orthostatic hypotension, especially with parenteral administration. Keep the patient in a supine position for

---

15 minutes afterward, and supervise ambulation. Have patient get up slowly.
• Watch for sensitivity reactions, such as fever and skin eruptions.
• Have epinephrine, antihistamines, and corticosteroids available.
• Monitor CBC periodically during prolonged therapy.

☑ **PATIENT TEACHING**
• Instruct patient to take drug with food or milk.
• Tell patient that urine may turn green, black, or brown.
• Advise patient to follow the doctor's orders regarding physical activity.
• Warn patient to avoid activities that require alertness until drug's CNS effects are known.
• Advise patient to avoid combining drug with alcohol or other CNS depressants.

▼ *NEW DRUG*

tizanidine hydrochloride
Zanaflex

Pregnancy Risk Category: C

HOW SUPPIED
Tablets: 4 mg

ACTION
Unknown. Acts as an alpha$_2$-adrenergic agonist. Thought to reduce spasticity by increasing presynaptic inhibition of motor neurons.

ONSET, PEAK, DURATION
Onset unknown after oral administration. Plasma levels peak in 1 to 2 hours and the effect dissipates in 3 to 6 hours.

INDICATIONS & DOSAGE
Acute and intermittent management of increased muscle tone associated with spasticity—
Adults: initially, 4 mg P.O. q 6 to 8 hours p.r.n. to maximum of three doses

in 24 hours. Dosage can be increased gradually in 2- to 4-mg increments. Maximum daily dose is 36 mg.

ADVERSE REACTIONS
CNS: *somnolence, sedation, asthenia, dizziness,* speech disorder, dyskinesia, nervousness, hallucinations.
CV: *hypotension, bradycardia.*
EENT: amblyopia.
GI: *dry mouth,* constipation, vomiting.
GU: *UTI,* urinary frequency.
Hepatic: elevations of liver function tests, hepatic injury.
Respiratory: pharyngitis, rhinitis.
Other: infection, flu syndrome.

INTERACTIONS
Alcohol, baclofen, benzodiazepines, other CNS depressants: additive CNS depressant effects. Avoid concomitant use.
Antihypertensives, other alpha$_2$- adrenergic agonists: may cause hypotension. Monitor patient closely. Do not use with other alpha$_2$-adrenergic agonists.
Oral contraceptives: decreased clearance of tizanidine. Dose of tizanidine may be reduced.

EFFECTS ON DIAGNOSTIC TESTS
Drug may increase LFTs.

CONTRAINDICATIONS
Contraindicated in patients with known hypersensitivity to the drug.

NURSING CONSIDERATIONS
• Use cautiously in patients who are currently taking antihypertensives, in those with renal and hepatic impairment, and in the elderly.
• Know that dosages will be reduced in patients with renal impairment. If higher dosages are needed, the individual doses rather than frequency should be increased.
• Know that tizanidine should be used in pregnancy only if the benefit justifies the risk to the fetus. Women taking the drug should not breast-feed.
• Know that safety and effectiveness in

pediatric patients have not been established.

● Obtain baseline liver function tests as ordered before treatment; during treatment at 1, 3, and 6 months; and then periodically thereafter.

☑ **PATIENT TEACHING**

● The patient should be advised of the limited clinical experience with tizanidine (duration of use and higher doses).

● Caution the patient that the drug may cause drowsiness and to avoid alcohol and activities, such as driving and operating machinery, that require alertness.

● Inform the patient that orthostatic hypotension can be minimized by rising slowly and avoiding sudden position changes.

atracurium besylate
cisatracurium besylate
doxacurium chloride
metocurine iodide
mivacurium chloride
pancuronium bromide
pipecuronium bromide
rocuronium bromide
succinylcholine chloride
tubocurarine chloride
vecuronium bromide

COMBINATION PRODUCTS
None.

---

atracurium besylate
Tracrium

Pregnancy Risk Category: C

HOW SUPPLIED
Injection: 10 mg/ml

ACTION
Prevents acetylcholine from binding to receptors on muscle end plate, thus blocking depolarization.

ONSET, PEAK, DURATION
Onset occurs in 2 minutes. Peak occurs in 3 to 5 minutes. About 25% of muscle twitch strength returns in 35 to 45 minutes; 95% in 60 to 70 minutes.

INDICATIONS & DOSAGE
Adjunct to general anesthesia to facilitate endotracheal intubation and to provide skeletal muscle relaxation during surgery or mechanical ventilation—
Dosage depends on anesthetic used, individual needs, and response. Dosages given here are representative only.
Adults and children over 2 years: 0.4 to 0.5 mg/kg by I.V. bolus. Maintenance dosage of 0.08 to 0.10 mg/kg within 20

to 45 minutes should be given during prolonged surgery. Maintenance dosages may be given q 12 to 25 minutes in patients receiving balanced anesthesia. For prolonged procedures, a constant infusion of 5 to 9 mcg/kg/minute may be used.
Children 1 month to 2 years: initial dose, 0.3 to 0.4 mg/kg. Frequent maintenance doses may be needed.

ADVERSE REACTIONS
CV: bradycardia, hypotension, tachycardia.
Respiratory: *prolonged dose-related apnea,* wheezing, increased bronchial secretions, dyspnea, bronchospasm, laryngospasm.
Skin: *skin flushing,* erythema, pruritus, urticaria, rash.
Other: *anaphylaxis.*

INTERACTIONS
Aminoglycoside antibiotics (amikacin, gentamicin, kanamycin, neomycin, streptomycin); polymyxin antibiotics (polymyxin B sulfate, colistin); clindamycin; quinidine; general anesthetics (halothane, enflurane, isoflurane): potentiated neuromuscular blockade, leading to increased skeletal muscle relaxation and prolonged effect. Use cautiously during and after surgery.
Lithium, magnesium salts, opioid analgesics: potentiated neuromuscular blockade, leading to increased skeletal muscle relaxation and possible respiratory paralysis. Reduce dose of atracurium.
Neostigmine, edrophonium, pyridostigmine: inhibition of drug and reversed neuromuscular block.

EFFECTS ON DIAGNOSTIC TESTS
None significant.

CONTRAINDICATIONS

Contraindicated in patients with hypersensitivity to the drug.

NURSING CONSIDERATIONS

● Use cautiously in those with CV disease; severe electrolyte disorder; bronchogenic carcinoma; hepatic, renal, or pulmonary impairment; neuromuscular disease; or myasthenia gravis and in elderly or debilitated patients.
● Administer sedatives or general anesthetics before neuromuscular blockers, which don't obtund consciousness or alter pain threshold.
● Administer analgesics, as ordered, for pain. Remember that patient may have pain but not be able to express it.
● Use this drug only under direct medical supervision by personnel skilled in the use of neuromuscular blockers and techniques for maintaining a patent airway. Have emergency respiratory support equipment (endotracheal equipment, ventilator, oxygen, atropine, edrophonium, neostigmine, and epinephrine) available.
● **I.V. use:** Drug usually is administered by rapid I.V. bolus injection but may be given by intermittent infusion or continuous infusion. At concentrations of 0.2 mg/ml to 0.5 mg/ml, atracurium is compatible for 24 hours in D_5W, 0.9% sodium chloride for injection, or dextrose 5% in 0.9% sodium chloride for injection.
● Do not use lactated Ringer's solution. In lactated Ringer's injection, atracurium is stable for 8 hours at a concentration of 0.5 mg/ml. However, because of increased degradation in this solution, it is not recommended.
● Do not give by I.M. injection.
● Do not mix with alkaline solutions (precipitate may form).
● Once spontaneous recovery starts, be prepared to reverse atracurium-induced neuromuscular blockade with an anticholinesterase agent (such as neostigmine or edrophonium), as ordered. Usually given together with an anticholinergic (such as atropine).
● Monitor respirations closely until patient is fully recovered from neuromuscular blockade, as evidenced by tests of muscle strength (hand grip, head lift, and ability to cough).
● A nerve stimulator and train-of-four monitoring are recommended to confirm antagonism of neuromuscular blockade and recovery of muscle strength. Evidence of spontaneous recovery should be seen before attempting reversal with neostigmine.
● Know that prior administration of succinylcholine doesn't prolong duration of action but quickens onset and may deepen neuromuscular blockade.

☑ **PATIENT TEACHING**
● Explain all events and procedures to the patient because he can still hear.

---

cisatracurium besylate
Nimbex

Pregnancy Risk Category: B

HOW SUPPLIED
Injection: 2 mg/ml, 10 mg/ml

ACTION
A nondepolarizing agent that binds to cholinergic receptors on the motor end plate, antagonizing acetylcholine and blocking neuromuscular transmission.

ONSET, PEAK, DURATION
Onset occurs in 1 to 3.3 minutes. Peak levels occur in 2 to 5 minutes. About 95% of muscle twitch strength returns in 46 to 121 minutes.

INDICATIONS & DOSAGE
Note: Dosage requirements vary widely among patients.
Adjunct to general anesthesia, to facilitate tracheal intubation, and to provide skeletal muscle relaxation during surgery —
Adults: initial dose of 0.15 mg/kg I.V.,

Reactions may be *common*, uncommon, *life-threatening*, or COMMON AND LIFE-THREATENING.

followed by maintenance doses of 0.03 mg/kg I.V. q 40 to 50 minutes p.r.n. (or initial dose of 0.20 mg/kg I.V., followed by maintenance doses of 0.03 mg/kg I.V. q 50 to 60 minutes p.r.n.). Alternatively, after initial dose, a maintenance infusion may be given at 3 mcg/kg/minute, reduced to 1 to 2 mcg/kg/minute p.r.n.

Children 2 to 12 years: 0.1 mg/kg I.V. over 5 to 10 seconds. After initial dose, a maintenance infusion may be given at 3 mcg/kg/minute, reduced to 1 to 2 mcg/kg/minute as needed.

Maintenance of neuromuscular blockade during mechanical ventilation in ICU—

Adults: After initial dose, 3 mcg/kg/minute (range: 0.5 to 10.2 mcg/kg/minute) I.V. infusion.

ADVERSE REACTIONS
CV: bradycardia, hypotension.
Respiratory: bronchospasm.
Skin: flushing, rash.

INTERACTIONS
Aminoglycosides, bacitracin, clindamycin, colistin, lincomycin, lithium, local anesthetics, magnesium salts, polymyxins, procainamide, quinidine, tetracyclines, sodium colistimethate: may enhance neuromuscular blocking action of cisatracurium. Use together cautiously.

Carbamazepine, phenytoin: may cause slightly shorter duration of neuromuscular block, requiring higher infusion rate. Monitor closely.

Isoflurane or enflurane administered with nitrous oxide/oxygen: may prolong duration of action of cisatracurium. Be aware that patient may require less frequent maintenance dosing, lower maintenance doses, or reduced infusion rate of cisatracurium.

EFFECTS ON DIAGNOSTIC TESTS
None known.

CONTRAINDICATIONS
Contraindicated in patients with hyper-sensitivity to drug, other bis-benzylisoquinolinium agents, or benzyl alcohol (found in 10 ml vial).

NURSING CONSIDERATIONS
● Drug is not recommended for rapid-sequence endotracheal intubation because of its intermediate onset.
● Use cautiously in pregnant or breast-feeding women.
● Cisatracurium has no known effect on consciousness, pain threshold, or cerebration. To avoid patient distress, neuromuscular block should not be induced before unconsciousness.
● **I.V. use:** 20-ml vial is intended for ICU use only. Drug is not compatible with propofol injection or ketorolac injection for Y-site administration. Drug is acidic and may not be compatible with an alkaline solution having a pH greater than 8.5 (such as barbiturate solutions for Y-site administration). Drug should not be diluted in lactated Ringer's injection because of chemical instability.
● Drug is colorless to slightly yellow or green-yellow. Inspect vials for particulate and discoloration before administration. Unclear solutions or those with visible particulate should not be used.
● Neuromuscular function should be monitored with nerve stimulator during administration. If stimulation does not elicit a response, infusion should be stopped until a response returns.
● To avoid inaccurate dosing, neuromuscular monitoring should be performed on a nonparetic limb in patients with hemiparesis or paraparesis.
● In patients with neuromuscular disease (myasthenia gravis and myasthenic syndrome), prolonged neuromuscular block is possible. Use of a peripheral nerve stimulator and a dose of not more than 0.02 mg/kg is recommended to assess the level of neuromuscular block and to monitor dosage requirements.
● Because patients with burns have been shown to develop resistance to nonde-polarizing neuromuscular blocking agents, they may require increased dos-

ing. Monitor closely.
• Monitor acid-base balance and electrolyte levels, as ordered. Abnormalities may potentiate or antagonize the action of cisatracurium.
• Monitor patient for malignant hyperthermia.
• Administer analgesics, if appropriate. Patient can feel pain but cannot indicate its presence.

☑ **PATIENT TEACHING**
• Explain the drug's purpose.
• Assure the patient that monitoring will be continuous.
• Explain all procedures and events; the drug does not interfere with the patient's ability to hear.

doxacurium chloride
Nuromax

Pregnancy Risk Category: C

HOW SUPPLIED
Injection: 1 mg/ml

ACTION
A nondepolarizing neuromuscular blocking agent that competes with acetylcholine for receptor sites at the motor end plate; because this action may be antagonized by cholinesterase inhibitors, doxacurium is considered a competitive antagonist.

ONSET, PEAK, DURATION
Onset occurs within 5 minutes. Peak effects are dose-dependent and occur within 3 to 9 minutes. Effects persist for 1 to 4 hours.

INDICATIONS & DOSAGE
To provide skeletal muscle relaxation during surgery as an adjunct to general anesthesia—
Dosage is highly individualized. All times of onset and duration are averages; considerable individual variation is normal.

Adults: 0.05 mg/kg rapid I.V. produces adequate conditions for endotracheal intubation in 5 minutes in about 90% of patients when used as part of a thiopental-narcotic induction technique. Lower doses may require longer delay before intubation is possible. Neuromuscular blockade at this dose lasts for an average of 100 minutes.
Children over 2 years: an initial dose of 0.03 mg/kg I.V. given during halothane anesthesia produces effective blockade in 7 minutes with duration of 30 minutes. Under the same conditions, 0.05 mg/kg produces blockade in 4 minutes with duration of 45 minutes.
Maintenance of neuromuscular blockade during long procedures—
Adults: after initial dose of 0.05 mg/kg I.V., maintenance doses of 0.005 to 0.01 mg/kg will prolong neuromuscular blockade for an average of 30 to 45 minutes.

ADVERSE REACTIONS
Respiratory: dyspnea, respiratory depression, *respiratory insufficiency or apnea.*
Other: prolonged muscle weakness.

INTERACTIONS
Alkaline solutions: physically incompatible; precipitate may form. Do not administer through same I.V. line.
Aminoglycosides (gentamicin, kanamycin, neomycin, and streptomycin), bacitracin, colistimethate, colistin, polymyxin B, tetracyclines: potentiated neuromuscular blockade leading to increased skeletal muscle relaxation and prolonged effect. Use together cautiously.
Carbamazepine, phenytoin: may prolong the time to maximal block or shorten the duration of block with neuromuscular blockers.
Inhalation anesthetics, quinidine: may enhance or prolong action of nondepolarizing neuromuscular blockers.
Magnesium salts: may enhance neuromuscular blockade. Monitor for excessive weakness.

Reactions may be *common*, uncommon, *life-threatening*, or COMMON AND LIFE-THREATENING.

EFFECTS ON DIAGNOSTIC TESTS
No information available.

CONTRAINDICATIONS
Contraindicated in patients with hypersensitivity to the drug and in neonates. The drug contains benzyl alcohol, which has been associated with fatalities in newborns.

NURSING CONSIDERATIONS
● Use cautiously, possibly at reduced dosage, in debilitated patients; in patients with metastatic cancer, severe electrolyte disturbances, or neuromuscular diseases; and in those in whom potentiation or difficulty in reversal of neuromuscular blockade is anticipated. Patients with myasthenia gravis or myasthenic syndrome (Eaton-Lambert syndrome) are particularly sensitive to the effects of nondepolarizing relaxants. Shorter-acting agents are recommended for use in such patients.
● Because of the lack of data supporting the drug's safety, be aware that it is not recommended for use in patients requiring prolonged mechanical ventilation in the intensive care unit, before or after administration of nondepolarizing neuromuscular blocking agents, or during cesarean section.
● Use drug only under direct medical supervision by personnel skilled in the use of neuromuscular blockers and techniques for maintaining a patent airway. Do not use unless facilities and equipment for mechanical ventilation, oxygen therapy, and intubation and an antagonist are within reach.
● To avoid distress to the patient, do not give the drug until the patient's consciousness is obtunded by general anesthetic. Doxacurium has no effect on consciousness or pain threshold.
● Drug is not metabolized; it is excreted in urine and bile. Patients with renal or hepatic insufficiency may require dosage adjustment.
● Keep in mind that the dosage should be adjusted to ideal body weight in obese patients (patients 30% or more above their ideal weight) to avoid prolonged neuromuscular blockade.
● Know that higher initial doses may be required in patients with severe burns and in some patients with severe liver disease. Higher doses (0.8 mg/kg) will produce intubating conditions more rapidly (4 minutes), with neuromuscular blockade for 160 minutes or more. Consequently, these higher doses should be reserved for long procedures. Administration during steady-state anesthesia with enflurane, halothane, or isoflurane may allow 33% reduction of dose.
● **I.V. use:** Prepare drug for I.V. use with D_5W, 0.9% sodium chloride for injection, dextrose 5% in 0.9% sodium chloride for injection, lactated Ringer's injection, and dextrose 5% in lactated Ringer's injection.
● When diluted as directed, remember that doxacurium is compatible with alfentanil, fentanyl, and sufentanil.
● Recommend that the product be administered immediately after reconstitution. Diluted solutions are stable for 24 hours at room temperature; however, because reconstitution dilutes the preservative, risk of contamination increases. Unused solutions should be discarded after 8 hours.
● Be aware that a nerve stimulator and train-of-four monitoring are recommended to document antagonism of neuromuscular blockade and recovery of muscle strength. Before attempting pharmacologic reversal with neostigmine, some evidence of spontaneous recovery should be present.
● Because the drug has minimal vagolytic action, monitor for bradycardia, which may occur during anesthesia.
● Monitor respirations until the patient is fully recovered from neuromuscular blockade, as evidenced by tests of muscle strength (hand grip, head lift, and ability to cough).
● Know that experimental evidence sug-

gests that acid-base and electrolyte balance may influence the actions of nondepolarizing neuromuscular blockers. Alkalosis may counteract paralysis; acidosis may enhance it.

☑ **PATIENT TEACHING**
● Inform the patient of need for drug.
● Reassure the patient and family that he'll be monitored at all times.

---

metocurine iodide
Metubine Iodide

Pregnancy Risk Category: C

HOW SUPPLIED
Injection: 2 mg/ml

ACTION
Prevents acetylcholine from binding to receptors on the muscle end plate, thus blocking depolarization.

ONSET, PEAK, DURATION
Onset occurs in 1 to 4 minutes. Peak effects occur in 3 to 5 minutes. Effects persist for 35 to 60 minutes; may take more than 6 hours for more than 50% of muscle twitch strength to return.

INDICATIONS & DOSAGE
Adjunct to anesthesia to induce skeletal muscle relaxation; to facilitate intubation—
Adults: 0.2 to 0.4 mg/kg for endotracheal intubation; supplemented with 0.5 to 1 mg for further relaxation.
To lessen muscle contractions in pharmacologically or electrically induced seizures—
Adults: 1.75 to 5.5 mg I.V.

ADVERSE REACTIONS
CV: hypotension secondary to histamine release, ganglionic blockade and histamine release, arrhythmias, *cardiac arrest*, bradycardia.
Respiratory: *dose-related prolonged apnea, bronchospasm.*

Other: residual muscle weakness, increased oropharyngeal secretions, allergic or idiosyncratic hypersensitivity reactions.

INTERACTIONS
Alkaline solutions, such as barbiturates, meperidine, or morphine: instability when combined in same syringe. Do not administer in same syringe.
Aminoglycoside antibiotics (including amikacin, gentamicin, kanamycin, neomycin, streptomycin); polymyxin antibiotics (polymyxin B sulfate, colistin); clindamycin; quinidine; general anesthetics (such as halothane, enflurane, isoflurane); furosemide; thiazide diuretics; beta-adrenergic blockers: potentiated neuromuscular blockade, leading to increased skeletal muscle relaxation and possible respiratory paralysis. Use cautiously during and after surgery.
Opioid analgesics: potentiated neuromuscular blockade, leading to increased skeletal muscle relaxation and possible respiratory paralysis. Use with extreme caution, and reduce dose of metocurine iodide.

EFFECTS ON DIAGNOSTIC TESTS
None reported.

CONTRAINDICATIONS
Contraindicated in patients with hypersensitivity to iodides or in whom histamine release is a hazard (asthmatic or atopic patients).

NURSING CONSIDERATIONS
● Use cautiously in elderly or debilitated patients. Also use cautiously in patients with cardiac, renal, hepatic, or pulmonary impairment; respiratory depression; myasthenia gravis; myasthenic syndrome of lung cancer or bronchogenic cancer; dehydration; thyroid disorders; collagen diseases; porphyria; electrolyte disturbances; hyperthermia; hypotension; or shock. Also use large doses cautiously in patients undergoing cesarean section.

Reactions may be *common*, uncommon, *life-threatening*, or COMMON AND LIFE-THREATENING.

• Know that metocurine should only be used by personnel skilled in airway management.

• Administer sedatives or general anesthetics before neuromuscular blockers, as ordered. Neuromuscular blockers do not obtund consciousness or alter pain threshold.

• Keep airway clear. Have emergency respiratory support equipment (endotracheal equipment, ventilator, oxygen, atropine, edrophonium, epinephrine, and neostigmine) available.

• **I.V. use:** Give by direct I.V. injection over 30 to 60 seconds. Dosage depends on anesthetic used, individual needs, and response. Dosages given are representative and must be adjusted. Administer as sustained injection over 30 to 60 seconds. Adults given cyclopropane, 2 to 4 mg I.V. (2.68 mg average); ether, 1.5 to 3 mg I.V. (2.1 mg average); nitrous oxide, 4 to 7 mg I.V. (4.79 mg average) with supplemental injections of 0.5 to 1 mg in 25 to 90 minutes, repeated p.r.n.

• Do not administer I.M.

• Store solution away from heat and sunlight. Do not mix with barbiturates (precipitate will form). Use fresh solutions only.

• Know that a nerve stimulator and train-of-four monitoring are recommended to document antagonism of neuromuscular blockade and recovery of muscle strength. Before attempting pharmacologic reversal with neostigmine, some evidence of spontaneous recovery should be seen.

• Monitor baseline electrolyte determinations (electrolyte imbalance, especially potassium, calcium, and magnesium levels as ordered, can potentiate neuromuscular effects) and vital signs, especially respirations.

• Monitor respirations closely until patient is fully recovered from neuromuscular blockade, as evidenced by tests of muscle strength (hand grip, head lift, and ability to cough).

• Measure fluid intake and output; renal dysfunction prolongs duration of action because drug is mainly unchanged before excretion.

• Give analgesics, as ordered, for pain.

☑ **PATIENT TEACHING**
• Explain all events and procedures to the patient because he can still hear.

mivacurium chloride
Mivacron

Pregnancy Risk Category: C

HOW SUPPLIED
Injection: 2 mg/ml in 5-ml and 10-ml vials
Infusion: 0.5 mg/ml in 50 ml of D_5W

ACTION
Competes with acetylcholine for receptor sites at the motor end plate. Because this action may be antagonized by cholinesterase inhibitors, mivacurium is considered a competitive antagonist.
The drug is a mixture of three stereoisomers, each possessing neuromuscular blocking activity.

ONSET, PEAK, DURATION
Onset occurs within 1 to 2 minutes. Peak effects occur in 2 to 5 minutes. 95% muscle twitch strength recovery within 20 to 35 minutes.

INDICATIONS & DOSAGE
Adjunct to general anesthesia, to facilitate endotracheal intubation, and to relax skeletal muscles during surgery or mechanical ventilation—
Adults: dosage is highly individualized. Usually, 0.15 mg/kg I.V. push over 5 to 15 seconds provides adequate muscle relaxation within 2½ minutes for endotracheal intubation. Supplemental doses of 0.1 mg/kg I.V. q 15 minutes are usually sufficient to maintain muscle relaxation.

Alternatively, maintain neuromuscular blockade with a continuous infusion of 4 mcg/kg/minute begun simultaneously with the initial dose, or 9 to 10 mcg/kg/minute started after spontaneous recovery caused by the initial dose is evident. When used with isoflurane or enflurane anesthesia, dosage usually is reduced up to 40%.

Children 2 to 12 years: 0.20 mg/kg I.V. push administered over 5 to 15 seconds. Neuromuscular blockade is usually evident in less than 2 minutes. Maintenance doses are generally required more frequently in children.

Alternatively, neuromuscular blockade can be maintained with a continuous I.V. infusion titrated to effect. Most children respond to 5 to 31 mcg/kg/minute (average 14 mcg/kg/minute).

ADVERSE REACTIONS
CNS: dizziness.
CV: *flushing,* tachycardia, bradycardia, arrhythmias, hypotension.
Respiratory: *bronchospasm,* wheezing, ***respiratory insufficiency or apnea.***
Skin: rash, urticaria, erythema.
Other: prolonged muscle weakness, phlebitis, muscle spasms.

INTERACTIONS
Alkaline solutions (such as barbiturate solutions): physically incompatible; precipitate may form. Do not administer through the same I.V. line.
Aminoglycosides (gentamicin, kanamycin, neomycin, and streptomycin), bacitracin, colistin, colistimethate, polymyxin B sulfate, tetracyclines: potentiated neuromuscular blockade, leading to increased skeletal muscle relaxation and prolonged effect. Use together cautiously.
Carbamazepine, phenytoin: may prolong the time to maximal blockade or shorten the duration of blockade with neuromuscular blockers.
Inhalation anesthetics (especially isoflurane or enflurane), quinidine: may enhance or prolong action of nondepolarizing neuromuscular blockers. Monitor for excessive weakness.

Magnesium salts: may enhance neuromuscular blockade. Monitor for excessive weakness.

EFFECTS ON DIAGNOSTIC TESTS
None reported.

CONTRAINDICATIONS
Contraindicated in patients with hypersensitivity to the drug.

NURSING CONSIDERATIONS
● Use cautiously in patients with significant CV disease and in patients who may be adversely affected by release of histamine (such as asthmatic patients). To avoid hypotension, initial dose of the drug should be lower or drug should be given over longer period (60 seconds).
● Also use cautiously, possibly at reduced dosage, in debilitated patients; in patients with metastatic cancer, severe electrolyte disturbances, or neuromuscular diseases; and in those in whom potentiation or difficulty in reversal of neuromuscular blockade is anticipated. Patients with myasthenia gravis or myasthenic syndrome (Eaton-Lambert syndrome) are particularly sensitive to effects of nondepolarizing relaxants. Test dose of 0.015 to 0.02 mg/kg may be used to assess the patient's sensitivity to the drug.
Alert: Use very cautiously, if at all, in patients who are homozygous for the atypical plasma pseudocholinesterase gene. Drug is metabolized to inactive compound by plasma pseudocholinesterase.
● Use only under direct medical supervision by personnel skilled in the use of neuromuscular blockers and techniques for maintaining a patent airway. Do not use unless facilities and equipment for artificial respiration, mechanical ventilation, oxygen therapy, and intubation and an antagonist are within reach.
● To avoid patient distress, do not administer until the patient's consciousness is obtunded by the general anesthetic because drug has no effect on

consciousness or pain threshold.

• Administer a test dose to assess the patient's sensitivity to the drug. Patients with severe burns are known to develop resistance to nondepolarizing neuromuscular blockers; however, they also may have reduced plasma pseudocholinesterase activity.

• Keep in mind that dosage should be adjusted to ideal body weight in obese patients (patients 30% or more above their ideal weight) to avoid prolonged neuromuscular blockade.

• Be aware that like other neuromuscular blockers, dosage requirements for children are higher on a mg/kg basis than those for adults. Onset and recovery of neuromuscular blockade occur more rapidly in children.

• **I.V. use:** Prepare drug for I.V. use with D_5W, 0.9% sodium chloride for injection, dextrose 5% in 0.9% sodium chloride for injection, lactated Ringer's injection, and dextrose 5% in lactated Ringer's injection. Diluted solutions are stable for 24 hours at room temperature.

• Remember that when diluted as directed, mivacurium is compatible with alfentanil, fentanyl, sufentanil, droperidol, and midazolam.

• For drug available as premixed infusion in D_5W, remove the protective outer wrap, then check container for minor leaks by squeezing the bag before administering. Do not add any other drugs to the container, and do not use the container in series connections.

• A nerve stimulator and train-of-four monitoring are recommended to document antagonism of neuromuscular blockade and recovery of muscle strength. Before attempting pharmacologic reversal with neostigmine or edrophonium, some signs of spontaneous recovery should be evident.

• Monitor respirations closely until patient is fully recovered from neuromuscular blockade, as evidenced by tests of muscle strength (hand grip, head lift, and ability to cough).

• Know that experimental evidence suggests that acid-base and electrolyte balances may influence the actions of nondepolarizing neuromuscular blockers. Alkalosis may counteract the paralysis; acidosis may enhance it.

• Know that duration of drug effect is increased about 150% in patients with end-stage renal disease and 300% in patients with hepatic dysfunction.

☑ **PATIENT TEACHING**
• Explain the drug's purpose.
• Reassure the patient and family that he'll be monitored at all times.

---

pancuronium bromide
Pavulon

Pregnancy Risk Category: C

HOW SUPPLIED
Injection: 1 mg/ml, 2 mg/ml

ACTION
Prevents acetylcholine from binding to receptors on the muscle end plate, thus blocking depolarization.

ONSET, PEAK, DURATION
Onset occurs in 30 to 45 seconds. Peak effects occur in 3 to $4\frac{1}{2}$ minutes. Effects persist for 35 to 45 minutes; 90% of muscle twitch strength returns within 1 hour.

INDICATIONS & DOSAGE
Adjunct to anesthesia to induce skeletal muscle relaxation; to facilitate intubation; to lessen muscle contractions in pharmacologically or electrically induced seizures; to assist with mechanical ventilation—
Dosage depends on anesthetic used, individual needs, and response. Dosages are representative only.
Adults and children 1 month and over: initially, 0.04 to 0.1 mg/kg I.V.; then 0.01 mg/kg q 30 to 60 minutes.
Neonates: individualized.

ADVERSE REACTIONS
CV: tachycardia, increased blood pressure.
Respiratory: *prolonged, dose-related respiratory insufficiency or apnea.*
Skin: transient rashes.
Other: excessive salivation, residual muscle weakness, allergic or idiosyncratic hypersensitivity reactions.

INTERACTIONS
Aminoglycoside antibiotics (including amikacin, gentamicin, kanamycin, neomycin, streptomycin); polymyxin antibiotics (polymyxin B sulfate, colistin); clindamycin; lincomycin; quinidine; general anesthetics (such as halothane, enflurane, isoflurane): potentiated neuromuscular blockade, leading to increased skeletal muscle relaxation and prolonged effect. Use cautiously during surgical and postoperative periods.
Lithium, opioid analgesics: potentiated neuromuscular blockade, leading to increased skeletal muscle relaxation and possible respiratory paralysis. Use with extreme caution, and reduce dose of pancuronium.
Succinylcholine: increased intensity and duration of neuromuscular blockade. Allow effects of succinylcholine to subside before administering pancuronium.

EFFECTS ON DIAGNOSTIC TESTS
None significant.

CONTRAINDICATIONS
Contraindicated in patients with hypersensitivity to bromides or preexisting tachycardia and in patients for whom even a minor increase in heart rate is undesirable.

NURSING CONSIDERATIONS
● Use cautiously in elderly or debilitated patients; in patients with renal, hepatic, or pulmonary impairment; and in those with respiratory depression, myasthenia gravis, myasthenic syndrome of lung cancer or bronchogenic carcinoma, dehydration, thyroid disorders, collagen diseases, porphyria, electrolyte disturbances, hyperthermia, and toxemic states. Also use large doses cautiously in patients undergoing cesarean section.
● Administer sedatives or general anesthetics before neuromuscular blockers, as ordered. Neuromuscular blockers do not obtund consciousness or alter the pain threshold.
● Know that pancuronium should be used only by personnel skilled in airway management.
● Have emergency respiratory support equipment (endotracheal equipment, ventilator, oxygen, atropine, edrophonium, epinephrine, and neostigmine) immediately available.
● **I.V. use:** Do not mix with alkaline solutions, such as barbiturate solutions, because precipitate will form; use only fresh solutions.
● Allow succinylcholine effects to subside before giving pancuronium.
● Store in refrigerator. Do not store in plastic containers or syringes, although plastic syringes may be used for administration.
● Monitor baseline electrolyte determinations (electrolyte imbalance can potentiate neuromuscular effects) and vital signs, especially respirations and heart rate.
● Measure fluid intake and output; renal dysfunction may prolong duration of action because 25% of the drug is unchanged before excretion.
● Keep in mind that a nerve stimulator and train-of-four monitoring are recommended to confirm antagonism of neuromuscular blockade and recovery of muscle strength. Before attempting pharmacologic reversal with neostigmine, some evidence of spontaneous recovery should be seen.
● Monitor respirations closely until patient is fully recovered from neuromuscular blockade, as evidenced by tests of muscle strength (hand grip, head lift, and ability to cough).
● Once spontaneous recovery starts, pancuronium-induced neuromuscular

blockade may be reversed with an anti-cholinesterase agent (such as neostigmine or edrophonium), which is usually administered with an anticholinergic (such as atropine).
● Know that drug does not cause histamine release or hypotension but may raise heart rate and blood pressure.
● Give analgesics, as ordered, for pain.

☑ **PATIENT TEACHING**
● Explain all events and procedures to the patient because he can still hear.

---

pipecuronium bromide
Arduan

Pregnancy Risk Category: C

HOW SUPPLIED
Powder for injection: 10-mg vial

ACTION
A nondepolarizing neuromuscular blocking agent that competes with acetylcholine for receptor sites at the motor end plate. Because this action may be antagonized by cholinesterase inhibitors, pipecuronium is considered a competitive antagonist.

ONSET, PEAK, DURATION
Onset occurs in 1 to 2 minutes. Peak effects occur within 5 minutes; 25% to 50% of muscle twitch strength returns within 24 minutes.

INDICATIONS & DOSAGE
To provide skeletal muscle relaxation during surgery as adjunct to general anesthesia—
Dosage is highly individualized. The following doses may serve as a guide for use in nonobese patients with normal renal function.
Adults and children: initially, 70 to 85 mcg/kg I.V. provides conditions considered ideal for endotracheal intubation and maintains paralysis for 1 to 2 hours. If succinylcholine is used for endotra-

cheal intubation, initial dose of 50 mcg/kg I.V. provides good relaxation for 45 minutes or more. Maintenance dose of 10 to 15 mcg/kg provides relaxation for about 50 minutes.

ADVERSE REACTIONS
CV: *hypotension,* bradycardia, hypertension, myocardial ischemia, *CVA,* thrombosis, atrial fibrillation, *ventricular extrasystole.*
GU: anuria.
Respiratory: dyspnea, respiratory depression, *respiratory insufficiency or apnea.*
Skin: rash, urticaria.
Other: prolonged muscle weakness, increased creatinine levels.

INTERACTIONS
Aminoglycosides (gentamicin, kanamycin, neomycin, and streptomycin), bacitracin, colistimethate, colistin, polymyxin B sulfate, tetracyclines: potentiated neuromuscular blockade, leading to increased skeletal muscle relaxation and prolonged effect. Use together cautiously.
Inhalation anesthetics, quinidine: enhances or prolongs action of nondepolarizing neuromuscular blockers.
Magnesium salts: may enhance neuromuscular blockade. Monitor for excessive weakness.

EFFECTS ON DIAGNOSTIC TESTS
None reported.

CONTRAINDICATIONS
Contraindicated in patients with hypersensitivity to the drug.

NURSING CONSIDERATIONS
● Use cautiously and with dosage adjustments in patients with renal failure because the drug is excreted by the kidneys. No information is available regarding use of the drug in patients with hepatic disease.
● Because of the lack of data supporting the drug's safety, know that it is not rec-

---

ommended for use in patients requiring prolonged mechanical ventilation in the intensive care unit, before or after administration of other nondepolarizing neuromuscular blockers, or during cesarean section.

• Be aware that patients with myasthenia gravis or myasthenic syndrome (Eaton-Lambert syndrome) are particularly sensitive to the effects of nondepolarizing relaxants. Shorter-acting agents are recommended.

• Keep in mind that the drug is not recommended for use in neonates and infants younger than 3 months. Limited evidence suggests that infants and children (ages 1 to 14) under balanced anesthesia or halothane anesthesia may be less sensitive than adults.

• Know that dosage should be adjusted to ideal body weight in obese patients (30% or more over their ideal weight) to avoid prolonged neuromuscular blockade.

• Use drug under direct medical supervision by personnel skilled in use of neuromuscular blockers and techniques for maintaining a patent airway. Do not use drug unless facilities and equipment for artificial respiration, mechanical ventilation, oxygen therapy, and intubation and an antagonist are within reach. *Alert:* Because of its prolonged duration of action, keep in mind that pipecuronium is recommended only for procedures that take 90 minutes or longer.

• Administer pipecuronium after succinylcholine when the latter is used to facilitate intubation.

• Give patients sedatives or general anesthetics before neuromuscular blockers are administered, as ordered. Neuromuscular blockers do not obtund consciousness or alter pain threshold.

• **I.V. use:** Reconstitute with 10 ml solution before use to yield a solution of 1 mg/ml. Using a large volume of diluent or adding the drug to a hanging I.V. solution is not recommended.

• After reconstitution with sterile water for injection or other compatible I.V. so-

lutions (such as 0.9% sodium chloride for injection, D_5W, lactated Ringer's injection, dextrose 5% in 0.9% sodium chloride for injection), drug is stable for 24 hours if refrigerated.

• After reconstitution with any solution other than bacteriostatic water for injection, discard unused drug.

• Know that after reconstitution with bacteriostatic water for injection, drug is stable for 5 days at room temperature or in the refrigerator. Bacteriostatic water contains benzyl alcohol and is not intended for use in neonates.

• Store powder at room temperature or in refrigerator (36° to 86° F [2° to 30° C]).

• Monitor respirations closely until patient is fully recovered from neuromuscular blockade, as evidenced by tests of muscle strength (hand grip, head lift, and ability to cough).

• Monitor for bradycardia during anesthesia.

• Know that a nerve stimulator and train-of-four monitoring are recommended to document antagonism of neuromuscular blockade and recovery of muscle strength. Before attempting pharmacologic reversal with neostigmine, some evidence of spontaneous recovery should be present.

• Be aware that experimental evidence suggests that acid-base and electrolyte balances may influence the actions of nondepolarizing neuromuscular blockers. Alkalosis may counteract the paralysis, and acidosis may enhance it.

☑ **PATIENT TEACHING**
• Explain the drug's purpose.
• Reassure the patient and family that he'll be monitored at all times.

rocuronium bromide
Zemuron

Pregnancy Risk Category: B

HOW SUPPLIED
Injection: 10 mg/ml

ACTION
Prevents acetylcholine from binding to receptors on the muscle end plate, thus blocking depolarization.

ONSET, PEAK, DURATION
Onset occurs within 1 minute. Peak effects occur within 2 minutes in most patients. Duration is dose-dependent; 25% recovery of muscle twitch strength occurs within 22 to 67 minutes.

INDICATIONS & DOSAGE
Adjunct to general anesthesia to facilitate endotracheal intubation and to provide skeletal muscle relaxation during surgery or mechanical ventilation— Dosage depends on anesthetic used, individual needs, and response. Dosages are representative and must be adjusted. **Adults:** initially, 0.6 mg/kg I.V. bolus. In most patients, tracheal intubation may be performed within 2 minutes; muscle paralysis should last about 22 minutes. A maintenance dosage of 0.1 mg/kg should provide an additional 12 minutes of muscle relaxation; 0.15 mg/kg will add 17 minutes; or 0.2 mg/kg will add 24 minutes to the duration of effect.

ADVERSE REACTIONS
CV: tachycardia, abnormal ECG, arrhythmias (rare), transient hypotension and hypertension.
GI: nausea, vomiting.
Respiratory: asthma.
Skin: rash, edema, pruritus.
Other: hiccups.

INTERACTIONS
Aminoglycoside antibiotics (including amikacin, gentamicin, kanamycin, neomycin, streptomycin); polymyxin antibiotics (polymyxin B sulfate, colistin); anticonvulsants; clindamycin; tetracyclines; quinidine; general anesthetics (such as halothane, enflurane, isoflu-rane); opiate analgesics; succinyl-choline: potentiated neuromuscular blockade, leading to increased skeletal muscle relaxation and potentiated effect. Use cautiously during surgical and postoperative periods.

EFFECTS ON DIAGNOSTIC TESTS
None known.

CONTRAINDICATIONS
Contraindicated in patients with hypersensitivity to bromides.

NURSING CONSIDERATIONS
● Use cautiously in patients with altered circulation time caused by CV disease, old age, and edematous states; hepatic disease; severe obesity; bronchogenic carcinoma; electrolyte disturbances; and neuromuscular disease.
● Administer sedatives or general anesthetics before neuromuscular blockers, as ordered. Neuromuscular blockers do not obtund consciousness or alter the pain threshold.
● Drug is not recommended for use during rapid sequence induction for cesarean section.
● Know that rocuronium should be used only by personnel skilled in airway management.
● Keep airway clear. Have emergency respiratory support equipment (endotracheal equipment, ventilator, oxygen, atropine, edrophonium, epinephrine, and neostigmine) available.
● **I.V. use:** Administer by rapid I.V. injection. Alternatively, give by continuous I.V. infusion. Infusion rates are highly individualized but have ranged from 0.004 to 0.16 mg/kg/minute. Compatible solutions include D_5W, 0.9% sodium chloride for injection, dextrose 5% in 0.9% sodium chloride for injection, sterile water for injection, and lactated Ringer's injection.
● Store reconstituted solution in refrig-

erator. Discard after 24 hours.
● Be alert that rocuronium provides conditions for intubation within 3 minutes. Effects last 25 to 40 minutes.
● Know that a nerve stimulator and train-of-four monitoring are recommended to confirm antagonism of neuromuscular blockade and recovery of muscle strength. Before attempting pharmacologic reversal with neostigmine, some evidence of spontaneous recovery should be present.
● Keep in mind that prior administration of succinylcholine may enhance neuromuscular blocking effect and duration of action.
● Monitor patients with liver disease because they may require higher doses of the drug to achieve adequate muscle relaxation. However, such patients exhibit prolonged effects from the drug.
● Monitor respirations closely until patient is fully recovered from neuromuscular blockade, as evidenced by tests of muscle strength (hand grip, head lift, and ability to cough).
● Know that rocuronium is well tolerated in patients with renal failure.
● Give analgesics, as ordered, for pain.

☑ **PATIENT TEACHING**
● Explain all events and procedures to the patient because he can still hear.

---

succinylcholine chloride (suxamethonium chloride)
Anectine, Anectine Flo-Pack, Quelicin, Scoline‡, Sucostrin

Pregnancy Risk Category: C

HOW SUPPLIED
Injection: 20 mg/ml, 50 mg/ml, 100 mg/ml; 100-mg vial, 500-mg vial, 1-g vial

ACTION
Prolongs depolarization of the muscle end plate.

ONSET, PEAK, DURATION
Onset occurs in 30 seconds to 1 minute after I.V. use; 2 to 3 minutes after I.M. use. Peak effects occur in 1 to 2 minutes after I.V. use. Effects persist for 4 to 10 minutes after I.V. use, 10 to 30 minutes after I.M. use.

INDICATIONS & DOSAGE
Adjunct to anesthesia to induce skeletal muscle relaxation; to facilitate intubation and assist with mechanical ventilation; to lessen muscle contractions in pharmacologically or electrically induced seizures—
Dosage depends on anesthetic used, individual needs, and response. Dosages are representative only.
Adults: 25 to 75 mg I.V., then 2.5 mg/minute p.r.n., or 2.5 mg/kg I.M. up to maximum of 150 mg I.M. in deltoid muscle.
Children: 1 to 2 mg/kg I.M. or I.V. Maximum I.M. dosage is 150 mg. (Children may be less sensitive to succinylcholine than adults.)

ADVERSE REACTIONS
CV: bradycardia, tachycardia, hypertension, hypotension, *arrhythmias,* flushing, *cardiac arrest.*
EENT: increased intraocular pressure.
Respiratory: *prolonged respiratory depression, apnea,* bronchrestriction.
Other: *malignant hyperthermia,* muscle fasciculation, *postoperative muscle pain,* myoglobinemia, allergic or idiosyncratic hypersensitivity reactions *(anaphylaxis).*

INTERACTIONS
Aminoglycoside antibiotics (including amikacin, gentamicin, kanamycin, neomycin, streptomycin); polymyxin antibiotics (polymyxin B sulfate, colistin); cholinesterase inhibitors (such as neostigmine, pyridostigmine, edrophonium, physostigmine, or echothiophate); general anesthetics (such as halothane, enflurane, isoflurane): potentiated neuromuscular blockade, leading to increased

---

skeletal muscle relaxation and potentiated effect. Use cautiously during and after surgery.

Cyclophosphamide, lithium, MAO inhibitors: prolonged apnea. Use with caution.

Digitalis glycosides: may cause arrhythmias. Use together cautiously.

Methotrimeprazine, opioid analgesics: potentiated neuromuscular blockade, leading to increased skeletal muscle relaxation and possible respiratory paralysis. Use with extreme caution.

Parenteral magnesium sulfate: potentiated neuromuscular blockade, increased skeletal muscle relaxation, and possible respiratory paralysis. Use with caution, preferably with reduced doses.

EFFECTS ON DIAGNOSTIC TESTS
Use of succinylcholine may increase serum potassium concentrations.

CONTRAINDICATIONS
Contraindicated in patients with hypersensitivity to the drug and in patients with abnormally low plasma pseudocholinesterase, angle-closure glaucoma, malignant hyperthermia, or penetrating eye injuries.

NURSING CONSIDERATIONS
● Use cautiously in elderly or debilitated patients; in patients receiving quinidine or digitalis glycoside therapy; in patients with hepatic, renal, or pulmonary impairment; in those with respiratory depression, severe burns or trauma, electrolyte imbalances, hyperkalemia, paraplegia, spinal neuraxis injury, CVA, degenerative or dystrophic neuromuscular disease, myasthenia gravis, myasthenic syndrome of lung cancer or bronchogenic carcinoma, dehydration, thyroid disorders, collagen diseases, porphyria, fractures, muscle spasms, eye surgery, and pheochromocytoma. Also use large doses cautiously in patients undergoing cesarean section.
● Know that succinylcholine is the drug of choice for short procedures (less than 3 minutes) and for orthopedic manipulations; use caution in fractures or dislocations.
● Administer sedatives or general anesthetics before neuromuscular blockers, which do not obtund consciousness or alter the pain threshold.
● Be aware that succinylcholine should be used only by personnel skilled in airway management.
● Keep airway clear. Have emergency respiratory support equipment (endotracheal equipment, ventilator, oxygen, atropine, and epinephrine) immediately available.
● **I.V. use:** Give test dose (5 to 10 mg I.V.) after patient has been anesthetized. Normal response (no respiratory depression or transient depression for up to 5 minutes) indicates drug may be given. Do not give if patient develops respiratory paralysis sufficient to permit endotracheal intubation. (Recovery within 30 to 60 minutes.)
● When giving drug I.M., inject deeply, preferably high into deltoid muscle.
● Store injectable form in refrigerator. Store powder form at room temperature in tightly closed container. Use immediately after reconstitution. Do not mix with alkaline solutions (thiopental sodium, sodium bicarbonate, or barbiturates).
● Monitor baseline electrolyte determinations and vital signs (check respirations every 5 to 10 minutes during infusion).
● Monitor respirations closely until patient is fully recovered from neuromuscular blockade, as evidenced by tests of muscle strength (hand grip, head lift, and ability to cough).
Alert: Don't use reversing agents. Unlike nondepolarizing agents, neostigmine or edrophonium may worsen neuromuscular blockade.
● Know that repeated or continuous infusions of succinylcholine are not advisable; they may cause reduced response or prolonged muscle relaxation and apnea.
● Give analgesics, as ordered, for pain.

☑ **PATIENT TEACHING**
● Explain all events and procedures to the patient because he can still hear.
● Reassure the patient that postoperative stiffness is normal and will soon subside.

---

tubocurarine chloride
Tubarine†

Pregnancy Risk Category: C

HOW SUPPLIED
Injection: 3 mg (20 units)/ml; 10 mg/ml‡

ACTION
A nondepolarizing neuromuscular blocking agent that prevents acetylcholine from binding to receptors on the muscle end plate, thus blocking depolarization.

ONSET, PEAK, DURATION
Onset occurs within 1 minute. Peak effects occur in 2 to 5 minutes. Effects persist for 20 to 40 minutes; 50% recovery of muscle twitch strength within 50 minutes, 90% recovery within 75 to 90 minutes.

INDICATIONS & DOSAGE
Adjunct to anesthesia to induce skeletal muscle relaxation; to facilitate intubation, orthopedic manipulations—
Dosage depends on anesthetic used, individual needs, and response. Dosages listed are representative and must be adjusted.
Adults: 1.1 unit/kg or 0.165 mg/kg I.V. slowly over 60 to 90 seconds. Average dose is initially 40 to 60 units I.V. May give 20 to 30 units in 3 to 5 minutes. For longer procedures, give 20 units p.r.n.
To assist with mechanical ventilation—
Adults and children: initially, 0.0165 mg/kg I.V. (average: 1 mg or 7 units); then adjust subsequent doses to patient response.
To lessen muscle contractions in phar-

macologically or electrically induced seizures—
Adults and children: 1.1 unit/kg or 0.165 mg/kg over 60 to 90 seconds. Initial dose is 20 units (3 mg) less than calculated dose.
Diagnosis of myasthenia gravis—
Adults: 4 to 33 mcg/kg as a single I.V. dose.

ADVERSE REACTIONS
CV: hypotension, arrhythmias, *cardiac arrest,* bradycardia.
Respiratory: *respiratory depression or apnea, bronchospasm.*
Other: profound and prolonged muscle relaxation, hypersensitivity reactions, idiosyncrasy, residual muscle weakness, increased salivation.

INTERACTIONS
Aminoglycoside antibiotics (including amikacin, gentamicin, kanamycin, neomycin, streptomycin); polymyxin antibiotics (polymyxin B sulfate, colistin); general anesthetics (such as halothane, enflurane, isoflurane): potentiated neuromuscular blockade, leading to increased skeletal muscle relaxation and potentiated effect. Use cautiously during and after surgery.
Amphotericin B, ethacrynic acid, furosemide, methotrimeprazine, opioid analgesics, propranolol, thiazide diuretics: potentiated neuromuscular blockade, leading to increased skeletal muscle relaxation and possible respiratory paralysis. Use with extreme caution during surgical and postoperative periods.
Quinidine: prolonged neuromuscular blockade. Use together with caution. Monitor closely.

EFFECTS ON DIAGNOSTIC TESTS
None significant.

CONTRAINDICATIONS
Contraindicated in patients with hypersensitivity to the drug and in patients for whom histamine release is a hazard (asthmatic patients).

Reactions may be *common,* uncommon, *life-threatening,* or COMMON AND LIFE-THREATENING.

NURSING CONSIDERATIONS

● Use cautiously in elderly or debilitated patients and in those with hepatic or pulmonary impairment, hypothermia, respiratory depression, myasthenia gravis, myasthenic syndrome of lung cancer or bronchogenic carcinoma, dehydration, thyroid disorders, collagen diseases, porphyria, electrolyte disturbances, fractures, and muscle spasms. Also use large doses cautiously in patients undergoing cesarean section.

● Keep airway clear. Have emergency respiratory support equipment (endotracheal equipment, ventilator, oxygen, atropine, edrophonium, epinephrine, and neostigmine) available.

● Know that only personnel skilled in airway management should administer tubocurarine.

● Allow succinylcholine effects to subside before giving tubocurarine.

● Administer sedatives or general anesthetics before neuromuscular blockers, which do not obtund consciousness or alter the pain threshold.

● Assess baseline electrolyte determinations (electrolyte imbalance can potentiate neuromuscular blocking effects).

● I.V. use: Give I.V. over 60 to 90 seconds.

● Do not mix with barbiturates (precipitate will form). Use only fresh solutions and discard if discolored.

● Check vital signs every 15 minutes. Notify the doctor at once of changes.

● Measure fluid intake and output; renal dysfunction prolongs duration of action because much of drug is unchanged before excretion.

● Know that a nerve stimulator and train-of-four monitoring are recommended to confirm antagonism of neuromuscular blockade and recovery of muscle strength. Before attempting pharmacologic reversal with neostigmine, some evidence of spontaneous recovery should be present.

● Monitor respirations closely until patient is fully recovered from neuromuscular blockade, as evidenced by tests of muscle strength (hand grip, head lift, and ability to cough).

● Give analgesics, as ordered, for pain.

☑ PATIENT TEACHING

● Explain all events and procedures to the patient because he still can hear.

---

vecuronium bromide
Norcuron

Pregnancy Risk Category: C

HOW SUPPLIED
Injection: 10- and 20-mg vials

ACTION
Prevents acetylcholine from binding to receptors on the muscle end plate, thus blocking depolarization.

ONSET, PEAK, DURATION
Onset occurs within 1 minute. Peak effects occur in 3 to 5 minutes. Effects persist for 25 to 30 minutes; 25% recovery of muscle twitch strength within 24 to 40 minutes, 95% recovery in 45 to 65 minutes.

INDICATIONS & DOSAGE
Adjunct to general anesthesia to facilitate endotracheal intubation and to provide skeletal muscle relaxation during surgery or mechanical ventilation—
Dosage depends on anesthetic used, individual needs, and response. Dosages are representative and must be adjusted. **Adults and children over 9 years:** initially, 0.08 to 0.1 mg/kg I.V. bolus. Maintenance doses of 0.01 to 0.015 mg/kg within 25 to 40 minutes of initial dose should be administered during prolonged surgical procedures. Maintenance doses may be given q 12 to 15 minutes in patients receiving balanced anesthesia.
Children under 9 years: may require a slightly higher initial dose and also may require supplementation slightly more often than adults. Alternatively, drug

---

may be given by continuous I.V. infusion of 1 mcg/kg/minute initially, then 0.8 to 1.2 mcg/kg/minute.

ADVERSE REACTIONS
Respiratory: *prolonged, dose-related respiratory insufficiency or apnea.*
Other: skeletal muscle weakness.

INTERACTIONS
Aminoglycoside antibiotics (including amikacin, gentamicin, kanamycin, neomycin, streptomycin); polymyxin antibiotics (polymyxin B sulfate, colistin); clindamycin; bacitracin; tetracyclines; quinidine; general anesthetics (such as halothane, enflurane, isoflurane); other skeletal muscle relaxants: potentiated neuromuscular blockade, leading to increased skeletal muscle relaxation and potentiated effect. Use cautiously during and after surgery.
Opioid analgesics: potentiated neuromuscular blockade, leading to increased skeletal muscle relaxation and possible respiratory paralysis. Use with extreme caution, and reduce dose of vecuronium.

EFFECTS ON DIAGNOSTIC TESTS
None significant.

CONTRAINDICATIONS
Contraindicated in patients with hypersensitivity to bromides.

NURSING CONSIDERATIONS
● Use cautiously in elderly patients; in patients with altered circulation caused by CV disease and edematous states; and in those with hepatic disease, severe obesity, bronchogenic carcinoma, electrolyte disturbances, and neuromuscular disease.
● Keep airway clear. Have emergency respiratory support equipment (endotracheal equipment, ventilator, oxygen, atropine, edrophonium, epinephrine, and neostigmine) available.
● Know that the drug should be used only by personnel skilled in airway management.

● Administer sedatives or general anesthetics before neuromuscular blockers, which do not obtund consciousness or alter the pain threshold.
● **I.V. use:** Administer by rapid I.V. injection. Alternatively, 10 to 20 mg may be added to 100 ml of a compatible solution and given by I.V. infusion. Compatible solutions include D_5W, 0.9% sodium chloride for injection, dextrose 5% in 0.9% sodium chloride for injection, and lactated Ringer's injection.
● Do not mix with alkaline solutions.
● Store reconstituted solution in refrigerator. Discard after 24 hours.
● Know that a nerve stimulator and train-of-four monitoring are recommended to confirm antagonism of neuromuscular blockade and recovery of muscle strength. Before attempting pharmacologic reversal with neostigmine, some evidence of spontaneous recovery should be seen.
● Monitor respirations closely until patient is fully recovered from neuromuscular blockade as evidenced by tests of muscle strength (hand grip, head lift, and ability to cough).
● Keep in mind that prior administration of succinylcholine may enhance the neuromuscular blocking effect and duration of action.
● Know that vecuronium is well tolerated in patients with renal failure.
● Give analgesics, as ordered, for pain.

☑ **PATIENT TEACHING**
● Explain all events and procedures to the patient because he can still hear.

43
Antihistamines

astemizole
azatadine maleate
azelastine hydrochloride
(See Chapter 86, NASAL DRUGS)
brompheniramine maleate
cetirizine hydrochloride
chlorpheniramine maleate
clemastine fumarate
cyproheptadine hydrochloride
dexchlorpheniramine maleate
diphenhydramine hydrochloride
fexofenadine hydrochloride
loratadine
promethazine hydrochloride
promethazine theoclate
triprolidine hydrochloride

COMBINATION PRODUCTS

ALLEREST MAXIMUM STRENGTH TABLETS ◊ : pseudoephedrine hydrochloride 30 mg and chlorpheniramine maleate 2 mg.

CHLOR-TRIMETON ALLERGY DECONGESTANT ◊ : chlorpheniramine maleate 4 mg and pseudoephedrine sulfate 60 mg.

CHLOR-TRIMETON DECONGESTANT REPETABS ◊ : chlorpheniramine maleate 8 mg and pseudoephedrine sulfate 120 mg.

CLARITIN-D: loratadine 5 mg and pseudoephedrine sulfate 120 mg.

CONDRIN-LA: phenylpropanolamine hydrochloride 75 mg and chlorpheniramine maleate 12 mg.

CONTACT CAPSULES ◊ : phenylpropanolamine 75 mg and chlorpheniramine maleate 8 mg.

CONTAC 12-HOUR CAPLETS ◊ : phenylpropanolamine 75 mg and chlorpheniramine maleate 8 mg.

CORICIDIN "D" TABLETS ◊ : chlorpheniramine maleate 2 mg, acetaminophen 325 mg, and phenylpropranolamine hydrochloride 12.5 mg.

DECONAMINE: pseudoephedrine hydrochloride 60 mg and chlorpheniramine maleate 4 mg.

DIMETAPP EXTENTABS: brompheniramine maleate 12 mg and phenylpropanolamine hydrochloride 75 mg.

DRIZE: phenylpropanolamine hydrochloride 75 mg and chlorpheniramine maleate 12 mg.

FEDAHIST: pseudoephedrine hydrochloride 60 mg and chlorpheniramine maleate 4 mg.

NALDECON: phenylephrine hydrochloride 10 mg, phenylpropanolamine hydrochloride 40 mg, phenyltoloxamine citrate 15 mg, and chlorpheniramine maleate 5 mg.

NOLAMINE: chlorpheniramine maleate 4 mg, phenindamine tartrate 24 mg, and phenylpropanolamine hydrochloride 50 mg.

NOVAFED A: pseudoephedrine hydrochloride 120 mg and chlorpheniramine maleate 8 mg.

NOVAHISTINE ELIXIR ◊ *: phenylephrine 5 mg, chlorpheniramine maleate 2 mg, and alcohol 5% per 5 ml.

ORNADE SPANSULES: phenylpropanolamine hydrochloride 75 mg and chlorpheniramine maleate 12 mg.

P-V-TUSSIN SYRUP*: chlorpheniramine maleate 2 mg/5 ml, phenindamine tartrate 5 mg/5 ml, phenylephrine hydrochloride 5 mg/ 5 ml, and pyrilamine maleate 6 mg/5 ml.

SUDAFED PLUS ◊ : pseudoephedrine hydrochloride 60 mg and chlorpheniramine maleate 4 mg.

TAVIST-D ◊ : clemastine fumarate 1.34 mg and phenylpropanolamine 75 mg.

TRIAMINIC-12: phenylpropanolamine hydrochloride 75 mg and chlorpheniramine maleate 12 mg.

TRINALIN REPETABS: azatadine maleate 1 mg and pseudoephedrine sulfate 120 mg.

---

*Liquid contains alcohol.   **May contain tartrazine.   †Canada only.   ‡Australia only.   ◊ OTC.

astemizole
Hismanal

Pregnancy Risk Category: C

HOW SUPPLIED
Tablets: 10 mg
Oral suspension: 2 mg/ml*‡

ACTION
Blocks effects of histamine at H_1 receptors. Astemizole is a nonsedating antihistamine; its chemical structure prevents entry into the CNS.

ONSET, PEAK, DURATION
Onset is slow although exact time is unknown. Serum levels peak within 1 hour. Effects last up to 24 hours.

INDICATIONS & DOSAGE
Relief of symptoms associated with chronic idiopathic urticaria and seasonal allergic rhinitis—
Adults and children over 12 years: 10 mg P.O. daily.

ADVERSE REACTIONS
CNS: headache, nervousness, dizziness, drowsiness.
CV: *arrhythmias* (with high plasma levels).
EENT: dry mouth, pharyngitis, conjunctivitis.
GI: abdominal pain, increased appetite, nausea, diarrhea.
Other: arthralgia, weight gain, cholestatic jaundice.

INTERACTIONS
Fluvoxamine: may alter astemizole's therapeutic effect. Monitor closely.
Itraconazole, ketoconazole, macrolide antibiotics (such as erythromycin): risk of serious adverse cardiac reactions. Don't use together.

EFFECTS ON DIAGNOSTIC TESTS
None reported.

CONTRAINDICATIONS
Contraindicated in patients with hepatic failure or hypersensitivity to astemizole and in patients taking the antifungal agents itraconazole or ketoconazole or macrolide antibiotics, including erythromycin.

NURSING CONSIDERATIONS
● Avoid use in patients with hepatic disease. Use cautiously in patients with renal disease. Also use cautiously in patients with lower respiratory tract diseases (including asthma); drying effects can increase the risk of bronchial mucus plug formation.
● See package insert for events causing serious CV adverse effects.

☑ PATIENT TEACHING
● Instruct patient to take astemizole only once a day. Warn patient not to increase dosage without consulting doctor. High doses may increase risk of arrhythmias.
● Instruct patient to take drug on an empty stomach at least 2 hours after a meal and to avoid eating for at least 1 hour after dosing.
● Warn patient to stop drug 4 to 6 weeks before allergy skin tests to preserve accuracy of tests.

azatadine maleate
Optimine, Zadine‡

Pregnancy Risk Category: B

HOW SUPPLIED
Tablets: 1 mg
Syrup: 0.5 mg/5 ml‡

ACTION
Competes with histamine for H_1-receptor sites on effector cells. Prevents, but does not reverse, histamine-mediated responses.

ONSET, PEAK, DURATION
Onset occurs within 15 to 60 minutes.

Reactions may be *common,* uncommon, *life-threatening,* or COMMON AND LIFE-THREATENING.

Plasma levels peak within 4 hours. Effects persist for 12 hours.

INDICATIONS & DOSAGE
Rhinitis, allergy symptoms, chronic urticaria—
Adults and children 12 years and older: 1 to 2 mg P.O. b.i.d. Maximum dosage is 4 mg daily.

ADVERSE REACTIONS
CNS: *drowsiness, dizziness,* vertigo, disturbed coordination.
CV: hypotension, palpitations.
GI: anorexia, nausea, vomiting, *dry mouth and throat,* epigastric distress.
GU: urine retention.
Hematologic: *thrombocytopenia.*
Respiratory: thick bronchial secretions.
Skin: urticaria, rash.

INTERACTIONS
CNS depressants: increased sedation. Use together cautiously.
MAO inhibitors: increased anticholinergic effects. Don't use together.

EFFECTS ON DIAGNOSTIC TESTS
Discontinue azatadine 4 days before performing diagnostic skin tests; antihistamines can prevent or reduce positive skin reactions, thereby masking a response to the test.

CONTRAINDICATIONS
Contraindicated in patients with acute asthmatic attacks and in breast-feeding patients.

NURSING CONSIDERATIONS
● Use cautiously in elderly patients and in patients with increased intraocular pressure, hyperthyroidism, CV or renal disease, hypertension, bronchial asthma, urine retention, prostatic hyperplasia, bladder-neck obstruction, and stenosing peptic ulcerations.
● Monitor blood counts (including platelets) during long-term therapy, as ordered; watch for signs of blood dyscrasias.

☑ **PATIENT TEACHING**
● Instruct patient to reduce GI distress by taking drug with food or milk.
● Warn patient to avoid alcohol and activities that require alertness until drug's CNS effects are known.
● Inform patient that coffee or tea may reduce drowsiness. Sugarless gum, sugarless sour hard candy, or ice chips may relieve dry mouth.
● Tell patient to notify doctor if tolerance develops because a different antihistamine may need to be prescribed.

---

brompheniramine maleate
Bromphen*◇, Chlorphed◇, Codimal-A, Conjec-B◇, Cophene-B, Dehist, Diamine T.D., Dimetane*◇, Dimetane Extentabs◇, Histaject Modified, Nasahist B, ND-Stat Revised, Oraminic II, Sinusol-B, Veltane

Pregnancy Risk Category: C

HOW SUPPLIED
Tablets: 4 mg◇, 8 mg, 12 mg
Tablets (extended-release): 8 mg◇, 12 mg◇
Elixir: 2 mg/5 ml*◇
Injection: 10 mg/ml

ACTION
Competes with histamine for H_1-receptor sites on effector cells. Prevents, but does not reverse, histamine-mediated responses.

ONSET, PEAK, DURATION
Onset occurs in 15 to 60 minutes. Peak levels occur within 2 to 5 hours. Peak effects occur in 3 to 9 hours. Effects persist for 4 to 8 hours for regular release preparations, longer for extended-release preparations.

INDICATIONS & DOSAGE
Rhinitis, allergy symptoms—
Adults: 4 to 8 mg P.O. t.i.d. or q.i.d.; or 8 to 12 mg extended-release P.O. b.i.d. or t.i.d. Maximum oral dosage is 24 mg

daily. Or, 5 to 20 mg q 6 to 12 hours I.M., I.V., or S.C. Maximum parenteral dosage is 40 mg daily.

Children 6 to 12 years: 2 to 4 mg P.O. t.i.d. or q.i.d.; or 8 to 12 mg extended-release P.O. q 12 hours; or 0.5 mg/kg I.M., I.V., or S.C. daily in divided doses t.i.d. or q.i.d.

Children under 6 years: 0.5 mg/kg P.O., I.M., I.V., or S.C. daily in divided doses t.i.d. or q.i.d.

Note: Children under 12 years should use only as directed by doctor.

ADVERSE REACTIONS
CNS: dizziness, tremors, irritability, insomnia, *drowsiness, stimulation.*
CV: hypotension, palpitations.
GI: anorexia, nausea, vomiting, *dry mouth and throat.*
GU: urine retention.
Hematologic: *thrombocytopenia, agranulocytosis.*
Skin: urticaria, rash.
Other: (after parenteral administration) local stinging, diaphoresis, syncope.

INTERACTIONS
CNS depressants: increased sedation. Use together cautiously.
MAO inhibitors: increased anticholinergic effects. Don't use together.

EFFECTS ON DIAGNOSTIC TESTS
Brompheniramine should be discontinued 4 days before performing diagnostic skin tests; it can prevent, reduce, or mask positive skin test response.

CONTRAINDICATIONS
Contraindicated in patients with hypersensitivity to any of the drug's ingredients; in those with acute asthma, severe hypertension or coronary artery disease, angle-closure glaucoma, urine retention, and peptic ulcer; and within 14 days of MAO inhibitor therapy.

NURSING CONSIDERATIONS
● Use cautiously in elderly patients and in those with increased intraocular pres-

sure, diabetes, ischemic heart disease, hyperthyroidism, hypertension, bronchial asthma, and prostatic hyperplasia.
● **I.V. use:** Injectable form containing 10 mg/ml can be given diluted or undiluted very slowly I.V.
Alert: Do not give the 100 mg/ml injection I.V.
● Monitor blood count during long-term therapy, as ordered; observe for signs of blood dyscrasias.

☑ **PATIENT TEACHING**
● Instruct patient to reduce GI distress by taking drug with food or milk.
● Warn patient to avoid alcohol and activities that require alertness until drug's CNS effects are known.
● Tell patient that coffee or tea may reduce drowsiness. Causes less drowsiness than some other antihistamines.
● Inform patient that sugarless gum, sugarless sour hard candy, or ice chips may relieve dry mouth.
● Tell patient to notify doctor if tolerance develops because a different antihistamine may need to be prescribed.

---

cetirizine hydrochloride
Zyrtec

Pregnancy Risk Category: B

HOW SUPPLIED
Tablets: 5 mg, 10 mg

ACTION
Selectively inhibits peripheral histamine-1 receptors.

ONSET, PEAK, DURATION
Onset is 20 minutes to 1 hour. Peak plasma levels occur in ½ to 1½ hours. Duration is at least 24 hours.

INDICATIONS & DOSAGE
Seasonal allergic rhinitis, perennial allergic rhinitis, chronic urticaria—
Adults and children 12 years and old-

Reactions may be *common,* uncommon, *life-threatening,* or COMMON AND LIFE-THREATENING.

er: 5 or 10 mg P.O. daily depending on symptom severity; 5 mg P.O. daily in those with renal or hepatic impairment.
✳ *New indication:* Seasonal allergic rhinitis, perennial allergic rhinitis, chronic urticaria—
Children 6 to 11 years: 5 or 10 mg (1 or 2 tsp) P.O. once daily depending on symptom severity.

ADVERSE REACTIONS
CNS: *somnolence,* fatigue, dizziness.
GI: dry mouth.
Other: pharyngitis.

INTERACTIONS
Ethanol and other CNS depressants: possible additive effect. Avoid concomitant use.
Theophylline: may cause decreased clearance of cetirizine. Monitor patient closely.

EFFECTS ON DIAGNOSTIC TESTS
None reported.

CONTRAINDICATIONS
Contraindicated in patients with hypersensitivity to the drug or to hydroxyzine.

NURSING CONSIDERATIONS
● Use cautiously in patients with renal impairment.
● Drug is not recommended for use in breast-feeding women.
● Safety of drug has not been established in children under age 12.

☑ PATIENT TEACHING
● Warn the patient not to drive or perform hazardous activities if he experiences somnolence, a common adverse reaction.
● Advise the patient not to use alcohol or other CNS depressants while taking the drug.

chlorpheniramine maleate
Aller-Chlor*L, Allergex‡, Chlo-Amine◇, Chlor-100◇, Chlorate◇, Chlor-Niramine◇, Chlor-Pro, Chlor-Pro 10, Chlorspan-12, Chlortab-4, Chlortab-8, Chlor-Trimeton*◇, Chlor-Trimeton 12 Hour Allergy◇, Chlor-Tripolon†◇, GenAllerate◇, Novopheniram‡◇, Pfeiffer's Allergy◇, Phenetron*, Piriton‡, Pyranistan◇, Telachlor, Teldrin◇, Trymegen◇

Pregnancy Risk Category: B

HOW SUPPLIED
Tablets: 4 mg◇, 8 mg◇, 12 mg◇
Tablets (chewable): 2 mg◇
Tablets (timed-release): 8 mg◇, 12 mg◇
Capsules (timed-release): 6 mg◇, 8 mg◇, 12 mg◇
Syrup: 2 mg/5 ml*◇
Injection: 10 mg/ml, 100 mg/ml

ACTION
Competes with histamine for H_1-receptor sites on effector cells. Prevents, but does not reverse, histamine-mediated responses.

ONSET, PEAK, DURATION
Onset occurs in 15 to 60 minutes. Peak concentrations occur 2 to 6 hours after oral dose, immediately after I.V. injection, unknown after I.M. administration. Effects persist up to 24 hours.

INDICATIONS & DOSAGE
Rhinitis, allergy symptoms—
Adults: 4 mg P.O. q 4 to 6 hours, not to exceed 24 mg/day; or 8 to 12 mg timed-release P.O. every 8 to 12 hours, not to exceed 24 mg daily. Alternatively, 5 to 20 mg I.M., I.V., or S.C. as a single dose. Maximum recommended parenteral dosage is 40 mg per 24 hours.
Children 6 to 12 years: 2 mg P.O. q 4 to 6 hours, not to exceed 12 mg/day. Alternatively, may give 8 mg timed-re-

lease P.O. h.s.
Children 2 to 6 years: 1 mg P.O. q 4 to 6 hours, not to exceed 4 mg daily.

ADVERSE REACTIONS
CNS: *stimulation,* sedation, *drowsiness,* excitability (in children).
CV: hypotension, palpitations.
GI: epigastric distress, *dry mouth.*
GU: urine retention.
Respiratory: thick bronchial secretions.
Skin: rash, urticaria.
Other: local stinging, burning sensation (after parenteral administration), pallor, weak pulse, transient hypotension.

INTERACTIONS
CNS depressants: increased sedation. Use together cautiously.
MAO inhibitors: increased anticholinergic effects. Don't use together.

EFFECTS ON DIAGNOSTIC TESTS
Discontinue chlorpheniramine 4 days before diagnostic skin tests; antihistamines can prevent, reduce, or mask positive skin test response.

CONTRAINDICATIONS
● Contraindicated in patients having acute asthmatic attacks.
● Antihistamines are not recommended for breast-feeding patients because small amounts of drug are excreted in breast milk.

NURSING CONSIDERATIONS
● Use cautiously in elderly patients and in those with increased intraocular pressure, hyperthyroidism, CV or renal disease, hypertension, bronchial asthma, urine retention, prostatic hyperplasia, bladder-neck obstruction, and stenosing peptic ulcerations.
● **I.V. use:** Drug is available in 10 mg/ml ampules for I.V. use.
Alert: Do not give the 100 mg/ml strength I.V. Chlorpheniramine is compatible with most I.V. solutions. Check with pharmacist before mixing with I.V. solutions to verify specific compatibili-

ties. Give injection over 1 minute.
● If symptoms occur during or after parenteral dose, discontinue drug. Notify the doctor.

☑ PATIENT TEACHING
● Warn patient to avoid alcohol and other CNS depressants and driving and other activities that require alertness until drug's CNS effects are known.
● Tell patient that coffee or tea may reduce drowsiness. Sugarless gum, sugarless sour hard candy, or ice chips may relieve dry mouth.
● Tell patient to notify doctor if tolerance develops because a different antihistamine may need to be prescribed.
● Tell parent that drug, including extended-release products, should not be used in children under 12 years unless directed by doctor.

---

clemastine fumarate
Tavist, Tavist-1 ◊

Pregnancy Risk Category: C

HOW SUPPLIED
Tablets: 1.34 mg ◊, 2.68 mg
Syrup: 0.67 mg per 5 ml

ACTION
Competes with histamine for H_1-receptor sites on effector cells. Prevents, but does not reverse, histamine-mediated responses.

ONSET, PEAK, DURATION
Onset occurs in 15 to 60 minutes. Peak levels occur in 2 to 4 hours; peak effects occur in 5 to 7 hours. Effects persist for 12 hours.

INDICATIONS & DOSAGE
Rhinitis, allergy symptoms—
Adults and children 12 years and over: 1.34 mg P.O. q 12 hours, or 2.68 mg P.O. once daily to t.i.d. as needed. Dosage should not exceed 8.04 mg/day.
Children 6 to 12 years: 0.67 to 1.34

mg P.O. b.i.d. Dosage should not exceed 4.02 mg/day.

ADVERSE REACTIONS
CNS: *sedation, drowsiness, seizures,* nervousness, tremor, confusion, restlessness, vertigo, headache, *sleepiness, dizziness, incoordination,* fatigue.
CV: hypotension, palpitations, tachycardia.
GI: *epigastric distress,* anorexia, diarrhea, nausea, vomiting, constipation, *dry mouth.*
GU: urine retention, urinary frequency.
Hematologic: hemolytic anemia, ***thrombocytopenia, agranulocytosis.***
Respiratory: *thick bronchial secretions.*
Skin: rash, urticaria, photosensitivity, diaphoresis.
Other: *anaphylactic shock.*

INTERACTIONS
CNS depressants: increased sedation. Use together cautiously.
MAO inhibitors: increased anticholinergic effects. Don't use together.

EFFECTS ON DIAGNOSTIC TESTS
Discontinue clemastine 4 days before diagnostic skin tests; antihistamines can prevent, reduce, or mask positive skin test response.

CONTRAINDICATIONS
Contraindicated in patients with hypersensitivity to drug or other antihistamines of similar chemical structure, in those with acute asthma, and in neonates or premature infants and breastfeeding patients.

NURSING CONSIDERATIONS
• Use cautiously in elderly patients and in those with angle-closure glaucoma, increased intraocular pressure, hyperthyroidism, CV disease, hypertension, bronchial asthma, prostatic hyperplasia, bladder-neck obstruction, pyloroduodenal obstruction, and stenosing peptic ulcerations.
• Know that children under 12 years should use only as directed by a doctor.
• Monitor blood counts during long-term therapy, as ordered; observe for signs of blood dyscrasias.

☑ PATIENT TEACHING
• Warn patient to avoid alcohol and driving or other activities that require alertness until drug's CNS effects are known.
• Tell patient that coffee or tea may reduce drowsiness. Sugarless gum, sugarless sour hard candy, or ice chips may relieve dry mouth.
• Tell patient to notify doctor if tolerance develops because a different antihistamine may need to be prescribed.

---

cyproheptadine hydrochloride
Periactin

Pregnancy Risk Category: B

HOW SUPPLIED
Tablets: 4 mg
Syrup: 2 mg/5 ml

ACTION
Competes with histamine for H_1-receptor sites on effector cells. Prevents, but does not reverse, histamine-mediated responses.

ONSET, PEAK, DURATION
Onset occurs in 15 to 60 minutes. Serum levels peak in 6 to 9 hours. Effects persist for 8 hours.

INDICATIONS & DOSAGE
Allergy symptoms, pruritus—
Adults: 4 to 20 mg P.O. daily in divided doses. Maximum dosage is 0.5 mg/kg daily.
Children 7 to 14 years: 4 mg P.O. b.i.d. or t.i.d. Maximum dosage is 16 mg/day.
Children 2 to 6 years: 2 mg P.O. b.i.d. or t.i.d. Maximum dosage is 12 mg daily.

ADVERSE REACTIONS
CNS: *drowsiness,* dizziness, headache, fatigue, sedation, sleepiness, incoordination, confusion, restlessness, insomnia, nervousness, tremor, *seizures.*
CV: hypotension, palpitations, tachycardia.
GI: nausea, vomiting, epigastric distress, *dry mouth,* diarrhea, constipation.
GU: urine retention, urinary frequency.
Hematologic: hemolytic anemia, leukopenia, *agranulocytosis, thrombocytopenia.*
Skin: rash, urticaria, photosensitivity.
Other: weight gain, *anaphylactic shock.*

INTERACTIONS
CNS depressants: increased sedation. Use together cautiously.
MAO inhibitors: increased anticholinergic effects. Don't use together.

EFFECTS ON DIAGNOSTIC TESTS
Discontinue cyproheptadine 4 days before diagnostic skin tests; antihistamines can prevent, reduce, or mask positive skin test response.

CONTRAINDICATIONS
Contraindicated in patients with hypersensitivity to drug or other drugs of similar chemical structure; in those with acute asthma, angle-closure glaucoma, stenosing peptic ulcer, symptomatic prostatic hyperplasia, bladder-neck obstruction, and pyloroduodenal obstruction; in concurrent therapy with MAO inhibitors; in neonates or premature infants; in elderly or debilitated patients, and in breast-feeding patients.

NURSING CONSIDERATIONS
● Use cautiously in patients with increased intraocular pressure, hyperthyroidism, CV disease, hypertension, or bronchial asthma.
● Know that children under 14 years should use only as directed by a doctor.

☑ PATIENT TEACHING
● Tell patient that GI distress can be reduced by taking drug with food or milk.
● Warn patient to avoid alcohol and driving or other activities that require alertness until drug's CNS effects are known.
● Tell patient that coffee or tea may reduce drowsiness. Sugarless gum, sugarless sour hard candy, or ice chips may relieve dry mouth.
● Instruct patient to notify doctor if tolerance develops because a different antihistamine may need to be prescribed.

---

dexchlorpheniramine maleate
Dexchlor, Poladex, Poladex T.D., Polaramine*, Polaramine Repetabs, Polargen

Pregnancy Risk Category: B

HOW SUPPLIED
Tablets: 2 mg
Tablets (timed-release): 4 mg, 6 mg
Syrup: 2 mg/5 ml*

ACTION
Competes with histamine for H_1-receptor sites on effector cells. Prevents, but does not reverse, histamine-mediated responses.

ONSET, PEAK, DURATION
Onset occurs in 15 to 60 minutes. Peak unknown. Effects persist for 4 to 8 hours.

INDICATIONS & DOSAGE
Rhinitis, allergy symptoms, contact dermatitis, pruritus—
Adults and children over 12 years: 2 mg P.O. q 4 to 6 hours, not to exceed 12 mg/day; or 4 to 6 mg timed-release P.O. q 8 to 10 hours.
Children 6 to 12 years: 1 mg P.O. q 4 to 6 hours, not to exceed 6 mg/day; or 4 mg timed-release tablet P.O. h.s.
Children 2 to 6 years: 0.5 mg P.O. q 4 to 6 hours, not to exceed 3 mg/day. Do

---

Reactions may be *common*, uncommon, *life-threatening*, or COMMON AND LIFE-THREATENING.

not use timed-release form.

ADVERSE REACTIONS
CNS: *drowsiness,* dizziness, *stimulation.*
GI: nausea, *dry mouth.*
GU: polyuria, dysuria, urine retention.

INTERACTIONS
CNS depressants: increased sedation.
Use together cautiously.
MAO inhibitors: increased anticholinergic effects. Don't use together.

EFFECTS ON DIAGNOSTIC TESTS
Antihistamines can prevent, reduce, or mask positive skin test response. Discontinue drug 4 days before diagnostic skin tests.

CONTRAINDICATIONS
● Contraindicated in patients with acute asthmatic attacks.
● Antihistamines are not recommended for use in breast-feeding patients because small amounts of drug are excreted in breast milk.

NURSING CONSIDERATIONS
● Use cautiously in elderly patients and in patients with increased intraocular pressure, hyperthyroidism, CV or renal disease, hypertension, bronchial asthma, urine retention, prostatic hyperplasia, bladder-neck obstruction, and stenosing peptic ulcer.
● Know that children under 6 years should use only as directed by a doctor. Timed-release tablets should not be used for children younger than 6 years.

☑ **PATIENT TEACHING**
● Warn patient to avoid alcohol and driving or other activities that require alertness until drug's CNS effects are known.
● Tell patient that coffee or tea may reduce drowsiness. Sugarless gum, sugarless sour hard candy, or ice chips may relieve dry mouth.
● Tell patient to notify doctor if toler-

ance develops because a different antihistamine may need to be prescribed.

---

diphenhydramine hydrochloride

Allerdryl† ◇, AllerMax Caplets ◇, Aller-med ◇, Banophen ◇, Banophen Caplets ◇, Beldin ◇, Belix ◇, Bena-D 10, Bena-D 50, Benadryl ◇, Benadryl 25 ◇, Benadryl Kapseals ◇, Benahist 10, Benahist 50, Ben-Allergin-50, Benoject-10, Benoject-50, Benylin Cough ◇, Bydramine Cough ◇, Compoz ◇, Diphenacen-50, Diphenadryl ◇, Diphen Cough ◇, Diphenhist ◇, Diphenhist Captabs ◇, Dormarex 2 ◇, Fynex ◇, Genahist ◇, Gen-D-phen ◇, Hydramine ◇, Hydramine Cough ◇, Hydramyn ◇, Hydril ◇, Hyrexin-50, Insomnal† ◇, Nervine Nighttime Sleep-Aid ◇, Nidryl ◇, Noradryl ◇, Nordryl ◇, Nordryl Cough ◇, Nytol Maximum Strength ◇, Nytol with DPH ◇, Phendry ◇, Phendry Children's Allergy Medicine ◇, Sleep-Eze 3 ◇, Sominex Formula 2 ◇, Tusstat ◇, Twilite Caplets ◇, Uni-Bent Cough ◇, Wehdryl-10, Wehdryl-50

Pregnancy Risk Category: B

HOW SUPPLIED
Tablets: 25 mg ◇, 50 mg ◇
Capsules: 25 mg ◇, 50 mg ◇
Elixir: 12.5 mg/5 ml (14% alcohol)* ◇
Syrup: 12.5 mg/5 ml ◇
Injection: 10 mg/ml, 50 mg/ml

ACTION
Competes with histamine for H_1-receptor sites on effector cells. Prevents, but does not reverse, histamine-mediated responses, particularly histamine's effects on the smooth muscle of the bronchial tubes, GI tract, uterus, and blood vessels. Structurally related to local anesthetics, diphenhydramine provides local anesthesia by preventing initiation and transmission of nerve impulses. Also

---

*Liquid contains alcohol.   **May contain tartrazine.   †Canada only.   ‡Australia only.   ◇ OTC.

suppresses cough reflex by a direct effect in the medulla of the brain.

ONSET, PEAK, DURATION
Onset occurs within 15 minutes of oral administration, immediately after I.V. administration, unknown after I.M. administration. Serum levels peak and drug effects occur 1 to 4 hours after administration. Effects persist for 6 to 8 hours.

INDICATIONS & DOSAGE
Rhinitis, allergy symptoms, motion sickness, Parkinson's disease—
Adults and children 12 years and over: 25 to 50 mg P.O. t.i.d. or q.i.d.; or 10 to 50 mg deep I.M. or I.V. Maximum I.M. or I.V. dosage is 400 mg daily.
Children under 12 years: 5 mg/kg daily P.O., deep I.M., or I.V. in divided doses q.i.d. Maximum dosage is 300 mg daily.
Sedation—
Adults: 25 to 50 mg P.O., or deep I.M., p.r.n.
Nighttime sleep aid—
Adults: 25 to 50 mg P.O. h.s.
Nonproductive cough—
Adults: 25 mg P.O. q 4 to 6 hours (not to exceed 150 mg daily).
Children 6 to 12 years: 12.5 mg P.O. q 4 to 6 hours (not to exceed 75 mg daily).
Children 2 to 6 years: 6.25 mg P.O. q 4 to 6 hours (not to exceed 25 mg/day).

ADVERSE REACTIONS
CNS: *drowsiness,* confusion, insomnia, headache, vertigo, *sedation, sleepiness, dizziness, incoordination,* fatigue, restlessness, tremor, nervousness, **seizures.**
CV: palpitations, hypotension, tachycardia.
EENT: diplopia, blurred vision, tinnitus.
GI: *nausea,* vomiting, diarrhea, *dry mouth,* constipation, *epigastric distress,* anorexia.
GU: dysuria, urine retention, urinary frequency.
Hematologic: hemolytic anemia,

thrombocytopenia, agranulocytosis.
Respiratory: nasal congestion, *thickening of bronchial secretions.*
Skin: urticaria, photosensitivity, rash.
Other: *anaphylactic shock.*

INTERACTIONS
CNS depressants: increased sedation. Use together cautiously.
MAO inhibitors: increased anticholinergic effects. Don't use together.

EFFECTS ON DIAGNOSTIC TESTS
Discontinue diphenhydramine 4 days before diagnostic skin tests; antihistamines can prevent, reduce, or mask positive skin test response.

CONTRAINDICATIONS
Contraindicated in patients with hypersensitivity to the drug, during acute asthmatic attacks, and in newborns or premature neonates and breast-feeding patients.

NURSING CONSIDERATIONS
● Use with extreme caution in patients with angle-closure glaucoma, prostatic hyperplasia, pyloroduodenal and bladder-neck obstruction, asthma or COPD, increased intraocular pressure, hyperthyroidism, CV disease, hypertension, and stenosing peptic ulcer.
● Know that children under 12 years should use only as directed by a doctor.
● Alternate injection sites to prevent irritation. Administer I.M. injection deeply into large muscle.

☑ PATIENT TEACHING
● Instruct patient to take 30 minutes before travel to prevent motion sickness.
● Tell the patient to take diphenhydramine with food or milk to reduce GI distress.
● Warn patient to avoid alcohol and driving or other hazardous activities that require alertness until drug's effect on the central nervous system is known.
● Tell patient that coffee or tea may reduce drowsiness. Sugarless gum, sugar-

---

*Reactions may be common, uncommon, **life-threatening**, or COMMON AND LIFE-THREATENING.*

less sour hard candy, or ice chips may relieve dry mouth.
● Tell patient to notify doctor if tolerance develops because a different antihistamine may need to be prescribed.
● Warn patient of possible photosensitivity reactions. Advise use of a sunblock.

▼ NEW DRUG

fexofenadine hydrochloride
Allegra

Pregnancy Risk Category: C

HOW SUPPLIED
Capsules: 60 mg

ACTION
Fexofenadine's principal effects are mediated through a selective inhibition of peripheral H_1 receptors.

ONSET, PEAK, DURATION
Following oral administration, peak fexofenadine plasma concentrations are reached within 3 hours. The mean half-life of the drug is 14.4 hours.

INDICATIONS & DOSAGE
Seasonal allergic rhinitis—
Adults and children age 12 and over: 60 mg P.O. b.i.d.; initially 60 mg P.O. once daily in patients with impaired renal function.

ADVERSE REACTIONS
CNS: fatigue, drowsiness.
GI: nausea, dyspepsia.
Other: viral infection, dysmenorrhea.

INTERACTIONS
None reported.

EFFECTS ON DIAGNOSTIC TESTS
None reported.

CONTRAINDICATIONS
Contraindicated in patients with hypersensitivity to drug or its components.

NURSING CONSIDERATIONS
● Use cautiously in patients with impaired renal function.
● Safety and effectiveness in children under age 12 have not been established.
● It is not known whether drug is excreted in breast milk; caution is recommended when administering drug to breast-feeding women. Advise women taking the drug to avoid breast-feeding.

☑ PATIENT TEACHING
● Caution patients not to perform hazardous activities if drowsiness occurs as a result of drug use.
● Instruct patient not to exceed prescribed dosage and to take drug only when needed.

loratadine
Claratyne‡, Claritin

Pregnancy Risk Category: B

HOW SUPPLIED
Tablets: 10 mg

ACTION
Blocks effects of histamine at H_1-receptor sites. Loratadine is a nonsedating antihistamine; its chemical structure prevents entry into the CNS.

ONSET, PEAK, DURATION
Onset occurs in 1 hour. Peak effects occur in 4 to 6 hours. Effects of loratadine persist for at least 24 hours.

INDICATIONS & DOSAGE
Symptomatic treatment of seasonal allergic rhinitis—
Adults and children 12 years and over: 10 mg P.O. daily. Dosage for patients with hepatic failure or renal insufficiency is 10 mg P.O. every other day.
Children 2 to 12 years and under 30 kg body weight: 5 mg daily.

ADVERSE REACTIONS
CNS: headache, somnolence (with high

*Liquid contains alcohol.   **May contain tartrazine.   †Canada only.   ‡Australia only.   ◇OTC.

doses), fatigue, drowsiness.
GI: dry mouth.

INTERACTIONS
Erythromycin: increased loratadine plasma concentrations. Monitor patient closely.

EFFECTS ON DIAGNOSTIC TESTS
None reported.

CONTRAINDICATIONS
Contraindicated in patients with hypersensitivity to the drug.

NURSING CONSIDERATIONS
• Use cautiously in patients with liver impairment and in breast-feeding patients.
• Be aware that administration of loratadine can affect the results of allergy skin tests.

☑ PATIENT TEACHING
• Make sure that the patient knows that he should take the drug only once daily. If his symptoms persist or worsen, he should contact the doctor.
• Advise patient to stop taking loratadine 7 days before allergy skin tests to preserve accuracy of the tests.

---

promethazine hydrochloride
Anergan 25, Anergan 50, Histantil†, Pentazine, Phenameth, Phenazine 25, Phenazine 50, Phencen-50, Phenergan*, Phenergan Fortis*, Phenergan Plain*, Phenoject-50, PMS-Promethazine†, Pro-50, Prometh-25, Prometh-50, Promethegan, Prorex-25, Prorex-50, Prothazine†*, Prothazine Plain, V-Gan-25, V-Gan-50

promethazine theoclate
Avomine‡

Pregnancy Risk Category: C

HOW SUPPLIED
promethazine hydrochloride
Tablets: 12.5 mg, 25 mg, 50 mg
Syrup: 5 mg/5 ml‡*, 6.25 mg/5 ml*, 10 mg/5 ml†*, 25 mg/5 ml*
Injection: 25 mg/ml, 50 mg/ml
Suppositories: 12.5 mg, 25 mg, 50 mg
promethazine theoclate
Tablets: 25 mg‡

ACTION
Competes with histamine for H_1-receptor sites on effector cells. Prevents, but does not reverse, histamine-mediated responses. A phenothiazine derivative.

ONSET, PEAK, DURATION
Onset occurs in 15 to 60 minutes after oral administration, 20 minutes after I.M. injection and P.R. administration, 3 to 5 minutes after I.V. administration. Peak unknown. Effects persist up to 12 hours.

INDICATIONS & DOSAGE
Motion sickness—
Adults: 25 mg P.O. b.i.d.
Children: 12.5 to 25 mg P.O., I.M., or P.R. b.i.d.
Nausea—
Adults: 12.5 to 25 mg P.O., I.M., or P.R. q 4 to 6 hours, p.r.n.
Children: 12.5 to 25 mg I.M. or P.R. q 4 to 6 hours, p.r.n.
Rhinitis, allergy symptoms—
Adults: 12.5 mg P.O. q.i.d.; or 25 mg P.O. h.s.
Children: 6.25 to 12.5 mg P.O. t.i.d. or 25 mg P.O. or P.R. h.s.
Sedation—
Adults: 25 to 50 mg P.O. or I.M. h.s. or p.r.n.
Children: 12.5 to 25 mg P.O., I.M., or P.R. h.s.
Routine preoperative or postoperative sedation or adjunct to analgesics—
Adults: 25 to 50 mg I.M., I.V., or P.O.
Children: 12.5 to 25 mg I.M., I.V., or P.O.

ADVERSE REACTIONS

CNS: *sedation,* confusion, sleepiness, dizziness, disorientation, extrapyramidal symptoms, *drowsiness.*
CV: hypotension, hypertension.
EENT: blurred vision.
GI: nausea, vomiting, *dry mouth.*
GU: urine retention.
Hematologic: leukopenia, *agranulocytosis, thrombocytopenia.*
Other: photosensitivity, rash.

INTERACTIONS

Anticholinergics, phenothiazines, tricyclic antidepressants: increased effects. Don't give together.
CNS depressants, ethanol: increased sedation. Use together cautiously.
Epinephrine: promethazine may block or reverse the effects of epinephrine. Use other pressor agents instead.
Levodopa: promethazine may decrease levodopa's antiparkinsonian action. Avoid concomitant use.
Lithium: promethazine may reduce GI absorption or enhance renal elimination of lithium. Avoid concomitant use.
MAO inhibitors: increased extrapyramidal effects. Don't use together.

EFFECTS ON DIAGNOSTIC TESTS

Discontinue promethazine 4 days before diagnostic skin tests; antihistamines can prevent, reduce, or mask positive skin test response. Drug may cause hyperglycemia and either false-positive or false-negative pregnancy test results. It may also interfere with blood grouping in the ABO system.

CONTRAINDICATIONS

Contraindicated in patients with hypersensitivity to the drug; in those with intestinal obstruction, prostatic hyperplasia, bladder-neck obstruction, seizure disorders, coma, CNS depression, and stenosing peptic ulcerations; and in newborns and premature neonates, and breast-feeding patients; and in acutely ill or dehydrated children.

NURSING CONSIDERATIONS

● Use cautiously in patients with pulmonary, hepatic, CV disease, or asthma.
● Know that pronounced sedative effect limits use in many ambulatory patients.
● Know that promethazine is used as an adjunct to analgesics (usually to increase sedation) and that it has no analgesic activity.
● Reduce GI distress by giving drug with food or milk.
● **I.V. use:** Don't give in a concentration greater than 25 mg/ml or at a rate exceeding 25 mg/minute. Shield I.V. infusion from direct light.
● Inject deep I.M. into large muscle mass. Rotate injection sites.
Alert: Don't administer via S.C. route.
● Be aware that drug may be mixed with meperidine in same syringe.
● In patients scheduled for a myelogram, discontinue drug 48 hours before procedure and do not resume drug until 24 hours after procedure, as ordered, because of the risk of seizures.

☑ PATIENT TEACHING

● Tell patient to take oral form with food or milk.
● When treating motion sickness, tell patient to take first dose 30 to 60 minutes before travel. On succeeding days of travel, patient should take dose upon rising and with evening meal.
● Warn patient to avoid alcohol and driving or other activities that require alertness until drug's CNS effects are known.
● Tell patient that coffee or tea may reduce drowsiness. Sugarless gum, sugarless sour hard candy, or ice chips may relieve dry mouth.
● Warn patient about possible photosensitivity and precautions to avoid it.

---

triprolidine hydrochloride
Actidil ◇, Alleract ◇, Myidyl

Pregnancy Risk Category: C

HOW SUPPLIED
Tablets: 2.5 mg ◊
Syrup*: 1.25 mg/5 ml ◊

ACTION
Competes with histamine for H_1-receptor sites on effector cells. Prevents, but does not reverse, histamine-mediated responses.

ONSET, PEAK, DURATION
Onset occurs in 15 to 60 minutes. Peak levels occur in about 2 hours. Peak effects occur in 2 to 3 hours. Effects persist for 4 to 8 hours.

INDICATIONS & DOSAGE
Colds and allergy symptoms—
Adults and children 12 years and over: 2.5 mg P.O. q 4 to 6 hours. Maximum dosage is 10 mg/day.
Children 6 to 12 years: 1.25 mg P.O. q 4 to 6 hours. Maximum dosage is 5 mg/day.
Children 4 to 6 years: 0.938 mg P.O. q 4 to 6 hours. Maximum dosage is 3.744 mg/day.
Children 2 to 4 years: 0.625 mg P.O. q 4 to 6 hours. Maximum dosage is 2.5 mg/day.
Children 4 months to 2 years: 0.313 mg P.O. q 4 to 6 hours. Maximum dosage is 1.252 mg/day.

ADVERSE REACTIONS
CNS: *drowsiness, dizziness,* confusion, restlessness, insomnia, headache, *sedation, sleepiness, incoordination,* fatigue, anxiety, nervousness, tremor, **seizures, stimulation.**
CV: hypotension, palpitations, tachycardia.
EENT: *dry nose and throat.*
GI: anorexia, diarrhea or constipation, nausea, vomiting, *dry mouth,* epigastric distress.
GU: urinary frequency, urine retention.
Hematologic: hemolytic anemia, **thrombocytopenia, agranulocytosis.**
Skin: urticaria, rash, photosensitivity, diaphoresis.

Other: **anaphylactic shock,** chills, thickening of bronchial secretions.

INTERACTIONS
CNS depressants: increased sedation. Use together cautiously.
MAO inhibitors: increased anticholinergic effects. Don't use together.

EFFECTS ON DIAGNOSTIC TESTS
Discontinue triprolidine 4 days before diagnostic skin tests; antihistamines can prevent, reduce, or mask positive skin test response.

CONTRAINDICATIONS
Contraindicated in patients with hypersensitivity to the drug, in those with acute asthma, and in neonates, premature infants, and breast-feeding patients.

NURSING CONSIDERATIONS
● Use with extreme caution in patients with increased intraocular pressure, angle-closure glaucoma, hyperthyroidism, CV disease, hypertension, bronchial asthma, prostatic hyperplasia, bladder-neck obstruction, and stenosing peptic ulcerations.
● Know that children under 12 years should use only as directed by a doctor.

☑ PATIENT TEACHING
● Tell patient to take drug with food or milk to reduce GI distress.
● Warn patient to avoid alcohol and driving or other activities that require alertness until drug's CNS effects are known.
● Tell patient that coffee or tea may reduce drowsiness. Sugarless gum, sugarless sour hard candy, or ice chips may relieve dry mouth.

Reactions may be *common,* uncommon, **life-threatening,** or COMMON AND LIFE-THREATENING.

albuterol
albuterol sulfate
aminophylline
atropine sulfate
    (See Chapter 21, antiarrhythmics.)
bitolterol mesylate
ephedrine sulfate
epinephrine
epinephrine bitartrate
epinephrine hydrochloride
ipratropium bromide
isoetharine hydrochloride
isoetharine mesylate
isoproterenol
isoproterenol hydrochloride
isoproterenol sulfate
metaproterenol sulfate
oxtriphylline
pirbuterol
salmeterol xinafoate
terbutaline sulfate
theophylline
theophylline sodium glycinate

COMBINATION PRODUCTS
Inhalants
DUO-MEDIHALER: isoproterenol hydrochloride 0.16 mg and phenylephrine bitartrate 0.24 mg per dose.
Oral bronchodilators
BRONCHIAL CAPSULES: 150 mg theophylline and 90 mg guaifenesin.
DILOR-G TABLETS: 200 mg dyphylline and 200 mg guaifenesin.
DYFLEX-G TABLETS: 200 mg dyphylline and 200 mg guaifenesin.
DYLINE-GG TABLETS: 200 mg dyphylline and 200 mg guaifenesin.
GLYCERYL-T CAPSULES: 150 mg theophylline and 90 mg guaifenesin.
MARAX*: theophylline 130 mg, ephedrine sulfate 25 mg, and hydroxyzine hydrochloride 10 mg.
NEOTHYLLINE-GG TABLETS: 200 mg dyphylline and 200 mg guaifenesin.

QUIBRON CAPSULES: 150 mg theophylline and 90 mg guaifenesin.
SYNOPHYLATE-GG SYRUP*: 33.3 mg/5 ml guaifenesin and 100 mg/ml theophylline sodium glycinate.
THALFED ◊: theophylline 120 mg, ephedrine hydrochloride 25 mg, and phenobarbital 8 mg.
Decongestants
ACTIFED ◊: pseudoephedrine hydrochloride 60 mg and triprolidine hydrochloride 2.5 mg.
CONGESPIRIN ◊: phenylephrine hydrochloride 1.25 mg and acetaminophen 81 mg.
DRISTAN ◊: phenylephrine hydrochloride 5 mg, chlorpheniramine maleate 2 mg, and acetaminophen 325 mg.
ELIXOPHYLLINE KI ELIXIR: theophylline 80 mg, potassium iodide 130 mg.
MARAX DF SYRUP: theophylline 97.5 mg, ephedrine sulfate 18.75 mg, hydroxyzine hydrochloride 7.5 mg.
NALDECON: phenylpropanolamine hydrochloride 40 mg, phenylephrine hydrochloride 10 mg, chlorpheniramine maleate 5 mg, and phenyltoloxamine citrate 15 mg.
SEMPREX-D: acrivastine 8 mg and pseudoephedrine hydrochloride 60 mg.
SLOPHYLLIN GG SYRUP: theophylline 150 mg and guaifenesin 90 mg.

---

albuterol (salbutamol)
Asmol‡, Proventil, Ventolin

albuterol sulfate (salbutamol sulphate)
Proventil, Proventil Repetabs, Respolin Autohaler Inhalation Device‡, Respolin Inhaler‡, Respolin Respirator Solution‡, Ventolin, Ventolin Obstetric Injection‡, Ventolin Rotacaps

Pregnancy Risk Category: C

HOW SUPPLIED
albuterol
Aerosol inhaler: 90 mcg/metered spray, 100 mcg/metered spray‡
albuterol sulfate
Capsules for inhalation: 200 mcg
Tablets: 2 mg, 4 mg
Tablets (extended-release): 4 mg, 8 mg
Syrup: 2 mg/5 ml
Solution for inhalation: 0.083%, 0.5%
Injection: 1 mg/ml‡

ACTION
Relaxes bronchial and uterine smooth muscle by acting on beta$_2$-adrenergic receptors.

ONSET, PEAK, DURATION
Onset occurs within 5 to 15 minutes after inhalation, within 15 to 30 minutes after oral administration. Peak effect occurs 1 to 1½ hours after inhalation, 2 to 3 hours after oral administration. Effects persist for 3 to 6 hours after inhalation, up to 6 hours for syrup, up to 8 hours for tablets, about 12 hours for extended-release preparations.

INDICATIONS & DOSAGE
To prevent or treat bronchospasm in patients with reversible obstructive airway disease and the prevention of bronchospasm due to exercise—
Adults and children 12 years and older: dosage and frequency vary with dosage form.
Aerosol inhalation—1 to 2 inhalations q 4 to 6 hours. More frequent administration or a greater number of inhalations is not recommended.
Solution for inhalation—2.5 mg t.i.d. or q.i.d. by nebulizer. To prepare solution, use 0.5 ml of the 0.5% solution diluted with 2.5 ml of 0.9% sodium chloride. Alternatively, use 3 ml of the 0.083% solution.
Capsules for inhalation—200 mcg inhaled q 4 to 6 hours using a Rotahaler inhalation device. Some patients may need 400 mcg q 4 to 6 hours.

Oral tablets—2 to 4 mg P.O. t.i.d. or q.i.d. Maximum dosage is 8 mg q.i.d.
Extended-release tablets—4 to 8 mg P.O. q 12 hours. Maximum dosage is 16 mg b.i.d.
Children 6 to 13 years: 2 mg (1 tsp) P.O. t.i.d. or q.i.d.
Children 2 to 5 years: 0.1 mg/kg P.O. t.i.d., not to exceed 2 mg (1 tsp) t.i.d.
Adults over 65 years: 2 mg P.O. t.i.d. or q.i.d.
To prevent exercise-induced asthma—
Adults: 2 inhalations 15 minutes before exercise.
Prevention of premature labor‡—
Adults: initially, 10 mcg/minute by continuous I.V. infusion (via an infusion pump). Dosage should be increased at 10-minute intervals until desired response is achieved.

ADVERSE REACTIONS
CNS: *tremor, nervousness,* dizziness, insomnia, *headache, hyperactivity,* weakness, CNS stimulation, malaise.
CV: *tachycardia, palpitations,* hypertension.
EENT: dry and irritated nose and throat (with inhaled form), nasal congestion, epistaxis, hoarseness, bad taste.
GI: heartburn, *nausea, vomiting,* anorexia.
Respiratory: bronchospasm, cough, wheezing, dyspnea, bronchitis, increased sputum.
Other: muscle cramps, hypokalemia (with high doses), increased appetite, hypersensitivity reactions.

INTERACTIONS
CNS stimulants: increased CNS stimulation. Avoid concomitant use.
MAO inhibitors, tricyclic antidepressants: increased adverse CV effects. Monitor patient closely.
Propranolol and other beta blockers: mutual antagonism. Monitor patient carefully.

Reactions may be *common,* uncommon, ***life-threatening,*** or **COMMON AND LIFE-THREATENING.**

EFFECTS ON DIAGNOSTIC TESTS
Albuterol may decrease the sensitivity of spirometry used for the diagnosis of asthma.

CONTRAINDICATIONS
Contraindicated in patients with hypersensitivity to the drug or any component of the formulation.

NURSING CONSIDERATIONS
• Use cautiously in patients with CV disorders, including coronary insufficiency and hypertension; in patients with hyperthyroidism or diabetes mellitus; and in those who are unusually responsive to adrenergics.
• Use extended-release tablets cautiously in patients with preexisting GI narrowing.
• Know that pleasant-tasting syrup may be taken by children as young as 2 years. Contains no alcohol or sugar.
• Know that aerosol form may be prescribed for use 15 minutes before exercise to prevent exercise-induced bronchospasm.
• Know that patients may use tablets and aerosol concomitantly. Monitor closely for toxicity.
• **I.V. use:** Where available, I.V. form may be used to prepare infusion using sodium chloride for injection, dextrose for injection, or sodium chloride and dextrose for injection. Do not administer drug without dilution. Do not mix with any other medication. Discard unused diluted solution after 24 hours.
• When used to prevent premature labor, monitor maternal heart rate closely. It should not exceed 140 beats/minute.
• After uterine contractions have ceased, drip rate of drug should be maintained for 1 hour, then gradually tapered at 50% increments in six hourly intervals. Do not continue infusions for more than 48 hours. If therapy needs to continue over 48 hours, doctor may prescribe 4 to 8 mg P.O. q.i.d.

☑ **PATIENT TEACHING**
• Warn patient about possibility of paradoxical bronchospasm. If this occurs, discontinue drug immediately.
• Teach patient to perform oral inhalation correctly. Give the following instructions for using metered-dose inhaler:
    —Shake the inhaler.
    —Clear nasal passages and throat.
    —Breathe out, expelling as much air from lungs as possible.
    —Place mouthpiece well into mouth as dose from inhaler is released, and inhale deeply.
    —Hold breath for several seconds, remove mouthpiece, and exhale slowly.
• If more than one inhalation is ordered, advise patient to wait at least 2 minutes before repeating procedure.
• Tell patient who is also using a steroid inhaler to use the bronchodilator first; then wait about 5 minutes before using the steroid. This allows bronchodilator to open air passages for maximum effectiveness.

---

aminophylline (theophylline ethylenediamine)
Aminophyllin, Cardophyllin‡, Corophyllin†, Phyllocontin, Phyllocontin-350, Somophyllin, Somophyllin-DF, Truphylline

Pregnancy Risk Category: C

HOW SUPPLIED
Tablets: 100 mg, 200 mg
Tablets (extended-release): 225 mg, 350 mg†
Oral liquid: 105 mg/5 ml
Injection: 250 mg/10 ml, 500 mg/20 ml, 100 mg/100 ml in 0.45% sodium chloride, 200 mg/100 ml in 0.45% sodium chloride
Rectal suppositories: 250 mg, 500 mg

ACTION
Inhibits phosphodiesterase, the enzyme that degrades cAMP. Results in relaxation of smooth muscle of the bronchial airways and pulmonary blood vessels.

ONSET, PEAK, DURATION
Onset occurs in 15 minutes after I.V. injection, 15 to 60 minutes after oral solution or tablets. Peak serum levels occur immediately after I.V. infusion; within 1 hour of oral solution; 2 hours after oral, uncoated tablets; 4 to 7 hours after extended-release capsules or tablets. Effects persist for variable lengths of time, depending on patient's age, concurrent illnesses, and smoking status.

INDICATIONS & DOSAGE
Symptomatic relief of bronchospasm—
Patients not currently receiving theophylline products who require rapid relief of symptoms: loading dose is 6 mg/kg (equivalent to 4.7 mg/kg anhydrous theophylline) I.V. (less than or equal to 25 mg/minute); then maintenance infusion.
Adults (nonsmokers): 0.7 mg/kg/hour I.V. for 12 hours; then 0.5 mg/kg/hour.
Otherwise healthy adult smokers: 1 mg/kg/hour I.V. for 12 hours; then 0.8 mg/kg/hour.
Older patients and adults with cor pulmonale: 0.6 mg/kg/hour I.V. for 12 hours; then 0.3 mg/kg/hour.
Adults with CHF or liver disease: 0.5 mg/kg/hour I.V. for 12 hours; then 0.1 to 0.2 mg/kg/hour.
Children 9 to 16 years: 1 mg/kg/hour I.V. for 12 hours; then 0.8 mg/kg/hour.
Children 6 months to 9 years: 1.2 mg/kg/hour for 12 hours; then 1 mg/kg/hour.
Patients currently receiving theophylline products: first determine the time, amount, route of administration, and dosage form of the patient's last dose of theophylline. Aminophylline infusions of 0.63 mg/kg (0.5 mg/kg anhydrous theophylline) will increase plasma levels of theophylline by 1 mcg/ml.

Some clinicians recommend a dose of 3.1 mg/kg (2.5 mg/kg anhydrous theophylline) if no obvious signs of theophylline toxicity are present.
Chronic bronchial asthma—
Dosage is highly individualized.
Adults and children: usual initial oral dose is 16 mg/kg or 400 mg (whichever is less) P.O. daily in three or four divided doses q 6 to 8 hours if using rapidly absorbed dosage forms. Dosage may be increased, if tolerated, in increments of 25% q 2 to 3 days. Alternatively, 12 mg/kg or 400 mg (whichever is less) P.O. daily in two to three divided doses q 8 to 12 hours if using extended-release preparations. Dosage may be increased, if tolerated, by 2 to 3 mg/kg daily q 3 days.

When the recommended maximum dosage is reached, dosage adjustment should be based on measurement of peak serum theophylline concentrations.

Note: Rectal dosage is the same as that recommended for oral dosage.

ADVERSE REACTIONS
CNS: *nervousness, restlessness,* headache, *insomnia, seizures,* muscle twitching, irritability.
CV: *palpitations, sinus tachycardia,* extrasystoles, flushing, marked hypotension, arrhythmias.
GI: *nausea, vomiting,* diarrhea, epigastric pain, hematemesis.
Respiratory: tachypnea, *respiratory arrest.*
Skin: urticaria.
Other: irritation (with rectal suppositories), hyperglycemia, fever.

INTERACTIONS
Adenosine: decreased antiarrhythmic effectiveness. Higher doses of adenosine may be necessary.
Alkali-sensitive drugs: reduced activity. Do not add to I.V. fluids containing aminophylline.
Barbiturates, carbamazepine, nicotine, phenytoin, rifampin: enhanced metabolism and decreased theophylline blood

---

levels. Monitor for decreased aminophylline effect.

Beta-adrenergic blockers: antagonism. Propranolol and nadolol, especially, may cause bronchospasm in sensitive patients. Use together cautiously.

Calcium channel blockers, cimetidine, disulfiram, influenza virus vaccine, interferon, macrolide antibiotics (such as erythromycin), oral contraceptives, quinolone antibiotics (such as ciprofloxacin): decreased hepatic clearance of theophylline; elevated theophylline levels. Monitor for signs of toxicity.

Ephedrine, other sympathomimetics: theophylline may exhibit synergistic toxicity with these agents, predisposing patients to cardiac arrhythmias. Monitor patient closely.

Lithium: theophylline may increase excretion of lithium. Monitor patient closely.

EFFECTS ON DIAGNOSTIC TESTS
Aminophylline may alter the assay for uric acid, depending on method used, and increases plasma-free fatty acids and urinary catecholamines. Theophylline levels are falsely elevated in the presence of furosemide, phenylbutazone, probenecid, theobromine, caffeine, tea, chocolate, cola beverages, and acetaminophen, depending on type of assay used.

CONTRAINDICATIONS
Contraindicated in patients with hypersensitivity to xanthine compounds (caffeine, theobromine) and ethylenediamine and in patients with active peptic ulcer disease and seizure disorders (unless adequate anticonvulsant therapy is given). Rectal suppositories are also contraindicated in patients who have an irritation or infection of the rectum or lower colon.

NURSING CONSIDERATIONS
● Use cautiously in neonates and infants under age 1, young children, and elderly patients; also use cautiously in patients

with CHF or other cardiac or circulatory impairment, COPD, cor pulmonale, renal or hepatic disease, hyperthyroidism, diabetes mellitus, peptic ulcer, severe hypoxemia, and hypertension.
● Relieve GI symptoms by giving oral drug with full glass of water at meals, although food in stomach delays absorption. No evidence exists that antacids reduce adverse GI reactions. Know that enteric-coated tablets also may delay and impair absorption.
Alert: Before giving loading dose, ensure that patient has not had recent theophylline therapy.
● **I.V. use:** I.V. drug administration can cause burning; dilute with compatible I.V. solution, and inject at a rate no faster than 25 mg/minute. Drug is compatible with most I.V. solutions except invert sugar, fructose, and fat emulsions.
● Suppositories are slowly and erratically absorbed. Administer rectal suppository if patients cannot take drug orally, as ordered. Schedule after evacuation, if possible; may be retained better if given before meal. Have patients remain recumbent 15 to 20 minutes after insertion.
● Monitor vital signs; measure and record fluid intake and output. Expected clinical effects include improved quality of pulse and respirations.
● Aminophylline is a soluble salt of theophylline. Know that dosage is adjusted by monitoring response, tolerance, pulmonary function, and serum theophylline levels. Monitor serum theophylline levels as ordered. Theophylline concentrations should range from 10 to 20 mcg/ml; toxicity has been reported with levels above 20 mcg/ml.
● Be aware that patients who experience urticaria may still tolerate other theophylline preparations. Urticaria may be caused by the ethylenediamine salt.

☑ **PATIENT TEACHING**
● Supply instructions for home care administration of form prescribed and dosage schedule. Some patients may re-

---

quire an around-the-clock dosage schedule.

• Warn elderly patient that dizziness, a common adverse reaction at start of therapy, may occur.

• Warn patient to check with the doctor or pharmacist before combining aminophylline with other drugs. Prescription or OTC remedies may contain ephedrine in combination with theophylline salts; excessive CNS stimulation may result.

• Advise patient to avoid switching brand without first checking with the doctor.

---

bitolterol mesylate
Tornalate

Pregnancy Risk Category: C

HOW SUPPLIED
Aerosol inhaler: 370 mcg/metered spray

ACTION
Relaxes bronchial smooth muscle by acting on beta$_2$-adrenergic receptors.

ONSET, PEAK, DURATION
Onset occurs in 3 to 4 minutes. Peak effects occur within ½ to 1 hour. Effects persist for 5 to 8 hours, may be only 2½ to 5 hours in steroid-dependent patients.

INDICATIONS & DOSAGE
To prevent or treat bronchial asthma and reversible bronchospasm—
Adults and children over 12 years: to treat bronchospasm, two inhalations with an interval of at least 1 to 3 minutes, followed by a third inhalation, if needed. To prevent bronchospasm, the usual dosage is two inhalations q 8 hours. In either case, dosage should never exceed three inhalations q 6 hours or two inhalations q 4 hours.

ADVERSE REACTIONS
CNS: *tremor,* nervousness, headache, dizziness, light-headedness.
CV: palpitations, chest discomfort, tachycardia.
EENT: throat irritation, cough.
GI: nausea, vomiting.
Other: dyspnea, hypersensitivity reactions.

INTERACTIONS
Adrenergic agents: may cause serious CV effects. Use together cautiously.
Other sympathomimetic bronchodilators: additive sympathomimetic effects. Avoid concurrent administration.
MAO inhibitors, tricyclic antidepressants: increased adverse CV effects.
Beta blockers: mutual antagonism. Monitor the patient carefully.

EFFECTS ON DIAGNOSTIC TESTS
Bitolterol therapy may increase AST levels and decrease platelet or leukocyte count. Proteinuria may also occur. Drug may also render spirometry insensitive for the diagnosis of asthma.

CONTRAINDICATIONS
Contraindicated in patients with hypersensitivity to the drug.

NURSING CONSIDERATIONS
• Use cautiously in patients with ischemic heart disease or hypertension, hyperthyroidism, diabetes mellitus, arrhythmias, seizure disorders, and history of unusual responsiveness to beta-adrenergic agonists.
• Monitor blood pressure regularly.

☑ PATIENT TEACHING
• Advise patient not to exceed recommended dosages. Too frequent use may cause tachycardia.
• Remind patient that beneficial effects last for up to 8 hours, longer than most other similar bronchodilators.
• Teach patient to perform oral inhalation correctly. Give the following instructions for using a metered-dose inhaler:
    —Shake the canister.
    —Clear nasal passages and throat.

Reactions may be *common,* uncommon, *life-threatening,* or COMMON AND LIFE-THREATENING.

—Breathe out, expelling as much air from lungs as possible.

—Place mouthpiece well into mouth as dose from inhaler is released, and inhale deeply and slowly for about 10 seconds.

—Hold breath for several seconds, remove mouthpiece, and exhale slowly.

● If the patient has trouble using a metered-dose inhaler, explain that a spacing device can help ensure proper drug delivery.

● If more than one inhalation is ordered, tell patient to wait at least 2 minutes before repeating procedure.

● Tell patient who is also using a steroid inhaler to use bronchodilator first, then wait about 5 minutes before using steroid. This allows the bronchodilator to open air passages for maximum effectiveness.

● Tell patient that manufacturer recommends rinsing plastic mouthpiece daily with warm tap water, then drying it to ensure proper delivery of drug.

---

ephedrine sulfate
Ectasule, Efedron, Ephedsol, Vicks Vatronol

Pregnancy Risk Category: C

HOW SUPPLIED
Tablets: 30 mg‡
Capsules: 25 mg, 50 mg
Injection: 25 mg/ml, 50 mg/ml

ACTION
Stimulates alpha- and beta-adrenergic receptors; a direct- and indirect-acting sympathomimetic.

ONSET, PEAK, DURATION
Onset occurs within 5 minutes of I.V. use, 10 to 20 minutes of I.M. use, 15 to 60 minutes after oral use. Peak unknown. Effects persist for 30 minutes to 1 hour after I.M. or S.C. use, 3 to 5 hours after oral use.

INDICATIONS & DOSAGE
To correct hypotension—
Adults: 25 mg 1 to 4 times daily P.O., 25 to 50 mg I.M. or S.C., or 10 to 25 mg I.V. p.r.n. to maximum of 150 mg/24 hours.
Children: 3 mg/kg or 25 to 100 mg/m² S.C. or I.V. daily, in four to six divided doses.
Bronchodilation or nasal decongestion—
Adults and children over 12 years: 12.5 to 25 mg P.O. b.i.d., t.i.d., or q.i.d. Maximum dosage is 150 mg daily in four to six divided doses.
Children 6 to 12 years: 6.25 to 12.5 mg q 4 hours, not to exceed 75 mg in 24 hours.
Children over 2 years: 2 to 3 mg/kg P.O. daily in four to six divided doses.

ADVERSE REACTIONS
CNS: *insomnia, nervousness,* dizziness, headache, muscle weakness, diaphoresis, euphoria, confusion, delirium.
CV: *palpitations,* tachycardia, hypertension, precordial pain.
EENT: dry nose and throat.
GI: nausea, vomiting, anorexia.
GU: urine retention, painful urination due to visceral sphincter spasm.

INTERACTIONS
Acetazolamide: increased serum ephedrine levels. Monitor for toxicity.
Alpha-adrenergic blockers: unopposed beta-adrenergic effects, resulting in hypotension. Avoid concomitant use.
Antihypertensives: decreased effects. Monitor blood pressure.
Beta-adrenergic blockers: unopposed alpha-adrenergic effects, resulting in hypertension. Monitor blood pressure.
Digitalis glycosides, general anesthetics (halogenated hydrocarbons): increased risk of ventricular arrhythmias. Monitor ECG closely.
Ergot alkaloids: enhanced vasoconstrictor activity. Monitor patient closely.

---

*Liquid contains alcohol.   **May contain tartrazine.   †Canada only.   ‡Australia only.   ◊ OTC.

Guanadrel, guanethidine: enhanced pressor effects of ephedrine. Monitor patient closely.

Levodopa: enhanced risk of ventricular arrhythmias. Monitor ECG closely.

MAO inhibitors, tricyclic antidepressants: when given with sympathomimetics, may cause severe hypertension (hypertensive crisis). Monitor patient and blood pressure closely.

Methyldopa, reserpine: may inhibit effects of ephedrine. Use together cautiously.

EFFECTS ON DIAGNOSTIC TESTS
None reported.

CONTRAINDICATIONS
Contraindicated in patients with hypersensitivity to ephedrine and other sympathomimetics; in those with porphyria, severe coronary artery disease, arrhythmias, angle-closure glaucoma, psychoneurosis, angina pectoris, substantial organic heart disease, and CV disease; and in those taking MAO inhibitors.

NURSING CONSIDERATIONS
● Use with extreme caution in elderly men and in those with hypertension, hyperthyroidism, nervous or excitable states, diabetes, and prostatic hyperplasia.

Alert: Know that hypoxia, hypercapnia, and acidosis, which may reduce effectiveness or increase the incidence of adverse reactions, must be identified and corrected before or during ephedrine administration.

● This drug is not a substitute for blood or fluid volume replenishment. Know that volume deficit must be corrected before administering vasopressors.

● **I.V. use:** Give 10 to 25 mg by I.V. injection slowly; repeat in 5 to 10 minutes if necessary. Compatible with most common I.V. solutions.

● To prevent insomnia, avoid giving within 2 hours of bedtime.

● Effectiveness decreases after 2 to 3 weeks, as tolerance develops. Doctor

may need to increase dosage. Drug is not addictive.

☑ **PATIENT TEACHING**
● Tell patient taking oral form of drug at home to take last dose of day at least 2 hours before bedtime.
● Warn patient not to take OTC drugs that contain ephedrine without informing the doctor.

---

epinephrine (adrenaline)
Adrenalin◇, Bronkaid Mist◇, Bronkaid Mistometer†, Primatene Mist◇

epinephrine bitartrate
AsthmaHaler◇, Broniten Mist◇, Bronkaid Mist Suspension◇, Medihaler-Epi◇, Primatene Mist*, Primatene Mist Suspension◇

epinephrine hydrochloride
Adrenalin Chloride◇, Asthma-Nefrin †◇, Epi-Pen, Epi-Pen Jr., Micro-Nefrin †◇, Nephron †◇, Racepinephrine †◇, Sus-Phrine, Vaponefrine

Pregnancy Risk Category: C

HOW SUPPLIED
Aerosol inhaler: 160 mcg◇, 200 mcg◇, 220 mcg◇, 250 mcg/metered spray◇
Nebulizer inhaler: 1% (1:100)†◇, 1.25%†◇, 2.25%†◇
Injection: 0.01 mg/ml (1:100,000), 0.1 mg/ml (1:10,000), 0.5 mg/ml (1:2,000), 1 mg/ml (1:1,000) parenteral; 5 mg/ml (1:200) parenteral suspension

ACTION
Stimulates alpha- and beta-adrenergic receptors within the sympathetic nervous system.

ONSET, PEAK, DURATION
Onset occurs immediately after I.V. injection, 3 to 5 minutes after inhalation, 6 to 15 minutes after S.C. injection,

---

variable after I.M. use. Peak effects occur within 5 minutes of I.V. administration, within 30 minutes of S.C. injection. Effects persist for 1 to 3 hours after inhalation, less than 1 to about 4 hours after parenteral use.

INDICATIONS & DOSAGE

Bronchospasm, hypersensitivity reactions, anaphylaxis—
Adults: 0.1 to 0.5 ml of 1:1,000 S.C. or I.M. Repeated q 10 to 15 minutes, p.r.n. Or 0.1 to 0.25 ml of 1:1,000 (1 to 2.5 ml of a commercially available 1:10,000 injection or of a 1:10,000 dilution prepared by diluting 1 ml of a commercially available 1:1,000 injection with 10 ml of water for injection or 0.9% sodium chloride for injection) I.V. slowly over 5 to 10 minutes.
Children: 0.01 ml (10 mcg) of 1:1,000/kg S.C.; repeated q 20 minutes to 4 hours p.r.n. Or, 0.004 to 0.005 ml/kg of 1:200 (Sus-Phrine) S.C.; repeated q 8 to 12 hours p.r.n.
Hemostasis—
Adults: 1:50,000 to 1:1,000, sprayed or applied topically.
Acute asthmatic attacks—
Adults and children 4 years and over: 160 to 250 mcg (metered aerosol) which is equivalent to one inhalation, repeated once if necessary after at least 1 minute; subsequent doses should not be administered for at least 3 hours. Alternatively, 1% (1:100) solution of epinephrine or 2.25% solution of racepinephrine administered with a hand-bulb nebulizer as one to three deep inhalations, repeated q 3 hours as needed.
To prolong local anesthetic effect—
Adults and children: in conjunction with local anesthetics, may be used in concentrations of 1:500,000 to 1:50,000. The most frequently used concentration is 1:200,000.
To restore cardiac rhythm in cardiac arrest—
Adults: usual adult dose is 0.5 to 1 mg I.V. Doses may be repeated q 3 to 5 minutes if needed. Higher dose epineph-

rine may be used if 1-mg doses fail: 3 to 5 mg (approximately 0.1 mg/kg) doses of epinephrine repeated q 3 to 5 minutes.
Children: usual pediatric dose is 0.01 mg/kg (0.1 ml/kg of 1:10,000 injection) I.V. Usual initial dose through an endotracheal tube is 0.1 mg/kg (0.1 ml/kg of a 1:1,000 injection) diluted in 1 to 2 ml of 0.45% or 0.9% sodium chloride solution. Subsequent I.V. or intratracheal doses range from 0.1 to 0.2 mg/kg (0.1 to 0.2 ml/kg of a 1:1,000 injection). I.V. or intratracheal doses may be repeated q 3 to 5 minutes if needed.
Note: 1 mg equals 1 ml of 1:1,000 or 10 ml of 1:10,000.

ADVERSE REACTIONS
CNS: *nervousness, tremor,* vertigo, *headache,* disorientation, agitation, *drowsiness,* fear, pallor, dizziness, weakness, ***cerebral hemorrhage, CVA.*** In patients with Parkinson's disease, the drug increases rigidity and tremor.
CV: *palpitations;* widened pulse pressure; ***hypertension; tachycardia; ventricular fibrillation; shock;*** anginal pain; ECG changes, including a decreased T-wave amplitude.
GI: *nausea, vomiting.*
Respiratory: dyspnea.
Skin: urticaria, pain, hemorrhage at injection site.

INTERACTIONS
Alpha-adrenergic blockers: hypotension due to unopposed beta-adrenergic effects. Avoid concomitant use.
Antihistamines, thyroid hormones, tricyclic antidepressants: when given with sympathomimetics, may cause severe adverse cardiac effects. Avoid giving together.
Beta blockers, such as propranolol: may cause vasoconstriction and reflex bradycardia. Monitor patient carefully.
Digitalis glycosides, general anesthetics (halogenated hydrocarbons): increased risk of ventricular arrhythmias. Monitor ECG closely.

---

*Liquid contains alcohol.   **May contain tartrazine.   †Canada only.   ‡Australia only.   ◇OTC.

Doxapram, mazindol, methylphenidate: enhanced CNS stimulation or pressor effects. Monitor patient closely.

Ergot alkaloids: enhanced vasoconstrictor activity. Monitor patient closely.

Guanadrel, guanethidine: enhanced pressor effects of epinephrine. Monitor patient closely.

Levodopa: enhanced risk of cardiac arrhythmias. Monitor ECG closely.

MAO inhibitors: increased risk of hypertensive crisis. Monitor blood pressure closely.

EFFECTS ON DIAGNOSTIC TESTS
Epinephrine therapy alters blood glucose and serum lactic acid levels (both may be increased), increases BUN levels, and interferes with tests for urinary catecholamines.

CONTRAINDICATIONS
● Contraindicated in patients with angle-closure glaucoma, shock (other than anaphylactic shock), organic brain damage, cardiac dilation, arrhythmias, coronary insufficiency, or cerebral arteriosclerosis. Also contraindicated in patients during general anesthesia with halogenated hydrocarbons or cyclopropane and in patients in labor (may delay second stage).

● Some commercial products contain sulfites: contraindicated in patients with sulfite allergies except when epinephrine is being used for treatment of serious allergic reactions or other emergency situations.

● In conjunction with local anesthetics, epinephrine is contraindicated for use in fingers, toes, ears, nose, or genitalia.

NURSING CONSIDERATIONS
● Use with extreme caution in patients with long-standing bronchial asthma and emphysema who have developed degenerative heart disease. Also use cautiously in elderly patients and in those with hyperthyroidism, CV disease, hypertension, psychoneurosis, and diabetes.

● Be aware that epinephrine is the drug of choice in emergency treatment of acute anaphylactic reactions.

● Discard epinephrine solutions after 24 hours or if solution is discolored or contains precipitate. Keep solution in light-resistant container, and don't remove before use.

● **I.V. use:** Don't mix with alkaline solutions. Use D_5W, 0.9% sodium chloride for injection, lactated Ringer's injection, or combinations of dextrose in sodium chloride. Mix just before use.

● When administering I.V., monitor blood pressure, heart rate, and ECG when therapy is initiated and frequently thereafter.

Alert: Avoid I.M. administration of parenteral suspension into buttocks. Gas gangrene may occur because epinephrine reduces oxygen tension of the tissues, encouraging the growth of contaminating organisms.

● Massage site after I.M. injection to counteract possible vasoconstriction. Repeated local injection can cause necrosis resulting from vasoconstriction at injection site.

● Observe patients closely for adverse reactions. Notify doctor if adverse reactions develop; he may adjust dosage or discontinue drug.

● Know that if a sharp blood pressure rise occurs, rapid-acting vasodilators, such as nitrites or alpha-adrenergic blockers, can be given to counteract the marked pressor effect of large doses of epinephrine.

● Know that epinephrine is rapidly destroyed by oxidizing agents, such as iodine, chromates, nitrates, nitrites, oxygen, and salts of easily reducible metals (such as iron).

☑ **PATIENT TEACHING**
● Teach patient to perform oral inhalation correctly. Give the following instructions for using a metered-dose inhaler:

　—Clear nasal passages and throat.

—Breathe out, expelling as much air from lungs as possible.

—Place mouthpiece well into mouth as dose from inhaler is released, and inhale deeply.

—Hold breath for several seconds, remove mouthpiece, and exhale slowly.

• If more than one inhalation is ordered, tell patient to wait at least 2 minutes before repeating procedure.

• Tell patient who is also using a steroid inhaler to use the bronchodilator first, then wait about 5 minutes before using steroid. This allows the bronchodilator to open air passages for maximum effectiveness.

• If patient has acute hypersensitivity reactions, such as to bee stings, it may be necessary to instruct him to self-inject epinephrine at home.

ipratropium bromide
Atrovent

Pregnancy Risk Category: B

HOW SUPPLIED
Inhaler: each metered dose supplies 18 mcg

Solution (for inhalation): 0.02% (500 mg/vial)

Solution (for nebulizer): 0.025% (250 mcg/ml)‡

Nasal spray: 0.03% (each metered dose supplies 21 mcg), 0.06% (each metered dose supplies 42 mcg)

ACTION
Inhibits vagally mediated reflexes by antagonizing acetylcholine.

ONSET, PEAK, DURATION
Onset occurs in 5 to 15 minutes. Peak effects occur in 1 to 2 hours. Effects persist usually 3 to 4 hours; up to 6 hours in some patients.

INDICATIONS & DOSAGE
Bronchospasm associated with COPD—

Adults: 1 to 2 inhalations q.i.d. Additional inhalations may be needed. However, total inhalations should not exceed 12 in 24 hours. Alternatively, use inhalation solution. Give 500 mcg dissolved in 0.9% sodium chloride and administer by nebulizer q 6 to 8 hours.

Children 5 to 12 years: give 125 to 250 mcg nebulizer solution dissolved in 0.9% sodium chloride and administer by nebulizer q 6 to 8 hours.

Perennial rhinitis—

Adults and children over 12 years: usual dosage of 0.03% nasal spray is 2 sprays (42 mcg) per nostril two to three times daily.

Common cold-induced rhinorrhea—

Adults and children over 12 years: usual dosage of 0.06% nasal spray is 2 sprays (84 mcg) per nostril three or four times daily.

ADVERSE REACTIONS
CNS: dizziness, headache, nervousness.
CV: palpitations.
EENT: cough, blurred vision, rhinitis, sinusitis.
GI: nausea, GI distress, dry mouth.
Respiratory: *upper respiratory tract infection, bronchitis,* cough, dyspnea, pharyngitis, bronchospasm, increased sputum.
Skin: rash.
Other: pain, back pain, chest pain, flu-like symptoms.

INTERACTIONS
Anticholinergics: increased anticholinergic effects. Avoid concomitant use.

EFFECTS ON DIAGNOSTIC TESTS
None reported.

CONTRAINDICATIONS
Contraindicated in patients with hypersensitivity to the drug or to atropine or any of its derivatives and in those with a history of hypersensitivity to soyalecithin or related food products, such as soybeans and peanuts.

---

*Liquid contains alcohol.   **May contain tartrazine.   †Canada only.   ‡Australia only.   ◊ OTC.

NURSING CONSIDERATIONS

• Use cautiously in patients with angle-closure glaucoma, prostatic hyperplasia, and bladder-neck obstruction.

• If using a face mask for a nebulizer, take care to avoid leakage around the mask; temporary blurring of vision or eye pain may occur.

☑ **PATIENT TEACHING**

• Warn patient that ipratropium bromide is not effective for treating acute episodes of bronchospasm where rapid response is required.

• Teach patient to perform oral inhalation correctly. Give the following instructions for using a metered-dose inhaler:

—Clear nasal passages and throat.

—Breathe out, expelling as much air from lungs as possible.

—Place mouthpiece well into mouth as dose from inhaler is released, and inhale deeply.

—Hold breath for several seconds, remove mouthpiece, and exhale slowly.

• Tell patient to avoid accidentally spraying into eyes. Temporary blurring of vision may result.

• If more than one inhalation is ordered, tell patient to wait at least 2 minutes before repeating procedure.

• Tell patient who is also using a steroid inhaler to use ipratropium first, then wait about 5 minutes before using the steroid. This allows the bronchodilator to open air passages for maximum effectiveness.

• Tell patient to take missed dose as soon as remembered unless it's almost time for the next dose. In that case, he should skip the missed dose and never double dose.

---

isoetharine hydrochloride
Arm-a-Med Isoetharine, Bronkosol, Dey-Dose Isoetharine, Dey-Dose Isoetharine S/F, Dey-Lute Isoetharine S/F, Dispos-a-Med Isoetharine

isoetharine mesylate
Bronkometer

Pregnancy Risk Category: C

HOW SUPPLIED

Aerosol inhaler: 340 mcg/metered spray
Nebulizer inhaler: 0.062%, 0.08%, 0.1%, 0.125%, 0.167%, 0.17%, 0.2%, 0.25%, 0.5%, 1% solution

ACTION

Relaxes bronchial smooth muscle by acting on beta$_2$-adrenergic receptors.

ONSET, PEAK, DURATION

Onset occurs in 1 to 6 minutes. Peak effects occur within 15 to 60 minutes. Effects persist 1 to 4 hours.

INDICATIONS & DOSAGE

Bronchial asthma and reversible bronchospasm that may occur with bronchitis and emphysema—

Adults: *hydrochloride form*—administered by hand nebulizer, oxygen aerosolization, or IPPB. Dosage must be carefully adjusted according to individual requirements and response. Usual adult dose administered through oxygen aerosolization is 0.5 ml (range: 0.25 to 0.5 ml) of a 1% solution, diluted 1:3. Alternatively, undiluted solutions may be given through oxygen aerosolization; usual adult dose is 4 ml (range: 2 to 4 ml) of a 0.125% solution, 2.5 ml of a 0.2% solution, or 2 ml of a 0.25% solution. Usual adult dosage through hand-bulb nebulizer of undiluted 1% solution is 4 inhalations (range: 3 to 7 inhalations).

mesylate form—1 to 2 inhalations. Occasionally, more may be required.

ADVERSE REACTIONS

CNS: *tremor, headache,* dizziness, excitement, anxiety.
CV: *palpitations,* increased heart rate, alterations in blood pressure.
GI: nausea, vomiting.

Reactions may be *common*, uncommon, *life-threatening*, or COMMON AND LIFE-THREATENING.

INTERACTIONS
Cyclopropane, digitalis glycosides, halogenated inhalation anesthetics, levodopa: increased risk of arrhythmias. Monitor closely.
Epinephrine, other sympathomimetics: may cause excessive tachycardia. Don't use together with isoetharine.
Propranolol and other beta blockers: blocked bronchodilating effect of isoetharine. Monitor patient carefully if used together.

EFFECTS ON DIAGNOSTIC TESTS
None reported.

CONTRAINDICATIONS
Contraindicated in patients with hypersensitivity to the drug.

NURSING CONSIDERATIONS
● Use cautiously in patients with hyperthyroidism, hypertension, or coronary disease and in those with hypersensitivity to sympathomimetics.
● Although isoetharine has minimal effects on the heart, know that it should be used cautiously in patients receiving general anesthetics that sensitize the myocardium to sympathomimetic drugs.
Alert: Monitor for severe paradoxical bronchoconstriction after excessive use. If bronchoconstriction occurs, discontinue immediately and notify doctor.

☑ PATIENT TEACHING
● Teach patient to perform oral inhalation correctly. Give the following instructions for using a metered-dose inhaler:
— Shake canister.
— Clear nasal passages and throat.
— Breathe out, expelling as much air from lungs as possible.
— Place mouthpiece well into mouth as dose from inhaler is released, and inhale deeply.
— Hold breath for several seconds, remove mouthpiece, and exhale slowly.
● If more than one inhalation is ordered,

tell patient to wait at least 2 minutes before repeating procedure.
● Tell patient who is also using a steroid inhaler to use the bronchodilator first, then wait about 5 minutes before using the steroid. This allows the bronchodilator to open air passages for maximum effectiveness.
● Because of oxidation of drug when diluted with water, pink sputum mimicking hemoptysis may occur after inhaling isoetharine solution. Tell patient not to be concerned.
● Warn patient that excessive use can lead to decreased effectiveness.

---

isoproterenol (isoprenaline)
Aerolone, Dey-Dose Isoproterenol, Dispos-a-Med Isoproterenol, Isuprel, Medihaler Iso, Vapo-Iso

isoproterenol hydrochloride
Isuprel, Isuprel Glossets, Isuprel Mistometer, Norisodrine Aerotrol

isoproterenol sulfate
Medihaler-Iso

Pregnancy Risk Category: C

HOW SUPPLIED
isoproterenol
Nebulizer inhaler: 0.25%, 0.5%, 1%
isoproterenol hydrochloride
Tablets (sublingual): 10 mg, 15 mg
Aerosol inhaler: 120 mcg or 131 mcg/metered spray
Injection: 20 mcg/ml, 200 mcg/ml
isoproterenol sulfate
Aerosol inhaler: 80 mcg/metered spray

ACTION
Relaxes bronchial smooth muscle by acting on beta$_2$-adrenergic receptors. As a cardiac stimulant, acts on beta$_1$-adrenergic receptors in the heart.

ONSET, PEAK, DURATION
Onset occurs immediately after I.V. use, 2 to 5 minutes after inhalation, 15 to 30

---

*Liquid contains alcohol.   **May contain tartrazine.   †Canada only.   ‡Australia only.   ◇OTC.

minutes after S.L. use. Peak unknown. Effects persist for ½ to 2 hours after inhalation, less than 1 hour after I.V. use, 1 to 2 hours after S.L. use.

INDICATIONS & DOSAGE
Bronchial asthma and reversible bronchospasm—
Adults: 10 to 15 mg hydrochloride S.L. t.i.d. or q.i.d. Daily S.L. dosage should not exceed 60 mg.
Children: 5 to 10 mg hydrochloride S.L. t.i.d. Daily S.L. dosage should not exceed 30 mg.
Bronchospasm—
Adults and children: acute dyspneic episodes: one inhalation of sulfate form initially. Repeated if needed after 2 to 5 minutes. No more than 6 inhalations should be taken during any single hour in a 24-hour period.

Maintenance dosage is one to two inhalations q.i.d. to six times daily.
Bronchospasm in COPD—
Administered via IPPB or for nebulization by compressed air or oxygen.
Adults: 2 ml of 0.125% or 2.5 ml of 0.1% solution (prepared by diluting 0.5 ml of 0.5% solution to 2 or 2.5 ml or by diluting 0.25 ml of 1% solution to 2 or 2.5 ml with water or 0.45% or 0.9% sodium chloride solution) up to five times daily.
Children: 2 ml of a 0.0625% solution or 2.5 ml of 0.05% solution (prepared by diluting 0.25 ml of 0.5% solution to 2 or 2.5 ml with water or 0.45% or 0.9% sodium chloride solution) up to five times daily.
Heart block and ventricular arrhythmias—
Adults: (hydrochloride) initially, 0.02 to 0.06 mg I.V. Subsequent doses 0.01 to 0.2 mg I.V. or 5 mcg/minute I.V.; or 0.2 mg I.M. initially, then 0.02 to 1 mg, p.r.n.
Children: (hydrochloride) I.V. infusion of 2.5 mcg/minute or 0.1 mcg/kg/minute. Dosage is adjusted based on patient's response.

Shock—
Adults and children: (hydrochloride) 0.5 to 5 mcg/minute by continuous I.V. infusion. Usual concentration is 1 mg (5 ml) in 500 ml D_5W. Rate adjusted according to heart rate, central venous pressure (CVP), blood pressure, and urine flow.

ADVERSE REACTIONS
CNS: *headache, mild tremor,* weakness, dizziness, *nervousness,* insomnia, ***Adams-Stokes seizures.***
CV: *palpitations, tachycardia, anginal pain, arrhythmias,* **cardiac arrest,** *rapid rise and fall in blood pressure.*
GI: *nausea, vomiting, heartburn.*
Respiratory: *bronchospasm,* bronchitis, sputum increase, pulmonary edema.
Other: diaphoresis, hyperglycemia; swelling of parotid glands with prolonged use.

INTERACTIONS
Epinephrine, other sympathomimetics: increased risk of arrhythmias. Use together cautiously.
Propranolol and other beta blockers: blocked bronchodilating effect of isoproterenol. Monitor patient carefully if used together.

EFFECTS ON DIAGNOSTIC TESTS
Isoproterenol may reduce sensitivity of spirometry in the diagnosis of asthma.

CONTRAINDICATIONS
Contraindicated in patients with tachycardia caused by digitalis intoxication, in patients with preexisting arrhythmias (other than those that may respond to treatment with isoproterenol), and in those with angina pectoris.

NURSING CONSIDERATIONS
● Use cautiously in elderly patients and in patients with renal or CV disease, coronary insufficiency, diabetes, hyperthyroidism, or history of sensitivity to sympathomimetic amines.
● Know that drug is not a substitute for

blood or fluid volume deficit. Volume deficit should be corrected before administering vasopressors.

● Do not use injection or inhalation solution if it's discolored or contains precipitate.

● **I.V. use:** Give by direct injection or I.V. infusion. For infusion, drug may be diluted with most common I.V. solutions. However, do not use with sodium bicarbonate injection; drug decomposes rapidly in alkaline solutions.

Alert: If heart rate exceeds 110 beats/minute with I.V. infusion, notify the doctor. Doses sufficient to increase the heart rate to more than 130 beats/minute may induce ventricular arrhythmias.

● When administering I.V. isoproterenol to treat shock, closely monitor blood pressure, CVP, ECG, arterial blood gas measurements, and urine output. Carefully adjust infusion rate according to these measurements, as ordered. Use a continuous infusion pump to regulate flow rate.

● If drug is administered via inhalation with oxygen, be sure oxygen concentration will not suppress respiratory drive.

● Follow same instructions for metered powder nebulizer, although deep inhalation is not necessary.

● Be aware that drug may aggravate ventilation-perfusion abnormalities; even while ease of breathing is improved, arterial oxygen tension may fall paradoxically.

● Be aware that isoproterenol may cause a slight rise in systolic blood pressure and a slight to marked drop in diastolic blood pressure.

● Monitor patient for adverse reactions.

☑ **PATIENT TEACHING**
● Teach patient to perform oral inhalation correctly. Give the following instructions for using a metered-dose inhaler:

—Clear nasal passages and throat.
—Breathe out, expelling as much air from lungs as possible.

—Place mouthpiece well into mouth as dose from inhaler is released, and inhale deeply.
—Hold breath for several seconds, remove mouthpiece, and exhale slowly.

● If more than one inhalation is ordered, tell patient to wait at least 2 minutes before repeating procedure.

● Tell patient who is also using a steroid inhaler to use the bronchodilator first, then wait about 5 minutes before using the steroid. This allows the bronchodilator to open air passages for maximum effectiveness.

● Warn patient using oral inhalant that drug may turn sputum and saliva pink.

● Teach patient to take S.L. tablet properly. Instruct patient to hold tablet under tongue and not to swallow saliva until tablet dissolves and is absorbed. Instruct him to rinse mouth with water between doses to help prevent oropharyngeal dryness.

● Caution patient that prolonged use of S.L. tablets can cause tooth decay.

● Tell patient not to use drug at bedtime if possible; it interrupts sleep patterns.

● Tell patient to discontinue drug immediately and notify doctor if drug causes precordial distress or anginal pain or if an increase in chest tightness or dyspnea occurs.

● Patient may develop a tolerance to this drug; warn against overuse.

---

metaproterenol sulfate
Alupent, Arm-A-Med Metaproterenol, Dey-Dose Metaproterenol, Dey-Lute Metaproterenol, Metaprel

Pregnancy Risk Category: C

HOW SUPPLIED
Tablets: 10 mg, 20 mg
Syrup: 10 mg/5 ml
Aerosol inhaler: 0.65 mg/metered spray
Nebulizer inhaler: 0.4%, 0.6%, 5% solution

ACTION
Relaxes bronchial smooth muscle by acting on beta₂-adrenergic receptors.

ONSET, PEAK, DURATION
Onset occurs in 1 minute with oral inhalation, in 5 to 30 minutes with aerosol nebulization, and in 15 minutes with oral administration. Peak effects occur within 1 hour. Effects persist for 1½ hours after inhalation, 1 to 4 hours after oral use.

INDICATIONS & DOSAGE
Acute episodes of bronchial asthma—
Adults and children 12 years and over: 2 to 3 inhalations. Do not repeat inhalations more often than q 3 to 4 hours. Do not exceed 12 inhalations daily.
Bronchial asthma and reversible bronchospasm—
Adults: 20 mg P.O. q 6 to 8 hours.
Children over 9 years or over 27 kg: 20 mg P.O. q 6 to 8 hours.
Children 6 to 9 years or less than 27 kg: 10 mg P.O. q 6 to 8 hours.
Children under 6 years: 1.3 to 2.6 mg/kg/day in divided doses of syrup.
   Alternatively, via IPPB or nebulizer:
Adults and children 12 years and over: 0.2 to 0.3 ml of 5% solution diluted in approximately 2.5 ml of 0.45% or 0.9% sodium chloride or 2.5 ml of a commercially available 0.4% or 0.6% solution q 4 hours p.r.n.
Children 6 to 12 years: 0.1 to 0.2 ml of a 5% solution diluted in 0.9% sodium chloride to final volume of 3 ml q 4 hours p.r.n.

ADVERSE REACTIONS
CNS: *nervousness,* weakness, drowsiness, *tremor,* vertigo, headache.
CV: *tachycardia,* hypertension, palpitations; *cardiac arrest* (with excessive use).
GI: *vomiting, nausea,* heartburn, dry mouth.

Respiratory: paradoxical bronchiolar constriction with excessive use, cough, dry and irritated throat.
Skin: rash, hypersensitivity reactions.

INTERACTIONS
Levodopa: risk of arrhythmias. Avoid concomitant use.
Propranolol, other beta blockers: blocked bronchodilating effect of metaproterenol. Monitor patient carefully if used together.

EFFECTS ON DIAGNOSTIC TESTS
Metaproterenol may reduce the sensitivity of spirometry in the diagnosis of asthma.

CONTRAINDICATIONS
Contraindicated in patients with hypersensitivity to the drug or any of its ingredients and in use during anesthesia with cyclopropane or halogenated hydrocarbon general anesthetics and in those with tachycardia and arrhythmias associated with tachycardia, peripheral or mesenteric vascular thrombosis, profound hypoxia or hypercapnia.

NURSING CONSIDERATIONS
● Use cautiously in patients with hypertension, hyperthyroidism, heart disease, diabetes, or cirrhosis and in those who are receiving digitalis glycosides.
● Be aware that patients may use tablets and aerosol concomitantly. Monitor closely for toxicity.
● Know that inhalant solution can be administered by IPPB with drug diluted in 0.9% sodium chloride solution or with a hand nebulizer at full strength.

☑ PATIENT TEACHING
● Teach patient to perform oral inhalation correctly. Give the following instructions for using a metered-dose inhaler:
   —Shake canister.
   —Clear nasal passages and throat.
   —Breathe out, expelling as much air from lungs as possible.

Reactions may be *common,* uncommon, *life-threatening,* or COMMON AND LIFE-THREATENING.

—Place mouthpiece well into mouth as dose from inhaler is released, and inhale deeply.

—Hold breath for several seconds, remove mouthpiece, and exhale slowly. Allow two minutes between inhalations.

● Store drug in light-resistant container.
● Tell patient that metaproterenol inhalations should precede steroid inhalations (when prescribed) by 10 to 15 minutes to maximize therapy.
● Tell patient who is also using a steroid inhaler to use the bronchodilator first, then wait about 5 minutes before using the steroid. This allows bronchodilator to open air passages for maximum effectiveness.
● If more than one inhalation is ordered, tell patient to wait at least 2 minutes before repeating procedure.
● Warn patient to discontinue immediately if paradoxical bronchospasm occurs and to notify doctor.
● Warn patient to notify doctor if no response is derived from dosage or to request dosage adjustment.

---

oxtriphylline (choline salt of theophyllinate)
Choledyl*

Pregnancy Risk Category: C

HOW SUPPLIED
Tablets: 100 mg, 200 mg
Tablets (extended-release): 400 mg, 600 mg
Tablets (delayed-release): 200 mg
Elixir:* 100 mg/5 ml
Syrup: 50 mg/5 ml

ACTION
Inhibits phosphodiesterase, the enzyme that degrades cAMP. Results in relaxation of smooth muscle of the bronchial airways and pulmonary blood vessels. Oxtriphylline is equivalent to 64% anhydrous theophylline.

ONSET, PEAK, DURATION
Onset and duration unknown. Peak effects occur within 1 hour after oral solution, within 2 hours of oral tablets.

INDICATIONS & DOSAGE
Acute bronchial asthma and reversible bronchospasm associated with chronic bronchitis and emphysema—
Adults (nonsmokers): 4.7 mg/kg P.O. q 8 hours.
Adults (smokers) and children 9 to 16 years: 4.7 mg/kg q 6 hours.
Children 1 to 9 years: 6.2 mg/kg P.O. q 6 hours.
    If total daily maintenance dosage is established at approximately 800 to 1,200 mg, one sustained-action tablet q 12 hours may be substituted.

ADVERSE REACTIONS
CNS: *restlessness, dizziness,* headache, *insomnia,* irritability, *seizures,* muscle twitching.
CV: *palpitations, sinus tachycardia,* extrasystoles, flushing, marked hypotension, arrhythmias.
GI: *nausea, vomiting,* epigastric pain, diarrhea.
Respiratory: tachypnea, *respiratory arrest.*

INTERACTIONS
Adenosine: decreased antiarrhythmic effectiveness. Higher doses of adenosine may be necessary.
Allopurinol (high-dose): increased serum theophylline levels. Monitor for toxicity.
Barbiturates, carbamazepine, nicotine, phenytoin, rifampin: enhanced metabolism and decreased theophylline blood levels. Monitor for decreased effect.
Beta-adrenergic blockers: antagonism. Propranolol and nadolol, especially, may cause bronchospasm in sensitive patients. Use together cautiously.
Cimetidine, influenza virus vaccine, macrolide antibiotics (such as erythromycin), oral contraceptives, quinolone antibiotics (such as ciprofloxacin): de-

---

*Liquid contains alcohol.   **May contain tartrazine.   †Canada only.   ‡Australia only.   ◊OTC.

creased hepatic clearance of theophylline; elevated theophylline levels. Monitor for signs of toxicity.
Lithium: increased renal excretion of lithium. Monitor for decreased effect.

EFFECTS ON DIAGNOSTIC TESTS
Oxtriphylline may falsely elevate serum uric acid levels measured by colorimetric methods. Theophylline levels may be falsely elevated in patients using furosemide, phenylbutazone, probenecid, some cephalosporins, sulfa medications, theobromine, caffeine, tea, chocolate, cola beverages, and acetaminophen, depending on assay method used.

CONTRAINDICATIONS
Contraindicated in patients with hypersensitivity to xanthines (caffeine, theobromine) and in patients with preexisting arrhythmias, especially tachyarrhythmias.

NURSING CONSIDERATIONS
● Use cautiously in young children, in elderly patients, and in those with peptic ulceration, COPD, cardiac failure, cor pulmonale, renal or hepatic impairment, glaucoma, severe hypoxemia, hypertension, compromised cardiac or circulatory function, angina, acute MI, sulfite sensitivity, hyperthyroidism, and diabetes mellitus.
● Do not combine with products containing ephedrine; excessive CNS stimulation (nervousness, tremor, akathisia) may result.
● Administer drug after meals and at bedtime.
● Know that oxtriphylline is a soluble salt of theophylline. Dosage is adjusted by monitoring response, tolerance, pulmonary function, and serum theophylline levels. Ensure that theophylline concentrations range from 10 to 20 mcg/ml; toxicity has been reported with levels above 20 mcg/ml.
● Monitor therapy carefully. Individuals metabolize theophyllines at different rates. Dosage adjustments are necessary

in elderly patients; in those with CHF, cor pulmonale, and hepatic disease; and in smokers.
● Store at 15° to 30° C (59° to 86° F). Protect elixir from light and tablets from moisture.

☑ PATIENT TEACHING
● Tell patient to report GI distress, palpitations, irritability, restlessness, nervousness, or insomnia; may indicate excessive CNS stimulation.
● Tell patient that tablets should not be chewed, crushed, or dissolved. Instruct him when to take drug.

pirbuterol
Maxair, Maxair Autohaler

Pregnancy Risk Category: C

HOW SUPPLIED
Inhaler: 0.2 mg/metered dose

ACTION
Relaxes bronchial smooth muscle by acting on beta₂-adrenergic receptors.

ONSET, PEAK, DURATION
Onset occurs within 5 minutes. Peak effects occur in 30 to 60 minutes. Effects persist for 5 hours.

INDICATIONS & DOSAGE
Prevention and reversal of bronchospasm, asthma—
Adults and children 12 years and over: 1 or 2 inhalations (0.2 to 0.4 mg) repeated q 4 to 6 hours. Not to exceed 12 inhalations daily.

ADVERSE REACTIONS
CNS: tremor, nervousness, dizziness, insomnia, headache, vertigo.
CV: tachycardia, palpitations, chest tightness.
EENT: dry or irritated throat, dry mouth, cough.
GI: nausea, vomiting, diarrhea.

Reactions may be *common,* uncommon, *life-threatening,* or COMMON AND LIFE-THREATENING.

INTERACTIONS
MAO inhibitors, tricyclic antidepressants: may potentiate action of beta-adrenergic agonist on vascular system. Use together cautiously.
Propranolol, beta-adrenergic blockers: decreased bronchodilating effects. Avoid concomitant use.

EFFECTS ON DIAGNOSTIC TESTS
None reported.

CONTRAINDICATIONS
Contraindicated in patients with hypersensitivity to pirbuterol.

NURSING CONSIDERATION
Use cautiously in patients with CV disorders, hyperthyroidism, diabetes, and seizure disorders or in those who are unusually responsive to sympathomimetic amines.

☑ PATIENT TEACHING
● Teach patient to perform oral inhalation correctly. Give the following instructions for using a metered-dose inhaler:
—Clear nasal passages and throat.
—Breathe out, expelling as much air from lungs as possible.
—Place mouthpiece well into mouth as dose from inhaler is released, and inhale deeply.
—Hold breath for several seconds, remove mouthpiece, and exhale slowly.
● If more than one inhalation is ordered, tell patient to wait at least 2 minutes before repeating procedure.
● Give the following instructions for using an autohaler:
—Remove mouthpiece cover by pulling down lip on back cover. Inspect mouthpiece for foreign objects. Locate "Up" arrows and air vents.
—Hold autohaler upright so arrows point up while raising lever until it snaps into place.
—Hold autohaler around the middle, and shake gently several times.
—Continue to hold upright and not block air vents at bottom. Exhale normally before use.
—Seal lips around mouthpiece. Inhale deeply through mouthpiece with steady, moderate force. A click will be heard and a soft puff will be felt when inhaling triggers the release of medication. Continue to take a full, deep breath.
—Take autohaler away from mouth when done inhaling. Hold breath for 10 seconds; then exhale slowly.
—Continue to hold autohaler upright while lowering lever. Lower lever after each puff. If additional puffs are ordered, wait one minute between each puff and repeat process.
● Tell patient who is also using a steroid inhaler to use the bronchodilator first, then wait about 5 minutes before using the steroid. This allows the bronchodilator to open air passages for maximum effectiveness.
● Tell patient who experiences increased bronchospasm after using drug to call the doctor.
● Advise patient to seek medical attention if a previously effective dosage does not control symptoms; this may signify worsening of the disease.

salmeterol xinafoate
Serevent

Pregnancy Risk Category: C

HOW SUPPLIED
Inhalation aerosol: 21 mcg/metered spray

ACTION
Not clearly defined. Selectively activates beta$_2$-adrenergic receptors, which results in bronchodilation. Also blocks the release of allergic mediators from mast cells lining the respiratory tract.

ONSET, PEAK, DURATION
Onset occurs in 10 to 20 minutes. Peak effects occur after about 3 hours; plasma levels peak within 45 minutes, but drug acts locally in the lung and its action is not dependent on plasma levels. Effects persist about 12 hours.

INDICATIONS & DOSAGE
Long-term maintenance treatment of asthma; prevention of bronchospasm in patients with nocturnal asthma or reversible obstructive airway disease who require regular treatment with short-acting beta agonists—
Adults and children over 12 years: 2 inhalations q 12 hours, 1 in the morning and 1 in the evening.

    Not for use to treat acute symptoms.
Prevention of exercise-induced bronchospasm—
Adults and children 12 years and over: 2 inhalations at least 30 to 60 minutes before exercise.

ADVERSE REACTIONS
CNS: *headache,* sinus headache, tremor, nervousness, giddiness.
CV: tachycardia, palpitations, ventricular arrhythmias.
EENT: *upper respiratory infection, nasopharyngitis,* nasal cavity or sinus disorder.
GI: nausea, vomiting, diarrhea, heartburn.
Respiratory: cough, lower respiratory infection, ***bronchospasm.***
Other: hypersensitivity reactions (rash, urticaria), joint and back pain, myalgia.

INTERACTIONS
Beta-adrenergic agonists, theophylline, other methylxanthines: possible adverse cardiac effects with excessive use. Monitor closely.
MAO inhibitors: risk of severe adverse CV effects. Avoid use within 14 days of MAO therapy.
Tricyclic antidepressants: risk of moderate to severe adverse CV effects. Use with extreme caution.

EFFECTS ON DIAGNOSTIC TESTS
None reported.

CONTRAINDICATIONS
Contraindicated in patients with hypersensitivity to the drug or any component of the formulation.

NURSING CONSIDERATION
Use cautiously in patients with coronary insufficiency, arrhythmias, hypertension, other CV disorders, thyrotoxicosis, or seizure disorders and in patients who are unusually responsive to sympathomimetics.

☑ PATIENT TEACHING
● Remind patient to take drug at approximately 12-hour intervals for optimum effect and to take the drug even when feeling better.
● If the patient is taking the drug to prevent exercise-induced bronchospasm, tell him he should take it 30 to 60 minutes before exercise.
Alert: Tell patient that although this drug is a beta agonist, it should not be used to treat acute bronchospasm. He must be provided with a short-acting beta agonist (such as albuterol) to treat such exacerbations.
● Tell patient to contact the doctor if the short-acting agonist no longer provides sufficient relief or if more than four inhalations are needed per day. This may be a sign that the asthma symptoms are worsening. Tell him not to increase the dosage of salmeterol.
● If patient is taking an inhaled corticosteroid, he should continue to use it on a regular basis. Warn patient not to take any other medications without the doctor's consent.

---

terbutaline sulfate
Brethaire, Brethine, Bricanyl

Pregnancy Risk Category: B

HOW SUPPLIED
Tablets: 2.5 mg, 5 mg
Aerosol inhaler: 200 mcg/metered spray
Injection: 1 mg/ml

ACTION
Relaxes bronchial smooth muscle by acting on beta$_2$-adrenergic receptors. Also relaxes uterine muscle.

ONSET, PEAK, DURATION
Onset occurs within 15 minutes of S.C. injection, 5 to 30 minutes after inhalation, 1 to 2 hours after oral use. Peak effects occur within 30 minutes to 1 hour of S.C. injection, 1 to 2 hours after inhalation, or 2 to 3 hours after oral use. Effects persist about 1½ to 4 hours after S.C. injection, 3 to 6 hours after inhalation, or 4 to 8 hours after oral use.

INDICATIONS & DOSAGE
Bronchospasm in patients with reversible obstructive airway disease—
Adults and children 12 years and older: dosage varies with dosage form.
Aerosol inhaler—2 inhalations separated by 60-second interval, repeated q 4 to 6 hours.
Injection—0.25 mg S.C. May be repeated in 15 to 30 minutes p.r.n. Dosage should not exceed 0.5 mg in 4 hours.
Tablets in adults—2.5 to 5 mg P.O. q 6 hours t.i.d. during waking hours. Maximum dosage is 15 mg/day.
Tablets in children 12 to 15 years—2.5 mg P.O. q 6 hours t.i.d. during waking hours. Maximum dosage is 7.5 mg/day. Not recommended for children under age 12.

ADVERSE REACTIONS
CNS: *nervousness, tremor, drowsiness, dizziness, headache,* weakness.
CV: *palpitations,* tachycardia, arrhythmias, flushing.
EENT: dry and irritated nose and throat (with inhaled form).
GI: *vomiting, nausea,* heartburn.

Respiratory: *paradoxical bronchospasm with prolonged usage,* dyspnea.
Other: hypokalemia (with high doses), diaphoresis.

INTERACTIONS
CNS stimulants: increased CNS stimulation. Avoid concomitant use.
Cyclopropane, digitalis glycosides, halogenated inhalation anesthetics, levodopa: increased risk of arrhythmias. Monitor closely, and avoid concomitant use with levodopa.
MAO inhibitors: when given with sympathomimetics, may cause severe hypertension (hypertensive crisis). Don't use together.
Propranolol, other beta blockers: blocked bronchodilating effects of terbutaline. Avoid concomitant use.

EFFECTS ON DIAGNOSTIC TESTS
Terbutaline may reduce the sensitivity of spirometry for the diagnosis of bronchospasm.

CONTRAINDICATIONS
Contraindicated in patients with hypersensitivity to the drug or sympathomimetic amines.

NURSING CONSIDERATIONS
● Use cautiously in patient with CV disorders, hyperthyroidism, diabetes, or seizure disorders.
● Give S.C. injections in lateral deltoid area.
● Protect injection from light. Do not use if discolored.
● Know that patients may use tablets and aerosol concomitantly. Monitor closely for toxicity.

☑ PATIENT TEACHING
● Ensure that patient and caregivers understand why drug is necessary.
● Teach patient to perform oral inhalation correctly. Give the following instructions for using a metered-dose inhaler:

---

*Liquid contains alcohol.   **May contain tartrazine.   †Canada only.   ‡Australia only.   ◇OTC.

—Clear nasal passages and throat.
—Breathe out, expelling as much air from lungs as possible.
—Place mouthpiece well into mouth as dose from inhaler is released, and inhale deeply.
—Hold breath for several seconds, remove mouthpiece, and exhale slowly.

• If more than one inhalation is ordered, tell patient to wait at least 2 minutes before repeating procedure.

• Tell patient who is also using a steroid inhaler to use bronchodilator first, then wait about 5 minutes before using steroid. This allows bronchodilator to open air passages for maximum effectiveness.

• Warn patient to discontinue the drug immediately and notify doctor if paradoxical bronchospasm occurs.

• Warn patient that tolerance may develop with prolonged use.

---

theophylline

Immediate-release liquids: Accurbron*, Aquaphyllin, Asmalix*, Bronkodyl*, Elixicon, Elixomin*, Elixophyllin*, Lanophyllin*, Lixolin, Slo-Phyllin, Theolair Liquid, Theon*

Immediate-release tablets and capsules: Bronkodyl, Elixophyllin, Nuelin‡, Slo-Phyllin, Somophyllin-T

Timed-release tablets: Constant-T, Duraphyl, Quibron-T/SR, Respbid, Sustaire, Theo-Dur, Theolair-SR, Theo-Time, Uniphyl

Timed-release capsules: Aerolate, Elixophyllin SR, Nuelin-SR‡, Slo-bid Gyrocaps, Slo-Phyllin, Somophyllin-CRT, Theo-24, Theobid Duracaps, Theobid Jr. Duracaps, Theochron, Theo-Dur Sprinkle, Theospan-SR, Theovent Long-Acting

theophylline sodium glycinate
Acet-Am†

Pregnancy Risk Category: C

HOW SUPPLIED
theophylline
Tablets: 100 mg, 125 mg, 200 mg, 250 mg, 300 mg
Tablets (chewable): 100 mg
Tablets (extended-release): 100 mg, 200 mg, 250 mg, 300 mg, 400 mg, 450 mg, 500 mg
Capsules: 100 mg, 200 mg
Capsules (extended-release): 50 mg, 60 mg, 65 mg, 75 mg, 100 mg, 125 mg, 130 mg, 200 mg, 250 mg, 260 mg, 300 mg
Elixir: 27 mg/5 ml, 50 mg/5 ml*
Oral solution: 27 mg/5 ml, 50 mg/5 ml
Syrup: 27 mg/5 ml, 50 mg/5 ml
Dextrose 5% injection: 200 mg in 50 ml or 100 ml; 400 mg in 100 ml, 250 ml, 500 ml, or 1,000 ml; 800 mg in 500 ml or 1,000 ml
theophylline sodium glycinate
Elixir: 110 mg/5 ml (equivalent to 55 mg anhydrous theophylline/5 ml)

ACTION
Inhibits phosphodiesterase, the enzyme that degrades cAMP. Results in relaxation of smooth muscle of the bronchial airways and pulmonary blood vessels.

ONSET, PEAK, DURATION
Onset occurs within 15 minutes of I.V. use, 15 minutes to 1 hour after oral use. Peak effects occur 15 to 30 minutes after I.V. use; 1 to 2 hours after oral use, except for enteric-coated tablets (peak in about 5 hours) and extended-release capsules and tablets (peak in 4 to 7 hours). Duration unknown.

INDICATIONS & DOSAGE
Extended-release preparations should not be used for the treatment of acute bronchospasm.

Reactions may be *common,* uncommon, ***life-threatening,*** or COMMON AND LIFE-THREATENING.

Oral theophylline for acute bronchospasm in patients not currently receiving theophylline—

Adults (nonsmokers): 6 mg/kg P.O., followed by 2 to 3 mg/kg q 6 hours for 2 doses. Maintenance dosage is 3 mg/kg q 8 hours.

Otherwise healthy adult smokers: 6 mg/kg P.O., followed by 3 mg/kg q 4 hours for 3 doses. Maintenance dosage is 3 mg/kg q 6 hours.

Older adults with cor pulmonale: 6 mg/kg P.O., followed by 2 mg/kg q 6 hours for 2 doses. Maintenance dosage is 2 mg/kg q 8 hours.

Adults with CHF or liver disease: 6 mg/kg P.O., followed by 2 mg/kg q 8 hours for 2 doses. Maintenance dosage is 1 to 2 mg/kg q 12 hours.

Children 9 to 16 years: 6 mg/kg P.O., followed by 3 mg/kg q 4 hours for 3 doses. Maintenance dosage is 3 mg/kg q 6 hours.

Children 6 months to 9 years: 6 mg/kg P.O., followed by 4 mg/kg q 4 hours for 3 doses. Maintenance dosage is 4 mg/kg q 6 hours.

Parenteral theophylline for patients not currently receiving theophylline—

Loading dose: 4.7 mg/kg I.V. slowly; then maintenance infusion.

Adults (nonsmokers): 0.55 mg/kg/hour I.V. for 12 hours, then 0.39 mg/kg/hour.

Otherwise healthy adult smokers: 0.79 mg/kg/hour I.V. for 12 hours; then 0.63 mg/kg/hour.

Older adults with cor pulmonale: 0.47 mg/kg/hour I.V. for 12 hours; then 0.24 mg/kg/hour.

Adults with CHF or liver disease: 0.39 mg/kg/hour I.V. for 12 hours; then 0.08 to 0.16 mg/kg/hour.

Children 9 to 16 years: 0.79 mg/kg/hour I.V. for 12 hours; then 0.63 mg/kg/hour.

Children 6 months to 9 years: 0.95 mg/kg/hour I.V. for 12 hours; then 0.79 mg/kg/hour.

Oral and parenteral theophylline for acute bronchospasm in patients currently receiving theophylline—

Adults and children: each 0.5 mg/kg I.V. or P.O. (loading dose) will increase plasma levels by 1 mcg/ml. Ideally, dose is based on current theophylline level. In emergency situations, some clinicians recommend a 2.5 mg/kg P.O. dose of rapidly absorbed form if no obvious signs of theophylline toxicity are present.

Chronic bronchospasm—

Adults and children: Initial dosage is 16 mg/kg or 400 mg P.O. daily (whichever is less) given in three or four divided doses at 6- to 8- hour intervals. Alternatively, 12 mg/kg or 400 mg P.O. daily (whichever is less) in an extended-release preparation given in two or three divided doses at 8- or 12-hour intervals. Dosage increased as tolerated at 2- to 3-day intervals to maximum dosage as follows:

Adults and children 16 years and over: 13 mg/kg or 900 mg P.O. daily (whichever is less).

Children 12 to 16 years: 18 mg/kg P.O. daily.

Children 9 to 12 years: 20 mg/kg P.O. daily.

Children under 9 years: 24 mg/kg P.O. daily.

ADVERSE REACTIONS

CNS: *restlessness, dizziness,* headache, *insomnia,* irritability, *seizures,* muscle twitching.

CV: *palpitations, sinus tachycardia,* extrasystoles, flushing, marked hypotension, arrhythmias.

GI: *nausea, vomiting,* diarrhea, epigastric pain.

Respiratory: tachypnea, *respiratory arrest.*

INTERACTIONS

Adenosine: decreased antiarrhythmic effectiveness. Higher doses of adenosine may be necessary.

Barbiturates, carbamazepine, nicotine, phenytoin, rifampin: enhanced metabolism and decreased theophylline blood levels. Monitor for decreased effect.
Beta-adrenergic blockers: antagonism. Propranolol and nadolol, especially, may cause bronchospasm in sensitive patients. Use together cautiously.
Calcium channel blockers, cimetidine, disulfiram, influenza virus vaccine, interferon, macrolide antibiotics (such as erythromycin), oral contraceptives, quinolone antibiotics (such as ciprofloxacin), caffeine: decreased hepatic clearance of theophylline; elevated theophylline levels. Monitor for signs of toxicity.

Patients taking Theo-24 should take it on an empty stomach because food accelerates the drug's absorption.

EFFECTS ON DIAGNOSTIC TESTS
Theophylline increases plasm-free fatty acids and urinary catecholamines. Depending on assay used, theophylline levels may be falsely elevated in the presence of furosemide, phenylbutazone, probenecid, theobromine, caffeine, tea, chocolate, cola beverages, and acetaminophen.

CONTRAINDICATIONS
Contraindicated in patients with hypersensitivity to xanthine compounds (caffeine, theobromine) and in those with active peptic ulcer and seizure disorders.

NURSING CONSIDERATIONS
● Use cautiously in young children, infants under 1 year, and neonates; in elderly patients; and in those with COPD, cardiac failure, cor pulmonale, renal or hepatic disease, peptic ulceration, hyperthyroidism, diabetes mellitus, glaucoma, severe hypoxemia, hypertension, compromised cardiac or circulatory function, angina, acute MI, or sulfite sensitivity.
● Be careful not to confuse extended-release dosage forms with regular-release dosage forms.
● **I.V. use:** Use commercially available infusion solution, or mix in D_5W. Use infusion pump for continuous infusion.
● Know that drug dosage may need to be increased in cigarette smokers and in habitual marijuana smokers because smoking causes the drug to be metabolized faster.
● Give drug around-the-clock, using extended-release product at bedtime, as ordered.
● Monitor vital signs; measure and record fluid intake and output. Expected clinical effects include improved quality of pulse and respirations.
● Know that individuals metabolize xanthines at different rates; dosage is determined by monitoring response, tolerance, pulmonary function, and serum theophylline levels. Serum theophylline concentrations should range from 10 to 20 mcg/ml; toxicity has been reported with levels above 20 mcg/ml.

☑ **PATIENT TEACHING**
● Supply instructions for home care and dosage schedule.
● Warn patient not to dissolve, crush, or chew extended-release products. Small children unable to swallow these can ingest (without chewing) the contents of capsules sprinkled over soft food.
● Tell patient to relieve GI symptoms by taking oral drug with full glass of water after meals, although food in stomach delays absorption.
● Warn patient to take the drug regularly, as directed. Patients tend to want to take extra "breathing pills."
● Warn elderly patient that dizziness, a common adverse reaction at start of therapy, may occur.
● Warn patient to check with the doctor or pharmacist about *any* other drugs used. OTC remedies may contain ephedrine in combination with theophylline salts; excessive CNS stimulation may result.

Expectorants and antitussives

benzonatate
codeine phosphate
  (See Chapter 28, NARCOTIC AND OPI-
  OID ANALGESICS.)
codeine sulfate
  (See Chapter 28, NARCOTIC AND OPI-
  OID ANALGESICS.)
**dextromethorphan hydrobro-
mide**
diphenhydramine hydrochloride
  (See Chapter 43, ANTIHISTAMINES.)
guaifenesin
hydromorphone hydrochloride
  (See Chapter 28, NARCOTIC AND OPI-
  OID ANALGESICS.)

COMBINATION PRODUCTS
Preparations are available in the following combinations:
● expectorants with decongestants or
antihistamines, or both
● antitussives with decongestants or antihistamines, or both
● expectorants and antitussives
● expectorants and antitussives with decongestants or antihistamines, or both

---

benzonatate
Tessalon

Pregnancy Risk Category: C

HOW SUPPLIED
Capsules: 100 mg

ACTION
Suppresses the cough reflex by direct
action on the cough center in the medulla through an anesthetic action.

ONSET, PEAK, DURATION
Onset occurs in 15 to 20 minutes. Peak
unknown. Effects persist for up to 8
hours.

INDICATIONS & DOSAGE
Symptomatic relief of cough—
Adults and children over 10 years:
100 P.O. t.i.d.; up to 600 mg daily may
be needed.

ADVERSE REACTIONS
CNS: dizziness, headache, sedation.
EENT: nasal congestion, burning sensa-
tion in eyes.
GI: nausea, constipation, GI upset.
Skin: hypersensitivity reactions (rash).
Other: chills.

INTERACTIONS
None significant.

EFFECTS ON DIAGNOSTIC TESTS
None reported.

CONTRAINDICATIONS
Contraindicated in patients hypersensitive to the drug or related compounds.
Use cautiously in patients hypersensitive to paraminobenzoic acid anesthetics
(procaine, tetracaine) because cross-sensitivity reactions may occur.

NURSING CONSIDERATIONS
● Don't use benzonatate when cough is
a valuable diagnostic sign or is beneficial (as after thoracic surgery).
● Monitor cough type and frequency.
● Use with percussion and chest vibration.

☑ PATIENT TEACHING
● Warn patient not to chew capsules or
dissolve in mouth. Produces either local
anesthesia that may result in aspiration
or CNS stimulation that may cause restlessness, tremor, and seizures.
● Instruct patient to report adverse reactions.

---

*Liquid contains alcohol.   **May contain tartrazine.   †Canada only.   ‡Australia only.   ◇OTC.

dextromethorphan hydrobromide

Balminil D.M.◊, Benylin DM◊, Broncho-Grippol-DM†, Children's Hold◊, DM Syrup◊, Hold◊, Koffex†, Mediquell◊, Neo-DM†, Ornex-DM 15◊, Ornex-DM 30◊, Pertussin Cough Suppressant◊, Pertussin CS◊, Pertussin ES◊, Robidex†, Robitussin Pediatric◊, Sedatuss†, St. Joseph Cough Suppressant for Children◊, Sucrets Cough Control Formula◊, Trocal◊, Vicks Formula 44 Pediatric Formula◊.

More commonly available in combination products, such as:
Anti-Tuss DM Expectorant◊, Baytussin DM◊, Benylin Expectorant Cough Formula◊, Cheracol D Cough◊, Codistan No. 1◊, Efficol Cough Whip◊, 2/G-DM Cough◊, Glycotuss dM◊, Guiamid D.M. Liquid◊, Guiatuss-DM◊, Halotussin-DM Expectorant◊, Kolephrin GG/DM◊, Mytussin DM◊, Naldecon Senior DX◊, Pertussin All-Night CS◊, Rhinosyn-DMX Expectorant◊, Robitussin-DM◊, Scot-Tussin DM Cough Chaser◊, Silexin Cough◊, Tolu-Sed DM◊, Tuss-DM◊, Unproco◊, Vicks Pediatric Formula 44E◊

Pregnancy Risk Category: C

HOW SUPPLIED
Liquid (extended-release): 30 mg/5 ml◊
Lozenges: 5 mg◊, 7.5 mg◊
Solution: 3.5 mg/5 ml, 5 mg/5 ml*◊, 7.5 mg/5 ml*◊, 10 mg/5 ml*◊, 15 mg/5 ml*◊, 15 mg/15 ml*◊

ACTION
An antitussive that suppresses the cough reflex by direct action on the cough center in the medulla.

ONSET, PEAK, DURATION
Onset occurs within 30 minutes. Peak unknown. Effects persist 3 to 6 hours with conventional dosage forms; up to 12 hours with extended-release forms.

INDICATIONS & DOSAGE
Nonproductive cough—
Adults and children 12 years and over: 10 to 20 mg P.O. q 4 hours, or 30 mg q 6 to 8 hours. Or, 60 mg extended-release liquid b.i.d. Maximum dosage is 120 mg daily.
Children 6 to 12 years: 5 to 10 mg P.O. q 4 hours, or 15 mg q 6 to 8 hours. Or, 30 mg extended-release liquid b.i.d. Maximum dosage is 60 mg daily.
Children 2 to 6 years: 2.5 to 5 mg P.O. q 4 hours, or 7.5 mg q 6 to 8 hours. Or, 15 mg extended-release liquid b.i.d. Maximum dosage is 30 mg daily.
  Dosages for children under 2 years must be individualized.

ADVERSE REACTIONS
CNS: drowsiness, dizziness.
GI: nausea, vomiting, stomach pain.

INTERACTIONS
MAO inhibitors: risk of hypotension, coma, hyperpyrexia, and death. Avoid concomitant use.

EFFECTS ON DIAGNOSTIC TESTS
None reported.

CONTRAINDICATIONS
Contraindicated in patients currently taking MAO inhibitors or within 2 weeks of discontinuing MAO inhibitors.

NURSING CONSIDERATIONS
● Use with caution in atopic children, sedated or debilitated patients, and in patients confined to the supine position. Also, use cautiously in patients with aspirin sensitivity.
● Don't use dextromethorphan when cough is a valuable diagnostic sign or is beneficial (as after thoracic surgery).
● Know that dextromethorphan 15 to 30 mg is equivalent to 8 to 15 mg codeine as an antitussive.

Reactions may be *common*, uncommon, ***life-threatening***, or COMMON AND LIFE-THREATENING.

• Be aware that drug produces no analgesia or addiction and little or no CNS depression.
• Use drug with chest percussion and vibration.
• Monitor cough type and frequency.

☑ PATIENT TEACHING
• Instruct patient to take exactly as prescribed.
• Tell patient to report adverse reactions.

---

guaifenesin (glyceryl guaiacolate)

Anti-Tuss*◇, Balminil Expectorant†, Baytussin◇, Breonesin◇, Cremacoat 2◇, Gee-Gee◇, GG-CEN*◇, Glyate*◇, Glycotuss◇, Glytuss◇, Guiatuss*◇, Halotussin, Humibid L.A.◇, Hytussin◇, Hytuss-2X◇, Naldecon Senior EX◇, Neo-Spec†, Nortussin◇, Resyl†◇, Robafen◇, Robitussin*◇, S-T Expectorant◇

Pregnancy Risk Category: C

HOW SUPPLIED
Tablets: 100 mg◇, 200 mg◇
Tablets (extended-release): 600 mg
Capsules: 200 mg◇
Capsules (extended-release): 300 mg
Solution: 100 mg/5 ml*◇, 200 mg/5 ml*◇

ACTION
Increases production of respiratory tract fluids to help liquefy and reduce the viscosity of tenacious secretions.

ONSET, PEAK, DURATION
Unknown.

INDICATIONS & DOSAGE
Expectorant—
Adults and children 12 years and over: 200 to 400 mg P.O. q 4 hours, or 600 to 1,200 mg extended-release capsules q 12 hours. Maximum dosage is 2,400 mg daily.

Children 2 to 6 years: 50 to 100 mg P.O. q 4 hours. Maximum dosage is 600 mg daily.
Children 6 to 12 years: 100 to 200 mg P.O. q 4 hours. Maximum dosage is 1,200 mg daily.

ADVERSE REACTIONS
CNS: dizziness, headache.
GI: vomiting and nausea (with large doses).
Skin: rash.

INTERACTIONS
None significant.

EFFECTS ON DIAGNOSTIC TESTS
Guaifenesin may cause color interference with tests for 5-hydroxyindoleacetic acid and vanillylmandelic acid.

CONTRAINDICATIONS
Contraindicated in patients hypersensitive to the drug.

NURSING CONSIDERATIONS
• Be aware that drug is used to liquefy thick, tenacious sputum. Evidence that guaifenesin is effective as expectorant but no evidence to support role an antitussive.
• Monitor cough type and frequency.

☑ PATIENT TEACHING
Alert: Ensure that patient understands that persistent cough may indicate a serious condition and that he should contact a doctor if cough lasts longer than 1 week, recurs frequently, or is associated with high fever, rash, or severe headache.
• Advise patient to take each dose with a glass of water; increasing fluid intake may prove beneficial.
• Encourage deep-breathing exercises.

46

Miscellaneous respiratory drugs

acetylcysteine
alpha₁ proteinase inhibitor
  (human)
beclomethasone dipropionate
beractant
colfosceril palmitate
cromolyn sodium
dexamethasone sodium
  phosphate inhalation
dornase alfa
epoprostenol sodium
flunisolide
nedocromil sodium
triamcinolone acetonide
zafirlukast
zileuton

COMBINATION PRODUCTS
None.

acetylcysteine
Airbront, Mucomyst, Mucomyst-10,
Mucosil-10, Mucosil-20, Parvolext‡

Pregnancy Risk Category: NR

HOW SUPPLIED
Solution: 10%, 20%
Injection: 200 mg/ml†‡

ACTION
A mucolytic that increases production
of respiratory tract fluids to help liquefy
and reduce the viscosity of tenacious secretions. Also restores liver stores of
glutathione to treat acetaminophen toxicity.

ONSET, PEAK, DURATION
Unknown.

INDICATIONS & DOSAGE
*Adjuvant therapy for abnormal viscid or
inspissated mucus secretions in patients
with pneumonia, bronchitis, tuberculo-*

*sis, cystic fibrosis, emphysema, atelecta-
sis (adjunct), pulmonary complications
of thoracic surgery and CV surgery—*
Adults and children: 1 to 2 ml 10% or
20% solution by direct instillation into
trachea as often as every hour; or 1 to
10 ml of 20% solution or 2 to 20 ml of
10% solution by nebulization q 2 to 6
hours p.r.n.
Acetaminophen toxicity—
Adults and children: initially, 140
mg/kg P.O., followed by 70 mg/kg P.O.
q 4 hours for 17 doses.

ADVERSE REACTIONS
CV: tachycardia, hypotension, hyper-
tension.
EENT: *rhinorrhea.*
GI: *stomatitis, nausea, vomiting.*
Respiratory: *bronchospasm* (especial-
ly in asthmatic patients).
Other: fever, clamminess, chest tight-
ness.

INTERACTIONS
Activated charcoal: limits acetylcysteine's effectiveness. Avoid concomitant
use in treating acetaminophen toxicity.

EFFECTS ON DIAGNOSTIC TESTS
None reported.

CONTRAINDICATIONS
Contraindicated in patients hypersensitive to the drug.

NURSING CONSIDERATIONS
● Use cautiously in elderly or debilitated patients with severe respiratory insufficiency.
● Use plastic, glass, stainless steel, or
another nonreactive metal when administering by nebulization. Hand-bulb nebulizers are not recommended because
output is too small and particle size too
large.

• Physically or chemically incompatible with tetracyclines, erythromycin lactobionate, amphotericin B, and ampicillin sodium. If administered by aerosol inhalation, these drugs should be nebulized separately. Iodized oil, trypsin, and hydrogen peroxide are physically incompatible with acetylcysteine; don't add to nebulizer.

• Monitor cough type and frequency.

• **I.V. use:** To prepare I.V. infusion, dilute calculated dose in D_5W. Dilute initial dose (150 mg/kg) in 200 ml of D_5W and infuse over 15 minutes. Dilute second dose of 50 mg/kg in 500 ml of D_5W and give over 4 hours. Dilute final dose of 100 mg/kg in 1,000 ml of D_5W and infuse over 16 hours.

• After opening, store in refrigerator; use within 96 hours.

Alert: Acetylcysteine is administered to treat acetaminophen overdose within 24 hours after ingestion. Start treatment immediately as prescribed; do not wait for results of acetaminophen blood levels.

• When used orally to treat acetaminophen overdose, dilute oral doses with cola, fruit juice, or water before administering. Dilute the 20% solution to a concentration of 5% (add 3 ml of diluent to each ml of acetylcysteine). If patient vomits within 1 hour of receiving loading or maintenance dose, repeat dose.

☑ **PATIENT TEACHING**
• Warn patient that drug may have a foul taste or smell that some patients find distressing.
• For maximum effect, instruct patient to clear his airway by coughing before aerosol administration.

---

alpha₁ proteinase inhibitor (human)
Prolastin

Pregnancy Risk Category: C

HOW SUPPLIED
Injection: 500 mg, 1,000 mg

ACTION
Replaces alpha₁-proteinase in patients with alpha₁-antitrypsin deficiency.

ONSET, PEAK, DURATION
Onset occurs within a few weeks. Serum levels peak immediately after I.V. infusion. Duration unknown.

INDICATIONS & DOSAGE
Chronic replacement therapy in patients with congenital alpha₁-antitrypsin deficiency and demonstrable panacinar emphysema—
Adults: 60 mg/kg I.V. once weekly. May give at a rate of 0.08 ml/kg/minute or greater.

ADVERSE REACTIONS
CNS: dizziness, light-headedness.
Hematologic: possible viral transmission, transient leukocytosis.
Other: delayed fever (transient).

INTERACTIONS
Cigarette smoke: blocks drug's effects. Patients should not smoke.

EFFECTS ON DIAGNOSTIC TESTS
None reported.

CONTRAINDICATIONS
Contraindicated in patients with selective immunoglobulin A (IgA) deficiency who have known antibodies against IgA.

NURSING CONSIDERATIONS
• Use cautiously in patients at risk for circulatory overload.
• **I.V. use:** Store powder for injection in the refrigerator (36° to 46° F [2° to 8° C]). Reconstitute using the supplied diluent (sterile water for injection). After reconstitution, administer within 3 hours. Inject directly into vein; intermittent or continuous infusion is not recommended. Do not refrigerate after reconstitution. Discard unused solution.
• Be aware that many commercial as-

---

*Liquid contains alcohol.   **May contain tartrazine.   †Canada only.   ‡Australia only.   ◇OTC.

says for alpha₁-proteinase inhibitor measure immunoreactivity of the protein and not inhibitor activity. Thus, monitoring serum level of the drug may not accurately reflect clinical response.

☑ PATIENT TEACHING
● Explain to patient that product has been treated to minimize the risk of transmission of hepatitis and AIDS. However, immunization against heptatitis B is recommended prior to drug therapy.
● Instruct patient to report adverse reactions promptly.
● Warn patient not to smoke throughout therapy.

---

beclomethasone dipropionate
Aldecin Inhaler‡, Beclodisk†, Becloforte Inhaler‡, Beclovent, Beclovent Rotacaps†, Vanceril

Pregnancy Risk Category: C

HOW SUPPLIED
Oral inhalation aerosol: 42 mcg/metered spray, 50 mcg/metered spray‡

ACTION
Unknown. Probably decreases inflammation, mainly by stabilizing leukocyte lysosomal membranes.

ONSET, PEAK, DURATION
Onset occurs in 1 to 4 weeks. Peak and duration unknown.

INDICATIONS & DOSAGE
Steroid-dependent asthma—
Adults and children 12 years and over: 2 inhalations t.i.d. or q.i.d. or 4 inhalations b.i.d. Maximum dosage is 20 inhalations daily (840 mcg).
Children 6 to 12 years: 1 to 2 inhalations t.i.d. or q.i.d. or 2 to 4 inhalations b.i.d. Maximum dosage is 10 inhalations daily (420 mcg).

ADVERSE REACTIONS
EENT: *hoarseness,* fungal infection of throat, *throat irritation.*
GI: dry mouth, *fungal infection of mouth.*
Skin: hypersensitivity reactions (urticaria, rash).
Other: angioedema, bronchospasm, suppression of hypothalmic-pituitary-adrenal function, *adrenal insufficiency,* facial edema, wheezing.

INTERACTIONS
None significant.

EFFECTS ON DIAGNOSTIC TESTS
None reported.

CONTRAINDICATIONS
Contraindicated in patients hypersensitive to any component of the formulation (fluorocarbons, oleic acid) and in those with status asthmaticus.

NURSING CONSIDERATIONS
● Use with extreme caution, if at all, in a patient with tuberculosis, fungal or bacterial infections, ocular herpes simplex or systemic viral infections.
● Not for use in patients with asthma controlled by bronchodilators or other noncorticosteroids alone or for those with nonasthmatic bronchial diseases.
● Use with caution in patients receiving systemic corticosteroid therapy.
● Be aware a spacer device may help ensure delivery of the proper dose and decrease local (oral) adverse effects.
● Check mucous membranes frequently for signs of fungal infection.
● Keep in mind that during times of stress (trauma, surgery, or infection) systemic corticosteroids may be needed to prevent adrenal insufficiency in previously steroid-dependent patients.
● Know that periodic measurement of growth and development may be necessary during high-dose or prolonged therapy in children.
Alert: Taper oral glucocorticoid therapy slowly as ordered. Acute adrenal insuffi-

ciency and death have occurred in asthmatics who changed abruptly from oral corticosteroids to beclomethasone.

☑ PATIENT TEACHING
● Inform patient that beclomethasone doesn't provide relief for acute asthma attacks.
● Tell patient requiring a bronchodilator to use it several minutes before beclomethasone.
● Instruct patient to carry a medical identification card indicating his need for supplemental systemic glucocorticoids during stress.
● If using a metered-dose inhaler, instruct the patient to shake the canister well before use.
● Advise patient to allow 1 minute to elapse before taking subsequent puffs of medication and to hold his breath for a few seconds to enhance action of drug.
● Instruct patient to contact his doctor if response to therapy decreases or if symptoms don't improve within 3 weeks; dosage may need to be adjusted. Tell patient not to exceed recommended dosage on his own.
● Tell patient to keep inhaler clean and unobstructed. He should wash it with warm water and dry it thoroughly.
● Tell patient to prevent oral fungal infections by gargling or rinsing mouth with water after each use, but not to swallow the water.
● Tell patient to report symptoms associated with corticosteroid withdrawal, including fatigue, weakness, arthralgia, orthostatic hypotension, and dyspnea.
● Tell patient to store medication between 36° and 86° F (2° and 30° C). Advise patient to ensure delivery of the proper dose by gently warming canister to room temperature before using.

beractant (natural lung surfactant)
Survanta

Pregnancy Category: NR

HOW SUPPLIED
Suspension for intratracheal instillation: 25 mg/ml

ACTION
Lowers the surface tension on alveolar surfaces during respiration and stabilizes the alveoli against collapse. An extract of bovine lung containing neutral lipids, fatty acids, surfactant-associated proteins, and phospholipids, which mimics naturally occurring surfactant; palmitic acid, tripalmitin, and colfosceril palmitate are added to standardize the solution's composition.

ONSET, PEAK, DURATION
Onset occurs in ½ to 2 hours. Peak unknown. Effects persist for 2 to 3 days.

INDICATIONS & DOSAGE
Prevention of respiratory distress syndrome (RDS), also known as hyaline membrane disease, in premature neonates weighing 1,250 g or less at birth or having symptoms consistent with surfactant deficiency—
Neonates: 4 ml/kg intratracheally; administer each dose in four quarter-doses; between quarter-doses, use a hand-held resuscitation bag at a rate of 60 breaths/minute and sufficient oxygen to prevent cyanosis. Give drug as soon as possible, preferably within 15 minutes of birth. Repeat in 6 hours if respiratory distress continues. Give no more than four doses in 48 hours.
Rescue treatment of RDS in premature infants—
Neonates: 4 ml/kg intratracheally; before administering, increase ventilator rate to 60 breaths/minute with an inspiratory time of 0.5 second and a fraction of inspired oxygen of 1. Administer each dose in four quarter-doses; between quarter-doses, continue mechanical ventilation for at least 30 seconds or until stable. Give dose as soon as RDS

is confirmed by X-ray, preferably within 8 hours of birth. Repeat in 6 hours if respiratory distress continues. Give no more than four doses in 48 hours.

ADVERSE REACTIONS
CV: *transient bradycardia,* vasoconstriction, hypotension.
Hematologic: decreased oxygen saturation, hypocapnia, hypercapnia.
Other: endotracheal tube reflux or blockage, pallor, *apnea.*

INTERACTIONS
None significant.

EFFECTS ON DIAGNOSTIC TESTS
None reported.

CONTRAINDICATIONS
None known.

NURSING CONSIDERATIONS
● Beractant should be administered only by personnel experienced in the care of clinically unstable premature neonates. Such personnel should have knowledge of neonatal intubation and airway management.
● Accurate determination of weight is essential to proper measurement of dosage.
● Continuously monitor the neonate before, during, and after beractant administration. The endotracheal (ET) tube may be suctioned before giving the drug; allow the neonate to stabilize before proceeding with administration.
● Refrigerate at 36° to 46° F (2° to 8°C). Warm before administration by allowing drug to stand at room temperature for at least 20 minutes or by holding in hand for at least 8 minutes. Do not use artificial warming methods. Unopened vials that have been warmed to room temperature may be returned to the refrigerator within 8 hours; however, warm and return drug to the refrigerator only once. Vials are for single use only—discard unused drug.
● Beractant does not require sonication

or reconstitution before use. Inspect contents before giving; ensure that the color is off-white to light brown and the contents are uniform. If settling occurs, swirl vial gently; do not shake. Some foaming is normal.
● Use a large-bore needle (20G or larger) to draw up drug; do not use a filter. Administer the drug using a #5 French end-hole catheter. Premeasure and shorten the catheter before use. Fill the catheter with beractant and discard any excess drug so that only the total dose to be given remains in the syringe. Insert catheter into the neonate's ET tube; make sure the catheter tip protrudes just beyond the end of the tube above the neonate's carina. Do not instill drug into a mainstem bronchus.
● Homogeneous distribution of the drug is important. In clinical trials, each dose of the drug was given in four quarter-doses, with the patient positioned differently after each administration. Each quarter-dose was given over 2 to 3 seconds; the catheter was removed and the patient ventilated between quarter-doses. With the head and body inclined slightly downward, the first quarter-dose was given with the head turned to the right; the second quarter-dose, with the head turned to the left. Then the head and body were inclined slightly upward; the third quarter-dose was given with the head turned to the right; the fourth quarter-dose, with the head turned to the left.
● Immediately after administration, moist breath sounds and crackles can occur. *Do not* suction the neonate for 1 hour unless other signs of airway obstruction are evident.
● Continuous monitoring of ECG and transcutaneous oxygen saturation are essential; frequent arterial blood pressure monitoring and frequent arterial blood gas sampling are highly desirable.
● Transient bradycardia and oxygen desaturation are common after dosing.
Alert: Know that beractant can rapidly affect oxygenation and lung compli-

ance. Peak ventilator inspiratory pressures may need to be adjusted if chest expansion improves substantially after drug administration. Notify doctor and adjust immediately as directed because lung overdistention and fatal pulmonary air leakage may result.

• Know that audiovisual materials that describe dosage and administration procedures are available from the manufacturer.

☑ **PATIENT TEACHING**
• Inform parents of need for drug and explain drug action and administration.
• Encourage parents to ask questions and address any concerns raised by them.

---

colfosceril palmitate
Exosurf Neonatal

Pregnancy Category: NR

HOW SUPPLIED
Suspension for intratracheal instillation: 10 ml

ACTION
Replaces a major component of naturally occurring lung surfactant (dipalmitoylphosphatidylcholine), which is deficient in premature neonates. The mixture also contains cetyl ethanol (which acts as a spreading agent between the air-fluid interface) and tyloxapol, a long chain ethanol polymer (which acts as a dispersant).

ONSET, PEAK, DURATION
Unknown.

INDICATIONS & DOSAGE
Prevention of respiratory distress syndrome (RDS) in neonates weighing less than 1,350 g at risk for developing RDS; prophylactic treatment of neonates weighing more than 1,350 g with evidence of pulmonary insufficiency—
Neonates: administer 5 ml/kg intratra-

cheally as soon as possible after delivery. If neonate is maintained on a mechanical ventilator, repeat dosage 12 and 24 hours later.
Rescue treatment of neonates with RDS—
Neonates: administer 5 ml/kg intratracheally as soon as possible after diagnosis of RDS. If the neonate is still mechanically ventilated, administer a second dose of 5 ml/kg 12 hours later.

ADVERSE REACTIONS
CNS: *seizures.*
CV: *intraventricular hemorrhage, patent ductus arteriosus, hypotension.*
Hematologic: *thrombocytopenia.*
Respiratory: *pulmonary hemmorrage, apnea, pulmonary air leak, pneumonia.*
Other: *hyperbilirubinemia, sepsis, meningitis, death from sepsis.*

INTERACTIONS
None significant.

EFFECTS ON DIAGNOSTIC TESTS
Abnormal laboratory values are common in critically ill, mechanically ventilated patients. No higher incidence was seen in colfosceril-treated patients.

CONTRAINDICATIONS
None known.

NURSING CONSIDERATIONS
• Colfosceril should be administered only by personnel experienced in the care of clinically unstable premature neonates. Such personnel should have knowledge of neonatal intubation and airway management.
• Accurate determination of weight is essential to proper measurement of dosage.
• Know that colfosceril can rapidly affect oxygenation and lung compliance. Peak ventilator inspiratory pressures may need to be adjusted if chest expansion improves substantially after drug administration. Notify doctor and adjust

---

immediately as directed because lung overdistention and fatal pulmonary air leakage may result.

● Continuous monitoring of ECG and transcutaneous oxygen saturation are essential; frequent arterial blood pressure monitoring and arterial blood gas sampling are highly desirable. Continuously monitor the neonate before, during, and after drug administration.

● Reconstitute drug immediately before use with the supplied preservative-free sterile water for injection. Do not use solutions that contain antibacterial preservatives. After reconstitution, drug is stable for up to 12 hours at 36° to 86° F (2° to 30°C). Fill a 10-ml syringe with the supplied 8 ml of diluent, using an 18G or 19G needle. Then, pierce the top of the vial and allow the vacuum to draw in the sterile water. Do not use vials without a vacuum. Aspirate as much of the 8 ml as possible out of the vial while maintaining vacuum. Quickly release the syringe plunger. Repeat this final step at least three or four times to ensure adequate mixing of the vial contents.

● When drawing up the dose, use liquid below the froth. Each 8-ml vial contains sufficient material to administer a 5 ml/kg dose to a neonate weighing up to 1,600 g.

● Note that the suspension should have a homogeneous, milky white appearance. Do not use vials that appear to contain large flakes. If the suspension appears to separate, the vial may be shaken gently or swirled to resuspend the material.

● Suction the neonate before administering drug. Do not suction for 2 hours after dosing unless it is necessary.

● Special endotracheal (ET) tube adapters are available with each kit of surfactant. Ensure that adapter used corresponds to the inside diameter of the neonate's ET tube. Insert the adapter into the tube with a twisting motion and connect it to the ventilator circuit. To administer the drug (in half-doses of 2.5

ml), remove the cap from side port of the adapter and attach syringe; do not interrupt mechanical ventilation. After dosing, remember to reattach cap.

● Instill each half-dose slowly over 1 to 2 minutes (30 to 50 mechanical breaths) in small bursts timed with inspiration. Administer first half-dose with the neonate in the midline position; then turn the neonate's head and torso 45 degrees to the right for 30 seconds to assist distribution of drug. Return the neonate to the midline position for the second half-dose, and again administer over 1 to 2 minutes. After the second half-dose, turn the neonate's head and torso 45 degrees to the left for 30 seconds.

● When administering, monitor the neonate's facial expressions, skin color, chest expansion, heart rate, and ET-tube patency and position. If the neonate becomes dusky or agitated, heart rate slows, drug backs up in the ET tube, or oxygen saturation decreases by more than 15%, discontinue the drug and modify peak inspiratory pressure, ventilator rate, or fraction of inspired oxygen (FIO_2) as ordered. Note that rapid improvements in lung function may require rapid reductions in peak inspiratory pressure, ventilator rate, or FIO_2. *Alert:* Reduce ventilator rate immediately if the transcutaneous or arterial carbon dioxide measurements are less than 30 mm Hg. Failure to reduce the rate may result in hypocapnia, which can reduce blood flow to the brain.

● If the neonate becomes pink and the transcutaneous oxygen saturation exceeds 95%, reduce FIO_2 in a stepwise fashion until the saturation is 90% to 95%. Do so immediately because hyperoxia (an excess of systemic oxygen) may result.

● Monitor neonates for pulmonary hemorrhage.

☑ **PATIENT TEACHING**
● Inform parents of need for drug and explain drug action and administration.

Reactions may be *common*, uncommon, *life-threatening*, or COMMON AND LIFE-THREATENING.

• Encourage parents to ask questions and address any concerns raised by them.

---

cromolyn sodium (sodium cromoglycate)

Crolom, Gastrocrom, Intal, Intal Aerosol Spray, Intal Nebulizer Solution, Nalcrom, Nasalcrom, Rynacrom†

Pregnancy Risk Category: B

HOW SUPPLIED

Capsules (for oral solution): 100 mg
Aerosol: 800 mcg/metered spray
Nasal solution: 5.2 mg/metered spray (40 mg/ml)
Solution (for nebulization): 20 mg/2 ml
Ophthalmic solution: 4%

ACTION

Inhibits the degranulation of sensitized mast cells that occurs after a patient's exposure to specific antigens. Also inhibits release of histamine and slow-reacting substance of anaphylaxis.

ONSET, PEAK, DURATION

Unknown.

INDICATIONS & DOSAGE

Mild to moderate persistent asthma—
Adults and children 5 years and over: 2 metered sprays using inhaler q.i.d. at regular intervals. Alternatively, 20 mg via nebulization q.i.d. at regular intervals.
Prevention and treatment of seasonal and perennial allergic rhinitis—
Adults and children over 5 years: 1 spray in each nostril t.i.d. or q.i.d. Maximal administration is six times daily.
Prevention of exercise-induced bronchospasm—
Adults and children 5 years or over: 2 metered sprays inhaled no more than 1 hour before anticipated exercise.
Conjunctivitis—
Adults and children 4 years and older: 1 to 2 drops in each eye four to six times daily at regular intervals.
Systemic mastocytosis—
Adults and children over 12 years: 200 P.O. q.i.d. before meals and h.s.
Children 2 to 12 years: 100 mg P.O. q.i.d. 30 minutes before meals or h.s.

ADVERSE REACTIONS

CNS: dizziness, headache.
EENT: *irritated throat and trachea,* nasal congestion, pharyngeal irritation, *sneezing,* nasal burning and irritation, epistaxis.
GI: nausea, esophagitis, abdominal pain.
GU: dysuria, urinary frequency.
Respiratory: ***bronchospasm*** (after inhalation of dry powder), *cough,* wheezing, eosinophilic pneumonia.
Skin: rash, urticaria.
Other: joint swelling and pain, lacrimation, swollen parotid gland, ***angioedema,*** *bad taste in mouth.*

INTERACTIONS

None significant.

EFFECTS ON DIAGNOSTIC TESTS

None reported.

CONTRAINDICATIONS

Contraindicated in patients experiencing acute asthma attacks and status asthmaticus and in patients with hypersensitivity to drug.

NURSING CONSIDERATIONS

• Administer with caution in children. Use of cromolyn oral inhalation solution is *not* recommended in children under 2 years; cromolyn powder or aerosol for oral inhalation, not recommended in children under 5 years; cromolyn ophthalmic solution, not recommended in children under 4 years; and cromolyn nasal solution, not recommended in children under 6 years.
• Use inhalation form cautiously in patients with coronary artery disease or a history of arrhythmias.

• Know that drug (except for ophthalmic solution) should be used only when acute episode of asthma has been controlled, airway is cleared, and the patient can breathe independently.

• Be aware that oral cromolyn sodium should be used in full-term neonates and infants *only* for a severe, incapacitating disease, that is, when benefits clearly outweigh the risks.

• Dissolve powder in capsules for oral dose in hot water, and further dilute with cold water before ingestion. Do not mix with fruit juice, milk, or food.

• Discontinue drug if the patient develops eosinophilic pneumonia, indicated by eosinophilia and infiltrates on chest X-ray film.

• Watch for recurrence of asthmatic symptoms when dosage is decreased, especially when corticosteroids are also used.

☑ **PATIENT TEACHING**
• Instruct patient how to administer form of drug prescribed.
• Instruct patient that full effects of drug may not be noted for 4 weeks.
• Tell patient that esophagitis may be relieved by antacids or a glass of milk.
• Warn patient who is using the nasal solution that stinging or sneezing may occur upon administration.

---

dexamethasone sodium phosphate inhalation
Decadron Phosphate Respihaler

Pregnancy Risk Category: C

HOW SUPPLIED
Inhalation aerosol: 84 mcg dexamethasone/metered spray

ACTION
Unknown. Probably decreases inflammation, mainly by stabilizing leukocyte lysosomal membranes.

ONSET, PEAK, DURATION
Onset occurs in 1 to 4 weeks. Peak and duration unknown.

INDICATIONS & DOSAGE
Persistent asthma—
Adults: initially, 3 inhalations t.i.d. or q.i.d. Decreased as needed and tolerated; most patients respond to 2 inhalations b.i.d. Maximum dosage is 12 inhalations daily.
Children: 2 inhalations t.i.d. or q.i.d. Decreased as needed and tolerated; most patients respond to 2 inhalations b.i.d. Maximum dosage is 8 inhalations daily.

ADVERSE REACTIONS
EENT: *hoarseness,* fungal infection of throat, *throat irritation.*
GI: dry mouth, *fungal infection of mouth.*
Other: rash, wheezing, facial edema.

INTERACTIONS
None significant.

EFFECTS ON DIAGNOSTIC TESTS
None reported.

CONTRAINDICATIONS
Contraindicated in patients hypersensitive to any component of the formulation (fluorocarbons, ethanol) and in those with status asthmaticus, persistent positive sputum cultures for *Candida albicans,* or systemic fungal infections.

NURSING CONSIDERATIONS
• Not for use in patients with asthma controlled by bronchodilators or other noncorticosteroids alone or for those with nonasthmatic bronchial diseases.
• Use cautiously in patients with ocular herpes simplex, nonspecific ulcerative colitis, diverticulitis, fresh intestinal anastomoses, peptic ulcer, renal insufficiency, hypertension, osteoporosis, and myasthenia gravis.
• Know that a spacer device may help ensure delivery of the proper dose of

---

Reactions may be *common,* uncommon, *life-threatening,* or COMMON AND LIFE-THREATENING.

medication and decrease local (oral) adverse effects.

● Check mucous membranes frequently for signs of fungal infection.

● Monitor patient for adverse effects. With prolonged use of high doses, systemic effects are likely because up to 50% of a dose is absorbed.

● Conduct periodic measurements of growth and development during high-dose or prolonged therapy in children.

● Know that during times of stress (trauma, surgery, or infection), systemic corticosteroids may be needed to prevent adrenal insufficiency in previously steroid-dependent patients.

Alert: Taper oral glucocorticoid therapy slowly as ordered. Acute adrenal insufficiency and death have occurred in asthmatics who switched abruptly from oral corticosteroids to inhaled steroids. Be sure patients report symptoms associated with corticosteroid withdrawal, including fatigue, weakness, arthralgia, orthostatic hypotension, and dyspnea.

☑ **PATIENT TEACHING**
● Inform patient that dexamethasone doesn't provide relief for acute asthma attacks.

● Instruct patient to store medication between 36° and 86° F (2° and 30°C). Tell patient that this medication needs to be at room temperature when used. If the canister is cold, the proper dose may not be delivered.

● Advise patient to ensure delivery of the proper dose by gently warming the canister to room temperature before using. Some patients carry the canister in a pocket to keep it warm.

● Advise patient requiring bronchodilator to use it several minutes before dexamethasone.

● Tell patient to allow 1 minute to elapse before taking subsequent puffs of medication and to hold his breath for a few seconds to enhance action of drug.

● Instruct patient to contact the doctor if response to therapy decreases or if symptoms don't improve within 3

weeks of initiating therapy; the doctor may need to adjust the dosage. Tell patient not to exceed recommended dosage on his own.

● Advise patient to prevent oral fungal infection by gargling or rinsing mouth with water after each use, but not to swallow water.

● Teach patient to keep inhaler clean and unobstructed. He should wash it with warm water and dry it thoroughly.

● Instruct patient to carry a card indicating need for supplemental systemic glucocorticoids during stress.

---

dornase alfa
Pulmozyme

Pregnancy Risk Category: B

HOW SUPPLIED
Inhalation solution: 2.5-mg ampule (1 mg/ml)

ACTION
Hydrolyzes DNA in sputum of cystic fibrosis patients, causing decreased viscosity and elasticity of pulmonary secretions.

ONSET, PEAK, DURATION
Significant improvement in lung function occurs within 3 days to 1 week. Reduction in respiratory tract infections takes weeks to months. Peak increases in baseline measurement of amount of air exhaled in first second of expiration occur after about 9 days of therapy. Duration unknown.

INDICATIONS & DOSAGE
To improve pulmonary function and decrease the frequency of moderate to severe respiratory infections in patients with cystic fibrosis—
Adults and children 5 years and over: 1 ampule (2.5 mg) inhaled once daily. Treatment usually takes 10 to 15 minutes. Use drug only with an approved nebulizer.

---

*Liquid contains alcohol.   **May contain tartrazine.   †Canada only.   ‡Australia only.   ◇OTC.

ADVERSE REACTIONS
EENT: *pharyngitis, voice alteration,* laryngitis, conjunctivitis.
Skin: *rash,* urticaria.
Other: *chest pain.*

INTERACTIONS
None significant.

EFFECTS ON DIAGNOSTIC TESTS
None reported.

CONTRAINDICATIONS
Contraindicated in patients hypersensitive to the drug or Chinese hamster ovary cell-derived products.

NURSING CONSIDERATIONS
● Know that drug is used in conjunction with other standard therapies for cystic fibrosis.
● Be aware that safety and efficacy in children under 5 years or with forced vital capacity of less than 40% of normal value have not been established.
● Administer only with the following nebulizers and compressors: the Hudson T Up-draft II disposable jet nebulizer and the Marquest Acorn II disposable jet nebulizer along with the Pulmo-Aide compressor or the PARI LC Jet⁺ reusable nebulizer along with the PARI PRONEB compressor.
● Discard cloudy or discolored solution.
● Do not mix with other drugs in the nebulizer. Doing so could lead to a physical or chemical reaction that may inactivate dornase alfa.
● Refrigerate drug in its protective foil pouch to protect it from strong light.

☑ PATIENT TEACHING
● Instruct patient how to administer drug at home.
● Remind the patient to breathe only through his mouth when using the nebulizer. If this is difficult, suggest use of a nose clip.
● Tell the patient that if he begins coughing during treatment to turn off the nebulizer without spilling the drug.

To resume, he should turn on the nebulizer and continue breathing through the mouthpiece until the nebulizer cup is empty or mist is no longer produced.

---

epoprostenol sodium
Flolan

Pregnancy Risk Category: B

HOW SUPPLIED
Injection: 0.5 mg (500,000 ng)/17 ml, 1.5 mg (1,500,000 ng)/17 ml

ACTION
Causes direct vasodilation of pulmonary and systemic arterial vascular beds and inhibits platelet aggregation.

ONSET, PEAK, DURATION
Unknown.

INDICATIONS & DOSAGE
Long-term I.V. treatment of primary pulmonary hypertension in New York Heart Association (NYHA) Class III and Class IV patients—
Adults: initially, 2 ng/kg/minute as I.V. infusion, increased in increments of 2 ng/kg/minute q 15 minutes or longer until dose-limiting pharmacologic effects are elicited. Maintenance dosing is begun with 4 ng/kg/minute less than the maximum tolerated rate determined during initial dosing. If the maximum rate is less than 5 ng/kg/minute, the maintenance infusion is started at one-half the maximum rate. Subsequent adjustments are made based on persistence, recurrence, or worsening of symptoms; such increases should be made gradually in 1- to 2-ng/kg/minute increments q 15 minutes or longer. Occurrence of adverse events from excessive doses may necessitate a gradual decrease in dosage in 2-ng/kg/minute increments q 15 minutes or longer.

ADVERSE REACTIONS
After initial dosing—

CNS: *headache, anxiety, nervousness, agitation,* dizziness, hypesthesia, paresthesia.
CV: *hypotension, chest pain,* bradycardia, tachycardia.
GI: *nausea, vomiting,* abdominal pain, dyspepsia.
Respiratory: dyspnea.
Skin: *flushing.*
Other: musculoskeletal pain, back pain, sweating.
During maintenance dosing—
CNS: *headache, anxiety, nervousness, dizziness, hypesthesia, hyperesthesia, paresthesia, tremor.*
CV: *tachycardia.*
GI: *nausea, vomiting, diarrhea.*
Hematologic: thrombocytopenia.
Skin: *flushing.*
Other: *jaw pain, flulike symptoms, chills, fever, sepsis, myalgia, nonspecific musculoskeletal pain.*

INTERACTIONS

Antihypertensive agents, diuretics, or other vasodilators: additional reductions in blood pressure may occur. Monitor blood pressure closely.
Anticoagulants, antiplatelet agents: may increase risk of bleeding. Monitor closely for bleeding.

EFFECTS ON DIAGNOSTIC TESTS
None reported.

CONTRAINDICATIONS
Contraindicated in patients with hypersensitivity to drug or structurally related compounds. Also contraindicated in patients with respiratory distress syndrome, hyaline membrane disease, or persistent fetal circulation and when a left-to-right shunt is present. Chronic use is contraindicated in patients with CHF due to severe left ventricular systolic dysfunction and in patients who develop pulmonary edema during initial dosing.

NURSING CONSIDERATIONS
● Use cautiously in elderly patients and in pregnant or breast-feeding women.
● Safety and efficacy in children have not been established.

● Drug should be used only by clinicians experienced in diagnosis and treatment of primary pulmonary hypertension. The appropriate dose must be determined in a setting with adequate personnel and equipment for physiologic monitoring and emergency care.
● **I.V. use:** Drug must be reconstituted only as directed, using sterile diluent for Flolan. Drug must not be reconstituted or mixed with any other parenteral medications or solutions before or during administration.
● Follow manufacturer guidelines for reconstituting drug. The prescribed concentration should be compatible with the infusion pump's minimum and maximum flow rates and reservoir capacity and with other criteria recommended by manufacturer. When used for maintenance infusion, drug should be prepared in a drug delivery reservoir appropriate for the infusion pump, with a total reservoir volume of at least 100 ml. Drug should be prepared using 2 vials of sterile diluent for use during 24 hours.
● Reconstituted solutions must be protected from light and refrigerated at 36° to 46° F (2° to 8° C) if not used immediately. Do not freeze reconstituted solutions. Discard frozen solution or solution that has been refrigerated for more than 48 hours.
● Maintenance dosing should be given by continuous I.V. infusion via a permanent indwelling central venous catheter using an ambulatory infusion pump. During establishment of dosing range, drug may be administered peripherally.
● To facilitate extended use at ambient temperatures above 77° F (25° C), a cold pouch with frozen gel packs can be used. The pouch must be able to maintain the drug at a temperature of 36° to 46° F for 12 hours. When such a pouch is used, the reconstituted solution should be used for no longer than 24 hours.

• After establishment of a maintenance infusion rate, observe the patient closely and monitor standing and supine blood pressure and heart rate for several hours to ensure tolerance.

• Avoid abrupt withdrawal of drug or sudden, large reductions in infusion rate. Ensure that a backup infusion pump and I.V. infusion set are available to avoid potential interruptions in drug delivery. A multilumen catheter should be considered if other I.V. therapies are routinely administered.

• Infusion rates should be adjusted only under a doctor's direction, except in life-threatening situations.

• Anticoagulant therapy should be administered during maintenance infusion, unless contraindicated. Monitor PT closely.

• To reduce risk of infection, aseptic technique must be used when reconstituting and administering the drug and when performing routine catheter care.

• All orders for epoprostenol are distributed only by Quantum Healthcare, Inc. To order the drug or request reimbursement assistance, call 800-622-1820.

☑ **PATIENT TEACHING**
• Discuss the patient's long-term need for epoprostenol. Ensure that the patient or a family member can care for a permanent I.V. catheter and infusion pump.

• Show the patient and family how to reconstitute, administer, and store the drug; how to use the infusion pump; and how to switch to a new pump in the event of pump failure. Stress the importance of maintaining continuous drug therapy.

• Urge the patient to report adverse reactions immediately; dosage adjustments may be necessary.

• Provide the patient with the telephone number of an organization that offers 24-hour support.

flunisolide
AeroBid, AeroBid-M

Pregnancy Risk Category: C

HOW SUPPLIED
Oral inhalant: 250 mcg/metered spray (at least 100 metered inhalations/container)

ACTION
Unknown. Probably decreases inflammation, mainly by stabilizing leukocyte lysosomal membranes.

ONSET, PEAK, DURATION
Onset occurs after 1 to 4 weeks of therapy. Peak and duration unknown.

INDICATIONS & DOSAGE
Persistent asthma—
Adults: 2 inhalations (500 mcg) b.i.d. Maximum total daily dose is 2,000 mcg (8 inhalations/day).
Children 6 to 15 years: 2 inhalations (500 mcg) b.i.d. Higher dosages have not been studied. Maximum total daily dose is 1,000 mcg.

ADVERSE REACTIONS
CNS: dizziness, irritability, nervousness.
CV: palpitations.
EENT: throat irritation, hoarseness, nasopharyngeal fungal infections, *sore throat, nasal congestion.*
GI: nausea, vomiting, dry mouth, *diarrhea, upset stomach,* abdominal pain, decreased appetite.
Other: *upper respiratory tract infection, cold symptoms, flu,* edema, fever, chest pain, rash, pruritus, *unpleasant taste.*

INTERACTIONS
None significant.

EFFECTS ON DIAGNOSTIC TESTS
None reported.

Reactions may be *common*, uncommon, *life-threatening*, or COMMON AND LIFE-THREATENING.

CONTRAINDICATIONS

Contraindicated in patients hypersensitive to the drug and in those with status asthmaticus or respiratory infections.

NURSING CONSIDERATIONS

● Not recommended for use in patients with asthma controlled by bronchodilators or other noncorticosteroids alone or for those with nonasthmatic bronchial diseases.

● Know that a spacer device may help to ensure proper dosage administration and decrease local (oral) adverse effects.

● Store medication between 36° and 86° F (2° and 30° C).

● Withdraw drug slowly as ordered in patients who have received long-term oral corticosteroid therapy.

● Be aware that after withdrawal of systemic corticosteroids, patient may still need supplementation of systemic steroids if patient show signs and symptoms of adrenal insufficiency when exposed to trauma, surgery, or infections.

☑ PATIENT TEACHING

● Warn patient that flunisolide doesn't relieve emergency asthma attacks.

● Advise patient to ensure delivery of the proper dose by gently warming the canister to room temperature before using. Some patients carry the canister in a pocket to keep it warm.

● Tell patient who also is using a bronchodilator to use it several minutes before he uses flunisolide.

● Instruct patient to allow 1 minute to elapse before repeating inhalations and to hold his breath for a few seconds to enhance drug action.

● Teach patient to keep inhaler clean and unobstructed. He should wash it with warm water and dry it thoroughly after use.

● Teach patient to check mucous membranes frequently for signs of fungal infection.

● The patient can prevent oral fungal infections by gargling or rinsing mouth with water after each inhaler use. Caution patient not to swallow the water.

● Advise parents of children receiving long-term therapy that the child should have periodic growth measurements and be checked for evidence of hypothalamic-pituitary-adrenal axis suppression.

---

nedocromil sodium
Tilade

Pregnancy Risk Category: B

HOW SUPPLIED

Inhalation aerosol: 1.75 mg/activation

ACTION

Reduces inflammatory changes in the airway by blocking the release of inflammation mediators (such as leukotrienes, histamine, and prostaglandins) from mast cells, eosinophils, monocytes, neutrophils, macrophages, and other immune cells.

ONSET, PEAK, DURATION

Onset occurs within days to 4 weeks. Time to peak concentration in an asthmatic patient occurs in 5 to 90 minutes. Effects persist for 6 to 12 hours.

INDICATIONS & DOSAGE

Maintenance in mild to moderate bronchial asthma—
Adults and children 12 years and over: 2 inhalations q.i.d. at regular intervals.

ADVERSE REACTIONS

CNS: headache, dysphagia, fatigue.
GI: nausea, vomiting, dyspepsia, abdominal pain, dry mouth.
Respiratory: upper respiratory tract infection, rhinitis, cough, pharyngitis, increased sputum, bronchitis, dyspnea, bronchospasm.
Other: *unpleasant taste,* chest pain.

INTERACTIONS

None significant.

---

*Liquid contains alcohol.   **May contain tartrazine.   †Canada only.   ‡Australia only.   ◊OTC.

EFFECTS ON DIAGNOSTIC TESTS
None reported.

CONTRAINDICATIONS
Contraindicated in patients hypersensitive to the formulation or in patients experiencing an acute asthmatic attack or acute bronchospasm.

NURSING CONSIDERATION
Know that drug should not be used during acute bronchospasm because drug action has a slow onset and is not therapeutic in aborting an acute attack.

☑ **PATIENT TEACHING**
• Warn the patient that nedocromil has no direct bronchodilating action and cannot replace bronchodilators during an acute asthmatic attack.
• Tell the patient that drug is an adjunct to the regular bronchodilator regimen and may reduce the need for corticosteroids or bronchodilators.
• Emphasize to the patient that regular use of the drug will help him feel better. Most patients report benefits after 1 week of use; some require longer treatment before any improvement.
• Teach the patient how to use the inhaler. Instruct him to shake canister immediately before use and to invert it just before actuation.
• Advise patient to clean inhaler at least twice a week and to remove canister before rinsing inhaler in hot running water. Then let inhaler air-dry overnight.

---

triamcinolone acetonide
Azmacort

Pregnancy Risk Category: C

HOW SUPPLIED
Inhalation aerosol: 100 mcg/metered spray

ACTION
Unknown. Probably decreases inflammation, mainly by stabilizing leukocyte lysosomal membranes.

ONSET, PEAK, DURATION
Onset occurs in 1 to 4 weeks. Peak and duration unknown.

INDICATIONS & DOSAGE
Persistent asthma—
Adults: 2 inhalations t.i.d. to q.i.d. Maximum dosage is 16 inhalations daily. In some patients, maintenance can be accomplished when total daily dosage is given b.i.d.
Children 6 to 12 years: 1 to 2 inhalations t.i.d. to q.i.d. Maximum dosage is 12 inhalations daily.

ADVERSE REACTIONS
Most adverse reactions to corticosteroids are dose- or duration-dependent.
EENT: dry or irritated nose or throat, hoarseness.
Respiratory: cough, wheezing.
Other: *oral candidiasis,* dry or irritated tongue or mouth, facial edema, hypothalamic pituitary adrenal function suppression, adrenal insufficiency.

INTERACTIONS
None significant.

EFFECTS ON DIAGNOSTIC TESTS
None reported.

CONTRAINDICATIONS
Contraindicated in patients hypersensitive to any component of the formulation and in those with status asthmaticus.

NURSING CONSIDERATIONS
• It is not known if drug is excreted in breast milk. Because of the risk of severe adverse effects, breast-feeding is not recommended.
• Use with extreme caution, if at all, in patients with tuberculosis of the respiratory tract; untreated fungal, bacterial, or systemic viral infections; or ocular herpes simplex.
• Unlike other available corticosteroids,

Reactions may be *common,* uncommon, ***life-threatening,*** or COMMON AND LIFE-THREATENING.

Azmacort has a spacer built into the drug-delivery device.

• Use cautiously in patients receiving systemic corticosteroids.

• Know that patients who have recently been switched from systemic administration of steroids to oral inhaled steroids may need to resume systemic steroid therapy during periods of stress or severe asthma attacks.

• Taper oral therapy slowly as ordered.

• Store medication between 36° and 86° F (2° and 30° C).

☑ PATIENT TEACHING

• Inform patient that inhaled corticosteroids don't provide relief for emergency asthma attacks.

• Advise patient to ensure delivery of the proper dose of medication by gently warming the canister to room temperature before using. Some patients carry the canister in a pocket to keep it warm.

• The patient requiring a bronchodilator should use it several minutes before triamcinolone. Tell patient to allow 1 minute to elapse before repeat inhalations and to hold breath for a few seconds to enhance drug action.

• Teach patient to check mucous membranes frequently for signs of fungal infection.

• Tell patient to prevent oral fungal infections by gargling or rinsing mouth with water after each use of the inhaler, but not to swallow the water.

• Tell patient to keep inhaler clean and unobstructed. He should wash it with warm water and dry it thoroughly after use.

• Instruct patient to contact the doctor if response to therapy decreases; the doctor may need to adjust the dosage. Tell patient not to exceed recommended dosage on his own.

• Instruct patient to carry a card indicating his need for supplemental systemic glucocorticoids during periods of stress.

▼ NEW DRUG

zafirlukast
Accolate

Pregnancy Risk Category: B

HOW SUPPLIED
Tablets: 20 mg

ACTION
Selectively competes for leukotriene receptor sites, blocking inflammatory action.

ONSET, PEAK, DURATION
Zafirlukast is rapidly absorbed after oral administration. Plasma levels peak within 3 hours after oral administration. Duration unknown.

INDICATIONS & DOSAGE
Prophylaxis and chronic treatment of asthma—
Adults and children 12 years and older: 20 mg P.O. b.i.d. taken 1 hour before or 2 hours after meals.

ADVERSE REACTIONS
CNS: *headache,* asthenia, dizziness.
GI: nausea, diarrhea, abdominal pain, vomiting, dyspepsia.
Musculoskeletal: myalgia, back pain.
Other: infection, pain, accidental injury, fever.

INTERACTIONS
Aspirin: increased plasma levels of zafirlukast. Monitor patient.
Terfenadine, erythromycin, theophylline: decreased plasma levels of zafirlukast. Monitor patient.
Warfarin: increased PT. Monitor PT and INR levels, and adjust dosage of anticoagulant, as ordered.

EFFECTS ON DIAGNOSTIC TESTS
Drug may elevate liver enzymes.

CONTRAINDICATIONS
Contraindicated in patients with known

hypersensitivity to the drug.

NURSING CONSIDERATIONS

● Know that drug is not indicated for use in the reversal of bronchospasm in acute asthma attacks.
● Administer with caution in patients with hepatic impairment and in the elderly.
● Know that drug should be used in pregnancy only if clearly needed. Breast-feeding women should not take the drug.
● Know that safety and effectiveness in patients under 12 years have not been established.

☑ **PATIENT TEACHING**
● Tell patient that drug is used for chronic treatment of asthma and to keep taking drug even if symptoms disappear.
● Advise patient to continue taking other antiasthma drugs as ordered.
● Instruct patient not to take drug with food. Drug should be taken 1 hour before or 2 hours after meals.

▼ *NEW DRUG*

zileuton
Zyflo

Pregnancy Risk Category: C

HOW SUPPLIED
Tablets: 600 mg

ACTION
Inhibits enzyme responsible for the formation of leukotrienes, thus reducing inflammatory response.

ONSET, PEAK, DURATION
Drug is rapidly absorbed after oral administration. Plasma levels peak in about 2 hours. Duration unknown.

INDICATIONS & DOSAGE
Prophylaxis and chronic treatment of asthma—

Adults and children 12 years and older: 600 mg P.O. q.i.d.

ADVERSE REACTIONS
CNS: *headache,* asthenia, dizziness, insomnia, nervousness, somnolence.
CV: chest pain.
EENT: conjunctivitis.
GI: dyspepsia, nausea, abdominal pain, constipation, flatulence, vomiting.
GU: UTI, vaginitis.
Hematologic: leukopenia.
Musculoskeletal: myalgia, arthralgia, hypertonia, neck pain and rigidity.
Skin: pruritus.
Other: pain, accidental injury, fever, lymphadenopathy, malaise.

INTERACTIONS
Propranolol and other beta-blockers: increased beta-blocker effect. Monitor patient and reduce dosage of beta blocker as needed.
Terfenadine: decreased clearance and increased plasma concentration of terfenadine. Do not administer concurrently.
Theophylline: decreased theophylline clearance (on average, serum theophylline concentrations double). Reduce theophylline dose, as ordered, and monitor serum levels.
Warfarin: increased PT. Monitor PT and INR and adjust dosage of anticoagulant, as ordered.

EFFECTS ON DIAGNOSTIC TESTS
Drug may elevate liver enzymes and temporarily lower WBC count.

CONTRAINDICATIONS
Contraindicated in patients with known hypersensitivity to the drug and in patients with active liver disease or transaminase elevations at least 3 times the upper limit of normal.

NURSING CONSIDERATIONS
● Know that drug is not indicated for

Reactions may be *common*, uncommon, *life-threatening*, or COMMON AND LIFE-THREATENING.

use in the reversal of bronchospasm in acute asthma attacks.

• Administer with caution in patients with hepatic impairment and in patients with a history of heavy alcohol use.

• Know that drug should be used in pregnancy only if the benefit of use outweighs the potential risk to the fetus. Breast-feeding women should not take the drug.

• Know that safety and effectiveness in patients under 12 years have not been established.

• Obtain baseline and periodic liver enzyme levels, as ordered.

☑ PATIENT TEACHING

• Tell patient that drug is used for chronic treatment of asthma and to keep taking drug even if symptoms disappear.

• Caution patient that drug is not a bronchodilator and should not be used to treat an acute asthma attack.

• Advise patient to continue taking other antiasthma drugs, as ordered.

• Instruct patient to notify the doctor if patient's short-acting bronchodilator doesn't relieve symptoms.

• Tell patient he'll regularly need to have tests done for liver enzyme levels.

• Tell patient to notify doctor immediately if he develops signs and symptoms of liver dysfunction (right upper quadrant pain, nausea, fatigue, pruritus, jaundice, malaise).

• Tell patient to avoid alcohol and to consult his doctor first before taking any OTC or new prescription drugs.

---

aluminum carbonate
aluminum hydroxide
aluminum phosphate
calcium carbonate
dihydroxyaluminum sodium carbonate
magaldrate
magnesium oxide
magnesium hydroxide
    (See Chapter 50, LAXATIVES.)
simethicone
sodium bicarbonate
    (See Chapter 64, acidifier and alkalinizers.)

COMBINATION PRODUCTS

ALKA-SELTZER WITH ASPIRIN ◇ : sodium bicarbonate 1,916 mg, aspirin 325 mg, and citric acid 1,000 mg.
ALKA-SELTZER WITHOUT ASPIRIN ◇ : sodium bicarbonate 958 mg, citric acid 832 mg, and potassium bicarbonate 312 mg.
ALUDROX SUSPENSION ◇ : aluminum hydroxide 307 mg and magnesium hydroxide 103 mg.
CAMALOX TABLETS ◇ : Aluminum hydroxide 225 mg, magnesium hydroxide 200 mg, and calcium carbonate 250 mg.
DI-GEL LIQUID ◇ : aluminum hydroxide 200 mg, magnesium hydroxide 200 mg, and simethicone 20 mg.
FLATULEX: simethicone 80 mg and activated charcoal 250 mg.
GAVISCON ◇ : aluminum hydroxide 31.7 mg and magnesium carbonate 137 mg.
GELUSIL ◇ : aluminum hydroxide 200mg, magnesium hydroxide 200 mg, and simethicone 25 mg.
GELUSIL-II ◇ : aluminum hydroxide 400 mg, magnesium hydroxide 400 mg, and simethicone 30 mg.
MAALOX ◇ : aluminum hydroxide 225 mg and magnesium hydroxide 200 mg.
MAALOX EXTRA STRENGTH TABLETS ◇ : aluminum hydroxide 400 mg and magnesium hydroxide 400 mg.
MAALOX PLUS TABLETS ◇ : aluminum hydroxide 200 mg, magnesium hydroxide 200 mg, and simethicone 25 mg.
MAALOX TC TABLETS ◇ : aluminum hydroxide 600 mg and magnesium hydroxide 300 mg.
MYLANTA TABLETS ◇ : aluminum hydroxide 200mg, magnesium hydroxide 200 mg, and simethicone 20 mg.
MYLANTA-II TABLETS ◇ : aluminum hydroxide 400 mg, magnesium hydroxide 400 mg, and simethicone 40 mg.
RIOPAN PLUS CHEWABLE TABLETS ◇ : magaldrate 540 mg and simethicone 20 mg.
RIOPAN PLUS SUSPENSION ◇ : magaldrate 540 mg and simethicone 20 mg/5 ml.
TITRALAC PLUS SUSPENSION ◇ : calcium carbonate 500 mg and simethicone 20 mg.
TITRALAC TABLETS ◇ : calcium carbonate 420 mg and glycine 150 mg.
UNIVOL† ◇ : aluminum hydroxide and magnesium carbonate co-dried gel 300 mg and magnesium hydroxide 100 mg.
WINGEL ◇ : aluminum hydroxide 180 mg and magnesium hydroxide 160 mg.

---

aluminum carbonate
Basaljel ◇

Pregnancy Risk Category: B

HOW SUPPLIED

Tablets or capsules: equivalent to aluminum hydroxide 500 mg ◇
Oral suspension: equivalent to aluminum hydroxide 400 mg/5 ml ◇

ACTION

An antacid that reduces total acid load in the GI tract, elevates gastric pH to reduce pepsin activity, strengthens the gastric mucosal barrier, and increases esophageal sphincter tone.

ONSET, PEAK, DURATION
Onset occurs in 20 minutes. Peak unknown. Effects persist for about 20 to 60 minutes in a fasting period and up to 3 hours if taken 1 hour after a meal.

INDICATIONS & DOSAGE
Antacid—
Adults: 5 to 10 ml of suspension P.O. q 2 hours p.r.n.; or 1 to 2 tablets or capsules P.O. q 2 hours p.r.n. Maximum dosage is 24 capsules, tablets, or teaspoonfuls per 24 hours.
To prevent formation of urinary phosphate stones (in conjunction with low-phosphate diet)—
Adults: 15 to 30 ml of suspension in water or juice P.O. 1 hour after meals and h.s.; or 2 to 6 tablets or capsules 1 hour after meals and h.s.

ADVERSE REACTIONS
CNS: encephalopathy.
GI: *constipation,* intestinal obstruction.
Other: hypophosphatemia, osteomalacia.

INTERACTIONS
Allopurinol, antibiotics (including quinolones and tetracyclines), corticosteroids, diflunisal, digoxin, ethambutol, histamine-2 antagonists, iron salts, isoniazid, penicillamine, phenothiazines, thyroid hormones, ticlopidine: decreased pharmacologic effect because of possible impaired absorption. Separate administration times by 1 to 2 hours.
Enteric-coated drugs: may be released prematurely in stomach. Separate doses by at least 1 hour.

EFFECTS ON DIAGNOSTIC TESTS
Aluminum carbonate may interfere with imaging techniques using sodium pertechnetate Tc99m and thus impair evaluation of Meckel's diverticulum. It may also interfere with reticuloendothelial imaging of liver, spleen, or bone marrow using technetium Tc99m sulfur colloid. It may antagonize pentagastrin's effect during gastric acid secretion tests. Drug may increase serum gastrin levels and decrease serum phosphate levels.

CONTRAINDICATIONS
None known.

NURSING CONSIDERATIONS
● Use cautiously in patients with chronic renal disease.
● When administering through nasogastric tube, make sure tube is placed correctly and is patent; after instilling, flush tube with water to ensure passage to stomach and to clear tube.
● Monitor long-term, high-dose use in patients on restricted sodium intake. Each tablet, capsule, or 5 ml of suspension contains about 3 mg of sodium.
● Record amount and consistency of stools. Manage constipation with laxatives or stool softeners as ordered. Alternate with magnesium-containing antacids (if the patient does not have renal disease).
● Monitor serum phosphate levels.
● Watch for symptoms of hypophosphatemia with prolonged use (anorexia, malaise, muscle weakness); can also lead to resorption of calcium and bone demineralization.
● Because drug contains aluminum, keep in mind that it is used in patients with renal failure to help control hyperphosphatemia by binding with phosphate in the GI tract.
● Know that Basaljel liquid contains no sugar.

☑ PATIENT TEACHING
● Warn patient not to take aluminum carbonate indiscriminately or to switch antacids without the doctor's advice.
● Instruct patient to shake suspension well and to take with small amount of water or fruit juice to facilitate passage.

---

aluminum hydroxide

AlternaGEL◇, Alu-Cap◇, Aluminum Hydroxide Gel◇, Aluminum Hydroxide Gel Concentrated◇, Alu-Tab◇, Amphojel◇, Dialume◇, Nephrox◇

Pregnancy Risk Category: C

HOW SUPPLIED

Tablets: 300 mg◇, 500 mg◇, 600 mg◇
Capsules: 475 mg◇, 500 mg◇
Oral suspension: 320 mg/5 ml◇, 450 mg/5ml◇, 600 mg/5 ml◇, 675 mg/5 ml◇

ACTION

An antacid that reduces total acid load in the GI tract, elevates gastric pH to reduce pepsin activity, strengthens the gastric mucosal barrier, and increases esophageal sphincter tone.

ONSET, PEAK, DURATION

Onset varies by dosage form; liquids are more rapid-acting than tablets or capsules. Peak unknown. Duration varies with gastric emptying time; 20 to 60 minutes in fasting patients, 3 hours when taken after meals.

INDICATIONS & DOSAGE

Antacid—
Adults: 500 to 1,500 mg P.O. (5 to 30 ml of most suspension products) 1 hour after meals and h.s.; alternatively, 300-mg tablet or 600-mg tablet (chewed before swallowing) taken with milk or water five to six times daily after meals and h.s.

ADVERSE REACTIONS

CNS: encephalopathy.
GI: *constipation,* intestinal obstruction.
Other: hypophosphatemia, osteomalacia.

INTERACTIONS

Allopurinol, antibiotics (including quinolones and tetracyclines), corticosteroids, diflunisal, digoxin, ethambutol, *histamine-$_2$ antagonists, iron salts, isoniazid, penicillamine, phenothiazines, thyroid hormones, ticlopidine:* decreased pharmacologic effect because of possible impaired absorption. Separate administration times.
Enteric-coated drugs: may be released prematurely in stomach. Separate doses by at least 1 hour.

EFFECTS ON DIAGNOSTIC TESTS

Aluminum hydroxide therapy may interfere with imaging techniques using sodium pertechnetate Tc99m and thus impair evaluation of Meckel's diverticulum. It may also interfere with reticuloendothelial imaging of liver, spleen, or bone marrow using technetium Tc99m sulfur colloid. It may antagonize pentagastrin's effect during gastric acid secretion tests. Drug may increase serum gastrin levels and decrease serum phosphate levels.

CONTRAINDICATIONS

None known.

NURSING CONSIDERATIONS

● Use cautiously in patients with chronic renal disease.
● When administering through nasogastric tube, make sure tube is placed correctly and is patent; after instilling, flush tube with water to ensure passage to stomach and to clear tube.
● Monitor long-term, high-dose use in patient on restricted sodium intake. Each tablet, capsule, or 5 ml of suspension contains 2 to 3 mg of sodium.
● Record amount and consistency of stools. Manage constipation with laxatives or stool softeners as ordered; alternate with magnesium-containing antacids (if the patient does not have renal disease).
● Monitor serum phosphate levels.
● Watch for symptoms of hypophosphatemia with prolonged use (anorexia, malaise, and muscle weakness); can also lead to resorption of calcium and bone demineralization.

Reactions may be *common*, uncommon, ***life-threatening***, or COMMON AND LIFE-THREATENING.

• Because drug contains aluminum, keep in mind that it is used in patients with renal failure to help control hyperphosphatemia by binding with phosphate in the GI tract.

☑ **PATIENT TEACHING**
• Instruct patient to shake suspension well and to follow with small amount of milk or water to facilitate passage.
• Advise patient not to take aluminum hydroxide indiscriminately or to switch antacids without the doctor's advice.

aluminum phosphate
Phosphaljel ◊

Pregnancy Risk Category: NR

HOW SUPPLIED
Oral suspension: 233 mg/5 ml ◊

ACTION
Provides supplemental phosphate.

ONSET, PEAK, DURATION
Onset occurs in about 20 minutes. Peak unknown. Effects persist for 20 to 60 minutes in fasting patients, 3 hours when taken after meals.

INDICATIONS & DOSAGE
To reduce fecal elimination of phosphorus—
Adults: 15 to 30 ml undiluted P.O. q 2 hours between meals and h.s.

ADVERSE REACTIONS
CNS: encephalopathy.
GI: *constipation,* intestinal obstruction.
Other: hypophosphatemia, osteomalacia.

INTERACTIONS
Ciprofloxacin and other quinolones, tetracyclines: decreased antibiotic effect. Separate administration times.
Enteric-coated drugs: may be released prematurely in stomach. Separate doses by at least 1 hour.

EFFECTS ON DIAGNOSTIC TESTS
Aluminum phosphate may interfere with imaging techniques using sodium pertechnetate Tc99m and thus impair evaluation of Meckel's diverticulum. It may also interfere with reticuloendothelial imaging of liver, spleen, or bone marrow using technetium Tc99m sulfur colloid. It may antagonize pentagastrin's effect during gastric acid secretion tests.

CONTRAINDICATIONS
None known.

NURSING CONSIDERATIONS
• Use cautiously in patients with chronic renal disease.
• When administering through nasogastric tube, make sure tube is placed correctly and is patent; after instilling, flush tube with water to ensure passage to stomach and to clear tube.
• Record amount and consistency of stools. Manage constipation with laxatives or stool softeners as ordered; alternate with magnesium-containing antacids (if the patient does not have renal disease).
• Monitor patient closely, especially with long-term use. Also monitor long-term, high-dose use in patients on restricted sodium intake.
Alert: Know that the drug can reverse hypophosphatemia induced by aluminum hydroxide.
• Be aware that Phosphaljel contains no sugar.

☑ **PATIENT TEACHING**
• Instruct patient to shake suspension well; it may be taken alone or with small amount of milk or water.
• Advise patient not to take aluminum phosphate indiscriminately or to switch antacids without the doctor's advice.

calcium carbonate
Alka-Mints ◊ , Amitone ◊ , Calcilac ◊ , Calcimax‡, Calglycine ◊ , Cal-Sup‡,

*Liquid contains alcohol. **May contain tartrazine. †Canada only. ‡Australia only. ◊OTC.

Chooz ◇, Dicarbosil ◇, Effercal-600‡, Equilet ◇, Gencalc ◇, Mallamint ◇, Rolaids Calcium Rich ◇, Titracid ◇, Titralac ◇, Titralac Extra Strength ◇, Titralac Plus ◇, Tums ◇, Tums E-X ◇, Tums Liquid Extra Strength ◇

Pregnancy Risk Category: NR

HOW SUPPLIED
Calcium carbonate contains 40% calcium; 20 mEq calcium per gram.
Tablets (chewable): 350 mg ◇, 420 mg ◇, 500 mg ◇, 750 mg, 850 mg, 1,000 mg, 1,250 mg‡
Tablets: 500 mg ◇, 600 mg ◇, 650 mg ◇, 1,000 mg ◇, 1,250 mg ◇
Chewing gum: 500 mg/piece
Oral suspension: 1 g/5 ml ◇, 250 mg/5 ml
Lozenges: 600 mg ◇

ACTION
An antacid that reduces total acid load in the GI tract, elevates gastric pH to reduce pepsin activity, strengthens the gastric mucosal barrier, and increases esophageal sphincter tone.

ONSET, PEAK, DURATION
Onset occurs within 20 minutes. Peak unknown. Effects persist for 20 to 60 minutes in fasting patients, 3 hours when taken after meals.

INDICATIONS & DOSAGE
Antacid, calcium supplement—
Adults: 350 mg to 1.5 g P.O. or 2 pieces of chewing gum 1 hour after meals and h.s. p.r.n.

ADVERSE REACTIONS
CNS: headache, irritability, weakness.
GI: rebound hyperacidity, *nausea.*

INTERACTIONS
Antibiotics (including quinolones and tetracyclines), hydantoins, iron salts, isoniazid, salicylates: decreased pharmacologic effect because of possible impaired absorption. Separate administration times.
Enteric-coated drugs: may be released prematurely in stomach. Separate doses by at least 1 hour.
Milk and other foods high in vitamin D: possible milk-alkali syndrome (headache, confusion, distaste for food, nausea, vomiting, hypercalcemia, hypercalciuria, calcinosis, hypophosphatemia). Avoid concomitant use.

EFFECTS ON DIAGNOSTIC TESTS
Drug may alter serum phosphate levels.

CONTRAINDICATIONS
Contraindicated in patients with ventricular fibrillation or hypercalcemia.

NURSING CONSIDERATIONS
● Use cautiously, if at all, in patients with sarcoidosis, renal or cardiac disease, and in patients receiving cardiac glycosides.
● Record amount and consistency of stools. Manage constipation with laxatives or stool softeners as ordered.
● Monitor serum calcium levels, especially in patients with mild renal impairment.
● Watch for symptoms of hypercalcemia (nausea, vomiting, headache, mental confusion, and anorexia).

☑ PATIENT TEACHING
● Advise patient not to take calcium carbonate indiscriminately or to switch antacids without the doctor's advice.
● Tell patient taking chewable tablets to chew thoroughly before swallowing and follow with a glass of water.
● Tell patient using suspension form to shake well and take with a small amount of water to facilitate passage.

dihydroxyaluminum sodium carbonate
Rolaids ◇

Pregnancy Risk Category: NR

HOW SUPPLIED
Tablets: 334 mg ◇

ACTION
An antacid that reduces total acid load in the GI tract, elevates gastric pH to reduce pepsin activity, strengthens the gastric mucosal barrier, and increases esophageal sphincter tone.

ONSET, PEAK, DURATION
Onset occurs in 20 minutes. Peak unknown. Effects persist for 20 to 60 minutes in fasting patients, 3 hours when taken after meals.

INDICATIONS & DOSAGE
Antacid—
Adults: 1 to 2 tablets (334 to 668 mg) P.O., chewed well, p.r.n.

ADVERSE REACTIONS
CNS: encephalopathy.
GI: *constipation,* intestinal obstruction.
Other: hypophosphatemia, osteomalacia.

INTERACTIONS
Allopurinol, antibiotics (including quinolones and tetracyclines), diflunisal, digoxin, iron, isoniazid, penicillamine, phenothiazines, quinidine: decreased pharmacologic effect because of possible impaired absorption. Separate administration times.
Enteric-coated drugs: may be released prematurely in stomach. Separate doses by at least 1 hour.

EFFECTS ON DIAGNOSTIC TESTS
Drug may interfere with evaluation of Meckel's diverticulum, reticuloendothelial imaging, and other tests using radiopaque media. It may also increase serum gastrin levels.

CONTRAINDICATIONS
None known.

NURSING CONSIDERATIONS
● Use cautiously in patients with renal disease.
● Record amount and consistency of stools. Manage constipation with laxatives or stool softeners as ordered; alternate with magnesium-containing antacids (if the patient does not have renal disease).
● Monitor long-term, high-dose use in patients on restricted sodium intake. Has high sodium content (53 mg/tablet) and may increase sodium and water retention.

☑ PATIENT TEACHING
● Advise patient not to take dihydroxyaluminum sodium carbonate indiscriminately.
● Encourage patient to follow his prescribed diet, if applicable.

---

magaldrate (aluminum-magnesium complex)
Antiflux†, Iosopan ◇, Lowsium ◇, Riopan ◇

Pregnancy Risk Category: NR

HOW SUPPLIED
Tablets: 480 mg ◇
Tablets (chewable): 480 mg ◇
Oral suspension: 540 mg/5 ml ◇

ACTION
An antacid that reduces total acid load in the GI tract, elevates gastric pH to reduce pepsin activity, strengthens the gastric mucosal barrier, and increases esophageal sphincter tone.

ONSET, PEAK, DURATION
Onset occurs within 20 minutes. Peak unknown. Effects persist for 20 to 60 minutes in fasting patients, 3 hours when taken after meals.

INDICATIONS & DOSAGE
Antacid—
Adults: 540 to 1,080 mg (5 to 10 ml) of suspension P.O. with water between meals and h.s.; or 480 to 960 mg tablets

(1 to 2 tablets) P.O. with water between meals and h.s.; or 480 to 960 mg chewable tablets (1 to 2 tablets) P.O., chewed before swallowing, between meals and h.s.

ADVERSE REACTIONS
GI: mild constipation or diarrhea.

INTERACTIONS
Allopurinol, antibiotics (including quinolones and tetracyclines), diflunisal, digoxin, iron salts, isoniazid, penicillamine, phenothiazines, quinidine, ticlopidine: decreased pharmacologic effect because of possible impaired absorption. Separate administration times by 1 to 2 hours.
Enteric-coated drugs: may be released prematurely in stomach. Separate doses by at least 1 hour.

EFFECTS ON DIAGNOSTIC TESTS
Magaldrate may antagonize pentagastrin's effect during gastric acid secretion tests; drug may decrease serum potassium levels and increase serum gastrin and urine pH levels.

CONTRAINDICATIONS
Contraindicated in patients with severe renal disease.

NURSING CONSIDERATIONS
● Use cautiously in patients with mild kidney impairment.
● When giving through nasogastric tube, make sure tube is placed properly and is patent. After instilling, flush tube with water to ensure passage to stomach and to clear tube.
● Monitor serum magnesium level in patients with mild kidney impairment. Symptomatic hypermagnesemia usually occurs only in severe renal failure.
Alert: Keep in mind that drug is not typically used in patients with renal failure to help control hypophosphatemia because it contains magnesium, which may accumulate.
● Be aware that the drug has a very low

sodium content and is good for patients on restricted sodium intake.

☑ PATIENT TEACHING
● Instruct patient to shake suspension well and to follow with water.
● Tell patient taking chewable tablets to chew thoroughly and to follow with a glass of water.
● Advise patient not to take magaldrate indiscriminately or to switch antacids without the doctor's advice.

---

magnesium oxide
Mag-Ox 400 ◇ , Maox-420 ◇ , Uro-Mag ◇

Pregnancy Risk Category: NR

HOW SUPPLIED
Tablets: 400 mg ◇ , 420 mg ◇
Capsules: 140 mg ◇

ACTION
Reduces total acid load in the GI tract, elevates gastric pH, strengthens the gastric mucosal barrier, and increases esophageal sphincter tone.

ONSET, PEAK, DURATION
Onset occurs within 20 minutes. Peak unknown. Effects persist for 20 to 60 minutes in fasting patients, 3 hours when taken after meals.

INDICATIONS & DOSAGE
Antacid—
Adults: 140 mg P.O. with water or milk after meals and h.s.
Laxative—
Adults: 4 g P.O. with water or milk, usually h.s.
Oral replacement therapy in mild hypomagnesemia—
Adults: 400 to 840 mg P.O. daily. Monitor serum magnesium level.

ADVERSE REACTIONS
GI: *diarrhea,* nausea, abdominal pain.
Other: hypermagnesemia.

Reactions may be *common,* uncommon, *life-threatening,* or COMMON AND LIFE-THREATENING.

INTERACTIONS
Allopurinol, antibiotics, digoxin, iron salts, penicillamine, phenothiazines: decreased effect because of possible impaired absorption. Separate administration times by 1 to 2 hours.
Enteric-coated drugs: may be released prematurely in stomach. Separate doses by at least 1 hour.

EFFECTS ON DIAGNOSTIC TESTS
No information available.

CONTRAINDICATIONS
Contraindicated in patients with severe renal disease.

NURSING CONSIDERATIONS
• Use cautiously in patients with mild renal impairment.
• When used as laxative, do not give other oral drugs 1 to 2 hours before or after treatment.
• Monitor serum magnesium levels. With prolonged use and some degree of renal impairment, watch for symptoms of hypermagnesemia (hypotension, nausea, vomiting, depressed reflexes, respiratory depression, and coma).
• If diarrhea occurs, be prepared to suggest alternative preparation.

☑ **PATIENT TEACHING**
• Advise patient not to take magnesium oxide indiscriminately or to switch antacids without the doctor's advice.

---

simethicone
Extra Strength Gas-X ◇, Gas-Relief ◇, Gas-X ◇, Maximum Strength Phazyme 125 Softgels ◇, Mylanta Gas ◇, Mylanta Gas Maximum Strength ◇, Mylanta Gas Regular Strength ◇, Mylicon ◇, Ovol†, Ovol-40†, Ovol-80†, Phazyme ◇, Phazyme 55† ◇, Phazyme 95 ◇

Pregnancy Risk Category: NR

HOW SUPPLIED
Tablets: 40 mg ◇, 55 mg† ◇, 60 mg ◇, 80 mg ◇, 95 mg ◇, 125 mg ◇
Capsules: 125 mg
Drops: 40 mg/0.6 ml ◇

ACTION
By its defoaming action, disperses or prevents formation of mucus-surrounded gas pockets in the GI tract.

ONSET, PEAK, DURATION
Onset and peak is immediate. Duration unknown.

INDICATIONS & DOSAGE
Flatulence, functional gastric bloating—
Adults and children over 12 years: 40 to 160 mg after each meal and h.s.

ADVERSE REACTIONS
GI: expulsion of excessive liberated gas as belching, rectal flatus.

INTERACTIONS
None significant.

EFFECTS ON DIAGNOSTIC TESTS
None reported.

CONTRAINDICATIONS
Contraindicated in patients hypersensitive to the drug.

NURSING CONSIDERATIONS
• Know that drug is not recommended for the treatment of infant colic because of limited information on its safety in infants and children.
• Be aware that medication does not prevent formation of gas.

☑ **PATIENT TEACHING**
• Tell patient to chew tablet before swallowing.
• Encourage patient to change positions frequently and ambulate to aid in passing flatus.

monoctanoin
pancreatin
pancrelipase
ursodiol

COMBINATION PRODUCTS
DONNAZYME TABLETS: pancreatin 300 mg, pepsin 150 mg, bile salts 150 mg, hyoscyamine sulfate 0.0518 mg, atropine sulfate 0.0097 mg, scopolamine hydrobromide 0.0033 mg, and phenobarbital 8.1 mg.
ENTOZYME TABLETS: pancreatin 300 mg, pepsin 250 mg, and bile salts 150 mg.
PANCREASE CAPSULES: lipase 4,000 units, protease 25,000 units, and amylase 20,000 units in enteric-coated microspheres.

---

monoctanoin
Moctanin

Pregnancy Risk Category: C

HOW SUPPLIED
Infusion: 120-ml bottles

ACTION
Dissolves gallstones by rendering them more soluble.

ONSET, PEAK, DURATION
Onset usually occurs within 72 hours. Peak and duration unknown.

INDICATIONS & DOSAGE
To solubilize cholesterol (radiolucent) gallstones retained in the biliary tract after cholecystectomy—
Adults: administered as a continuous infusion for 2 to 10 days (for elimination or size reduction of stones) through a catheter inserted directly into common bile duct at a rate of 3 to 5 ml/hour and at a pressure of 10 cm H_2O.

ADVERSE REACTIONS
GI: *pain, abdominal discomfort, nausea, vomiting, diarrhea,* anorexia, indigestion.
Other: fever.

INTERACTIONS
None significant.

EFFECTS ON DIAGNOSTIC TESTS
None reported.

CONTRAINDICATIONS
Contraindicated in patients with impaired hepatic function, biliary tract infection, or a history of recent duodenal ulceration or jejunitis; porto-systemic shunting; acute pancreatitis, or any active life-threatening problems that would be complicated by perfusion into the biliary tract.

NURSING CONSIDERATIONS
● Be aware monoctanoin therapy should be initiated only by individuals experienced in infusion therapy.
● Because impaired liver function may lead to metabolic acidosis during monoctanoin administration, obtain routine liver function tests as ordered before perfusion therapy begins.
Alert: Do not administer parenterally; for biliary tract infusion only.
● Dilute each vial with sterile water for injection. Dilution will reduce solution viscosity and enhance bathing of stone.
● Warm the solution to 60° to 80° F (16° to 27° C) before perfusion. Temperature should not fall below 65° F (18° C) during administration.
● Use a peristaltic infusion pump to regulate the infusion. Outpatients may use a battery-operated portable pump.
● Keep pump pressure at 10 cm H_2O to minimize GI and biliary tract irritation. Pressure must be below 15 cm H_2O.

Reactions may be *common,* uncommon, *life-threatening,* or COMMON AND LIFE-THREATENING.

● Reduce GI symptoms by slowing the infusion rate or discontinuing infusion during meals, as ordered.

☑ **PATIENT TEACHING**
● Instruct outpatient on use of pump and drug administration.
● Inform patient of need for follow-up care and diagnostic studies.
● Tell patient to report adverse effects.

pancreatin
Bioglan Panazyme‡, Dizymes TabletsL, Entozyme, 4X Pancreatin 600 mg ◊ , Hi-Vegi-Lip Tablets ◊ , Pancrezyme 4X Tablets ◊

Pregnancy Risk Category: C

HOW SUPPLIED
Bioglan Panazyme‡
Tablets: 468 mg pancreatin, 7,200 units lipase, 656 units protease, and 9,200 units amylase
Dizymes
Tablets (enteric-coated): 250 mg pancreatin, 6,750 units lipase, 41,250 units protease, and 43,750 units amylase ◊
Donnazyme
Tablets: 500 mg pancreatin, 1,000 units lipase, 12,500 units protease, and 12,500 units amylase
8X Pancreatin 900 mg
Tablets (enteric-coated): 7,200 mg pancreatin, 22,500 units lipase, 180,000 units protease, and 180,000 units amylase ◊
Entozyme
Tablets: 500 mg pancreatin, 600 units lipase, 7,500 units protease, and 7,500 units amylase
4X Pancreatin 600 mg
Tablets (enteric-coated): 2,400 mg pancreatin, 12,000 units lipase, 60,000 units protease, and 60,000 units amylase ◊
Hi-Vegi-Lip
Tablets (enteric-coated): 2,400 mg pancreatin, 4,800 units lipase, 60,000 units protease, and 60,000 units amylase ◊
Pancrezyme 4X

Tablets (enteric-coated): 2,400 mg pancreatin, 12,000 units lipase, 60,000 units protease, and 60,000 units amylase ◊

ACTION
Replaces endogenous exocrine pancreatic enzymes and aids digestion of starches, fats, and proteins.

ONSET, PEAK, DURATION
Onset and peak unknown. Effects persist for 1 to 2 hours.

INDICATIONS & DOSAGE
Exocrine pancreatic secretion insufficiency; digestive aid in diseases associated with deficiency of pancreatic enzymes, such as cystic fibrosis—
Adults and children: dosage varies with condition being treated. Usual initial dosage is 8,000 to 24,000 units of lipase activity before or with each meal or snack. The total daily dose may also be given in divided doses at 1 to 2 hour intervals throughout the day.

ADVERSE REACTIONS
GI: nausea, diarrhea (with high doses).
Other: allergic reactions, perianal irritation.

INTERACTIONS
Antacids: may negate pancreatin's beneficial effect. Avoid concomitant use.
Oral iron: may decrease serum iron response. Monitor for decreased effectiveness.

EFFECTS ON DIAGNOSTIC TESTS
Pancreatin, particularly in large doses, increases serum uric acid concentrations.

CONTRAINDICATIONS
Contraindicated in patients with hypersensitivity to the drug, or to pork protein or enzymes, acute pancreatitis, and acute exacerbations of chronic pancreatitis.

NURSING CONSIDERATIONS

• Use with caution in pregnant or breast-feeding patients.

• Be aware that minimal USP standards dictate that each milligram of bovine or porcine pancreatin contain lipase 2 units, protease 25 units, and amylase 25 units.

• To avoid indigestion, monitor patient's dietary intake to ensure a proper balance of fat, protein, and starch intake. Dosage varies according to degree of maldigestion and malabsorption, amount of fat in diet, and enzyme activity of individual preparations.

• Keep in mind that fewer bowel movements and improved stool consistency indicate effective therapy.

• Know that the drug is not effective in GI disorders unrelated to pancreatic enzyme deficiency.

• Know that enteric coating on some products may reduce available enzyme in upper portion of jejunum.

☑ **PATIENT TEACHING**

• Instruct patient to take before or with meals and snacks.

• Tell patient not to crush or chew enteric-coated forms. Capsules containing enteric-coated microspheres may be opened and sprinkled on a small quantity of cooled, soft food. Stress importance of swallowing immediately without chewing and following with glass of water or juice.

• Warn patient not to inhale powder form or powder from capsules; may irritate skin or mucous membranes.

• Tell patient to store in airtight containers at room temperature.

• Instruct patient not to change brands without consulting doctor.

---

pancrelipase

Cotazym Capsules, Cotazym-S Capsules, Creon 5 Capsules, Creon 10 Capsules, Creon 20 Capsules, Ilozyme Tablets, Ku-Zyme HP Capsules, Pancrease Capsules, Pancrease MT 4, Pancrease MT 10, Pancrease MT 16, Pancrease MT 20, Pancrelipase Capsules, Protilase Capsules, Ultrase MT 12, Ultrase MT 20, Ultrase MT 24, Viokase Powder, Viokase Tablets, Zymase Capsules

Pregnancy Risk Category: C

HOW SUPPLIED

Cotazym
Capsules: 8,000 units lipase, 30,000 units protease, 30,000 units amylase, and 25 mg calcium carbonate

Cotazym-S
Capsules (enteric-coated spheres): 5,000 units lipase, 20,000 units protease, and 20,000 units amylase

Creon 5
Capsules (delayed-release): 5,000 units lipase, 18,750 units protease, and 16,600 units amylase

Creon 10
Capsules (delayed-release): 10,000 units lipase, 37,500 units protease, and 33,200 units amylase

Creon 20
Capsules (delayed-release): 20,000 units lipase, 75,000 units protease, and 66,400 units amylase

Ilozyme
Tablets: 11,000 units lipase, 30,000 units protease, and 30,000 units amylase

Ku-Zyme HP
Capsules: 8,000 units lipase, 30,000 units protease, and 30,000 units amylase

Pancrease
Capsules (enteric-coated microspheres): 4,000 units lipase, 25,000 units protease, and 20,000 units amylase

Pancrease MT 4
Capsules (enteric-coated microtablets): 4,500 units lipase, 12,000 units protease, and 12,000 units amylase

Pancrease MT 10
Capsules (enteric-coated microtablets): 10,000 units lipase, 30,000 units protease, and 30,000 units amylase

Pancrease MT 16
Capsules (enteric-coated microtablets): 16,000 units lipase, 48,000 units pro-

tease, and 48,000 units amylase

Pancrease MT 20
Capsules (enteric-coated microtablets):
20,000 units lipase, 44,000 units protease, and 56,000 units amylase

Pancrelipase
Capsules (enteric-coated pellets): 4,000 units lipase, 25,000 units protease, and 20,000 units amylase

Protilase
Capsules (enteric-coated spheres):
4,000 units lipase, 25,000 units protease, and 20,000 units amylase

Ultrase MT 12
Capsules (delayed-release): 12,000 units lipase, 39,000 units protease, and 39,000 units amylase

Ultrase MT 20
Capsules (delayed-release): 20,000 units lipase, 65,000 units protease, and 65,000 units amylase

Ultrase MT 24
Capsules (delayed-release): 24,000 units lipase, 78,000 units protease, and 78,000 units amylase

Viokase
Powder: 16,800 units lipase, 70,000 units protease, and 70,000 units amylase per 0.7 g powder
Tablets: 8,000 units lipase, 30,000 units protease, and 30,000 units amylase

Zymase
Capsules (enteric-coated spheres):
12,000 units lipase, 24,000 units protease, and 24,000 units amylase

ACTION
Replaces endogenous exocrine pancreatic enzymes and aids digestion of starches, fats, and proteins.

ONSET, PEAK, DURATION
Variable.

INDICATIONS & DOSAGE
Exocrine pancreatic secretion insufficiency, cystic fibrosis in adults and children, steatorrhea and other disorders of fat metabolism secondary to insufficient pancreatic enzymes—
Adults and children 12 years and old-
er: dosage titrated to patient's response. Usual initial dosage 4,000 to 48,000 units of lipase with each meal.
Children 7 to 12 years: 4,000 to 12,000 units (more, if needed) of lipase activity with each meal or snack.
Children 1 to 6 years: 4,000 to 8,000 units of lipase with each meal and 4,000 units of lipase with each snack.
Children 6 months to 1 year: 2,000 units of lipase with each meal.
Children under 6 months: dosage not established.

ADVERSE REACTIONS
GI: *nausea,* cramping, diarrhea (high doses).

INTERACTIONS
Antacids: may destroy enteric coating and result in enhanced degradation of pancrelipase. Avoid concomitant use.
Oral iron: may decrease serum iron response. Monitor for decreased effectiveness.

EFFECTS ON DIAGNOSTIC TESTS
Pancrelipase, particularly in large doses, increases serum uric acid concentrations.

CONTRAINDICATIONS
Contraindicated in patients with severe hypersensitivity to pork, acute pancreatitis, or acute exacerbations of chronic pancreatic diseases.

NURSING CONSIDERATIONS
● Know that drug should be used only after confirmed diagnosis of exocrine pancreatic insufficiency. It's not effective in GI disorders unrelated to enzyme deficiency.
● Know that lipase activity is greater than with other pancreatic enzymes.
● For infants, mix powder with applesauce and give with meals. Avoid contact with or inhalation of powder because it may be very irritating. Older children may take capsules with food.
● Monitor patient's stools. Adequate re-

placement decreases number of bowel movements and improves stool consistency.

• Know that minimal USP standards dictate that each milligram of pancrelipase contain 24 units lipase, 100 units protease, and 100 units amylase.

• Know that dosage varies with degree of maldigestion and malabsorption, amount of fat in diet, and enzyme activity of individual preparations.

• Know that enteric coating on some products may reduce available enzyme in upper portion of jejunum.

☑ **PATIENT TEACHING**
• Instruct patient to take before or with meals and snacks.

• Advise patient not to crush or chew enteric-coated forms. Capsules containing enteric-coated microspheres may be opened and sprinkled on a small quantity of cooled, soft food. Stress importance of swallowing immediately without chewing and following with glass of water or juice.

• Warn patient not to inhale powder form or powder from capsules; it may irritate skin or mucous membranes.

• Tell patient to store in airtight containers at room temperature.

• Instruct patient not to change brands without consulting doctor.

---

ursodiol
Actigall

Pregnancy Risk Category: B

HOW SUPPLIED
Capsules:: 300 mg

ACTION
Unknown. A naturally occurring bile acid that probably suppresses hepatic synthesis and secretion of cholesterol as well as intestinal cholesterol absorption. After long-term use, ursodiol can solubilize cholesterol from gallstones.

ONSET, PEAK, DURATION
Onset and duration unknown. Peak levels occur 1 to 3 hours after dose.

INDICATIONS & DOSAGE
Dissolution of gallstones less than 20 mm in diameter when surgery precluded—
Adults: 8 to 10 mg/kg P.O. daily in two or three divided doses.

ADVERSE REACTIONS
CNS: headache, fatigue, anxiety, depression, sleep disorders.
EENT: rhinitis.
GI: nausea, vomiting, dyspepsia, metallic taste, abdominal pain, biliary pain, cholecystitis, diarrhea, constipation, stomatitis, flatulence.
Respiratory: cough.
Skin: pruritus, rash, dry skin, urticaria, hair thinning, diaphoresis.
Other: arthralgia, myalgia, back pain.

INTERACTIONS
Aluminum-containing antacids, cholestyramine, colestipol: bind ursodiol and prevent its absorption. Avoid concomitant use.
Clofibrate, estrogens, oral contraceptives: increased hepatic cholesterol secretion; may counteract the effects of ursodiol. Avoid concomitant use.

EFFECTS ON DIAGNOSTIC TESTS
None reported.

CONTRAINDICATIONS
Contraindicated in patients hypersensitive to ursodiol or other bile acids and in those with chronic hepatic disease, unremitting acute cholecystitis, cholangitis, biliary obstruction, gallstone-induced pancreatitis, or biliary fistula.

NURSING CONSIDERATIONS
• Know that drug won't dissolve calcified cholesterol stones, radiolucent bile pigment stones, or radiopaque stones.
Alert: Monitor liver function test results, including AST and ALT, at the start of

---

therapy and after 1 month, 3 months, and then every 6 months during therapy, as ordered. Abnormal tests may indicate a worsening of the disease. A theoretical risk exists that a hepatotoxic metabolite of ursodiol may form in some patients.

• Know that therapy usually is long-term, with ultrasound images of the gallbladder taken every 6 months. If partial stone dissolution does not occur within 12 months, eventual success is unlikely. Safety of use for longer than 24 months has not been established.

☑ **PATIENT TEACHING**

• Tell patient about alternative therapies, including "watchful waiting" (no intervention) and cholecystectomy because the relapse rate may be as high as 50% after 5 years.

• Tell patient to report adverse effects.

attapulgite
bismuth subsalicylate
calcium polycarbophil
(See Chapter 50, LAXATIVES.)
kaolin and pectin mixtures
loperamide
octreotide acetate
opium tincture
opium tincture, camphorated

COMBINATION PRODUCTS
K-C ◊: 5.2 g kaolin, 260 mg pectin, 260 mg bismuth subsalicylate in 30-ml suspension.
KAODENE NON-NARCOTIC ◊: 3.9 g kaolin and 194.4 mg pectin in 30-ml bismuth subsalicylate liquid.

---

attapulgite
Children's Kaopectate, Diasorb, Donnagel, Fowler's†, Kaopectate Advanced Formula, Kaopectate Maximum Strength, K-Pek, Parepectolin, Rheaban Maximum Strength

Pregnancy Risk Category: NR

HOW SUPPLIED
Tablets: 300 mg, 600 mg†, 630 mg†, 750 mg
Chewable tablets: 300 mg, 600 mg
Oral suspension: 600 mg/15 ml, 750 ml/5ml, 750 mg/15 ml†, 900 mg/15 ml†

ACTION
A hydrated magnesium aluminum silicate that is thought to adsorb large numbers of bacteria and toxins and reduce water loss.

ONSET, PEAK, DURATION
Unknown.

INDICATIONS & DOSAGE
Acute, nonspecific diarrhea—

Adults and adolescents: 1.2 to 1.5 g (up to 3 g if using Diasorb) P.O. after each loose bowel movement, not to exceed 9 g in 24 hours.
Children 6 to 12 years: 600 mg (suspension) or 750 mg (tablet) P.O. after each loose bowel movement, not to exceed 4.2 g (suspension) or 4.5 g (tablet) in 24 hours.
Children 3 to 6 years: 300 mg P.O. after each loose bowel movement, not to exceed 2.1 g in 24 hours.

ADVERSE REACTIONS
GI: constipation.

INTERACTIONS
Oral medications: potential for impaired absorption of oral medications when administered concurrently with attapulgite. Administer attapulgite not less than 2 hours before or 3 hours after these medications, and monitor for decreased effectiveness.

EFFECTS ON DIAGNOSTIC TESTS
None reported.

CONTRAINDICATIONS
Contraindicated in patients with dysentery or suspected bowel obstruction.

NURSING CONSIDERATIONS
● Use cautiously in patients with dehydration. Promote adequate fluid intake to compensate for fluid loss from diarrhea.
● Be aware that drug should not be used if diarrhea is accompanied by fever or by blood or mucus in the stool. If these signs occur during treatment, withhold drug and notify doctor.

☑ PATIENT TEACHING
● Tell the patient to take the drug after each loose bowel movement until diar-

---

Reactions may be *common*, uncommon, *life-threatening*, or COMMON AND LIFE-THREATENING.

rhea is controlled.
● Instruct the patient to notify the doctor if diarrhea is not controlled within 48 hours or if fever develops.

---

bismuth subsalicylate
Bismatrol ◊, Bismatrol Extra Strength ◊, Maximum Strength Pepto-Bismol Liquid ◊, Pepto-Bismol ◊, Pink Bismuth ◊

Pregnancy Risk Category: NR

HOW SUPPLIED
Tablets (chewable): 262 mg ◊
Caplets: 262 mg
Oral suspension: 262 mg/15 ml ◊, 524 mg/15 ml ◊

ACTION
Unknown. Has a mild water-binding capacity; also may adsorb toxins and provide protective coating for mucosa.

ONSET, PEAK, DURATION
Onset occurs within 1 hour. Peak and duration unknown.

INDICATIONS & DOSAGE
Mild, nonspecific diarrhea—
Adults: 30 ml or 2 tablets P.O. q ½ to 1 hour, up to a maximum of eight doses and for no longer than 2 days.
Children 3 to 6 years: 5 ml or ⅓ tablet P.O.
Children 6 to 9 years: 10 ml or ⅔ tablet P.O.
Children 9 to 12 years: 15 ml or 1 tablet P.O.

ADVERSE REACTIONS
GI: temporary darkening of tongue and stools.
Other: salicylism (with high doses).

INTERACTIONS
Aspirin, other salicylates: risk of salicylate toxicity. Monitor closely.
Oral anticoagulants, oral antidiabetic agents: theoretical risk of increased ef-

fects of these agents after high doses of bismuth subsalicylate. Monitor the patient closely.
Tetracycline: decreased tetracycline absorption. Separate administration times by at least 2 hours.

EFFECTS ON DIAGNOSTIC TESTS
Because bismuth is radiopaque, it may interfere with radiologic examination of the GI tract.

CONTRAINDICATIONS
Contraindicated in patients hypersensitive to salicylates.

NURSING CONSIDERATIONS
● Use cautiously in patients taking aspirin. Discontinue if tinnitus occurs.
● Avoid use before GI radiologic procedures because bismuth is radiopaque and may interfere with X-rays.

☑ PATIENT TEACHING
● Advise patient that bismuth subsalicylate contains salicylate (each tablet has 102 mg salicylate; the regular-strength liquid has 130 mg/15 ml, and the extra-strength liquid has 230 mg/15 ml).
● Instruct patient to chew tablets well before swallowing or to shake liquid before measuring dose.
● Tell patient to call the doctor if diarrhea persists for more than 2 days or is accompanied by high fever.
● Tell patient to consult with the doctor before giving bismuth subsalicylate to children or teenagers during or after recovery from the flu or chickenpox.
● Inform patient that all forms of Pepto-Bismol are effective against traveler's diarrhea. Tablets and caplets may be more convenient to carry.

---

kaolin and pectin mixtures
Kaolin with Pectin ◊, Kao-Spen ◊, Kaodene Non-Narcotic ◊, Kapectolin ◊, K-C ◊

Pregnancy Risk Category: NR

HOW SUPPLIED
Oral suspension: 5.2 mg kaolin and 260 mg pectin per 30 ml ◇ (Kao-Spen ◇); 90 g kaolin, 2 g pectin per 30 ml ◇ (Kaolin with Pectin ◇, Kapectolin ◇)

ACTION
Decreases fluid content of stools, although *total* water loss seems to remain the same.

ONSET, PEAK, DURATION
Unknown.

INDICATIONS & DOSAGE
Mild, nonspecific diarrhea—
Adults and children 12 years and older: 60 to 120 ml P.O. after each bowel movement.
Children 3 to 6 years: 15 to 30 ml P.O. after each bowel movement.
Children 6 to 12 years: 30 to 60 ml P.O. after each bowel movement.

ADVERSE REACTIONS
GI: drug absorption of nutrients, other drugs, and enzymes; fecal impaction or ulceration in infants and elderly or debilitated patients after chronic use; constipation.

INTERACTIONS
Orally administered drugs: adsorption may occur. Separate administration times by at least 2 to 3 hours.

EFFECTS ON DIAGNOSTIC TESTS
None reported.

CONTRAINDICATIONS
None known.

NURSING CONSIDERATION
Administer other oral drugs 2 to 3 hours before or after administration of a kaolin and pectin mixture.

☑ PATIENT TEACHING
● Warn patient not to use drug to replace specific therapy for underlying cause.

● Advise patient not to use drug for more than 2 days.

---

loperamide
Imodium, Imodium A-D ◇, Kaopectate II Caplets ◇, Maalox Anti-Diarrheal Caplets ◇, Pepto Diarrhea Control ◇

Pregnancy Risk Category: B

HOW SUPPLIED
Caplets: 2 mg ◇
Capsules: 2 mg
Oral liquid: 1 mg/5 ml ◇

ACTION
Inhibits peristaltic activity, prolonging transit of intestinal contents.

ONSET, PEAK, DURATION
Onset unknown. Peak plasma levels occur about 2½ hours after oral liquid, 4 to 5 hours after capsules. Effects persist for about 24 hours.

INDICATIONS & DOSAGE
Acute, nonspecific diarrhea—
Adults: initially, 4 mg P.O., then 2 mg after each unformed stool. Maximum dosage is 16 mg daily.
Children 2 to 5 years: 5 ml P.O. t.i.d. on first day. If diarrhea persists, contact doctor.
Children 6 to 8 years: 10 ml (2 mg) P.O. b.i.d. on first day. If diarrhea persists, contact doctor. Do not exceed 4 mg daily.
Children 9 to 11 years: 10 ml (2 mg) t.i.d. P.O. on first day. (Subsequent doses of 5 ml (1 mg)/10 kg of body weight may be administered after each unformed stool.) Maximum dosage is 6 mg daily.
Chronic diarrhea—
Adults: initially, 4 mg P.O., then 2 mg after each unformed stool until diarrhea subsides. Dosage adjusted to individual response.

Reactions may be *common,* uncommon, *life-threatening,* or COMMON AND LIFE-THREATENING.

ADVERSE REACTIONS
CNS: drowsiness, fatigue, dizziness.
GI: dry mouth; abdominal pain, distention, or discomfort; *constipation;* nausea; vomiting.
Skin: rash, hypersensitivity reactions.

INTERACTIONS
None significant.

EFFECTS ON DIAGNOSTIC TESTS
None reported.

CONTRAINDICATIONS
Contraindicated in patients with hypersensitivity and when constipation must be avoided. Also contraindicated in children under 2 years.

NURSING CONSIDERATIONS
● Use cautiously in patients with hepatic disease.
● Be aware that the drug produces antidiarrheal action similar to diphenoxylate but without as many adverse CNS effects.
Alert: Monitor children closely for CNS effects; they may be more sensitive to CNS effects of drug than adults.

☑ PATIENT TEACHING
● Advise patient not to exceed recommended dosage.
● In acute diarrhea, tell patient to discontinue drug and seek medical attention if no improvement occurs within 48 hours; in chronic diarrhea, he should notify doctor and discontinue drug if no improvement occurs after taking 16 mg daily for at least 10 days.
● Advise patient with acute colitis to stop drug immediately if abdominal distention or other symptoms develop and notify the doctor.

---

octreotide acetate
Sandostatin

Pregnancy Risk Category: B

HOW SUPPLIED
Injection ampules: 0.05 mg, 0.1 mg, 0.5 mg
Injection-multidose vials: 0.2 mg/ml, 1 mg/ml

ACTION
Mimics the action of naturally occurring somatostatin.

ONSET, PEAK, DURATION
Onset occurs within 30 minutes. Peak levels occur within ½ hour. Effects persist up to 12 hours.

INDICATIONS & DOSAGE
Flushing and diarrhea associated with carcinoid tumors—
Adults: 0.1 to 0.6 mg daily S.C. in two to four divided doses for the first 2 weeks of therapy (usual daily dosage is 0.3 mg). Subsequent dosage based on individual response.
Watery diarrhea associated with vasoactive intestinal polypeptide secreting tumors (VIPomas)—
Adults: 0.2 to 0.3 mg daily S.C. in two to four divided doses for the first 2 weeks of therapy. Subsequent dosage based on individual response; typically, don't exceed 0.45 mg daily.
Acromegaly—
Adults: initially, 50 mcg S.C. t.i.d., then adjusted according to somatomedin C levels q 2 weeks.

ADVERSE REACTIONS
CNS: dizziness, light-headedness, fatigue, headache.
CV: sinus bradycardia, conduction abnormalities, arrhythmias.
EENT: blurred vision.
GI: *nausea, diarrhea, abdominal pain or discomfort, loose stools,* vomiting, fat malabsorption, gallbladder abnormalities, flatulence, constipation.
GU: pollakiuria, urinary tract infection.
Skin: flushing, edema, wheal, erythema or pain at injection site, alopecia.
Other: hyperglycemia, hypoglycemia, hypothyroidism, and pain, and/or burn-

---

ing at the S.C. injection site, cold symptoms, backache, joint pain, flulike symptoms.

INTERACTIONS
Cyclosporine: may decrease plasma levels of cyclosporine. Monitor patient closely.

EFFECTS ON DIAGNOSTIC TESTS
Ocreotide suppresses secretion of growth hormone and of the gastroenterohepatic peptides gastrin, VIP, insulin, glucagon, secretin, motilin, and pancreatic polypeptide.

CONTRAINDICATIONS
Contraindicated in patients hypersensitive to the drug or any of its components.

NURSING CONSIDERATIONS
• Monitor baseline thyroid function tests as ordered.
• Monitor somatomedin C levels every 2 weeks as ordered. Know that dosage adjustments are based on this level.
• Monitor laboratory tests periodically, such as thyroid function tests, urine 5-hydroxyindoleacetic acid, plasma serotonin, and plasma substance P (for carcinoid tumors).
• Monitor patients regularly for gallbladder disease. Octreotide therapy may be associated with development of cholelithiasis because of its effect on gallbladder motility or fat absorption.
• Monitor closely for symptoms of glucose imbalance. Be alert that insulin-dependent diabetic patients and patients receiving oral antidiabetic agents or oral diazoxide may require dosage adjustments during therapy.
• Keep in mind that octreotide therapy may alter fluid and electrolyte balance and may require adjustment of other drugs used to control symptoms of the disease, such as beta blockers.
• Be aware that half-life may be altered in patients in end-stage renal failure who are receiving dialysis.

☑ **PATIENT TEACHING**
• Instruct patient to report any signs of abdominal discomfort immediately.
• Stress importance of need for periodic laboratory testing during octreotide therapy.

---

opium tincture*

Controlled Substance Schedule II

opium tincture, camphorated* (paregoric)

Controlled Substance Schedule III
Pregnancy Risk Category: NR

HOW SUPPLIED
opium tincture
Oral solution: equivalent to morphine 10 mg/ml*
opium tincture, camphorated
Oral solution: Each 5 ml contains morphine, 2 mg; anise oil, 0.2 ml; benzoic acid, 20 mg; camphor, 20 mg; glycerin, 0.2 ml; and ethanol to make 5 ml*

ACTION
Increases smooth muscle tone in the GI tract, inhibits motility and propulsion, and diminishes secretions.

ONSET, PEAK, DURATION
Unknown.

INDICATIONS & DOSAGE
Acute, nonspecific diarrhea—
Note: Do not confuse opium tincture with camphorated opium tincture.
Opium tincture:
Adults: 0.6 ml (range 0.3 to 1 ml) P.O. q.i.d. Maximum dosage is 6 ml daily.
Camphorated opium tincture
Adults: 5 to 10 ml P.O. once daily, b.i.d., t.i.d., or q.i.d. until diarrhea subsides.
Children: 0.25 to 0.5 ml/kg camphorated opium tincture P.O. once daily, b.i.d., t.i.d., or q.i.d. until diarrhea subsides.

Reactions may be *common*, uncommon, *life-threatening*, or COMMON AND LIFE-THREATENING.

ADVERSE REACTIONS
CNS: dizziness, light-headedness.
GI: nausea, vomiting, physical dependence after long-term use.

INTERACTIONS
None significant.

EFFECTS ON DIAGNOSTIC TESTS
Opium tincture and camphorated opium tincture may prevent delivery of technitium-99m disofenin to the small intestine during hepatobiliary imaging tests; delay test until 24 hours after last dose. The drugs also may increase serum amylase and lipase levels by inducing contractions of the sphincter of Oddi and increasing biliary tract pressure.

CONTRAINDICATIONS
Contraindicated in patients with acute diarrhea caused by poisoning until toxic material is removed from GI tract or in those with diarrhea caused by organisms that penetrate intestinal mucosa.

NURSING CONSIDERATIONS
● Use cautiously in patients with asthma, prostatic hyperplasia, hepatic disease, and history of opioid dependence.
● Mix with sufficient water to ensure passage to stomach.
● Know that a milky fluid forms when camphorated opium tincture is added to water.
Alert: For overdose, use the narcotic antagonist naloxone, as ordered, to reverse respiratory depression.
Alert: Keep in mind that opium content of opium tincture is 25 times greater than camphorated opium tincture. Camphorated opium tincture is more dilute, and teaspoonful doses are easier to measure than dropper quantities of opium tincture.
● Keep in mind that the drug is an effective and prompt-acting antidiarrheal, but unique because dosage can be adjusted precisely to patient's needs.
● Store in tightly capped, light-resistant container.

☑ **PATIENT TEACHING**
● Advise patient against using drug for more than 2 days; risk of physical dependence increases with long-term use.
● Instruct patient to measure dosage carefully to avoid overdose which can have serious consequences.

---

*Liquid contains alcohol. **May contain tartrazine. †Canada only. ‡Australia only. ◇ OTC.

50

Laxatives

bisacodyl
calcium polycarbophil
cascara sagrada
cascara sagrada aromatic
    fluidextract
cascara sagrada fluidextract
castor oil
docusate calcium
docusate sodium
glycerin
lactulose
magnesium citrate
magnesium hydroxide
magnesium sulfate
methylcellulose
mineral oil
phenolphthalein, white
phenolphthalein, yellow
polyethylene glycol and elec-
    trolyte solution
psyllium
senna
sodium phosphates

COMBINATION PRODUCTS

AGORAL ◊ : mineral oil 28% and white phenolphthalein 1.3% in emulsion, with tragacanth, agar, egg albumin, acacia, and glycerin.
DIALOSE PLUS ◊ : docusate sodium 100 mg and casanthranol 30 mg.
DOXIDAN ◊ : docusate calcium 60 mg and phenolphthalein 65 mg.
D-S-S PLUS ◊ : docusate sodium 100 mg and casanthranol 30 mg.
HALEY'S M-O ◊ : mineral oil (25%) and magnesium hydroxide.
KONDREMUL WITH PHENOLPHTHALEIN ◊ : heavy mineral oil 55%, white phenolphthalein 150 mg/15 ml, and Irish moss as emulsifier.
MODANE PLUS ◊ : docusate sodium 100 mg and white phenolphthalein 65 mg.
PERI-COLACE-CAPSULES ◊ : docusate sodium 100 mg and casanthranol 30 mg.

PERI-COLACE-SYRUP ◊ : docusate sodium 60 mg and casanthranol 30 mg/15 ml.
SENOKOT-S ◊ : docusate sodium 50 mg and standardized senna concentrate 187 mg.
UNILAX SOFTGEL ◊ : docusate sodium 230 mg and yellow phenolphthalein 130 mg.

---

bisacodyl

Bisac-Evac ◊ , Bisacolax† ◊ , Bisalax‡ ◊ , Bisco-Lax** ◊ , Carter's Little Pills ◊ , Dacodyl ◊ , Deficol ◊ , Dulcagen ◊ , Dulcolax ◊ , Durolax‡, Fleet Bisacodyl ◊ , Fleet Bisacodyl Prep ◊ , Fleet Laxative ◊ , Laxit† ◊ , Theralax ◊

Pregnancy Risk Category: B

HOW SUPPLIED
Tablets (enteric-coated): 5 mg ◊
Enema: 0.33 mg/ml ◊ , 10 mg/5 ml (microenema)‡
Powder for rectal solution (bisacodyl tannex): 1.5 mg bisacodyl and 2.5 g tannic acid
Suppositories: 5 mg ◊ , 10 mg ◊

ACTION
Unknown. A stimulant laxative that increases peristalsis probably by direct effect on the smooth muscle of the intestine. Thought to either irritate the musculature or stimulate the colonic intramural plexus. Also promotes fluid accumulation in the colon and small intestine.

ONSET, PEAK, DURATION
Onset occurs 15 to 60 minutes after suppository, 6 to 12 hours after oral administration. Peak and duration variable.

Reactions may be *common*, uncommon, ***life-threatening***, or **COMMON AND LIFE-THREATENING**.

Photoguide to tablets and capsules

One of the most critical responsibilities of any nurse is to ensure that the patient receives the right medication. This task becomes easier when the nurse can verify the appearance of drugs prescribed for the patient. The following photoguide provides full-color photographs of some of the most commonly prescribed tablets and capsules in the United States. Shown here in actual size, the tablets and capsules are organized alphabetically for quick reference.

Accupril

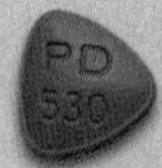

10 mg

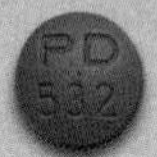

20 mg

acetaminophen and codeine

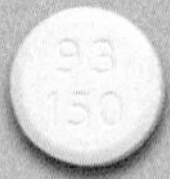

300 mg/30 mg

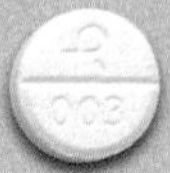

300 mg/60 mg

Adalat

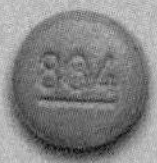

30 mg (extended-release)

Altace

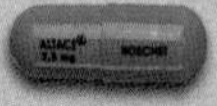

2.5 mg

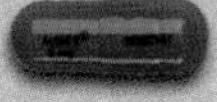

5 mg

Ambien

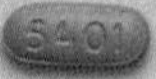

5 mg   10 mg

amitriptyline hydrochloride

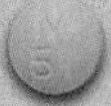

25 mg

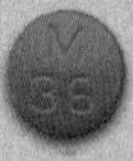

50 mg

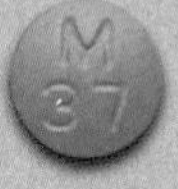

75 mg

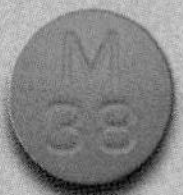

100 mg

amoxicillin trihydrate

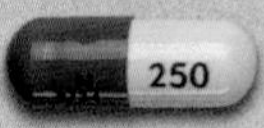

250 mg

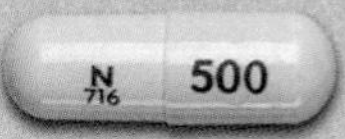

500 mg

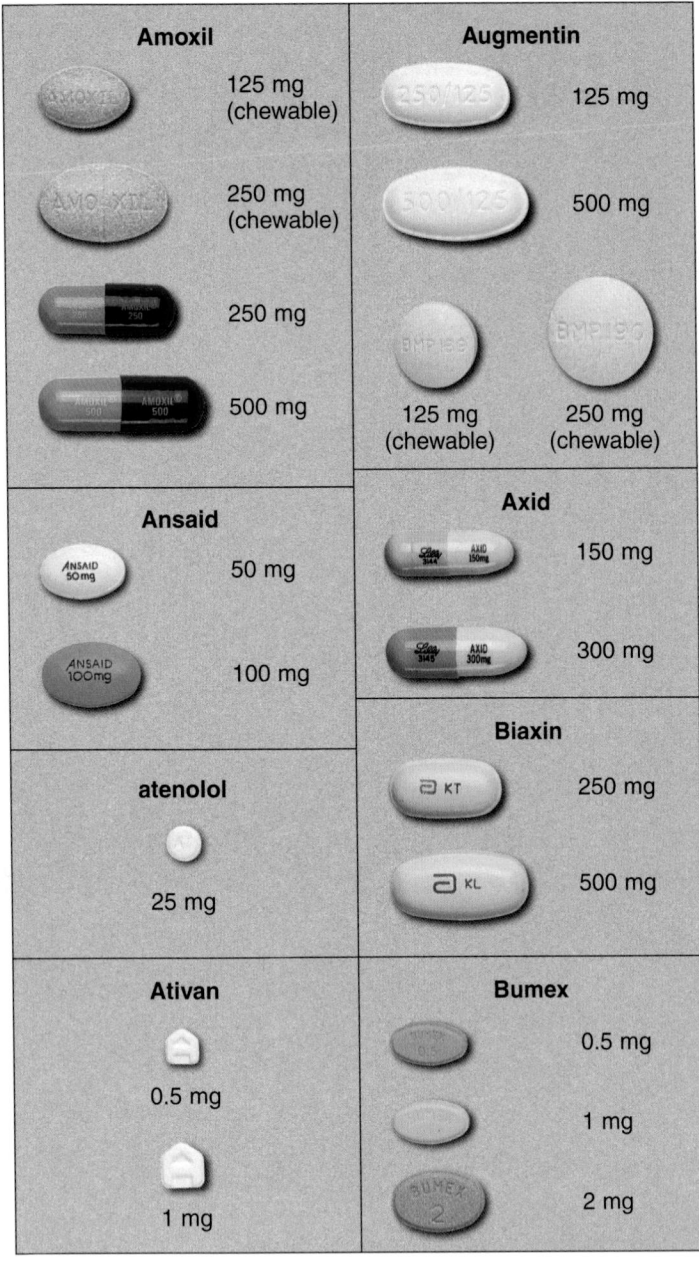

Amoxil	
	125 mg (chewable)
	250 mg (chewable)
	250 mg
	500 mg

Ansaid	
ANSAID 50 mg	50 mg
ANSAID 100mg	100 mg

atenolol

25 mg

Ativan	
	0.5 mg
	1 mg

Augmentin	
250/125	125 mg
500/125	500 mg
BMP 189 125 mg (chewable)	BMP 190 250 mg (chewable)

Axid	
Lilly 3144 AXID 150mg	150 mg
Lilly 3145 AXID 300mg	300 mg

Biaxin	
a KT	250 mg
a KL	500 mg

Bumex	
	0.5 mg
	1 mg
BUMEX 2	2 mg

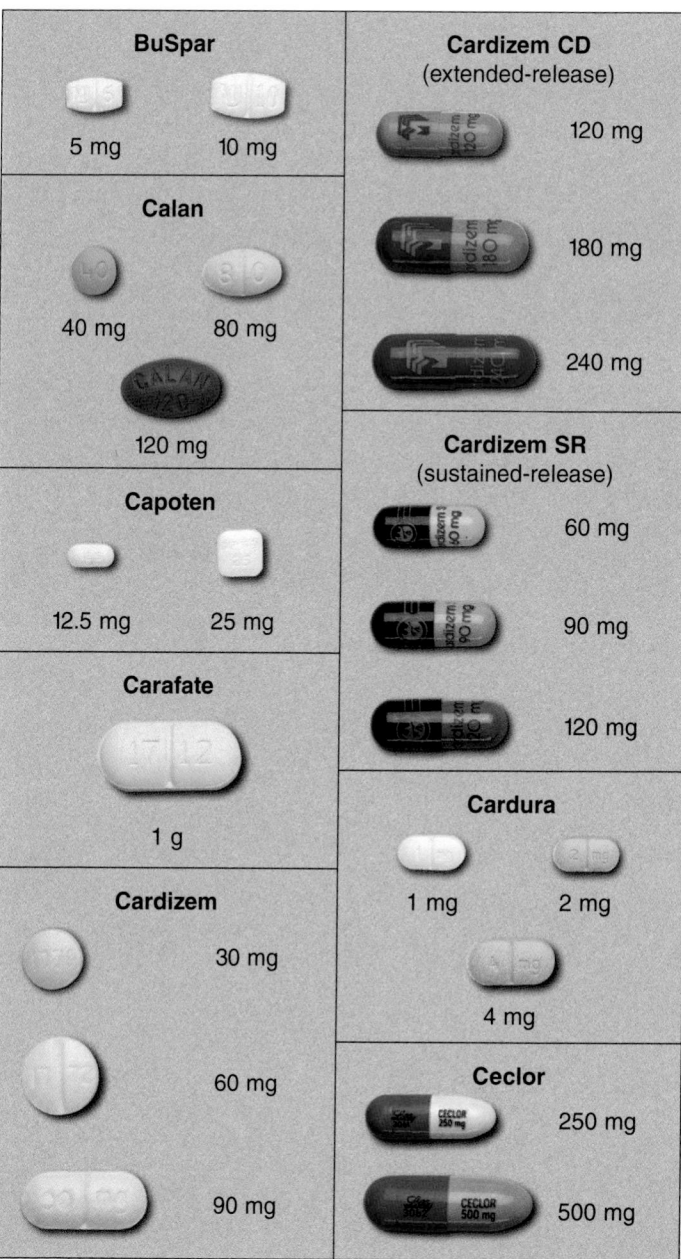

BuSpar

5 mg   10 mg

Calan

40 mg   80 mg

120 mg

Capoten

12.5 mg   25 mg

Carafate

1 g

Cardizem

30 mg

60 mg

90 mg

Cardizem CD
(extended-release)

120 mg

180 mg

240 mg

Cardizem SR
(sustained-release)

60 mg

90 mg

120 mg

Cardura

1 mg   2 mg

4 mg

Ceclor

250 mg

500 mg

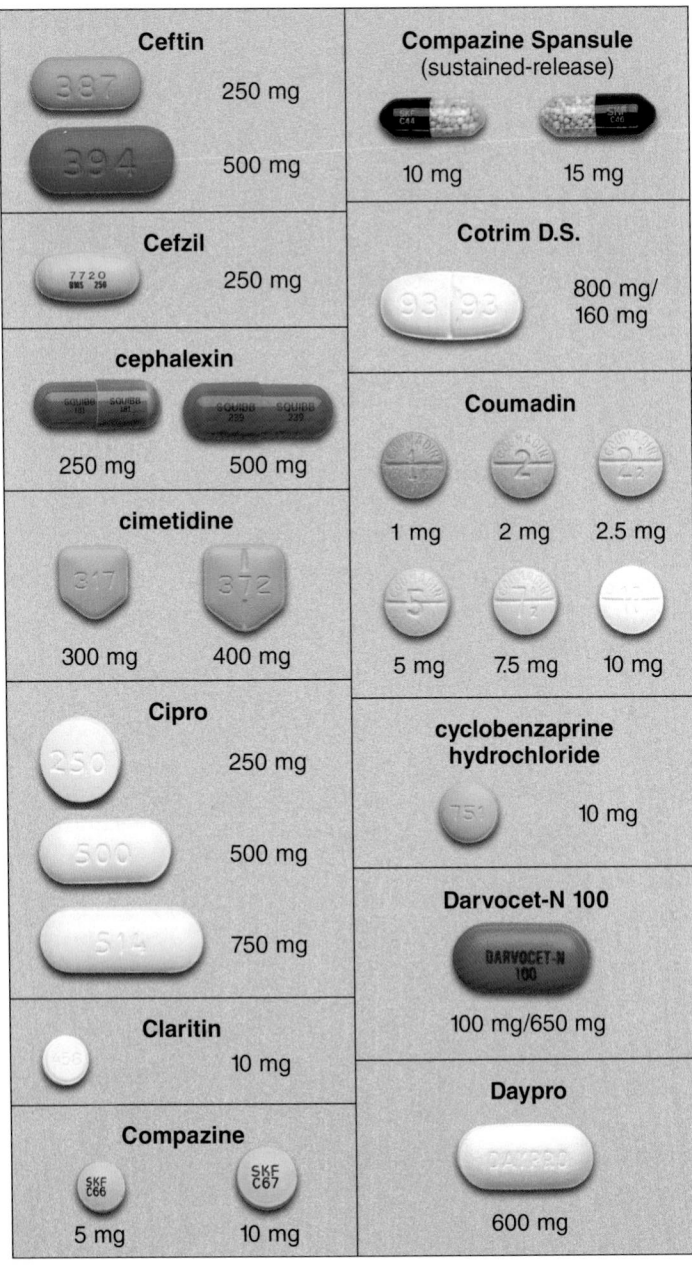

Ceftin

387 — 250 mg

394 — 500 mg

Cefzil

7720 BMS 250 — 250 mg

cephalexin

250 mg   500 mg

cimetidine

317   372

300 mg   400 mg

Cipro

250 — 250 mg

500 — 500 mg

514 — 750 mg

Claritin

10 mg

Compazine

SKF C66   SKF C67

5 mg   10 mg

Compazine Spansule
(sustained-release)

10 mg   15 mg

Cotrim D.S.

93 93 — 800 mg/160 mg

Coumadin

1 mg   2 mg   2.5 mg

5 mg   7.5 mg   10 mg

cyclobenzaprine hydrochloride

751 — 10 mg

Darvocet-N 100

DARVOCET-N 100

100 mg/650 mg

Daypro

DAYPRO

600 mg

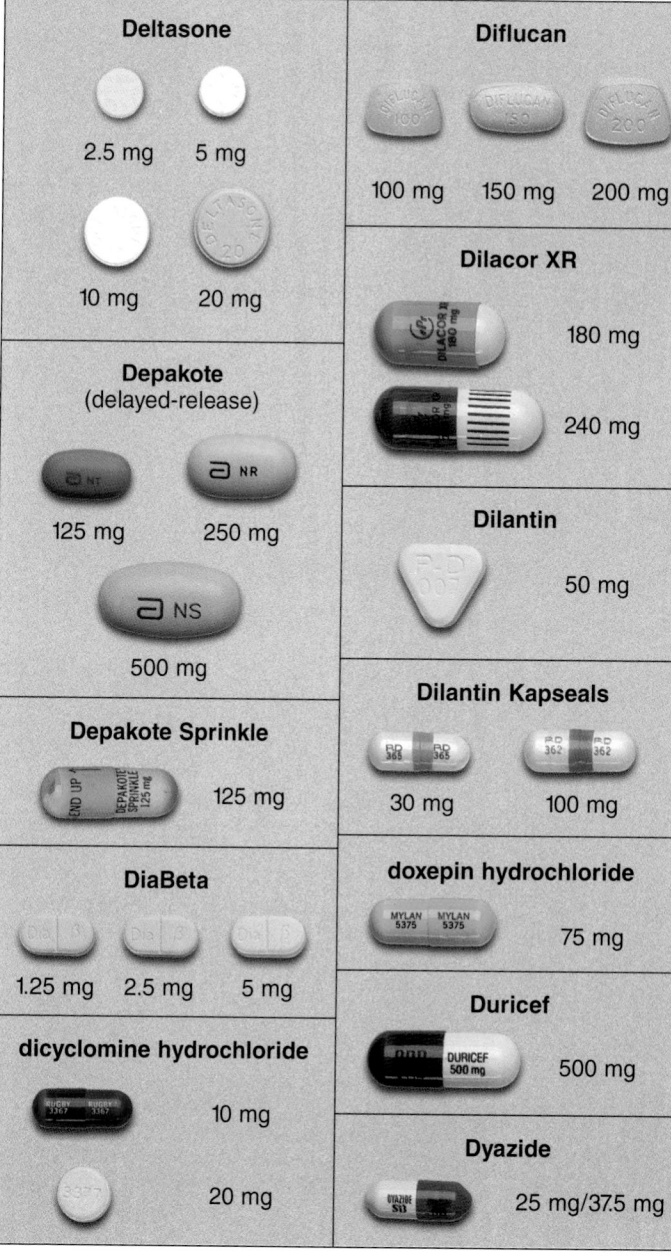

Deltasone

2.5 mg 5 mg

10 mg 20 mg

Depakote
(delayed-release)

125 mg 250 mg

500 mg

Depakote Sprinkle

125 mg

DiaBeta

1.25 mg 2.5 mg 5 mg

dicyclomine hydrochloride

10 mg

20 mg

Diflucan

100 mg 150 mg 200 mg

Dilacor XR

180 mg

240 mg

Dilantin

50 mg

Dilantin Kapseals

30 mg 100 mg

doxepin hydrochloride

75 mg

Duricef

500 mg

Dyazide

25 mg/37.5 mg

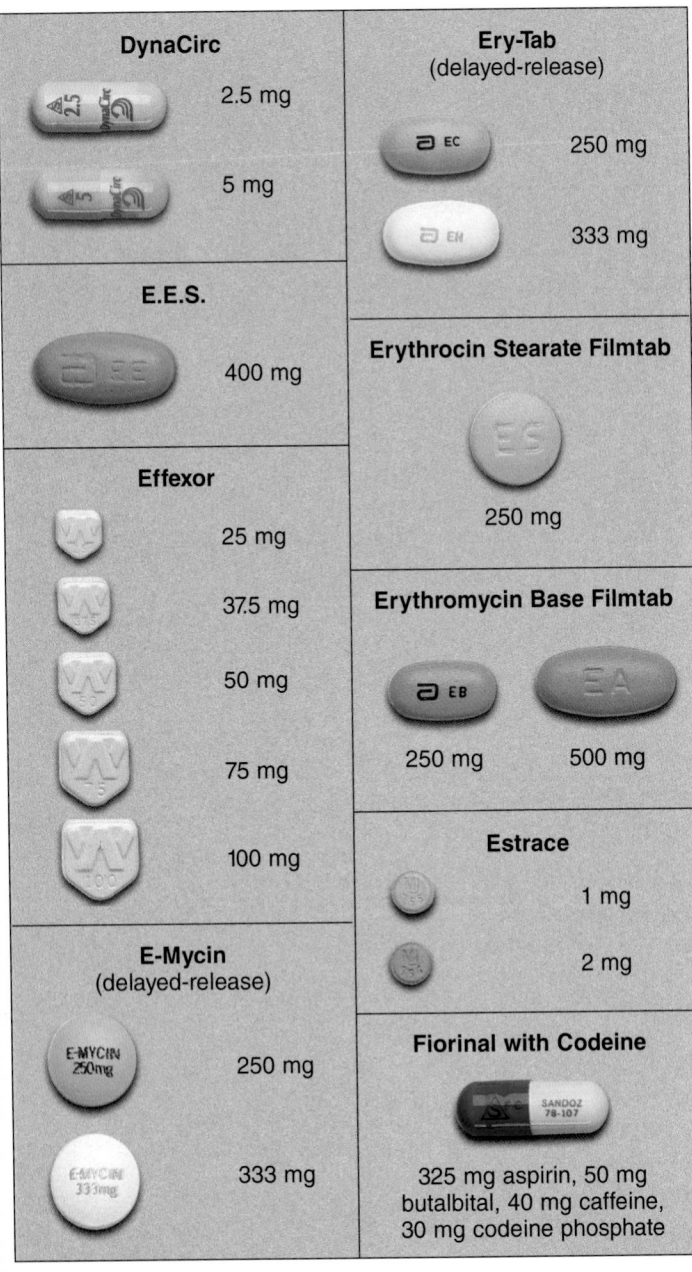

DynaCirc

2.5 mg

5 mg

E.E.S.

400 mg

Effexor

25 mg

37.5 mg

50 mg

75 mg

100 mg

E-Mycin
(delayed-release)

250 mg

333 mg

Ery-Tab
(delayed-release)

250 mg

333 mg

Erythrocin Stearate Filmtab

250 mg

Erythromycin Base Filmtab

250 mg   500 mg

Estrace

1 mg

2 mg

Fiorinal with Codeine

325 mg aspirin, 50 mg
butalbital, 40 mg caffeine,
30 mg codeine phosphate

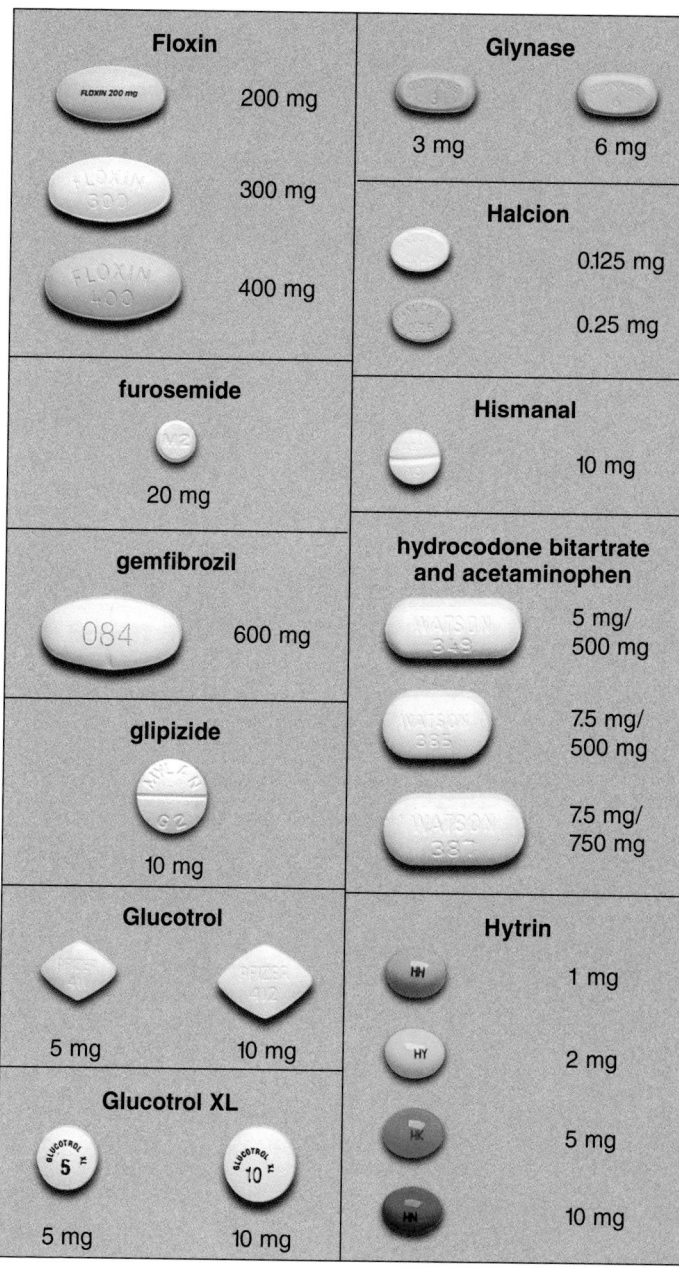

Floxin

200 mg

300 mg

400 mg

furosemide

20 mg

gemfibrozil

600 mg

glipizide

10 mg

Glucotrol

5 mg   10 mg

Glucotrol XL

5 mg   10 mg

Glynase

3 mg   6 mg

Halcion

0.125 mg

0.25 mg

Hismanal

10 mg

**hydrocodone bitartrate
and acetaminophen**

5 mg/
500 mg

7.5 mg/
500 mg

7.5 mg/
750 mg

Hytrin

1 mg

2 mg

5 mg

10 mg

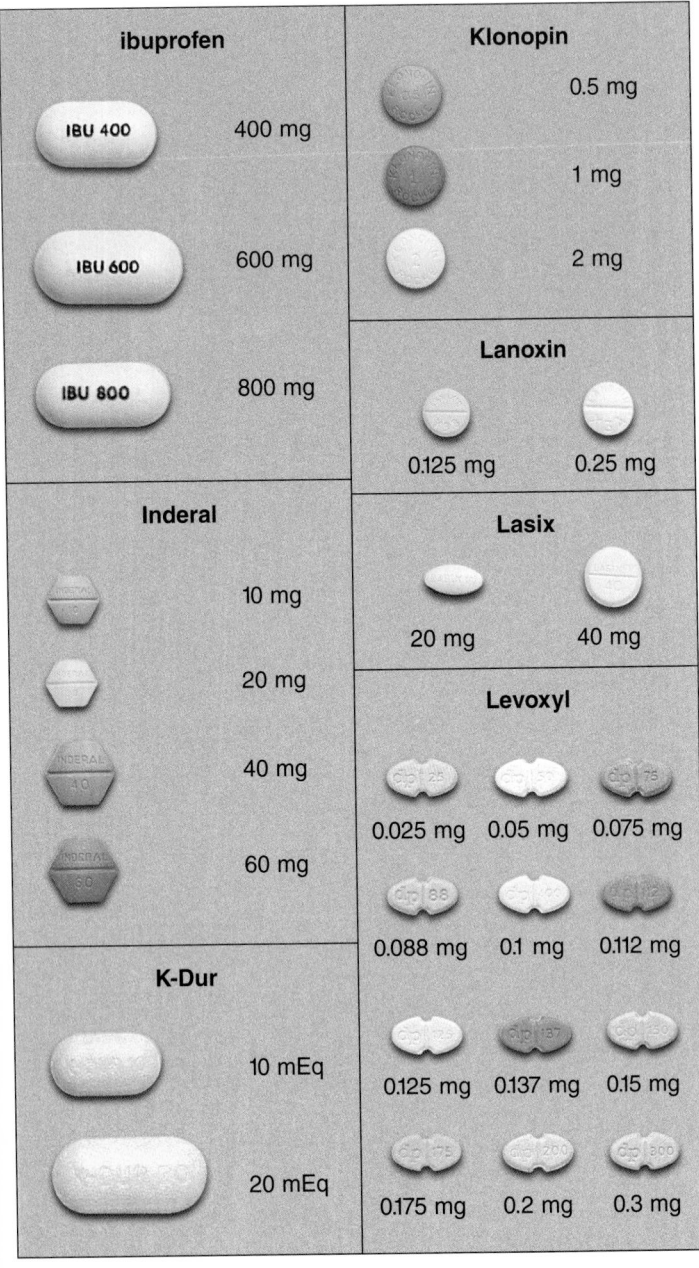

ibuprofen

IBU 400 — 400 mg

IBU 600 — 600 mg

IBU 800 — 800 mg

Inderal

10 mg

20 mg

40 mg

60 mg

K-Dur

10 mEq

20 mEq

Klonopin

0.5 mg

1 mg

2 mg

Lanoxin

0.125 mg   0.25 mg

Lasix

20 mg   40 mg

Levoxyl

0.025 mg   0.05 mg   0.075 mg

0.088 mg   0.1 mg   0.112 mg

0.125 mg   0.137 mg   0.15 mg

0.175 mg   0.2 mg   0.3 mg

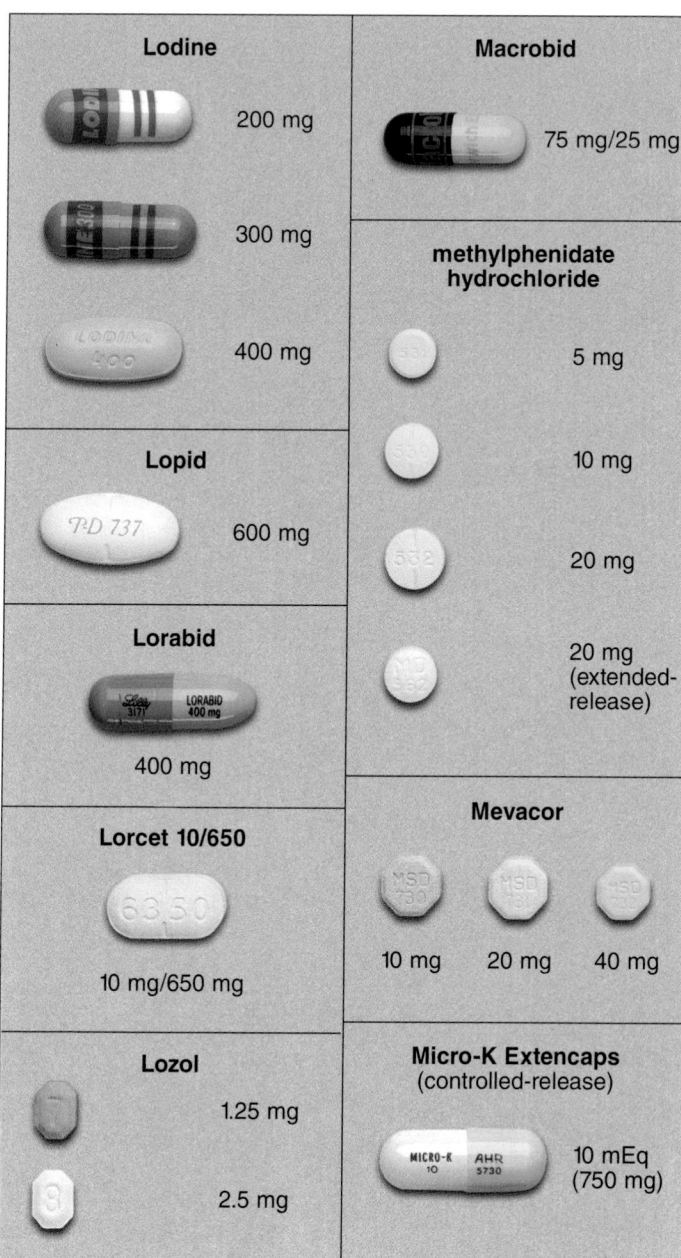

Iodine

200 mg

300 mg

400 mg

Lopid

7-D 737

600 mg

Lorabid

400 mg

Lorcet 10/650

10 mg/650 mg

Lozol

1.25 mg

2.5 mg

Macrobid

75 mg/25 mg

methylphenidate hydrochloride

5 mg

10 mg

20 mg

20 mg (extended-release)

Mevacor

10 mg   20 mg   40 mg

Micro-K Extencaps
(controlled-release)

10 mEq (750 mg)

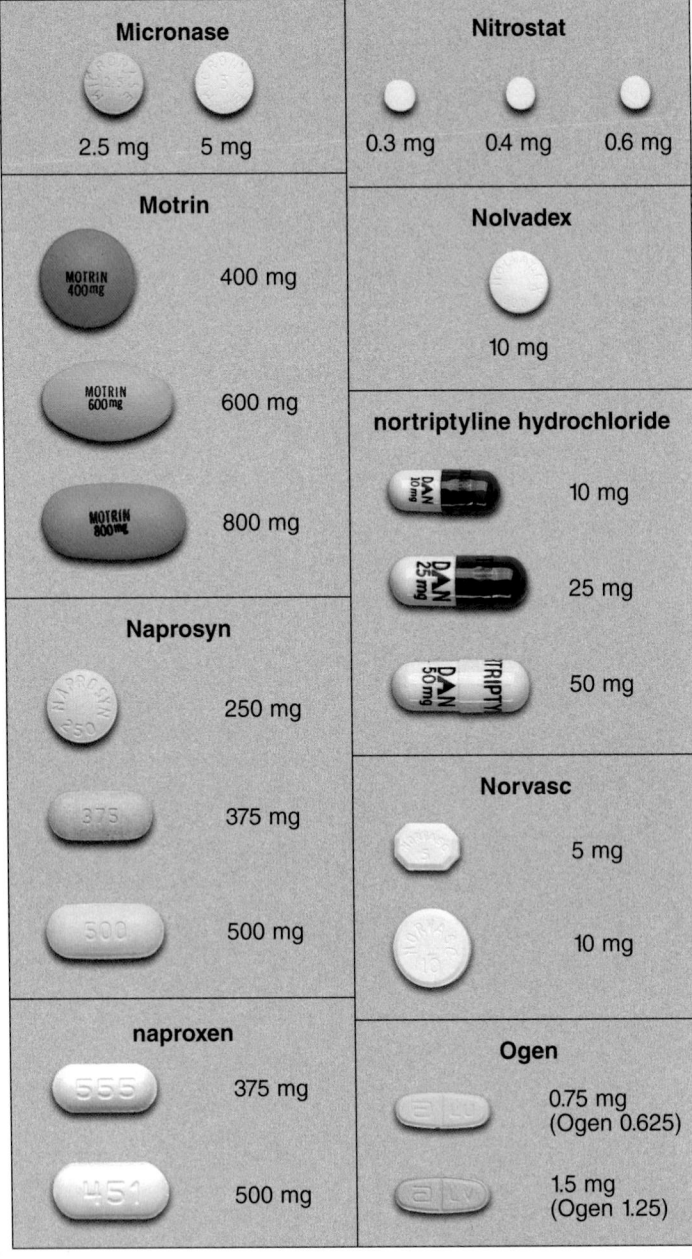

Micronase

2.5 mg   5 mg

Motrin

MOTRIN 400 mg   400 mg

MOTRIN 600 mg   600 mg

MOTRIN 800 mg   800 mg

Naprosyn

NAPROSYN 250   250 mg

375   375 mg

500   500 mg

naproxen

555   375 mg

451   500 mg

Nitrostat

0.3 mg   0.4 mg   0.6 mg

Nolvadex

10 mg

nortriptyline hydrochloride

DAN 10mg   10 mg

DAN 25mg   25 mg

DAN 50mg NTRIPTY   50 mg

Norvasc

5 mg

10 mg

Ogen

0.75 mg (Ogen 0.625)

1.5 mg (Ogen 1.25)

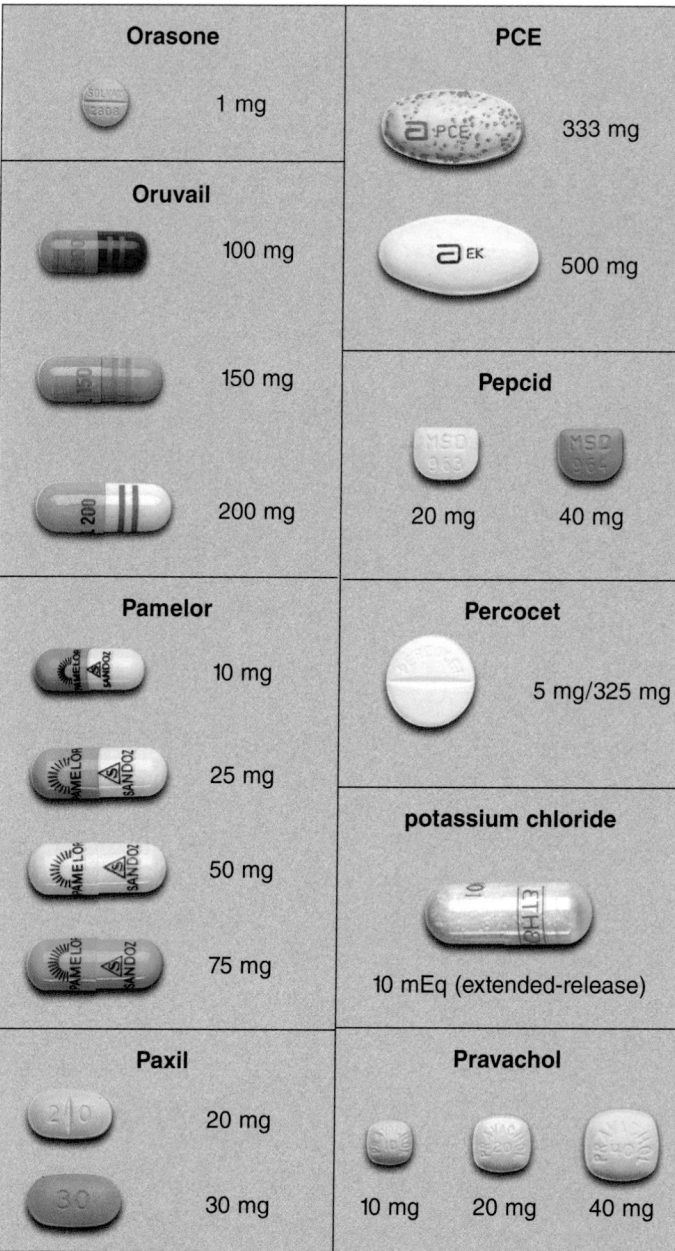

Orasone	**PCE**
1 mg	333 mg
Oruvail	500 mg
100 mg	**Pepcid**
150 mg	20 mg · 40 mg
200 mg	**Percocet**
Pamelor	5 mg/325 mg
10 mg	**potassium chloride**
25 mg	10 mEq (extended-release)
50 mg	
75 mg	
Paxil	**Pravachol**
20 mg	
30 mg	10 mg · 20 mg · 40 mg

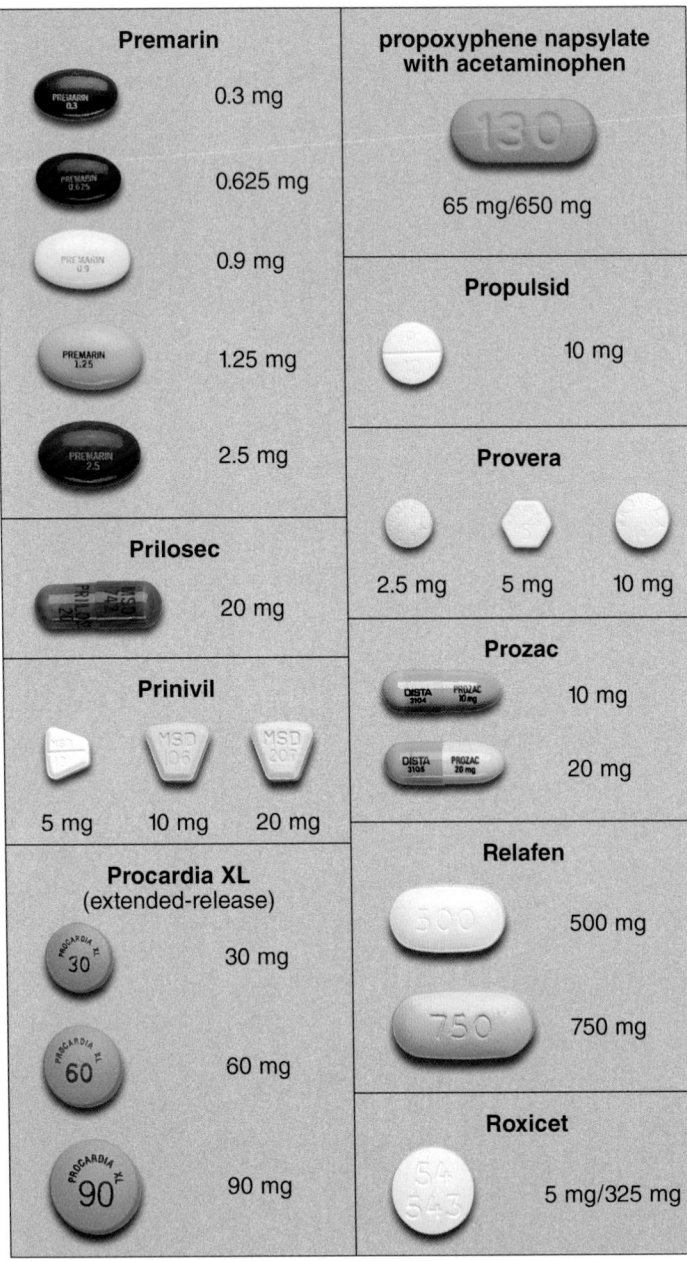

Premarin

0.3 mg

0.625 mg

0.9 mg

1.25 mg

2.5 mg

Prilosec

20 mg

Prinivil

5 mg   10 mg   20 mg

Procardia XL
(extended-release)

30 mg

60 mg

90 mg

**propoxyphene napsylate
with acetaminophen**

65 mg/650 mg

Propulsid

10 mg

Provera

2.5 mg   5 mg   10 mg

Prozac

10 mg

20 mg

Relafen

500 mg

750 mg

Roxicet

5 mg/325 mg

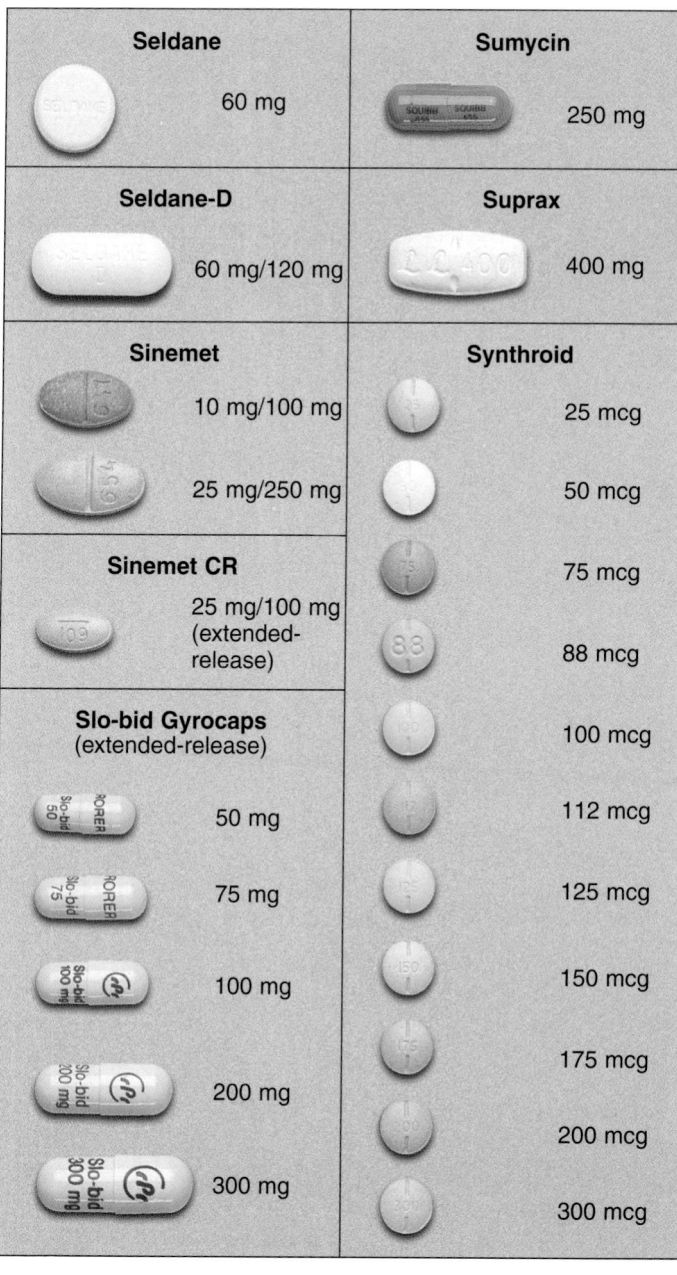

Seldane	**Sumycin**
60 mg	250 mg
Seldane-D	**Suprax**
60 mg/120 mg	400 mg
Sinemet	**Synthroid**
10 mg/100 mg	25 mcg
25 mg/250 mg	50 mcg
Sinemet CR	75 mcg
25 mg/100 mg (extended-release)	88 mcg
Slo-bid Gyrocaps (extended-release)	100 mcg
50 mg	112 mcg
75 mg	125 mcg
100 mg	150 mcg
200 mg	175 mcg
300 mg	200 mcg
	300 mcg

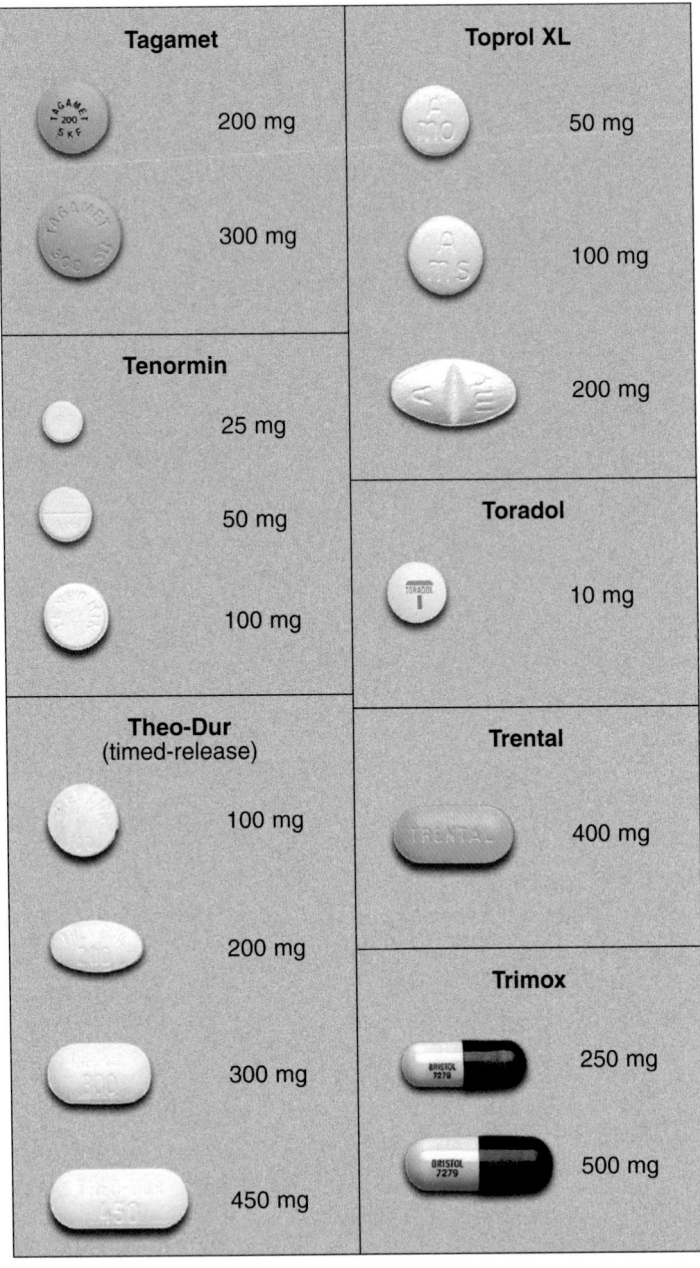

Tagamet

200 mg

300 mg

Tenormin

25 mg

50 mg

100 mg

Theo-Dur
(timed-release)

100 mg

200 mg

300 mg

450 mg

Toprol XL

50 mg

100 mg

200 mg

Toradol

10 mg

Trental

400 mg

Trimox

250 mg

500 mg

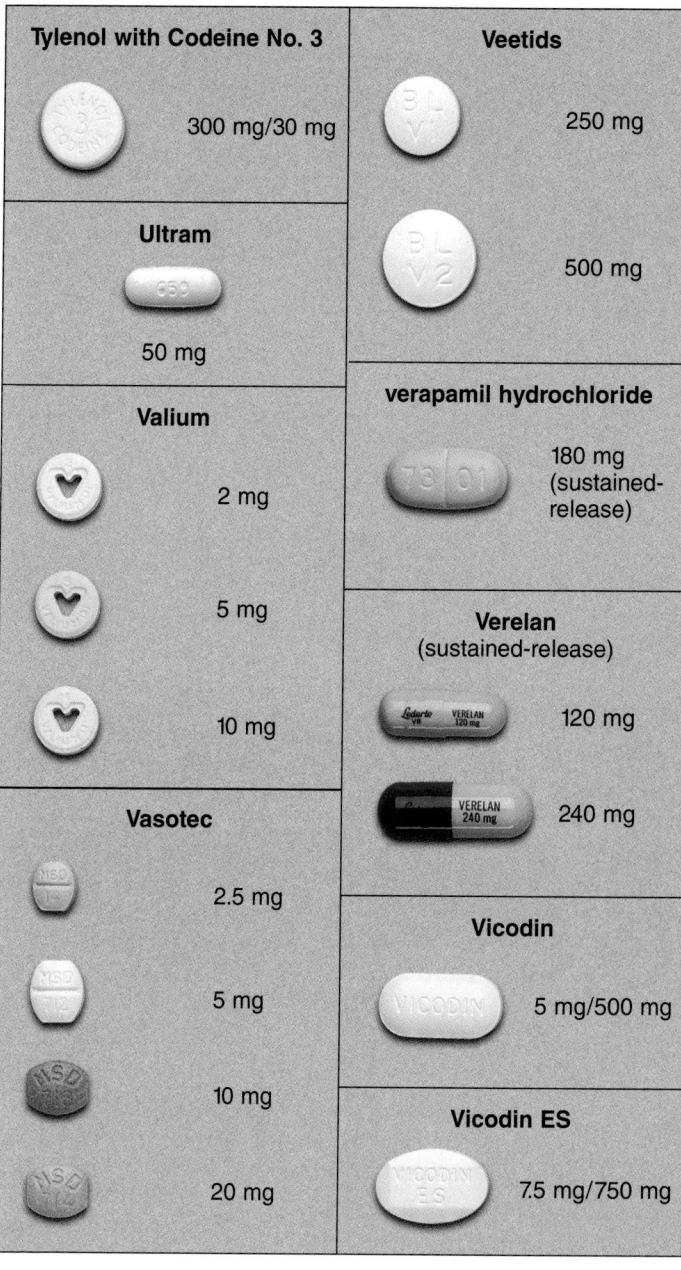

Tylenol with Codeine No. 3

300 mg/30 mg

Ultram

50 mg

Valium

2 mg

5 mg

10 mg

Vasotec

2.5 mg

5 mg

10 mg

20 mg

Veetids

250 mg

500 mg

verapamil hydrochloride

180 mg (sustained-release)

Verelan
(sustained-release)

120 mg

240 mg

Vicodin

5 mg/500 mg

Vicodin ES

7.5 mg/750 mg

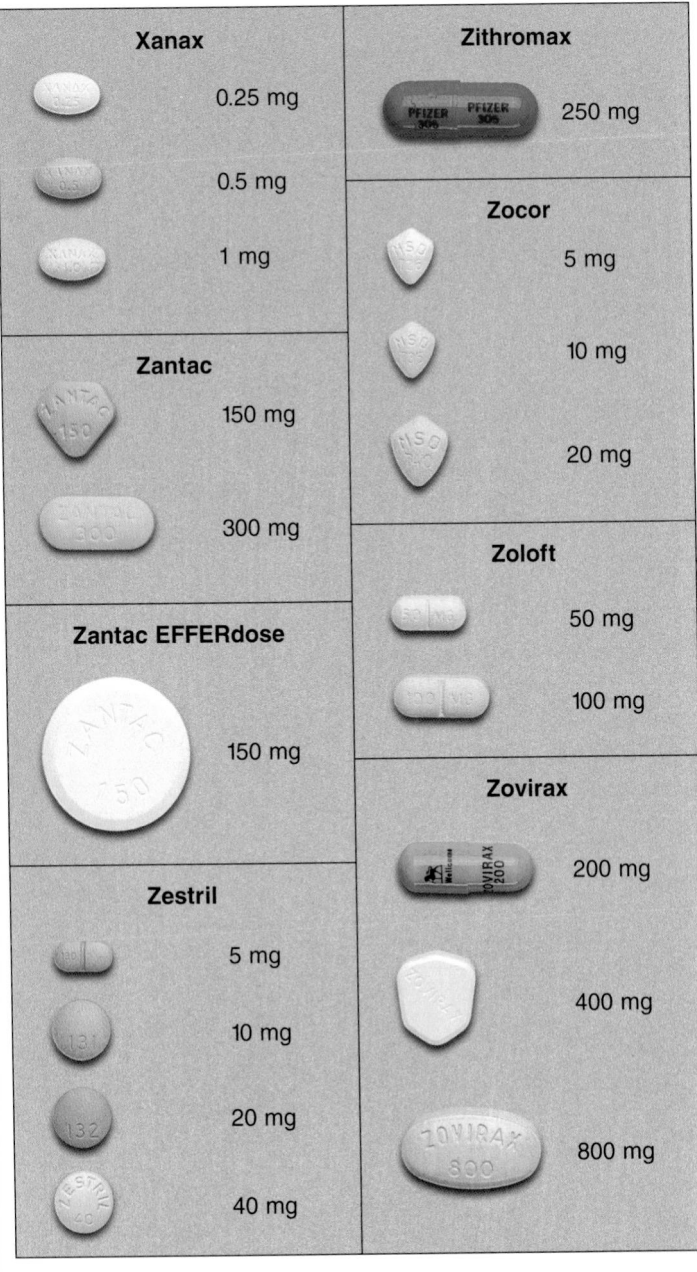

Xanax

0.25 mg

0.5 mg

1 mg

Zantac

150 mg

300 mg

Zantac EFFERdose

150 mg

Zestril

5 mg

10 mg

20 mg

40 mg

Zithromax

250 mg

Zocor

5 mg

10 mg

20 mg

Zoloft

50 mg

100 mg

Zovirax

200 mg

400 mg

800 mg

INDICATIONS & DOSAGE
Chronic constipation; preparation for delivery, surgery, or rectal or bowel examination—
Adults and children 12 years and over: 10 to 15 mg P.O. in evening or before breakfast. Up to 30 mg P.O. as needed and ordered, or 10 mg P.R. for evacuation before examination or surgery.
Children 6 to 12 years: 5 mg P.O. or P.R. h.s. or before breakfast. Oral dose is not recommended if child cannot swallow tablet whole.

ADVERSE REACTIONS
CNS: muscle weakness with excessive use, dizziness, faintness.
GI: *nausea, vomiting, abdominal cramps,* diarrhea (with high doses), *burning sensation in rectum* (with suppositories), laxative dependence with long-term or excessive use.
Other: alkalosis, hypokalemia, tetany, protein-losing enteropathy in excessive use, fluid and electrolyte imbalance.

INTERACTIONS
Milk or antacids: gastric irritation or dyspepsia from premature dissolution of enteric coating. Do not administer together.

EFFECTS ON DIAGNOSTIC TESTS
None reported.

CONTRAINDICATIONS
Contraindicated in patients with hypersensitivity, abdominal pain, nausea, vomiting, or other symptoms of appendicitis or acute surgical abdomen and in those with rectal bleeding, gastroenteritis, or intestinal obstruction.

NURSING CONSIDERATIONS
● Time administration of drug so as not to interfere with scheduled activities or sleep. Soft, formed stools are usually produced 15 to 60 minutes after rectal administration.
● Before giving for constipation, determine if the patient has adequate fluid in-take, exercise, and diet.
● Know that tablets and suppositories are used together to clean the colon before and after surgery and before barium enema.
● Insert suppository as high as possible into the rectum, and try to position the suppository against the rectal wall. Avoid embedding within fecal material because this may delay the onset of action.
● Store tablets and suppositories at a temperature below 86° F (30° C).

☑ PATIENT TEACHING
● Advise the patient to swallow enteric-coated tablet whole to avoid GI irritation. Don't give within 1 hour of milk or antacid intake.
● Tell patient drug is for short-term treatment only (a stimulant laxative, this type is frequently abused). Discourage excessive use.
● Advise the patient to report adverse effects to the doctor.
● Teach the patient about dietary sources of bulk which include bran and other cereals, fresh fruit, and vegetables.

---

calcium polycarbophil
Equalactin ◇, Fiberall ◇, FiberCon ◇, FiberLax ◇, FiberNorm ◇, Mitrolan ◇

Pregnancy Risk Category: NR

HOW SUPPLIED
Tablets: 500 mg ◇, 625 mg ◇
Tablets (chewable): 500 mg ◇, 1,250 mg ◇

ACTION
A bulk-forming laxative that absorbs water and expands to increase bulk and moisture content of stools. The increased bulk encourages peristalsis and bowel movement. As an antidiarrheal, absorbs free fecal water, thereby producing formed stools.

ONSET, PEAK, DURATION
Onset occurs in 12 to 24 hours. Peak effects may not occur for up to 3 days. Duration variable.

INDICATIONS & DOSAGE
Constipation—
Adults: 1 g P.O. q.i.d. as required. Maximum dosage is 6 g in 24-hour period.
Children 2 to 6 years: use must be directed by doctor. 500 mg P.O. b.i.d. as required. Maximum dosage is 1.5 g in 24-hour period.
Children 6 to 12 years: 500 mg P.O. 1 to 3 times daily as required. Maximum dosage is 3 g in 24-hour period.
Diarrhea associated with irritable bowel syndrome, as well as acute nonspecific diarrhea—
Adults: 1 g P.O. q.i.d. as required. Maximum dosage is 6 g in 24-hour period.
Children 2 to 6 years: use must be directed by doctor. 500 mg P.O. b.i.d. as required. Maximum dosage is 1.5 g in 24-hour period.
Children 6 to 12 years: 500 mg P.O. t.i.d. as required. Maximum dosage is 3 g in 24-hour period.

ADVERSE REACTIONS
GI: abdominal fullness and increased flatus, intestinal obstruction.
Other: laxative dependence (with long-term or excessive use).

INTERACTIONS
Tetracyclines: impaired absorption of tetracyclines. Avoid using together.

EFFECTS ON DIAGNOSTIC TESTS
None reported.

CONTRAINDICATIONS
Contraindicated in patients with signs of GI obstruction.

NURSING CONSIDERATIONS
● Before giving for constipation, determine if the patient has adequate fluid intake, exercise, and diet.
Alert: Be aware that rectal bleeding or

failure to respond to therapy may indicate need for surgery.

☑ **PATIENT TEACHING**
● Advise the patient to chew Equalactin or Mitrolan tablets thoroughly before swallowing and to drink a full glass of water with each dose. When used as an antidiarrheal, tell the patient not to drink a glass of water.
● Teach the patient about dietary sources of bulk, which include bran and other cereals, fresh fruit, and vegetables.
● For severe diarrhea, advise the patient to repeat dose every half hour, but not to exceed maximum daily dosage.

---

cascara sagrada ◊

cascara sagrada aromatic fluidextract * ◊

cascara sagrada fluidextract * ◊

Pregnancy Risk Category: C

HOW SUPPLIED
Tablets: 325 mg ◊
Aromatic fluidextract: 1 g/ml* ◊
Fluidextract: 1 g/ml* ◊

ACTION
Unknown. A stimulant laxative that increases peristalsis probably by direct effect on the smooth muscle of the intestine. Thought to either irritate the musculature or stimulate the colonic intramural plexus. Also promotes fluid accumulation in the colon and small intestine.

ONSET, PEAK, DURATION
Onset occurs in 6 to 10 hours. Peak and duration variable.

INDICATIONS & DOSAGE
Acute constipation; preparation for bowel or rectal examination—
Adults and children 12 years and

over: one 325 mg tablet of cascara sagrada P.O. once daily h.s.; 200 to 400 mg of cascara sagrada extract P.O. once daily; 0.5 to 1.5 ml of cascara sagrada fluidextract P.O. once daily or 5 ml of aromatic cascara fluidextract P.O. once daily.

Children under 2 years: one-quarter adult dosage.

Children 2 to 12 years: one-half adult dosage.

ADVERSE REACTIONS
GI: *nausea;* vomiting; diarrhea; loss of normal el function with excessive use; *abdominal cramps,* especially in severe constipation; malabsorption of nutrients; "cathartic colon" (syndrome resembling ulcerative colitis radiologically and pathologically) with chronic misuse; discoloration of rectal mucosa after long-term use.
Other: hypokalemia, protein enteropathy, electrolyte imbalance (with excessive use), laxative dependence (with long-term or excessive use).

INTERACTIONS
None significant.

EFFECTS ON DIAGNOSTIC TESTS
Drug turns alkaline urine pink to red, red to violet, or red to brown and turns acidic urine yellow to brown in the phenolsulfonphthalein excretion test.

CONTRAINDICATIONS
Contraindicated in patients with abdominal pain, nausea, vomiting, or other symptoms of appendicitis or acute surgical abdomen; acute surgical delirium; fecal impaction; and intestinal obstruction or perforation.

NURSING CONSIDERATIONS
● Use cautiously when rectal bleeding is present.
● Before giving for constipation, determine if the patient has adequate fluid intake, exercise, and diet.
● Monitor serum electrolytes during

prolonged use.
● Be aware that cascara aromatic fluidextract is less active and less bitter than the nonaromatic fluidextract.
● Know that liquid preparations are more reliable than solid dosage forms.

☑ PATIENT TEACHING
● Warn patient that drug may turn alkaline urine red-pink and acidic urine yellow-brown.
● Teach the patient about dietary sources of bulk, which include bran and other cereals, fresh fruit, and vegetables.

---

castor oil
Alphamul◇, Castor Oil Capsules, Emulsoil◇, Fleet Flavored Castor Oil◇, Kellogg's Tasteless Castor Oil◇, Minims Castor Oil‡◇, Neoloid◇, Purge◇

Pregnancy Risk Category: NR

HOW SUPPLIED
Capsules: 0.62 ml
Oral liquid: 36.4% (Neoloid◇), 60% (Alphamul◇), 67% (Fleet◇), 95% (Emulsoil◇, Purge◇), 100% (Kellogg's◇, Minims◇)

ACTION
Unknown. A stimulant laxative that increases peristalsis probably by direct effect on the smooth muscle of the intestine. Thought to either irritate the musculature or stimulate the colonic intramural plexus. Also promotes fluid accumulation in the colon and small intestine.

ONSET, PEAK, DURATION
Onset occurs in 2 to 6 hours. Peak and duration variable.

INDICATIONS & DOSAGE
Preparation for rectal or bowel examination or for surgery—
Adults and children 12 years and older: 15 to 60 ml P.O.

---

*Liquid contains alcohol.   **May contain tartrazine.   †Canada only.   ‡Australia only.   ◇OTC.

Children under 2 years: 2.5 to 7.5 ml P.O. Increased dose produces no greater effect.

Children 2 to 12 years: 5 to 15 ml P.O.

For all patients, administered as a single dose about 16 hours before surgery or procedure.

ADVERSE REACTIONS

GI: *nausea;* vomiting; diarrhea; loss of normal bowel function with excessive use; *abdominal cramps,* especially in severe constipation; malabsorption of nutrients; "cathartic colon" (syndrome resembling ulcerative colitis radiologically and pathologically) with chronic misuse; laxative dependence with long-term or excessive use. May cause constipation after catharsis.

Other: hypokalemia, protein-losing enteropathy, other electrolyte imbalances (with excessive use).

INTERACTIONS
None significant.

EFFECTS ON DIAGNOSTIC TESTS
None reported.

CONTRAINDICATIONS
Contraindicated in patients with ulcerative bowel lesions; abdominal pain, nausea, vomiting, or other symptoms of appendicitis or acute surgical abdomen; and anal or rectal fissures, fecal impaction, or intestinal obstruction or perforation; and during menstruation or pregnancy.

NURSING CONSIDERATIONS
● Use cautiously in patients with rectal bleeding.
● Give castor oil with juice or carbonated beverage to mask oily taste. Have the patient stir mixture and drink it promptly. Ice held in the mouth before taking drug will help prevent tasting it.
● Shake emulsion well before measuring dose. Emulsion is better tolerated but is more expensive. Store below 40° F (4.4° C). Don't freeze.

● Give on empty stomach for best results.
● Time drug administration so that it doesn't interfere with scheduled activities or sleep.
● Know that increased intestinal motility lessens absorption of concomitantly administered oral drugs. Separate administration times.
Alert: Be aware that failure to respond to drug may indicate acute condition requiring surgery.

☑ **PATIENT TEACHING**
● Tell the patient not to expect another bowel movement for 1 to 2 days after castor oil has emptied bowel.
● Warn patient about potential adverse reactions.

---

docusate calcium (dioctyl calcium sulfosuccinate)

DC 240◇, DC Softgels◇, Dioctocal◇, Pro-Cal-Sof◇, Sulfalax Calcium◇, Surfak◇

docusate sodium (dioctyl sodium sulfosuccinate)

Afko-Lube◇, Colace◇, Coloxyl‡, Coloxyl Enema Concentrate‡, Dialose◇, Diocto◇, Dioeze◇, Dionex◇, Diosuccin◇, Dio-Sul◇, Disonate◇, Di-Sosul◇, DOS◇, Doss◇, Doxinate◇, D-S-S◇, Duosol◇, Genasoft◇, Laxinate 100◇, Modane Soft◇, Molatoc◇, Pro-Sof◇, Pro-Sof Liquid Concentrate◇, Pro-Sof Liquid Plus◇, Regulax SS◇, Regulex†◇, Regutol◇, Stulex◇, Therevac Plus◇, Therevac-SB◇

Pregnancy Risk Category: C

HOW SUPPLIED
docusate calcium
Capsules: 50 mg◇, 240 mg◇
docusate sodium
Tablets: 100 mg◇

EFFECTS ON DIAGNOSTIC TESTS
None reported.

CONTRAINDICATIONS
Contraindicated in patients on a low-galactose diet.

NURSING CONSIDERATIONS
● Use cautiously in patients with diabetes mellitus.
● To minimize sweet taste, dilute with water or fruit juice or give with food.
● Prepare enema (not commercially available) by adding 200 g (300 ml) to 700 ml of water or 0.9% sodium chloride solution. The diluted solution is administered as a retention enema for 30 to 60 minutes. Use a rectal balloon catheter.
● If the enema is not retained for at least 30 minutes, be prepared to repeat dose.
● Monitor serum sodium level for possible hypernatremia, especially when giving in higher doses to treat hepatic encephalopathy.
● Be prepared to replace fluid loss.
● Store at room temperature, preferably below 86° F (30° C). Don't freeze.

☑ **PATIENT TEACHING**
● Instruct home care patient how to mix and then administer drug.
● Inform patient about adverse reactions and tell him to notify doctor if they become bothersome or if diarrhea occurs.
● Instruct patient not to take other laxatives while on lactulose therapy.

---

magnesium citrate (citrate of magnesia)
Citroma ◊ , Citro-Mag† , Citro-Nesia ◊ , Evac-Q-Mag

magnesium hydroxide (milk of magnesia)
Milk of Magnesia ◊ , Milk of Magnesia Concentrate ◊ , Phillips' Milk of Magnesia ◊

magnesium sulfate (epsom salts) ◊

Pregnancy Risk Category: NR

HOW SUPPLIED
magnesium citrate
Oral solution: approximately 168 mEq magnesium/240 ml ◊
magnesium hydroxide
Oral suspension: 7% to 8.5% (approximately 80 mEq magnesium/30 ml) ◊
magnesium sulfate
Granules: approximately 40 mEq magnesium/5 g ◊

ACTION
A saline laxative that produces an osmotic effect in the small intestine by drawing water into the intestinal lumen.

ONSET, PEAK, DURATION
Onset occurs in ½ to 3 hours. Peak and duration variable.

INDICATIONS & DOSAGE
Constipation; to evacuate bowel before surgery—
Adults and children 12 years and older: 11 to 25 g magnesium citrate P.O. daily as a single dose or divided; 2.4 to 4.8 g (30 to 60 ml) magnesium hydroxide P.O. daily as a single dose or divided; 10 to 30 g magnesium sulfate P.O. daily as a single dose or divided.
Children 6 to 12 years: 5.5 to 12.5 g magnesium citrate P.O. daily as a single dose or divided; 1.2 to 2.4 g (15 to 30 ml) magnesium hydroxide P.O. daily as a single dose or divided; 5 to 10 g magnesium sulfate P.O. daily as a single dose or divided.
Children 2 to 6 years: 2.7 to 6.25 g magnesium citrate P.O. daily as a single dose or divided; 0.4 to 1.2 g (5 to 15 ml) magnesium hydroxide P.O. daily as a single dose or divided; 2.5 to 5 g magnesium sulfate P.O. daily as a single dose or divided.
Antacid—

Adults: 5 to 15 ml milk of magnesia P.O. t.i.d. or q.i.d.

ADVERSE REACTIONS
GI: *abdominal cramping, nausea, diarrhea,* laxative dependence with long-term or excessive use.
Other: fluid and electrolyte disturbances with daily use.

INTERACTIONS
Orally administered drugs: impaired absorption. Separate administration times.

EFFECTS ON DIAGNOSTIC TESTS
No information available.

CONTRAINDICATIONS
Contraindicated in patients with abdominal pain, nausea, vomiting, or other symptoms of appendicitis or acute surgical abdomen and in those with myocardial damage, heart block, fecal impaction, rectal fissures, intestinal obstruction or perforation, renal disease, and patients about to deliver.

NURSING CONSIDERATIONS
● Use cautiously in patients with rectal bleeding.
● Time drug administration so that it doesn't interfere with scheduled activities or sleep. Drug produces watery stools in 3 to 6 hours.
● Before giving for constipation, determine if the patient has adequate fluid intake, exercise, and diet.
● Chill magnesium citrate before use to make it more palatable.
● Shake suspension well; give with large amount of water when used as laxative. When administering through nasogastric tube, make sure tube is placed properly and is patent. After instilling, flush tube with water to ensure passage to stomach and maintain tube patency.
Alert: Monitor serum electrolytes as ordered during prolonged use. Magnesium may accumulate in patients with renal insufficiency.

● Keep in mind that drug is for short-term therapy only.
● Know that magnesium sulfate is more potent than other saline laxatives.

☑ **PATIENT TEACHING**
● Instruct patient on drug administration.
● Teach patient about dietary sources of bulk, which include bran and other cereals, fresh fruit, and vegetables.
● Warn patient that frequent or prolonged use as a laxative may cause dependence.

methylcellulose
Citrucel ◇, Citrucel Orange Flavor ◇,
Citrucel Sugar-Free Orange Flavor ◇,
Cologel ◇

Pregnancy Risk Category: NR

HOW SUPPLIED
Powder: 2 g/tbs (heaping) ◇
Tablets: 500 mg ◇

ACTION
A bulk-forming laxative that absorbs water and expands to increase bulk and moisture content of stools. The increased bulk encourages peristalsis and bowel movement.

ONSET, PEAK, DURATION
Onset occurs in 12 to 24 hours. Peak effects may not occur for up to 3 days. Duration variable.

INDICATIONS & DOSAGE
Chronic constipation—
Adults: 1 to 3 tbs (heaping) in 8 oz (240 ml) of cold water daily to t.i.d. Usual dose up to 6 g daily (3 tbs).
Children 6 to 12 years: 1 to 1½ level tbs in 4 oz (120 ml) of cold water daily to t.i.d. Usual dose up to 3 g daily (1½ tbs).

ADVERSE REACTIONS
GI: *nausea,* vomiting, diarrhea (with

excessive use); esophageal, gastric, small intestinal, or colonic strictures when drug is chewed or taken in dry form; *abdominal cramps,* especially in severe constipation; laxative dependence (with long-term or excessive use).

INTERACTIONS
None significant.

EFFECTS ON DIAGNOSTIC TESTS
None reported.

CONTRAINDICATIONS
Contraindicated in patients with abdominal pain, nausea, vomiting, or other symptoms of appendicitis or acute surgical abdomen and in those with intestinal obstruction or ulceration, disabling adhesions, or difficulty swallowing.

NURSING CONSIDERATIONS
• Before giving for constipation, determine if the patient has adequate fluid intake, exercise, and diet.
• Be aware that the drug is especially useful in debilitated patients and in those with postpartum constipation, irritable bowel syndrome, diverticulitis, and colostomies. It's also used to treat laxative abuse and to empty colon before barium enema examinations.
• Know that the drug is not absorbed systemically and is nontoxic.

☑ **PATIENT TEACHING**
• Tell patient to take drug with at least 8 oz of liquid to mask grittiness.
• Teach patient about food sources of bulk: bran, cereals, fruits, vegetables.

mineral oil (liquid petrolatum)
Agoral Plain ◇ , Fleet Mineral Oil Enema ◇ , Kondremul ◇ , Kondremul Plain ◇ , Lansöoyl† , Liqui-Doss ◇ , Milkinol ◇ , Neo-Cultol ◇ , Petrogalar Plain ◇

Pregnancy Risk Category: C

HOW SUPPLIED
Emulsion: 50% ◇
Oral liquid: in pints, quarts, gallons ◇
Enema: 120 ml ◇ , 133 ml ◇

ACTION
A lubricant laxative that increases water retention in stools by creating a barrier between colon wall and feces that prevents colonic reabsorption of fecal water.

ONSET, PEAK, DURATION
Onset occurs in 6 to 8 hours. Peak and duration variable.

INDICATIONS & DOSAGE
Constipation; preparation for bowel studies or surgery—
Adults and children 12 years and older: 5 to 45 ml P.O. h.s.; or 120 ml P.R. (as enema).
Children 6 to 12 years: 5 to 20 ml P.O. h.s.; or 30 to 60 ml P.R. (as enema).
Children 2 to 6 years: 30 to 60 ml P.R. (as enema).

ADVERSE REACTIONS
GI: *nausea;* vomiting; diarrhea (with excessive use); *abdominal cramps,* especially in severe constipation; decreased absorption of nutrients and fat-soluble vitamins, resulting in deficiency; slowed healing after hemorrhoidectomy.
Other: laxative dependence (with long-term or excessive use), anal pruritus, anal irritation, hemorrhoids, perianal discomfort, *lipid pneumonia.*

INTERACTIONS
Docusate salts: may increase mineral oil absorption and cause lipid pneumonia. Separate administration times.
Fat-soluble vitamins (A,D,E, and K): possible decreased absorption after prolonged administration. Monitor for vitamin deficiency.

EFFECTS ON DIAGNOSTIC TESTS
None reported.

CONTRAINDICATIONS
Contraindicated in patients with abdominal pain, nausea, vomiting, or other symptoms of appendicitis or acute surgical abdomen and in those with fecal impaction or intestinal obstruction or perforation.

NURSING CONSIDERATIONS
● Use cautiously in young children; in elderly or debilitated patients because of susceptibility to lipid pneumonia through aspiration, absorption, and transport from intestinal mucosa; and in patients with rectal bleeding.
● Before giving for constipation, determine if the patient has adequate fluid intake, exercise, and diet.
● Give drug on an empty stomach because it delays passage of food from stomach; drug is more active on an empty stomach.
● Give with fruit juice or carbonated drink to disguise taste.
● Keep in mind that drug may be used when the patient needs to ease the strain of evacuation.

☑ **PATIENT TEACHING**
● Advise the patient to take drug only at bedtime on an empty stomach and not to take it for more than 1 week. Tell him to take drug with fruit juice or carbonated drink to disguise taste.
● To avoid soiling clothing, advise the patient of possible rectal leakage from excessive dosages.
● Teach the patient about dietary sources of bulk, which include bran and other cereals, fresh fruit, and vegetables.

---

phenolphthalein, white
Alophen ◇ , Medilax ◇ , Modane ◇ , Phenolax Wafers** ◇ , Prulet ◇

phenolphthalein, yellow
Espotabs ◇ , Evac-U-Gen ◇ , Evac-U-Lax ◇ , Ex-Lax ◇ , Ex-Lax Chocolated ◇ , Ex-Lax Maximum Relief Formula ◇ , Ex-Lax Pills ◇ , Feen-A-Mint ◇ , Feen-A-Mint Chocolated ◇ , Feen-A-Mint Gum ◇ , Lax-Pills ◇

Pregnancy Risk Category: NR

HOW SUPPLIED
phenolphthalein, white
Tablets: 60 mg ◇ , 65 mg ◇ , 120 mg, 130 mg ◇
Tablets (chewable): 60 mg ◇ , 64.8 mg ◇ , 120 mg ◇
phenolphthalein, yellow
Tablets: 90 mg, 135 mg
Tablets (chewable): 80 mg ◇ , 90 mg ◇ , 97.2 mg ◇
Chewing gum: 97.2 mg ◇

ACTION
Unknown. A stimulant laxative that increases peristalsis probably by direct effect on the smooth muscle of the intestine. Thought either to irritate the musculature or stimulate the colonic intramural plexus. Also promotes fluid accumulation in the colon and small intestine.

ONSET, PEAK, DURATION
Onset occurs in 6 to 10 hours. Peak unknown. Effects persist for 3 to 4 days.

INDICATIONS & DOSAGE
Constipation—
Adults and children 12 years and over: 30 to 270 mg P.O., preferably h.s.
Children 6 to 12 years: 30 to 60 mg P.O. h.s.
Children 2 to 6 years: 15 to 30 mg P.O. h.s.

ADVERSE REACTIONS
GI: diarrhea; *colic (with large doses):* factitious nausea; vomiting; loss of normal bowel function (with excessive use); *abdominal cramps,* especially in

---

Reactions may be *common,* uncommon, *life-threatening,* or COMMON AND LIFE-THREATENING.

severe constipation; malabsorption of nutrients; "cathartic colon" (syndrome resembling ulcerative colitis radiologically and pathologically) with chronic misuse; reddish discoloration in alkaline feces or urine, laxative dependence (with long-term or excessive use).

Skin: dermatitis, pruritus, rash, increased pigmentation.

Other: hypersensitivity reactions.

INTERACTIONS
None significant.

EFFECTS ON DIAGNOSTIC TESTS
Drug may increase rate of phenolsulfonphthalein (PSP) excretion during PSP excretion tests and may cause false-positive results on urine urobilinogen and estrogen tests using Kolber procedure.

CONTRAINDICATIONS
Contraindicated in patients with abdominal pain, nausea, vomiting, or other symptoms of appendicitis or acute surgical abdomen; in patients with fecal impaction or intestinal obstruction or perforation.

NURSING CONSIDERATIONS
● Use cautiously in patients with rectal bleeding.
● Before giving for constipation, determine if the patient has adequate fluid intake, exercise, and diet.
● Time drug administration so that it doesn't interfere with scheduled activities or sleep.
● Be aware that yellow phenolphthalein has been reported to be two to three times as potent as white phenolphthalein, although this has not been proved in clinical studies.

☑ PATIENT TEACHING
● Tell parents that children may mistake for candy. Keep out of reach.
● Warn the patient to avoid excessive sun exposure, not to use drug with any other product containing phenolphthalein, and to discontinue use if dermatoses occur.
● Warn the patient that the drug may discolor alkaline urine red-pink and acidic urine yellow-brown.
● Teach the patient about dietary sources of bulk, which include bran and other cereals, fresh fruit, and vegetables.

---

polyethylene glycol and electrolyte solution
Colovage, CoLyte, Co-Lav, Glycoprep‡, GoLYTELY, Go-Evac, Nulytely, OCL

Pregnancy Risk Category: C

HOW SUPPLIED
Powder for oral solution: polyethylene glycol (PEG) 3350 (6 g), anhydrous sodium sulfate (568 mg), sodium chloride (146 mg), potassium chloride (74.5 mg) per 100 ml (Colovage); PEG 3350 (120 g), sodium sulfate (3.36 g), sodium chloride (2.92 g), potassium chloride (1.49 g) per 2 liters (CoLyte); PEG 3350 (60 g), sodium chloride (1.46 g), potassium chloride (0.745 g), sodium bicarbonate (1.68 g), sodium sulfate (5.68 g) per liter (Co-Lav); PEG 3350 (60 g), sodium chloride (1.46 g), potassium chloride (745 mg), sodium bicarbonate (1.68 g), sodium sulfate (5.68 g) per liter (Glycoprep‡); PEG 3350 (236 g), sodium sulfate (22.74 g), sodium bicarbonate (6.74g), sodium chloride (5.86 g), potassium chloride (2.97 g) per 4.8 liter (GoLYTELY); PEG 3350 (59 g), sodium sulfate (5.685 g), sodium bicarbonate (1.685 g), sodium chloride (1.465 g), potassium chloride (0.743 g) per liter (Go-Evac); PEG 3350 (420 g), sodium bicarbonate (5.72 g), sodium chloride (11.2 g), potassium chloride (1.48 g) per 4 liters (Nulytely); PEG 3350 (6 g), sodium sulfate decahydrate (1.29 g), sodium chloride (146 mg), potassium chloride (75 mg), polysorbate-80 (30 mg) per 100 ml (OCL)

ACTION
PEG 3350, a nonabsorbable solution, acts as an osmotic agent. Sodium sulfate greatly reduces sodium absorption. The electrolyte concentration causes virtually no net absorption or secretion of ions.

ONSET, PEAK, DURATION
Onset occurs within 1 hour. Peak and duration variable.

INDICATIONS & DOSAGE
Bowel preparation before GI examination—
Adults: 240 ml P.O. q 10 minutes until 4 liters are consumed or until the watery stool is clear. Typically, administer 4 hours before examination, allowing 3 hours for drinking and 1 hour for bowel evacuation.

ADVERSE REACTIONS
GI: *nausea, bloating, cramps, vomiting, abdominal fullness.*
Skin: urticaria, dermatitis, allergic reaction.
Other: anal irritation, rhinorrhea.

INTERACTIONS
Orally administered drugs: decreased absorption if administered within 1 hour of starting therapy. Administer at least 2 to 3 hours before starting therapy.

EFFECTS ON DIAGNOSTIC TESTS
Patient preparation for barium enema may be less satisfactory with this solution as it may interfere with the barium coating of the colonic mucosa using the double-contrast technique.

CONTRAINDICATIONS
Contraindicated in patients with GI obstruction or perforation, gastric retention, toxic colitis, or megacolon.

NURSING CONSIDERATIONS
● Use tap water to reconstitute powder. Shake vigorously to ensure that all powder is dissolved. Refrigerate reconstituted solution but use within 48 hours.

Alert: Do not add flavoring or additional ingredients to the solution or administer chilled solution. Hypothermia has been reported after ingestion of large amounts of chilled solution.
● Administer solution early in the morning if the patient is scheduled for a mid-morning examination. Orally administered solution induces diarrhea (onset 30 to 60 minutes) that rapidly cleans the bowel, usually within 4 hours.
● When used as preparation for barium enema, administer solution the evening before the examination to avoid interfering with barium coating of the colonic mucosa.
● If administered to semiconscious patients or to patients with impaired gag reflex, take care to prevent aspiration.
● Be aware that no major shifts in fluid or electrolyte balance have been reported.

☑ **PATIENT TEACHING**
● Tell the patient to fast for 3 to 4 hours before taking the solution and thereafter ingest only clear fluids until the examination is complete.
● Warn the patient about adverse reactions.

psyllium
Cillium ◇, Effer-Syllium Instant Mix ◇, Fiberall ◇, Fibrepur† ◇, Genfiber ◇, Hydrocil Instant ◇, Karacil† ◇, Konsyl ◇, Konsyl-D ◇, Maalox Daily Fiber Therapy ◇, Metamucil ◇, Metamucil Effervescent Sugar Free ◇, Metamucil Instant Mix ◇, Metamucil Sugar-Free ◇, Modane Bulk ◇, Muci-Lax ◇, Mylanta Natural Fiber Supplement ◇, Naturacil ◇, Perdiem Fiber ◇, Prodiem Plain† ◇, Pro-Lax ◇, Reguloid Natural ◇, Restore ◇, Serutan ◇, Siblin ◇, Syllact ◇, Uni Laxative ◇, Versabran ◇, V-Lax ◇

Pregnancy Risk Category: NR

HOW SUPPLIED
Chewable pieces: 1.7 g/piece ◇
Effervescent powder: 3.4 g/packet ◇, 3.7 g/packet ◇
Granules: 2.5 g/tsp ◇, 4.03 g/tsp ◇
Powder: 3.3 g/tsp ◇, 3.4 g/tsp ◇, 3.5 g/tsp ◇, 4.94 g/tsp ◇
Wafers: 3.4 g/wafer ◇

ACTION
A bulk-forming laxative that absorbs water and expands to increase bulk and moisture content of the stool, thus encouraging peristalsis and bowel movement.

ONSET, PEAK, DURATION
Onset occurs in 12 to 24 hours. Peak effects may not occur for 3 days. Duration variable.

INDICATIONS & DOSAGE
Constipation; bowel management—
Adults: 1 to 2 tsp (rounded) P.O. in full glass of liquid once daily, b.i.d., or t.i.d., followed by second glass of liquid; or 1 packet dissolved in water once daily, b.i.d., or t.i.d.
Children over 6 years: 1 tsp (level) P.O. in half a glass of liquid h.s.

ADVERSE REACTIONS
GI: nausea, vomiting, diarrhea (with excessive use); esophageal, gastric, small intestinal, and rectal obstruction when drug is taken in dry form; abdominal cramps, especially in severe constipation.

INTERACTIONS
None significant.

EFFECTS ON DIAGNOSTIC TESTS
None reported.

CONTRAINDICATIONS
Contraindicated in patients with hypersensitivity to drug, abdominal pain, nausea, vomiting, or other symptoms of appendicitis and in those with intestinal obstruction or ulceration, disabling adhesions, or difficulty swallowing.

NURSING CONSIDERATIONS
● Before giving for constipation, determine if the patient has adequate fluid intake, exercise, and diet.
● Mix with at least 8 oz (240 ml) of cold, pleasant-tasting liquid, such as orange juice, to mask grittiness, and stir only a few seconds. Have the patient drink mixture immediately so it does not congeal. Follow with additional glass of liquid.
● For dosages in children under 6 years, consult the doctor.
● Know that drug may reduce appetite if taken before meals.
● Be aware that the drug is not absorbed systemically and is nontoxic. It is especially useful in debilitated patients and those with postpartum constipation, irritable bowel syndrome, and diverticular disease. It's also used to treat chronic laxative abuse and in combination with other laxatives to empty colon before barium enema examinations.

☑ PATIENT TEACHING
● Teach the patient how to properly mix medication. Tell him to take drug with plenty of water. Advise the patient that inhaling powder may cause allergic reactions.
● Tell the patient that laxative effect usually occurs in 12 to 24 hours but may be delayed 3 days.
● Advise the diabetic patient to check the label and use brand of psyllium that does not contain sugar.
● Teach patient about food sources of bulk: bran, cereals, fruit, vegetables.

senna
Black-Draught ◇, Fletcher's Castoria ◇, Senexon ◇, Senna-Gen ◇, Senokot ◇, SenokotXTRA ◇, Senolax ◇, X-Prep Liquid* ◇

Pregnancy Risk Category: C

HOW SUPPLIED
Tablets: 187 mg ◊, 217 mg ◊, 600 mg ◊
Granules: 326 mg/tsp ◊, 1.65 g/½ tsp ◊
Suppositories: 652 mg ◊
Syrup: 218 mg/5 ml ◊

ACTION
Unknown. A stimulant laxative that increases peristalsis probably by direct effect on the smooth muscle of the intestine. Thought to either irritate the musculature or stimulate the colonic intramural plexus. Also promotes fluid accumulation in the colon and small intestine.

ONSET, PEAK, DURATION
Onset occurs in 6 to 10 hours. Peak and duration variable.

INDICATIONS & DOSAGE
Acute constipation; preparation for bowel or rectal examination—
Adults: dosage range for Senokot is 1 to 8 tablets P.O.; ½ to 4 tsp of granules added to liquid P.O.; 1 to 2 suppositories P.R. h.s.; or 1 to 4 tsp syrup P.O. h.s. Dosage for Black-Draught is 2 tablets or ¼ to ½ tsp (level) of granules mixed with water.

X-Prep Liquid used solely as single dose for preradiographic bowel evacuation. Give 20 g powder dissolved in juice or 75 ml liquid P.O. between 2 p.m. and 4 p.m. on day before X-ray procedure. Use in divided doses, if needed, for elderly or debilitated patients.
Children over 27 kg: one-half adult dose of tablets, granules, or syrup (except Black-Draught tablets and granules—not recommended for children).
Children 1 month to 1 year: 1.25 to 2.5 ml Senokot syrup P.O. h.s.

ADVERSE REACTIONS
GI: *nausea;* vomiting; diarrhea; loss of normal bowel function with excessive use; *abdominal cramps,* especially in severe constipation; malabsorption of nutrients; "cathartic colon" (syndrome resembling ulcerative colitis radiologically) with chronic misuse; possible

constipation after catharsis; yellow or yellow-green cast to feces; diarrhea in breast-feeding infants of mothers receiving senna; darkened pigmentation of rectal mucosa with long-term use (usually reversible within 4 to 12 months after stopping drug); laxative dependence with excessive use.
GU: red-pink discoloration in alkaline urine; yellow-brown color to acidic urine.
Other: protein-losing enteropathy, electrolyte imbalance (such as hypokalemia).

INTERACTIONS
None significant.

EFFECTS ON DIAGNOSTIC TESTS
In the phenolsulfonphthalein excretion test, senna may turn urine pink to red, red to violet, or red to brown.

CONTRAINDICATIONS
Contraindicated in patients with ulcerative bowel lesions; nausea, vomiting, abdominal pain, or other symptoms of appendicitis or acute surgical abdomen; fecal impaction; or intestinal obstruction or perforation.

NURSING CONSIDERATIONS
● Before giving for constipation, determine if the patient has adequate fluid intake, exercise, and diet.
● Limit diet to clear liquids after X-Prep Liquid is taken.
● Avoid exposing product to excessive heat or light.
● Know that drug is used for short-term therapy.
● Know that senna is one of the most effective laxatives for counteracting constipation caused by narcotic analgesics.

☑ PATIENT TEACHING
● Teach the patient about dietary sources of bulk, including bran and other cereals, fresh fruit, and vegetables.

Reactions may be *common,* uncommon, *life-threatening,* or COMMON AND LIFE-THREATENING.

● Tell the patient to report persistent or severe reactions.

---

sodium phosphates
Fleet Phospho-Soda ◇

Pregnancy Risk Category: NR

HOW SUPPLIED
Liquid: 2.4 g/5 ml sodium phosphate and 900 mg sodium biphosphate/5 ml ◇
Enema: 160 mg/ml sodium phosphate and 60 mg/ml sodium biphosphate ◇

ACTION
A saline laxative that produces an osmotic effect in the small intestine by drawing water into the intestinal lumen.

ONSET, PEAK, DURATION
Onset occurs in ½ to 3 hours after oral use, 5 to 10 minutes after enema. Peak and duration variable after oral dose, complete upon evacuation following enema.

INDICATIONS & DOSAGE
Constipation—
Adults: 20 to 30 ml solution mixed with 120 ml cold water P.O.; or 60 to 135 ml P.R. (as enema).
Children: 5 to 15 ml solution mixed with 120 ml of cold water P.O.; or 67.5 ml P.R. (as enema).

ADVERSE REACTIONS
GI: *abdominal cramping.*
Other: fluid and electrolyte disturbances (hypernatremia, hyperphosphatemia) with daily use; laxative dependence with long-term or excessive use.

INTERACTIONS
None significant.

EFFECTS ON DIAGNOSTIC TESTS
None reported.

CONTRAINDICATIONS
Contraindicated in patients with abdom-inal pain, nausea, vomiting, or other symptoms of appendicitis or acute surgical abdomen; intestinal obstruction or perforation; edema; CHF; megacolon; or impaired renal function and in patients on sodium-restricted diets.

NURSING CONSIDERATIONS
● Use cautiously in patients with large hemorrhoids or anal excoriations.
● Before giving for constipation, determine if the patient has adequate fluid intake, exercise, and diet.
Alert: Be aware that up to 10% of sodium content of drug may be absorbed.

☑ PATIENT TEACHING
● Teach patient about dietary sources of bulk, which include bran and other cereals, fresh fruit, and vegetables.
● Warn patient about adverse reactions and stress importance of using only for short-term therapy.

51

Antiemetics

chlorpromazine hydrochloride
(See Chapter 33, ANTIPSYCHOTICS.)
dimenhydrinate
diphenidol hydrochloride
dronabinol
granisetron hydrochloride
meclizine hydrochloride
metoclopramide hydrochloride
ondansetron hydrochloride
perphenazine
(See Chapter 33, ANTIPSYCHOTICS.)
prochlorperazine
prochlorperazine edisylate
prochlorperazine maleate
promethazine hydrochloride
(See Chapter 43, ANTIHISTAMINES.)
scopolamine
(See Chapter 38, ANTICHOLINERGICS.)
thiethylperazine maleate
trimethobenzamide
hydrochloride

COMBINATION PRODUCTS
None.

---

dimenhydrinate

Andrumin‡, Apo-Dimenhydrinate†, Calm X ◇, Children's Dramamine ◇, Dimetabs, Dinate, Dommanate, Dramamine ◇ *, Dramamine Chewable ◇ **, Dramamine Liquid ◇ *, Dramanate, Dramilin, Dramocen, Dramoject, Dymenate, Gravol†, Gravol L/A†, Hydrate, Marmine ◇, Nauseatol†, Nico-Vert ◇, Novo-Dimenate†, PMS-Dimenhydrinate†, Tega-Vert ◇, Travamine†, Travs‡, Triptone Caplets ◇, Wehamine*

Pregnancy Risk Category: B

HOW SUPPLIED
Tablets: 50 mg ◇
Tablets (chewable): 50 mg ◇
Capsules: 50 mg ◇

Elixir: 15 mg/5 ml†
Syrup: 12.5 mg/4 ml* ◇, 15.62 mg/5 ml
Injection: 50 mg/ml

ACTION
Unknown. An antihistamine that may affect neural pathways originating in the labyrinth to inhibit nausea and vomiting.

ONSET, PEAK, DURATION
Onset occurs right after I.V. administration, within 15 to 20 minutes of I.M. injection, within 20 to 30 minutes of oral administration. Peak unknown. Effects last for 3 to 6 hours.

INDICATIONS & DOSAGE
Prevention and treatment of motion sickness—
Adults and children 12 years and over: 50 to 100 mg P.O. q 4 to 6 hours; 50 mg I.M., p.r.n.; or 50 mg I.V. diluted in 10 ml sodium chloride for injection, injected over 2 minutes. Maximum dosage is 400 mg daily.
Children 6 to 12 years: 25 to 50 mg P.O. q 6 to 8 hours, not to exceed 150 mg in 24 hours.
Children 2 to 6 years: 12.5 to 25 mg P.O. q 6 to 8 hours, not to exceed 75 mg in 24 hours.
Children over 2 years: 1.25 mg/kg or 37.5 mg/m^2 I.M. q.i.d. Maximum dosage is 300 mg daily.

ADVERSE REACTIONS
CNS: *drowsiness,* headache, dizziness, confusion, nervousness, insomnia (especially in children), vertigo, tingling and weakness of hands, lassitude, excitation.
CV: palpitations, hypotension, tachycardia.
EENT: blurred vision, dry respiratory passages, diplopia, nasal congestion.
GI: dry mouth, nausea, vomiting, diar-

Reactions may be *common*, uncommon, ***life-threatening***, or COMMON AND LIFE-THREATENING.

rhea, epigastric distress, constipation, anorexia.
Respiratory: wheezing, thickened bronchial secretions.
Skin: photosensitivity, urticaria, rash.
Other: *anaphylaxis,* tightness of chest.

INTERACTIONS
CNS depressants, ethanol: additive CNS effects. Avoid concomitant use.

EFFECTS ON DIAGNOSTIC TESTS
Drug may alter or confuse test results for xanthines (caffeine, aminophylline) because of its 8-chlorotheophylline content; discontinue drug 4 days before diagnostic skin tests to avoid preventing, reducing, or masking test response.

CONTRAINDICATIONS
Contraindicated in patients hypersensitive to drug or its components.

NURSING CONSIDERATIONS
• Use cautiously in patients with seizures, acute angle-closure glaucoma, or enlarged prostate gland or in patients receiving ototoxic drugs.
• **I.V. use:** Before administration, dilute each ml of drug with 10 ml of sterile water for injection, D_5W, or 0.9% sodium chloride for injection. Give by direct injection over not less than 2 minutes.
• Know that undiluted solution irritates veins and may cause sclerosis.
• Because incompatibilities are common, avoid mixing parenteral preparation with other drugs.
Alert: Be aware that most I.V. products contain benzyl alcohol, which has been associated with a fatal "gasping syndrome" in premature infants and low birth weight infants.
• Like other antiemetics, know that drug may mask symptoms of ototoxicity, brain tumor, or intestinal obstruction.

☑ PATIENT TEACHING
• Advise patient to avoid activities that require alertness until CNS effects of the drug are known.

• Instruct patient to report adverse reactions promptly.

---

diphenidol hydrochloride
Vontrol**

Pregnancy Risk Category: NR

HOW SUPPLIED
Tablets: 25 mg

ACTION
Unknown. Probably diminishes labyrinthine function and vestibular stimulation and influences the chemoreceptor trigger zone to inhibit nausea and vomiting.

ONSET, PEAK, DURATION
Onset and duration unknown. Blood levels peak in 1½ to 3 hours.

INDICATIONS & DOSAGE
Peripheral (labyrinthine) vertigo—
Adults: 25 to 50 mg P.O. q 4 hours, p.r.n.
Nausea and vomiting—
Adults: 25 to 50 mg P.O. q 4 hours, p.r.n. Maximum dosage is 300 mg/day.
Children over 6 months weighing more than 11 kg: 0.88 mg/kg P.O. q 4 hours, not to exceed 5.5 mg/kg/24 hours.

ADVERSE REACTIONS
CNS: *drowsiness,* dizziness, sleep disturbances, *confusion,* auditory and visual hallucinations, depression, malaise, headache, disorientation.
CV: transient hypotension.
GI: dry mouth, nausea, indigestion, heartburn.
Skin: urticaria.

INTERACTIONS
None significant.

EFFECTS ON DIAGNOSTIC TESTS
No information available.

CONTRAINDICATIONS
Contraindicated in patients with anuria

and hypersensitivity to drug.

NURSING CONSIDERATIONS
● Use cautiously in patients with glaucoma, pyloric stenosis, pylorospasm, obstructive lesions of GI or GU tract, prostatic hyperplasia, or organic cardiospasm (achalasia).
● Closely supervise patients. Patients usually are hospitalized when receiving drug. Monitor fluid intake and output; report any changes.
● Like other antiemetics, be alert that drug may mask symptoms of ototoxicity, brain tumor, intestinal obstruction, or other conditions.
Alert: Stop drug if auditory or visual hallucinations, disorientation, or confusion occur and notify doctor.

☑ **PATIENT TEACHING**
● Advise patient to ask for assistance when getting out of bed or during ambulation because of potential adverse CNS reactions.
● Instruct patient to report adverse reactions promptly.

---

dronabinol (delta-g-tetrahydrocannabinol)
Marinol

Controlled Substance Schedule II
Pregnancy Risk Category: C

HOW SUPPLIED
Capsules: 2.5 mg, 5 mg, 10 mg

ACTION
Unknown. A derivative of marijuana.

ONSET, PEAK, DURATION
Onset unknown. Serum levels peak in 2 to 4 hours. Effects last 4 to 6 hours.

INDICATIONS & DOSAGE
Nausea and vomiting associated with cancer chemotherapy—
Adults: 5 mg/m^2 P.O. 1 to 3 hours before administration of chemotherapy.

Then same dose q 2 to 4 hours after chemotherapy for a total of four to six doses per day. If needed, dosage increased in 2.5-mg/m$_2$ increments to a maximum of 15 mg/m$_2$ per dose.
Anorexia and weight loss in patients with AIDS—
Adults: 2.5 mg P.O. b.i.d. before lunch and dinner. If unable to tolerate, decrease dose to 2.5 mg P.O. given as a single dose daily in the evening or at bedtime. May gradually increase dosage to maximum of 20 mg/day.

ADVERSE REACTIONS
CNS: *dizziness, drowsiness, euphoria, ataxia,* depersonalization, hallucinations, somnolence, headache, muddled thinking, asthenia, amnesia, confusion, *paranoia.*
CV: tachycardia, orthostatic hypotension, palpitations, vasodilation.
GI: *dry mouth, nausea, vomiting,* diarrhea.
Other: visual disturbances.

INTERACTIONS
CNS depressants, ethanol, psychotomimetic substances, sedatives: additive effects. Avoid concomitant use.

EFFECTS ON DIAGNOSTIC TESTS
None reported.

CONTRAINDICATIONS
Contraindicated in patients hypersensitive to sesame oil or cannabinoids.

NURSING CONSIDERATIONS
● Use cautiously in elderly, pregnant, or lactating patients and in those with heart disease, psychiatric illness, and history of drug abuse.
● Expect drug to be prescribed only for patients who have not responded satisfactorily to other antiemetics.
● Know that dronabinol is the principal active substance present in *Cannabis sativa* (marijuana). This substance can produce both physical and psychological dependence and has a high potential

---

for abuse.
• Keep in mind that CNS effects are intensified at higher drug dosages.
• Be aware that drug's effects may persist for days after treatment ends.

☑ **PATIENT TEACHING**
• Tell the patient drug may induce unusual changes in mood or other adverse behavioral effects.
• Advise the patient against activities that require alertness until the CNS effects of the drug are known.
• Warn caregivers to supervise the patient during and immediately after treatment.

---

granisetron hydrochloride
Kytril

Pregnancy Risk Category: B

HOW SUPPLIED
Injection: 1 mg/ml
Tablets: 1 mg

ACTION
A selective antagonist of a specific type of serotonin receptor (5-HT₃) located in the CNS in the chemoreceptor trigger zone and in the peripheral nervous system on nerve terminals of the vagus nerve. Drug's blocking action may occur at both sites.

ONSET, PEAK, DURATION
Unknown.

INDICATIONS & DOSAGE
Prevention of nausea and vomiting associated with emetogenic cancer chemotherapy—
Adults and children 2 to 16 years: 10 mcg/kg I.V. infused over 5 minutes. Begin infusion within 30 minutes before administration of chemotherapy. Alternatively, 1 mg P.O. up to 1 hour before chemotherapy and dosage repeated 12 hours later.

ADVERSE REACTIONS
CNS: *headache, asthenia,* somnolence, dizziness, anxiety.
CV: hypertension.
GI: diarrhea, *constipation,* abdominal pain, *nausea,* vomiting, decreased appetite.
Hematologic: *leukopenia,* anemia, *thrombocytopenia.*
Other: fever, alopecia, elevated liver function tests.

INTERACTIONS
None significant.

EFFECTS ON DIAGNOSTIC TESTS
None reported.

CONTRAINDICATIONS
Contraindicated in patients hypersensitive to the drug.

NURSING CONSIDERATIONS
• I.V. use: Dilute drug with 0.9% sodium chloride for injection or D₅W to a volume of 20 to 50 ml. Infuse over 5 minutes, beginning within 30 minutes before initiating chemotherapy, and only on the days chemotherapy is given. Diluted solutions are stable for 24 hours at room temperature.
• Do not mix with other drugs; data regarding compatibility are limited.

☑ **PATIENT TEACHING**
• Stress to patient the importance of taking second dose of oral drug 12 hours later for maximum effectiveness.
• Instruct patient to report adverse reactions immediately.

**meclizine hydrochloride
(meclozine hydrochloride)**
Ancolan‡, Antivert, Antivert/25◇, Antivert/50, Bonamine†, Bonine◇, Dizmiss◇, D-Vert 15, D-Vert 30, Meni-D, Ru-Vert M, Vergon◇

Pregnancy Risk Category: B

HOW SUPPLIED
Tablets: 12.5 mg, 25 mg ◇, 50 mg
Tablets (chewable): 25 mg ◇
Capsules: 15 mg, 25 mg, 30 mg

ACTION
Unknown. An antihistamine that may affect neural pathways originating in the labyrinth to inhibit nausea and vomiting.

ONSET, PEAK, DURATION
Onset occurs in about 1 hour. Peak unknown. Effects persist 8 to 24 hours.

INDICATIONS & DOSAGE
Vertigo—
Adults: 25 to 100 mg P.O. daily in divided doses. Dosage varies with response.
Motion sickness—
Adults: 25 to 50 mg P.O. 1 hour before travel, then daily for duration of trip.

ADVERSE REACTIONS
CNS: *drowsiness,* restlessness, excitation, nervousness, auditory and visual hallucinations.
CV: hypotension, palpitations, tachycardia.
EENT: blurred vision, diplopia, tinnitus, dry nose and throat.
GI: dry mouth, constipation, anorexia, nausea, vomiting, diarrhea.
GU: urine retention, urinary frequency.
Skin: urticaria, rash.

INTERACTIONS
CNS depressants: increased drowsiness. Use together cautiously.

EFFECTS ON DIAGNOSTIC TESTS
Drug should be discontinued 4 days before diagnostic skin tests to avoid preventing, reducing, or masking test response.

CONTRAINDICATIONS
Contraindicated in patients hypersensitive to the drug.

NURSING CONSIDERATIONS
● Use cautiously in patients with asthma, glaucoma, or prostatic hyperplasia.
● Like other antiemetics, be alert that drug may mask symptoms of ototoxicity, brain tumor, or intestinal obstruction.

☑ PATIENT TEACHING
● Advise patient to avoid hazardous activities that require alertness until CNS effects of the drug are known.
● Instruct patient to report persistent or serious adverse reactions promptly.

---

metoclopramide hydrochloride
Apo-Metoclop†, Clopra, Emex†, Maxeran†, Maxolon, Maxolon High Dose‡, Octamide, Octamide PFS, Pramin‡, Reclomide, Reglan

Pregnancy Risk Category: B

HOW SUPPLIED
Tablets: 5 mg, 10 mg
Syrup: 5 mg/5 ml
Injection: 5 mg/ml

ACTION
Stimulates motility of the upper GI tract by increasing lower esophageal sphincter tone and blocks dopamine receptors at the chemoreceptor trigger zone.

ONSET, PEAK, DURATION
Onset occurs within 1 to 3 minutes of I.V. administration, 10 to 15 minutes after I.M. injection, 30 to 60 minutes after oral ingestion. Peak occurs in 1 to 2 hours after oral administration, unknown for parenteral administration. Effects persist for 1 to 2 hours.

INDICATIONS & DOSAGE
Prevention or reduction of nausea and vomiting associated with emetogenic cancer chemotherapy—
Adults: 1 to 2 mg/kg I.V. 30 minutes before cancer chemotherapy, then repeated q 2 hours for two doses, then q 3

hours for three doses.

Prevention or reduction of postoperative nausea and vomiting—
Adults: 10 to 20 mg I.M. near the end of the surgical procedure, repeated q 4 to 6 hours p.r.n.

To facilitate small-bowel intubation and to aid in radiologic examinations—
Adults and children over 14 years: 10 mg (2 ml) I.V. as a single dose over 1 to 2 minutes.
Children under 6 years: 0.1 mg/kg I.V.
Children 6 to 14 years: 2.5 to 5 mg I.V. (0.5 to 1 ml).

Delayed gastric emptying secondary to diabetic gastroparesis—
Adults: 10 mg P.O. for mild symptoms, slow I.V. (1 to 2 minutes) for severe symptoms 30 minutes before meals and h.s. I.V. dose may be necessary for up to 10 days, then P.O. dose may be started to continue for rest of 2 to 8 weeks.

Gastroesophageal reflux disease—
Adults: 10 to 15 mg P.O. q.i.d., p.r.n., 30 minutes before meals and h.s.

In patients with impaired renal function: If creatinine clearance is below 40 ml/minute, decrease initial dosage by half the recommended dose.

ADVERSE REACTIONS
CNS: *restlessness, anxiety, drowsiness, fatigue, lassitude,* depression, akathisia, insomnia, confusion, ***suicide ideation, seizures,*** hallucinations, headache, dizziness, extrapyramidal symptoms, tardive dyskinesia, dystonic reactions.
CV: transient hypertension, hypotension.
GI: nausea, bowel disturbances, diarrhea.
Hematologic: neutropenia, ***agranulocytosis.***
Skin: rash, urticaria.
Other: fever, prolactin secretion, loss of libido, urinary frequency, incontinence.

INTERACTIONS
Anticholinergics, opioid analgesics: antagonized GI motility effects of metoclopramide. Use together cautiously.

Butyrophenones, phenothiazines: increased risk of extrapyramidal effects. Monitor closely.
CNS depressants, ethanol: additive CNS effects. Avoid concomitant use.

EFFECTS ON DIAGNOSTIC TESTS
Drug may increase serum aldosterone and prolactin levels.

CONTRAINDICATIONS
Contraindicated in patients in which stimulation of GI motility might be dangerous (for example, those with hemorrhage, obstruction, or perforation) and in those with hypersensitivity to drug, pheochromocytoma, or seizure disorders.

NURSING CONSIDERATIONS
● Use cautiously in patients with history of depression, Parkinson's disease, and hypertension.
● **I.V. use:** Give lower doses (10 mg or less) by direct injection over 1 to 2 minutes. Dilute doses larger than 10 mg in 50 ml of a compatible diluent, and infuse over at least 15 minutes. Protection from light is unnecessary if the infusion mixture is administered within 24 hours.
● Know that the drug is compatible with D_5W, 0.9% sodium chloride for injection, and dextrose 5% in sodium chloride 0.45%.
● Closely monitor blood pressure in patients receiving I.V. form of the drug.
Alert: Use diphenhydramine 25 mg I.V. as ordered to counteract the extrapyramidal adverse effects associated with high metoclopramide doses.
● Know that safety and effectiveness have not been established for therapy that continues longer than 12 weeks.

☑ PATIENT TEACHING
● Advise patient to avoid activities requiring alertness for 2 hours after taking each dose.
● Instruct patient to report persistent or serious adverse reactions promptly.

---

*Liquid contains alcohol.　　**May contain tartrazine.　　†Canada only.　　‡Australia only.　　◇ OTC.

ondansetron hydrochloride
Zofran

Pregnancy Risk Category: B

HOW SUPPLIED
Tablets: 4 mg, 8 mg
Injection: 2 mg/ml, 4mg/ml
Premixed injection: 32 mg/50 ml

ACTION
A selective antagonist of a specific type of serotonin receptor ($5\text{-}HT_3$) located in the CNS at the area postrema (chemoreceptor trigger zone) and in the peripheral nervous system on nerve terminals of the vagus nerve. Drug's blocking action may occur at both sites.

ONSET, PEAK, DURATION
Unknown.

INDICATIONS & DOSAGE
Prevention of nausea and vomiting associated with emetogenic chemotherapy—
Adults and children 12 years and over: 8 mg P.O. 30 minutes before start of chemotherapy. Follow with 8 mg P.O. 8 hours after first dose. Then follow with 8 mg q 12 hours for 1 to 2 days. Alternatively, administer a single dose of 32 mg by I.V. infusion over 15 minutes beginning 30 minutes before chemotherapy; or three divided doses of 0.15 mg/kg I.V. (first dose given 30 minutes before chemotherapy; subsequent doses given 4 and 8 hours after first dose). Infuse drug over 15 minutes.
Children 4 to 12 years: 4 mg P.O. 30 minutes before start of chemotherapy. Follow with 4 mg P.O. 4 and 8 hours after first dose. Then follow with 4 mg q 8 hours for 1 to 2 days. Alternatively, three doses of 0.15 mg/kg I.V. Give first dose 30 minutes before chemotherapy; administer subsequent doses 4 and 8 hours after first dose. Infuse drug over 15 minutes.
Prevention of postoperative nausea and

vomiting—
Adults: 4 mg I.V. (undiluted) over 2 to 5 minutes. Alternatively, 16 mg P.O. 1 hour before induction of anesthesia.
Prevention of nausea and vomiting associated with radiotherapy in patients receiving either total body irradiation, single high-dose fraction to the abdomen, or daily fractions to the abdomen—
Adults: 8 mg P.O. t.i.d.

ADVERSE REACTIONS
CNS: *headache, malaise, fatigue, dizziness, sedation.*
GI: *diarrhea, constipation,* abdominal pain, xerostomia.
Hepatic: transient elevations in AST and ALT levels.
Skin: rash.
Other: *musculoskeletal pain,* chills, urine retention, chest pain, injection-site reaction, fever, hypoxia, gynecologic disorders.

INTERACTIONS
Drugs that alter hepatic drug metabolizing enzymes, such as phenobarbital or cimetidine: may alter pharmacokinetics of ondansetron. No dosage adjustment appears necessary.

EFFECTS ON DIAGNOSTIC TESTS
Drug may increase serum levels of ALT and AST.

CONTRAINDICATIONS
Contraindicated in patients hypersensitive to the drug.

NURSING CONSIDERATIONS
● Use cautiously in patients with liver failure.
● **I.V. use:** Dilute drug in 50 ml of D_5W injection or 0.9% sodium chloride for injection before administration.
Alert: Administer as I.V. infusion over 15 minutes.
● Know that drug is also stable for up to 48 hours after dilution in 5% dextrose in 0.9% sodium chloride for injection, 5%

dextrose in 0.45% sodium chloride for injection, and 3% sodium chloride for injection.

☑ **PATIENT TEACHING**
● Instruct patient to alert nurse immediately if difficulty breathing occurs after drug administration.
● Tell patient receiving drug I.V. to report discomfort at insertion site promptly.

prochlorperazine
Compazine, PMS Prochlorperazine†, Prorazin†, Stemetil†

prochlorperazine edisylate
Compa-Z, Compazine, Compazine Syrup, Cotranzine, Ultrazine-10

prochlorperazine maleate
Anti-Naus‡, Compazine, Compazine Spansule, PMS Prochlorperazine†, Prorazin†, Stemetil†

Pregnancy Risk Category: NR

HOW SUPPLIED
prochlorperazine
Tablets: 5 mg, 10 mg
Injection: 5 mg/ml
Suppositories: 2.5 mg, 5 mg, 25 mg
prochlorperazine edisylate
Syrup: 5 mg/5 ml
Injection: 5 mg/ml
prochlorperazine maleate
Tablets: 5 mg, 10 mg, 25 mg
Capsules (sustained-release): 10 mg, 15 mg, 30 mg

ACTION
Acts on the chemoreceptor trigger zone to inhibit nausea and vomiting; in larger doses, partially depresses the vomiting center.

ONSET, PEAK, DURATION
Onset 30 to 40 minutes after oral use, 60 minutes after rectal use, 10 to 20 minutes after I.M. use. Peak unknown.

Effects persist 3 to 4 hours after regular-release preparations, 10 to 12 hours after sustained-release preparations, 3 to 4 hours after rectal or I.M. use.

INDICATIONS & DOSAGE
Preoperative nausea control—
Adults: 5 to 10 mg I.M. 1 to 2 hours before induction of anesthesia; repeat once in 30 minutes, if necessary. Or, 5 to 10 mg I.V. 15 to 30 minutes before induction of anesthesia; repeat once if necessary.
Severe nausea and vomiting—
Adults: 5 to 10 mg P.O., t.i.d. or q.i.d.; 15 mg sustained-release form P.O. on rising; 10 mg sustained-release form P.O. q 12 hours; 25 mg P.R., b.i.d.; or 5 to 10 mg I.M. repeated q 3 to 4 hours, p.r.n. Maximum I.M. dosage is 40 mg daily. Alternatively, 2.5 to 10 mg I.V. at a rate not to exceed 5 mg/minute.
Children 9 to 13 kg: 2.5 mg P.O. or P.R. once daily or b.i.d. Maximum dosage is 7.5 mg daily. Or give 0.132 mg/kg by deep I.M. injection. Control usually is obtained with one dose.
Children 14 to 17 kg: 2.5 mg P.O. or P.R., b.i.d. or t.i.d. Maximum dosage is 10 mg daily. Or give 0.132 mg/kg by deep I.M. injection. Control usually is obtained with one dose.
Children 18 to 39 kg: 2.5 mg P.O. or P.R., t.i.d.; or 5 mg P.O. or P.R., b.i.d. Maximum dosage is 15 mg daily. Or, give 0.132 mg/kg by deep I.M. injection. Control usually is obtained with one dose.
To manage symptoms of psychotic disorders—
Adults: 5 to 10 mg P.O., t.i.d. or q.i.d.
Children 2 to 12 years: 2.5 mg P.O. or P.R., b.i.d. or t.i.d. Do not exceed 10 mg on day 1. Increase dosage gradually to recommended maximum (if necessary). In children 2 to 5 years, maximum daily dosage is 25 mg. In children 6 to 10 years, maximum daily dosage is 25 mg.
To manage symptoms of severe psychoses—
Adults: 10 to 20 mg I.M. repeated in 1

to 4 hours, if needed. Rarely, patients may receive 10 to 20 mg q 4 to 6 hours. Institute oral therapy after symptoms are controlled.

Children 2 to 12 years: 0.13 mg/kg I.M.

Nonpsychotic anxiety—

Adults: 5 to 10 mg by deep I.M. injection q 3 to 4 hours, not to exceed 20 mg daily or for longer than 12 weeks; or 5 to 10 mg P.O., t.i.d. or q.i.d. Alternatively, give 15 mg extended-release capsule once daily or 10 mg extended-release capsule q 12 hours.

ADVERSE REACTIONS

CNS: *extrapyramidal reactions,* sedation, pseudoparkinsonism, EEG changes, dizziness.
CV: *orthostatic hypotension,* tachycardia, ECG changes.
EENT: *ocular changes, blurred vision.*
GI: *dry mouth, constipation.*
GU: *urine retention,* dark urine, menstrual irregularities, inhibited ejaculation.
Hematologic: *transient leukopenia, agranulocytosis.*
Hepatic: *cholestatic jaundice.*
Skin: *mild photosensitivity,* allergic reactions, *exfoliative dermatitis.*
Other: hyperprolactinemia, gynecomastia, weight gain, increased appetite.

INTERACTIONS

Antacids: inhibited absorption of oral phenothiazines. Separate antacid and phenothiazine doses by at least 2 hours.
Anticholinergics, including antidepressants and antiparkinsonian agents: increased anticholinergic activity and aggravated parkinsonian symptoms. Use together cautiously.
Barbiturates: may decrease phenothiazine effect. Monitor patient for decreased antiemetic effect.

EFFECTS ON DIAGNOSTIC TESTS

Drug causes false-positive test results for urinary porphyrins, urobilinogen, amylase, and 5-hydroxyindoleacetic acid (5-HIAA) because of darkening of urine by metabolites; it also causes false-positive urine pregnancy test results in tests using human chorionic gonadotrophin. Drug elevates test results for liver enzymes and protein-bound iodine and causes quinidine-like ECG effects.

CONTRAINDICATIONS

Contraindicated in patients hypersensitive to phenothiazines and in those with CNS depression including coma; during pediatric surgery; when using spinal or epidural anesthetic, adrenergic blockers, or ethanol; and in children under 2 years.

NURSING CONSIDERATIONS

● Use cautiously in patients with impaired CV function, glaucoma, seizure disorders; in those who have been exposed to extreme heat; and in children with acute illness.
● Dilute oral solution with tomato or fruit juice, milk, coffee, carbonated beverage, tea, water, or soup or mix with pudding.
● **I.V. use:** 15 to 30 minutes before induction, add 20 mg of prochlorperazine per liter of D_5W and 0.9% sodium chloride solution. Infusion rate should not exceed 5 mg/minute. Maximum parenteral dosage is 40 mg daily. Infuse slowly, never as a bolus.
● For I.M. use, inject deeply into upper outer quadrant of gluteal region.
● Do not give S.C. or mix in syringe with another drug.
● To prevent contact dermatitis, avoid getting concentrate or injection solution on hands or clothing.
● Watch for orthostatic hypotension, especially when giving drug I.V.
● Monitor CBC and liver function studies during long-term therapy as ordered.
Alert: Know that the drug is used only when vomiting can't be controlled by other measures or when only a few doses are required. If more than four doses are needed in 24 hours, notify the doctor.
● Store in light-resistant container. Slight yellowing does not affect potency;

discard extremely discolored solutions.

☑ PATIENT TEACHING
● Teach patient what to use to dilute oral solution.
● Advise patient to wear protective clothing when exposed to sunlight.
● Tell patient to call doctor if more than four doses are needed within 24 hours.

---

thiethylperazine maleate
Norzine, Torecan**

Pregnancy Risk Category: X

HOW SUPPLIED
Tablets: 10 mg
Injection: 5 mg/ml
Suppositories: 10 mg

ACTION
Unknown. Probably acts on the chemoreceptor trigger zone to inhibit nausea and vomiting.

ONSET, PEAK, DURATION
Onset occurs in 30 minutes. Peak unknown. Effects persist 4 hours.

INDICATIONS & DOSAGE
Nausea and vomiting—
Adults: 10 mg P.O., I.M., or P.R. once daily, b.i.d. or t.i.d.

ADVERSE REACTIONS
CNS: *extrapyramidal reactions* (high incidence), sedation (low incidence), pseudoparkinsonism, EEG changes, dizziness, confusion (especially in elderly patients).
CV: *orthostatic hypotension,* tachycardia, ECG changes.
EENT: *ocular changes, blurred vision.*
GI: *dry mouth, constipation.*
GU: *urine retention,* dark urine, menstrual irregularities, inhibited ejaculation, gynecomastia.
Hematologic: *transient leukopenia,* **agranulocytosis.**
Hepatic: *cholestatic jaundice.*

Skin: *mild photosensitivity,* allergic reactions.
Other: hyperprolactinemia, weight gain, increased appetite.

INTERACTIONS
Antacids: inhibited absorption of oral phenothiazines. Separate antacid and phenothiazine doses by at least 2 hours.
Anticholinergics, including antidepressants and antiparkinsonian agents: increased anticholinergic activity and increased risk of parkinsonian-like symptoms. Use together cautiously.
Barbiturates: may decrease phenothiazine effect. Monitor patient for decreased antiemetic effect.

EFFECTS ON DIAGNOSTIC TESTS
Drug may alter immunologic urine pregnancy test results.

CONTRAINDICATIONS
Contraindicated in patients hypersensitive to phenothiazines, in those with severe CNS depression or hepatic disease, in patients experiencing coma, and in pregnancy.

NURSING CONSIDERATIONS
● Use cautiously in patients with aspirin or tartrazine hypersensitivity.
Alert: Don't give I.V. May cause severe hypotension.
● For nausea and vomiting associated with anesthesia and surgery, give deep I.M. injection shortly before or when terminating anesthesia.
● If drug gets on skin, wash off at once to prevent contact dermatitis.
● Use only when vomiting can't be controlled by other measures or when only a few doses are required.
● Store suppositories in tightly covered container and at temperatures below 77° F (25° C).

☑ PATIENT TEACHING
● Warn patient about hypotension and suggest that he stay in bed for 1 hour after receiving drug.

---

*Liquid contains alcohol.   **May contain tartrazine.   †Canada only.   ‡Australia only.   ◇OTC.

● Instruct patient to report decreased urine output, visual changes, and any CNS effects immediately.

---

trimethobenzamide hydrochloride

Arrestin, Benzacot, Bio-Gan, Stemetic, Tebamide, Tegamide, T-Gen, Ticon, Tigan, Triban, Tribenzagan, Trimazide

Pregnancy Risk Category: NR

HOW SUPPLIED
Capsules: 100 mg, 250 mg
Injection: 100 mg/ml
Suppositories: 100 mg, 200 mg

ACTION
Unknown. Probably acts on the chemoreceptor trigger zone to inhibit nausea and vomiting.

ONSET, PEAK, DURATION
Onset occurs 10 to 20 minutes after oral administration, 15 to 35 minutes after I.M. administration. Peak unknown. Effects persist for 2 to 3 hours after I.M. administration, 3 to 4 hours after oral administration.

INDICATIONS & DOSAGE
Nausea and vomiting—
Adults: 250 mg P.O., t.i.d. or q.i.d.; or 200 mg I.M. or P.R., t.i.d. or q.i.d.
Children under 13 kg: 100 mg P.R. t.i.d. or q.i.d.
Children 13 to 40 kg: 100 to 200 mg P.O. or P.R. t.i.d. or q.i.d.

ADVERSE REACTIONS
CNS: *drowsiness,* dizziness (in large doses), headache, disorientation, depression, parkinsonion-like symptoms, ***coma, seizures.***
CV: hypotension.
GI: diarrhea.
Hepatic: jaundice.
Other: hypersensitivity reactions (pain, stinging, burning, redness, swelling at

I.M. injection site); blurred vision; muscle cramps.

INTERACTIONS
CNS depressants, ethanol: additive CNS depression. Avoid concomitant use.

EFFECTS ON DIAGNOSTIC TESTS
None reported.

CONTRAINDICATIONS
Contraindicated in patients with hypersensitivity to drug. Suppositories are contraindicated in patients hypersensitive to benzocaine hydrochloride or similar local anesthetic.

NURSING CONSIDERATIONS
● Use cautiously in children; drug may be associated with Reye's syndrome.
● For I.M. administration, inject deeply into upper outer quadrant of gluteal region to reduce pain and local irritation.
● Like other antiemetics, drug may mask signs of overdose of toxic agents or symptoms of intestinal obstruction, brain tumor, or other conditions.
● Withhold drug if skin hypersensitivity reaction occurs.

☑ PATIENT TEACHING
● Instruct patient to refrigerate suppositories.
● Advise patient of the possibility of drowsiness and dizziness, and caution against driving or other activities requiring alertness until CNS effects of the drug are known.

Reactions may be *common,* uncommon, *life-threatening,* or COMMON AND LIFE-THREATENING.

52
Antiulcer drugs

cimetidine
famotidine
lansoprazole
misoprostol
nizatidine
omeprazole
ranitidine hydrochloride
sucralfate

COMBINATION PRODUCTS
None.

cimetidine
Tagamet, Tagamet HB◊, Tagamet
HCl, Tagamet Tiltab

Pregnancy Risk Category: B

HOW SUPPLIED
Tablets: 100 mg◊, 200 mg, 300 mg,
400 mg, 800 mg
Oral liquid: 300 mg/5 ml
Effervescent tablets: 800 mg‡
Injection: 100 mg/ml‡, 300 mg/2 ml;
300 mg in 50 ml 0.9% sodium chloride
solution

ACTION
Competitively inhibits the action of hist-
amine-2 at receptor sites of the parietal
cells, decreasing gastric acid secretion.

ONSET, PEAK, DURATION
Onset unknown. Peak levels occur right
after I.V. administration, unknown for
I.M. administration, 45 to 90 minutes
after oral dose. Effects last 4 to 5 hours
after oral dose, unknown after parenteral administration. Therapeutic effects
last 4 to 5 hours.

INDICATIONS & DOSAGE
*Duodenal ulcer (short-term treatment
and maintenance)—*
Adults and children 16 years and

over: 800 mg P.O. h.s. Alternatively,
400 mg P.O. b.i.d. or 300 mg q.i.d. (with
meals and h.s.). Treatment continued for
4 to 6 weeks unless endoscopy shows
healing. For maintenance therapy, 400
mg h.s. For parenteral therapy, 300 mg
diluted to 20 ml with 0.9% sodium
chloride solution or other compatible
I.V. solution by I.V. push over at least 5
minutes q 6 hours; or 300 mg diluted in
50 ml D_5W or other compatible I.V. solution by I.V. infusion over 15 to 20
minutes q 6 hours; or 300 mg I.M. q 6
hours (no dilution necessary). Parenteral
dosage increased by giving 300-mg doses more frequently to maximum daily
dosage of 2,400 mg as needed. Alternatively, 900 mg/day (37.5 mg/hour) I.V.
diluted in 100 to 1,000 ml of compatible
solution by continuous I.V. infusion.
Active benign gastric ulceration—
Adults: 800 mg P.O. h.s., or 300 mg
P.O. q.i.d. (with meals and h.s.) for up
to 6 weeks.
*Pathologic hypersecretory conditions
(such as Zollinger-Ellison syndrome,
systemic mastocytosis, and multiple endocrine adenomas)—*
**Adults and children 16 years and
over:** 300 mg P.O. q.i.d. with meals and
h.s.; adjusted to individual needs. Maximum oral daily dosage is 2,400 mg.
For parenteral therapy, 300 mg diluted to 20 ml with 0.9% sodium chloride
solution or other compatible I.V. solution by I.V. push over at least 5 minutes
q 6 hours; or 300 mg diluted in 50 ml
dextrose 5% solution or other compatible I.V. solution by I.V. infusion over 15
to 20 minutes q 6 hours. Parenteral
dosage increased by giving 300-mg doses more frequently to maximum daily
dosage of 2,400 mg as needed.
Gastroesophageal reflux disease—
Adults: 800 mg P.O. b.i.d. or 400 mg
q.i.d. before meals and h.s. for up to 12

weeks.

Prevention of upper GI bleeding in critically ill patients—

Adults: 50 mg/hour by continuous I.V. infusion for up to 7 days; 25 mg/hour to patients with creatinine clearance below 30 ml/minute.

Heartburn—

Adults: 200 mg (Tagament HB only) P.O. with water as symptoms occur, or as directed, up to b.i.d. Maximum dosage 400 mg daily. Drug shouldn't be taken daily for longer than 2 weeks.

ADVERSE REACTIONS

CNS: confusion, dizziness, headache, peripheral neuropathy, somnolence, hallucinations.

GI: *mild and transient diarrhea.*

GU: transient elevations in serum creatinine levels, impotence, mild gynecomastia if used longer than 1 month.

Hematologic: *agranulocytosis* (rare), *neutropenia, thrombocytopenia* (rare), *aplastic anemia* (rare).

Hepatic: jaundice (rare).

Other: hypersensitivity reactions, muscle pain, arthralgia.

INTERACTIONS

Antacids: interference with cimetidine absorption. Separate administration by at least 1 hour if possible.

Lidocaine, phenytoin, propranolol, some benzodiazepines, theophylline, warfarin: inhibited hepatic microsomal enzyme metabolism of these drugs; monitor serum levels.

EFFECTS ON DIAGNOSTIC TESTS

Drug may antagonize pentagastrin's effect during gastric acid secretion tests; it may cause false-negative results in skin tests using allergan extracts. Drug therapy increases prolactin levels and serum alkaline phosphatase and creatinine levels.

FD and C blue dye #2 used in Tagamet tablets may impair interpretation of Hemoccult and Gastroccult tests on gastric content aspirate. Wait at least 15 minutes after tablet administration before drawing the sample and follow test manufacturer's instructions closely.

CONTRAINDICATIONS

Contraindicated in patients hypersensitive to the drug.

NURSING CONSIDERATIONS

● Use cautiously in elderly or debilitated patients because they may be more susceptible to cimetidine-induced confusion.

● Identify tablet strength when obtaining a drug history.

● **I.V. use:** Dilute I.V. solutions with 0.9% sodium chloride solution, D_5W and dextrose 10% in water (and combinations of these), lactated Ringer's solution, or 5% sodium bicarbonate injection. Do not dilute with sterile water for injection.

Alert: Don't infuse I.V. too rapidly; bradycardia may occur. When giving I.V. in 100 ml of diluent solution, don't infuse so rapidly that circulatory overload results. Some authorities recommend infusing drug over at least 30 minutes, to minimize risk of adverse cardiac effects. Sometimes given as continuous I.V. infusion. Use infusion pump if given in a total volume of 250 ml over 24 hours or less.

● Schedule cimetidine dose at end of hemodialysis treatment. Hemodialysis reduces blood levels of cimetidine. Adjust dosage as ordered in patients with renal failure.

● Keep in mind that effectiveness for treatment of gastric ulcer is not as great as for duodenal ulcer.

● Know that up to 10 g overdose can occur without adverse reactions.

☑ PATIENT TEACHING

● Remind patient taking cimetidine once daily to take it at bedtime. If drug is being taken more than once a day, instruct him to take it with meals.

● Instruct patient taking Tagament HB not to exceed recommended dosage and not to take daily for longer than 14 days.

● Warn patient receiving drug I.M. that injection may be painful.

● Urge patient to avoid cigarette smoking because it may increase gastric acid secretion and worsen disease.

---

famotidine
Pepcid, Pepcid AC ◇, Pepcidine‡

Pregnancy Risk Category: B

HOW SUPPLIED
Tablets: 10 mg, 20 mg, 40 mg
Powder for oral suspension: 40 mg/5 ml after reconstitution
Injection: 10 mg/ml
Premixed injection: 20 mg/50 ml in 0.9% sodium chloride

ACTION
Competitively inhibits the action of histamine-2 at receptor sites of the parietal cells, decreasing gastric acid secretion.

ONSET, PEAK, DURATION
Onset occurs within 1 hour after oral or I.V. dose. Peak levels occur within 20 minutes of I.V. injection, 1 to 3 hours after oral dose. Effects persist up to 12 hours.

INDICATIONS & DOSAGE
Duodenal ulcer (short-term treatment)—
Adults: For acute therapy, 40 mg P.O. once daily h.s. or 20 mg P.O. b.i.d. For maintenance therapy, give 20 mg P.O. once daily h.s.
Benign gastric ulcer (short-term treatment)—
Adults: 40 mg P.O. daily h.s. for 8 weeks.
Pathologic hypersecretory conditions (such as Zollinger-Ellison syndrome)—
Adults: 20 mg P.O. q 6 hours up to 160 mg q 6 hours.
Hospitalized patients with intractable ulcerations or hypersecretory conditions or patients who cannot take oral medication—
Adults: 20 mg I.V. q 12 hours.
Gastroesophageal reflux disease (GERD)—
Adults: 20 mg P.O. b.i.d. for up to 6 weeks. For esophagitis caused by GERD, 20 to 40 mg b.i.d. for up to 12 weeks.
Prevention or treatment of heartburn—
Adults: 10 mg (Pepcid AC only) P.O. 1 hour before meals (prevention) or 10 mg (Pepcid AC only) P.O. with water when symptoms occur. Maximum dosage is 20 mg daily. Drug should not be taken daily for longer than 2 weeks.

In patients with severe renal insufficiency: If creatinine clearance is less than 10 ml/minute, give 20 mg I.V. or P.O. h.s. or prolong dosing interval to q 36 to 48 hours.

ADVERSE REACTIONS
CNS: *headache,* dizziness, vertigo, malaise, paresthesia.
EENT: tinnitus, taste disorder, orbital edema.
GI: diarrhea, constipation, anorexia, dry mouth.
GU: increased BUN and creatinine levels.
Skin: acne, dry skin, flushing.
Other: transient irritation at I.V. site, musculoskeletal pain, palpitations, fever.

INTERACTIONS
None significant.

EFFECTS ON DIAGNOSTIC TESTS
Drug may antagonize pentagastrin during gastric acid secretion tests. It may also elevate hepatic enzyme levels. In skin tests using allergan extracts, drug may cause false-negative results.

CONTRAINDICATIONS
Contraindicated in patients hypersensitive to the drug.

NURSING CONSIDERATIONS

• **I.V. use:** To prepare I.V. injection, dilute 2 ml (20 mg) famotidine with compatible I.V. solution to a total volume of either 5 or 10 ml, and inject over at least 2 minutes. Compatible solutions include sterile water for injection, 0.9% sodium chloride for injection, D_5W or $D_{10}W$ injection, 5% sodium bicarbonate injection, and lactated Ringer's injection.

• Alternatively, give famotidine by intermittent I.V. infusion. Dilute 20 mg (2 ml) famotidine in 100 ml of compatible solution, and infuse over 15 to 30 minutes. Solution is stable for 48 hours at room temperature after dilution.

• Store I.V. injection in refrigerator at 36° to 46° F (2° to 8° C).

• Store reconstituted suspension below 86° F (30° C). Discard after 30 days.

☑ PATIENT TEACHING

• Instruct the patient on proper use of OTC product (Pepcid AC), if appropriate.

• Tell the patient to take prescription drug with a snack if desired.

• Remind patient that the prescription drug is most effective if taken at bedtime. Tell patients taking 20 mg b.i.d. to take at least one dose at bedtime.

• Advise him not to take prescription drug for more than 8 weeks, unless ordered by the doctors, and to limit use of OTC drug to no more than 2 weeks.

• With doctor's knowledge, allow the patient to take antacids concomitantly, especially at the beginning of therapy when pain is severe.

• Urge the patient to avoid cigarette smoking because it may increase gastric acid secretion and worsen disease.

---

lansoprazole
Prevacid

Pregnancy Risk Category: B

HOW SUPPLIED
Capsules (delayed-release): 15 mg, 30 mg

ACTION
Inhibits the activity of the proton pump and binds to hydrogen-potassium adenosine triphosphatase, located at the secretory surface of the gastric parietal cells, to block the formation of gastric acid.

ONSET, PEAK, DURATION
Onset and duration unknown. Peak effects occur in 1.7 hours.

INDICATIONS & DOSAGE
Short-term treatment of active duodenal ulcer—
Adults: 15 mg P.O. daily before eating for 4 weeks.
Short-term treatment of erosive esophagitis—
Adults: 30 mg P.O. daily before eating for up to 8 weeks. If healing doesn't occur, 8 more weeks of therapy may be given. Maintenance dose for healing is 15 mg P.O. daily.
Long-term treatment of pathologic hypersecretory conditions, including Zollinger-Ellison syndrome—
Adults: initially, 60 mg P.O. once daily. Dosage increased as needed. Daily dosages of more than 120 mg should be given in divided doses.

ADVERSE REACTIONS
CNS: headache, agitation, amnesia, anxiety, apathy, confusion, depression, dizziness or syncope, hallucinations, hemiplegia, aggravated hostility, decreased libido, nervousness, paresthesia, thinking abnormality.
CV: chest pain, edema, angina, CVA, hypertension or hypotension, *MI*, palpitations, *shock,* vasodilation, cardiospasm.
EENT: amblyopia, deafness, eye pain, visual field deficits, otitis media, taste perversion, tinnitus.
GI: *diarrhea, nausea, abdominal pain,* halitosis, melena, anorexia, cholelithiasis, constipation, dry mouth, thirst, dys-

---

Reactions may be *common,* uncommon, *life-threatening,* or COMMON AND LIFE-THREATENING.

pepsia, dysphagia, eructation, esophageal stenosis, esophageal ulcer, esophagitis, fecal discoloration, flatulence, gastric nodules, fundic gland polyps, gastroenteritis, GI hemorrhage, hematemesis, increased appetite, increased salivation, rectal hemorrhage, stomatitis, tenesmus, ulcerative colitis.
GU: hematuria, impotence, renal calculi, albuminuria, abnormal menses, gynecomastia, breast tenderness.
Hematologic: anemia, hemolysis.
Metabolic: diabetes mellitus, goiter, hyperglycemia, hypoglycemia, gout, weight gain or loss.
Musculoskeletal: arthritis or arthralgia, musculoskeletal pain, myalgia.
Respiratory: asthma, bronchitis, increased cough, dyspnea, epistaxis, hemoptysis, hiccups, pneumonia, upper respiratory tract inflammation.
Skin: acne, alopecia, pruritus, rash, urticaria.
Other: asthenia, candidiasis, fever, flu-like syndrome, infection, malaise.

INTERACTIONS
Ampicillin esters, digoxin, iron salts, ketoconazole: lansoprazole may inhibit absorption. Monitor patient closely.
Sucralfate: delayed lansoprazole absorption. Give lansoprazole at least 30 minutes prior to sucralfate.
Theophylline: may cause mild increase in theophylline clearance. Use together cautiously. Dosage adjustment of theophylline may be needed when lansoprazole is started or stopped.

EFFECTS ON DIAGNOSTIC TESTS
None reported.

CONTRAINDICATIONS
Contraindicated in patients hypersensitive to the drug.

NURSING CONSIDERATIONS
● Know that no dosage adjustment is necessary in patients with renal insufficiency or in elderly patients. For patients with severe liver disease, dosage

adjustment may be necessary.
● Be aware that lansoprazole should not to be used as maintenance therapy for treatment of patients with duodenal ulcer or erosive esophagitis.
● Because it is not known if lansoprazole is excreted in breast milk, be aware that a decision to discontinue breast-feeding or the drug should be made when drug is prescribed for breast-feeding women.

☑ **PATIENT TEACHING**
● Instruct patient to take the drug before eating.
● Tell patient who has trouble swallowing capsules to open and sprinkle contents over applesauce.

---

misoprostol
Cytotec

Pregnancy Risk Category: X

HOW SUPPLIED
Tablets: 100 mcg, 200 mcg

ACTION
A synthetic prostaglandin E_1 analogue that replaces gastric prostaglandins depleted by NSAID therapy. Misoprostol also decreases basal and stimulated gastric acid secretion and may increase gastric mucus and bicarbonate production.

ONSET, PEAK, DURATION
Onset occurs in 30 minutes. Plasma levels peak within 10 to 15 minutes. Effects persist about 3 hours.

INDICATIONS & DOSAGE
Prevention of NSAID-induced gastric ulcer in elderly or debilitated patients at high risk for complications from gastric ulcer and in patients with a history of NSAID-induced ulcer—
Adults: 200 mcg P.O. q.i.d. with food; if not tolerated, may be decreased to 100 mcg P.O. q.i.d. Dosage should be given for duration of NSAID therapy.

Last dose should be given h.s.

ADVERSE REACTIONS
CNS: headache.
GI: *diarrhea, abdominal pain,* nausea, flatulence, dyspepsia, vomiting, constipation.
Other: hypermenorrhea, dysmenorrhea, spotting, cramps, menstrual disorders.

INTERACTIONS
Antacids: reduced plasma levels when administered concomitantly. Not considered significant.

EFFECTS ON DIAGNOSTIC TESTS
Drug causes a modest decrease in basal pepsin secretion.

CONTRAINDICATIONS
Contraindicated in pregnant or lactating patients.

NURSING CONSIDERATIONS
● Know that drug should not be routinely given to women of childbearing age unless they are at high risk for developing ulcers or complications from NSAID-induced ulcers.
Alert: Take special precautions to prevent use of drug during pregnancy. Make sure the patient understands the dangers of misoprostol to a fetus and that she receives both oral and written warnings about these dangers. Also ensure that she can comply with effective contraception and that she has a negative serum pregnancy test within 2 weeks of initiating therapy.

☑ PATIENT TEACHING
● Instruct all patients not to share misoprostol. Remind them that when taken by a pregnant patient this drug may cause miscarriage, often with potentially life-threatening bleeding.
● Advise patient not to begin misoprostol therapy until the second or third day of the next normal menstrual period.

nizatidine
Axid, Tazac‡

Pregnancy Risk Category: C

HOW SUPPLIED
Capsules: 150 mg, 300 mg

ACTION
Competitively inhibits the action of histamine-2 (H_2) at receptor sites of the parietal cells, decreasing gastric acid secretion.

ONSET, PEAK, DURATION
Onset occurs within 30 minutes. Peak levels occur in ½ to 3 hours. Effects persist up to 12 hours.

INDICATIONS & DOSAGE
Active duodenal ulcer—
Adults: 300 mg P.O. daily h.s. Alternatively, 150 mg P.O. b.i.d.
Maintenance therapy for duodenal ulcer—
Adults: 150 mg P.O. daily h.s.
Benign gastric ulcer—
Adults: 150 mg P.O. b.i.d. or 300 mg h.s. for 8 weeks.
Gastroesophageal reflux disease—
Adults: 150 mg P.O. b.i.d.
    In patients with impaired renal function: If creatinine clearance is 20 to 50 ml/minute, 150 mg P.O. daily for treatment of active duodenal ulcer, or 150 mg every other day for maintenance therapy; if creatinine clearance is below 20 ml/minute, 150 mg P.O. every other day for treatment, or 150 mg every third day for maintenance.

ADVERSE REACTIONS
CNS: *somnolence.*
CV: arrhythmias.
Hematologic: eosinophilia.
Skin: *diaphoresis,*rash, urticaria.
Other: hyperuricemia, fever, hepatocellular injury, elevated liver function tests.

INTERACTIONS
Aspirin: possibly elevated serum salicylate levels (with high doses).
Tomato-based mixed-vegetable juices: may decrease potency of the drug when used concomitantly.

EFFECTS ON DIAGNOSTIC TESTS
False-positive test results for urobilinogen may occur during drug therapy.

CONTRAINDICATIONS
Contraindicated in patients hypersensitive to H_2-receptor antagonists.

NURSING CONSIDERATIONS
• Use cautiously and in reduced dosages in patients with renal impairment.
• If necessary, open capsules and mix contents with apple juice. However, be aware that drug loses some potency when combined with tomato-based mixed-vegetable juices. Ask pharmacist about compatibility.

☑ PATIENT TEACHING
• Tell patient who has difficulty swallowing capsules that contents may be mixed with apple juice but not with tomato-based mixed vegetable juices.
• Urge patient to avoid cigarette smoking because it may increase gastric acid secretion and worsen disease.

---

omeprazole
Losec†‡], Prilosec

Pregnancy Risk Category: C

HOW SUPPLIED
Capsules (delayed-release): 10 mg, 20 mg

ACTION
Inhibits the activity of the acid (proton) pump, and binds to hydrogen-potassium adenosine triphosphatase, located at the secretory surface of the gastric parietal cells to block the formation of gastric acid.

ONSET, PEAK, DURATION
Onset occurs within 1 hour. Peak effects occur within 2 hours. Effects persist 3 days or more; may take 4 days for gastric acid production to return to normal.

INDICATIONS & DOSAGE
Severe erosive esophagitis; poorly responsive gastroesophageal reflux disease (GERD)—
Adults: 20 mg P.O. daily for 4 to 8 weeks. Patients with GERD should have failed initial therapy with a histamine-2 antagonist.
Maintenance of healing erosive esophagitis—
Adults: 20 mg P.O. daily.
Pathologic hypersecretory conditions (such as Zollinger-Ellison syndrome)—
Adults: initially, 60 mg P.O. daily; dosage titrated according to patient response. If daily dosage exceeds 80 mg, administer in divided doses. Dosages up to 120 mg t.i.d. have been given. Continue therapy as long as clinically indicated.
Duodenal ulcer (short-term treatment)—
Adults: 20 mg P.O. daily for 4 to 8 weeks.
Treatment of Helicobacter pylori *infection or ulcers caused by* H. pylori—
Adults: 40 mg every morning in combination with 500 mg clarithromycin t.i.d for days 1 to 14; then, 20 mg daily for days 15 to 28.
✽ *New indication: Short-term treatment of active benign gastric ulcer—*
Adults: 40 mg P.O. once daily for 4 to 8 weeks.

ADVERSE REACTIONS
CNS: headache, dizziness, asthenia.
GI: diarrhea, abdominal pain, nausea, vomiting, constipation, flatulence.
Respiratory: cough, upper respiratory infection.
Skin: rash.
Other: back pain.

INTERACTIONS

Ampicillin esters, iron derivatives, keto-conazole: may exhibit poor bioavailability in patients taking omeprazole because optimal absorption of these drugs requires a low gastric pH. Avoid concomitant use.

Diazepam, phenytoin, warfarin: decreased hepatic clearance, possibly leading to increased serum levels. Monitor closely.

EFFECTS ON DIAGNOSTIC TESTS

Serum gastrin levels rise in most patients during the first 2 weeks of therapy.

CONTRAINDICATIONS

Contraindicated in patients hypersensitive to the drug or any component of the formulation.

NURSING CONSIDERATIONS

● Know that dosage adjustments aren't needed for renal or hepatic impairment.
● Know that omeprazole increases its own bioavailability with repeated dosages. Drug is labile in gastric acid; less drug is lost to hydrolysis because the drug increases gastric pH.

☑ PATIENT TEACHING

● Tell the patient to swallow capsules whole and not to open or crush them.
● Caution patient not to perform hazardous activities if dizziness occurs.

---

ranitidine hydrochloride

Apo-Ranitidine†, Zantac*, Zantac-C†, Zantac 75 ◊, Zantac 150, Zantac 150 EFFERdose, Zantac 150 GELdose, Zantac 300, Zantac 300 GELdose

Pregnancy Risk Category: B

HOW SUPPLIED

Tablets: 75 mg ◊ , 150 mg, 300 mg
Dispersible tablets: 150 mg‡
Effervescent tablets: 150 mg
Effervescent granules: 150 mg
Syrup: 15 mg/ml*

Injection: 25 mg/ml
Infusion: 0.5 mg/ml in 100-ml containers

ACTION

Competitively inhibits the action of histamine-2 at receptor sites of the parietal cells, decreasing gastric acid secretion.

ONSET, PEAK, DURATION

Onset occurs within 1 hour. Peak effects occur in 1 to 3 hours. Effects persist up to 13 hours.

INDICATIONS & DOSAGE

Duodenal and gastric ulcer (short-term treatment); pathologic hypersecretory conditions, such as Zollinger-Ellison syndrome—
Adults: 150 mg P.O. b.i.d. or 300 mg daily h.s. Alternatively, 50 mg I.V. or I.M. q 6 to 8 hours. Patients with Zollinger-Ellison syndrome may require dosages up to 6 g P.O. daily.
Maintenance therapy for duodenal or gastric ulcer—
Adults: 150 mg P.O. h.s.
Gastroesophageal reflux disease—
Adults: 150 mg P.O. b.i.d.
Erosive esophagitis—
Adults: 150 mg P.O. q.i.d. Maintenance therapy is 150 mg P.O. b.i.d.
Treatment for heartburn—
Adults: 75 mg (Zantac 75 only) P.O. as symptoms occur, not to exceed 150 mg daily.

In patients with impaired renal function: If creatinine clearance is below 50 ml/minute, 150 mg P.O. q 24 hours or 50 mg I.V. q 18 to 24 hours.

ADVERSE REACTIONS

CNS: vertigo, malaise.
EENT: blurred vision.
Hematologic: reversible leukopenia, pancytopenia.
Hepatic: elevated liver enzymes, jaundice.
Other: burning and itching at injection site, ***anaphylaxis***, angioneurotic edema.

Reactions may be *common*, uncommon, *life-threatening*, or COMMON AND LIFE-THREATENING.

INTERACTIONS
Antacids: may interfere with ranitidine absorption. Stagger doses if possible.
Diazepam: decreased absorption of diazepam. Monitor closely.
Glipizide: possible increased hypoglycemic effect. Adjust glipizide dosage as necessary.
Procainamide: possible decreased renal clearance of procainamide. Monitor patient closely for toxicity.
Warfarin: possible interference with warfarin clearance. Monitor closely.

EFFECTS ON DIAGNOSTIC TESTS
Drug may cause false-positive results in urine protein tests using Multistix. It may increase serum creatinine, lactate dehydrogenase, alkaline phosphatase, AST, ALT, and total bilirubin levels. Drug may also decrease WBC, RBC, and platelet counts.

CONTRAINDICATIONS
Contraindicated in patients hypersensitive to the drug.

NURSING CONSIDERATIONS
● Use cautiously in patients with hepatic dysfunction. Adjust dosage in patients with impaired renal function as ordered.
● Avoid using aluminum-based needles or other equipment when mixing or administering drug. Drug is incompatible with aluminum.
● **I.V. use:** When administering by I.V. push, dilute to a total volume of 20 ml, and inject over a period of 5 minutes. No dilution is necessary when administering I.M.
● To prepare I.V. injection, dilute 50 mg (2 ml) in 100 ml of compatible solution, and infuse over 15 to 20 minutes. Compatible solutions include 0.9% sodium chloride for injection, D_5W or $D_{10}W$ injection, 5% sodium bicarbonate injection, or lactated Ringer's injection.
● When giving by intermittent I.V. infusion, dilute 50 mg ranitidine in 100 ml of D_5W, and infuse over 15 to 20 minutes. Or, give by continuous I.V. infu-

sion: 150 mg in 250 ml of compatible solution. Administer at 6.25 mg/hour using an infusion pump.
● When administering premixed I.V. infusion, give by slow I.V. drip (over 15 to 20 minutes). Don't add other drugs to the solution. If used with a primary I.V. fluid system, discontinue the primary solution during the infusion.

☑ PATIENT TEACHING
● Instruct patient on proper use of OTC preparation, as indicated.
● Remind patient taking prescription drug once daily to take it at bedtime for best results.
● Instruct patient to take without regard to meals because absorption is not affected by food.
● Tell patient taking EFFERdose to dissolve drug in 6 to 8 ounces of water before taking it.
● Urge patient to avoid cigarette smoking because it may increase gastric acid secretion and worsen disease.

---

sucralfate
Carafate, SCF‡, Sulcrate†

Pregnancy Risk Category: B

HOW SUPPLIED
Tablets: 1 g
Suspension: 1 g/10 ml

ACTION
Unknown. Probably adheres to and protects the ulcer's surface by forming a barrier.

ONSET, PEAK, DURATION
Onset and peak unknown. Effects persist for up to 6 hours.

INDICATIONS & DOSAGE
Short-term (up to 8 weeks) treatment of duodenal ulcer—
Adults: 1 g P.O. q.i.d. 1 hour before meals and h.s.
Maintenance therapy for duodenal ul-

cer—
Adults: 1 g P.O. b.i.d.

ADVERSE REACTIONS
CNS: dizziness, sleepiness, headache, vertigo.
GI: *constipation,* nausea, gastric discomfort, diarrhea, bezoar formation, vomiting, flatulence, dry mouth, indigestion.
Skin: rash, pruritus.
Other: back pain.

INTERACTIONS
Antacids: may decrease binding of drug to gastroduodenal mucosa, impairing effectiveness. Don't administer within 30 minutes of each other.
Cimetidine, ciprofloxacin, digoxin, ketoconazole, norfloxacin, phenytoin, quinidine, ranitidine, tetracycline, theophylline: decreased absorption. Separate administration times by at least 2 hours.

EFFECTS ON DIAGNOSTIC TESTS
None reported.

CONTRAINDICATIONS
None known.

NURSING CONSIDERATIONS
• Use with caution in patients with chronic renal failure.
• Know that drug is minimally absorbed and has a low incidence of adverse reactions.
• Monitor for severe, persistent constipation.
• Be aware that studies suggest that sucralfate is as effective as cimetidine in healing duodenal ulcer.
• Know that drug contains aluminum but isn't classified as an antacid.

☑ **PATIENT TEACHING**
• Tell patient to take sucralfate on an empty stomach (1 hour before each meal and at bedtime).
• Tell patient to continue prescribed regimen to ensure complete healing. Pain and ulcerative symptoms may sub-

side within first few weeks of therapy.
• Urge patient to avoid cigarette smoking because it may increase gastric acid secretion and worsen disease.

---

betamethasone
betamethasone acetate and
   betamethasone sodium
   phosphate
betamethasone sodium
   phosphate
cortisone acetate
dexamethasone
dexamethasone acetate
dexamethasone sodium
   phosphate
fludrocortisone acetate
hydrocortisone
hydrocortisone acetate
hydrocortisone sodium
   phosphate
hydrocortisone sodium
   succinate
methylprednisolone
methylprednisolone acetate
methylprednisolone sodium
   succinate
prednisolone
prednisolone sodium phosphate
prednisolone steaglate
prednisolone tebutate
prednisone
triamcinolone
triamcinolone acetonide

COMBINATION PRODUCTS
DECADRON PHOSPHATE WITH
XYLOCAINE: dexamethasone phosphate
4 mg and lidocaine hydrochloride 10
mg per ml.
PREDNISOLONE ACETATE AND PRED-
NISOLONE SODIUM PHOSPHATE: prednisolone acetate 80 mg/ml and prednisolone sodium phosphate 20 mg/ml

---

betamethasone
Betnelan†, Betnesol†, Celestone*

betamethasone acetate and betamethasone sodium phosphate
Celestone Chronodose‡, Celestone
Soluspan

betamethasone sodium phosphate
Celestone Phosphate, Selestoject

Pregnancy Risk Category: C

HOW SUPPLIED
betamethasone
Tablets: 600 mcg
Tablets (effervescent): 500 mcg†
Syrup: 600 mcg/5 ml
**betamethasone acetate and be-
tamethasone sodium phosphate**
Injection (suspension): betamethasone
acetate 3 mg and betamethasone sodium
phosphate (equivalent to 3-mg base) per
ml
betamethasone sodium phosphate
Injection: 4 mg (equivalent to 3-mg
base)/ml in 5-ml vials

ACTION
Not completely defined. Decreases inflammation, mainly by stabilizing
leukocyte lysosomal membranes; suppresses the immune response; stimulates
bone marrow; and influences protein,
fat, and carbohydrate metabolism.

ONSET, PEAK, DURATION
Onset prompt. Peak unknown. Duration
variable but thought to persist for 3.25
days after oral administration, 7 to 14
days after parenteral administration.

INDICATIONS & DOSAGE
Betamethasone sodium phosphate and
betamethasone acetate suspension combination product should *not* be used for
I.V. administration.

Conditions with severe inflammation; conditions requiring immunosuppression—
Adults: 0.6 to 7.2 mg P.O. daily; or 0.5 to 9 mg I.M., I.V., or into joint or soft tissue daily. Betamethasone sodium phosphate-acetate suspension 6 to 12 mg injected into large joints or 1.5 to 6 mg injected into smaller joints. Both injections may be given q 1 to 2 weeks p.r.n.

ADVERSE REACTIONS
Most adverse reactions to corticosteroids are dose- or duration-dependent.
CNS: *euphoria, insomnia,* psychotic behavior, pseudotumor cerebri, vertigo, headache, paresthesia, *seizures.*
CV: *CHF,* hypertension, edema, arrhythmias, thrombophlebitis, ***thromboembolism.***
EENT: cataracts, glaucoma.
Endocrine: menstrual irregularities, cushingoid state (moonface, buffalo hump, central obesity).
GI: *peptic ulceration,* GI irritation, increased appetite, pancreatitis, nausea, vomiting.
Skin: delayed wound healing, acne, various skin eruptions.
Other: muscle weakness, osteoporosis, hirsutism, susceptibility to infections; hypokalemia, hyperglycemia, and carbohydrate intolerance; growth suppression in children; *acute adrenal insufficiency may follow increased stress (infection, surgery, or trauma) or abrupt withdrawal after long-term therapy.*
After abrupt withdrawal: rebound inflammation, fatigue, weakness, arthralgia, fever, dizziness, lethargy, depression, fainting, orthostatic hypotension, dyspnea, anorexia, hypoglycemia. *After prolonged use, sudden withdrawal may be fatal.*

INTERACTIONS
Aspirin, indomethacin, and other NSAIDs: increased risk of GI distress and bleeding. Give together cautiously.

Barbiturates, phenytoin, rifampin: decreased corticosteroid effect. Corticosteroid dosage may need to be increased.
Corticosteroids: reduce serum salicylate levels.
Oral anticoagulants: altered dosage requirements. Monitor PT closely.
Potassium-depleting drugs, such as thiazide diuretics: enhanced potassium-wasting effects of betamethasone. Monitor serum potassium levels.
Skin-test antigens: decreased response. Defer skin testing until therapy is completed.
Toxoids and vaccines: decreased antibody response and increased risk of neurologic complications. Avoid concomitant use.

EFFECTS ON DIAGNOSTIC TESTS
Adrenocorticoid therapy suppresses reactions to skin tests, causes false-negative results in the nitroblue tetrazolium tests for systemic bacterial infections, and decreases ^{131}I uptake and protein-bound iodine concentrations in thyroid function tests. It may increase serum glucose and cholesterol levels; decrease serum potassium, calcium, thyroxine, and triiodothyronine levels; and increase urine glucose and calcium levels.

CONTRAINDICATIONS
Contraindicated in patients hypersensitive to the drug and in those with viral or bacterial infections (except in life-threatening situations) or systemic fungal infections.

NURSING CONSIDERATIONS
● Use with extreme caution in a patient with recent MI or peptic ulcer (used only in life-threatening situations).
● Use cautiously in patients with renal disease, hypertension, osteoporosis, diabetes mellitus, hypothyroidism, cirrhosis, diverticulitis, nonspecific ulcerative colitis, recent intestinal anastomoses, thromboembolic disorders, seizures, myasthenia gravis, CHF, tuberculosis, ocular herpes simplex, emotional insta-

bility, and psychotic tendencies. Because some formulations contain sulfite preservatives, also use cautiously in patients with hypersensitivity to sulfites.
Alert: Know that drug should not be used for alternate-day therapy.

● Obtain baseline weight before starting therapy, and weigh patients daily; report any sudden weight gain to the doctor.

● For better results and less toxicity, give a once-daily dose in the morning.

● To reduce GI irritation, give with milk or food.

● To prevent muscle atrophy, give I.M. injection deeply. Rotate injection sites.

● **I.V. use:** Compatible with 0.9% sodium chloride, D_5W, lactated Ringer's injection, dextrose 5% in lactated Ringer's injection, and dextrose 5% in Ringer's injection.

● Be aware that drug should always be titrated to lowest effective dose.

● Monitor blood glucose and serum potassium levels regularly, as ordered. Diabetic patients may require adjustments in insulin dosage.

● Monitor for depression or mood changes, especially in patients receiving long-term therapy.

● A calorie- or sodium-restricted diet with protein supplementation may be necessary for patients receiving long-term therapy.

● Know that elderly patients may be more susceptible to osteoporosis.

● Adrenal suppression may last up to 1 year after drug is stopped.

● Gradually reduce drug dosage after long-term therapy, as ordered.

● Observe for signs of infection, especially after steroid withdrawal.

☑ PATIENT TEACHING
● Tell patient not to stop drug abruptly or without the doctor's consent.

● Tell patient to take drug with food or milk; tell patient using effervescent tablets to dissolve them in water immediately before ingestion.

● Teach patient about the drug's effects. Warn patient on long-term therapy

about cushingoid symptoms and to report sudden weight gain or swelling to the doctor.

● Make sure patient reports symptoms associated with corticosteroid withdrawal, including fatigue, weakness, arthralgia, orthostatic hypotension, and dyspnea.

● Make sure patient understands to contact the doctor if symptoms are worsening or the medication is no longer effective. Tell patient not to increase dosage without the doctor's consent.

● Advise elderly patient receiving long-term therapy to consider exercise or physical therapy. Also tell him to ask his doctor about vitamin D or calcium supplement.

● Advise patients receiving prolonged therapy to have periodic ophthalmic examinations.

● Tell patient to report slow healing.

● Instruct patient to carry a card indicating his need for supplemental glucocorticoids during stress.

---

cortisone acetate
Cortate‡, Cortone Acetate

Pregnancy Risk Category: C

HOW SUPPLIED
Tablets: 5 mg, 10 mg, 25 mg
Injection (suspension): 50 mg/ml

ACTION
Not completely defined. Decreases inflammation, mainly by stabilizing leukocyte lysosomal membranes; suppresses the immune response; stimulates bone marrow; and influences protein, fat, and carbohydrate metabolism.

ONSET, PEAK, DURATION
Highly variable.

INDICATIONS & DOSAGE
Adrenal insufficiency, allergy, inflammation—
Adults: 25 to 300 mg P.O. or 20 to 300

---

mg I.M. daily. Dosages are highly individualized, depending on severity of disease.

ADVERSE REACTIONS
Most adverse reactions to corticosteroids are dose- or duration-dependent.
CNS: *euphoria, insomnia,* psychotic behavior, pseudotumor cerebri, vertigo, headache, paresthesia, *seizures.*
CV: *CHF,* hypertension, edema, arrhythmias, thrombophlebitis, *thromboembolism.*
EENT: cataracts, glaucoma.
Endocrine: menstrual irregularities, cushingoid state (moonface, buffalo hump, central obesity).
GI: *peptic ulceration,* GI irritation, increased appetite, pancreatitis, nausea, vomiting.
Skin: delayed wound healing, acne, various skin eruptions; atrophy at I.M. injection sites.
Other: muscle weakness, osteoporosis, hirsutism, susceptibility to infections; possible hypokalemia, hyperglycemia, and carbohydrate intolerance; growth suppression in children; *acute adrenal insufficiency may follow increased stress (infection, surgery, or trauma) or abrupt withdrawal after long-term therapy.*
After abrupt withdrawal: rebound inflammation, fatigue, weakness, arthralgia, fever, dizziness, lethargy, depression, fainting, orthostatic hypotension, dyspnea, anorexia, hypoglycemia. *After prolonged use, sudden withdrawal may be fatal.*

INTERACTIONS
Aspirin, indomethacin, and other NSAIDs: increased risk of GI distress and bleeding. Give together cautiously.
Barbiturates, phenytoin, rifampin: decreased corticosteroid effect. Increase corticosteroid dosage, as ordered.
Live attenuated virus vaccines, other toxoids and vaccines: decreased antibody response and increased risk of neurologic complications. Avoid concomitant use.
Oral anticoagulants: altered dosage requirements. Monitor PT and INR closely.
Potassium-depleting drugs, such as thiazide diuretics: enhanced potassium-wasting effects of cortisone. Monitor serum potassium levels.
Salicylates: decreased serum salicylate levels with corticosteroids.
Skin-test antigens: decreased response. Defer skin testing until therapy is completed.

EFFECTS ON DIAGNOSTIC TESTS
Cortisone therapy suppresses reactions to skin tests, causes false-negative results in the nitroblue tetrazolium test for systemic bacterial infections, and decreases ^{131}I uptake and protein-bound iodine concentrations in thyroid function tests. It may increase serum glucose and cholesterol levels; decrease serum potassium, calcium, thyroxine, and triiodothyronine levels; and increase urine glucose and calcium levels.

CONTRAINDICATIONS
Contraindicated in patients with hypersensitivity to drug or any of its ingredients or systemic fungal infections.

NURSING CONSIDERATIONS
● Use with extreme caution in a patient with recent MI.
● Use cautiously in patients with GI ulcer, renal disease, hypertension, osteoporosis, diabetes mellitus, hypothyroidism, cirrhosis, diverticulitis, nonspecific ulcerative colitis, recent intestinal anastomoses, thromboembolic disorders, seizures, myasthenia gravis, CHF, tuberculosis, ocular herpes simplex, emotional instability, and psychotic tendencies.
● To reduce GI irritation, give with milk or food.
● For better results and less toxicity, give a once-daily dose in the morning.
● I.M. route causes slow onset of action. Should not be used in acute conditions

where a rapid effect is required. May be used on a twice-daily schedule matching diurnal variation. Rotate injection sites to prevent muscle atrophy.

• Mixing or diluting parenteral suspension may alter absorption rate and decrease the drug's effectiveness.

Alert: Know that drug is not for I.V. use.

• Know that drug should always be titrated to lowest effective dose.

• Monitor serum electrolyte and blood glucose levels as ordered.

• Monitor patient for fluid and electrolyte imbalances. Patients may need low-sodium diet and potassium supplements.

• Know that elderly patients may be more susceptible to osteoporosis.

• Gradually reduce drug dosage after long-term therapy, as ordered.

• Observe for signs of infection, especially after steroid withdrawal.

☑ **PATIENT TEACHING**

• Tell patient not to discontinue drug abruptly or without the doctor's consent.

• Instruct patient to take drug with milk or food.

• Advise patient receiving long-term therapy to consider exercise or physical therapy. Also tell him to ask his doctor about vitamin D or calcium supplement.

• Tell patient to report slow healing.

• Warn patient on long-term therapy about cushingoid symptoms and to report sudden weight gain or swelling to the doctor.

• Instruct patient to carry a card indicating his need for supplemental glucocorticoids during stress.

---

dexamethasone

Decadron*, Deronil†, Dexameth, Dexamethasone Intensol*, Dexasone†, Dexone 0.5, Dexone 0.75, Dexone 1.5, Dexone 4, Hexadrol*, Mymethasone*

dexamethasone acetate

Dalalone D.P., Dalalone L.A., Decadron-LA, Decaject-L.A., Dexacen LA-8, Dexasone-LA, Dexone LA, Solurex-LA

dexamethasone sodium phosphate

Dalalone, Decadron Phosphate, Decaject, Dexacen-4, Dexasone, Dexone, Hexadrol Phosphate, Solurex

Pregnancy Risk Category: C

HOW SUPPLIED
dexamethasone
Tablets: 0.25 mg, 0.5 mg, 0.75 mg, 1 mg, 1.5 mg, 2 mg, 4 mg, 6 mg
Oral solution: 0.5 mg/5 ml, 1 mg/ml
Elixir: 0.5 mg/5 ml*
dexamethasone acetate
Injection: 8 mg/ml, 16 mg/ml suspension
dexamethasone sodium phosphate
Injection: 4 mg/ml, 10 mg/ml, 20 mg/ml, 24 mg/ml

ACTION
Not clearly defined. Decreases inflammation, mainly by stabilizing leukocyte lysosomal membranes; suppresses the immune response; stimulates bone marrow; and influences protein, fat, and carbohydrate metabolism.

ONSET, PEAK, DURATION
Onset occurs within 1 hour after I.M. or I.V. administration; 1 to 2 hours after oral administration. Peak effects occur within 1 hour after I.M. or I.V. administration, within 1 to 2 hours after oral administration, or within 8 hours after use of the injectable suspension (acetate). Effects persist about 2½ days after oral use, 6 days after I.M. use (acetate), and up to 3 weeks after intralesional or intra-articular use (acetate or sodium phosphate).

INDICATIONS & DOSAGE
Cerebral edema—
Adults: initially, 10 mg (phosphate) I.V.; then 4 to 6 mg I.M. q 6 hours until symptoms subside (usually 2 to 4 days); then tapered over 5 to 7 days.
Inflammatory conditions, allergic reactions, neoplasias—
Adults: 0.75 to 9 mg/day P.O. or 0.5 to 9 mg/day (phosphate) I.M.; or 4 to 16 mg (acetate) I.M. into joint or soft tissue q 1 to 3 weeks; or 0.8 to 1.6 mg (acetate) into lesions q 1 to 3 weeks.
Shock—
Adults: 1 to 6 mg/kg (phosphate) I.V. as a single dose; or 40 mg I.V. q 2 to 6 hours, p.r.n.; continued only until patient is stabilized (usually not longer than 48 to 72 hours).
Dexamethasone suppression test for Cushing's syndrome—
Adults: after determining baseline 24-hour urine levels of 17-hydroxycorticosteroids, 0.5 mg P.O. q 6 hours for 48 hours; 24-hour urine collection made for determination of 17-hydroxycorticosteroid excretion again during second 24 hours of dexamethasone administration.

ADVERSE REACTIONS
Most adverse reactions to corticosteroids are dose- or duration-dependent.
CNS: *euphoria, insomnia,* psychotic behavior, pseudotumor cerebri, vertigo, headache, paresthesia, *seizures.*
CV: *CHF,* hypertension, edema, arrhythmias, thrombophlebitis, ***thromboembolism.***
EENT: cataracts, glaucoma.
Endocrine: menstrual irregularities, cushingoid state (moonface, buffalo hump, central obesity).
GI: *peptic ulceration,* GI irritation, increased appetite, pancreatitis, nausea, vomiting.
Skin: delayed wound healing, acne, various skin eruptions; atrophy at I.M. injection sites.
Other: muscle weakness, osteoporosis, hirsutism, susceptibility to infections;

hypokalemia, hyperglycemia, and carbohydrate intolerance; growth suppression in children; ***acute adrenal insufficiency may follow increased stress (infection, surgery, or trauma) or abrupt withdrawal after long-term therapy.***
After abrupt withdrawal: rebound inflammation, fatigue, weakness, arthralgia, fever, dizziness, lethargy, depression, fainting, orthostatic hypotension, dyspnea, anorexia, hypoglycemia. *After prolonged use, sudden withdrawal may be fatal.*

INTERACTIONS
Aspirin, indomethacin, and other NSAIDs: increased risk of GI distress and bleeding. Give together cautiously.
Barbiturates, phenytoin, rifampin: decreased corticosteroid effect. Increase corticosteroid dosage, as ordered.
Oral anticoagulants: altered dosage requirements. Monitor PT and INR closely.
Potassium-depleting drugs, such as thiazide diuretics: enhanced potassium-wasting effects of dexamethasone. Monitor serum potassium levels.
Salicylates: decreased serum salicylate levels
Skin-test antigens: decreased response. Defer skin testing until therapy is completed.
Toxoids and vaccines: decreased antibody response and increased risk of neurologic complications. Avoid concomitant use.

EFFECTS ON DIAGNOSTIC TESTS
Dexamethasone suppresses reactions to skin tests, causes false-negative results in the nitroblue tetrazolium test for systemic bacterial infections, and decreases ^{131}I uptake and protein-bound iodine concentrations in thyroid function tests. It may increase serum glucose and cholesterol levels; decrease serum potassium, calcium, thyroxine, and triiodothyronine levels; and increase urine glucose and calcium levels.

CONTRAINDICATIONS
Contraindicated in patients hypersensitive to any component of the drug and in those with systemic fungal infections.

NURSING CONSIDERATIONS
• Use with extreme caution in patient with recent MI.
• Use cautiously in patients with GI ulcer, renal disease, hypertension, osteoporosis, diabetes mellitus, hypothyroidism, cirrhosis, diverticulitis, nonspecific ulcerative colitis, recent intestinal anastomoses, thromboembolic disorders, seizures, myasthenia gravis, CHF, tuberculosis, ocular herpes simplex, emotional instability, and psychotic tendencies. Because some formulations contain sulfite preservatives, also use cautiously in patients sensitive to sulfites.
• For better results and less toxicity, give a once-daily dose in the morning.
• Give oral dose with food when possible.
• Give I.M. injection deeply into gluteal muscle. Rotate injection sites to prevent muscle atrophy. Avoid S.C. injection because atrophy and sterile abscesses may occur.
• **I.V. use:** When administering as direct injection, inject undiluted over at least 1 minute. When administering as an intermittent or continuous infusion, dilute solution according to the manufacturer's instructions and give over the prescribed duration. If used for continuous infusion, change solution every 24 hours.
• Always titrate to lowest effective dose as ordered.
• Monitor patients' weight, blood pressure, and serum electrolyte levels.
• Watch for depression or psychotic episodes, especially in high-dose therapy.
• Diabetic patients may need increased insulin; monitor blood glucose levels.
• Know that drug may mask or exacerbate infections, including latent amebiasis.
• Know that elderly patients may be more susceptible to osteoporosis.
• Inspect patient's skin for petechiae.

• Gradually reduce drug dosage after long-term therapy as ordered.

☑ **PATIENT TEACHING**
• Tell patient not to discontinue drug abruptly or without the doctor's consent.
• Instruct patient to take drug with food or milk.
• Teach patient the signs of early adrenal insufficiency: fatigue, muscular weakness, joint pain, fever, anorexia, nausea, dyspnea, dizziness, and fainting.
• Instruct patient to carry a card indicating his need for supplemental systemic glucocorticoids during stress, especially when dosage is decreased.
• Warn patient on long-term therapy about cushingoid symptoms and to report sudden weight gain or swelling to the doctor.
• Warn patient about easy bruising.
• Advise patient receiving long-term therapy to consider exercise or physical therapy. Give vitamin D or calcium supplement as ordered.
• Advise patient receiving long-term therapy to have periodic ophthalmic examinations.

---

fludrocortisone acetate
Florinef

Pregnancy Risk Category: C

HOW SUPPLIED
Tablets: 0.1 mg

ACTION
Increases sodium reabsorption and potassium and hydrogen secretion at the nephrons' distal convoluted tubules.

ONSET, PEAK, DURATION
Onset variable. Peak levels occur in 1.7 hours. Effects persist for 1 to 2 days.

INDICATIONS & DOSAGE
Salt-losing adrenogenital syndrome—
Adults: 0.1 to 0.2 mg P.O. daily. Decrease dosage to 0.05 mg daily if tran-

sient hypertension develops as a result of drug therapy.

ADVERSE REACTIONS
CV: *sodium and water retention,* hypertension, cardiac hypertrophy, edema, CHF.
Skin: bruising, diaphoresis, urticaria, or allergic rash.
Other: hypokalemia.

INTERACTIONS
Barbiturates, phenytoin, rifampin: increased clearance of fludrocortisone acetate.
Potassium-depleting drugs, such as thiazide diuretics: enhanced potassium-wasting effects of fludrocortisone. Monitor serum potassium levels.

EFFECTS ON DIAGNOSTIC TESTS
Fludrocortisone therapy increases serum sodium levels and decreases serum potassium levels. Glucose tolerance tests should be performed only if necessary, because addisonian patients tend to develop severe hypoglycemia within 3 hours of the test.

CONTRAINDICATIONS
Contraindicated in patients with hypersensitivity to drug or in patients with systemic fungal infections.

NURSING CONSIDERATIONS
● Use cautiously in patients with hypothyroidism, cirrhosis, ocular herpes simplex, emotional instability, and psychotic tendencies, nonspecific ulcerative colitis, diverticulitis, fresh intestinal anastomoses, active or latent peptic ulcer, renal insufficiency, hypertension, osteoporosis, and myasthenia gravis.
● Be aware that drug is used with cortisone or hydrocortisone in adrenal insufficiency.
Alert: Monitor patient's blood pressure and serum electrolyte levels. If hypertension occurs, notify doctor and expect dosage to be decreased by 50%.
● Weigh patients daily; report sudden

weight gain to the doctor.
● Unless contraindicated, give low-sodium diet that's high in potassium and protein. Be aware that potassium supplements may be needed.

☑ PATIENT TEACHING
● Tell patients to report worsening symptoms, such as hypotension, weakness, cramping, and palpitations, to the doctor.
● Warn patient that mild peripheral edema is common.

---

hydrocortisone
Cortef, Cortenema, Hydrocortone

hydrocortisone acetate
Cortifoam, Hydrocortone Acetate

hydrocortisone sodium phosphate
Hydrocortone Phosphate

hydrocortisone sodium succinate
A-hydroCort, Solu-Cortef

Pregnancy Risk Category: C

HOW SUPPLIED
hydrocortisone
Tablets: 5 mg, 10 mg, 20 mg
Enema: 100 mg/60 ml
hydrocortisone acetate
Injection: 25 mg/ml*, 50 mg/ml* suspension
Enema: 10% aerosol foam (provides 90 mg/application)
Suppositories: 25 mg
hydrocortisone sodium phosphate
Injection: 50 mg/ml solution
hydrocortisone sodium succinate
Injection: 100-mg vial*, 250-mg vial*, 500-mg vial*, 1,000-mg vial*

ACTION
Not clearly defined. Decreases inflammation, mainly by stabilizing leukocyte lysosomal membranes; suppresses the

immune response; stimulates bone marrow; and influences protein, fat, and carbohydrate metabolism.

ONSET, PEAK, DURATION
Highly variable.

INDICATIONS & DOSAGE
Severe inflammation, adrenal insufficiency—
Adults: 5 to 30 mg P.O. b.i.d., t.i.d., or q.i.d. (as much as 80 mg q.i.d. may be given in acute situations); or initially, 100 to 500 mg succinate I.M. or I.V., and then 50 to 100 mg I.M., as indicated; or 15 to 240 mg phosphate I.M. or I.V. daily in divided doses q 12 hours; or 5 to 75 mg acetate into joints or soft tissue. Dosage varies with size of joint. Local anesthetics often are injected with dose.
Shock—
Adults: initially, 50 mg/kg succinate I.V., repeated in 4 hours. Repeat dosage q 24 hours as needed. Alternatively, 100 to 500 mg to 2 g q 2 to 6 hours; continued until patient is stabilized (usually not longer than 48 to 72 hours).
Children: phosphate (I.M.) or succinate (I.M. or I.V.) 0.16 to 1 mg/kg or 6 to 30 mg/m^2 once daily or b.i.d.
Adjunct for ulcerative colitis and proctitis—
Adults: 1 enema (100 mg) P.R. nightly for 21 days. Alternatively, 1 applicator (90-mg foam) P.R. daily or b.i.d. for 14 to 21 days.

ADVERSE REACTIONS
Most adverse reactions to corticosteroids are dose- or duration-dependent.
CNS: *euphoria, insomnia,* psychotic behavior, pseudotumor cerebri, vertigo, headache, paresthesia, *seizures.*
CV: *CHF,* hypertension, edema, arrhythmias, thrombophlebitis, thromboembolism.
EENT: cataracts, glaucoma.
Endocrine: menstrual irregularities, cushingoid state (moonface, buffalo hump, central obesity).
GI: *peptic ulceration,* GI irritation, increased appetite, pancreatitis, nausea, vomiting.
Skin: delayed wound healing, acne, various skin eruptions, easy bruising.
Other: muscle weakness, osteoporosis, hirsutism, susceptibility to infections; possible hypokalemia, hyperglycemia, and carbohydrate intolerance; growth suppression in children; *acute adrenal insufficiency may occur with increased stress (infection, surgery, or trauma) or abrupt withdrawal after long-term therapy.*
After abrupt withdrawal: rebound inflammation, fatigue, weakness, arthralgia, fever, dizziness, lethargy, depression, fainting, orthostatic hypotension, dyspnea, anorexia, hypoglycemia. *After prolonged use, sudden withdrawal may be fatal.*

INTERACTIONS
Aspirin, indomethacin, and other NSAIDs: increased risk of GI distress and bleeding. Give together cautiously.
Barbiturates, phenytoin, rifampin: decreased corticosteroid effect. Increase corticosteroid dosage, as ordered.
Live attenuated virus vaccines, other toxoids and vaccines: decreased antibody response and increased risk of neurologic complications. Avoid concomitant use.
Oral anticoagulants: altered dosage requirements. Monitor PT and INR closely.
Potassium-depleting drugs, such as thiazide diuretics: enhanced potassium-wasting effects of hydrocortisone. Monitor serum potassium levels.
Skin-test antigens: decreased response. Defer skin testing until after therapy.

EFFECTS ON DIAGNOSTIC TESTS
Hydrocortisone suppresses reactions to skin tests, causes false-negative results in the nitroblue tetrazolium test for systemic bacterial infections, and decreases ^{131}I uptake and protein-bound iodine

---

*Liquid contains alcohol.   **May contain tartrazine.   †Canada only.   ‡Australia only.   ◊OTC.

concentrations in thyroid function tests. It may increase serum glucose and cholesterol levels; decrease serum potassium, calcium, thyroxine, and triiodothyronine levels; and increase urine glucose and calcium levels.

CONTRAINDICATIONS
Contraindicated in patients allergic to any component of the formulation, in those with systemic fungal infections, and in premature infants (succinate).

NURSING CONSIDERATIONS
• Use with extreme caution in patient with recent MI.
• Use cautiously in patients with GI ulcer, renal disease, hypertension, osteoporosis, diabetes mellitus, hypothyroidism, cirrhosis, diverticulitis, nonspecific ulcerative colitis, recent intestinal anastomoses, thromboembolic disorders, seizures, myasthenia gravis, CHF, tuberculosis, ocular herpes simplex, emotional instability, and psychotic tendencies.
• For better results and less toxicity, give a once-daily dose in the morning.
• Give oral dose with food when possible.
• **I.V. use:** Do not use the acetate or suspension form for I.V. use. When administering as direct injection, inject directly into vein or an I.V. line containing a free-flowing compatible solution over 30 seconds to several minutes. When administering as an intermittent or continuous infusion, dilute solution according to manufacturer's instructions, and give over the prescribed duration. If used for continuous infusion, change solution every 24 hours.
• Hydrocortisone sodium phosphate may be added directly to D₅W or 0.9% sodium chloride for I.V. administration.
• Reconstitute hydrocortisone sodium succinate with bacteriostatic water or bacteriostatic sodium chloride solution before adding to I.V. solutions. When giving by direct I.V. injection, inject over at least 30 seconds. For infusion,

dilute with D_5W, 0.9% sodium chloride, or dextrose 5% in 0.9% sodium chloride to a concentration of 1 mg/ml or less.
• Give I.M. injection deeply into gluteal muscle. Rotate injection sites to prevent muscle atrophy. Avoid S.C. injection because atrophy and sterile abscesses may occur.
Alert: Do not confuse Solu-Cortef with Solu-Medrol (methylprednisolone sodium succinate).
• Know that injectable forms are not used for alternate-day therapy.
• Enema may produce same systemic effects as other forms of hydrocortisone. If enema therapy must exceed 21 days, discontinue gradually by reducing administration to every other night for 2 or 3 weeks, as ordered.
• Be aware high-dose therapy is usually not continued beyond 48 hours.
• Always titrate to lowest effective dose as ordered.
• Monitor patients' weight, blood pressure, and serum electrolyte levels.
• Unless contraindicated, give low-sodium diet that's high in potassium and protein. Administer potassium supplements as ordered.
• Know that drug may mask or exacerbate infections, including latent amebiasis.
• Stress (fever, trauma, surgery, and emotional problems) may increase adrenal insufficiency. Increase dosage, as ordered.
• Watch for depression or psychotic episodes, especially during high-dose therapy.
• Inspect patients' skin for petechiae.
• Diabetic patients may need increased insulin; monitor blood glucose levels.
• Periodic measurement of growth and development may be necessary during high-dose or prolonged therapy in children.
• Know that elderly patients may be more susceptible to osteoporosis.
• Gradually reduce drug dosage after long-term therapy, as ordered.

☑ **PATIENT TEACHING**
- Tell patient not to discontinue the drug abruptly or without the doctor's consent.
- Instruct patient to take oral form of drug with milk or food.
- Warn patient on long-term therapy about cushingoid symptoms and to report sudden weight gain or swelling to the doctor.
- Teach patient the signs of early adrenal insufficiency: fatigue, muscular weakness, joint pain, fever, anorexia, nausea, dyspnea, dizziness, and fainting.
- Instruct patient to carry a card identifying his need for supplemental systemic glucocorticoids during stress.
- Warn patient about easy bruising.
- Advise patient receiving long-term therapy to consider exercise or physical therapy. Also tell him to ask his doctor about vitamin D or calcium supplement.
- Advise patient receiving long-term therapy to have periodic ophthalmic examinations.

---

methylprednisolone
Medrol**

methylprednisolone acetate
depMedalone-40, depMedalone-80, Depoject-40, Depoject-80, Depo-Medrol, Depopred-40, Depopred-80, Depo-Predate 40, Depo-Predate 80, Duralone-40, Duralone-80, Medralone-40, Medralone-80, Rep-pred 40, Rep-pred 80

methylprednisolone sodium succinate
A-methaPred, Solu-Medrol

Pregnancy Risk Category: C

HOW SUPPLIED
methylprednisolone
Tablets: 2 mg, 4 mg, 8 mg, 16 mg, 24 mg, 32 mg
methylprednisolone acetate
Injection (suspension): 20 mg/ml, 40

mg/ml, 80 mg/ml
methylprednisolone sodium succinate
Injection: 40-mg vial, 125-mg vial, 500-mg vial, 1,000-mg vial, 2,000-mg vial

ACTION
Not clearly defined. Decreases inflammation, mainly by stabilizing leukocyte lysosomal membranes; suppresses the immune response; stimulates bone marrow; and influences protein, fat, and carbohydrate metabolism.

ONSET, PEAK, DURATION
Onset occurs rapidly after I.V. or oral administration; slowly (6 to 48 hours) after I.M. injection of acetate suspension. Peak effects occur immediately after I.V. injection, within 1 to 2 hours after oral administration, 4 to 8 days after I.M. use, or 7 days after intralesional or intra-articular administration. Effects persist for 30 to 36 hours after oral administration, 1 to 4 weeks after I.M. use, or 1 to 5 weeks after intralesional or intra-articular administration.

INDICATIONS & DOSAGE
Severe inflammation or immunosuppression—
Adults: 2 to 60 mg P.O. daily in four divided doses; 10 to 80 mg acetate I.M. daily, or 10 to 250 mg succinate I.M. or I.V. up to q 4 hours; or 4 to 40 mg acetate into smaller joints or 20 to 80 mg acetate into larger joints. Intralesional administration is usually 20 to 60 mg acetate. Intralesional and intra-articular injections may be repeated q 1 to 5 weeks.
Children: succinate 0.03 to 0.2 mg/kg or 1 to 6.25 mg/m² I.M. once daily or b.i.d.
Shock—
Adults: 100 to 250 mg succinate I.V. at 2- to 6-hour intervals; or 30 mg/kg I.V. initially, repeated q 4 to 6 hours p.r.n. Continue therapy for 2 to 3 days or until the patient is stable.

---

*Liquid contains alcohol.   **May contain tartrazine.   †Canada only.   ‡Australia only.   ◇OTC.

ADVERSE REACTIONS
Most adverse reactions to corticosteroids are dose- or duration-dependent.

CNS: *euphoria, insomnia,* psychotic behavior, pseudotumor cerebri, vertigo, headache, paresthesia, *seizures.*

CV: *CHF,* hypertension, edema, arrhythmias, thrombophlebitis, ***thromboembolism, fatal arrest or circulatory collapse*** (following rapid administration of large I.V. doses).

EENT: cataracts, glaucoma.

Endocrine: menstrual irregularities, cushingoid state (moonface, buffalo hump, central obesity).

GI: *peptic ulceration,* GI irritation, increased appetite, pancreatitis, nausea, vomiting.

Skin: delayed wound healing, acne, various skin eruptions.

Other: muscle weakness, osteoporosis, hirsutism, susceptibility to infections; hypokalemia, hyperglycemia, and carbohydrate intolerance; growth suppression in children; *acute adrenal insufficiency may occur with increased stress (infection, surgery, or trauma) or abrupt withdrawal after long-term therapy.*

After abrupt withdrawal: rebound inflammation, fatigue, weakness, arthralgia, fever, dizziness, lethargy, depression, fainting, orthostatic hypotension, dyspnea, anorexia, hypoglycemia. *After prolonged use, sudden withdrawal may be fatal.*

INTERACTIONS
Aspirin, indomethacin, and other NSAIDs: increased risk of GI distress and bleeding. Give together cautiously.

Barbiturates, phenytoin, rifampin: decreased corticosteroid effect. Increase corticosteroid dosage, as ordered.

Oral anticoagulants: altered dosage requirements. Monitor PT and INR closely.

Potassium-depleting drugs, such as thiazide diuretics: enhanced potassium-wasting effects of methylprednisolone. Monitor serum potassium levels.

Salicylates: decreased serum salicylate levels.

Skin-test antigens: decreased response. Defer skin testing until after therapy.

Toxoids and vaccines: decreased antibody response and increased risk of neurologic complications. Avoid concomitant use.

EFFECTS ON DIAGNOSTIC TESTS
Methylprednisolone suppresses reactions to skin tests, causes false-negative results in the nitroblue tetrazolium test for systemic bacterial infections, and decreases ^{131}I uptake and protein-bound iodine concentrations in thyroid function tests. It may increase serum glucose and cholesterol levels; may decrease serum potassium, calcium, thyroxine, and triiodothyronine levels; and may increase urine glucose and calcium levels.

CONTRAINDICATIONS
Contraindicated in patients allergic to any component of the formulation, in those with systemic fungal infections and in premature infants (acetate and succinate).

NURSING CONSIDERATIONS
● Use cautiously in patients with GI ulceration or renal disease, hypertension, osteoporosis, diabetes mellitus, hypothyroidism, cirrhosis, diverticulitis, nonspecific ulcerative colitis, recent intestinal anastomoses, thromboembolic disorders, seizures, myasthenia gravis, CHF, tuberculosis, ocular herpes simplex, emotional instability, and psychotic tendencies.

● Know that drug may be used for alternate-day therapy.

● For better results and less toxicity, give a once-daily dose in the morning.

● Give oral dose with food when possible. Know that critically ill patients may require concomitant antacid or histamine-2-receptor antagonist therapy.

● **I.V. use:** Use only methylprednisolone sodium succinate; never use

---

Reactions may be *common*, uncommon, *life-threatening*, or COMMON AND LIFE-THREATENING.

acetate form for I.V. use. Reconstitute according to the manufacturer's directions using the supplied diluent, or use bacteriostatic water for injection with benzyl alcohol.

● When administering as direct injection, inject diluted drug into a vein or free-flowing compatible I.V. solution over at least 1 minute. For treatment of shock, give massive doses over at least 10 minutes to prevent arrhythmias and circulatory collapse. When administering as an intermittent or continuous infusion, dilute solution according to the manufacturer's instructions, and give over the prescribed duration. If used for continuous infusion, change solution every 24 hours.

● Compatible solutions include D_5W, 0.9% sodium chloride, and dextrose 5% in 0.9% sodium chloride.

● Do not confuse Solu-Medrol with Solu-Cortef (hydrocortisone sodium succinate).

Alert: The manufacturers of Solu-Medrol state that the drug should not be given intrathecally because severe adverse reactions have been reported.

● Give I.M. injection deeply into gluteal muscle. Avoid S.C. injection because atrophy and sterile abscesses may occur.

● Dermal atrophy may occur with large doses of acetate salt. Use multiple small injections rather than a single large dose and rotate injection sites.

● Don't use acetate salt when immediate onset of action is needed.

● Discard reconstituted solutions after 48 hours.

● Always titrate to lowest effective dose, as ordered.

● Monitor patients' weight, blood pressure, serum electrolyte levels, and sleep patterns. Euphoria may initially interfere with sleep, but patients generally adjust to the medication after 1 to 3 weeks.

● Know that drug may mask or exacerbate infections, including latent amebiasis.

● Watch for depression or psychotic episodes, especially in high-dose therapy.

● Diabetic patients may need increased insulin; monitor blood glucose levels.

● Watch for an enhanced response to drug in patients with hypothyroidism or cirrhosis.

● Watch for allergic reaction to the dye tartrazine in patients with sensitivity to aspirin.

● Unless contraindicated, give low-sodium diet that's high in potassium and protein. Administer potassium supplements as needed.

● Know that elderly patients may be more susceptible to osteoporosis.

● Gradually reduce drug dosage after long-term therapy, as ordered.

☑ **PATIENT TEACHING**
● Tell patient not to discontinue drug abruptly or without the doctor's consent.

● Instruct patient to take oral form of drug with milk or food.

● Teach patient the signs of early adrenal insufficiency: fatigue, muscular weakness, joint pain, fever, anorexia, nausea, dyspnea, dizziness, and fainting.

● Instruct patient to carry a card identifying his need for supplemental systemic glucocorticoids during stress.

● Warn patient on long-term therapy about cushingoid symptoms and to report sudden weight gain or swelling to the doctor.

● Advise patient receiving long-term therapy to consider exercise or physical therapy. Also tell patient to ask doctor about vitamin D or calcium supplement.

prednisolone
Cortalone**, Delta-Cortef, Delta-solone‡, Panafcortelone‡, Prelone, Solone‡

prednisolone sodium phosphate
Hydeltrasol, Key-Pred-SP, Pediapred, Predate-S, Predicort RP, Predsol Re-

tention Enema‡, Predsol Suppositories‡

prednisolone steaglate
Sintisone‡

prednisolone tebutate
Hydeltra-TBA, Nor-Pred TBA, Predalone TBA, Predate TBA, Predcor TBA

Pregnancy Risk Category: C

HOW SUPPLIED
prednisolone
Tablets: 1 mg‡, 5 mg, 25 mg‡
Syrup: 15 mg/5 ml
prednisolone sodium phosphate
Oral solution: 5 mg/5 ml
Injection: 20 mg/ml
Retention enema: 20 mg/100 ml‡
Suppositories: 5 mg‡
prednisolone steaglate
Tablets: 6.65 mg (equal to 3.5 mg prednisolone)‡
prednisolone tebutate
Injection (suspension): 20 mg/ml

ACTION
Not clearly defined. Decreases inflammation, mainly by stabilizing leukocyte lysosomal membranes; suppresses the immune response; stimulates bone marrow; and influences protein, fat, and carbohydrate metabolism.

ONSET, PEAK, DURATION
Onset occurs rapidly after I.V., I.M., or oral administration; 1 to 2 days after intralesional or intra-articular use of tebutate suspension. Peak levels occur within 1 hour after I.M. or I.V. injection or within 1 to 2 hours after oral administration. Effects persist for 30 to 36 hours after oral use; up to 4 weeks after I.M. use, or 3 days to 4 weeks after intralesional or intra-articular use.

INDICATIONS & DOSAGE
Severe inflammation or immunosuppression—

Adults: 2.5 to 15 mg P.O. b.i.d., t.i.d., or q.i.d.; 2 to 30 mg I.M. (phosphate) or I.V. (phosphate) q 12 hours; or 2 to 30 mg (phosphate) into joints (depending on joint size), lesions, or soft tissue; or 4 to 40 mg (tebutate) into joints (depending on joint size) and lesions p.r.n.
Proctitis‡—
Adults: 1 suppository b.i.d., preferably in the morning and h.s.
Ulcerative colitis‡—
Adults: 1 retention enema h.s. nightly for 2 to 4 weeks. The contents of the enema should be retained overnight.

ADVERSE REACTIONS
Most adverse reactions to corticosteroids are dose- or duration-dependent.
CNS: *euphoria, insomnia,* psychotic behavior, pseudotumor cerebri, vertigo, headache, paresthesia, *seizures.*
CV: *CHF,* hypertension, edema, arrhythmias, thrombophlebitis, ***thromboembolism.***
EENT: cataracts, glaucoma.
Endocrine: menstrual irregularities, cushingoid state (moonface, buffalo hump, central obesity).
GI: *peptic ulceration,* GI irritation, increased appetite, pancreatitis, nausea, vomiting.
Skin: delayed wound healing, acne, various skin eruptions.
Other: muscle weakness, osteoporosis, hirsutism, susceptibility to infections; hypokalemia, hyperglycemia, and carbohydrate intolerance; growth suppression in children; *acute adrenal insufficiency may occur with increased stress (infection, surgery, or trauma) or abrupt withdrawal after long-term therapy.*
After abrupt withdrawal: rebound inflammation, fatigue, weakness, arthralgia, fever, dizziness, lethargy, depression, fainting, orthostatic hypotension, dyspnea, anorexia, hypoglycemia. *After prolonged use, sudden withdrawal may be fatal.*

Reactions may be *common,* uncommon, *life-threatening,* or COMMON AND LIFE-THREATENING.

INTERACTIONS

Aspirin, indomethacin, and other NSAIDs: increased risk of GI distress and bleeding. Give together cautiously.

Barbiturates, phenytoin, rifampin: decreased corticosteroid effect. Increase corticosteroid dosage, as ordered.

Oral anticoagulants: altered dosage requirements. Monitor PT and INR closely.

Potassium-depleting drugs, such as thiazide diuretics: enhanced potassium-wasting effects of prednisolone. Monitor serum potassium levels.

Salicylates: decreased serum salicylate levels.

Skin-test antigens: decreased response. Defer skin testing until therapy is completed.

Toxoids and vaccines: decreased antibody response and increased risk of neurologic complications. Avoid concomitant use.

EFFECTS ON DIAGNOSTIC TESTS

Prednisolone suppresses reactions to skin tests, causes false-negative results in the nitroblue tetrazolium test for systemic bacterial infections, and decreases ^{131}I uptake and protein-bound iodine concentrations in thyroid function tests. It may increase serum glucose and cholesterol levels; may decrease serum potassium, calcium, thyroxine, and tri-iodothyronine levels; and may increase urine glucose and calcium levels.

CONTRAINDICATIONS

Contraindicated in patients with hypersensitivity to drug or any of its ingredients and systemic fungal infections.

NURSING CONSIDERATIONS

• Use with extreme caution in a patient with recent MI.

• Use cautiously in patients with GI ulcer, renal disease, hypertension, osteoporosis, diabetes mellitus, hypothyroidism, cirrhosis, diverticulitis, nonspecific ulcerative colitis, recent intestinal anastomoses, thromboembolic disorders, seizures, myasthenia gravis, CHF, tuberculosis, ocular herpes simplex, emotional instability, and psychotic tendencies.

Alert: Don't confuse with prednisone.

• Always titrate to lowest effective dose, as ordered.

• Be aware that prednisolone salts (sodium phosphate, and tebutate) are used parenterally less often than other corticosteroids that have more potent anti-inflammatory action.

• Know that drug may be used for alternate-day therapy.

• Give oral dose with food when possible to reduce GI irritation.

• Give I.M. injection deeply into gluteal muscle. Rotate injection sites to prevent muscle atrophy. Avoid S.C. injection because atrophy and sterile abscesses may occur.

• **I.V. use:** Use only prednisolone sodium phosphate. When administering as direct injection, inject undiluted over at least 1 minute. When administering as an intermittent or continuous infusion, dilute solution according to the manufacturer's instructions, and give over the prescribed duration. D_5W or 0.9% sodium chloride is recommended as diluent for I.V. infusion.

• Monitor patients' weight, blood pressure, and serum electrolyte levels.

• Watch for depression or psychotic episodes, especially in high-dose therapy.

• Watch for allergic reaction to the dye tartrazine in patients with sensitivity to aspirin.

• Diabetic patients may need increased insulin; monitor blood glucose levels.

• Unless contraindicated, give low-sodium diet that's high in potassium and protein. Administer potassium supplements as needed.

• Know that drug may mask or exacerbate infections, including latent amebiasis.

• Know that elderly patients may be more susceptible to osteoporosis.

• Gradually reduce drug dosage after long-term therapy as ordered.

☑ **PATIENT TEACHING**
• Tell patient not to discontinue drug abruptly or without the doctor's consent.
• Instruct patient to take oral form of drug with food or milk.
• Teach patient the signs of early adrenal insufficiency: fatigue, muscular weakness, joint pain, fever, anorexia, nausea, dyspnea, dizziness, and fainting.
• Instruct patient to carry a card identifying his need for supplemental systemic glucocorticoids during stress.
• Warn patient on long-term therapy about cushingoid symptoms and to report sudden weight gain or swelling to the doctor.
• Tell patient to report slow healing.
• Advise patient receiving long-term therapy to consider exercise or physical therapy. Also tell patient to ask doctor about vitamin D or calcium supplement.

---

prednisone
Apo-Prednisone†, Deltasone, Liquid Pred*, Meticorten, Novo-prednisone†, Orasone, Panafcort‡, Panasol, Prednicen-M, Prednisone Intensol*, Sone‡, Sterapred, Winpred†

Pregnancy Risk Category: C

HOW SUPPLIED
Tablets: 1 mg, 2.5 mg, 5 mg, 10 mg, 20 mg, 25 mg, 50 mg
Oral solution: 5 mg/5 ml*, 5 mg/ml (concentrate)*
Syrup: 5 mg/5 ml*

ACTION
Not clearly defined. Decreases inflammation, mainly by stabilizing leukocyte lysosomal membranes; suppresses the immune response; stimulates bone marrow; and influences protein, fat, and carbohydrate metabolism.

ONSET, PEAK, DURATION
Variable.

INDICATIONS & DOSAGE
Severe inflammation or immunosuppression—
Adults: 5 to 60 mg P.O. daily in two to four divided doses. Maintenance dosage given once daily or every other day. Dosage must be individualized.
Children: 0.14 to 2 mg/kg or 4 to 60 mg/m^2 daily P.O. in four divided doses.

ADVERSE REACTIONS
Most adverse reactions to corticosteroids are dose- or duration-dependent.
CNS: *euphoria, insomnia,* psychotic behavior, pseudotumor cerebri, vertigo, headache, paresthesia, *seizures.*
CV: *CHF,* hypertension, edema, arrhythmias, thrombophlebitis, *thromboembolism.*
EENT: cataracts, glaucoma.
Endocrine: menstrual irregularities, cushingoid state (moonface, buffalo hump, central obesity).
GI: *peptic ulceration,* GI irritation, increased appetite, pancreatitis, nausea, vomiting.
Skin: delayed wound healing, acne, various skin eruptions.
Other: muscle weakness, osteoporosis, hirsutism, susceptibility to infections; hypokalemia, hyperglycemia, and carbohydrate intolerance; growth suppression in children; *acute adrenal insufficiency may occur with increased stress (infection, surgery, or trauma) or abrupt withdrawal after long-term therapy.*
After abrupt withdrawal: rebound inflammation, fatigue, weakness, arthralgia, fever, dizziness, lethargy, depression, fainting, orthostatic hypotension, dyspnea, anorexia, hypoglycemia. *After prolonged use, sudden withdrawal may be fatal.*

INTERACTIONS
Aspirin, indomethacin, and other NSAIDs: increased risk of GI distress and bleeding. Give together cautiously.
Barbiturates, phenytoin, rifampin: decreased corticosteroid effect. Increase

---

corticosteroid dosage, as ordered.

Oral anticoagulants: altered dosage requirements. Monitor PT and INR closely.

Potassium-depleting drugs, such as thiazide diuretics: enhanced potassium-wasting effects of prednisone. Monitor serum potassium levels.

Salicylates: decreased serum salicylate levels.

Skin-test antigens: decreased response. Defer skin testing until therapy is completed.

Toxoids and vaccines: decreased antibody response and increased risk of neurologic complications. Avoid concomitant use.

EFFECTS ON DIAGNOSTIC TESTS
Prednisone suppresses reactions to skin tests, causes false-negative results in the nitroblue tetrazolium test for systemic bacterial infections, and decreases ^{131}I uptake and protein-bound iodine concentrations in thyroid function tests. It may increase serum glucose and cholesterol levels; may decrease serum potassium, calcium, thyroxine, and triiodothyronine levels; and may increase urine glucose and calcium levels.

CONTRAINDICATIONS
Contraindicated in patients with hypersensitivity to drug or systemic fungal infections.

NURSING CONSIDERATIONS
● Use cautiously in patients with GI ulcer, renal disease, hypertension, osteoporosis, diabetes mellitus, hypothyroidism, cirrhosis, diverticulitis, nonspecific ulcerative colitis, recent intestinal anastomoses, thromboembolic disorders, seizures, myasthenia gravis, CHF, tuberculosis, ocular herpes simplex, emotional instability, and psychotic tendencies.
Alert: Don't confuse with prednisolone.
● Know that drug may be used for alternate-day therapy.
● Always titrate to lowest effective dose as ordered.

● For better results and less toxicity, give a once-daily dose in the morning.
● Unless contraindicated, give oral dose with food when possible to reduce GI irritation.
● Monitor patient's blood pressure, sleep patterns, and serum potassium levels.
● Weigh patients daily; report sudden weight gain to the doctor.
● Watch for depression or psychotic episodes, especially in high-dose therapy.
● Diabetic patients may need increased insulin; monitor blood glucose levels.
● Know that elderly patients may be more susceptible to osteoporosis.
● Know that drug may mask or exacerbate infections, including latent amebiasis.
● Unless contraindicated, give low-sodium diet that's high in potassium and protein. Administer potassium supplements as needed.
● Gradually reduce drug dosage after long-term therapy, as ordered.

☑ **PATIENT TEACHING**
● Tell patient not to discontinue drug abruptly or without the doctor's consent.
● Instruct patient to take drug with food or milk.
● Teach patient signs of early adrenal insufficiency: fatigue, muscular weakness, joint pain, fever, anorexia, nausea, dyspnea, dizziness, and fainting.
● Instruct patient to carry a card identifying his need for supplemental systemic glucocorticoids during stress.
● Warn patient on long-term therapy about cushingoid symptoms and to report sudden weight gain or swelling to the doctor.
● Advise patient receiving long-term therapy to consider exercise or physical therapy. Also tell patient to ask doctor about vitamin D or calcium supplement.
● Tell patient to report slow healing.
● Advise patient receiving long-term therapy to have periodic ophthalmic examinations.

---

triamcinolone
Aristocort, Atolone, Kenacort**

triamcinolone acetonide
Cenocort A-40, Cinonide 40, Kenaject-40, Kenalog-10, Kenalog-40, Tac-3, Triam-A, Triamonide 40, Tri-Kort, Trilog

Pregnancy Risk Category: C

HOW SUPPLIED
triamcinolone
Tablets: 1 mg, 2 mg, 4 mg, 8 mg
triamcinolone acetonide
Injection (suspension): 3 mg/ml, 10 mg/ml, 40 mg/ml

ACTION
Not clearly defined. Decreases inflammation, mainly by stabilizing leukocyte lysosomal membranes; suppresses the immune response; stimulates bone marrow; and influences protein, fat, and carbohydrate metabolism.

ONSET, PEAK, DURATION
Highly variable.

INDICATIONS & DOSAGE
Severe inflammation or immunosuppression—
Adults: 4 to 48 mg P.O. daily in divided doses; 40 mg I.M. (acetonide) weekly; 1 mg (acetonide) into lesions; 2.5 to 40 mg (acetonide) into joints (depending on joint size) or soft tissue. A local anesthetic often is injected along with triamcinolone into the joint.

ADVERSE REACTIONS
Most adverse reactions to corticosteroids are dose- or duration-dependent.
CNS: *euphoria, insomnia,* psychotic behavior, pseudotumor cerebri, vertigo, headache, paresthesia, *seizures.*
CV: *CHF,* hypertension, edema, arrhythmias, thrombophlebitis, *thromboembolism.*
EENT: cataracts, glaucoma.

Endocrine: menstrual irregularities, cushingoid state (moonface, buffalo hump, central obesity).
GI: *peptic ulceration,* GI irritation, increased appetite, pancreatitis, nausea, vomiting.
Skin: delayed wound healing, acne, various skin eruptions.
Other: muscle weakness, osteoporosis, hirsutism, susceptibility to infections; hypokalemia, hyperglycemia, and carbohydrate intolerance; growth suppression in children; *acute adrenal insufficiency may occur with increased stress (infection, surgery, or trauma) or abrupt withdrawal after long-term therapy.*
After abrupt withdrawal: rebound inflammation, fatigue, weakness, arthralgia, fever, dizziness, lethargy, depression, fainting, orthostatic hypotension, dyspnea, anorexia, hypoglycemia. *After prolonged use, sudden withdrawal may be fatal.*

INTERACTIONS
Aspirin, indomethacin, and other NSAIDs: increased risk of GI distress and bleeding. Give together cautiously.
Barbiturates, phenytoin, rifampin: decreased corticosteroid effect. Increase corticosteroid dosage, as ordered.
Oral anticoagulants: altered dosage requirements. Monitor PT and INR closely.
Potassium-depleting drugs, such as thiazide diuretics: enhanced potassium-wasting effects of triamcinolone. Monitor serum potassium levels.
Salicylates: decreased serum salicylate levels.
Skin-test antigens: decreased response. Defer skin testing until after therapy.
Toxoids and vaccines: decreased antibody response and increased risk of neurologic complications. Avoid concomitant use.

EFFECTS ON DIAGNOSTIC TESTS
Triamcinolone suppresses reactions to skin tests, causes false-negative results

---

Reactions may be *common,* uncommon, *life-threatening,* or COMMON AND LIFE-THREATENING.

in the nitroblue tetrazolium test for systemic bacterial infections, and decreases ^{131}I uptake and protein-bound iodine concentrations in thyroid function tests. It may increase serum glucose and cholesterol levels; may decrease serum potassium, calcium, thyroxine, and triiodothyronine levels; and may increase urine glucose and calcium levels.

CONTRAINDICATIONS
Contraindicated in patients hypersensitive to any component of the formulation or in those with systemic fungal infections.

NURSING CONSIDERATIONS
• Use cautiously in patients with GI ulcer, renal disease, hypertension, osteoporosis, diabetes mellitus, hypothyroidism, cirrhosis, diverticulitis, nonspecific ulcerative colitis, recent intestinal anastomoses, thromboembolic disorders, seizures, myasthenia gravis, CHF, tuberculosis, ocular herpes simplex, emotional instability, and psychotic tendencies.
• Know that drug is not used for alternate-day therapy.
• Always titrate to lowest effective dose, as ordered.
• For better results and less toxicity, give a once-daily dose in the morning.
• Give oral dose with food when possible to reduce GI irritation.
• Parenteral form is *not* for I.V. use.
• Don't use diluents that contain preservatives; flocculation may occur.
• Give I.M. injection deeply into gluteal muscle. Rotate injection sites to prevent muscle atrophy.
• Monitor patients' weight, blood pressure, and serum electrolyte levels.
• Watch for allergic reaction to the dye tartrazine in patients with sensitivity to aspirin.
• Watch for depression or psychotic episodes, especially in high-dose therapy.
• Diabetic patients may need increased insulin; monitor blood glucose levels.

• Know that drug may mask or exacerbate infections, including latent amebiasis.
• Know that elderly patients may be more susceptible to osteoporosis.
• Unless contraindicated, give low-sodium diet that's high in potassium and protein. Administer potassium supplements as needed.
• Gradually reduce drug dosage after long-term therapy, as ordered.

☑ **PATIENT TEACHING**
• Tell patient not to discontinue drug abruptly or without the doctor's consent.
• Instruct patient to take drug with food or milk.
• Teach patient the signs of early adrenal insufficiency: fatigue, muscular weakness, joint pain, fever, anorexia, nausea, dyspnea, dizziness, and fainting.
• Instruct patient to carry a card identifying his need for supplemental systemic glucocorticoids during stress.
• Warn patient on long-term therapy about cushingoid symptoms and to report sudden weight gain and swelling to the doctor.
• Tell patient to report slow healing.
• Advise patient receiving long-term therapy to consider exercise or physical therapy. Also tell patient to ask doctor about vitamin D or calcium supplement.

danazol
fluoxymesterone
methyltestosterone
nandrolone decanoate
nandrolone phenpropionate
stanozolol
testosterone
testosterone cypionate
testosterone propionate
testosterone transdermal system

COMBINATION PRODUCTS

ANDROGYN L.A., DELADUMONE, VALERTEST NO. 1: testosterone enanthate 90 mg/ml and estradiol valerate 4 mg/ml in sesame oil.

DEPANDROGEN, DEPO-TESTADIOL, DEPOTESTOGEN, DUO-CYP, DURATESTRIN, TEST EST CYP (oil): testosterone cypionate 50 mg and estradiol cypionate 2 mg.

ESTRATEST: esterified estrogens 1.25 mg and methyltestosterone 2.5 mg.

ESTRATEST H.S.: esterified estrogens 0.625 mg and methyltestosterone 1.25 mg.

HALODRIN: fluoxymesterone 1 mg with ethinyl estradiol 0.02 mg.

PREMARIN WITH METHYLTESTOSTERONE: conjugated estrogens 0.625 mg and methyltestosterone 5 mg; or conjugated estrogens 1.25 mg and methyltestosterone 10 mg.

---

danazol
Cycloment†, Danocrine

Pregnancy Risk Category: X

HOW SUPPLIED
Capsules: 50 mg, 100 mg, 200 mg

ACTION
Not clearly defined. Gonadotropin inhibitor that suppresses the pituitary-ovarian axis and inhibits estrogenic effects.

ONSET, PEAK, DURATION
Onset for pain relief in fibrocystic breast disease occurs within 1 month. Unknown for other indications. Peak effects occur in 6 to 8 weeks when treating endometriosis and in 2 to 3 months when treating fibrocystic breast disease. Unknown for treatment of angioedema. Duration variable.

INDICATIONS & DOSAGE
Mild endometriosis—
Women: initially, 100 to 200 mg P.O. b.i.d. uninterrupted for 3 to 6 months; may be continued for 9 months. Subsequent dosage based on patient response.
Moderate to severe endometriosis—
Women: 400 mg P.O. b.i.d. uninterrupted for 3 to 6 months; may be continued for 9 months.
Fibrocystic breast disease—
Women: 100 to 400 mg P.O. daily in two divided doses uninterrupted for 2 to 6 months.
Prevention of hereditary angioedema—
Adults: 200 mg P.O. b.i.d. to t.i.d., continued until favorable response is achieved. Then dosage decreased by 50% at 1- to 3-month intervals.

ADVERSE REACTIONS
CNS: dizziness, headache, sleep disorders, fatigue, tremor, irritability, excitation, lethargy, mental depression, chills, paresthesia.
CV: elevated blood pressure.
EENT: visual disturbances.
GI: gastric irritation, nausea, vomiting, diarrhea, constipation, change in appetite.
GU: hematuria, *hypoestrogenic effects (flushing, diaphoresis, vaginitis [including itching, dryness, and burning];*

Reactions may be *common*, uncommon, *life-threatening*, or COMMON AND LIFE-THREATENING.

vaginal bleeding, nervousness, emotional lability, menstrual irregularities).
Hepatic: reversible jaundice, elevated liver enzyme levels, hepatic dysfunction.
Other: muscle cramps or spasms; androgenic effects in women *(weight gain, hirsutism,* hoarseness, *clitoral enlargement, decreased breast size,* acne, edema, changes in libido, *oily skin or hair,* voice deepening); *allergic reactions.*

INTERACTIONS
Carbamazepine: May increase carbamazepine levels. Monitor closely.
Warfarin: May prolong PT in patients stabilized on warfarin. Monitor PT and INR.

EFFECTS ON DIAGNOSTIC TESTS
Glucose tolerance test results may be abnormal. Total serum thyroxine (T_4) may be decreased; triiodothyronine (T_3) may be increased. PT (especially in patients on anticoagulant therapy) may be prolonged.

CONTRAINDICATIONS
Contraindicated in patients with undiagnosed abnormal genital bleeding; porphyria; or impaired renal, cardiac, or hepatic function; during pregnancy; and in breast-feeding patients.

NURSING CONSIDERATIONS
● Use cautiously in patients with seizure disorders or migraine headache.
Alert: Avoid use in women of childbearing age until pregnancy is ruled out.
● Unless contraindicated, use with diet high in calories and protein.
● Monitor closely for signs of virilization. Some androgenic effects, such as deepening of voice, may not be reversible upon discontinuation of drug.
● Periodically evaluate hepatic function as ordered. Semen evaluation is routinely performed every 3 to 4 months, especially in adolescent boys.
● Know that periodic dosage decreases or gradual drug withdrawal is best.

● After withdrawal of treatment, ovulation and cyclic menstrual bleeding usually return in 2 to 3 months; fibrocystic disease symptoms return within 1 year for 50% of patients.

☑ PATIENT TEACHING
● Advise patient taking danazol for fibrocystic breast disease to examine breasts regularly and to call the doctor immediately if breast nodules enlarge.
● Make sure patient understands the importance of using an effective nonhormonal contraceptive during therapy.
● Instruct patient to report adverse reactions, especially signs of virilization, promptly.
● Advise washing after intercourse to decrease the risk of vaginitis. Instruct patient to wear only cotton underwear.

fluoxymesterone
Android-F, Halotestin**

Controlled Substance Schedule III
Pregnancy Risk Category: X

HOW SUPPLIED
Tablets: 2 mg, 5 mg, 10 mg

ACTION
Stimulates target tissues to develop normally in androgen-deficient men.

ONSET, PEAK, DURATION
Unknown.

INDICATIONS & DOSAGE
Hypogonadism caused by testicular deficiency—
Adults: 5 to 20 mg P.O. daily.
Delayed puberty—
Adolescent: highly individualized; duration of therapy 4 to 6 months.
Palliation of breast cancer in women—
Adults: 10 to 40 mg P.O. daily in divided doses. All dosages are individualized and reduced to minimum when effect is noted.

---

*Liquid contains alcohol.   **May contain tartrazine.   †Canada only.   ‡Australia only.   ◇OTC.

ADVERSE REACTIONS

CNS: headache, anxiety, depression, paresthesia, sleep apnea syndrome.
CV: edema.
GI: nausea.
GU: *hypoestrogenic effects in women (flushing; diaphoresis; vaginitis, including itching, dryness, and burning; vaginal bleeding; nervousness; emotional lability; menstrual irregularities); excessive hormonal effects in men (prepubertal—premature epiphyseal closure,* acne, priapism, *growth of body and facial hair,* phallic enlargement; postpubertal—testicular atrophy, oligospermia, decreased ejaculatory volume, impotence, gynecomastia, epididymitis).*
Hematologic: polycythemia, elevated serum lipid levels, suppression of clotting factors.
Hepatic: reversible jaundice, peliosis hepatis, elevated liver enzyme levels, *liver cell tumors.*
Other: hypercalcemia; hypersensitivity skin manifestations; androgenic effects in women (acne, edema, *weight gain, hirsutism,* hoarseness, clitoral enlargement, deepening voice, *decreased breast size,* changes in libido, male-pattern baldness, *oily skin or hair*).

INTERACTIONS

Hepatotoxic medications: increased risk of hepatotoxicity. Monitor closely.
Insulin, oral antidiabetic agents: altered dosage requirements. Monitor blood glucose levels in diabetic patients.
Oral anticoagulants: altered dosage requirements. Monitor PT and INR.

EFFECTS ON DIAGNOSTIC TESTS

Fluoxymesterone may cause abnormal results of the glucose tolerance test. Thyroid function test results (protein-bound iodine, radioactive iodine uptake, thyroid-binding capacity) may decrease. PT may be prolonged. Abnormal liver function test may occur. Because of this agent's anabolic activity, serum sodium, potassium, calcium, phosphate, and cholesterol levels may all rise.

CONTRAINDICATIONS

Contraindicated in patients with hypersensitivity to drug, in males with breast cancer or prostate cancer, in those with cardiac, hepatic, or renal decompensation; during pregnancy; and in breast-feeding patients.

NURSING CONSIDERATIONS

● Use cautiously in prepubertal males, benign prostatic hyperplasia, and aspirin sensitivity.
Alert: Avoid use in women of childbearing age until pregnancy is ruled out.
● Unless contraindicated, use with diet high in calories and protein. Give small, frequent feedings.
● Watch for symptoms of jaundice and periodically evaluate hepatic function, as ordered. Dosage adjustment may reverse condition. If liver function test results are abnormal, notify doctor because therapy should be stopped.
● Know that edema can be controlled with sodium restriction or diuretics. Monitor weight routinely.
● Monitor male patients for signs of excessive sexual stimulation or priapism.
● Be aware that semen evaluation is routinely performed every 3 to 4 months, especially in adolescent boys.
Alert: Know that hypercalcemia symptoms may be difficult to distinguish from symptoms associated with condition being treated, unless anticipated and thought of as a symptom cluster. Hypercalcemia is particularly likely to occur in patients with metastatic breast cancer and may indicate bone metastases.
Alert: Know that the drug should not be used for enhancement of athletic performance or physique.
● Watch for symptoms of hypoglycemia in diabetic patients. Check blood glucose levels. Dosage of antidiabetic drug may need adjustment.
● When used in breast cancer, subjec-

tive effects may not occur for about 1 month; objective effects on clinical symptoms may take 3 months.

☑ PATIENT TEACHING
● If GI upset occurs, tell patient to take drug with food or meals.
● Make sure patient understands the importance of using an effective nonhormonal contraceptive during therapy.
● Advise washing after intercourse to decrease the risk of vaginitis. Instruct patient to wear only cotton underwear.
● Tell women to report menstrual irregularities and to discontinue therapy pending etiologic determination.
● Explain to patient taking drug for palliation of breast cancer that virilization usually occurs. Give emotional support. Tell patient to report androgenic effects immediately. Stopping drug will prevent further androgenic changes but will probably not reverse existing effects.

---

methyltestosterone
Android, Metandren**, Metandren†, Oreton Methyl, Testomet‡, Testred, Virilon

Controlled Substance Schedule III
Pregnancy Risk Category: X

HOW SUPPLIED
Tablets: 5 mg‡, 10 mg, 25 mg, 50 mg‡
Tablets (buccal): 10 mg, 25 mg†
Capsules: 10 mg

ACTION
Stimulates target tissues to develop normally in androgen-deficient men.

ONSET, PEAK, DURATION
Onset and duration unknown. Serum levels peak in 1 hour after buccal administration and 2 hours after oral administration.

INDICATIONS & DOSAGE
Postpartum breast engorgement in non-breast-feeding women—

Adults: 80 mg P.O. daily, or 40 mg buccally daily for 3 to 5 days.
Breast cancer in women 1 to 5 years postmenopausal—
Adults: 50 to 200 mg P.O. daily; or 25 to 100 mg buccally daily.
Male hypogonadism—
Adults: 10 to 40 mg P.O. daily; or 5 to 25 mg buccally daily.
Postpubertal cryptorchidism—
Adults: 30 mg P.O. daily; or 15 mg buccally daily.

ADVERSE REACTIONS
CNS: headache, anxiety, depression, paresthesia, sleep apnea syndrome.
CV: edema.
EENT: irritation of oral mucosa (with buccal administration).
GI: nausea.
GU: *hypoestrogenic effects in women (flushing; diaphoresis; vaginitis, including itching, dryness, and burning; vaginal bleeding; nervousness; emotional lability; menstrual irregularities); excessive hormonal effects in men (prepubertal—premature epiphyseal closure,* acne, priapism, *growth of body and facial hair,* phallic enlargement; postpubertal—testicular atrophy, oligospermia, decreased ejaculatory volume, impotence, gynecomastia, epididymitis).
Hepatic: reversible jaundice, cholestatic hepatitis, abnormal liver enzyme levels.
Other: hypercalcemia; polycythemia; hypersensitivity skin manifestations; suppression of clotting factors; muscle cramps or spasms; androgenic effects in women (acne, edema, *weight gain, hirsutism,* hoarseness, clitoral enlargement, *decreased breast size,* deepening voice, changes in libido, male-pattern baldness, *oily skin or hair*).

INTERACTIONS
Hepatotoxic medications: increased risk of hepatotoxicity. Monitor closely.
Insulin, oral antidiabetic agents: altered dosage requirements. Monitor blood glucose levels in diabetic patients.
Oral anticoagulants: altered dosage re-

---

quirements. Monitor PT and INR.

EFFECTS ON DIAGNOSTIC TESTS
Methyltestosterone may cause abnormal results of the glucose tolerance test. Thyroid function test results (protein-bound iodine, radioactive iodine uptake, thyroid-binding capacity) may decrease. PT (especially in patients on anticoagulant therapy) may be prolonged. Abnormal liver function test may occur. Because of this agent's anabolic activity, serum sodium, potassium, calcium, phosphate, and cholesterol levels may all rise.

CONTRAINDICATIONS
Contraindicated in pregnant and breast-feeding patients or in males with breast cancer or prostate cancer.

NURSING CONSIDERATIONS
● Use cautiously in elderly patients; patients with cardiac, renal, or hepatic disease; or healthy males with delayed puberty.
● Avoid use in women of childbearing age until pregnancy is ruled out.
● In children, X-rays of the wrist bones should be taken before therapy begins to establish the level of bone maturation. During treatment, bone maturation may proceed more rapidly than linear growth; ensure intermittent dosage and periodically review X-ray results to monitor bone maturation.
● Typically used only for intermittent therapy. Because of potential hepatotoxicity, watch closely for jaundice.
● Promptly report signs of virilization in women.
● Unless contraindicated, use with diet high in calories and protein. Give small, frequent feedings.
● Periodically check hemoglobin and hematocrit values, serum cholesterol and calcium levels, and cardiac and liver function test results, as ordered.
● Check weight regularly. Edema can be controlled with sodium restriction or diuretics.

Alert: Therapeutic response in breast cancer is usually apparent within 3 months. Know therapy should be stopped if signs of disease progression appear.
● Report signs of hypercalcemia. In metastatic breast cancer, hypercalcemia may indicate progression of bone metastases.
● Know that semen evaluation is routinely performed every 3 to 4 months, especially in adolescent boys.
Alert: Know that the drug should not be used for enhancement of athletic performance or physique.

☑ **PATIENT TEACHING**
● Make sure patient understands the importance of using an effective nonhormonal contraceptive during therapy.
● Buccal tablets are twice as potent as oral tablets. Tell patient to avoid eating, drinking, chewing, or smoking while buccal tablet is in place and not to swallow tablet. Place in upper or lower buccal pouch between cheek and gum; tablet requires 30 to 60 minutes to dissolve. Instruct patient to change tablet absorption site with each dose to minimize risk of buccal irritation.
● Review signs and symptoms of virilization with female patient and instruct her to notify doctor immediately if any occur.
● Drug enhances hypoglycemia; teach patient the signs of hypoglycemia and method for checking blood glucose level. Instruct patient to report hypoglycemia immediately.
● Advise washing after intercourse to decrease the risk of vaginitis. Instruct patient to wear only cotton underwear.

nandrolone decanoate
Anabolin LA, Androlone-D, Deca-Durabolin, Decolone, Hybolin Decanoate, Kabolin, Nandrobolic L.A., Neo-Durabolic

Reactions may be *common*, uncommon, *life-threatening*, or COMMON AND LIFE-THREATENING.

nandrolone phenpropionate
Anabolin IM, Androlone, Durabolin, Hybolin Improved, Nandrobolic

Controlled Substance Schedule III
Pregnancy Risk Category: X

HOW SUPPLIED
nandrolone decanoate
Injection (in oil): 50 mg/ml, 100 mg/ml, 200 mg/ml
nandrolone phenpropionate
Injection (in oil): 25 mg/ml, 50 mg/ml

ACTION
Anabolic steroid that promotes tissue-building processes, reverses catabolism, and stimulates erythropoiesis.

ONSET, PEAK, DURATION
Onset and duration unknown. Serum levels peak in 1 to 2 days (phenpropionate) or 3 to 6 days (decanoate).

INDICATIONS & DOSAGE
Severe debility or disease states, refractory anemias—
Adults: 50 to 100 mg decanoate I.M. at 1 to 4 week intervals for females; 50 to 200 mg decanoate I.M. at 1 to 4 week intervals for males. Therapy should be intermittent.
Children 2 to 13 years: 25 to 50 mg decanoate I.M. q 3 to 4 weeks.
Control of metastatic breast cancer—
Adults: 25 to 100 mg phenpropionate I.M. weekly.

ADVERSE REACTIONS
CNS: excitation, insomnia, habituation, depression.
CV: edema.
GI: nausea, vomiting, diarrhea.
GU: bladder irritability, *hypoestrogenic effects in women (flushing; diaphoresis; vaginitis, including itching, dryness, and burning; vaginal bleeding; nervousness; emotional lability; menstrual irregularities); excessive hormonal effects in men (prepubertal—premature epiphyseal closure, acne, priapism, growth of body and facial hair,* phallic enlargement; postpubertal—testicular atrophy, oligospermia, decreased ejaculatory volume, impotence, gynecomastia, epididymitis).
Hematologic: elevated serum lipid levels, suppression of clotting factors.
Hepatic: reversible jaundice, peliosis hepatis, elevated liver enzyme levels, *liver cell tumors.*
Skin: pain and induration at injection site.
Other: androgenic effects in women (acne, edema, *weight gain, hirsutism,* hoarseness, clitoral enlargement, *decreased breast size,* changes in libido, male-pattern baldness, *oily skin or hair).*

INTERACTIONS
Hepatotoxic medications: increased risk of hepatotoxicity. Monitor closely.
Insulin, oral antidiabetic agents: altered dosage requirements. Monitor blood glucose levels in diabetic patients.
Oral anticoagulants: altered dosage requirements. Monitor PT and INR.

EFFECTS ON DIAGNOSTIC TESTS
Nandrolone may cause abnormal results of fasting plasma glucose, glucose tolerance, and metyrapone tests. Thyroid function test results (protein-bound iodine, radioactive iodine uptake, thyroid-binding capacity) and 17-ketosteroid levels may decrease. Liver function test results, prothrombin time (especially in patients receiving anticoagulant therapy), and serum-creatinine levels may be elevated. Because of this agent's anabolic activity, serum sodium, potassium, calcium, phosphate, and cholesterol levels may all rise.

CONTRAINDICATIONS
Contraindicated in patients with hypersensitivity to anabolic steroids, in males with breast cancer or prostate cancer, in those with nephrosis, in those experiencing the nephrotic phase of nephritis, in women with breast cancer and hyper-

calcemia, during pregnancy, or in breast-feeding patients.

NURSING CONSIDERATIONS

● Use cautiously in patients with diabetes; cardiac, renal, or hepatic disease; epilepsy; or migraine or other conditions that may be aggravated by fluid retention.

● Avoid use in women of childbearing age until pregnancy is ruled out.

● In children, X-rays of the wrist bones should be taken before surgery to establish the level of bone maturation. During treatment, bone maturation may proceed more rapidly than linear growth; ensure intermittent dosage and periodically review X-ray results to monitor bone maturation.

● Inject I.M. drug deeply, preferably into upper outer quadrant of gluteal muscle in adults. Rotate injection sites to prevent muscle atrophy.

● Unless contraindicated, use with diet high in calories and protein. Give small, frequent feedings.

● Watch for signs of virilization, which may be irreversible despite prompt discontinuation of therapy.

● Closely observe boys under 7 years for precocious development of male sexual characteristics.

● Know that semen evaluation is routinely performed every 3 to 4 months, especially in adolescent boys.

Alert: Periodically evaluate hepatic function, as ordered. Watch for jaundice; dosage adjustment may reverse condition. If liver function test results are abnormal, therapy should be stopped.

● Check weight regularly. Edema generally can be controlled with sodium restrictions or diuretics.

● Watch for symptoms of hypoglycemia in diabetic patients. Check blood glucose levels. Adjust dosage of antidiabetic agent, as ordered.

● Check quantitative urine and serum calcium levels. Hypercalcemia is most likely to occur in patients with breast cancer.

● When used to promote erythropoiesis in refractory anemias, make sure patients have adequate daily iron intake.

● Be aware that anabolic steroids may alter results of laboratory studies performed during therapy and for 2 to 3 weeks after therapy ends.

☑ PATIENT TEACHING

● Make sure patient understands the importance of using an effective nonhormonal contraceptive during therapy.

● Review signs and symptoms of virilization with female patient, and instruct her to notify doctor immediately if any occur.

● Advise washing after intercourse to decrease the risk of vaginitis. Instruct patients to wear only cotton underwear.

● Tell women to report menstrual irregularities and to discontinue therapy pending etiologic determination.

---

stanozolol
Winstrol

Controlled Substance Schedule III
Pregnancy Risk Category: X

HOW SUPPLIED
Tablets: 2 mg

ACTION
Anabolic steroid that promotes tissue-building processes, reverses catabolism, and stimulates erythropoiesis.

ONSET, PEAK, DURATION
Unknown.

INDICATIONS & DOSAGE
Prevention of hereditary angioedema—
Adults: initially, 2 mg P.O. t.i.d. Following a favorable response, dosage is gradually reduced at 1- to 3-month intervals to a dosage of 2 mg P.O. daily. Some patients may be maintained on 2 mg every other day.
Children under 6 years: 1 mg P.O. daily during an attack only.

Reactions may be *common*, uncommon, *life-threatening*, or COMMON AND LIFE-THREATENING.

Children 6 to 12 years: up to 2 mg P.O. daily during an attack only.

Note: Stanozolol is used in children only during an acute attack.

ADVERSE REACTIONS
CNS: excitation, insomnia, habituation, depression.
CV: edema.
GI: nausea, vomiting, constipation, diarrhea.
GU: bladder irritability, hypoestrogenic effects in women (flushing; diaphoresis; vaginitis, including itching, dryness, and burning; vaginal bleeding; nervousness; emotional lability; menstrual irregularities); excessive hormonal effects in men (prepubertal—premature epiphyseal closure, *acne,* priapism, *growth of body and facial hair,* phallic enlargement; postpubertal—testicular atrophy, oligospermia, decreased ejaculatory volume, impotence, gynecomastia, epididymitis).
Hematologic: elevated serum lipid levels, suppression of clotting factors.
Hepatic: reversible jaundice, peliosis hepatis, elevated liver enzyme levels, *liver cell tumors.*
Other: androgenic effects in women (acne, edema, *weight gain, hirsutism,* hoarseness, clitoral enlargement, *decreased breast size,* changes in libido, male-pattern baldness, *oily skin or hair*).

INTERACTIONS
Hepatotoxic medications: increased risk of hepatotoxicity. Monitor closely.
Insulin, oral antidiabetic agents: altered dosage requirements. Monitor blood glucose levels in diabetic patients.
Oral anticoagulants: altered dosage requirements. Monitor PT and INR.

EFFECTS ON DIAGNOSTIC TESTS
Stanozolol may cause abnormal results of fasting plasma glucose, glucose tolerance, and metyrapone tests. It may increase sulfobromophthalein retention. Thyroid function test results (protein-bound iodine, radioactive iodine uptake, thyroid-binding capacity) and 15-ketosteroid levels may decrease. Liver function test results, PT (especially in patients receiving anticoagulant therapy), and serum creatinine levels may be elevated. Because of the agent's anabolic activity, serum sodium, potassium, calcium, phosphate, and cholesterol levels may all rise.

CONTRAINDICATIONS
Contraindicated in patients with hypersensitivity to anabolic steroids; in males with breast cancer or prostate cancer; in nephrosis or nephrotic phase of nephritis; in women with breast cancer and with hypercalcemia; during pregnancy; and in breast-feeding patients.

NURSING CONSIDERATIONS
● Use cautiously in patients with diabetes; cardiac, renal, or hepatic disease; epilepsy; or migraine or other conditions that may be aggravated by fluid retention.
● Avoid use in women of childbearing age until pregnancy is ruled out.
● In children, X-rays of the wrist bones should be taken before therapy begins to establish the level of bone maturation. During treatment, bone maturation may proceed more rapidly than linear growth; ensure intermittent dosage and review X-ray results periodically to monitor bone maturation.
● Know that a lower dosage in young women (2 mg b.i.d.) is recommended to avoid virilization. Watch for signs of virilization, which may be irreversible despite prompt discontinuation of therapy. Doctor must decide if benefits of therapy outweigh adverse effects.
● To minimize GI distress, administer before or with meals.
● Unless contraindicated, use with diet high in calories and protein. Give small, frequent feedings.
● Closely observe boys under 7 years for precocious development of male sexual characteristics.

● Know that semen evaluation is routinely performed every 3 to 4 months, especially in adolescent boys.
● Monitor weight routinely. Edema is generally controllable with sodium restriction or diuretics.
Alert: Periodically evaluate hepatic function. Watch for symptoms of jaundice; dosage adjustment may reverse condition. Check liver function test results regularly; if they are abnormal, therapy should be discontinued.
● Monitor serum cholesterol levels.
● Watch for symptoms of hypoglycemia in diabetic patients. Check blood glucose levels. Adjust dosage of antidiabetic agent, as ordered.
● Know that anabolic steroids may alter results of laboratory studies performed during therapy and for 2 to 3 weeks after therapy ends.

☑ **PATIENT TEACHING**
● Make sure patient understands the importance of using an effective nonhormonal contraceptive during therapy.
● Instruct patient to take drug before or with meals.
● Review signs and symptoms of virilization with female patient, and instruct her to notify doctor immediately if any occur.
● Advise washing after intercourse to decrease the risk of vaginitis. Instruct patients to wear only cotton underwear.
● Tell women to report menstrual irregularities and to discontinue therapy pending etiologic determination.

testosterone
Andro 100, Andronaq-50, Histerone-50, Histerone-100, Tesamone 100, Testaqua, Testoject-50

testosterone cypionate
Andro-Cyp 100, Andro-Cyp 200, Andronaq-LA, Andronate 100, Andronate 200, depAndro 100, depAndro 200, Depotest, Depo-Testosterone, Duratest-100, MDuratest-200,

T-Cypionate, Testa-C, Testoject-LA, Testred Cypionate 200, Virilon IM

testosterone propionate
Malogen†, Testex

Controlled Substance Schedule III
Pregnancy Risk Category: X

HOW SUPPLIED
testosterone
Injection (aqueous suspension): 25 mg/ml, 50 mg/ml, 100 mg/ml
testosterone cypionate
Injection (in oil): 50 mg/ml, 100 mg/ml, 200 mg/ml
testosterone propionate
Injection (in oil): 25 mg/ml, 50 mg/ml, 100 mg/ml

ACTION
Stimulates target tissues to develop normally in androgen-deficient men. Testosterone may have some antiestrogen properties, making it useful to treat certain estrogen-dependent breast cancers. Its action in postpartum breast engorgement is not known because testosterone does not suppress lactation.

ONSET, PEAK, DURATION
Unknown.

INDICATIONS & DOSAGE
Male hypogonadism—
Adults: 10 to 25 mg (testosterone or propionate) I.M. two to three times weekly, or 50 to 400 mg (cypionate) I.M. q 2 to 4 weeks.
Metastatic breast cancer in women 1 to 5 years postmenopausal—
Adults: 100 mg I.M. three times weekly; 50 to 100 mg (propionate) I.M. three times weekly; or 200 to 400 mg (cypionate) I.M. q 2 to 4 weeks.
Postpartum breast pain and engorgement—
Adults: 25 to 50 mg I.M. of testosterone or testosterone propionate daily for 3 to 4 days.

ADVERSE REACTIONS

CNS: headache, anxiety, depression, paresthesia, sleep apnea syndrome.
GU: hypoestrogenic effects in women (flushing; diaphoresis; vaginitis, including itching, drying, and burning; vaginal bleeding; menstrual irregularities); excessive hormonal effects in men (prepubertal—premature epiphyseal closure, *acne,* priapism, *growth of body and facial hair,* phallic enlargement; postpubertal—testicular atrophy, oligospermia, decreased ejaculatory volume, impotence, gynecomastia, epididymitis).
Hepatic: reversible jaundice, cholestatic hepatitis, abnormal liver enzyme levels.
Skin: pain and induration at injection site, local edema.
Other: edema, nausea, hypercalcemia; polycythemia; hypersensitivity skin manifestations; suppression of clotting factors; androgenic effects in women.

INTERACTIONS

Hepatotoxic medications: increased risk of hepatotoxicity. Monitor closely.
Insulin, oral antidiabetic agents: altered dosage requirements. Monitor blood glucose levels in diabetic patients.
Oral anticoagulants: altered dosage requirements. Monitor PT and INR.

EFFECTS ON DIAGNOSTIC TESTS

Testosterone may cause abnormal results of glucose tolerance tests. Thyroid function test results and serum 17-ketosteroid levels may decrease. Liver function test results, PT, and serum creatinine levels may be elevated. Increased serum sodium, potassium, calcium, phosphate, and cholesterol levels may occur.

CONTRAINDICATIONS

Contraindicated in male patients with breast or prostate cancer; in patients with hypercalcemia; in those with cardiac, hepatic, or renal decompensation; during pregnancy, and in breast-feeding patients.

NURSING CONSIDERATIONS

• Use cautiously in elderly patients.
• Avoid use in women of childbearing age until pregnancy is ruled out.
• Administer daily dosage requirement in divided doses for best results.
• Store I.M. preparations at room temperature. If crystals appear, warm and shake the bottle to disperse them.
• Inject deep into upper outer quadrant of gluteal muscle. Rotate injection sites. Report soreness at site.
• Unless contraindicated, use with diet high in calories and protein. Give small, frequent feedings.
• Monitor liver function test results.
• In patients with metastatic breast cancer, hypercalcemia usually indicates progression of bone metastases. Report signs of hypercalcemia.
• Report signs of virilization in women.
• Monitor weight routinely.
• Monitor prepubertal boys by X-ray for rate of bone maturation.
Alert: Therapeutic response in breast cancer is usually apparent within 3 months. Know that therapy should be stopped if disease progresses.
• Know that androgens may alter results of laboratory studies during therapy and for 2 to 3 weeks after therapy ends.

☑ **PATIENT TEACHING**
• Make sure patient understands the importance of using an effective nonhormonal contraceptive during therapy.
• Review signs and symptoms of virilization with female patient and instruct her to notify doctor if any occur.
• Advise washing after intercourse to decrease the risk of vaginitis. Instruct patients to wear cotton underwear.
• Instruct men to report priapism, reduced ejaculatory volume, and gynecomastia. Notify doctor if these occur.
• Teach patient to recognize and immediately report signs of hypoglycemia.

testosterone transdermal system

Androderm, Testoderm

Controlled Substance Schedule III
Pregnancy Risk Category: X

HOW SUPPLIED

Transdermal system: 2.5 mg/day, 4 mg/day, 6 mg/day

ACTION

Releases testosterone, which stimulates target tissues to develop normally in androgen-deficient men.

ONSET, PEAK, DURATION

Onset unknown. Serum levels peak within 2 to 4 hours after application. Steady-state levels are reached after 3 to 4 weeks of therapy. Testosterone levels decline toward baseline within 2 hours after removal.

INDICATIONS & DOSAGE

Primary or hypogonadotropic hypogonadism in men—
Adults: (Testoderm) one 6-mg/day patch applied to the scrotal area daily. If scrotal area is too small for the 6-mg/day patch, therapy started with the smaller sized 4 mg/day patch. Patch worn for 22 to 24 hours daily.
Adults: (Androderm) 2 systems applied nightly for a total dose of 5 mg/day. Apply to clean, dry skin on back, abdomen, upper arms, or thigh.

ADVERSE REACTIONS

CNS: *CVA,* headache, depression.
GU: *gynecomastia,* prostatitis, prostate abnormalities, urinary tract infection, breast tenderness.
Skin: acne irritation, *blister under system,* allergic contact dermatitis, or burning and induration at site.
Other: *pruritus,* GI bleeding

INTERACTIONS

Insulin: altered insulin dosage requirements. Monitor blood glucose levels.
Oral anticoagulants: altered anticoagulant dosage requirements. Monitor PT and INR.
Oxyphenbutazone: may increase oxyphenbutazone levels. Monitor patient.

EFFECTS ON DIAGNOSTIC TESTS

Androgens may decrease levels of thyroxin-binding globulin, resulting in decreased total T_4 serum levels and increased resin uptake of T_3 and T_4.

CONTRAINDICATIONS

Contraindicated in patients hypersensitive to the drug, in women, and in men with known or suspected breast or prostate cancer.

NURSING CONSIDERATIONS

● Use cautiously in elderly men. Use cautiously in patients with preexisting renal, hepatic, or cardiac disease.
● Periodically assess liver function tests, serum lipid profiles, hemoglobin and hematocrit (with chronic use), prostatic acid phosphatase and prostate-specific antigen levels, as ordered.

☑ PATIENT TEACHING

● Teach patient how to apply the transdermal system. Warn patient using Testoderm that adequate serum levels will not be attained if the patch is not applied to genital skin. Tell patient using Androderm that patch is *not* to be applied to scotum. Application site should be rotated with an interval of 7 days between applications to the same site. Avoid bony prominences.
● Tell male patient that topical testosterone has caused virilization in female partners, who should report acne or changes in body hair distribution.
● Advise patient to report persistent erections, nausea, vomiting, changes in skin color, or ankle edema to the doctor.
● Tell patient that Androderm does not have to be removed during sexual intercourse or while showering.

Reactions may be *common,* uncommon, *life-threatening,* or COMMON AND LIFE-THREATENING.

chlorotrianisene
dienestrol
diethylstilbestrol
diethylstilbestrol diphosphate
esterified estrogens
estradiol
estradiol cypionate
estradiol valerate
estrogens, conjugated
estropipate
ethinyl estradiol
ethinyl estradiol and desogestrel
ethinyl estradiol and
    ethynodiol diacetate
ethinyl estradiol and
    levonorgestrel
ethinyl estradiol and
    norethindrone
ethinyl estradiol and norethin-
    drone acetate
ethinyl estradiol and
    norgestimate
ethinyl estradiol and norgestrel
ethinyl estradiol, norethindrone
    acetate, and ferrous fumarate
mestranol and norethindrone
mestranol and norethynodrel
hydroxyprogesterone caproate
levonorgestrel
medroxyprogesterone acetate
norethindrone
norethindrone acetate
norgestrel
progesterone

COMBINATION PRODUCTS

MENRIUM 5-2: chlordiazepoxide 5 mg
and esterified estrogens 0.2 mg.
MENRIUM 5-4: chlordiazepoxide 5 mg
and esterified estrogens 0.4 mg.
MENRIUM 10-4: chlordiazepoxide 10 mg
and esterified estrogens 0.4 mg.
PMB-200: conjugated estrogens 0.45
mg and meprobamate 200 mg.
PMB-400: conjugated estrogens 0.45
mg and meprobamate 400 mg.

chlorotrianisene
TACE**

Pregnancy Risk Category: X

HOW SUPPLIED
Capsules: 12 mg, 25 mg

ACTION
Increases the synthesis of DNA, RNA,
and protein in responsive tissues and reduces release of follicle-stimulating hormone and luteinizing hormone from the
pituitary gland.

ONSET, PEAK, DURATION
Onset and peak unknown. Effects persist for about 24 hours.

INDICATIONS & DOSAGE
Prostate cancer—
Adults: 12 to 25 mg P.O. daily.
Female hypogonadism—
Adults: 12 to 25 mg P.O. for 21 days,
followed by one dose of progesterone
100 mg I.M. or 5 days of oral progesto-
gen concurrently with last 5 days of
chlorotrianisene (for example, medroxyprogesterone 5 to 10 mg).
*Vasomotor symptoms associated with
menopausal symptoms, atrophic vaginitis, kraurosis vulvae—*
Adults: 12 to 25 mg P.O. daily for 30
days or cyclic (3 weeks on, 1 week off).

ADVERSE REACTIONS
CNS: headache, dizziness, chorea, migraine, depression, *seizures.*
CV: thrombophlebitis; *thromboembolism;* hypertension; edema; *increased
risk of CVA, pulmonary embolism, MI.*
EENT: worsening of myopia or astigmatism, intolerance of contact lenses.
GI: *nausea,* vomiting, abdominal
cramps, bloating, colitis, acute pancre-

atitis, anorexia, increased appetite, excessive thirst, weight changes.

GU: in women—breakthrough bleeding, altered menstrual flow, dysmenorrhea, *increased risk of endometrial cancer, possibility of increased risk of breast cancer,* amenorrhea, cervical erosion or abnormal secretions, enlargement of uterine fibromas, vaginal candidiasis; in men—*gynecomastia, testicular atrophy, impotence.*

Hepatic: cholestatic jaundice, *hepatic adenoma.*

Skin: melasma, urticaria, hirsutism or hair loss, erythema nodosum, dermatitis.

Other: breast changes (tenderness, enlargement, secretion), hypercalcemia, gallbladder disease.

INTERACTIONS

Carbamazepine, phenobarbital, rifampin: decreased effectiveness of estrogen therapy. Monitor closely.

Corticosteroids: possible enhanced effects of corticosteroids. Monitor closely.

Cyclosporine: increased risk of toxicity. Use together with caution and frequently monitor cyclosporine levels.

Dantrolene, other hepatotoxic medications: increased risk of hepatotoxicity. Monitor closely.

Oral anticoagulants: dosage adjustments may be necessary. Monitor PT and INR

Tamoxifen: estrogens may interfere with effectiveness of tamoxifen. Avoid concomitant use.

EFFECTS ON DIAGNOSTIC TESTS

In patients with diabetes, chlorotrianisene may increase blood glucose levels, necessitating dosage adjustment of insulin or oral hypoglycemic drugs.

Chlorotrianisene has the potential to decrease the effects of warfarin-type anticoagulants.

CONTRAINDICATIONS

Contraindicated in patients with thrombophlebitis or thromboembolic disorders; in those with breast, reproductive organ, or genital cancer; in those with undiagnosed abnormal genital bleeding; and during pregnancy.

NURSING CONSIDERATIONS

● Use cautiously in patients with cerebrovascular or coronary artery disease; asthma; bone disease; migraine; seizures; cardiac, hepatic, or renal dysfunction; hypercalcemia from metastatic breast disease; and family history (mother, grandmother, sister) of breast or genital tract cancer, or who have breast nodules, fibrocystic disease, or abnormal mammographic findings.

● Ensure that patients have a thorough physical examination before initiating estrogen therapy. Periodically monitor blood pressure, hepatic function, and serum lipid levels.

● Monitor weight regularly and recommend sodium restriction, as needed. May cause fluid retention and edema.

● Notify the pathologist about any patients receiving estrogen therapy when specimens are obtained and sent to pathology for evaluation.

● Because of the risk of thromboembolism, know that therapy should be stopped at least 1 month before procedures associated with prolonged immobilization or thromboembolism, such as knee or hip surgery.

☑ PATIENT TEACHING

● Tell patient that package insert describing estrogen's adverse effects is available; also explain effects.

Alert: Warn patient to immediately report suspected pregnancy; abdominal pain; pain, numbness, or stiffness in legs or buttocks; pressure or pain in chest; shortness of breath; severe headaches; visual disturbances, such as blind spots, flashing lights, or blurriness; vaginal bleeding or discharge; breast lumps; swelling of hands or feet; yellow skin and sclera; dark urine; and light-colored stools.

● Explain to patient on cyclic therapy for postmenopausal symptoms that, although withdrawal bleeding may occur during week off drug, fertility is not restored. Pregnancy cannot occur because patient does not ovulate.

• Teach women how to perform routine breast self-examination.

• Tell diabetic patient to report elevated blood glucose test results so that antidiabetic medication dosage can be adjusted.

• Emphasize the importance of regular physical examinations. Studies suggest that postmenopausal women who use estrogen replacement for more than 5 years to treat menopausal symptoms may be at increased risk for endometrial cancer. This risk is reduced by using cyclic rather than continuous therapy and the lowest possible dosages of estrogen. Adding progestins to the regimen decreases the incidence of endometrial hyperplasia; however, it isn't known if progestins affect the incidence of endometrial cancer. Most studies show no increased risk of breast cancer.

---

dienestrol (dienoestrol)
DV, Ortho Dienestrol

Pregnancy Risk Category: X

HOW SUPPLIED
Vaginal cream: 0.01%

ACTION
Unknown.

ONSET, PEAK, DURATION
Unknown.

INDICATIONS & DOSAGE
Atrophic vaginitis and kraurosis vulvae (short-term)—
Postmenopausal women: 1 to 2 intravaginal applications of vaginal cream daily for 1 to 2 weeks (as directed); then half that dose for the same period. Doctor may prescribe a maintenance dosage of 1 applicatorful one to three times a week.

ADVERSE REACTIONS
GU: vaginal discharge, increased intravaginal discomfort, uterine bleeding (with excessive use), burning sensation.
Other: systemic effects (breast tenderness, peripheral edema).

INTERACTIONS
Carbamazepine, phenobarbital, rifampin: decreased effectiveness of estrogen therapy. Monitor closely.
Corticosteroids: possible enhanced effects of corticosteroids. Monitor closely.
Cyclosporine: increased risk of toxicity. Use together with caution and frequently monitor cyclosporine levels.
Dantrolene, other hepatotoxic medications: increased risk of hepatotoxicity. Monitor closely.
Oral anticoagulants: dosage adjustments may be necessary. Monitor PT and INR.
Tamoxifen: estrogens may interfere with effectiveness of tamoxifen. Avoid concomitant use.

EFFECTS ON DIAGNOSTIC TESTS
Dienestrol increases sulfobromophthalein retention, PT and clotting factors VII to X, and norepinephrine-induced platelet aggregability. It decreases antithrombin III concentration.

Drug increases thyroid-binding globulin concentration; as a result, total thyroid concentration (measured by protein-bound iodine or total thyroxine) increases, and free triiodothyronine resin uptake decreases. Serum folate and pyridoxine concentrations may decrease; triglyceride, glucose, and phospholipid levels may increase. Glucose tolerance may be impaired. Pregnanediol excretion may decrease.

CONTRAINDICATIONS
Contraindicated in patients with active thrombophlebitis or thromboembolic disorders associated with estrogen therapy or past history of such events; in those with breast, reproductive organ, or genital cancer; or in those with undiag-

---

nosed abnormal genital bleeding and during pregnancy.

NURSING CONSIDERATIONS
● Use cautiously in patients with cerebral vascular or coronary artery disease, diabetes, hypertension, epilepsy, migraine; strong family history of breast cancer or who have breast nodules, fibrocystic disease, or abnormal mammograms; cardiac or renal dysfunction; history of depression; liver dysfunction; metabolic bone diseases; and young patients in whom bone growth is not complete.
● Ensure that patients have a thorough physical examination before initiating estrogen therapy. Patients receiving long-term therapy should have examinations yearly. Periodically monitor body weight, blood pressure, hepatic function, and serum lipid levels as ordered.
● Monitor closely. Systemic reactions may occur with normal intravaginal use.

☑ PATIENT TEACHING
● Tell patient that patient package insert that describes estrogen's adverse effects is available; however, also give patient verbal explanation.
● Instruct patient to apply drug at bedtime to increase effectiveness.
● Teach patient how to insert suppositories or cream, and tell her to wash vaginal area with soap and water before application.
● Instruct patient to remain recumbent for 30 minutes after administration to prevent loss of drug.
● Tell patient not to wear a tampon while receiving vaginal therapy. She may need to wear a sanitary pad to protect clothing.
● Instruct patient to report systemic reactions (breast pain or tenderness, swelling of the hands or feet) or vaginal discharge or bleeding.
● Teach women how to perform routine breast self-examination.
● Warn patient not to exceed the prescribed dosage.

● Inform patient withdrawal bleeding may occur if estrogen is suddenly stopped.

---

diethylstilbestrol (stilboestrol)
DES

diethylstilbestrol diphosphate
DES, Honvol†, Stilphostrol

Pregnancy Risk Category: X

HOW SUPPLIED
diethylstilbestrol
Tablets: 1 mg, 5 mg
diethylstilbestrol diphosphate
Tablets: 50 mg, 83 mg†
Injection: 50 mg/ml†

ACTION
Increases the synthesis of DNA, RNA, and protein in responsive tissues. Also reduces release of follicle-stimulating hormone and luteinizing hormone from the pituitary gland.

ONSET, PEAK, DURATION
Unknown.

INDICATIONS & DOSAGE
Prostate cancer—
Men: initially, 1 to 3 mg P.O. daily; may be reduced to 1 mg daily, or 50 mg P.O. diphosphate t.i.d. Then increased up to 200 mg or more as needed t.i.d. or 0.5 g I.V., followed by 1 g daily for 5 or more days as needed. Maintenance dosage 0.25 to 0.5 g I.V. once or twice weekly.
Metastatic, advanced breast cancer—
Men and postmenopausal women: 15 mg P.O. daily.

ADVERSE REACTIONS
CNS: headache, dizziness, chorea, depression, *seizures.*
CV: thrombophlebitis; *thromboembolism;* hypertension; edema; *increased*

---

risk of CVA, pulmonary embolism, MI.
EENT: worsening of myopia or astigmatism, intolerance of contact lenses.
GI: *nausea,* vomiting, abdominal cramps, bloating, anorexia, increased appetite, excessive thirst, weight changes, pancreatitis.
GU: in women—breakthrough bleeding, altered menstrual flow, dysmenorrhea, amenorrhea, cervical erosion, *increased risk of endometrial cancer, possibility of increased risk of breast cancer,* altered cervical secretions, enlargement of uterine fibromas, vaginal candidiasis, loss of libido; in men—gynecomastia, testicular atrophy, impotence.
Hepatic: cholestatic jaundice, *hepatic adenoma.*
Skin: melasma, urticaria, hirsutism or hair loss, erythema nodosum, dermatitis.
Other: breast tenderness or enlargement, hypercalcemia, gallbladder disease.

INTERACTIONS
Carbamazepine, phenobarbital, rifampin: decreased effectiveness of estrogen therapy. Monitor closely.
Corticosteroids: possible enhanced effects of corticosteroids. Monitor closely.
Cyclosporine: increased risk of toxicity. Use together with caution and frequently monitor cyclosporine levels.
Dantrolene, other hepatotoxic medications: increased risk of hepatotoxicity. Monitor closely.
Oral anticoagulants: dosage adjustments may be necessary. Monitor PT.
Tamoxifen: estrogens may interfere with effectiveness of tamoxifen. Avoid concomitant use.

EFFECTS ON DIAGNOSTIC TESTS
Diethylstilbestrol may cause increases in blood glucose levels, necessitating dosage adjustment of insulin or oral hypoglycemic drugs. Diethylstilbestrol increases sulfobromophthalein retention, prothrombin and clotting factors VII to X, and norepinephrine-induced platelet aggregability. Increases in thyroid-binding globulin concentrations may occur, resulting in increased total thyroid concentrations (measured by protein-bound iodine or total thyroxine) and decreased uptake of free triiodothyronine resin. Antithrombin III concentrations decrease; serum folate and pyridoxine concentrations and pregnanediol excretion may decrease; triglyceride, glucose, and phospholipid levels may increase. Glucose tolerance may be impaired.

CONTRAINDICATIONS
Contraindicated in men with known or suspected breast cancer except in selected patients being treated for metastatic disease, in patients with active thrombophlebitis or thromboembolic disorders, estrogen-dependent neoplasia, undiagnosed abnormal genital bleeding, during pregnancy, and history of thrombophlebitis, thrombosis, or thromboembolic disorders associated with estrogen use.

NURSING CONSIDERATIONS
● Use cautiously in patients with hypertension, mental depression, bone disease, migraine, seizures, diabetes mellitus, cardiac, hepatic, or renal dysfunction, and cerebrovascular or coronary artery disease.
● Ensure that patients have a physical examination before initiating therapy. Patients receiving long-term therapy should be examined yearly. Monitor weight, BP, hepatic function, and serum lipid levels.
Alert: Know that high incidence of gross nonmalignant genital changes may occur in offspring of women taking drug during pregnancy. Female offspring have a higher than normal risk of developing cervical and vaginal adenocarcinoma. Male offspring may have a higher than normal risk of developing testicular tumors, epididymal cysts, and impaired fertility.
● If patients experience GI upset, give

drug with or immediately after meals.
- **I.V. use:** Mix ordered dose in 250 to 500 ml of D₅W or 0.9% sodium chloride. Infuse at 1 to 2 ml/minute for the first 15 minutes; if no adverse reactions occur, increase infusion rate to administer entire dose within 1 hour.
- Notify the pathologist about any patients receiving estrogen therapy when specimens are obtained and sent to pathology for evaluation.
- Know that increased number of CV deaths reported in men taking diethylstilbestrol tablet (5 mg daily) for prostate cancer for a long time. This effect is not associated with 1-mg daily dose.
- Because of the risk of thromboembolism, know that therapy should be discontinued at least 1 month before procedures associated with prolonged immobilization or thromboembolism, such as knee or hip surgery.

☑ **PATIENT TEACHING**
- Tell patient that patient package insert that describes estrogen's adverse effects is available; however, also give patient verbal explanation.
- Tell patient not to crush, break, or chew enteric-coated tablets. Instruct patient to take with food if stomach upset occurs.

Alert: Warn patient to immediately report abdominal pain; pain, numbness, or stiffness in legs or buttocks; pressure or pain in chest; shortness of breath; severe headache; visual disturbances, such as blind spots, flashing lights, or blurriness; vaginal bleeding or discharge; breast lumps; sudden weight gain; swelling of hands or feet; yellow sclera or skin; dark urine; and light-colored stools.
- Teach women how to perform routine breast self-examination.
- Tell diabetic patient to report elevated blood glucose test results so that antidiabetic medication dosage can be adjusted.

esterified estrogens
Estratab, Menest, Neo-Estrone†

Pregnancy Risk Category: X

HOW SUPPLIED
Tablets: 0.3 mg, 0.625 mg, 1.25 mg, 2.5 mg
Tablets (film-coated): 0.3 mg, 0.625 mg, 1.25 mg, 2.5 mg

ACTION
Increases the synthesis of DNA, RNA, and protein in responsive tissues. Also reduces release of follicle-stimulating hormone and luteinizing hormone from the pituitary gland.

ONSET, PEAK, DURATION
Unknown.

INDICATIONS & DOSAGE
Inoperable prostate cancer—
Men: 1.25 to 2.5 mg P.O. t.i.d.
Breast cancer—
Men and postmenopausal women: 10 mg P.O. t.i.d. for 3 or more months.
Female hypogonadism—
Women: 2.5 to 7.5 mg a day in divided doses in cycles of 20 days on, 10 days off.
Castration, primary ovarian failure—
Women: 1.25 mg daily in cycles of 3 weeks on, 1 week off. Adjust for symptoms.
Vasomotor menopausal symptoms—
Women: average dosage is 1.25 mg P.O. daily in cycles of 3 weeks on, 1 week off.
Atrophic vaginitis and atrophic urethritis—
Women: 0.3 to 1.25 mg or more P.O. daily in cycles of 3 weeks on, 1 week off.

ADVERSE REACTIONS
CNS: headache, dizziness, chorea, depression, *seizures.*
CV: thrombophlebitis; *thromboembolism;* hypertension; edema; *increased*

risk of CVA, pulmonary embolism, MI.
EENT: worsening of myopia or astigmatism, intolerance of contact lenses.
GI: *nausea,* vomiting, abdominal cramps, bloating, anorexia, increased appetite, weight changes, pancreatitis.
GU: in women—breakthrough bleeding, altered menstrual flow, dysmenorrhea, amenorrhea, *increased risk of endometrial cancer, possibility of increased risk of breast cancer,* cervical erosion, altered cervical secretions, enlargement of uterine fibromas, vaginal candidiasis; in men—gynecomastia, testicular atrophy, impotence.
Hepatic: cholestatic jaundice, *hepatic adenoma.*
Skin: melasma, rash, hirsutism or hair loss, erythema nodosum, dermatitis.
Other: breast changes (tenderness, enlargement, secretion), gallbladder disease, hypercalcemia.

INTERACTIONS
Carbamazepine, phenobarbital, rifampin: decreased effectiveness of estrogen therapy. Monitor closely.
Corticosteroids: possible enhanced effects. Monitor closely.
Cyclosporine: increased risk of toxicity. Use together with caution and frequently monitor cyclosporine levels.
Dantrolene, other hepatotoxic medications: increased risk of hepatotoxicity. Monitor closely.
Oral anticoagulants: dosage adjustments may be necessary. Monitor PT and INR.
Tamoxifen: estrogens may interfere with effectiveness of tamoxifen. Avoid concomitant use.

EFFECTS ON DIAGNOSTIC TESTS
Therapy with esterified estrogens increases sulfobromophthalein retention, PT and clotting factors VII to X, and norepinephrine-induced platelet aggregability. Increases in the thyroid-binding globulin concentration may occur, resulting in increased total thyroid concentrations (measured by protein-bound iodine or total thyroxine) and decreased uptake of free triiodothyronine resin. Serum folate, pyridoxine, and antithrombin III concentrations may decrease; triglyceride, glucose, and phospholipid levels may increase. Glucose tolerance may be impaired. Pregnanediol excretion may decrease.

CONTRAINDICATIONS
Contraindicated in patients with breast cancer (except metastatic disease), estrogen-dependent neoplasia, active thrombophlebitis or thromboembolic disorders, undiagnosed abnormal genital bleeding, hypersensitivity to drug, history of thromboembolic disease, or during pregnancy.

NURSING CONSIDERATIONS
• Use cautiously in patients with history of hypertension, mental depression, cardiac or renal dysfunction, liver impairment, or bone diseases, migraine, seizures, or diabetes mellitus.
• Ensure that patients have a thorough physical examination before initiating estrogen therapy. Patients receiving long-term therapy should have repeat examinations yearly. Periodically monitor body weight, blood pressure, serum lipid levels, and hepatic function.
• Notify the pathologist about any patients receiving estrogen therapy when specimens are obtained and sent to pathology for evaluation.
• Because of the risk of thromboembolism, know that therapy should be discontinued at least 1 month before procedures associated with prolonged immobilization or thromboembolism, such as knee or hip surgery.

☑ **PATIENT TEACHING**
• Tell patient that patient package insert that describes estrogen's adverse effects is available; however, also give patient verbal explanation.
• Emphasize the importance of regular physical examinations. Studies suggest that postmenopausal women who use

---

estrogen replacement for more than 5 years to treat menopausal symptoms may be at increased risk for endometrial cancer. This risk is reduced by using cyclic rather than continuous therapy and the lowest possible dosages of estrogen. Adding progestins to the regimen decreases the incidence of endometrial hyperplasia; however, it isn't known if progestins affect the incidence of endometrial cancer. Most studies show no increased risk of breast cancer.

Alert: Warn patient to immediately report abdominal pain; pain, numbness, or stiffness in legs or buttocks; pressure or pain in chest; shortness of breath; severe headaches; visual disturbances, such as blind spots, flashing lights, or blurriness; vaginal bleeding or discharge; breast lumps; swelling of hands or feet; yellow skin or sclera; dark urine; and light-colored stools.

• Tell diabetic patient to report elevated blood glucose test results so that antidiabetic medication dosage can be adjusted.

• Explain to patient on cyclic therapy for postmenopausal symptoms that, although she may experience withdrawal bleeding during week off drug, fertility is not restored. Pregnancy cannot occur because patient does not ovulate.

• Teach women how to perform routine breast self-examination.

---

estradiol (oestradiol)
Climara, Estrace**, Estrace Vaginal Cream, Estraderm

estradiol cypionate
depGynogen, Depo-Estradiol, Dura-Estrin, E-Cypionate, Estro-Cyp, Estrofem, Estroject-L.A.

estradiol valerate (oestradiol valerate)
Climara Patch, Delestrogen, Dioval, Duragen-10, Duragen-20, Duragen-40, Estradiol L.A., Estra-L 20, Estra-L 40, Estraval, Estraval P.A., Feminate, Femogex, Gynogen L.A., L.A.E., Menaval, Primogyn Depot‡, Ru-Est-Span 20, Ru-Est-Span 40, Valergen-10, Valergen-20, Valergen-40

Pregnancy Risk Category: X

HOW SUPPLIED
estradiol
Tablets (micronized): 0.5 mg, 1 mg, 2 mg
Transdermal: 4 mg/10 cm² (delivers 0.05 mg/24 hours); 8 mg/20 cm² (delivers 0.1 mg/24 hours)
Vaginal cream (in nonliquefying base): 0.1 mg/g
estradiol cypionate
Injection (in oil): 1 mg/ml, 5 mg/ml
estradiol valerate
Injection (in oil): 10 mg/ml, 20 mg/ml, 40 mg/ml

ACTION
Increases the synthesis of DNA, RNA, and protein in responsive tissues. Also reduces release of follicle-stimulating hormone and luteinizing hormone from the pituitary gland.

ONSET, PEAK, DURATION
Unknown.

INDICATIONS & DOSAGE
Vasomotor menopausal symptoms, female hypogonadism, female castration, primary ovarian failure—
Adults: 1 to 2 mg P.O. (estradiol) daily in cycles of 21 days on and 7 days off, or cycles of 5 days on and 2 days off; or 1 transdermal system (Estraderm) delivering 0.05 mg/24 hours or as a system (Climara) delivering either 0.05 mg/24 hours or 0.1 mg/24 hours and applied once weekly in cycles of 3 weeks on and 1 week off. Alternatively, 1 to 5 mg (cypionate) I.M. q 3 to 4 weeks or 10 to 20 mg (valerate) I.M. q 4 weeks p.r.n.
Atrophic vaginitis, kraurosis vulvae—
Adults: 0.05 mg/24 hours (Estraderm) applied twice weekly in a cyclic regimen; or 0.05 mg/24 hours (Climara) applied weekly in a cyclic regimen; or 2 to

---

4 g intravaginal applications of cream daily for 1 to 2 weeks. When vaginal mucosa is restored, maintenance dosage is 1 g one to three times weekly in a cyclic regimen. Alternatively, 10 to 20 mg (valerate) I.M. q 4 weeks p.r.n.

Palliative treatment of advanced, inoperable breast cancer—

Men and postmenopausal women: 10 mg P.O. (estradiol) t.i.d. for 3 months.

Palliative treatment of advanced inoperable prostate cancer—

Men: 30 mg (valerate) I.M. q 1 to 2 weeks, or 1 to 2 mg P.O. (estradiol) t.i.d.

ADVERSE REACTIONS

CNS: headache, dizziness, chorea, depression, *seizures.*

CV: thrombophlebitis, *thromboembolism,* hypertension, edema.

EENT: worsening of myopia or astigmatism, intolerance of contact lenses.

GI: *nausea,* vomiting, abdominal cramps, bloating, increased appetite, weight changes, pancreatitis.

GU: in women—breakthrough bleeding, altered menstrual flow, dysmenorrhea, amenorrhea, *increased risk of endometrial cancer, possibility of increased risk of breast cancer,* cervical erosion, altered cervical secretions, enlargement of uterine fibromas, vaginal candidiasis; in men—gynecomastia, testicular atrophy, impotence.

Hepatic: cholestatic jaundice, *hepatic adenoma.*

Skin: melasma, urticaria, erythema nodosum, dermatitis, hair loss.

Other: breast changes (tenderness, enlargement, secretion), gallbladder disease, hypercalcemia.

INTERACTIONS

Carbamazepine, phenobarbital, rifampin: decreased effectiveness of estrogen therapy. Monitor closely.

Corticosteroids: possible enhanced effects of corticosteroids. Monitor closely.

Cyclosporine: increased risk of toxicity. Use together with caution and monitor cyclosporine levels frequently.

Dantrolene, other hepatotoxic medications: increased risk of hepatotoxicity. Monitor closely.

Oral anticoagulants: dosage adjustments may be necessary. Monitor PT and INR.

Tamoxifen: estrogens may interfere with effectiveness of tamoxifen. Avoid concomitant use.

EFFECTS ON DIAGNOSTIC TESTS

Estradiol increases sulfobromophthalein retention, PT and clotting factors VII to X, and norepinephrine-induced platelet aggregability, Increases in thyroid-binding globulin concentrations may occur, resulting in increased total thyroid concentrations (measured by protein-bound iodine or total thyroxine) and decreased uptake of free triiodothyronine resin. Serum folate, pyridoxine, and antithrombin III concentrations may decrease; triglyceride, glucose, and phospholipid levels may increase. Glucose tolerance may be impaired. Pregnanediol excretion may decrease.

CONTRAINDICATIONS

Contraindicated in patients with thrombophlebitis or thromboembolic disorders, estrogen-dependent neoplasia, breast or reproductive organ cancer (except for palliative treatment), or undiagnosed abnormal genital bleeding and during pregnancy. Also contraindicated in patients with history of thrombophlebitis or thromboembolic disorders associated with previous estrogen use (except for palliative treatment of breast and prostate cancer).

NURSING CONSIDERATIONS

● Use cautiously in patients with cerebrovascular or coronary artery disease; asthma; bone diseases; migraine; seizures; cardiac, hepatic or renal dysfunction; or in women with a strong family history of breast cancer or who have breast nodules, fibrocystic disease, or abnormal mammographic findings.

● Ensure that patients have a physical

examination before initiating therapy. Patients receiving long-term therapy should be examined yearly. Monitor serum lipid levels, BP, body weight, and hepatic function as ordered.

● Ask patients about allergies, especially to foods or plants. Estradiol is available as an aqueous solution or as a solution in peanut oil; estradiol cypionate, as a solution in cottonseed oil or vegetable oil; estradiol valerate, as a solution in castor oil, sesame oil, or vegetable oil.

● To administer as an I.M. injection, make sure drug is well dispersed in solution by rolling vial between palms. Inject deep I.M. into large muscle. Rotate injection sites to prevent muscle atrophy. Never give drug I.V.

● Apply the transdermal patch to clean, dry, hairless, intact skin on abdomen or buttocks. Do not apply it to breasts, waistline, or other areas where clothing can loosen the patch. When applying, ensure good contact with the skin, especially around the edges, and hold in place with the palm for about 10 seconds. Rotate application sites.

● Know that in women who are currently taking oral estrogen, treatment with the Estraderm transdermal patch can begin 1 week after withdrawal of oral therapy or sooner if menopausal symptoms appear before the end of the week.

● Because of the risk of thromboembolism, know that therapy should be discontinued at least 1 month before procedures associated with prolonged immobilization or thromboembolism, such as knee or hip surgery.

● Notify the pathologist about any patients receiving estrogen therapy when specimens are obtained and sent to pathology for evaluation.

☑ **PATIENT TEACHING**
● Tell patient that patient package insert that describes estrogen's adverse effects is available; however, also give patient verbal explanation.

● Emphasize the importance of regular physical examinations. Postmenopausal women who use estrogen replacement for more than 5 years may be at increased risk for endometrial cancer. This risk is reduced by using cyclic rather than continuous therapy and the lowest possible dosages of estrogen. Adding progestins to the regimen decreases the incidence of endometrial hyperplasia; however, it isn't known if progestins affect the incidence of endometrial cancer. Most studies show no increased risk of breast cancer.

● Tell patient how to use cream. Patient should wash vaginal area with soap and water before applying and take drug at bedtime or lie flat for 30 minutes after instillation to minimize drug loss.

Alert: Warn patient to immediately report abdominal pain; pain, numbness, or stiffness in legs or buttocks; pressure or pain in chest; shortness of breath; severe headaches; visual disturbances; vaginal bleeding or discharge; breast lumps; swelling of hands or feet; yellow skin or sclera; dark urine; and light-colored stools.

● Explain to patient on cyclic therapy for postmenopausal symptoms that, although withdrawal bleeding may occur during week off drug, fertility is not restored. Pregnancy cannot occur because patient does not ovulate.

● Tell diabetic patient to report elevated blood glucose test results so that antidiabetic medication dosage can be adjusted.

● Teach women how to perform routine breast self-examination.

---

estrogens, conjugated (estrogenic substances, conjugated; oestrogens, conjugated)
C.E.S.†, Premarin, Premarin Intravenous

Pregnancy Risk Category: X

HOW SUPPLIED
Tablets: 0.3 mg, 0.625 mg, 0.9 mg, 1.25 mg, 2.5 mg

Injection: 25 mg/5 ml
Vaginal cream: 0.625 mg/g

ACTION
Increases the synthesis of DNA, RNA, and protein in responsive tissues. Also reduces release of follicle-stimulating hormone and luteinizing hormone from the pituitary gland.

ONSET, PEAK, DURATION
Unknown.

INDICATIONS & DOSAGE
Abnormal uterine bleeding (hormonal imbalance)—
Women: 25 mg I.V. or I.M., repeated in 6 to 12 hours as needed.
Palliative treatment of breast cancer (at least 5 years after menopause)—
Men and postmenopausal women: 10 mg P.O. t.i.d. for 3 months or more.
Female castration, primary ovarian failure—
Women: 1.25 mg P.O. daily in cycles of 3 weeks on and 1 week off.
Osteoporosis—
Postmenopausal women: 0.625 mg P.O. daily in cyclic regimen (3 weeks on, 1 week off)
Hypogonadism—
Women: 2.5 mg P.O. daily, b.i.d., or t.i.d. for 20 consecutive days each month.
Vasomotor menopausal symptoms—
Women: 0.3 to 1.25 mg P.O. daily in cycles of 3 weeks on and 1 week off.
Atrophic vaginitis, kraurosis vulvae—
Women: 0.5 to 2 g intravaginally once daily on a cyclical basis (3 weeks on and 1 week off).
Palliative treatment of inoperable prostate cancer—
Men: 1.25 to 2.5 mg P.O. t.i.d.

ADVERSE REACTIONS
CNS: headache, dizziness, chorea, depression, *seizures.*
CV: thrombophlebitis; *thromboembolism;* hypertension; edema; *increased risk of CVA, pulmonary embolism, MI.*

EENT: worsening of myopia or astigmatism, intolerance of contact lenses.
GI: *nausea,* vomiting, abdominal cramps, bloating, anorexia, increased appetite, weight changes, pancreatitis.
GU: in women—breakthrough bleeding, altered menstrual flow, dysmenorrhea, amenorrhea, *increased risk of endometrial cancer, possibility of increased risk of breast cancer,* cervical erosion, altered cervical secretions, enlargement of uterine fibromas, vaginal candidiasis; in men—gynecomastia, testicular atrophy, impotence.
Hepatic: cholestatic jaundice, *hepatic adenoma.*
Skin: melasma, urticaria, flushing (with rapid I.V. administration), hirsutism or hair loss, erythema nodosum, dermatitis.
Other: breast changes (tenderness, enlargement, secretion), hypercalcemia, gallbladder disease.

INTERACTIONS
Carbamazepine, phenobarbital, rifampin: decreased effectiveness of estrogen therapy. Monitor closely.
Corticosteroids: possible enhanced effects of corticosteroids. Monitor closely.
Cyclosporine: increased risk of toxicity. Use together with caution and frequently monitor cyclosporine levels.
Dantrolene, other hepatotoxic medications: increased risk of hepatotoxicity. Monitor closely.
Oral anticoagulants: dosage adjustments may be necessary. Monitor PT and INR.
Tamoxifen: estrogens may interfere with effectiveness of tamoxifen. Avoid concomitant use.

EFFECTS ON DIAGNOSTIC TESTS
Therapy with estrogens increases sulfobromophthalein retention, PT and clotting factors VII to X, and norepinephrine-induced platelet aggregability. Increases in thyroid-binding globulin concentration may occur, resulting in increased total thyroid concentration (measured by protein-bound iodine or

---

total thyroxine) and decreased uptake of free triiodothyronine resin. Serum folate, pyridoxine, and antithrombin III concentrations may decrease; triglyceride, glucose, and phospholipid levels may increase. Glucose tolerance may be impaired. Pregnanediol excretion may decrease.

CONTRAINDICATIONS
Contraindicated in patients with thrombophlebitis or thromboembolic disorders, estrogen-dependent neoplasia, breast or reproductive organ cancer (except for palliative treatment), or undiagnosed abnormal genital bleeding and during pregnancy.

NURSING CONSIDERATIONS
• Use cautiously in patients with cerebrovascular or coronary artery disease; asthma; bone disease; migraine; seizures; cardiac, hepatic, or renal dysfunction; or in women with family history (mother, grandmother, sister) of breast or genital tract cancer or who have breast nodules, fibrocystic disease, or abnormal mammographic findings.
• Ensure that patients have a thorough physical examination before initiating estrogen therapy. Patients receiving long-term therapy should have examinations yearly. Periodically monitor serum lipid levels, blood pressure, body weight, and hepatic function, as ordered.
• Know that I.M. or I.V. use preferred for rapid treatment of dysfunctional uterine bleeding or reduction of surgical bleeding.
• Refrigerate before reconstituting. Agitate gently after adding diluent.
• **I.V. use:** When giving by direct I.V. injection, administer slowly to avoid flushing reaction. For infusion, mix with D_5W, 0.9% sodium chloride for injection, or invert sugar solutions. Avoid mixing with solutions of acidic pH to prevent incompatibility.
• When administering by I.M. injection, inject deeply into large muscle. Rotate injection sites to prevent muscle atrophy.

• Notify the pathologist about any patients receiving estrogen therapy when specimens are obtained and sent to pathology for evaluation.
• Because of the risk of thromboembolism, know that therapy should be discontinued at least 1 month before procedures associated with prolonged immobilization or thromboembolism, such as knee or hip surgery.

☑ PATIENT TEACHING
• Tell patient that package insert describing estrogen's adverse effects is available; also explain effects.
• Emphasize the importance of regular physical examinations. Studies suggest that postmenopausal women who use estrogen replacement for more than 5 years to treat menopausal symptoms may be at increased risk for endometrial cancer. This risk is reduced by using cyclic rather than continuous therapy and the lowest possible dosages of estrogen. Adding progestins to the regimen decreases the incidence of endometrial hyperplasia; however, it isn't known if progestins affect the incidence of endometrial cancer. Most studies show no increased risk of breast cancer.
• Teach patient how to use vaginal cream. Patient should wash the vaginal area with soap and water before applying. Tell her to use drug at bedtime or to lie flat for 30 minutes after instillation to minimize drug loss.
• Explain to patient on cyclic therapy for postmenopausal symptoms that, although withdrawal bleeding may occur during week off drug, fertility is not restored. Pregnancy cannot occur because she does not ovulate.
Alert: Warn patient to immediately report abdominal pain; pain, numbness, or stiffness in legs or buttocks; pressure or pain in chest; shortness of breath; severe headaches; visual disturbances, such as blind spots, flashing lights, or blurriness; vaginal bleeding or discharge; breast lumps; swelling of hands or feet; yellow skin or sclera; dark urine; and

---

Reactions may be *common*, uncommon, *life-threatening*, or COMMON AND LIFE-THREATENING.

light-colored stools.
● Tell diabetic patient to report elevated blood glucose test results so that antidiabetic medication dosage can be adjusted.
● Teach women how to perform routine breast self-examination.

estropipate (piperazine estrone sulfate)
Ogen, OrthoEST

Pregnancy Risk Category: X

HOW SUPPLIED
Tablets: 0.75 mg, 1.5 mg, 3 mg, 6 mg
Vaginal cream: 1.5 mg/g

ACTION
Increases the synthesis of DNA, RNA, and proteins in responsive tissues. Also reduces release of follicle-stimulating hormone and luteinizing hormone from the pituitary gland.

ONSET, PEAK, DURATION
Unknown.

INDICATIONS & DOSAGE
Vulval and vaginal atrophy—
Women: 0.625 to 5 mg P.O. daily 3 weeks on, 1 week off, or 2 to 4 g of vaginal cream daily. Typically, dosage given on a cyclical, short-term basis.
Primary ovarian failure, female castration, female hypogonadism—
Women: administered on a cyclical basis—1.5 to 7.5 mg P.O. daily for the first 3 weeks, followed by a rest period of 8 to 10 days. If bleeding does not occur by the end of the rest period, cycle repeated.
Vasomotor menopausal symptoms—
Women: 0.625 mg to 5 mg P.O. daily in cyclic method of 3 weeks on, 1 week off.
Prevention of osteoporosis—
Women: 0.625 mg P.O. daily for 25 days of a 31-day cycle.

ADVERSE REACTIONS
CNS: depression, headache, dizziness, migraine, *seizures.*
CV: edema; thrombophlebitis; *increased risk of CVA, pulmonary embolism, MI; thromboembolism.*
GI: nausea, vomiting, abdominal cramps, bloating, weight changes.
GU: increased size of uterine fibromas, *increased risk of endometrial cancer, possibility of increased risk of breast cancer,* vaginal candidiasis, cystitis-like syndrome, dysmenorrhea, amenorrhea, breakthrough bleeding, condition resembling premenstrual syndrome.
Hepatic: cholestatic jaundice, *hepatic adenoma.*
Skin: hemorrhagic eruption, erythema nodosum, *erythema multiforme,* hirsutism, melasma, hair loss.
Other: breast engorgement or enlargement, hypercalcemia, gallbladder disease, aggravation of porphyria, libido changes.

INTERACTIONS
Carbamazepine, phenobarbital, rifampin: decreased effectiveness of estrogen therapy. Monitor closely.
Corticosteroids: possible enhanced effects of corticosteroids. Monitor closely.
Cyclosporine: increased risk of toxicity. Use together with caution and frequently monitor cyclosporine levels.
Dantrolene, other hepatotoxic medications: increased risk of hepatotoxicity. Monitor closely.
Oral anticoagulants: dosage adjustments may be necessary. Monitor PT and INR.
Tamoxifen: estrogens may interfere with effectiveness of tamoxifen. Avoid concomitant use.

EFFECTS ON DIAGNOSTIC TESTS
Therapy with estrogens increases sulfobromophthalein retention, PT and clotting factors VII to X, and norepinephrine-induced platelet aggregability. Increases in thyroid-binding globulin concentration may occur, resulting in increased total thyroid concentration (measured by protein-bound iodine or

total thyroxine) and decreased uptake of free triiodothyronine resin. Serum folate, pyridoxine, and antithrombin III concentrations may decrease; triglyceride, glucose, and phospholipid levels may increase. Glucose tolerance may be impaired. Pregnanediol excretion may decrease.

CONTRAINDICATIONS
Contraindicated in patients with active thrombophlebitis or thromboembolic disorders; in those with estrogen-dependent neoplasia, breast, reproductive organ, or genital cancer; in those with undiagnosed genital bleeding; and during pregnancy.

NURSING CONSIDERATIONS
● Use cautiously in patients with cerebrovascular or coronary artery disease; asthma; mental depression; bone disease; migraine; seizures; cardiac, hepatic, or renal dysfunction; and in women with a family history (mother, grandmother, sister) of breast or genital tract cancer or who have breast nodules, fibrocystic disease, or abnormal mammographic findings.
● Ensure that patients have a thorough physical examination before initiating estrogen therapy. Patients receiving long-term therapy should have examinations yearly. Periodically monitor serum lipid levels, blood pressure, body weight, and hepatic function as ordered.
● Know that when used to treat hypogonadism, the duration of therapy necessary to produce withdrawal bleeding depends on the patient's endometrial response to the drug. If satisfactory withdrawal bleeding does not occur, an oral progestin is added to the regimen, as ordered. Explain to the patient that, despite the return of withdrawal bleeding, pregnancy cannot occur because she does not ovulate.
● Be aware of the following estropipate/estrone equivalents:

0.75 mg estropipate	=	0.625 mg estrone
1.5 mg estropipate	=	1.25 mg estrone
3 mg estropipate	=	2.5 mg estrone
6 mg estropipate	=	5 mg estrone

● Because of the risk of thromboembolism, know that therapy should be discontinued at least 1 month before procedures associated with prolonged immobilization or thromboembolism, such as knee or hip surgery.

☑ PATIENT TEACHING
● Tell patient that package insert describing estrogen's adverse effects is available; also explain effects.
● Stress the importance of regular physical examinations. Postmenopausal women who use estrogen replacement for more than 5 years may be at increased risk for endometrial cancer. This risk is reduced by using cyclic rather than continuous therapy and the lowest possible dosages of estrogen. Adding progestins to the regimen decreases the incidence of endometrial hyperplasia; however, it isn't known if progestins affect the incidence of endometrial cancer. Most studies show no increased risk of breast cancer.
Alert: Warn patient to immediately report abdominal pain; pain, stiffness, or numbness in the legs or buttocks; pressure or pain in the chest; shortness of breath; severe headaches; visual disturbances, such as blind spots or flashing lights; vaginal bleeding or discharge; breast lumps; swelling of the hands or feet; yellow skin or sclera; dark urine; and light-colored stools.
● Teach women how to perform routine breast self-examination.

ethinyl estradiol (ethinyloestradiol)
Estinyl**, Feminone

Pregnancy Risk Category: X

HOW SUPPLIED
Tablets: 0.02 mg, 0.05 mg, 0.5 mg

ACTION
Increases the synthesis of DNA, RNA, and protein in responsive tissues. Also reduces release of follicle-stimulating hormone and luteinizing hormone from the pituitary gland.

ONSET, PEAK, DURATION
Unknown.

INDICATIONS & DOSAGE
Palliative treatment of metastatic breast cancer (at least 5 years after menopause)—
Women: 1 mg P.O. t.i.d. for at least 3 months.
Female hypogonadism—
Women: 0.05 mg P.O. once daily to t.i.d. 2 weeks a month, followed by 2 weeks of progesterone therapy; continued for three to six monthly dosing cycles, followed by 2 months off.
Vasomotor menopausal symptoms—
Women: 0.02 to 0.05 mg P.O. daily for cycles of 3 weeks on and 1 week off.
Palliative treatment of metastatic inoperable prostate cancer—
Men: 0.15 to 2 mg P.O. daily.

ADVERSE REACTIONS
CNS: headache, dizziness, chorea, depression, *seizures.*
CV: thrombophlebitis; *thromboembolism;* hypertension; edema, *increased risk of CVA, pulmonary embolism, MI.*
EENT: worsening of myopia or astigmatism, intolerance to contact lenses.
GI: *nausea,* vomiting, abdominal cramps, bloating, anorexia, increased appetite, weight changes.
GU: in women—breakthrough bleeding, altered menstrual flow, dysmenorrhea, amenorrhea, cervical erosion, *increased risk of endometrial cancer, possibility of increased risk of breast cancer,* altered cervical secretions, enlargement of uterine fibromas, vaginal candidiasis; in men—gynecomastia, tes-

ticular atrophy, impotence.
Hepatic: cholestatic jaundice, *hepatic adenoma.*
Skin: melasma, urticaria, acne, seborrhea, oily skin, hirsutism or hair loss, erythema nodosum, dermatitis.
Other: breast changes (tenderness, enlargement, secretion), hypercalcemia, gallbladder disease.

INTERACTIONS
Carbamazepine, phenobarbital, rifampin: decreased effectiveness of estrogen therapy. Monitor closely.
Corticosteroids: possible enhanced effects of corticosteroids. Monitor closely.
Cyclosporine: increased risk of toxicity. Use together with caution and frequently monitor cyclosporine levels.
Dantrolene, other hepatotoxic medications: increased risk of hepatotoxicity. Monitor closely.
Oral anticoagulants: dosage adjustments may be necessary. Monitor PT and INR.
Tamoxifen: estrogens may interfere with effectiveness of tamoxifen. Avoid concomitant use.

EFFECTS ON DIAGNOSTIC TESTS
Therapy with ethinyl estradiol increases sulfobromophthalein retention, PT and clotting factors VII to X, and norepinephrine-induced platelet aggregability. Increases in thyroid-binding globulin concentration may occur, resulting in increased total thyroid concentration (measured by protein-bound iodine or total thyroxine) and decreased uptake of free triiodothyronine resin. Serum folate, pyridoxine, and antithrombin III concentrations may decrease; triglyceride, glucose, and phospholipid levels may increase. Glucose tolerance may be impaired. Pregnanediol excretion may decrease.

CONTRAINDICATIONS
Contraindicated in patients with throm-

bophlebitis or thromboembolic disorders, estrogen-dependent neoplasia, breast or reproductive organ cancer (except for palliative treatment), or undiagnosed abnormal genital bleeding and during pregnancy.

NURSING CONSIDERATIONS
● Use cautiously in patients with cerebrovascular or coronary artery disease; asthma; mental depression; bone disease; cardiac, hepatic, or renal dysfunction; or in women with a family history (mother, grandmother, sister) of breast or genital tract cancer, or who have breast nodules, fibrocystic disease, or abnormal mammographic findings.
● Ensure that patients have a thorough physical examination before initiating estrogen therapy. Patients receiving long-term therapy should have examinations yearly. Periodically monitor serum lipid levels, blood pressure, body weight, and hepatic function as ordered.
● Because of the risk of thromboembolism, know that therapy should be discontinued at least 1 month before procedures associated with prolonged immobilization or thromboembolism, such as knee or hip surgery.
● Notify the pathologist about any patients receiving estrogen therapy when specimens are obtained and sent to pathology for evaluation.

☑ PATIENT TEACHING
● Tell patient that patient package insert that describes estrogen's adverse effects is available; however, also give patient verbal explanation.
● Emphasize the importance of regular physical examinations. Studies suggest that postmenopausal women who use estrogen replacement for more than 5 years to treat menopausal symptoms may be at increased risk for endometrial cancer. This risk is reduced by using cyclic rather than continuous therapy and the lowest possible dosages of estrogen. Adding progestins to the regimen decreases the incidence of endome-

trial hyperplasia; however, it isn't known if progestins affect the incidence of endometrial cancer. Most studies show no increased risk of breast cancer.
● Explain to patient on cyclic therapy for postmenopausal symptoms that, although withdrawal bleeding may occur during week off drug, fertility is not restored. Pregnancy cannot occur because patient does not ovulate.
Alert: Warn patient to immediately report abdominal pain; pain, numbness, or stiffness in legs or buttocks; pressure or pain in chest; shortness of breath; severe headaches; visual disturbances, such as blind spots, flashing lights, or blurriness; vaginal bleeding or discharge; breast lumps; swelling of hands or feet; yellow skin or sclera; dark urine; or light-colored stools.
● Tell diabetic patient to report elevated blood glucose test results so that antidiabetic medication dosage can be adjusted.
● Teach women how to perform routine breast self-examination.

ethinyl estradiol and desogestrel
monophasic: Desogen, Ortho-Cept

ethinyl estradiol and ethynodiol diacetate
monophasic: Demulen 1/35, Demulen 1/50

ethinyl estradiol and levonorgestrel
monophasic: Levlen, Nordette
triphasic: Tri-Levlen, Triphasil

ethinyl estradiol and norethindrone
monophasic: Brevicon, Genora 0.5/35, Genora 1/35, ModiCon, N.E.E. 1/35, Nelova 0.5/35 E, Nelova 1/35 E, Norcept-E 1/35, Norethin 1/35 E, Norinyl 1+35, Ortho-Novum 1/35, Ovcon-35, Ovcon-50
biphasic: Jenset-28, Nelova 10/11, Ortho-Novum 10/11

triphasic: Ortho-Novum 7/7/7, Tri-Norinyl

ethinyl estradiol and norethindrone acetate
monophasic: Loestrin 21 1/20, Loestrin 21 1.5/30, Norlestrin 21 1/50, Norlestrin 21 2.5/50

ethinyl estradiol and norgestimate
monophasic: Ortho Cyclen
triphasic: Ortho Tri-Cyclen

ethinyl estradiol and norgestrel
monophasic: Lo/Ovral, Ovral

ethinyl estradiol, norethindrone acetate, and ferrous fumarate
monophasic: Loestrin Fe 1/20, Loestrin Fe 1.5/30, Norlestrin Fe 1 50, Norlestrin Fe 2.5/50

mestranol and norethindrone
monophasic: Genora 1/50, Nelova 1/50 M, Norethin 1/50 M, Norinyl 1+50, Ortho-Novum 1/50

mestranol and norethynodrel
monophasic: Enovid 5 mg, Enovid 10 mg

Pregnancy Risk Category: X

HOW SUPPLIED
Monophasic oral contraceptives
ethinyl estradiol and desogestrel
Tablets: ethinyl estradiol 30 mcg and desogestrel 0.15 mg (Desogen, Ortho-Cept)
ethinyl estradiol and ethynodiol diacetate
Tablets: ethinyl estradiol 35 mcg and ethynodiol diacetate 1 mg (Demulen 1/35); ethinyl estradiol 50 mcg and ethynodiol diacetate 1 mg (Demulen 1/50)
ethinyl estradiol and levonorgestrel
Tablets: ethinyl estradiol 30 mcg and

levonorgestrel 0.15 mg (Levlen, Nordette)
ethinyl estradiol and norethindrone
Tablets: ethinyl estradiol 35 mcg and norethindrone 0.4 mg (Ovcon-35); ethinyl estradiol 35 mcg and norethindrone 0.5 mg (Brevicon, Genora 0.5|35, ModiCon, Nelova 0.5/35 E); ethinyl estradiol 35 mcg and norethindrone 1 mg (Genora 1/35, N.E.E. 1/35, Nelova 1/35 E, Norcept-E 1/35, Norethin 1/35 E, Norinyl 1+35, Ortho-Novum 1/35); ethinyl estradiol 50 mcg and norethindrone 1 mg (Ovcon-50)
ethinyl estradiol and norethindrone acetate
Tablets: ethinyl estradiol 20 mcg and norethindrone acetate 1 mg (Loestrin 21 1/20); ethinyl estradiol 30 mcg and norethindrone acetate 1.5 mg (Loestrin 21 1.5/30); ethinyl estradiol 50 mcg and norethindrone acetate 1 mg (Norlestrin 21 1/50); ethinyl estradiol 50 mcg and norethindrone acetate 2.5 mg (Norlestrin 21 2.5/50)
ethinyl estradiol and norgestimate
Tablets: ethinyl estradiol 35 mcg and norgestimate 0.25 mg (Ortho Cyclen)
ethinyl estradiol and norgestrel
Tablets: ethinyl estradiol 30 mcg and norgestrel 0.3 mg (Lo/Ovral); ethinyl estradiol 50 mcg and norgestrel 0.5 mg (Ovral)
ethinyl estradiol, norethindrone acetate, and ferrous fumarate
Tablets: ethinyl estradiol 20 mcg, norethindrone acetate 1 mg, and ferrous fumarate 75 mg (Loestrin Fe 1/20); ethinyl estradiol 30 mcg, norethindrone acetate 1.5 mg, and ferrous fumarate 75 mg (Loestrin Fe 1.5/30); ethinyl estradiol 50 mcg, norethindrone acetate 1 mg, and ferrous fumarate 75 mg (Norlestrin Fe 1/50); ethinyl estradiol 50 mcg, norethindrone acetate 2.5 mg, and ferrous fumarate 75 mg (Norlestrin Fe 2.5/50)
mestranol and norethindrone
Tablets: mestranol 50 mcg and norethindrone 1 mg (Genora 1/50, Nelova 1/50 M, Norethin 1/50 M, Norinyl 1+50, Or-

---

*Liquid contains alcohol.   **May contain tartrazine.   †Canada only.   ‡Australia only.   ◊ OTC.

tho-Novum 1/50)

mestranol and norethynodrel

Tablets: mestranol 75 mg and norethynodrel 5 mg (Enovid 5 mg); mestranol 150 mg and norethynodrel 9.85 mg (Enovid 10 mg).

Biphasic oral contraceptives
ethinyl estradiol and norethindrone

Tablets: ethinyl estradiol 35 mcg and norethindrone 0.5 mg during phase 1 [10 days]; ethinyl estradiol 35 mcg and norethindrone 1 mg during phase 2 [11 days] (Jenset-28, Nelova 10/11, Ortho-Novum 10/11)

Triphasic oral contraceptives
ethinyl estradiol and levonorgestrel

Tablets: (Tri-Levlen, Triphasil) ethinyl estradiol 35 mcg and levonorgestrel 0.05 mg during phase 1 [6 days]; ethinyl estradiol 35 mcg and levonorgestrel 0.075 mg during phase 2 [5 days]; ethinyl estradiol 35 mcg and levonorgestrel 0.125 mg during phase 3 [10 days]

ethinyl estradiol and norethindrone

Tablets: (Tri-Norinyl) ethinyl estradiol 35 mcg and norethindrone 0.5 mg during phase 1 [7 days]; ethinyl estradiol 35 mcg and norethindrone 1 mg during phase 2 [9 days]; ethinyl estradiol 35 mcg and norethindrone 0.5 mg during phase 3 [5 days]; (Ortho-Novum 7/7/7) ethinyl estradiol 35 mcg and norethindrone 0.5 mg during phase 1 [7 days]; ethinyl estradiol 35 mcg and norethindrone 0.75 mg during phase 2 [7 days]; ethinyl estradiol 35 mcg and norethindrone 1 mg during phase 3 [7 days]

Tablets: (Ortho Tri-Cyclen) ethinyl estradiol 35 mcg and norgestimate 0.18 mg during phase 1 [7 days]; ethinyl estradiol 35 mcg and norgestimate 0.215 mg during phase 2 [7 days]; ethinyl estradiol 35 mcg and norgestimate 0.25 mg during phase 3 [7 days]

ACTION

Oral contraceptives inhibit ovulation through a negative feedback mechanism directed at the hypothalamus. They also may prevent transport of the ovum through the fallopian tubes.

Estrogen suppresses secretion of follicle-stimulating hormone, blocking follicular development and ovulation.

Progestin suppresses secretion of luteinizing hormone so ovulation cannot occur even if the follicle develops. Progestin thickens cervical mucus, which interferes with sperm migration, and also causes endometrial changes that prevent implantation of the fertilized ovum.

ONSET, PEAK, DURATION

Onset and duration unknown. Plasma levels of ethinyl estradiol peak within 1 to 2 hours; of norethindrone, within ½ to 4 hours.

INDICATIONS & DOSAGE

Contraception—

Adults: *Monophasic oral contraceptives—*1 tablet P.O. daily, beginning on day 5 of menstrual cycle (first day of menstrual flow is day 1). With 20- and 21-tablet packages, new dosing cycle begins 7 days after last tablet taken. With 28-tablet packages, dosage is 1 tablet daily without interruption; extra tablets are placebos or contain iron.

Biphasic oral contraceptives—
1 color tablet P.O. daily for 10 days; then next color tablet for 11 days. With 21-tablet packages, new dosing cycle begins 7 days after last tablet taken. With 28-tablet packages, dosage is 1 tablet daily without interruption.

*Triphasic oral contraceptives—*1 tablet P.O. daily in the sequence specified by the brand. With 21-tablet packages, new dosing cycle begins 7 days after last tablet taken. With 28-tablet packages, dosage is 1 tablet daily without interruption.

Endometriosis—

Adults: 1 tablet Enovid 5 mg or 10 mg P.O. daily for 2 weeks starting on day 5 of menstrual cycle. Continued without interruption for 6 to 9 months, increasing dosage by 5 to 10 mg q 2 weeks, up to 20 mg daily; up to 40 mg daily as needed and ordered if breakthrough bleeding occurs.

ADVERSE REACTIONS

CNS: *headache, dizziness,* depression, lethargy, migraine.
CV: *thromboembolism,* hypertension, edema, *pulmonary embolism, CVA.*
EENT: worsening of myopia or astigmatism, intolerance of contact lenses, exophthalmos, diplopia.
GI: *nausea,* vomiting, abdominal cramps, bloating, anorexia, changes in appetite, weight gain, *bowel ischemia,* pancreatitis.
GU: *breakthrough bleeding,* granulomatous colitis, dysmenorrhea, amenorrhea, cervical erosion or abnormal secretions, enlargement of uterine fibromas, vaginal candidiasis.
Hepatic: gallbladder disease, cholestatic jaundice, *liver tumors.*
Skin: rash, acne, *erythema multiforme.*
Other: breast changes tenderness, enlargement, secretion); hypercalcemia.

INTERACTIONS

Carbamazepine, phenobarbital, phenytoin, rifampin: decreased effectiveness of estrogen therapy. Monitor closely.
Corticosteroids: possible enhanced effects of corticosteroids. Monitor closely.
Griseofulvin, penicillins, sulfonamides, tetracyclines: may decrease effectiveness of oral contraceptives. Avoid concomitant use, if possible.
Oral anticoagulants: dosage adjustments may be necessary. Monitor PT and INR.
Tamoxifen: estrogens may interfere with effectiveness of tamoxifen. Avoid concomitant use.

EFFECTS ON DIAGNOSTIC TESTS

Therapy with ethinyl estradiol increases sulfobromophthalein retention, PT and clotting factors VII to X, and norepinephrine-induced platelet aggregability. Increases in thyroid-binding globulin concentration may occur, resulting in increased total thyroid concentration (measured by protein-bound iodine or total thyroxine) and decreased uptake of free triiodothyronine resin. Serum folate, pyridoxine, and antithrombin III concentrations may decrease; triglyceride, glucose, and phospholipid levels may increase. Glucose tolerance may be impaired. Pregnanediol excretion may decrease.

CONTRAINDICATIONS

Contraindicated in patients with thromboembolic disorders, cerebrovascular or coronary artery disease, diplopia or any ocular lesion arising from ophthalmic vascular disease, classical migraine, MI, known or suspected breast cancer, known or suspected estrogen-dependent neoplasia, benign or malignant liver tumors, active liver disease or history of cholestatic jaundice with pregnancy or prior use of oral contraceptives, and undiagnosed abnormal vaginal bleeding; in known or suspected pregnancy; and in breast-feeding patients.

NURSING CONSIDERATIONS

● Use cautiously in patients with cardiac, renal, or hepatic insufficiency; hyperlipidemia; hypertension; migraine; seizure disorders; or asthma.
● Be aware that triphasic oral contraceptives may cause fewer adverse reactions, such as breakthrough bleeding and spotting.
● Know that the Centers for Disease Control and Prevention reports that the use of oral contraceptives *may decrease* the incidence of ovarian and endometrial cancers. Also, oral contraceptives do not appear to increase a woman's risk of breast cancer. However, the FDA reports that oral contraceptives may be linked to an increased risk of cervical cancer.
● Monitor serum lipid levels, BP, body weight, and hepatic function as ordered.
● Know that many laboratory tests are affected by oral contraceptives.
● Estrogens and progestins may alter glucose tolerance, thus changing dosage requirements for antidiabetic drugs. Monitor blood glucose levels.
● Discontinue if patients develop granulomatous colitis while on oral contra-

ceptives and notify doctor.

• Know that drug should be discontinued at least 1 week before surgery to decrease risk of thromboembolism. Tell patient to use an alternative method of birth control.

☑ **PATIENT TEACHING**

• Tell patient to take tablets at same time each day; nighttime dosing may reduce nausea and headaches.

• Advise patient to use an additional method of birth control, such as condoms or a diaphragm with spermicide, for the first week of administration in the initial cycle.

• Tell patient missed doses in midcycle greatly increase likelihood of pregnancy.

• If one tablet is missed, tell patient to take it as soon as she remembers or to take two tablets the next day and continue regular schedule. If patient misses 2 consecutive days, instruct her to take two tablets daily for 2 days and then resume normal schedule. Also advise her to use an additional method of birth control for 7 days after two missed doses. If three or more doses are missed, tell patient to discard remaining tablets in monthly package and to substitute another contraceptive method. If next menstrual period doesn't begin on schedule, warn patient to rule out pregnancy before starting new dosing cycle. If menstrual period begins, have patient start new dosing cycle 7 days after last tablet was taken.

• Warn patient that headache, nausea, dizziness, breast tenderness, spotting, and breakthrough bleeding are common at first. These effects should diminish after three to six dosing cycles (months).

• Instruct patient to weigh herself at least twice a week and to report any sudden weight gain or edema to the doctor.

• Warn patient to avoid exposure to ultraviolet light or prolonged exposure to sunlight.

Alert: Warn patient to immediately report abdominal pain; numbness, stiffness, or pain in legs or buttocks; pressure or pain in chest; shortness of breath; severe headache; visual disturbances, such as blind spots, blurriness, or flashing lights; undiagnosed vaginal bleeding or discharge; two consecutive, missed menstrual periods; lumps in the breast; swelling of hands or feet; or severe pain in the abdomen (tumor rupture in the liver).

• Advise patient of increased risks associated with simultaneous use of cigarettes and oral contraceptives.

• If one menstrual period is missed and tablets have been taken on schedule, tell patient to continue taking them. If two consecutive menstrual periods are missed, tell patient to stop drug and have pregnancy test. Progestins may cause birth defects if taken early in pregnancy.

• Advise patient not to take same drug for longer than 12 months without consulting the doctor. Stress importance of Papanicolaou tests and annual gynecologic examinations.

• Advise patient to check with the doctor about how soon pregnancy may be attempted after hormonal therapy is stopped. Many doctors recommend that women not become pregnant within 2 months after stopping drug.

• Warn patient of possible delay in achieving pregnancy when drug is discontinued.

• Tell patient many doctors advise women on long-term therapy (5 years or longer) to stop drug and use other birth control methods. Periodically reassess patient while off hormone therapy.

• Teach patient how to perform routine breast self-examination.

---

hydroxyprogesterone caproate

Delta-Lutin, Duralutin, Gesterol L.A. 250, Hy/Gestrone, Hylutin, Hyprogest 250, Pro-Depo, Prodrox 250, Pro-Span

Pregnancy Risk Category: X

HOW SUPPLIED
Injection: 125 mg/ml, 250 mg/ml

ACTION
Suppresses ovulation, possibly by inhibiting pituitary gonadotropin secretion, and forms thick cervical mucus.

ONSET, PEAK, DURATION
Onset and peak unknown. Effects persist for 9 to 17 days.

INDICATIONS & DOSAGE
Amenorrhea, uterine bleeding—
Adults: 375 mg I.M. q 4 weeks. Stop after four cycles.
Palliative treatment of advanced inoperable endometrial cancer—
Adults: 1 to 7 g I.M. weekly.

ADVERSE REACTIONS
CNS: depression.
CV: thrombophlebitis, *thromboembolism, CVA, pulmonary embolism,* edema.
EENT: exophthalmos, diplopia.
GU: breakthrough bleeding, dysmenorrhea, amenorrhea, cervical erosion, abnormal secretions.
Hepatic: cholestatic jaundice.
Skin: rash, acne, pruritus, melasma, irritation and pain at injection site.
Other: breast tenderness, enlargement, or secretion; changes in weight.

INTERACTIONS
None significant.

EFFECTS ON DIAGNOSTIC TESTS
Glucose tolerance has been shown to decrease in a small percentage of patients receiving this drug. Abnormal thyroid or liver function tests may occur; the metyrapone test may be altered and pregnanediol excretion may decrease.

CONTRAINDICATIONS
Contraindicated in patients with hypersensitivity to drug, thromboembolic disorders, cerebral apoplexy, breast or genital organ cancer, undiagnosed abnormal vaginal bleeding, severe hepatic disease, or missed abortion and during pregnancy.

NURSING CONSIDERATIONS
● Use cautiously in patients with diabetes mellitus, seizures, migraine, cardiac or renal disease, asthma, mental depression, or impaired liver function.
● Know that drug should not be used to induce withdrawal bleeding or as a test for pregnancy; drug may cause birth defects and masculinization of female fetus.
● Give oil solutions (sesame oil and castor oil) via deep I.M. injection in gluteal muscle. Rotate injection sites to prevent muscle atrophy.

☑ PATIENT TEACHING
● FDA regulations require that, before receiving first dose, patient reads package insert explaining possible adverse effects of progestin. Also give patient verbal explanation.
Alert: Tell patient to report any unusual symptoms immediately and to stop drug and call the doctor if visual disturbances or migraine occur.
● Warn patient that edema and weight gain are likely. Tell her to monitor weight routinely, and recommend sodium-restricted diet as needed.
● Instruct patient to report breast pain or tenderness, vaginal discharge or bleeding, and swelling of the hands or feet.
● Teach patient how to perform routine breast self-examination.
● Instruct patient that normal menstrual cycles may not resume for 2 to 3 months after drug is stopped.

levonorgestrel
Norplant System

Pregnancy Risk Category: X

HOW SUPPLIED
Implants: 36 mg per capsule; each kit

---

contains six capsules

ACTION
Slowly releases the synthetic progestin levonorgestrel into the bloodstream. How progestins provide contraception is not fully understood, but they alter the mucus covering the cervix, prevent implantation of the egg, and, in some patients, prevent ovulation.

ONSET, PEAK, DURATION
Onset and peak levels occur within 24 hours. Effects persist about 5 years.

INDICATIONS & DOSAGE
Prevention of pregnancy—
Women: six capsules implanted subdermally in the midportion of the upper arm, about 8 cm above the elbow crease, during the first 7 days of the onset of menses. Capsules are placed in fanlike position, 15 degrees apart (total of 75 degrees). Contraceptive efficacy lasts for 5 years.

ADVERSE REACTIONS
CNS: headache, nervousness, dizziness.
GI: nausea, *abdominal discomfort,* appetite change.
GU: *amenorrhea, many days of bleeding or prolonged bleeding, spotting, irregular onset of bleeding, frequent onset of bleeding, scanty bleeding, cervicitis, vaginitis, leukorrhea.*
Skin: dermatitis, acne, hirsutism, hypertrichosis, alopecia, infection at implant site, transient pain or itching at implant site.
Other: adnexal enlargement, mastalgia, weight gain, *musculoskeletal pain, removal difficulty, breast discharge.*

INTERACTIONS
Carbamazepine, phenytoin, rifampin: may reduce the contraceptive efficacy of levonorgestrel implants. Monitor closely.

EFFECTS ON DIAGNOSTIC TESTS
Decreased sex hormone–binding globulin and thyroxine concentrations and increased triiodothyronine uptake have been reported.

CONTRAINDICATIONS
Contraindicated in patients with active thrombophlebitis or thromboembolic disorders, undiagnosed abnormal genital bleeding, acute liver disease, malignant or benign liver tumors, known or suspected breast cancer, and in known or suspected pregnancy.

NURSING CONSIDERATIONS
● Use cautiously in patients with a history of depression, in diabetic and prediabetic patients, and in patients with hyperlipidemia.
● Know that most patients develop variations in menstrual bleeding patterns, including irregular bleeding, prolonged bleeding, spotting, and amenorrhea. In most patients, these irregularities diminish over time.
● Be aware that irregular bleeding may mask symptoms of cervical or endometrial cancer.
● Closely monitor patients with conditions that may be aggravated by fluid retention because steroid hormones may cause fluid retention.
● Be aware laboratory tests for sex hormone-binding globulin and thyroxine (T_4) concentrations may show decreased values; for triiodothyronine (T_3) uptake, increased values.
● Know implants do not contain estrogen. Levonorgestrel is a totally synthetic progestin.
● Expect implants to be removed if patients develop active thrombophlebitis or thromboembolic disease or will be immobilized for a significant length of time because of illness or some other factor.
● If jaundice develops, expect implants to be removed because steroid hormone metabolism is impaired in patients with liver failure.
● Although retinal thrombosis after use of oral contraceptives has been reported, no similar incidents have been documented after use of the implant system.

Reactions may be *common,* uncommon, *life-threatening,* or COMMON AND LIFE-THREATENING.

However, patients with sudden unexplained vision problems, including users of contact lenses who develop vision changes or changes in lens tolerance, should be immediately evaluated by an ophthalmologist.

☑ **PATIENT TEACHING**
Alert: Tell patient to report to the doctor immediately if one of the implanted capsules falls out (before the skin heals over the implant). Contraceptive efficacy may be impaired.
● Warn patient that missed menstrual periods are not an accurate indicator of early pregnancy because drug may induce amenorrhea. Advise patient that 6 weeks or more of amenorrhea (after a pattern of regular menstrual periods) could indicate pregnancy. If pregnancy is confirmed, the implants must be removed.
● Encourage regular (at least annual) physical examinations.

---

medroxyprogesterone acetate
Amen, Curretab, Cycrin, Depo-Provera, Provera

Pregnancy Risk Category: X

HOW SUPPLIED
Tablets: 2.5 mg, 5 mg, 10 mg
Injection (suspension): 100 mg/ml, 150 mg/ml, 400 mg/ml

ACTION
Suppresses ovulation, possibly by inhibiting pituitary gonadotropin secretion, thus preventing follicular maturation and causing endometrial thinning.

ONSET, PEAK, DURATION
Unknown.

INDICATIONS & DOSAGE
Abnormal uterine bleeding caused by hormonal imbalance—
Adults: 5 to 10 mg P.O. daily for 5 to 10 days beginning on 16th day of menstrual cycle. If the patient also has received estrogen—10 mg P.O. daily for 10 days beginning on 16th day of cycle.
Secondary amenorrhea—
Adults: 5 to 10 mg P.O. daily for 5 to 10 days.
Endometrial or renal cancer—
Adults: 400 to 1,000 mg I.M. weekly.
Contraception in women—
Adults: 150 mg I.M. once q 3 months.

ADVERSE REACTIONS
CNS: depression.
CV: thrombophlebitis, *pulmonary embolism,* edema, *thromboembolism, CVA.*
EENT: exophthalmos, diplopia.
GU: breakthrough bleeding, dysmenorrhea, amenorrhea, cervical erosion, abnormal secretions.
Hepatic: cholestatic jaundice.
Skin: rash, pain, induration, sterile abscesses, acne, pruritus, melasma, alopecia, hirsutism.
Other: breast tenderness, enlargement, or secretion; changes in weight.

INTERACTIONS
Aminoglutethimide, rifampin: decreased progestin effects. Monitor for diminished therapeutic response. Patient should use a nonhormonal contraceptive during therapy with these drugs.

EFFECTS ON DIAGNOSTIC TESTS
Pregnanediol excretion may decrease; serum alkaline phosphatase and amino acid levels may increase. Glucose tolerance has been shown to decrease in a small percentage of patients receiving this drug.

CONTRAINDICATIONS
Contraindicated in patients with hypersensitivity to drug, active thromboembolic disorders, or past history of thromboembolic disorders or of cerebral vascular disease or apoplexy, breast cancer, undiagnosed abnormal vaginal bleeding, missed abortion, or hepatic dysfunction

and during pregnancy. Tablets are also contraindicated in patients with liver dysfunction or known or suspected malignant disease of the genital organs.

NURSING CONSIDERATIONS
● Use cautiously in patients with diabetes mellitus, seizures, migraine, cardiac or renal disease, asthma, and mental depression.
● Know that the drug should not be used as test for pregnancy; drug may cause birth defects and masculinization of female fetus.
● I.M. injection may be painful. Monitor sites for evidence of sterile abscess. Rotate injection sites to prevent muscle atrophy.

☑ **PATIENT TEACHING**
● FDA regulations require that, before receiving first dose, patient reads package insert explaining possible adverse effects of progestins. Also, give patient verbal explanation.
Alert: Tell patient to report any unusual symptoms immediately and to stop drug and call the doctor if visual disturbances or migraine occurs.
● Teach patient how to perform routine monthly breast self-examination.

---

norethindrone
Micronor, Norlutin, Nor-Q.D.

norethindrone acetate
Aygestin, Aygestin Cycle Pack, Norlutate

Pregnancy Risk Category: X

HOW SUPPLIED
norethindrone
Tablets: 0.35 mg, 5 mg
norethindrone acetate
Tablets: 5 mg

ACTION
Suppresses ovulation, possibly by inhibiting pituitary gonadotropin secre-

tion, and forms thick cervical mucus.

ONSET, PEAK, DURATION
Unknown.

INDICATIONS & DOSAGE
Amenorrhea, abnormal uterine bleeding—
Adults: 5 to 20 mg norethindrone or 2.5 to 10 mg norethindrone acetate P.O. daily on days 5 to 25 of menstrual cycle.
Endometriosis—
Adults: 10 mg norethindrone P.O. daily for 14 days; then increased by 5 mg daily q 2 weeks up to 30 mg daily. Or 5 mg norethindrone acetate P.O. daily for 14 days; then increased by 2.5 mg daily q 2 weeks, up to 15 mg daily.
Contraception in women—
Adults: initially, 0.35 mg norethindrone P.O. on the first day of menstruation; then 0.35 mg daily.

ADVERSE REACTIONS
CNS: depression.
CV: thrombophlebitis, *pulmonary embolism,* edema, *thromboembolism, CVA.*
EENT: exophthalmos, diplopia.
GU: breakthrough bleeding, dysmenorrhea, amenorrhea, cervical erosion, abnormal secretions.
Hepatic: cholestatic jaundice.
Skin: melasma, rash, acne, pruritus.
Other: breast tenderness, enlargement, or secretion; changes in weight.

INTERACTIONS
Barbiturates, carbamazepine, rifampin: decreased progestin effects. Monitor for diminished therapeutic response.

EFFECTS ON DIAGNOSTIC TESTS
Pregnanediol excretion may decrease; serum alkaline phosphatase and amino acid levels may increase. Glucose tolerance has been shown to decrease in a small percentage of patients receiving this drug.

Reactions may be *common,* uncommon, *life-threatening,* or COMMON AND LIFE-THREATENING.

CONTRAINDICATIONS

Contraindicated in patients with thromboembolic disorders, cerebral apoplexy, or history of these conditions; hypersensitivity to drug; breast cancer, undiagnosed abnormal vaginal bleeding, severe hepatic disease, or missed abortion and during pregnancy.

NURSING CONSIDERATIONS

• Use cautiously in patients with diabetes mellitus, seizures, migraine, cardiac or renal disease, asthma, and mental depression.
• Norethindrone acetate is twice as potent as norethindrone. Know that norethindrone acetate should not be used for contraception.
• Know that use as test for pregnancy is not appropriate; drug may cause birth defects and masculinization of female fetus.
• Know that preliminary estrogen treatment is usually needed in menstrual disorders.
• Watch patients carefully for signs of edema.

☑ PATIENT TEACHING

• FDA regulations require that, before receiving first dose, patient reads package insert explaining possible adverse effects of progestin. Also give patient verbal explanation.
Alert: Tell patient to report any unusual symptoms immediately and to stop drug and call the doctor if visual disturbances or migraine occurs.
• Teach patient how to perform routine monthly breast self-examination.

norgestrel
Ovrette**

Pregnancy Risk Category: X

HOW SUPPLIED
Tablets: 0.075 mg

ACTION
Unknown. Probably suppresses ovulation, possibly by inhibiting pituitary gonadotropin secretion, and forms thick cervical mucus.

ONSET, PEAK, DURATION
Unknown.

INDICATIONS & DOSAGE
Contraception in women—
Adults: 0.075 mg P.O. daily.

ADVERSE REACTIONS
CNS: cerebral thrombosis or hemorrhage, migraine, depression.
CV: thrombophlebitis, *pulmonary embolism,* edema, *thromboembolism, CVA.*
EENT: exophthalmos, diplopia.
GU: *breakthrough bleeding, change in menstrual flow,* dysmenorrhea, spotting, amenorrhea, cervical erosion.
Hepatic: cholestatic jaundice.
Skin: melasma, rash, acne, pruritus.
Other: breast tenderness, enlargement, or secretion; changes in weight.

INTERACTIONS
Barbiturates, carbamazepine, rifampin: decreased progestin effects. Monitor for diminished therapeutic response.

EFFECTS ON DIAGNOSTIC TESTS
Pregnanediol excretion may decrease; serum alkaline phosphatase and amino acid levels may increase. Glucose tolerance has been shown to decrease in a small percentage of patients receiving this drug.

CONTRAINDICATIONS
Contraindicated in patients with thromboembolic disorders, cerebral apoplexy, or history of these conditions; hypersensitivity to drug; breast cancer, undiagnosed abnormal vaginal bleeding, severe hepatic disease, and missed abortion, and during pregnancy.

NURSING CONSIDERATIONS
● Use cautiously in patients with diabetes mellitus, seizures, migraine, cardiac or renal disease, asthma, and mental depression.
● Be aware that norgestrel is a progestin-only oral contraceptive known as the "minipill."

☑ PATIENT TEACHING
● FDA regulations require that, before receiving first dose, patient reads package insert explaining possible adverse effects of progestins. Also provide verbal explanation.
● Tell patient to take pill every day, at the same time, even if menstruating.
● Risk of pregnancy increases with each tablet missed. Tell patient who misses one tablet to take it as soon as she remembers and then to take the next tablet at the regular time. Advise patient who misses two tablets to take one as soon as she remembers and then to take the next regular dose at the usual time and also to use a nonhormonal method of contraception in addition to norgestrel until 14 tablets have been taken. Instruct patient who misses three or more tablets to discontinue drug and use a nonhormonal method of contraception until after menses. If menstrual period does not occur within 45 days, pregnancy testing is necessary.
● Advise patient using oral contraceptives of the increased risk of serious adverse CV reactions associated with heavy cigarette smoking (15 or more cigarettes per day). These risks are quite marked in women over age 35.
● Instruct patient to immediately report excessive bleeding or bleeding between menstrual cycles, breast pain or tenderness, vaginal discharge, or swelling of the hands or feet.
Alert: Tell patient to report any unusual symptoms immediately and to stop drug and call the doctor if visual disturbances, migraine, or numbness or tingling in limbs occurs.
● Teach patient how to perform routine breast self-examination.

progesterone
Gesterol 50, Progestilin†

Pregnancy Risk Category: X

HOW SUPPLIED
Injection (in oil): 50 mg/ml

ACTION
Suppresses ovulation, possibly by inhibiting pituitary gonadotropin secretion, and forms thick cervical mucus.

ONSET, PEAK, DURATION
Unknown.

INDICATIONS & DOSAGE
Amenorrhea—
Adults: 5 to 10 mg I.M. daily for 6 to 8 days, usually beginning 8 to 10 days before the anticipated start of menstruation.
Dysfunctional uterine bleeding—
Adults: 5 to 10 mg I.M. daily for six doses.

ADVERSE REACTIONS
CNS: depression.
CV: thrombophlebitis, *thromboembolism, CVA, pulmonary embolism,* edema.
GU: breakthrough bleeding, dysmenorrhea, amenorrhea, cervical erosion, abnormal secretions.
Hepatic: cholestatic jaundice.
Skin: melasma, rash, acne, pruritus, pain at injection site.
Other: breast tenderness, enlargement, or secretion.

INTERACTIONS
Barbiturates, carbamazepine, rifampin: decreased progestin effects. Monitor for diminished therapeutic response.

EFFECTS ON DIAGNOSTIC TESTS
Pregnanediol excretion may decrease; serum alkaline phosphatase and amino

acid levels may increase. Glucose tolerance has been shown to decrease in a small percentage of patients receiving this drug.

CONTRAINDICATIONS
Contraindicated in patients with thromboembolic disorders, cerebral apoplexy, or history of these conditions; hypersensitivity to drug; breast cancer, undiagnosed abnormal vaginal bleeding, severe hepatic disease, and missed abortion.

NURSING CONSIDERATIONS
● Use cautiously in patients with diabetes mellitus, seizures, migraine, cardiac or renal disease, asthma, and mental depression.
● Know preliminary estrogen treatment is usually needed in menstrual disorders.
● Give oil solutions (peanut oil or sesame oil) via deep I.M. injection. Check sites frequently for irritation. Rotate injection sites.

☑ PATIENT TEACHING
● FDA regulations require that, before receiving first dose, patient reads package insert explaining possible adverse effects of progestins. Also give patient verbal explanation.
Alert: Tell patient to report any unusual symptoms immediately and to stop drug and call the doctor if visual disturbances or migraine occurs.
Alert: Tell patient to report increased depression immediately; drug may need to be discontinued.
● Teach patient how to perform routine breast self-examination.

56
Gonadotropins

gonadorelin acetate
histrelin acetate
menotropins
nafarelin acetate

COMBINATION PRODUCTS
None.

---

gonadorelin acetate
Lutrepulse

Pregnancy Risk Category: B

HOW SUPPLIED
Injection: 0.8 mg/10 ml, 3.2 mg/10 ml vials; supplied as kit with I.V. supplies and ambulatory infusion pump

ACTION
Mimics action of gonadotropin-releasing hormone, resulting in the synthesis and release of luteinizing hormone (LH) from anterior pituitary gland. LH then acts upon reproductive organs to regulate hormone synthesis.

ONSET, PEAK, DURATION
Unknown.

INDICATIONS & DOSAGE
Induction of ovulation in women with primary hypothalamic amenorrhea—
Adults: 5 mcg I.V. q 90 minutes for 21 days. If no response follows three treatment intervals, increase dosage as ordered.

ADVERSE REACTIONS
Skin: hematoma, local infection, inflammation, mild phlebitis.
Other: multiple pregnancy, ovarian hyperstimulation.

INTERACTIONS
Other ovulation stimulators: Additive effects. Avoid concomitant use.

EFFECTS ON DIAGNOSTIC TESTS
None reported.

CONTRAINDICATIONS
Contraindicated in patients hypersensitive to the drug, in women with conditions that could be complicated by pregnancy (such as prolactinoma), in those who are anovulatory from any cause other than a hypothalamic disorder, and in those with ovarian cysts.

NURSING CONSIDERATIONS
● **I.V. use:** To mimic the naturally occurring hormone, administer gonadorelin in a pulsatile fashion with the available ambulatory infusion pump. Set the pulse period at 1 minute (infuse drug over 1 minute) and the pulse interval at 90 minutes.
● To give 2.5 mcg/pulse, reconstitute the 0.8-mg vial with 8 ml of supplied diluent, and set the pump to deliver 25 microliters/pulse. To administer 5 mcg/pulse, use the same dosage strength and dilution, but set the pump to deliver 50 microliters/pulse.
● Some patients may need higher I.V. doses. To give 10 mcg/pulse, reconstitute the 3.2-mg vial with 8 ml of supplied diluent, and set pump to deliver 25 microliters/pulse. To give 20 mcg/pulse, use same dosage strength and dilution, but set pump to deliver 50 microliters/pulse.
● Inspect the I.V. site at each visit.
● Know that patients usually need pelvic ultrasound on days 7 and 14 after a baseline scan. Some doctors prefer shorter intervals between scans.

☑ PATIENT TEACHING
● Ensure that patient understands that multiple pregnancy is possible (inci-

---

Reactions may be *common*, uncommon, ***life-threatening***, or **COMMON AND LIFE-THREATENING**.

dence is about 12%). Monitoring of dosage and ovarian ultrasonography to monitor drug response are needed.

• Instruct patient about proper aseptic technique and care of the I.V. site. Cannula and I.V. site should be changed every 48 hours. Written instructions are available for patient.

• Anaphylaxis has been reported with similar drugs. Teach patient symptoms of hypersensitivity reactions (rash, hives, wheezing, difficulty breathing, rapid heartbeat), and encourage her to report these at once.

• Tell patient to report signs of infection, hematoma, inflammation, or phlebitis at injection site. She also should report severe abdominal pain, bloating, swelling of the hands or feet, nausea, vomiting, diarrhea, substantial weight gain, or shortness of breath.

• Encourage patient to adhere to the close monitoring schedule required by the therapy. Regular pelvic examinations, midluteal-phase serum progesterone determinations, and multiple ovarian ultrasound scans are necessary.

---

histrelin acetate
Supprelin

Pregnancy Risk Category: X

HOW SUPPLIED
Injection: 120 mcg/0.6 ml, 300 mcg/0.6 ml, 600 mcg/0.6 ml

ACTION
An agonist that mimics the effects of gonadotropin-releasing hormone (GnRH; also called luteinizing hormone-releasing hormone, or LHRH) but is more potent. Chronic administration desensitizes responsiveness of the pituitary gonadotropin, decreasing sex hormone production by the testes or ovaries.

ONSET, PEAK, DURATION
Unknown.

INDICATIONS & DOSAGE
Centrally mediated (idiopathic or neurogenic) precocious puberty—
Children (girls 2 to 8 years; boys 2 to 9½ years): 10 mcg/kg S.C. daily.

ADVERSE REACTIONS
CNS: *mood changes, nervousness, dizziness, depression, headache, libido changes, insomnia, anxiety,* paresthesia, cognitive changes, syncope, somnolence, lethargy, impaired consciousness, tremor, hyperkinesia, *seizures,* hot flashes, conduct disorder, fatigue.
CV: *vasodilation,* edema, palpitations, pallor, tachycardia, hypertension.
EENT: epistaxis, ear congestion, abnormal pupillary function, otalgia, visual disturbances, hearing loss, polyopia, photophobia, rhinorrhea, sinusitis, nasal infections,.
GI: *abdominal pain, nausea, vomiting, diarrhea, flatulence, decreased appetite, dyspepsia,* cramps, constipation, thirst, gastritis, GI distress.
GU: *menstrual changes, vaginal dryness, leukorrhea, hypermenorrhea, vaginal bleeding, vaginitis, dysmenorrhea,* polyuria, incontinence, dysuria, hematuria, nocturia, tenderness of female genitalia, glycosuria.
Hematologic: hyperlipidemia, anemia.
Respiratory: *upper respiratory infection, respiratory congestion, cough,* asthma, breathing disorder, bronchitis, hyperventilation.
Skin: *redness, swelling, acne, rash, diaphoresis,* urticaria, pruritus, alopecia.
Other: *fever, arthralgia, muscle stiffness, muscle cramps, breast pain or edema,* breast discharge, decreased breast size, *weight gain, body pains,* chills, malaise, purpura, acute hypersensitivity reactions *(anaphylaxis, angioedema).*

INTERACTIONS
None significant.

EFFECTS ON DIAGNOSTIC TESTS
None reported.

CONTRAINDICATIONS

Contraindicated in patients hypersensitive to any component of drug and in pregnant or breast-feeding patients. Safety and efficacy haven't been established in children under 2 years.

NURSING CONSIDERATIONS

• Be aware drug is indicated only for patients who will comply with the daily schedule. Noncompliance or inadequate dosing may result in inadequate control of the pubertal process, which can result in recurrence of symptoms, including onset of menses, breast development, or testicular growth; long-term consequences may involve decreased adult height.

• A complete physical and endocrinologic evaluation should be performed before initiating drug therapy; several indices should be reexamined at 3 months, then every 6 to 12 months thereafter. Such evaluations should include determinations of height and weight, hand and wrist X-rays for bone-age determination, sex steroid (estradiol or testosterone) levels, and GnRH stimulation test. Monitor these tests periodically to determine effectiveness of therapy.

• Further tests to rule out other causes of precocious puberty include beta human chorionic gonadotropin levels (to detect chorionic gonadotropin-secreting tumor); pelvic/adrenal/testicular ultrasound (to detect steroid-secreting tumor); and computed tomography scan of the head (to detect any previously undiagnosed intracranial tumor). Workup also sets baseline of gonad size for serial monitoring.

• Refrigerate drug (36° to 46° F [2° to 8° C]) and protect from light in its original container. Use vials only once because drug does not contain preservatives. Allow drug to reach room temperature before giving.

• Give S.C. and rotate injection sites to minimize local reactions.

• Know that decreases in follicle-stimulating hormone, luteinizing hormone, and sex steroid levels occur within 3 months.

• Patients should be reevaluated if prepubertal levels of sex steroids or GnRH test responses are not achieved within 3 months of therapy.

☑ PATIENT TEACHING

• Before therapy, make sure patient and caregivers understand the importance of adhering to the daily schedules. Tell parents to give drug at the same time each day to aid compliance and ensure adequate dosing.

• Drug is dispensed as a 30-day kit that contains a patient information leaflet. Ensure that caregivers read and understand the leaflet.

• Inform patient that because drug is a peptide, it's destroyed in the GI tract and so must be given parenterally.

• Explain importance of rotating injection sites daily. Sites should include upper arms, thighs, and abdomen.

• Warn patient of the potential risks of therapy and potential adverse effects. During the first month of treatment, girls commonly experience a slight menstrual flow, which probably is related to decreasing estrogen levels brought on by treatment. As estrogen levels drop, menses begins because estrogens support the endometrium.

• Advise patient to seek medical attention at once if any signs of hypersensitivity reactions occur—sudden development of skin rash, difficulty in breathing or swallowing, or rapid heartbeat. Notify the doctor if severe or persistent swelling, redness, or irritation appears at the injection site.

menotropins
Personal

Pregnancy Risk Category: X

HOW SUPPLIED

Injection: 75 international units of luteinizing hormone (LH) and 75 units of follicle-stimulating hormone (FSH) activity per ampule; 150 units of LH and 150 units of FSH activity per ampule

ACTION
When given to women who have not had primary ovarian failure, mimics FSH in inducing follicular growth and LH in aiding follicular maturation; induces spermatogenesis in men.

ONSET, PEAK, DURATION
Onset for follicular growth and maturation, 9 to 12 days. Peak and duration unknown.

INDICATIONS & DOSAGE
Anovulation—
Women: 75 units each of FSH and LH I.M. daily for 7 to 12 days, followed by 5,000 to 10,000 units of human chorionic gonadotropin (HCG) I.M. 1 day after last dose of menotropins. Repeated for one to three menstrual cycles until ovulation occurs.
Infertility with ovulation—
Women: 75 units each of FSH and LH I.M. daily for 7 to 12 days, then 5,000 to 10,000 units HCG I.M. 1 day after last dose of menotropins. Repeated for two menstrual cycles, then 150 units each of FSH and LH daily for 7 to 12 days, followed by 5,000 to 10,000 units HCG I.M. 1 day after last dose of menotropins. Repeated for two menstrual cycles.
Infertility in men—
Men: prior treatment with HCG of 5,000 units three times a week for 4 to 6 months; then 75 units each of FSH and LH I.M. three times weekly (given with 2,000 units of HCG twice weekly) for at least 4 months. If increased spermatogenesis does not occur, increase to 150 units each of FSH and LH three times weekly (dosage of HCG remains unchanged).

ADVERSE REACTIONS
CNS: headache, malaise, dizziness.
CV: *stroke,* tachycardia.
GI: nausea, vomiting, diarrhea, abdominal cramps, bloating.
GU: *ovarian enlargement with pain and abdominal distention,* multiple births, ovarian hyperstimulation syndrome, ovarian cysts.
Respiratory: *atelectasis, acute respiratory distress syndrome, pulmonary embolism, pulmonary infarction, arterial occlusion,* dyspnea, tachypnea.
Other: fever, *gynecomastia, hypersensitivity and anaphylactic reactions,* chills, musculoskeletal aches, joint pains, rash, ectopic pregnancy.

INTERACTIONS
None significant.

EFFECTS ON DIAGNOSTIC TESTS
None reported.

CONTRAINDICATIONS
Contraindicated in patients hypersensitive to the drug; in women with primary ovarian failure, uncontrolled thyroid or adrenal dysfunction, pituitary tumor, abnormal uterine bleeding, uterine fibromas, or ovarian cysts or enlargement; in pregnant patients; and in men with normal pituitary function, primary testicular failure, or infertility disorders other than hypogonadotropic hypogonadism.

NURSING CONSIDERATIONS
• Monitor closely to ensure adequate ovarian stimulation without hyperstimulation.
• Reconstitute with 1 to 2 ml of sterile 0.9% sodium chloride for injection. Use immediately.
• Rotate injection sites.

☑ PATIENT TEACHING
• Tell patient about possibility of multiple births.
• In infertility, encourage daily intercourse from day before HCG is given until ovulation occurs.
• Tell patient that pregnancy usually occurs 4 to 6 weeks after therapy.
• Instruct patient to immediately report severe abdominal pain, bloating,

swelling of the hands or feet, nausea, vomiting, diarrhea, substantial weight gain, or shortness of breath.

---

nafarelin acetate
Synarel

Pregnancy Risk Category: X

HOW SUPPLIED
Nasal solution: 200 mcg/spray in metered-dose spray bottle (2 mg/ml)

ACTION
A gonadotropin-releasing hormone (GnRH) analogue that acts on the pituitary to decrease release of follicle-stimulating hormone and luteinizing hormone, thus decreasing ovarian stimulation, lowering circulating estrogens, and improving symptoms associated with endometriosis.

ONSET, PEAK, DURATION
Decreased levels of sex hormones occur after 4 weeks. Serum levels peak 10 to 40 minutes after dose. Effects persist for up to 3 to 6 months.

INDICATIONS & DOSAGE
Management of endometriosis—
Women 18 years and older: 1 spray in one nostril b.i.d. Treatment begun on day 2, 3, or 4 of menstrual cycle. Maximum duration of therapy is 6 months.
Central precocious puberty—
Children: 2 sprays in each nostril in the morning and evening. Total daily dosage is 8 sprays (1,600 mcg).

ADVERSE REACTIONS
CNS: *headaches, emotional lability, insomnia,* depression.
EENT: *nasal irritation.*
Skin: *acne,* seborrhea, hirsutism.
Other: edema, *hot flushes, decreased libido, myalgia, reduced breast size,* weight gain or loss, increased libido, decreased bone density, *vaginal dryness.*

INTERACTIONS
Topical nasal decongestant: possible interference with nafarelin absorption; use at least 30 minutes after nafarelin.

EFFECTS ON DIAGNOSTIC TESTS
Tests of pituitary gonadotropin and gonadal functions may be misleading during treatment and for as long as 4 to 8 weeks after treatment.

CONTRAINDICATIONS
Contraindicated in patients hypersensitive to GnRH analogs or any components of the formulation (benzalkonium chloride, sorbitol, purified water, glacial acetic acid, hydrochloric acid, or sodium hydroxide), in those with undiagnosed vaginal bleeding, in breast-feeding patients, and during pregnancy.

NURSING CONSIDERATIONS
● Be aware that studies have confirmed a small loss in bone density after 6 months of therapy, probably caused by drug-induced hypoestrogenic state. Patients with chronic alcohol or tobacco use, strong family history of osteoporosis, or use of drugs that may reduce bone mass should not receive additional therapy and should weigh risks and benefits before an initial trial of drug.

☑ PATIENT TEACHING
● Teach patient that menstruation will stop with regular use of drug and to call the doctor if menstruation persists or breakthrough bleeding occurs.
● Advise patient to use a nonhormonal form of contraception. Drug is not a reliable contraceptive, particularly if patient misses doses. Tell patient to stop the drug and call the doctor if she thinks she is pregnant.
● Instruct patient to immediately report severe abdominal pain, bloating, swelling of the hands or feet, nausea, vomiting, diarrhea, substantial weight gain, or shortness of breath.
● Tell patient who develops a cold or rhinitis during therapy to call the doctor.

Reactions may be *common*, uncommon, *life-threatening*, or COMMON AND LIFE-THREATENING.

57

Antidiabetic drugs and glucagon

acarbose
acetohexamide
chlorpropamide
glimepiride
glipizide
glucagon
glyburide
insulins
metformin hydrochloride
tolazamide
tolbutamide
troglitazone

COMBINATION PRODUCTS
HUMULIN 50/50 ◊: isophane insulin suspension (human) 50% and insulin injection (human) 50%, 100 units/ml.
HUMULIN 70/30 ◊, MIXTARD HUMAN‡, NOVOLIN 70/30 ◊): isophane insulin suspension (human) 70% and insulin injection (human) 30%, 100 units/ml.

---

acarbose
Precose

Pregnancy Risk Category: B

HOW SUPPLIED
Tablets: 50 mg, 100 mg

ACTION
An alpha-glucosidase inhibitor that delays digestion of carbohydrates, resulting in a smaller rise in blood glucose concentration.

ONSET, PEAK, DURATION
Onset and duration are unknown. Plasma level peaks in 1 hour.

INDICATIONS & DOSAGE
Adjunct to diet to lower blood glucose in patients with non-insulin-dependent diabetes mellitus whose hyperglycemia cannot be managed by diet alone or by

diet and a sulfonylurea—
Adults: Individualized. Initially, 25 mg P.O. t.i.d. at start of each main meal. Subsequent dosage adjustment made q 4 to 8 weeks, based on 1-hour postprandial glucose level and tolerance. Maintenance dosage is 50 mg to 100 mg P.O. t.i.d.; patients weighing less than 60 kg should not exceed 50 mg P.O. t.i.d.

ADVERSE REACTIONS
GI: *abdominal pain, diarrhea, flatulence.*
Other: elevated serum transaminase level.

INTERACTIONS
Calcium channel blockers, corticosteroids, estrogens, isoniazid, nicotinic acid, oral contraceptives, phenothiazines, phenytoin, sympathomimetics, thiazides and other diuretics, thyroid products: may cause hyperglycemia during concomitant use or hypoglycemia when withdrawn. Monitor blood glucose level.
Intestinal adsorbents (such as activated charcoal) and digestive enzyme preparations containing carbohydrate-splitting enzymes (such as amylase and pancreatin): may reduce the effect of acarbose. Do not administer concomitantly.

EFFECTS ON DIAGNOSTIC TESTS
Acarbose therapy, particularly in doses exceeding 50 mg t.i.d., may cause elevations of serum transaminase and, in rare cases, bilirubin levels.

CONTRAINDICATIONS
Contraindicated in patients with hypersensitivity to the drug, diabetic ketoacidosis, cirrhosis, inflammatory bowel disease, colonic ulceration, partial intestinal obstruction, predisposition to in-

---

*Liquid contains alcohol.   **May contain tartrazine.   †Canada only.   ‡Australia only.   ◊OTC.

testinal obstruction, chronic intestinal disease associated with marked disorder of digestion or absorption, and any condition that may deteriorate because of increased intestinal gas formation.

NURSING CONSIDERATIONS
● Drug is not recommended for use in patients with serum creatinine levels greater than 2.0 mg/dl and in pregnant or breast-feeding women.
● Use cautiously in patients with mild to moderate renal impairment and in those receiving a sulfonylurea or insulin. Acarbose may increase hypoglycemic potential of the sulfonylurea. Monitor a patient receiving both drugs closely. If hypoglycemia occurs, treat patient with oral glucose (dextrose). Severe hypoglycemia may require I.V. glucose infusion or glucagon administration. Dosage adjustments may be needed to prevent further hypoglycemia, so report hypoglycemia and treatment required to the doctor. Insulin therapy may be needed in times of increased stress (infection, fever, surgery, or trauma). Monitor the patient closely for hyperglycemia.
● Safety and efficacy of drug have not been established in children.
● Monitor the patient's 1-hour postprandial plasma glucose level to determine therapeutic effectiveness of acarbose and to identify appropriate dose. Report hyperglycemia to the doctor. Thereafter, glycosylated hemoglobin should be measured every 3 months.
● Monitor serum transaminase level every 3 months in the first year of therapy and periodically thereafter in patients receiving doses in excess of 50 mg t.i.d. Report abnormalities; dosage adjustment or drug withdrawal may be needed.

☑ **PATIENT TEACHING**
● Have patient take the drug daily with first bite of each of three main meals.
● Explain to patient that therapy relieves symptoms but doesn't cure the disease.
● Stress importance of adhering to specific diet, weight reduction, exercise, and hygiene programs. Show the patient how to monitor blood glucose level and how to recognize and treat hyperglycemia.
● Teach patient taking a sulfonylurea how to recognize hypoglycemia, and to treat symptoms with a form of dextrose rather than with a product containing table sugar.
● Urge patient to carry medical identification at all times.

---

acetohexamide
Dimelor†, Dymelor

Pregnancy Risk Category: NR

HOW SUPPLIED
Tablets: 250 mg, 500 mg

ACTION
Unknown. A sulfonylurea that probably stimulates insulin release from the pancreatic beta cells and reduces glucose output by the liver. An extrapancreatic effect increases peripheral sensitivity to insulin.

ONSET, PEAK, DURATION
Onset within 1 hour. Plasma levels of acetohexamide peak within 2 hours; plasma levels of insulin, within 1 to 2 hours. Effects last 12 to 24 hours.

INDICATIONS & DOSAGE
Adjunct to diet to lower blood glucose level in patients with type II diabetes (non-insulin-dependent)—
Adults: initially, 250 mg P.O. daily before breakfast; dosage increased q 5 to 7 days (by 250 to 500 mg), as needed, to maximum of 1.5 g daily in divided doses b.i.d. or t.i.d. before meals.
To replace insulin therapy in patients with type II diabetes—
Adults: if insulin dosage is less than 20 units daily, insulin is stopped and oral therapy started with 250 mg P.O. daily before breakfast, increased as above, if needed. If insulin dosage is 20 or more

units daily, oral therapy is started with 250 mg P.O. daily before breakfast, while insulin dosage is reduced by 25% to 30% daily or every other day, depending on response to oral therapy.

ADVERSE REACTIONS
CNS: paresthesia, fatigue, dizziness, vertigo, malaise, headache.
EENT: tinnitus.
GI: nausea, heartburn, epigastric distress.
Hematologic: leukopenia, *thrombocytopenia, aplastic anemia, agranulocytosis,* hemolytic anemia.
Skin: rash, pruritus, erythema, urticaria.
Other: *hypersensitivity reactions, hypoglycemia*

INTERACTIONS
Anabolic steroids, chloramphenicol, clofibrate, guanethidine, MAO inhibitors, phenylbutazone, salicylates, sulfonamides: increased hypoglycemic activity. Monitor blood glucose level.
Beta blockers, clonidine: prolonged hypoglycemic effect and masked symptoms of hypoglycemia. Use together cautiously.
Corticosteroids, glucagon, rifampin, thiazide diuretics: decreased hypoglycemic response. Monitor blood glucose level.
Ethanol: possible disulfiram-like reaction. Avoid concomitant use.
Hydantoins: increased blood levels of hydantoins. Monitor blood levels.
Oral anticoagulants: increased hypoglycemic activity or enhanced anticoagulant effect. Monitor blood glucose level and PT.

EFFECTS ON DIAGNOSTIC TESTS
Acetohexamide therapy alters serum uric acid concentration, cholesterol, alkaline phosphatase, bilirubin, and BUN levels.

CONTRAINDICATIONS
Contraindicated for treating patients with type I diabetes (insulin-dependent) or diabetes that can be adequately controlled by diet. Also contraindicated in patients with type II diabetes complicated by ketosis, acidosis, diabetic coma; hyperglycemia associated with primary renal disease; pregnancy or lactation; major surgery; severe infections; severe trauma; or hypersensitivity to sulfonylureas.

NURSING CONSIDERATIONS
• Use cautiously in patients with a history of porphyria, impaired hepatic or renal function, or in debilitated, malnourished, or elderly patients.
• During periods of increased stress, such as infection, fever, surgery, or trauma, patients may require insulin therapy. Monitor patients closely for hyperglycemia in these situations.
• Know that patients transferring from another oral agent usually need no transition period.
• Be aware that patients transferring from insulin therapy to an oral antidiabetic agent require blood glucose monitoring at least three times a day before meals. Patients may require hospitalization during transition.

☑ **PATIENT TEACHING**
• Instruct patient about nature of disease, importance of following therapeutic regimen, adhering to specific diet, weight reduction, exercise, and personal hygiene programs and about avoiding infection. Explain how and when to perform self-monitoring of blood glucose level, and teach recognition of and intervention for hypoglycemia and hyperglycemia.
• Make sure patient understands that therapy only relieves symptoms.
• Tell patient not to change drug dosage without the doctor's consent and to report abnormal blood or urine glucose test results.
• Teach patient to carry candy or other simple sugars to treat mild hypoglycemic episodes. Severe episodes may require hospital treatment.

- Advise patient not to take any other medication, including OTC drugs, without checking with the doctor.
- Advise patient to avoid moderate to large intake of alcohol because of possible disulfiram-like reaction.
- Advise patient to carry medical identification at all times.

chlorpropamide
Apo-Chlorpropamide†, Diabinese, Glucamide, Novo-Propamide†

Pregnancy Risk Category: C

HOW SUPPLIED
Tablets: 100 mg, 250 mg

ACTION
Unknown. A sulfonylurea that probably stimulates insulin release from the pancreatic beta cells and reduces glucose output by the liver. An extrapancreatic effect increases peripheral sensitivity to insulin. Also exerts an antidiuretic effect in patients with diabetes insipidus.

ONSET, PEAK, DURATION
Onset occurs within 1 hour. Peak levels occur in 2 to 4 hours; peak hypoglycemic effect, within 3 to 6 hours. Effects persist for up to 60 hours.

INDICATIONS & DOSAGE
Adjunct to diet to lower blood glucose level in patients with type II diabetes (non-insulin-dependent)—
Adults: 250 mg P.O. daily with breakfast. Initial dosage increased after 5 to 7 days because of extended duration of action; then increased q 3 to 5 days by 50 to 125 mg, if needed, to a maximum of 750 mg daily. On the other hand, some patients with mild diabetes respond well to dosages of 100 mg or less daily.
Adults over 65 years: initially, 100 to 125 mg P.O. daily.
To change from insulin to oral therapy—
Adults: if insulin dosage is less than 40 units daily, insulin is stopped and oral

therapy started as above. If insulin dosage is 40 units or more daily, oral therapy started as above with insulin reduced 50%. Insulin dosage reduced further according to response.

ADVERSE REACTIONS
CNS: paresthesia, fatigue, dizziness, vertigo, malaise, headache.
EENT: tinnitus.
GI: nausea, heartburn, epigastric distress.
GU: tea-colored urine.
Hematologic: leukopenia, ***thrombocytopenia, aplastic anemia, agranulocytosis,*** hemolytic anemia.
Skin: rash, pruritus, erythema, urticaria.
Other: *hypersensitivity reactions, prolonged hypoglycemia, dilutional hyponatremia.*

INTERACTIONS
Anabolic steroids, chloramphenicol, clofibrate, guanethidine, MAO inhibitors, salicylates, sulfonamides: increased hypoglycemic activity. Monitor blood glucose level.
Beta blockers: prolonged hypoglycemic effect and masked symptoms of hypoglycemia. Use together cautiously.
Corticosteroids, glucagon, rifampin, thiazide diuretics: decreased hypoglycemic response. Monitor blood glucose level.
Ethanol: possible disulfiram-like reaction. Avoid concomitant use.
Hydantoins: increased blood levels of hydantoins. Monitor blood levels.
Oral anticoagulants: increased hypoglycemic activity or enhanced anticoagulant effect. Monitor blood glucose level and PT.

EFFECTS ON DIAGNOSTIC TESTS
Chlorpropamide therapy alters cholesterol, alkaline phosphatase, bilirubin, urine phenylketone, porphyrias, protein levels and cephalin flocculation (thymol turbidity).

CONTRAINDICATIONS
Contraindicated for treating type I dia-

betes (insulin-dependent) or diabetes that can be adequately controlled by diet. Also contraindicated in patients with type II diabetes complicated by ketosis, acidosis, diabetic coma, major surgery, severe infections, severe trauma, during pregnancy or breast-feeding; and in patients with hypersensitivity to the drug.

NURSING CONSIDERATIONS
● Use cautiously in patients with porphyria, impaired hepatic or renal function or in debilitated, malnourished or elderly patients.
● Know that elderly patients may be more sensitive to adverse effects.
● Know that drug may accumulate in patients with renal insufficiency. Watch for and report signs of impending renal insufficiency, such as dysuria, anuria, and hematuria.
Alert: Know adverse effects of chlorpropamide, especially hypoglycemia, may be more frequent or severe than with some other sulfonylureas because of its long duration of action. If hypoglycemia occurs, monitor patients closely for a minimum of 3 to 5 days.
● Monitor serum alkaline phosphatase levels routinely, as ordered. Progressive increases may indicate the need to discontinue drug.
● Patients transferring from another oral antidiabetic agent usually need no transition period.
● Patients may require hospitalization during transition from insulin therapy to an oral antidiabetic agent. Monitor patients' blood glucose levels at least three times a day before meals.

☑ PATIENT TEACHING
● Instruct patient about nature of the disease, importance of following therapeutic regimen, adhering to specific diet, weight reduction, exercise, and personal hygiene programs, and about avoiding infection. Explain how and when to perform self-monitoring of blood glucose level, and teach recogni-

tion of and intervention for hypoglycemia and hyperglycemia.
● Make sure patient understands that therapy only relieves symptoms.
● Tell patient not to change drug dosage without the doctor's consent and to report abnormal blood or urine glucose test results.
● Teach patient to carry candy or other simple sugars to treat mild hypoglycemic episodes. Severe episodes may require hospital treatment.
● Advise patient not to take any other drugs, including OTC drugs, without checking with the doctor.
● Advise patient to avoid intake of alcohol. Chlorpropamide-alcohol flush is characterized by facial flushing, lightheadedness, headache, and occasional breathlessness. Even very small amounts of alcohol can produce this reaction.
● Advise patient to carry medical identification at all times.
Alert: Tell patient to report rash, skin eruptions, and other signs and symptoms of hypersensitivity to the doctor immediately.

▼ NEW DRUG

---

glimepiride
Amaryl

Pregnancy Risk Category: C

HOW SUPPLIED
Tablets: 1 mg, 2 mg, 4 mg

ACTION
The exact mechanism of glimepiride's ability to lower blood glucose may depend on stimulating the release of insulin from functioning pancreatic beta cells. Drug can also lead to increased sensitivity of peripheral tissues to insulin.

ONSET, PEAK, DURATION
Significant absorption occurs within 1 hour after administration; peak drug lev-

---

*Liquid contains alcohol.   **May contain tartrazine.   †Canada only.   ‡Australia only.   ◇ OTC.

els occur 2 to 3 hours after administration. Duration is unknown.

INDICATIONS & DOSAGE

Adjunct to diet and exercise to lower blood glucose in patients with non-insulin-dependent (type II) diabetes mellitus whose hyperglycemia can't be managed by diet and exercise alone—
Adults: Initially, 1 to 2 mg P.O. once daily with first main meal of the day; usual maintenance dosage is 1 to 4 mg P.O. once daily. After reaching a dosage of 2 mg, dosage is increased in increments not exceeding 2 mg q 1 to 2 weeks, based on patient's blood glucose response. Maximum dose is 8 mg/day.
Adjunct to insulin therapy in patients with non-insulin-dependent diabetes mellitus whose hyperglycemia can't be managed by diet and exercise in conjunction with oral hypoglycemic agents—
Adults: 8 mg P.O. once daily with first main meal of the day; used in combination with low-dose insulin. Insulin adjusted upward weekly as needed, guided by patient's blood glucose response.
Adults with renal impairment—
Adults: Suggested starting dose of 1 mg P.O. once daily with first main meal of the day, followed by appropriate dose titrated as needed.

ADVERSE REACTIONS

CNS: dizziness, asthenia, headache.
EENT: changes in accommodation.
GI: nausea.
Hematologic: leukopenia, hemolytic anemia, agranulocytosis, ***thrombocytopenia, aplastic anemia, pancytopenia.***
Hepatic: cholestatic jaundice.
Skin: allergic skin reactions (pruritus, erythema, urticaria, and morbilliform or maculopapular eruptions).
Other: hypoglycemia.

INTERACTIONS

NSAIDs and other drugs that are highly protein-bound (such as salicylates, sul-

fonamides, chloramphenicol, coumarins, probenecid, MAO inhibitors and beta-adrenergic blocking agents): may potentiate hypoglycemic action of sulfonylureas like glimepiride.
Drugs that tend to produce hyperglycemia, such as estrogens, oral contraceptives, corticosteroids, phenothiazines, thyroid products, phenytoin, nicotinic acid, isoniazid, and sympathomimetics thiazides and other diuretics: may lead to loss of glucose control. Adjust dosage as ordered.
Beta-adrenergic blocking agents: may mask symptoms of hypoglycemia.
Insulin: concomitant use may increase potential for hypoglycemia.

EFFECTS ON DIAGNOSTIC TESTS

Drug may elevate transaminase levels.

CONTRAINDICATIONS

Contraindicated in patients with hypersensitivity to the drug and in patients with diabetic ketoacidosis, which should be treated with insulin.

NURSING CONSIDERATIONS

● Use cautiously in debilitated or malnourished patients and in those with adrenal, pituitary, hepatic, or renal insufficiency; these patients are more susceptible to the hypoglycemic action of glucose-lowering drugs. Its use is not recommended in elderly patients.
● Glimepiride and insulin may be used concurrently in secondary failure patients (those who lose glucose control after initially responding to therapy).
● Fasting blood glucose should be monitored periodically to determine therapeutic response. Glycosylated hemoglobin should also be monitored, usually every 3 to 6 months to more precisely assess long-term glycemic control.
● Know that oral hypoglycemic agents have been associated with an increased risk of cardiovascular mortality compared with diet alone or with diet and insulin therapy.

• Know that safety and effectiveness in pediatric patients have not been established.
• It is not known whether glimepiride is excreted in breast milk. Drug should not be administered to breast-feeding women due to the potential for hypoglycemia in nursing infants.

☑ **PATIENT TEACHING**
• Tell patient to take drug with the first meal of the day.
• Make sure patient understands that therapy relieves symptoms but doesn't cure the disease. He should also understand the potential risks and advantages of taking this drug and other treatment methods.
• Stress importance of adhering to diet, weight-reduction, exercise, and personal-hygiene programs. Explain to patient and family how and when to perform self-monitoring of blood glucose levels, and teach recognition of and intervention for signs and symptoms of hyperglycemia and hypoglycemia.
• Advise patient to carry medical identification about his condition.
• Advise women planning a pregnancy to consult a doctor prior to becoming pregnant. Insulin may be required during pregnancy and breast-feeding.

---

glipizide
Glucotrol, Glucotrol XL, Minidiab‡

Pregnancy Risk Category: C

HOW SUPPLIED
Tablets: 5 mg, 10 mg
Tablets (extended-release): 5 mg, 10 mg

ACTION
Unknown. A sulfonylurea that probably stimulates insulin release from the pancreatic beta cells and reduces glucose output by the liver. An extrapancreatic effect increases peripheral sensitivity to insulin.

ONSET, PEAK, DURATION
Onset occurs within 15 to 30 minutes. Serum drug levels peak 1 to 3 hours after oral dose; peak insulin levels occur in ½ to 2 hours. Effects persist for 10 to 16 hours.

INDICATIONS & DOSAGE
Adjunct to diet to lower blood glucose level in patients with type II diabetes (non-insulin-dependent)—
Adults: initially, 5 mg P.O. daily 30 minutes before breakfast. Elderly patients or those with liver disease may be started on 2.5 mg. Maximum once-daily dose is 15 mg. Doses above 15 mg should be divided; maximum total daily dosage is 40 mg for immediate release tablets.
Extended-release tablets: initially, 5 mg P.O. daily. Titrate in 5-mg increments q 3 months depending on level of glycemic control. Maximum daily dosage is 20 mg.
To replace insulin therapy—
Adults: if insulin dosage is more than 20 units daily, the patient is started at usual dosage in addition to 50% of the insulin. If insulin dosage is less than 20 units, insulin may be discontinued on initiation of glipizide.

ADVERSE REACTIONS
CNS: dizziness, drowsiness, headache.
GI: nausea, constipation, diarrhea.
Hematologic: leukopenia, hemolytic anemia, *agranulocytosis, thrombocytopenia, aplastic anemia.*
Hepatic: cholestatic jaundice.
Skin: rash, pruritus.
Other: *hypoglycemia.*

INTERACTIONS
Anabolic steroids, chloramphenicol, clofibrate, guanethidine, MAO inhibitors, probenecid, salicylates, sulfonamides: increased hypoglycemic activity. Monitor blood glucose level.
Beta blockers: prolonged hypoglycemic effect and masked symptoms of hypoglycemia. Use together cautiously.

Corticosteroids, glucagon, rifampin, thiazide diuretics: decreased hypoglycemic response. Monitor blood glucose level.
Ethanol: possible disulfiram-like reaction. Avoid concomitant use.
Hydantoins: increased blood levels of hydantoins. Monitor blood levels.
Oral anticoagulants: increased hypoglycemic activity or enhanced anticoagulant effect. Monitor blood glucose levels and PT.

EFFECTS ON DIAGNOSTIC TESTS
Glipizide therapy alters cholesterol, alkaline phophatase, AST, lactate dehydrogenase, and BUN levels.

CONTRAINDICATIONS
Contraindicated in patients with hypersensitivity to drug, diabetic ketoacidosis with or without coma, and during pregnancy or breast-feeding.

NURSING CONSIDERATIONS
● Use cautiously in patients with renal and hepatic disease and in debilitated, malnourished, or elderly patients.
● Give about 30 minutes before meals.
● Some patients may attain effective control on a once-daily regimen, whereas others respond better with divided dosing.
● Be aware that glipizide is a second-generation sulfonylurea. The frequency of adverse reactions appears to be lower than with first-generation drugs, such as chlorpropamide.
● During periods of increased stress, patients may require insulin therapy. Monitor patients closely for hyperglycemia in these situations.
● Patients transferring from insulin therapy to an oral antidiabetic agent require blood glucose monitoring at least three times daily before meals. Patients may require hospitalization during transition.

☑ PATIENT TEACHING
● Instruct patient about disease, importance of following therapeutic regimen, adhering to diet, weight reduction, exercise, personal hygiene programs, and avoiding infection. Explain how and when to perform self-monitoring of blood glucose level, and teach recognition of hypoglycemia and hyperglycemia.
● Tell patient not to change drug dosage without the doctor's consent and to report abnormal blood or urine glucose test results.
● Tell patient not to take any other medication, including OTC drugs, without checking with the doctor.
● Advise patient to carry medical identification at all times.

glucagon

Pregnancy Risk Category: B

HOW SUPPLIED
Powder for injection: 1 mg (1 unit)-vial, 10 mg (10 units)-vial

ACTION
Raises blood glucose level by promoting catalytic depolymerization of hepatic glycogen to glucose.

ONSET, PEAK, DURATION
Onset almost immediate after parenteral administration. Peak hyperglycemic effect occurs within 30 minutes. Hyperglycemic effects persist 1 to 2 hours. Onset, peak and duration variable when used to relax GI smooth muscle but occur more quickly and last for shorter duration.

INDICATIONS & DOSAGE
Hypoglycemia—
Adults and children weighing more than 20 kg: 1 mg S.C., I.M., or I.V.
Children weighing 20 kg or less: 0.5 mg S.C., I.M., or I.V.
Note: May repeat in 15 minutes, if necessary. I.V. glucose must be given if patient fails to respond. When patient responds, supplemental carbohydrate

needs to be given immediately.
Diagnostic aid for radiologic examination—
Adults: 0.25 to 2 mg I.V. or I.M. before radiologic procedure.

ADVERSE REACTIONS
CV: hypotension.
GI: nausea, vomiting.
Respiratory: respiratory distress.
Other: hypersensitivity reactions (***bronchospasm,*** rash, dizziness, light-headedness).

INTERACTIONS
Phenytoin: inhibited glucagon-induced insulin release. Use cautiously.

EFFECTS ON DIAGNOSTIC TESTS
Glucagon lowers serum potassium levels.

CONTRAINDICATIONS
Contraindicated in patients with hypersensitivity to drug or with pheochromocytoma.

NURSING CONSIDERATIONS
● Use cautiously in those with history of insulinoma or pheochromocytoma.
● **I.V. use:** Reconstitute 1-unit vial with 1 ml of diluent; reconstitute 10-unit vial with 10 ml of diluent. Use only the diluent supplied by the manufacturer when preparing doses of 2 mg or less. For larger doses, dilute with sterile water for injection.
● For I.V. drip infusion, use dextrose solution, which is compatible with glucagon (drug forms a precipitate in chloride solutions). Inject directly into vein or into I.V. tubing of a free-flowing compatible solution over 2 to 5 minutes. Interrupt primary infusion during glucagon injection if using the same I.V. line.
Alert: Arouse patients from coma as quickly as possible and give additional carbohydrates orally to prevent secondary hypoglycemic reactions.
● Unstable hypoglycemic diabetic patients may not respond to glucagon;

give dextrose I.V. instead as ordered.

☑ **PATIENT TEACHING**
● Instruct patient and caregivers in proper glucagon administration and recognition of hypoglycemia.
● Explain importance of calling the doctor at once in emergencies.

glyburide (glibenclamide)
DiaBeta**, Euglucon†, Glynase PresTab, Micronase

Pregnancy Risk Category: B

HOW SUPPLIED
Tablets: 1.25 mg, 2.5 mg, 5 mg
Tablets (micronized): 1.5 mg, 3 mg, 5 mg

ACTION
Unknown. A sulfonylurea that probably stimulates insulin release from the pancreatic beta cells and reduces glucose output by the liver. An extrapancreatic effect increases peripheral sensitivity to insulin and causes a mild diuretic effect.

ONSET, PEAK, DURATION
Onset occurs in 1 hour for micronized form, 2 to 4 hours for nonmicronized form. Peak levels of glyburide occur in 2 to 4 hours; maximum increases in insulin levels are seen in 1 to 2 hours. Effects persist for 24 hours.

INDICATIONS & DOSAGE
Adjunct to diet to lower blood glucose level in patients with type II diabetes (non-insulin-dependent)—
Adults: initially, 2.5 to 5 mg regular tablets P.O. once daily with breakfast. Patients who are more sensitive to antidiabetic agents should be started at 1.25 mg daily. Usual maintenance dosage is 1.25 to 20 mg daily as a single dose or in divided doses.
Alternatively, micronized formulation may be used. Initial dosage is 1.5 to 3 mg daily. Patients who are more sensi-

tive to antidiabetic agents should be started at 0.75 mg daily. Usual maintenance dosage of the micronized formulation is 0.75 to 12 mg/day. Patients receiving above 6 mg/day may have a better response with b.i.d. dosing.
To replace insulin therapy—
Adults: if insulin dosage is below 40 units/day, the patient may be switched directly to glyburide when insulin is discontinued. If insulin dosage is 40 or more units/day, patient is started on 5 mg regular tablets or 3 mg micronized formulation P.O. once daily in addition to 50% of the insulin dosage.

ADVERSE REACTIONS
EENT: changes in accommodation or blurred vision.
GI: nausea, epigastric fullness, heartburn.
Hematologic: leukopenia, hemolytic anemia, *agranulocytosis, thrombocytopenia, aplastic anemia.*
Hepatic: cholestatic jaundice, hepatitis, abnormal liver function.
Skin: rash, pruritus, other allergic reactions.
Other: *hypoglycemia,* arthralgia, myalgia, angioedema.

INTERACTIONS
Anabolic steroids, chloramphenicol, clofibrate, guanethidine, MAO inhibitors, salicylates, sulfonamides: increased hypoglycemic activity. Monitor blood glucose level.
Beta blockers: prolonged hypoglycemic effect and masked symptoms of hypoglycemia. Use together cautiously.
Corticosteroids, glucagon, rifampin, thiazide diuretics: decreased hypoglycemic response. Monitor blood glucose level.
Ethanol: possible disulfiram-like reaction. Avoid concomitant use.
Hydantoins: increased blood levels of hydantoins. Monitor blood levels.
Oral anticoagulants: increased hypoglycemic activity or enhanced anticoagulant effect. Monitor blood glucose level and PT.

EFFECTS ON DIAGNOSTIC TESTS
Glyburide therapy alters cholesterol, alkaline phophatase, and BUN levels.

CONTRAINDICATIONS
Contraindicated in patients with hypersensitivity to the drug or diabetic ketoacidosis with or without coma, and during pregnancy or breast-feeding.

NURSING CONSIDERATIONS
• Use cautiously in patients with hepatic or renal impairment, or in debilitated, malnourished, or elderly patients.
• Know that elderly patients may be more sensitive to adverse effects.
Alert: Know that micronized glyburide (Glynase PresTab) contains drug in a smaller particle size and is not bioequivalent to regular glyburide tablets. Patients who have been taking Micronase or DiaBeta need to be retitrated.
• Know that although most patients may take glyburide once daily, those taking more than 10 mg daily may achieve better results with twice-daily dosage.
• Know that glyburide is a second-generation sulfonylurea. The frequency of adverse effects appears to be lower than with first-generation drugs, such as chlorpropamide.
• During periods of increased stress, such as infection, fever, surgery, or trauma, patients may require insulin therapy. Monitor patients closely for hyperglycemia in these situations.
• Patients transferring from insulin to an oral antidiabetic agent require blood glucose monitoring at least three times a day before meals. Patients may require hospitalization during transition.

☑ PATIENT TEACHING
• Instruct patient about nature of disease, importance of following therapeutic regimen, adhering to specific diet, weight reduction, exercise, and personal hygiene programs, and about avoiding infection. Explain how and when to perform self-monitoring of blood glucose levels, and teach recognition of and in-

tervention for hypoglycemia and hyperglycemia.

• Tell patient not to change drug dosage without the doctor's consent and to report abnormal blood or urine glucose test results.

• Teach patient to carry candy or other simple sugars to treat mild hypoglycemic episodes. Severe episodes may require hospital treatment.

• Advise patient not to take any other medication, including OTC drugs, without first checking with the doctor.

• Advise patient to carry medical identification at all times.

Alert: Instruct patient to report any episode of hypoglycemia to the doctor immediately; severe hypoglycemia is sometimes fatal in patients receiving as little as 2.5 to 5 mg glyburide daily.

insulins
insulin injection (regular insulin, crystalline zinc insulin)
Actrapid HM‡, Actrapid HM Penfill‡, Actrapid MC‡, Actrapid MC Penfill‡, Humulin R◊, Hypurin

Neutral‡, Insulin 2‡, Novolin R◊, Novolin R PenFill◊, Pork Regular Iletin II◊, Regular (Concentrated) Iletin II, Regular Iletin I◊, Regular Purified Pork Insulin◊, Velosulin Human‡, Velosulin Insuject‡

insulin zinc suspension, prompt (semilente)
Semilente MC‡

isophane insulin suspension (neutral protamine Hagedorn insulin, NPH)
Humulin N◊, Humulin NPH‡, Hypurin Isophane‡, Insulatard‡, Insulatard Human†, Isotard MC‡, Novolin N◊, Novolin N PenFill◊, NPH Insulin◊, NPH Purified Pork◊, Pork NPH Iletin II◊, Protaphane HM‡,

Protaphane HM Penfill‡, Protaphane MC‡

isophane insulin suspension with insulin injection
Actraphane HM‡, Actraphane HM Penfill‡, Actraphane MC‡, Humulin 50/50◊, Humulin 70/30◊, Novolin 70/30, Novolin 70/30 PenFill◊

insulin zinc suspension (lente)
Humulin L◊, Lente Iletin II◊, Lente Insulin◊, Lente MC‡, Lente Purified Pork Insulin◊, Monotard HM‡, Monotard MC‡, Novolin L◊

protamine zinc suspension (PZI)
Protamine Zinc Insulin MC‡

insulin zinc suspension, extended (ultralente)
Humulin U◊, Ultralente Insulin◊, Ultratard HM‡, Ultratard MC‡

Pregnancy Risk Category: NR

HOW SUPPLIED
insulin injection
Injection (human): 100 units/ml (Actrapid HM‡, Humulin R◊, Novolin R◊, Velosulin Human‡); 100 units/ml in 1.5-ml cartridge system◊ (Actrapid HM Penfill‡, Novolin R PenFill◊)
Injection (from pork): 100 units/ml◊
Injection (purified beef): 100 units/ml (Hypurin Neutral‡, Insulin 2‡)
Injection (purified pork): 100 units/ml (Actrapid MC‡, Pork Regular Iletin II◊, Regular Purified Pork Insulin◊); 100 units/ml in 1.5-ml cartridge system‡ (Actrapid MC Penfill‡); 100 units/ml in 2-ml cartridge system‡; 500 units/ml (Regular [Concentrated] Iletin II)
insulin zinc suspension, prompt
Injection (purified pork): 100 units/ml◊ (Semilente MC‡)
isophane insulin suspension
Injection (from beef): 100 units/ml◊ (NPH Insulin◊)

Injection (human, recombinant): 100 units/ml (Humulin N ◊, Humulin NPH‡, Insulatard Human†, Novolin N ◊, Protaphane HM‡); 100 units/ml in 1.5-ml cartridge system (Protaphane HM PenFill‡, Novolin N PenFill ◊)
Injection (purified beef): 100 units/ml (Hypurin Isophane‡, Isotard MC‡)
Injection (purified pork): 100 units/ml (Insulatard‡, NPH Purified Pork ◊, Pork NPH Iletin II, Protaphane MC‡)

isophane insulin suspension 50% with insulin injection 50%
Injection (human): 100 units/ml (Humulin 50/50 ◊)

isophane insulin suspension 70% with insulin injection 30%
Injection (human): 100 units/ml (Actraphane HM‡, Humulin 70/30 ◊, Novolin 70/30 ◊); 100 units/ml in 1.5-ml cartridge system (Actraphane HM PenFill‡, Novolin 70/30 PenFill ◊)
Injection (purified pork): 100 units/ml (Actraphane MC‡)

insulin zinc suspension
Injection (from beef): 100 units/ml (Lente Insulin ◊, Lente MC‡)
Injection (purified beef): 100 units/ml (Lente MC‡)
Injection (purified pork): 100 units/ml (Lente Iletin II, Monotard MC‡, Lente Purified Pork Insulin ◊)
Injection (human): 100 units/ml ◊ (Humulin L ◊, Monotard HM‡, Novolin I ◊)

protamine zinc suspension
Injection (purified pork): 100 units/ml Protamine Zinc Insulin MC‡

insulin zinc suspension, extended
Injection (from beef): 100 units/ml ◊ (Ultralente Insulin ◊)
Injection (human): 100 units/ml (Ultratard HM‡, Humulin U ◊)
Injection (purified pork): 100 units/ml‡ (Ultratard MC‡)

ACTION
Increases glucose transport across muscle and fat cell membranes to reduce blood glucose level. Promotes conversion of glucose to its storage form, glycogen; triggers amino acid uptake and conversion to protein in muscle cells and inhibits protein degradation; stimulates triglyceride formation and inhibits release of free fatty acids from adipose tissue; and stimulates lipoprotein lipase activity, which converts circulating lipoproteins to fatty acids.

ONSET, PEAK, DURATION
Highly variable. Onset occurs within ½ to 1½ hours with S.C. rapid-acting insulin, 1 to 2½ hours with S.C. intermediate-acting insulins, and 4 to 8 hours with S.C. long-acting insulins. Serum levels peak in 2 to 3 hours with S.C. rapid-acting regular insulins, 4 to 10 hours with S.C. rapid-acting semilente insulin, 4 to 15 hours with S.C. intermediate-acting insulins, and 10 to 30 hours with S.C. long-acting insulins. Effects persist for 5 to 7 hours with S.C. rapid-acting regular insulin, 12 to 16 hours with S.C. rapid-acting semilente insulin, 18 to 24 hours with S.C. intermediate-acting insulins, and 36 hours for S.C. long-acting insulins.

INDICATIONS & DOSAGE
Diabetic ketoacidosis (use regular insulin only)—
Adults: 0.33 units/kg as an I.V. bolus, followed by 0.1 units/kg/hour by continuous infusion. Continue infusion until blood glucose level drops to 250 mg/dl; then S.C. insulin is begun with dosage and dosage interval adjusted according to patient's blood glucose concentration.

Alternatively, 50 to 100 units I.V. and 50 to 100 units S.C. stat; then additional doses q 2 to 6 hours based on blood glucose levels.

To prepare infusion, add 100 units of regular insulin and 1 g of albumin to 100 ml of 0.9% sodium chloride solution. Insulin concentration will be 1 unit/ml. (The albumin will adhere to plastic, preventing insulin from adhering to plastic.)
Children: 0.1 unit/kg as an I.V. bolus, then 0.1 unit/kg hourly by continuous

infusion until blood glucose level drops to 250 mg/dl; then S.C. insulin started. Alternatively, 1 to 2 units/kg in two divided doses, one I.V. and the other S.C., followed by 0.5 to 1 unit/kg I.V. q 1 to 2 hours based on blood glucose levels.

Type I diabetes (insulin-dependent), adjunct to type II diabetes (noninsulin-dependent) inadequately controlled by diet and oral antidiabetic agents—
Adults and children: therapeutic regimen is prescribed by the doctor and adjusted according to patient's blood glucose concentrations.

ADVERSE REACTIONS
Skin: urticaria, pruritus, swelling, redness, stinging, warmth at injection site.
Other: *lipoatrophy, lipohypertrophy,* hypersensitivity reactions (***anaphylaxis,*** rash), ***hypoglycemia,*** hyperglycemia (rebound, or Somogyi, effect).

INTERACTIONS
Anabolic steroids, beta blockers, clofibrate, ethanol, fenfluramine, guanethidine, MAO inhibitors, salicylates, tetracycline: prolonged hypoglycemic effect. Monitor blood glucose level carefully.
Corticosteroids, dextrothyroxine, epinephrine, smoking, thiazide diuretics, thyroid hormone: diminished insulin response. Monitor for hyperglycemia.
Diazoxide, phenytoin (high doses): may inhibit endogenous insulin secretion and cause hypoglycemia in diabetic patients. Carefully adjust insulin dosage when using with these drugs.
Oral contraceptives: may decrease glucose tolerance in diabetic patients. Monitor blood glucose levels and adjust insulin dosage carefully.

EFFECTS ON DIAGNOSTIC TESTS
The physiologic effects of insulin may decrease serum magnesium, potassium, or inorganic phosphate concentrations.

CONTRAINDICATIONS
Contraindicated in patients with a history of systemic allergic reaction to pork.

NURSING CONSIDERATIONS
● Know that insulin is the drug of choice to treat diabetes during pregnancy. Insulin requirements increase in pregnant diabetic patients and then decline immediately postpartum. Monitor patient closely.
● Dosage is always expressed in USP units. Remember to use only the syringes calibrated for the particular concentration of insulin administered. U-500 insulin must be administered with a U-100 syringe because no syringes are made for this strength.
● Be aware some patients may develop insulin resistance and require large insulin doses to control symptoms of diabetes. U-500 insulin is available as Regular (Concentrated) Iletin II for such patients. Although every pharmacy may not stock it, it is available. Nurses should give the hospital pharmacy sufficient notice before requesting refill of in-house prescription. Never store U-500 insulin in same area with other insulin preparations because of danger of severe overdose if given accidentally to other patients.
● To mix insulin suspension, swirl vial gently or rotate between palms or between palm and thigh. Don't shake vigorously: this causes bubbling and air in syringe.
● Know that lente, semilente, and ultralente insulins may be mixed in any proportion. Regular insulin may be mixed with NPH or lente insulins in any proportion. When mixing regular insulin with intermediate or long acting insulin, always draw up regular insulin into syringe first.
● Note that switching from separate injections to a prepared mixture may alter patient response. Whenever NPH or lente is mixed with regular insulin in the same syringe, give it immediately to avoid loss of potency.
● Don't use insulin that changes color or becomes clumped or granular in appearance.

● Check expiration date on vial before using contents.

● Know that usual administration route is S.C. For proper S.C. administration, remember to pinch a fold of skin with the fingers at least 3″ (7.6 cm) apart, and insert the needle at a 45- to 90-degree angle.

● Press but do not rub site after injection. Rotate injection sites and chart to avoid overuse of one area. Know that diabetic patients may achieve better control if injection site is rotated within same anatomic region.

Alert: Know that regular insulin is used in patients with circulatory collapse, diabetic ketoacidosis, or hyperkalemia. Do not use regular insulin (Concentrated), 500 units/ml, I.V. Do not use intermediate or long-acting insulins for coma or other emergency requiring rapid drug action. Also know that ketosis-prone type I severely ill, and newly diagnosed diabetic patients with very high blood glucose levels may require hospitalization and I.V. treatment with regular fast-acting insulin.

● **I.V. use:** Only administer regular insulin I.V. Inject directly, at ordered rate, into vein through an intermittent infusion device or into a port close to I.V. access site. Intermittent infusion is not recommended. If given by continuous infusion, infuse drug diluted in 0.9% sodium chloride at the prescribed rate.

● Store insulin in cool area. Refrigeration is desirable but not essential, except with regular insulin concentrated.

☑ PATIENT TEACHING

● Make sure patient knows that therapy only relieves symptoms.

● Instruct patient about nature of disease, importance of following the therapeutic regimen, adhering to specific diet, weight reduction, exercise, and personal hygiene program, and about avoiding infection. Emphasize the importance of the timing of injections and eating and that meals must not be omitted.

● Stress to patient that accuracy of measurement is important, especially with concentrated regular insulin. Aids, such as magnifying sleeve or dose magnifier, may improve accuracy. Instruct patient and caregivers how to measure and administer insulin.

● Advise patient not to alter the order of mixing insulins or change the model or brand of insulin, syringe, or needle.

● Teach that self-monitoring of blood glucose levels and urine ketone tests are essential guides to dosage and success of therapy. It's important to recognize hypoglycemic symptoms because insulin-induced hypoglycemia is hazardous and may cause brain damage if prolonged; most adverse effects are self-limiting and temporary.

● Instruct patient on proper use of equipment for performing self-monitoring of blood glucose levels.

● Advise patient not to smoke within 30 minutes after insulin injection. Cigarette smoking decreases the amount of absorption of insulin administered subcutaneously.

● Tell patient that marijuana use may increase insulin requirements.

● Advise patient to wear a medical identification bracelet at all times, to carry ample insulin and syringes on trips, to have carbohydrates (lump of sugar or candy) on hand for emergencies, and to note time zone changes for dosage schedule when traveling.

---

metformin hydrochloride
Glucophage

Pregnancy Risk Category: B

HOW SUPPLIED
Tablets: 500 mg, 850 mg

ACTION
Decreases hepatic glucose production and intestinal absorption of glucose and improves insulin sensitivity (increases peripheral glucose uptake and utilization).

ONSET, PEAK, DURATION
Not clearly defined, although food does delay onset and peak of the drug.

INDICATIONS & DOSAGE
Adjunct to diet to lower blood glucose level in patients with type II diabetes (non-insulin-dependent)—
Adults: initially, 500 mg P.O. b.i.d. given with morning and evening meals, or 850 mg P.O. once daily given with morning meal. When 500-mg dose form used, dosage increased 500 mg weekly to maximum dosage of 2,500 mg P.O. daily in divided doses as needed. When 850-mg dose form used, dosage increased 850 mg every other week to a maximum dosage of 2,550 mg P.O. daily in divided doses as needed. Elderly and debilitated patients should be conservatively dosed due to the potential decrease in renal function.

ADVERSE REACTIONS
GI: diarrhea, nausea, vomiting, abdominal bloating, flatulence, anorexia.
Hematologic: megaloblastic anemia.
Other: *lactic acidosis,* unpleasant or metallic taste.

INTERACTIONS
Calcium channel blockers, corticosteroids, estrogens, isoniazid, nicotinic acid, oral contraceptives, phenothiazines, phenytoin, sympathomimetics, thiazide and other diuretics, thyroid agents: may produce hyperglycemia. Monitor patient's glycemic control. Metformin dosage may need to be increased.
Cationic drugs, such as amiloride, cimetidine, digoxin, morphine, procainamide, quinidine, quinine, ranitidine, triamterene, trimethoprim, vancomycin: have the potential to compete for common renal tubular transport systems, which may increase metformin plasma levels. Monitor patient's blood glucose level.
Nifedipine: increased metformin plasma levels. Monitor patient closely. Metformin dosage may need to be decreased.

EFFECTS ON DIAGNOSTIC TESTS
None reported.

CONTRAINDICATIONS
Contraindicated in patients with hypersensitivity to the drug, renal disease, or metabolic acidosis. Metformin should be temporarily withheld in patients undergoing radiologic studies involving parenteral administration of iodinated contrast materials because use of such products may result in acute renal dysfunction. The drug should also be promptly discontinued if the patient enters a hypoxic state. Metformin generally should be avoided in patients with hepatic disease.

NURSING CONSIDERATIONS
• Use caution when giving drug to elderly, debilitated, or malnourished patients and to those with adrenal or pituitary insufficiency because of increased risk of hypoglycemia.
• Know that before therapy begins, the patient's renal function should be assessed and then assessed at least annually thereafter. If renal impairment is detected, expect the doctor to switch the patient to a different antidiabetic agent.
• Administer with meals; once-daily dosage should be given with breakfast and twice-daily dosage with breakfast and dinner.
• Know that when transferring patients from standard oral hypoglycemic agents (except chlorpropamide) to metformin, no transition period generally is necessary. When switching patients from chlorpropamide to metformin, care should be exercised during the first 2 weeks of metformin therapy because the prolonged retention of chlorpropamide increases the risk of hypoglycemia during this time.
• Monitor patient's blood glucose levels regularly to evaluate effectiveness of therapy. Notify doctor if blood glucose

levels become elevated despite therapy.
• Be aware that if the patient has not responded to 4 weeks of therapy using the maximum dosage, the doctor may add an oral sulfonylurea while continuing metformin at the maximum dosage. If the patient still does not respond after several months of concomitant therapy at maximum dosages, the doctor may discontinue both agents and institute insulin therapy.
• Monitor patient closely during times of increased stress, such as infection, fever, surgery, or trauma. Insulin therapy may be needed in these situations.
• Be aware that the incidence of metformin-induced lactic acidosis is very low. Reported cases have occurred primarily in diabetic patients with significant renal insufficiency; with multiple, concomitant medical or surgical problems; and with multiple, concomitant drug regimens. The risk increases with the degree of renal impairment and the patient's age.
Alert: Know that metformin should be discontinued immediately and the doctor notified if the patient develops any condition associated with hypoxemia or dehydration because of the risk of lactic acidosis associated with these conditions.
• Expect metformin therapy to be temporarily suspended for any surgical procedure (except minor procedures not associated with restricted intake of food and fluids) and should not be restarted until the patient's oral intake has resumed and renal function has been evaluated as normal.
• Monitor the patient's hematologic status for evidence of megaloblastic anemia. Patients with inadequate vitamin B_{12} or calcium intake or absorption appear to be predisposed to developing subnormal vitamin B_{12} levels. These patients should have routine serum vitamin B_{12} level determinations every 2 to 3 years.

☑ **PATIENT TEACHING**
Alert: Instruct patient about nature of diabetes, importance of following therapeutic regimen, adhering to specific diet, weight reduction, exercise, personal hygiene programs, and avoiding infection. Explain how and when to perform self-monitoring of blood glucose level, and teach signs of hypoglycemia and hyperglycemia.
• Instruct patient to discontinue drug and notify the doctor immediately if unexplained hyperventilation, myalgia, malaise, unusual somnolence, or other nonspecific symptoms of early lactic acidosis occur.
• Warn patient not to consume excessive alcohol while taking metformin.
• Tell patient not to change drug dosage without the doctor's consent. Encourage patient to report abnormal blood glucose results.
• Advise patient not to take any other medication, including OTC drugs, without checking with the doctor.
• Instruct patient to carry medical identification at all times.

---

tolazamide
Tolamide, Tolinase

Pregnancy Risk Category: C

HOW SUPPLIED
Tablets: 100 mg, 250 mg, 500 mg

ACTION
Unknown. A sulfonylurea that probably stimulates insulin release from the pancreatic beta cells and reduces glucose output by the liver. An extrapancreatic effect increases peripheral sensitivity to insulin.

ONSET, PEAK, DURATION
Onset occurs in 4 to 6 hours. Peak hypoglycemic effect within 4 to 6 hours. Effects persist for 12 to 24 hours.

INDICATIONS & DOSAGE

Adjunct to diet to lower blood glucose levels in patients with type II diabetes mellitus (non-insulin-dependent) whose hyperglycemia is inadequately controlled with insulin therapy of over 30 units/day give as multiple injections—
Adults: initially, 100 mg P.O. daily with breakfast if fasting blood sugar (FBS) is under 200 mg/dl, or 250 mg P.O. if FBS is over 200 mg/dl. Dosage adjusted at weekly intervals by 100 to 250 mg as needed. Maximum daily dosage is 500 mg b.i.d. before meals.
Adults over 65 years: 100 mg P.O. once daily.

To change from insulin to oral therapy—
Adults: if insulin dosage is under 20 units daily, insulin is stopped and oral therapy started at 100 mg P.O. daily with breakfast. If insulin dosage is 20 to 40 units daily, insulin is stopped and oral therapy started at 250 mg P.O. daily with breakfast. If insulin dosage is over 40 units daily, insulin is decreased by 50% and oral therapy started at 250 mg P.O. daily with breakfast. Dosage may be adjusted by 100 to 250 mg.

ADVERSE REACTIONS

CNS: paresthesia, fatigue, dizziness, vertigo, malaise, headache.
GI: nausea, vomiting, epigastric distress.
Hematologic: leukopenia, hemolytic anemia, *thrombocytopenia, aplastic anemia, agranulocytosis.*
Skin: rash, urticaria, pruritus, erythema.
Other: *hypersensitivity reactions, hypoglycemia.*

INTERACTIONS

Anabolic steroids, chloramphenicol, clofibrate, guanethidine, MAO inhibitors, salicylates, sulfonamides: increased hypoglycemic activity. Monitor blood glucose level.
Beta blockers: prolonged hypoglycemic effect and masked symptoms of hypoglycemia. Use together cautiously.
Corticosteroids, glucagon, rifampin,
thiazide diuretics: decreased hypoglycemic response. Monitor blood glucose level.
Ethanol: possible disulfiram-like reaction. Avoid concomitant use of moderate to large amounts of ethanol.
Hydantoins: increased blood levels of hydantoins. Monitor blood levels.
Oral anticoagulants: increased hypoglycemic activity or enhanced anticoagulant effect. Monitor blood glucose levels and PT.

EFFECTS ON DIAGNOSTIC TESTS

Tolazamide therapy alters alkaline phosphatase and cholesterol levels.

CONTRAINDICATIONS

Contraindicated for treating type I diabetes (insulin-dependent) or diabetes that can be adequately controlled by diet. Also contraindicated in patients with type II diabetes complicated by ketosis, acidosis, coma, or other acute complications such as major surgery, severe infection, or severe trauma; in patients with uremia or hypersensitivity to drug; and during pregnancy or breastfeeding.

NURSING CONSIDERATIONS

● Use cautiously in elderly, debilitated, or malnourished patients or patients with impaired hepatic or renal function or porphyria.
● Know that elderly patients may be more sensitive to adverse effects.
● Be aware that patients transferring from another oral antidiabetic agent usually need no transition period.
● Patients transferring from insulin therapy to an oral antidiabetic agent require blood glucose level testing at least three times a day before meals. Hospitalization may be required during the transition.

☑ PATIENT TEACHING

● Make sure patient knows that therapy relieves symptoms but doesn't cure disease.

---

*Liquid contains alcohol.   **May contain tartrazine.   †Canada only.   ‡Australia only.   ◇OTC.

● Instruct patient about nature of disease, importance of following therapeutic regimen, adhering to specific diet, weight reduction, exercise, and personal hygiene programs, and about avoiding infection. Explain how and when to perform self-monitoring of blood glucose levels, and teach recognition of and intervention for hypoglycemia and hyperglycemia.

● Tell patient not to change drug dosage without the doctor's consent and to report abnormal blood or urine glucose test results.

● Teach patient to carry candy or other simple sugars to treat mild hypoglycemic episodes. Severe episodes may require hospital treatment.

● Advise patient not to take any other medication, including OTC drugs, without checking with the doctor.

● Advise patient to avoid moderate to large intake of alcohol because of possible disulfiram-like reaction.

● Advise patient to carry medical identification at all times.

---

tolbutamide
Apo-Tolbutamide, Mobenol†, Novo-Butamide†, Oramide, Orinase

Pregnancy Risk Category: C

HOW SUPPLIED
Tablets: 250 mg, 500 mg

ACTION
Unknown. A sulfonylurea that probably stimulates insulin release from the pancreatic beta cells and reduces glucose output by the liver. An extrapancreatic effect increases peripheral sensitivity to insulin.

ONSET, PEAK, DURATION
Onset occurs within 1 hour. Plasma levels peak in 3 to 5 hours; peak hypoglycemic effects within 5 to 8 hours. Effects persist for 6 to 12 hours.

INDICATIONS & DOSAGE
Adjunct to diet to lower blood glucose levels in patients with type II diabetes (non-insulin-dependent)—
Adults: initially, 1 to 2 g P.O. daily as a single dose or in divided doses b.i.d. to t.i.d. Dosage adjusted, if necessary, to maximum of 3 g daily; however, the manufacturer states that little benefit occurs with doses greater than 2 g daily.
To change from insulin to oral therapy—
Adults: if insulin dosage is under 20 units daily, insulin is stopped and oral therapy started at 1 to 2 g P.O. daily. If insulin dosage is 20 to 40 units daily, insulin is reduced by 30% to 50% and oral therapy started as above. If insulin dosage is over 40 units daily, insulin is reduced by 20% and oral therapy started as above. Further reductions are based on patient's response to oral therapy.

ADVERSE REACTIONS
CNS: paresthesia, fatigue, dizziness, vertigo, malaise, headache.
GI: nausea, heartburn, epigastric distress.
Hematologic: leukopenia, hemolytic anemia, *thrombocytopenia, aplastic anemia, agranulocytosis.*
Skin: rash, pruritus, erythema, urticaria.
Other: *hypersensitivity reactions, hypoglycemia, dilutional hyponatremia.*

INTERACTIONS
Anabolic steroids, chloramphenicol, clofibrate, guanethidine, MAO inhibitors, salicylates, sulfonamides: increased hypoglycemic activity. Monitor blood glucose level.
Beta blockers: prolonged hypoglycemic effect and masked symptoms of hypoglycemia. Use together cautiously.
Corticosteroids, glucagon, rifampin, thiazide diuretics: decreased hypoglycemic response. Monitor blood glucose level.
Ethanol: possible disulfiram-like reaction. Avoid concomitant use of moderate to large amount of ethanol.
Hydantoins: increased blood levels of

---

hydantoins. Monitor blood levels closely.
Oral anticoagulants: increased hypoglycemic activity or enhanced anticoagulant effect. Monitor blood glucose levels and PT.

EFFECTS ON DIAGNOSTIC TESTS
Tolbutamide therapy alters alkaline
phosphatase, bilirubin, cholesterol, total
protein, and urine porphyrins and protein levels; it also alters cephalin flocculation (thymol turbidity) and ^{131}I thyroid
uptake.

CONTRAINDICATIONS
Contraindicated for treating type I diabetes (insulin-dependent) or diabetes
that can be adequately controlled by
diet. Also contraindicated in patients
with type II diabetes complicated by
fever, ketosis, acidosis, coma, or other
acute complications such as major
surgery, severe infection, or severe trauma; in patients with hypersensitivity to
drug or severe renal insufficiency; and
during pregnancy or breast-feeding.

NURSING CONSIDERATIONS
• Use cautiously in elderly, debilitated,
or malnourished patients or patients
with impaired hepatic or renal function
or porphyria.
• Know that elderly patients may be
more sensitive to adverse effects.
• Know that patients transferring from
another oral antidiabetic agent usually
need no transition period.
• Be aware that patients transferring
from insulin therapy to an oral antidiabetic agent require blood glucose level
testing at least three times a day before
meals. Hospitalization may be required
during the transition.

☑ PATIENT TEACHING
• Instruct patient about nature of disease, importance of following therapeutic regimen, adhering to specific diet,
weight reduction, exercise, and personal
hygiene program, and about avoiding

infection. Explain how and when to perform self-monitoring of blood glucose
levels, and teach recognition of and intervention for hypoglycemia and hyperglycemia.
• Tell him that therapy relieves symptoms but doesn't cure disease.
• Tell patient not to change dosage
without doctor's consent and to report
abnormal glucose test results.
• Teach patient to carry candy or other
simple sugars to treat mild hypoglycemic episodes.
• Advise patient not to take any other
medication, including OTC drugs, without checking with the doctor.
• Advise patient to avoid moderate to
large intake of alcohol because of possible disulfiram-like reaction.
• Advise patient to carry medical identification at all times.

▼ NEW DRUG

troglitazone
Rezulin

Pregnancy Risk Category: B

HOW SUPPLIED
Tablets: 200 mg, 400 mg

ACTION
Inhibits hepatic glucose production and
enhances effects of circulating insulin.

ONSET, PEAK, DURATION
Drug is rapidly absorbed. Plasma levels
peak within 2 to 3 hours after oral administration. Steady-state plasma levels
are reached in 3 to 5 days. Duration unknown.

INDICATIONS & DOSAGE
*Adjunct to diet and insulin therapy in
patients with type II (noninsulin-dependent) diabetes mellitus whose hyperglycemia is inadequately controlled
with insulin therapy of over 30 units/day
given as multiple injections—*
Adults: initially, for patients on insulin

therapy, continue with current insulin dose and begin concomitant therapy with 200 mg P.O. once daily, taken with a meal. Dosage may be increased after 2 to 4 weeks if needed. Usual daily dose is 400 mg; maximum daily dose is 600 mg. The insulin dose may be decreased by 10% to 25% when fasting glucose levels are below 120 mg/dl in patients receiving both troglitazone and insulin.

ADVERSE REACTIONS
CNS: *headache,* asthenia, dizziness.
CV: peripheral edema.
GI: nausea, diarrhea.
GU: UTI.
Musculoskeletal: back pain.
Respiratory: rhinitis, pharyngitis.
Other: *infection, pain,* accidental injury.

INTERACTIONS
Cholestyramine: reduced absorption of troglitazone. Avoid concomitant use.
Oral contraceptives: may reduce plasma concentrations of hormones, resulting in loss of contraceptive properties. Additional form of contraception is recommended.
Terfenadine: decreased terfenadine efficacy. Monitor patient.

EFFECTS ON DIAGNOSTIC TESTS
Drug may cause transient elevations in AST and ALT levels, small increases in serum lipid levels, and small decreases in hemoglobin, hematocrit, and nuetrophil counts.

CONTRAINDICATIONS
Contraindicated in patients with known hypersensitivity to the drug.

NURSING CONSIDERATIONS
● Use cautiously in patients with hepatic disease and heart failure patients with Class III and IV status.
● Know that drug should be used in pregnancy only if the benefit justifies the potential risk to the fetus. The preferred antidiabetic agent to be used during pregnancy is insulin. Breast-feeding women should not take troglitazone.
● The safety and effectiveness in pediatric patients have not been established.
● Be aware that troglitazone does not stimulate insulin secretion, so should not be used to treat patients with type I diabetes or ketoacidosis.
● When used concomitantly with insulin, monitor patient for hypoglycemia. Know that dose of insulin may need to be reduced.
● Before starting therapy with troglitazone, investigate and address secondary causes of poor glycemic control (including infection and poor injection technique.)
● Monitor glucose levels, especially during times of increased stress, such as infection, fever, surgery, and trauma.

☑ PATIENT TEACHING
● Instruct patient about nature of diabetes, importance of following treatment, avoiding infection, and adhering to specific diet, weight reduction, exercise, and personal hygiene programs. Explain how and when to perform self-monitoring of blood glucose level, teach signs of hypoglycemia and hyperglycemia, and explain what to do if those conditions occur. Include responsible family members in teaching.
● Tell patient that drug should be taken with a meal. If a dose is missed, take it with the next meal. Tell him not to take two doses the next day.
● Tell patient that drug may cause resumption of ovulation in premenopausal anovulatory women, causing an increased risk for pregnancy.
● Instruct patient to carry medical identification at all times.

Reactions may be *common,* uncommon, *life-threatening,* or COMMON AND LIFE-THREATENING.

levothyroxine sodium
liothyronine sodium
liotrix
thyroid
thyrotropin

COMBINATION PRODUCTS
None.

---

levothyroxine sodium (T₄ or L-thyroxine sodium)

Eltroxin†, Levo-T, Levothroid, Levoxine, Levoxyl, Oroxine‡, Synthroid**

Pregnancy Risk Category: A

HOW SUPPLIED
Tablets: 25 mcg, 50 mcg, 75 mcg, 88 mcg, 100 mcg, 112 mcg, 125 mcg, 137 mcg, 150 mcg, 175 mcg, 200 mcg, 300 mcg
Injection: 200 mcg-vial, 500 mcg-vial

ACTION
Not completely defined. Stimulates metabolism of all body tissues by accelerating rate of cellular oxidation.

ONSET, PEAK, DURATION
Onset in 24 hours. Time to peak therapeutic effect is 3 to 4 weeks. Effects persist for 1 to 3 weeks.

INDICATIONS & DOSAGE
Cretinism—
Children 0 to 6 months: 25 to 50 mcg or 10 to 15 mcg/kg P.O. daily.
Children 6 to 12 months: 50 to 75 mcg or 6 to 8 mcg/kg P.O. daily.
Children 1 to 5 years: 75 to 100 mcg or 5 to 6 mcg/kg P.O. daily.
Children 6 to 12 years: 100 to 150 mcg or 4 to 5 mcg/kg P.O. daily.
Children over 12 years: >150 mcg or 2 to 3 mcg/kg P.O. daily.

Myxedema coma—
Adults: 200 to 500 mcg I.V.; then 100 to 300 mcg given on second day, followed by parenteral maintenance dosage of 50 to 200 mcg I.V. daily. Patient should be switched to oral maintenance as soon as possible.
Thyroid hormone replacement—
Adults: initially, 25 to 50 mcg P.O. daily, increased by 25 mcg P.O. q 2 to 4 weeks until desired response occurs. Maintenance dosage is 100 to 200 mcg P.O. daily. May administer I.V. or I.M. when P.O. ingestion is precluded for long periods. However, dosage adjustment is necessary.
Adults over 65 years: 12.5 to 50 mcg P.O. daily. Increased by 12.5 to 25 mcg at 3- to 8-week intervals depending on response.
Children: initially, 25 to 50 mcg in children younger than 1 year or 3 to 5 mcg/kg in children 1 year and older P.O. daily, gradually increased by 25 to 50 mcg q 2 to 4 weeks until desired response occurs.

ADVERSE REACTIONS
CNS: *nervousness, insomnia, tremor,* headache.
CV: *tachycardia, palpitations, **arrhythmias,** angina pectoris, **cardiac arrest.***
GI: diarrhea, vomiting.
Other: weight loss, diaphoresis, heat intolerance, fever, menstrual irregularities, allergic skin reactions.

INTERACTIONS
Cholestyramine, colestipol: impaired levothyroxine absorption. Separate doses by 4 to 5 hours.
Insulin, oral antidiabetic agents: altered serum glucose levels. Monitor blood glucose levels. Dosage adjustments may be necessary.
I.V. phenytoin: free thyroid released.

---

*Liquid contains alcohol.   **May contain tartrazine.   †Canada only.   ‡Australia only.   ◇OTC.

Monitor for tachycardia.
Oral anticoagulants: altered PT. Monitor PT. Dosage adjustments may be necessary.
Sympathomimetics, such as epinephrine: increased risk of coronary insufficiency. Monitor closely.

EFFECTS ON DIAGNOSTIC TESTS
Levothyroxine therapy alters radioactive iodine (^{131}I) thyroid uptake, protein-bound iodine levels, and liothyronine uptake.

CONTRAINDICATIONS
Contraindicated in patients with hypersensitivity to drug, acute MI uncomplicated by hypothyroidism, untreated thyrotoxicosis, or uncorrected adrenal insufficiency.

NURSING CONSIDERATIONS
• Use with extreme caution in elderly patients and those with angina pectoris, hypertension, other CV disorders, renal insufficiency, or ischemia.
• Use cautiously in those with diabetes mellitus or insipidus or myxedema.
• Rapid replacement in patients with arteriosclerosis may precipitate angina, coronary occlusion, or CVA. Use cautiously in these patients. Also, in patients with coronary artery disease who must receive thyroid hormone, observe carefully for possible coronary insufficiency.
• Know that thyroid hormone replacement requirements are about 25% lower in patients over age 60 than in young adults.
• Also know that patients with adult hypothyroidism are unusually sensitive to thyroid hormone. Patient should be started at lowest dosage and titrated to higher dosages according to patients' symptoms and laboratory data until euthyroid state is reached.
• **I.V. use:** Prepare I.V. dose immediately before injection. Do not mix with other solutions. Inject into vein over 1 to 2 minutes.

• When changing from levothyroxine to liothyronine (T_3), levothyroxine should be stopped and liothyronine begun. Dosage should be increased in small increments after residual effects of levothyroxine have disappeared. When changing from liothyronine to levothyroxine, levothyroxine is started several days before withdrawing liothyronine to avoid relapse.
• Monitor blood pressure and heart rate closely. High initial I.V. dosage is usually well tolerated by patients in myxedema coma. Normal serum levels of T_4 should occur within 24 hours, followed by a threefold increase in serum T_3 in 3 days.
• Know that thyroid hormones alter thyroid function test results.
• Know that patients taking levothyroxine who need to have radioactive iodine uptake studies performed must discontinue drug 4 weeks before test.

☑ **PATIENT TEACHING**
• Make sure patient understands the importance of compliance. Tell patient to take thyroid hormones at the same time each day, preferably before breakfast, to maintain constant hormone levels. Suggest morning dosage to prevent insomnia.
• Warn patient (especially elderly patient) to tell the doctor at once if chest pain, palpitations, sweating, nervousness, shortness of breath, or other signs of overdose or aggravated CV disease occur.
• Advise patient who has achieved stable response not to change brands.
• Tell patient to report unusual bleeding and bruising.

liothyronine sodium (T_3)
Cyronine, Cytomel, Tertroxin‡, Triostat

Pregnancy Risk Category: A

HOW SUPPLIED
Tablets: 5 mcg, 25 mcg, 50 mcg
Injection: 10 mcg/ml

ACTION
Not clearly defined. Enhances oxygen consumption by most tissues of the body, increases the basal metabolic rate and the metabolism of carbohydrates, lipids, and proteins.

ONSET, PEAK, DURATION
Onset unknown. Peak occurs in 2 to 3 days. Effects persist about 3 days.

INDICATIONS & DOSAGE
Congenital hypothyroidism—
Children: 5 mcg P.O. daily with a 5-mcg increase q 3 to 4 days until desired response achieved.
Myxedema—
Adults: initially, 5 mcg P.O. daily, increased by 5 to 10 mcg q 1 or 2 weeks until daily dosage reaches 25 mcg. Then, increased by 12.5 to 25 mcg daily q 1 to 2 weeks. Maintenance dosage is 50 to 100 mcg daily.
Myxedema coma, premyxedema coma—
Adults: initially, 10 to 20 mcg I.V. for patients with known or suspected CV disease; 25 to 50 mcg I.V. for patients not known to have CV disease. Subsequent dosage adjustments made as indicated by patient's condition and response. Patient should be switched to oral therapy as soon as possible.
Nontoxic goiter—
Adults: initially, 5 mcg P.O. daily; may increase by 5 to 10 mcg daily q 1 to 2 weeks, until daily dosage reaches 25 mcg. Then, increase by 12.5 to 25 mcg daily q 1 to 2 weeks. Usual maintenance dosage is 75 mcg daily.
Thyroid hormone replacement—
Adults: initially, 25 mcg P.O. daily, increased by 12.5 to 25 mcg q 1 to 2 weeks until satisfactory response occurs. Usual maintenance dosage is 25 to 75 mcg daily.
Geriatric patients: 5 mcg daily, increased in 5-mcg daily increments.

T_3 suppression test to differentiate hyperthyroidism from euthyroidism—
Adults: 75 to 100 mcg P.O. daily for 7 days.

ADVERSE REACTIONS
CNS: *nervousness, insomnia, tremor,* headache.
CV: *tachycardia,* **arrhythmias,** angina pectoris, **cardiac decompensation and collapse.**
GI: diarrhea, vomiting.
Other: weight loss, heat intolerance, diaphoresis, accelerated bone maturation in infants and children, menstrual irregularities, skin reactions.

INTERACTIONS
Cholestyramine, colestipol: impaired liothyronine absorption. Separate doses by 4 to 5 hours.
Insulin, oral antidiabetic agents: initial thyroid replacement therapy may cause increases in insulin or oral hypoglycemic requirements. Monitor blood glucose levels. Dosage adjustments may be necessary.
Oral anticoagulants: altered PT. Monitor PT. Dosage adjustments may be necessary.
Sympathomimetics, such as epinephrine: increased risk of coronary insufficiency. Monitor closely.

EFFECTS ON DIAGNOSTIC TESTS
Liothyronine therapy alters radioactive iodine (^{131}I) uptake, protein-bound iodine levels, and liothyronine uptake.

CONTRAINDICATIONS
Contraindicated in patients with hypersensitivity to drug, acute MI uncomplicated by hypothyroidism, untreated thyrotoxicosis, or uncorrected adrenal insufficiency.

NURSING CONSIDERATIONS
● Use with extreme caution in elderly patients and those with angina pectoris, hypertension, other CV disorders, renal insufficiency, or ischemia.

---

*Liquid contains alcohol.   **May contain tartrazine.   †Canada only.   ‡Australia only.   ◇OTC.

- Use cautiously in patients with diabetes mellitus or insipidus or myxedema.
- Rapid replacement in patients with arteriosclerosis may precipitate angina, coronary occlusion, or CVA. Use cautiously in these patients. In patients with coronary artery disease who must receive thyroid hormones, observe carefully for possible coronary insufficiency. *Alert:* Know that levothyroxine is usually the preferred agent for thyroid hormone replacement therapy. Liothyronine may be used when a rapid onset or a rapidly reversible agent is desirable or in patients with impaired peripheral conversion of levothyroxine to liothyronine.
- Be aware that regulation of liothyronine dosage is difficult.
- Know that thyroid hormone replacement requirements are about 25% lower in patients over age 60 than in young adults.
- **I.V. use:** Repeat dosages should be administered longer than 4 hours apart but less than 12 hours apart. Do not administer injection I.M. or S.C.
- Monitor pulse and blood pressure.
- Know that thyroid hormones alter thyroid function tests. Monitor PT; patients taking these hormones usually require decreased anticoagulant dosage.
- When changing from levothyroxine to liothyronine, levothyroxine should be stopped and liothyronine begun at a low dosage. Dosage should be increased in small increments after residual effects of levothyroxine have disappeared. When changing from liothyronine to levothyroxine, levothyroxine is started several days before withdrawing liothyronine to avoid relapse.
- Know that patients taking liothyronine who need radioactive iodine uptake studies done must discontinue drug 7 to 10 days before test.

☑ **PATIENT TEACHING**
- Make sure patient understands the importance of compliance. Tell patient to take thyroid hormones at the same time

each day, preferably before breakfast, to maintain constant hormone levels. Suggest morning dosage to prevent insomnia.
- Advise patient who has achieved a stable response not to change brands.
- Warn patient (especially elderly patient) to tell the doctor at once if chest pain, palpitations, sweating, nervousness, or other signs of overdose or aggravated CV disease occur.
- Tell patient to report unusual bleeding and bruising.

liotrix
Euthroid**, Thyrolar

Pregnancy Risk Category: A

HOW SUPPLIED
Tablets: levothyroxine sodium (T_4) 30 mcg and liothyronine sodium (T_3) 7.5 mcg (Euthroid-½); levothyroxine sodium 60 mcg and liothyronine sodium 15 mcg (Euthroid-1); levothyroxine sodium 120 mcg and liothyronine sodium 30 mcg (Euthroid-2); levothyroxine sodium 180 mcg and liothyronine sodium 45 mcg (Euthroid-3); levothyroxine sodium 12.5 mcg and liothyronine sodium 3.1 mcg (Thyrolar-¼); levothyroxine sodium 25 mcg and liothyronine sodium 6.25 mcg (Thyrolar-½); levothyroxine sodium 50 mcg and liothyronine sodium 12.5 mcg (Thyrolar-1); levothyroxine sodium 100 mcg and liothyronine sodium 25 mcg (Thyrolar-2); levothyroxine sodium 150 mcg and liothyronine sodium 37.5 mcg (Thyrolar-3)

ACTION
Not clearly defined. Stimulates metabolism of all body tissues by accelerating the rate of cellular oxidation and provides both T_3 and T_4 to the tissues.

ONSET, PEAK, DURATION
Unknown.

INDICATIONS & DOSAGE

Hypothyroidism—
Dosages are expressed in thyroid equivalents and must be individualized to approximate the deficit in the patient's thyroid secretion.
Adults: initially, a single dose of Thyrolar-¼, Thyrolar-½, or Euthroid-½. Dosage is adjusted at 2-week intervals.

ADVERSE REACTIONS

CNS: *nervousness, insomnia, tremor,* headache.
CV: *tachycardia, **arrhythmias,** angina pectoris, **cardiac decompensation and collapse.***
GI: diarrhea, vomiting.
Other: weight loss, heat intolerance, diaphoresis, accelerated rate of bone maturation in infants and children, menstrual irregularities, allergic skin reactions.

INTERACTIONS

Cholestyramine, colestipol: impaired liotrix absorption. Separate doses by 4 to 5 hours.
Insulin, oral antidiabetic agents: altered serum glucose levels. Monitor blood glucose levels. Dosage adjustments may be necessary.
I.V. phenytoin: free thyroid released. Monitor for tachycardia.
Oral anticoagulants: altered PT. Monitor PT. Dosage adjustments may be necessary.
Sympathomimetics, such as epinephrine: increased risk of coronary insufficiency. Monitor closely.

EFFECTS ON DIAGNOSTIC TESTS

Liotrix therapy alters radioactive iodine (^{131}I) thyroid uptake, protein-bound iodine levels, and T_3 uptake.

CONTRAINDICATIONS

Contraindicated in patients with hypersensitivity to drug, acute MI uncomplicated by hypothyroidism, untreated thyrotoxicosis, or uncorrected adrenal insufficiency.

NURSING CONSIDERATIONS

● Use with extreme caution in elderly patients and those with angina pectoris, hypertension, other CV disorders, renal insufficiency, or ischemia.
● Use cautiously in patients with myxedema or diabetes mellitus or insipidus.
● Rapid replacement in arteriosclerosis may precipitate angina, coronary occlusion, or CVA. Use cautiously in these patients.
● In patients with coronary artery disease who must receive thyroid hormones, observe carefully for possible coronary insufficiency. Also observe carefully during surgery because arrhythmias can be precipitated.
● Know that thyroid hormone replacement requirements are about 25% lower in patients over age 60 than in young adults.
● Monitor pulse and blood pressure.
● Know that thyroid hormones alter thyroid function test results.

☑ PATIENT TEACHING

● Make sure patient understands importance of compliance. Patient should take thyroid hormones at the same time each day, preferably before breakfast, to maintain constant hormone levels. Morning dosage may prevent insomnia.
● Warn patient (especially elderly patient) to tell the doctor at once if chest pain, palpitations, sweating, nervousness, or other signs of overdose or aggravated CV disease occur.
● The two commercially prepared liotrix drugs contain different amounts of each ingredient; tell patient not to change from one brand to the other.
● Tell patient to report unusual bleeding and bruising.

thyroid

Armour Thyroid, S-P-T, Thyrar, Thyroid Strong, Thyroid USP Enseals, Thyro-Teric, Westhroid

Pregnancy Risk Category: A

HOW SUPPLIED
Tablets: 15 mg, 30 mg, 60 mg, 65 mg, 90 mg, 120 mg, 130 mg, 180 mg, 240 mg, 300 mg
Tablets (bovine origin): 30 mg, 60 mg, 120 mg
Tablets (pork origin): 15 mg, 30 mg, 60 mg, 120 mg, 200 mg, 250 mg, 300 mg
Tablets (enteric-coated): 60 mg, 120 mg
Strong tablets (50% stronger than thyroid USP, and containing 0.3% iodine): 32.5 mg, 65 mg, 130 mg, 200 mg
Capsules (porcine origin): 60 mg, 120 mg, 180 mg, 300 mg

ACTION
Not clearly defined. Stimulates metabolism of all body tissues by accelerating the rate of cellular oxidation.

ONSET, PEAK, DURATION
Unknown.

INDICATIONS & DOSAGE
Mild hypothyroidism—
Adults: initially, 60 mg P.O. daily, increased by 60 mg q 30 days until desired response occurs. Usual maintenance dosage is 60 to 180 mg daily as a single dose.
Severe hypothyroidism—
Adults: initially, 15 mg P.O. daily, increased by 30 mg daily after 2 weeks, and 2 weeks later increased to 60 mg daily. After 2 months, increased to 120 mg daily, as needed, for 2 months; then to 180 mg daily as needed.
Congenital or severe hypothyroidism in children—
Children: same as adults with severe hypothyroidism.

ADVERSE REACTIONS
CNS: *nervousness, insomnia, tremor,* headache.
CV: *tachycardia, **arrhythmias,** angina pectoris, **cardiac decompensation and collapse.***
GI: diarrhea, vomiting.
Other: weight loss, heat intolerance, diaphoresis, accelerated rate of bone maturation in infants and children, menstrual irregularities, allergic skin reactions.

INTERACTIONS
Cholestyramine: impaired thyroid absorption. Separate doses by 4 to 5 hours.
Insulin, oral antidiabetic agents: altered serum glucose levels. Monitor glucose levels, and adjust dosage as needed.
Oral anticoagulants: altered PT. Monitor PT and adjust dosage as needed.
Sympathomimetics, such as epinephrine: increased risk of coronary insufficiency. Monitor closely.

EFFECTS ON DIAGNOSTIC TESTS
Thyroid USP therapy alters ^{131}I thyroid uptake, protein-bound iodine levels, and liothyronine uptake.

CONTRAINDICATIONS
Contraindicated in patients with hypersensitivity to drug, acute MI uncomplicated by hypothyroidism, untreated thyrotoxicosis, or uncorrected adrenal insufficiency.

NURSING CONSIDERATIONS
● Use with extreme caution in elderly patients and those with angina pectoris, hypertension, other CV disorders, renal insufficiency, or ischemia.
● Use cautiously in patients with myxedema or diabetes mellitus or insipidus.
● In patients with coronary artery disease, observe carefully for possible coronary insufficiency.
● Know that thyroid hormone replacement requirements are about 25% lower in patients over age 60.
● Monitor pulse and blood pressure.
● Know that in children, sleeping pulse rate and basal morning temperature guide treatment.
● Know that thyroid hormones alter thyroid function test results.

☑ **PATIENT TEACHING**
● Tell patient to take thyroid hormones at the same time each day, preferably

---

before breakfast, to maintain constant hormone levels. Suggest morning dosage to prevent insomnia.

• Advise patient who has achieved stable response not to change brands.

• Warn patient (especially elderly patient) to tell the doctor at once if chest pain, palpitations, sweating, nervousness, or other signs of overdose or aggravated CV disease occur.

• Tell patient to report unusual bleeding and bruising.

---

thyrotropin (thyroid-stimulating hormone, or TSH)
Thytropar

Pregnancy Risk Category: C

HOW SUPPLIED
Powder for injection: 10 IU-vial

ACTION
Stimulates uptake of radioactive iodine (^{131}I) in patients with thyroid cancer and promotes thyroid hormone production by the anterior pituitary gland.

ONSET, PEAK, DURATION
Onset occurs in minutes. Hypertrophy and hyperplasia of the thyroid gland occur within 24 hours. Effects rapidly reverse after withdrawal.

INDICATIONS & DOSAGE
Diagnosis of thyroid cancer remnant with ^{131}I after surgery—
Adults: 10 IU I.M. or S.C. for 3 to 7 days.
Differential diagnosis of primary and secondary hypothyroidism—
Adults: 10 IU I.M. or S.C. for 1 to 3 days.
In protein-bound iodine or ^{131}I uptake determinations for differential diagnosis of subclinical hypothyroidism or low thyroid reserve—
Adults: 10 IU I.M. or S.C.
Therapy for thyroid cancer (local or metastatic) with ^{131}I—

Adults: 10 IU I.M. or S.C. for 3 to 8 days.
To determine thyroid status of patient receiving thyroid hormone—
Adults: 10 units I.M. or S.C. for 1 to 3 days.

ADVERSE REACTIONS
CNS: headache.
CV: *tachycardia,* hypotension.
GI: nausea, vomiting.
Other: thyroid hyperplasia (with large doses), hypersensitivity reactions (postinjection flare, urticaria, ***anaphylaxis***).

INTERACTIONS
Insulin, oral antidiabetic agents: altered serum glucose levels. Monitor glucose levels, and adjust dosage as needed.
Oral anticoagulants: altered PT. Monitor PT. Dosage adjustments may be necessary.
Sympathomimetics such as epinephrine: increased risk of coronary insufficiency. Monitor closely.

EFFECTS ON DIAGNOSTIC TESTS
Thyrotropin therapy alters ^{131}I thyroid uptake.

CONTRAINDICATIONS
Contraindicated in patients with hypersensitivity to the drug, coronary thrombosis, or untreated Addison's disease.

NURSING CONSIDERATIONS
• Use cautiously in patients with angina pectoris, CHF, hypopituitarism, and adrenocortical suppression.
• Know that 3-day dosage schedule may be used in long-standing pituitary myxedema or with prolonged use of thyroid medication.

☑ PATIENT TEACHING
• Explain to patient how drug is used.
• Instruct patient to report adverse reactions promptly

---

methimazole
potassium iodide
**potassium iodide, saturated
    solution**
strong iodine solution
propylthiouracil
**radioactive iodine (sodium
    iodide)** [131]I

COMBINATION PRODUCTS
None.

methimazole
Tapazole

Pregnancy Risk Category: D

HOW SUPPLIED
Tablets: 5 mg, 10 mg

ACTION
Inhibits oxidation of iodine in thyroid
gland, blocking iodine's ability to combine with tyrosine to form thyroxine.
Also may prevent coupling of monoiodotyrosine and diiodotyrosine to form
thyroxine and triiodothyronine.

ONSET, PEAK, DURATION
Onset occurs within 5 days. Plasma levels peak in ½ to 1 hour. Duration unknown.

INDICATIONS & DOSAGE
Hyperthyroidism—
Adults: if mild, 15 mg P.O. daily; if
moderately severe, 30 to 45 mg daily ; if
severe, 60 mg daily. Daily dose divided
into three doses at 8-hour intervals.
Maintenance dosage is 5 to 15 mg daily.
Children: 0.4 mg/kg P.O. daily in divided doses q 8 hours. Maintenance
dosage is 0.2 mg/kg daily in divided
doses q 8 hours.

ADVERSE REACTIONS
CNS: headache, drowsiness, vertigo,
paresthesia, neuritis, neuropathies, CNS
stimulation, depression.
EENT: loss of taste.
GI: diarrhea, nausea, vomiting (may be
dose-related), salivary gland enlargement, epigastric distress.
GU: nephritis.
Hematologic: *agranulocytosis,*
leukopenia, *thrombocytopenia, aplastic
anemia.*
Hepatic: jaundice, hepatic dysfunction,
hepatitis.
Skin: rash, urticaria, discoloration, pruritus, erythema nodosum, exfoliative
dermatitis, lupuslike syndrome.
Other: arthralgia, myalgia, fever, lymphadenopathy, hypothyroidism (mental
depression; cold intolerance; hard, nonpitting edema; hypoprothrombinemia
and bleeding).

INTERACTIONS
None significant.

EFFECTS ON DIAGNOSTIC TESTS
Methimazole therapy alters selenomethionine (^{75}Se) uptake by the pancreas
and ^{123}I or ^{131}I uptake by the thyroid.
Hepatotoxicity may be evident by elevations of PT, ALT, and AST, bilirubin, alkaline phosphatase, and lactate dehydrogenase levels.

CONTRAINDICATIONS
Contraindicated in patients with hypersensitivity to drug and in breast-feeding
patients.

NURSING CONSIDERATIONS
● Use with extreme caution during pregnancy. Pregnant women may require
less drug as pregnancy progresses.
Monitor thyroid function studies closely. Thyroid may be added to regimen.

Drug may be stopped during last few weeks of pregnancy.

• Monitor CBC periodically as ordered to detect impending leukopenia, thrombocytopenia, and agranulocytosis. Also monitor hepatic function.

Alert: Dosages over 30 mg/day increase the risk of agranulocytosis.

Alert: Patients over 40 years may have an increased risk of developing methimazole-induced agranulocytosis.

• Watch for signs of hypothyroidism (mental depression; cold intolerance; hard, nonpitting edema); notify doctor because dosage may need to be adjusted as necessary.

• Discontinue drug and notify doctor if severe rash or enlarged cervical lymph nodes develop.

☑ **PATIENT TEACHING**

• Tell patient to take drug with meals to reduce adverse GI reactions.

• Warn patient to report fever, sore throat, mouth sores, skin eruptions, anorexia, pruritus, right upper quadrant pain, yellow skin or sclera.

• Tell him to ask the doctor about using iodized salt and eating shellfish.

• Warn patient against OTC cough medicines; many contain iodine.

• Instruct patient to store drug in light-resistant container.

---

potassium iodide
Iostat, Pima, Thyro-Block

potassium iodide, saturated solution (SSKI)

strong iodine solution (Lugol's solution)

Pregnancy Risk Category: D

HOW SUPPLIED
potassium iodide
Tablets: 130 mg
Tablets (enteric-coated): 300 mg
Oral solution: 500 mg/15 ml

Syrup: 325 mg/5 ml
potassium iodide, saturated solution
Oral solution: 1 g/ml
strong iodine solution
Oral solution: iodine 50 mg/ml and potassium iodide 100 mg/ml

ACTION
Inhibits thyroid hormone formation, limits iodide transport into the thyroid gland, and blocks thyroid hormone release.

ONSET, PEAK, DURATION
Onset occurs within 24 hours. Peak occurs in 10 to 15 days. Duration unknown.

INDICATIONS & DOSAGE
Preparation for thyroidectomy—
Adults and children: strong iodine solution (USP), 0.1 to 0.3 ml P.O. t.i.d., or potassium iodide, saturated solution (SSKI), 1 to 5 drops in water P.O. t.i.d. after meals for 10 to 14 days before surgery.
Thyrotoxic crisis—
Adults and children: 500 mg P.O. q 4 hours (about 10 drops of SSKI) or 1 ml of strong iodine solution t.i.d.
Radiation protectant for thyroid gland—
Adults and children 1 year and over: 130 mg P.O. daily for 7 to 14 days after radiation exposure.
Children up to 1 year: 65 mg P.O. daily for 7 to 14 days after exposure.

ADVERSE REACTIONS
EENT: inflammation of salivary glands, periorbital edema.
GI: diarrhea, burning mouth and throat, sore teeth and gums, *metallic taste.*
Skin: acneiform rash.
Other: fever; *hypersensitivity reactions.*

INTERACTIONS
ACE inhibitors, potassium-sparing diuretics: risk of hyperkalemia. Avoid concomitant use.
Antithyroid medications: potassium io-

---

dide may potentiate hypothyroid or goitrogenic effects. Monitor closely. *Lithium carbonate:* hypothyroidism may occur. Use with caution.

EFFECTS ON DIAGNOSTIC TESTS
Potassium iodide may alter the results of thyroid function tests.

CONTRAINDICATIONS
Contraindicated in patients with tuberculosis, acute bronchitis, iodide hypersensitivity, or hyperkalemia. Some formulations contain sulfites, which may precipitate allergic reactions in hypersensitive individuals.

NURSING CONSIDERATIONS
● Use cautiously in patients with hypocomplementemic vasculitis, goiter, or autoimmune thyroid disease.
● Know that drug is usually given with other antithyroid drugs.
● Know that doctor may avoid prescribing enteric-coated tablets, which have been associated with small-bowel lesions and can lead to serious complications, including perforation, hemorrhage, or obstruction.
● Dilute oral solutions in water, milk, or fruit juice, and give after meals to prevent gastric irritation, to hydrate the patient, and to mask salty taste.
● Give iodides through straw to avoid tooth discoloration.
Alert: Know that earliest signs of delayed hypersensitivity reactions caused by iodides are irritation and swollen eyelids.
● Store in light-resistant container.

☑ **PATIENT TEACHING**
● Instruct patient how to mask salty taste of oral solution. Tell him to take all forms of the drug after meals.
● Warn patient that sudden withdrawal may precipitate thyroid crisis.
● Tell him to ask the doctor about using iodized salt and eating shellfish.

propylthiouracil (PTU)
Propyl-Thyracil†

Pregnancy Risk Category: D

HOW SUPPLIED
Tablets: 50 mg, 100 mg†

ACTION
Inhibits oxidation of iodine in thyroid gland, blocking iodine's ability to combine with tyrosine to form thyroxine, and may prevent coupling of monoiodotyrosine and diiodotyrosine to form thyroxine and triiodothyronine.

ONSET, PEAK, DURATION
Onset and duration unknown. Plasma levels peak 1 to 1½ hours after oral administration.

INDICATIONS & DOSAGE
Hyperthyroidism—
Adults: 100 to 150 mg P.O. t.i.d.; up to 1,200 mg daily have been used in severe cases. Maintenance dosage is 100 to 150 mg daily in divided doses t.i.d.
Children over 10 years: 150 to 300 mg P.O. daily in divided doses t.i.d. Maintenance dosage determined by patient response.
Children 6 to 10 years: 50 to 150 mg P.O. daily in divided doses t.i.d. Maintenance dosage determined by patient's response.
Thyrotoxic crisis—
Adults and children: 200 mg P.O. q 4 to 6 hours on first day; once full control of symptoms is achieved, dosage is gradually reduced to usual maintenance levels.

ADVERSE REACTIONS
CNS: headache, drowsiness, vertigo, paresthesia, neuritis, neuropathies, CNS stimulation, depression.
CV: vasculitis.
EENT: visual disturbances.
GI: diarrhea, *nausea, vomiting* (may be dose-related), epigastric distress, sali-

---

vary gland enlargement, loss of taste.
GU: nephritis.
Hematologic: *agranulocytosis,*
leukopenia, *thrombocytopenia, aplastic
anemia.*
Hepatic: jaundice, *hepatotoxicity.*
Skin: rash, urticaria, skin discoloration,
pruritus, erythema nodosum, exfoliative
dermatitis, lupuslike syndrome.
Other: arthralgia, myalgia, fever, lymphadenopathy; dose-related hypothyroidism (mental depression; hypoprothrombinemia and bleeding; cold intolerance; hard, nonpitting edema).

INTERACTIONS
Anticoagulants: anticoagulant effects
may be increased. Monitor PT and INR.

EFFECTS ON DIAGNOSTIC TESTS
PTU therapy alters selenomethionine
(^{75}Se) levels and PT; it also alters AST,
ALT, and lactate dehydrogenase levels,
as well as liothyronine uptake.

CONTRAINDICATIONS
Contraindicated in patients with hypersensitivity to drug and in breast-feeding
patients.

NURSING CONSIDERATIONS
● Use cautiously in pregnant patients.
Pregnant women may require less drug
as pregnancy progresses. Monitor thyroid function studies closely. Thyroid
may be added to regimen. Drug may be
stopped during last few weeks of pregnancy.
● Give drug with meals to reduce adverse GI reactions.
● Watch for signs of hypothyroidism
(mental depression; cold intolerance;
hard, nonpitting edema); adjust dosage
as ordered.
● Monitor CBC periodically to detect
impending leukopenia, thrombocytopenia, and agranulocytosis.
Alert: Discontinue drug and notify doctor if severe rash or enlarged cervical
lymph nodes develop.
Alert: Patients older than 40 years may

have an increased risk of developing
propylthiouracil-induced agranulocytosis.
● Store drug in light-resistant container.

☑ **PATIENT TEACHING**
● Instruct patient to take drug with
meals.
● Warn patient to report fever, sore
throat, mouth sores, and skin eruptions.
● Tell him to ask the doctor about using
iodized salt and eating shellfish.
● Warn patient against taking OTC
cough medicines; many contain iodine.

radioactive iodine (sodium iodide) ^{131}I
Iodotope Therapeutic, Sodium Iodide
^{131}I Therapeutic

Pregnancy Risk Category: X

HOW SUPPLIED
All radioactivity concentrations are determined at the time of calibration.
Iodotope Therapeutic
Capsules: radioactivity range is 1 to 50
millicuries (mCi)/capsule at time of calibration
Oral solution: radioactivity concentration is 7.05 mCi/ml at time of calibration; in vials containing approximately
7, 14, 28, 70, or 106 mCi at time of calibration
Sodium Iodide ^{131}I Therapeutic
Capsules: radioactivity range is 0.8 to
100 mCi/capsule at the time of calibration
Oral solution: radioactivity range is 3.5
to 150 mCi/vial at the time of calibration

ACTION
Limits thyroid hormone secretion by de-
stroying thyroid tissue. The affinity of
thyroid tissue for radioactive iodine facilitates uptake of drug by cancerous
thyroid tissue that has metastasized to
other sites in the body.

ONSET, PEAK, DURATION
Onset occurs in 2 to 4 weeks. Peak effect occurs in 2 to 4 months. Duration unknown.

INDICATIONS & DOSAGE
Hyperthyroidism—
Adults: usual dosage is 4 to 10 mCi P.O. Dosage is based on estimated weight of thyroid gland and thyroid uptake. Treatment repeated after 6 weeks, based on serum thyroxine level.
Thyroid cancer—
Adults: initially, 50 mCi P.O. with subsequent doses of 100 to 150 mCi. Dosage is based on estimated malignant thyroid tissue and metastatic tissue as determined by total body scan. Treatment repeated according to clinical status.

ADVERSE REACTIONS
CV: chest pain, tachycardia.
EENT: *fullness in neck,* pain on swallowing, sore throat, cough.
Hematologic: anemia; blood dyscrasia; leukopenia; *thrombocytopenia;* possible increased risk of *leukemia* later (after sufficient ^{131}I dose for thyroid ablation following cancer surgery).
Skin: rash, pruritus, urticaria.
Other: hypothyroidism; radiation-induced thyroiditis; radiation sickness (nausea, vomiting); *death;* temporary thinning of hair; allergic type reactions; possible increased risk of birth defects in offspring after sufficient ^{131}I dose for thyroid ablation after cancer surgery.

INTERACTIONS
Lithium carbonate: hypothyroidism may occur. Use with caution.
   The following drugs can interfere with the action of ^{131}I and should be withheld the specified time before administering the ^{131}I dose:
   Adrenocorticoids: 1 week.
   Benzodiazepines: 1 month.
   Cholecystographic agents: 6 to 9 months.
   Contrast media containing iodine: 1
to 2 months.
   Iodine-containing products, including vitamins, expectorants, antitussives, and topical agents: 2 weeks.
   Salicylates: 1 to 2 weeks.

EFFECTS ON DIAGNOSTIC TESTS
[131]I therapy alters ^{131}I thyroid uptake and protein-bound iodine levels.

CONTRAINDICATIONS
Contraindicated in pregnant patients except to treat thyroid cancer and in breast-feeding patients.

NURSING CONSIDERATIONS
● Know that all antithyroid medications and thyroid preparations need to be stopped 1 week before ^{131}I dose. If medications are not stopped, patients may receive thyroid-stimulating hormone for 3 days before ^{131}I dose. When treating women of childbearing age, give dose during menstruation or within 7 days after menstruation.
● Know that after therapy for hyperthyroidism, patients should not resume antithyroid drugs, but should continue propranolol or other drugs used to treat symptoms of hyperthyroidism until onset of full ^{131}I effect occurs (usually 6 weeks).
● Monitor thyroid function via serum thyroxine levels, as ordered.
● Institute full radiation precautions. Have patient use disposal methods when coughing and expectorating. After dose for hyperthyroidism, patient's urine and saliva are slightly radioactive for 24 hours; vomitus is highly radioactive for 6 to 8 hours.
● After dose for thyroid cancer, patient's urine, saliva, and perspiration are radioactive for 3 days. Isolate patient and observe these precautions: Do not allow pregnant personnel to care for patient, use disposable eating utensils and linens; instruct patient to save urine in lead container for 24 to 48 hours so that amount of radioactive material can be determined. Limit contact with patient

THYROID HORMONE ANTAGONISTS   793

to 30 minutes per shift per person the first day, and increase time, as necessary, to 1 hour second day and longer on third day.

☑ **PATIENT TEACHING**
● Tell patient to fast overnight before administration and to drink as much fluid as possible for 48 hours after administration.
● Instruct patient on radiation precautions to use after drug administration.
● Warn patient who is discharged less than 7 days after ^{131}I dose for thyroid cancer to avoid close contact with small children and not to sleep in the same room with spouse for 7 days after treatment.

corticotropin
repository corticotropin
cosyntropin
desmopressin acetate
leuprolide acetate
(See Chapter 72, ANTINEOPLASTICS
THAT ALTER HORMONE BALANCE.)
somatrem
somatropin
vasopressin

COMBINATION PRODUCTS
None.

---

corticotropin
(adrenocorticotropic
hormone, ACTH)
ACTH, Acthar

repository corticotropin
Acthar Gel (H.P.)†, ACTH Gel, H.P.
Acthar Gel

Pregnancy Risk Category: C

HOW SUPPLIED
Aqueous injection: 25 unit-vial, 40
units/vial
Repository injection: 40 units/ml, 80
units/ml

ACTION
By replacing the body's own tropic hormone, stimulates the adrenal cortex to
secrete its entire spectrum of hormones.

ONSET, PEAK, DURATION
Variable.

INDICATIONS & DOSAGE
*Diagnostic test of adrenocortical func-
tion—*
Adults: 40 units I.V. infusion q 12
hours for 48 hours or I.M. q 12 hours
for 1 to 2 days; or 10 to 25 units aque-

ous form in 500 ml of D_5W I.V. over 8
hours, between blood samplings.
   Individual dosages generally vary
with adrenal glands' sensitivity to stimulation as well as with specific disease.
Infants and younger children require
larger doses per kilogram than do older
children and adults.
For therapeutic use—
Adults: 40 units aqueous form S.C. or
I.M. in four divided doses; or 40 to 80
units q 24 to 72 hours (repository form).

ADVERSE REACTIONS
CNS: *seizures,* dizziness, vertigo, increased intracranial pressure with papilledema, pseudotumor cerebri.
CV: hypertension, CHF, necrotizing
angiitis, ***shock.***
EENT: cataracts, glaucoma.
GI: peptic ulceration with perforation
and hemorrhage, pancreatitis, abdominal distention, ulcerative esophagitis,
nausea, vomiting.
Skin: impaired wound healing, thin
fragile skin, petechiae, ecchymoses, facial erythema, diaphoresis, acne, hyperpigmentation, allergic reactions, hirsutism.
Other: muscle weakness, steroid myopathy, loss of muscle mass, osteoporosis, vertebral compression fractures,
pneumonia, abscess and septic infection, cushingoid symptoms, suppression
of growth in children, activation of latent diabetes mellitus, progressive increase in antibodies, loss of corticotropin stimulatory effect, hypersensitivity
reactions (rash, ***bronchospasm***), *sodium
and fluid retention,* calcium and potassium loss, hypokalemic alkalosis, negative nitrogen balance, menstrual irregularities.

INTERACTIONS
Anticonvulsants, barbiturates, rifampin:

Reactions may be *common,* uncommon, *life-threatening,* or COMMON AND LIFE-THREATENING.

increased metabolism of corticotropin and decreased effectiveness. Monitor for lack of effect.

Antidiabetic agents: may increase requirements of antidiabetic agents due to intrinsic hyperglycemic activity of corticotropin. Monitor blood glucose levels closely.

Estrogens: may potentiate the effects of cortisol. Dosage adjustments may be necessary.

NSAIDs, salicylates: increased risk of GI bleeding. Avoid concomitant use.

Oral anticoagulants: altered PT. Monitor PT. Dosage adjustments may be necessary.

Potassium-wasting diuretics, amphotericin B: increased risk of hypokalemia. Monitor serum potassium levels.

EFFECTS ON DIAGNOSTIC TESTS

Corticotropin therapy alters blood and urinary glucose levels; sodium and potassium levels; protein-bound iodine levels; radioactive iodine (^{131}I) uptake and liothyronine (T_3) uptake; total protein values; serum amylase, urine amino acid, serotonin, uric acid, calcium and 17-ketosteroid levels; and leukocyte counts.

High plasma cortisol concentrations may be reported erroneously in patients receiving spironolactone, cortisone, or hydrocortisone when fluorometric analysis is used. This does not occur with the radioimmunoassay or competitive protein-binding method. However, therapy can be maintained with prednisone, dexamethasone, or betamethasone because they are not detectable by the fluorometric method.

CONTRAINDICATIONS

Contraindicated in patients with peptic ulcer, scleroderma, osteoporosis, systemic fungal infections, ocular herpes simplex, peptic ulceration, CHF, hypertension, sensitivity to pork and pork products, adrenocortical hyperfunction or primary insufficiency, or Cushing's syndrome. Also contraindicated in those who have had recent surgery.

NURSING CONSIDERATIONS

● Use cautiously in pregnant patients and in women of childbearing age. Also use cautiously in patients being immunized and in those patients with latent tuberculosis or tuberculin reactivity, hypothyroidism, cirrhosis, acute gouty arthritis, psychotic tendencies, renal insufficiency, diverticulitis, nonspecific ulcerative colitis, thromboembolic disorders, seizures, uncontrolled hypertension, or myasthenia gravis.

● Know that corticotropin treatment should be preceded by verification of adrenal responsiveness and test for hypersensitivity and allergic reactions.

● **I.V. use:** Use only the aqueous form for I.V. administration. Dilute in 500 ml of D_5W and infuse over 8 hours.

● If administering gel, warm it to room temperature, draw into large needle, and give slowly as deep I.M. injection with 21G or 22G needle.

● Refrigerate reconstituted solution and use within 24 hours.

● Know that corticotropin may mask signs of chronic disease and decrease host resistance and ability to localize infection.

● Note and record weight changes, fluid exchange, and resting blood pressures until minimal effective dosage is achieved.

● Watch neonates of corticotropin-treated mothers for signs of hypoadrenalism.

● Unusual stress may require additional use of rapidly acting corticosteroids. When possible, gradually reduce corticotropin dosage to smallest effective dose as ordered to minimize induced adrenocortical insufficiency. Know that therapy can be reinstituted if stressful situation (trauma, surgery, severe illness) occurs shortly after stopping drug.

☑ **PATIENT TEACHING**
● Warn patient that injection is painful.
● Stress importance of informing all members of health care team about ther-

apeutic use of drug because unusual stress may require additional use of rapidly acting corticosteroids.

• Instruct patient how to handle troublesome adverse reactions, such as limiting sodium intake to reduce severity of edema and increasing protein intake to combat nitrogen loss.

• Advise patient about need for close follow up care.

cosyntropin
Cortrosyn

Pregnancy Risk Category: C

HOW SUPPLIED
Injection: 0.25 mg-vial

ACTION
By replacing the body's own tropic hormone, stimulates the adrenal cortex to secrete its entire spectrum of hormones.

ONSET, PEAK, DURATION
Onset occurs within 5 minutes of I.V. use. Peak cortisol levels occur within 1 hour of I.M. or I.V. use. Duration unknown.

INDICATIONS & DOSAGE
Diagnostic test of adrenocortical function—
Adults and children 2 years and over: 0.25 I.M. or I.V. (unless label prohibits I.V. administration) between blood samplings.
Children under 2 years: 0.125 mg I.M. or I.V.

ADVERSE REACTIONS
CNS: *seizures,* dizziness, vertigo, increased intracranial pressure with papilledema, pseudotumor cerebri.
EENT: cataracts, glaucoma.
GI: peptic ulceration, pancreatitis, abdominal distension, ulcerative esophagitis, nausea, vomiting.
Skin: pruritus; impaired wound healing; thin, fragile skin; petechiae; ecchy-

moses; facial erythema; diaphoresis; acne; hyperpigmentation; hirsutism.
Other: flushing, hypersensitivity reactions, muscle weakness, steroid myopathy, loss of muscle mass, osteoporosis, vertebral compression, fractures, cushingoid symptoms, menstrual irregularities.

INTERACTIONS
Cortisone, hydrocortisone: may interfere with test results of cortisol levels if administered on test day.
Spironolactone: may interfere with fluorometric analysis of cortisol levels. Avoid concomitant use.

EFFECTS ON DIAGNOSTIC TESTS
Cosyntropin therapy alters blood glucose levels.

CONTRAINDICATIONS
Contraindicated in patients with hypersensitivity to drug.

NURSING CONSIDERATIONS
• Use cautiously in patients hypersensitive to natural corticotropin.
• **I.V. use:** Reconstitute with 1 ml of supplied diluent. For direct injection, administer over at least 2 minutes. May be further diluted with D_5W or 0.9% sodium chloride and infused over 6 hours. Solution is stable for 12 hours at room temperature.
• Know that drug is synthetic duplication of the biologically active part of the corticotropin molecule. It is less likely to produce sensitivity than natural corticotropin derived from animal sources.
• Monitor patients for allergic reactions, rashes, dyspnea, wheezing, or evidence of anaphylaxis.

☑ PATIENT TEACHING
• Explain test procedure to patient.
• Tell patient to report adverse reactions immediately.

Reactions may be *common,* uncommon, *life-threatening,* or COMMON AND LIFE-THREATENING.

desmopressin acetate
DDAVP, Minirin‡, Stimate

Pregnancy Risk Category: B

HOW SUPPLIED
Nasal solution: 0.1 mg/ml
Injection: 4 mcg/ml

ACTION
Increases the permeability of the renal tubular epithelium to adenosine monophosphate and water; the epithelium promotes reabsorption of water and produces a concentrated urine (ADH effect). Desmopressin also increases factor VIII activity by releasing endogenous factor VIII from plasma storage sites.

ONSET, PEAK, DURATION
Onset occurs within 1 hour for antidiuretic action, within 15 to 30 minutes for antihemorrhagic action. Peak antidiuretic effects occur within 1 to 5 hours, peak antihemorrhagic action in 1½ to 2 hours. Antidiuretic effects persist for 8 to 12 hours, antihemorrhagic effects for 4 to 12 hours.

INDICATIONS & DOSAGE
Nonnephrogenic diabetes insipidus, temporary polyuria and polydipsia associated with pituitary trauma—
Adults: 0.1 to 0.4 ml intranasally daily in one to three doses. Morning and evening doses adjusted separately for adequate diurnal rhythm of water turnover. Alternatively, injectable form administered in dosage of 0.5 to 1 ml I.V. or S.C. daily, usually in two divided doses.
Children 3 months to 12 years: 0.05 to 0.3 ml intranasally daily in one or two doses.
Hemophilia A and von Willebrand's disease—
Adults and children: 0.3 mcg/kg diluted in 0.9% sodium chloride and infused I.V. over 15 to 30 minutes. Dose repeated if necessary as indicated by laboratory response and the patient's clinical condition.
Primary nocturnal enuresis—
Children 6 years and over: initially, 20 mcg intranasally h.s. Dosage adjusted according to response. Maximum recommended dosage is 40 mcg daily.

ADVERSE REACTIONS
CNS: headache.
CV: slight rise in blood pressure at high dosage.
EENT: rhinitis, epistaxis, sore throat, cough.
GI: nausea, abdominal cramps.
GU: vulval pain.
Other: flushing, local erythema, swelling or burning after injection.

INTERACTIONS
Clofibrate: enhanced and prolonged effects of desmopressin. Monitor carefully.
Demeclocycline, epinephrine, ethanol, heparin, lithium: increased risk of adverse effects. Monitor closely.

EFFECTS ON DIAGNOSTIC TESTS
None reported.

CONTRAINDICATIONS
Contraindicated in patients hypersensitive to the drug, and in patients with Type IIB von Willebrand's disease.

NURSING CONSIDERATIONS
● Use cautiously in nursing women; it is not known whether desmopressin is distributed into milk.
● Use cautiously in patients with coronary artery insufficiency or hypertensive CV disease or in patients with conditions associated with fluid and electrolyte imbalances, such as cystic fibrosis, because these patients are prone to hyponatremia.
● Know that desmopressin injection should not be used to treat hemophilia A with factor VIII levels of 0% to 5% or severe cases of von Willebrand's disease.

---

*Liquid contains alcohol.   **May contain tartrazine.   †Canada only.   ‡Australia only.   ◇OTC.

• Intranasal use can cause changes in the nasal mucosa resulting in erratic, unreliable absorption. Report a worsening condition to the doctor, who may prescribe injectable DDAVP.

• Adjust fluid intake to reduce risk of water intoxication and sodium depletion, especially in children or elderly patients.

Alert: Overdose may cause oxytocic or vasopressor activity. Withhold drug and notify doctor. Use furosemide if fluid retention is excessive, as ordered.

☑ **PATIENT TEACHING**

• Instruct patient to clear nasal passages before administering drug.

• Some patients may have difficulty measuring and inhaling drug into nostrils. Teach patient and caregivers correct method of administration.

• Nasal congestion, allergic rhinitis, or upper respiratory infections may impair drug absorption. Advise patient to report such conditions to the doctor; they may require a dosage adjustment.

• Teach patient using S.C. desmopressin to rotate injection sites to prevent tissue damage.

• Warn patient to drink only enough water to satisfy thirst.

• Inform patient that, when treating hemophilia A and von Willebrand's disease, taking desmopressin may avoid the hazards of using blood products.

• Advise patient to wear medical identification indicating his use of this drug.

---

somatrem
Protropin

Pregnancy Risk Category: C

HOW SUPPLIED
Injectable lyophilized powder: 5-mg (about 15-IU) vial, 10-mg (about 30-IU) vial

ACTION
Purified growth hormone (GH) of recombinant DNA origin that stimulates linear, skeletal muscle, and organ growth.

ONSET, PEAK, DURATION
Peak levels occur in about 7.5 hours. Effects persist for 12 to 48 hours.

INDICATIONS & DOSAGE
Long-term treatment of children who have growth failure because of lack of adequate endogenous GH secretion—
Children (prepuberty): highly individualized; up to 0.1 mg/kg I.M. or S.C. three times weekly.

ADVERSE REACTIONS
Other: hypothyroidism, hyperglycemia, *antibodies to GH.*

INTERACTIONS
Glucocorticoids: may inhibit growth-promoting action of somatrem. Adjust glucocorticoid dosage as necessary.

EFFECTS ON DIAGNOSTIC TESTS
Somatrem therapy alters glucose tolerance test (reduced with high doses) and total protein and thyroid function tests (thyroxine-binding capacity and radioactive uptake may be decreased).

CONTRAINDICATIONS
Contraindicated in patients with epiphyseal closure, active neoplasia, or hypersensitivity to benzyl alcohol.

NURSING CONSIDERATIONS

• Use cautiously in patients with hypothyroidism and in those whose GH deficiency is caused by an intracranial lesion.

• Be sure to check this product's expiration date.

• To prepare the solution, inject the supplied bacteriostatic water for injection into the vial containing the drug. Then swirl the vial with a gentle rotary motion until the contents are completely dissolved. Don't shake the vial.

• After reconstitution, vial solution

Reactions may be *common,* uncommon, *life-threatening,* or COMMON AND LIFE-THREATENING.

should be clear. Don't inject solution if it is cloudy or contains any particles.
● If drug is administered to neonates, reconstitute immediately before use with sterile water for injection (without bacteriostat). Use the vial once; then discard.
● Store reconstituted vial in refrigerator; use within 7 days.
Alert: Know that toxicity in neonates has occurred from exposure to benzyl alcohol used in the drug as a preservative.
● Know that regular checkups, including monitoring of height and of blood and radiologic studies, are necessary.
● Observe patients for signs of glucose intolerance and hyperglycemia.
● Monitor periodic thyroid function tests for hypothyroidism as ordered, which may require treatment with a thyroid hormone.

☑ **PATIENT TEACHING**
● Reassure patient and caregivers that somatrem is *pure* and *safe.* Drug replaces pituitary-derived human GH, which was removed from the market in 1985 because of its association with a rare but fatal viral infection (Jakob-Creutzfeldt disease).
● Review the signs and symptoms of hypothyroidism and hyperglycemia. Instruct patient and parents to report any such signs or symptoms promptly.

---

somatropin
Humatrope, Nutropin

Pregnancy Risk Category: C

HOW SUPPLIED
Injection: 2-mg (about 6-IU [Humatrope]) vial†, 5-mg (about 15-IU [Humatrope]) vial, 10-mg (about 30-IU [Nutropin]) vial

ACTION
Purified growth hormone (GH) of recombinant DNA origin that stimulates skeletal, linear, muscle, and organ growth.

ONSET, PEAK, DURATION
Onset and duration unknown. Plasma levels peak in about 7.5 hours.

INDICATIONS & DOSAGE
Long-term treatment of growth failure in children with inadequate secretion of endogenous GH—
Children: up to 0.06 mg/kg body weight S.C. or I.M. three times weekly using Humatrope or 0.30 mg/kg body weight S.C. weekly in daily divided doses using Nutropin.
Growth failure in children associated with chronic renal insufficiency up to the time of renal transplantation (Nutropin only)—
Children: 0.35 mg/kg body weight S.C. weekly in daily divided doses.
✳ *New indication: Long-term treatment of short stature associated with Turner's syndrome—*
Children: up to 0.375 mg/kg/week (approximately 1.125 IU/kg/week) S.C. divided into equal doses given three to seven times a week.

ADVERSE REACTIONS
CNS: headache, weakness.
CV: mild, transient edema.
Hematologic: *leukemia.*
Metabolic: mild hyperglycemia, hypothyroidism.
Other: injection site pain, localized muscle pain, antibodies to GH.

INTERACTIONS
None significant.

EFFECTS ON DIAGNOSTIC TESTS
Serum levels of inorganic phosphorus, alkaline phosphatase, and parathyroid hormone may increase with somatropin therapy. Laboratory measurements of thyroid hormone may also change.

CONTRAINDICATIONS
Contraindicated in patients with closed epiphyses or an active underlying intracranial lesion. Humatrope should not be reconstituted with the supplied dilu-

---

*Liquid contains alcohol.   **May contain tartrazine.   †Canada only.   ‡Australia only.   ◇OTC.

ent for patients with a known sensitivity to either *m*-cresol or glycerin.

NURSING CONSIDERATIONS
● Use cautiously in children with hypothyroidism and in those whose GH deficiency is caused by an intracranial lesion. Be aware that these children should be examined frequently for progression or recurrence of the underlying disease.
● To prepare the solution, inject the supplied diluent into the vial containing the drug by aiming the stream of the liquid against the glass wall of the vial. Then swirl the vial with a gentle rotary motion until the contents are completely dissolved. *Don't shake* the vial.
● After reconstitution, vial solution should be clear. Don't inject solution if it is cloudy or contains particles.
● Know that patients on dialysis require changes in drug administration schedule as follows:
—Hemodialysis: administer prior to bedtime or 3 to 4 hours after dialysis.
—Chronic Cycling Peritoneal dialysis: administer in the morning after completion of dialysis.
—Chronic Ambulatory Peritoneal Dialysis: administer in the evening at the time of the overnight exchange.
● Store reconstituted vial in refrigerator; use within 14 days.
● If sensitivity to the diluent should occur, the vials may be reconstituted with sterile water for injection. When drug is reconstituted in this manner, use only 1 reconstituted dose per vial, refrigerate the solution if it is not used immediately after reconstitution, use the reconstituted dose within 24 hours, and discard the unused portion.
● Monitor child's height regularly. Know that regular checkups, including monitoring of blood and radiologic studies, also are necessary.
● Monitor patient's blood glucose levels regularly because GH may induce a state of insulin resistance.
● Know that excessive glucocorticoid therapy will inhibit the growth-promoting effect of somatropin. Patients with a coexisting corticotropin deficiency should have their glucocorticoid replacement dosage carefully adjusted to avoid an inhibitory effect on growth.
● Monitor periodic thyroid function tests, as ordered, for hypothyroidism, which may require treatment with a thyroid hormone.

☑ PATIENT TEACHING
● Inform parents that child with endocrine disorders (including GH deficiency) may develop slipped capital epiphyses more frequently. Tell them that if they notice their child is limping, they should notify the doctor.
● Stress importance of close follow-up care.

---

vasopressin (ADH)
Pitressin

Pregnancy Risk Category: C

HOW SUPPLIED
Injection: 0.5-ml and 1-ml ampules, 20 units/ml

ACTION
Increases the permeability of the renal tubular epithelium to adenosine monophosphate and water; the epithelium promotes reabsorption of water and produces a concentrated urine (ADH effect).

ONSET, PEAK, DURATION
Onset and peak unknown. Effects persist for 2 to 8 hours.

INDICATIONS & DOSAGE
Nonnephrogenic, nonpsychogenic diabetes insipidus—
Adults: 5 to 10 units I.M. or S.C. b.i.d. to q.i.d., p.r.n.; or intranasally (aqueous solution used as spray or applied to cot-

ton balls) in individualized dosages, based on response.

Children: 2.5 to 10 units I.M. or S.C. b.i.d. to q.i.d., p.r.n.; or intranasally (aqueous solution used as spray or applied to cotton balls) in individualized doses.

Postoperative abdominal distention—
Adults: initially, 5 units (aqueous) I.M.; then q 3 to 4 hours, increased to 10 units, if needed. Dosage reduced proportionately for children.

To expel gas before abdominal X-ray—
Adults: 5 to 15 units S.C. at 2 hours; then again at 30 minutes before X-ray.

ADVERSE REACTIONS
CNS: tremor, headache, vertigo.
CV: angina in patients with vascular disease; vasoconstriction, *arrhythmias, cardiac arrest,* myocardial ischemia, circumoral pallor, decreased cardiac output.
GI: abdominal cramps, nausea, vomiting, flatulence.
Other: water intoxication (drowsiness, listlessness, headache, confusion, weight gain, *seizures, coma*), hypersensitivity reactions (urticaria, angioedema, *bronchoconstriction, anaphylaxis*), diaphoresis, cutaneous gangrene.

INTERACTIONS
Carbamazepine, chlorpropamide, clofibrate, fludrocortisone, tricyclic antidepressants: increased antidiuretic response. Use together cautiously.
Demeclocycline, ethanol, heparin, lithium, norepinephrine: reduced antidiuretic activity. Use together cautiously.

EFFECTS ON DIAGNOSTIC TESTS
None reported.

CONTRAINDICATIONS
Contraindicated in patients with chronic nephritis accompanied by nitrogen retention.

NURSING CONSIDERATIONS
● Use cautiously in children, elderly pa-

tients, pregnant patients, preoperative and postoperative polyuric patients, and in those with seizure disorders, migraine headache, asthma, CV disease, heart failure, renal disease, goiter with cardiac complications, arteriosclerosis, or fluid overload.
● Know that synthetic desmopressin is sometimes preferred because of its longer duration of action and less frequent adverse reactions. Desmopressin also is commercially available as a nasal solution.
● May be used for transient polyuria resulting from ADH deficiency related to neurosurgery or head injury.
Alert: Never inject during first stage of labor; may cause ruptured uterus.
● Know that minimum effective dosage should be used to reduce adverse reactions.
● Give with 1 to 2 glasses of water to reduce adverse reactions and to improve therapeutic response.
● Monitor specific gravity of urine and fluid intake and output to aid evaluation of drug effectiveness.
● To prevent possible seizures, coma, and death, observe patients closely for early signs of water intoxication.
● Monitor blood pressure of patients taking vasopressin twice daily. Watch for excessively elevated blood pressure or lack of response to drug, which may be indicated by hypotension. Also monitor daily weight.
● A rectal tube will facilitate gas expulsion after vasopressin injection.

☑ **PATIENT TEACHING**
● Instruct patient to rotate injection sites to prevent tissue damage.
● Tell patient to report adverse reactions promptly.

61

Parathyroid-like drugs

calcifediol
calcitonin (human)
calcitonin (salmon)
calcitriol
dihydrotachysterol
etidronate disodium

COMBINATION PRODUCTS
None.

---

calcifediol
Calderol

Pregnancy Risk Category: C

HOW SUPPLIED
Capsules: 20 mcg, 50 mcg

ACTION
A vitamin D analogue that stimulates calcium absorption from the GI tract and promotes secretion of calcium from bone to blood.

ONSET, PEAK, DURATION
Onset unknown. Peak levels occur in 4 hours. Effects persist for 15 to 20 days.

INDICATIONS & DOSAGE
Metabolic bone disease and hypocalcemia associated with chronic renal failure—
Adults: initially, 300 to 350 mcg P.O. weekly. Dosage increased at 4-week intervals if necessary.

ADVERSE REACTIONS
Vitamin D intoxication associated with hypercalcemia
CNS: headache, somnolence, weakness, irritability, psychosis (rare).
CV: hypertension, arrhythmias.
EENT: conjunctivitis, photosensitivity reactions, rhinorrhea.
GI: constipation, nausea, vomiting,

polydipsia, pancreatitis, metallic taste, dry mouth, anorexia, diarrhea.
GU: polyuria, nocturia.
Skin: pruritus.
Other: bone and muscle pain, weight loss, hyperthermia, nephrocalcinosis, decreased libido.

INTERACTIONS
Cholestyramine, colestipol: decreased absorption of orally administered vitamin D analogues. Avoid concomitant use.
Corticosteroids: counteract vitamin D analogue effects. Don't use together.
Digitalis glycosides: increased risk of arrhythmias. Avoid concomitant use.
Magnesium-containing antacids: possible hypermagnesemia, especially in patients with chronic renal failure. Avoid concomitant use.
Other vitamin D analogues: increased toxicity. Avoid concomitant use.

EFFECTS ON DIAGNOSTIC TESTS
Calcifediol may falsely elevate cholesterol determinations made using the Zlatkis-Zak reaction. Alters concentrations of serum alkaline phosphatase concentrations and may alter electrolytes, such as magnesium, phosphate, and calcium, in the serum and urine.

CONTRAINDICATIONS
Contraindicated in patients with hypercalcemia or vitamin D toxicity.

NURSING CONSIDERATIONS
● Monitor serum calcium level as ordered; serum calcium level multiplied by serum phosphate level should not exceed 70. During titration, serum calcium level should be determined at least weekly.
● If hypercalcemia occurs, discontinue calcifediol and notify doctor. Drug may

---

be resumed after serum calcium level returns to normal.

☑ **PATIENT TEACHING**
• Teach the patient to report signs and symptoms of hypercalcemia.
• Instruct the patient about importance of getting an adequate daily intake of calcium. Inform the patient about foods high in calcium and how much should be consumed daily to meet RDA.

---

calcitonin (human)
Cibacalcin

calcitonin (salmon)
Calcimar, Miacalcin, Miacalcin Nasal Spray, Salmonine Osteocalcin

Pregnancy Risk Category: C

HOW SUPPLIED
calcitonin human
Injection: 0.5 mg/vial
calcitonin salmon
Injection: 100 IU/ml, 1-ml ampules; 200 IU/ml, 2-ml ampules
Nasal spray: 200 I.U./activation in 2-ml bottle

ACTION
Decreases osteoclastic activity by inhibiting osteocytic osteolysis and decreases mineral release and matrix or collagen breakdown in bone.

ONSET, PEAK, DURATION
Onset immediate after I.V. injection, within 15 minutes after I.M. or S.C. injection. Plasma levels peak immediately after I.V. injection, within 4 hours after I.M. or S.C. injection. Effects persist for 30 minutes to 12 hours after I.V. administration, 8 to 24 hours after I.M. or S.C. injection.

INDICATIONS & DOSAGE
Paget's disease of bone (osteitis deformans)—
Adults: initially, 100 IU of calcitonin

(salmon) daily S.C. or I.M.; maintenance dosage is 50 to 100 IU daily or every other day. Alternatively, calcitonin (human) 0.5 mg two or three times weekly or 0.25 mg daily. Some patients may need as much as 0.5 mg twice daily.
Hypercalcemia—
Adults: 4 IU/kg of calcitonin (salmon) q 12 hours I.M. If response inadequate after 1 or 2 days dose increased to 8 IU/kg I.M. q 12 hours. If response remains unsatisfactory after 2 more days, dosage increased to maximum of 8 IU/kg I.M. q 6 hours.
Postmenopausal osteoporosis—
Adults: 100 IU of calcitonin (salmon) daily I.M. or S.C. Alternatively, 200 IU (1 activation) of calcitonin (salmon) daily intranasally, alternating nostrils daily. Patients should receive adequate vitamin D and calcium supplements.

ADVERSE REACTIONS
CNS: headache, weakness, dizziness, paresthesia.
EENT: eye pain, nasal congestion.
GI: transient *nausea*, unusual taste, diarrhea, anorexia, *vomiting*, epigastric discomfort, abdominal pain.
GU: *increased urinary frequency*, nocturia.
Skin: *facial flushing*, rashes, pruritus of ear lobes, *inflammation at injection site*.
Other: hypersensitivity reactions *(anaphylaxis)*, edema of feet, chills, chest pressure, shortness of breath, tender palms and soles.

INTERACTIONS
None significant.

EFFECTS ON DIAGNOSTIC TESTS
None reported.

CONTRAINDICATIONS
Contraindicated in patients hypersensitive to salmon calcitonin. Human calcitonin has no contraindications.

NURSING CONSIDERATIONS
• Be aware that skin test is usually done

---

before therapy.
• Systemic allergic reactions possible because hormone is protein. Keep epinephrine handy.
• Know that calcitonin (human) is especially indicated in patients who have developed resistance to calcitonin (salmon). Calcitonin (human) is associated with risk of diminishing efficacy caused by antibody formation or hypersensitivity reactions.
• Administer at bedtime when possible to minimize nausea and vomiting.
• I.M. route is preferred if volume of dose to be administered exceeds 2 ml.
• Use freshly reconstituted solution within 2 hours.
• Observe the patient for signs of hypocalcemic tetany during therapy (muscle twitching, tetanic spasms, and seizures when hypocalcemia is severe).
• Monitor serum calcium level closely. Watch for signs of hypercalcemia relapse: bone pain, renal calculi, polyuria, anorexia, nausea, vomiting, thirst, constipation, lethargy, bradycardia, muscle hypotonicity, pathologic fracture, psychosis, and coma.
• Know that periodic examinations of urine sediment are advisable.
• Monitor periodic serum alkaline phosphatase and 24-hour urine hydroxyproline levels to evaluate drug effect as ordered.
• In patients with good initial clinical response to calcitonin who suffer relapse, expect to evaluate for antibody response to the hormone protein.
• If symptoms have been relieved after 6 months, know that treatment may be discontinued until symptoms or radiologic signs recur.
• Store calcitonin (human) at room temperature (77° F [25° C]); refrigerate calcitonin (salmon) at 36° to 46° F (2° to 8° C).
• When administered for postmenopausal osteoporosis, remind the patient to take adequate calcium and vitamin D supplements.

☑ **PATIENT TEACHING**
• Instruct the home care patient or family member on how to administer drug. Tell them to administer drug at bedtime if only one dose is required daily. If nasal spray is prescribed, tell patient to alternate nostrils daily.
• Facial flushing and warmth occur in 20% to 30% of all patients within minutes of injection and usually last about 1 hour. Reassure the patient that this is a transient effect.
• Tell patient to report signs and symptoms of hypercalcemia promptly. Inform him that if calcitonin loses its hypocalcemic activity, other drugs or increased dosages will not help.

---

calcitriol (1,25-dihydroxy-cholecalciferol)
Calcijex, Delta D, Rocaltrol

Pregnancy Risk Category: C

HOW SUPPLIED
Capsules: 0.25 mcg, 0.5 mcg
Injection: 1 mcg/ml, 2 mcg/ml

ACTION
A vitamin D analogue that stimulates calcium absorption from the GI tract and promotes secretion of calcium from bone to blood.

ONSET, PEAK, DURATION
Onset occurs within 2 to 6 hours. Plasma levels peak in 3 to 6 hours. Effects persist for 3 to 5 days.

INDICATIONS & DOSAGE
Hypocalcemia in patients undergoing chronic dialysis—
Adults: initially, 0.25 mcg P.O. daily. Dosage may be increased by 0.25 mcg daily at 4- to 8-week intervals. Maintenance dosage is 0.25 mcg every other day, up to 1.25 mcg daily.
Hypoparathyroidism and pseudohypoparathyroidism—
Adults and children 6 years and over:

initially, 0.25 mcg P.O. daily. Dosage may be increased at 2- to 4-week intervals. Maintenance dosage is 0.25 to 2 mcg daily.

Hypoparathyroidism—
Children 1 to 6 years: 0.25 to 0.75 mcg P.O. daily.

ADVERSE REACTIONS

Vitamin D intoxication associated with hypercalcemia
CNS: headache, somnolence, weakness, irritability, psychosis (rare).
CV: hypertension, arrhythmias.
EENT: conjunctivitis, photophobia, rhinorrhea.
GI: nausea, vomiting, constipation, polydipsia, pancreatitis, metallic taste, dry mouth, anorexia.
GU: polyuria, nocturia.
Skin: pruritus.
Other: bone and muscle pain, weight loss, hyperthermia, nephrocalcinosis, decreased libido.

INTERACTIONS

Cholestyramine, colestipol, excessive use of mineral oil: decreased absorption of orally administered vitamin D analogues. Avoid concomitant use.
Corticosteroids: counteract vitamin D analogue effects. Don't use together.
Digitalis glycosides: increased risk of arrhythmias. Avoid concomitant use.
Magnesium-containing antacids: may induce hypermagnesemia, especially in patients with chronic renal failure. Avoid concomitant use.

EFFECTS ON DIAGNOSTIC TESTS

Calcitriol therapy may falsely elevate cholesterol determinations made using the Zlatkis-Zak reaction. It also alters serum alkaline phosphatase concentrations and may alter electrolytes, such as magnesium, phosphate, and calcium in serum and urine.

CONTRAINDICATIONS

Contraindicated in patients with hypercalcemia or vitamin D toxicity. Withhold all preparations containing vitamin D.

NURSING CONSIDERATIONS

● Monitor serum calcium level; serum calcium level multiplied by the serum phosphate level should not exceed 70. During titration, determine serum calcium level twice weekly. Discontinue if hypercalcemia occurs and notify doctor, but resume after serum calcium level returns to normal. Patient should receive adequate daily intake of calcium. Observe for hypocalcemia, bone pain, and weakness prior to and throughout therapy.
● Use cautiously in patients receiving digitalis glycosides and in those with sarcoidosis or hyperparathyroidism.
● Protect from heat and light.

☑ PATIENT TEACHING

● Tell the patient to immediately report early symptoms of vitamin D intoxication: weakness, nausea, vomiting, dry mouth, constipation, muscle or bone pain, or metallic taste.
● Instruct the patient to adhere to diet and calcium supplementation and to avoid unapproved OTC drugs and magnesium-containing antacids.
Alert: Tell the patient that this drug must not be taken by anyone for whom it was not prescribed. It is the most potent form of vitamin D available.

---

dihydrotachysterol
AT-10‡, DHT Intensol*, Hytakerol

Pregnancy Risk Category: C

HOW SUPPLIED

Tablets: 0.125 mg, 0.2 mg, 0.4 mg
Capsules: 0.125 mg
Oral solution: 0.2 mg/5 ml, 0.2 mg/ml* (DHT Intensol*), 0.25 mg/ml (in sesame oil)

Note: 1 mg of dihydrotachysterol is equal to 120,000 units ergocalciferol (vitamin D_2).

ACTION
A vitamin D analogue that stimulates calcium absorption from the GI tract and promotes secretion of calcium from bone to blood.

ONSET, PEAK, DURATION
Onset occurs in several hours. Peak effects occur in 1 to 2 weeks. Effects persist up to 9 weeks.

INDICATIONS & DOSAGE
Hypocalcemia associated with hypoparathyroidism and pseudohypoparathyroidism—
Adults: initially, 0.75 to 2.5 mg P.O. daily for 4 days. Maintenance dosage is 0.2 to 1.5 mg daily.
Children: initially, 1 to 5 mg P.O. for 4 days. Maintenance dosage is 0.5 to 1.5 mg daily.
Prophylaxis of hypocalcemic tetany following thyroid surgery—
Adults: 0.25 mg P.O. daily (with calcium supplements).

ADVERSE REACTIONS
Vitamin D intoxication associated with hypercalcemia
CNS: headache, somnolence, irritability, psychosis (rare).
CV: hypertension, arrhythmias.
EENT: conjunctivitis, photophobia, rhinorrhea.
GI: nausea, vomiting, constipation, polydipsia, pancreatitis, metallic taste, dry mouth, anorexia, diarrhea.
GU: polyuria, nocturia.
Other: weakness, bone and muscle pain, thirst, weight loss, hyperthermia, decreased libido, nephrocalcinosis.

INTERACTIONS
Cholestyramine, colestipol, excessive use of mineral oil: decreased absorption of orally administered vitamin D analogues. Avoid concomitant use.
Corticosteroids: counteract vitamin D analogue effects. Don't use together.
Digitalis glycosides: increased risk of arrhythmias. Avoid concomitant use.
Magnesium-containing antacids: possible hypermagnesemia, especially in patients with chronic renal failure. Avoid concomitant use.
Other vitamin D analogues: increased toxicity. Avoid concomitant use.
Thiazide diuretics: may cause hypercalcemia.

EFFECTS ON DIAGNOSTIC TESTS
Drug alters serum alkaline phosphatase concentrations and cholesterol levels and may alter electrolyte levels, such as magnesium, phosphate, and calcium, in serum and urine.

CONTRAINDICATIONS
Contraindicated in patients with hypercalcemia or vitamin D toxicity.

NURSING CONSIDERATIONS
● Monitor serum calcium level as ordered; the serum calcium level multiplied by serum phosphate level should not exceed 70. During titration, determine serum calcium level twice weekly. Discontinue if hypercalcemia occurs and notify doctor. Know that drug can be resumed after serum calcium level returns to normal. Adequate daily intake of calcium is 1,000 mg.
● Monitor urine calcium level.
● Store in tightly closed, light-resistant container. Don't refrigerate.

☑ PATIENT TEACHING
● Tell the patient to report any early signs of hypercalcemia: thirst, headache, vertigo, tinnitus, or anorexia promptly.
● Instruct the patient to adhere to diet and calcium supplementation and to avoid unapproved OTC drugs and magnesium-containing antacids.

---

etidronate disodium
Didronel

Pregnancy Risk Category: C

HOW SUPPLIED
Tablets: 200 mg, 400 mg
Injection: 50 mg/ml

ACTION
Decreases osteoclastic activity by inhibiting osteocytic osteolysis and decreases mineral release and matrix or collagen breakdown in bone.

ONSET, PEAK, DURATION
Highly variable.

INDICATIONS & DOSAGE
Symptomatic Paget's disease of bone (osteitis deformans)—
Adults: 5 to 10 mg/kg P.O. daily (not to exceed 6 months of therapy) or 11 to 20 mg/kg P.O. daily (not to exceed 3 months of therapy) in single dose 2 hours before a meal with water or juice. Treatment is initiated only after an etidronate-free period of at least 90 days, and when there is specific evidence of active disease process.
Heterotopic ossification in spinal cord injuries—
Adults: 20 mg/kg P.O. daily for 2 weeks, then 10 mg/kg daily for 10 weeks. Total treatment period is 12 weeks.
Heterotopic ossification after total hip replacement—
Adults: 20 mg/kg P.O. daily for 1 month before total hip replacement and for 3 months afterward.
Malignancy-associated hypercalcemia—
Adults: 7.5 mg/kg I.V. daily for 3 consecutive days; a period of at least 7 days should elapse between courses of I.V. therapy. Maintenance dosage is 20 mg/kg P.O. daily for 30 days, initiated the day following the last I.V. dosage. May be used for a maximum of 90 days.

ADVERSE REACTIONS
GI: occur most frequently at dosage of 20 mg/kg daily—diarrhea, increased frequency of bowel movements, nausea, constipation, stomatitis.
Other: increased or recurrent bone pain, pain at previously asymptomatic sites, increased risk of fracture, *elevated serum phosphate level,* fever, fluid overload, dyspnea, **seizures,** abnormal hepatic function, hypersensitivity reactions.

INTERACTIONS
None significant.

EFFECTS ON DIAGNOSTIC TESTS
May elevate serum phosphate levels.

CONTRAINDICATIONS
Contraindicated in patients with known hypersensitivity to drug or in patients with clinically overt osteomalacia. Also, I.V. etidronate disodium is contraindicated in patients with serum creatinine concentrations of 5 mg/dl or greater.

NURSING CONSIDERATIONS
● Use cautiously in patients with impaired renal function.
● Know that some patients may receive I.V. drug for up to 7 days. Risk of hypokalemia increases after 3 days.
● Monitor renal function before and during therapy as ordered.
● Don't give drug with food, milk, or antacids; may reduce absorption.
● **I.V. use:** Dilute daily dose in at least 250 ml of 0.9% sodium chloride solution or D_5W, and infuse over at least 2 hours.
● To monitor drug effect, review serum alkaline phosphatase and urinary hydroxyproline excretion.
● Be aware that elevated serum phosphate level may occur, especially in patients receiving higher doses. Phosphate level usually returns to normal 2 to 4 weeks after drug is discontinued.

☑ PATIENT TEACHING
● Stress importance of a diet high in calcium and vitamin D.
● Tell patient not to eat for 2 hours after daily dose.
● Tell patient that improvement may not occur for up to 3 months and may continue for months after drug is stopped.

62
Diuretics

acetazolamide
acetazolamide sodium
amiloride hydrochloride
bumetanide
chlorothiazide
chlorothiazide sodium
chlorthalidone
ethacrynate sodium
ethacrynic acid
furosemide
hydrochlorothiazide
indapamide
mannitol
methazolamide
metolazone
spironolactone
torsemide
triamterene
urea

COMBINATION PRODUCTS
ALDACTAZIDE 25/25: spironolactone 25 mg and hydrochlorothiazide 25 mg.
ALDACTAZIDE 50/50: spironolactone 50 mg and hydrochlorothiazide 50 mg.
DYAZIDE: triamterene 37.5 mg and hydrochlorothiazide 25 mg.
MAXZIDE: triamterene 75 mg and hydrochlorothiazide 50 mg.
MAXZIDE-25MG: triamterene 37.5 mg and hydrochlorothiazide 25 mg.
MODURETIC: amiloride hydrochloride 5 mg and hydrochlorothiazide 50 mg.
SPIROZIDE: spironolactone 25 mg and hydrochlorothiazide 25 mg.
ZIAC 2.5: bisoprolol fumarate 2.5 mg and hydrochlorthiazide 6.25 mg.
ZIAC 5: bisoprolol fumarate 5 mg and hydrochlorthiazide 6.25 mg.
ZIAC 10: bisoprolol fumarate 10 mg and hydrochlorthiazide 6.25 mg.

---

acetazolamide
Acetazolam†, AK-Zol, Apo-Acetazolamide†, Dazamide, Diamox, Diamox Sequels

acetazolamide sodium
Diamox Parenteral, Diamox Sodium†

Pregnancy Risk Category: C

HOW SUPPLIED
acetazolamide
Tablets: 125 mg, 250 mg
Capsules (extended-release): 500 mg
acetazolamide sodium
Injection: 500 mg-vial

ACTION
Blocks the action of carbonic anhydrase, promoting renal excretion of sodium, potassium, bicarbonate, and water, and decreases secretion of aqueous humor in the eye, thereby lowering intraocular pressure. As an anticonvulsant, may inhibit carbonic anhydrase in the CNS and decrease abnormal paroxysmal or excessive neuronal discharge. In acute mountain sickness, carbonic anhydrase inhibitors produce a respiratory and metabolic acidosis that may stimulate ventilation, increase cerebral blood flow, promote the release of oxygen from hemoglobin, and increase ventilation.

ONSET, PEAK, DURATION
Onset occurs 1 to 1½ hours after tablets, 2 hours after capsules, 2 minutes after I.V. injection. Peak effects occur 2 to 4 hours after tablets, 8 to 12 hours after capsules, 15 minutes after I.V. injection. Effects persist for 8 to 12 hours after tablets, 18 to 24 hours after capsules, 4 to 5 hours after I.V. injection.

Reactions may be *common,* uncommon, *life-threatening,* or COMMON AND LIFE-THREATENING.

INDICATIONS & DOSAGE

Secondary glaucoma and preoperative treatment of acute angle-closure glaucoma—

Adults: 250 mg P.O. q 4 hours; or 250 mg P.O. b.i.d. for short-term therapy. To rapidly lower intraocular pressure, initially, 500 mg I.V., then 125 to 250 mg I.V. q 4 hours.

Edema in CHF—

Adults: 250 to 375 mg P.O., or I.V. daily in the morning.

Chronic open-angle glaucoma—

Adults: 250 mg to 1 g P.O. daily in divided doses q.i.d., or 500 mg (extended-release) P.O. b.i.d.

Prevention or amelioration of acute mountain sickness—

Adults: 500 mg to 1 g P.O. daily in divided doses q 8 to 12 hours, or 500 mg (extended-release) P.O. b.i.d. Treatment started 24 to 48 hours before ascent, and continued for 48 hours while at high altitude.

Adjunctive treatment of myoclonic, refractory generalized tonic-clonic, absence, or mixed seizures—

Adults and children: 8 to 30 mg/kg P.O. daily in divided doses. For adults, the optimum dosage range is 375 mg to 1 g daily. Usually given with other anticonvulsants.

ADVERSE REACTIONS

CNS: drowsiness, paresthesia, confusion.

EENT: transient myopia, hearing dysfunction, tinnitus.

GI: nausea, vomiting, anorexia, altered taste, diarrhea.

GU: polyuria, hematuria.

Hematologic: *aplastic anemia,* hemolytic anemia, leukopenia.

Skin: rash.

Other: *pain at injection site,* sterile abscesses, hyperchloremic acidosis, hypokalemia, asymptomatic hyperuricemia, glycosuria.

INTERACTIONS

Amphetamines, anticholinergics, *mecamylamine, procainamide, quinidine:* decreased renal clearance of these agents, increasing toxicity. Monitor closely.

Cyclosporine: increased cyclosporine levels which may cause nephrotoxicity and neurotoxicity. Monitor closely.

Lithium: increased excretion of lithium resulting in decreased effectiveness. Monitor closely.

Methenamine: reduced effectiveness of acetazolamide. Avoid concomitant use.

Primidone: serum and urine concentrations of primidone may be decreased. Monitor patient closely.

Salicylates: possible accumulation and toxicity of acetazolamide, including CNS depression and metabolic acidosis. Monitor closely.

EFFECTS ON DIAGNOSTIC TESTS

Because it alkalinizes urine, acetazolamide may cause false-positive proteinuria in Albustix or Albutest. Acetazolamide may also decrease thyroid iodine uptake.

CONTRAINDICATIONS

Contraindicated in patients with hypersensitivity to the drug; in long-term therapy for chronic noncongestive angle-closure glaucoma; and in those with hyponatremia or hypokalemia, renal or hepatic disease or dysfunction, adrenal gland failure, and hyperchloremic acidosis.

NURSING CONSIDERATIONS

• Use cautiously in patients with respiratory acidosis, emphysema, or chronic pulmonary disease, and in patients receiving other diuretics.

• Reconstitute 500-mg vial with at least 5 ml of sterile water for injection. Use within 24 hours of reconstitution.

• **I.V. use:** Inject 100 to 500 mg/minute into a large vein using a 21G or 23G needle. Intermittent or continuous infusion is not recommended.

• If the patient is unable to swallow oral forms, check with the pharmacist. He

---

may make a suspension using crushed acetazolamide tablets in a highly flavored syrup, such as cherry, raspberry, or chocolate. Although concentrations up to 500 mg/5 ml are feasible, concentrations of 250 mg/5 ml are more palatable. Refrigeration improves palatability but doesn't improve stability. Suspensions are stable for 1 week.

• Monitor fluid intake and output, glucose, and electrolytes, especially serum potassium, bicarbonate, and chloride. When used in diuretic therapy, consult the doctor and dietitian about providing a high-potassium diet.

• Monitor elderly patients closely because they are especially susceptible to excessive diuresis.

• Weigh the patient daily. Rapid or excessive fluid loss causes weight loss and hypotension.

• Keep in mind that the diuretic effect decreases when acidosis occurs but can be reestablished by withdrawing drug, as ordered, for several days and then restarting, or by using intermittent administration schedules.

• Because bicarbonate ion excretion makes the patient's urine alkaline, be aware that the drug may cause false-positive urine protein tests.

• Know that drug may increase blood glucose and cause glycosuria.

☑ **PATIENT TEACHING**
• Tell patient to take oral form with food if GI upset occurs.

• Caution patient not to perform hazardous activities if adverse CNS reactions occur.

• Tell patient to monitor blood glucose and urine for sugar.

---

amiloride hydrochloride
Kaluril‡, Midamor

Pregnancy Risk Category: B

HOW SUPPLIED
Tablets: 5 mg

ACTION
A potassium-sparing diuretic that inhibits sodium reabsorption and potassium excretion in the distal tubules.

ONSET, PEAK, DURATION
Onset occurs within 2 hours. Peak effects occur in 6 to 10 hours. Effects persist for 24 hours.

INDICATIONS & DOSAGE
Hypertension; edema associated with CHF, usually in patients also taking thiazide or other potassium-wasting diuretics—
Adults: usual dosage is 5 mg P.O. daily. Increased to 10 mg daily, if necessary. Maximum dosage is 20 mg daily.

ADVERSE REACTIONS
CNS: *headache,* weakness, dizziness, encephalopathy.
CV: orthostatic hypotension.
GI: *nausea, anorexia, diarrhea, vomiting,* abdominal pain, constipation, appetite changes.
GU: impotence.
Hematologic: *aplastic anemia,* neutropenia.
Other: hyperkalemia, fatigue, muscle cramps, dyspnea.

INTERACTIONS
ACE inhibitors, potassium-containing salt substitutes, potassium-sparing diuretics, potassium supplements: possible hyperkalemia. Avoid concomitant use.
Lithium: decreased lithium clearance, increasing risk of lithium toxicity. Monitor lithium level.
NSAIDs: decreased diuretic effectiveness. Avoid concomitant use.

EFFECTS ON DIAGNOSTIC TESTS
Transient abnormal renal and hepatic function tests have been noted. Amiloride therapy causes severe hyperkalemia in diabetic patients following I.V. glucose tolerance testing; discontinue amiloride at least 3 days before testing.

Reactions may be *common,* uncommon, *life-threatening,* or COMMON AND LIFE-THREATENING.

CONTRAINDICATIONS

Contraindicated in patients with elevated serum potassium level (greater than 5.5 mEq/L). Don't administer to patients receiving other potassium-sparing diuretics, such as spironolactone and triamterene. Also contraindicated in patients with anuria, acute or chronic renal insufficiency, diabetic nephropathy, and hypersensitivity to the drug.

NURSING CONSIDERATIONS

● Use cautiously in patients with diabetes mellitus, cardiopulmonary disease, and severe, existing hepatic insufficiency and in elderly or debilitated patients.

● To prevent nausea, administer amiloride with meals.

● If amiloride is not taken concurrently with a potassium-wasting drug, monitor potassium level because of increased risk of hyperkalemia. Alert doctor immediately if potassium level exceeds 6.5 mEq/L, and expect drug to be discontinued.

☑ PATIENT TEACHING

● Advise the patient to avoid sudden posture changes and to rise slowly to avoid orthostatic hypotension.

● Caution the patient not to perform hazardous activities if adverse CNS reactions occur.

● To prevent serious hyperkalemia, warn the patient to avoid excessive ingestion of potassium-rich foods, potassium-containing salt substitutes, and potassium supplements.

---

bumetanide
Bumex, Burinex‡

Pregnancy Risk Category: C

HOW SUPPLIED
Tablets: 0.5 mg, 1 mg, 2 mg
Injection: 0.25 mg/ml

ACTION

A potent loop diuretic that inhibits sodium and chloride reabsorption at the ascending portion of the loop of Henle.

ONSET, PEAK, DURATION

Onset occurs within minutes after I.V. administration, 40 minutes after I.M. injection, 30 to 60 minutes after oral use. Peak effects occur 15 to 30 minutes after I.V. administration, 1 to 2 hours after oral use. Effects persist for 4 to 6 hours after oral use, 3½ to 4 hours after I.V. administration.

INDICATIONS & DOSAGE
Edema in CHF, or hepatic or renal disease—

Adults: 0.5 to 2 mg P.O. once daily. If diuretic response is not adequate, a second or third dose may be given at 4- to 5-hour intervals. Maximum dosage is 10 mg/day. May be administered parenterally if P.O. not feasible. Usual initial dose is 0.5 to 1 mg given I.V. or I.M. If response is not adequate, a second or third dose may be given at 2- to 3-hour intervals. Maximum dosage is 10 mg/day.

ADVERSE REACTIONS

CNS: dizziness, headache, vertigo.
CV: volume depletion and dehydration, orthostatic hypotension, ECG changes, chest pain, increased cholesterol.
EENT: transient deafness, tinnitus.
GI: nausea, vomiting, upset stomach, dry mouth, diarrhea, pain.
GU: *renal failure,* premature ejaculation, difficulty maintaining erection, oliguria.
Hematologic: azotemia, *thrombocytopenia.*
Skin: rash, pruritus, diaphoresis.
Other: hypokalemia; hypochloremic alkalosis; hypomagnesemia, asymptomatic hyperuricemia; weakness; arthritic pain; fluid and electrolyte imbalances, including dilutional hyponatremia, hypocalcemia, hyperglycemia, and glucose intolerance impairment;

---

muscle pain and tenderness.

INTERACTIONS

Aminoglycoside antibiotics: potentiated ototoxicity. Use together cautiously.

Antihypertensives: increased risk of hypotension. Use together cautiously.

Digitalis glycosides: increased risk of digitalis toxicity from bumetanide-induced hypokalemia. Monitor potassium and digitalis levels.

Indomethacin, NSAIDs, probenecid: inhibited diuretic response. Use together cautiously.

Lithium: decreased lithium clearance, increasing risk of lithium toxicity. Monitor lithium level.

Metolazone: profound diuresis and potential electrolyte loss. Monitor the patient for fluid and electrolyte disorders.

Other potassium-wasting drugs, such as corticosteroids, amphotericin-B: increased risk of hypokalemia. Use together cautiously.

EFFECTS ON DIAGNOSTIC TESTS

Bumetanide therapy alters electrolyte balance and liver and renal function tests.

CONTRAINDICATIONS

Contraindicated in patients with hypersensitivity to the drug or to sulfonamides (possible cross-sensitivity), in those with anuria or hepatic coma, and in patients in states of severe electrolyte depletion.

NURSING CONSIDERATIONS

● Use cautiously in patients with hepatic cirrhosis and ascites, in the elderly, and in those with depressed renal function.

● **I.V. use:** Give I.V. doses directly, using a 21G or 23G needle over 1 to 2 minutes. For intermittent infusion, give diluted drug through an intermittent infusion device or piggyback into an I.V. line containing a free-flowing, compatible solution. Infuse at ordered rate. Continuous infusion not recommended.

● To prevent nocturia, give in the morning. If second dose is necessary, give in early afternoon.

● Be aware that the safest and most effective dosage schedule for control of edema is intermittent dosage given on alternate days, or for 3 to 4 days with 1 or 2 days of rest periods.

● Monitor fluid intake and output, weight, and serum electrolyte, BUN, creatinine, and carbon dioxide levels frequently.

● Watch for signs of hypokalemia, such as muscle weakness and cramps.

● Consult the doctor and dietitian about providing a high-potassium diet. Foods rich in potassium include citrus fruits, tomatoes, bananas, dates, and apricots.

● Monitor blood glucose levels in diabetic patients.

● Monitor blood uric acid levels, especially in patients with a history of gout.

● Monitor blood pressure and pulse rate during rapid diuresis. Bumetanide can lead to profound water and electrolyte depletion.

● If oliguria or azotemia develops or increases, know that the doctor may stop drug.

● Keep in mind that bumetanide can be safely used in patients allergic to furosemide; 1 mg of bumetanide equals 40 mg of furosemide.

☑ PATIENT TEACHING

● Tell patient to take drug in morning to prevent nocturia and if second dose is prescribed to take it in early afternoon. Also instruct patient to take drug with food or milk if adverse GI reactions occur.

● Advise patient to stand up slowly to prevent dizziness, and to limit alcohol intake and strenuous exercise in hot weather to avoid exacerbating orthostatic hypotension.

chlorothiazide
Azide‡, Chlotride‡, Diuret‡, Diurigen, Diuril

chlorothiazide sodium
Sodium Diuril

Pregnancy Risk Category: C

HOW SUPPLIED
chlorothiazide
Tablets: 250 mg, 500 mg
Oral suspension: 250 mg/5 ml
chlorothiazide sodium
Injection: 500-mg vial

ACTION
A thiazide diuretic that increases sodium and water excretion by inhibiting sodium reabsorption in the nephron's cortical diluting site.

ONSET, PEAK, DURATION
Onset occurs 2 hours after an oral dose, 15 minutes after I.V. use. Peak effects occur in about 4 hours after an oral dose, 30 minutes after I.V. use. Effects persist for 6 to 12 hours.

INDICATIONS & DOSAGE
Edema, hypertension—
Adults: 500 mg to 1 g P.O. or I.V. daily or twice a day.
Diuresis, hypertension—
Children 6 months to 12 years: 10 to 20 mg/kg P.O. daily or in two divided doses. Do not exceed 1,000 mg/day in children over 2 years; in children under 2 years, maximum dose is 375 mg/day.
Children under 6 months: up to 30 mg/kg P.O. daily in two divided doses.

ADVERSE REACTIONS
CNS: dizziness, vertigo, headache, paresthesia, weakness, restlessness.
CV: volume depletion and dehydration, orthostatic hypotension, vasculitis, increased cholesterol and triglyceride levels.
GI: anorexia, nausea, pancreatitis, vomiting, epigastric distress, abdominal pain, diarrhea, constipation.
GU: impotence, *renal failure,* interstitial nephritis, hematuria.

Hematologic: *aplastic anemia,* agranulocytosis, leukopenia, *thrombocytopenia,* hemolytic anemia.
Hepatic: jaundice.
Skin: dermatitis, photosensitivity, rash, urticaria, alopecia.
Other: impotence, hypersensitivity reactions; *hypokalemia;* asymptomatic hyperuricemia; hyperglycemia and impairment of glucose tolerance; fluid and electrolyte imbalances, including dilutional hyponatremia and hypochloremia, metabolic alkalosis, hypercalcemia; gout; *anaphylaxis,* pneumonitis.

INTERACTIONS
Amphotericin B: increased risk of hypokalemia.
Antidiabetic agents: decreased effectiveness; dosage adjustments may be necessary. Monitor blood glucose levels.
Cholestyramine, colestipol: decreased intestinal absorption of thiazides. Separate doses.
Corticosteroids: increased risk of hypokalemia.
Diazoxide: increased antihypertensive, hyperglycemic, and hyperuricemic effects. Use together cautiously.
Digitalis glycosides: increased risk of digitalis toxicity from chlorothiazide-induced hypokalemia. Monitor potassium and digitalis levels.
Ethanol, barbiturates, opiates: increased orthostatic hypotensive effect. Monitor closely.
Lithium: decreased lithium clearance, increasing risk of lithium toxicity. Monitor lithium level.
NSAIDs: increased risk of NSAID-induced renal failure. Monitor the patient for renal failure.

EFFECTS ON DIAGNOSTIC TESTS
Chlorothiazide therapy may alter serum electrolyte levels and may increase serum urate, glucose, cholesterol, and triglyceride levels. It may also interfere with tests for parathyroid function and should be dicontinued before such tests.

CONTRAINDICATIONS
Contraindicated in patients with anuria or hypersensitivity to other thiazides or other sulfonamide-derived drugs.

NURSING CONSIDERATIONS
● Use cautiously in patients with severe renal disease and impaired hepatic function.
● To prevent nocturia, give in the morning. If second dose is necessary give in early afternoon.
● Administer oral form with food to enhance absorption.
● **I.V. use:** Reconstitute 500 mg with 18 ml of sterile water for injection. Inject reconstituted drug directly into vein, through an I.V. line containing a free-flowing, compatible solution, or through an intermittent infusion device. Store reconstituted solutions at room temperature up to 24 hours. Compatible with I.V. dextrose or sodium chloride solutions.
● Never inject I.M. or S.C.
● Avoid I.V. infiltration; can be very painful.
● Avoid simultaneous administration with whole blood and its derivatives.
● Monitor fluid intake and output, weight, blood pressure, and serum electrolyte levels.
● Watch for signs of hypokalemia, such as muscle weakness and cramps. Drug may be used with potassium-sparing diuretic to prevent potassium loss.
● Consult the doctor and dietitian about providing a high-potassium diet. Foods rich in potassium include citrus fruits, tomatoes, bananas, dates, and apricots.
● Monitor blood glucose levels, and check insulin requirements in diabetic patients.
● Monitor serum creatinine and BUN regularly. Cumulative effects of the drug may occur with impaired renal function.
● Monitor blood uric acid level, especially in patients with a history of gout.
● Monitor serum calcium and watch for progressive renal impairment.
● Monitor elderly patients, who are especially susceptible to excessive diuresis.
● As ordered, discontinue thiazides and thiazide-like diuretics before parathyroid function tests.
● In patients with hypertension, be aware that therapeutic response may be delayed several weeks.

☑ PATIENT TEACHING
● Instruct the patient to take drug with food and in morning to prevent nocturia. If second dose is necessary tell the patient to take it in early afternoon.
● Advise the patient to avoid sudden posture changes and to rise slowly to avoid orthostatic hypotension.
● Advise the patient to use a sunblock to prevent photosensitivity reactions.

---

chlorthalidone
Apo-Chlorthalidone†, Hygroton, Novo-Thalidone†, Thalitone, Uridon†

Pregnancy Risk Category: B

HOW SUPPLIED
Tablets: 15 mg, 25 mg, 50 mg, 100 mg

ACTION
Although not a thiazide, chlorthalidone acts similarly, increasing sodium and water excretion by inhibiting sodium and chloride reabsorption in the nephron's distal segment.

ONSET, PEAK, DURATION
Onset occurs in 2 to 3 hours. Peak effects occur in 2 to 6 hours. Effects persist for 2 to 3 days.

INDICATIONS & DOSAGE
Edema, hypertension—
Adults: initially, 25 to 100 mg P.O. daily, or up to 200 mg P.O. on alternate days.
Children: 2 mg/kg or 60 mg/m^2 P.O. three times weekly.

ADVERSE REACTIONS
CNS: dizziness, vertigo, headache, paresthesia, weakness, restlessness.
CV: volume depletion and dehydration, vasculitis, increased cholesterol and triglyceride levels.
GI: anorexia, nausea, pancreatitis, vomiting, abdominal pain, diarrhea, constipation.
GU: impotence.
Hematologic: *aplastic anemia, agranulocytosis,* leukopenia, thrombocytopenia.
Hepatic: jaundice.
Skin: dermatitis, photosensitivity, rash, purpura, urticaria.
Other: hypersensitivity reactions; *hypokalemia;* asymptomatic hyperuricemia; hyperglycemia and impairment of glucose tolerance; fluid and electrolyte imbalances, including dilutional hyponatremia and hypochloremia, metabolic alkalosis, hypercalcemia; gout.

INTERACTIONS
Amphotericin B: increased risk of hypokalemia.
Antidiabetic agents: decreased effectiveness; dosage adjustments may be necessary. Monitor blood glucose levels.
Cholestyramine, colestipol: decreased intestinal absorption of thiazides. Separate doses.
Corticosteroids: increased risk of hypokalemia.
Diazoxide: increased antihypertensive, hyperglycemic, and hyperuricemic effects. Use together cautiously.
Digitalis glycosides: increased risk of digitalis toxicity from chlorthalidone-induced hypokalemia. Monitor potassium and digitalis levels.
Ethanol, barbiturates, opiates: increased orthostatic hypotensive effect. Monitor closely.
Lithium: decreased lithium clearance, increasing risk of lithium toxicity. Monitor lithium level.
NSAIDs: increased risk of NSAID-induced renal failure. Monitor closely.

EFFECTS ON DIAGNOSTIC TESTS
Chlorthalidone therapy may alter serum electrolyte levels and may increase serum urate, glucose, cholesterol, and triglyceride levels.
Chlorthalidone may interfere with tests for parathyroid functions and should be discontinued before such tests.

CONTRAINDICATIONS
Contraindicated in patients with anuria or hypersensitivity to thiazides or other sulfonamide-derived drugs.

NURSING CONSIDERATIONS
● Use cautiously in patients with severe renal disease and impaired hepatic function.
● To prevent nocturia, give in the morning.
● Monitor fluid intake and output, weight, blood pressure, and serum electrolyte levels.
● Watch for signs of hypokalemia, such as muscle weakness, and cramps. Know that drug may be used with potassium-sparing diuretic to prevent potassium loss.
● Consult the doctor and dietitian about a high-potassium diet. Foods rich in potassium include citrus fruits, tomatoes, bananas, and dates.
● Monitor serum creatinine and BUN levels regularly. Cumulative effects of the drug may occur with impaired renal function.
● Monitor blood uric acid levels, especially in patients with a history of gout.
● Monitor blood glucose levels, and check insulin requirements in diabetic patients.
● Monitor elderly patients, who are especially susceptible to excessive diuresis.
Alert: Do not use Hygroton and Thalitone interchangeably; they have different strengths and dosages.
● As ordered, discontinue thiazides and thiazide-like diuretics before parathyroid function tests.
● In patients with hypertension, be

aware that therapeutic response may be delayed several weeks.

Alert: Do not confuse Uridon tablets (available in Canada only) with the urinary anti-infective Uridon Modified (available in the United States).

☑ **PATIENT TEACHING**
• Instruct the patient to take in morning to prevent nocturia.
• Advise the patient to avoid sudden posture changes and to rise slowly to avoid orthostatic hypotension.
• Advise the patient to use a sunblock to prevent photosensitivity reactions.

---

ethacrynate sodium
Sodium Edecrin

ethacrynic acid
Edecril‡, Edecrin

Pregnancy Risk Category: B

HOW SUPPLIED
ethacrynic acid
Tablets: 25 mg, 50 mg
ethacrynate sodium
Injection: 50 mg (with 62.5 mg of mannitol and 0.1 mg of thimerosal)

ACTION
A potent loop diuretic that inhibits sodium and chloride reabsorption at the proximal and distal tubules and the ascending loop of Henle.

ONSET, PEAK, DURATION
Onset occurs in 5 minutes after I.V. use, 30 minutes after oral use. Peak effects occur 15 to 30 minutes after I.V. use, 2 hours after oral use. Effects persist for 2 hours after I.V use, 6 to 8 hours after oral use.

INDICATIONS & DOSAGE
Acute pulmonary edema—
Adults: 50 mg or 0.5 to 1 mg/kg I.V. Usually only one dose is necessary, though a second dose may be required.

Edema—
Adults: 50 to 200 mg P.O. daily. Refractory cases may require up to 200 mg b.i.d.
Children: initial dose is 25 mg P.O., increased cautiously in 25-mg increments daily until desired effect is achieved.

ADVERSE REACTIONS
CNS: confusion, fatigue, vertigo, headache.
CV: volume depletion and dehydration, orthostatic hypotension.
EENT: transient or permanent deafness with too-rapid I.V. injection, blurred vision, tinnitus, hearing loss.
GI: diarrhea, anorexia, nausea, vomiting, *GI bleeding*, pancreatitis.
GU: oliguria, hematuria, nocturia, polyuria, frequent urination.
Hematologic: *agranulocytosis*, neutropenia, *thrombocytopenia*, azotemia.
Other: hypokalemia; hypochloremic alkalosis; asymptomatic hyperuricemia; fever; chills; malaise; fluid and electrolyte imbalances, including dilutional hyponatremia, hypocalcemia, hypomagnesemia; hyperglycemia and impaired glucose tolerance.

INTERACTIONS
Aminoglycoside antibiotics: potentiated ototoxic adverse reactions of both drugs. Use together cautiously.
Antihypertensives: increased risk of hypotension. Use together cautiously.
Cisplatin: increased risk of ototoxicity. Avoid concomitant use.
Digitalis glycosides: increased risk of digitalis toxicity from ethacrynate-induced hypokalemia. Monitor potassium and digitalis levels.
Lithium: decreased lithium clearance, increasing risk of lithium toxicity. Monitor lithium level.
Metolazone: profound diuresis and enhanced electrolyte loss. Use together cautiously.
NSAIDs: decreased diuretic effectiveness. Use together cautiously.

Reactions may be *common*, uncommon, *life-threatening*, or COMMON AND LIFE-THREATENING.

Warfarin: potentiated anticoagulant effect. Use together cautiously.

EFFECTS ON DIAGNOSTIC TESTS
Ethacrynic acid therapy alters electrolyte balance and liver and renal function tests.

CONTRAINDICATIONS
Contraindicated in patients with hypersensitivity to the drug, in those with anuria, and in infants.

NURSING CONSIDERATIONS
● Use cautiously in patients with electrolyte abnormalities or hepatic impairment.
● To prevent nocturia, give oral doses in the morning.
● **I.V. use:** Reconstitute vacuum vial with 50 ml of D₅W or 0.9% sodium chloride solution. Give slowly through tubing of running infusion over several minutes. Discard unused solution after 24 hours. Don't use cloudy or opalescent solutions.
● If more than one I.V. dose is necessary, use a new injection site to avoid thrombophlebitis.
● Don't mix with whole blood or its derivatives.
● Don't give S.C. or I.M. because of local pain and irritation.
● Monitor fluid intake and output, weight, blood pressure, and serum electrolyte levels.
● Watch for signs of hypokalemia, such as muscle weakness and cramps.
● Consult the doctor and dietitian about providing a high-potassium diet. Foods rich in potassium include citrus fruits, tomatoes, bananas, dates, and apricots. Know that potassium chloride and sodium supplements may be needed.
● Monitor elderly patients, who are especially susceptible to excessive diuresis.
● Monitor blood uric acid levels, especially in patients with a history of gout.
Alert: Be aware that severe diarrhea will necessitate discontinuing drug. Know

that patient should not receive drug again after diarrhea has resolved.

☑ **PATIENT TEACHING**
● Instruct patient to take oral form of drug in morning to prevent nocturia and if second dose is required to take it in early afternoon. Also tell patient to take drug with food or milk if adverse GI reactions occur.
● Advise patient to avoid sudden posture changes and to rise slowly to avoid orthostatic hypotension.
● Caution patient not to perform hazardous activities if drowsiness occurs.
● Advise diabetic patient to closely monitor blood glucose levels.

---

furosemide (frusemide†‡)
Apo-Furosemide†, Furoside†, Lasix*, Lasix Special†, Myrosemide*, Novosemide†, Urex‡, Urex-M‡, Uritol†

Pregnancy Risk Category: C

HOW SUPPLIED
Tablets: 20 mg, 40 mg, 80 mg, 500 mg†‡
Oral solution: 8 mg/ml, 10 mg/ml, 40 mg/5 ml
Injection: 10 mg/ml

ACTION
A potent loop diuretic that inhibits sodium and chloride reabsorption at the proximal and distal tubules and the ascending loop of Henle.

ONSET, PEAK, DURATION
Onset occurs about 5 minutes after I.V. administration, about 20 to 60 minutes after oral administration. Peak effects occur within 30 minutes of I.V. administration, within 1 to 2 hours of oral administration. Effects persist about 2 hours after I.V. administration, 6 to 8 hours after oral administration.

INDICATIONS & DOSAGE

Acute pulmonary edema—
Adults: 40 mg I.V. injected slowly over 1 to 2 minutes; then 80 mg I.V. in 1 to 1½ hours if needed.
Edema—
Adults: 20 to 80 mg P.O. daily in the morning, second dose in 6 to 8 hours; carefully titrated up to 600 mg daily if needed. Or, 20 to 40 mg I.M. or I.V., increased by 20 mg q 2 hours until desired response is achieved. Give I.V. dose slowly over 1 to 2 minutes.
Infants and children: 2 mg/kg P.O. daily, increased by 1 to 2 mg/kg in 6 to 8 hours if needed; carefully titrated up to 6 mg/kg daily if needed.
Hypertension—
Adults: 40 mg P.O. b.i.d. Dosage adjusted according to response.

ADVERSE REACTIONS

CNS: vertigo, headache, dizziness, paresthesia, restlessness.
CV: volume depletion and dehydration, orthostatic hypotension, increased cholesterol levels.
EENT: transient deafness with too rapid I.V. injection, blurred vision.
GI: abdominal discomfort and pain, diarrhea, anorexia, nausea, vomiting, constipation, pancreatitis.
GU: nocturia, polyuria, frequent urination, oliguria.
Hematologic: *agranulocytosis,* leukopenia, *thrombocytopenia,* azotemia, anemia, *aplastic anemia.*
Skin: dermatitis, purpura.
Other: hypokalemia; hypochloremic alkalosis; asymptomatic hyperuricemia; fever; muscle spasm; weakness; fluid and electrolyte imbalances, including dilutional hyponatremia, hypocalcemia, hypomagnesemia; hyperglycemia and impaired glucose tolerance; transient pain at injection site with I.M. administration; thrombophlebitis with I.V. administration.

INTERACTIONS

Aminoglycoside antibiotics, cisplatin: potentiated ototoxicity. Use together cautiously.
Antidiabetic agents: decreased hypoglycemic effects. Monitor blood glucose levels.
Antihypertensives: increased risk of hypotension. Use together cautiously.
Corticosteroids, corticotropin, amphotericin B, metolazone: increased risk of hypokalemia. Monitor potassium levels closely.
Digitalis glycosides, neuromuscular blockers: increased toxicity of these agents from furosemide-induced hypokalemia. Monitor potassium levels.
Ethacrynic acid: may increase risk of ototoxicity. Do not use concomitantly.
Lithium: decreased lithium excretion, resulting in lithium toxicity. Monitor lithium level.
NSAIDs: inhibited diuretic response. Use together cautiously.
Salicylates: may cause salicylate toxicity.
Sucralfate: may reduce diuretic and antihypertensive effect.

EFFECTS ON DIAGNOSTIC TESTS

Furosemide therapy alters electrolyte balance and liver and renal function tests.

CONTRAINDICATIONS

Contraindicated in patients with anuria or in patients with a history of hypersensitivity to the drug.

NURSING CONSIDERATIONS

● Use cautiously in patients with hepatic cirrhosis. Know that furosemide should be used during pregnancy only if potential benefits clearly outweigh possible risks to fetus.
● To prevent nocturia, give P.O. and I.M. preparations in the morning. Give second doses in early afternoon.
● **I.V. use:** Given by direct injection over 1 to 2 minutes. Alternatively, dilute with D_5W, 0.9% sodium chloride solution, or lactated Ringer's solution, and infuse no faster than 4 mg/minute to

avoid ototoxicity. Use prepared infusion solution within 24 hours.

Alert: Monitor weight, blood pressure, and pulse rate routinely with chronic use and during rapid diuresis. Furosemide can lead to profound water and electrolyte depletion.

• Be aware that if oliguria or azotemia develops or increases, it may require stopping drug.

• Monitor fluid intake and output and serum electrolyte, BUN, and carbon dioxide levels frequently.

• Watch for signs of hypokalemia, such as muscle weakness and cramps.

• Consult the doctor and dietitian about a high-potassium diet. Foods rich in potassium include citrus fruits, tomatoes, bananas, and dates.

• Monitor blood glucose levels in diabetic patients.

• Know that furosemide may not be well absorbed orally in severe CHF. Drug may need to be given I.V. even if patient is taking other oral medications.

• Monitor blood uric acid, especially in patients with a history of gout.

• Monitor elderly patients, who are especially susceptible to excessive diuresis, with potential for circulatory collapse and thromboembolic complications.

• Store tablets in light-resistant container to prevent discoloration (doesn't affect potency). Don't use discolored (yellow) injectable preparation. Refrigerate oral furosemide solution to ensure drug stability.

☑ **PATIENT TEACHING**

• Advise patient to take the drug with food to prevent GI upset. Also tell patient to take drug in morning to prevent nocturia; if second dose is required, tell patient to take the second dose in early afternoon.

• Advise patient to stand slowly to prevent dizziness and to limit alcohol intake and strenuous exercise in hot weather to avoid exacerbating orthostatic hypotension.

• Advise patient to immediately report ringing in ears, severe abdominal pain, or sore throat and fever; may indicate furosemide toxicity.

• Discourage patient taking furosemide at home from storing different types of medication in the same container, increasing the risk of drug errors. The most popular strengths of furosemide and digoxin are white tablets approximately equal in size.

• Tell patient to check with the doctor or pharmacist before taking any OTC medications.

• Teach patient to avoid direct sunlight and use protective clothing and a sunblock; there is a risk of photosensitivity.

---

hydrochlorothiazide
Apo-Hydro†, Aquazide-H, Diaqua, Dichlotride‡, Diuchlor H†, Esidrix, Ezide, Hydro-D, HydroDIURIL, Hydro-Par, Mictrin, Neo-Codema†, Novo-Hydrazide†, Oretic, Urozide†

Pregnancy Risk Category: B

HOW SUPPLIED
Tablets: 25 mg, 50 mg, 100 mg
Oral solution: 10 mg/ml, 50 mg/5 ml, 100 mg/ml

ACTION
A thiazide diuretic that increases sodium and water excretion by inhibiting sodium and chloride reabsorption in the nephron's distal segment.

ONSET, PEAK, DURATION
Onset occurs in 2 hours. Peak effects occur within 4 to 6 hours. Effects persist for 6 to 12 hours.

INDICATIONS & DOSAGE
Edema—
Adults: 25 to 100 mg P.O. daily or intermittently.
Children 2 to 12 years: 37.5 to 100 mg P.O. daily in two divided doses.
Children 6 months to 2 years: 12.5 to

37.5 mg P.O. daily in two divided doses.
Infants under 6 months: up to 3 mg/kg
P.O. daily in two divided doses. Total
daily dosage may range from 12.5 to
37.5 mg.
Hypertension—
Adults: 25 to 50 mg P.O. daily as a single dose or divided b.i.d. Daily dosage
increased or decreased according to
blood pressure.

Doses greater than 50 mg/day are not
required when combined with other antihypertensives.

ADVERSE REACTIONS
CNS: dizziness, vertigo, headache,
paresthesia, weakness, restlessness.
CV: volume depletion and dehydration,
orthostatic hypotension, allergic myocarditis, vasculitis.
GI: anorexia, nausea, pancreatitis, epigastric distress, vomiting, abdominal
pain, diarrhea, constipation.
GU: polyuria, frequent urination, *renal
failure,* interstitial nephritis.
Hematologic: *aplastic anemia, agranulocytosis,* leukopenia, *thrombocytopenia,* hemolytic anemia.
Hepatic: jaundice.
Respiratory: respiratory distress, pneumonitis.
Skin: dermatitis, photosensitivity, rash,
purpura, alopecia.
Other: hypersensitivity reactions; hypokalemia; asymptomatic hyperuricemia; hyperglycemia and impaired
glucose tolerance; fluid and electrolyte
imbalances, including dilutional hyponatremia and hypochloremia, metabolic alkalosis, hypercalcemia; gout;
muscle cramps; *anaphylactic reactions.*

INTERACTIONS
Antidiabetic agents: decreased effectiveness of hypoglycemic agents;
dosage adjustments may be necessary.
Monitor blood glucose levels.
Antihypertensives: additive antihypertensive effect. Use together cautiously.
Cholestyramine, colestipol: decreased
intestinal absorption of thiazides. Sepa-

rate doses.
Corticosteroids and amphotericin B: increased risk of hypokalemia.
Diazoxide: increased antihypertensive,
hyperglycemic, and hyperuricemic effects. Use together cautiously.
Digitalis glycosides: increased risk of
digitalis toxicity from hydrochloroth-
iazide-induced hypokalemia. Monitor
potassium and digitalis levels.
Ethanol, barbiturates, opiates: increased orthostatic hypotensive effect.
Monitor closely.
Lithium: decreased lithium excretion,
increasing risk of lithium toxicity. Monitor lithium level.
NSAIDs: increased risk of NSAID-induced renal failure. Monitor closely.

EFFECTS ON DIAGNOSTIC TESTS
Hydrochlorothiazide therapy may alter
serum electrolyte levels and may increase serum urate, glucose, cholesterol,
and triglyceride levels. It also may interfere with tests for parathyroid function
and should be discontinued before such
tests.

CONTRAINDICATIONS
Contraindicated in patients with anuria
or hypersensitivity to other thiazides or
other sulfonamide derivatives.

NURSING CONSIDERATIONS
● Use cautiously in children and in patients with severe renal disease, impaired hepatic function, and progressive
hepatic disease.
● To prevent nocturia, give in the morning.
● Monitor fluid intake and output,
weight, blood pressure, and serum electrolyte levels.
● Watch for signs of hypokalemia, such
as muscle weakness and cramps. Drug
may be used with potassium-sparing diuretics to prevent potassium loss.
● Consult the doctor and dietitian about
a high-potassium diet. Foods rich in
potassium include citrus fruits, tomatoes, bananas, and dates.

- Monitor serum creatinine and BUN levels regularly. Cumulative effects of the drug may occur with impaired renal function.
- Monitor blood uric acid levels, especially in patients with a history of gout.
- Monitor blood glucose levels, especially in diabetic patients.
- Monitor elderly patients, who are especially susceptible to excessive diuresis.
- As ordered, discontinue thiazides and thiazide-like diuretics before parathyroid function tests.
- In patients with hypertension, know that therapeutic response may be delayed several weeks.

✓ **PATIENT TEACHING**
- Advise the patient to take the drug with food to minimize GI upset. Also tell him to take drug in morning to avoid nocturia; if second dose is needed, have him take it in early afternoon.
- Advise the patient to avoid sudden posture changes and to rise slowly to avoid orthostatic hypotension.
- Advise the patient to use a sunblock to prevent photosensitivity reactions.
- Tell the patient to check with the doctor or pharmacist before taking any OTC medications.

---

indapamide
Lozide†, Lozol, Natrilix‡

Pregnancy Risk Category: B

HOW SUPPLIED
Tablets: 1.25 mg, 2.5 mg

ACTION
Unknown. A thiazide-like diuretic that probably inhibits sodium reabsorption in the nephron's distal segment. Also has a direct vasodilating effect that may be a result of calcium channel-blocking action.

ONSET, PEAK, DURATION
Onset occurs in 1 to 2 hours. Peak effects occur within 2 hours. Effects persist for up to 36 hours.

INDICATIONS & DOSAGE
Edema—
Adults: initially, 2.5 mg P.O. daily in the morning. Increased to 5 mg daily after 1 week, if needed.
Hypertension—
Adults: initially, 1.25 mg P.O. daily in a.m. Increased to 2.5 mg daily after 4 weeks, if needed. Increased to 5 mg daily after 4 more weeks, if needed.

ADVERSE REACTIONS
CNS: headache, nervousness, dizziness, light-headedness, weakness, vertigo, restlessness, drowsiness, fatigue, anxiety, depression, numbness of extremities, irritability, agitation.
CV: volume depletion and dehydration, orthostatic hypotension, palpitations, premature ventricular contractions, irregular heartbeat, vasculitis.
GI: anorexia, nausea, epigastric distress, vomiting, abdominal pain, diarrhea, constipation.
GU: nocturia, polyuria, frequent urination, impotence.
Skin: rash, pruritus, urticaria, flushing.
Other: muscle cramps and spasms; asymptomatic hyperuricemia; fluid and electrolyte imbalances, including dilutional hyponatremia and hypochloremia, metabolic alkalosis, hypokalemia; gout; rhinorrhea; weight loss.

INTERACTIONS
Amphotericin B: increased risk of hypokalemia.
Corticosteroids: increased risk of hypokalemia.
Diazoxide: increased antihypertensive, hyperglycemic, and hyperuricemic effects. Use together cautiously.
Digitalis glycosides: increased risk of digitalis toxicity from indapamide-induced hypokalemia. Monitor potassium and digitalis levels.

Lithium: decreased lithium clearance which may increase lithium toxicity. Should not be administered concomitantly.

NSAIDs: increased risk of NSAID-induced renal failure. Monitor the patient for signs of renal failure.

EFFECTS ON DIAGNOSTIC TESTS
Indapamide therapy may alter serum electrolyte levels and may increase serum urate, glucose, cholesterol, and triglyceride levels. It also may interfere with tests for parathyroid function and should be discontinued before such tests.

CONTRAINDICATIONS
Contraindicated in patients with anuria or hypersensitivity to other sulfonamide-derived drugs.

NURSING CONSIDERATIONS
● Use cautiously in patients with severe renal disease, impaired hepatic function, and progressive hepatic disease.
● To prevent nocturia, give in the morning.
● Monitor fluid intake and output, weight, blood pressure, and serum electrolyte levels.
● Watch for signs of hypokalemia, such as muscle weakness and cramps. Know that drug may be used with potassium-sparing diuretic to prevent potassium loss.
● Consult the doctor and dietitian about a high-potassium diet. Foods rich in potassium include citrus fruits, tomatoes, bananas, and dates.
● Monitor serum creatinine and BUN levels regularly. Cumulative effects of the drug may occur with impaired renal function.
● Monitor blood uric acid levels, especially in patients with a history of gout.
● Monitor blood glucose levels, especially in diabetic patients.
● Monitor elderly patients, who are especially susceptible to excessive diuresis.

● As ordered, discontinue thiazides and thiazide-like diuretics before parathyroid function tests.
● In patients with hypertension, be aware that therapeutic response may be delayed several weeks.

☑ **PATIENT TEACHING**
● Instruct the patient to take drug in morning to prevent nocturia and with food if GI upset occurs.
● Advise the patient to avoid sudden posture changes and to rise slowly to avoid orthostatic hypotension.

---

mannitol
Osmitrol

Pregnancy Risk Category: B

HOW SUPPLIED
Injection: 5%, 10%, 15%, 20%, 25%

ACTION
An osmotic diuretic that increases the osmotic pressure of glomerular filtrate, inhibiting tubular reabsorption of water and electrolytes, and that elevates blood plasma osmolality, resulting in enhanced water flow into extracellular fluid.

ONSET, PEAK, DURATION
Onset occurs in 30 to 60 minutes. Peak effects occur within 1 hour. Effects persist for 6 to 8 hours.

INDICATIONS & DOSAGE
Test dose for marked oliguria or suspected inadequate renal function—
Adults and children over 12 years: 200 mg/kg or 12.5 g as a 25% I.V. solution over 3 to 5 minutes. Response is adequate if 30 to 50 ml urine/hour is excreted over 2 to 3 hours; if response is inadequate, a second test dose is given. If still no response after the second dose, mannitol should not be continued.
Oliguria—
Adults and children over 12 years: 50 to 100 g I.V. as a 5% to 25% solution

over 1½ to several hours.

Prevention of oliguria or acute renal failure—

Adults and children over 12 years: 50 to 100 g I.V. of a concentrated solution, followed by a 5% to 10% solution. Exact concentration determined by fluid requirements.

Reduction of intraocular or intracranial pressure—

Adults and children over 12 years: 1.5 to 2 g/kg as a 15% to 25% I.V. solution over 30 to 60 minutes.

Diuresis in drug intoxication—

Adults and children over 12 years: 5% to 10% solution continuously up to 200 g I.V., while maintaining 100 to 500 ml urine output/hour and a positive fluid balance.

Irrigating solution during transurethral resection of the prostate gland—

Adults: 2.5% to 5% solution as needed.

ADVERSE REACTIONS

CNS: *seizures,* dizziness, headache.
CV: edema, thrombophlebitis, hypotension, hypertension, CHF, tachycardia, angina-like chest pain, vascular overload.
EENT: blurred vision, rhinitis, dry mouth.
GI: thirst, nausea, vomiting, *diarrhea.*
GU: urine retention.
Other: fluid and electrolyte imbalance, dehydration, local pain, fever, chills, urticaria.

INTERACTIONS

Lithium: increased urinary excretion of lithium. Monitor closely.

EFFECTS ON DIAGNOSTIC TESTS

Mannitol therapy alters electrolyte balance. It also may interfere with tests for inorganic phosphorus concentration or blood ethylene glycol.

CONTRAINDICATIONS

Contraindicated in patients with hypersensitivity to the drug and in those with anuria, severe pulmonary congestion, frank pulmonary edema, severe CHF, severe dehydration, metabolic edema, progressive renal disease or dysfunction, or active intracranial bleeding except during craniotomy.

NURSING CONSIDERATIONS

● To redissolve crystallized solution (occurs at low temperatures or in concentrations greater than 15%), warm bottle in hot water bath and shake vigorously. Cool to body temperature before giving. Do not use solution with undissolved crystals.
● **I.V. use:** Administer as intermittent or continuous infusion at prescribed rate, using an in-line filter and an infusion pump. Direct injection is not recommended. Check I.V. line patency at infusion site before and during administration.
● Avoid infiltration; if it occurs, observe for inflammation, edema, and necrosis.
● For maximum intraocular pressure reduction before surgery, give 1 to 1½ hours preoperatively, as ordered.
● Monitor vital signs, including central venous pressure, and fluid intake and output hourly. Report increasing oliguria. Check weight, renal function, fluid balance, and serum and urine sodium and potassium levels daily.
● Insert urethral catheter in comatose or incontinent patients because therapy is based on strict evaluation of fluid intake and output. In patients with urethral catheters, use an hourly urometer collection bag to facilitate accurate evaluation of output.
● Be aware that drug can be used to measure glomerular filtration rate.
● To relieve thirst, give frequent mouth care or fluids as permitted.
● When used as an irrigating solution for prostate surgery, keep in mind that concentrations of 3.5% or greater are needed to avoid hemolysis.

☑ PATIENT TEACHING

● Tell patient that he may feel thirsty or experience mouth dryness, and emphasize importance of drinking only the amount of fluids ordered.

• Instruct patient to report adverse reactions promptly and to alert nurse if discomfort occurs at I.V. site.

methazolamide
Neptazane

Pregnancy Risk Category: C

HOW SUPPLIED
Tablets: 25 mg, 50 mg

ACTION
A carbonic anhydrase inhibitor that decreases secretion of aqueous humor, lowering intraocular pressure.

ONSET, PEAK, DURATION
Onset occurs in 2 to 4 hours. Peak effects occur in 6 to 8 hours. Effects persist for 10 to 18 hours.

INDICATIONS & DOSAGE
Glaucoma (chronic open-angle or secondary, or preoperatively in obstructive or acute angle-closure)—
Adults: 50 to 100 mg P.O. b.i.d. or t.i.d.

ADVERSE REACTIONS
CNS: drowsiness, paresthesia, fatigue, malaise, confusion.
EENT: transient myopia, hearing dysfunction, tinnitus.
GI: nausea, vomiting, anorexia, taste alteration, diarrhea.
GU: crystalluria, renal calculi.
Skin: urticaria.
Other: metabolic acidosis, electrolyte imbalance.

INTERACTIONS
Amphetamines, anticholinergics, mecamylamine, procainamide, quinidine: decreased renal clearance of these agents, increasing the risk of toxicity. Avoid concomitant use.
Methenamine compounds: reduced methenamine effectiveness. Avoid con-

comitant use.
Salicylates: accumulation and toxicity of methazolamide may occur. Monitor closely.

EFFECTS ON DIAGNOSTIC TESTS
Because methazolamide alkalizes urine, it may cause false-positive proteinuria when Albustix or Albutest test is performed. Methazolamide also may decrease iodine uptake by the thyroid.

CONTRAINDICATIONS
Contraindicated for long-term use in patients with angle-closure glaucoma, depressed serum sodium or potassium levels, renal or hepatic disease or dysfunction, adrenal gland dysfunction, or hyperchloremic acidosis.

NURSING CONSIDERATIONS
• Use cautiously in patients with emphysema and pulmonary obstruction.
• Monitor fluid intake and output, weight, and serum electrolyte levels.
• Monitor elderly patients, who are especially susceptible to excessive diuresis.
• Know that this drug may cause false-positive urine protein tests by alkalinizing urine.
• Evaluate the patient for eye pain to ensure drug is effective in decreasing intraocular pressure.

☑ PATIENT TEACHING
• Caution the patient to comply with prescribed dosage to lessen risk of metabolic acidosis. Effects may decrease in acidosis.
• Warn the patient not to perform hazardous activities if adverse CNS reactions occur.

metolazone
Diulo, Mykrox, Zaroxolyn**

Pregnancy Risk Category: B

HOW SUPPLIED
Tablets (extended-release): 2.5 mg, 5 mg, 10 mg
Tablets (prompt-release): 0.5 mg

ACTION
Increases sodium and water excretion by inhibiting sodium reabsorption in the cortical diluting site of the ascending loop of Henle.

ONSET, PEAK, DURATION
Onset occurs in 1 hour. Peak effects occur in about 2 to 4 hours after prompt-release tablets, 8 hours after extended-release tablets. Effects persist for 12 to 24 hours.

INDICATIONS & DOSAGE
Edema in CHF or renal disease—
Adults: 5 to 20 mg (extended-release) P.O. daily.
Hypertension—
Adults: 2.5 to 5 mg (extended-release) P.O. daily. Maintenance dosage based on patient's blood pressure. Or 0.5 mg (prompt-release) P.O. once daily in a.m., increased to 1 mg P.O. daily as needed. If response is inadequate, another antihypertensive is added.

ADVERSE REACTIONS
CNS: *dizziness,* headache, fatigue, vertigo, paresthesia, weakness, restlessness, drowsiness, anxiety, depression, nervousness, blurred vision.
CV: volume depletion and dehydration, orthostatic hypotension, palpitations, vasculitis, increased cholesterol levels.
GI: anorexia, nausea, pancreatitis, epigastric distress, vomiting, abdominal pain, diarrhea, constipation, dry mouth.
GU: nocturia, polyuria, frequent urination, impotence.
Hematologic: *aplastic anemia, agranulocytosis,* leukopenia.
Hepatic: jaundice, hepatitis.
Skin: dermatitis, photosensitivity, rash, purpura, pruritus, urticaria.
Other: hyperglycemia and glucose tolerance impairment; fluid and electrolyte imbalances, including hypokalemia, hypomagnesemia, dilutional hyponatremia and hypochloremia, metabolic alkalosis, hypercalcemia; muscle cramps.

INTERACTIONS
Amphotericin B: increased risk of hypokalemia.
Anticoagulants: may affect hypoprothrombinemic response. Monitor PT.
Antidiabetic agents: may alter blood glucose level requiring dosage adjustment of antidiabetic agents. Monitor blood glucose levels.
Cholestyramine, colestipol: decreased intestinal absorption of thiazides. Separate doses.
Corticosteroids: increased risk of hypokalemia.
Diazoxide: increased antihypertensive, hyperglycemic, and hyperuricemic effects. Use together cautiously.
Digitalis glycosides: increased risk of digitalis toxicity from metolazone-induced hypokalemia. Monitor potassium and digitalis levels.
Ethanol, barbiturates, opiates: increased orthostatic hypotensive effect. Monitor closely.
Lithium: decreased lithium clearance, increasing risk of lithium toxicity. Monitor lithium level.
NSAIDs: increased risk of NSAID-induced renal failure. Monitor the patient for signs of renal failure.
Other antihypertensives: may have additive effects. Use together cautiously.

EFFECTS ON DIAGNOSTIC TESTS
Metolazone therapy may alter serum electrolyte levels and may increase serum urate, glucose, cholesterol, and triglyceride levels. It also may interfere with tests for parathyroid function and should be discontinued before such tests.

CONTRAINDICATIONS
Contraindicated in patients with anuria, hepatic coma or precoma, or hypersensitivity to thiazides or other sulfon-

amide-derived drugs.

NURSING CONSIDERATIONS
• Use cautiously in patients with impaired renal or hepatic function.
• To prevent nocturia, give in the morning.
• Keep in mind that Mykrox (prompt-release) tablets are more rapidly and completely absorbed than other brands, mimicking an oral solution. Do not interchange Mykrox with Diulo (extended-release) or Zaroxolyn (extended-release) tablets.
• Monitor fluid intake and output, weight, blood pressure, and serum electrolyte levels.
• Watch for signs of hypokalemia, such as muscle weakness and cramps. Know that drug may be used with potassium-sparing diuretic to prevent potassium loss.
• Consult the doctor and dietitian about providing a high-potassium diet. Foods rich in potassium include citrus fruits, tomatoes, bananas, dates, and apricots.
• Monitor blood glucose levels, especially in diabetic patients.
• Monitor blood uric acid levels, especially in patients with a history of gout.
• Monitor elderly patients, who are especially susceptible to excessive diuresis.
• In patients with hypertension, know that the therapeutic response may be delayed several weeks.
• Keep in mind that unlike thiazide diuretics, metolazone is effective in patients with decreased renal function.
• Be aware that drug is used as an adjunct in furosemide-resistant edema.
• As ordered, discontinue thiazides and thiazide-like diuretics before parathyroid function tests.

☑ PATIENT TEACHING
• Tell the patient to take drug in morning to prevent nocturia.
• Advise the patient to avoid sudden posture changes and to rise slowly to avoid orthostatic hypotension.

• Advise the patient to use a sunblock to prevent photosensitivity reactions.

---

spironolactone
Aldactone, Novospiroton†, Spirotone‡

Pregnancy Risk Category: NR

HOW SUPPLIED
Tablets: 25 mg, 50 mg, 100 mg

ACTION
A potassium-sparing diuretic that antagonizes aldosterone in the distal tubules, increasing sodium and water excretion.

ONSET, PEAK, DURATION
Onset occurs in 1 to 2 days. Peak effects occur within 2 to 3 days. Effects persist for 2 to 3 days.

INDICATIONS & DOSAGE
Edema—
Adults: 25 to 200 mg P.O. daily or in divided doses.
Children: 3.3 mg/kg P.O. daily or in divided doses.
Hypertension—
Adults: 50 to 100 mg P.O. daily or in divided doses.
Diuretic-induced hypokalemia—
Adults: 25 to 100 mg P.O. daily.
Detection of primary hyperaldosteronism—
Adults: 400 mg P.O. daily for 4 days (short test) or 3 to 4 weeks (long test). If hypokalemia and hypertension are corrected, a presumptive diagnosis of primary hyperaldosteronism is made.
Management of primary hyperaldosteronism—
Adults: 100 to 400 mg P.O. daily.

ADVERSE REACTIONS
CNS: headache, drowsiness, lethargy, confusion, ataxia.
GI: diarrhea, gastric bleeding, ulceration, cramping, gastritis, vomiting.
Skin: urticaria, maculopapular

Reactions may be *common*, uncommon, *life-threatening*, or COMMON AND LIFE-THREATENING.

eruptions.
Other: *hyperkalemia,* dehydration, hyponatremia, transient elevation in BUN, mild acidosis, inability to maintain erection, hirsutism, gynecomastia, breast soreness and menstrual disturbances in women, drug fever, *agranulocytosis.*

INTERACTIONS

ACE inhibitors, indomethacin, potassium-containing salt substitutes, potassium-rich foods, other potassium-sparing diuretics, potassium supplements: increased risk of hyperkalemia. Use together cautiously, especially in patients with renal impairment.
Aspirin: possible blocked diuretic effect of spironolactone. Watch for diminished spironolactone response.
Digoxin: may alter digoxin clearance, increasing risk of digoxin toxicity. Monitor digoxin levels.

EFFECTS ON DIAGNOSTIC TESTS

Spironolactone therapy alters fluorometric determinations of plasma and urinary 17-hydroxycorticosteroid levels and may cause false elevations on radioimmunoassay of serum digoxin.

CONTRAINDICATIONS

Contraindicated in patients with known hypersensitivity to drug, anuria, acute or progressive renal insufficiency, or hyperkalemia.

NURSING CONSIDERATIONS

● Use cautiously in patients with fluid or electrolyte imbalances, impaired renal function, and hepatic disease.
● To enhance absorption, give drug with meals.
● Protect drug from light.
● Monitor serum electrolytes, fluid intake and output, weight, and blood pressure.
● Monitor elderly patients, who are more susceptible to excessive diuresis.
● Inform the laboratory that patient is taking spironolactone because it may interfere with some laboratory tests that measure digoxin levels.
● Be aware that drug is less potent than thiazide and loop diuretics; useful as an adjunct to other diuretic therapy. Diuretic effect delayed 2 to 3 days when used alone.
● Keep in mind that maximum antihypertensive response may be delayed for up to 2 weeks.
● Watch for hyperchloremic metabolic acidosis, which may occur during therapy, because of danger in patients with hepatic cirrhosis.
● Know that breast cancer has been reported in some patients taking spironolactone.

☑ PATIENT TEACHING

● Instruct the patient to take drug in morning to prevent nocturia; if second dose is needed, tell the patient to take it in early afternoon. Also tell the patient to take it with food.
Alert: Warn the patient to avoid excessive ingestion of potassium-rich foods, potassium-containing salt substitutes, and potassium supplements to prevent serious hyperkalemia.
● Caution the patient not to perform hazardous activities if adverse CNS reactions occur.

---

torsemide
Demadex

Pregnancy Risk Category: B

HOW SUPPLIED

Injection: 10 mg/ml
Tablets: 5 mg, 10 mg, 20 mg, 100 mg

ACTION

A loop diuretic that enhances excretion of sodium, chloride, and water by acting on the ascending portion of the loop of Henle.

ONSET, PEAK, DURATION

Onset occurs within 10 minutes of I.V. use, 1 hour after oral use. Peak effects

---

occur within 1 hour of I.V. use, 1 to 2 hours after oral use. Effects persist for 6 to 8 hours.

INDICATIONS & DOSAGE

Diuresis in patients with CHF—
Adults: initially, 10 to 20 mg P.O. or I.V. once daily. If response is inadequate, the dose is doubled until a response is obtained. Maximum dosage is 200 mg daily.

Diuresis in patients with chronic renal failure—
Adults: initially, 20 mg P.O. or I.V. once daily. If response is inadequate, the dose is doubled until a response is obtained. Maximum dosage is 200 mg daily.

Diuresis in patients with hepatic cirrhosis—
Adults: initially, 5 to 10 mg P.O. or I.V. once daily with an aldosterone antagonist or a potassium-sparing diuretic. If response is inadequate, the dose is doubled until a response is obtained. Maximum dosage is 40 mg daily.

Hypertension—
Adults: initially, 5 mg P.O. daily. Increased to 10 mg if needed and tolerated. If response is still inadequate, another antihypertensive should be added.

ADVERSE REACTIONS

CNS: dizziness, headache, nervousness, insomnia, syncope.
CV: ECG abnormalities, chest pain, edema, increased cholesterol level, *dehydration.*
EENT: rhinitis, cough, sore throat.
GI: diarrhea, constipation, nausea, dyspepsia.
GU: *excessive urination,* impotence.
Other: asthenia, arthralgia, myalgia, rash, *electrolyte imbalances including hypokalemia and hypomagnesemia,* increased uric acid, *excessive thirst.*

INTERACTIONS

Cholestyramine: decreased absorption of torsemide. Separate administration times by at least 3 hours.

Digoxin: decreased torsemide clearance. No dosage adjustments are necessary.
Indomethacin: decreased diuretic effectiveness in sodium-restricted patients. Avoid concomitant use.
Lithium, ototoxic drugs such as aminoglycosides or ethacrynic acid: possible increased toxicity of these agents. Avoid concomitant use.
NSAIDs: may potentiate nephrotoxicity of NSAIDs. Use together cautiously.
Probenecid: decreased diuretic effectiveness. Avoid concomitant use.
Salicylates: decreased excretion, possibly leading to salicylate toxicity. Avoid concomitant use.
Spironolactone: decreased renal clearance of spironolactone. No dosage adjustments are necessary.

EFFECTS ON DIAGNOSTIC TESTS

Torsemide therapy alters electrolyte balance and renal function tests. It also may mildly affect glucose, serum lipid, and alkaline phosphatase levels, CBC, and platelet count.

CONTRAINDICATIONS

Contraindicated in patients with anuria or hypersensitivity to the drug or other sulfonylurea derivatives.

NURSING CONSIDERATIONS

● Use cautiously in patients with hepatic disease and associated cirrhosis and ascites; sudden changes in fluid and electrolyte balance may precipitate hepatic coma in these patients.
● To prevent nocturia, give in the morning.
● Inspect ampules for precipitate or discoloration before use.
● **I.V. use:** May be given by direct injection over at least 2 minutes. Rapid injection may cause ototoxicity. Don't give more than 200 mg at once.
● Monitor fluid intake and output, serum electrolyte levels, blood pressure, weight, and pulse rate during rapid diuresis and routinely with chronic use. Drug can cause profound diuresis and

water and electrolyte depletion.
• Watch for signs of hypokalemia, such as muscle weakness and cramps.
• Consult the doctor and dietitian about providing a high-potassium diet. Foods rich in potassium include citrus fruits, tomatoes, bananas, dates, and apricots.
• Monitor elderly patients, who are especially susceptible to excessive diuresis with potential for circulatory collapse and thromboembolic complications.

☑ **PATIENT TEACHING**
• Tell the patient to take drug in morning to prevent nocturia.
• To prevent orthostatic hypotension, advise the patient to change positions slowly to prevent dizziness, and to limit alcohol intake and strenuous exercise in hot weather to prevent orthostatic hypotension.
• Advise the patient to immediately report ringing in ears. May indicate toxicity.
• Tell the patient to check with the doctor or pharmacist before taking any OTC medications.

---

triamterene
Dyrenium, Dytac‡

Pregnancy Risk Category: B

HOW SUPPLIED
Tablets†: 50 mg, 100 mg
Capsules: 50 mg, 100 mg

ACTION
A potassium-sparing diuretic that inhibits sodium reabsorption and potassium and hydrogen excretion by direct action on the distal tubules.

ONSET, PEAK, DURATION
Onset occurs in 2 to 4 hours. Peak effects occur in several days. Effects persist for 7 to 9 hours.

INDICATIONS & DOSAGE
Edema—
Adults: initially, 100 mg P.O. b.i.d. after meals. Total dosage should not exceed 300 mg daily.

ADVERSE REACTIONS
CNS: dizziness, weakness, fatigue, headache.
CV: hypotension.
GI: dry mouth, nausea, vomiting, diarrhea.
Hematologic: megaloblastic anemia related to low folic acid levels, *thrombocytopenia.*
Skin: photosensitivity, rash.
Other: *anaphylaxis, hyperkalemia,* muscle cramps, transient elevation in BUNs or creatinine levels, acidosis, interstitial nephritis, hypokalemia, hyperglycemia, azotemia, renal stones, jaundice, increased liver enzyme abnormalities.

INTERACTIONS
ACE inhibitors, potassium-containing salt substitutes, potassium-rich foods, potassium supplements: increased risk of hyperkalemia. Use together as long as serum potassium is monitored.
Amantadine: increased risk of amantadine toxicity. Don't use together.
Lithium: decreased lithium clearance, increasing risk of lithium toxicity. Monitor lithium level.
NSAIDs: may enhance risk of nephrotoxicity. Use together cautiously.
Quinidine: may interfere with some laboratory tests that measure quinidine levels. Inform laboratory that patient is taking triamterene.

EFFECTS ON DIAGNOSTIC TESTS
Triamterene therapy may interfere with enzyme assays that use fluorometry, such as serum quinidine determinations.

CONTRAINDICATIONS
Contraindicated in patients with hypersensitivity to the drug and in those with anuria, severe or progressive renal dis-

ease or dysfunction, severe hepatic disease, or hyperkalemia.

NURSING CONSIDERATIONS
● Use cautiously in patients with impaired hepatic function or diabetes mellitus and in elderly or debilitated patients.
● To minimize nausea, give medication after meals.
● Monitor blood pressure, blood uric acid, CBC, blood glucose, BUN, and serum electrolyte levels.
● Watch for blood dyscrasia.
● To minimize excessive rebound potassium excretion, withdraw drug gradually, as ordered.
● Know that drug is less potent than thiazides and loop diuretics and is useful as an adjunct to other diuretic therapy. Usually used with potassium-wasting diuretics. Full effect is delayed 2 to 3 days when used alone.

☑ PATIENT TEACHING
● Tell the patient to take drug after meals to minimize nausea.
Alert: Warn the patient to avoid excessive ingestion of potassium-rich foods, potassium-containing salt substitutes, and potassium supplements to prevent serious hyperkalemia.
Teach the patient to avoid direct sunlight, wear protective clothing, and use a sunblock to prevent photosensitivity reactions.
● Tell patient urine may turn blue.

---

urea (carbamide)
Ureaphil

Pregnancy Risk Category: C

HOW SUPPLIED
Injection: 40 g/150 ml

ACTION
An osmotic diuretic that increases the osmotic pressure of glomerular filtrate, inhibiting tubular reabsorption of water

and electrolytes. Also elevates blood plasma osmolality, resulting in enhanced water flow into extracellular fluid.

ONSET, PEAK, DURATION
Onset occurs in 30 to 45 minutes. Peak effects occur in 1 to 2 hours. Diuresis and decreased CSF pressure last for 3 to 10 hours; decreased intraocular pressure lasts 5 to 6 hours.

INDICATIONS & DOSAGE
Elevated intracranial or intraocular pressure—
Adults: 1 to 1.5 g/kg as a 30% solution by slow I.V. infusion over 1 to 2½ hours. Rate should not exceed 4 ml/minute. Maximum dosage is 120 g daily.
Children: 0.5 to 1.5 g/kg by slow I.V. infusion (rate not to exceed 4 ml/minute) or 35 g/m² in 24 hours. Children under 2 years may receive as little as 0.1 g/kg by slow I.V. infusion.

ADVERSE REACTIONS
CNS: *headache,* syncope, disorientation.
CV: hypotension, tachycardia, dizziness, ECG changes.
GI: *nausea, vomiting.*
Other: irritation or necrotic sloughing with extravasation, hemolysis (with rapid administration), fluid overload, **hyponatremia,** hypokalemia.

INTERACTIONS
Lithium: increased lithium clearance and decreased lithium effectiveness. Monitor lithium level.

EFFECTS ON DIAGNOSTIC TESTS
Urea therapy alters electrolyte balance.

CONTRAINDICATIONS
Contraindicated in patients with severely impaired renal function, marked dehydration, frank hepatic failure, active intracranial bleeding, and sickle-cell disease with CNS involvement.

Reactions may be *common,* uncommon, *life-threatening,* or COMMON AND LIFE-THREATENING.

NURSING CONSIDERATIONS
● Use cautiously in patients with cardiac disease or hepatic or renal impairment and during pregnancy and breastfeeding.

● **I.V. use:** Avoid rapid I.V. infusion; may cause hemolysis or increased capillary bleeding. Maximum infusion rate is 4 ml/minute.

Alert: Avoid extravasation; may cause reactions ranging from mild irritation to necrosis.

● To prepare 135 ml of 30% solution, mix contents of 40-g vial of urea with 105 ml of D_5W or dextrose 10% in water or 10% invert sugar in water. Each ml of 30% solution provides 300 mg urea.

● Use freshly reconstituted urea only for I.V. infusion; solution becomes ammonia upon standing. Use within minutes of reconstitution and discard within 24 hours.

● Assess breath sounds for crackles, indicating pulmonary edema.

● Watch for signs of hyponatremia (nausea, vomiting, tachycardia) or hypokalemia (muscle weakness, lethargy); may indicate electrolyte depletion before serum levels are reduced.

● Maintain adequate hydration; monitor blood pressure, fluid intake and output, and serum electrolyte levels.

● In patients with renal disease, monitor BUN level.

● To ensure bladder emptying in comatose patients, use an indwelling urinary catheter, and use an hourly urometer collection bag for accurate evaluation of diuresis.

● If satisfactory diuresis does not occur in 6 to 12 hours, be aware that urea should be discontinued and renal function reevaluated.

☑ PATIENT TEACHING
● Instruct patient to report adverse reactions promptly.

● Tell patient to alert nurse if discomfort occurs at I.V. insertion site.

---

*Liquid contains alcohol.   **May contain tartrazine.   †Canada only.   ‡Australia only.   ◇ OTC.

63
Electrolytes and replacement solutions

calcium acetate
calcium carbonate
calcium chloride
calcium citrate
calcium glubionate
calcium gluceptate
calcium gluconate
calcium lactate
calcium phosphate, dibasic
calcium phosphate, tribasic
dextran, low molecular weight
dextran, high molecular weight
hetastarch
magnesium chloride
magnesium sulfate
potassium acetate
potassium bicarbonate
potassium chloride
potassium gluconate
Ringer's injection
Ringer's injection, lactated
sodium chloride

COMBINATION PRODUCTS
KLORVESS*: 20 mEq each potassium
and chloride (from potassium chloride,
potassium bicarbonate, and l-lysine
monohydrochloride).
K-LYTE-CL: 25 mEq potassium, 25
mEq chloride (from potassium chloride,
potassium bicarbonate, and lysine hydrochloride).
NEUTRA-PHOS: phosphorus 250 mg,
sodium 164 mg, potassium 278 mg
(from dibasic and monobasic sodium
and potassium phosphate).
TWIN-K: 15 ml supplies 20 mEq of potassium ions as a combination of potassium gluconate and calcium citrate.

---

calcium acetate
Phos-Ex ◇, Phos-Lo

calcium carbonate
Apo-Cal† ◇, BioCal ◇, Calcarb
600 ◇, Cal-Carb-HD ◇, Calci-
Chew ◇, Calciday 667 ◇, Calcilac ◇,
Calci-Mix ◇, Calcite 500† ◇, Calcium
500† ◇, Calcium 600 ◇,
Calglycine ◇, Cal-Guard Softgels,
Cal-Plus ◇, Calsan† ◇, Caltrate
300† ◇, Caltrate 600† ◇, Caltrate
Chewable† ◇, Chooz ◇, Dicarbosil ◇,
Gencalc 600 ◇, Mallamint ◇, Mega-
Cal† ◇, Nephro-Calci ◇, Nu-Cal† ◇,
Os-Cal† ◇, Os-Cal 500 ◇, Os-Cal
Chewable† ◇, Oysco ◇, Oysco 500
Chewable ◇, Oyst-Cal 500 ◇, Oyst-
Cal 500 Chewable ◇, Oystercal
500 ◇, Oyster Shell Calcium-500 ◇,
Rolaids Calcium Rich ◇, Super Calci-
um 1200 ◇, Titralac ◇, Tums ◇, Tums
E-X ◇

calcium chloride ◇
Calciject†

calcium citrate ◇
Citrical ◇, Citrical Liquitabs† ◇

calcium glubionate ◇
Calcium-Sandoz†, Neo-Calglucon

calcium gluceptate ◇

calcium gluconate ◇
Kalcinate

calcium lactate ◇

calcium phosphate, dibasic ◇

calcium phosphate, tribasic
Posture ◇

Pregnancy Risk Category: C

HOW SUPPLIED
calcium acetate

Reactions may be *common*, uncommon, *life-threatening*, or COMMON AND LIFE-THREATENING.

Contains 253 mg or 12.7 mEq of elemental calcium/g

Tablets: 250 mg ◇, 500 mg ◇, 667 mg, 668 mg ◇, 1,000 mg ◇

Injection: 0.5 mEq Ca^{++} per ml

calcium carbonate

Contains 400 mg or 20 mEq of elemental calcium/g

Tablets: 650 mg ◇, 667 mg ◇, 750 mg ◇, 1.25 g ◇, 1.5 g ◇

Tablets (chewable): 350 mg ◇, 420 mg ◇, 500 mg ◇, 625 mg ◇ †, 750 mg ◇, 850 mg ◇, 1.25 g ◇

Capsules: 600 mg ◇, 1.25 g ◇

Oral suspension: 1.25 g/5 ml ◇

Powder packets: 6.5 g (2,400 mg calcium) per packet ◇

calcium chloride

Contains 270 mg or 13.5 mEq of elemental calcium/g

Injection: 10% solution in 10-ml ampules, vials, and syringes

calcium citrate

Contains 211 mg or 10.6 mEq of elemental calcium/g

Tablets: 950 mg ◇

Effervescent tablets: 2376 mg ◇

calcium glubionate

Contains 64 mg or 3.2 mEq elemental calcium/g

Syrup: 1.8 g/5 ml

calcium glucepate

Contains 82 mg or 4.1 mEq elemental calcium/g

Injection: 1.1 g/5 ml in 5-ml ampules or 10-ml vials

calcium gluconate

Contains 90 mg or 4.5 mEq of elemental calcium/g

Tablets: 500 mg ◇, 650 mg ◇, 975 mg ◇, 1 g ◇

Injection: 10% solution in 10-ml ampules and vials, 10-ml or 50-ml vials

Pharmacy bulk vials: 100 ml, 200 ml

calcium lactate

Contains 130 mg or 6.5 mEq of elemental calcium/g

Tablets: 325 mg, 650 mg

calcium phosphate, dibasic

Contains 230 mg or 11.5 mEq of elemental calcium/g

Tablets: 500 mg ◇

calcium phosphate, tribasic

Contains 400 mg or 20 mEq of elemental calcium/g

Tablets: 300 mg ◇, 600 mg ◇

ACTION

Replaces and maintains calcium.

ONSET, PEAK, DURATION

Onset and peak effects occur immediately after I.V. injection, return to normal within ½ to 2 hours.

INDICATIONS & DOSAGE

Hypocalcemic emergency—

Adults: 7 to 14 mEq calcium I.V. May be given as a 10% calcium gluconate solution, 2% to 10% calcium chloride solution, or a 22% calcium gluceptate solution.

Children: 1 to 7 mEq calcium I.V.

Infants: up to 1 mEq calcium I.V.

Hypocalcemic tetany—

Adults: 4.5 to 16 mEq calcium I.V. Repeated until tetany is controlled.

Children: 0.5 to 0.7 mEq/kg calcium I.V. three to four times a day until tetany is controlled.

Neonates: 2.4 mEq/kg I.V. daily in divided doses.

Adjunctive treatment of cardiac arrest—

Adults: 0.027 to 0.054 mEq/kg calcium chloride I.V., 4.5 to 6.3 mEq calcium gluceptate I.V., or 2.3 to 3.7 mEq calcium gluconate I.V.

Children: 0.27 mEq/kg calcium chloride I.V. Repeated in 10 minutes if necessary; determine serum calcium levels before administering further doses.

Adjunctive treatment of magnesium intoxication—

Adults: initially, 7 mEq I.V. Subsequent doses must be based upon the patient's response.

During exchange transfusions—

Adults: 1.35 mEq I.V. concurrently with each 100 ml citrated blood.

Neonates: 0.45 mEq I.V. after each 100 ml citrated blood.

Hyperphosphatemia—

---

*Liquid contains alcohol.   **May contain tartrazine.   †Canada only.   ‡Australia only.   ◇ OTC.

Adults: 1,334 to 2,000 mg P.O. calcium acetate t.i.d. with meals. Most dialysis patients will require three to four tablets with each meal.
Dietary supplement—
Adults: 500 mg to 2 g P.O. daily.

ADVERSE REACTIONS

CNS: with I.V. use—tingling sensations, sense of oppression or heat waves; with rapid I.V. injection—syncope.
CV: mild fall in blood pressure; with rapid I.V. injection—vasodilation, bradycardia, *arrhythmias, cardiac arrest.*
GI: with oral use—irritation, hemorrhage, *constipation;* with I.V. use—chalky taste; with oral calcium chloride—hemorrhage, nausea, vomiting, thirst, abdominal pain.
GU: hypercalcemia, polyuria, renal calculi.
Skin: with I.M. use—local reactions including burning, necrosis, tissue sloughing, cellulitis, soft tissue calcification.
Other: with S.C. injection—pain and irritation; with I.V. use—*vein irritation.*

INTERACTIONS

Atenolol, tetracyclines, fluoroquinolones: decreased bioavailability of these agents and calcium when oral preparations are taken together. Separate administration times.
Calcium channel blockers: decreased calcium effectiveness. Avoid concomitant use.
Digitalis glycosides: increased digitalis toxicity; give calcium cautiously (if at all) to digitalized patients.
Sodium polystyrene sulfonate: risk of metabolic acidosis in patients with renal disease. Avoid concomitant use.
Thiazide diuretics: risk of hypercalcemia. Avoid concomitant use.
Foods containing oxalic acid (found in rhubarb and spinach), phytic acid (bran and whole cereals), and phosphorus (milk and dairy products): may interfere with calcium absorption.

EFFECTS ON DIAGNOSTIC TESTS

I.V. calcium may produce transient elevation of plasma 11-hydroxycorticosteroid concentrations (Glen-Nelson technique) and false-negative values for serum and urine magnesium as measured by the Titan yellow method.

CONTRAINDICATIONS

Contraindicated in patients with ventricular fibrillation, hypercalcemia, hypophosphatemia, or renal calculi and in cancer patients with bone metastases.

NURSING CONSIDERATIONS

● Use all calcium products with extreme caution in patients with sarcoidosis and renal or cardiac disease, and in digitalized patients. Use calcium chloride cautiously in patients with cor pulmonale, respiratory acidosis, and respiratory failure.
● Warm solutions to body temperature before administration.
● **I.V. use (direct injection):** Administer slowly through a small needle into a large vein or through an I.V. line containing a free-flowing, compatible solution at a rate not exceeding 1 ml/minute (1.5 mEq/minute) for calcium chloride, 1.5 to 5 ml/minute for calcium gluconate, and 2 ml/minute for calcium gluceptate. Do not use scalp veins in children.
● **I.V. use (intermittent infusion):** Infuse diluted solution through an I.V. line containing a compatible solution. Maximum rate of 200 mg/minute suggested for calcium gluceptate and calcium gluconate.
● Give calcium chloride I.V. only. When adding to parenteral solutions that contain other additives (especially phosphorus or phosphate), watch for precipitate. Use an in-line filter.
● Know that drug will precipitate if administered I.V. with sodium bicarbonate or other alkaline drugs.
● Give calcium gluconate I.V. only.
● Monitor ECG when giving calcium I.V. Stop if the patient complains of dis-

comfort and notify doctor. Following
I.V. injection, the patient should remain
recumbent for 15 minutes.
● Give I.M. injection in the gluteal region in adults; lateral thigh in infants.
Use I.M. route only in emergencies
when no I.V. route available.
● Ensure that the doctor specifies the
form of calcium he wants given; crash
carts usually contain both calcium gluconate and calcium chloride.
● Monitor blood calcium levels frequently. Hypercalcemia may result after
large doses in chronic renal failure. Report abnormalities.
Alert: Be aware that severe necrosis and
tissue sloughing can occur after extravasation. Calcium gluconate is less irritating to veins and tissues than calcium
chloride.

☑ **PATIENT TEACHING**
● Tell patient to take oral calcium 1 to
1½ hours after meals if GI upset occurs.
● Warn patient to avoid oxalic acid
(found in rhubarb and spinach), phytic
acid (in bran and whole cereals), and
phosphorus (in dairy products) in the
meal preceding calcium consumption;
these substances may interfere with calcium absorption.

**dextran, low molecular
weight (dextran 40)**
Dextran 40, Gentran 40, 10% LMD,
Rheomacrodex

Pregnancy Risk Category: C

HOW SUPPLIED
Injection: 10% dextran 40 in D_5W or
0.9% sodium chloride solution

ACTION
Expands plasma volume via colloidal
osmotic effect, drawing fluid from interstitial to intravascular space, providing
fluid replacement.

ONSET, PEAK, DURATION
Onset and peak effects occur immediately after an I.V. infusion. Effects persist up to 3 hours.

INDICATIONS & DOSAGE
Plasma volume expansion—
Adults: dosage by I.V. infusion depends
on amount of fluid loss. First 10 ml/kg
of dextran infused rapidly with central
venous pressure monitoring, the remaining dose slowly. Total dosage not to exceed 20 ml/kg body weight daily. If
therapy continues longer than 24 hours,
do not exceed 10 ml/kg daily—continued for no longer than 5 days.
Prophylaxis of venous thrombosis—
Adults: 10 ml/kg (500 to 1,000 ml) I.V.
on the day of the procedure; 500 ml on
days 2 and 3.
*Hemodiluent in extracorporeal circula-
tion—*
Adults: 10 to 20 ml/kg added to the
perfusion circuit, not to exceed total
dosage of 20 ml/kg.

ADVERSE REACTIONS
GI: nausea, vomiting.
GU: tubular stasis and blocking, in-
creased urine viscosity.
Hematologic: *decreased hemoglobin
and hematocrit levels;* increased bleed-
ing time (with higher doses).
Hepatic: increased AST and ALT lev-
els.
Skin: hypersensitivity reactions, ur-
ticaria.
Other: *anaphylaxis,* thrombophlebitis.

INTERACTIONS
None significant.

EFFECTS ON DIAGNOSTIC TESTS
Falsely elevated blood glucose levels
may occur in patients receiving dextran
40 or 70 if the test uses high concentrations of acid. Dextran may cause turbidity, which interferes with bilirubin assays that use alcohol, total protein levels
using biuret reagent, and blood glucose
levels using the orthotoluidine method.

Blood typing and cross-matching using enzyme techniques may give unreliable readings if the samples are taken after the dextran infusion.

Dextran 40 administration has been associated with abnormal renal and hepatic function test results.

CONTRAINDICATIONS
Contraindicated in patients with hypersensitivity to the drug and in those with marked hemostatic defects, marked cardiac decompensation, and renal disease with severe oliguria or anuria.

NURSING CONSIDERATIONS
● Use cautiously in patients with active hemorrhage, thrombocytopenia, or diabetes mellitus.
● Assess hydration before starting therapy; otherwise, use urine or serum osmolality because urine specific gravity is affected by urine dextran concentration.
● **I.V. use:** Observe the patient closely during early phase of infusion when most anaphylactic reactions occur.
● Watch for circulatory overload and a rise in central venous pressure. Provides plasma expansion slightly greater than volume infused.
● Monitor urine flow rate during administration. If oliguria or anuria occurs or is not relieved, stop dextran and give loop diuretic as ordered.
● Check hemoglobin and hematocrit levels; if values fall below 30% by volume, notify the doctor.
● As ordered, use D_5W solution instead of 0.9% sodium chloride solution for patients with heart failure.
● Be aware the doctor may order dextran 1 to protect against dextran-induced anaphylaxis. Administer 20 ml of dextran 1 (containing 150 mg/ml) I.V. over 60 seconds, 1 to 2 minutes before the I.V. infusion of dextran.
● Be aware that drug may interfere with analyses of blood grouping, crossmatching, bilirubin, blood glucose, and protein.
● Store at constant 77° F (25° C). May

precipitate in storage but can be heated to dissolve if necessary.
● Monitor blood glucose levels before and during infusion. Know that the drug metabolizes to glucose.

☑ PATIENT TEACHING
● Explain use and administration of dextran to patient and family.
● Tell patient to report adverse effects.

---

dextran, high molecular weight (dextran 70, dextran 75)
Dextran 75, Gendex 75, Gentran 70, Gentran 75, Macrodex

Pregnancy Risk Category: C

HOW SUPPLIED
Injection: 6% dextran 70 in 0.9% sodium chloride solution or dextrose 5%; 6% dextran 75 in 0.9% sodium chloride solution or dextrose 5%

ACTION
Expands plasma volume via colloidal osmotic effect, drawing fluid from interstitial to intravascular space, providing fluid replacement.

ONSET, PEAK, DURATION
Onset and peak effects occur right after infusion. Duration unknown.

INDICATIONS & DOSAGE
Plasma expander—
Adults: 30 g (500 ml of 6% solution) I.V. In emergencies, may be given at 1.2 to 2.4 g (20 to 40 ml) per minute. In normovolemic or nearly normovolemic patients, rate of infusion should not exceed 240 mg (4 ml)/minute.

Total dosage during first 24 hours not to exceed 1.2 g/kg; actual dosage depends on amount of fluid loss and resultant hemoconcentration and must be determined for each patient.

ADVERSE REACTIONS

GI: nausea, vomiting.

GU: increased specific gravity and viscosity of urine, tubular stasis and blocking. oliguria, anuria.

Hematologic: *decreased hemoglobin and hematocrit levels;* with doses of 15 ml/kg body weight, prolonged bleeding time and significant suppression of platelet function.

Hepatic: increased AST and ALT levels.

Skin: hypersensitivity reactions, urticaria.

Other: fever, arthralgia, nasal congestion, fluid overload, *anaphylaxis, thrombophlebitis.*

INTERACTIONS

Will increase bleeding if given in combination with other antithrombotics, such as aspirin, heparin, warfarin, thrombolytics, or abciximab. Use together with extreme caution.

EFFECTS ON DIAGNOSTIC TESTS

Falsely elevated blood glucose levels may occur in patients receiving dextran 40 or 70 if the test uses high concentrations of acid. Dextran may cause turbidity, which interferes with bilirubin assays that use alcohol, total protein levels using biuret reagent, and blood glucose levels using the orthotoluidine method. Blood typing and cross-matching using enzyme techniques may give unreliable readings if the samples are taken after the dextran infusion.

Dextran 40 administration has been associated with abnormal renal and hepatic function test results.

CONTRAINDICATIONS

Contraindicated in patients with hypersensitivity to dextran and in those with marked hemostatic defects, marked cardiac decompensation, renal disease with severe oliguria or anuria, hypervolemic conditions, and severe bleeding disorders.

NURSING CONSIDERATIONS

● Use cautiously in patients with active hemorrhage, thrombocytopenia, impaired renal clearance, chronic liver disease, and abdominal conditions or in patients undergoing bowel surgery.

● Assess hydration before starting therapy; otherwise, use urine or serum osmolality because urine specific gravity is affected by the urine dextran concentration.

● Have blood samples drawn *before* starting infusion.

Alert: **I.V. use:** Observe patient closely during early phase of infusion when most anaphylactic reactions occur.

● As ordered, use D_5W solution instead of 0.9% sodium chloride solution for patients with heart failure.

● Monitor urine flow rate during administration. If oliguria or anuria occurs or is not relieved by infusion, stop dextran and give loop diuretic.

● Watch for circulatory overload. Provides plasma expansion slightly greater than volume infused.

● Monitor hemoglobin and hematocrit levels; if values fall below 30% by volume, notify the doctor.

● Be aware that the doctor may order dextran 1 to protect against dextran-induced anaphylaxis. Give 20 ml of dextran 1 (containing 150 mg/ml) I.V. over 60 seconds, 1 to 2 minutes before I.V. infusion of dextran 70.

● Be aware that the drug may interfere with analyses of blood grouping, cross-matching, bilirubin, blood glucose, and protein.

● Know that the drug may precipitate in storage but can be heated to dissolve if necessary.

● Monitor blood glucose levels before and during infusion. Know that the drug metabolizes to glucose.

☑ PATIENT TEACHING

● Explain use and administration of dextran to patient and family.
● Tell patient to report adverse effects.

hetastarch
Hespan

Pregnancy Risk Category: C

HOW SUPPLIED
Injection: 500 ml (6 g/100 ml in 0.9% sodium chloride solution)

ACTION
Expands plasma volume and provides fluid replacement.

ONSET, PEAK, DURATION
Onset and peak effects occur immediately after I.V. infusion. Duration unknown.

INDICATIONS & DOSAGE
Plasma expander—
Adults: 500 to 1,000 ml I.V., depending on amount of blood lost and resultant hemoconcentration. Total dosage usually not to exceed 1,500 ml/day. Up to 20 ml/kg hourly may be used in hemorrhagic shock.

ADVERSE REACTIONS
CNS: headache.
CV: peripheral edema of lower extremities.
EENT: periorbital edema.
GI: nausea, vomiting.
Respiratory: wheezing.
Skin: urticaria.
Other: wheezing, mild fever, chills, muscle pain, fluid overload, dilution of clotting factors.

INTERACTIONS
None significant.

EFFECTS ON DIAGNOSTIC TESTS
When added to whole blood, hetastarch increases the erythrocyte sedimentation rate.

CONTRAINDICATIONS
Contraindicated in patients with known hypersensitivity, severe bleeding disorders, severe CHF, or renal failure with oliguria and anuria.

NURSING CONSIDERATIONS
● Know that hetastarch is *not* a substitute for blood or plasma.
● To avoid circulatory overload, monitor patients with impaired renal function carefully.
● When used in continuous-flow centrifugation, know that leukapheresis ratio is usually one part hetastarch to eight parts venous whole blood.
● Discontinue if allergic or sensitivity reactions occur and notify doctor. If necessary, administer an antihistamine as ordered.
● Discard partially used bottles.
● Use cautiously in patients with liver disease.

☑ PATIENT TEACHING
● Explain use and administration of drug to patient and family.
● Tell patient to report adverse reactions promptly.

magnesium chloride
Slow-Mag ◇

magnesium sulfate

Pregnancy Risk Category: NR

HOW SUPPLIED
magnesium chloride
Tablets (delayed-release): 64 mg
magnesium sulfate
Injectable solutions: 10%, 12.5%, 25%, 50% in 2-ml, 5-ml, 10-ml, 20-ml, and 30-ml ampules, vials, and prefilled syringes

ACTION
Replaces and maintains magnesium levels; as an anticonvulsant, reduces muscle contractions by interfering with release of acetylcholine at myoneural junction.

ONSET, PEAK, DURATION
Onset is immediate after I.V. administration; about 1 hour after I.M. administration; and unknown after oral administration. Serum levels peak within 4 hours of oral dose; unknown after I.V. and I.M. administration. Effects persist for about 30 minutes after I.V. administration; 3 to 4 hours after I.M. administration; and 4 to 6 hours after oral administration.

INDICATIONS & DOSAGE
Mild hypomagnesemia—
Adults: 1 g I.V. by piggyback or I.M. q 6 hours for four doses, depending on serum magnesium level. Alternatively, 3 g P.O. q 6 hours for four doses.
Severe hypomagnesemia (serum magnesium 0.8 mEq/L or less, with symptoms)—
Adults: 2 to 5 g I.V. in 1 liter of solution over 3 hours.
Subsequent doses depend on serum magnesium levels.
Magnesium supplementation—
Adults: 64 mg (one tablet) P.O. t.i.d.
Magnesium supplementation in total parenteral nutrition (TPN)—
Adults: 4 to 24 mEq I.V. daily added to TPN solution.
Infants: 2 to 10 mEq I.V. daily added to TPN solution.
Each 2 ml of 50% solution contains 1 g, or 8.12 mEq, magnesium sulfate.
Acute treatment of preeclampsia and eclampsia—
Adults: loading dose: 2 to 4 g (4 to 8 ml of 50% solution), given by slow I.V. bolus (over 5 minutes). Maintenance dosage is 1 to 2 g hourly by constant infusion. Prepare by adding 8 ml of 50% solution to 250 ml D_5W.
Hypomagnesemic seizures—
Adults: 1 to 4 g by I.V. infusion, then 4 to 5 g I.M. of a 50% solution q 4 to 6 hours, based on the patient's response and magnesium blood level.
Seizures secondary to hypomagnesemia in acute nephritis—
Children: 20 to 40 mg/kg in 20% solution I.M. q 4 to 6 hours p.r.n., or 100 mg/kg of 1% to 3% solution I.V. very slowly. Titrate dosage based on magnesium blood level and seizure response.
Paroxysmal atrial tachycardia unresponsive to other treatments—
Adults: 3 to 4 g I.V. of 10% solution over 30 seconds, with close monitoring of ECG.

ADVERSE REACTIONS
CNS: toxicity—*weak or absent deep tendon reflexes,* flaccid paralysis, hypothermia, drowsiness, stupor.
CV: slow, weak pulse; arrhythmias (caused by hypocalcemia); *hypotension; circulatory collapse* (with toxicity).
Respiratory: *respiratory paralysis*
Skin: flushing, diaphoresis.
Other: hypocalcemia.

INTERACTIONS
Digitalis glycosides: possible serious cardiac conduction changes. Administer with extreme caution.
Neuromuscular blockers: possible increased neuromuscular blockage. Use cautiously.
Nitrofurantoin, tetracyclines, penicillamine, alendronate, quinolones: decreased bioavailability with oral magnesium supplements. Separate administration by 2 to 3 hours.

EFFECTS ON DIAGNOSTIC TESTS
None reported.

CONTRAINDICATIONS
Contraindicated in patients with myocardial damage or heart block and in actively progressing labor.

NURSING CONSIDERATIONS
● Use parenteral magnesium with extreme caution in patients with impaired renal function.
● **I.V. use:** Inject I.V. bolus dose slowly, using infusion pump for continuous infusion, if available, to avoid respiratory or cardiac arrest. Maximum infusion rate is 150 mg/minute. Rapid drip

causes feeling of heat.

Alert: When giving I.V. for severe hypomagnesemia, watch for respiratory depression and signs of heart block. Respirations should be over 16 breaths/minute before dose is given.

● Be aware that undiluted 50% solutions may be given by deep I.M. injection to adults. Dilute solutions to 20% or less for use in children.

● Keep I.V. calcium available to reverse magnesium intoxication.

● Know that drug is incompatible with alkalis, including carbonates and bicarbonates. Precipitate may form if mixed with solutions containing ethanol, arsenates, barium, calcium, clindamycin, heavy metals, hydrocortisone sodium succinate, phosphates, polymyxin B sulfate, procaine, salicylates, or tartrates.

● Test knee-jerk and patellar reflexes before each additional dose. If absent, notify doctor and give no more magnesium until reflexes return; otherwise, the patient may develop temporary respiratory failure and need cardiopulmonary resuscitation or I.V. administration of calcium.

● Check magnesium level after repeated doses.

● Monitor fluid intake and output. Output should be 100 ml or more during 4-hour period before dose.

● After giving to toxemic patients within 24 hours before delivery, watch neonate for signs of magnesium toxicity, including neuromuscular and respiratory depression.

☑ **PATIENT TEACHING**
● Explain use and administration of drug to patient and family.
● Tell patient to report adverse effects.

---

potassium acetate

Pregnancy Risk Category: C

HOW SUPPLIED
Injection: 2 mEq/ml in 20-ml, 30-ml vials; 4 mEq/ml in 50-ml vials.

ACTION
Replaces and maintains potassium level.

ONSET, PEAK, DURATION
Onset and peak levels occur right after I.V. infusion. Duration unknown.

INDICATIONS & DOSAGE
Treatment of hypokalemia—
Adults: no more than 20 mEq hourly in concentration of 40 mEq/liter or less. Total 24-hour dosage should not exceed 150 mEq (3 mEq/kg in children). Potassium replacement should be done with ECG monitoring and frequent serum potassium determinations. I.V. route should be used only for life-threatening hypokalemia or when oral replacement not feasible.
Prevention of hypokalemia—
Adults: dosage is individualized to the patient's needs, not to exceed 150 mEq/day. Administered as an additive to I.V. infusions. Usual dose is 20 mEq/liter infused at a rate not to exceed 20 mEq/hour.
Children: individualized dosage not to exceed 3 mEq/kg/day. Administered as an additive to I.V. infusions.

ADVERSE REACTIONS
Signs of hyperkalemia—
CNS: paresthesia of the extremities, listlessness, mental confusion, weakness or heaviness of legs, flaccid paralysis.
CV: hypotension, *arrhythmias, heart block,* ECG changes, *cardiac arrest.*
GI: nausea, vomiting, abdominal pain, diarrhea.
Respiratory: *respiratory paralysis.*
Other: pain and redness at infusion site, fever, hyperkalemia.

INTERACTIONS
ACE inhibitors, potassium-sparing diuretics: increased risk of hyperkalemia. Use with extreme caution.

EFFECTS ON DIAGNOSTIC TESTS
None reported.

CONTRAINDICATIONS
Contraindicated in patients with severe renal impairment with oliguria, anuria, or azotemia; in those with untreated Addison's disease; and in those with acute dehydration, heat cramps, hyperkalemia, hyperkalemic form of familial periodic paralysis, and conditions associated with extensive tissue breakdown.

NURSING CONSIDERATIONS
● Use cautiously in patients with cardiac disease and in those with renal impairment.
● **I.V. use:** Give by I.V. infusion only, never I.V. push or I.M. Always dilute before administering. Watch for pain and redness at infusion site. Large-bore needle reduces local irritation.
Alert: Give slowly as diluted solution; potentially fatal hyperkalemia may result from too-rapid infusion.
● During therapy, monitor ECG, renal function, fluid intake and output, and serum potassium, serum creatinine, and BUN levels. Never give potassium postoperatively until urine flow is established.

☑ **PATIENT TEACHING**
● Explain use and administration to patient and family.
● Tell patient to report adverse effects.

---

potassium bicarbonate
K⁺Care ET, K-Electrolyte Effervescent Tablets, K-Gen ET, K-Ide, Klor-Con/EF, K-Lyte

Pregnancy Risk Category: NR

HOW SUPPLIED
Effervescent tablets: 6.5 mEq, 25 mEq

ACTION
Replaces and maintains potassium.

ONSET, PEAK, DURATION
Onset and duration unknown. Peak levels occur within 4 hours.

INDICATIONS & DOSAGE
Hypokalemia—
Adults: 25 to 50 mEq dissolved in one-half to a full glass of water (120 to 240 ml) once daily to q.i.d.

ADVERSE REACTIONS
CNS: paresthesia of the extremities, listlessness, mental confusion, weakness or heaviness of legs, flaccid paralysis.
CV: *arrhythmias*, ECG changes, hypotension, *heart block, cardiac arrest*.
GI: *nausea, vomiting, abdominal pain,* diarrhea.

INTERACTIONS
ACE inhibitors, potassium-sparing diuretics: risk of hyperkalemia. Use with extreme caution.

EFFECTS ON DIAGNOSTIC TESTS
None reported.

CONTRAINDICATIONS
Contraindicated in patients with severe renal impairment with oliguria, anuria, or azotemia; in those with untreated Addison's disease; and in patients with acute dehydration, heat cramps, hyperkalemia, hyperkalemic form of familial periodic paralysis, and other conditions associated with extensive tissue breakdown.

NURSING CONSIDERATIONS
● Use cautiously in patients with cardiac disease and in those with renal impairment.
● Dissolve potassium bicarbonate tablets completely in 6 to 8 oz (180 to 240 ml) of cold water.
● Ask the patient's flavor preference. Available in lime and orange flavors.
● Don't administer potassium supplements postoperatively until urine flow has been established.
● Never switch potassium products

---

without a doctor's order. Potassium chloride cannot be given instead of potassium bicarbonate.
● Monitor BUN, serum potassium, and creatinine levels; and fluid intake and output.

☑ **PATIENT TEACHING**
● Tell patient to take drug with meals and sip slowly over 5 to 10 minutes.
● Tell patient to report adverse effects.
● Warn patients not to use salt substitutes concurrently, except with doctor's permission.

---

potassium chloride

Cena-K, K+10, Kaochlor 10%*, Kaochlor S-F 10%*, Kaon-Cl, Kaon-Cl 20%*, Kato Powder, Kay Ciel*, K+Care, K-Dur, K-Lease, K-Lor, Klor-10%*, Klor-Con, Klorvess, Klotrix, K-Lyte/Cl, K-Norm, K-Tab, Micro-K Extencaps, Rum-K, Slow-K, Ten-K

Pregnancy Risk Category: C

HOW SUPPLIED
Tablets (controlled-release): 6.7 mEq (500 mg), 8 mEq (600 mg), 10 mEq (750 mg), 20 mEq (1,500 mg)
Tablets (film-coated): 2.5 mEq (200 mg), 8 mEq (600 mg), 10 mEq (750 mg)
Capsules (controlled-release): 8 mEq (600 mg), 10 mEq (750 mg)
Oral liquid: 5% (10 mEq/15 ml), 7.5% (15 mEq/15 ml), 10% (20 mEq/15 ml), 15% (30 mEq/15 ml), 20% (40 mEq/15 ml)
Powder for oral use: 15-mEq packet, 20-mEq packet, 25-mEq packet, 25-mEq dose
Injection: 20-mEq, 40-mEq ampules; additive syringes containing 30-mEq or 40-mEq; 10-mEq, 20-mEq, 30-mEq, 40-mEq, 60-mEq, 100-mEq, 200-mEq, 400-mEq, or 1,000-mEq vials

ACTION
Replaces and maintains potassium level.

ONSET, PEAK, DURATION
Onset and serum levels peak immediately after I.V. infusion. Duration unknown.

INDICATIONS & DOSAGE
Hypokalemia—
Adults: 40 to 100 mEq P.O. daily in three or four divided doses for treatment; 10 to 20 mEq for prevention. Further dosage based on serum potassium level.
Children: 3 mEq/kg daily. Total daily dosage not to exceed 40 mEq/m^2.

Use I.V. route only when oral replacement is not feasible or when hypokalemia is life-threatening. If serum potassium is less than 2 mEq/ml, maximum infusion rate is 40 mEq/hour; maximum infusion concentration is 80 mEq/L; and maximum 24-hour dose is 400 mEq. If serum potassium level is greater than 2 mEq/ml, maximum infusion rate is 10 mEq/hour; maximum infusion concentration is 40 mEq/L; and maximum 24-hour dose is 200 mEq. For routine supplementation, the usual dose is 10 to 20 mEq hourly in concentration of 40 mEq/L or less.

ADVERSE REACTIONS
Signs of hyperkalemia—
CNS: paresthesia of the extremities, listlessness, mental confusion, weakness or heaviness of limbs, flaccid paralysis.
CV: *arrhythmias, heart block, possible cardiac arrest,* ECG changes, hypotension.
GI: *nausea, vomiting, abdominal pain,* diarrhea.
Respiratory: *respiratory paralysis.*
Other: *postinfusion phlebitis,* hyperkalemia.

INTERACTIONS
ACE inhibitors, potassium-sparing diuretics: risk of hyperkalemia. Use with extreme caution.

EFFECTS ON DIAGNOSTIC TESTS
None reported.

Reactions may be *common,* uncommon, *life-threatening,* or COMMON AND LIFE-THREATENING.

CONTRAINDICATIONS
Contraindicated in patients with severe renal impairment with oliguria, anuria, or azotemia; in those with untreated Addison's disease; and in patients with acute dehydration, heat cramps, hyperkalemia, hyperkalemic form of familial periodic paralysis, and other conditions associated with extensive tissue breakdown.

NURSING CONSIDERATIONS
● Use cautiously in patients with cardiac disease and in those with renal impairment.
Alert: **I.V. use:** Give by infusion only, never I.V. push or I.M. Give slowly as dilute solution; potentially fatal hyperkalemia may result from too-rapid infusion.
● Give oral potassium supplements with extreme caution because different forms deliver varying amounts of potassium. Never switch products without a doctor's order.
● Make sure powders are completely dissolved before administering.
● Know that enteric-coated tablets are not recommended because of increased potential for GI bleeding and small-bowel ulcerations.
● Know that tablets in wax matrix sometimes lodge in esophagus and cause ulceration in cardiac patients who have esophageal compression from enlarged left atrium. Use liquid form in such patients and in those with esophageal stasis or obstruction.
● Know that drug is often used orally with potassium-wasting diuretics to maintain potassium levels.
● Be aware that sugar-free liquid is available (Kaochlor S-F 10%); use if tablet or capsule passage is likely to be delayed, such as in GI obstruction. Have patients sip slowly to minimize GI irritation.
● Don't crush sustained-release potassium products.
● Monitor ECG and serum electrolyte levels during therapy.
● Monitor renal function. Potassium should not be given during immediate postoperative period until urine flow is established.

☑ PATIENT TEACHING
● Instruct patient how to prepare (powders) and administer drug form prescribed. Tell patient to take with or after meals with full glass of water or fruit juice to lessen GI distress.
● Teach patient the signs and symptoms of hyperkalemia, and tell patient to notify doctor if they occur.
● Tell patient to alert nurse if discomfort occurs at I.V. insertion site.
● Warn patient not to use salt substitutes concurrently, except with the doctor's permission.

potassium gluconate
Glu-K, Kaon Liquid*, Kaon Tablets, Kaylixir*, K-G Elixir*, Potassium-Rougier†

Pregnancy Risk Category: C

HOW SUPPLIED
Tablets: 500 mg (2 mEq K+), 1,170 mg (5 mEq K+)
Elixir: 4.68 g (20 mEq K+)/15 ml*

ACTION
Replaces and maintains intracellular and extracellular potassium.

ONSET, PEAK, DURATION
Onset and duration unknown. Peak levels occur within 4 hours of oral dose.

INDICATIONS & DOSAGE
Hypokalemia—
Adults: 40 to 100 mEq P.O. daily in three or four divided doses for treatment; 10 to 20 mEq daily for prevention. Further dosage adjustments are based on serum potassium determinations.

ADVERSE REACTIONS
CNS: paresthesia of the extremities,

listlessness, mental confusion, weakness or heaviness of legs, flaccid paralysis. **CV:** *arrhythmias,* ECG changes. **GI:** *nausea, vomiting, abdominal pain,* diarrhea.

INTERACTIONS
ACE inhibitors, potassium-sparing diuretics: risk of hyperkalemia. Use with extreme caution.

EFFECTS ON DIAGNOSTIC TESTS
None reported.

CONTRAINDICATIONS
Contraindicated in patients with severe renal impairment with oliguria, anuria, or azotemia; in those with untreated Addison's disease; and in patients with acute dehydration, heat cramps, hyperkalemia, hyperkalemic form of familial periodic paralysis, and other conditions associated with extensive tissue breakdown.

NURSING CONSIDERATIONS
● Give oral potassium supplements with extreme caution because different forms deliver varying amounts of potassium. Never switch products without a doctor's order.
● Use cautiously in patients with cardiac disease and in those with renal impairment.
● Don't administer potassium supplements postoperatively until urine flow has been established.
● Monitor ECG, serum potassium and creatinine levels, BUN, and fluid intake and output.

☑ PATIENT TEACHING
● Advise the patient to sip liquid potassium slowly to minimize GI irritation. Also tell patient to take drug with or after meals with a full glass of water or fruit juice.
● Warn the patient not to use salt substitutes concurrently, except with the doctor's permission.

Ringer's injection

Pregnancy Risk Category: NR

HOW SUPPLIED
Injection: 250 ml, 500 ml, 1,000 ml

ACTION
Replaces fluids and electrolytes.

ONSET, PEAK, DURATION
Onset and serum levels peak immediately after I.V. infusion. Duration unknown.

INDICATIONS & DOSAGE
Fluid and electrolyte replacement—
Adults and children: dosage highly individualized, but usually 1.5 to 3 liters (2% to 6% body weight), infused I.V. over 18 to 24 hours.

ADVERSE REACTIONS
CV: fluid overload.

INTERACTIONS
None significant.

EFFECTS ON DIAGNOSTIC TESTS
None reported.

CONTRAINDICATIONS
Contraindicated in patients with renal failure, except as emergency volume expander.

NURSING CONSIDERATIONS
● Use cautiously in patients with CHF, circulatory insufficiency, renal dysfunction, hypoproteinemia, and pulmonary edema.
● Know that Ringer's injection contains sodium, 147 mEq/liter; potassium, 4 mEq/liter; calcium, 4.5 mEq/liter; and chloride, 155.5 mEq/liter.
● Be aware that electrolyte content is insufficient for treating severe electrolyte deficiencies, but it does provide electrolytes in levels approximately equal to those of the blood.

PATIENT TEACHING
● Explain use and administration of drug to patient and family.
● Tell patient to report any unusual signs or symptoms promptly.

Ringer's injection, lactated (Hartmann's solution, Ringer's lactate solution)

Pregnancy Risk Category: NR

HOW SUPPLIED
Injection: 150 ml, 250 ml, 500 ml, 1,000 ml

ACTION
Replaces fluids and electrolytes.

ONSET, PEAK, DURATION
Onset and serum levels peak immediately after I.V. infusion. Duration unknown.

INDICATIONS & DOSAGE
Fluid and electrolyte replacement—
Adults and children: dosage highly individualized, but usually 1.5 to 3 liters (2% to 6% body weight) infused I.V. over 18 to 24 hours.

ADVERSE REACTIONS
CV: fluid overload.

INTERACTIONS
None significant.

EFFECTS ON DIAGNOSTIC TESTS
None reported.

CONTRAINDICATIONS
Contraindicated in patients with renal failure, except as emergency volume expander.

NURSING CONSIDERATIONS
● Use cautiously in patients with CHF, circulatory insufficiency, renal dysfunction, hypoproteinemia, and pulmonary edema.

● Know that lactated Ringer's injection contains sodium, 130 mEq/L; potassium, 4 mEq/L; calcium, 3 mEq/L; chloride, 109.7 mEq/L; and lactate, 28 mEq/L.
● Be aware that lactated Ringer's injection more closely approximates the electrolyte concentration in blood plasma.

☑ **PATIENT TEACHING**
● Explain use and administration of drug to patient and family.
● Tell patient to report any unusual signs or symptoms promptly.

---

sodium chloride

Pregnancy Risk Category: C

HOW SUPPLIED
Tablets: 650 mg
Tablets (slow-release): 600 mg
Injection: 0.45% sodium chloride solution 25 ml, 50 ml, 150 ml, 250 ml, 500 ml, 1,000 ml; 0.9% sodium chloride solution 2 ml, 3 ml, 5 ml, 10 ml, 20 ml, 25 ml, 30 ml, 50 ml, 100 ml, 150 ml, 250 ml, 500 ml, 1,000 ml; 3% sodium chloride solution 500 ml; 5% sodium chloride solution 500 ml; 14.6% sodium chloride solution 20 ml, 40 ml, 200 ml; 23.4% sodium chloride solution 30 ml, 50 ml, and 200 ml.

ACTION
Replaces and maintains sodium and chloride levels.

ONSET, PEAK, DURATION
Onset and serum levels peak immediately after I.V. infusion. Duration unknown.

INDICATIONS & DOSAGE
Fluid and electrolyte replacement in hyponatremia caused by electrolyte loss or in severe salt depletion—
Adults: dosage is highly individualized. 3% or 5% solution used only with fre-

---

quent electrolyte determination and given only slow I.V. With 0.45% solution: 3% to 8% of body weight, according to deficiencies, over 18 to 24 hours; with 0.9% solution: 2% to 6% of body weight, according to deficiencies, over 18 to 24 hours.

Management of heat cramp caused by excessive perspiration—
Adults: 1 g P.O. with every glass of water.

ADVERSE REACTIONS
CV: aggravation of CHF; edema if given too rapidly or in excess.
Respiratory: *pulmonary edema* if given too rapidly or in excess.
Other: hypernatremia and aggravation of existing metabolic acidosis with excessive infusion; serious electrolyte disturbances, loss of potassium; local tenderness, abscess, tissue necrosis at injection site; thrombophlebitis.

INTERACTIONS
None significant.

EFFECTS ON DIAGNOSTIC TESTS
None reported.

CONTRAINDICATIONS
Contraindicated in patients with conditions in which sodium and chloride administration is detrimental. Sodium chloride 3% and 5% injections are contraindicated in patients with increased, normal, or only slightly decreased serum electrolyte concentrations.

NURSING CONSIDERATIONS
● Use cautiously in patients with CHF, circulatory insufficiency, renal dysfunction, and hypoproteinemia and in elderly or postoperative patients.
● Never use bacteriostatic sodium chloride injection with newborns.
Alert: **I.V. use:** Infuse 3% and 5% solutions slowly and cautiously to avoid pulmonary edema. Use only for critical situations, and observe the patient continually.

● Don't confuse concentrates (14.6%, 23.4%) available to add to parenteral nutrient solutions with 0.9% sodium chloride injection, and never give without diluting. Read labels carefully.
● Monitor serum electrolyte levels.

☑ **PATIENT TEACHING**
● Explain use and administration of drug to patient and family.
● Tell patient to report adverse reactions promptly.

ammonium chloride
sodium bicarbonate
sodium lactate
tromethamine

COMBINATION PRODUCTS
None.

---

ammonium chloride ◇

Pregnancy Risk Category: C

HOW SUPPLIED
Tablets: 500 mg ◇
Tablets (enteric-coated): 500 mg ◇
Injection: 2.14% (0.4 mEq/ml), 26.75%
(5 mEq/ml)

ACTION
Increases free hydrogen ion concentration, resulting in acidosis, and acts as an expectorant by causing reflex stimulation of bronchial mucous glands.

ONSET, PEAK, DURATION
Onset and serum levels peak immediately after I.V. infusion. Duration unknown.

INDICATIONS & DOSAGE
Metabolic alkalosis; chloride replacement—
Adults and children: I.V. dose (in mEq) is equal to the serum chloride deficit (in mEq/L) multiplied by the extracellular fluid volume (estimated as 20% of the body weight in kilograms). One-half the calculated volume should be given, then the patient reassessed.
Acidifier—
Adults: 4 to 12 g P.O. daily in divided doses q 4 to 6 hours.
Children: 75 mg/kg P.O. daily in four divided doses.

ADVERSE REACTIONS
Adverse reactions usually result from ammonia toxicity or too-rapid I.V. administration.
CNS: *coma,* twitching, *tonic convulsions.*
CV: bradycardia, cardiac arrhythmias.
Skin: rash, pallor, diaphoresis.
Respiratory: irregular respirations with periods of apnea.
Other: *metabolic acidosis,* pain at injection site, hypokalemia.

INTERACTIONS
Spironolactone: increased systemic acidosis. Use together cautiously.

EFFECTS ON DIAGNOSTIC TESTS
None reported.

CONTRAINDICATIONS
Contraindicated in patients with primary respiratory acidosis and high total carbon dioxide (CO_2) and buffer base and in those with severe hepatic or renal dysfunction (as self-medication).

NURSING CONSIDERATIONS
● Use cautiously in patients with pulmonary insufficiency or cardiac edema and in infants.
● Determine CO_2 combining power and serum electrolytes before and during therapy to prevent acidosis. Each gram of ammonium chloride will reduce the CO_2 combining power by 1.1 volume percent.
● **I.V. use:** Dilute concentrated form (26.75%) before administration. Add 100 to 200 mEq (20 to 40 ml of the 26.75% solution) to 500 or 1,000 ml of 0.9% sodium chloride for injection. Administer via infusion pump, not exceeding 5 ml/minute in adults.
● Lessen pain of I.V. injection by decreasing infusion rate.

• To decrease GI adverse reactions, give oral form after meals. Enteric-coated tablets may also minimize GI symptoms but are absorbed erratically.

• Do not administer drug with milk or other alkaline solutions; they are incompatible.

• Monitor urine pH and output. Diuresis is normal for first 2 days.

• Monitor rate and depth of respirations frequently.

• Observe for signs of ammonia toxicity: pallor, sweating, irregular breathing, and twitching. Notify doctor at once.

☑ **PATIENT TEACHING**

• Instruct patient to take oral form after meals. Tell him not to ingest milk or milk-based products at the meal preceding drug administration.

• Tell patient to report adverse reactions promptly.

---

sodium bicarbonate ◊
Arm and Hammer Pure Baking Soda, Bell/ans, Citrocarbonate, Soda Mint

Pregnancy Risk Category: C

HOW SUPPLIED
Tablets ◊ : 325 mg, 520 mg, 650 mg
Injection: 4% (2.4 mEq/5 ml), 4.2% (5 mEq/10 ml), 5% (297.5 mEq/500 ml), 7.5% (8.92 mEq/10 ml and 44.6 mEq/50 ml), 8.4% (10 mEq/10 ml and 50 mEq/50 ml)

ACTION
Restores body's buffering capacity of the body and neutralizes excess acid.

ONSET, PEAK, DURATION
Onset and peak serum levels occur immediately after I.V. infusion. Duration unknown after I.V. infusion. Onset, peak, and duration unknown after oral administration.

INDICATIONS & DOSAGE
Cardiac arrest—

Adults and children: 1 mEq/kg I.V. of 7.5% or 8.4% solution, followed by 0.5 mEq/kg I.V. every 10 minutes, depending on arterial blood gases (ABGs). Further dosages based on results of ABG analysis. If ABG results are unavailable, use 0.5 mEq/kg I.V. every 10 minutes until spontaneous circulation returns.

Infants up to 2 years: not to exceed 8 mEq/kg I.V. daily of 4.2% solution.
Metabolic acidosis—
Adults and children: dosage depends on blood CO_2 content, pH, and the patient's clinical condition. Generally, 2 to 5 mEq/kg infused over 4- to 8-hour period.
Systemic or urinary alkalinization—
Adults: initially, 4 g P.O., followed by 1 to 2 g q 4 hours.
Children: 84 to 840 mg/kg P.O. daily.
Antacid—
Adults: 300 mg to 2 g P.O. up to q.i.d. taken with glass of water.

ADVERSE REACTIONS
GI: gastric distention, belching, flatulence.
Other: with overdose—*metabolic alkalosis,* hypernatremia, hyperosmolarity; local pain and irritation at injection site.

INTERACTIONS
Anorexiants, flecainide, mecamylamine, quinidine, sympathomimetics: urine alkalinization causes decreased renal clearance of these drugs and increased risk of toxicity. Monitor closely.
Chlorpropamide, lithium, methotrexate, salicylates, tetracycline: increased urine alkalinization causes increased renal clearance of these drugs and reduced effectiveness. Monitor closely.
Enteric-coated drugs: may be released prematurely in stomach. Avoid concomitant use.

EFFECTS ON DIAGNOSTIC TESTS
Sodium bicarbonate therapy may alter serum electrolyte levels and may increase serum lactate levels.

Reactions may be *common,* uncommon, *life-threatening,* or COMMON AND LIFE-THREATENING.

CONTRAINDICATIONS

Contraindicated in patients with metabolic or respiratory alkalosis, in patients who are losing chlorides by vomiting or from continuous GI suction, in those receiving diuretics known to produce hypochloremic alkalosis; and in those with hypocalcemia in which alkalosis may produce tetany, hypertension, seizures, or CHF. Orally administered sodium bicarbonate is contraindicated in patients with acute ingestion of strong mineral acids.

NURSING CONSIDERATIONS

• Use with extreme caution in patients with CHF or other edematous or sodium-retaining conditions or renal insufficiency.

• **I.V. use:** May be added to other I.V. fluids. Sodium bicarbonate inactivates such catecholamines as norepinephrine and dopamine, and forms precipitate with calcium. Do not mix sodium bicarbonate with I.V. solutions of these agents, and flush I.V. line adequately.

• To avoid risk of alkalosis, obtain blood pH, PaO_2, $PaCO_2$, and serum electrolytes. Keep the doctor informed of serum laboratory results.

Alert: Be aware that sodium bicarbonate is not routinely recommended for use in cardiac arrest because it may produce a paradoxical acidosis from CO_2 production. It should not be routinely administered during the early stages of resuscitation unless preexisting acidosis is clearly present.

☑ PATIENT TEACHING

• Tell the patient not to take with milk. May cause hypercalcemia, alkalosis, and possibly renal calculi.

---

sodium lactate

Pregnancy Risk Category: NR

HOW SUPPLIED

Injection: ⅙ molar solution (167 mEq/L)

Injection: 5 mEq/ml

ACTION

Metabolized to sodium bicarbonate, producing buffering effect.

ONSET, PEAK, DURATION

Onset and serum levels peak right after infusion. Conversion of sodium lactate to bicarbonate requires 1 to 2 hours. Duration unknown.

INDICATIONS & DOSAGE

Alkalinize urine—
Adults: 30 ml of ⅙ molar solution/kg of body weight I.V., given in divided doses over 24 hours.
Metabolic acidosis—
Adults: ⅙ molar injection (167 mEq lactate/L I.V.); dosage depends on degree of bicarbonate deficit.

ADVERSE REACTIONS

Other: fever, infection or thrombophlebitis at injection site; with overdose— *metabolic alkalosis,* hypernatremia, hyperosmolarity.

INTERACTIONS

None significant.

EFFECTS ON DIAGNOSTIC TESTS

None reported.

CONTRAINDICATIONS

Contraindicated in patients with hypernatremia, lactic acidosis, or conditions in which sodium administration is detrimental.

NURSING CONSIDERATIONS

• Use with extreme caution in patients with metabolic or respiratory alkalosis, severe hepatic or renal disease, shock, hypoxia, or beriberi.

• **I.V. use:** Add sodium lactate to other I.V. solutions, or give as an isotonic ⅙ molar solution. Drug is compatible with most common I.V. solutions.

• Do not mix with sodium bicarbonate; the drugs are incompatible.

● Monitor serum electrolyte levels to avoid alkalosis.

☑ **PATIENT TEACHING**
● Explain use and administration of drug to patient and family.
● Tell patient to report any unusual signs and symptoms.

---

tromethamine
Tham

Pregnancy Risk Category: C

HOW SUPPLIED
Injection: 18 g/500 ml

ACTION
Combines with hydrogen ions and associated acid anions; resulting salts are excreted. Also has osmotic diuretic effect.

ONSET, PEAK, DURATION
Onset and peak are immediately after I.V. infusion. Duration unknown.

INDICATIONS & DOSAGE
Metabolic acidosis associated with cardiac bypass surgery or with cardiac arrest—
Adults: dosage depends on bicarbonate deficit. Calculate as follows: Each ml of 0.3 M tromethamine solution required = weight in kg × bicarbonate deficit (mEq/L). Additional therapy based on serial determinations of existing bicarbonate deficit. Administer over at least 1 hour; individual doses should not exceed 500 mg/kg.

Acidosis during bypass surgery: Average dose of 9 ml/kg (2.7 mEq/kg or 0.32 g/kg); total single dose of 500 ml (150 mEq or 18 g) is adequate for most adults; not to exceed 500 mg/kg over a period of less than 1 hour.

Cardiac arrest: 3.6 to 10.8 g (111 to 333 ml) injected into large peripheral vein.

ADVERSE REACTIONS
Respiratory: *respiratory depression.*
Other: hypoglycemia, *hyperkalemia* (with decreased urine output), venospasm; I.V. thrombosis; inflammation, necrosis, and sloughing (if extravasation occurs); hemorrhagic hepatic necrosis.

INTERACTIONS
None significant.

EFFECTS ON DIAGNOSTIC TESTS
Tromethamine alters serum electrolyte levels. Transient decreases in blood glucose concentrations may occur.

CONTRAINDICATIONS
Contraindicated in patients with anuria, uremia, or chronic respiratory acidosis, or during pregnancy (except in acute, life-threatening situations).

NURSING CONSIDERATIONS
● Use cautiously in patients with renal disease and poor urine output. Monitor ECG and serum potassium levels.
● Make these determinations before, during, and after therapy: blood pH; carbon dioxide tension; bicarbonate, glucose, and electrolyte levels.
● I.V. use: Give slowly through 18G to 20G needle into largest antecubital vein, or by indwelling I.V. catheter.
● In patients with associated respiratory acidosis, have mechanical ventilation available.
● To prevent blood pH from rising above normal, be prepared to adjust dosage carefully, as ordered.
● If extravasation occurs, infiltrate area with 1% procaine and 150 units hyaluronidase, as ordered.

☑ **PATIENT TEACHING**
● Explain use of drug to patient and family.
● Tell them to report reactions.

---

ferrous fumarate
ferrous gluconate
ferrous sulfate
ferrous sulfate, dried
iron dextran
iron sorbitol
polysaccharide iron complex

COMBINATION PRODUCTS
FERGON PLUS: ferrous gluconate 58 mg, vitamin B$_{12}$ ½ NF unit with intrinsic factor, and vitamin C 75 mg.
FEROCYL ◊ : ferrous fumarate/150 mg and docusate sodium 100 mg.
FERRO-DOCUSATE-T.R., FERRO-DOK TR, FERRO-DSS: ferrous fumarate 150 mg and docusate sodium 100 mg.
FERRO-SEQUELS ◊ : ferrous fumarate 150 mg and docusate sodium 100 mg.

---

ferrous fumarate
Femiron ◊ , Feostat ◊ , Feostat Drops ◊ , Fumasorb ◊ , Fumerin ◊ , Hemocyte ◊ , Ircon ◊ , Nephro-Fer ◊ , Novofumar†, Palafer†, Palafer Pediatric Drops†, Span-FF ◊

Pregnancy Risk Category: A

HOW SUPPLIED
Each 100 mg of ferrous fumarate provides 33 mg of elemental iron.
Tablets ◊ : 63 mg, 195 mg, 200 mg, 300 mg, 324 mg, 325 mg, 350 mg
Tablets (chewable): 100 mg ◊
Capsules (extended-release): 325 mg ◊
Oral suspension: 100 mg/5 ml ◊
Drops: 45 mg/0.6 ml ◊

ACTION
Provides elemental iron, an essential component in the formation of hemoglobin.

ONSET, PEAK, DURATION
Onset occurs within 4 days. Peak effects occur in 7 to 10 days. Effects persist for 2 to 4 months.

INDICATIONS & DOSAGE
Iron deficiency—
Adults: 50 to 100 mg of elemental iron three times daily.
Children: 4 to 6 mg/kg/day of elemental iron in three divided doses.

ADVERSE REACTIONS
GI: *nausea, epigastric pain, vomiting, constipation, diarrhea,* black stools, anorexia.
Other: suspension and drops may temporarily stain teeth.

INTERACTIONS
Antacids, cimetidine, calcium supplements, penicillamine, dimercaprol: decreased iron absorption. Separate doses by 2 to 4 hours.
L-thyroxine, fluoroquinolones, methyldopa, levodopa, etidronate, tetracycline: iron may decrease absorption of these drugs. Separate iron administration from these drug doses by 2 hours. Monitor thyroid function of patients on L-thyroxine.
Vitamin C: may increase iron absorption. Beneficial drug interaction.
Yogurt, cheese, eggs, milk, whole-grain breads and cereals, tea, and coffee: may impair oral iron absorption.

EFFECTS ON DIAGNOSTIC TESTS
Ferrous fumarate blackens feces and may interfere with tests for occult blood in the stool; the guaiac test and ortho-toluidine test may yield false-positive results, but benzidine test is usually not affected. Iron overload may decrease uptake of technetium 99m and thus interfere with skeletal imaging.

CONTRAINDICATIONS

Contraindicated in patients with primary hemochromatosis or hemosiderosis, in patients with hemolytic anemia unless iron deficiency anemia is also present, in those receiving repeated blood transfusions, and in patients with peptic ulcer disease, regional enteritis, or ulcerative colitis.

NURSING CONSIDERATIONS

• Use cautiously on long-term basis.
• Keep in mind that GI upset may be related to dose. Between-meal doses are preferable, but can be given with some foods, although absorption may be decreased. Enteric-coated products reduce GI upset but also reduce amount of iron absorbed.
• Check for constipation; record color and amount of stools.
• Be aware that oral iron may turn stools black. Although this unabsorbed iron is harmless, it could mask the presence of melena.
• Monitor hemoglobin and hematocrit levels and reticulocyte count during therapy, as ordered.
• Know that combination products, such as Ferro-Sequels and Ferocyl, contain stool softeners, which help prevent constipation, a common adverse reaction.

☑ PATIENT TEACHING

• Tell patient to take tablets with juice (preferably orange juice) or water, but not with milk or antacids.
• To avoid staining teeth, tell patient to take suspension with straw and place drops at back of throat.
• Caution patient not to crush tablets, or allow the patient to chew extended-release iron preparations.
• Caution patient not to substitute one iron salt for another; the amount of elemental iron may vary.
• Inform parents that as little as three or four tablets can cause serious poisoning in children.

ferrous gluconate
Fergon*◊, Fertinic†, Novoferrogluc†, Simron◊

Pregnancy Risk Category: A

HOW SUPPLIED

Each 100 mg of ferrous gluconate provides 11.6 mg of elemental iron.
Tablets: 300 mg◊, 320 mg◊, 325 mg◊
Capsules: 86 mg◊
Elixir: 300 mg/5 ml*◊

ACTION

Provides elemental iron, an essential component in the formation of hemoglobin.

ONSET, PEAK, DURATION

Onset occurs in 4 days. Peak effects occur in 7 to 10 days. Effects persist for 2 to 4 months.

INDICATIONS & DOSAGE

Iron deficiency—
Adults: 50 to 100 mg of elemental iron t.i.d.
Children: 4 to 6 mg/kg/day of elemental iron in three divided doses.

ADVERSE REACTIONS

GI: *nausea,* epigastric pain, vomiting, *constipation,* diarrhea, *black stools,* anorexia.
Other: elixir may temporarily stain teeth.

INTERACTIONS

Antacids, cholestyramine resin, cimetidine, vitamin E: decreased iron absorption. Separate doses by at least 2 hours.
Chloramphenicol: delayed response to iron therapy. Monitor patient.
Fluoroquinolones, penicillamine, tetracyclines: decreased GI absorption, possibly resulting in decreased serum levels or efficacy. Separate doses by 2 to 4 hours.
L-thyroxine: decreased L-thyroxine ab-

sorption. Separate doses by at least 2 hours. Monitor thyroid function.
Levodopa, methyldopa: decreased absorption and efficacy of levodopa and methyldopa. Monitor for decreased effect of these agents.
Vitamin C: may increase iron absorption. A beneficial drug interaction.
Yogurt, cheese, eggs, milk, whole-grain breads and cereals, tea, and coffee: may impair oral iron absorption.

EFFECTS ON DIAGNOSTIC TESTS
Ferrous gluconate blackens feces and may interfere with test for occult blood in the stools; the guaiac test and ortho-toluidine test may yield false-positive results, but benzidine test is usually not affected.

Iron overload may decrease uptake of technetium 99m and thus interfere with skeletal imaging.

CONTRAINDICATIONS
Contraindicated in patients with peptic ulceration, regional enteritis, ulcerative colitis, hemosiderosis, and primary hemochromatosis; in patients with hemolytic anemia unless an iron deficiency anemia is also present; and in patients receiving repeated blood transfusions.

NURSING CONSIDERATIONS
• Use cautiously on long-term basis.
• Keep in mind that GI upset may be related to dose. Between-meal doses are preferable, but can be given with some foods, although absorption may be decreased. Enteric-coated products reduce GI upset but also reduce amount of iron absorbed.
• Check for constipation; record color and amount of stools.
• Be aware that oral iron may turn stools black. This unabsorbed iron is harmless; however, it could mask melena.
• Monitor hemoglobin and hematocrit levels and reticulocyte count during therapy.

☑ **PATIENT TEACHING**
• Instruct patient to dilute liquid preparations in juice (preferably orange juice) or water, but not in milk or antacids. To promote absorption, tell patient to take tablets with orange juice.
• To avoid staining teeth, tell patient to take elixir with straw.
• Inform parents that as few as three or four tablets can cause serious iron poisoning in children.
• Caution patient not to substitute one iron salt for another as the amounts of elemental iron vary.

---

ferrous sulfate
Apo-Ferrous Sulfate†, Feosol*◇, Fer-In-Sol Drops*◇, Fer-In-Sol Syrup*◇, Fer-Iron Drops◇, Feritard‡, Fero-Grad†, Fero-Gradumet◇, Ferospace◇, Mol-Iron*◇

ferrous sulfate, dried
Feosol◇, Fer-In-Sol◇, Ferra-TD◇, Ferralyn Lanacaps◇, Mol-Iron*◇, Novoferrosulfa†, PMS Ferrous Sulfate†, Slow-Fe◇

Pregnancy Risk Category: A

HOW SUPPLIED
Ferrous sulfate is 20% elemental iron; dried and powdered, about 32% elemental iron.
Tablets: 195 mg◇, 300 mg◇, 324 mg◇; 200 mg (dried)
Tablets (extended-release): 159 mg (dried)◇, 525 mg
Capsules: 190 mg (dried), 250 mg◇
Capsules (extended-release): 150 mg (dried)◇, 159 mg (dried)◇
Elixir: 220 mg/5 ml*◇
Syrup: 90 mg/5 ml◇
Solution: 300 mg/5 ml
Drops: 125 mg/ml

ACTION
Provides elemental iron, an essential component in the formation of hemoglobin.

---

*Liquid contains alcohol.   **May contain tartrazine.   †Canada only.   ‡Australia only.   ◇OTC.

ONSET, PEAK, DURATION
Onset occurs within 4 days. Peak effects occur within 7 to 10 days. Effects persist for 2 to 4 months.

INDICATIONS & DOSAGE
Iron deficiency—
Adults: 50 to 100 mg of elemental iron t.i.d.
Children: 4 to 6 mg/kg/day of elemental iron in three divided doses.

ADVERSE REACTIONS
GI: *nausea,* epigastric pain, vomiting, *constipation, black stools,* diarrhea, anorexia.
Other: liquid forms may temporarily stain teeth.

INTERACTIONS
Antacids, cholestyramine resin, cimetidine, vitamin E: decreased iron absorption. Separate doses if possible.
Chloramphenicol: delayed response to iron therapy. Monitor patient.
Fluoroquinolones, penicillamine, tetracyclines: decreased GI absorption, possibly resulting in decreased serum levels or efficacy. Separate doses by 2 to 4 hours.
Levodopa, methyldopa: decreased absorption and efficacy of levodopa and methyldopa. Monitor for decreased effect of these agents.
L-thyroxine: decreased L-thyroxine absorption. Separate doses by at least 2 hours. Monitor thyroid function.
Vitamin C: may increase iron absorption. A beneficial drug interaction.
Yogurt, cheese, eggs, milk, whole-grain breads and cereals, tea, and coffee: may impair oral iron absorption.

EFFECTS ON DIAGNOSTIC TESTS
Ferrous sulfate blackens feces and may interfere with tests for occult blood in the stool; the guaiac test and orthotoluidine test may yield false-positive results, but benzidine test is usually not affected.

Iron overload may decrease uptake of technetium 99m and thus interfere with skeletal imaging.

CONTRAINDICATIONS
Contraindicated in patients with hemosiderosis and primary hemochromatosis; in those with hemolytic anemia unless iron deficiency anemia is also present; in those with peptic ulceration, ulcerative colitis, and regional enteritis; and in patients receiving repeated blood transfusions.

NURSING CONSIDERATIONS
● Use cautiously on long-term basis.
● Keep in mind that GI upset may be related to dose. Between-meal doses are preferable, but can be given with some foods, although absorption may be decreased. Enteric-coated products reduce GI upset but also reduce amount of iron absorbed.
● Be aware that oral iron may turn stools black. Although this unabsorbed iron is harmless, it could mask melena.
● Monitor hemoglobin and hematocrit levels and reticulocyte count during therapy, as ordered.

☑ PATIENT TEACHING
● Tell patient to take with juice.
● Instruct patient not to crush or chew extended-release preparations.
● Inform parents that as little as three to four tablets can cause serious iron poisoning in children.
● Caution patient not to substitute one iron salt for another as the amounts of elemental iron vary.

iron dextran
Imferon†, InFeD

iron sorbitol

Pregnancy Risk Category: C

HOW SUPPLIED
1 ml iron dextran provides 50 mg elemental iron.

66

Anticoagulants

dalteparin sodium
danaparoid sodium
enoxaparin sodium
heparin calcium
heparin sodium
warfarin sodium

COMBINATION PRODUCTS
None.

dalteparin sodium
Fragmin

Pregnancy Risk Category: B

HOW SUPPLIED
Syringe: 2,500 anti-factor Xa IU/0.2 ml

ACTION
A low-molecular-weight heparin derivative that enhances the inhibition of factor Xa and thrombin by antithrombin.

ONSET, PEAK, DURATION
Onset and duration unknown. Peak anti-factor Xa activity in about 4 hours.

INDICATIONS & DOSAGE
Prophylaxis against deep vein thrombosis in patients undergoing abdominal surgery who are at risk for thromboembolic complications—
Adults: 2,500 IU S.C. daily, starting 1 to 2 hours prior to surgery and repeated once daily for 5 to 10 days postoperatively.

ADVERSE REACTIONS
Hematologic: *thrombocytopenia.*
Skin: pruritus, rash, *hematoma at injection site,* pain or skin necrosis (rare) at injection site.
Other: hemorrhage, ecchymoses, bleeding complications, fever, *anaphylactoid reactions* (rare).

INTERACTIONS
Oral anticoagulants, antiplatelet agents: May increase risk of bleeding. Use together cautiously.

EFFECTS ON DIAGNOSTIC TESTS
Dalteparin may falsely elevate transaminase levels (AST, ALT).

CONTRAINDICATIONS
Contraindicated in patients with hypersensitivity to the drug, heparin, or pork products; active major bleeding; or thrombocytopenia associated with positive in vitro tests for antiplatelet antibody in the presence of the drug.

NURSING CONSIDERATIONS
● Use with extreme caution in patients with history of heparin-induced thrombocytopenia and in those at increased risk for hemorrhage, such as those with severe uncontrolled hypertension, bacterial endocarditis, congenital or acquired bleeding disorders, active ulceration and angiodysplastic GI disease, or hemorrhagic stroke or shortly after brain, spinal, or ophthalmologic surgery.
● Use with caution in patients with bleeding diathesis, thrombocytopenia, platelet defects, severe liver or kidney insufficiency, hypertensive or diabetic retinopathy, and recent GI bleeding.
● Know that patients who are candidates for dalteparin therapy are those who are at risk for deep vein thrombosis, including patients who are over age 40, obese, undergoing surgery under general anesthesia lasting longer than 30 minutes, or have additional risk factors (such as malignancy or a history of deep vein thrombosis or pulmonary embolism).
● Have patient assume a sitting or supine position when administering the drug. Give S.C. injection deeply. Injection sites include a U-shaped area

---

*Liquid contains alcohol. **May contain tartrazine. †Canada only. ‡Australia only. ◊OTC.

around the navel, upper outer side of thigh, and upper outer quadrangle of buttock. Rotate sites daily. When the area around the navel or the thigh is used, use thumb and forefinger to lift up a fold of skin while giving the injection. The entire length of the needle should be inserted at a 45- to 90-degree angle.

• Never administer the drug I.M.

• Do not mix with other injections or infusions unless specific compatibility data support such mixing.

Alert: Be aware that drug is not interchangeable (unit for unit) with unfractionated heparin or other low-molecular-weight heparin.

• Know that periodic, routine CBCs and fecal occult blood tests are recommended during the course of treatment. Patients do not require regular monitoring of PT or activated PTT.

• Monitor patient closely for thrombocytopenia.

• Be aware that the drug should be discontinued if a thromboembolic event occurs despite dalteparin prophylaxis.

☑ **PATIENT TEACHING**

• Instruct the patient and family to watch for and report signs of bleeding.

• Tell patient to avoid OTC drugs containing aspirin or other salicylates.

▼ **NEW DRUG**

danaparoid sodium
Orgaran

Pregnancy Risk Category: B

HOW SUPPLIED
Ampule: 750 anti-Xa units/0.6 ml
Syringe: 750 anti-Xa units/0.6 ml

ACTION
Prevents fibrin formation by inhibiting generation of thrombin by factor Xa and factor IIa.

ONSET, PEAK, DURATION
Onset and duration unknown. Peak anti-Xa activity occurs in 2 to 5 hours.

INDICATIONS & DOSAGE
Prophylaxis against postoperative deep vein thrombosis (DVT) in patients undergoing elective hip replacement surgery—
Adults: 750 anti-Xa units S.C. b.i.d. starting 1 to 4 hours preoperatively, and then not sooner than 2 hours after surgery. Treatment continued for 7 to 10 days postoperatively or until risk of DVT has diminished.

ADVERSE REACTIONS
CNS: insomnia, headache, asthenia, dizziness.
CV: peripheral edema, *hemorrhage.*
GI: *nausea, constipation,* vomiting.
GU: UTI, urinary retention.
Hematologic: anemia.
Musculoskeletal: joint disorder.
Skin: rash, pruritus.
Other: *fever, injection site pain,* infection.

INTERACTIONS
Oral anticoagulants, platelet inhibitors: May increase risk of bleeding; use together cautiously. .

EFFECTS ON DIAGNOSTIC TESTS
Danaparoid may cause unreliable PT and Thrombotest results within 5 hours after administration.

CONTRAINDICATIONS
Contraindicated in patients with hypersensitivity to the drug or to pork products, severe hemorrhagic diathesis (such as hemophilia or idiopathic thrombocytopenic purpura), active major bleeding, or thrombocytopenia associated with positive in vitro tests for antiplatelet antibody in the presence of the drug.

Reactions may be *common*, uncommon, *life-threatening*, or COMMON AND LIFE-THREATENING.

NURSING CONSIDERATIONS

● Use with extreme caution in patients at increased risk of hemorrhage, such as in severe uncontrolled hypertension, acute bacterial endocarditis, congenital or acquired bleeding disorders, active ulcerative and angiodysplastic GI disease, non-hemorrhagic stroke, postoperative use of indwelling epidural catheter, or shortly after brain, spinal, or ophthalmic surgery.

● Know that drug contains sodium sulfite, which can cause allergic reactions in some people, especially asthmatics.

● Use with caution in patients with impaired renal function.

● Know that drug should be used in pregnancy only if clearly needed. Caution should be used when giving the drug to breast-feeding women.

● Know that the safety and effectiveness of drug in pediatric patients have not been established.

● Danaparoid should never be given I.M. To administer drug, have the patient lie down. Give S.C. injection deeply, using a 25 to 26-gauge needle. Injection sites should be alternated between the left and right anterolateral and posterolateral abdominal wall. Gently pull up a skin fold with thumb and forefinger and insert entire length of the needle into tissue. Don't rub afterward.
Alert: Be aware that drug is not interchangeable (unit for unit) with heparin or low molecular weight heparin.

● Know that periodic, routine CBCs (including platelet count) and fecal occult blood tests are recommended during therapy. Patients don't require regular monitoring of PT and PTT.

● Know that the drug has little effect on PT, PTT, fibrinolytic activity, and bleeding time.
Alert: Monitor the patient's hematocrit and blood pressure closely; a decrease in either may signal hemorrhage.

● In the event of serious bleeding, danaparoid should be stopped and blood products transfused as ordered.

● Store ampules at room temperature; syringes should be refrigerated at 2° to 8° C (36° to 46° F). Protect drug from light.

☑ **PATIENT TEACHING**
● Instruct patient and family to watch for and report signs of bleeding.
● Tell patient to avoid OTC drugs containing aspirin or other salicylates.

---

enoxaparin sodium
Lovenox

Pregnancy Risk Category: B

HOW SUPPLIED
Injection: 30 mg per 0.3 ml

ACTION
A low-molecular weight heparin derivative that accelerates formation of antithrombin III-thrombin complex and deactivates thrombin, preventing conversion of fibrinogen to fibrin. Enoxaparin has a higher anti-factor Xa-to anti-factor IIa-activity ratio.

ONSET, PEAK, DURATION
Onset unknown. Peak effects occur 3 to 5 hours after S.C. injection. Effects persist up to 24 hours.

INDICATIONS & DOSAGE
To prevent pulmonary embolism and deep vein thrombosis after hip or knee replacement surgery—
Adults: 30 mg S.C. q 12 hours for 7 to 10 days. Initial dose given between 12 and 24 hours postoperatively provided hemostasis has been established.

ADVERSE REACTIONS
CNS: confusion.
CV: edema, peripheral edema, *cardiovascular toxicity* (chest pain, dizziness, irregular heartbeat).
GI: nausea.
Hematologic: hypochromic anemia, *thrombocytopenia.*

Other: irritation, pain, hematoma, or erythema at the injection site; fever; pain; *hemorrhage;* ecchymoses; bleeding complications, **angioedema,** *rash or hives.*

INTERACTIONS

Anticoagulants, antiplatelet agents: increased risk of bleeding. Don't use together.

Plicamycin and valproic acid: may cause hypoprothrombinemia and inhibit platelet aggregation.

EFFECTS ON DIAGNOSTIC TESTS

Enoxaparin therapy may decrease the patient's platelet count and may increase transaminase levels (AST and ALT).

CONTRAINDICATIONS

Contraindicated in patients with hypersensitivity to the drug or to heparin or pork products; in patients with active, major bleeding or thrombocytopenia; and in those who demonstrate antiplatelet antibodies in the presence of the drug.

NURSING CONSIDERATIONS

● Use with extreme caution in patients with a history of heparin-induced thrombocytopenia and in patients with threatened abortion, aneurysms, cerebrovascular hemorrhage, or uncontrolled hypertension.

● Use cautiously in the elderly and in patients with conditions that put them at increased risk for hemorrhage, such as bacterial endocarditis; congenital or acquired bleeding disorders; ulcer disease; angiodysplastic GI disease; hemorrhagic stroke; or recent spinal, eye, or brain surgery. Also use cautiously in patients with regional or lumbar block anesthesia, blood dyscrasias, recent childbirth, pericarditis or pericardial effusion, renal insufficiency, or severe CNS trauma.

● Draw blood to establish baseline coagulation parameters before therapy.

● Never administer the drug I.M.

● Don't massage after S.C. injection. Watch for signs of bleeding at site. Rotate sites and keep record.

● Avoid excessive I.M. injections of other drugs to prevent or minimize hematomas. If possible, don't give I.M. injections at all.

● Monitor platelet counts regularly. Patients with normal coagulation won't require close monitoring of PT or PTT.

● Regularly inspect the patient for bleeding gums, bruises on arms or legs, petechiae, nosebleeds, melena, tarry stools, hematuria, hematemesis.

● To treat severe overdose, give protamine sulfate (a heparin antagonist) by slow I.V. infusion at a concentration of 1% to equal the dosage of enoxaparin injected, as ordered.

☑ PATIENT TEACHING

● Instruct the patient and his family to watch for signs of bleeding and to notify the doctor immediately.

● Tell patient to avoid OTC drugs containing aspirin or other salicylates.

heparin calcium
Calcilean†, Calciparine, Caprin‡, Uniparin-Ca‡

heparin sodium
Hepalean†, Heparin Leo†, Heparin Lock Flush Solution (with Tubex), Hep-Lock, Liquaemin Sodium, Uniparin‡

Pregnancy Risk Category: C

HOW SUPPLIED

Products are derived from beef lung or porcine intestinal mucosa.

heparin calcium
Ampule: 12,500 units/0.5 ml; 20,000 units/0.8 ml
Syringe: 5,000 units/0.2 ml

heparin sodium
Carpuject: 5,000 units/ml
Disposable syringes: 1,000 units/ml, 2,500 units/ml, 5,000 units/ml, 7,500

---

units/ml, 10,000 units/ml, 15,000 units/ml, 20,000 units/ml, 40,000 units/ml

Premixed I.V. solutions: 1,000 units in 500 ml of 0.9% sodium chloride solution; 2,000 units in 1,000 ml of 0.9% sodium chloride solution; 12,500 units in 250 ml of 0.45% sodium chloride solution; 25,000 units in 250 ml of 0.45% sodium chloride solution; 25,000 units in 500 ml of 0.45% sodium chloride solution; 10,000 units in 100 ml of D₅W; 12,500 units in 250 ml of D₅W 25,000 units in 250 ml D₅W; 25,000 units in 500 ml D₅W; 20,000 units in 500 ml of D₅W

Unit-dose ampules: 1,000 units/ml, 5,000 units/ml, 10,000 units/ml

Vials: 1,000 units/ml, 2,500 units/ml, 5,000 units/ml, 7,500 units/ml, 10,000 units/ml, 15,000 units/ml, 20,000 units/ml, 40,000 units/ml

heparin sodium flush

Disposable syringes: 10 units/ml, 100 units/ml

Vials: 10 units/ml, 100 units/ml

ACTION

Accelerates formation of antithrombin III-thrombin complex and deactivates thrombin, preventing conversion of fibrinogen to fibrin.

ONSET, PEAK, DURATION

Onset occurs in 20 to 60 minutes after S.C. administration, immediately after I.V. injection. Plasma levels peak 2 to 4 hours after S.C. injection. Correlation between plasma level and drug effect is poor; heparin is rapidly cleared from plasma within ½ to 3 hours, but its duration of action is dose-dependent.

INDICATIONS & DOSAGE

Heparin dosage is highly individualized, depending upon disease state, age, and renal and hepatic status.

Full-dose continuous I.V. infusion therapy for deep vein thrombosis, MI, pulmonary embolism—

Adults: initially, 5,000 units by I.V. bo-

lus, followed by 750 to 1,500 units/hour by I.V. infusion with pump. Hourly rate adjusted 8 hours after bolus dose and according to results of PTT.

Children: initially, 50 units/kg I.V. followed by 25 units/kg/hour or 20,000 units/m² daily by I.V. infusion pump. Dosage adjusted according to PTT.

Full-dose S.C. therapy for deep vein thrombosis, MI, pulmonary embolism—

Adults: initially, 5,000 units I.V. bolus and 10,000 to 20,000 units in a concentrated solution S.C., followed by 8,000 to 10,000 units S.C. q 8 hours or 15,000 to 20,000 units in a concentrated solution q 12 hours.

Full-dose intermittent I.V. therapy for deep vein thrombosis, MI, pulmonary embolism—

Adults: initially, 10,000 units by I.V. bolus and then adjusted according to PTT, and 5,000 to 10,000 units I.V. q 4 to 6 hours.

Children: initially, 100 units/kg by I.V. bolus followed by 50 to 100 units/kg q 4 hours.

Fixed low-dose therapy for venous thrombosis, pulmonary embolism, atrial fibrillation with embolism, postoperative deep vein thrombosis, and prevention of embolism—

Adults: 5,000 units S.C. q 12 hours. In surgical patients, first dose given 2 hours before procedure, followed by 5,000 units S.C. q 8 to 12 hours for 5 to 7 days or until patient can walk.

Consumptive coagulopathy (such as disseminated intravascular coagulation)—

Adults: 50 to 100 units/kg by I.V. bolus or continuous I.V. infusion q 4 hours.

Children: 25 to 50 units/kg by I.V. bolus or continuous I.V. infusion q 4 hours. If no improvement within 4 to 8 hours, discontinue heparin.

Open-heart surgery—

Adults: (total body perfusion) 150 to 300 units/kg continuous I.V infusion.

Patency maintenance of I.V. indwelling catheters—

Adults: 10 to 100 units I.V. flush. Use sufficient volume to fill the device. Not intended for therapeutic use.

ADVERSE REACTIONS
Hematologic: *hemorrhage* (with excessive dosage), *overly prolonged clotting time, thrombocytopenia.*
Other: irritation; mild pain; hematoma; ulceration; cutaneous or subcutaneous necrosis; *"white clot" syndrome;* hypersensitivity reactions, including chills, fever, pruritus, rhinitis, urticaria, anaphylactoid reactions.

INTERACTIONS
Oral anticoagulants: increased additive anticoagulation. Monitor PT and PTT.
Salicylates, other antiplatelet agents: increased anticoagulant effect. Don't use together.
Thrombolytics: increased risk of hemorrhage. Monitor closely.

EFFECTS ON DIAGNOSTIC TESTS
Heparin therapy prolongs PT, may falsely elevate AST and serum ALT levels, and may cause false elevations in some tests for serum thyroxine levels.

CONTRAINDICATIONS
Contraindicated in patients hypersensitive to the drug. Conditionally contraindicated in patients with active bleeding; blood dyscrasia; or bleeding tendencies, such as hemophilia, thrombocytopenia, or hepatic disease with hypoprothrombinemia; suspected intracranial hemorrhage; suppurative thrombophlebitis; inaccessible ulcerative lesions (especially of GI tract) and open ulcerative wounds; extensive denudation of skin; ascorbic acid deficiency and other conditions that cause increased capillary permeability; during or after brain, eye, or spinal cord surgery; during spinal tap or spinal anesthesia; during continuous tube drainage of stomach or small intestine; in subacute bacterial endocarditis; shock; advanced renal disease; threatened abortion; severe hypertension.

Although heparin use is clearly haz-

ardous in these conditions, its risks and its benefits must be evaluated.

NURSING CONSIDERATIONS
● Use cautiously during menses; in patients with mild hepatic or renal disease, alcoholism, occupations with high risk of physical injury; immediately postpartum; and in patients with history of allergies, asthma, or GI ulcerations.
● Draw blood to establish baseline coagulation parameters before therapy.
● Know that when the patient requires anticoagulation during pregnancy, most clinicians use heparin.
● Keep in mind that drug requirements are higher in early phases of thrombogenic diseases and febrile states; lower when the patient's condition stabilizes.
● Be aware that elderly patients should usually start at lower doses.
● Check order and vial carefully. Heparin comes in various concentrations.
● Give low-dose injections sequentially between iliac crests in lower abdomen deep into S.C. fat. Inject drug S.C. slowly into fat pad. Leave needle in place for 10 seconds after injection; then withdraw needle. Don't massage after S.C. injection, and watch for signs of bleeding at injection site. Alternate sites every 12 hours—right for morning, left for evening.
● **I.V. use:** Administer I.V. using infusion pump to provide maximum safety because of long-term effect and irregular absorption when given S.C. Check constant I.V. infusions regularly, even when pumps are in good working order, to prevent overdosage or underdosage. Place notice above the patient's bed to inform I.V. team or laboratory personnel to apply pressure dressings after taking blood.
● During intermittent I.V. therapy, always draw blood ½ hour before next scheduled dose to avoid falsely elevated PTT. Blood for PTT may be drawn any time after 8 hours of initiation of continuous I.V. heparin therapy. Blood for

PTT should never be drawn from the
I.V. tubing of the heparin infusion or
from the infused vein. Falsely elevated
PTT will result. Always draw blood
from the opposite arm.
• Don't skip a dose or "catch up" with
an I.V. containing heparin. If I.V. runs
out, restart it as soon as possible, and
reschedule bolus dose immediately.
• Know that concentrated heparin solutions (greater than 100 units/ml) can irritate blood vessels.
• Never piggyback other drugs into an
infusion line while the heparin infusion
is running. Never mix another drug and
heparin in the same syringe when giving
a bolus.
• Avoid excessive I.M. injections of
other drugs to prevent or minimize
hematomas. If possible, don't give I.M.
injections at all.
• Measure PTT carefully and regularly.
Anticoagulation is present when PTT
values are one and one-half to two times
the control values.
• Monitor platelet count regularly.
Thrombocytopenia caused by heparin
may be associated with a type of arterial
thrombosis known as "white clot" syndrome.
• Regularly inspect the patient for
bleeding gums, bruises on arms or legs,
petechiae, nosebleeds, melena, tarry
stools, hematuria, hematemesis.
Alert: To treat severe heparin calcium or
heparin sodium overdose, use protamine
sulfate, a heparin antagonist, as ordered.
Dosage is based on the dose of heparin,
its route of administration, and the time
elapsed since it was given. As a general
rule, 1 to 1.5 mg of protamine/100 units
of heparin is given if only a few minutes
have elapsed; 0.5 to 0.75 mg prota-
mine/100 units heparin if 30 to 60 minutes have elapsed, 0.25 to 0.375 mg pro-
tamine/100 units heparin if 2 hours or
more have elapsed. Do not give more
than 50 mg protamine in a 10-minute
period.
• Know that abrupt withdrawal may
cause increased coagulability, and he-

parin therapy is usually followed by oral
anticoagulants for prophylaxis.

☑ **PATIENT TEACHING**
• Instruct the patient and his family to
watch for signs of bleeding and notify
the doctor immediately.
• Tell the patient to avoid OTC medications containing aspirin, other salicylates, or drugs that may interact with heparin.

---

warfarin sodium
Coumadin, Panwarfin, Sofarin,
Warfilone Sodium†

Pregnancy Risk Category: X

HOW SUPPLIED
Tablets: 1 mg, 2 mg, 2.5 mg, 4 mg,
5 mg, 7.5 mg, 10 mg

ACTION
Inhibits vitamin K-dependent activation
of clotting factors II, VII, IX, and X,
formed in the liver.

ONSET, PEAK, DURATION
Onset occurs in ½ to 3 days. Peak unknown. Effects persist for 2 to 5 days.

INDICATIONS & DOSAGE
*Pulmonary embolism associated with
deep vein thrombosis, M.I., rheumatic
heart disease with heart valve damage,
prosthetic heart valves, chronic atrial
fibrillation—*
Adults: 2 to 5 mg P.O. daily for 2 to 4
days, then dosage based on daily PT.
Usual maintenance dosage is 2 to 10 mg
P.O. daily.

ADVERSE REACTIONS
GI: anorexia, nausea, vomiting, cramps,
diarrhea, mouth ulcerations, sore
mouth, melena.
GU: hematuria, excessive menstrual
bleeding.
Hematologic: *hemorrhage* (with excessive dosage).

Hepatic: hepatitis, elevated liver function tests, jaundice.
Skin: dermatitis, urticaria, necrosis, gangrene, alopecia, *rash.*
Other: *fever,* headache.

INTERACTIONS
Acetaminophen: may increase bleeding with long-term (longer than 2 weeks) therapy with high doses (more than 2 g/day) of acetaminophen. Monitor very carefully.
Allopurinol, amiodarone, anabolic steroids, cephalosporins, chloramphenicol, cimetidine, ciprofloxacin, clofibrate, danazol, diazoxide, diflunisal, disulfiram, erythromycin, ethacrynic acid, fenoprofen calcium, fluconazole, fluoroquinolones, glucagon, heparin, ibuprofen, influenza virus vaccine, isoniazid, itraconazole, ketoprofen, lovastatin, meclofenamate, methimazole, methylthiouracil, metronidazole, miconazole, nalidixic acid, neomycin (oral), norfloxacin, ofloxacin, omeprazole, pentoxifylline, propafenone, propoxyphene, propylthiouracil, quinidine, simvastatin, streptokinase, sulfinpyrazone, sulfonamides, sulindac, tamoxifen, tetracyclines, thiazides, thyroid drugs, tricyclic antidepressants, urokinase, vitamin E: increased PT. Monitor the patient carefully for bleeding. Consider anticoagulant dosage reduction.
Anticonvulsants: increased serum levels of phenytoin and phenobarbital. Monitor closely.
Barbiturates, carbamazepine, corticosteroids, corticotropin, dicloxacillin, ethchlorvynol, griseofulvin, haloperidol, meprobanate, mercaptopurine, methaqualone, nafcillin, oral contraceptives containing estrogen, rifampin, spironolactone, sucralfate, trazodone: decreased PT with reduced anticoagulant effect. Monitor patient carefully.
Chloral hydrate, glutethimide, propylthiouracil, sulfinpyrazone, triclofos sodium: increased or decreased PT. Avoid use if possible, and monitor the patient carefully.

Cholestyramine: decreased response when administered too close together. Administer 6 hours after oral anticoagulants.
Nonsteroidal anti-inflammatory agents and salicylates: increased PT; ulcerogenic effects. Don't use together.
Sulfonylureas (oral antidiabetic agents): increased hypoglycemic response. Monitor blood glucose levels.
Foods or enteral products containing vitamin K: may impair anticoagulation. Patient should maintain consistent daily intake of leafy green vegetables.

EFFECTS ON DIAGNOSTIC TESTS
Warfarin prolongs both PT and PTT; it may enhance uric acid excretion, elevate serum transaminase levels, increase lactate dehydrogenase activity, and cause false-negative serum theophylline levels.

CONTRAINDICATIONS
Contraindicated in known hypersensitivity; pregnancy, threatened abortion, eclampsia, or preeclampsia; blood dyscrasias or hemorrhagic tendencies; recent surgery involving large open areas, eye, brain, or spinal cord; recent prostatectomy; major regional lumbar block anesthesia, spinal puncture, diagnostic or therapeutic invasive procedures; bleeding from the GI, GU, or respiratory tracts; aneurysm; cerebrovascular hemorrhage; severe or malignant hypertension; severe renal or hepatic disease; subacute bacterial endocarditis, pericarditis, or pericardial effusion; a history of warfarin-induced necrosis; unsupervised patients with senility, alcoholism, or psychosis; or situations where there are inadequate laboratory facilities for coagulation testing.

NURSING CONSIDERATIONS
● Use cautiously in patients with diverticulitis, colitis, mild or moderate hypertension, mild or moderate hepatic or renal disease, with drainage tubes in any orifice; with regional or lumbar block

anesthesia; or in any condition that increases risk of hemorrhage and during lactation.

• Draw blood to establish baseline coagulation parameters before therapy.

• Know that PT determinations are essential for proper control. Doctors typically try to maintain PT at one and one-half to two times normal; high incidence of bleeding when PT exceeds two and one-half times the control values.

• Give warfarin at the same time daily.

• Be aware that I.V. form may be obtained from manufacturer in the rare instances that oral therapy cannot be given. Follow manufacturer guidelines carefully regarding preparation and administration.

• Because onset of action is delayed, keep in mind that heparin sodium is often given during first few days of treatment. When heparin is being given simultaneously, blood for PT should not be drawn within 5 hours of intermittent I.V. heparin administration. However, blood for PT may be drawn at any time during continuous heparin infusion.

• Regularly inspect the patient for bleeding gums, bruises on arms or legs, petechiae, nosebleeds, melena, tarry stools, hematuria, and hematemesis.

• Observe breast-feeding infants of patients on drug for unexpected bleeding.

Alert: Withhold drug and call the doctor at once if fever or rash (signal severe adverse reactions) occurs.

• Be aware that half-life of warfarin's anticoagulant effect is 36 to 44 hours. Effect can be neutralized by vitamin K injections.

• Know that the drug is the best oral anticoagulant for the patient taking antacids or phenytoin.

• Know that elderly patients and patients with renal or hepatic failure are especially sensitive to warfarin effect.

☑ **PATIENT TEACHING**

• Stress importance of complying with prescribed dosage and follow-up appointments. The patient should carry a card that identifies him as a potential bleeder.

• Tell the patient and his family to watch for signs of bleeding and to call the doctor at once if they occur.

• Warn the patient to avoid OTC products containing aspirin, other salicylates, or drugs that may interact with warfarin.

• Tell the patient to notify the doctor if menses is heavier than usual; may require dosage adjustment.

• Tell the patient to use electric razor when shaving to avoid scratching skin and to use a soft toothbrush.

• Warn the patient to read food labels. Food and enteral feedings that contain vitamin K may impair anticoagulation.

• Tell the patient to eat a daily, consistent amount of leafy green vegetables, which contain vitamin K. Eating different amounts daily may alter anticoagulant effects.

albumin 5%
albumin 25%
antihemophilic factor
anti-inhibitor coagulant complex
antithrombin III, human
factor IX (human)
factor IX complex
plasma protein fraction

COMBINATION PRODUCTS
None.

___

albumin 5%
Albuminar 5%, Albutein 5%, Buminate 5%, Plasbumin 5%

albumin 25%
Albuminar 25%, Albutein 25%, Buminate 25%, Plasbumin 25%

Pregnancy Risk Category: C

HOW SUPPLIED
albumin 5%
Injection: 50-ml, 250-ml, 500-ml, 1,000-ml vials
albumin 25%
Injection: 10-ml, 20-ml, 50-ml, 100-ml vials

ACTION
Albumin 5% supplies colloid to the blood and expands plasma volume. Albumin 25% provides intravascular oncotic pressure in a 5:1 ratio, causing a fluid shift from interstitial spaces to the circulation and slightly increasing plasma protein concentration.

ONSET, PEAK, DURATION
Onset and peak occur immediately to within 15 minutes if patient well hydrated. Duration of action depends on the initial blood volume of the patient. If blood volume is reduced, volume expansion persists for many hours; however, if blood volume is normal, the effect lasts a shorter time.

INDICATIONS & DOSAGE
Hypovolemic shock—
Adults: initially, 500 to 750 ml 5% solution by I.V. infusion, repeated q 30 minutes, p.r.n. Alternatively, 100 to 200 ml I.V. of 25% solution, repeated after 10 to 30 minutes, if needed. Dosage varies with the patient's condition and response.
Children: 12 to 20 ml 5% solution/kg by I.V. infusion, repeated in 15 to 30 minutes if response is not adequate. Alternatively, 2.5 to 5 ml I.V. of 25% solution/kg, repeated after 10 to 30 minutes if needed.
Hypoproteinemia—
Adults: 200 to 300 ml of 25% albumin. Dosage varies with the patient's condition and response.
Hyperbilirubinemia—
Infants: 1 g albumin (4 ml 25%)/kg during or 1 to 2 hours before exchange transfusion.

ADVERSE REACTIONS
CNS: headache.
CV: *vascular overload after rapid infusion,* hypotension, tachycardia.
GI: increased salivation, nausea, vomiting.
Respiratory: altered respiration, dyspnea, pulmonary edema.
Skin: urticaria, rash.
Other: chills, fever, back pain.

INTERACTIONS
None significant.

EFFECTS ON DIAGNOSTIC TESTS
Preparations of albumin derived from placental tissue may increase serum alkaline phosphatase level; all products

___

Reactions may be *common,* uncommon, *life-threatening,* or COMMON AND LIFE-THREATENING.

may slightly increase plasma albumin levels.

CONTRAINDICATIONS
Contraindicated in patients with hypersensitivity to the drug, severe anemia, or cardiac failure.

NURSING CONSIDERATIONS
● Use with extreme caution in patients with hypertension, low cardiac reserve, hypervolemia, pulmonary edema, or hypoalbuminemia with peripheral edema.
● Make sure the patient is properly hydrated before infusion.
● Take care when preparing and administering drug to minimize waste. This product is expensive, and random supply shortages occur often.
● **I.V. use:** Avoid rapid I.V. infusion. Specific rate is individualized according to the patient's age, condition, and diagnosis. Know that 5% albumin is infused undiluted; 25% albumin may be infused undiluted or diluted with sterile water for injection, 0.9% sodium chloride solution, or D_5W injection. Use solution promptly. Discard unused solution. Don't use cloudy solutions or those containing sediment. Solution should be clear amber color.
Alert: Do not give more than 250 g in 48 hours.
● Watch for hemorrhage or shock after surgery or injury. Rapid rise in blood pressure may cause bleeding from sites that are not apparent at lower pressures.
● Monitor vital signs carefully.
● Watch for signs of vascular overload (heart failure or pulmonary edema).
● Monitor fluid intake and output and hemoglobin, hematocrit, serum protein, and electrolyte levels during therapy.
● Follow storage instructions on bottle. Freezing may cause bottle to break.

☑ PATIENT TEACHING
● Explain to patient and family the use and administration of albumin.
● Tell patient to report adverse reactions promptly.

antihemophilic factor (AHF)
Hemofil M, Humate-P, Hyate:C, Koate-HP, Koate-HS, Monoclate, Monoclate-P, Profilate OSD

Pregnancy Risk Category: C

HOW SUPPLIED
Injection: vials, with diluent. Units specified on label.

ACTION
Directly replaces deficient clotting factor.

ONSET, PEAK, DURATION
Onset immediate after I.V. administration. Time to peak effect is 1 to 2 hours after I.V. administration. Duration unknown.

INDICATIONS & DOSAGE
Spontaneous hemorrhage in patients with hemophilia A (factor VIII deficiency)—
Adults and children: calculate dosage using this formula:

$$\text{AHF required (IU)} = \text{body weight (kg)} \times \text{desired factor VIII increase (\% of normal)} \times 0.5$$

To prevent spontaneous hemorrhage, the desired level of factor VIII is 5% of normal; for mild hemorrhage, 30% of normal; for moderate hemorrhage and minor surgery, 30% to 50% of normal; for severe hemorrhage, 80% to 100% of normal.
Treatment of bleeding in patients with hemophilia A (factor VIII deficiency)—
Adults and children: for minor hemorrhage into muscle and joints, 8 to 10 IU/kg I.V. (or calculated dose to raise plasma factor VIII levels to 20% to 40% of normal) q 8 to 12 hours for 1 to 3 days as needed. For overt bleeding, an initial dose of 15 to 25 IU/kg I.V., followed by 8 to 15 IU/kg q 8 to 12 hours for 3 to 4 days. To treat massive bleed-

---

ing or hemorrhage involving major organs, an initial dose of 40 to 50 IU/kg I.V., followed by 20 to 25 IU/kg I.V. q 8 to 12 hours.

Prevention of bleeding in hemophilic patients requiring surgery—

Adults: 25 to 30 IU/kg I.V. 1 hour before surgery, followed by one-half of the initial dosage 5 hours later. Dosage adjusted to achieve a level of AHF 80% to 100% of normal during surgery and maintained at 30% to 60% of normal for at least 10 to 14 days postoperatively.

ADVERSE REACTIONS
CV: tightness in chest.
GI: nausea.
Respiratory: wheezing.
Skin: *urticaria.*
Other: *chills, fever, thrombosis, hemolytic anemia, thrombocytopenia,* hypersensitivity reactions, (stinging at injection site, fever, *anaphylaxis*), risk of hepatitis B and HIV.

INTERACTIONS
None significant.

EFFECTS ON DIAGNOSTIC TESTS
None reported.

CONTRAINDICATIONS
Contraindicated in patients with hypersensitivity to murine (mouse) protein or to the drug.

NURSING CONSIDERATIONS
● Use cautiously in neonates, infants, and patients with hepatic disease because of their susceptibility to hepatitis, which may be transmitted in antihemophilic factor.
● Monitor coagulation studies before therapy.
● Monitor patients with blood types A, B, and AB for possible hemolysis.
● Know that a change in urine color to an orange or red hue can signify a hemolytic reaction.
● As ordered, administer hepatitis B vaccine before administering antihe-

mophilic factor.
● Refrigerate concentrate until ready to use. Warm concentrate and diluent bottles to room temperature before reconstituting. To mix drug, gently roll vial between hands.
● Use reconstituted solution within 3 hours. Store away from heat and do not refrigerate. Refrigeration after reconstitution may cause the active ingredient to precipitate. Don't shake or mix with other I.V. solutions. Solution should be filtered before administration.
● **I.V. use:** Take baseline pulse rate before I.V. administration. Use plastic syringe; drug may interact with glass syringe and bind to its surface. If pulse rate increases significantly, flow rate should be reduced or administration stopped.
● Do not use S.C. or I.M.
● Monitor vital signs regularly.
● Monitor coagulation studies frequently during therapy.
● Monitor the patient for allergic reactions.
● Be aware that some patients develop inhibitors to factor VIII, resulting in decreased response to the drug.
● Keep in mind that risk of hepatitis, including non-A and non-B hepatitis, must be weighed against risk of the patient not receiving the drug.
● Because of the manufacturing process, be aware that the risk of HIV transmission is extremely low.

☑ **PATIENT TEACHING**
● Explain to patient and family the use and administration of antihemophilic factor.
● Tell patient to report adverse reactions promptly.
● Patient should wear medical identification tag.
● Tell patient to notify doctor if medication seems less effective; a change may signify the development of antibodies.

anti-inhibitor coagulant complex
Autoplex T, Feiba VH Immuno

Pregnancy Risk Category: C

HOW SUPPLIED
Injection: number of units of factor VIII correctional activity indicated on label of vial

ACTION
Unknown. It has been suggested that efficacy may be related in part to the presence of the activated factors, which leads to more complete factor X activation in conjunction with tissue factor, phospholipid, and ionic calcium and allows the coagulation process to proceed beyond those stages where factor VIII is needed.

ONSET, PEAK, DURATION
Onset occurs within 10 to 30 minutes. Peak and duration unknown.

INDICATIONS & DOSAGE
Prevention and control of hemorrhagic episodes in certain patients with hemophilia A who have developed inhibitor antibodies to antihemophilic factor; management of bleeding in patients with acquired hemophilia who have spontaneously acquired inhibitors to factor VIII—
Adults and children: highly individualized and varies among manufacturers. For Autoplex T, 25 to 100 units/kg I.V., depending on the severity of hemorrhage. If no hemostatic improvement occurs within 6 hours after initial administration, dosage repeated. For Feiba VH Immuno, 50 to 100 units/kg I.V. q 6 or 12 hours until clear signs of improvement. Maximum daily dosage is 200 units/kg.

ADVERSE REACTIONS
CNS: headache.
CV: changes in blood pressure, *acute MI, thromboembolic events.*
GI: nausea, vomiting.
Hematologic: *disseminated intravascular coagulation (DIC).*
Skin: flushing, rash, urticaria.
Other: fever, chills, hypersensitivity reactions, risk of hepatitis B and HIV.

INTERACTIONS
Antifibrinolytic agents: may alter effects of anti-inhibitor coagulant complex. Do not use together.

EFFECTS ON DIAGNOSTIC TESTS
None reported.

CONTRAINDICATIONS
Contraindicated in patients with signs of fibrinolysis, in those with DIC, and in those with a normal coagulation mechanism.

NURSING CONSIDERATIONS
● Use with caution in patients with liver disease.
● As ordered, administer hepatitis B vaccine before administering drug.
● Keep epinephrine available to treat anaphylaxis.
● Know that Feiba VH Immuno should not be used with newborns, but Autoplex T can be used with caution.
● **I.V. use:** Warm the drug and diluent to room temperature prior to reconstitution. Reconstitute according to manufacturer's directions. Use the filter needle provided by the manufacturer to withdraw the reconstituted solution from the vial into the syringe; the filter needle should then be replaced with a sterile injection needle for administration. Administer as soon as possible. If drug is given as an I.V. infusion, the administration set must contain a filter. Autoplex T infusions should be completed within 1 hour after reconstitution; Feiba VH Immuno infusions, within 3 hours.
● The rate of administration should be individualized according to the patient's response. Autoplex T infusions may be-

gin at a rate of 2 ml/minute; if well tolerated, the infusion rate may be increased gradually to 10 ml/minute. Feiba VH Immuno infusion rate should not exceed 2 units/kg/minute.

Alert: If flushing, lethargy, headache, transient chest discomfort, or changes in blood pressure or pulse rate develop because of a rapid rate of infusion, stop the drug and notify the doctor. Know that these symptoms usually disappear with cessation of the infusion. The infusion may then be resumed at a slower rate, as ordered.

• Monitor the patient closely for hypersensitivity reactions.
• Monitor vital signs regularly, and report significant changes to the doctor.
• Reassure patient that because of the manufacturing process, the risk of HIV transmission is extremely low.

☑ **PATIENT TEACHING**
• Explain to patient and family the use and administration of anti-inhibitor coagulant complex.
• Tell patient to report adverse reactions promptly.

---

antithrombin III, human (AT-III, heparin cofactor I)
ATnativ, Thrombate III

Pregnancy Risk Category: C

HOW SUPPLIED
Injection: 500 IU

ACTION
Replaces deficient AT-III in patients with hereditary AT-III deficiency, normalizing coagulation inhibition and inhibiting thromboembolism formation. Also deactivates plasmin (to lesser extent than the clotting factor).

ONSET, PEAK, DURATION
Onset immediate after I.V. administration. Peak unknown. Effects persist about 4 days.

INDICATIONS & DOSAGE
Thromboembolism associated with hereditary AT-III deficiency—
Adults and children: initial dose is individualized to quantity required to increase AT-III activity to 120% of normal activity as determined 30 minutes after administration. Usual dose is 50 to 100 IU/minute I.V., not to exceed 100 IU/minute. Dose is calculated based on anticipated 1% increase in plasma AT-III activity produced by 1 IU/kg of body weight using the formula:

$$\text{Dose required (IU)} = \frac{(\text{desired activity [\%]} - \text{baseline activity [\%]}) \times \text{weight (kg)}}{1.4}$$

Maintenance dosage is individualized to quantity required to increase AT-III activity to 80% of normal activity and is administered at 24-hour intervals.

To calculate subsequent dosages, multiply the desired AT-III activity (as percentage of normal) minus the baseline AT-III activity (as percentage of normal) by body weight (in kg). Divide by actual increase in AT-III activity (as percentage) produced by 1 IU/kg as determined 30 minutes after administration of initial dose.

Treatment is usually continued for 2 to 8 days but may be prolonged in pregnancy or when used with surgery or immobilization.

ADVERSE REACTIONS
CV: vasodilation, lowered blood pressure.
GU: diuresis.

INTERACTIONS
Heparin: increased anticoagulant effect of both drugs. Heparin dosage reduction may be necessary.

EFFECTS ON DIAGNOSTIC TESTS
Plasma levels of antithrombin III may be measured with clotting assays or amidolytic assays using synthetic chromogenic substrates. Immunoassays may not detect all congenital antithrombin III deficiencies.

Reactions may be *common*, uncommon, *life-threatening*, or COMMON AND LIFE-THREATENING.

CONTRAINDICATIONS
None known.

NURSING CONSIDERATIONS
• Use with extreme caution in children and neonates because safety and efficacy have not been established.
• Use drug cautiously. It is prepared from pooled plasma from human donors and carries with it a minimal risk of transmission of viruses, including hepatitis and HIV.
Alert: Because of the risk of neonatal thromboembolism (sometimes fatal) in children of parents with hereditary AT-III deficiency, anticipate obtaining AT-III levels immediately after birth.
• **I.V. use:** Reconstitute using 10 ml of sterile water (provided), 0.9% sodium chloride solution, or D_5W. Do not shake vial. Dilute further in same diluent solution if desired.
• Obtain AT-III activity levels twice daily until the dosage requirement has stabilized, then daily immediately before dose. Functional assays are preferred because quantitative immunologic test results may be normal despite decreased AT-III activity.
• Monitor for dyspnea and increased blood pressure, which may occur if administration rate is too rapid.
• Keep in mind that 1 IU is equivalent to the quantity of endogenous AT-III present in 1 ml of normal human plasma.
• Keep in mind that heparin binds to AT-III lysine binding sites, resulting in increased efficacy of heparin.
• Know that drug is not recommended for long-term prophylaxis of thrombotic episodes.
• Store at 36° to 46° F (2° to 8° C).

☑ **PATIENT TEACHING**
• Explain to patient and parents the use and administration of antithrombin III, human.
• Instruct patient to report adverse reactions promptly.

factor IX (human)
AlphaNine, AlphaNine SD, Mononine

factor IX complex
Bebulin VH Immuno, Konyne-80, Profilnine Heat-Treated, Proplex T

Pregnancy Risk Category: C

HOW SUPPLIED
Injection: vials, with diluent. Units specified on label.

ACTION
Directly replaces deficient clotting factor.

ONSET, PEAK, DURATION
Onset immediate after I.V. administration. Time to peak effect is 10 to 30 minutes after I.V. administration. Duration unknown.

INDICATIONS & DOSAGE
Factor IX deficiency (hemophilia B or Christmas disease), anticoagulant overdosage—
Adults and children: approximate units required factor IX = 1 unit/kg × body weight in kilograms × percentage of desired increase of factor IX level. Infusion rates vary according to the product and the comfort of the patient. Dosage is highly individualized, depending on degree of deficiency, level of factor IX desired, weight of the patient, and severity of bleeding.

ADVERSE REACTIONS
CNS: headache.
CV: *thromboembolic reactions, MI, disseminated intravascular coagulation, pulmonary embolism,* changes in blood pressure.
GI: nausea, vomiting.
Skin: urticaria.
Other: *transient fever, chills, flushing, tingling.*

INTERACTIONS

Aminocaproic acid: increased risk of thrombosis. Avoid concomitant use.

EFFECTS ON DIAGNOSTIC TESTS

None reported.

CONTRAINDICATIONS

Contraindicated in patients with hepatic disease in whom there is any suspicion of intravascular coagulation or fibrinolysis. Mononine is contraindicated in patients with hypersensitivity to murine (mouse) protein.

NURSING CONSIDERATIONS

● Use cautiously in neonates and infants because of susceptibility to hepatitis, which may be transmitted with factor IX complex.
● As ordered, administer hepatitis B vaccine before administering factor IX complex.
● Reconstitute with 20 ml of sterile water for injection for each vial of lyophilized drug. Keep refrigerated until ready to use; warm to room temperature before reconstituting. Use within 3 hours of reconstitution. Unstable in solution. Don't shake, refrigerate, or mix solution with other I.V. solutions. Store away from heat.
● **I.V. use:** Avoid rapid infusion. If tingling sensation, fever, chills, or headache develops, decrease flow rate and notify the doctor.
● Observe the patient for allergic reactions, and monitor vital signs regularly.
● Keep in mind that risk of hepatitis, including non-A and non-B hepatitis, must be weighed against risk of not receiving the drug.
● Because of the manufacturing process, be aware that the risk of HIV transmission is extremely low.

☑ **PATIENT TEACHING**
● Explain to family and patient the use and administration of factor IX.
● Tell patient to report adverse reactions promptly.

plasma protein fraction

Plasmanate, Plasma-Plex, Plasmatein, Protenate

Pregnancy Risk Category: C

HOW SUPPLIED

Injection: 5% solution in 50-ml, 250-ml, 500-ml vials

ACTION

Supplies colloid to the blood and expands plasma volume.

ONSET, PEAK, DURATION

Onset and serum levels peak immediately after I.V. infusion. Duration unknown.

INDICATIONS & DOSAGE

Shock—
Adults: varies with the patient's condition and response, but usual dose is 250 to 500 ml I.V. (12.5 to 25 g protein), usually no faster than 10 ml/minute.
Children: 6.6 to 33 ml/kg (0.33 to 1.65 g/kg of protein) I.V., 5 to 10 ml/minute.
Hypoproteinemia—
Adults: 1,000 to 1,500 ml I.V. daily. Maximum infusion rate is 8 ml/minute.

ADVERSE REACTIONS

CNS: headache.
CV: hypotension (after rapid infusion or intra-arterial administration); *vascular overload* (after rapid infusion); tachycardia.
GI: nausea, vomiting, hypersalivation.
Respiratory: dyspnea, pulmonary edema.
Skin: rash.
Other: flushing, chills, fever, back pain.

INTERACTIONS

None significant.

EFFECTS ON DIAGNOSTIC TESTS

PPF slightly increases plasma protein levels.

Reactions may be *common*, uncommon, *life-threatening*, or COMMON AND LIFE-THREATENING.

CONTRAINDICATIONS

Contraindicated in patients with severe anemia or heart failure and in those undergoing cardiac bypass.

NURSING CONSIDERATIONS

● Use cautiously in patients with hepatic or renal failure, low cardiac reserve, and restricted sodium intake.

● **I.V. use:** Check expiration date before using. Don't use solutions that are cloudy, contain sediment, or have been frozen. Discard solutions in containers opened for more than 4 hours because it contains no preservatives.

● Know that solutions containing amino acids or alcohol may not be infused through the same I.V. line because the proteins may precipitate.

● If the patient is dehydrated, give additional fluids either P.O. or I.V., as ordered.

● Do not give more than 250 g or 5,000 ml in 48 hours.

● Monitor blood pressure. Be prepared to slow or stop infusion if hypotension suddenly occurs. Vital signs should return to normal gradually; monitor hourly.

● Watch for signs of vascular overload (heart failure or pulmonary edema).

● Watch for hemorrhage or shock after surgery or injury. A rapid rise in blood pressure may cause bleeding from sites that are not apparent at lower pressures.

● Monitor intake and output. Watch for and report decreased urine output.

● Keep in mind that drug contains 130 to 160 mEq sodium/liter.

☑ **PATIENT TEACHING**

● Explain to patient and family the use and administration of plasma protein fraction.

● Tell patient to report adverse reactions promptly.

---

*Liquid contains alcohol.   **May contain tartrazine.   †Canada only.   ‡Australia only.   ◇ OTC.

68

Thrombolytic enzymes

alteplase
anistreplase
reteplase, recombinant
streptokinase
urokinase

COMBINATION PRODUCTS
None.

---

alteplase (tissue plasminogen activator, recombinant; tPA)
Actilyse‡, Activase

Pregnancy Risk Category: C

HOW SUPPLIED
Injection: 50-mg (29 million–IU), 100 mg (58 million–IU) vials

ACTION
Binds to fibrin in a thrombus, and locally converts plasminogen to plasmin, which initiates local fibrinolysis.

ONSET, PEAK, DURATION
Onset immediate. Peak effects occur in about 45 minutes. Effects persist for about 4 hours.

INDICATIONS & DOSAGE
Lysis of thrombi obstructing coronary arteries in acute MI—
Adults: 100 mg I.V. infusion over 3 hours as follows: 60 mg in the first hour, of which 6 to 10 mg is given as a bolus over the first 1 to 2 minutes. Then 20 mg/hour infusion for 2 hours. Smaller adults (under 65 kg) should receive 1.25 mg/kg in a similar fashion (60% in the first hour, 10% as a bolus; then 20% of the total dose per hour for 2 hours).
Management of acute massive pulmonary embolism—
Adults: 100 mg I.V. infusion over 2

hours. Heparin begun at the end of the infusion when PTT or thrombin time returns to twice normal or less.
Do not exceed 100-mg dose. Higher doses may increase risk of intracranial bleeding.
✳ *New indication: Acute ischemic stroke—*
Adults: 0.9 mg/kg I.V. infusion over 1 hour with 10% of the total dose administered as an initial I.V. bolus over 1 minute. Maximum total dosage is 90 mg.
Note: Administer within 3 hours after symptoms occur and only when an intracranial bleed has been ruled out.

ADVERSE REACTIONS
CNS: *cerebral hemorrhage,* fever.
CV: hypotension, arrhythmias, edema.
GI: nausea, vomiting.
Hematologic: *severe, spontaneous bleeding* (cerebral, retroperitoneal, GU, GI).
Other: bleeding at puncture sites, hypersensitivity reactions (*anaphylaxis*), CHOLESTEROL EMBOLIZATION.

INTERACTIONS
Aspirin, coumarin anticoagulants, dipyridamole, heparin: increased risk of bleeding. Monitor the patient carefully.

EFFECTS ON DIAGNOSTIC TESTS
Altered results may be expected in coagulation and fibrinolytic tests. The use of aprotinin (150 to 200 units/ml) in the blood sample may attenuate this interference.

CONTRAINDICATIONS
Contraindicated in patients with active internal bleeding, intracranial neoplasm, arteriovenous malformation, aneurysm, and severe uncontrolled hypertension. Also contraindicated in patients with a history of CVA, recent (within 2

Reactions may be *common,* uncommon, *life-threatening,* or COMMON AND LIFE-THREATENING.

months) intraspinal or intracranial trauma or surgery, or known bleeding diathesis. Also contraindicated in patients with history or current evidence of intracranial hemorrhage, suspicion of subarachnoid hemorrhage, or seizure at onset of stroke when used for acute ischemic stroke.

NURSING CONSIDERATIONS
• Use cautiously in patients with recent (within 10 days) major surgery when bleeding is difficult to control because of its location; in pregnancy and first 10 days postpartum; organ biopsy; trauma (including cardiopulmonary resuscitation); GI or GU bleeding; cerebrovascular disease; hypertension (systolic pressure of 180 mm Hg or higher or diastolic pressure of 110 mm Hg or higher); mitral stenosis, atrial fibrillation, or other condition that may lead to left heart thrombus; acute pericarditis or subacute bacterial endocarditis; hemostatic defects due to hepatic or renal impairment; septic thrombophlebitis; diabetic hemorrhagic retinopathy; in patients receiving anticoagulants; and in patients age 75 and older.
• Know that recanalization of occluded coronary arteries and improvement of heart function require initiation of treatment with alteplase as soon as possible after the onset of symptoms.
• Administer alteplase I.V. only, using a controlled infusion device.
• **I.V. use:** Reconstitute drug with sterile water for injection (without preservatives) only. (Check manufacturer's labeling for specific information.) Do not use vial if the vacuum is not present in 50-mg vials, but know that 100-mg vials don't have a vacuum. Reconstitute with a large-bore (18G) needle, directing the stream of sterile water at the lyophilized cake. Do not shake. Slight foaming is common (allow foaming to settle before use), and solution should be clear or pale yellow.
• Keep in mind that drug may be administered as reconstituted (1 mg/ml) or

diluted with an equal volume of 0.9% sodium chloride solution or D_5W to make a 0.5 mg/ml solution. Adding other drugs to the infusion is not recommended.
• Reconstitute alteplase solution immediately before use, and administer it within 8 hours.
• Be aware that anticoagulant and antiplatelet therapy is frequently initiated during or after treatment with alteplase to decrease the risk of rethrombosis.
• Monitor vital signs and neurologic status carefully. Patient should be kept on strict bed rest.
• Have antiarrhythmics readily available, and carefully monitor ECG. Coronary thrombolysis is associated with arrhythmias induced by reperfusion of ischemic myocardium. Such arrhythmias do not differ from those commonly associated with MI.
• Avoid invasive procedures during thrombolytic therapy. Carefully monitor the patient for signs of internal bleeding, and frequently check all puncture sites. Bleeding is the most common adverse effect and may occur internally and at external puncture sites.
• If uncontrollable bleeding occurs, stop infusion (and concomitant heparin) and notify doctor.

☑ PATIENT TEACHING
• Explain to patient and family use and administration of alteplase.
• Tell patient to report adverse reactions promptly.

---

anistreplase (anisoylated plasminogen-streptokinase activator complex; APSAC)
Eminase

Pregnancy Risk Category: C

HOW SUPPLIED
Injection: 30 units-vial

ACTION

Anistreplase, derived from Lys-plasminogen and streptokinase, is formulated into a fibrinolytic enzyme plus activator complex with the activator temporarily blocked by an anisoyl group. The drug is activated in vivo by a nonenzymatic process that removes the anisoyl group. The active drug converts plasminogen to plasmin, resulting in thrombolysis.

ONSET, PEAK, DURATION

Onset immediate after I.V. administration. Peak effects occur in about 45 minutes. Effects persist for 6 hours to 2 days.

INDICATIONS & DOSAGE

Lysis of coronary artery thrombi following acute MI—
Adults: 30 units I.V. over 2 to 5 minutes. Administered by direct injection.

ADVERSE REACTIONS

CNS: *intracranial hemorrhage.*
CV: *arrhythmias, conduction disorders, hypotension.*
EENT: hemoptysis, gum or mouth hemorrhage.
GI: hemorrhage.
GU: hematuria.
Hematologic: *bleeding tendency,* eosinophilia.
Skin: hematoma, urticaria, pruritus, flushing, delayed (2 weeks after therapy) purpuric rash.
Other: bleeding at puncture sites, *anaphylaxis or anaphylactoid reactions* (rare), arthralgia.

INTERACTIONS

Heparin, oral anticoagulants, drugs that alter platelet function (including aspirin and dipyridamole): may increase the risk of bleeding. Use together cautiously.

EFFECTS ON DIAGNOSTIC TESTS

Drug prolongs activated partial thromboplastin time (APTT), PT, and thrombin time; it remains active in vivo and can cause degeneration of fibrinogen in blood samples drawn for analysis. Decreases in alpha$_2$-antiplasmin, factor V, factor VIII, fibrinogen, and plasminogen activities have been reported, as well as moderate reductions in hematocrit and hemoglobin. Concentrations of fibrinogen- and fibrin-degeneration products are increased.

CONTRAINDICATIONS

Contraindicated in patients with a history of severe allergic reaction to anistreplase or streptokinase; active internal bleeding, CVA, recent (within the past 2 months) intraspinal or intracranial surgery or trauma, aneurysm, arteriovenous malformation, intracranial neoplasm, uncontrolled hypertension, or known bleeding diathesis.

NURSING CONSIDERATIONS

● Use cautiously in patients with recent (within 10 days) major surgery (when bleeding is difficult to control because of its location); trauma (including cardiopulmonary resuscitation); GI or GU bleeding; cerebrovascular disease; hypertension (systolic pressure of 180 mm Hg or higher or diastolic pressure of 110 mm Hg or higher); mitral stenosis, atrial fibrillation, or other conditions that may lead to left heart thrombus; acute pericarditis or subacute bacterial endocarditis; hemostatic defects due to hepatic or renal impairment; septic thrombophlebitis; diabetic hemorrhagic retinopathy; in pregnancy and first 10 days postpartum; in patients receiving anticoagulants; and in patients 75 years and older.
● **I.V. use:** Unlike other thrombolytics that must be infused, administer anistreplase by direct injection into an I.V. line over 2 to 5 minutes.
● Reconstitute the drug by slowly adding 5 ml of sterile water for injection. Direct the stream against the side of the vial, not at the drug itself. Gently roll the vial to mix the dry powder and water. To avoid excessive foaming,

don't shake the vial. The reconstituted solution should be colorless to pale yellow. Inspect for precipitate. If the drug is not administered within 30 minutes of reconstituting, discard the vial.

● Do not mix the drug with other medications; do not dilute the solution after reconstitution.

● Carefully monitor ECG during treatment. Be prepared to treat bradycardia or ventricular irritability. Thrombolytic therapy is associated with reperfusion arrhythmias that may signify successful thrombolysis. These arrhythmias are similar to those seen in the course of an acute MI and may include sinus bradycardia, accelerated idioventricular rhythm, ventricular tachycardia, or premature ventricular depolarizations.

● Carefully monitor the patient; avoid I.M. injections and nonessential handling or moving of patient. Bleeding is the most common adverse reaction and may occur internally and at external puncture sites.

● Be aware that anticoagulant or antiplatelet therapy may be used with drug treatment to decrease the risk of rethrombosis.

● Be aware that anistreplase is derived from human plasma. No cases of hepatitis or HIV infection have been reported to date. The manufacturing process is designed to purify the plasma used in preparation of the drug.

Alert: Keep in mind the efficacy of drug may be limited if antistreptokinase antibodies are present. Antibody levels may be elevated if more than 5 days has elapsed since previous treatment with anistreplase or streptokinase, or if the patient has had a recent streptococcal infection.

● Be aware that in vitro coagulation tests will be affected by the presence of anistreplase. This can be attenuated if blood samples are collected in the presence of aprotinin (150 to 200 units/ml).

☑ PATIENT TEACHING
● Explain to patient and family the use and administration of anistreplase.
● Tell patient to report adverse reactions promptly.

▼ *NEW DRUG*

reteplase, recombinant
Retavase

Pregnancy Risk Category: C

HOW SUPPLIED
Injection: 10.8 units (18.8 mg)/vial
Supplied in a kit with components for reconstitution for two single-use vials.

ACTION
Enhances the cleavage of plasminogen to generate plasmin, which leads to fibrinolysis.

ONSET, PEAK, DURATION
Unknown. Effective elimination half-life is 13 to 16 minutes.

INDICATIONS & DOSAGE
Management of acute myocardial infarction—
Adults: double-bolus injection of 10 + 10 U. Give each bolus I.V. over 2 minutes. If complications, such as serious bleeding or an anaphylactoid reaction, do not occur after first bolus, give second bolus 30 minutes after the start of first bolus.

ADVERSE REACTIONS
CNS: *intracranial hemorrhage.*
CV: *arrhythmias, cholesterol embolization, hemorrhage.*
GI: *hemorrhage.*
GU: hematuria.
Hematologic: *bleeding tendency*, anemia.
Other: bleeding at puncture sites.

INTERACTIONS
Heparin, oral anticoagulants, platelet inhibitors (aspirin, dipyridamole, and abciximab): may increase risk of bleed-

ing. Use together cautiously.

EFFECTS ON DIAGNOSTIC TESTS
Retaplase may alter coagulation studies; drug remains active in vitro and can lead to degradation of fibrinogen in sample. Collect blood samples in the presence of PPACK (chloromethylketone) at 2-μM concentrations.

CONTRAINDICATIONS
Contraindicated in patients with active internal bleeding, known bleeding diathesis, history of cerebrovascular accident, recent intracranial or intraspinal surgery or trauma, severe uncontrolled hypertension, intracranial neoplasm, arteriovenous malformation, or aneurysm.

NURSING CONSIDERATIONS
● Use cautiously in patients with recent (within 10 days) major surgery, obstetric delivery, organ biopsy, or trauma; previous puncture of noncompressible vessels; cerebrovascular disease; recent GI or GU bleeding; hypertension (systolic pressure of 180 mm Hg or more or a diastolic pressure of 110 mm Hg or more); conditions that may lead to left heart thrombus including mitral stenosis; acute pericarditis or subacute bacterial endocarditis; hemostatic defects; diabetic hemorrhagic retinopathy; septic thrombophlebitis; any other condition in which bleeding would be difficult to manage; and in patients 75 years or older. Use cautiously in breast-feeding women.
● Carefully monitor ECG during treatment. Coronary thrombolysis may result in arrhythmias associated with reperfusion. Be prepared to treat bradycardia or ventricular irritability.
● Carefully monitor the patient for bleeding. Avoid I.M. injections, invasive procedures, and nonessential handling of the patient. Bleeding is the most common adverse reaction and may occur internally or at external puncture sites. Should local measures not control serious bleeding, discontinue concomi-

tant anticoagulation therapy and notify the doctor. Withhold the second bolus of reteplase.
● Know that drug should be used in pregnancy only if the benefit justifies the potential risk to the fetus.
● Know that safety and effectiveness in children have not been established.
● **I.V. use:** Know that reteplase is administered I.V. as a double-bolus injection. If bleeding or anaphylactoid reactions occur after the first bolus, notify doctor; second bolus may be withheld.
● Reconstitute drug according to manufacturer's instructions using items provided in the kit. Reconstitute with sterile water for injection, USP (without preservatives). Reconstituted solution should be colorless; the resulting concentration will be 1 U/ml. If foaming occurs, allow the vial to stand for several minutes. Inspect for precipitation. Use within 4 hours of reconstitution; discard unused portions.
● Do not administer drug with other I.V. medications through the same I.V. line. Note that heparin and reteplase are incompatible in solution.
● Be aware that potency is expressed in terms of units specific for reteplase and not comparable to other thrombolytic agents.
● Use of noncompressible pressure sites should be avoided during therapy. If an arterial puncture is needed, an upper extremity vessel that can be compressed manually should be used. Apply pressure for at least 30 minutes; then apply a pressure dressing. Check site frequently.

☑ **PATIENT TEACHING**
● Explain to patient and family about the use and administration of reteplase.
● Tell patient to report adverse reactions immediately.

---

streptokinase
Kabikinase, Streptase

Pregnancy Risk Category: C

HOW SUPPLIED
Injection: 250,000 IU, 600,000 IU, 750,000 IU, 1,500,000 IU in vials for reconstitution

ACTION
Activates plasminogen in two steps: Plasminogen and streptokinase form a complex that exposes the plasminogen-activating site; plasminogen is then converted to plasmin by cleavage of the peptide bond, leading to fibrinolysis.

ONSET, PEAK, DURATION
Onset immediate after I.V. administration. Peak effects occur in 20 minutes to 2 hours. Effects persist for about 4 hours.

INDICATIONS & DOSAGE
Arteriovenous cannula occlusion—
Adults: 250,000 IU in 2 ml I.V. solution by I.V. pump infusion into each occluded limb of the cannula over 25 to 35 minutes. Clamp off cannula for 2 hours. Then aspirate contents of cannula; flush with sodium chloride solution and reconnect.
Venous thrombosis, pulmonary embolism, and arterial thrombosis and embolism—
Adults: loading dose is 250,000 IU I.V. infusion over 30 minutes. Sustaining dose is 100,000 IU/hour I.V. infusion for 72 hours for deep vein thrombosis and 100,000 IU/hour over 24 to 72 hours by I.V. infusion pump for pulmonary embolism and arterial thrombosis or embolism.
Lysis of coronary artery thrombi following acute MI—
Adults: loading dose is 20,000 IU bolus via coronary catheter, followed by infusion of maintenance dose of 2,000 IU/minute over 60 minutes. Alternatively, may be administered as an I.V. infusion. Usual adult dose is 1.5 million IU infused I.V. over 60 minutes.

ADVERSE REACTIONS
CNS: polyradiculoneuropathy, headache.
CV: reperfusion arrhythmias, *hypotension,* vasculitis.
EENT: periorbital edema.
GI: nausea.
Hematologic: *bleeding.*
Respiratory: minor breathing difficulty, *bronchospasm, pulmonary edema.*
Skin: urticaria, pruritus, flushing.
Other: phlebitis at injection site, hypersensitivity reactions *(anaphylaxis),* delayed hypersensitivity reactions (interstitial nephritis, serum sickness-like reactions), musculoskeletal pain, *angioedema, fever.*

INTERACTIONS
Anticoagulants: increased risk of bleeding. Monitor the patient closely.
Antifibrinolytic agents: streptokinase activity is inhibited and reversed by antifibrinolytic agents such as aminocaproic acid.
Aspirin, dipyridamole, indomethacin, phenylbutazone, drugs affecting platelet activity: increased risk of bleeding. Monitor patients closely. Combined therapy with low-dose aspirin (162.5 mg) or dipyridamole has improved acute and long-term results.

EFFECTS ON DIAGNOSTIC TESTS
Drug increases thrombin time, activated partial thromboplastin time, and PT; it moderately decreases hematocrit.

CONTRAINDICATIONS
● Contraindicated in patients with ulcerative wounds, active internal bleeding, and recent CVA; recent trauma with possible internal injuries; visceral or intracranial malignant neoplasms; ulcerative colitis; diverticulitis; severe hypertension; acute or chronic hepatic or renal insufficiency; uncontrolled hypocoagulation; chronic pulmonary disease with cavitation; subacute bacterial endocarditis or rheumatic valvular disease; recent cerebral embolism,

thrombosis, hemorrhage; or severe allergic reaction to streptokinase.

● Also contraindicated within 10 days after intra-arterial diagnostic procedure or any surgery, including liver or kidney biopsy, lumbar puncture, thoracentesis, paracentesis, or extensive or multiple cutdowns.

● I.M. injections and other invasive procedures are contraindicated during streptokinase therapy.

NURSING CONSIDERATIONS

● Use cautiously when treating arterial embolism that originates from left side of heart because of danger of cerebral infarction.

● Know that only doctors with wide experience in thrombotic disease management, where clinical and laboratory monitoring can be performed, should use streptokinase.

● Before using streptokinase to clear an occluded arteriovenous cannula, try flushing with heparinized sodium chloride solution, as ordered.

● Keep aminocaproic acid available to treat bleeding, and corticosteroids to treat allergic reactions.

● Before initiating therapy, draw blood for coagulation studies, hematocrit, platelet count, and type and crossmatching. Rate of I.V. infusion depends on thrombin time and streptokinase resistance.

● To check for hypersensitivity reactions, give 100 IU intradermally as ordered; a wheal and flare response within 20 minutes means the patient is probably allergic. Monitor vital signs frequently.

● Be aware that if the patient has had either a recent streptococcal infection or recent treatment with streptokinase, a higher loading dose may be necessary.

● **I.V. use:** Reconstitute each vial with 5 ml of 0.9% sodium chloride solution for injection or D$_5$W solution. Further dilute to 45 ml (if necessary, total volume may be increased to 500 ml in a glass or 50 ml in a plastic container). Don't shake; roll gently to mix. Some flocculation may be present after reconstituting; discard if large amounts are present. Filter solution with 0.8-micron or larger filter. Use within 8 hours. Store powder at room temperature and refrigerate after reconstitution.

● Do not mix with other medications or give other drugs through the same I.V. line.

● Monitor the patient for excessive bleeding every 15 minutes for the 1st hour, every 30 minutes for the 2nd through 8th hours, then every 4 hours. If bleeding is evident, stop therapy and notify doctor. Know that pretreatment with heparin or drugs that affect platelets causes high risk of bleeding, but may improve long-term results. Monitor closely.

● Monitor pulses, color, and sensation of extremities every hour.

● Maintain the involved extremity in straight alignment to prevent bleeding from the infusion site.

● Avoid unnecessary handling of patients; pad side rails. Bruising is more likely during therapy.

● Keep a laboratory flow sheet on the patient's chart to monitor PTT, PT, thrombin time, and hemoglobin and hematocrit levels. Monitor vital signs and neurologic status.

● Avoid IM injection. Keep venipuncture sites to a minimum; use pressure dressing on puncture sites for at least 15 minutes.

Alert: Watch for signs of hypersensitivity. Notify the doctor immediately. Antihistamines or corticosteroids may be used to treat mild allergic reactions. If a severe reaction occurs, the infusion should be stopped immediately and the doctor notified.

● Be aware that heparin by continuous infusion is usually started within 1 to 4 hours after stopping streptokinase. Use infusion pump to administer heparin.

● Keep in mind that thrombolytic therapy in patients with acute MI may decrease infarct size, improve ventricular function, and decrease incidence of CHF. Streptokinase must be administered within 6 hours of the onset of symptoms for optimal effect.

☑ **PATIENT TEACHING**
● Explain to patient and family the use and administration of streptokinase.
● Tell patient to report adverse reactions promptly.

urokinase
Abbokinase, Abbokinase Open-Cath, Ukidan‡

Pregnancy Risk Category: B

HOW SUPPLIED
Injection: 5,000 units (IU) per unit-dose vial; 9,000 units (IU) per unit-dose vial; 250,000-IU vial

ACTION
Activates plasminogen to plasmin by directly cleaving peptide bonds at two different sites, causing fibrolysis.

ONSET, PEAK, DURATION
Onset immediate after I.V. administration. Peak effects occur in 20 minutes to 2 hours. Effects persist for about 4 hours.

INDICATIONS & DOSAGE
Lysis of acute massive pulmonary embolism and lysis of pulmonary embolism accompanied by unstable hemodynamics—
Adults: for I.V. infusion *only* by constant infusion pump.
Priming dose: 4,400 IU/kg of urokinase–0.9% sodium chloride or D_5W solution admixture, given over 10 minutes. Followed with 4,400 IU/kg/hour for 12 hours. Therapy followed with continuous I.V. infusion of heparin, then oral anticoagulants.
Coronary artery thrombosis—
Adults: after a bolus dose of heparin ranging from 2,500 to 10,000 units,

6,000 IU/minute of urokinase is infused into the occluded artery for up to 2 hours. Average total dosage is 500,000 IU. Urokinase therapy should be initiated within 6 hours of onset of symptoms.
Venous catheter occlusion—
Adults: solution containing 5,000 IU/ml is instilled into occluded line and, after 5 minutes, is aspirated. Aspiration attempts repeated q 5 minutes for 30 minutes. If not patent after 30 minutes, the line is capped and urokinase left to work for 30 to 60 minutes before aspirating again. May require second instillation.

ADVERSE REACTIONS
CV: reperfusion arrhythmias, hypotension.
Hematologic: *bleeding.*
Respiratory: bronchospasm, minor breathing difficulties.
Other: phlebitis at injection site, fever, chills, nausea, vomiting, hypersensitivity reaction.

INTERACTIONS
Anticoagulants: increased risk of bleeding. Monitor the patient closely.
Aspirin, dipyridamole, indomethacin, phenylbutazone, other drugs affecting platelet activity: increased risk of bleeding.

EFFECTS ON DIAGNOSTIC TESTS
Drug increases thrombin time, activated partial thromboplastin time, and PT; it sometimes moderately decreases hematocrit.

CONTRAINDICATIONS
● Contraindicated in patients with active internal bleeding, history of CVA, aneurysm, arteriovenous malformation, known bleeding diathesis, recent trauma with possible internal injuries, visceral or intracranial malignancy, pregnancy and first 10 days postpartum, ulcerative colitis, diverticulitis, severe hypertension, hemostatic defects including those secondary to severe hepatic or renal in-

sufficiency, uncontrolled hypocoagulation, chronic pulmonary disease with cavitation, subacute bacterial endocarditis or rheumatic valvular disease, and recent cerebral embolism, thrombosis, or hemorrhage.

• Also contraindicated within 10 days after intra-arterial diagnostic procedure or any surgery (liver or kidney biopsy, lumbar puncture, thoracentesis, paracentesis, or extensive or multiple cutdowns) or within two months after intracranial or intraspinal surgery.

• I.M. injections and other invasive procedures are contraindicated during urokinase therapy.

NURSING CONSIDERATIONS

• Have typed and crossmatched RBCs, whole blood, plasma expanders (other than dextran), and aminocaproic acid available to treat bleeding, and corticosteroids, epinephrine, and antihistamines to treat allergic reactions.

• Know that only doctors with extensive experience in thrombotic disease management should use urokinase in institutions where clinical and laboratory monitoring can be performed.

• **I.V. use:** Reconstitute according to manufacturer's directions. Gently roll vial; do not shake. Don't use bacteriostatic water for injection to reconstitute; it contains preservatives. Dilute further with 0.9% sodium chloride solution or D_5W solution before infusion. Urokinase solutions may be filtered through a 0.45-micron or smaller cellulose-membrane filter before administration. Discard unused solution.

• Do not mix with other medications. Administer through separate I.V. line.

• Monitor the patient for excessive bleeding every 15 minutes for the 1st hour; every 30 minutes for the 2nd through 8th hours; then once every 4 hours. Pretreatment with drugs affecting platelets places patient at high risk of bleeding.

• Monitor pulses, color, and sensation of extremities every hour.

• Although the incidence of hypersensitivity reactions is low, watch for signs of this reaction.

• Keep a laboratory flow sheet on the patient's chart to monitor partial thromboplastin time, PT, thrombin time, and hemoglobin and hematocrit levels.

• Monitor vital signs and neurologic status. Don't take blood pressure in lower extremities because this could dislodge a clot.

• Keep venipuncture sites to a minimum; use pressure dressing on puncture sites for at least 15 minutes.

• Maintain the involved extremity in straight alignment to prevent bleeding from the infusion site.

• Avoid unnecessary handling of patients; pad side rails. Bruising is more likely during therapy.

• Be aware that heparin by continuous infusion is usually started within 3 to 4 hours after urokinase has been stopped to prevent recurrent thrombosis.

☑ PATIENT TEACHING

• Explain to patient and family the use and administration of urokinase.

• Instruct the patient to report adverse reactions promptly.

Reactions may be *common*, uncommon, *life-threatening*, or COMMON AND LIFE-THREATENING.

69

Alkylating drugs

busulfan
carboplatin
carmustine
chlorambucil
cisplatin
cyclophosphamide
ifosfamide
lomustine
mechlorethamine hydrochloride
melphalan
streptozocin
thiotepa
uracil mustard

COMBINATION PRODUCTS
None.

---

busulfan
Mylaran

Pregnancy Risk Category: D

HOW SUPPLIED
Tablets: 2 mg

ACTION
Unknown. Thought to cross-link strands of cellular DNA and interferes with RNA transcription, causing an imbalance of growth that leads to cell death. Cell cycle-nonspecific.

ONSET, PEAK, DURATION
Onset of disease response occurs in 1 to 2 weeks. Peak and duration undefined.

INDICATIONS & DOSAGE
Chronic myelocytic (granulocytic) leukemia—
Adults: 4 to 8 mg P.O. daily, up to 12 mg P.O. daily, until WBC count falls to 15,000/mm^3; drug stopped until WBC count rises to 50,000/mm^3, and then resumed as before; or 4 to 8 mg P.O. daily until WBC count falls to 10,000 to

20,000/mm^3; then daily dosage reduced as needed to maintain WBC count at this level (usually 1 to 3 mg daily).
Children: 0.06 to 0.12 mg/kg/day or 1.8 to 4.6 mg/m^2/day P.O.; dosage adjusted to maintain WBC count at 20,000/mm^3, but never less than 10,000/mm^3.

ADVERSE REACTIONS
CNS: unusual tiredness or weakness, fatigue.
GI: cheilosis, dry mouth, anorexia.
Hematologic: leukopenia (WBC count falling after about 10 days and continuing to fall for 2 weeks after stopping drug), *thrombocytopenia, anemia, severe pancytopenia.*
Respiratory: *irreversible pulmonary fibrosis (commonly called "busulfan lung").*
Skin: *transient hyperpigmentation,* rash, urticaria, anhidrosis.
Other: gynecomastia, alopecia, Addison-like wasting syndrome, profound hyperuricemia caused by increased cell lysis, cataracts, jaundice.

INTERACTIONS
Anticoagulants, aspirin: increased risk of bleeding. Avoid concomitant use.
Thioguanine: may cause hepatotoxicity, esophageal varices, or portal hypertension. Use together cautiously.

EFFECTS ON DIAGNOSTIC TESTS
Drug-induced cellular dysplasia may interfere with interpretation of cytologic studies. Busulfan therapy may increase blood and urine levels of uric acid as a result of increased purine catabolism that accompanies cell destruction.

CONTRAINDICATIONS
Contraindicated in patients with chronic myelogenous leukemia that has demon-

---

*Liquid contains alcohol.   **May contain tartrazine.   †Canada only.   ‡Australia only.   ◇ OTC.

strated prior resistance to the drug. Not useful with chronic lymphocytic leukemia or acute leukemia or in the blastic crisis of chronic myelogenous leukemia.

NURSING CONSIDERATIONS
• Use cautiously in patients recently given other myelosuppressants or radiation treatment and in those with depressed neutrophil or platelet count. Because high-dose therapy has been associated with seizures, use such therapy cautiously in patients with a history of head trauma or seizures or in patients receiving other drugs that lower the seizure threshold.
• Follow institutional policy regarding preparation and handling of drug. Label as a hazardous drug.
• Know that therapeutic effects are often accompanied by toxicity.
• To prevent bleeding, avoid all I.M. injections when platelet count is below 100,000/mm³.
• Monitor patient response (increased appetite and sense of well-being, decreased total WBC count, reduced size of spleen), which usually begins within 1 to 2 weeks.
• Monitor serum uric acid. To prevent hyperuricemia with resulting uric acid nephropathy, know that allopurinol may be ordered in addition to keeping patient adequately hydrated.
• Anticipate possible blood transfusion during treatment because of cumulative anemia.
Alert: Be aware that pulmonary fibrosis may occur as late as 8 months to 10 years after treatment with busulfan.

☑ PATIENT TEACHING
• Advise patient to watch for signs of infection (fever, sore throat, fatigue) and bleeding (easy bruising, nosebleeds, bleeding gums, melena). Tell patient to take temperature daily.
• Instruct patient to report symptoms of toxicity so dosage adjustments can be made. Persistent cough and progressive dyspnea with alveolar exudate, sugges-

tive of pneumonia, may be the result of drug toxicity.
• Instruct patient to avoid any OTC product containing aspirin.
• Inform patient that drug may cause darkening of skin.
• Advise women of childbearing age to avoid becoming pregnant during therapy. Recommend patient consult with doctor before becoming pregnant.
• Warn breast-feeding patient to discontinue breast-feeding because of the possibility of infant toxicity.
• Instruct patient to take drug on an empty stomach to decrease nausea and vomiting.
• Because of the incidence of impotence and male sterility, advise men of child-bearing potential about sperm banking.

carboplatin
Paraplatin, Paraplatin-AQ†

Pregnancy Risk Category: D

HOW SUPPLIED
Injection: 50-mg, 150-mg, 450-mg vials

ACTION
Unknown. An alkylating agent that probably produces cross-linking of DNA strands. Cell cycle-nonspecific.

ONSET, PEAK, DURATION
Undefined.

INDICATIONS & DOSAGE
Palliative treatment of ovarian cancer—
Adults: 360 mg/m² I.V. on day 1 q 4 weeks; doses should not be repeated until platelet count exceeds 100,000/mm³ and neutrophil count exceeds 2,000/mm³. Subsequent doses are based on blood counts.
Patients with renal dysfunction: patients with a creatinine clearance of 41 to 59 ml/minute should receive a starting dose of 250 mg/m²; patients with a creatinine clearance of 16 to 40 ml/min-

Reactions may be *common*, uncommon, *life-threatening*, or COMMON AND LIFE-THREATENING.

ute should receive a starting dose of 200 mg/m². Recommended dosage adjustments are not available for patients with a creatinine clearance of 15 ml/minute or less.

ADVERSE REACTIONS
CNS: dizziness, confusion, peripheral neuropathy, ototoxicity, central neurotoxicity, paresthesia, *CVA.*
CV: *cardiac failure; embolism.*
EENT: visual disturbances; change in taste.
GI: constipation, diarrhea, *nausea, vomiting.*
Hematologic: THROMBOCYTOPENIA, *leukopenia,* neutropenia, anemia, BONE MARROW SUPPRESSION.
Other: alopecia; hypersensitivity reactions; *increased BUN, creatinine, AST, or alkaline phosphatase levels; pain; asthenia; anaphylaxis; decreased serum electrolyte levels.*

INTERACTIONS
Bone marrow suppressants (including radiation therapy): increased hematologic toxicity. Monitor closely.
Nephrotoxic agents: enhanced nephrotoxicity of carboplatin. Use cautiously.

EFFECTS ON DIAGNOSTIC TESTS
High doses may cause elevated bilirubin, alkaline phosphatase, AST, serum creatinine, and BUN levels.

CONTRAINDICATIONS
Contraindicated in patients with a history of hypersensitivity to cisplatin, platinum-containing compounds, or mannitol or with severe bone marrow suppression or bleeding.

NURSING CONSIDERATIONS
● Determine serum electrolyte, creatinine, and BUN levels; CBC; and creatinine clearance before the first infusion and before each course of treatment.
● Keep in mind that bone marrow suppression may be more severe in patients with creatinine clearance below 60

ml/minute; dosage adjustments are recommended for such patients.
● Follow institutional policy to reduce risks because preparation and administration of parenteral form of this drug is associated with mutagenic, teratogenic, and carcinogenic risks for personnel.
● Check ordered dose against laboratory test results carefully. Only one increase in dosage is recommended. Subsequent doses should not exceed 125% of starting dose.
Alert: Have epinephrine, corticosteroids, and antihistamines available when administering carboplatin because anaphylactoid reactions may occur within minutes of administration.
● **I.V. use:** Reconstitute with D_5W, 0.9% sodium chloride solution, or sterile water for injection to make a concentration of 10 mg/ml. Add 5 ml of diluent to the 50-mg vial, 15 ml of diluent to the 150-mg vial, or 45 ml of diluent to the 450-mg vial. It can then be further diluted for infusion with 0.9% sodium chloride solution or D_5W. A concentration as low as 0.5 mg/ml can be prepared. Give drug by continuous or intermittent infusion over at least 15 minutes.
● Do not use needles or I.V. administration sets containing aluminum to administer carboplatin; precipitation and loss of drug's potency may occur.
● Know that therapeutic effects are often accompanied by toxicity.
● To prevent bleeding, avoid all I.M. injections when platelet count is below 100,000/mm³.
● Monitor vital signs during infusion.
● Monitor CBC and platelet count frequently during therapy and, when indicated, until recovery. WBC and platelet count nadirs usually occur by day 21. Levels usually return to baseline by day 28. Know that dose should not be repeated unless platelet count exceeds 100,000/mm³.
● Administer antiemetic therapy as ordered. Carboplatin can produce severe vomiting.
● Anticipate possible blood transfusions

during treatment because of cumulative anemia.

● Know that hydration or diuresis before or after treatment is not necessary.
● Be aware that patients over age 65 are at greater risk for neurotoxicity.
● Store unopened vials at room temperature. Once reconstituted and diluted as directed, drug is stable at room temperature for 8 hours. Because the drug does not contain antibacterial preservatives, discard unused drug after 8 hours.

☑ PATIENT TEACHING

● Advise patient to watch for signs of infection (fever, sore throat, fatigue) and bleeding (easy bruising, nose bleeds, bleeding gums, melena). Tell patient to take temperature daily.
● Instruct patient to avoid OTC products containing aspirin.
● Because of incidence of impotence, sterility, and amenorrhea, advise patients (male and female) of childbearing age before initiating therapy. Also recommend women patients consult with the doctor before becoming pregnant.
● Because of the possibility of infant toxicity, advise breast-feeding patient taking carboplatin to discontinue breast-feeding.

---

carmustine (BCNU)
BiCNU

Pregnancy Risk Category: D

HOW SUPPLIED
Injection: 100-mg vial (lyophilized), with a 3-ml vial of absolute alcohol supplied as a diluent

ACTION
Inhibits enzymatic reactions involved with DNA synthesis, cross-links strands of cellular DNA, and interferes with RNA transcription, causing an imbalance of growth that leads to cell death. Cell cycle-nonspecific.

ONSET, PEAK, DURATION
Undefined.

INDICATIONS & DOSAGE
Brain tumors, Hodgkin's disease, malignant lymphoma, and multiple myeloma—
Adults: 75 to 100 mg/m^2 I.V. by slow infusion daily for 2 days; repeated q 6 weeks if platelet count is above 100,000/mm^3 and WBC count is above 4,000/mm^3. Dosage is reduced by 30% when WBC count is 2,000 to 3,000/mm^3 and platelet count is 25,000 to 75,000/mm^3. Dosage is reduced by 50% when WBC count is less than 2,000/mm^3 and platelet count is less than 25,000/mm^3.

Alternative therapy: 150 to 200 mg/m^2 I.V. by slow infusion as a single dose, repeated q 6 weeks.

ADVERSE REACTIONS
CNS: ataxia, drowsiness.
EENT: ocular toxicities.
GI: *nausea* beginning in 2 to 6 hours (can be severe), *vomiting.*
GU: nephrotoxicity, azotemia, *renal failure.*
Hematologic: *cumulative bone marrow suppression,* delayed 4 to 6 weeks, lasting 1 to 2 weeks; *leukopenia; thrombocytopenia; acute leukemia or bone marrow dysplasia* may occur after long-term use; anemia.
Hepatic: hepatotoxicity.
Respiratory: *pulmonary fibrosis.*
Skin: facial flushing, hyperpigmentation.
Other: *intense pain at infusion site from venous spasm;* possible hyperuricemia in lymphoma patients when rapid cell lysis occurs.

INTERACTIONS
Anticoagulants, aspirin: increased risk of bleeding. Avoid concomitant use.
Cimetidine: may increase carmustine's bone marrow toxicity. Avoid combination if possible.

EFFECTS ON DIAGNOSTIC TESTS
Drug may increase BUN, serum alkaline phosphatase, AST, and bilirubin levels.

CONTRAINDICATIONS
Contraindicated in patients with hypersensitivity to drug.

NURSING CONSIDERATIONS
● Be aware that pulmonary toxicity appears to be dose-related and may occur 9 days to 15 years after treatment. Obtain pulmonary function tests as ordered before and during therapy.
● Follow institutional policy to reduce risks because preparation and administration of parenteral form of this drug is associated with carcinogenic, mutagenic, and teratogenic risks for personnel.
● To reduce nausea, give antiemetic before administering drug, as ordered.
● **I.V. use:** To reconstitute, dissolve 100 mg of carmustine in the 3 ml of absolute alcohol provided by the manufacturer. Dilute solution with 27 ml of sterile water for injection. Resultant solution contains 3.3 mg of carmustine/ml in 10% alcohol. Dilute in 0.9% sodium chloride solution or D_5W for I.V. infusion. Give at least 250 ml over 1 to 2 hours. To reduce pain on infusion, dilute further or slow infusion rate.
● Discard drug if powder liquefies or appears oily (decomposition has occurred).
● Administer only in glass containers. Solution is unstable in plastic I.V. bags.
● Don't mix with other drugs during administration.
● Avoid contact with skin because carmustine will cause a brown stain. If drug comes into contact with skin, wash off thoroughly.
● Perform liver, renal function, and pulmonary function tests periodically, as ordered.
● Monitor CBC, as ordered.
● Monitor serum uric acid level, as ordered. To prevent hyperuricemia with resulting uric acid nephropathy, know that allopurinol may be used with adequate hydration.

● Be aware that therapeutic effects are often accompanied by toxicity.
● To prevent bleeding, avoid all I.M. injections when platelet count is below 100,000/mm³.
● Anticipate possible blood transfusions during treatment because of cumulative anemia.
● Store reconstituted solution in refrigerator for 48 hours or at room temperature for 8 hours. May decompose at temperatures above 80° F (26.6° C).

☑ **PATIENT TEACHING**
● Advise patient to watch for signs of infection (fever, sore throat, fatigue) and bleeding (easy bruising, nosebleeds, bleeding gums, melena). Tell patient to take temperature daily.
● Instruct patient to avoid any OTC product containing aspirin.
● Advise breast-feeding patient to discontinue breast-feeding during therapy because of possible infant toxicity.
● Advise women of childbearing age to avoid becoming pregnant during therapy. Recommend patient consult with doctor before becoming pregnant.

---

chlorambucil
Leukeran

Pregnancy Risk Category: D

HOW SUPPLIED
Tablets: 2 mg

ACTION
Cross-links strands of cellular DNA and interferes with RNA transcription, causing an imbalance of growth that leads to cell death. Cell cycle-nonspecific.

ONSET, PEAK, DURATION
Clinical onset occurs within 3 to 4 weeks. Peak plasma concentration occurs in 1 hour. Duration undefined.

INDICATIONS & DOSAGE
Chronic lymphocytic leukemia; malig-

---

nant lymphomas including lymphosar-coma, giant follicular lymphoma, and Hodgkin's disease—
Adults: 0.1 to 0.2 mg/kg P.O. daily for 3 to 6 weeks; then adjusted for maintenance (usually 4 to 10 mg daily).

ADVERSE REACTIONS
CNS: *seizures,* peripheral neuropathy, tremor, muscle twitching, confusion, agitation, ataxia, flaccid paresis.
GI: *nausea, vomiting,* stomatitis, diarrhea.
GU: *azoospermia, infertility,* sterile cystitis.
Hematologic: *neutropenia,* delayed up to 3 weeks, lasting up to 10 days after last dose; *bone marrow suppression; thrombocytopenia; anemia;* myelosuppression (usually moderate, gradual, and rapidly reversible).
Hepatic: hepatotoxicity.
Respiratory: interstitial pneumonitis, *pulmonary fibrosis* (rare).
Skin: rash, hypersensitivity.
Other: allergic febrile reaction.

INTERACTIONS
Anticoagulants, aspirin: increased risk of bleeding. Avoid concomitant use.

EFFECTS ON DIAGNOSTIC TESTS
Drug may increase concentrations of serum alkaline phosphatase, AST, and blood and urine uric acid.

CONTRAINDICATIONS
Contraindicated in patients with hypersensitivity or resistance to previous therapy. Patients hypersensitive to other alkylating agents may also be hypersensitive to chlorambucil.

NURSING CONSIDERATIONS
● Use cautiously in patients with a history of head trauma or seizures or in patients receiving other drugs that lower the seizure threshold. Also use cautiously within 4 weeks of a full course of radiation or chemotherapy.
● Monitor CBC, as ordered.

● Monitor serum uric acid level, as ordered. To prevent hyperuricemia with resulting uric acid nephropathy, know that allopurinol may be used with adequate hydration.
● If WBC count falls below 2,000/mm³ or granulocyte count falls below 1,000/mm³, follow institutional policy for infection control in immunocompromised patients. Severe neutropenia is reversible up to cumulative dosage of 6.5 mg/kg in a single course.
● Be aware that therapeutic effects are often accompanied by toxicity.
● To prevent bleeding, avoid all I.M. injections when platelet count is below 100,000/mm³.
● Anticipate possible blood transfusions during treatment because of cumulative anemia.

☑ **PATIENT TEACHING**
● Advise patient to watch for signs of infection (fever, sore throat, fatigue) and bleeding (easy bruising, nosebleeds, bleeding gums, melena). Tell patient to take temperature daily.
● Instruct patient to avoid OTC products containing aspirin.
● Advise breast-feeding patient to discontinue breast-feeding during therapy because of possible infant toxicity.
● Advise women of childbearing age to avoid becoming pregnant during therapy and to notify doctor immediately if pregnancy is suspected.

cisplatin (cis-platinum, CDDP)
Platamine‡, Platinol, Platinol AQ

Pregnancy Risk Category: D

HOW SUPPLIED
Injection: 0.5 mg/ml†, 1 mg/ml

ACTION
Unknown. Probably cross-links strands of cellular DNA and interferes with RNA transcription, causing an imbal-

ance of growth that leads to cell death. Cell cycle-nonspecific.

ONSET, PEAK, DURATION
Onset and peak undefined. Effects persist for several days after administration.

INDICATIONS & DOSAGE
Adjunctive therapy in metastatic testicular cancer—
Adults: 20 mg/m^2 I.V. daily for 5 days. Repeated q 3 weeks for three cycles or longer.
Adjunctive therapy in metastatic ovarian cancer—
Adults: 100 mg/m^2 I.V.; repeated q 4 weeks. Or 75 to 100 mg/m^2 I.V. once q 4 weeks in combination with cyclophosphamide.
Advanced bladder cancer—
Adults: 50 to 70 mg/m^2 I.V. q 3 to 4 weeks. Patients who have received other antineoplastic agents or radiation therapy should receive 50 mg/m^2 q 4 weeks.
Note: Prehydration and mannitol diuresis may reduce renal toxicity and ototoxicity significantly.

ADVERSE REACTIONS
CNS: *peripheral neuritis,* loss of taste, *seizures.*
EENT: *tinnitus, hearing loss, ototoxicity,* vestibular toxicity, optic neuritis, papilledema, cerebral blindness, blurred vision.
GI: *nausea, vomiting* (beginning 1 to 4 hours after dose and lasting 24 hours).
GU: more prolonged and SEVERE RENAL TOXICITY with repeated courses of therapy.
Hematologic: MYELOSUPPRESSION; *leukopenia, thrombocytopenia, anemia;* nadirs in circulating platelet and WBC counts on days 18 to 23, with recovery by day 39.
Other: *anaphylactoid reaction, hypomagnesemia,* hypokalemia, hypocalcemia, hyponatremia, hypophosphatemia, hyperuricemia.

INTERACTIONS
Aminoglycoside antibiotics: additive nephrotoxicity. Monitor renal function studies very carefully.
umetanide, ethacrynic acid, furosemide: additive ototoxicity. Avoid concomitant use.
Phenytoin: decreased serum phenytoin levels. Monitor serum levels.

EFFECTS ON DIAGNOSTIC TESTS
Drug may increase BUN, serum creatinine, and serum uric acid levels. It may decrease creatinine clearance, serum calcium, magnesium, phosphate, and potassium levels, indicating nephrotoxicity.

CONTRAINDICATIONS
Contraindicated in patients with hypersensitivity to the drug or to other platinum-containing compounds and in those with severe renal disease, hearing impairment, or myelosuppression.

NURSING CONSIDERATIONS
● Use cautiously in patients previously treated with radiation or cytotoxic agents, in those with preexisting peripheral neuropathies, and with other ototoxic and nephrotoxic drugs.
● Monitor CBC, electrolyte levels (especially potassium and magnesium), platelet count, and renal function studies before initial and subsequent dosages, as ordered.
● To detect hearing loss, perform audiometry before initial dosage and subsequent courses, as ordered.
● Administer mannitol at 12.5-g I.V. bolus before starting cisplatin infusion, as ordered. Follow, if ordered, by infusion of mannitol at rate of up to 10 g/hour p.r.n. to maintain urine output during and 6 to 24 hours after cisplatin infusion.
● Hydrate patient with 0.9% sodium chloride solution before giving drug, as ordered. Maintain urine output of at least 100 ml/hour for 4 consecutive hours before therapy and for 24 hours after therapy.

---

*Liquid contains alcohol.   **May contain tartrazine.   †Canada only.   ‡Australia only.   ◊ OTC.

• Follow institutional policy to reduce risks because preparation and administration of parenteral form of this drug is associated with carcinogenic, mutagenic, and teratogenic risks for personnel.

• **I.V. use:** Reconstitute powder using sterile water for injection. Add 10 ml to the 10-mg vial or 50 ml to the 50-mg vial to make a solution containing 1 mg/ml. If necessary, further dilute with dextrose 5% in 0.3% sodium chloride injection or dextrose 5% in 0.45% sodium chloride injection. Solutions are stable for 20 hours at room temperature. Don't refrigerate.

• Keep in mind that infusions are most stable in chloride-containing solutions (such as 0.9% sodium chloride, 0.45% sodium chloride, and 0.22% sodium chloride).

• Be aware that the manufacturer recommends administering the drug as an I.V. infusion in 2 liters of 0.9% sodium chloride solution with 37.5 g of mannitol over 6 to 8 hours.

• Do not use needles or I.V. administration sets that contain aluminum because it will displace the platinum, causing a loss of potency and formation of a black precipitate.

• Know that therapeutic effects are often accompanied by toxicity.

• Check current protocol. Some clinicians use I.V. sodium thiosulfate to minimize toxicity.

• Administer antiemetics, as ordered. Nausea and vomiting may be severe and protracted. Monitor intake and output. Continue I.V. hydration until patient can tolerate adequate oral intake.

• Keep in mind that ondansetron, granisetron, or high-dose metoclopramide has been used very effectively to treat and prevent nausea and vomiting. Some clinicians combine metoclopramide with dexamethasone and antihistamines, or ondansetron or granisetron with dexamethasone.

• Be alert that delayed-onset vomiting (3 to 5 days after treatment) has been reported. Patients may need prolonged antiemetic treatment.

• Know that renal toxicity is cumulative. Renal function must return to normal before next dose can be given.

• Know that dosage should not be repeated unless platelet count is over 100,000/mm^3, WBC count is over 4,000/mm^3, creatinine level is under 1.5 mg/dl, or BUN level is under 25 mg/dl.

• To prevent bleeding, avoid all I.M. injections when platelet counts are below 100,000/mm^3.

• Anticipate blood transfusions during treatment because of cumulative anemia.

• To prevent hypokalemia, know that potassium chloride (10 to 20 mEq/L) is frequently added to I.V. fluids before and after cisplatin therapy.

Alert: Immediately administer epinephrine, corticosteroids, or antihistamines for anaphylactoid reactions, as ordered.

☑ **PATIENT TEACHING**
• Advise patient to watch for signs of infection (fever, sore throat, fatigue) and bleeding (easy bruising, nosebleeds, bleeding gums, melena). Tell patient to take temperature daily.

• Tell patient to report tinnitus or numbness in hands or feet immediately.

• Instruct patient to avoid any OTC products containing aspirin.

• Advise breast-feeding patient taking this drug to discontinue breast-feeding because of the possibility of infant toxicity.

• Advise women of childbearing age to avoid becoming pregnant during therapy. Also recommend consulting with doctor before becoming pregnant.

cyclophosphamide
Cycoblastin‡, Cytoxan**, Cytoxan Lyophilized, Endoxan-Asta‡, Neosar, Procytox†

Pregnancy Risk Category: D

HOW SUPPLIED
Tablets: 25 mg, 50 mg
Injection: 100-mg, 200-mg, 500-mg,
1-g, 2-g vials

ACTION
Cross-links strands of cellular DNA and
interferes with RNA transcription, causing an imbalance of growth that leads to
cell death. Cell cycle-nonspecific.

ONSET, PEAK, DURATION
Undefined.

INDICATIONS & DOSAGE
*Breast and ovarian cancers; Hodgkin's
disease; chronic lymphocytic leukemia;
chronic myelocytic leukemia; acute lymphoblastic leukemia; acute myelocytic
and monocytic leukemia; neuroblastoma; retinoblastoma; malignant lymphoma; multiple myeloma; mycosis fungoides; sarcoma—*
Adults and children: initially, 40 to 50
mg/kg I.V. in divided doses over 2 to 5
days. Alternatively, 10 to 15 mg/kg I.V.
q 7 to 10 days, 3 to 5 mg/kg I.V. twice
weekly, or 1 to 5 mg/kg P.O. daily, depending on patient tolerance. Subsequent dosages adjusted according to evidence of antitumor activity or leukopenia.
*"Minimal change" nephrotic syndrome
in children—*
Children: 2.5 to 3 mg/kg P.O. daily for
60 to 90 days.

ADVERSE REACTIONS
CV: *cardiotoxicity* (with very high doses and in combination with doxorubicin).
GI: anorexia, *nausea and vomiting* (beginning within 6 hours), abdominal
pain, stomatitis, mucositis.
GU: HEMORRHAGIC CYSTITIS, fertility
impairment.
Hematologic: *leukopenia,* nadir between days 8 to 15, recovery in 17 to 28
days; *thrombocytopenia; anemia.*
Respiratory: *pulmonary fibrosis* (high
doses).

Skin: *reversible alopecia,* rash, pigmentation, nail changes.
Other: *secondary malignant disease,
anaphylaxis,* hypersensitivity reactions,
hepatotoxicity.

INTERACTIONS
Barbiturates: increased pharmacologic
effect and enhanced cyclophosphamide
toxicity due to induction of hepatic enzymes. Monitor patient closely.
Cardiotoxic drugs: additive adverse cardiac effects. Monitor for toxicity.
Chloramphenicol, corticosteroids: reduced activity of cyclophosphamide.
Use cautiously.
Digoxin: may decrease serum digoxin
levels. Monitor levels closely.
Succinylcholine: prolonged neuromuscular blockade. Don't use together.

EFFECTS ON DIAGNOSTIC TESTS
Drug may suppress positive reaction to
Candida, mumps , triciphyton, and tuberculin TB skin test. A false-positive
result for the Papanicolaou test may occur. Drug therapy may also increase
serum uric acid levels and decrease
serum pseudocholinesterase levels.

CONTRAINDICATIONS
Contraindicated in patients with hypersensitivity to the drug or with severe
bone marrow suppression.

NURSING CONSIDERATIONS
● Use cautiously in patients with
leukopenia, thrombocytopenia, malignant cell infiltration of bone marrow, or
hepatic or renal disease and in those
who have recently undergone radiation
therapy or chemotherapy.
● Follow institutional policy to reduce
risks. Preparation and administration of
parenteral form of this drug is associated with carcinogenic, mutagenic, and
teratogenic risks for personnel.
● **I.V. use:** Reconstitute powder using
sterile water for injection or bacteriostatic water for injection containing only
parabens. For the nonlyophilized prod-

---

*Liquid contains alcohol.   **May contain tartrazine.   †Canada only.   ‡Australia only.   ◇OTC.

uct, add 5 ml to the 100-mg vial, 10 ml
to the 200-mg vial, 25 ml to the 500-mg
vial, 50 ml to the 1-g vial, or 100 ml to
the 2-g vial to produce a solution containing 20 mg/ml. Shake to dissolve;
this may take up to 6 minutes, and it
may be difficult to completely dissolve
drug. Lyophilized preparation is much
easier to reconstitute; check package insert for quantity of diluent needed to reconstitute drug.
● After reconstitution, administer as ordered by direct I.V. injection or infusion. For I.V. infusion, further dilute
with D₅W, dextrose 5% in 0.9% sodium
chloride injection, dextrose 5% in
Ringer's injection, lactated Ringer's injection, sodium lactate injection, or
0.45% sodium chloride injection.
● Check reconstituted solution for small
particles. Filter solution if necessary.
● Know that reconstituted solution is
stable for 6 days refrigerated or 24
hours at room temperature. However,
use stored solutions cautiously because
the drug contains no preservatives.
● Don't give the drug at bedtime; infrequent urination during the night may increase the possibility of cystitis. If cystitis occurs, discontinue drug and notify
doctor. Cystitis can occur months after
therapy ceases. Mesna may be given to
lower the incidence and severity of
bladder toxicity.
● Monitor CBC and renal and liver
function tests, as ordered.
● Monitor serum uric acid level, as ordered. To prevent hyperuricemia with
resulting uric acid nephropathy, know
that allopurinol may be used with adequate hydration.
Alert: Monitor for cyclophosphamide
toxicity if patient's corticosteroid therapy is discontinued.
● To prevent bleeding, avoid all I.M. injections when platelet count is below
100,000/mm³.
● Anticipate possible blood transfusions
because of cumulative anemia.
● Know that therapeutic effects are often accompanied by toxicity.

☑ **PATIENT TEACHING**
● Warn patient that alopecia is likely to
occur but that it is reversible.
● Advise patient to watch for signs of
infection (fever, sore throat, fatigue) and
bleeding (easy bruising, nosebleeds,
bleeding gums, melena). Tell patient to
take temperature daily.
● Instruct patient to avoid OTC products
containing aspirin.
● To minimize the risk of hemorrhagic
cystitis, encourage patient to void every
1 to 2 hours while awake and to drink at
least 3 liters of fluid daily. If patient is
taking oral form of drug, instruct him to
avoid taking it at bedtime because infrequent urination increases risk of cystitis.
● Advise male and female patients to
practice contraception while taking this
drug and for 4 months after; drug is potentially teratogenic.
● Advise breast-feeding patient taking
this drug to discontinue breast-feeding
because of the possibility of infant toxicity.
● Drug can cause irreversible sterility in
both male and female patients. Counsel
patients of childbearing potential before
initiating therapy. Also recommend female patient consults with doctor before
becoming pregnant.

ifosfamide
IFEX

Pregnancy Risk Category: D

HOW SUPPLIED
Injection: 1 g, 2 g†, 3 g

ACTION
Cross-links strands of cellular DNA and
interferes with RNA transcription, causing an imbalance of growth that leads to
cell death. Cell cycle-nonspecific.

ONSET, PEAK, DURATION
Undefined.

INDICATIONS & DOSAGE
Testicular cancer—
Adults: 1.2 g/m^2/day I.V. for 5 consecutive days. Treatment is repeated q 3 weeks or after the patient recovers from hematologic toxicity.

ADVERSE REACTIONS
CNS: *somnolence, confusion,* **coma, seizures,** *ataxia, hallucinations, depressive psychosis, dizziness, disorientation, cranial nerve dysfunction.*
GI: *nausea, vomiting.*
GU: *hemorrhagic cystitis, hematuria, nephrotoxicity.*
Hematologic: *leukopenia, thrombocytopenia, myelosuppression.*
Hepatic: elevated liver enzyme levels, liver dysfunction.
Other: *alopecia, metabolic acidosis,* infection, phlebitis.

INTERACTIONS
Allopurinol: may produce excessive ifosfamide effect by prolonging half-life. Monitor for enhanced toxicity.
Anticoagulants, aspirin: increased risk of bleeding. Avoid concomitant use.
Barbiturates, chloral hydrate, phenytoin: may increase ifosfamide toxicity by inducing hepatic enzymes that hasten the formation of toxic metabolites. Monitor patient closely.
Corticosteroids: may inhibit hepatic enzymes, reducing ifosfamide's effect. Monitor for enhanced ifosfamide toxicity if concurrent steroid dosage is suddenly reduced or discontinued.
Myelosuppressants: enhanced hematologic toxicity. Dosage adjustment may be necessary.

EFFECTS ON DIAGNOSTIC TESTS
Drug therapy may increase serum levels of AST, ALT, bilirubin, lactic dehydrogenase, creatinine, BUN, and alkaline phosphatase.

CONTRAINDICATIONS
Contraindicated in patients with hypersensitivity to the drug and in those with severe bone marrow suppression.

NURSING CONSIDERATIONS
● Use cautiously in patients with renal impairment or compromised bone marrow reserve as indicated by leukopenia, granulocytopenia, extensive bone marrow metastases, prior radiation therapy, or prior therapy with cytotoxic agents.
● Administer antiemetics, as ordered, before giving ifosfamide to help decrease nausea.
● Follow institutional policy to reduce risks. Preparation and administration of parenteral form of this drug is associated with carcinogenic, mutagenic, and teratogenic risks for personnel.
● **I.V. use:** Reconstitute each gram of drug with 20 ml of diluent to yield a solution of 50 mg/ml. Use sterile water for injection or bacteriostatic water for injection. Solutions may then be further diluted with sterile water, dextrose 2.5% or 5% in water, 0.45% or 0.9% sodium chloride for injection, 5% dextrose and 0.9% sodium chloride for injection, or lactated Ringer's injection.
● Infuse each dose over at least 30 minutes.
● As ordered, administer ifosfamide with a protecting agent (mesna) to prevent hemorrhagic cystitis. Obtain urinalysis before each dose. If microscopic hematuria is present, mesna must be given concomitantly with or before ifosfamide to prevent cystitis. (Dosage adjustments of mesna given concomitantly may be necessary.) Adequate fluid intake (2 liters/day, either P.O. or I.V.) is essential before and 72 hours after therapy.
● Assess patients for mental status changes; dosage may have to be decreased.
● Know that ifosfamide and mesna are physically compatible and may be mixed in the same I.V. solution.
● Keep in mind that reconstituted solution is stable for 1 week at room temperature or 6 weeks if refrigerated. However, use solution within 6 hours if

drug was reconstituted with sterile water without a preservative (such as benzyl alcohol or parabens).
● Don't give the drug at bedtime; infrequent voiding during the night may increase the possibility of cystitis. If cystitis develops, discontinue drug and notify doctor.
● Be aware that bladder irrigation with 0.9% sodium chloride solution may decrease the possibility of cystitis.
● Monitor CBC and renal and liver function tests, as ordered.
● To prevent bleeding, avoid all I.M. injections when platelet count is below 100,000/mm^3.
● Anticipate possible blood transfusions because of cumulative anemia.

☑ **PATIENT TEACHING**
● To minimize contact of ifosfamide and its metabolites with the bladder mucosa, remind patient to void frequently.
● Advise patient to watch for signs of infection (fever, sore throat, fatigue) and bleeding (easy bruising, nosebleeds, bleeding gums, melena). Tell patient to take temperature daily.
● Instruct patient to avoid OTC products containing aspirin.
● Advise breast-feeding patient to discontinue breast-feeding during therapy because of possible infant toxicity.
● Advise women of childbearing age to avoid becoming pregnant during therapy. Also recommend consulting with doctor before becoming pregnant.

lomustine (CCNU)
CeeNU

Pregnancy Risk Category: D

HOW SUPPLIED
Capsules: 10 mg, 40 mg, 100 mg, dose pack (two 10-mg, two 40-mg, two 100-mg capsules)

ACTION
Cross-links strands of cellular DNA and

interferes with RNA transcription, causing an imbalance of growth that leads to cell death. Cell cycle-nonspecific.

ONSET, PEAK, DURATION
Undefined.

INDICATIONS & DOSAGE
Brain tumor, Hodgkin's disease—
Adults and children: 100 to 130 mg/m^2 P.O. as a single dose q 6 weeks. Dosage reduced according to degree of bone marrow suppression. Repeat doses should not be given until WBC count is more than 4,000/mm^3 and platelet count is more than 100,000/mm^3.

ADVERSE REACTIONS
CNS: disorientation, lethargy, ataxia.
GI: *nausea, vomiting,* stomatitis.
GU: nephrotoxicity, progressive azotemia, *renal failure.*
Hematologic: *anemia, leukopenia,* delayed up to 6 weeks, lasting 1 to 2 weeks; thrombocytopenia, delayed up to 4 weeks, lasting 1 to 2 weeks; *bone marrow suppression,* delayed up to 4 to 6 weeks.
Other: hepatotoxicity, *secondary malignant disease,* pulmonary fibrosis, alopecia.

INTERACTIONS
Anticoagulants, aspirin: increased risk of bleeding. Avoid concomitant use.

EFFECTS ON DIAGNOSTIC TESTS
Drug therapy may cause transient increases in liver function tests.

CONTRAINDICATIONS
Contraindicated in patients with hypersensitivity to the drug.

NURSING CONSIDERATIONS
● Use cautiously in patients with decreased platelet, WBC, or RBC counts and in those receiving other myelosuppressants.
● To avoid nausea, give antiemetic before administering, as ordered.

• Give 2 to 4 hours after meals; drug will be more completely absorbed if taken when the stomach is empty.

• Monitor CBC weekly, as ordered. Usually not administered more often than every 6 weeks; bone marrow toxicity is cumulative and delayed, usually occuring in 4 to 6 weeks after drug administration.

• Periodically monitor liver function tests, as ordered.

• To prevent bleeding, avoid all I.M. injections when platelet count is below 100,000/mm³.

• Anticipate possible blood transfusions because of cumulative anemia.

• Know that therapeutic effects are often accompanied by toxicity.

• Store capsules at room temperature. Avoid exposure to moisture and protect from temperatures above 40° C.

☑ **PATIENT TEACHING**
• Advise patient to watch for signs of infection (fever, sore throat, fatigue) and bleeding (easy bruising, nosebleeds, bleeding gums, melena). Tell patient to take temperature daily.

• Instruct patient to avoid OTC products containing aspirin.

• Advise breast-feeding patients to discontinue breast-feeding during therapy because of possible infant toxicity.

• Advise women of childbearing age to avoid becoming pregnant during therapy. Also recommend consulting with doctor before becoming pregnant.

---

mechlorethamine hydrochloride (nitrogen mustard)
Mustargen

Pregnancy Risk Category: D

HOW SUPPLIED
Injection: 10-mg vials

ACTION
Cross-links strands of cellular DNA and interferes with RNA transcription, causing an imbalance of growth that leads to cell death. Cell cycle-nonspecific.

ONSET, PEAK, DURATION
Onset occurs in seconds to minutes. Peak and duration undefined.

INDICATIONS & DOSAGE
Polycythemia vera, chronic lymphocytic leukemia, chronic myelocytic leukemia, malignant effusions (pericardial, peritoneal, pleural), mycosis fungoides, Hodgkin's disease, lymphosarcoma, bronchogenic cancer—
Adults: 0.4 mg/kg I.V. as a single dose or in divided doses of 0.1 to 0.2 mg/kg/day. Given through running I.V. infusion. Subsequent courses of therapy given when patient has recovered hematologically from previous course (usually 3 to 6 weeks).
Malignant effusions—
Adults: 0.4 mg/kg intracavitarily, although 0.2 mg/kg has been used intrapericardially.

ADVERSE REACTIONS
CNS: weakness, vertigo.
EENT: tinnitus; deafness with high doses.
GI: *nausea, vomiting,* and *anorexia* beginning within minutes, lasting 8 to 24 hours.
Hematologic: *thrombocytopenia,* lymphocytopenia, *agranulocytosis,* nadir of myelosuppression occurring by days 4 to 10 and lasting 10 to 21 days; mild anemia begins in 2 to 3 weeks.
Skin: rash, sloughing, severe irritation if drug extravasates or touches skin.
Other: *alopecia,* precipitation of herpes zoster, *anaphylaxis, secondary malignant disease,* hyperuricemia; *thrombophlebitis,* amyloidosis, jaundice, menstrual irregularities, impaired spermatogenesis.

INTERACTIONS
Anticoagulants, aspirin: increased risk of bleeding. Avoid concomitant use.

EFFECTS ON DIAGNOSTIC TESTS
Drug therapy increases blood and urine uric acid levels. Renal, hepatic, and bone marrow function abnormalities have been reported.

CONTRAINDICATIONS
Contraindicated in patients with hypersensitivity to the drug and with known infectious diseases.

NURSING CONSIDERATIONS
• Use cautiously in patients with severe anemia, depressed neutrophil or platelet count, or in those who have recently undergone radiation therapy or chemotherapy. Monitor CBC.
• Follow institutional policy to reduce risks. Preparation and administration of parenteral form of this drug is associated with carcinogenic, mutagenic, and teratogenic risks for personnel.
• **I.V. use:** Reconstitute the drug using 10 ml of sterile water for injection or 0.9% sodium chloride injection. The resulting solution contains 1 mg/ml of mechlorethamine. Give by direct injection into a vein or into the tubing of a free-flowing I.V. solution.
• Prepare immediately before infusion. Very unstable solution. Visually inspect before using; use within 15 minutes, and discard unused solution.
• Dispose of any equipment used in the preparation and administration of mechlorethamine properly and according to institutional policy. Neutralize unused solution with an equal volume of 5% sodium bicarbonate and 5% sodium thiosulfate for 45 minutes.
Alert: Make sure I.V. solution doesn't infiltrate. Mechlorethamine is a potent vesicant. If drug extravasates, apply cold compresses and infiltrate the area with isotonic sodium thiosulfate, as ordered.
• When given intracavitarily for sclerosing effect, dilute using up to 100 ml of 0.9% sodium chloride for injection. Turn patient from side to side every 15 minutes to 1 hour to distribute drug.

• Monitor serum uric acid level, as ordered. To prevent hyperuricemia with resulting uric acid nephropathy, know that mechlorethamine may be used with adequate hydration.
• Know that therapeutic effects are often accompanied by toxicity.
• Be aware that neurotoxicity increases with dose and patient age.
• To prevent bleeding, avoid all I.M. injections when platelet count is below 100,000/mm^3.
• Anticipate possible blood transfusions because of cumulative anemia.

☑ **PATIENT TEACHING**
• Advise patient to watch for signs of infection (fever, sore throat, fatigue) and bleeding (easy bruising, nosebleeds, bleeding gums, melena). Tell patient to take temperature daily.
• Instruct patient to avoid OTC products containing aspirin.
• Advise women of childbearing age to avoid becoming pregnant during therapy. Suggest consulting with doctor before becoming pregnant.
• Advise breast-feeding patient taking this drug to discontinue breastfeeding because of the possibility of infant toxicity.

melphalan (L-phenylalanine mustard)
Alkeran

Pregnancy Risk Category: D

HOW SUPPLIED
Tablets (scored): 2 mg
Injection: 50 mg

ACTION
Cross-links strands of cellular DNA and interferes with RNA transcription, causing an imbalance of growth that leads to cell death. Cell cycle-nonspecific.

ONSET, PEAK, DURATION
Undefined.

INDICATIONS & DOSAGE

Multiple myeloma—
Adults: initially, 6 mg P.O. daily for 2 to 3 weeks; then drug is stopped for up to 4 weeks or until WBC and platelet counts stop dropping and begin to rise again; maintenance dosage of 2 mg daily then given. Alternative therapy: 0.15 mg/kg P.O. daily for 7 days, or 0.25 mg/kg for 4 days; repeated q 4 to 6 weeks.

Alternatively, administered I.V. to patients who can't tolerate oral therapy. 16 mg/m^2 given by infusion over 15 to 20 minutes at 2-week intervals for four doses. After patient has recovered from toxicity, drug given at 4-week intervals. Dose reduction of up to 50% should be considered in patients with renal insufficiency.

Nonresectable advanced ovarian cancer—
Adults: 0.2 mg/kg P.O. daily for 5 days. Repeated q 4 to 6 weeks, depending on bone marrow recovery.

ADVERSE REACTIONS

CV: hypotension, tachycardia, edema.
GI: nausea, vomiting, diarrhea, oral ulceration.
Hematologic: *thrombocytopenia, leukopenia, bone marrow suppression,* hemolytic anemia.
Respiratory: *pneumonitis, pulmonary fibrosis,* dyspnea, bronchospasm.
Skin: pruritus, alopecia, urticaria, ulceration at injection site.
Other: *anaphylaxis,* hypersensitivity, hepatotoxicity.

INTERACTIONS

Anticoagulants, aspirin: increased risk of bleeding. Avoid concomitant use.
Antigout agents: decreased effectiveness. Dosage adjustments may be necessary.
Bone marrow suppressants: additive toxicity. Monitor closely.
Cyclosporine: severe renal failure may occur. Monitor closely.
Vaccines: decreased effectiveness of killed-virus vaccines and increased risk

of toxicity from live-virus vaccines. Postpone routine immunization for at least 3 months after last dose of melphalan.

EFFECTS ON DIAGNOSTIC TESTS

Drug therapy may increase blood and urine levels of uric acid.

CONTRAINDICATIONS

Contraindicated in patients with hypersensitivity to the drug and in those whose disease is known to be resistant to the drug. Patients hypersensitive to chlorambucil may have cross-sensitivity to melphalan.

NURSING CONSIDERATIONS

● Be aware that drug is not recommended in patients with severe leukopenia, thrombocytopenia, or anemia or in those with chronic lymphocytic leukemia. Use cautiously in patients receiving concurrent radiation and chemotherapy.
● Keep in mind that dosage may need to be reduced in patients with renal impairment.
● Know that melphalan is the drug of choice in combination with prednisone in patients with multiple myeloma.
● Follow institutional policy to reduce risks. Preparation and administration of parenteral form of the drug is associated with carcinogenic, mutagenic, and teratogenic risks for personnel.
● **I.V. use:** Because drug isn't stable in solution, reconstitute immediately before administering with the 10 ml of sterile diluent supplied by the manufacturer. Shake vigorously until a solution is clear. The resultant solution will contain 5 mg/ml of melphalan. Immediately dilute the required dose in 0.9% sodium chloride for injection. Final concentration shouldn't exceed 0.45 mg/ml. Give infusion over 15 to 20 minutes.
● Promptly dilute and administer; the reconstituted product begins to degrade within 30 minutes. After final dilution, nearly 1% of the drug degrades every 10 minutes. Don't refrigerate the reconsti-

tuted product because a precipitate will form.
• Give oral form on empty stomach. Food decreases drug absorption.
• Monitor serum uric acid level and CBC, as ordered.
• To prevent bleeding, avoid all I.M. injections when platelet count is below 100,000/mm³.
• Anticipate possible blood transfusions because of cumulative anemia.

☑ **PATIENT TEACHING**
• Advise patient to watch for signs of infection (fever, sore throat, fatigue) and bleeding (easy bruising, nosebleeds, bleeding gums, melena). Tell patient to take temperature daily.
• Instruct patient to avoid OTC products containing aspirin.
• Advise women of childbearing age to avoid becoming pregnant during therapy. Suggest consulting with the doctor before becoming pregnant.
• Advise breast-feeding patient taking this drug to discontinue breast-feeding because of the possibility of infant toxicity.

---

streptozocin
Zanosar

Pregnancy Risk Category: C

HOW SUPPLIED
Injection: 1-g vials

ACTION
Unknown. Probably cross-links strands of cellular DNA and interferes with RNA transcription, causing an imbalance of growth that leads to cell death. Cell cycle-nonspecific.

ONSET, PEAK, DURATION
Undefined.

INDICATIONS & DOSAGE
Metastatic islet cell carcinoma of the pancreas—

Adults and children: 500 mg/m² I.V. for 5 consecutive days q 6 weeks until maximum benefit or toxicity is observed. Alternatively, 1,000 mg/m² at weekly intervals for the first 2 weeks. Not to exceed a single dose of 1,500 mg/m².

ADVERSE REACTIONS
CNS: confusion, lethargy, depression.
GI: *nausea, vomiting,* diarrhea.
GU: *renal toxicity* (evidenced by azotemia, glycosuria, and renal tubular acidosis), mild proteinuria.
Hematologic: *anemia, leukopenia, thrombocytopenia.*
Hepatic: elevated liver enzyme levels, jaundice, *liver dysfunction.*
Other: hyperglycemia, hypoglycemia, diabetes mellitus.

INTERACTIONS
Doxorubicin: prolonged elimination half-life of doxorubicin. Dose of doxorubicin should be reduced.
Other potentially nephrotoxic drugs, such as aminoglycosides: increased risk of renal toxicity. Use cautiously.
Phenytoin: may decrease effectiveness of streptozocin in patients with pancreatic cancer. Monitor carefully.

EFFECTS ON DIAGNOSTIC TESTS
Drug therapy may decrease serum albumin and increase liver function test values; these increases are a sign of hepatotoxicity. BUN and serum creatinine levels may be increased, indicating nephrotoxicity. Drug may decrease blood glucose levels because of a sudden release of insulin.

CONTRAINDICATIONS
None known.

NURSING CONSIDERATIONS
• Use cautiously in patients with renal disease.
• Obtain renal function tests before therapy, as ordered.

• Follow institutional policy to reduce risks. Preparation and administration of parenteral form of this drug is associated with carcinogenic, mutagenic, and teratogenic risks for personnel.

• **I.V. use:** Reconstitute streptozocin powder with 9.5 ml of D$_5$W or 0.9% sodium chloride for injection. This will produce a pale gold solution. May be further diluted with D$_5$W or 0.9% sodium chloride for injection. Infuse over at least 15 minutes to minimize the risk of phlebitis.

Alert: If extravasation occurs, stop infusion at once and notify doctor.

• Use within 12 hours of reconstitution. The product contains no preservatives and is not intended as a multiple-dose vial.

• Monitor renal function tests after each course of therapy, as ordered. Renal toxicity resulting from streptozocin therapy is dose-related and cumulative. Urinalysis; BUN, creatinine, and serum electrolyte levels; and creatinine clearance should be obtained at least weekly during drug therapy. Weekly monitoring should continue for 4 weeks after each course.

• Test urine for protein and glucose levels each nursing shift. Mild proteinuria is one of the first signs of renal toxicity; notify the doctor, who may reduce the dosage.

• Monitor CBC and liver function studies at least weekly, as ordered.

• Make sure patients are being treated with an antiemetic. Nausea and vomiting occur in most patients.

• Know that therapeutic effects are often accompanied by toxicity.

☑ **PATIENT TEACHING**
• Advise patient to watch for signs of infection (fever, sore throat, fatigue) and bleeding (easy bruising, nosebleeds, bleeding gums, melena). Tell patient to take temperature daily.

• Advise breast-feeding patient taking drug to discontinue breast-feeding due to the possibility of infant toxicity.

thiotepa (TESPA, triethylenethiophosphoramide, TSPA)
Thioplex

Pregnancy Risk Category: D

HOW SUPPLIED
Injection: 15-mg vials

ACTION
Cross-links strands of cellular DNA and interferes with RNA transcription, causing an imbalance of growth that leads to cell death. Cell cycle-nonspecific.

ONSET, PEAK, DURATION
Undefined.

INDICATIONS & DOSAGE
Breast and ovarian cancers, lymphoma, Hodgkin's disease—
Adults and children over 12 years: 0.3 to 0.4 mg/kg I.V. q 1 to 4 weeks or 0.2 mg/kg for 4 to 5 days at intervals of 2 to 4 weeks.
Bladder tumor—
Adults and children over 12 years: 60 mg in 30 to 60 ml of sterile water instilled in bladder for 2 hours once weekly for 4 weeks.
Neoplastic effusions—
Adults and children over 12 years: 0.6 to 0.8 mg/kg intracavitarily.

ADVERSE REACTIONS
CNS: headache, dizziness, fatigue, weakness.
EENT: blurred vision, laryngeal edema, conjunctivitis.
GI: *nausea, vomiting,* abdominal pain, anorexia.
GU: amenorrhea, decreased spermatogenesis, dysuria, urine retention, hemorrhagic cystitis.
Hematologic: *leukopenia* begins within 5 to 10 days; *thrombocytopenia; neutropenia; anemia.*
Respiratory: asthma.
Skin: hives, rash, dermatitis.

Other: fever, alopecia, hypersensitivity, *anaphylactic shock.*

INTERACTIONS
Anticoagulants, aspirin: increased risk of bleeding. Avoid concomitant use.
Neuromuscular blocking agents: may prolong muscular paralysis.
Alert: Succinylcholine: increased apnea with concomitant use.

EFFECTS ON DIAGNOSTIC TESTS
Drug therapy may increase blood and urine levels of uric acid and decrease plasma pseudocholinesterase concentrations.

CONTRAINDICATIONS
Contraindicated in patients with hypersensitivity to the drug and in those with severe bone marrow, hepatic, or renal dysfunction.

NURSING CONSIDERATIONS
● Know that use in pregnancy is not recommended except in situations where the benefits outweigh the risk of teratogenicity involved.
● Use cautiously in patients with mild bone marrow suppression and renal or hepatic dysfunction.
● Follow institutional policy to minimize risks. Preparation and administration of parenteral form of this drug is linked with mutagenic, teratogenic, and carcinogenic risks to personnel.
● I.V. use: Reconstitute with 1.5 ml of sterile water for injection. Do not reconstitute with any other solution. Further dilute with 0.9% sodium chloride for injection, D₅W, dextrose 5% in 0.9% sodium chloride for injection, Ringer's injection, or lactated Ringer's injection. Solutions are stable for up to 5 days if refrigerated.
● If pain occurs at insertion site, dilute the drug further or use a local anesthetic, as ordered, to reduce pain. Make sure drug does not infiltrate.
● Discard if solution appears grossly opaque or has a precipitate. Solutions

should be clear to slightly opaque. To eliminate haze, filter solutions through a 0.22-micron filter before administration.
● For bladder instillation: Dehydrate patients 8 to 10 hours before therapy. Instill drug into bladder by catheter; ask patients to retain solution for 2 hours. Know that volume may be reduced to 30 ml if discomfort is too great with 60 ml. Reposition patients every 15 minutes for maximum area contact.
● Monitor CBC weekly for at least 3 weeks after last dose, as ordered.
● Know that drug should be discontinued if WBC count is below 3,000/mm³ or if platelet count is below 150,000/mm³. If that occurs, notify doctor.
● Monitor serum uric acid levels, as ordered. To prevent hyperuricemia with resulting uric acid nephropathy, know that allopurinol may be used with adequate hydration.
● Know that therapeutic effects are often accompanied by toxicity.
● To prevent bleeding, avoid all I.M. injections when platelet count is below 100,000/mm³.
● Anticipate blood transfusions because of cumulative anemia.
● Refrigerate and protect dry powder from direct sunlight to avoid possible drug breakdown.

☑ **PATIENT TEACHING**
● Advise patient to watch for signs of infection (fever, sore throat, fatigue) and bleeding (easy bruising, nosebleeds, bleeding gums, melena). Tell patient to take temperature daily. Tell patients to report even mild infections.
● Instruct patient to avoid OTC products containing aspirin.
● Advise breast-feeding patient to stop breast-feeding during therapy because of possible infant toxicity.
● Advise women of childbearing age to avoid becoming pregnant during therapy. Suggest consulting with doctor before becoming pregnant.

Reactions may be *common,* uncommon, *life-threatening,* or COMMON AND LIFE-THREATENING.

uracil mustard
Uracil Mustard Capsules**

Pregnancy Risk Category: D

HOW SUPPLIED
Capsules: 1 mg

ACTION
Cross-links strands of cellular DNA and interferes with RNA transcription, causing an imbalance of growth that leads to cell death. Cell cycle-nonspecific.

ONSET, PEAK, DURATION
Undefined.

INDICATIONS & DOSAGE
Chronic lymphocytic and myelocytic leukemia, Hodgkin's disease, malignant lymphoma of the histiocytic and lymphocytic types, reticulum cell sarcoma, mycosis fungoides, polycythemia vera—
Adults: 0.15 mg/kg P.O. as a single dose weekly for 4 weeks. If response occurs, weekly administration may continue. Alternatively, 1 to 2 mg P.O. daily for 3 months or until desired response or toxicity; maintenance dosage is 1 mg daily for 3 out of 4 weeks until optimum response or relapse; or 3 to 5 mg P.O. for 7 days, not to exceed total dosage of 0.5 mg/kg, then 1 mg daily until response, and then 1 mg daily for 3 to 4 weeks.
Children: 0.3 mg/kg P.O. as a single dose weekly for four weeks. If response occurs, weekly administration may continue.

ADVERSE REACTIONS
CNS: irritability, nervousness, depression.
GI: *nausea, vomiting, diarrhea.*
Hematologic: bone marrow suppression, delayed 2 to 4 weeks; ***thrombocytopenia; leukopenia; anemia.***
Skin: pruritus, dermatitis.
Other: fertility impairment, hepatotoxicity, amenorrhea, azoospermia.

INTERACTIONS
Anticoagulants, aspirin: increased risk of bleeding. Avoid concomitant use.

EFFECTS ON DIAGNOSTIC TESTS
Drug therapy may increase blood and urine levels of uric acid.

CONTRAINDICATIONS
Contraindicated in patients with hypersensitivity to the drug and in those with aplastic anemia, thrombocytopenia, or leukopenia.

NURSING CONSIDERATIONS
● Monitor platelet count. Check CBC once or twice weekly for 4 weeks; then 4 weeks after stopping drug, as ordered.
● Monitor serum uric acid level, as ordered. To prevent hyperuricemia and resulting uric acid nephropathy, know that allopurinol may be used with adequate hydration.
● Know that therapeutic effects are often accompanied by toxicity.
● To prevent bleeding, avoid all I.M. injections when platelet count is below 100,000/mm³.
● Anticipate possible blood transfusions because of cumulative anemia.

☑ PATIENT TEACHING
● Instruct patient to take drug at bedtime to minimize nausea.
● Advise patient to watch for signs of infection (fever, sore throat, fatigue) and bleeding (easy bruising, nosebleeds, bleeding gums, melena). Tell patient to take temperature daily.
● Instruct patients to avoid OTC products containing aspirin.
● Advise breast-feeding patients to stop breast-feeding during therapy because of possible infant toxicity.
● Advise women of childbearing age to avoid becoming pregnant during therapy. Suggest consulting with doctor before becoming pregnant. Drug should not be used in pregnancy unless potential benefits outweigh potential risks.

---

*Liquid contains alcohol.   **May contain tartrazine.   †Canada only.   ‡Australia only.   ◊OTC.

70

Antimetabolites

cladribine
cytarabine
floxuridine
fludarabine phosphate
fluorouracil
hydroxyurea
mercaptopurine
methotrexate
methotrexate sodium
thioguanine

COMBINATION PRODUCTS
None.

---

cladribine
(2-chlorodeoxyadenosine,
CdA)
Leustatin

Pregnancy Risk Category: D

HOW SUPPLIED
Injection: 1 mg/ml, 10-mg vial, preservative-free

ACTION
Unknown. A purine nucleoside analogue that enters tumor cells, is phosphorylated by deoxycytidine kinase, and is subsequently converted into an active triphosphate deoxynucleotide. This metabolite probably impairs synthesis of new DNA, inhibits repair of existing DNA, and disrupts cellular metabolism.

ONSET, PEAK, DURATION
Onset has a median time of approximately 4 months to response. Peak undefined. Median duration of response is greater than 8 months.

INDICATIONS & DOSAGE
Active hairy cell leukemia—
Adults: 0.09 mg/kg daily by continuous I.V. infusion for 7 days.

ADVERSE REACTIONS
CNS: *headache, fatigue,* dizziness, insomnia, asthenia.
CV: tachycardia, edema.
EENT: epistaxis.
GI: *nausea, decreased appetite, vomiting, diarrhea,* constipation, abdominal pain.
Hematologic: NEUTROPENIA, *anemia, thrombocytopenia.*
Respiratory: *abnormal breath or chest sounds, cough,* shortness of breath.
Skin: *rash, pruritus, erythema, purpura,* petechiae.
Other: *fever,* INFECTION, *local reaction at the injection site, chills, diaphoresis, malaise, trunk pain, myalgia, arthralgia,* hyperuricemia.

INTERACTIONS
None significant.

EFFECTS ON DIAGNOSTIC TESTS
Drug frequently alters hematologic studies because of its suppressive effect on bone marrow. It may increase blood and urine concentrations of uric acid.

CONTRAINDICATIONS
Contraindicated in patients hypersensitive to the drug.

NURSING CONSIDERATIONS
● Use cautiously in patients with renal or hepatic impairment.
● I.V. use: For a 24-hour infusion, add the calculated dose to a 500-ml infusion bag of 0.9% sodium chloride for injection. Once diluted, administer promptly or store in refrigerator for no more than 8 hours. Don't use solutions that contain dextrose because studies have shown increased degradation of the drug. Repeat preparation daily for 7 consecutive days.
Alert: Because the drug product doesn't

---

contain any bacteriostatic agents, use strict aseptic technique to prepare the daily admixture.

● Alternatively, prepare a 7-day infusion solution, using bacteriostatic sodium chloride for injection, which contains 0.9% benzyl alcohol. Studies have shown acceptable physical and chemical stability using Pharmacia Deltec medication cassettes. First, pass the calculated amount of drug through a disposable 0.22-micron hydrophilic syringe filter into a sterile infusion reservoir. Next, add sufficient bacteriostatic sodium chloride injection to bring the total volume to 100 ml. Clamp off the line; then disconnect and discard the filter. If necessary, aseptically aspirate air bubbles from the reservoir using a new filter or a sterile vent filter assembly.

● Be aware that because the calculated dose dilutes the benzyl alcohol preservative, 7-day infusion solutions prepared for patients weighing more than 187 lb (85 kg) may have reduced preservative effectiveness.

● Because of the risk of hyperuricemia from tumor lysis, administer allopurinol, as ordered, during therapy.

● Monitor hematologic function closely, as ordered, especially during the first 4 to 8 weeks of therapy. Cladribine is a toxic drug, and some toxicity is expected during treatment. Severe bone marrow suppression, including neutropenia, anemia, and thrombocytopenia, has commonly been observed in patients treated with this drug; many patients also have preexisting hematologic impairment from their disease.

● Keep in mind that fever is common during the 1st month of therapy. In clinical trials, virtually all patients received parenteral antibiotics.

● To prevent bleeding, avoid all I.M. injections when platelet count is below 100,000/mm^3.

● Anticipate possible blood transfusions because of cumulative anemia.

● Refrigerate unopened vials at 36° to 46° F (2° to 8° C) and protect from light.

Although freezing doesn't adversely affect the drug, a precipitate may form; this will disappear if the drug is allowed to warm to room temperature gradually and the vial is vigorously shaken. Don't heat or microwave; don't refreeze.

☑ **PATIENT TEACHING**
● Advise patient to watch for signs of infection (fever, sore throat, fatigue) and bleeding (easy bruising, nosebleeds, bleeding gums, melena). Tell patient to take temperature daily.
● Advise women of childbearing age to avoid becoming pregnant because of the risk of fetal malformations.
● Advise breast-feeding patient to discontinue breast-feeding during therapy because of possible infant toxicity.

cytarabine (ara-C, cytosine arabinoside)
Alexan‡, Cytosart†, Cytosar-U

Pregnancy Risk Category: D

HOW SUPPLIED
Injection: 100-mg, 500-mg, 1-g, 2-g vials

ACTION
Inhibits DNA synthesis.

ONSET, PEAK, DURATION
Onset and duration undefined. Levels peak 20 to 60 minutes after S.C. injection.

INDICATIONS & DOSAGE
Acute nonlymphocytic leukemia, acute lymphocytic leukemia, blast phase of chronic myelocytic leukemia—
Adults and children: 100 mg/m^2 daily by continuous I.V. infusion or 100 mg/m^2 I.V. q 12 hours. Given for 7 days and repeated q 2 weeks. For maintenance, 1 mg/kg S.C. once or twice a week.
Meningeal leukemia—
Adults and children: highly variable from 5 mg/m^2 to 75 mg/m^2 intrathecal-

---

ly. Frequency also varies from once a day for 4 days to once q 4 days. The most frequently used dosage is 30 mg/m², q 4 days until CSF fluid is normal, followed by one additional dose.

ADVERSE REACTIONS
CNS: neurotoxicity, malaise, dizziness, headache.
EENT: conjunctivitis.
GI: *nausea, vomiting, diarrhea, anorexia, anal ulceration,* abdominal pain; oral ulcers in 5 to 10 days; high dose given rapid I.V. may cause projectile vomiting, bowel necrosis.
GU: urine retention, renal dysfunction.
Hematologic: *leukopenia,* with initial WBC count nadir 7 to 9 days after drug is stopped and a second (more severe) nadir 15 to 24 days after drug is stopped; anemia; reticulocytopenia; *thrombocytopenia,* with platelet count nadir occurring on day 10; *megaloblastosis.*
Hepatic: *hepatotoxicity* (usually mild and reversible), jaundice.
Skin: *rash,* pruritus, alopecia.
Other: flulike syndrome, hyperuricemia, infection, *fever, thrombophlebitis,* myalgia, bone pain, *anaphylaxis,* edema.

INTERACTIONS
Digoxin: may decrease digoxin absorption. Monitor closely. Digoxin oral liquid and liquid-filled capsules may not be affected.
Flucytosine: decreased flucytosine activity.
Gentamicin: decreased activity against *Klebsiella pneumoniae.*

EFFECTS ON DIAGNOSTIC TESTS
Drug therapy may increase blood and urine levels of uric acid. It may also increase serum alkaline phosphatase, AST, and bilirubin concentrations, which indicate drug-induced hepatotoxicity.

CONTRAINDICATIONS
Contraindicated in patients hypersensitive to the drug.

NURSING CONSIDERATIONS
● Use cautiously in patients with hepatic or renal compromise, gout, or myelosuppression.
● To reduce nausea, give antiemetic before administering, as ordered. Nausea and vomiting are more frequent when large doses are administered rapidly by I.V. push. These reactions are less frequent when given by infusion.
● Follow institutional policy to reduce risks. Preparation and administration of parenteral form of this drug is associated with carcinogenic, mutagenic, and teratogenic risks for personnel.
● **I.V. use:** Reconstitute drug using the provided diluent, which is bacteriostatic water for injection containing benzyl alcohol. Avoid this diluent when preparing drug for neonates or for intrathecal use. Reconstitute 100-mg vial with 5 ml of diluent or 500-mg vial with 10 ml of diluent. Reconstituted solution is stable for 48 hours. Discard cloudy reconstituted solution.
● For I.V. infusion, further dilute using 0.9% sodium chloride for injection or D₅W.
● For intrathecal administration, use preservative-free 0.9% sodium chloride. Add 5 ml to the 100-mg vial or 10 ml to the 500-mg vial. Use immediately after reconstitution. Discard unused drug.
● Monitor fluid intake and output carefully. Maintain high fluid intake and give allopurinol, if ordered, to avoid urate nephropathy in leukemia induction therapy. Monitor serum uric acid level, as ordered.
● Monitor hepatic and renal function studies and CBC, as ordered.
● Know that therapy may be modified or stopped if granulocyte count is below 1,000/mm³ or if platelet count is below 50,000/mm³.
● Know that corticosteroid eyedrops are prescribed to prevent drug-induced keratitis.
● Provide diligent mouth care to help prevent stomatitis.
Alert: Assess patients receiving high

doses for neurotoxicity, which may first appear as nystagmus, but can progress to ataxia and cerebellar dysfunction.
● To prevent bleeding, avoid all I.M. injections when platelet count is below 100,000/mm³.
● Anticipate possible blood transfusions because of cumulative anemia.
● Know that therapeutic effects are often accompanied by toxicity.

☑ **PATIENT TEACHING**
● Advise patient to watch for signs of infection (fever, sore throat, fatigue) and bleeding (easy bruising, nosebleeds, bleeding gums, melena). Tell patients to take temperature daily.
● Advise breast-feeding patient to discontinue breast-feeding during therapy because of possible infant toxicity.
● Advise women of childbearing age to avoid becoming pregnant during therapy. Also recommend consulting with doctor before becoming pregnant. Drug may harm the fetus.

---

floxuridine
FUDR

Pregnancy Risk Category: D

HOW SUPPLIED
Powder for injection: 500 mg for reconstitution (5-ml, 10-ml vials)
Preservative-free injection: 100 mg/ml (5-ml vials)

ACTION
Inhibits DNA synthesis.

ONSET, PEAK, DURATION
Undefined.

INDICATIONS & DOSAGE
GI adenocarcinoma metastatic to the liver—
Adults: 0.1 to 0.6 mg/kg daily by intra-arterial infusion for 14 to 21 days or until toxicity occurs; or 0.4 to 0.6 mg/kg daily into hepatic artery.

ADVERSE REACTIONS
CNS: malaise, weakness, headache, lethargy, disorientation, confusion, euphoria.
CV: myocardial ischemia, angina.
EENT: blurred vision, nystagmus, photophobia, epistaxis.
GI: *anorexia, stomatitis, nausea, vomiting, diarrhea, bleeding, abdominal pain, enteritis,* GI ulceration, intra- and extrahepatic biliary sclerosis, acalculous cholycystitis.
Hematologic: *leukopenia, anemia, thrombocytopenia, agranulocytosis.*
Skin: *erythema,* dermatitis, pruritus, rash, alopecia, photosensitivity.
Other: thrombophlebitis, *anaphylaxis,* fever.

INTERACTIONS
None significant.

EFFECTS ON DIAGNOSTIC TESTS
Drug therapy may increase serum concentrations of ALT, AST, alkaline phosphatase, bilirubin, and lactic dehydrogenase; these increases indicate drug-induced hepatotoxicity.

CONTRAINDICATIONS
Contraindicated in patients with poor nutritional state, bone marrow suppression, or serious infection.

NURSING CONSIDERATIONS
● Use cautiously following high-dose pelvic radiation therapy or use of alkylating agents and in patients with impaired hepatic or renal function.
● Follow institutional policy to reduce risks. Preparation and administration of parenteral form of this drug is associated with carcinogenic, mutagenic, and teratogenic risks for personnel.
● Reconstitute with sterile water for injection. To prepare infusion, dilute in D₅W or 0.9% sodium chloride solution.
● Refrigerated solution is stable for no more than 2 weeks.
● Use an infusion pump with intra-arterial infusions.

- Check line for bleeding, blockage, displacement, or leakage.
- Monitor fluid intake and output, CBC, and renal and hepatic function, as ordered.
- Know that use of antacid eases but won't prevent GI distress. An H$_2$ antihistamine is recommended to prevent peptic ulcer disease during drug therapy.
- Provide diligent mouth care to help prevent stomatitis.
- Be alert that severe skin and adverse GI reactions require stopping drug.
- Know that drug should be discontinued if WBC count falls below 3,500/mm^3 or if platelet count falls below 100,000/mm^3. If either occurs, notify doctor.
- To prevent bleeding, avoid all I.M. injections when platelet count is below 100,000/mm^3.
- Anticipate possible blood transfusions because of cumulative anemia.

☑ **PATIENT TEACHING**
- Inform patient that therapeutic effect may be delayed 1 to 6 weeks.
- Advise patient to watch for signs of infection (fever, sore throat, fatigue) and bleeding (easy bruising, nosebleeds, bleeding gums, melena). Tell patient to take temperature daily.
- Inform patient that exposure to sun may initiate or intensify skin reaction.
- Advise breast-feeding patient to discontinue breast-feeding during therapy because of possible infant toxicity.
- Advise women of childbearing age to avoid becoming pregnant during therapy. Also recommend consulting with the doctor before becoming pregnant.

fludarabine phosphate
Fludara

Pregnancy Risk Category: D

HOW SUPPLIED
Powder for injection: 50 mg

ACTION
Unknown. An antineoplastic antimetabolite that may have multifaceted actions. After conversion to its active metabolite, fludarabine interferes with DNA synthesis by inhibiting DNA polymerase alpha, ribonucleotide reductase, and DNA primase.

ONSET, PEAK, DURATION
Median time to respond is 7 to 21 weeks. Peak and duration undefined.

INDICATIONS & DOSAGE
B-cell chronic lymphocytic leukemia in patients who have either not responded or responded inadequately to at least one standard alkylating agent regimen—
Adults: 25 mg/m^2 I.V. over 30 minutes for 5 consecutive days. Cycle repeated q 28 days.

ADVERSE REACTIONS
CNS: *fatigue, malaise, weakness, paresthesia,* peripheral neuropathy, headache, sleep disorder, depression, cerebellar syndrome, *CVA,* transient ischemic attack, agitation, *confusion; coma, death* (with very high doses).
CV: *edema,* angina, phlebitis, ***arrhythmias, CHF, MI,*** supraventricular tachycardia, deep venous thrombosis, ***aneurysm,*** hemorrhage.
EENT: *visual disturbances,* hearing loss, delayed blindness (with high doses), sinusitis, pharyngitis, epistaxis.
GI: *nausea, vomiting, diarrhea,* constipation, *anorexia,* stomatitis, *GI bleeding,* esophagitis, mucositis.
GU: dysuria, *urinary infection* or hesitancy, proteinuria, hematuria, ***renal failure.***
Hematologic: ***hemolytic anemia,*** MYELOSUPPRESSION.
Hepatic: liver failure, cholelithiasis.
Respiratory: *cough, pneumonia, dyspnea, upper respiratory tract infection,* allergic pneumonitis, hemoptysis, hypoxia, bronchitis, sinusitis, pharyngitis.
Skin: *rash,* pruritus, alopecia, sebor-

Reactions may be *common,* uncommon, ***life-threatening,*** or COMMON AND LIFE-THREATENING.

rhea.

Other: *fever, chills, pain, myalgia,* tumor lysis syndrome, INFECTION, *anaphylaxis,* diaphoresis, hypocalcemia, hyperkalemia, hyperglycemia, dehydration, hyperuricemia, hyperphosphatemia.

INTERACTIONS
Other myelosuppressants: increased toxicity. Avoid concomitant use.
Pentostatin: concurrent use increases risk of pulmonary toxicity. Avoid concomitant administration.

EFFECTS ON DIAGNOSTIC TESTS
None reported.

CONTRAINDICATIONS
Contraindicated in patients hypersensitive to the drug or its components.

NURSING CONSIDERATIONS
● Use cautiously in patients with renal insufficiency.
● Follow institutional policy to reduce risks. Preparation and administration of parenteral form of this drug is associated with mutagenic, teratogenic, and carcinogenic risks for personnel.
● **I.V. use:** To prepare solution, add 2 ml of sterile water for injection to the solid cake of fludarabine. Dissolution should occur within 15 seconds; each milliliter will contain 25 mg of drug. Dilute further in 100 or 125 ml of D_5W or 0.9% sodium chloride for injection. Use within 8 hours of reconstitution.
Alert: Monitor patients closely and expect modified dosage based on toxicity. Most toxic effects are dose-dependent. Advanced age, renal insufficiency, and bone marrow impairment may predispose patients to increased or excessive toxicity.
● Know that careful hematologic monitoring is required, especially of neutrophil and platelet counts. Bone marrow suppression can be severe.
● To prevent bleeding, avoid all I.M. injections when platelet count is below

$100,00/mm^3$.
● Anticipate possible blood transfusions because of cumulative anemia.
● Know that optimal duration of therapy is not yet determined. Current recommendations suggest three additional cycles after achieving maximal response before discontinuing therapy.
● Take preventive measures before starting drug treatment. Hyperuricemia, hypocalcemia, hyperkalemia, and renal failure may result from rapid lysis of tumor cells.
● Store drug in refrigerator at 36° to 46° F (2° to 8° C).

☑ **PATIENT TEACHING**
● Advise patient to watch for signs of infection (fever, sore throat, fatigue) and bleeding (easy bruising, nosebleeds, bleeding gums, melena). Tell patient to take temperature daily.
● Advise women of childbearing age to avoid becoming pregnant during therapy. Also recommend consulting with doctor before becoming pregnant.
● Advise breast-feeding patient to discontinue beast-feeding during therapy because of possible infant toxicity.

---

fluorouracil (5-fluorouracil, 5-FU)
Adrucil, Efudex, Fluoroplex

Pregnancy Risk Category: D (injection), X (topical form)

HOW SUPPLIED
Injection: 50 mg/ml
Cream: 1%, 5%
Topical solution: 1%, 2%, 5%

ACTION
Thought to inhibit DNA and RNA synthesis.

ONSET, PEAK, DURATION
Undefined.

INDICATIONS & DOSAGE
Colon, rectal, breast, stomach, and pancreatic cancers—
Adults: 12 mg/kg I.V. daily for 4 days; if no toxicity, 6 mg/kg given on the 6th, 8th, 10th, and 12th day; then a single weekly maintenance dose of 10 to 15 mg/kg I.V. begun after toxicity (if any) from initial course has subsided. (Dosages recommended based on actual body weight unless patient is obese or retaining fluid.) Maximum single recommended dose is 800 mg/day.
Palliative treatment of advanced colorectal cancer—
Adults: 425 mg/m² I.V. daily for 5 consecutive days. Given with 20 mg/m² of leucovorin I.V. Repeated at 4-week intervals for two additional courses; then repeated at intervals of 4 to 5 weeks if tolerated.
Multiple actinic (solar) keratoses; superficial basal cell carcinoma—
Adults: apply cream or topical solution b.i.d. Usual duration of treatment is 2 to 6 weeks.

ADVERSE REACTIONS
CNS: acute cerebellar syndrome, confusion, disorientation, euphoria, ataxia, headache, nystagmus, *weakness, malaise.*
CV: myocardial ischemia, angina.
EENT: epistaxis, photophobia, lacrimation, lacrimal duct stenosis, visual changes.
GI: *stomatitis, GI ulcer* (may precede leukopenia), *nausea and vomiting* (in 30% to 50% of patients), *diarrhea, anorexia,* GI bleeding.
Hematologic: **leukopenia, thrombocytopenia, agranulocytosis,** anemia; WBC count nadir 9 to 14 days after first dose; platelet count nadir in 7 to 14 days.
Skin: *dermatitis; erythema; scaling; pruritus;* nail changes; pigmented palmar creases; erythematous, contact dermatitis, desquamative rash of hands and feet with long-term use ("hand-foot syndrome"); photosensitivity, *reversible alopecia in 5% to 20% of patients.*

Other: *pain, burning,* soreness, suppuration, swelling (with topical use), **anaphylaxis,** thrombophlebitis.

INTERACTIONS
Leucovorin calcium, prior treatment with alkylating agents: increased toxicity of fluorouracil. Use with extreme caution.

EFFECTS ON DIAGNOSTIC TESTS
Drug may decrease plasma albumin concentrations because of drug-induced protein malabsorption.

CONTRAINDICATIONS
Contraindicated in patients hypersensitive to the drug; patients who are in a poor nutritional state; patients with bone marrow suppression (WBC counts of 5,000/mm³ or less or platelet counts of 100,000/mm³ or less); patients with potentially serious infections; and those who have had major surgery within the previous month.

NURSING CONSIDERATIONS
● Use cautiously after high-dose pelvic radiation therapy or use of alkylating agents or in patients with impaired hepatic or renal function or widespread neoplastic infiltration of bone marrow.
● Follow institutional policy to reduce risks. Preparation and administration of parenteral form of this drug is associated with carcinogenic, mutagenic, and teratogenic risks for personnel.
● Give antiemetic, as ordered, before administering drug to reduce nausea.
● **I.V. use:** Know that drug may be administered by direct injection without dilution. For I.V. infusion, drug may be diluted with D₅W, sterile water for injection, or 0.9% sodium chloride for injection.
● Don't use cloudy solution. If crystals form, redissolve by warming.
● Use plastic I.V. containers for administering continuous infusions. Solution is more stable in plastic I.V. bags than in glass bottles.

Reactions may be *common*, uncommon, **life-threatening**, or COMMON AND LIFE-THREATENING.

• Don't refrigerate fluorouracil. Protect drug from sunlight.
• Apply topical form with caution near eyes, nose, and mouth.
• Avoid occlusive dressings with topical dressings because they increase the risk of inflammatory reactions in adjacent normal skin.
• Wash hands immediately after handling topical form of medication. Apply topical form with a nonmetal applicator or suitable gloves.
• Expect to use 1% topical concentration on the face. Higher concentrations are used for thicker-skinned areas or resistant lesions.
• Expect to use 5% topical strength for superficial basal cell carcinoma confirmed by biopsy.
• Be aware that ingestion and systemic absorption of topical form may cause leukopenia, thrombocytopenia, stomatitis, diarrhea, or GI ulceration, bleeding, and hemorrhage. Application to large ulcerated areas may cause systemic toxicity.
• Watch for stomatitis or diarrhea (signs of toxicity). May use topical oral anesthetic to soothe lesions, as ordered. Discontinue drug if diarrhea occurs and notify doctor.
• Encourage diligent oral hygiene to prevent superinfection of denuded mucosa.
• Monitor WBC and platelet counts daily, as ordered. Watch for ecchymoses, petechiae, easy bruising, and anemia.
• Monitor fluid intake and output, CBC, and renal and hepatic function tests, as ordered.
• Be aware that dermatologic adverse effects are reversible when drug is stopped.
• To prevent bleeding, avoid all I.M. injections when platelet count is below 100,000/mm³.
• Anticipate possible blood transfusions because of cumulative anemia.
Alert: Be alert that fluorouracil toxicity may be delayed for 1 to 3 weeks.
• Know that the drug is sometimes ordered as 5-fluorouracil or 5-FU. The numeral 5 is part of the drug name and should not be confused with dosage units.

☑ **PATIENT TEACHING**
• Warn patient that alopecia may occur, but that it's reversible.
• Caution patient to avoid prolonged exposure to sunlight or ultraviolet light when topical form is used.
• Tell patient to use highly protective sunblock to avoid inflammatory erythematous dermatitis. Long-term use of the drug is associated with erythematous, desquamative rash of the hands and feet. May be treated with pyridoxine (50 to 150 mg P.O. daily) for 5 to 7 days.
• Warn patient that topically treated area may be unsightly during therapy and for several weeks after therapy. Complete healing may take 1 or 2 months.
• Advise women of childbearing age to avoid becoming pregnant during therapy. Also recommend consulting with doctor before becoming pregnant.
• Advise breast-feeding patients to discontinue breast-feeding during therapy because of possible infant toxicity.

hydroxyurea
Hydrea**

Pregnancy Risk Category: NR

HOW SUPPLIED
Capsules: 500 mg

ACTION
Unknown. Thought to inhibit DNA synthesis.

ONSET, PEAK, DURATION
Onset and duration unknown. Serum levels peak in 2 hours.

INDICATIONS & DOSAGE
Melanoma; resistant chronic myelocytic leukemia; recurrent, metastatic, or inoperable ovarian cancer; head and neck

cancers—
Adults: 80 mg/kg P.O. as single dose q 3 days; or 20 to 30 mg/kg P.O. as a single daily dose.

ADVERSE REACTIONS
CNS: hallucinations, headache, dizziness, disorientation, *seizures,* malaise.
GI: *anorexia, nausea, vomiting, diarrhea,* stomatitis, constipation.
GU: increased BUN and serum creatinine levels.
Hematologic: *leukopenia, thrombocytopenia,* anemia, megaloblastosis; *dose-limiting and dose-related bone marrow suppression,* with rapid recovery.
Skin: alopecia (rare).
Other: fever, chills.

INTERACTIONS
Cytotoxic drugs, radiation therapy: enhanced toxicity of hydroxyurea. Use together cautiously.

EFFECTS ON DIAGNOSTIC TESTS
Drug therapy elevates BUN, serum creatinine, and serum uric acid levels.

CONTRAINDICATIONS
Contraindicated in patients hypersensitive to the drug and with marked bone marrow depression (leukopenia [less than 2,500/mm³ WBCs], thrombocytopenia [less than 100,000/mm³ platelets], or severe anemia).

NURSING CONSIDERATIONS
● Use cautiously in patients with renal dysfunction.
● Routinely measure BUN, uric acid, and serum creatinine levels, as ordered.
● Monitor fluid intake and output; keep patients hydrated.
● To prevent bleeding, avoid all I.M. injections when platelet count is below 100,000/mm³.
● Anticipate possible blood transfusions because of cumulative anemia.
● Be aware that dosage modification may be required after chemotherapy or radiation therapy.

● Be aware that auditory and visual hallucinations and hematologic toxicity increase when decreased renal function exists.
● Know that the drug crosses blood-brain barrier.
● Be alert that concomitant radiation therapy may increase incidence or severity of GI distress or stomatitis.

☑ **PATIENT TEACHING**
● Tell patient who can't swallow capsules that he may empty contents into water and take immediately.
● Advise patient to watch for signs of infection (fever, sore throat, fatigue) and bleeding (easy bruising, nosebleeds, bleeding gums, melena). He should also take his temperature daily.
● Advise women of childbearing age to avoid becoming pregnant during therapy. Also recommend consulting with doctor before becoming pregnant.

mercaptopurine
(6-mercaptopurine, 6-MP)
Purinethol

Pregnancy Risk Category: D

HOW SUPPLIED
Tablets (scored): 50 mg

ACTION
Inhibits RNA and DNA synthesis.

ONSET, PEAK, DURATION
Undefined.

INDICATIONS & DOSAGE
Acute myeloblastic leukemia, chronic myelocytic leukemia—
Adults: 80 to 100 mg/m² (rounded to the nearest 25 mg) P.O. daily as a single dose up to 5 mg/kg/day.
Children: 70 mg/m² (rounded to the nearest 25 mg) P.O. daily.
Acute lymphoblastic leukemia—
Children: 70 mg/m² (rounded to the nearest 25 mg) P.O. daily.

Usual maintenance for adults and children: 1.5 to 2.5 mg/kg/day.

ADVERSE REACTIONS
GI: nausea, vomiting, anorexia, painful oral ulcers, diarrhea, pancreatitis, GI ulceration.
Hematologic: *leukopenia, thrombocytopenia,* anemia—all may persist several days after drug is stopped.
Hepatic: *jaundice,* hepatotoxicity.
Skin: rash, hyperpigmentation.
Other: hyperuricemia.

INTERACTIONS
Allopurinol: slowed inactivation of mercaptopurine. Decrease mercaptopurine to one-quarter or one-third normal dose.
Hepatotoxic drugs: may enhance hepatotoxicity of mercaptopurine. Monitor for hepatotoxicity.
Nondepolarizing neuromuscular blockers: antagonized muscle relaxant effect. Notify the anesthesiologist that the patient is receiving mercaptopurine.
Warfarin: antagonized or potentiated anticoagulant effect. Monitor PT.

EFFECTS ON DIAGNOSTIC TESTS
Drug therapy may cause falsely elevated serum glucose and uric acid values when sequential multiple analyzer is used.

CONTRAINDICATIONS
Contraindicated in patients whose disease has shown resistance to the drug.

NURSING CONSIDERATIONS
● Be aware that dosage modifications may be required after chemotherapy or radiation therapy in patients with depressed neutrophil or platelet counts and in those with impaired hepatic or renal function.
● Be aware that drug is sometimes ordered as 6-mercaptopurine or 6-MP. The numeral 6 is part of drug name and does not signify number of dosage units.
● Monitor blood counts and serum transaminase, alkaline phosphatase, and bilirubin levels weekly during induction and monthly during maintenance, as ordered.
● Observe for signs of bleeding and infection.
● Monitor fluid intake and output. Encourage adequate fluid intake (3 liters daily).
Alert: Watch for jaundice, clay-colored stools, and frothy dark urine. Hepatic dysfunction is reversible when drug is stopped. If hepatic tenderness occurs, drug should be stopped and doctor notified.
● Monitor serum uric acid level, as ordered. If allopurinol is ordered, use cautiously.
● To prevent bleeding, avoid all I.M. injections when platelet count is below 100,000/mm^3.
● Anticipate possible blood transfusions because of cumulative anemia.
● Be alert that GI adverse reactions are less common in children than in adults.

☑ **PATIENT TEACHING**
● Advise patient to watch for signs of infection (fever, sore throat, fatigue) and bleeding (easy bruising, nosebleeds, bleeding gums, melena). Tell patient to take temperature daily.
● Advise women of childbearing age to avoid becoming pregnant during therapy. Also recommend consulting with the doctor before becoming pregnant.
● Advise breast-feeding patients to discontinue breast-feeding during therapy because of possible infant toxicity.

---

methotrexate (Amethopterin, MTX)

methotrexate sodium
Folex, Folex PFS, Mexate-AQ, Rheumatrex

Pregnancy Risk Category: X

HOW SUPPLIED
Tablets (scored): 2.5 mg
Injection: 20-mg, 25-mg, 50-mg, 100-

---

mg, 250-mg vials, lyophilized powder, preservative-free; 25-mg/ml vials, preservative-free solution; 2.5-mg/ml, 25-mg/ml vials, lyophilized powder, preserved

ACTION

Prevents reduction of folic acid to tetra-hydrofolate by binding to dihydrofolate reductase.

ONSET, PEAK, DURATION

Onset and duration undefined. Serum concentrations peak immediately after I.V. injection, within ½ to 1 hour after I.M. injection, or 1 to 2 hours after oral dose.

INDICATIONS & DOSAGE

Trophoblastic tumors (choriocarcinoma, hydatidiform mole)—
Adults: 15 to 30 mg P.O. or I.M. daily for 5 days. Repeated after 1 or more weeks, according to response or toxicity.
Acute lymphocytic leukemia—
Adults and children: 3.3 mg/m^2/day P.O., I.M., or I.V. for 4 to 6 weeks or until remission occurs; then 20 to 30 mg/m^2 P.O. or I.M. weekly in two divided doses or 2.5 mg/kg I.V. q 14 days.
Meningeal leukemia—
Adults and children: 12 mg/m^2 or less (maximum 15 mg) intrathecally q 2 to 5 days until CSF is normal, then one additional dose.
Burkitt's lymphoma (Stage I, II, or III)—
Adults: 10 to 25 mg P.O. daily for 4 to 8 days with 1-week rest intervals.
Lymphosarcoma (Stage III)—
Adults: 0.625 to 2.5 mg/kg daily P.O., I.M., or I.V.
Osteosarcoma—
Adults: initially, 12 g/m^2 I.V. as 4-hour infusion. Subsequent doses 12 to 15 g/m^2 I.V. as 4-hour I.V. infusion given at 4th, 5th, 6th, 7th, 11th, 12th, 15th, 16th, 29th, 30th, 44th, 45th weeks after surgery. Given with leucovorin, 15 mg P.O., I.M., or I.V. q 6 hours for 10 doses, beginning 24 hours after start of methotrexate infusion.

Mycosis fungoides—
Adults: 2.5 to 10 mg P.O. daily, or 50 mg I.M. weekly, or 25 mg I.M. twice weekly.
Psoriasis—
Adults: 10 to 25 mg P.O., I.M., or I.V. as single weekly dose.
Rheumatoid arthritis—
Adults: initially, 7.5 mg P.O. weekly, either in a single dose or divided as 2.5 mg P.O. q 12 hours for three doses once a week. Dosage may be gradually increased to a maximum of 20 mg weekly.

ADVERSE REACTIONS

CNS: *arachnoiditis* within hours of intrathecal use; subacute neurotoxicity, which may begin a few weeks later; *leukoencephalopathy;* demyelination; malaise; fatigue; dizziness; headache; aphasia; hemiparesis; drowsiness; *seizures.*
EENT: pharyngitis, gingivitis, blurred vision.
GI: *stomatitis, diarrhea,* abdominal distress, anorexia, GI ulceration and bleeding, enteritis, *nausea, vomiting.*
GU: nephropathy, *tubular necrosis, renal failure,* hematuria, menstrual dysfunction, defective spermatogenesis, infertility, abortion, cystitis.
Hematologic: WBC and platelet count nadirs occurring on day 7; *anemia, leukopenia, thrombocytopenia* (all dose-related).
Hepatic: acute toxicity (elevated transaminase level), *chronic toxicity* (cirrhosis, *hepatic fibrosis*).
Respiratory: *pulmonary fibrosis; pulmonary interstitial infiltrates;* pneumonitis; dry, nonproductive cough.
Skin: *urticaria,* pruritus, hyperpigmentation, erythematous rashes, ecchymoses; psoriatic lesions (aggravated by exposure to sun), rash, photosensitivity, alopecia, acne.
Other: osteoporosis (in children, with long-term use), fever, chills, reduced resistance to infection, septicemia, hyperuricemia, arthralgia, myalgia, diabetes, *sudden death.*

Reactions may be *common,* uncommon, *life-threatening,* or COMMON AND LIFE-THREATENING.

INTERACTIONS

Digoxin: may decrease serum digoxin levels. Monitor closely.

Folic acid derivatives: antagonized methotrexate effect. Avoid concomitant use, except for leucovorin rescue with high-dose methotrexate therapy.

NSAIDs, phenylbutazone, probenecid, salicylates, sulfonamides: increased methotrexate toxicity; don't use together if possible.

Oral antibiotics: may decrease absorption of methotrexate.

Phenytoin: may decrease serum phenytoin levels. Monitor closely.

Theophylline: may increase level of theophylline. Monitor closely.

Vaccines: immunizations may be ineffective; risk of disseminated infection with live-virus vaccines. Defer immunization, if possible.

EFFECTS ON DIAGNOSTIC TESTS

Drug therapy may increase blood and urine levels of uric acid. Methotrexate may alter results of laboratory assay for folate, thus interfering with the detection of folic acid deficiency.

CONTRAINDICATIONS

Contraindicated in patients hypersensitive to the drug and during pregnancy or breast-feeding. It also is contraindicated in patients with psoriasis or rheumatoid arthritis who also have alcoholism, alcoholic liver, chronic liver disease, immunodeficiency syndromes, or preexisting blood dyscrasias.

NURSING CONSIDERATIONS

● Use cautiously and at modified dosage in patients with impaired hepatic or renal function, bone marrow suppression, aplasia, leukopenia, thrombocytopenia, or anemia. Also use cautiously in patients with infection, peptic ulceration, and ulcerative colitis and in very young, elderly, or debilitated patients.

● Follow institutional policy to reduce risks. Preparation and administration of parenteral form of this drug is associated with carcinogenic, mutagenic, and teratogenic risks for personnel.

● **I.V. use:** Know that dilution of drug depends on product and that infusion guidelines vary, depending on dose.

● Reconstitute solutions without preservatives immediately before use, and discard any unused drug.

● Monitor pulmonary function tests periodically, as ordered, and fluid intake and output daily. Encourage fluid intake of 2 to 3 liters daily.

● Monitor serum uric acid level, as ordered.

Alert: Alkalinize urine as ordered by giving sodium bicarbonate tablets to prevent precipitation of drug, especially with high doses. Maintain urine pH at more than 6.5. Reduce dosage as ordered if BUN level reaches 20 to 30 mg/dl or creatinine level reaches 1.2 to 2 mg/dl. Stop drug if BUN level is greater than 30 mg/dl or creatinine level is greater than 2 mg/dl and notify doctor.

● Use preservative-free formulation for intrathecal administration.

● Watch for increases in AST, ALT, and alkaline phosphatase levels, which may signal hepatic dysfunction.

● Watch for signs of bleeding (especially GI) and infection.

● To prevent bleeding, avoid all I.M. injections when platelet count is below 100,000/mm³.

● Anticipate blood transfusions because of cumulative anemia.

● Know that rash, redness, or ulcerations in mouth or adverse pulmonary reactions may signal serious complications.

● Know that leucovorin rescue is necessary with high-dose (greater than 100 mg) protocols and is started 24 hours after beginning methotrexate therapy.

Monitor methotrexate levels and adjust leucovorin dose as ordered.

☑ PATIENT TEACHING

● Advise patient to watch for signs of infection (fever, sore throat, fatigue) and bleeding (easy bruising, nosebleeds, bleeding gums, melena). Tell patient to take temperature daily.

● Teach and encourage diligent mouth care to reduce the risk of superinfection in the mouth.

● Tell patient to use highly protective sunblock when exposed to sunlight.

● Warn patient to avoid conception during and immediately after therapy because of possible abortion or congenital anomalies.

● Advise breast-feeding patient to discontinue breast-feeding during therapy because of possible infant toxicity.

thioguanine (6-thioguanine, 6-TG)
Lanvis†

Pregnancy Risk Category: D

HOW SUPPLIED
Tablets (scored): 40 mg

ACTION
Inhibits purine synthesis.

ONSET, PEAK, DURATION
Undefined.

INDICATIONS & DOSAGE
Acute nonlymphocytic leukemia, chronic myelogenous leukemia—
Adults and children: initially, 2 mg/kg P.O. daily (usually calculated to nearest 20 mg). If necessary, dose is then increased gradually to 3 mg/kg/day as tolerated.

ADVERSE REACTIONS
GI: nausea, vomiting, stomatitis, diarrhea, anorexia.
Hematologic: *leukopenia, anemia, thrombocytopenia* (occurs slowly over 2 to 4 weeks).
Hepatic: *hepatotoxicity,* jaundice.
Other: hyperuricemia.

INTERACTIONS
Myelosuppressants: increased risk of

toxicity, especially myelosuppression, bleeding, and hepatotoxicity. Use together cautiously.

EFFECTS ON DIAGNOSTIC TESTS
Drug therapy may increase blood and urine levels of uric acid.

CONTRAINDICATIONS
Contraindicated in patients whose disease has shown resistance to the drug. There is usually complete cross-resistance between mercaptopurine and thioguanine.

NURSING CONSIDERATIONS
● Use cautiously and with dosage modification in patients with renal or hepatic dysfunction.

● Monitor CBC daily during induction and then weekly during maintenance therapy, as ordered.

● Monitor serum uric acid level, as ordered. Hyperuricemia can be minimized by increased urine alkalization and the administration of allopurinol.

● Watch for jaundice; may be reversible if drug is stopped promptly

● To prevent bleeding, avoid all I.M. injections when platelet count is below 100,000/mm^3.

● Anticipate possible blood transfusions because of cumulative anemia.

● Know that drug is sometimes ordered as 6-thioguanine. The numeral 6 is part of drug name and does not signify dosage units.

☑ PATIENT TEACHING
● Advise patient to watch for signs of infection (fever, sore throat, fatigue) and bleeding (easy bruising, nosebleeds, bleeding gums, melena). Tell patient to take temperature daily.

● Advise women of childbearing age to avoid becoming pregnant during therapy. Also recommend consulting with doctor before becoming pregnant.

● Advise breast-feeding patient to discontinue breast-feeding during therapy because of possible infant toxicity.

71

Antibiotic antineoplastic drugs

bleomycin sulfate
dactinomycin
daunorubicin hydrochloride
doxorubicin hydrochloride
idarubicin hydrochloride
mitomycin
pentostatin
plicamycin

COMBINATION PRODUCTS
None.

---

bleomycin sulfate
Blenoxane

Pregnancy Risk Category: D

HOW SUPPLIED
Injection: 15-unit vials

ACTION
Unknown. Thought to inhibit DNA synthesis and cause scission of single- and double-stranded DNA.

ONSET, PEAK, DURATION
Undefined.

INDICATIONS & DOSAGE
Dosage and indications may vary. Check the treatment protocol with the doctor.
Squamous cell carcinoma (head and neck, skin, penis, cervix, and vulva), lymphosarcoma, reticulum cell carcinoma, testicular carcinoma—
Adults: 10 to 20 units/m² I.V., I.M., or S.C. one or two times weekly to total of 300 to 400 units.
Hodgkin's disease—
Adults: 10 to 20 units/m² I.V., I.M., or S.C. one or two times weekly. After 50% response, maintenance dosage is 1 unit I.M. or I.V. daily or 5 units I.M. or I.V. weekly.

✳ **New indication:** *Treatment of malignant pleural effusion; prevention of recurrent pleural effusions—*
Adults: 60 units administered as a single-dose bolus intrapleural injection.

ADVERSE REACTIONS
GI: *stomatitis, anorexia, nausea, vomiting,* diarrhea.
Respiratory: pulmonary toxicity such as PNEUMONITIS, *pulmonary fibrosis.*
Skin: *erythema, hyperpigmentation, acne, rash, striae, skin tenderness, pruritus, reversible alopecia,* hyperkeratosis, nail changes.
Other: *chills,* weight loss, fever, *anaphylactoid reactions.*

INTERACTIONS
Digitalis glycosides: decreased serum digoxin levels. Monitor closely.
Phenytoin: decreased serum phenytoin levels. Monitor closely.

EFFECTS ON DIAGNOSTIC TESTS
Drug therapy may increase blood and urine concentrations of uric acid.

CONTRAINDICATIONS
Contraindicated in patients hypersensitive to the drug.

NURSING CONSIDERATIONS
● Use cautiously in patients with renal or pulmonary impairment.
● Obtain pulmonary function tests as ordered. Drug should be stopped if tests show a marked decline.
● Follow institutional policy to reduce risks. Preparation and administration of parenteral form of this drug is associated with carcinogenic, mutagenic, and teratogenic risks for personnel.
● **I.V. use:** Reconstitute drug with 5 ml or more of 0.9% sodium chloride for injection. For I.V. infusion, dilute with 50

---

to 100 ml 0.9% sodium chloride for injection. Administer over 10 minutes.

● For I.M. use, dilute drug in 1 to 5 ml of sterile water for injection, bacteriostatic water for injection, 0.9% sodium chloride for injection.

● For intrapleural use, dissolve drug in 50 to 100 ml 0.9% sodium chloride injection and administer through a thoracotomy tube after drainage of excess pleural fluid and confirmation of complete lung expansion.

● Monitor injection site for irritation.

Alert: Adverse pulmonary reactions are more common in patients over age 70. Pulmonary fibrosis is fatal in 1% of patients, especially when cumulative dosage exceeds 400 units. Also, pulmonary toxic adverse effects may be increased in patients receiving radiation therapy.

● Monitor chest X-ray, as ordered, and listen to lungs regularly.

● If patient's condition requires sclerosis, drug may be instilled when chest tube drainage is 100 to 300 ml/24 hours before therapy; ideally, drainage should be under 100 ml. Following instillation, thoracotomy tube is clamped and patient is moved alternately from the supine to left and right lateral positions for the next 4 hours. The clamp is then removed and suction reestablished. The amount of time the chest tube is left in place after sclerosis depends on the patient's condition.

● Monitor for fever, which may be treated with antipyretics. This reaction usually occurs within 3 to 6 hours of administration.

● Watch for hypersensitivity reactions, which may be delayed for several hours, especially in patients with lymphoma (test dose of 1 to 2 units should be given before first two doses in these patients. If no reaction occurs, regular dosage is followed).

● Don't use adhesive dressings on skin.

● Refrigerate unopened vials containing dry powder. Refrigerated, reconstituted solution is stable for 4 weeks; at room temperature, for 2 weeks. Bleomycin may adsorb to plastic I.V. bags. For prolonged stability, use glass containers.

☑ **PATIENT TEACHING**

● Warn patient that alopecia may occur, but that it's usually reversible.

● Tell patient to report adverse reactions promptly and to take infection-control and bleeding precautions.

● Instruct patient that if he is to ever receive anesthesia, he must inform the anesthesiologist of prior treatment with bleomycin. The pulmonary toxicity of drug may be enhanced by the high intraoperative forced inspiratory oxygen.

dactinomycin (actinomycin D)
Cosmegen

Pregnancy Risk Category: C

HOW SUPPLIED
Injection: 500 mcg-vial

ACTION
Unknown. May interfere with DNA-dependent RNA synthesis by intercalation.

ONSET, PEAK, DURATION
Undefined.

INDICATIONS & DOSAGE
Dosage and indications vary. Check treatment protocol with the doctor.
Sarcoma, trophoblastic tumors in women, testicular cancer—
Adults: 500 mcg (0.5 mg) I.V. daily for 5 days. Maximum dosage is 15 mcg/kg or 400 to 600 mcg/m²/day for 5 days. After bone marrow recovery, course may be repeated.
Wilms' tumor, rhabdomyosarcoma, Ewing's sarcoma—
Children: 10 to 15 mcg/kg or 450 mcg/m²/day I.V. for 5 days. Maximum dosage is 500 mcg/day. Or 2.5 mg/m² I.V. in equally divided daily doses over 7 days. After bone marrow recovery,

course may be repeated.

ADVERSE REACTIONS
GI: *anorexia, nausea, vomiting,* abdominal pain, diarrhea, *stomatitis,* ulceration, proctitis.
Hematologic: *anemia, leukopenia, thrombocytopenia, pancytopenia, aplastic anemia, agranulocytosis.*
Hepatic: *hepatotoxicity.*
Skin: *erythema;* desquamation; *hyperpigmentation of skin, especially in previously irradiated areas; acnelike eruptions (reversible);* "radiation recall effect."
Other: phlebitis and severe damage to soft tissue at injection site, reversible alopecia, malaise, fatigue, lethargy, fever, myalgia, hypocalcemia, *anaphylactoid reaction, death.*

INTERACTIONS
Bone marrow suppressants: additive toxicity. Monitor closely.
Vitamin K derivatives: decreased effectiveness. Monitor closely.

EFFECTS ON DIAGNOSTIC TESTS
Drug therapy may increase blood and urine concentrations of uric acid; it may also interfere with determination of antibiotic drug levels (peak and trough).

CONTRAINDICATIONS
Contraindicated in patients with chickenpox or herpes zoster.

NURSING CONSIDERATIONS
● To reduce nausea, give antiemetic before drug, as ordered.
● Follow institutional policy to reduce risks. Preparation and administration of parenteral form of this drug is associated with carcinogenic, mutagenic, and teratogenic risks for personnel.
● **I.V. use:** Use only sterile water (without preservatives) as diluent for reconstitution. Add 1.1 ml to vial to yield gold-colored solution containing 0.5 mg/ml. Give by direct injection into a vein or through tubing of a free-flowing

I.V. solution of 0.9% sodium chloride for injection or D₅W.
● For I.V. infusion, dilute with up to 50 ml of D₅W or 0.9% sodium chloride for injection; infuse over 15 minutes.
● Administer through a running I.V. line with good blood return. Drug is a vesicant; if extravasation occurs, severe tissue necrosis may result. If infiltration occurs, apply cold compresses to area and notify doctor.
● If skin contact occurs, irrigate with water for at least 15 minutes.
Alert: Be aware that dosage must be reduced in patients who have recently been treated with, or who will receive concomitant treatment with, radiation therapy or other chemotherapy drugs.
● In the event of a spill, use a solution of trisodium phosphate 5% to inactivate the drug.
● Monitor CBC and platelet counts and renal and hepatic functions, as ordered.
● Monitor for stomatitis, diarrhea, leukopenia, or thrombocytopenia.
● Discard unused solutions.

☑ **PATIENT TEACHING**
● Advise patient to watch for signs of infection (fever, sore throat, fatigue) and bleeding (easy bruising, nosebleeds, bleeding gums, melena) and to take temperature daily.
● Tell patient that alopecia may occur, but that it's usually reversible.
● Tell patient who received a course of radiation therapy that he may experience a "radiation recall effect" in the prior treatment field.

---

daunorubicin hydrochloride
Cerubidin‡, Cerubidine

Pregnancy Risk Category: D

HOW SUPPLIED
Injection: 20 mg-vial

ACTION
May interfere with DNA-dependent

RNA synthesis by intercalation.

ONSET, PEAK, DURATION
Undefined.

INDICATIONS & DOSAGE
Dosage and indications vary. Check treatment protocol with the doctor.
Remission induction in acute nonlymphocytic (myelogenous, monocytic, erythroid) leukemia—
Adults: in combination, 30 to 45 mg/m²/day I.V. on days 1, 2, and 3 of the first course and on days 1 and 2 of subsequent courses with cytarabine infusions.
Remission induction in acute lymphocytic leukemia—
Adults: in combination 45 mg/m²/day I.V. on days 1, 2, and 3 of the first course.
Children 2 years and older: 25 mg/m² I.V. on day 1 every week, for up to 6 weeks, if needed.
Children under 2 years or body surface area under 0.5 m²: dose calculated based on body weight (1 mg/kg).

ADVERSE REACTIONS
CV: *irreversible cardiomyopathy* (dose-related), ECG changes.
GI: *nausea, vomiting,* diarrhea.
GU: red urine (transient).
Hematologic: *bone marrow suppression* (lowest blood counts 10 to 14 days after administration).
Hepatic: *hepatotoxicity.*
Skin: rash, *reversible alopecia.*
Other: *severe cellulitis or tissue sloughing if drug extravasates,* **anaphylactoid reaction,** fever, chills, hyperuricemia.

INTERACTIONS
Dexamethasone, heparin: don't mix. May form a precipitate.
Doxorubicin: additive cardiotoxicity. Monitor closely.
Hepatotoxic drugs: increased risk of additive hepatotoxicity. Monitor closely.

EFFECTS ON DIAGNOSTIC TESTS
Drug therapy may increase blood and urine concentration of uric acid; it may also cause an increase in serum alkaline phosphatase, AST, and bilirubin levels, indicating drug-induced hepatotoxicity.

CONTRAINDICATIONS
None reported.

NURSING CONSIDERATIONS
● Use cautiously in patients with myelosuppression or impaired cardiac, renal, or hepatic function.
● Take preventive measures (including adequate hydration) before starting treatment. Hyperuricemia may result from rapid lysis of leukemic cells. Allopurinol may be ordered.
● Know that cardiac function studies (including ECG) should be performed before treatment and then periodically throughout therapy.
● Follow institutional policy to reduce risks. Preparation and administration of parenteral form of this drug is associated with carcinogenic, mutagenic, and teratogenic risks for personnel.
● **I.V. use:** Reconstitute drug using 4 ml of sterile water for injection to produce a 5 mg/ml solution.
● Withdraw the desired dose into a syringe containing 10 to 15 ml of 0.9% sodium chloride for injection. Inject into the tubing of a free-flowing I.V. solution of D_5W or 0.9% sodium chloride for injection over 2 to 3 minutes. Alternatively, dilute in 50 ml of 0.9% sodium chloride for injection, and infuse over 10 to 15 minutes, or dilute in 100 ml, and infuse over 30 to 45 minutes.
● Inject into tubing of free-flowing I.V. line. If extravasation occurs, discontinue I.V. infusion immediately, apply ice to area for 24 to 48 hours, and notify doctor. Drug is a vesicant; if extravasation occurs, severe tissue necrosis may result.
● Never give drug I.M. or S.C.
● Be aware that cumulative adult dosage is limited to 500 to 600 mg/m² (450 mg/

Reactions may be *common*, uncommon, *life-threatening*, or COMMON AND LIFE-THREATENING.

m² when patients are also receiving or have received cyclophosphamide or radiation therapy to cardiac area).
● Know that therapeutic effects are often accompanied by toxicity.
● Monitor CBC and hepatic function tests, as ordered; monitor ECG every month during therapy.
● Monitor pulse rate closely. Light resting pulse rate is a sign of cardiac adverse reactions. Notify the doctor if this occurs.
Alert: Stop drug immediately and notify doctor if signs of CHF or cardiomyopathy develop.
● Monitor for nausea and vomiting which may last 24 to 48 hours.
● Anticipate the need for blood transfusions to combat anemia.
● Know that reddish color is similar to that of doxorubicin. Take care to avoid confusing the two drugs.
● Optimally, use within 8 hours of preparation. Reconstituted solution is stable for 24 hours at room temperature or 48 hours if refrigerated.

☑ **PATIENT TEACHING**
● Advise patient to watch for signs of infection (fever, sore throat, fatigue) and bleeding (easy bruising, nosebleeds, bleeding gums, melena) and to take temperature daily.
● Advise patient that red urine for 1 to 2 days is normal and does not indicate the presence of blood in urine.
● Advise patient that alopecia may occur, but that it's usually reversible.
● Advise women of childbearing age to avoid becoming pregnant during therapy and to consult with doctor before becoming pregnant.

---

doxorubicin hydrochloride
Adriamycin‡, Adriamycin PFS, Adriamycin RDF, Rubex

Pregnancy Risk Category: D

HOW SUPPLIED
Injection (preservative-free): 2 mg/ml
Powder for injection: 10-mg, 20-mg, 50-mg, 100-mg, 150-mg vials

ACTION
Unknown. May interfere with DNA-dependent RNA synthesis by intercalation.

ONSET, PEAK, DURATION
Undefined.

INDICATIONS & DOSAGE
Dosage and indications vary. Check treatment protocol with the doctor.
Bladder, breast, lung, ovarian, stomach, and thyroid cancers; Hodgkin's disease; acute lymphoblastic and myeloblastic leukemia; Wilms' tumor; neuroblastoma; lymphoma; sarcoma—
Adults: 60 to 75 mg/m² I.V. as single dose q 3 weeks; or 30 mg/m² I.V. in single daily dose, days 1 to 3 of 4-week cycle. Alternatively, 20 mg/m² I.V. once weekly. Maximum cumulative dosage is 550 mg/m².

ADVERSE REACTIONS
CV: cardiac depression, seen in such ECG changes as sinus tachycardia, T-wave flattening, ST-segment depression, voltage reduction; *arrhythmias; acute left ventricular failure; irreversible cardiomyopathy.*
EENT: conjunctivitis.
GI: nausea, vomiting, diarrhea, *stomatitis,* esophagitis, anorexia.
GU: red urine (transient).
Hematologic: leukopenia during days 10 to 15 with recovery by day 21; *thrombocytopenia;* MYELOSUPPRESSION.
Skin: urticaria, facial flushing, *complete alopecia within 3 to 4 weeks* (hair may regrow 2 to 5 months after drug is stopped), hyperpigmentation of nailbeds and dermal creases, "radiation recall effect."
Other: *severe cellulitis or tissue sloughing* (if drug extravasates); hyperuricemia; fever; chills; *anaphylaxis.*

INTERACTIONS

Aminophylline, cephalothin, dexamethasone, fluorouracil, heparin, hydrocortisone: may form a precipitate. Don't mix together.

Digoxin: may decrease serum digoxin levels. Monitor closely.

Streptozocin: increased and prolonged blood levels. Dosage may have to be adjusted.

EFFECTS ON DIAGNOSTIC TESTS

Drug therapy may increase blood and urine concentrations of uric acid.

CONTRAINDICATIONS

Contraindicated in patients with marked myelosuppression induced by previous treatment with other antitumor agents or by radiotherapy and in patients who have received lifetime cumulative dosage of 550 mg/m² of doxorubicin or daunorubicin.

NURSING CONSIDERATIONS

● Know that cardiac function studies (including ECG) should be performed before treatment and then periodically throughout therapy. Be aware that dexrazoxane may be administered concomitantly with doxorubicin if the accumulated dose of doxorubicin has reached 300 mg/m².

● Take preventive measures (including adequate hydration) before starting treatment. Hyperuricemia may result from rapid lysis of leukemic cells. Allopurinol may be ordered.

● Premedicate with antiemetic, as ordered, to reduce nausea.

● Follow institutional policy to reduce risks. Preparation and administration of parenteral form of this drug is associated with carcinogenic, mutagenic, and teratogenic risks for personnel.

● **I.V. use:** Reconstitute using preservative-free 0.9% sodium chloride for injection. Add 5 ml to the 10-mg vial, 10 ml to the 20-mg vial, or 25 ml to the 50-mg vial. Shake vial and allow drug to dissolve; final concentration will be 2

mg/ml. Give by direct injection into the tubing of a free-flowing I.V. solution containing D₅W or 0.9% sodium chloride for injection. Administration rate should not be less than 3 minutes. Drug is a severe vesicant; if extravasation occurs, tissue necrosis may result.

● Don't place I.V. line over joints or in extremities with poor venous or lymphatic drainage. If extravasation occurs, discontinue I.V. infusion immediately, apply ice to area for 24 to 48 hours, and notify doctor. Monitor area closely because extravasation may be progressive. Early consultation with a plastic surgeon may be advisable.

● If vein streaking occurs, slow administration rate. However, if welts occur, stop administration and report this to the doctor.

● If skin or mucosal contact occurs, immediately wash with soap and water.

● In the event of a leak or spill, inactivate drug with 5% sodium hypochlorite solution (household bleach).

● Never give this drug I.M. or S.C.

● Know that dosage modification may be required in patients with myelosuppression and in those with impaired cardiac or hepatic function, and in elderly patients.

● Be prepared to decrease dosage if serum bilirubin level rises: 50% of the dosage should be given when bilirubin is 1.2 to 3 mg/100 ml; 25% when it's greater than 3 mg/100 ml.

● Monitor CBC and hepatic function tests, as ordered; monitor ECG monthly during therapy.

● Be prepared to stop drug or slow rate of infusion if tachycardia develops and notify the doctor.

Alert: If signs of CHF develop, stop the drug and notify the doctor. In many instances, CHF can be prevented by limiting cumulative dosage to 550 mg/m² (400 mg/m²) when patients are also receiving or have received cyclophosphamide or radiation therapy to cardiac area).

● Know that reddish color is similar to

that of daunorubicin. Take care to avoid confusing the two drugs.
● Keep in mind that esophagitis is very common in patients who have also received radiation therapy.
● Know that refrigerated, reconstituted solution is stable for 48 hours; at room temperature, it's stable for 24 hours.

☑ **PATIENT TEACHING**
● Advise patient to watch for signs of infection (fever, sore throat, fatigue) and bleeding (easy bruising, nosebleeds, bleeding gums, melena) and to take temperature daily.
● Advise patient that orange to red urine for 1 to 2 days is normal and does not indicate presence of blood.
● Warn patient that alopecia may occur, but that it's usually reversible.

---

idarubicin hydrochloride
Idamycin

Pregnancy Risk Category: D

HOW SUPPLIED
Powder for injection: 5 mg, 10 mg, 20 mg

ACTION
Unknown Probably inhibits nucleic acid synthesis by intercalation and interacts with the enzyme topoisomerase II. It is highly lipophilic, which results in an increased rate of cellular uptake.

ONSET, PEAK, DURATION
Onset and duration undefined. Intracellular drug levels peak within a few minutes after injection.

INDICATIONS & DOSAGE
Dosage and indications vary. Check treatment protocol with the doctor.
Acute myeloid leukemia, including FAB (French-American-British) classifications M1 through M7, in combination with other approved antileukemic agents—

Adults: 12 mg/m²/day for 3 days by slow I.V. injection (over 10 to 15 minutes) in combination with 100 mg/m²/day of cytarabine for 7 days by continuous I.V. infusion; or as a 25 mg/m² bolus (cytarabine), followed by 200 mg/m²/day (cytarabine) for 5 days by continuous infusion.

A second course may be administered if needed. If patients experience severe mucositis, administration is delayed until recovery is complete and dosage reduced by 25%. Dosage should also be reduced in patients with hepatic or renal impairment. Idarubicin should not be given if bilirubin level is above 5 mg/dl.

ADVERSE REACTIONS
CNS: *headache, changed mental status,* peripheral neuropathy, *seizures.*
CV: *CHF,* atrial fibrillation, chest pain, *MI,* asymptomatic decline in left ventricular ejection fraction, *myocardial insufficiency, arrhythmias,* HEMORRHAGE, *myocardial toxicity.*
GI: *nausea, vomiting, cramps, diarrhea, mucositis, severe enterocolitis with perforation* (rare).
GU: decreased renal function.
Hematologic: *myelosuppression.*
Hepatic: changes in hepatic function.
Skin: *rash, urticaria, bullous erythrodermatous rash on palms and soles,* hives at injection site, erythema at previously irradiated sites, tissue necrosis at injection site (if extravasation occurs).
Other: INFECTION, *alopecia, fever,* hyperuricemia, hypersensitivity reactions.

INTERACTIONS
Alkaline solutions, heparin: incompatibility. Idarubicin should not be mixed with other drugs unless specific compatibility data is available.

EFFECTS ON DIAGNOSTIC TESTS
None reported.

CONTRAINDICATIONS
None reported.

NURSING CONSIDERATIONS

• Use with extreme caution in patients with bone marrow suppression induced by previous drug therapy or radiotherapy, impaired hepatic or renal function, prior treatment with anthracyclines or cardiotoxic agents, or a preexisting cardiac condition.

• Cardiotoxicity is the dose-limiting toxicity of this drug.

• Take preventive measures (including adequate hydration) before starting treatment. Hyperuricemia may result from rapid lysis of leukemic cells. Allopurinol may be ordered.

• Assess patient for systemic infection and ensure that it's controlled before therapy begins.

• Give antiemetics, as ordered, to prevent or treat nausea and vomiting.

• Follow institutional policy to reduce risks. Preparation and administration of parenteral form of this drug is associated with carcinogenic, mutagenic, and teratogenic risks for personnel.

• **I.V. use:** Reconstitute to a final concentration of 1 mg/ml using 0.9% sodium chloride for injection without preservatives. Add 5 ml to the 5-mg vial, 10 ml to the 10-mg vial, or 20 ml to the 20-mg vial. Do *not* use bacteriostatic sodium chloride. Vial is under negative pressure.

• Administer over 10 to 15 minutes into a free-flowing I.V. infusion of 0.9% sodium chloride or 5% dextrose solution running into a large vein.

• Drug is a vesicant; tissue necrosis may result. If extravasation occurs, discontinue infusion immediately and notify doctor. Treat with intermittent ice packs—for ½ hour immediately, and then for ½ hour four times daily for 4 days.

• Know that reconstituted solutions are stable for 3 days (72 hours) at room temperature (59° to 86° F [15° to 30° C]); 7 days if refrigerated. Label any unused solutions with CHEMOTHERAPY HAZARD label.

• Monitor hepatic and renal function tests and CBC frequently, as ordered.

• To prevent bleeding, avoid all I.M. injections when platelet count is below 100,000/mm³.

• Anticipate the need for blood transfusions to combat anemia.

• Notify doctor if signs or symptoms of CHF occur.

☑ PATIENT TEACHING

• Instruct patient to recognize signs and symptoms of extravasation and to call the doctor or nurse if these occur.

• Warn patient to watch for signs of infection (fever, sore throat, fatigue) and bleeding (easy bruising, nosebleeds, bleeding gums, melena).

• Advise patient that red urine for several days is normal and does not indicate presence of blood.

• Advise women of childbearing age to avoid becoming pregnant during therapy and to consult with doctor before becoming pregnant.

---

mitomycin (mitomycin-C)
Mutamycin

Pregnancy Risk Category: NR

HOW SUPPLIED
Injection: 5-mg, 20-mg, 40-mg vials

ACTION
Acts like an alkylating agent, cross-linking strands of DNA. This causes an imbalance of cell growth, leading to cell death.

ONSET, PEAK, DURATION
Undefined.

INDICATIONS & DOSAGE
Dosage and indications vary. Check treatment protocol with the doctor.
Disseminated adenocarcinoma of stomach or pancreas—
Adults: 20 mg/m² as an I.V. single dose. Cycle repeated after 6 to 8 weeks when WBC and platelet counts have returned to normal.

ADVERSE REACTIONS

CNS: headache, neurologic abnormalities, confusion, drowsiness, fatigue.
GI: *nausea, vomiting, anorexia, diarrhea.*
Hematologic: THROMBOCYTOPENIA, LEUKOPENIA (may be delayed up to 8 weeks and may be cumulative with successive doses).
Respiratory: *interstitial pneumonitis,* pulmonary edema, dyspnea, nonproductive cough, adult respiratory distress syndrome.
Other: desquamation, induration, pruritus, *pain at injection site; septicemia;* cellulitis, ulceration, sloughing with extravasation; *reversible alopecia; fever; microangiopathic hemolytic anemia, characterized by thrombocytopenia, renal failure, and hypertension;* blurred vision, pain.

INTERACTIONS

Vinca alkaloids: may cause acute respiratory distress when administered concomitantly. Monitor closely.

EFFECTS ON DIAGNOSTIC TESTS

Drug therapy, through drug-induced renal toxicity, may increase serum creatinine and BUN concentrations.

CONTRAINDICATIONS

Contraindicated in patients hypersensitive to the drug and in those with thrombocytopenia, coagulation disorders, or an increase in bleeding tendency due to other causes.

NURSING CONSIDERATIONS

● Follow institutional policy to reduce risks. Preparation and administration of parenteral form of this drug is associated with mutagenic, teratogenic, and carcinogenic risks to personnel.
● **I.V. use:** Using sterile water for injection, reconstitute the 5-mg vials with 10 ml, the 20-mg vials with 40 ml, and the 40-mg vials with 80 ml.
● For infusion, dilute with 0.9% sodium

chloride for injection, D_5W, or sodium lactate for injection. After dilution, drug is stable for 3 hours in D_5W, 12 hours in 0.9% sodium chloride for injection, and 24 hours in sodium lactate for injection at room temperature.
● Avoid extravasation. Stop infusion immediately if extravasation occurs because of the potential for severe ulceration and necrosis, and notify doctor.
● Never give this drug I.M. or S.C.
● Continue CBC and blood studies, as ordered, at least 8 weeks after therapy is stopped. Leukopenia and thrombocytopenia are cumulative.
● To prevent bleeding, avoid all I.M. injections when platelet count is below 100,000/mm³.
● Anticipate the need for blood transfusions to combat anemia.
● Monitor patient for dyspnea with nonproductive cough; chest x-ray may show infiltrates.
● Monitor renal function tests, as ordered.

☑ PATIENT TEACHING
● Warn patient to watch for signs of infection (fever, sore throat, fatigue) and bleeding (easy bruising, nosebleeds, bleeding gums, melena). Tell patient to take temperature daily.
● Warn patient that alopecia may occur, but that it's usually reversible.

pentostatin (2´-deoxycoformycin)
Nipent

Pregnancy Risk Category: D

HOW SUPPLIED
Powder for injection: 10 mg-vial

ACTION
Inhibits the enzyme adenosine deaminase (ADA), causing an increase in intracellular levels of deoxyadenosine triphosphate. This leads to cell damage and death. Because the greatest activity

of ADA is in cells of the lymphoid system (especially malignant T cells), pentostatin is useful in treating leukemias.

ONSET, PEAK, DURATION
Undefined.

INDICATIONS & DOSAGE
Alpha-interferon–refractory hairy-cell leukemia—
Adults: 4 mg/m^2 I.V. every other week.

ADVERSE REACTIONS
CNS: *headache, neurologic symptoms, anxiety, confusion, depression, dizziness, insomnia, nervousness, paresthesia, somnolence, abnormal thinking, fatigue.*
CV: *arrhythmias, abnormal ECG, thrombophlebitis, peripheral edema, hemorrhage.*
EENT: *abnormal vision, conjunctivitis, ear pain, eye pain, epistaxis, pharyngitis, rhinitis, sinusitis.*
GI: *nausea, vomiting, anorexia, diarrhea, constipation, flatulence, stomatitis.*
GU: *hematuria, dysuria, increased BUN and creatinine levels.*
Hematologic: *myelosuppression,* LEUKOPENIA, *anemia,* **thrombocytopenia,** *lymphadenopathy.*
Hepatic: *elevated liver enzyme levels.*
Respiratory: *cough, bronchitis, dyspnea, lung edema, pneumonia.*
Skin: *ecchymosis, petechiae, rash, eczema, dry skin, herpes simplex or zoster, maculopapular rash, vesiculobullous rash, pruritus, seborrhea, discoloration, diaphoresis.*
Other: *fever,* INFECTION, *pain, hypersensitivity reactions, chills, sepsis,* DEATH, NEOPLASM, *chest pain, abdominal pain, back pain, flulike syndrome, asthenia, malaise, myalgia, arthralgia, weight loss.*

INTERACTIONS
Cytarabine or vidarabine: increased incidence or severity of adverse effects associated with either drug. Avoid con-

comitant use.
Fludarabine: risk of severe or fatal pulmonary toxicity. Don't use together.

EFFECTS ON DIAGNOSTIC TESTS
None reported.

CONTRAINDICATIONS
Contraindicated in patients hypersensitive to the drug.

NURSING CONSIDERATIONS
● Use cautiously and only under the supervision of a doctor qualified and experienced in the use of chemotherapeutic agents. Adverse reactions after pentostatin therapy are common.
● Know that use in patients with renal damage (creatinine clearance of 60 ml/minute or less) should be avoided.
● Make sure patients are adequately hydrated before therapy. Administer 500 to 1,000 ml of D$_5$W in 0.45% sodium chloride solution, as ordered, for hydration. Ensure at least 2 liters of urine output daily while on therapy.
● Follow institutional policy to reduce risks. Preparation and administration of parenteral form of this drug is associated with mutagenic, teratogenic, and carcinogenic risks to personnel.
● I.V. use: Add 5 ml of sterile water for injection to the vial containing pentostatin powder for injection. Mix thoroughly to make a solution of 2 mg/ml. Drug may be administered by I.V. bolus injection or diluted further in 25 or 50 ml of D$_5$W or 0.9% sodium chloride for injection and infused over 20 to 30 minutes.
● Use reconstituted solution within 8 hours; it contains no preservatives.
● Treat all spills and waste products with 5% sodium hypochlorite (household bleach).
● Give an additional 500 ml of D$_5$W, as ordered, for hydration after drug is administered.
● Know that the optimal duration of therapy is unknown. Current recommendations suggest two additional courses

of therapy after a complete response. If a partial response is not evident after 6 months of therapy, drug will be discontinued. If a partial response is evident, drug will be continued for another 6 months.

Alert: Withhold or discontinue drug in patients with evidence of CNS toxicity, a severe rash, or an active infection, and notify the doctor. Drug may be resumed when the infection clears.

• Temporarily withhold drug if the absolute neutrophil count falls below 200/mm³ and the pretreatment level was over 500/mm³, and notify the doctor. No recommendations exist regarding dosage adjustments in patients with anemia, neutropenia, or thrombocytopenia.

• Be aware that drug should be used only in patients who have hairy-cell leukemia refractory to alpha-interferon. This is defined as disease that progresses after a minimum of 3 months of treatment with alpha-interferon or disease that does not exhibit a response after 6 months of therapy.

• Monitor renal function.

☑ **PATIENT TEACHING**
• Advise patient to watch for signs of infection (fever, sore throat, fatigue) and bleeding (easy bruising, nosebleeds, bleeding gums, melena) and to take temperature daily.

• Advise women of childbearing age to avoid becoming pregnant during therapy and to consult with doctor before becoming pregnant.

---

plicamycin (mithramycin)
Mithracin

Pregnancy Risk Category: X

HOW SUPPLIED
Injection: 2.5-mg vials

ACTION
Unknown. Thought to form a complex with DNA, thus inhibiting RNA synthe-

sis. Also inhibits osteocytic activity, blocking calcium and phosphorus resorption from bone.

ONSET, PEAK, DURATION
Onset occurs in 1 to 2 days. Effects peak 3 days after single dose and persist for 7 to 10 days.

INDICATIONS & DOSAGE
Dosage and indications vary. Check treatment protocol with the doctor.
Hypercalcemia and hypercalciuria associated with advanced malignant disease—
Adults: 25 mcg/kg/day I.V. for 3 to 4 days. Dosage repeated at weekly intervals until desired response is obtained.
Testicular cancer—
Adults: 25 to 30 mcg/kg/day I.V. for 8 to 10 days or until toxicity occurs.

ADVERSE REACTIONS
CNS: drowsiness, weakness, lethargy, depression, headache, malaise.
GI: *nausea, vomiting,* anorexia, diarrhea, stomatitis.
GU: increased BUN and serum creatinine levels.
Hematologic: *leukopenia, thrombocytopenia; bleeding syndrome* (from epistaxis to generalized hemorrhage).
Hepatic: *elevated liver enzymes levels,* hepatotoxicity.
Skin: facial flushing, rash.
Other: *decreased serum calcium,* potassium, and phosphorus levels; *death,* fever, cellulitis with extravasation, phlebitis.

INTERACTIONS
None significant.

EFFECTS ON DIAGNOSTIC TESTS
Because of drug-induced toxicity, drug therapy may increase serum concentrations of alkaline phosphatase, AST, ALT, lactate dehydrogenase, and bilirubin; it may also increase serum creatinine and BUN levels through nephrotoxicity.

CONTRAINDICATIONS

Contraindicated in patients with thrombocytopenia, bone marrow suppression, or coagulation and bleeding disorders and in women who are or who may become pregnant.

NURSING CONSIDERATIONS

● Use with extreme caution in patients with significant renal or hepatic impairment.

● Obtain baseline platelet count and PT before therapy, as ordered.

● To reduce nausea, give antiemetic before administering, as ordered.

● Follow institutional policy to reduce risks. Preparation and administration of parenteral form of this drug is associated with carcinogenic, mutagenic, and teratogenic risks for personnel.

● **I.V. use:** To prepare solution, add 4.9 ml of sterile water for injection to vial and shake to dissolve. Then dilute for I.V infusion in 1,000 ml of D_5W or 0.9% sodium chloride. Administer by infusion over 4 to 6 hours. Discard unused drug.

● Be aware that slow infusion reduces nausea that develops with I.V. push.

● Avoid extravasation. Plicamycin is a vesicant and tissue necrosis may result. If I.V. solution infiltrates, stop immediately, notify doctor, and use ice packs. Restart I.V. line.

● Avoid contact with skin or mucous membranes.

● Monitor platelet count and PT during therapy, as ordered. Discontinue drug if WBC count is less than 4,000/mm³, if platelet count falls to less than 150,000/mm³, or if PT is prolonged more than 4 seconds longer than control, and notify doctor.

Alert: Know that facial flushing is an early indicator of bleeding.

● To prevent bleeding, avoid all I.M. injections when platelet count is below 100,000/mm³.

● Anticipate the need for blood transfusions to combat anemia.

● Monitor lactate dehydrogenase, AST, ALT, alkaline phosphatase, BUN, creatinine, potassium, calcium, and phosphorus levels, as ordered.

● Monitor patients for tetany, carpopedal spasm, Chvostek's sign, and muscle cramps; check serum calcium level. Precipitous drop in calcium level is possible.

● Store lyophilized powder in refrigerator and protect from light.

● Be aware that patients receiving drug for treatment testicular cancer may require calcium supplementation.

☑ **PATIENT TEACHING**

● Advise patient to watch for signs of infection (fever, sore throat, fatigue) and bleeding (easy bruising, nosebleeds, bleeding gums, melena) and to take temperature daily.

● Advise women of childbearing age to avoid becoming pregnant during therapy and to consult with doctor before becoming pregnant.

72

Antineoplastics that alter hormone balance

anastrozole
bicalutamide
diethylstilbestrol
(See Chapter 55, ESTROGENS AND PROGESTINS)
estramustine phosphate sodium
flutamide
goserelin acetate
leuprolide acetate
megestrol acetate
nilutamide
tamoxifen citrate
testolactone

COMBINATION PRODUCTS
None.

anastrozole
Arimidex

Pregnancy Risk Category: D

HOW SUPPLIED
Tablets: 1 mg

ACTION
Selective nonsteroidal aromatase inhibitor that significantly lowers serum estradiol concentrations, thereby inhibiting stimulation of breast cancer cell growth in postmenopausal women.

ONSET, PEAK, DURATION
Unknown.

INDICATIONS & DOSAGE
Treatment of advanced breast cancer in postmenopausal women with disease progression after tamoxifen therapy—
Adults: 1 mg P.O. daily.

ADVERSE REACTIONS
CNS: *headache,* dizziness, depression, paresthesia.
CV: chest pain, edema.
GI: *nausea,* vomiting, diarrhea, constipation, abdominal pain, anorexia, dry mouth.
GU: vaginal hemorrhage, vaginal dryness.
Respiratory: dyspnea, increased cough, pharyngitis.
Skin: *hot flushes,* rash, sweating.
Other: *asthenia, pain, back pain,* bone pain, peripheral edema, pelvic pain, thromboembolic disease, weight gain.

INTERACTIONS
None.

EFFECTS ON DIAGNOSTIC TESTS
None reported.

CONTRAINDICATIONS
None known.

NURSING CONSIDERATIONS
- Use cautiously in breast-feeding women.
- Know that pregnancy must be ruled out before treatment.
- Be aware that drug should be administered under the supervision of a qualified doctor experienced in the use of anticancer drugs.

☑ **PATIENT TEACHING**
- Instruct the patient to report adverse reactions.
- Stress need for follow-up care.
- Counsel patient of childbearing age about potential risks to pregnancy during therapy.

bicalutamide
Casodex

Pregnancy Risk Category: X

HOW SUPPLIED
Tablets: 50 mg

ACTION
A nonsteroidal antiandrogen that binds to cytosol androgen receptors in target tissue.

ONSET, PEAK, DURATION
Unknown.

INDICATIONS & DOSAGE
Adjunct therapy in combination with a leutinizing hormone-releasing hormone (LHRH) analog for treatment of advanced prostate cancer—
Adults: 50 mg P.O. once daily in morning or evening.

ADVERSE REACTIONS
CNS: anxiety, depression, headache, dizziness, paresthesia, insomnia.
CV: *hot flashes,* hypertension, chest pain, peripheral edema.
GI: *constipation, nausea, diarrhea,* abdominal pain, flatulence, increased liver enzymes, vomiting.
GU: nocturia, hematuria, urinary tract infection, impotence, *gynecomastia,* urinary incontinence.
Hematologic: hypochromic anemia, iron deficiency anemia.
Respiratory: dyspnea.
Skin: rash, sweating, dry skin, pruritis.
Other: *general pain, back pain, breast pain, pelvic pain, asthenia, infection,* flu syndrome, hyperglycemia, bone pain, weight loss.

INTERACTIONS
Coumarin anticoagulants: displacement of these drugs from their protein-binding sites. Monitor prothrombin times closely, and know that the anticoagulant dose may need adjustment.

EFFECTS ON DIAGNOSTIC TESTS
Drug may elevate AST, ALT, bilirubin, BUN, and creatinine levels and decrease hemoglobin and WBC counts.

CONTRAINDICATIONS
Contraindicated in patients with hypersensitivity to the drug or any component and during pregnancy.

NURSING CONSIDERATIONS
● Use cautiously in patients with moderate-to-severe hepatic impairment (drug is extensively metabolized by the liver).
● Bicalutamide is used in combination with a LHRH analogue. Treatment should be started at the same time for both drugs.
● Give drug at same time each day.
● Regularly monitor serum prostate specific antigen (PSA) levels, as ordered. PSA levels help in assessing response to therapy. Report elevated levels to the doctor, who should evaluate the patient to determine disease progression.
● Monitor liver function studies, as ordered. When a patient develops jaundice or exhibits laboratory evidence of liver injury in the absence of liver metastases, drug should be discontinued. Abnormalities are usually reversible on discontinuation.

☑ PATIENT TEACHING
● Tell the patient to take drug at the same time each day, without regard to meals.
● Urge him not to stop drug therapy without consulting the doctor.

---

estramustine phosphate sodium
Emcyt, Estracyst‡

Pregnancy Risk Category: NR

HOW SUPPLIED
Capsules: 140 mg

ACTION
Unknown. A combination of estrogen and an alkylating agent; probably acts

by its ability to bind selectively to a protein present in the prostate gland.

ONSET, PEAK, DURATION
Unknown.

INDICATIONS & DOSAGE
Palliative treatment of metastatic or progressive prostate cancer—
Adults: 10 to 16 mg/kg/day P.O. in three or four divided doses. Usual dosage is 14 mg/kg daily. Therapy continued for up to 3 months and, if successful, maintained as long as the patient responds.

ADVERSE REACTIONS
CNS: lethargy, insomnia, headache, anxiety.
CV: *MI,* sodium and fluid retention, chest pain, thrombophlebitis, *CHF, stroke.*
GI: *nausea, vomiting,* diarrhea, anorexia, flatulence, GI bleeding, thirst.
Hematologic: *leukopenia, thrombocytopenia.*
Respiratory: *edema, pulmonary embolism,* dyspnea.
Skin: rash, pruritus, dry skin, thinning of hair, flushing.
Other: *painful gynecomastia and breast tenderness,* leg cramps.

INTERACTIONS
Calcium-rich foods (milk and dairy products) and calcium containing drugs such as antacids: impaired absorption of estramustine. Do not administer at same time.

EFFECTS ON DIAGNOSTIC TESTS
Drug therapy may increase norephinephrine-induced platelet aggregability and may reduce response to the metyrapone test. Glucose tolerance may be decreased.

CONTRAINDICATIONS
Contraindicated in patients hypersensitive to estradiol and nitrogen mustard. Also contraindicated in those with active thrombophlebitis or thromboembolic disorders, except when the actual tumor mass is the cause of the thromboembolic phenomenon.

NURSING CONSIDERATIONS
● Use cautiously in patients with history of thrombophlebitis or thromboembolic disorders and cerebrovascular or coronary artery disease. Monitor weight regularly in these patients. Estramustine may exaggerate preexisting peripheral edema or CHF.
● Also use cautiously in patients with impaired liver function. Monitor liver function periodically throughout therapy.
● Be aware that each 140-mg capsule contains 12.5 mg of sodium.
● Monitor blood pressure and blood glucose periodically throughout therapy. Drug may increase blood pressure and decrease blood glucose.
● Keep in mind that estramustine is a combination of estrogen estradiol and a nitrogen mustard, shown to be effective in patients refractory to estrogen therapy alone.
● Be aware that patients may continue therapy as long as response is favorable. Some patients have taken the drug for more than 3 years.
● Store capsules in refrigerator.

☑ **PATIENT TEACHING**
● Tell patient to take this drug on an empty stomach (1 hour before or 2 hours after meals) and to avoid taking with milk or dairy products.
● Because of the possibility of mutagenic effects, advise patient and partner to use contraception if woman is of childbearing age.

flutamide
Euflex†, Eulexin

Pregnancy Risk Category: D

HOW SUPPLIED
Capsules: 125 mg, 250 mg†

ACTION
Inhibits androgen uptake or prevents binding of androgens in nucleus of cells within target tissues.

ONSET, PEAK, DURATION
Onset and duration unknown. Plasma levels peak 2 hours after dose.

INDICATIONS & DOSAGE
Metastatic prostate cancer (stage B_2, C, D_2) in combination with luteinizing hormone-releasing hormone analogues such as leuprolide acetate—
Adults: 250 mg P.O. q 8 hours.

ADVERSE REACTIONS
CNS: drowsiness, confusion, depression, anxiety, nervousness.
CV: peripheral edema, hypertension.
GI: *diarrhea, nausea, vomiting,* anorexia.
GU: *impotence, loss of libido.*
Hematologic: anemia, leukopenia, *thrombocytopenia,* hemolytic anemia.
Hepatic: elevated liver enzyme levels, hepatitis, encephalopathy.
Skin: rash, photosensitivity.
Other: *hot flashes,* gynecomastia.

INTERACTIONS
None significant.

EFFECTS ON DIAGNOSTIC TESTS
Elevation of plasma testosterone and estradiol levels has been reported. Serum ALT, AST, bilirubin, and creatinine levels may be increased.

CONTRAINDICATIONS
Contraindicated in patients hypersensitive to the drug.

NURSING CONSIDERATIONS
● Monitor liver function tests and CBC periodically, as ordered.
● Know that flutamide must be taken continuously with the agent used for medical castration (such as leuprolide acetate) to allow the full benefit of therapy. Leuprolide suppresses testosterone production while flutamide inhibits testosterone action at the cellular level. Together, they can impair the growth of androgen-responsive tumors.

☑ PATIENT TEACHING
● Advise patient not to discontinue drug therapy without consulting the doctor.
● Instruct patient to report adverse reactions promptly.

---

goserelin acetate
Zoladex

Pregnancy Risk Category: X (endometriosis); D (breast cancer)

HOW SUPPLIED
Implants: 3.6 mg, 10.8 mg

ACTION
A luteinizing hormone-releasing hormone (LHRH) analogue that acts on the pituitary to decrease the release of follicle-stimulating hormone and luteinizing hormone, resulting in dramatically lowered serum levels of sex hormones.

ONSET, PEAK, DURATION
Onset occurs in 2 to 4 weeks. Serum levels peak after 12 to 15 days. Suppression of hormone production to castration levels persists throughout therapy.

INDICATIONS & DOSAGE
Endometriosis, palliative treatment of advanced prostate cancer—
Adults: 3.6 mg S.C. q 28 days into the upper abdominal wall. For endometriosis, maximum duration of therapy is 6 months. For prostate cancer, 10.8 mg S.C. q 12 weeks into upper abdominal wall.
✴*New indication: Palliative treatment of advanced breast cancer in pre- and perimenopausal women—*
Adults: 3.6 mg S.C. q 28 days into the upper abdominal wall.

ADVERSE REACTIONS

CNS: lethargy, pain (worsened in the first 30 days), dizziness, *insomnia*, anxiety, *depression, headache,* chills, *emotional lability.*

CV: edema, ***CHF, arrhythmias,*** *peripheral edema,* ***CVA,*** hypertension, ***MI,*** peripheral vascular disorder, chest pain.

GI: nausea, vomiting, diarrhea, constipation, ulcer, anorexia, abdominal pain.

GU: *impotence, sexual dysfunction, lower urinary tract symptoms,* renal insufficiency, urinary obstruction, *vaginitis,* urinary tract infection, amenorrhea.

Hematologic: anemia.

Respiratory: COPD, upper respiratory infection.

Skin: rash, *diaphoresis, acne, seborrhea,* hirsutism.

Other: *hot flashes,* gout, hyperglycemia, weight increase, breast swelling and tenderness, *changes in breast size, pain, changes in libido, asthenia, infection,* breast pain, back pain, hypercalcemia.

INTERACTIONS
None significant.

EFFECTS ON DIAGNOSTIC TESTS
Serum testosterone levels increase during the first week of therapy and then decrease. Serum acid phosphatase may increase initially and will decrease by week 4.

CONTRAINDICATIONS
Contraindicated in patients with hypersensitivity to LHRH, LHRH agonist analogues, or to goserelin acetate. Also contraindicated during pregnancy or breast-feeding.

NURSING CONSIDERATIONS
● Because use of the drug is associated with a loss of bone mineral density in women, use cautiously in patients with other risk factors for osteoporosis, such as family history of osteoporosis, chronic alcohol or tobacco abuse, or the use of drugs such as corticosteroids or anti-convulsants that affect bone density.

● Before administering to female patients, rule out pregnancy.

● Administer drug into the upper abdominal wall using aseptic technique. After cleaning the area with an alcohol swab (and injecting a local anesthetic), stretch the patient's skin with one hand while grasping the barrel of the syringe with the other. Insert the needle into the subcutaneous fat; then change direction of the needle so that it parallels the abdominal wall. The needle should then be pushed in until the hub touches the patient's skin; then withdrawn about 1 cm (this creates a gap for the drug to be injected) before depressing the plunger completely.

● To avoid the need for a new syringe and injection site, do not aspirate after inserting the needle.

Alert: Know that the implant comes in a preloaded syringe. If the package is damaged, do not use the syringe. Make sure that the drug is visible in the translucent chamber of the syringe.

● When used for prostate cancer, be aware that LHRH analogues such as goserelin may initially cause a worsening of prostatic cancer symptoms because the drug initially increases testosterone serum levels. A few patients may experience increased bone pain. Rarely, disease exacerbation (either spinal cord compression or ureteral obstruction) has occurred.

☑ PATIENT TEACHING
● Advise patient to report every 28 days for a new implant. A delay of a couple of days is permissible.

● Tell women to use a nonhormonal form of contraception during treatment. Caution patient about the significant risks to the fetus should pregnancy occur.

● Tell patient to call the doctor if menstruation persists or if breakthrough bleeding occurs. Menstruation should stop during treatment.

● After therapy ends, inform patient that

---

*Liquid contains alcohol.   **May contain tartrazine.   †Canada only.   ‡Australia only.   ◇OTC.

she may experience a delayed return of menses. Persistent amenorrhea is rare.

---

leuprolide acetate

Lucrin‡, Lupron, Lupron Depot, Lupron Depot-Ped, Lupron Depot-3 Month

Pregnancy Risk Category: X

HOW SUPPLIED

Injection: 1 mg/0.2 ml (5 mg/ml) in 2.8-ml multiple-dose vials
Depot injection: 3.75 mg, 7.5 mg, 11.5 mg, 15 mg, 22.5 mg

ACTION

Initially stimulates but then inhibits the release of follicle-stimulating hormone and luteinizing hormone, resulting in testosterone suppression.

ONSET, PEAK, DURATION

Testosterone concentrations decline to castrate levels within 2 to 4 weeks. Time to peak effect for amenorrhea usually occurs after 1 to 2 months of therapy. Normal pituitary-gonadal system function is usually restored within 4 to 12 weeks after therapy is withdrawn. Cyclic bleeding in females usually returns within 60 to 90 days after therapy is withdrawn.

INDICATIONS & DOSAGE

Advanced prostate cancer—
Adults: 1 mg S.C. daily. Alternatively, 7.5 mg I.M. (depot injection) monthly or 22.5 mg I.M. q 3 months (depot injection).
Endometriosis—
Adults: 3.75 mg I.M (depot injection only) as a single injection once a month for up to 6 months.
Central precocious puberty—
Children: initially, 0.3 mg/kg (minimum 7.5 mg) I.M. (depot injection only) as a single injection q 4 weeks. Dosage may be increased in increments of 3.75 mg q 4 weeks, if needed. Thera-

py should be discontinued before female child reaches age 11 and before male child reaches age 12.

ADVERSE REACTIONS

CNS: *dizziness, depression, headache, pain,* insomnia.
CV: arrhythmias, angina, *MI, peripheral edema, ECG changes,* hypotension, hypertension, murmur.
GI: *nausea, vomiting,* anorexia, constipation.
GU: *impotence, vaginitis,* urinary frequency, hematuria, urinary tract infection, gynecomastia.
Hepatic: elevated liver enzyme levels.
Respiratory: dyspnea, sinus congestion, pulmonary fibrosis.
Other: transient bone pain during first week of treatment, *hot flashes,* skin reactions at injection site, androgen-like effects, joint disorder, myalgia, neuromuscular disorder, *weight gain or loss,* anemia, dermatitis, *asthenia.*

INTERACTIONS

None significant.

EFFECTS ON DIAGNOSTIC TESTS

Serum acid phosphatase and testosterone levels initially increase, then decrease with continued therapy.

CONTRAINDICATIONS

Contraindicated in patients hypersensitive to the drug or other gonadotropin-releasing hormone analogues, during pregnancy or lactation, and in women with undiagnosed vaginal bleeding.

NURSING CONSIDERATIONS

● Use cautiously in patients hypersensitive to benzyl alcohol.
● Never administer by I.V. injection.
● Know that depot injections should be administered under medical supervision. Use supplied diluent to reconstitute drug. Draw 1 ml into a syringe with a 22G needle (extra diluent is provided and should be discarded). Withdraw 1.5 ml from ampule for the 3-month formu-

---

lation. Inject into vial; then shake well. Suspension will appear milky. Although the suspension is stable for 24 hours after reconstitution, it contains no bacteriostatic agent. Use immediately.
● Be aware that response to the treatment of central precocious puberty should be monitored q 1 to 2 months after the start of therapy with a GnRH stimulation test and sex steroid levels. Measurement of bone age for advancement should be done q 6 to 12 months.
● Know that drug use may cause an increase in the signs and symptoms being treated during first few weeks of therapy.

☑ **PATIENT TEACHING**
● Prior to starting a child on treatment of central precocious puberty, ensure that parents understand the importance of continuous therapy.
● Carefully instruct patient who will self-administer S.C. injection about proper administration techniques and advise them to use only the syringes provided by the manufacturer.
● Advise patient that if another syringe must be substituted, a low-dose insulin syringe (U-100, 0.5 ml) may be an appropriate choice but that needle gauge should not be smaller than 22G.
● Advise patient to store the drug at room temperature, protected from light and sources of heat.
● Reassure patient with history of undesirable effects from other endocrine therapies that drug is easier to tolerate.
● Reassure patient that effects disappear after about 1 week. Worsening of prostate cancer symptoms or central precocious puberty symptoms may occur initially.
● Advise female patient of childbearing age to use a nonhormonal form of contraception during treatment.

---

megestrol acetate
Megace, Megostat‡

Pregnancy Risk Category: D

HOW SUPPLIED
Tablets: 20 mg, 40 mg
Oral suspension: 40 mg/ml

ACTION
A progestin that changes the tumor's hormonal environment and alters the neoplastic process. Mechanism responsible for appetite stimulation is unknown.

ONSET, PEAK, DURATION
Unknown.

INDICATIONS & DOSAGE
Breast cancer—
Adults: 40 mg P.O. q.i.d.
Endometrial cancer—
Adults: 40 to 320 mg P.O. daily in divided doses.
Treatment of anorexia, cachexia, or unexplained significant weight loss in patients with AIDS—
Adults: 800 mg P.O. (oral suspension) daily.

ADVERSE REACTIONS
CV: thrombophlebitis.
GI: nausea, vomiting.
GU: breakthrough menstrual bleeding.
Respiratory: *pulmonary embolism,* dyspnea.
Skin: rash.
Other: weight gain, increased appetite, carpal tunnel syndrome, alopecia, hyperglycemia, tumor flare.

INTERACTIONS
None significant.

EFFECTS ON DIAGNOSTIC TESTS
Pregnanediol excretion may decrease; serum alkaline phosphatase and amino acid concentrations may increase. Glucose tolerance has been shown to decrease in a small percentage of patients.

CONTRAINDICATIONS

Contraindicated in patients hypersensitive to the drug or as a diagnostic test for pregnancy.

NURSING CONSIDERATIONS

● Use cautiously in patients with history of thrombophlebitis.
● Know that megestrol is a relatively nontoxic drug with a low incidence of adverse effects.
● Be aware that 2 months is an adequate trial when treating patients with cancer.

☑ PATIENT TEACHING

● Inform patient that therapeutic response isn't immediate.
● Advise breast-feeding patient to discontinue breast-feeding during therapy because of possible infant toxicity.
● Advise women of childbearing age to use an effective form of contraception while receiving this drug.

▼ NEW DRUG

nilutamide
Nilandron

Pregnancy Risk Category: C

HOW SUPPLIED
Tablets: 50 mg

ACTION
This nonsteroidal antiandrogen interacts with the androgen receptor and prevents normal androgenic response.

ONSET, PEAK, DURATION
Unknown.

INDICATIONS & DOSAGE
Adjunct therapy with surgical castration for the treatment of metastatic prostate cancer—
Adults: 6 tablets (50 mg each) P.O. once a day for a total of 300 mg/day for 30 days; then 3 tablets once a day for a total of 150 mg/day thereafter.

ADVERSE REACTIONS
CNS: dizziness.
CV: hypertension.
EENT: *impaired adaptation to darkness,* abnormal vision.
GI: nausea, constipation.
GU: UTI.
Hepatic: elevated liver enzymes.
Respiratory: dyspnea, interstitial pneumonitis.
Other: *hot flushes.*

INTERACTIONS
Vitamin K antagonists, phenytoin, and theophylline: possible delayed elimination and toxicity. Doses should be modified accordingly.

EFFECTS ON DIAGNOSTIC TESTS
None reported.

CONTRAINDICATIONS
Contraindicated in patients with hypersensitivity to the drug and in patients with severe hepatic and respiratory disease.

NURSING CONSIDERATIONS
● Nilutamide is used in combination with surgical castration and should begin on the same day or on the day after surgery for maximum benefit.
● Safety for use in breast-feeding women has not been determined. Drug should be given to pregnant women only if clearly needed.
● Know that safety and effectiveness in pediatric patients have not been determined.
● Obtain baseline liver enzymes and periodically, at 3-month intervals, as ordered. Know that the drug should be discontinued if transaminase levels exceed 3 times the upper limit of normal.
● A baseline chest X-ray should be obtained before therapy begins. Monitor patient, especially if he is Asian, for signs of interstitial pneumonitis, and notify the doctor if they occur. Obtain chest X-ray, as ordered.

☑ PATIENT TEACHING
● Explain purpose of drug, how it is given, and the importance of not stopping treatment without consulting the doctor.
● Tell patient to report dyspnea or aggravation of pre-existing dyspnea immediately.
● Inform patient of the possibility of developing hepatitis and to report symptoms of nausea, vomiting, abdominal pain, or jaundice to doctor. Tell patient to avoid alcohol.
● Warn patient that visual disturbances such as a delay in the ability to adapt to darkness may affect driving at night or through tunnels.

---

tamoxifen citrate
Alpha-Tamoxifen†, Nolvadex, Nolvadex-D†‡, Novo-Tamoxifen†, Tamofen†, Tamone†, Tamoplex†

Pregnancy Risk Category: D

HOW SUPPLIED
Tablets: 10 mg, 20 mg
Tablets (enteric-coated)†: 10 mg, 20 mg

ACTION
Exact antineoplastic action is unknown; acts as an estrogen antagonist.

ONSET, PEAK, DURATION
Onset occurs in 4 to 10 weeks, but may take several months. Peak unknown. Estrogen antagonism may persist for several weeks after drug is discontinued.

INDICATIONS & DOSAGE
Advanced premenopausal and postmenopausal breast cancers—
Adults: 10 to 20 mg P.O. b.i.d.

ADVERSE REACTIONS
EENT: corneal changes, cataracts, retinopathy.
GI: *nausea, vomiting, diarrhea.*
GU: *vaginal discharge* and bleeding, *irregular menses, increased BUN, amenorrhea.*

Hematologic: transient fall in WBC or platelet counts, leukopenia, ***thrombocytopenia.***
Hepatic: changes in liver enzymes, fatty liver, cholestasis, ***hepatic necrosis.***
Skin: *skin changes.*
Other: temporary bone or tumor pain, *hot flashes,* brief exacerbation of pain from osseous metastases, *weight gain or loss, fluid retention, hypercalcemia.*

INTERACTIONS
Bromocriptine: may elevate tamoxifen levels.
Coumarin-type anticoagulants: may cause significant increase in anticoagulant effect. Monitor patient and PT closely.

EFFECTS ON DIAGNOSTIC TESTS
Drug therapy may increase levels of serum calcium, usually in patients with bone metastases. Serum triglycerides, cholesterol, T_4, and hepatic enzymes may be increased. Variations on karyopknotic index in vaginal smears and various degrees of estrogen effect on Papanicolaou smears have been infrequently seen in postmenopausal patients.

CONTRAINDICATIONS
Contraindicated in patients hypersensitive to the drug.

NURSING CONSIDERATIONS
● Use cautiously in patients with existing leukopenia or thrombocytopenia. Monitor CBC closely in these patients, as ordered.
● Monitor serum lipid levels, as ordered, during long-term therapy in patients with preexisting hyperlipidemia.
● Monitor serum calcium levels, as ordered. Drug may compound hypercalcemia related to bone metastases during initiation of therapy.
● Know that the drug acts as an "antiestrogen." Best results have been reported in patients with positive estrogen receptors.
● Be aware that adverse reactions are

---

usually minor and well tolerated.

☑ PATIENT TEACHING
● Tell patient taking enteric-coated tablets (Nolvadex-D†‡) to swallow the tablets whole without crushing or chewing. Tell her not to take antacids within 2 hours of a dose.
● Reassure patient that acute exacerbation of bone pain during tamoxifen therapy usually indicates drug will produce good response. Use analgesic to relieve pain.
● Strongly encourage a woman who's taking or has taken tamoxifen to have regular gynecologic examinations because of increased risk of uterine cancer associated with its use.
● Advise patient to use barrier form of contraception because short-term therapy induces ovulation in premenopausal women.
● Advise women of childbearing age to avoid becoming pregnant during therapy. Also recommend consulting with doctor before becoming pregnant.

---

testolactone
Teslac

Controlled Substance Schedule III
Pregnancy Risk Category: C

HOW SUPPLIED
Tablets: 50 mg

ACTION
Exact antineoplastic action is unknown. Appears to inhibit aromatase activity and decrease estrone synthesis.

ONSET, PEAK, DURATION
Onset occurs in 6 to 12 weeks. Peak and duration unknown.

INDICATIONS & DOSAGE
Advanced postmenopausal breast cancer; advanced premenopausal breast cancer in women whose ovarian func-

tion has been terminated—
Women: 250 mg P.O. q.i.d.

ADVERSE REACTIONS
CNS: paresthesia, peripheral neuropathy.
CV: increased blood pressure, edema.
GI: nausea, vomiting, diarrhea, anorexia, glossitis.
Skin: alopecia, erythema, nail changes.

INTERACTIONS
Oral anticoagulants: increased pharmacologic effects. Monitor patient and PT carefully.

EFFECTS ON DIAGNOSTIC TESTS
Drug therapy may increase levels of serum calcium, urinary creatinine, and urinary 17-ketosteroids. Estradiol levels measured by radioimmunoassay may be decreased.

CONTRAINDICATIONS
Contraindicated in patients hypersensitive to the drug and in males with breast cancer.

NURSING CONSIDERATIONS
● Monitor fluid and electrolyte levels, especially calcium level.
● Force fluids to aid calcium excretion and encourage exercise to prevent hypercalcemia. Immobilized patients are prone to hypercalcemia.
● Know that higher-than-recommended doses may increase incidence of remission in patients with visceral metastases.

☑ PATIENT TEACHING
● Inform patient that therapeutic response isn't immediate. Three months is an adequate trial for this drug.
● Tell patient to notify doctor if numbness or tingling occurs in fingers, toes, or face.

Reactions may be *common,* uncommon, *life-threatening,* or COMMON AND LIFE-THREATENING.

73
Miscellaneous antineoplastic drugs

altretamine
amifostine
asparaginase
bacillus Calmette-Guérin (BCG),
    live intravesical
dacarbazine
docetaxel
etoposide
etoposide phosphate
gemcitabine hydrochloride
irinotecan hydrochloride
mitotane
mitoxantrone hydrochloride
paclitaxel
pegaspargase
porfimer sodium
procarbazine hydrochloride
teniposide
topotecan hydrochloride
tretinoin
vinblastine sulfate
vincristine sulfate
vinorelbine tartrate

COMBINATION PRODUCTS
None.

---

altretamine
(hexamethylmelamine; HMM)
Hexalen

Pregnancy Risk Category: D

HOW SUPPLIED
Capsules: 50 mg

ACTION
Unknown. Structurally similar to triethylenemelamine, but not an alkylating agent. Metabolism is important for antitumor activity.

ONSET, PEAK, DURATION
Onset and duration undefined. Plasma levels peak in ½ to 3 hours.

INDICATIONS & DOSAGE
Palliative treatment of persistent or recurrent ovarian cancer after first-line therapy with cisplatin or alkylating agent–based combination therapy—
Adults: 260 mg/m² P.O. daily in four divided doses with meals and h.s. for 14 or 21 consecutive days in a 28-day cycle.

ADVERSE REACTIONS
CNS: *peripheral neuropathy,* ataxia, paresthesia, fatigue, *seizures,* dizziness, mood disorders, vertigo.
GI: *nausea and vomiting,* anorexia.
Hematologic: *leukopenia, thrombocytopenia, anemia.*
Renal: increased serum creatinine and BUN levels.
Skin: erythematous maculopapular eczema, alopecia.

INTERACTIONS
Cimetidine: may increase half-life of altretamine. Monitor for toxicity.
MAO inhibitors: severe orthostatic hypotension. Avoid concomitant use.

EFFECTS ON DIAGNOSTIC TESTS
Alkaline phosphatase, serum creatinine and BUN levels may be increased.

CONTRAINDICATIONS
Contraindicated in patients hypersensitive to the drug and in those with preexisting severe bone marrow suppression or severe neurologic toxicity.

NURSING CONSIDERATIONS
● Obtain baseline CBC and platelet count, as ordered, before each course of therapy, and monitor monthly.
● Perform a careful neurologic assessment before each course of therapy.
● Know that continuous high-dose daily treatment is associated with a higher incidence of mild to moderate neurotoxici-

---

*Liquid contains alcohol.   **May contain tartrazine.   †Canada only.   ‡Australia only.   ◇OTC.

ty. It appears to be reversible when therapy is discontinued. Drug may be given with pyridoxine to reduce neurotoxicity.

Alert: Be prepared to discontinue drug temporarily for at least 14 days if laboratory tests show a platelet count below 75,000/mm^3, WBC count below 2,000/mm^3, or granulocyte count below 1,000/mm^3. Also discontinue temporarily, as ordered, if patients experience severe GI distress that is unresponsive to symptomatic treatment or develop signs of progressive neuropathy. Drug should be discontinued, as ordered, if neurologic symptoms fail to stabilize.

• Continuous daily use of this drug is associated with nausea and vomiting, which is usually treatable with antiemetics. If nausea and vomiting is severe, dosage reduction or temporary discontinuation may be necessary.

☑ **PATIENT TEACHING**
• Tell patient to take drug with meals to minimize nausea and vomiting.
• Tell patient to watch for signs of infection (fever, sore throat, fatigue) and bleeding (easy bruising, nosebleeds, bleeding gums, melena) and to take temperature daily.
• Advise patient to use contraception; drug may harm fetus.

▼ **NEW DRUG**

amifostine
Ethyol

Pregnancy Risk Category: C

HOW SUPPLIED
Injection: 500 mg anhydrous base and 500 mg mannitol in 10-ml vial

ACTION
Dephosphorylated by alkaline phosphatase in tissue to a pharmacologically active free thiol metabolite. Free thiol in normal tissues binds and detoxifies reactive metabolites of cisplatin, reducing the toxic effects of cisplatin on renal tissue. Free thiol can also act as a scavenger of free radicals that may be generated in tissues exposed to cisplatin.

ONSET, PEAK, DURATION
Amifostine has been found in bone marrow cells 5 to 8 minutes following administration. Drug is rapidly cleared from the plasma with an elimination half-life of approximately 8 minutes.

INDICATIONS & DOSAGE
Reduction of the cumulative renal toxicity associated with repeated administration of cisplatin in patients with advanced ovarian cancer or non-small cell lung cancer—
Adults: 910 mg/m^2 daily as a 15-minute I.V. infusion, starting 30 minutes before chemotherapy. If hypotension occurs and blood pressure doesn't return to normal within 5 minutes after stopping treatment, subsequent cycles should use a dose of 740 mg/m^2.

ADVERSE REACTIONS
CNS: dizziness, somnolence.
CV: *hypotension.*
GI: *nausea, vomiting.*
Other: flushing or feeling of warmth, chills or feeling of coldness, hiccups, sneezing, hypocalcemia, allergic reactions ranging from rash to rigors.

INTERACTIONS
None known, although special consideration should be given to the administration of amifostine in patients receiving antihypertensive drugs or other drugs that could potentiate hypotension.

EFFECTS ON DIAGNOSTIC TESTS
None reported.

CONTRAINDICATIONS
Contraindicated in patients hypersensitive to aminothiol compounds or mannitol. Amifostine should not be used in patients receiving chemotherapy for potentially curable malignancies (includ-

ing certain malignancies of germ cell origin), except for patients involved in clinical studies. Also contraindicated in hypotensive or dehydrated patients and in those receiving antihypertensive drugs that can't be stopped during the 24 hours preceding amifostine administration.

NURSING CONSIDERATIONS

• Use cautiously in the elderly and in patients with ischemic heart disease, arrhythmias, CHF, or history of stroke or transient ischemic attacks.

• Use cautiously in patients in whom the common adverse effects of nausea, vomiting, and hypotension are likely to have serious consequences.

• Reconstitute each single-dose vial with 9.5 ml of sterile 0.9% sodium chloride injection. Use of other solutions to reconstitute the drug is not recommended. Reconstituted solution (500 mg amifostine/10 ml) is chemically stable for 5 hours at room temperature (about 77° F [25° C]) or 24 hours if refrigerated (35° to 46° F [2° to 8° C]).

• Amifostine can be prepared in polyvinyl chloride bags in concentrations of 5 to 40 mg/ml and has the same stability as when the drug is reconstituted in a single-use vial.

• Inspect vial for particulate matter and discoloration before administration; discard drug if cloudiness or precipitation noted.

• If possible and if ordered, stop antihypertensive therapy 24 hours preceding amifostine administration.

• Patients receiving amifostine should be adequately hydrated before administration. Keep patient supine during infusion.

• Monitor blood pressure every 5 minutes during infusion. If hypotension occurs and requires interrupting therapy, notify doctor and keep patient supine with his legs elevated. Then give an infusion of normal saline solution, as ordered, using a separate I.V. line. If blood pressure returns to normal within 5 minutes and patient is asymptomatic, infusion may be restarted so the full dose of the drug can be given. If the full dose can't be given, subsequent doses should be limited to 740 mg/m^2.

• Don't infuse for more than 15 minutes; a longer infusion has been associated with a higher incidence of adverse reactions.

• Know that antiemetic medication, including dexamethasone 20 mg I.V. and a serotonin 5HT$_3$ receptor antagonist, should be administered before, and concurrent with, amifostine administration. Additional antiemetics may be needed, based on chemotherapeutic drugs administered.

• Monitor patient's fluid balance if drug used with highly emetogenic chemotherapy.

• Monitor serum calcium level in patients at risk for hypocalcemia such as those with nephrotic syndrome. If necessary, calcium supplements should be administered, as ordered.

• Safety and effectiveness in pediatric patients have not been established.

☑ PATIENT TEACHING

• Instruct patient to remain in a supine position throughout infusion.

• Advise patient not to breast-feed; it is unknown if the drug or its metabolites are excreted in breast milk.

---

asparaginase
(L-asparaginase)
Elspar, Kidrolase†

Pregnancy Risk Category: C

HOW SUPPLIED
Injection: 10,000-unit vial

ACTION
Destroys the amino acid asparagine, which is needed for protein synthesis in acute lymphocytic leukemia. This leads to death of the leukemic cell.

ONSET, PEAK, DURATION
Onset almost immediate. Time to peak plasma concentration is almost immediate after I.V. administration; 4 to 24 hours after I.M. administration. Effects persist for 23 to 33 days after withdrawal of therapy.

INDICATIONS & DOSAGE
Acute lymphocytic leukemia (in combination with other drugs)—
Adults and children: 1,000 IU/kg I.V. daily for 10 days, injected over 30 minutes; or 6,000 IU/m² I.M. at intervals specified in protocol.
Sole induction agent for acute lymphocytic leukemia—
Adults: 200 IU/kg I.V. daily for 28 days.

ADVERSE REACTIONS
CNS: confusion, drowsiness, depression, hallucinations, *intracranial hemorrhage,* fatigue, *coma,* agitation, headache, lethargy, somnolence.
GI: *vomiting, anorexia, nausea,* cramps.
GU: *azotemia, renal failure,* glycosuria, polyuria.
Hematologic: *anemia, hypofibrinogenemia,* depression of other clotting factors, *leukopenia.*
Hepatic: elevated AST and ALT levels, *hepatotoxicity.*
Skin: *rash, urticaria,* hypersensitivity reactions.
Other: weight loss, HEMORRHAGIC PANCREATITIS AND ANAPHYLAXIS, chills, *death, fatal hyperthermia,* fever, *hyperglycemia.*

INTERACTIONS
Methotrexate: decreased methotrexate effectiveness. Avoid concomitant use.
Prednisone, vincristine: increased toxicity. Monitor patient closely.

EFFECTS ON DIAGNOSTIC TESTS
Drug therapy alters results of thyroid function tests by decreasing concentrations of serum thyroxine-binding globulin.

CONTRAINDICATIONS
Contraindicated in patients with pancreatitis or history of pancreatitis and previous hypersensitivity unless desensitized.

NURSING CONSIDERATIONS
● Use cautiously in patients with preexisting hepatic dysfunction. Drug should be given in hospital setting with close supervision.
● Monitor blood and urine glucose before and during therapy. Watch for signs of hyperglycemia.
● Be aware that allopurinol should be started before therapy begins to help prevent uric acid nephropathy.
Alert: Know that risk of hypersensitivity increases with repeated dosages. An intradermal skin test should be performed prior to initial dose and when drug is given after an interval of 1 week or more between doses. Give 2 IU asparaginase as intradermal injection, as ordered. Observe site for at least 1 hour for erythema or a wheal, which indicate a positive response. Know that a patient with a negative skin test may still develop an allergic reaction to the drug. Desensitization may need to be performed before giving the first treatment dose and on retreatment of any patient. One IU of the drug may be ordered I.V. The dose is then doubled q 10 minutes provided no reaction has occurred, until the total amount given equals the patient's total dose for that day.
● Know drug should not be used alone to induce remission unless combination therapy is inappropriate. Not recommended for maintenance therapy.
● Follow institutional policy to reduce risks. Preparation and administration of parenteral form of this drug is associated with carcinogenic, mutagenic, and teratogenic risks for personnel.
● **I.V. use:** Give I.V. injection over 30 minutes through a running infusion of 0.9% sodium chloride solution or 5% dextrose solution.
● For I.M. injection, limit dose at single

injection site to 2 ml.

• Reconstitute with 2 to 5 ml of either sterile water for injection or sodium chloride for injection.

• Don't use cloudy solutions.

• If drug contacts skin or mucous membranes, wash with copious amounts of water for at least 15 minutes.

• Refrigerate unopened dry powder. Reconstituted solution is stable for 8 hours if refrigerated.

• Keep epinephrine, diphenhydramine, and I.V. corticosteroids available for treating anaphylaxis.

• Monitor CBC and bone marrow function tests, as ordered.

• Obtain serum amylase level determinations, as ordered, to check pancreatic status. If elevated, asparaginase should be discontinued.

• Help prevent occurrence of tumor lysis which can result in uric acid nephropathy by increasing fluid intake.

• Know that drug may affect clotting factors, leading to thrombosis or, more commonly, severe bleeding. Monitor patient and bleeding studies closely.

• Because of vomiting, administer parenteral fluids, as ordered, for 24 hours or until oral fluids are tolerated.

• Know that some patients may develop hypersensitivity to asparaginase, derived from cultures of *Escherichia coli. Erwinia* asparaginase, derived from cultures of *Erwinia carotovora*, has been used in these patients without cross-sensitivity.

☑ **PATIENT TEACHING**

• Tell patient to watch for signs of infection (fever, sore throat, fatigue) and bleeding (easy bruising, nosebleeds, bleeding gums, melena) and to take temperature daily.

• Stress importance of maintaining an adequate fluid intake to help prevent hyperuricemia. If adverse GI reactions prevent patient from drinking fluids, tell patient to notify doctor.

bacillus Calmette-Guérin (BCG), live intravesical
ImmuCyst†, TheraCys, TICE BCG

Pregnancy Risk Category: C

HOW SUPPLIED
TheraCys
Suspension (freeze-dried) for bladder instillation: 27 mg/vial
TICE BCG
Suspension (freeze-dried) for bladder instillation: about 50 mg/ampule

ACTION
Unknown. Instillation of the live bacterial suspension causes a local inflammatory response. Local infiltration of histiocytes and leukocytes is followed by a decrease in superficial tumors within the bladder.

ONSET, PEAK, DURATION
Undefined.

INDICATIONS & DOSAGE
In situ carcinoma of the urinary bladder (primary and relapsed)—
Adults: three reconstituted and diluted vials administered intravesically once weekly for 6 weeks (induction), followed by additional treatments at 3, 6, 12, 18, and 24 months (TheraCys); or, one bladder instillation (one ampule suspended in 50 ml of sterile, preservative-free sodium chloride solution) once weekly for 6 weeks, and then once monthly for 6 to 12 months (TICE BCG).

ADVERSE REACTIONS
GI: *nausea, vomiting, anorexia,* diarrhea.
GU: *dysuria, urinary frequency, hematuria, cystitis, urinary urgency, nocturia,* urinary incontinence, *urinary tract infection,* cramps, pain, decreased bladder capacity, renal toxicity, genital pain.
Hematologic: *anemia,* leukopenia.
Hepatic: elevated liver enzyme levels.

Other: hypersensitivity reaction, *malaise,* fever, chills, myalgia, arthralgia, *disseminated mycobacterial infection.*

INTERACTIONS
Antibiotics: may attenuate the response to BCG intravesical. Avoid concomitant use.

Bone marrow suppressants, immunosuppressants, and radiation therapy: may impair the response to BCG intravesical by decreasing the immune response; may also increase the risk of osteomyelitis or disseminated BCG infection. Avoid concomitant use.

EFFECTS ON DIAGNOSTIC TESTS
Tuberculin sensitivity may be rendered positive by BCG intravesical treatment. Determine patient's reactivity to tuberculin before initiating therapy.

CONTRAINDICATIONS
Contraindicated in immunocompromised patients, in those receiving immunosuppressive therapy or asymptomatic carriers with a positive HIV serology, and in those with urinary tract infection or fever of unknown origin. If fever is caused by infection, the drug should be withheld until patient recovers.

NURSING CONSIDERATIONS
● Determine patient's reactivity to tuberculin before therapy. Tuberculin sensitivity may be rendered positive by BCG intravesical treatment.
● Know that this drug should not be handled by a caregiver with a known immunologic deficiency.
● Be aware that BCG intravesical should not be administered within 7 to 14 days of transurethral resection or biopsy. Fatal disseminated BCG infection has occurred after traumatic catheterization.
● To administer TheraCys, reconstitute only with 1 ml of provided diluent per vial just before use. Do not remove rubber stopper to prepare solution. Use immediately. Add contents of three reconstituted vials to 50 ml of sterile, preservative-free sodium chloride solution (final volume, 53 ml). Instill a urethral catheter into bladder under aseptic conditions, drain bladder, and then infuse 53 ml of prepared solution by gravity feed. Remove catheter and properly dispose of unused drug.
● To administer TICE BCG, use thermosetting plastic or sterile glass containers and syringes. Draw 1 ml of sterile, preservative-free sodium chloride solution into a 3-ml syringe. Add to one ampule of drug; gently expel back into ampule three times to ensure thorough mixing. Use immediately. Dispense cloudy suspension into top end of a catheter-tipped syringe that contains 49 ml of sodium chloride solution. Gently rotate syringe. Properly dispose of unused drug.
● Handle drug and material used for instillation as infectious material because it contains live, attenuated mycobacteria. Dispose of associated equipment (syringes, catheters, and containers) as biohazardous waste.
● Use strict aseptic technique to administer the drug to minimize trauma to the GU tract and to prevent introducing other contaminants.
● If there is evidence of traumatic catheterization, do not administer the drug and alert doctor. Subsequent treatment may resume after 1 week as if no interruption occurred.
● Carefully monitor patient's urinary status because the drug causes an inflammatory response in the bladder.
● Closely monitor patients for evidence of systemic BCG infection. BCG infections are rarely detected by positive cultures. Know that therapy should be withheld if systemic infection is suspected (short-term high fever above 103° F [39.4° C] or persistent fever above 101° F [38.3° C] for longer than 2 days or with severe malaise). Contact an infectious disease specialist for initiation of fast-acting antituberculosis therapy, as ordered.

Reactions may be *common*, uncommon, *life-threatening*, or COMMON AND LIFE-THREATENING.

• Know that drug is not used as an immunizing agent to prevent cancer or tuberculosis; drug should not be confused with BCG vaccine.

• Keep in mind that drug has the potential to cause hypersensitivity. Manage symptomatically.

• Be aware that patients with a small bladder capacity may experience increased local irritation with the usual dose of BCG intravesical.

• Be prepared to treat bladder irritation symptomatically with phenazopyridine, acetaminophen, and propantheline, as ordered. Systemic hypersensitivity can be treated with diphenhydramine. In order to minimize the risk of systemic infection, some clinicians give isoniazid for 3 days starting on the first day of treatment.

☑ PATIENT TEACHING
• Tell patient to retain the drug in the bladder for 2 hours after instillation (if possible). For the first hour, have patient lie 15 minutes prone, 15 minutes supine, and 15 minutes on each side; the second hour may be spent in the sitting position.

• Tell patient to sit when voiding.

• Instruct patient to disinfect urine for 6 hours after instillation of drug. Tell him to pour undiluted household bleach (5% sodium hypochlorite solution) in equal volume to voided urine into the toilet and wait 15 minutes before flushing.

• Tell patient to notify doctor if symptoms worsen or if any of the following symptoms develops: blood in the urine, fever and chills, frequent urge to urinate, painful urination, nausea, vomiting, joint pain, or rash.

Alert: Caution patient that a cough that develops after therapy could indicate a life-threatening BCG infection. Tell him to report it immediately.

• Advise women of childbearing age not to become pregnant or breast-feed during drug therapy.

dacarbazine (DTIC)
DTIC†, DTIC-Dome

Pregnancy Risk Category: C

HOW SUPPLIED
Injection: 100-mg, 200-mg vials

ACTION
Unknown. Probably cross-links strands of cellular DNA and interferes with RNA transcription, causing an imbalance of growth that leads to cell death. Cell cycle-nonspecific.

ONSET, PEAK, DURATION
Undefined.

INDICATIONS & DOSAGE
Metastatic malignant melanoma—
Adults: 2 to 4.5 mg/kg I.V. daily for 10 days; then repeated q 4 weeks as tolerated. Or 250 mg/m^2 I.V. daily for 5 days, repeated at 3-week intervals.
Hodgkin's disease—
Adults: 150 mg/m^2 I.V. daily (in combination with other agents) for 5 days, repeated q 4 weeks; or 375 mg/m^2 on the first day of a combination regimen, repeated q 15 days.

ADVERSE REACTIONS
GI: *severe nausea and vomiting, anorexia.*
Hematologic: *leukopenia, thrombocytopenia.*
Hepatic: transient increase in liver enzyme levels, *hepatotoxicity* (rare).
Skin: phototoxicity, rash, facial flushing.
Other: *flulike syndrome* (fever, malaise; myalgia, beginning 7 days after treatment ends and lasts possibly 7 to 21 days), alopecia, *anaphylaxis;* severe pain if I.V. solution infiltrates or if solution is too concentrated; tissue damage; facial paresthesia.

INTERACTIONS
Anticoagulants, aspirin: increased risk

of bleeding. Avoid concomitant use.
Bone marrow suppressants: additive
toxicity. Monitor closely.
*Phenobarbital, phenytoin, other drugs
that induce hepatic metabolism:* enhanced dacarbazine activation and risk
of toxicity. Monitor closely.

EFFECTS ON DIAGNOSTIC TESTS
Drug therapy causes transient increases
in serum BUN, ALT, AST, and alkaline
phosphatase levels.

CONTRAINDICATIONS
Contraindicated in patients hypersensitive to the drug.

NURSING CONSIDERATIONS
● Use cautiously if bone marrow function is impaired.
● Administer antiemetics, as ordered,
before giving dacarbazine. Nausea and
vomiting may sometimes subside after
several doses.
● Follow institutional policy to reduce
risks. Preparation and administration of
parenteral form of this drug is associated with carcinogenic, mutagenic, and
teratogenic risks for personnel.
● **I.V. use:** Reconstitute drug using sterile water for injection. Add 9.9 ml to the
100-mg vial or 19.7 ml to the 200-mg
vial. The resulting solution will be colorless to clear yellow. For infusion, further dilute by using up to 250 ml of
0.9% sodium chloride solution or D₅W;
infuse over 30 minutes.
● May dilute further or slow infusion
rate to decrease pain at insertion site.
● Avoid extravasation during infusion.
If I.V. solution infiltrates, discontinue
immediately, apply ice to area for 24 to
48 hours, and notify doctor.
● Keep in mind that reconstituted solutions are stable for 8 hours at room temperature and normal lighting conditions,
or up to 3 days if refrigerated. Diluted
solutions are stable for 8 hours at normal room temperature and light, or up
to 24 hours if refrigerated. If solutions
turn pink, decomposition has occurred;

discard drug.
● Discard refrigerated solution after 72
hours and room temperature solution after 8 hours.
● To prevent bleeding, avoid all I.M. injections when platelet count is below
100,000/mm³.
● Anticipate the need for blood transfusions to combat anemia.
● Know that therapeutic effects are often accompanied by toxicity. Monitor
CBC and platelet count.
● For Hodgkin's disease, be aware that
drug is usually given with bleomycin,
vinblastine, and doxorubicin.

☑ **PATIENT TEACHING**
● Tell patient to watch for signs of infection (fever, sore throat, fatigue) and
bleeding (easy bruising, nosebleeds,
bleeding gums, melena) and to take
temperature daily.
● Instruct patient to avoid OTC products
containing aspirin.
● Advise patient to avoid sunlight and
sunlamps for first 2 days after treatment.
● Reassure patient that flulike syndrome
may be treated with mild antipyretics,
such as acetaminophen.
● Counsel female patient to avoid pregnancy and breast-feeding during drug
therapy.

▼ *NEW DRUG*

docetaxel
Taxotere

Pregnancy Risk Category: D

HOW SUPPLIED
Injection: 20 mg, 80 mg in single-dose
vials

ACTION
Disrupts microtubular network in cells
essential for mitotic and interphase cellular functions.

ONSET, PEAK, DURATION
Quickly distributed throughout the body after I.V. administration. Its terminal half-life is about 11 hours.

INDICATIONS & DOSAGE
Treatment of patients with locally advanced or metastatic breast cancer who have progressed during anthracycline-based therapy or have relapsed during anthracycline-based adjuvant therapy— **Adults:** 60 to 100 mg/m² I.V. over 1 hour q 3 weeks.

ADVERSE REACTIONS
CNS: *asthenia,* paresthesia, dysesthesia, pain (including burning sensation), weakness.
CV: *fluid retention,* hypotension
GI: *stomatitis, nausea, vomiting, diarrhea.*
Hematologic: *anemia,* NEUTROPENIA, FEBRILE NEUTROPENIA, MYELOSUPPRESSION (dose limiting), LEUKOPENIA, THROMBOCYTOPENIA, *septic and nonseptic death.*
Skin: *alopecia,* skin eruptions, desquamation, nail pigmentation alterations, nail pain, flushing, rash.
Other: HYPERSENSITIVITY REACTIONS, *infection,* chest tightness, back pain, dyspnea, drug fever, chills, *myalgia,* arthralgia, *increased liver function tests.*

INTERACTIONS
Compounds that induce, inhibit, or are metabolized by cytochrome P450 3A4 (such as cyclosporin, terfenadine, ketoconazole, erythromycin, and troleandomycin): metabolism of docetaxel may be modified by concomitant administration. Use cautiously when administering these agents with docetaxel.

EFFECTS ON DIAGNOSTIC TESTS
None reported.

CONTRAINDICATIONS
Contraindicated in patients with history of severe hypersensitivity to drug or to other formulations containing polysor-

bate 80 and in those with neutrophil counts below 1,500 cells/mm³.

NURSING CONSIDERATIONS
● Do not administer docetaxel in patients with bilirubin values above upper limits of normal. Patients with ALT or AST above 1.5 times upper limits of normal and alkaline phosphatase greater than 2.5 times upper limit of normal generally should not receive the drug.
● Premedicate all patients with oral corticosteroids, such as dexamethasone 16 mg P.O. (8 mg b.i.d.) daily for 5 days starting 1 day before docetaxel administration, to reduce incidence and severity of fluid retention and hypersensitivity reactions.
● Dilute docetaxel using the diluent supplied prior to administration. Allow drug and diluent to stand at room temperature for 5 minutes before mixing. After adding all the diluent to the drug vial, gently rotate vial for about 15 seconds. Allow solution to stand for a few minutes to enable foam to dissipate. All foam need not fully dissipate before proceeding to the next step.
● Prepare docetaxel infusion solution by withdrawing the required amount of premixed solution from the vial and injecting it into 250 ml normal saline or D₅W to produce a final concentration of 0.3 to 0.9 mg/ml. Doses exceeding 240 mg require a larger volume of infusion solution so as not to exceed a concentration of 0.9 mg/ml of docetaxel. Mix the infusion thoroughly by manual rotation.
● Wear gloves during preparation and administration of docetaxel. If solution contacts skin, wash immediately and thoroughly with soap and water. If drug contacts mucous membranes, they should be flushed thoroughly with water. Mark all waste materials with CHEMOTHERAPY HAZARD labels.
● Prepare and store infusion solutions in bottles (glass or polypropylene) or plastic bags, and administer through polyethylene-lined administration sets.

- Bone marrow toxicity is the most frequent and dose-limiting toxicity. Frequent blood count monitoring is necessary during therapy.
- Monitor patient closely for hypersensitivity reactions, especially during the first and second infusions.
- Safety and effectiveness in children have not been established.

☑ PATIENT TEACHING
- Advise patient of childbearing age to avoid pregnancy or breast-feeding during therapy.
- Warn patient that alopecia occurs in almost 80% of all patients.
- Tell patient to promptly report a sore throat, fever, or unusual bruising or bleeding, as well as signs of fluid retention, such as swelling or dyspnea.

etoposide (VP-16)
VePesid

etoposide phosphate
Etopophos

Pregnancy Risk Category: D

HOW SUPPLIED
etoposide
Capsules: 50 mg
Injection: 20 mg/ml in 5-ml and 50-ml vials
etoposide phosphate
Injection: 113.6-mg vials equivalent to 100 mg etoposide

ACTION
Unknown. It is thought to damage DNA and inhibit DNA synthesis. Appears to be cell-cycle specific.

ONSET, PEAK, DURATION
Undefined.

INDICATIONS & DOSAGE
Testicular cancer—
Adults: 50 to 100 mg/m^2 I.V. on 5 consecutive days q 3 to 4 weeks; or 100 mg/m^2 on days 1, 3, and 5 q 3 to 4 weeks.
Small-cell carcinoma of the lung—
Adults: 35 mg/m^2/day I.V. for 4 days; or 50 mg/m^2/day I.V. for 5 days. Oral dosage is two times the I.V. dose, rounded to the nearest 50 mg.

ADVERSE REACTIONS
CNS: peripheral neuropathy.
CV: hypotension (from too-rapid infusion).
GI: *nausea and vomiting, anorexia, diarrhea,* abdominal pain, *stomatitis.*
Hematologic: *anemia,* **myelosuppression** (dose-limiting), LEUKOPENIA, THROMBOCYTOPENIA.
Other: *reversible alopecia,* **anaphylaxis** (rare), phlebitis at injection site (infrequent).

INTERACTIONS
Warfarin: may further prolong PT. Monitor closely.

EFFECTS ON DIAGNOSTIC TESTS
None reported.

CONTRAINDICATIONS
Contraindicated in patients hypersensitive to the drug.

NURSING CONSIDERATIONS
- Use cautiously in patients who have had cytotoxic or radiation therapy.
- Obtain baseline blood pressure prior to therapy.
- Have diphenhydramine, hydrocortisone, epinephrine, and emergency equipment available to establish an airway in case of anaphylaxis.
- Follow institutional policy to reduce risks. Preparation and administration of parenteral form of this drug is associated with carcinogenic, mutagenic, and teratogenic risks for personnel.
- **I.V. use:** Give etoposide by slow I.V. infusion (over at least 30 minutes) to prevent severe hypotension. Etoposide phosphate may be given over 5 to 210 minutes.

Reactions may be *common,* uncommon, *life-threatening,* or COMMON AND LIFE-THREATENING.

• Dilute etoposide for infusion in either D_5W or 0.9% sodium chloride solution to a concentration of 0.2 or 0.4 mg/ml. Higher concentrations may crystallize. Etoposide phosphate may be given without further dilution or it may be diluted to concentrations as low as 0.1 mg/ml in either D_5W or 0.9% sodium chloride.

• Do not administer etoposide through a membrane-type in-line filter because the diluent may dissolve it.

• Know that etoposide diluted to 0.2 mg/ml is stable for 96 hours at room temperature in plastic or glass unprotected from light; solutions diluted to 0.4 mg/ml are stable for 48 hours under the same conditions. Diluted solutions of etoposide phosphate are stable at room temperature or under refrigeration for 24 hours.

• Store capsules in refrigerator.

Alert: Monitor blood pressure every 15 minutes during infusion. If systolic pressure falls below 90 mm Hg, stop infusion and notify the doctor.

• Monitor CBC, as ordered. Observe for signs of bone marrow suppression.

• Observe oral cavity for signs of ulceration.

• To prevent bleeding, avoid all I.M. injections when platelet count is below 100,000/mm³.

• Anticipate the need for blood transfusion to combat anemia.

• Know that etoposide has caused complete remissions in small-cell lung cancer and testicular cancer.

• Be aware that the dose of etoposide phosphate is expressed as etoposide equivalents; 113.6 mg of etoposide phosphate is equivalent to 100 mg of etoposide.

☑ **PATIENT TEACHING**

• Tell patient to watch for signs of infection (fever, sore throat, fatigue) and bleeding (easy bruising, nosebleeds, bleeding gums, melena) and to take temperature daily.

• Inform patient of need for frequent blood pressure readings during I.V. administration.

• Advise women of childbearing age to avoid pregnancy or breast-feeding during therapy.

▼ *NEW DRUG*

gemcitabine hydrochloride
Gemzar

Pregnancy Risk Category: D

HOW SUPPLIED
Powder for injection: 200-mg, 1-g vials

ACTION
Cytotoxic; cell-phase specific; inhibits DNA synthesis and blocks progression of cells through G1/S-phase boundary.

ONSET, PEAK, DURATION
Unknown.

INDICATIONS & DOSAGE
Locally advanced or metastatic adenocarcinoma of the pancreas and those treated previously with fluorouracil—
Adults: 1,000 mg/m² I.V. over 30 minutes once weekly for up to 7 weeks, unless toxicity occurs. Patients should be monitored prior to each dose with CBC (including differential) and platelet count. If bone marrow suppression is detected, therapy is adjusted. Full dose should be given if absolute granulocyte count (AGC) is 1,000/mm³ or more and platelet count is 100,000/mm³ or more. If AGC is 500/mm³ to 999/mm³, or if platelet count is 50,000/mm³ to 99,999/mm³, 75% of dose should be given. Dose should be held if AGC is below 500/mm³ or platelet count is below 50,000/mm³. Treatment course of 7 weeks is followed by 1 week rest. Subsequent dosage cycles consist of 1 infusion weekly for 3 out of 4 consecutive weeks. Dosage adjustments for subsequent cycles are based on AGC

and platelet count nadirs and the degree of nonhematologic toxicity.

ADVERSE REACTIONS
CNS: *somnolence, paresthesia.*
GI: *stomatitis, nausea, vomiting, constipation, diarrhea.*
GU: *proteinuria, hematuria,* elevated BUN and creatinine.
Hematologic: *anemia,* LEUKOPENIA, NEUTROPENIA, THROMBOCYTOPENIA.
Hepatic: *elevated liver enzymes.*
Respiratory: *dyspnea,* bronchospasm.
Other: *alopecia, pain, fever, rash, flu-like symtoms,* HEMORRHAGE, *infection, edema, peripheral edema.*

INTERACTIONS
None reported.

EFFECTS ON DIAGNOSTIC TESTS
None reported.

CONTRAINDICATIONS
Contraindicated in patients with hypersensitivity to the drug.

NURSING CONSIDERATIONS
● Use cautiously in patients with renal or hepatic impairment.
● Know that the drug is not recommended for use in pregnant or breast-feeding patients.
● Know that safety and effectiveness in children have not been determined.
● Follow institutional policy to reduce risks. Preparation and administration of parenteral form of drug is associated with mutagenic, teratogenic, and carcinogenic risks for personnel.
● **I.V. use:** To prepare solution, add 5 ml of 0.9% sodium chloride injection without preservatives to a 200-mg vial or 25 ml of diluent to a 1-g vial. Shake to dissolve. The resulting concentration is 40 mg/ml; reconstitution at greater concentrations is not recommended. Resulting concentration may be further diluted with 0.9% sodium chloride injection to a concentration as low as 0.1 mg/ml, if needed. Solution should be clear to a

light straw-colored, and be free of particulate matter. It is stable for 24 hours at room temperature. Do not refrigerate reconstituted drug because crystallization may occur.
● Be aware that prolonging infusion time beyond 60 minutes or administering drug more frequently than once weekly may increase toxicity.
● Monitor patient closely. Expect dosage modification according to toxicity and degree of myelosuppression. Age, gender, and presence of renal impairment may predispose patient to toxicity.
● Know that careful hematologic monitoring, especially of neutrophil and platelet counts, is required.
● Obtain baseline and periodic renal and hepatic laboratory tests, as ordered.

☑ PATIENT TEACHING
● Advise patient to watch for signs of infection (fever, sore throat, fatigue) and bleeding (easy bruising, nosebleeds, bleeding gums, melena). Tell patient to take temperature daily.
● Advise women of childbearing age to avoid pregnancy or breast-feeding during therapy.

▼ NEW DRUG

irinotecan hydrochloride
Camptosar

Pregnancy Risk Category: D

HOW SUPPLIED
Injection: 100-mg/5-ml vial

ACTION
Irinotecan is a derivative of camptothecin. Camptothecins interact specifically with the enzyme topoisomerase I, which relieves torsional strain in DNA by inducing reversible single-strand

breaks. Irinotecan and its active metabolite bind to the topoisomerase I-DNA complex and prevent religation of these single-strand breaks.

ONSET, PEAK, DURATION
Maximum concentration of the active metabolite generally occurs within 1 hour after the end of a 90-minute infusion. Terminal half-life of the active metabolite is about 10 hours.

INDICATIONS & DOSAGE
Treatment of metastatic carcinoma of the colon or rectum that has recurred or progressed following fluorouracil (5-FU) therapy—
Adults: initially, 125 mg/m^2 I.V. infusion over 90 minutes. Recommended treatment is 125 mg/m^2 I.V. once weekly for 4 weeks followed by a 2-week rest period. Thereafter, additional courses of treatment may be repeated q 6 weeks (4 weeks on therapy, followed by 2 weeks off therapy). Subsequent doses may be adjusted to a low of 50 mg/m^2 or to a maximum of 150 mg/m^2 in 25- to 50-mg/m^2 increments, depending on patient's tolerance. Treatment with additional courses may continue indefinitely in patients who respond favorably and in those whose disease remains stable, provided intolerable toxicity does not occur.

ADVERSE REACTIONS
CNS: *insomnia, dizziness, asthenia, headache, akathisia.*
CV: *vasodilation, edema.*
GI: DIARRHEA, *nausea, vomiting, anorexia, stomatitis, constipation, flatulence, dyspepsia, abdominal cramping and pain, abdominal enlargement.*
Hematologic: *leukopenia, anemia, **neutropenia.***
Metabolic: *weight loss, dehydration, increased alkaline phosphatase, increased AST levels.*
Respiratory: *dyspnea, increased coughing, rhinitis.*
Skin: *alopecia, sweating, rash.*
Other: *fever, pain, back pain, chills, minor infection.*

INTERACTIONS
Other antineoplastic agents: may cause additive adverse effects, such as myelosuppression and diarrhea. Monitor patient closely.
Pelvic/abdominal irradiation: increased risk of severe myelosuppression. Avoid concurrent use of drug with irradiation.

EFFECTS ON DIAGNOSTIC TESTS
None reported.

CONTRAINDICATIONS
Contraindicated in patients with hypersensitivity to the drug.

NURSING CONSIDERATIONS
● Use cautiously in elderly patients.
● Premedicate patient with antiemetic agents on the day of treatment starting at least 30 minutes before administering irinotecan.
● Drug is packaged in a plastic blister to protect against inadvertent breakage and leakage. Inspect vial for damage and visible signs of leakage before removing blister.
● Store vial at room temperature of 59° to 86° F (15° to 30° C), and protect from light.
● Wear gloves while handling and preparing infusion solutions. If drug contacts skin, wash thoroughly with soap and water. If drug contacts mucous membranes, flush thoroughly with water.
● Irinotecan must be diluted in 5% dextrose injection (preferred) or 0.9% sodium chloride injection before infusion. Final concentration range is 0.12 to 1.1 mg/ml.
● Irinotecan solution is stable for up to 24 hours at room temperature of 77° F (25° C) and in ambient fluorescent lighting. Solutions diluted in D$_5$W, stored at refrigerated temperatures of 3° to 46° F (2° to 8° C), and protected from light are stable for 48 hours. However, because of possible microbial con-

tamination during dilution, use the admixture within 24 hours if refrigerated or 6 hours if kept at room temperature. Refrigerating admixtures using 0.9% sodium chloride is not recommended because of a low and sporadic incidence of visible particulate. Do not freeze admixture because drug may precipitate.

• Do not add other drugs to irinotecan infusion.

• Extravasation of drug should be avoided. If extravasation occurs, site should be flushed with sterile water and ice applied. Notify the doctor.

• Diuretic therapy may be withheld during therapy and periods of active vomiting or diarrhea to decrease risk of dehydration.

• Know that drug can induce severe diarrhea. Diarrhea occurring within 24 hours of administration may be preceded by diaphoresis and abdominal cramping and may be relieved by 0.25 to 1 mg atropine I.V., unless contraindicated. Diarrhea occurring more than 24 hours after administration of irinotecan may be prolonged, leading to dehydration and electrolyte imbalances, and can be life-threatening. Late diarrhea occurring after 24 hours should be treated with loperamide, as ordered. Monitor patient's fluid status and serum electrolytes.

• Therapy should be temporarily discontinued if neutropenic fever occurs or if the absolute neutrophil count drops below 500/mm³. Dosage should be reduced, as ordered, especially if WBC count is below 2,000/mm³, neutrophil below 1,000/mm³, hemoglobin is below 8 g/dl, or platelet count is below 100,000/mm³.

• Routine administration of a colony-stimulating factor is not necessary but may be helpful in patients experiencing significant neutropenia.

• Monitor WBC count with differential, hemoglobin level, and platelet count before each dose of irinotecan.

• Safety and effectiveness in children have not been established.

☑ **PATIENT TEACHING**
• Advise women of childbearing age to avoid pregnancy or breast-feeding during therapy.

• Inform patient about risk of diarrhea and how to treat it; tell him to avoid laxatives.

• Tell patient to notify doctor if vomiting occurs, fever or evidence of infection develops, or symptoms of dehydration (fainting, light-headedness, or dizziness) occur following irinotecan administration.

• Warn patient that alopecia may occur.

---

mitotane (o,p´-DDD)
Lysodren

Pregnancy Risk Category: C

HOW SUPPLIED
Tablets (scored): 500 mg

ACTION
Unknown. May suppress function of adrenocortical tissue and hinder extraadrenal metabolism of cortisol.

ONSET, PEAK, DURATION
Steroid levels decrease within 2 to 4 weeks; tumor response, within 4 to 6 weeks. Levels peak 3 to 5 hours after dose. Median duration of regression has been 6 to 7 months.

INDICATIONS & DOSAGE
Inoperable adrenocortical cancer—
Adults: initially, 2 to 6 g P.O. daily in divided doses t.i.d. or q.i.d.; increased to 9 to 10 g P.O. daily, in divided doses t.i.d. or q.i.d. Dosage is adjusted until maximum tolerated dosage is achieved (varies from 2 to 16 g/day but is usually 8 to 10 g/day).

ADVERSE REACTIONS
CNS: *depression, somnolence, lethargy, vertigo;* brain damage and dysfunction in long-term, high-dose therapy.
CV: hypertension.

EENT: visual disturbances.
GI: *severe nausea, vomiting, diarrhea, anorexia.*
GU: hemorrhagic cystitis.
Skin: dermatitis, *maculopapular rash.*
Other: increased serum cholesterol level, adrenal insufficiency.

INTERACTIONS
Warfarin: increased metabolism, which may require higher warfarin doses. Monitor PT and INR closely.

EFFECTS ON DIAGNOSTIC TESTS
Drug therapy may increase concentrations of urinary 17-hydroxycorticosteroid, plasma cortisol, protein-bound iodine, and serum uric acid.

CONTRAINDICATIONS
Contraindicated in patients hypersensitive to the drug. Be aware that drug should not be used in patients in shock or who have suffered trauma.

NURSING CONSIDERATIONS
● Use cautiously in patients with hepatic disease.
● To reduce nausea, give antiemetic before mitotane, as ordered.
● Monitor effectiveness according to reduction in pain, weakness, and anorexia.
● Assess and record behavioral and neurologic signs daily. Prolonged therapy has been associated with significant neurologic impairment.
● Be aware that use of corticosteroids may avoid acute adrenocorticoid insufficiency and is usually required. Glucocorticoid dosage should be increased in periods of physiologic stress such as infection or trauma.
● Because drug distributes mostly to body fat, know that obese patients may need higher dosage and may have longer-lasting adverse reactions.
● Keep in mind that an adequate therapeutic trial is at least 3 months, but treatment can continue if clinical benefits are observed.

☑ **PATIENT TEACHING**
● Warn ambulatory patient to avoid activities that require alertness and good motor coordination until CNS effects of the drug are known.
● Instruct patient to notify doctor if severe adverse GI or skin reactions occur because dosage adjustment may be needed.
● Counsel female patient to avoid pregnancy or breast-feeding during therapy.

mitoxantrone hydrochloride
Novantrone

Pregnancy Risk Category: D

HOW SUPPLIED
Injection: 2 mg/ml in 10-ml, 12.5-ml, 15-ml vials

ACTION
Not fully understood; probably cell-cycle nonspecific. Reacts with DNA, producing cytotoxic effect.

ONSET, PEAK, DURATION
Undefined.

INDICATIONS & DOSAGE
Combination initial therapy for acute nonlymphocytic leukemia—
Adults: induction begins with 12 mg/m^2 I.V. daily on days 1 through 3, in combination with 100 mg/m^2 daily of cytarabine on days 1 through 7. A second induction may be given if response is not adequate. Maintenance therapy: 12 mg/m^2 on days 1 and 2, in combination with cytarabine on days 1 through 5.
✳ *New indication: Combination initial therapy for pain related to advanced hormone-refractory prostate cancer—*
Adults: 12 to 14 mg/m^2 I.V. infusion over 15 to 30 minutes q 21 days.

ADVERSE REACTIONS
CNS: *seizures,* headache.
CV: *CHF, arrhythmias,* tachycardia.

---

*Liquid contains alcohol.   **May contain tartrazine.   †Canada only.   ‡Australia only.   ◇OTC.

EENT: conjunctivitis.
GI: *bleeding, abdominal pain, diarrhea, nausea, mucositis, vomiting, stomatitis.*
GU: *renal failure.*
Hematologic: *myelosuppression.*
Hepatic: jaundice.
Respiratory: *dyspnea, cough.*
Skin: *alopecia, petechiae, ecchymoses.*
Other: hyperuricemia, *sepsis, fungal infections, fever.*

INTERACTIONS
Heparin: physically incompatible. Do not mix together.

EFFECTS ON DIAGNOSTIC TESTS
None reported.

CONTRAINDICATIONS
Contraindicated in patients hypersensitive to mitoxantrone.

NURSING CONSIDERATIONS
● Use cautiously in patients with prior exposure to anthracyclines or other cardiotoxic drugs, prior radiation therapy to the mediastinal area, and preexisting heart disease.
● Be aware that patients with significant myelosuppression should not receive mitoxantrone unless the benefits outweigh the risks.
● Follow institutional policy to minimize risks. Preparation and administration of parenteral form is associated with mutagenic, teratogenic, and carcinogenic risks to personnel.
● **I.V. use:** Dilute dose (available as an aqueous solution of 2 mg/ml in volumes of 10, 12.5, and 15 ml) in at least 50 ml of 0.9% sodium chloride injection or D_5W injection. Administer by direct injection into a free-flowing I.V. line of 0.9% sodium chloride or D_5W injection over at least 3 minutes, usually 15 to 30 minutes. Mixing with other drugs is not recommended.
● If drug extravasates, discontinue infusion immediately and notify doctor.
● Be prepared to administer allopurinol,

as ordered. Uric acid nephropathy can be avoided by hydrating the patient before and during therapy.
● Closely monitor hematologic and laboratory chemistry parameters.
● To prevent bleeding, avoid all I.M. injections if platelet count falls below $100,000/mm^3$.
● Anticipate the need for blood transfusion to combat anemia.
● Be aware that left ventricular ejection fraction should be monitored.
● Be prepared to treat infections with antibiotics, as ordered.
● If severe nonhematologic toxicity occurs during the first course, know that the second course should be delayed until patient recovers.
● Store undiluted solution at room temperature. Diluted mixture is stable for 7 days at room temperature.

☑ **PATIENT TEACHING**
● Inform patient that urine may appear blue-green within 24 hours after administration and some bluish discoloration of the sclera may occur. These effects are not harmful.
● Advise patient to watch for signs of bleeding and infection.
● Advise women of childbearing age to avoid pregnancy during therapy. Also recommend consulting doctor before becoming pregnant.

---

paclitaxel
Taxol

Pregnancy Risk Category: D

HOW SUPPLIED
Injection: 30 mg/5 ml, 100 mg/17 ml

ACTION
Prevents depolymerization of cellular microtubules, thus inhibiting the normal reorganization of the microtubule network necessary for mitosis and other vital cellular functions.

ONSET, PEAK, DURATION
Undefined.

INDICATIONS & DOSAGE
Metastatic ovarian cancer after failure of first-line or subsequent chemotherapy—
Adults: 135 mg/m^2 or 175 mg/m^2 I.V. over 3 hours q 3 weeks.
Breast cancer after failure of combination chemotherapy for metastatic disease or relapse within 6 months of adjuvant chemotherapy—
Adults: 175 mg/m^2 I.V. over 3 hours every 3 weeks.

ADVERSE REACTIONS
CNS: *peripheral neuropathy.*
CV: *bradycardia, hypotension, abnormal ECG.*
GI: *nausea, vomiting, diarrhea, mucositis.*
Hematologic: NEUTROPENIA, LEUKOPENIA, THROMBOCYTOPENIA, anemia, *bleeding.*
Hepatic: *elevated liver enzyme levels.*
Other: *hypersensitivity reactions (anaphylaxis), alopecia, myalgia, arthralgia, phlebitis, cellulitis at injection site, infections.*

INTERACTIONS
Cisplatin: possible additive myelosuppressive effects. When given together, paclitaxel should be given before cisplatin.
Ketoconazole: inhibited paclitaxel metabolism. Use together cautiously.

EFFECTS ON DIAGNOSTIC TESTS
Drug alters hematologic studies because of its suppressive effect on bone marrow.

CONTRAINDICATIONS
Contraindicated in patients hypersensitive to the drug or to polyoxyethylated castor oil, a vehicle used in drug solution, and in patients with baseline neutrophil counts below 1,500/mm^3.

NURSING CONSIDERATIONS
● Use cautiously in patients with hepatic impairment.
● Some patients experience peripheral neuropathies, which may be cumulative and dose-related. Severe symptoms may require dose reduction.
● To reduce the incidence or severity of hypersensitivity, anticipate pretreating patients with corticosteroids, such as dexamethasone, and antihistamines, as ordered. Both histamine-1 receptor antagonists, such as diphenhydramine, and histamine-2 receptor antagonists, such as cimetidine or ranitidine, may be used. Severe hypersensitivity reactions have occurred in as many as 2% of patients treated in early clinical trials.
● Follow institutional protocol for the safe handling, preparation, and administration of chemotherapeutic drugs. Preparation and administration of parenteral form of this drug is associated with carcinogenic, mutagenic, and teratogenic risks for personnel. Mark all waste materials with CHEMOTHERAPY HAZARD labels.
● **I.V. use:** Dilute concentrate before infusion. Compatible solutions include 0.9% sodium chloride injection, D$_5$W, 5% dextrose in 0.9% sodium chloride injection, and 5% dextrose in Ringer's lactate injection. Dilute to a final concentration of 0.3 to 1.2 mg/ml. Diluted solutions are stable for 27 hours at room temperature.
● Prepare and store infusion solutions in glass containers. The undiluted concentrate shouldn't contact polyvinylchloride I.V. bags or tubing. Prepared solution may appear hazy. Store diluted solution in glass or polypropylene bottles, or use polypropylene or polyolefin bags. Administer through polyethylene-lined administration sets, and use an in-line 0.22-micron filter.
● Take care to avoid extravasation.
● Continuously monitor patients for 30 minutes after initiating the infusion. Continue close monitoring throughout the infusion.

---

*Liquid contains alcohol. **May contain tartrazine. †Canada only. ‡Australia only. ◇OTC.

• Frequently monitor blood counts during therapy. Bone marrow toxicity is the most common and dose-limiting toxicity. Packed RBC or platelet transfusions may be necessary in severe cases. Institute bleeding precautions as appropriate.

• Avoid all I.M. injections when platelet count is below 100,000/mm^3.

• If patient develops significant cardiac conduction abnormalities, initiate appropriate therapy and continuous cardiac monitoring during therapy and subsequent infusions.

☑ **PATIENT TEACHING**

• Tell patient to watch for signs of infection (fever, sore throat, fatigue) and bleeding (easy bruising, nosebleeds, bleeding gums, melena), and to take temperature daily.

• Teach patient the signs and symptoms of peripheral neuropathy, such as a tingling or burning sensation or numbness in the extremities, and advise her to report these symptoms immediately.

• Warn patient that alopecia is common (up to 82% of patients).

• Advise women of childbearing age to avoid becoming pregnant during therapy and to consult with doctor before becoming pregnant.

---

pegaspargase
(PEG-L-**asparaginase**)
Oncaspar

Pregnancy Risk Category: C

HOW SUPPLIED
Injection: 750 IU/ml

ACTION
A modified version of the enzyme L-asparaginase that exerts its cytotoxic activity by inactivating the amino acid asparagine. Asparagine is required by tumor cells to synthesize proteins. Because the tumor cells cannot synthesize their own asparagine, protein synthesis and, eventually, synthesis of DNA and RNA is inhibited.

ONSET, PEAK, DURATION
Undefined.

INDICATIONS & DOSAGE
Acute lymphoblastic leukemia (ALL) in patients who require L-asparaginase but have developed hypersensitivity to the native forms of L-asparaginase —
Adults and children with body surface area (BSA) of at least 0.6 m^2:
2,500 IU/m^2 I.M. or I.V. q 14 days.
Children with BSA less than 0.6 m^2:
82.5 IU/kg I.M. or I.V. q 14 days.

ADVERSE REACTIONS
CNS: seizures, headache, paresthesia, *status epilepticus,* somnolence, coma, mental status changes, dizziness, emotional lability, mood changes, parkinsonism, confusion, disorientation, fatigue.
CV: hypotension, tachycardia, chest pain, subacute bacterial endocarditis, hypertension.
EENT: epistaxis.
Endocrine: hyperglycemia, hypoglycemia.
GI: nausea, vomiting, abdominal pain, anorexia, diarrhea, constipation, indigestion, flatulence, mucositis, *pancreatitis (sometimes fulminant and fatal),* increased serum amylase and lipase levels, severe colitis.
GU: increased BUN level, increased creatinine level, increased urinary frequency, hematuria, severe hemorrhagic cystitis, renal dysfunction, renal failure.
Hematologic: *thrombosis;* prolonged PTs, prolonged PTTs, decreased antithrombin III; disseminated intravascular coagulation; decreased fibrinogen; hemolytic anemia; *leukopenia; pancytopenia; agranulocytosis; thrombocytopenia;* increased thromboplastin; easy bruising; ecchymoses; *hemorrhage.*
Hepatic: jaundice, abnormal liver function test results, bilirubinemia, increased ALT and AST, ascites, hypoalbuminemia, fatty changes in liver, *liver failure.*

Reactions may be *common*, uncommon, *life-threatening*, or COMMON AND LIFE-THREATENING.

Metabolic: hyperuricemia, hyponatremia, uric acid nephropathy, hypoproteinemia, proteinuria, weight loss, metabolic acidosis, increased blood ammonia level, hyperglycemia, hypoglycemia.
Musculoskeletal: arthralgia, myalgia, musculoskeletal pain, joint stiffness, cramps.
Respiratory: cough, *severe bronchospasm,* upper respiratory tract infection.
Skin: itching, alopecia, fever blister, purpura, hand whiteness, fungal changes, nail whiteness and ridging, erythema simplex, petechial rash, injection pain or reaction, localized edema.
Other: hypersensitivity reactions, including *anaphylaxis,* rash, erythema, edema, pain, fever, chills, urticaria, dyspnea, or bronchospasm; pain in extremities; peripheral edema; malaise; night sweats; mouth tenderness; infection; *sepsis, septic shock.*

INTERACTIONS
Aspirin, dipyridamole, heparin, NSAIDs, warfarin: imbalances in coagulation factors may occur, predisposing the patient to bleeding or thrombosis. Use together cautiously.
Methotrexate: during the period of its inhibition of protein synthesis and cell replication, pegaspargase may interfere with the action of such drugs as methotrexate, which require cell replication for their lethal effects. Monitor for decreased effectiveness.
Protein-bound drugs: depletion of serum proteins by pegaspargase may increase toxicity of other drugs that bind to proteins. Monitor for toxicity. Pegaspargase also may interfere with enzymatic detoxification of other drugs, particularly in the liver. Administer concomitantly with caution.

EFFECTS ON DIAGNOSTIC TESTS
None reported.

CONTRAINDICATIONS
Contraindicated in patients with pancre-
atitis or a history of pancreatitis; in those who have had significant hemorrhagic events associated with prior L-asparaginase; and in those with previous serious allergic reactions, such as generalized urticaria, bronchospasm, laryngeal edema, hypotension, or other unacceptable adverse reactions to pegaspargase.

NURSING CONSIDERATIONS
● Use cautiously in pregnant patients and in patients with liver dysfunction.
● Know that pegaspargase should be used as the sole induction agent only when a combined regimen that uses other chemotherapeutic agents is inappropriate because of toxicity or other specific patient-related factors, or in patients refractory to other therapy.
● Be aware that I.M. route is preferred because it has the lowest incidence of hepatotoxicity, coagulopathy, and GI and renal disorders.
● Do not administer if drug has been frozen. Although there may not be a change in the appearance of the drug, pegaspargase's activity is destroyed after freezing. Obtain new dose from pharmacist.
● Avoid excessive agitation; do *not* shake. Keep refrigerated at 36° to 46° F (2° to 8° C). Do not use if cloudy or if precipitate is present. Do not use if stored at room temperature for more than 48 hours. Do not freeze. Discard unused portions. Use only one dose per vial; do not reenter the vial.
● The drug may be a contact irritant, and the solution must be handled and administered with care. Gloves are recommended. Inhalation of vapors and contact with skin or mucous membranes, especially those of the eyes, must be avoided. In case of contact, wash with copious amounts of water for at least 15 minutes.
● When administering I.M., limit the volume administered at a single injection site to 2 ml. If the volume to be administered is greater than 2 ml, use mul-

---

tiple injection sites.

• When administered I.V., give over a period of 1 to 2 hours in 100 ml of 0.9% sodium chloride or dextrose 5% injection through an infusion that is already running.

Alert: Monitor patient closely for hypersensitivity reactions. Hypersensitivity reactions, including life-threatening anaphylaxis, may occur during therapy, especially in patients with known hypersensitivity to the other forms of L-asparaginase. As a routine precaution, keep patients under observation for 1 hour and have resuscitation equipment and other agents necessary to treat anaphylaxis (such as epinephrine, oxygen, and I.V. steroids) readily available. Know that moderate to life-threatening hypersensitivity reactions require discontinuation of L-asparaginase.

• As a guide to the effects of therapy, monitor the patient's peripheral blood count and bone marrow, as ordered. A fall in circulating lymphoblasts is often noted after initiating therapy. This may be accompanied by a marked rise in serum uric acid levels.

• Take preventive measures (including adequate hydration) before starting treatment. Hyperuricemia may result from rapid lysis of leukemic cells. Allopurinol may be ordered.

• Obtain frequent serum amylase determinations, as ordered, to detect pancreatitis. Monitor patient's blood glucose during therapy to detect hyperglycemia.

• Monitor patient for liver dysfunction when pegaspargase is used in conjunction with hepatotoxic chemotherapeutic agents.

• Be aware that pegaspargase may affect a number of plasma proteins; therefore, monitoring of fibrinogen, PT, and PTT may be indicated. Question doctor if not ordered.

☑ **PATIENT TEACHING**
• Inform the patient of the possibility of hypersensitivity reactions and the importance of alerting the staff immediate-ly if any occur.

• Instruct patient not to take any other drugs, including OTC preparations, until approved by the doctor because the risk of bleeding is higher when pegaspargase is given concomitantly with certain drugs, such as aspirin, or because it may increase the toxicity of other medications.

• Instruct the patient to report signs and symptoms of infection (fever, chills, and malaise); drug may have immunosuppressant activity.

• Advise patient to avoid pregnancy or breast-feeding during therapy.

---

porfimer sodium
Photofrin

Pregnancy Risk Category: C

HOW SUPPLIED
Injection: 75 mg/vial

ACTION
A photosensitizing drug that damages cancer cells through propagation of radical reactions. Tumor death also occurs through ischemic necrosis secondary to vascular occlusion that appears to be partly mediated by release of thromboxane A_2. Cytotoxic and antitumor actions of porfimer depend on light and oxygen.

ONSET, PEAK, DURATION
Unknown.

INDICATIONS & DOSAGE
Palliative treatment for patients with completely obstructing esophageal cancer or for those with partially obstructing esophageal cancer who cannot be satisfactorily treated with Nd:YAG laser therapy—
Adults: 2 mg/kg I.V. for 3 to 5 minutes (first stage of therapy), followed by illumination with laser light 40 to 50 hours later (second stage). A second laser-light application may be given 96 to 120 hours after injection. A total of three

---

courses (each course consisting of both stages) may be given, separated by at least 30 days.

ADVERSE REACTIONS
CNS: anxiety, confusion, *insomnia.*
CV: hypotension, hypertension, cardiac failure, atrial fibrillation, tachycardia.
GI: *constipation, abdominal pain, nausea, vomiting,* diarrhea, dyspepsia, dysphagia, eructation, esophageal edema, esophageal tumor bleeding, esophageal stricture, esophagitis, hematemesis, melena, anorexia.
GU: urinary tract infection.
Hematologic: *anemia.*
Respiratory: coughing, *dyspnea, pharyngitis, pleural effusion, pneumonia,* respiratory insufficiency, tracheoesophageal fistula.
Skin: *photosensitivity.*
Other: *back or chest pain,* asthenia, substernal or general pain, edema, fever, surgical complication, dehydration, weight loss, moniliasis.

INTERACTIONS
Other photosensitizing drugs (tetracyclines, sulfonamides, phenothiazines, sulfonylurea hypoglycemic agents, thiazide diuretics, griseofulvin): may increase photosensitivity reaction. Use together cautiously.

EFFECTS ON DIAGNOSTIC TESTS
None reported.

CONTRAINDICATIONS
Contraindicated in patients with porphyria, tracheoesophageal or bronchoesophageal fistula, tumor eroding into major blood vessel, or hypersensitivity to porphyrins.

NURSING CONSIDERATIONS
● Women receiving porfimer must not breast-feed because it isn't known if drug is excreted in human milk.
● Safety and efficacy in children have not been established.
● Before each course of treatment, pa-

tients should be evaluated for a tracheoesophageal or bronchoesophageal fistula.
● **I.V. use:** Reconstitute each vial of porfimer with 31.8 ml of 5% dextrose solution or 0.9% sodium chloride solution for injection, resulting in final concentration of 2.5 mg/ml. Shake until dissolved. Do not mix porfimer with other drugs in same solution. Reconstituted drug is opaque. Inspect carefully for particulate and discoloration before administration. Protect reconstituted drug from bright light, and use immediately.
● Take precautions to prevent extravasation at injection site. If it occurs, protect the area from light.
● Don't allow drug to contact eyes or skin during preparation or administration. Protect an exposed person from bright light.
● Know that the patient must receive 630-nm wavelength laser-light therapy 40 to 50 hours after porfimer injection for drug to be effective. A second laser-light treatment (but not a second injection) may be given as early as 96 hours or as late as 120 hours after injection. Before a second treatment, the residual tumor should be debrided; be aware that vigorous debridement may cause tumor bleeding. Monitor patient closely.
● Know that inflammation of treatment area may cause substernal chest pain. Notify the doctor if this occurs; pain may be sufficiently intense to warrant short-term use of opiate analgesics.
● Monitor CBC regularly to detect anemia. Drug and laser therapy may cause tumor bleeding.

☑ **PATIENT TEACHING**
● Instruct patient to avoid direct sunlight and bright indoor light for 30 days after injection, but tell him to expose skin to ambient indoor light. After 30 days, he should expose a small area of skin (not face) to sunlight for 10 minutes. If he doesn't develop a photosensitivity reaction (erythema, edema, blistering) within 24 hours, he can gradually resume

---

outdoor activities while exercising caution. If photosensitivity occurs, he should avoid sunlight and bright indoor light for 2 weeks before retesting.
• Urge patient traveling to an area with stronger sun to retest his photosensitivity level.
• Warn patient that ultraviolet sunscreens do not protect against photosensitivity.
• Advise patient to wear dark sunglasses with an average white light transmittance of less than 4% when outdoors.
• Advise female patients of childbearing age to use an effective contraceptive method and to notify the doctor of suspected pregnancy.

---

procarbazine hydrochloride
Matulane, Natulan†

Pregnancy Risk Category: D

HOW SUPPLIED
Capsules: 50 mg

ACTION
Unknown. Thought to inhibit DNA, RNA, and protein synthesis.

ONSET, PEAK, DURATION
Unknown.

INDICATIONS & DOSAGE
Dosage and indications vary. Check treatment protocol with the doctor.
Adjunct treatment of Hodgkin's disease (stages III and IV), other cancers using MOPP (nitrogen mustard, vincristine, procarbazine, prednisone) regimen—
Adults: 2 to 4 mg/kg P.O. daily in a single dose or divided doses for the 1st week. Then, 4 to 6 mg/kg/day until WBC count falls below 4,000/mm³ or platelet count falls below 100,000/mm³. After bone marrow recovers, maintenance dosage of 1 to 2 mg/kg/day resumed. For MOPP regimen, 100 mg/m²/day P.O. for 14 days.
Children: 50 mg/m² P.O. daily for 1st

week; then 100 mg/m² until response or toxicity occurs. Maintenance dosage is 50 mg/m² P.O. daily after bone marrow recovery.

ADVERSE REACTIONS
CNS: nervousness, depression, headache, dizziness, *coma,* insomnia, nightmares, paresthesia, neuropathy, *hallucinations,* confusion, *seizures.*
CV: hypotension, tachycardia, syncope.
EENT: retinal hemorrhage, nystagmus, photophobia.
GI: *nausea, vomiting,* abdominal pain, hematemesis, melena, anorexia, stomatitis, dry mouth, dysphagia, diarrhea, constipation.
GU: hematuria, urinary frequency, nocturia.
Hematologic: *bleeding tendency, thrombocytopenia, leukopenia, anemia,* hemolytic anemia.
Respiratory: *pleural effusion,* cough, pneumonitis.
Skin: dermatitis, pruritus, rash, hyperpigmentation, flushing, herpes.
Other: reversible alopecia, gynecomastia.

INTERACTIONS
CNS depressants: additive depressant effects. Avoid concomitant use.
Digoxin: may decrease serum digoxin levels. Monitor closely.
Drugs and foods high in tyramine (Chianti wine, cheese), local anesthetics, sympathomimetics, tricyclic antidepressants: possible tremor, palpitations, increased blood pressure. Monitor closely.
Ethanol: mild disulfiram-like reaction. Warn patients not to drink alcoholic beverages.

EFFECTS ON DIAGNOSTIC TESTS
None reported.

CONTRAINDICATIONS
Contraindicated in patients hypersensitive to the drug and in those with inadequate bone marrow reserve as shown by

bone marrow aspiration.

NURSING CONSIDERATIONS
• Use cautiously in patients with impaired hepatic or renal function.
• Monitor CBC and platelet counts.
• To prevent bleeding, avoid all I.M. injections when platelet count is below 100,000/mm³.
• Anticipate the need for blood transfusions to combat anemia.
• Be prepared to discontinue drug if patient becomes confused or if paresthesia or other neuropathies develop. Notify doctor.

☑ PATIENT TEACHING
• To decrease nausea and vomiting, advise patient to take drug at bedtime and in divided doses.
• Tell patient to watch for signs of infection (fever, sore throat, fatigue) and bleeding (easy bruising, nosebleeds, bleeding gums, melena) and to take temperature daily.
• Warn patient to avoid alcohol while taking this drug. Urge him to stop medication and check with the doctor immediately if he experiences a disulfiram-like reaction (chest pains, rapid or irregular heartbeat, severe headache, stiff neck).
• Instruct patient to avoid foods high in tyramine, such as wine, cheese, and bananas, and OTC preparations containing sympathomimetics.
• Warn patient to avoid hazardous activities that require alertness and good motor coordination until the CNS effects are known.
• Advise women of childbearing age to avoid becoming pregnant during therapy and to consult with doctor before becoming pregnant.

---

teniposide (VM-26)
Vumon

Pregnancy Risk Category: D

HOW SUPPLIED
Injection: 10 mg/ml

ACTION
A phase-specific cytotoxic drug that acts in the late S or early G_2 phase of the cell cycle, thus preventing cells from entering mitosis.

ONSET, PEAK, DURATION
Undefined.

INDICATIONS & DOSAGE
Refractory childhood acute lymphoblastic leukemia—
Children: optimum dosage hasn't been established. In clinical trials, dosages ranged from 165 to 250 mg/m² I.V. once or twice weekly for 4 to 6 weeks. Usually used in combination with other agents.

ADVERSE REACTIONS
CV: hypotension from rapid infusion.
GI: *nausea and vomiting, mucositis, diarrhea.*
Hematologic: MYELOSUPPRESSION (dose-limiting), LEUKOPENIA, NEUTROPENIA, THROMBOCYTOPENIA, *anemia.*
Other: alopecia (rare), *anaphylaxis* (rare), rash, *infection,* bleeding, hypersensitivity reactions (chills, fever, urticaria, tachycardia, *bronchospasm,* dyspnea, hypotension, flushing); *phlebitis and extravasation* (at injection site).

INTERACTIONS
Heparin: physical incompatibility. Don't mix together.
Methotrexate: may increase clearance and intracellular levels of methotrexate.
Sodium salicylate, sulfamethazole, tolbutamide: may displace teniposide from protein-binding sites and increase toxicity.

EFFECTS ON DIAGNOSTIC TESTS
Drug therapy may increase blood and urine concentrations of uric acid.

CONTRAINDICATIONS

Contraindicated in patients hypersensitive to the drug or to polyoxyethylated castor oil, an injection vehicle.

NURSING CONSIDERATIONS

• Be aware that some clinicians may decide to use this drug despite a patient's history of hypersensitivity because the therapeutic benefits outweigh its risks. Such patients should be treated with antihistamines and corticosteroids before the infusion begins and should be closely watched during drug administration.
• Obtain baseline blood counts, renal and hepatic function tests, as ordered.
• Monitor blood pressure before therapy.
• Have on hand diphenhydramine, hydrocortisone, epinephrine, and emergency equipment to establish an airway in case of anaphylaxis.
• Follow institutional policy to reduce risks. Preparation and administration of parenteral form of this drug is associated with carcinogenic, mutagenic, and teratogenic risks for personnel.
• **I.V. use:** Dilute drug in either D_5W or 0.9% sodium chloride injection to a final concentration of 0.1, 0.2, 0.4, or 1 mg/ml. Don't agitate vigorously; precipitation of drug may occur. Discard cloudy solutions. Prepare and store the drug in glass containers. Infuse over 45 to 90 minutes to prevent hypotension.
• Don't mix with other drugs or solutions.
• Ensure careful placement of the I.V. catheter. Extravasation can result in local tissue necrosis or sloughing.
• Don't administer through a membrane-type in-line filter because the diluent may dissolve it.
• Monitor blood counts and renal and hepatic function tests, as ordered.
• Monitor blood pressure every 30 minutes during infusion. If systolic blood pressure falls below 90 mm Hg, stop infusion and notify the doctor.
• In normal saline or D_5W, concentrations of 0.1 to 0.4 mg/ml are chemically stable for at least 24 hours at room or refrigerated temperature in glass containers. In plastic containers, 0.1 mg/ml in normal saline is stable for 8 hours at room or refrigerated temperatures. Do not use D_5W and store in plastic containers.

☑ PATIENT TEACHING

• Tell patient to report signs and symptoms of infection (fever, sore throat, fatigue) and bleeding (easy bruising, nosebleeds, bleeding gums, melena) and to take temperature daily.
• Advise women of childbearing age to avoid becoming pregnant during therapy and to consult with doctor before becoming pregnant.

▼ *NEW DRUG*

topotecan hydrochloride
Hycamtin

Pregnancy Risk Category: D

HOW SUPPLIED

Injection: 4 mg single-dose vial

ACTION

Relieves torsional strain in DNA by inducing reversible single-strand breaks. Binds to the topoisomerase I-DNA complex and prevents religation of these single-strand breaks. Cytotoxicity of topotecan is thought to be due to double-strand DNA damage produced during DNA synthesis when replication enzymes interact with the ternary complex formed by topotecan, topoisomerase I, and DNA.

ONSET, PEAK, DURATION

Onset and peak unknown. Drug's terminal half-life is between 2 and 3 hours.

INDICATIONS & DOSAGE

Metastatic carcinoma of the ovary after failure of initial or subsequent chemotherapy—
Adults: 1.5 mg/m² I.V. infusion given

---

over 30 minutes daily for 5 consecutive days, starting on day 1 of a 21-day cycle. Minimum of four cycles should be given. For patients with creatinine clearance of 20 to 39 ml/minute, dosage should be decreased to 0.75 mg/m². If severe neutropenia occurs, dosage should be reduced by 0.25 mg/m² for subsequent courses. Alternatively, in the event of severe neutropenia, granulocyte-colony stimulating factor may be administered following the subsequent course (before resorting to dosage reduction) starting from day 6 of the course (24 hours after the completion of topotecan administration).

ADVERSE REACTIONS

CNS: *fatigue, asthenia, headache, paresthesia.*
GI: *nausea, vomiting, diarrhea, constipation, abdominal pain, stomatitis, anorexia.*
Hematologic: NEUTROPENIA, LEUKOPENIA, THROMBOCYTOPENIA, *anemia.*
Hepatic: transient elevation of AST, ALT, and bilirubin levels.
Respiratory: *dyspnea.*
Skin: *alopecia.*
Other: *sepsis, fever.*

INTERACTIONS

Granulocyte-colony stimulating factor: prolonged duration of neutropenia. If granulocyte-colony stimulating factor is to be used, do not start it until day 6 of the course, 24 hours after completion of topotecan treatment.
Cisplatin: increased severity of myelosuppression, if given together. Use both drugs with extreme caution.

EFFECTS ON DIAGNOSTIC TESTS
None reported.

CONTRAINDICATIONS
Contraindicated in patients with hypersensitivity to drug or any of its components, or severe bone marrow depression and in pregnant or breast-feeding women.

NURSING CONSIDERATIONS
Alert: Prior to administration of the first course of therapy, patients must have a baseline neutrophil count greater than 1,500 cells/mm³ and a platelet count above 100,000 cells/mm³.
● Be aware that topotecan should be prepared under a vertical laminar flow hood while wearing gloves and protective clothing. If drug solution contacts the skin, wash immediately and thoroughly with soap and water. If mucous membranes are affected, flush areas thoroughly with water.
● Each 4-mg vial should be reconstituted with 4 ml sterile water for injection. The appropriate volume of reconstituted solution is then diluted in either 0.9% sodium chloride solution or D_5W before administration.
● Because the lyophilized dosage form contains no antibacterial preservative, use reconstituted product immediately.
● Protect unopened vials of drug from light. Reconstituted vials stored at 68° to 77° F (20° to 25° C) and exposed to ambient lighting are stable for 24 hours.
● Know that bone marrow suppression (primarily neutropenia) is the dose-limiting toxicity of topotecan. The nadir occurs at about 11 days. Neutropenia is not cumulative over time.
● Know that the duration of thrombocytopenia is about 5 days, with nadir at 15 days. The nadir for anemia is 15 days. Blood or platelet transfusions may be necessary.
● Frequent monitoring of peripheral blood cell counts are necessary. Patients should not be treated with subsequent courses of topotecan until neutrophil counts recover to over 1,000 cells/mm³, platelet counts recover to over 100,000 cells/mm³, and hemoglobin levels recover to over 9 mg/dl (with transfusion if needed).
● Know that inadvertent extravasation of topotecan has been associated with mild local reactions, such as erythema and bruising.
● Be aware that safety and effectiveness

---

in children have not been established.

☑ **PATIENT TEACHING**
● Instruct patient to promptly report sore throat, fever, chills, or unusual bleeding or bruising.
● Advise patient of child-bearing age to avoid pregnancy and breast-feeding during therapy.
● Teach patient and family about adverse reactions to expect and the need for frequent monitoring of blood counts.

---

tretinoin
Vesanoid

Pregnancy Risk Category: D

HOW SUPPLIED
Capsules: 10 mg

ACTION
Unknown.

ONSET, PEAK, DURATION
Onset and duration unknown. Peak levels occur in 1 to 2 hours.

INDICATIONS & DOSAGE
Induction of remission in patients with acute promyelocytic leukemia (APL), French-American-British (FAB) classification M3 (including M3 variant), when anthracycline chemotherapy is contraindicated or unsuccessful—
Adults and children 1 year and older: 45 mg/m²/day P.O. in two even doses. Therapy should be discontinued 30 days after complete remission is documented or after 90 days of treatment, whichever occurs first.

ADVERSE REACTIONS
CNS: *headache,* dizziness, *paresthesia, anxiety, insomnia, depression, confusion,* **cerebral hemorrhage,** intracranial hypertension, agitation, hallucination, abnormal gait, agnosia, aphasia, asterixis, cerebellar edema, cerebellar disorders, **convulsions, coma,** CNS depression, dysarthria, encephalopathy, facial paralysis, hemiplegia, hyporeflexia, hypotaxia, no light reflex, neurologic reaction, spinal cord disorder, tremor, leg weakness, unconsciousness, dementia, forgetfulness, somnolence, slow speech.
CV: *chest discomfort, arrhythmias, hypotension, hypertension, phlebitis, edema, cardiac failure,* **cardiac arrest,** *myocardial infarction, pericardial effusions,* impaired myocardial contractility, progressive hypoxemia, enlarged heart, heart murmur, ischemia, stroke, myocarditis, pericarditis, secondary cardiomyopathy.
EENT: *earache, ear fullness,* hearing loss, *visual disturbances,* changed visual acuity, visual field defects, *ocular disorders.*
GI: *GI hemorrhage, nausea, vomiting, anorexia, abdominal pain, GI disorders, diarrhea, constipation, dyspepsia, abdominal distention,* hepatosplenomegaly, hepatitis, ulcer, unspecified liver disorder.
GU: *renal insufficiency,* dysuria, **acute renal failure,** micturition frequency, renal tubular necrosis, enlarged prostate.
Hematologic: *leukocytosis, hemorrhage, disseminated intravascular coagulation.*
Respiratory: *pneumonia, upper respiratory tract disorders, dyspnea, respiratory insufficiency, pleural effusion, rales, expiratory wheezing,* lower respiratory tract disorders, pulmonary infiltrates, bronchial asthma, pulmonary edema, laryngeal edema, unspecified pulmonary disease, pulmonary hypertension.
Skin: *flushing, rash, skin and mucous membrane dryness, pruritis, alopecia, increased sweating,* skin changes.
Other: **retinoic acid-APL syndrome** (see Nursing considerations), **septicemia, multiorgan failure,** *weakness, fatigue, fever, infections, malaise, shivering, peripheral edema, pain, injection site reactions, myalgia, bone pain, mucositis,* flank pain, cellulitis, facial edema, fluid imbalance, pallor, lymph dis-

---

Reactions may be *common,* uncommon, ***life-threatening,*** or **COMMON AND LIFE-THREATENING.**

order, acidosis, hypothermia, ascites, bone inflammation, *weight gain or loss, hypercholesterolemia, hypertriglyceridemia, elevated liver function studies.*

INTERACTIONS
None reported.

EFFECTS ON DIAGNOSTIC TESTS
None known.

CONTRAINDICATIONS
Contraindicated in patients with known hypersensitivity to retinoids. Do not give drug to patients who are sensitive to parabens, which are used as preservatives in gelatin capsule.

NURSING CONSIDERATIONS
● Drug is not recommended for use in pregnant or breast-feeding women.
● Patients with APL are at high risk and can have severe reactions, so give drug under supervision of doctor with experience managing such patients and in a facility able to monitor drug tolerance and protect and maintain patient compromised by toxicity.
● About 25% of patients in clinical trials experienced Retinoic Acid-APL Syndrome, characterized by fever, dyspnea, weight gain, radiographic pulmonary infiltrates, and pleural or pericardial effusions. Notify doctor immediately if any of these appears, because the syndrome has occasionally been accompanied by impaired myocardial contractility and episodic hypotension with or without concomitant leukocytosis. Some patients have died from progressive hypoxemia and multiorgan failure. The syndrome generally occurs during the first month of therapy. Prompt treatment with high-dose steroids appears to reduce morbidity and mortality.
● Monitor CBC and platelet counts regularly. Patients with high WBC counts at diagnosis are at increased risk for further, rapid elevations. Rapidly evolving leukocytosis is associated with a higher

risk of life-threatening complications.
● Monitor the patient (especially a child) for pseudotumor cerebri. Early signs and symptoms include papilledema, headache, nausea, vomiting, and visual disturbances. Notify the doctor immediately if any occurs.
● Monitor cholesterol and triglyceride levels and liver function studies. Notify the doctor of abnormalities.
● Maintain infection control and bleeding precautions, and provide prompt treatment, as ordered.
● Ensure that pregnancy testing and contraception counseling are repeated monthly throughout therapy and for 1 month after completion of therapy.

☑ PATIENT TEACHING
● Explain infection control and bleeding precautions. Tell the patient to notify the doctor of signs and symptoms of infection (fever, sore throat, fatigue) or bleeding (easy bruising, nosebleeds, bleeding gums, melena) and to take temperature daily.
● Inform a female patient that a pregnancy test is required 1 week before therapy begins and that therapy will be delayed, if possible, until a negative result is obtained.
● Instruct a female patient to use contraception during therapy and for 1 month after completion, despite history of infertility or menopause, unless a hysterectomy has been performed. Tell her to use two methods of contraception simultaneously, unless abstinence is the chosen method, and to notify the doctor if pregnancy is suspected.

---

vinblastine sulfate (VLB)
Alkaban-AQ, Velban, Velbe†‡, Velsar

Pregnancy Risk Category: D

HOW SUPPLIED
Injection: 10-mg vials (lyophilized powder), 1 mg/ml in 10-ml vials

---

ACTION
Arrests mitosis in metaphase, blocking cell division.

ONSET, PEAK, DURATION
Undefined.

INDICATIONS & DOSAGE
Breast or testicular cancer, Hodgkin's disease and malignant lymphoma, choriocarcinoma, lymphosarcoma, mycosis fungoides, Kaposi's sarcoma, histiocytosis—
Adults: 0.1 mg/kg or 3.7 mg/m² I.V. weekly or q 2 weeks. May increase to maximum dosage of 0.5 mg/kg or 18.5 mg/m² I.V. weekly according to response. Do not repeat dosage if WBC count is below 4,000/mm³.
Children: initial dose, 2.5 mg/m² I.V. weekly. Dosage increased by 1.25 mg/m² until WBC count is below 3,000/mm³ or tumor response is seen. Maximum dosage is 12.5 mg/m² I.V. weekly.

ADVERSE REACTIONS
CNS: depression, *paresthesia, peripheral neuropathy and neuritis, numbness, loss of deep tendon reflexes, muscle pain and weakness,* **seizures, CVA,** headache.
CV: hypertension, *MI.*
EENT: pharyngitis.
GI: *nausea, vomiting, ulcer, bleeding, constipation, ileus, anorexia,* diarrhea, abdominal pain, *stomatitis.*
Hematologic: *anemia, leukopenia* (nadir occurs days 4 to 10 and lasts another 7 to 14 days), **thrombocytopenia.**
Respiratory: *acute bronchospasm,* shortness of breath.
Skin: reversible alopecia, vesiculation.
Other: *irritation, phlebitis, weight loss,* cellulitis, necrosis with extravasation.

INTERACTIONS
Erythromycin and other drugs that inhibit the cytochrome P450 pathway: may increase toxicity of vinblastine.
Mitomycin: increased risk of bronchospasm and shortness of breath. Monitor patient's respiratory status.
Phenytoin: decreased plasma phenytoin levels. Monitor closely.

EFFECTS ON DIAGNOSTIC TESTS
Drug therapy may increase blood and urine concentrations of uric acid.

CONTRAINDICATIONS
Contraindicated in patients with severe leukopenia or bacterial infection.

NURSING CONSIDERATIONS
• Use cautiously in patients with hepatic dysfunction.
• To reduce nausea, give antiemetic before drug, as ordered.
• Follow institutional policy to reduce risks. Preparation and administration of parenteral form of this drug is associated with carcinogenic, mutagenic, and teratogenic risks for personnel.
• **I.V. use:** Inject directly into vein or tubing of running I.V. line over 1 minute. Drug is a vesicant; if extravasation occurs, stop infusion immediately and notify doctor. The manufacturer recommends that moderate heat be applied to area of leakage. Local injection of hyaluronidase may help disperse drug, as ordered. Some clinicians prefer to apply ice packs on and off every 2 hours for 24 hours, with local injection of hydrocortisone or 0.9% sodium chloride.
• Reconstitute 10-mg vial with 10 ml of sodium chloride injection or sterile water. This yields 1 mg/ml. Refrigerate reconstituted solution. Protect solution from light. and discard after 30 days.
• Do not administer into a limb with compromised circulation.
Alert: After administering, monitor for development of life-threatening acute bronchospasm. If this occurs, notify the doctor immediately. Reaction is most likely to occur in patients who are also receiving mitomycin.
• Monitor patient for stomatitis. Be prepared to stop drug if stomatitis occurs

---

Reactions may be *common,* uncommon, *life-threatening,* or COMMON AND LIFE-THREATENING.

and notify doctor.

• Assess bowel activity. Give laxatives as needed and ordered. May use stool softeners prophylactically.

• Know that dosage should not be repeated more frequently than every 7 days or severe leukopenia will occur.

• Assess for numbness and tingling in hands and feet. Assess gait for early evidence of footdrop.

• Take care to avoid confusing vinblastine with vincristine or vindesine.

• Know that the drug is less neurotoxic than vincristine.

• Anticipate a decrease in dosage by 50% if bilirubin levels are greater than 3 mg/100 ml.

• Drugs known to cause urine retention, particularly in elderly patients, should be discontinued for the first few days after vinblastine therapy.

☑ **PATIENT TEACHING**

• Tell patient to report signs and symptoms of infection (fever, sore throat, fatigue) and bleeding (easy bruising, nosebleeds, bleeding gums, melena) and to take temperature daily.

• Warn patient that alopecia may occur, but explain that it's usually reversible.

• Warn patient of childbearing age to avoid pregnancy during therapy.

---

vincristine sulfate (VCR)
Oncovin, Vincasar PFS

Pregnancy Risk Category: D

HOW SUPPLIED
Injection: 1 mg/ml in 1-ml, 2-ml, 5-ml multiple-dose vials; 1 mg/ml in 1-ml, 2-ml, 5-ml preservative-free vials

ACTION
Arrests mitosis in metaphase, blocking cell division.

ONSET, PEAK, DURATION
Undefined.

INDICATIONS & DOSAGE
Acute lymphoblastic and other leukemias, Hodgkin's disease, malignant lymphoma, neuroblastoma, rhabdomyosarcoma, Wilms' tumor—
Adults: 1.4 mg/m² I.V. weekly. Maximum weekly dosage is 2 mg.
Children over 10 kg: 2 mg/m² I.V. weekly.
Children 10 kg and under or with a body surface area below 1 m²: initially, 0.05 mg/kg I.V. weekly.

ADVERSE REACTIONS
CNS: *peripheral neuropathy,* sensory loss, *loss of deep tendon reflexes, paresthesia, wristdrop and footdrop,* **seizures, coma,** headache, ataxia, cranial nerve palsies, *jaw pain,* hoarseness, vocal cord paralysis, *muscle weakness and cramps*—some neurotoxicities may be permanent.
CV: hypotension, hypertension.
EENT: visual disturbances, blindness, diplopia, optic and extraocular neuropathy, ptosis.
GI: diarrhea, *constipation, cramps,* ileus that mimics surgical abdomen, paralytic ileus, *nausea, vomiting,* anorexia, dysphagia, *intestinal necrosis, stomatitis.*
GU: urine retention, SIADH, dysuria, acute uric acid neuropathy, polyuria.
Hematologic: anemia, *leukopenia, thrombocytopenia.*
Respiratory: *acute bronchospasm,* dyspnea.
Skin: rash, reversible alopecia.
Other: fever, weight loss, severe local reaction with extravasation, *phlebitis,* cellulitis at injection site, hyponatremia.

INTERACTIONS
Asparaginase: decreased hepatic clearance of vincristine. Monitor for toxicity.
Calcium channel blockers: enhanced vincristine accumulation in cells.
Digoxin: decreased digoxin effects. Monitor serum digoxin level.
Mitomycin: possibly increased frequency of bronchospasm and acute pul-

---

monary reactions. Monitor patient's respiratory status.

Phenytoin: may reduce phenytoin levels.

EFFECTS ON DIAGNOSTIC TESTS

Drug therapy may increase blood and urine concentrations of uric acid. Because WBC and platelet counts may decrease, frequently monitor blood counts.

CONTRAINDICATIONS

Contraindicated in patients who are hypersensitive to the drug or who have the demyelinating form of Charcot-Marie-Tooth syndrome. Do not give to patients who are concurrently receiving radiation therapy through ports that include the liver.

NURSING CONSIDERATIONS

● Use cautiously in patients with hepatic dysfunction, neuromuscular disease, or infection.

● Follow institutional policy to reduce risks. Preparation and administration of parenteral form of this drug is associated with carcinogenic, mutagenic, and teratogenic risks for personnel.

● **I.V. use:** Inject directly into vein or tubing of running I.V. line slowly over 1 minute. Vincristine is a vesicant; if drug extravasates, stop infusion immediately and notify doctor. Apply heat on and off every 2 hours for 24 hours. Administer 150 units hyalaronidase, as ordered, to area of infiltration.

● A 50% dose reduction is recommended if direct serum bilirubin level exceeds 3 mg/dl.

● Don't administer 5-mg vials to one patient as a single dose. The 5-mg vials are for multiple-dose use only.

Alert: After administering, monitor for development of life-threatening acute bronchospasm. If this occurs, notify the doctor immediately. This reaction is most likely to occur in those also receiving mitomycin.

● Monitor for hyperuricemia, especially in patients with leukemia or lymphoma.

Maintain hydration and administer allopurinol, as ordered, to prevent uric acid nephropathy. Monitor for toxicity.

● Monitor fluid intake and output. Fluid restriction may be necessary if SIADH develops.

● Because of the risk of neurotoxicity, know that drug should not be given more than once a week. Children are more resistant to neurotoxicity than adults. Neurotoxicity is dose-related and usually reversible.

● Check for depression of Achilles tendon reflex, numbness, tingling, footdrop or wristdrop, difficulty in walking, ataxia, and slapping gait. Also check ability to walk on heels. Support patients when walking.

● Monitor bowel function. Give stool softener or laxative, as ordered, or water before dosing. Constipation may be an early sign of neurotoxicity.

● Take care to avoid confusing vincristine with vinblastine or vindesine.

● Know that all vials (1-mg, 2-mg, 5-mg) contain 1 mg/ml solution and should be refrigerated.

● Discontinue drugs known to cause urine retention, particularly in elderly patients, for the first few days after vincristine therapy.

☑ PATIENT TEACHING

● Tell patient to report signs and symptoms of infection (fever, sore throat, fatigue) and bleeding (easy bruising, nosebleeds, bleeding gums, melena) and to take temperature daily.

● Warn patient that alopecia may occur, but explain that it's usually reversible.

● Advise women of childbearing age to avoid becoming pregnant during therapy and to consult with doctor before becoming pregnant.

---

vinorelbine tartrate
Navelbine

Pregnancy Risk Category: D

HOW SUPPLIED
Injection: 10 mg/ml, 50 mg/5 ml

ACTION
A semisynthetic vinca alkaloid that exerts its antineoplastic effect by disrupting microtubule assembly, which, in turn, disrupts spindle formation and prevents mitosis.

ONSET, PEAK, DURATION
Undefined.

INDICATIONS & DOSAGE
Alone or as adjunct therapy with cisplatin for first-line treatment of ambulatory patients with nonresectable advanced non–small-cell lung cancer (NSCLC); alone or with cisplatin in stage IV of NSCLC; with cisplatin in stage III of NSCLC—
Adults: 30 mg/m^2 I.V. weekly. In combination treatment, same dosage used along with 120 mg/m^2 of cisplatin, given on days 1 and 29, then q 6 weeks.

ADVERSE REACTIONS
GI: *nausea, vomiting, anorexia, diarrhea, constipation, stomatitis.*
Hematologic: *bone marrow suppression (agranulocytosis,* LEUKOPENIA, *thrombocytopenia, anemia).*
Hepatic: *abnormal liver function test results, bilirubinemia.*
Respiratory: dyspnea.
Skin: *alopecia,* rash,*injection pain or reaction.*
Other: *peripheral neuropathy, asthenia,* jaw pain, *fatigue,* myalgia, SIADH, chest pain, arthralgia, loss of deep tendon reflexes.

INTERACTIONS
Cisplatin: increased risk of bone marrow suppression when used concomitantly with cisplatin. Monitor patient's hematologic status closely.
Mitomycin: may cause pulmonary reactions. Monitor patient's respiratory status closely.

EFFECTS ON DIAGNOSTIC TESTS
None reported.

CONTRAINDICATIONS
Contraindicated in patients with pretreatment granulocyte counts less than 1,000 cells/mm^3.

NURSING CONSIDERATIONS
● Use with extreme caution in patients whose bone marrow may have been compromised by previous exposure to radiation therapy or chemotherapy or whose bone marrow is still recovering from chemotherapy.
● Use cautiously in patients with hepatic impairment. Monitor liver enzymes.
● Check patient's granulocyte count before administration. The count should be equal to or greater than 1,000 cells/mm^3 for drug to be administered. Withhold drug and notify doctor if count is less.
● Know that vinorelbine must be diluted before administration to a concentration of 1.5/ml to 3 mg/ml with D$_5$W or 0.9% sodium chloride solution in a syringe. Alternatively, dilute to a concentration of 0.5 mg/ml to 2 mg/ml in an I.V. bag. Administer the drug I.V. over 6 to 10 minutes into the side port of a free-flowing I.V. line that is closest to the I.V. bag, followed by flushing with at least 75 to 125 ml of D$_5$W or 0.9% sodium chloride solution.
● Avoid extravasation when administering vinorelbine because drug can cause considerable irritation, localized tissue necrosis, and thrombophlebitis. If extravasation occurs, drug administration should be stopped immediately and any remaining dosage portion injected into a different vein.
● Be aware that dosage adjustments are made according to hematologic toxicity or hepatic insufficiency, whichever results in the lower dosage. Expect dosage reduction of 50% if granulocyte count falls below 1,500 cells/mm^3 but is greater than 1,000 cells/mm^3. If three consecutive doses are skipped because

of agranulocytosis, further vinorelbine therapy should not be given.

● Know that the drug may be a contact irritant, and the solution must be handled and administered with care. Gloves are recommended. Inhalation of vapors and contact with skin or mucous membranes, especially those of the eyes, must be avoided. In case of contact, wash with copious amounts of water for at least 15 minutes.

Alert: Monitor deep tendon reflexes; loss may represent cumulative toxicity.

● Monitor patient closely for hypersensitivity reactions.

● As a guide to the effects of therapy, monitor patient's peripheral blood count and bone marrow, as ordered.

☑ **PATIENT TEACHING**

● Instruct patient not to take any other drugs, including OTC preparations, until approved by the doctor.

● Tell patient to report signs and symptoms of infection (fever, sore throat, fatigue) and bleeding (easy bruising, nosebleeds, bleeding gums, melena) and to take temperature daily.

● Advise women of childbearing age to avoid becoming pregnant during therapy.

azathioprine
cyclosporine
lymphocyte immune globulin
muromonab-CD3
mycophenolate mofetil
tacrolimus

COMBINATION PRODUCTS
None.

azathioprine
Imuran, Thioprine‡

Pregnancy Risk Category: D

HOW SUPPLIED
Tablets: 50 mg
Powder for injection: 100 mg

ACTION
Unknown.

ONSET, PEAK, DURATION
Onset occurs in 4 to 8 weeks. Serum levels peak in 1 to 2 hours. Clinical effects may persist for several days after the drug is discontinued.

INDICATIONS & DOSAGE
Immunosuppression in kidney transplantation—
Adults and children: initially, 3 to 5 mg/kg P.O. or I.V. daily, usually beginning on the day of transplantation. Maintained at 1 to 3 mg/kg daily (dosage varies considerably according to patient response).
Severe, refractory rheumatoid arthritis—
Adults: initially, 1 mg/kg P.O. as a single dose or divided into two doses. If patient response is not satisfactory after 6 to 8 weeks, dosage may be increased by 0.5 mg/kg daily (up to a maximum of 2.5 mg/kg daily) at 4-week intervals.

ADVERSE REACTIONS
GI: *nausea, vomiting, pancreatitis,* steatorrhea, diarrhea, abdominal pain.
Hematologic: LEUKOPENIA, bone marrow suppression, anemia, *pancytopenia, thrombocytopenia, immunosuppression* (possibly profound).
Hepatic: *hepatotoxicity,* jaundice.
Skin: rash.
Other: arthralgia, alopecia, *infections,* fever, myalgia, *increased risk of neoplasia.*

INTERACTIONS
Allopurinol: impaired inactivation of azathioprine. Decrease azathioprine dose to one-quarter or one-third normal dose.
Angiotensin converting enzyme inhibitors: combination may cause severe leukopenia. Monitor patient closely.
Nondepolarizing neuromuscular blockers: azathioprine may reverse the neuromuscular blockade.
Vaccines: decreased immune response. Postpone routine immunization.
Warfarin: azathioprine may decrease action of warfarin.

EFFECTS ON DIAGNOSTIC TESTS
Drug alters CBC and differentiated blood counts, decreases serum uric acid levels, and elevates liver enzyme test results.

CONTRAINDICATIONS
Contraindicated in patients hypersensitive to the drug.

NURSING CONSIDERATIONS
● Use cautiously in patients with hepatic or renal dysfunction.
● Administer drug after meals to minimize adverse GI effects.
● **I.V. use:** Reconstitute 100-mg vial with 10 ml of sterile water for injection.

---

*Liquid contains alcohol.   **May contain tartrazine.   †Canada only.   ‡Australia only.   ◊OTC.

Visually inspect for particles before giving. Drug may be administered by direct I.V. injection or further diluted in 0.9% sodium chloride for injection or D_5W and infused over 30 to 60 minutes. Use only for patients unable to tolerate oral medications.

● To prevent bleeding, avoid all I.M. injections when platelet count is below 100,000/mm³.

● Monitor hemoglobin and WBC and platelet counts at least once monthly, as ordered, more often at beginning of treatment. Notify doctor if counts drop suddenly or become dangerously low. The drug may need to be temporarily withheld.

● Watch for early signs of hepatotoxicity: clay-colored stools, dark urine, pruritus, and yellow skin and sclera; and for increased alkaline phosphatase, bilirubin, AST, and ALT levels.

● Be aware that therapeutic response usually occurs within 8 weeks.

● Keep in mind that the benefits must be weighed against the risk with systemic viral infections, such as chickenpox and herpes zoster.

● Be aware that patients with rheumatoid arthritis previously treated with alkylating agents, such as cyclophosphamide, chlorambucil, melphalan, or others may have a prohibitive risk of neoplasia if treated with the drug.

● Know that drug should not be used for treating rheumatoid arthritis in pregnant women.

☑ **PATIENT TEACHING**
● Warn patient to report even mild infections (colds, fever, sore throat, and malaise) because drug is a potent immunosuppressant.

● Instruct patient to avoid conception during therapy and for 4 months after stopping therapy.

● Warn patient that some thinning of hair is possible.

● Tell patient taking this drug for refractory rheumatoid arthritis that it may take up to 12 weeks to be effective.

cyclosporine (cyclosporin)
Neoral, Sandimmun‡, Sandimmune

Pregnancy Risk Category: C

HOW SUPPLIED
Oral solution: 100 mg/ml
Injection: 50 mg/ml
Capsules: 25 mg, 50 mg, 100 mg

ACTION
Unknown. Thought to inhibit the proliferation and function of T lymphocytes.

ONSET, PEAK, DURATION
Onset and duration unknown. Serum levels peak within 3½ hours after oral dose.

INDICATIONS & DOSAGE
Prophylaxis of organ rejection in kidney, liver, or heart transplantation—
Adults and children: 15 mg/kg P.O. 4 to 12 hours before transplantation and continued daily postoperatively for 1 to 2 weeks. Then dosage reduced by 5% each week to maintenance level of 5 to 10 mg/kg/day. Alternatively, 5 to 6 mg/kg I.V. concentrate 4 to 12 hours before transplantation. Postoperatively, dosage repeated daily until patients can tolerate oral forms.

ADVERSE REACTIONS
CNS: *tremor, headache, seizures,* confusion, paresthesia.
CV: *hypertension.*
EENT: *gum hyperplasia,* oral thrush, sinusitis.
GI: *nausea, vomiting,* diarrhea, abdominal discomfort.
GU: NEPHROTOXICITY.
Hematologic: anemia, *leukopenia, thrombocytopenia,* hemolytic anemia.
Hepatic: *hepatotoxicity.*
Skin: acne, flushing.
Other: increased low-density lipoprotein levels, *infections, hirsutism, anaphylaxis,* gynecomastia.

Reactions may be *common,* uncommon, *life-threatening,* or COMMON AND LIFE-THREATENING.

INTERACTIONS

Acyclovir, aminoglycosides, amphotericin B, co-trimoxazole, melphalan, NSAIDs, ranitidine, vancomycin: increased risk of nephrotoxicity. Avoid concomitant use.

Azathioprine, corticosteroids, cyclophosphamide, verapamil: increased immunosuppression. Monitor closely.

Carbamazepine, isoniazid, phenobarbital, phenytoin, rifabutin, rifampin: possible decreased immunosuppressant effect. Know that cyclosporine dosage may need to be increased.

Cimetidine, danazol, diltiazem, erythromycin, fluconazole, imipenem-cilastatin, ketoconazole, metoclopramide, methylprednisone, nicardipine, prednisolone: may increase blood levels of cyclosporine. Monitor for increased toxicity.

Digoxin: cyclosporine may elevate digoxin levels.

Potassium-sparing diuretics: cyclosporine may induce hyperkalemia.

Vaccines: decreased immune response. Postpone routine immunization.

EFFECTS ON DIAGNOSTIC TESTS

Drug therapy may alter CBC and differential blood tests and may increase serum lipid levels; drug elevation of serum BUN and creatinine and liver function tests may signal nephrotoxicity or hepatotoxicity.

CONTRAINDICATIONS

Contraindicated in patients hypersensitive to the drug or to polyoxyethylated castor oil (found in injectable form).

NURSING CONSIDERATIONS

● Measure oral solution doses carefully in an oral syringe. To increase palatability, mix with whole milk or fruit juice. Use a glass container.

● Give dosage once daily in the morning.

● Neoral has greater bioavailability than Sandimmune form. Less Neoral is needed to yield the same blood concentration derived from Sandimmune. Switch patients between these two brands using blood concentration monitoring, as ordered.

● **I.V. use:** Administer cyclosporine I.V. concentrate at one-third the oral dose and dilute before use. Dilute each milliliter of the concentrate in 20 to 100 ml of D_5W or 0.9% sodium chloride for injection. Dilute immediately before administration; infuse over 2 to 6 hours. Usually reserved for patients who cannot tolerate oral medications.

● Always give cyclosporine concomitantly with adrenal corticosteroids as ordered.

● Monitor cyclosporine blood levels at regular intervals. Absorption of cyclosporine oral solution can be erratic.

● Monitor BUN and serum creatinine levels. Nephrotoxicity may develop 2 to 3 months after transplant surgery, possibly requiring dosage reduction. Notify the doctor of any signs or symptoms of nephrotoxicity.

● Know that the doctor must differentiate between transplanted kidney rejection and cyclosporine-induced nephrotoxicity.

● Monitor liver function tests, as ordered, for hepatotoxicity.

☑ PATIENT TEACHING

● Encourage patient to take drug at same time each day, and teach him how to measure dosage and mask taste of oral solution, if prescribed. Tell him not to take cyclosporine with grapefruit juice, unless instructed to do so.

● Advise patient to take with meals if drug causes nausea.

● Advise patient to take Neoral on an empty stomach.

● Stress to patient that therapy should not be stopped without the doctor's approval.

● To prevent thrush, instruct patient to swish and swallow nystatin four times daily.

● Recommend use of mechanical contraceptive measures, such as a diaphragm or condom, while receiving cyclosporine therapy. Advise female patient not to use oral contraceptives.

---

lymphocyte immune globulin (antithymocyte globulin [equine], ATG)
Atgam

Pregnancy Risk Category: C

HOW SUPPLIED
Injection: 50 mg of equine IgG/ml in 5-ml ampules

ACTION
Unknown. Inhibits cell-mediated immune responses by either altering T cell function or eliminating antigen-reactive T cells.

ONSET, PEAK, DURATION
Onset and duration unknown. Plasma levels peak after 5 days.

INDICATIONS & DOSAGE
Prevention of acute renal allograft rejection—
Adults and children: 15 mg/kg I.V. daily for 14 days, followed by alternate-day dosing for 14 days; the first dose should be given within 24 hours of transplantation.
Treatment of acute renal allograft rejection—
Adults and children: 10 to 15 mg/kg I.V. daily for 14 days. Additional alternative-day therapy up to a total of 21 doses can be given. Therapy should be initiated when rejection is diagnosed.
Aplastic anemia—
Adults: 10 to 20 mg/kg I.V daily for 8 to 14 days. Additional alternative-day therapy up to a total of 21 doses can be administered.

ADVERSE REACTIONS
CNS: malaise, *seizures,* headache.
CV: *hypotension, chest pain,* thrombophlebitis, tachycardia, edema, iliac vein obstruction, renal artery stenosis.
EENT: *laryngospasm.*
GI: *nausea, vomiting, diarrhea,* hiccups, epigastric pain, abdominal distention, stomatitis.
Hematologic: LEUKOPENIA, THROMBOCYTOPENIA, *hemolysis, aplastic anemia.*
Hepatic: elevated liver enzyme level.
Respiratory: *dyspnea,* **pulmonary edema.**
Skin: *rash, pruritus, urticaria.*
Other: *febrile reactions, hypersensitivity reactions, serum sickness,* **anaphylaxis,** *infections, arthralgia,* night sweats, lymphadenopathy, hyperglycemia, *chills, myalgia, arthralgia.*

INTERACTIONS
Muromonab-CD3: increased risk of infection. Monitor closely.

EFFECTS ON DIAGNOSTIC TESTS
Elevations of hepatic serum enzymes have been reported.

CONTRAINDICATIONS
Contraindicated in patients hypersensitive to the drug. An intradermal skin test is recommended at least 1 hour before the first dose. Marked local swelling or erythema larger than 10 mm indicates an increased potential for severe systemic reaction, such as anaphylaxis. Severe reactions to the skin test, such as hypotension, tachycardia, dyspnea, generalized rash, or anaphylaxis, usually preclude further administration of the drug.

NURSING CONSIDERATIONS
● Use cautiously in patients receiving additional immunosuppressive therapy (such as corticosteroids or azathioprine) because of the increased potential for infection. Do not dilute ATG concentrate with dextrose solutions or solutions with a low salt concentration because a precipitate may form. The proteins in ATG can be denatured by air. ATG is unstable in acidic solutions.
● **I.V. use:** Dilute concentrated drug for

---

injection before administration. Dilute the required dose in 250 to 1,000 ml of 0.45% or 0.9% sodium chloride solution. The final concentration of drug should not exceed 1 mg/ml. When adding ATG to the infusion solution, make sure the container is inverted so that the drug does not contact air inside the container. Gently rotate or swirl the container to mix contents; do not shake because this may cause excessive foaming or denature the drug protein. Infuse with an in-line filter with a pore size of 0.2 to 1 micron over no less than 4 hours (most institutions infuse over 4 to 8 hours).

• Do not use solutions that are more than 12 hours old, including actual infusion time.

• Refrigerate at 35° to 47° F (2° to 8° C). ATG concentrate is heat-sensitive. Do not freeze.

• Monitor for signs of infection.

☑ **PATIENT TEACHING**
• Instruct patient to report adverse drug reactions promptly, especially signs of infection (fever, sore throat, fatigue).
• Tell patient to alert nurse immediately if discomfort occurs at I.V. insertion site because drug can cause a chemical phlebitis.
• Advise female patient to avoid pregnancy during drug therapy.

---

muromonab-CD3
Orthoclone OKT3

Pregnancy Risk Category: C

HOW SUPPLIED
Injection: 1 mg/1 ml in 5-ml ampules

ACTION
Muromonab-CD3 is an immunoglobulin G antibody that reacts in the T-lymphocyte membrane with a molecule (CD3) needed for antigen recognition. This drug depletes the blood of $CD3^+$ T cells, which leads to restoration of allograft

function and reversal of rejection.

ONSET, PEAK, DURATION
Onset almost immediate. Peak unknown. Number of circulating $CD3^+$ T cells returns to pretreatment levels within 1 week after drug is withdrawn.

INDICATIONS & DOSAGE
Acute allograft rejection in renal transplant patients; in steroid-resistant hepatic or cardiac allograft rejection—
Adults: 5 mg I.V. bolus once daily for 10 to 14 days.

ADVERSE REACTIONS
CNS: *tremor, headache, seizures, encephalopathy, cerebral edema.*
CV: *chest pain, tachycardia,* hypertension.
GI: *nausea, vomiting, diarrhea.*
Respiratory: *severe pulmonary edema, dyspnea, wheezing.*
Other: *fever, chills, tremors,* INFECTION, *anaphylaxis,* increased serum creatinine, *cytokine release syndrome* (from flulike symptoms to shock), *aseptic meningitis, risk of neoplasia.*

INTERACTIONS
Immunosuppressants: increased risk of infection. Monitor closely.
Indomethacin: increased muromonab-CD3 levels with encephalopathy and other CNS effects. Monitor patient closely.
Live virus vaccines: may potentiate replication and increase effects of virus vaccine.

EFFECTS ON DIAGNOSTIC TESTS
None reported.

CONTRAINDICATIONS
Contraindicated in pregnancy and lactation. Also contraindicated in patients with hypersensitivity to the drug or to any other product of murine (mouse) origin; who have anti-murine antibody titers equal to or greater than 1:1,000; who have fluid overload, as evidenced

---

*Liquid contains alcohol.   **May contain tartrazine.   †Canada only.   ‡Australia only.   ◊ OTC.

by chest X-ray or a weight gain greater than 3% within the week before treatment; or who have history of seizures or are predisposed to seizures.

NURSING CONSIDERATIONS
● Obtain chest X-ray within 24 hours before starting drug treatment, as ordered.
● Assess patients for signs of fluid overload before treatment.
● Keep in mind that treatment should begin in a facility that is equipped and staffed for cardiopulmonary resuscitation and where patients can be monitored closely.
● Be alert that most adverse reactions develop within ½ to 6 hours after the first dose.
● Administer an antipyretic, as ordered, before giving the drug to help lower incidence of expected pyrexia and chills. Corticosteroids may also be administered, as ordered, before first injection to help decrease the incidence of adverse reactions. Methylprednisolone sodium succinate (1 mg/kg) before injection, followed by hydrocortisone sodium succinate (100 mg) 30 minutes after injection, have been recommended to alleviate the severity of the first-dose reaction.
● Be aware that muromonab-CD3 is a monoclonal antibody preparation. Patients develop antibodies to this preparation that can lead to loss of effectiveness and more severe adverse reactions if a second course of therapy is attempted. Therefore, experts believe that this drug should be used for only a single course of treatment.
● **I.V. use:** Draw solution into a syringe through a low protein-binding 0.2- or 0.22-micron filter. Discard filter and attach needle for I.V. bolus injection.
● Do not add or infuse other drugs simultaneously through the same I.V. line. If the same I.V. line is used for sequential infusion of other drugs, flush with saline before and after infusion of muromonab-CD3.

☑ PATIENT TEACHING
● Inform patient of expected adverse reactions.
● Reassure him that reactions will be less severe as treatment progresses.
● Advise female patient to avoid pregnancy during drug therapy.

---

mycophenolate mofetil
CellCept

Pregnancy Risk Category: C

HOW SUPPLIED
Capsules: 250 mg

ACTION
Inhibits proliferative response of T- and B-lymphocytes, suppresses antibody formation by B-lymphocytes, and may inhibit recruitment of leukocytes into sites of inflammation and graft rejection.

ONSET, PEAK, DURATION
Onset and duration unknown. Peak levels occur in 30 to 75 minutes.

INDICATIONS & DOSAGE
Prophylaxis of organ rejection in patients receiving allogenic renal transplants—
Adults: 1 g P.O. b.i.d. within 72 hours after transplantation, together with corticosteroids and cyclosporine.

ADVERSE REACTIONS
CNS: *tremor,* insomnia, dizziness, *headache.*
CV: *chest pain, hypertension, edema.*
GI: *diarrhea, constipation, nausea, dyspepsia, vomiting, oral moniliasis, abdominal pain,* hemorrhage.
GU: *urinary tract infection, hematuria,* kidney tubular necrosis.
Hematologic: *anemia, leukopenia,* THROMBOCYTOPENIA, hypochromic anemia, leukocytosis.
Metabolic: *hypercholesteremia, hypophosphatemia, hypokalemia,* hyper-

kalemia, hyperglycemia.
Respiratory: *dyspnea, cough, infection,* pharyngitis, bronchitis, pneumonia.
Skin: *acne,* rash.
Other: *pain, fever, infection, sepsis, asthenia, back pain, peripheral edema.*

INTERACTIONS
Acyclovir, ganciclovir, and other drugs known to undergo renal tubular secretion: increased risk of toxicity for both drugs. Monitor patient closely.
Antacids with magnesium and aluminum hydroxides: decreased absorption of mycophenolate. Separate dosages.
Azathioprine: has not been clinically studied. Avoid concomitant use.
Cholestyramine: may interfere with enterohepatic recirculation, reducing mycophenolate bioavailability. Avoid concurrent use.
Oral contraceptives: may affect efficacy of oral contraceptives.

EFFECTS ON DIAGNOSTIC TESTS
None reported.

CONTRAINDICATIONS
Contraindicated in patients with hypersensitivity to the drug, mycophenolic acid, or any drug component.

NURSING CONSIDERATIONS
● Drug is not recommended for use in pregnant patients (unless benefits outweigh risks to fetus) or in breast-feeding women.
● Use cautiously in patients with gastrointestinal disorders.
● Safety of drug has not been established in children.
● Doses greater than 1 g b.i.d. should be avoided after immediate post-transplant period in patients with severe chronic renal impairment.
● Because of potential teratogenic effects, do not open or crush capsule. Avoid inhaling the powder in the capsule or having it contact skin or mucous membranes. If such contact occurs,

wash thoroughly with soap and water, and rinse eyes with plain water.
● Monitor CBC regularly, as ordered. If neutropenia develops, notify the doctor, who may interrupt therapy, reduce the dose, order diagnostic tests, or give additional treatment.

☑ PATIENT TEACHING
● Warn patient not to open or crush capsules but to swallow them whole, on an empty stomach.
● Stress the importance of not interrupting or stopping therapy without first consulting the doctor.
● Inform female patient that a pregnancy test is required 1 week before therapy begins.
● Instruct female patient to use contraception during therapy and for 6 weeks after discontinuation, even with a history of infertility, unless a hysterectomy has been performed. Tell her to use two methods of contraception simultaneously, unless abstinence is the chosen method, and to notify the doctor immediately of suspected pregnancy.

---

tacrolimus
Prograf

Pregnancy Risk Category: C

HOW SUPPLIED
Capsules: 1 mg, 5 mg
Injection: 5 mg/ml

ACTION
Precise mechanism unknown. Inhibits T-lymphocyte activation, which results in immunosuppression.

ONSET, PEAK, DURATION
Onset and duration unknown. Serum levels peak in 1.5 to 3.5 hours.

INDICATIONS & DOSAGE
Prophylaxis of organ rejection in allogenic liver transplantation—
Adults: 0.05 to 0.1 mg/kg/day I.V. as a

continuous infusion administered no sooner than 6 hours after transplantation. Oral therapy should be substituted as soon as possible, with the first oral dose given 8 to 12 hours after discontinuing the I.V. infusion. The recommended initial oral dosage is 0.15 to 0.3 mg/kg/day P.O. in two divided doses q 12 hours. Dosage should be titrated according to clinical response.

Children: initially, 0.1 mg/kg/day I.V., followed by 0.3 mg/kg/day P.O. on a schedule similar to that for adults, adjusted as needed.

ADVERSE REACTIONS

CNS: *headache, tremor, insomnia, paresthesia.*
CV: *hypertension, peripheral edema.*
GI: *diarrhea, nausea, constipation, abnormal liver function test, anorexia, vomiting, abdominal pain.*
GU: *abnormal renal function, increased creatinine or BUN levels, urinary tract infection, oliguria.*
Hematologic: *anemia, leukocytosis,* **thrombocytopenia**
Metabolic: *hyperkalemia, hypokalemia, hyperglycemia, hypomagnesemia.*
Respiratory: *pleural effusion, atelectasis, dyspnea.*
Skin: *pruritus, rash.*
Other: *pain, fever, asthenia, back pain, ascites,* **anaphylaxis.**

INTERACTIONS

Bromocriptine, cimetidine, clarithromycin, clotrimazole, cyclosporine, danazol, diltiazem, erythromycin, fluconazole, itraconazole, ketoconazole, methylprednisolone, metoclopramide, nicardipine, verapamil: may increase tacrolimus levels. Monitor for adverse effects.
Carbamazepine, phenobarbital, phenytoin, rifabutin, rifampin: may decrease tacrolimus levels. Monitor effectiveness of tacrolimus.
Cyclosporine: increased risk of excess nephrotoxicity. Do not administer together.

Immunosuppressants (except adrenal corticosteroids): may oversuppress the immune system. Monitor patient closely, especially during times of stress.
Inducers of cytochrome P-450 enzyme system: may increase tacrolimus metabolism and decrease plasma levels. Dosage adjustment may be needed.
Inhibitors of cytochrome P-450 enzyme system: may decrease tacrolimus metabolism and increase plasma levels. Dosage adjustment may be needed.
Nephrotoxic drugs, such as aminoglycosides, amphotericin B, cisplatin, cyclosporine: may cause additive or synergistic effects. Monitor closely.
Viral vaccines: tacrolimus may interfere with the immune response to live virus vaccines. Defer routine immunizations.

EFFECTS ON DIAGNOSTIC TESTS
None reported.

CONTRAINDICATIONS
Contraindicated in patients with hypersensitivity to the drug. The I.V. form is contraindicated in those who are hypersensitive to castor oil derivatives.

NURSING CONSIDERATIONS
Alert: Know that because of the risk of anaphylaxis, injection should be used only in patients who cannot take the oral form.
● Keep epinephrine 1:1,000 available to treat anaphylaxis.
● Be aware that children with normal renal and hepatic function may require higher dosages than adults.
● Also be aware that patients with hepatic or renal dysfunction should receive the lowest dosage possible.
● Expect to administer adrenal corticosteroids concomitantly with this drug.
● **I.V. use:** Dilute drug with 0.9% sodium chloride for injection or 5% dextrose injection to a concentration between 0.004 mg/ml and 0.02 mg/ml prior to use. Diluted infusion solution should be stored for no more than 24 hours in glass or polyethylene contain-

ers. The drug should not be stored in a polyvinyl chloride container because of decreased stability and the potential for extraction of phthalates.

• Monitor the patient continuously during the first 30 minutes of I.V. administration and frequently thereafter for signs and symptoms of anaphylaxis.

• Monitor the patient for signs of neurotoxicity and nephrotoxicity, especially in a patient receiving a high dosage or having renal dysfunction.

• Monitor the patient for signs and symptoms of hyperkalemia, and obtain serum potassium levels regularly, as ordered. Know that potassium-sparing diuretics should be avoided during tacrolimus therapy.

• Monitor the patient's blood glucose level regularly, as ordered, and the patient for signs and symptoms of hyperglycemia. Be aware that treatment of hyperglycemia may be necessary.

• Be aware that patients receiving this drug are at increased risk for infections, lymphomas, and other malignant diseases.

• Know that other immunosuppressants (except for adrenal corticosteroids) should not be used during tacrolimus therapy.

☑ **PATIENT TEACHING**
• Instruct the patient to check with the doctor before taking any other medication during tacrolimus therapy.
• Tell the patient to report adverse reactions promptly.

Vaccines and toxoids

BCG vaccine
cholera vaccine
diphtheria and tetanus toxoids,
 adsorbed
diphtheria and tetanus toxoids
 and pertussis vaccine
diphtheria and tetanus toxoids
 and acellular pertussis
 vaccine
Haemophilus b conjugate
 vaccines
hepatitis A vaccine, inactivated
hepatitis B vaccine, recombinant
influenza virus vaccine, 1995-
 1996 trivalent types A & B
 (purified surface antigen)
influenza virus vaccine, 1995-
 1996 trivalent types A & B
 (split or purified split virus)
influenza virus vaccine, 1995-
 1996 trivalent types A & B
 (whole virion)
Japanese encephalitis virus
 vaccine, inactivated
measles, mumps, and rubella
 virus vaccine, live
measles and rubella virus
 vaccine, live attenuated
measles virus vaccine, live
 attenuated
meningococcal polysaccharide
 vaccine
mumps virus vaccine, live
plague vaccine
pneumococcal vaccine, polyvalent
poliovirus vaccine, live, oral,
 trivalent
poliovirus vaccine, inactivated
rabies vaccine, adsorbed
rabies vaccine, human diploid
 cell
rubella and mumps virus
 vaccine, live
rubella virus vaccine, live attenuated

tetanus toxoid, adsorbed
tetanus toxoid, fluid
typhoid vaccine
typhoid vaccine, oral
typhoid Vi polysaccharide
 vaccine
varicella virus vaccine
yellow fever vaccine

COMBINATION PRODUCTS
AcTHIB/DTP: 10 mcg *Haemophilus* b
PRP conjugated to 24 mcg tetanus toxoid, 6.7 Lf (limit flocculation) units
diphtheria toxoid, 5 Lf units tetanus toxoid, and 4 units whole-cell pertussis
vaccine/0.5 ml.
COMVAX: 7.5 mcg *Haemophilus* b PRP,
125 mcg *Neisseria meningitidis* OMPC,
and 5 mcg hepatitis B surface antigen/
0.5 ml.
TETRAMUNE: 10 mcg purified
Haemophilus b saccharide and approximately 25 mcg CRM$_{197}$ protein, 12.5 Lf
units inactivated diphtheria, 5 Lf units
inactivated tetanus, and 4 protective
units pertussis/0.5 ml.

BCG vaccine
TICE BCG

Pregnancy Risk Category: C

HOW SUPPLIED
Percutaneous vaccine: 1 to 8×10^8
CFU/vial (Tice strain)

ACTION
A live, attenuated bacterial vaccine prepared from *Mycobacterium bovis* that
promotes active immunity to tuberculosis (TB).

ONSET, PEAK, DURATION
Unknown.

Reactions may be *common*, uncommon, *life-threatening*, or COMMON AND LIFE-THREATENING.

INDICATIONS & DOSAGE
TB exposure—
Adults and children 1 month and over: 0.2 to 0.3 ml (percutaneous vaccine) applied to cleaned skin followed by application of multiple-puncture disk.
Infants less than 1 month: dosage reduced by one-half by using 2 ml of sterile water without preservatives when reconstituting.

ADVERSE REACTIONS
Systemic: osteomyelitis, lymphadenopathy, allergic reaction, *anaphylaxis.*

INTERACTIONS
Immunosuppressants: may reduce response to BCG vaccine. Avoid if possible.
Isoniazid, rifampin, streptomycin: inhibited multiplication of BCG. Avoid using together.

EFFECTS ON DIAGNOSTIC TESTS
Tuberculin sensitivity may be rendered positive by BCG intravesical treatment. Determine patient's reactivity to tuberculin before initiating therapy.

CONTRAINDICATIONS
Contraindicated in patients with hypogammaglobulinemia, in the presence of a positive tuberculin reaction (when meant for use as immunoprophylactic after exposure to TB) in immunosuppressed patients, in those with fresh smallpox vaccinations, in those who have suffered burns, and in patients receiving corticosteroid therapy. Patients should avoid this vaccine during pregnancy.

NURSING CONSIDERATIONS
● Use cautiously in patients with chronic skin disease. Inject in area of healthy skin only.
● Obtain history of allergies and reaction to immunization.
● Keep epinephrine 1:1,000 available to treat anaphylaxis.

● Do not shake vial after reconstitution. Use within 2 hours.
● Keep in mind that recommended injection site is over the insertion point of deltoid muscle.
● Don't administer to febrile children.
● Know that expected lesion forms in 7 to 14 days. Papules reach a maximum diameter of 3 mm, then fade.
● Allow at least 6 to 8 weeks between BCG and live virus vaccines; administer killed virus vaccines 7 days before or 10 days after BCG, as ordered.
● Know that vaccine is of no value as immunoprophylactic in patients with positive tuberculin test.
● Destroy live vaccine by autoclaving or treating with formaldehyde solution before disposal.

☑ **PATIENT TEACHING**
● Advise patient to have tuberculin skin test 2 to 3 months after BCG vaccination.
● Tell patient to report unusual signs and symptoms after vaccination.

---

cholera vaccine

Pregnancy Risk Category: C

HOW SUPPLIED
Injection: suspension of killed *Vibrio cholerae* (each milliliter contains 8 units of Inaba and Ogawa serotypes) in 1.5-ml and 20-ml vials

ACTION
Promotes active immunity to cholera.

ONSET, PEAK, DURATION
Although onset and peak are not precisely known, most patients develop immunity after second dose. Effects persist for 3 to 6 months.

INDICATIONS & DOSAGE
Primary immunization for persons traveling to areas where cholera is endemic or epidemic—

Adults and children over 10 years: two doses of 0.5 ml I.M. or S.C., 1 week to 1 month apart, before traveling in cholera area. Booster is 0.5 ml q 6 months as needed.

Children 6 months to 4 years: 0.2 ml I.M. or S.C. Boosters of same dose should be given q 6 months as needed.

Children 5 to 10 years: 0.3 ml I.M. or S.C. Boosters of same dose should be given q 6 months as needed.

ADVERSE REACTIONS
Systemic: malaise, fever, headache.
Other: *erythema, swelling, pain, induration at injection site, **anaphylaxis**.*

INTERACTIONS
Plague, typhoid, or other vaccines with systemic adverse reactions: enhanced toxicity. Don't use together.
Yellow fever vaccine: simultaneous administration may interfere with immune response to both vaccines. Administer 3 weeks apart.

EFFECTS ON DIAGNOSTIC TESTS
None reported.

CONTRAINDICATIONS
Contraindicated in those with acute illness or a history of severe systemic reaction or allergic response to vaccine.

NURSING CONSIDERATIONS
● Obtain history of allergies and reaction to immunization.
● Keep epinephrine 1:1,000 available to treat anaphylaxis.
● Shake vial vigorously before withdrawing each dose.
● Do not administer I.M. to persons with thrombocytopenia or any coagulation disorder that would contraindicate I.M. injection.
● Administer I.M. in deltoid muscle in adults and children over 3 years.
● Keep in mind that I.M. and S.C. routes give higher levels of protection. May be given intradermally (preferably into the inner surface of the forearm) to

adults and children over 5 years, but the volume of injection is limited to 0.2 ml.
● Know that vaccine is about 50% effective in reducing clinical illness incidence for 3 to 6 months.

☑ **PATIENT TEACHING**
● Advise patients that pain, induration, and swelling are common at the injection site for 24 to 48 hours.
● Tell travelers to avoid food and water that may be contaminated.

---

diphtheria and tetanus toxoids, adsorbed

Pregnancy Risk Category: C

HOW SUPPLIED
Available in pediatric (DT) and adult (Td) strengths
Injection (for pediatric use): diphtheria toxoid 6.6 Lf (limit flocculation) units and tetanus toxoid 5 Lf units per 0.5 ml; diphtheria toxoid 7.5 Lf units and tetanus toxoid 7.5 Lf units per 0.5 ml; diphtheria toxoid 10 Lf units and tetanus toxoid 5 Lf units per 0.5 ml; diphtheria toxoid 12.5 Lf units and tetanus toxoid 5 Lf units per 0.5 ml.
Injection (for adult use): diphtheria toxoid 2 Lf units and tetanus toxoid 2 Lf units per 0.5 ml; diphtheria toxoid 2 Lf units and tetanus toxoid 5 Lf units per 0.5 ml.

ACTION
Promotes immunity to diphtheria and tetanus by inducing production of antitoxins.

ONSET, PEAK, DURATION
Onset and peak unknown. Effects persist for 10 years.

INDICATIONS & DOSAGE
Primary immunization—
Adults and children 7 years or over: adult strength; 0.5 ml I.M. 4 to 8 weeks apart for two doses and a third dose 6 to

12 months after the second dose. Booster is 0.5 ml I.M. q 10 years.
Infants 6 weeks to 1 year: pediatric strength; 0.5 ml I.M. at least 4 weeks apart for three doses. Give booster dose 6 to 12 months after third injection.
Children 1 to 6 years: use pediatric strength; 0.5 ml I.M. at least 4 weeks apart for two doses. Give booster dosage 6 to 12 months after the second injection. If the final immunizing dose is given after the seventh birthday, use the adult strength.

ADVERSE REACTIONS
Systemic: *anaphylaxis,* chills, fever, malaise, headache, tachycardia, hypotension.
Other: *pain, stinging, edema, erythema, induration at injection site,* flushing, urticaria, pruritus.

INTERACTIONS
None significant.

EFFECTS ON DIAGNOSTIC TESTS
None reported.

CONTRAINDICATIONS
Contraindicated in immunosuppressed patients and in those receiving radiation or corticosteroid therapy. Vaccination should be deferred in patients with respiratory illness and during polio outbreaks; also deferred in those with acute illness except during emergency. When polio is a risk, single antigen is used. Know that in children under 6 years, use only when diphtheria, tetanus, and pertussis combination is contraindicated because of pertussis component.

NURSING CONSIDERATIONS
● Obtain history of allergies and reaction to immunization.
● Before injection, verify strength (pediatric or adult) of toxoid used.
● Keep epinephrine 1:1,000 available to treat anaphylaxis.
● Give in site not recently used for vaccines or toxoids.

● Know that drug is not used to treat an acute diphtheria infection.

☑ PATIENT TEACHING
● Advise patient that local reactions such as pain and pruritus are common at the injection site.
● Review primary immunization schedule with patient or parents, and stress importance of compliance with subsequent injections.

---

diphtheria and tetanus toxoids and whole-cell pertussis vaccine (DTP, DPT)
DTwP, Tri-Immunol

diphtheria and tetanus toxoids and acellular pertussis vaccine
Acel-Imune, DTaP, Tripedia

Pergnancy Risk Category C

HOW SUPPLIED
whole-cell vaccine
Injection: 6.5 Lf (limit flocculation) units inactivated diphtheria, 5 Lf units inactivated tetanus, and 4 protective units pertussis per 0.5 ml, in 2.5, 5, and 7.5-ml vials; 10 Lf units inactivated diphtheria, 5.5 Lf units inactivated tetanus, and 4 protective units pertussis per 0.5 ml in 5= ml vials (DTwP); 12.5 Lf units inactivated diphtheria, 5 Lf units inactivated tetanus, and 4 protective units pertussis per 0.5 ml, in 7.5-ml vials (Tri-Immunol)
acellular vaccine
Injection: 5 Lf units inactivated diphtheria, 5 Lf units inactivated tetanus, and 300 hemagglutinating units of acellular pertussis vaccine per 0.5 ml; 66.7 Lf units inactivated diphtheria, 5 Lf units inactivated tetanus, and 46.8 pertussis antigens per 0.5 ml

ACTION
Promotes active immunity to diphtheria, tetanus, and pertussis (DTP) by induc-

ing production of antitoxins and antibodies.

ONSET, PEAK, DURATION
Most patients develop immunity about 2 weeks after the final dose. Effects persist for 4 to 6 years.

INDICATIONS & DOSAGE
Primary immunization—
Children 6 weeks to 6 years: 0.5 ml I.M. 4 to 8 weeks apart for three doses and a fourth dose 1 year later. Booster is 0.5 ml I.M. when starting school unless 4th dose in series was administered after child's fourth birthday; then, a booster is not necessary at time of school entrance.

Not advised for adults or children over 6 years.

Products containing acellular pertussis vaccine may now be used for any dose in DTP immunization.

ADVERSE REACTIONS
Systemic: *seizures, encephalopathy, anaphylaxis, shock,* peripheral neuropathy, thrombocytopenic purpura.
Other: *soreness, redness,* expected nodule remaining several weeks at injection site, *fever,* hypersensitivity reactions, urticaria.

INTERACTIONS
Immunosuppressants: may reduce response to DTP vaccine. Avoid if possible.

EFFECTS ON DIAGNOSTIC TESTS
None reported.

CONTRAINDICATIONS
Contraindicated in patients who developed an immediate anaphylactic reaction or encephalopathy within 7 days of a DTP dose, in immunosuppressed patients, in those on corticosteroid therapy, and in those with an evolving neurologic condition. Vaccination should be deferred in patients with acute febrile illness of unknown etiology. Children

with preexisting neurologic disorders should not receive pertussis component. Also, children who exhibit neurologic signs after DTP injection shouldn't receive pertussis component in any succeeding injections. Diphtheria and tetanus toxoids (called DT) should be given instead.

NURSING CONSIDERATIONS
● Obtain history of allergies and reaction to immunization.
● Keep epinephrine 1:1,000 available to treat anaphylaxis.
● Shake before using. Refrigerate.
● Administer only by deep I.M. injection, preferably in thigh or deltoid muscle. Don't give S.C.
● Keep in mind that DTP injection may be given at same time as trivalent oral polio vaccine.
● Know that acellular vaccine may be associated with a lower incidence of local pain and fever.
● Know that vaccine is not used for active infection.

☑ PATIENT TEACHING
● Make sure parents know the risks and benefits of this vaccine before it is administered.
● Tell parents to report systemic reactions promptly; remind them that local reactions are common.

Haemophilus **b conjugate vaccines**

Haemophilus **b conjugate vaccine, diphtheria CRM$_{197}$ protein conjugate (HbOC)**
HibTITER

Haemophilus **b conjugate vaccine, diphtheria toxoid conjugate (PRP-D)**
ProHIBiT

Haemophilus b conjugate vaccine, meningococcal protein conjugate (PRP-OMP)
PedvaxHIB

Pregnancy Risk Category: C

HOW SUPPLIED
Haemophilus b conjugate vaccine, diphtheria CRM_{197} protein conjugate
Injection: 10 mcg of purified *Haemophilus* b saccharide and approximately 25 mcg CRM_{197} protein per 0.5 ml
Haemophilus b conjugate vaccine, diphtheria toxoid conjugate
Injection: 25 mcg of *Haemophilus influenzae* type B (HIB) capsular polysaccharide and 18 mcg of diphtheria toxoid protein per 0.5 ml
Haemophilus b conjugate vaccine, meningococcal protein conjugate
Powder for injection: 15 mcg of *Haemophilus* b PRP, 250 mcg *Neisseria meningitidis* OMPC per dose
Injection: 7.5 mcg of *Haemophilus* bPRP and 125 mcg *Neisseria meningitidis* OMPC per 0.5 ml

ACTION
Promotes active immunity to HIB; is a polymer of ribose, ribitol, and phosphate (PRP) and is covalently linked to highly antigenic substances, enabling the vaccine to promote an immune response in infants.

ONSET, PEAK, DURATION
Most patients develop immunity about 2 weeks after final dose. Effects persist for several years.

INDICATIONS & DOSAGE
Immunization against HIB infection—conjugate vaccine, diphtheria CRM_{197} protein conjugate
Infants: 0.5 ml I.M. at age 2 months. Repeated at 4 months and 6 months. A= booster dose is required at age 15 months.
Previously unvaccinated infants 2 to 6 months: 0.5 ml I.M. Repeated in 2 months and again in 4 months for a total of three doses. Booster dose given at age 15 months.
Previously unvaccinated infants 7 to 11 months: 0.5 ml I.M. Repeated in 2 months, for a total of two doses. Booster dose given at age 15 months (but no sooner than 2 months after the last vaccination).
Previously unvaccinated infants 12 to 14 months: 0.5 ml I.M. Booster dose given at age 15 months (but no sooner than 2 months after the first vaccination).
Previously unvaccinated children 15 months to 5 years: 0.5 ml I.M. A booster dose is not required.
Conjugate vaccine, diphtheria toxoid conjugate
Previously unvaccinated children 15 months to 5 years: 0.5 ml I.M. A booster dose is not required. Not recommended for use in children under age 15 months.
Conjugate vaccine, meningococcal protein conjugate
Infants: 0.5 ml I.M. at age 2 months. Repeated at 4 months. Booster dose is required at age 12 months.
Previously unvaccinated infants 2 to 6 months: 0.5 ml I.M. Repeated in 2 months. Booster dose given at age 12 months.
Previously unvaccinated infants 7 to 11 months: 0.5 ml I.M. Repeated in 2 months. Booster dose given at 15 months (but no sooner than 2 months after the last vaccination).
Previously unvaccinated infants 12 to 14 months: 0.5 ml I.M. Booster dose given at age 15 months (but no sooner than 2 months after the first vaccination).
Previously unvaccinated children 15 months to 5 years: 0.5 ml I.M. A booster dose is not required.

ADVERSE REACTIONS
Systemic: *anaphylaxis,* fever.
Other: *erythema, pain at injection site,*

---

*Liquid contains alcohol.   **May contain tartrazine.   †Canada only.   ‡Australia only.   ◇OTC.

diarrhea, vomiting, crying.

INTERACTIONS
Immunosuppressants: may suppress antibody response to HIB vaccine. Know that immunization may need to be deferred.

EFFECTS ON DIAGNOSTIC TESTS
None reported.

CONTRAINDICATIONS
Contraindicated in patients with acute illness.

NURSING CONSIDERATIONS
● Keep epinephrine 1:1,000 available in case of anaphylaxis.
● Don't administer intradermally or I.V. Must administer I.M.
● Administer into anterolateral aspect of the upper thigh in small children. Injections may be made into the deltoid muscle of larger children if sufficient muscle mass is present.
● Know that vaccine is not routinely given to adults or children over 5 years unless they are at high risk for infection (including patients with chronic conditions such as functional asplenia, splenectomy, Hodgkin's disease, or sickle cell anemia).
Alert: Don't administer to febrile children.
● Know that immunization against HIB infection is recommended for children with HIV infections. The usual immunization schedule should be followed in these children.
● This vaccine and DTP may be given simultaneously. A combination product is commercially available.
● Know that diphtheria toxoid conjugate vaccine (ProHIBiT) is not recommended in children under 15 months.
● HIB is an important cause of meningitis in infants and preschool children.
● Keep in mind that this vaccine protects against HIB only and will not protect children against any other microorganisms that cause meningitis.

☑ PATIENT TEACHING
● Warn patient or parents that pain may occur at injection site.
● Tell patient or parents to notify doctor if adverse reactions persist or become severe.

---

hepatitis A vaccine, inactivated
Havrix, Vaqta

Pregnancy Risk Category: C

HOW SUPPLIED
Havrix
Injection: 360 ELISA units (EL.U.)/0.5 ml, 720 EL.U./0.5 ml; 1,440 EL.U./ml
Vaqta
Injection: 25 units/0.5 ml, 50 units/ml

ACTION
Promotes active immunity to hepatitis A virus.

ONSET, PEAK, DURATION
In clinical studies, 80% to 98% of adults vaccinated were seroconverted by day 15 and 96% were seroconverted in 1 month. When a booster was given 6 months after the first dose, 100% of patients were seropositive 1 month later. In clinical studies of children receiving the drug, 99% of those vaccinated were seroconverted following two doses. When a booster (third) dose was administered 6 months after the first dose, 100% of the children were seropositive 1 month later. Effects persist for at least 6 months. Duration beyond 6 months has not been established.

INDICATIONS & DOSAGE
Active immunization against hepatitis A virus—
Adults: 1,440 EL.U. (Havrix) or 50 units (Vaqta) I.M. as a single dose. For booster dose, 1,440 EL.U. (Havrix) or 50 units (Vaqta) I.M. given 6 months after initial dose. A booster dose is recommended if prolonged immunity is de-

sired.

Children 2 to 18 years: 720 EL.U. (Havrix) or 25 units (Vaqta) I.M. as a single dose, followed by a booster dose of 720 EL.U. (Havrix) or 25 units (Vaqta) I.M. given 6 to 12 months after initial dose. Booster dose is recommended if prolonged immunity is desired.

ADVERSE REACTIONS
CNS: episode of hypertonia, insomnia, photophobia, vertigo, *headache.*
GI: *anorexia, nausea,* abdominal pain, diarrhea, dysgeusia, vomiting.
Musculoskeletal: arthralgia, elevation of creatine phosphokinase level, myalgia.
Respiratory: pharyngitis, other upper respiratory tract infections.
Skin: pruritus, rash, urticaria, *induration, redness, swelling,* hematoma, *injection site soreness.*
Other: *fatigue, fever, malaise,* lymphadenopathy, ***anaphylaxis.***

INTERACTIONS
None significant.

EFFECTS ON DIAGNOSTIC TESTS
None reported.

CONTRAINDICATIONS
Contraindicated in patients with hypersensitivity to any component of the vaccine.

NURSING CONSIDERATIONS
● Use with caution in patients with thrombocytopenia or bleeding disorders and in those who are taking an anticoagulant because bleeding may occur following an I.M. injection.
● As with any vaccine, administration of hepatitis A vaccine should be delayed, if possible, in patients with any febrile illness.
● Keep epinephrine available to treat an anaphylactoid reaction.
● Be aware that if vaccine is administered to immunosuppressed persons or persons receiving immunosuppressants,

the expected immune response may not be obtained.
● Know that persons who should receive the vaccine include people traveling to or living in areas of higher endemicity for hepatitis A (Africa, Asia [except Japan] the Mediterranean basin, Eastern Europe, the Middle East, Central and South America, Mexico, and parts of the Caribbean), military personnel, native peoples of Alaska and the Americas, persons engaging in high-risk sexual activity, and users of illegal injectable drugs. Certain institutional workers, employees of child day-care centers, laboratory workers who handle live hepatitis A virus, and handlers of primate animals also may benefit.
● **I.M. use:** Shake vial or syringe well before withdrawal and use. After it has been agitated thoroughly, the vaccine is an opaque white suspension. Discard if it appears otherwise. No dilution or reconstitution is necessary.
● Administer as an I.M. injection into the deltoid region in adults. It should not be administered in the gluteal region; such injections may result in suboptimal response. Never inject I.V., S.C., or intradermally.
● Be aware that hepatitis A vaccine will not prevent infection in persons who have an unrecognized hepatitis A infection at the time of vaccination.

☑ **PATIENT TEACHING**
● Inform the patient that the vaccine will not prevent hepatitis caused by other agents or pathogens known to infect the liver.
● Warn the patient about local adverse reactions. Tell patient to report persistent or severe reactions promptly.

hepatitis B vaccine, recombinant
Engerix-B, Recombivax HB

Pregnancy Risk Category: C

HOW SUPPLIED

Injection: 2.5 mcg hepatitis B surface antigen (HBs)Ag/0.5ml (Recombivax HB, pediatric formulation); 5 mcg HBsAg/0.5 ml (Recombivax HB, adolescent/high-risk infant formulation); 10 mcg HBsAg/0.5 ml (Engerix-B, adolescent/pediatric formulation); 10 mcg HBsAg/ml (Recombivax HB, adult formulation); 20 mcg HBsAg/ml (Engerix-B, adult formulation); 40 mcg HBsAg/ml (Recombivax HB dialysis formulation)

ACTION

Promotes active immunity to hepatitis B.

ONSET, PEAK, DURATION

Most patients develop immunity about 2 weeks after final dose. Effects persist for many years. Booster doses are currently not recommended for this vaccine.

INDICATIONS & DOSAGE

Immunization against infection from all known subtypes of hepatitis B virus (HBV); primary preexposure prophylaxis against HBV; or postexposure prophylaxis (when given with hepatitis B immune globulin)—
Engerix-B
Adults: initially, 20 mcg (1-ml adult formulation) is given I.M., followed by a second dose of 20 mcg I.M. 30 days later. A third dose of 20 mcg I.M. is given 30 days after second dose. A fourth dose is given 12 months after the initial dose.

Adults undergoing dialysis or receiving immunosuppressants: initially, 40 mcg I.M. (divided into two 20-mcg doses and administered at different sites). Followed with a second dose of 40 mcg I.M. in 30 days, and a final dose of 40 mcg I.M. 6 months after the initial dose.

Note: Certain populations (neonates born to infected mothers, persons recently exposed to the virus, and travelers to high-risk areas) may receive the vaccine on an abbreviated schedule, with the initial dose followed by a second dose in 1 month, and the third dose after 2 months. For prolonged maintenance of protective antibody titers, a booster dose is recommended 12 months after the initial dose.

Adolescents 11 to 20 years of age: initially, 10 mcg (0.5-ml adolescent/pediatric formulation) I.M., followed by a second dose of 10 mcg I.M. 30 days later. A third dose of 10 mcg I.M. is given 6 months after the initial dose. Alternatively, 20 mcg (1-ml adult formulation) is given I.M., followed by a second dose of 20 mcg I.M. 30 days later. A third dose of 20 mcg I.M. is given 6 months after the initial dose.

Neonates and children up to 11 years: initially, 10 mcg (0.5-ml pediatric formulation) I.M., followed by a second dose of 10 mcg I.M. 30 days later. A third dose of 10 mcg I.M. is given 6 months after the initial dose.
Recombivax HB
Adults: initially, 10 mcg (1-ml adult formulation) I.M., followed by a second dose of 10 mcg I.M. 30 days later. A third dose of 10 mcg is given I.M. 6 months after the initial dose.

Adults undergoing dialysis: initially, 40 mcg I.M. (use dialysis formulation, which contains 40 mcg/ml). Followed with a second dose of 40 mcg I.M. in 30 days, and a final dose of 40 mcg I.M. 6 months after the initial dose.

Children 11 to 20 years: initially, 5 mcg (0.5-ml adolescent/high-risk infant formulation) I.M., followed by a second dose of 5 mcg I.M. 30 days later. A third dose of 5 mcg is given I.M. 6 months after the initial dose.

Children 1 to 11 years: initially, 2.5 mcg (0.5-ml pediatric formulation) I.M., followed by a second dose of 2.5 mcg I.M. 30 days later. A third dose of 2.5 mcg I.M. is given 6 months after the initial dose.

Infants born of HBsAg-negative mothers: initially, 2.5 mcg (0.5 ml pediatric formulation) I.M., followed by a second dose of 0.5 mcg 30 days later. A third dose of 0.5 mcg is given I.M. 6 months after the initial dose.

Infants born of HBsAg-positive mothers: initially, 5 mcg (0.5-ml adolescent/high-risk infant formulation) I.M., followed by a second dose of 5 mcg I.M. 30 days later. A third dose of 5 mcg is given I.M. 6 months after the initial dose.

ADVERSE REACTIONS
Systemic: *anaphylaxis,* headache, dizziness, nausea, insomnia, paresthesia, neuropathy, pharyngitis, anorexia, diarrhea, arthralgia, vomiting, slight fever, transient malaise, flulike symptoms, myalgia.
Other: local inflammation at injection site, *injection site soreness.*

INTERACTIONS
Immunosuppressants: may require larger than usual doses of hepatitis B vaccine (recombinant).

EFFECTS ON DIAGNOSTIC TESTS
None reported.

CONTRAINDICATIONS
Contraindicated in patients hypersensitive to yeast; recombinant vaccines are derived from yeast cultures.

NURSING CONSIDERATIONS
● Use cautiously in patients with serious, active infections or compromised cardiac or pulmonary status and in those for whom a febrile or systemic reaction could pose a risk.
● Know that the American Academy of Pediatrics recommends hepatitis B vaccination for all neonates and encourages immunization for adolescents when resources allow.
● Although anaphylaxis has not been reported, always keep epinephrine available when giving this vaccine to counteract possible reaction.
● Thoroughly agitate vial just before administration to restore suspension.

● Give adults and adolescents the vaccine in the deltoid muscle; give infants and young children the vaccine in the anterolateral aspect of the thigh. Never administer I.V.
● Administer S.C. in persons at risk for hemorrhage, such as hemophiliacs. Otherwise, do not use this route; it may lead to an increased incidence or severity of local reactions.
● Keep in mind that certain health care personnel (especially those working with dialysis patients, in blood banks, in emergency medicine, with selected patients and patient contacts, or among populations in which the infection is endemic [Indo-Chinese, native peoples of Alaska, and Haitian refugees]; certain military personnel, morticians and embalmers, sexually active homosexual men, prostitutes, prisoners, and users of illegal injectable drugs are at increased risk for infection and should be considered for the vaccine.
● Be aware that recombinant hepatitis B vaccine is not made with any human plasma products.
● Refrigerate both opened and unopened vials. Don't freeze.

☑ **PATIENT TEACHING**
● Warn patient or parents about local adverse reactions. Tell patient to report persistent or severe reactions promptly.
● Review immunization schedule with patient or parents, and stress importance of completing series.

influenza virus vaccine, 1995-1996 trivalent types A & B (purified surface antigen)
Fluvirin

influenza virus vaccine, 1995-1996 trivalent types A & B (split or purified split virus)
Fluogen, Flu-Shield, Fluzone

influenza virus vaccine, 1995-1996 trivalent types A & B (whole virion)
Fluzone (Whole)

Pregnancy Risk Category: C

HOW SUPPLIED
Injection: 15 mcg A/Texas/36/91-like (H1N1), 15 mcg A/Johannesburg/33/94-like (H3N2), and 15 mcg B/Beijing/184/93-like hemagglutinin antigens per 0.5 ml

ACTION
Promotes immunity to influenza by inducing production of antibodies.

ONSET, PEAK, DURATION
Although onset and peak not precisely known, most patients develop immunity in 2 to 4 weeks. Immunity declines following vaccination, possibly within 6 months.

INDICATIONS & DOSAGE
Influenza prophylaxis—
Adults and children 12 years and over: 0.5 ml whole virus, split virus, or purified split virus I.M. Only one dose is required.
Children 9 to 12 years: 0.5 ml split virus or purified split virus I.M. Only one dose is required.
Children 3 to 9 years: 0.5 ml split virus or purified split virus I.M. Repeated in 4 weeks unless child has been previously vaccinated.
Children 6 to 36 months: 0.25 ml split virus or purified split virus I.M. Repeated in 4 weeks unless child has been previously vaccinated.

ADVERSE REACTIONS
Systemic: *anaphylaxis,* fever, malaise, myalgia.
Other: erythema, induration, and *soreness at injection site.*
  Fever and malaise reactions occur most often in children and in others not

exposed to influenza viruses. Severe reactions in adults are rare.

INTERACTIONS
Immunosuppressants: may reduce the immune response to this vaccine.
Theophylline, warfarin: clearance may be impaired.

EFFECTS ON DIAGNOSTIC TESTS
No information available.

CONTRAINDICATIONS
Contraindicated in patients with hypersensitivity to eggs. Vaccination should be deferred in patients with acute respiratory or other active infection.

NURSING CONSIDERATIONS
● Use cautiously in patients with a history of sulfite allergy.
● Obtain history of allergies, especially to eggs, and reaction to immunization.
● Keep epinephrine 1:1,000 available to treat anaphylaxis.
● Note that the combination of antigens used to create influenza vaccine changes annually even though some antigens may be the same as previous years. Do not use leftover supplies to immunize patients for the current flu season.
● Thoroughly agitate vial just before administration to restore suspension.
● Give injections for adults and older children in deltoid muscle; for infants and children under 3 years, give in anterolateral aspect of thigh.
● Ideally, vaccinations should be performed in November because outbreaks of influenza generally don't occur until December. The vaccine should not be given too early in the season because antibody titers may begin to decline before the flu season.
● Know that children 12 years and under should be given their second dose in December, if possible.
● Vaccines may be given to both children and adults throughout the flu season, even as late as April.
● The American Academy of Pediatrics

Reactions may be *common,* uncommon, *life-threatening,* or COMMON AND LIFE-THREATENING.

recommends that influenza vaccine can be administered simultaneously (but at a different site and with a different syringe) with other routine vaccinations in children.

● Know that this vaccine is considered safe in pregnant patients. Vaccination shouldn't be postponed, regardless of the stage of pregnancy, in patients who have high-risk conditions and who will be in the first trimester of pregnancy when flu season begins.

● Keep in mind that immunodeficient patients may receive two doses 1 month apart; however, there is little evidence that booster doses improve the immunogenic response to the vaccine. Know that chemoprophylaxis with amantadine may be helpful.

● Know that vaccine is strongly recommended for anyone over 6 months; for patients with chronic disease, metabolic disorders, or medical conditions that put them at risk for complications from influenza; for health care workers, especially doctors, nurses, employees of nursing homes, volunteer workers, and other personnel in both hospital and outpatient settings; and for household members who may contact persons at high risk for medical complications of influenza. Also recommended for anyone who wishes to reduce the chance of infection.

● Keep in mind that allergic reactions, which usually occur immediately, are extremely rare.

● Be alert that paralysis ssociated with Guillain-BarrÉe syndrome is rare, and has only been associated with the 1976 vaccine.

● Remember that although there is little information regarding influenza in persons with HIV, it is recommended that these patients receive the vaccine. Patients with advanced disease may exhibit a low response; there is no evidence that a booster dose will improve the immune response.

☑ **PATIENT TEACHING**
● Advise patient about the risks of vaccination as compared with risk of influenza and its complications.

● Ensure that patient understands that annual vaccination with the current vaccine is necessary because immunity to influenza decreases in the year after the injection.

● Ensure that patient understands that the vaccine cannot cause influenza. Fever, malaise, and myalgia may begin 6 to 12 hours after vaccination and persist 1 to 2 days. Such systemic reactions are not common.

Japanese encephalitis virus vaccine, inactivated
JE-VAX

Pregnancy Risk Category: C

HOW SUPPLIED
Injection: 1-ml, 10-ml vials

ACTION
Provides active immunity against Japanese encephalitis (JE), a mosquito-borne arboviral flavivirus infection that's the leading cause of viral encephalitis in Asia.

ONSET, PEAK, DURATION
Not clearly defined. An immune response is thought to occur within 10 days. Duration of protection is thought to be at least 2 years in persons receiving three doses.

INDICATIONS & DOSAGE
Active immunization against JE—
Primary immunization schedule
Adults and children 3 years and over: 1 ml S.C. on days 0, 7, and 30.
Children 1 to 3 years: 0.5 ml S.C. on days 0, 7, and 30.
Booster doses
Adults and children 3 years and over: 1 ml S.C., 2 years after last dose.
Children 1 to 3 years: 0.5 ml S.C., 2

---

*Liquid contains alcohol.   **May contain tartrazine.   †Canada only.   ‡Australia only.   ◇OTC.

years after last dose.

ADVERSE REACTIONS

Systemic: *headache; dizziness; nausea; vomiting; abdominal pain; **respiratory distress; anaphylaxis;** rash;* generalized urticaria; *fever; malaise; chills; myalgia;* angioedema of the face, oropharynx, extremities, or lips.

Other: *local tenderness and swelling at injection site.*

INTERACTIONS
None significant.

EFFECTS ON DIAGNOSTIC TESTS
None reported.

CONTRAINDICATIONS
Contraindicated in patients hypersensitive to the drug or to thimerosal, a preservative, and in patients who exhibited severe adverse reactions, such as generalized urticaria or angioedema, to a prior dose of the vaccine. Because the vaccine is derived from mouse brain, its use is contraindicated in patients hypersensitive to substances of murine or neural origin.

NURSING CONSIDERATIONS
● Use cautiously in pregnant or breast-feeding patients, elderly patients, and those with a history of urticaria after vaccines, drugs, or insect stings. Advanced age may be a risk factor for developing symptomatic illness after JE infection. JE acquired during pregnancy can cause intrauterine infection and fetal death.

● Use vaccine to provide protection against JE in persons planning to travel or reside in areas where the virus is endemic. It's not indicated for all persons traveling to or residing in Asia. For most travelers to Asia, the risk for acquiring JE is extremely low. Contact the Centers for Disease Control and Prevention at (404) 332-4555 for current travel advisories.

● Keep epinephrine 1:1,000 and other resuscitation equipment and drugs available to treat anaphylaxis and other adverse reactions.

● To prepare vaccine for injection, use supplied diluent (sterile water for injection). Add 1.3 ml of diluent to the single-dose vial and 11 ml of diluent to the 10-dose vial. Shake vial thoroughly to ensure dissolution of vaccine. After reconstitution, refrigerate vaccine (36° to 46° F [2° to 8° C]) for up to 8 hours.

● Follow the recommended three-dose schedule for best results. Be aware that when time constraints prohibit the use of this schedule, an abbreviated schedule with injections on days 0, 7, and 14 may be used.

● Know that when it isn't possible to follow usual dose schedule, a two-dose regimen with injections on days 0 and 7 may be used. Antibodies will be induced in about 80% of patients with this schedule. A two-dose regimen should not be used unless circumstances are unusual.

● Monitor patients closely for 30 minutes after injection.

● Be aware that reactions to the first dose have occurred a median of 12 hours after injection (88% happened within 3 days). The delay between the second dose and adverse effects was usually longer, with a median of 3 days and some effects not seen for 2 weeks. Some patients exhibited adverse reactions to the second or third dose, even when the first or second dose was well tolerated.

☑ PATIENT TEACHING
● Warn patient about the possibility of delayed generalized urticaria or delayed angioedema of the extremities, face, oropharynx or (especially) the lips. Generalized urticaria or angioedema may occur within minutes of vaccination. Most reactions occur within 48 hours. However, reactions that may be related to the vaccine have occurred as late as 17 days after the injection.

● Because of the possibility of delayed

Reactions may be *common*, uncommon, *life-threatening*, or COMMON AND LIFE-THREATENING.

reactions, advise patient to remain in areas where medical care is available for 10 days after injection. Caution against international travel during this time. Advise patient to seek medical assistance as soon as any reaction appears.

• Encourage patient and parents to report adverse effects after vaccination. Health care providers should report these adverse effects to the U.S. Department of Health and Human Services Vaccine Adverse Event Reporting System (VAERS). Contact VAERS at (800) 822-7967 for information about the system and reporting forms.

• Teach patient about precautions that may limit exposure to mosquito bites, such as using insect repellents, wearing protective clothing, and avoiding outdoor activities, especially in the evening.

---

measles, mumps, and rubella virus vaccine, live
M-M-R II

Pregnancy Risk Category: C

HOW SUPPLIED
Injection: single-dose vial containing not less than 1,000 TCID$_{50}$ (tissue culture infective doses) of attenuated measles virus derived from Enders' attenuated Edmonston strain (grown in chick embryo culture), 20,000 TCID$_{50}$ of the Jeryl Lynn (B level) mumps strain (grown in chick embryo culture), and 1,000 TCID$_{50}$ of the Wistar RA 27/3 strain of rubella virus (propagated in human diploid cell culture) per 0.5-ml dose

ACTION
Promotes immunity to measles, mumps, and rubella virus by inducing production of antibodies.

ONSET, PEAK, DURATION
Although onset and peak are not precisely known, most patients develop immunity in 2 to 6 weeks. Effects have been shown to persist up to 11 years without decline.

INDICATIONS & DOSAGE
Routine immunization—
Children: one vial S.C. A two-dose schedule is recommended, with the first dose given at 15 months (12 months in high-risk areas) and the second dose given either at 4 to 6 years or at 11 or 12 years.
Adults: one vial S.C. People born after 1957 should receive two doses at least 1 month apart.

ADVERSE REACTIONS
Systemic: arthritis, arthralgia, urticaria, rash, fever, regional lymphadenopathy, diarrhea, *anaphylaxis.*
Other: erythema at injection site, arthralgia.

INTERACTIONS
Immune serum globulin, plasma, whole blood: antibodies in serum may interfere with immune response. Don't use vaccine within 3 to 11 months, depending on dose of antibody or blood given.
Immunosuppressants: may decrease immune response to vaccine.

EFFECTS ON DIAGNOSTIC TESTS
Vaccine may temporarily decrease response to tuberculin skin testing. If the skin test is necessary, administer it either before or simultaneously with the vaccine.

CONTRAINDICATIONS
Contraindicated in immunosuppressed patients; in those with cancer, blood dyscrasia, gamma globulin disorders, fever, active untreated tuberculosis, or anaphylactic or anaphylactoid reactions to neomycin or eggs; in those receiving corticosteroid or radiation therapy; and in pregnant patients.

NURSING CONSIDERATIONS
• Obtain history of allergies, especially

anaphylactic reactions to antibiotics, or reaction to immunization.

- Keep epinephrine 1:1,000 available to treat anaphylaxis.
- Inject into outer aspect of upper arm. Don't give I.V.
- Use only diluent supplied. Discard 8 hours after reconstituting.
- Refrigerate; protect from light. Solution may be used if red, pink, or yellow, but must be clear.
- Know that incidence of adverse effects is low (0.5% to 4%).
- Treat fever with antipyretics, such as acetaminophen.
- Be aware that presence of maternal antibodies may prevent response in children under 12 months.
- Keep in mind that the Immunization Practices Advisory Committee recommends that colleges and other postÐhigh school educational institutions, as well as medical institutions employing health care providers, obtain documentation of the receipt of two doses of vaccine after age 1 (or other proof of immunity, such as infection, documented by a doctor). Combined measles, mumps, and rubella vaccine is preferred.

Alert: The Centers for Disease Control and Prevention recommends that, during a measles outbreak in a health care facility, susceptible personnel exposed to the measles virus (whether or not they received measles vaccine or immunoglobulin) avoid patient contact for days 5 through 21 after such exposure. If they become ill, they should avoid patient contact for at least 7 days after developing rash.

☑ **PATIENT TEACHING**
- Warn parents about adverse reactions associated with the vaccine.
- Review immunization schedule with parents, and stress importance of receiving second injection at the appropriate time to maintain immunization.

measles and rubella virus vaccine, live attenuated
M-R-Vax II

Pregnancy Risk Category: C

HOW SUPPLIED
Injection: single-dose vial containing not less than 1,000 TCID$_{50}$ (tissue culture infective doses) per 0.5 ml of attenuated measles virus derived from Enders' attenuated Edmonston strain (grown in chick embryo culture); 1,000 TCID$_{50}$ of the Wistar RA 27/3 strain of rubella virus

ACTION
Promotes immunity to measles and rubella virus by inducing production of antibodies.

ONSET, PEAK, DURATION
Although onset and peak are not clearly defined, immunity for most patients occurs in 2 to 6 weeks. Effects have been shown to persist up to 11 years without decline.

INDICATIONS & DOSAGE
Immunization—
Adults and children 15 months and older: 0.5 ml (1,000 units) S.C.

ADVERSE REACTIONS
Systemic: rash, fever, arthralgia, lymphadenopathy, *anaphylaxis.*

INTERACTIONS
Immune serum globulin, plasma, whole blood: antibodies in serum may interfere with immune response. Don't use vaccine within 3 months of transfusion.
Immunosuppressants: may reduce immune response to vaccine.

EFFECTS ON DIAGNOSTIC TESTS
Vaccine may temporarily decrease response to tuberculin skin testing. If necessary, administer test either before or simultaneously with the vaccine.

Reactions may be *common*, uncommon, *life-threatening*, or COMMON AND LIFE-THREATENING.

CONTRAINDICATIONS
Contraindicated in immunosuppressed patients; in those with cancer, blood dyscrasia, gamma globulin disorders, fever, active untreated tuberculosis or anaphylactic or anaphylactoid reactions to eggs or neomycin; in those receiving corticosteroid or radiation therapy; and in pregnant patients.

NURSING CONSIDERATIONS
● Obtain history of allergies, especially anaphylactic reactions to antibiotics.
● Keep epinephrine 1:1,000 available to treat anaphylaxis.
● Use only diluent supplied. Discard 8 hours after reconstituting.
● Inject into outer upper arm. Don't inject I.V.
● Store in refrigerator and protect from light. Solution may be used if red, pink, or yellow, but must be clear (with no precipitation).
Alert: Vaccine should not be given within 1 month of other live virus vaccines, except oral poliovirus vaccine. Immunization should be deferred in patients with acute illness.
● Allow at least 3 weeks between BCG and rubella vaccines.

☑ **PATIENT TEACHING**
● Warn patient or parents about adverse reactions associated with vaccine.

---

measles virus vaccine, live attenuated
Attenuvax

Pregnancy Risk Category: C

HOW SUPPLIED
Injection: single-dose vial containing not less than 1,000 TCID$_{50}$ (tissue culture infective doses) of measles virus derived from the more attenuated line of Enders' attenuated Edmonston strain (grown in chick embryo culture)

ACTION
Promotes immunity to measles virus by inducing production of antibodies.

ONSET, PEAK, DURATION
Although exact onset and peak unknown, most patients develop immunity within 2 to 6 weeks. Vaccine-induced antibody levels have been shown to persist for at least 13 years without substantial decline.

INDICATIONS & DOSAGE
Immunization—
Adults and children age 15 months or over: 0.5 ml (1,000 units) S.C. A two-dose schedule is recommended, with the first dose given at age 15 months (age 12 months in high-risk areas) and the second dose given at age 4 to 6 or 11 to 12 years of age.
Measles outbreak control—
Children: if cases occur in children under age 1, children should be vaccinated as young as age 6 months. All students and siblings should be revaccinated if they are without documentation of measles immunity.
Adults: school personnel born in or after 1957 should be revaccinated if they are without proof of measles immunity. If the outbreak is in a medical facility, all workers born in or after 1957 should be revaccinated if they are without proof of immunity.

ADVERSE REACTIONS
Systemic: febrile seizures in susceptible children, anorexia, leukopenia, fever, rash, lymphadenopathy, *anaphylaxis.*
Other: erythema, swelling, and tenderness at injection site.

INTERACTIONS
Immune serum globulin, plasma, whole blood: antibodies in serum may interfere with immune response. Don't use vaccine for at least 3 months after administration of these products.

EFFECTS ON DIAGNOSTIC TESTS
Vaccine may temporarily decrease response to tuberculin skin test. If the skin test is necessary, administer it before, at the same time, or 6 weeks after immunization.

CONTRAINDICATIONS
Contraindicated in immunosuppressed patients; in those with cancer, blood dyscrasia, gamma globulin disorders, fever, active untreated tuberculosis, or anaphylactic or anaphylactoid reactions to neomycin or eggs; in those receiving corticosteroid or radiation therapy; and in pregnant patients.

NURSING CONSIDERATIONS
● Obtain history of allergies, especially anaphylactic reactions to antibiotics, or reaction to immunization. Immunization should be deferred in patients with acute illness or after administration of blood or plasma.
● Keep epinephrine 1:1,000 available to treat anaphylaxis.
● Use only diluent supplied. Discard 8 hours after reconstituting.
● Do not give I.V.
● Refrigerate and protect from light. Reconstituted solution is clear yellow with no precipitation. Do not use if discolored.
● Know that vaccine may be given with oral poliovirus vaccine.
● Keep in mind that the Immunization Practices Advisory Committee recommends that colleges and other post-high school educational institutions, as well as medical institutions employing health care providers, obtain documentation of the receipt of two doses of vaccine after age 1 (or other proof of immunity, such as infection, documented by a doctor). Combined measles, mumps, and rubella vaccine is preferred.
Alert: The Centers for Disease Control and Prevention recommends that, during a measles outbreak in a health care facility, susceptible personnel exposed to the measles virus (whether or not they received measles vaccine or immune globulin) avoid patient contact for days 5 through 21 after such exposure. If they become ill, they should avoid patient contact for at least 7 days after developing rash.
● Know that if attenuated measles vaccine is administered immediately after exposure to the disease, some protection may be provided. This level of protection is significantly increased if the vaccine is administered even a few days before exposure.

☑ PATIENT TEACHING
● Warn patient about adverse reactions associated with vaccine.
● Review immunization schedule with patient or parents and stress importance of receiving second injection at appropriate time.
● Stress the importance of avoiding pregnancy for 3 months after vaccination. Offer to provide contraception information.

---

meningococcal polysaccharide vaccine
Menomune-A/C/Y/W-135

Pregnancy Risk Category: C

HOW SUPPLIED
Injection: 1-dose, 10-dose, and 50-dose vials with vial of diluent

ACTION
Promotes active immunity to meningitis.

ONSET, PEAK, DURATION
Although exact onset and peak unknown, most patients develop immunity in 10 to 14 days. Antibody titers decline within 3 years.

INDICATIONS & DOSAGE
Meningococcal meningitis prophylaxis—
Adults and children 2 years and older: 0.5 ml S.C.

ADVERSE REACTIONS
Systemic: headache, malaise, chills, fever, muscle cramps, ***anaphylaxis.***
Other: *pain, tenderness, erythema, induration* (at injection site).

INTERACTIONS
Immunosuppressants: may reduce immune response to vaccine.

EFFECTS ON DIAGNOSTIC TESTS
None reported.

CONTRAINDICATIONS
Contraindicated in pregnant patients and patients with hypersensitivity to thimerosal. Vaccination should be deferred in patients with acute illness. Vaccine is not contraindicated in immunocompromise.

NURSING CONSIDERATIONS
● Obtain history of allergies and reaction to immunization.
● Keep epinephrine 1:1,000 available to treat anaphylaxis.
● Do not give I.V.
● Know that vaccine may be given with other immunizations.
● Know that routine vaccination is not recommended. Vaccine should be reserved for individuals at risk. These are individuals who live or are traveling to epidemic or highly endemic areas, household or institutional contacts of meningococcal disease as an adjunct to appropriate antibiotic chemoprophylaxis, medical and laboratory personnel at risk of exposure to meningococcal disease, presence of terminal complement component deficiency, and patients with anatomic or functional asplenia.
● Be aware that some clinicians will revaccinate children if they are at high risk and if they previously received vaccine before age 4 years.

☑ **PATIENT TEACHING**
● Warn patient or parents about adverse reactions associated with vaccine.
● Stress to patient the importance of avoiding pregnancy for 3 months after vaccination. Offer to provide contraception information.

---

mumps virus vaccine, live
Mumpsvax

Pregnancy Risk Category: C

HOW SUPPLIED
Injection: single-dose vial containing not less than 20,000 $TCID_{50}$ (tissue culture infective doses) of attenuated mumps virus derived from Jeryl Lynn mumps strain (grown in chick embryo culture) per 0.5 ml and vial of diluent; single-dose vial containing not less than 5,000 $TCID_{50}$(tissue culture infective doses) of the U.S. Reference Mumps Virus in each 0.5ml†

ACTION
Promotes active immunity to mumps.

ONSET, PEAK, DURATION
Although exact onset and peak unknown, most patients develop immunity in 2 to 3 weeks. Effects persist for at least 20 years; probably lifelong.

INDICATIONS & DOSAGE
Immunization—
Adults and children 1 year and older: 0.5 ml (20,000 units) S.C.

ADVERSE REACTIONS
CNS: *febrile seizures* (rare).
Other: *anaphylaxis, slight fever,* rash, malaise, mild allergic reactions, mild lymph adenopathy, diarrhea, injection-site reaction.

INTERACTIONS
Immune serum globulin, plasma, whole blood: antibodies in serum may interfere with immune response. Don't use vaccine for at least 3 months after administration of these products.

EFFECTS ON DIAGNOSTIC TESTS
Vaccine may temporarily decrease the response to tuberculin skin test. If the skin test is necessary, administer it before, at the same time, or 6 weeks after the vaccine.

CONTRAINDICATIONS
Contraindicated in immunosuppressed patients; in those with cancer, blood dyscrasia, gamma globulin disorders, fever, untreated active tuberculosis, or anaphylactic or anaphylactoid reactions to neomycin or eggs; in those receiving corticosteroid or radiation therapy; and in pregnant patients.

NURSING CONSIDERATIONS
● Obtain history of allergies, especially anaphylactic reactions to antibiotics, and reaction to immunization. Defer in patients with acute or febrile illness and for at least 3 months after transfusions or treatment with immune serum globulin.
● Keep epinephrine 1:1,000 available to treat anaphylaxis.
● Use only diluent supplied. Discard 8 hours after reconstituting.
● Do not give I.V.
● Refrigerate and protect from light. Reconstituted solution is clear yellow; do not use if discolored.
● Treat fever with antipyretics.
● Do not give this vaccine less than 1 month before or after immunization with other live virus vaccines; however, trivalent live, oral poliovirus vaccine may be administered simultaneously.
● Know that vaccine is not recommended for infants under 12 months because retained maternal mumps antibodies may interfere with the immune response.
● Do not use for delayed hypersensitivity (allergy) skin testing. Use mumps skin-test antigen, a killed viral product.

☑ PATIENT TEACHING
● Warn patient or parents about adverse reactions associated with vaccine.
● Stress to patient the importance of avoiding pregnancy for 3 months after

vaccination. Offer to provide contraception information.

---

plague vaccine

Pregnancy Risk Category: C

HOW SUPPLIED
Injection: 1.8 to 2.2 billion killed plague bacilli (*Yersinia pestis*)/ml in 20-ml vials

ACTION
Promotes active immunity to plague caused by *Y. pestis.*

ONSET, PEAK, DURATION
Onset and peak unknown. Effects persist for 6 to 12 months.

INDICATIONS & DOSAGE
Primary immunization and booster—
Adults and children 11 years and older: 1 ml I.M., followed by 0.2 ml in 4 to 12 weeks, then 0.2 ml 3 to 6 months after the second dose. Booster is 0.1 to 0.2 ml q 6 months while in plague area.
Children: Centers for Disease Control and Prevention does not recommend vaccination because data are insufficient.

ADVERSE REACTIONS
Systemic: headache, malaise, *slight fever, lymphadenopathy, **anaphylaxis,** arthralgia, myalgia, nausea, vomiting, leukocytosis.
Other: swelling, *induration, and erythema at injection site.*

INTERACTIONS
Cholera, typhoid vaccine: increased risk of adverse effects. Don't give at the same time.

EFFECTS ON DIAGNOSTIC TESTS
None reported.

CONTRAINDICATIONS
Contraindicated in immunosuppressed

or pregnant patients and in those hypersensitive to beef, soy, casein, phenol, or formaldehyde. Patients who have had severe local or systemic reactions to plague vaccine should not be revaccinated. Also contraindicated in patients with severe thrombocytopenia or any coagulation disorder that would contraindicate I.M. injections.

NURSING CONSIDERATIONS
● Obtain history of allergies and reaction to immunization. Know that immunization should be deferred in patients with respiratory infection.
● Keep epinephrine 1:1,000 available to treat anaphylaxis.
● Inject into the deltoid area, the preferred site.
● Recommended for all laboratory and field personnel working with *Yersinia pestis.*

☑ **PATIENT TEACHING**
● Warn patient about adverse reactions associated with vaccine.
● Caution women of childbearing age to notify doctor of suspected pregnancy before administration.

---

pneumococcal vaccine, polyvalent
Pneumovax 23, Pnu-Imune 23

Pregnancy Risk Category: C

HOW SUPPLIED
Injection: 25 mcg each of 23 polysaccharide isolates/0.5 ml

ACTION
Promotes active immunity to infections caused by *Streptococcus pneumoniae.*

ONSET, PEAK, DURATION
Onset occurs in 2 to 3 weeks. Peak unknown. Effects persist for 5 to 10 years in most patients.

INDICATIONS & DOSAGE
Pneumococcal immunization—
Adults and children 2 years and older: 0.5 ml I.M. or S.C.
Not recommended for children under 2 years.

ADVERSE REACTIONS
Systemic: *anaphylaxis, slight fever,* myalgia, rash, arthralgia.
Other: *soreness at injection site;* severe local reaction associated with revaccination within 3 years.

INTERACTIONS
Immunosuppressants: may reduce immune response to vaccine.

EFFECTS ON DIAGNOSTIC TESTS
None reported.

CONTRAINDICATIONS
Contraindicated in patients hypersensitive to the drug or its components (phenol). Also contraindicated in patients with Hodgkin's disease who have received extensive chemotherapy or nodal irradiation.

NURSING CONSIDERATIONS
● Check immunization history to avoid revaccination within 3 years.
● Obtain history of allergies and reaction to immunization. Eggs and egg protein are not used during the manufacture of the vaccine; contains phenol as a preservative.
● Keep epinephrine 1:1,000 available to treat anaphylaxis.
● Inject in deltoid or midlateral thigh. Don't inject I.V.
● When splenectomy is being considered, know that vaccine should be given at least 2 weeks before procedure to ensure adequate antibody response. This vaccine may be less effective in splenectomized patients.
● Vaccine protects against 23 pneumococcal types, accounting for 90% of pneumococcal disease.
● Know that the vaccine may be admin-

---

*Liquid contains alcohol.　　**May contain tartrazine.　　†Canada only.　　‡Australia only.　　◇OTC.

istered to children 2 years of age and over to prevent pneumococcal otitis media although the Centers for Disease Control and Prevention does not recommend otitis media as indicator for this vaccine.

● Vaccine is recommended for all adults over 65 years.

● Be aware that simultaneous administration with influenza virus vaccine is safe and effective.

● Keep refrigerated. Reconstitution or dilution not necessary.

☑ **PATIENT TEACHING**
● Warn patient about adverse reactions associated with this vaccine.

● Tell patient to treat fever with mild antipyretics.

poliovirus vaccine, live, oral, trivalent (TOPV)
Orimune

poliovirus vaccine, inactivated (IPV)
IPOL, Poliovax

Pregnancy Risk Category: C

HOW SUPPLIED
Oral vaccine: mixture of three live viruses (types 1, 2, and 3), grown in monkey kidney tissue culture, in 0.5-ml single-dose Dispettes
Inactivated virus vaccine injection: mixture of three types of poliovirus (types 1, 2, and 3) grown in tissue culture. IPOL uses monkey kidney cultures; Poliovax uses human diploid cell cultures. IPV comes in 0.5-ml prefilled syringes.

ACTION
Promotes immunity to poliomyelitis by inducing humoral antibodies and antibodies in the lymphatic tissue.

ONSET, PEAK, DURATION
An antibody response usually occurs within 7 to 10 days with TOPV; un-

known with IPV. Peak effects occur in 21 days with TOPV; unknown for IPV. Duration is thought to last for years.

INDICATIONS & DOSAGE
Poliovirus immunization—
Children and nonimmunized adults:
0.5 ml P.O. (TOPV), followed by a second dose of 0.5 ml in 6 to 8 weeks. A third 0.5-ml dose is given 6 to 12 months after second dose. A reinforcing dose of 0.5 ml should be given before entry to school.
Infants: 0.5 ml P.O. at 2 months, 4 months, and 18 months.
Poliovirus immunization (IPV) in persons who cannot receive TOPV—
Adults: 0.5 ml S.C., followed by a second dose in 4 to 8 weeks. A third dose is given in 6 to 12 months.
Children: 0.5 ml S.C. at 2 months and 4 months. A third dose is given at 15 to 18 months. A reinforcing dose of 0.5 ml S.C. should be given before entry into school.

ADVERSE REACTIONS
Systemic: *poliomyelitis* (TOPV only), *fever,* sleepiness, crying, decreased appetite, hypersensitivity reactions.
Other: erythema, induration, *pain* (at injection site).

INTERACTIONS
Immune serum globulin, plasma, whole blood: antibodies in serum may interfere with immune response. Don't use vaccine within 3 months of transfusion.
Immunosuppressants: may reduce immune response to vaccine.

EFFECTS ON DIAGNOSTIC TESTS
Vaccine may temporarily decrease the response to tuberculin skin test. If the skin test is necessary, administer it before, at the same time, or 6 weeks after immunization.

CONTRAINDICATIONS
Oral vaccine is contraindicated in immunosuppressed patients; in those with

Reactions may be *common,* uncommon, *life-threatening,* or COMMON AND LIFE-THREATENING.

cancer or immunoglobulin abnormalities; in those receiving radiation, antimetabolite, alkylating agent, or corticosteroid therapy; or in those who have a household contact who fits one of these preceding categories. These patients should receive IPV. Injectable vaccine is contraindicated in patients hypersensitive to neomycin, streptomycin, or polymixin B.

NURSING CONSIDERATIONS
• Do not use TOPV in siblings of child with known immunodeficiency syndrome. IPV is the preferred form.
• Obtain history of allergies and reaction to immunization.
• Do not administer oral form of vaccine parenterally.
• Keep TOPV frozen until used. Once thawed, if unopened, may refrigerate up to 30 days; if opened, up to 7 days. Thaw before administration.
• Know that color change of TOPV from pink to yellow has no effect on efficacy of the vaccine. Yellow color is caused by storage at low temperatures.
Alert: Know that parenteral form should be administered to immunodeficient patients or those with altered immune status because they may be at risk for developing the disease if live virus vaccine is administered.
• Oral vaccine should be deferred in patients with vomiting or diarrhea. Both forms of vaccine should be deferred in patients with acute illness.
• Do not administer to neonates under 6 weeks.
• Be aware that the highest risk of poliovirus infection occurs after the first dose of the oral vaccine.
• Know that adults at high risk for exposure who have completed a primary course may receive another dose.
• Keep in mind that vaccine is not effective in modifying or preventing existing or incubating poliomyelitis.

☑ PATIENT TEACHING
• Make sure parents know the risks and benefits of this vaccine before it's administered.
• Warn patient or parents about adverse reactions associated with this vaccine.

---

rabies vaccine, adsorbed

Pregnancy Risk Category: C

HOW SUPPLIED
Injection: single dose 1-ml vial

ACTION
Promotes active immunity to rabies.

ONSET, PEAK, DURATION
Onset unknown. Antibody levels peak within 2 weeks after the last of the three doses. Duration unknown, although at 9 to 12 months after immunization, 97% of patients continue to have antibody titers at or above a level of 0.1 IU (which is considered by the Centers for Disease Control and Prevention as the minimal acceptable antibody titer for complete rabies virus neutralization).

INDICATIONS & DOSAGE
Preexposure prophylaxis rabies immunization for persons in high-risk groups—
Adults and children: 1 ml I.M. at 0, 7, and 21 or 28 days for a total of three injections. Patients at increased risk for rabies should be checked q 6 months and given a booster vaccination, 1 ml I.M., as needed, to maintain adequate serum titer.
Postexposure rabies prophylaxis—
Adults and children not previously vaccinated against rabies: 20 IU/kg doses of human rabies immune globulin (HRIG) I.M. and five 1-ml injections of rabies vaccine adsorbed I.M. given on days 0, 3, 7, 14, and 28.
Adults and children previously vaccinated against rabies: two 1-ml injections of rabies vaccine adsorbed I.M. given on days 0 and 3. HRIG should not be given.

---

*Liquid contains alcohol.   **May contain tartrazine.   †Canada only.   ‡Australia only.   ◇ OTC.

ADVERSE REACTIONS

Systemic: *headache, nausea, slight fever, fatigue,* reaction resembling serum sickness, *abdominal pain, myalgia, dizziness.*

Other: *anaphylaxis; transient pain, erythema, swelling or itching at injection site;* aching of the injected muscle, mild inflammatory reaction at injection site.

INTERACTIONS

Antimalarial drugs, corticosteroids, immunosuppressants: decreased response to rabies vaccine. Avoid concomitant use.

EFFECTS ON DIAGNOSTIC TESTS

None reported.

CONTRAINDICATIONS

Contraindicated in patients who have experienced life-threatening allergic reactions to previous injections of this vaccine or to components of this vaccine, including thimerosal.

NURSING CONSIDERATIONS

● Use with caution in patients with a history of non-life-threatening allergic reactions to previous injections of the vaccine, in patients with hypersensitivity to monkey-derived proteins, and in children.
● Keep epinephrine 1:1,000 available to treat an anaphylactoid reaction.
● Administer as an I.M. injection into the deltoid region in adults and older children. For younger children, the midanterolateral aspect of the thigh also is acceptable. Know that this vaccine is not for use by the intradermal route. Take care not to inject the vaccine near a peripheral nerve or into adipose or subcutaneous tissue.
● Know that the vaccine is normally a light pink color because of the presence of phenol red in the suspension.
● Know that preexposure immunization should be delayed in persons with an acute illness.

Alert: If patient experiences a serious adverse reaction to the vaccine, report the reaction promptly to the manufacturer: Michigan Department of Public Health, 517-335-8050 during working hours or 517-335-9030 at other times.
● Don't confuse vaccine with rabies immune globulin. Both drugs may be given in some situations.

☑ PATIENT TEACHING

● Inform patient about adverse reactions associated with this vaccine and importance of alerting doctor so any serious adverse reaction can be reported.
● Caution patient not to perform hazardous activities if dizziness occurs.

rabies vaccine, human diploid cell (HDCV)
Imovax Rabies, Imovax Rabies I.D.

Pregnancy Risk Category: C

HOW SUPPLIED

Intradermal injection: 0.25 IU rabies antigen/dose
I.M. injection: 2.5 IU of rabies antigen/ml, in single-dose vial with diluent

ACTION

Promotes active immunity to rabies.

ONSET, PEAK, DURATION

Onset occurs within 1 week. Antibody levels peak after 1 to 2 months. Effects persist for 2 or more years.

INDICATIONS & DOSAGE

Postexposure antirabies immunization—
Adults and children: five 1-ml doses of HDCV I.M. (for example, in the deltoid region). First dose given as soon as possible after exposure; an additional dose given on each of days 3, 7, 14, and 28 after first dose. If no antibody response after this primary series occurs, a booster dose is recommended.
Preexposure prophylaxis immunization

Reactions may be *common*, uncommon, *life-threatening*, or COMMON AND LIFE-THREATENING.

for persons in high-risk groups—
Adults and children: three 1-ml injections administered I.M. First dose given on day 0 (the first day of therapy), second dose on day 7, and third dose on either day 21 or 28. Alternatively, 0.1 ml intradermally on the same dosage schedule.

ADVERSE REACTIONS
Systemic: *headache,* dizziness, *nausea,* abdominal pain, diarrhea, muscle aches, *fever, **anaphylaxis,** serum sickness, fatigue.*
Other: *pain, erythema, swelling, or itching at injection site.*

INTERACTIONS
Antimalarial drugs, corticosteroids, immunosuppressants: decreased response to rabies vaccine. Avoid concomitant use.

EFFECTS ON DIAGNOSTIC TESTS
None reported.

CONTRAINDICATIONS
No contraindications reported for persons after exposure. An acute febrile illness contraindicates use of vaccine for persons previously exposed.

NURSING CONSIDERATIONS
● Use cautiously in patients with a history of hypersensitivity.
● Keep epinephrine 1:1,000 available to treat anaphylaxis.
Alert: Do not use intradermal route for postexposure rabies vaccination.
● Know that the alternative regimen of 0.1-ml doses is only for preexposure prophylaxis. For postexposure prophylaxis, only use the 1-ml doses.
● Don't confuse vaccine with rabies immune globulin. Both drugs may be given in some situations.
● Be prepared to stop corticosteroid therapy during immunizing period unless therapy is essential for the treatment of other conditions.
● Keep in mind that some patients who

receive booster doses experience serum sickness-like hypersensitivity reactions. These reactions usually respond to antihistamines.

☑ **PATIENT TEACHING**
● Inform patient about adverse reactions associated with vaccine. Tell patient to report persistent or severe reactions to doctor.
● Stress importance of receiving booster, if appropriate for patient.

rubella and mumps virus vaccine, live
Biavax II

Pregnancy Risk Category: C

HOW SUPPLIED
Injection: single-dose vial containing not less than 1,000 TCID$_{50}$ (tissue culture infective doses) of the Wistar RA 27/3 rubella virus (propagated in human diploid cell culture) and not less than 20,000 TCID$_{50}$ of the Jeryl Lynn mumps strain (grown in chick embryo cell culture)

ACTION
Promotes immunity to rubella and mumps by inducing antibody production.

ONSET, PEAK, DURATION
Although onset and peak unknown, most people acquire immunity in 2 to 6 weeks. Effects persist for 10 years or longer.

INDICATIONS & DOSAGE
Rubella and mumps immunization—
Adults and children 1 year and older: 0.5 ml S.C.

ADVERSE REACTIONS
Systemic: polyneuritis, rash, thrombocytopenic purpura, urticaria, fever, diarrhea, arthritis, arthralgia, ***anaphylaxis,*** lymphadenopathy.

Other: pain, erythema, induration (at injection site).

INTERACTIONS
Immune serum globulin, plasma, whole blood: antibodies in serum may interfere with immune response. Don't give vaccine for at least 3 months after administration of these products.
Immunosupressants: may reduce immune response to vaccine.

EFFECTS ON DIAGNOSTIC TESTS
Vaccine may temporarily decrease response to tuberculin skin test. If the skin test is necessary, administer it before, at the same time, or 6 weeks after immunization.

CONTRAINDICATIONS
Contraindicated in pregnant or immunosuppressed patients; in those with cancer, blood dyscrasia, gamma globulin disorders, fever, or active untreated tuberculosis; history of anaphylaxis or anaphylactoid reactions to neomycin or eggs; and in those receiving corticosteroid (except those receiving corticosteroids as replacement therapy) or radiation therapy.

NURSING CONSIDERATIONS
● Obtain history of allergies, especially anaphylactic reaction to antibiotics, and reaction to immunization.
● Keep epinephrine 1:1,000 available to treat anaphylaxis.
● Know that in patients with acute illness and after administration of immune serum globulin, blood, or plasma, the vaccination should be deferred.
● Use only diluent supplied. Discard 8 hours after reconstituting.
● Inject into outer upper arm. Don't inject I.V.
● Allow an interval of at least 3 weeks between BCG and rubella vaccines.
● Refrigerate and protect from light. Reconstituted solution is clear yellow; don't use if discolored.

☑ PATIENT TEACHING
● Inform patient about adverse reactions associated with vaccine.
● Stress to patients the importance of avoiding pregnancy for 3 months after vaccination. Offer to provide contraception information.

---

rubella virus vaccine, live attenuated (RA 27/3)
Meruvax II

Pregnancy Risk Category: C

HOW SUPPLIED
Injection: single-dose vial containing not less than 1,000 $TCID_{50}$ (tissue culture infective doses) of the Wistar RA 27/3 strain of rubella virus (propagated in human diploid cell culture)

ACTION
Promotes immunity to rubella by inducing production of antibodies.

ONSET, PEAK, DURATION
Although the precise onset and peak unknown, most patients develop immunity in 2 to 6 weeks. Effects persist for 10 years or longer.

INDICATIONS & DOSAGE
Rubella immunization—
Adults and children 1 year and older: 0.5 ml (1,000 units) S.C.

ADVERSE REACTIONS
Systemic: polyneuritis, rash, thrombocytopenic purpura, urticaria, arthralgia, malaise, headache, sore throat, fever, arthritis, *anaphylaxis,* lymphadenopathy.
Other: pain, erythema, induration (at injection site).

INTERACTIONS
Immune serum globulin, plasma, whole blood: antibodies in serum may interfere with immune response. Don't use vaccine for at least 3 months after ad-

---

Reactions may be *common,* uncommon, *life-threatening*, or COMMON AND LIFE-THREATENING.

ministration of these products.
Immunosuppressants: may reduce immune response to vaccine.

EFFECTS ON DIAGNOSTIC TESTS
Vaccine may temporarily decrease response to tuberculin skin test. If the skin test is necessary, administer it before, at the same time, or 6 weeks after immunization.

CONTRAINDICATIONS
Contraindicated in pregnant or immunosuppressed patients; in those with cancer, blood dyscrasia, gamma globulin disorders, fever, or active untreated tuberculosis; in those with a history of hypersensitivity to neomycin; and in patients receiving corticosteroid (except those receiving corticosteroids as replacement therapy) or radiation therapy.

NURSING CONSIDERATIONS
● Obtain history of allergies and reaction to immunization.
● Keep epinephrine 1:1,000 available to treat anaphylaxis.
● Immunization should be deferred in patients with acute illness and after administration of human immune serum globulin, blood, or plasma.
● Use only diluent supplied. Discard 8 hours after reconstituting.
● Inject into outer upper arm. Don't inject I.V.
● Refrigerate and protect from light. Reconstituted solution is clear yellow; don't use if discolored.
● Allow at least 3 weeks between BCG and rubella vaccines.

☑ **PATIENT TEACHING**
● Inform patient about adverse reactions associated with vaccine.
● Stress to patient the importance of avoiding pregnancy for 3 months after vaccination. Offer to provide contraception information.

tetanus toxoid, adsorbed

tetanus toxoid, fluid

Pregnancy Risk Category: C

HOW SUPPLIED
tetanus toxoid, adsorbed
Injection: 5 to 10 Lf (limit flocculation) units of inactivated tetanus/0.5-ml dose, in 0.5-ml syringes and 5-ml vials
tetanus toxoid, fluid
Injection: 4 to 5 Lf units of inactivated tetanus/0.5-ml dose, in 0.5-ml syringes and 7.5-ml vials

ACTION
Promotes immunity to tetanus by inducing antitoxin production.

ONSET, PEAK, DURATION
Although exact onset and peak unknown, most patients possess immunity after two doses. Effects unknown but may persist for 10 years or more.

INDICATIONS & DOSAGE
Primary immunization—
Adults and children 6 years and over: 0.5 ml (adsorbed) I.M. 4 to 8 weeks apart for two doses; then third dose 6 to 12 months after the second. Alternatively, 0.5 ml (fluid) I.M. or S.C. 4 to 8 weeks apart for three doses; then fourth dose of 0.5 ml 6 to 12 months after third dose.
Children 6 weeks to 6 years: 0.5 ml (adsorbed) I.M. at ages 2, 4, and 6 months. A fourth dose is given at age 15 to 18 months. A fifth dose is given at age 4 to 6 years, just before entry into school, if indicated.
Booster doses—
Adults: 0.5 ml I.M. at 10-year intervals.

ADVERSE REACTIONS
Systemic: tachycardia, hypotension, urticaria, pruritus, slight fever, chills, malaise, aches and pains, flushing, *anaphylaxis.*

---

*Liquid contains alcohol.   **May contain tartrazine.   †Canada only.   ‡Australia only.   ◇OTC.

Other: erythema, induration, nodule (at injection site).

INTERACTIONS
Chloramphenicol: may interfere with response to tetanus toxoid.
Immunosuppressants: may reduce immune response to vaccine.

EFFECTS ON DIAGNOSTIC TESTS
None reported.

CONTRAINDICATIONS
Contraindicated in immunosuppressed patients and in those with immunoglobulin abnormalities or severe hypersensitivity or neurologic reactions to the toxoid or any ingredient in it, such as thimerosal. Also contraindicated in patients with thrombocytopenia or any coagulation disorder that would contraindicate I.M. injection unless the potential benefits outweigh the risks. Vaccination should be deferred in patients with acute illness and during polio outbreaks, except in emergencies.

NURSING CONSIDERATIONS
● Use cautiously (adsorbed form) in infants or children with cerebral damage, neurologic disorders, or a history of febrile seizures.
● Obtain history of allergies and reaction to immunization.
● Determine date of last tetanus immunization.
● Keep epinephrine 1:1,000 available to treat anaphylaxis.
● Know that vaccine is used for prevention, not treatment, of tetanus infections.
● Do not confuse this drug with tetanus immune globulin, human. Both drugs may be given in some situations.
● Be aware that adsorbed form produces longer duration of immunity. Fluid form provides quicker booster effect in patients actively immunized previously.

☑ **PATIENT TEACHING**
● Advise patient to avoid use of hot or cold compresses at injection site; this

may increase severity of local reaction.
● Instruct patient to report persistent or severe adverse reactions.

---

typhoid vaccine, parenteral

typhoid vaccine, oral
Vivotif Berna Vaccine

Pregnancy Risk Category: C

HOW SUPPLIED
Injection: suspension of killed Ty-2 strain of *Salmonella typhi;* 8 units/ml in 5-ml, 10-ml, and 20-ml vials
Capsules (enteric-coated): 2 to 6×10^9 colony-forming units of viable *Salmonella typhi* $Ty^{21}a$ and 5 to 50×10^9 bacterial cells of nonviable $Ty^{21}a2$

ACTION
Provides active immunity to typhoid fever.

ONSET, PEAK, DURATION
Immunity occurs at end of primary immunity immunization. Peak unknown. Effects persist for 3 to 5 years.

INDICATIONS & DOSAGE
Primary immunization—
Adults: one capsule (oral vaccine) on alternate days taken 1 hour before meals for four doses. Protocol repeated as booster q 5 years.
Adults and children over 10 years: 0.5 ml S.C. (injection); repeated in 4 weeks. Protocol repeated as booster q 3 years.
Children 6 months to 10 years: 0.25 ml S.C. (injection); repeated in 4 weeks. Protocol repeated as booster q 3 years.

ADVERSE REACTIONS
CNS: headache.
GI: nausea, abdominal cramps, vomiting.
Skin: rash, urticaria, swelling, pain, inflammation (at injection site).
Other: *fever,* malaise, *anaphylaxis,* myalgia.

Reactions may be *common,* uncommon, *life-threatening*, or COMMON AND LIFE-THREATENING.

INTERACTIONS

Sulfonamides, other antibiotics: may impair antibody response to oral vaccine. Don't use together.

EFFECTS ON DIAGNOSTIC TESTS

None reported.

CONTRAINDICATIONS

Contraindicated in immunosuppressed patients and in patients with hypersensitivity to the vaccine. Vaccination should be deferred in patients with acute illness.

NURSING CONSIDERATIONS

● Obtain history of allergies and reaction to immunization.
● Treat fever with antipyretics.
● Keep epinephrine 1:1,000 available to treat anaphylaxis.
● Shake thoroughly before withdrawing from vial.
● Do not give intradermally.
● Refrigerate vaccine at 35.5° to 50° F (2° to 10° C).

☑ **PATIENT TEACHING**
● When administering oral vaccine, ensure that patient understands the importance of taking all four doses and following the alternate-day regimen.
● Tell patient to take oral vaccine with cold or lukewarm water and not to chew or crush enteric-coated capsules.
● Inform patient about adverse reactions associated with vaccine.

---

typhoid Vi polysaccharide vaccine
Typhim Vi

Pregnancy Risk Category: C

HOW SUPPLIED

Injection: 0.5-ml syringe, 20-dose vial, 50-dose vial

ACTION

Promotes active immunity to typhoid fever.

ONSET, PEAK, DURATION

Most patients develop immunity about 2 weeks after vaccination. Protection lasts for about 2 years.

INDICATIONS & DOSAGE

Active immunization against typhoid fever—

Adults and children 2 years and older: 0.5 ml I.M. as a single dose. Reimmunization every 2 years with 0.5 ml I.M. as a single dose, if needed.

ADVERSE REACTIONS

CNS: *headache.*
GI: nausea, vomiting, abdominal cramps.
Skin: *pain or tenderness, induration, erythema* (at injection site), rash, urticaria.
Other: *anaphylaxis,* malaise, myalgia, fever.

INTERACTIONS

None significant.

EFFECTS ON DIAGNOSTIC TESTS

None reported.

CONTRAINDICATIONS

Contraindicated in patients with hypersensitivity to any component of the vaccine. The vaccine should not be used to treat a patient with typhoid fever or given to a patient who is a chronic typhoid carrier.

NURSING CONSIDERATIONS

● Use with caution in patients with thrombocytopenia or a bleeding disorder and those who are taking an anticoagulant because bleeding may occur following an I.M. injection in these individuals.
● As with any vaccine, administration should be delayed, if possible, in patients with any febrile illness.
● Although anaphylaxis is rare, keep epinephrine available to treat an anaphy-

---

*Liquid contains alcohol.   **May contain tartrazine.   †Canada only.   ‡Australia only.   ◇OTC.

lactoid reaction.

● **I.M. use:** Administer as an I.M. injection into the deltoid region in adults and into the deltoid or vastus lateralis in children. It should not be administered in the gluteal region or areas where there may be a nerve trunk. Never inject I.V.

☑ **PATIENT TEACHING**
● Advise the patient to take all necessary precautions to avoid contact with or ingestion of contaminated food and water.
● Inform the patient that immunization should be given at least 2 weeks prior to expected exposure. Although an optimal reimmunization schedule has not been established, recommended reimmunization consists of a single dose for U.S. travelers every 2 years if exposure to typhoid fever is possible.
● Inform the patient about the adverse reactions associated with vaccine.

---

varicella virus vaccine
Varivax

Pregnancy Risk Category: C

HOW SUPPLIED
Injection: single dose vial containing 1350 PFU of Oka/Merck varicella virus (live)

ACTION
Prevents chickenpox by inducing the production of antibodies to varicella-zoster virus.

ONSET, PEAK, DURATION
Although the precise onset and peak unknown, most patients develop immunity in 4 to 6 weeks. Effects persist for at least 2 years.

INDICATIONS & DOSAGE
Prevention of varicella-zoster (chickenpox) infections —
Adults and children 13 years and over: 0.5 ml S.C. followed by a second 0.5 ml dose 4 to 8 weeks later.

Children 1 to 12 years: 0.5 ml S.C.

ADVERSE REACTIONS
Other: *anaphylaxis,* fever, herpes zoster, injection site reactions (swelling, redness, pain, rash), varicella-like rash.

INTERACTIONS
Blood products, immune globulin: may inactivate vaccine. Defer vaccination for at least 5 months following blood or plasma transfusions or administration of immune globulin or varicella-zoster immune globulin.
Immunosuppressants: risk of severe reactions to live-virus vaccines. Postpone routine vaccination.
Salicylates: Reye's syndrome has been reported after natural varicella infection. Avoid use of salicylates for 6 weeks after varicella immunization.

EFFECTS ON DIAGNOSTIC TESTS
None reported.

CONTRAINDICATIONS
Contraindicated in patients hypersensitive to the drug; in those with history of anaphylactoid reaction to neomycin, blood dyscrasia, leukemia, lymphomas, neoplasms affecting bone marrow or lymphatic system, primary and acquired immunosuppressive states, active untreated tuberculosis, or any febrile respiratory illness or other active febrile infection; and in pregnant patients.

NURSING CONSIDERATIONS
● To reconstitute the vaccine, first withdraw 0.7 ml of diluent into the syringe to be used for reconstitution. Inject all the diluent in the syringe into the vial of lyophilized vaccine, and gently agitate to mix thoroughly. Administer immediately after reconstitution. Discard if not used within 30 minutes.
● Have epinephrine available for potential anaphylaxis reaction.
● Vaccine has been safely and effectively used in combination with measles, mumps, and rubella vaccine.

Alert: Know that the vaccine contains a live attenuated virus. There is some evidence that children who develop a rash may be capable of transmitting the virus.

☑ **PATIENT TEACHING**
● Inform patients or parents of adverse reactions associated with vaccine.
● Caution women of childbearing age to notify doctor of suspected pregnancy before administration.

---

yellow fever vaccine
YF-Vax

Pregnancy Risk Category: C

HOW SUPPLIED
Injection: live, attenuated 17D yellow fever virus in 1-, 5-, and 20-dose vials, with diluent; supplied only to designated yellow fever vaccination centers authorized to issue yellow fever vaccination certificates

ACTION
Provides active immunity to yellow fever.

ONSET, PEAK, DURATION
Effective immunity occurs in 7 to 10 days. Peak occurs within 28 days of vaccination. Immunity lasts more than 10 years and may persist for life.

INDICATIONS & DOSAGE
Primary vaccination—
Adults and children 9 months and over: 0.5 ml deep S.C.; booster is 0.5 ml S.C. q 10 years.

ADVERSE REACTIONS
Systemic: *anaphylaxis, fever, malaise,* myalgia, headache.
Other: mild swelling, pain (at injection site).

INTERACTIONS
Cholera vaccine: concurrent administration may interfere with immune response to both yellow fever and cholera vaccines. Administer 3 weeks apart.
Immunosuppressants: may increase viral replication and the development of infection with yellow fever virus. Immunization should be deferred until immunosuppressant is discontinued.

EFFECTS ON DIAGNOSTIC TESTS
None reported.

CONTRAINDICATIONS
Contraindicated in immunosuppressed patients; in those with cancer, gamma globulin deficiency, or hypersensitivity to eggs; or in those receiving corticosteroid or radiation therapy. Also contraindicated during pregnancy and in infants under 9 months, except in high-risk areas.

NURSING CONSIDERATIONS
● Obtain history of allergies, especially to eggs, and reaction to immunization.
● Keep epinephrine 1:1,000 available to treat anaphylaxis.
● Reconstitute with sodium chloride injection that contains no preservatives (they inactivate the yellow fever viruses).
● Keep frozen. Don't use unless shipping case contains some dry ice on arrival. Avoid vigorous shaking; carefully swirl mixture until suspension is uniform. Use within 1 hour after reconstituting. Discard remainder.
● Yellow fever vaccine should not be given within 1 month of other live virus vaccines; may be given concurrently with hepatitis B vaccine.

☑ **PATIENT TEACHING**
● Inform patient about adverse reactions associated with vaccine.
● Caution women of childbearing age to notify doctor of suspected pregnancy before administration.

---

black widow spider antivenin
Crotalidae antivenin, polyvalent
diphtheria antitoxin, equine
***Micrurus fulvius* antivenin**

COMBINATION PRODUCTS
None.

---

black widow spider antivenin
Antivenin *(Latrodectus mactans)*

Pregnancy Risk Category: C

HOW SUPPLIED
Injection: combination package—one
vial of antivenin (6,000-unit vial), one
2.5-ml vial of diluent (sterile water for
injection), and one 1-ml vial of normal
equine (horse) serum (1:10 dilution) for
sensitivity testing

ACTION
Unknown.

ONSET, PEAK, DURATION
Immediate response after I.V. administra-
tration. Concentrations peak up to 2
days after I.M. injection.

INDICATIONS & DOSAGE
Black widow spider bite—
Adults and children: 2.5 ml I.M. in anterolateral thigh. Second dose may be
needed. In severe cases, antivenin may
be given I.V.

ADVERSE REACTIONS
Systemic: *hypersensitivity reactions,*
anaphylaxis, serum sickness, neuro-
toxicity.

INTERACTIONS
None significant.

EFFECTS ON DIAGNOSTIC TESTS
None reported.

CONTRAINDICATIONS
Contraindicated in patients hypersensitive to the drug when desensitization is
not feasible.

NURSING CONSIDERATIONS
• Immobilize patient; splint the bitten
limb to prevent spread of venom.
• Obtain history of allergies, especially
to horses, and reaction to immunization.
Have epinephrine 1:1,000 available in
case of anaphylaxis.
• For best results, know that antivenin
should be given as soon as possible.
• Test for sensitivity before giving the
drug, as ordered. Use 0.2 ml of a 1:10
dilution in 0.9% sodium chloride solution.
Alert: Give I.M. dosage in anterolateral
thigh so that a tourniquet may be applied if a systemic reaction occurs.
• **I.V. use:** Dilute antivenin in 10 to 50
ml of 0.9% sodium chloride solution
and infuse over 15 minutes.
• Watch the patient for 2 to 3 days. Venom is neurotoxic and may cause respiratory paralysis and seizures.

☑ **PATIENT TEACHING**
• Explain to patient and family how
drug will be administered.
• Instruct patient to report adverse reactions promptly.

Crotalidae antivenin, polyvalent

Pregnancy Risk Category: C

HOW SUPPLIED
Injection: combination package—one
vial of lyophilized serum, one vial of

Reactions may be *common*, uncommon, *life-threatening*, or COMMON AND LIFE-THREATENING.

diluent (10 ml of bacteriostatic water for injection), and one 1-ml vial of normal horse serum (diluted 1:10) for sensitivity testing

ACTION
Neutralizes and binds venom of snakes of the species crotalids (pit vipers), including rattlesnakes, water moccasins, and copperheads.

ONSET, PEAK, DURATION
Immediate response after I.V. administration. Concentrations peak up to 2 days after I.M. injection.

INDICATIONS & DOSAGE
Crotalid (rattlesnake) bites—
Adults and children: initially, 20 to 150 ml I.V., depending on severity of bite and patient response. If large amount of venom, more than 150 ml may be given I.V. directly into superficial vein. Subsequent doses based on patient's response; may need another 10 to 50 ml if swelling progresses, if systemic symptoms increase, or if new manifestations appear.

ADVERSE REACTIONS
Systemic: *hypersensitivity reactions,* **anaphylaxis,** *serum sickness,* lymphadenopathy, arthralgia, fever.
Other: pain, erythema, urticaria.

INTERACTIONS
Antihistamines: enhanced toxicity of crotaline venoms. Don't use together.

EFFECTS ON DIAGNOSTIC TESTS
None reported.

CONTRAINDICATIONS
Contraindicated in patients hypersensitive to the drug.

NURSING CONSIDERATIONS
• Use cautiously. Studies indicate that 60% of patients treated with this antivenin develop hypersensitivity.
• Immobilize the patient immediately.

Splint the bitten extremity.
• Obtain history of allergies, especially to horses, and reaction to immunization. Have epinephrine 1:1,000 ready in case of hypersensitivity reaction.
Alert: Type and crossmatch blood as soon as possible; hemolysis from venom prevents accurate crossmatching.
• For best results, antivenin should be administered as soon as possible.
• Test for sensitivity before giving drug. Give 0.02 to 0.03 ml of a 1:10 dilution in 0.9% sodium chloride solution intradermally. Read results after 5 to 10 minutes. Watch carefully for delayed allergic reaction or relapse.
• Be aware that children, who have less resistance and less body fluid to dilute venom, may need twice the adult dose.
• Give corticosteroids as prescribed. If a large number of vials are administered, serum sickness may result.
• Discard unused portion.

☑ PATIENT TEACHING
• Explain to patient and family that a test dose will be given first to check for sensitivity to the drug.
• Instruct patient to report adverse reactions promptly.

---

diphtheria antitoxin, equine

Pregnancy Risk Category: C

HOW SUPPLIED
Injection: not less than 500 units/ml in 10,000-unit and 20,000-unit vials

ACTION
Binds with circulating toxin and prevents disease progression.

ONSET, PEAK, DURATION
Immediate response after I.V. administration. Concentrations peak up to 2 days after I.M. injection.

INDICATIONS & DOSAGE
Diphtheria prevention—

Adults and children: 5,000 to 10,000 units I.M.
Diphtheria treatment—
Adults and children: 20,000 to 80,000 units or more slow I.V. Additional doses may be given in 24 hours. I.M. route may be used in mild cases.

ADVERSE REACTIONS
Systemic: *hypersensitivity reactions,* anaphylaxis, serum sickness (urticaria, pruritus, fever, malaise, arthralgia) may occur in 7 to 12 days.
Other: pain, erythema, urticaria.

INTERACTIONS
None significant.

EFFECTS ON DIAGNOSTIC TESTS
None reported.

CONTRAINDICATIONS
Contraindicated in patients hypersensitive to the drug.

NURSING CONSIDERATIONS
● Obtain history of allergies, especially to horses, and reaction to immunization. Have epinephrine 1:1,000 ready in case of hypersensitivity reaction. Antitoxin should be used with extreme caution in patients with history of allergic disorders.
● Test for sensitivity before giving the drug, as ordered.
Alert: If patient has symptoms of diphtheria (sore throat, fever, tonsillar membrane), therapy should be started immediately, without waiting for culture reports.
● For storage, refrigerate antitoxin at 35.6° to 50° F (2° to 10° C). Before administering, warm to 90° to 95° F (32.2° to 35° C), never higher.

☑ **PATIENT TEACHING**
● Explain to patient and family that a test dose will be given first to check for sensitivity to the drug.
● Tell patient to report adverse reactions promptly.

Micrurus fulvius antivenin

Pregnancy Risk Category: C

HOW SUPPLIED
Injection: combination package with 10 ml of diluent

ACTION
Neutralizes and binds coral snake venom.

ONSET, PEAK, DURATION
Immediate response after I.V. administration. Concentrations peak up to 2 days after I.M. injection.

INDICATIONS & DOSAGE
Eastern and Texas coral snake bite—
Adults and children: 30 to 50 ml (3 to 5 vials) slow I.V. through running I.V. of 0.9% sodium chloride solution. First 1 to 2 ml given over 3 to 5 minutes, and signs of allergic reaction watched for. If no signs develop, injection is continued. 100 ml or more may be needed.
    Not effective for Sonoran or Arizona coral snake bites.

ADVERSE REACTIONS
Systemic: hypersensitivity reactions, *anaphylaxis,* fever, arthralgia, lymphadenopathy.
Other: pain, erythema, urticaria.

INTERACTIONS
None significant.

EFFECTS ON DIAGNOSTIC TESTS
No information available.

CONTRAINDICATIONS
Contraindicated in patients hypersensitive to the drug.

NURSING CONSIDERATIONS
● Immobilize the patient and splint bitten limb to prevent spread of venom.
● Obtain accurate patient history of allergies, especially to horses, and reac-

tion to immunization. Make sure epinephrine 1:1,000 is available in case of hypersensitivity reaction.

• Test for sensitivity before giving the drug, as ordered.

• Antivenin should be given as soon as possible (before onset of neurotoxic signs); asymptomatic patients should be treated because systemic signs usually develop later.

• Watch the patient carefully for 24 hours. Venom is neurotoxic and may cause respiratory paralysis.

☑ **PATIENT TEACHING**

• Explain to patient and family that a test dose will be given first to check for sensitivity to the drug.

• Tell patient to report adverse reactions promptly.

77
Immune serums

cytomegalovirus immune globulin, intravenous
hepatitis B immune globulin, human
immune globulin intramuscular
immune globulin intravenous
rabies immune globulin, human
respiratory syncytial virus immune globulin intravenous, human
Rh₀(D) immune globulin, human
Rh₀(D) immune globulin intravenous, human
tetanus immune globulin, human
varicella-zoster immune globulin

COMBINATION PRODUCTS
None.

---

cytomegalovirus immune globulin (human), intravenous (CMV-IGIV)
CytoGam

Pregnancy Risk Category: C

HOW SUPPLIED
Injection: 2.5 g/50 ml

ACTION
Provides passive immunity by supplying a relatively high concentration of immunoglobulin (Ig) G antibodies against CMV. Increasing these antibody levels in CMV-exposed patients may attenuate or reduce the incidence of serious CMV disease.

ONSET, PEAK, DURATION
Unknown.

INDICATIONS & DOSAGE
To attenuate primary CMV disease in seronegative kidney transplant recipients who receive a kidney from a CMV seropositive donor—
Adults: administered I.V. based on time after transplantation:
> within 72 hours: 150 mg/kg
> 2 weeks after: 100 mg/kg
> 4 weeks after: 100 mg/kg
> 6 weeks after: 100 mg/kg
> 8 weeks after: 100 mg/kg
> 12 weeks after: 50 mg/kg
> 16 weeks after: 50 mg/kg.

Initial dose given at 15 mg/kg/hour. Increased to 30 mg/kg/hour after 30 minutes if no untoward reactions occur, then to 60 mg/kg/hour after another 30 minutes if no reactions occur. Volume should not exceed 75 ml/hour. Subsequent doses may be given at 15 mg/kg/hour for 15 minutes, increasing q 15 minutes in a stepwise fashion to 60 mg/kg/hour.

ADVERSE REACTIONS
Systemic: hypotension, nausea, vomiting, wheezing, *anaphylaxis.*
Other: flushing, chills, muscle cramps, back pain, fever.

INTERACTIONS
Live virus vaccines: may interfere with the immune response to live virus vaccines. Vaccination should be deferred for at least 3 months.

EFFECTS ON DIAGNOSTIC TESTS
No information available.

CONTRAINDICATIONS
Contraindicated in patients with sensitivity to other human Ig preparations or with selective IgA deficiency.

NURSING CONSIDERATIONS
● Obtain vital signs before therapy.
● **I.V. use:** Prepare for administration as follows: Remove tab portion of vial cap and clean rubber stopper with 70%

Reactions may be *common*, uncommon, *life-threatening*, or COMMON AND LIFE-THREATENING.

alcohol or equivalent. To avoid foaming, do not shake vial. Inspect vial for clarity and particles.

• If possible, administer through a separate I.V. line, using a constant infusion pump. Filters are unnecessary. If unable to administer through separate line, piggyback into preexisting line of sodium chloride injection or one of the following dextrose solutions with or without sodium chloride: dextrose 2.5% in water, D_5W, dextrose 10% in water, or dextrose 20% in water. Do not dilute more than 1:2 with any of the above solutions.

• Begin infusion within 6 hours of entering the vial; finish within 12 hours.

• Monitor the patient's vital signs closely midinfusion, postinfusion, and before any increase in infusion rate.

Alert: If anaphylaxis or drop in blood pressure occurs, discontinue infusion, notify the doctor, and be prepared to administer CPR and such drugs as diphenhydramine and epinephrine.

• Refrigerate at 36° to 46° F (2° to 8° C).

☑ **PATIENT TEACHING**
• Review the drug therapy regimen with patient, and stress importance of compliance in follow-up visits.

• Instruct patient to report adverse reactions promptly.

---

hepatitis B immune globulin, human
H-BIG, Hep-B-Gammagee, Hyper-Hep

Pregnancy Risk Category: C

HOW SUPPLIED
Injection: 1-ml, 4-ml, 5-ml vials; 0.5-ml neonatal single-dose syringe

ACTION
Provides passive immunity to hepatitis B.

ONSET, PEAK, DURATION
Onset occurs in 1 to 6 days. Peak levels occur 3 to 11 days after I.M. administration. Protective for 2 months or more.

INDICATIONS & DOSAGE
Hepatitis B exposure in high-risk patients—
Adults and children: 0.06 ml/kg I.M. within 7 days after exposure. Dosage repeated 28 days after exposure if patient refuses hepatitis B vaccine.
Neonates born to patients who test positive for hepatitis B surface antigen (HbsAg): 0.5 ml within 12 hours of birth.

ADVERSE REACTIONS
Systemic: *anaphylaxis,* urticaria, angioedema.
Other: pain and tenderness at the injection site.

INTERACTIONS
Live virus vaccines: may interfere with response to live virus vaccines. Defer routine immunization for 3 months.

EFFECTS ON DIAGNOSTIC TESTS
None reported.

CONTRAINDICATIONS
Contraindicated in patients with a history of anaphylactic reactions to immune serum.

NURSING CONSIDERATIONS
• Obtain history of allergies and reaction to immunizations. Make sure epinephrine 1:1,000 is available.

• Inject into anterolateral aspect of thigh or deltoid muscle areas in older children and adults; inject into anterolateral aspect of thigh for neonates and children under 3 years.

• For postexposure prophylaxis (for example, needle stick, direct contact), know that drug is usually given with hepatitis B vaccine.

• This immune globulin provides passive immunity; do not confuse with he-

---

*Liquid contains alcohol.   **May contain tartrazine.   †Canada only.   ‡Australia only.   ◊ OTC.

patitis B vaccine. Both drugs may be given at the same time. Do not mix in the same syringe.

☑ **PATIENT TEACHING**
● Inform patient that pain and tenderness may occur at injection site.
● Tell patient to report any signs of hypersensitivity immediately.

---

immune globulin intramuscular (IGIM, IG, gamma globulin)
Gammar

immune globulin intravenous (IGIV)
Gamimune N, Gammagard S/D, Gammar-P IV, Iveegam, Polygam S/D, Sandoglobulin, Venoglobulin-I, Venoglobulin-S

Pregnancy Risk Category: C

HOW SUPPLIED
immune globulin intramuscular
Injection: 2-ml, 10-ml vials
immune globulin intravenous
Injection: 5% in 10-ml, 50-ml, 100-ml, 250-ml vials (Gamimune N)
5% in 2.5-g, 5-g, 10-g vials; 10% in 5-g, 10-g, 20-g vials (Venoglobulin-S)
Powder for injection: 50 mg protein/ml in 0.5-g, 2.5-g, 5-g, 10-g vials (Gammagard); 2.5-g vials (Gammar-IV); 500-mg, 1-g, 2.5-g, 5-g vials (Iveegam); 2.5-g, 5-g, 10-g vials (Polygam S/D); 1-g, 3-g, 6-g vials (Sandoglobulin); 500-mg, 2.5-g, 5-g, 10-g vials (Venoglobulin-I)

ACTION
Provides passive immunity by increasing antibody titer. The primary component is IgG.

ONSET, PEAK, DURATION
Onset and peak occur immediately after I.V. administration; peak occurs 2 to 5 days after I.M. injection. Duration unknown.

INDICATIONS & DOSAGE
Agammaglobulinemia or hypogammaglobulinemia—
Adults: initially, 1.2 ml/kg I.M., followed by 0.6 ml/kg once q 2 to 4 weeks. Maximum single dose is 30 to 50 ml. Alternatively, 100 to 400 mg/kg I.V. q 2 to 4 weeks. Infused at 0.01 to 0.02 ml/kg/minute for 30 minutes. If no discomfort, rate increased to maximum of 0.06 ml/kg/minute. For Sandoglobulin, 200 mg/kg I.V. monthly. Infused at 0.5 to 1 ml/minute. After 15 to 30 minutes, infusion rate increased to 1.5 to 2.5 ml/minute.
Children: 20 to 40 ml I.M. monthly.
Hepatitis A exposure—
Adults and children: 0.02 ml/kg I.M. as soon as possible after exposure. Up to 0.06 ml/kg may be given q 4 to 6 months if exposure will be 3 months or longer.
Modification or prevention of measles—
Adults and children: 0.25 ml/kg I.M. within 6 days after exposure.
Measles exposure in immunocompromised child—
Children: 0.5 ml/kg I.M. within 6 days after exposure.
Prophylaxis in primary immunodeficiencies—
Adults and children: 100 to 400 mg/kg by I.V. infusion monthly (Gamimune only). Infusion rate is 0.01 to 0.02 ml/kg/minute for 30 minutes. If no discomfort occurs, rate increased to maximum of 0.08 ml/kg/minute.
Idiopathic thrombocytopenic purpura—
Adults: 0.4 g/kg Gamimune N for 5 consecutive days or Sandoglobulin I.V. for 2 to 5 consecutive days. Additional doses may be given based on response. Up to three doses of Gammagard 1,000 mg/kg may be given (every other day) if necessary. Or, Venoglobulin-I 500 mg/kg (up to 2,000 mg/kg) daily for 2 to 7 days.
B-cell chronic lymphocytic leukemia (CLL)—
Adults: 400 mg/kg Gammagard S/D or Polygam S/D q 3 to 4 weeks.

Reactions may be *common*, uncommon, *life-threatening*, or COMMON AND LIFE-THREATENING.

Bone marrow transplantation—
Adults: 500 mg/kg Gamimune N (only) 7 and 2 days pretransplant, then weekly for 90 days post-transplant.
Pediatric HIV infection—
Children: 400 mg/kg Gamimune N (only) q 28 days.

ADVERSE REACTIONS
Systemic: headache, urticaria, malaise, fever, *anaphylaxis,* nausea, vomiting, chills, dyspnea, chest pain, hip pain, faintness, chest tightness, shortness of breath.
Other: pain, erythema, muscle stiffness at injection site.

INTERACTIONS
Live virus vaccines: length of time to wait before administering live virus vaccinations varies with dose of immune globulin given; see American Academy of Pediatrics recommendations.

EFFECTS ON DIAGNOSTIC TESTS
None reported.

CONTRAINDICATIONS
Contraindicated in patients hypersensitive to the drug.

NURSING CONSIDERATIONS
● Obtain history of allergies and reaction to immunizations. Make sure epinephrine 1:1,000 is available in case of anaphylaxis.
● **I.V. use:** Polygam S/D, Gammagard S/D, and Iveegam recommend use of 15-micron in-line filter.
● Know that most adverse effects are related to a rapid infusion rate.
● When giving I.M., use gluteal region. Doses over 10 ml should be divided and injected into several muscle sites to reduce pain and discomfort.
● Know that immune globulin should not be given for prophylaxis against hepatitis A if 6 weeks or more have elapsed since exposure or after onset of clinical illness.

☑ **PATIENT TEACHING**
● Explain to patient and family how drug will be administered.
● Tell patient that local reactions may occur at injection site. Instruct him to notify doctor promptly if adverse reactions persist or become severe.

---

rabies immune globulin, human
Hyperab, Imogam Rabies

Pregnancy Risk Category: C

HOW SUPPLIED
Injection: 150 IU/ml in 2-ml, 10-ml vials

ACTION
Provides passive immunity to rabies.

ONSET, PEAK, DURATION
Although onset and peak are not closely defined, an adequate titer of passive antibody is present 24 hours after injection. Exact duration unknown, but it is short.

INDICATIONS & DOSAGE
Rabies exposure—
Adults and children: 20 IU/kg I.M. at time of first dose of rabies vaccine. Half of dose is used to infiltrate wound area; the remainder is given I.M. in a different site.

ADVERSE REACTIONS
Systemic: slight fever, *anaphylaxis, angioedema, rash, nephrotic syndrome.*
Other: pain, redness, induration at injection site.

INTERACTIONS
Live virus vaccines (measles, mumps, rubella, or polio): interferes with response to vaccine. Delay immunization if possible.

EFFECTS ON DIAGNOSTIC TESTS
None reported.

CONTRAINDICATIONS
None known.

NURSING CONSIDERATIONS
● Use with caution in patients with history of prior systemic allergic reactions following the administration of human immunoglobulin preparations or in patients known to be hypersensitive to thimerosal or who have immunoglobulin A deficiency.
● Obtain history of animal bites, allergies, and reaction to immunizations. Have epinephrine 1:1,000 available to treat anaphylaxis.
● Ask patients when last tetanus immunization was received; many doctors order a booster at this time.
● Use only with rabies vaccine and immediate local treatment of wound. Don't give rabies vaccine and rabies immune globulin in same syringe or at same site. Give regardless of time between exposure and start of therapy.
● Don't administer live-virus vaccines within 3 months of rabies immune globulin.
● Don't administer more than 5 ml I.M. at one injection site; divide I.M. doses greater than 5 ml, and administer at different sites.
● Know that this immune serum provides passive immunity. Do not confuse this drug with rabies vaccine, which is a suspension of killed microorganisms used to confer active immunity. The two drugs are often given together prophylactically after exposure to rabid animals.
● Clean wound thoroughly with soap and water; this is the best prophylaxis against rabies.

☑ PATIENT TEACHING
● Inform patient that local reactions may occur at injection site. Instruct him to notify doctor promptly if reactions persist or become severe.
● Tell patient that a tetanus shot may also be necessary.

respiratory syncytial virus immune globulin intravenous, human (RSV-IGIV)
RespiGam

Pregnancy Risk Category: C

HOW SUPPLIED
Injection: 50 mg ±10 mg/ml in a 50-ml single-use vial

ACTION
Provides passive immunity to RSV.

ONSET, PEAK, DURATION
Unknown, although antibodies persist for at least 1 month.

INDICATIONS & DOSAGE
Prevention of serious lower respiratory tract infections caused by RSV in children with bronchopulmonary dysplasia (BPD) or history of premature birth—
Premature infants and children under 2 years: Single infusion monthly. Give 1.5 ml/kg/hour I.V. for 15 minutes; then, if clinical condition allows a higher rate, increase to 3 ml/kg/hour for 15 minutes and then to a maximum of 6 ml/kg/hour until infusion ends. Maximum recommended total dosage per monthly infusion is 750 mg/kg.

ADVERSE REACTIONS
CNS: dizziness, anxiety.
CV: fluid overload, tachycardia, hypertension, palpitations, chest tightness.
GI: vomiting, diarrhea, gastroenteritis, abdominal cramps.
Respiratory: respiratory distress, wheezing, rales, hypoxia, tachypnea, dyspnea.
Skin: rash, flushing, pruritus.
Other: fever, injection site inflammation, overdose effect, myalgia, arthralgia, *hypersensitivity reactions including anaphylaxis, angioneurotic edema.*

Reactions may be *common*, uncommon, *life-threatening*, or COMMON AND LIFE-THREATENING.

INTERACTIONS
Live-virus vaccines, such as mumps, rubella, and especially measles: may interfere with response. If such vaccines are given during or within 10 months after RSV-IGIV, be aware that reimmunization is recommended, if appropriate.

EFFECTS ON DIAGNOSTIC TESTS
None reported.

CONTRAINDICATIONS
Contraindicated in patients with history of severe hypersensitivity to drug or other human immunoglobulin and selective IgA deficiency.

NURSING CONSIDERATIONS
● Know that children with fluid overload should not receive drug.
● Safety and efficacy of drug have not been established in children with congenital heart disease (CHD). In clinical trials, children with CHD, especially those with right to left shunts, had an increased frequency of cardiac surgery and severe, life-threatening adverse reactions.
● Know that first dose should be given before RSV season begins and that subsequent doses should be given monthly throughout the RSV season to maintain protection. Children with RSV should continue to receive monthly doses for duration of RSV season.
● **I.V. use:** Drug does not contain a preservative. Single-use vial should be entered only once; do not shake, avoid foaming. Infusion should begin within 6 hours and be completed within 12 hours after vial is entered. Do not use if solution is turbid. Administer through I.V. line using a constant infusion pump. Predilution of drug before infusion is not recommended. Although filters are not necessary for the infusion, an in-line filter with a pore size larger than 15 micrometers may be used. Give the drug separately from other drugs.
● Adhere to infusion rate guidelines; most adverse reactions may be related

to the rate used. In especially ill children with BPD, slower rates may be indicated.
● Assess cardiopulmonary status and vital signs before beginning the infusion, before each rate increase, and every 30 minutes thereafter until 30 minutes after completion of the infusion.
● Monitor closely for signs of fluid overload. Children with BPD may be more prone to this condition. Report increases in heart rate, respiratory rate, retractions, or rales. Have a loop diuretic, such as furosemide or bumetanide, available.
Alert: If patient develops hypotension, anaphylaxis, or severe allergic reaction, stop infusion and administer epinephrine (1:1,000), as ordered. Know that patients with selective IgA deficiency can develop antibodies to IgA and have anaphylactic or allergic reactions to subsequent administration of blood products containing IgA, including RSV-IGIV.

☑ PATIENT TEACHING
● Explain to parents the importance of their child receiving drug monthly throughout the RSV season, even if already infected.
● Tell parents how drug is administered and which adverse reactions are associated with administration. Instruct parents to report adverse reactions promptly.

Rh₀(D) immune globulin, human

Gamulin Rh, HypRho-D, HypRho D-MiniDose, MICRhoGAM, Mini-Gamulin Rh, RhoGAM

Rh₀(D) immune globulin intravenous, human
WinRho SD

Pregnancy Risk Category: C

HOW SUPPLIED
Rh₀(D) immune globulin, human
Injection: 300 mcg of Rh₀(D) immune globulin/vial (standard dose); 50 mcg of

$Rh_o(D)$ immune globulin/vial (micro-dose)
$Rh_o(D)$ immune globulin I.V., human
Injection: 120 mcg, 300 mcg

ACTION
Suppresses the active antibody response and formation of anti-$Rh_o(D)$ antibodies in $Rh_o(D)$-negative, D^u-negative persons exposed to Rh-positive blood. $Rh_o(D)$ immune globulin I.V. may form complexes with RBCs blocking platelet destruction in adults who are $Rh_o(D)$ antigen-positive. However, the mechanism of action is not completely understoood.

ONSET, PEAK, DURATION
Unknown.

INDICATIONS & DOSAGE
$Rh_o(D)$ immune globulin, human
Rh exposure—
Adults (after abortion, miscarriage, ectopic pregnancy; or postpartum): transfusion unit or blood bank determines fetal packed RBC volume entering patient's blood; then one vial I.M. is given if fetal packed RBC volume is less than 15 ml. More than one vial I.M. may be required if large fetomaternal hemorrhage occurs; must be given within 72 hours after delivery or miscarriage.
Transfusion accidents—
Adults and children: consult blood bank or transfusion unit at once; must be given within 72 hours.
After postabortion or miscarriage to prevent Rh antibody formation—
Adults: consult transfusion unit or blood bank. One microdose vial will suppress immune reaction to 2.5 ml $Rh_o(D)$-positive RBCs. Ideally, should be given within 3 hours, but may be given up to 72 hours after abortion or miscarriage.
$Rh_o(D)$ immune globulin I.V., human
Rh exposure—
Adults (after abortion, aminocentesis [after 34 weeks gestation], or any other manipulation late in pregnancy [after 34 weeks gestation] associated with increased risk of Rh isoimmu-nization): 120 mcg I.M. or I.V.; must be given within 72 hours after delivery, miscarriage, or manipulation.
Pregnancy—
Adults: 300 mcg (WinRho SD) I.M. or I.V. at 28 weeks gestation. If administered early in the pregnancy, additional doses should be given at 12-week intervals to maintain adequate levels of passively acquired anti-Rh antibodies. Then, within 72 hours of delivery, 120 mcg should be given I.M. or I.V. If 72 hours have elapsed, drug should be given as soon as possible, up to 28 days.
Transfusion accidents—
Adults: 600 mcg I.V q 8 hours or 1200 mcg I.M. q 12 hours until total dose administered. Total dose depends on volume of packed red blood cells or whole blood infused.
Immune thrombocytopenic purpura (ITP) in adults who are $Rh_o(D)$ antigen-positive—
Adults: initially 50 mcg/kg I.V. If hemoglobin is less than 10 g/dl, initial dose is reduced to 25 to 40 mcg/kg. Initial dose may be administered as a single dose or divided into two doses and administered on separate days. Then, 25 to 60 mcg/kg I.V. may be administered, as needed, to elevate platelet counts with specific dosage that's determined individually.

ADVERSE REACTIONS
Systemic: slight fever.
Other: discomfort at injection site, ***anaphylaxis.***

INTERACTIONS
Live virus vaccines: may interfere with response. Delay immunization if possible.

EFFECTS ON DIAGNOSTIC TESTS
None reported.

CONTRAINDICATIONS
Contraindicated in $Rh_o(D)$-positive or D^u-positive patients and those previous-

---

ly immunized to $Rh_o(D)$ blood factor. Also contraindicated in patients with anaphylactic or severe systemic reaction to human globulin.

NURSING CONSIDERATIONS
● Use extreme caution when administering drug to patients with IgA deficiency. Because of risk of the patient developing IgA antibodies and having an anaphylactic reaction, the doctor must weigh the potential benefits of treatment against the potential for hypersensitivity reactions.
● Obtain history of allergies and reaction to immunization. Be sure epinephrine 1:1,000 is available in case of anaphylaxis.
Alert: Immediately after delivery, send a sample of neonate's cord blood to laboratory for typing and crossmatching. Confirm if mother is $Rh_o(D)$-negative and D^u-negative. Administer drug to mother as ordered only if infant is $Rh_o(D)$-positive or Du-positive.
● **I.V. use:** Reconstitute *only* with 0.9% sodium chloride solution. Do *not* administer with other products.
● Keep in mind that this immune serum provides passive immunity to the patient exposed to Rh_o-positive fetal blood during pregnancy. Prevents formation of maternal antibodies (active immunity), which would endanger future Rh_o-positive pregnancies.
● Know that vaccination with live virus vaccines should be deferred for 3 months after administration of $Rh_o(D)$ immune globulin.
● Know that mini-dose preparations are recommended for every patient undergoing abortion or miscarriage up to 12 weeks' gestation unless she is $Rh_o(D)$-positive or D^u-positive or has Rh antibodies, or unless the father or fetus is Rh-negative.
● Refrigerate at 36° to 46° F (2° to 8° C) and use within 4 hours of reconstitution. Discard unused drug.

☑ PATIENT TEACHING
● Explain to patient how drug protects future Rh_o-positive fetuses, if used because of pregnancy or explain to patient drug use in condition indicated.
● Warn patient about adverse reactions associated with drug.

---

tetanus immune globulin, human
Hyper-Tet

Pregnancy Risk Category: C

HOW SUPPLIED
Injection: 250-unit vial or syringe

ACTION
Provides passive immunity to tetanus.

ONSET, PEAK, DURATION
Onset unknown. Peak levels occur 2 to 3 days after I.M. injection. Protection lasts about 4 weeks.

INDICATIONS & DOSAGE
Tetanus exposure—
Adults and children: 250 units I.M.
Tetanus treatment—
Adults and children: single doses of 3,000 to 6,000 units I.M. have been used. Optimal dosage schedules have not been established.

ADVERSE REACTIONS
Systemic: slight fever, *hypersensitivity reactions, anaphylaxis,* angioedema, nephrotic syndrome.
Other: pain, stiffness, erythema at injection site.

INTERACTIONS
None significant.

EFFECTS ON DIAGNOSTIC TESTS
None reported.

CONTRAINDICATIONS
Contraindicated in patients with thrombocytopenia or any coagulation disorder

---

that would contraindicate I.M. injection unless potential benefits outweigh the risks.

NURSING CONSIDERATIONS
● Use cautiously in patients with history of prior systemic allergic reactions following administration of human immunoglobulin preparations or those allergic to thimerosal.
● Obtain history of injury, tetanus immunizations, last tetanus toxoid injection, allergies, and reaction to immunizations. Have epinephrine 1:1,000 available to treat hypersensitivity reaction.
● Know that tetanus immune globulin is used only if wound is more than 24 hours old or patient has had fewer than two tetanus toxoid injections.
● Thoroughly clean wound and remove all foreign matter.
● Inject into deltoid muscle for adults and children 3 years and over and into anterolateral aspect of the thigh in neonates and children under 3 years.
● Do not confuse this drug with tetanus toxoid. Tetanus immune globulin is not a substitute for tetanus toxoid, which should be given at the same time to produce active immunization. Don't give at same site as toxoid.
● Be aware that antibodies remain at effective levels for about 4 weeks, which is several times the duration of equine antitetanus antibodies. This protects patients for the incubation period of most tetanus cases.

☑ PATIENT TEACHING
● Warn patient about local adverse reactions associated with drug.
● Instruct patient to report serious adverse reactions promptly.
● Advise patient to complete full series of tetanus immunizations.

varicella-zoster immune globulin (VZIG)

Pregnancy Risk Category: C

HOW SUPPLIED
Injection: 10% to 18% solution of the globulin fraction of human plasma containing 125 units of varicella-zoster virus antibody (volume is about 1.25 ml)

ACTION
Provides passive immunity to varicella-zoster virus.

ONSET, PEAK, DURATION
Unknown, although antibodies persist for at least 1 month.

INDICATIONS & DOSAGE
Passive immunization of susceptible immunodeficient patients after exposure to varicella (chickenpox or herpes zoster)—
Adults and children over 40 kg: 625 units I.M.
Children 30.1 to 40 kg: 500 units I.M.
Children 20.1 to 30 kg: 375 units I.M.
Children 10.1 to 20 kg: 250 units I.M.
Children to 10 kg: 125 units I.M.

ADVERSE REACTIONS
Systemic: GI distress, malaise, headache, respiratory distress, *anaphylaxis.*
Other: discomfort at injection site, rash.

INTERACTIONS
Live virus vaccines: may interfere with response. Defer vaccination for 3 months after administration of VZIG.

EFFECTS ON DIAGNOSTIC TESTS
None reported.

CONTRAINDICATIONS
Contraindicated in those with history of severe reaction to human immune serum

---

Reactions may be *common*, uncommon, *life-threatening*, or COMMON AND LIFE-THREATENING.

globulin or thrombocytopenia.

NURSING CONSIDERATIONS
● Obtain accurate patient history of allergies and reaction to immunization. Make sure epinephrine 1:1,000 is available in case of anaphylaxis.
● For maximum benefit, administer as soon as possible after presumed exposure. May be of benefit when given as late as 96 hours after exposure.
● Administer only by deep I.M. injection into a large muscle mass such as the gluteal muscle. Never administer I.V.
● Refrigerate vial.
● Although usually restricted to children under 15 years, be aware that VZIG may be administered to adolescents and adults if necessary.
● VZIG is not recommended for nonimmunosuppressed patients.
● VZIG provides passive immunity; do not confuse with varicella vaccine. Do not use these two drugs in combination.
● Be alert that drug is not commercially distributed. Available only from 20 regional U.S. distribution centers. These centers will distribute to Canada and overseas. Contact the Massachusetts Public Health Biologic Laboratories or The Centers for Disease Control and Prevention for more information.

☑ PATIENT TEACHING
● Warn patient about local adverse reactions associated with drug.
● Instruct patient to report serious adverse reactions to doctor promptly.

aldesleukin
epoetin alfa
filgrastim
interferon alfa-2a, recombinant
interferon alfa-2b, recombinant
interferon alfa-n3
interferon beta-1a
interferon beta-1b, recombinant
interferon gamma-1b
levamisole hydrochloride
sargramostim

COMBINATION PRODUCTS
None.

---

aldesleukin (interleukin-2, IL-2)
Proleukin

Pregnancy Risk Category: C

HOW SUPPLIED
Powder for injection: 22 million IU/vial

ACTION
Unknown, although stimulation of an immunologic host reaction to the tumor may be involved.

ONSET, PEAK, DURATION
Unknown, although tumor regression may continue up to 12 months following initiation of therapy.

INDICATIONS & DOSAGE
Metastatic renal cell carcinoma—
Adults: 600,000 IU/kg (0.037 mg/kg) I.V. q 8 hours for 5 days (total of 14 doses). After a 9-day rest, the sequence is repeated for another 14 doses. Repeat courses may be given after a rest period of at least 7 weeks.

ADVERSE REACTIONS
CNS: *headache, mental status changes,*
dizziness, sensory dysfunction, special senses disorders, syncope, motor dysfunction, **coma,** fatigue.
CV: *hypotension, sinus tachycardia, arrhythmias, bradycardia,* **PVCs,** *premature atrial contractions, myocardial ischemia,* **MI, CHF, cardiac arrest,** *myocarditis, endocarditis,* **CVA,** *pericardial effusion, thrombosis,* **capillary leak syndrome (CLS).**
EENT: *conjunctivitis.*
GI: *nausea, vomiting, diarrhea, stomatitis, anorexia, bleeding, dyspepsia, constipation.*
GU: *oliguria, anuria, proteinuria, hematuria, dysuria,* urine retention, urinary frequency.
Hematologic: *anemia,* THROMBOCYTOPENIA, LEUKOPENIA, *coagulation disorders,* leukocytosis, eosinophilia.
Hepatic: *jaundice;* ascites; hepatomegaly; *elevated bilirubin, serum transaminase, alkaline phosphatase levels.*
Respiratory: *pulmonary congestion, dyspnea, pulmonary edema,* **respiratory failure, pleural effusion, apnea, pneumothorax,** *tachypnea.*
Skin: *pruritus, erythema, rash, dryness, exfoliative dermatitis,* purpura, alopecia, petechiae.
Other: *elevated BUN and serum creatinine levels; hypomagnesemia; acidosis; hypocalcemia; hypophosphatemia; hypokalemia; hyperuricemia; hypoalbuminemia;* hypoproteinemia; *hyponatremia;* hyperkalemia; arthralgia; myalgia; *fever; chills; abdominal, chest, or back pain; weakness; malaise;* edema; *infections of catheter tip, urinary tract, or injection site; phlebitis;* SEPSIS; *weight gain;* weight loss.

INTERACTIONS
Antihypertensives: increased risk of hypotension. Monitor closely.

Reactions may be *common,* uncommon, *life-threatening,* or COMMON AND LIFE-THREATENING.

Cardiotoxic, hepatotoxic, myelotoxic, or nephrotoxic drugs: enhanced toxicity. Avoid concomitant use.

Corticosteroids: decreased antitumor effectiveness of aldesleukin. Avoid concomitant use.

Psychotropic agents: unpredictable interaction. Because aldesleukin can alter CNS function, use together cautiously.

EFFECTS ON DIAGNOSTIC TESTS
No direct laboratory test interference has been reported. Toxic effects of drug may be seen in decreasing hepatic, renal, and thyroid function tests; abnormal serum electrolytes; or abnormal cardiac or pulmonary function tests.

CONTRAINDICATIONS
Contraindicated in patients hypersensitive to the drug or any component of the formulation and in patients with abnormal cardiac (thallium) stress test or pulmonary function tests or organ allografts. Retreatment is contraindicated in patients who experience any of the following adverse effects: pericardial tamponade; disturbances in cardiac rhythm that were uncontrolled or unresponsive to intervention; sustained ventricular tachycardia (five beats or more); chest pain accompanied by ECG changes, indicating MI or angina pectoris; renal dysfunction requiring dialysis for 72 hours or more; coma or toxic psychosis lasting 48 hours or more; seizures that were repetitive or difficult to control; ischemia or perforation of the bowel; GI bleeding requiring surgery.

NURSING CONSIDERATIONS
● This drug should not be used unless the patient has had definitive tests documenting normal cardiac and pulmonary function. Use with extreme caution in patients with normal test results if they have a history of cardiac or pulmonary disease and in patients with a history of seizure disorders.

● Use cautiously and with close clinical monitoring because severe adverse effects usually accompany therapy at the recommended dosage.

● Use cautiously in patients who require large volumes of fluid (such as patients with hypercalcemia).

● Know that drug should be administered only in a hospital under the direction of a doctor experienced in the use of chemotherapeutic agents. An intensive care facility and intensive care or cardiopulmonary specialists must be available.

● Monitor hematologic tests, including CBC, differential, and platelet counts; serum electrolyte levels; and renal and liver function tests, and obtain chest X-ray before therapy, as ordered. Repeat daily during therapy.

● Treat patients with bacterial infections before therapy, as ordered.

● **I.V. use:** To avoid altering the pharmacologic properties of the drug, reconstitute and dilute carefully, and follow manufacturer's recommendations. Do not mix with other drugs or albumin.

● Reconstitute the vial containing 22 million IU (1.3 mg) with 1.2 ml of sterile water for injection. Do not use bacteriostatic water or 0.9% sodium chloride for injection; these diluents increase aggregation of drug. Direct the stream at the sides of the vial and gently swirl to reconstitute. Do not shake. The reconstituted solution will have a concentration of 18 million IU (1.1 mg)/ml. It should be particle-free and colorless to slightly yellow.

● Add the ordered dose of reconstituted drug to 50 ml of D_5W and infuse over 15 minutes. Do not use an in-line filter. Plastic infusion bags are preferred because they provide consistent drug delivery.

● Discard unused portion. Vials are for single-dose use and contain no preservatives.

● Refrigerate powder for injection or reconstituted solutions. Return drug to room temperature before administering to patients. After reconstitution and dilution, administer within 48 hours.

• Be prepared to adjust dosage of other drugs as ordered to compensate for renal and hepatic impairment occurring during treatment. Know that dosage is modified by withholding a dose or interrupting therapy rather than by reducing the dose, as ordered.

• Withhold dose and notify doctor if patient develops moderate to severe lethargy or somnolence; continued administration can result in coma.

• Administer packed RBCs or platelets, as ordered. Severe anemia or thrombocytopenia may occur.

Alert: Know that this drug has been associated with CLS, a condition caused by the loss of vascular tone, in which plasma proteins and fluids escape into the extravascular space. Mean arterial blood pressure begins to drop within 2 to 12 hours of treatment; edema and effusions may be severe, and death can result from hypoperfusion of major organs. Other conditions that accompany CLS include arrhythmias, MI, angina, mental status changes, renal insufficiency, respiratory distress or failure, and GI bleeding or infarction.

• Therapy is associated with impaired neutrophil function, which can lead to disseminated infection. Many studies employed prophylactic antibiotic therapy with oxacillin, nafcillin, ciprofloxacin, or vancomycin; check protocol and administer antibiotics, as ordered. Monitor for infection.

• Know that patients should be neurologically stable with a negative computed tomography scan for CNS metastases. Drug may exacerbate symptoms in patients with unrecognized or undiagnosed CNS metastases.

☑ PATIENT TEACHING

• Explain administration schedule to patient and caregivers, and stress importance of compliance.

• Instruct patient to report adverse reactions promptly.

epoetin alfa (erythropoietin)
Epogen, Procrit

Pregnancy Risk Category: C

HOW SUPPLIED
Injection: 2,000 units/ml, 3,000 units/ml, 4,000 units/ml, 10,000 units/ml

ACTION
Mimics the effects of erythropoietin, a naturally occurring hormone produced by the kidneys. Epoetin alfa is one of the factors controlling the rate of RBC production. It acts on the erythroid tissues in the bone marrow, stimulating mitotic activity of erythroid progenitor cells and early precursor cells. It functions as a growth factor and as a differentiating factor, enhancing rate of RBC production.

ONSET, PEAK, DURATION
Increase in reticulocyte count occurs within 7 to 10 days; RBC count, hematocrit, and hemoglobin increase in 2 to 6 weeks. Serum levels peak immediately after I.V. infusion or within 4 to 24 hours after S.C. administration. Hematocrit level may begin to decrease about 2 weeks after discontinuation.

INDICATIONS & DOSAGE
Anemia due to reduced production of endogenous erythropoietin caused by end-stage renal disease—
Adults: dosage is individualized. Starting dose is 50 to 100 units/kg I.V. three times weekly. (Nondialysis patients with chronic renal failure or patients receiving continuous peritoneal dialysis may receive the drug by S.C. injection or I.V.) Dosage is reduced when target hematocrit level is reached or if the hematocrit rises more than 4 points in any 2-week period. Dosage is increased if hematocrit does not increase by 5 to 6 points after 8 weeks of therapy. Maintenance dosage is highly individualized.

Reactions may be *common,* uncommon, *life-threatening,* or COMMON AND LIFE-THREATENING.

Adjunctive treatment of HIV-infected patients with anemia secondary to zidovudine therapy—
Adults: 100 units/kg I.V. or S.C. three times weekly for 8 weeks or until target hemoglobin level is reached. If response is not satisfactory after 8 weeks, dose may be increased by 50 to 100 units/kg I.V. or S.C. three times weekly. After 4 to 8 weeks, dosage may be further increased in increments of 50 to 100 units/kg three times weekly, up to a maximum of 300 units/kg I.V. or S.C. three times weekly.

Anemia secondary to cancer chemotherapy—
Adults: 150 units/kg S.C. three times weekly for 8 weeks or until target hemoglobin level is reached. If response is not satisfactory after 8 weeks, dosage may be increased up to 300 units/kg S.C. three times weekly.

❋ *New indication: Reduction of need for allogeneic blood transfusion in anemic patients scheduled to undergo elective, noncardiac, nonvascular surgery—*
Adults: 300 units/kg/day S.C. daily for 10 days before surgery, on day of surgery, and for 4 days after surgery. Alternatively, 600 units/kg S.C. in once-weekly doses (21, 14, and 7 days before surgery), plus a fourth dose on day of surgery.

ADVERSE REACTIONS
CNS: *headache, seizures, paresthesia, fatigue,* dizziness.
CV: *hypertension, edema.*
GI: *nausea, vomiting, diarrhea.*
Respiratory: *cough, shortness of breath.*
Skin: *rash,* urticaria.
Other: increased clotting of arterio-venous grafts, *pyrexia, arthralgia, cough, injection site reactions, asthenia.*

INTERACTIONS
None significant.

EFFECTS ON DIAGNOSTIC TESTS
Moderate increases in BUN, uric acid, creatinine, phosphorous, and potassium levels have been reported.

CONTRAINDICATIONS
Contraindicated in patients with uncontrolled hypertension, hypersensitivity to mammalian cell-derived products or albumin (human).

NURSING CONSIDERATIONS
● Monitor blood pressure before therapy. Up to 80% of patients with chronic renal failure have hypertension. Blood pressure may rise, especially when the hematocrit level is increasing in the early part of therapy.
● **I.V. use:** Give by direct injection without dilution. Solution contains no preservatives. Discard unused portion. Do not mix with other drugs.
● When used in HIV-infected patients, be prepared to individualize dosage based on response, as ordered. Dosage recommendations are for patients with endogenous erythropoietin levels of 500 units/L or less and cumulative zidovudine doses of 4.2 g/week or less.
● Be aware that patients treated with epoetin alfa may require additional heparin to prevent clotting during dialysis treatments.
● Monitor blood count, as ordered. Hematocrit level may rise and cause excessive clotting.
● Institute diet restrictions or drug therapy to control blood pressure. Reduce dosage in patients who exhibit a rapid rise in hematocrit (more than 4 points in any 2-week period), as ordered, to prevent hypertension.
● Know that the patient's response to epoetin alfa depends on the amount of endogenous erythropoietin in the plasma. Patients with levels of 500 units/L or more usually have transfusion-dependent anemia and will probably not respond to the drug. Those with levels below 500 units/L usually respond well.
● Be aware that patients should receive adequate iron supplementation beginning no later than when epoetin

---

*Liquid contains alcohol.   **May contain tartrazine.   †Canada only.   ‡Australia only.   ◊ OTC.

alfa treatment starts and continuing throughout therapy.

● Keep in mind that patients with end-stage renal disease may experience an improved appetite and enhanced well-being as a result of increased hematocrit level.

☑ PATIENT TEACHING
● After injection (usually within 2 hours), inform patient that pain or discomfort in limbs (long bones) and pelvis and coldness and sweating are not uncommon. Symptoms may persist up to 12 hours and then disappear.
● Advise patient that blood specimens will be drawn weekly for blood counts and that dosage adjustments may be made based on the results.
● Advise patient to avoid driving or operating heavy machinery during initiation of therapy. A relationship between excessively rapid hematocrit rise and seizures may exist.

---

filgrastim (granulocyte colony-stimulating factor; G-CSF)
Neupogen

Pregnancy Risk Category: C

HOW SUPPLIED
Injection: 300 mcg/ml

ACTION
A glycoprotein that stimulates proliferation and differentiation of hematopoietic cells. Filgrastim is specific for neutrophils.

ONSET, PEAK, DURATION
Onset occurs in 5 to 60 minutes. Serum levels peak in 2 to 8 hours (S.C.) or 24 hours (I.V.). Effects decline by 50% in first 24 hours after drug is discontinued, and absolute neutrophil count returns to pretreatment levels within 1 to 7 days.

INDICATIONS & DOSAGE
To decrease incidence of infection in patients with nonmyeloid malignant disease receiving myelosuppressive antineoplastic agents—
Adults and children: 5 mcg/kg/day I.V. or S.C. as a single dose given no sooner than 24 hours after cytotoxic chemotherpy. Doses may be increased in increments of 5 mcg/kg for each chemotherapy cycle depending on the duration and severity of the nadir of the absolute neutrophil count (ANC).
To decrease incidence of infection in patients with nonmyeloid malignant disease receiving myelosuppressive antineoplastic agents followed by bone marrow transplantation—
Adults and children: 10 mcg/kg/day I.V. or S.C. at least 24 hours after cytotoxic chemotherapy and bone marrow infusion. Subsequent dosages adjusted according to the neutrophil response.
Congenital neutropenia—
Adults: 6 mcg/kg S.C. b.i.d. Dosage adjusted according to patient's response.
Idiopathic or cyclic neutropenia—
Adults: 5 mcg/kg S.C. daily. Dosage adjusted according to patient's response.
Peripheral blood progenitor cell (PBPC) collection and therapy in cancer patients—
Adults: 10 mcg/kg/day S.C. Give 4 days before leukapheresis and continue until last leukapheresis.

ADVERSE REACTIONS
CNS: headache, weakness.
CV: *MI,* arrhythmias, chest pain.
GI: *nausea, vomiting, diarrhea, mucositis,* stomatitis, constipation.
Hematologic: *thrombocytopenia,* leukocytosis.
Respiratory: dyspnea, cough.
Skin: *alopecia,* rash, cutaneous vasculitis.
Other: *skeletal pain, fever, fatigue, hypersensitivity reactions.*

INTERACTIONS
Chemotherapeutic agents: rapidly di-

---

viding myeloid cells are potentially sensitive to cytotoxic agents. Do not use within 24 hours before or after a dose of one of these agents.

EFFECTS ON DIAGNOSTIC TESTS
WBC counts may be increased to $100,000/mm^3$ or more. Transient increases in neutrophils, as well as reversible elevations in uric acid, lactate dehydrogenase, and alkaline phosphatase levels, have been noted. Transient decreases in blood pressure and increases in serum creatinine and aminotransferase levels were also reported.

CONTRAINDICATIONS
Contraindicated in patients hypersensitive to proteins derived from *Escherichia coli* or to the drug or its components.

NURSING CONSIDERATIONS
● Obtain baseline CBC and platelet count before therapy, as ordered.
● **I.V. use:** Dilute in 50 to 100 ml of D_5W and give by intermittent infusion over 15 to 60 minutes or continuous infusion over 24 hours. If the final concentration of the drug is going to be 2 to 15 mcg/ml, add albumin at a concentration of 2 mg/ml (0.2%) to minimize binding of the drug to plastic containers or tubing.
● Once a dose is withdrawn, do not reenter vial. Discard unused portion. Vials are for single-dose use and contain no preservatives.
● Refrigerate at 36° to 46° F (2° to 8° C). Do not freeze; avoid shaking. Store at room temperature for a maximum of 6 hours; discard after 6 hours.
● Obtain CBC and platelet count twice weekly during therapy, as ordered. Patients who receive this drug may potentially receive high doses of chemotherapy, which may increase the risk of toxicities.
● Be aware that a transiently increased neutrophil count is common 1 or 2 days after initiation of therapy. Give daily for

up to 2 weeks or until the ANC has returned to $10,000/mm^3$ after the expected chemotherapy-induced neutrophil nadir, as ordered.

☑ **PATIENT TEACHING**
● If patient will be self-administering the drug, teach him how to administer it and how to dispose of used needles, syringes, drug containers, and unused medicine.
● Instruct patient to report persistent or serious adverse reactions promptly.

---

interferon alfa-2a, recombinant (rIFN-A)
Roferon-A

Pregnancy Risk Category: C

HOW SUPPLIED
Injection: 3 million IU/vial; 18 and 36 million IU/multiple-dose vial

ACTION
Unknown. Appears to involve direct antiproliferative action against tumor cells or viral cells to inhibit replication and modulation of host immune response by enhancing the phagocytic activity of macrophages and by augmenting specific cytotoxicity of lymphocytes for target cells.

ONSET, PEAK, DURATION
Onset unknown. Peak levels occur 3.8 hours after I.M. administration or 7.3 hours after S.C. administration. Duration unknown.

INDICATIONS & DOSAGE
Hairy-cell leukemia—
Adults: for induction, 3 million IU S.C. or I.M. daily for 16 to 24 weeks. For maintenance, 3 million IU S.C. or I.M. three times a week.
AIDS-related Kaposi's sarcoma—
Adults: for induction, 36 million IU S.C. or I.M. daily for 10 to 12 weeks. For maintenance, 36 million IU S.C. or

I.M. three times a week.
Philadelphia chromosome-positive chronic myelogenous leukemia—
Adults: initially, 3 million IU daily for 3 days; then 6 million IU for 3 days, then 9 million IU for the duration of treatment.

ADVERSE REACTIONS
CNS: *dizziness, confusion,* paresthesia, numbness, lethargy, *depression, decreased mental status,* forgetfulness, **coma,** nervousness, insomnia, sedation, apathy, anxiety, irritability, fatigue, vertigo, gait disturbances, incoordination.
CV: hypotension, chest pain, arrhythmias, palpitations, syncope, **CHF,** hypertension, edema, **MI.**
EENT: *dryness or inflammation of the oropharynx,* rhinorrhea, sinusitis, conjunctivitis, earache, eye irritation.
GI: *anorexia, nausea, diarrhea, vomiting,* abdominal fullness, *abdominal pain,* flatulence, constipation, hypermotility, gastric distress, *weight loss, change in taste.*
GU: transient impotence.
Hematologic: *leukopenia,* mild **thrombocytopenia.**
Hepatic: *hepatitis.*
Respiratory: *cough, dyspnea.*
Skin: *rash, dryness, pruritus, partial alopecia,* urticaria, flushing.
Other: inflammation at injection site (rare), *flulike syndrome (fever, fatigue, myalgia, headache, chills, arthralgia),* diaphoresis, excessive salivation, cyanosis, night sweats, hot flashes.

INTERACTIONS
Aminophylline, theophylline: may reduce theophylline clearance. Monitor serum levels.
CNS depressants: enhanced CNS effects. Avoid concomitant use.
Live virus vaccine: increased risk of adverse reactions and decreased antibody response. Don't use together.

EFFECTS ON DIAGNOSTIC TESTS
Drug therapy may cause mild and transient changes in blood pressure (hypotension is likely). Interferons may decrease hemoglobin, hematocrit, leukocyte counts, platelets, and neutrophils (dose-related; recovery occurs within several days or weeks after drug withdrawal). Drug may increase PT and partial thromboplastin time (dose-related); ALT, AST, lactic dehydrogenase, and alkaline phosphatase levels (dose-related; reversibile on drug withdrawal); and serum calcium, serum phosphorous, and fasting blood glucose levels.

CONTRAINDICATIONS
Contraindicated in patients hypersensitive to the drug or to murine (mouse) immunoglobulin.

NURSING CONSIDERATIONS
● Use cautiously in patients with severe hepatic or renal function impairment, seizure disorders, compromised CNS function, cardiac disease, or myelosuppression.
● Obtain allergy history. Drug contains phenol as a preservative and serum albumin as a stabilizer.
● Use S.C. administration route in patients whose platelet count is below 50,000/mm^3.
● Administer at bedtime to minimize daytime drowsiness.
● Make sure patients are well hydrated, especially during initial stages of treatment.
● At the beginning of therapy, assess patients for flulike symptoms, which tend to diminish with continued therapy. Premedicate with acetaminophen to minimize symptoms.
● Monitor for CNS adverse reactions, such as decreased mental status and dizziness, during therapy.
● For patients who develop thrombocytopenia, exercise extreme care in performing invasive procedures; inspect injection site and skin frequently for signs of bruising; limit frequency of I.M. injections; test urine, emesis fluid, stool, and secretions for occult blood.

• Keep in mind that severe adverse reactions may require dosage reduction to one-half or discontinuation of therapy until reactions subside.

• Know that different brands of interferon may not be equivalent and may require different dosage.

Alert: Neurotoxicity and cardiotoxicity are more common in elderly patients, especially those with underlying CNS or cardiac impairment.

• Be alert that use with blood dyscrasia causing medications, bone marrow suppressant, or radiation therapy may increase bone marrow suppressant effects. Dosage reduction may be required.

• Refrigerate the drug.

☑ **PATIENT TEACHING**

• Advise patient that laboratory tests will be performed before and periodically during therapy. Tests include a CBC with differential, platelet count, blood chemistry and electrolyte studies, liver function tests, and, if he has a pre-existing cardiac disorder or advanced stages of cancer, ECGs.

• Instruct patient in proper oral hygiene during treatment because the bone marrow suppressant effects of interferon may lead to microbial infection, delayed healing, and gingival bleeding. This drug may also decrease salivary flow.

• Emphasize need to follow the doctor's instructions about taking and recording temperature and how and when to take acetaminophen.

• Advise patient to check with the doctor for instructions after missing a dose.

• Tell patient that drug may cause temporary loss of some hair, which should return when drug is withdrawn.

• If patient will be self-administering drug, teach him how to prepare and administer it and how to dispose of used needles, syringes, containers, and unused medication.

interferon alfa-2b, recombinant (IFN-alpha 2)
Intron A

Pregnancy Risk Category: C

HOW SUPPLIED
Powder for injection: 3 million IU/vial with diluent, 5 million IU/vial with diluent, 10 million IU/vial with diluent, 18 million IU/vial with diluent, 25 million IU/vial with diluent, 50 million IU/vial with diluent
Injection: 10 million IU/2-ml, 18 million IU/3-ml, 25 million IU/5-ml vials

ACTION
Unknown. Appears to involve direct antiproliferative action against tumor cells or viral cells to inhibit replication, and modulation of host immune response by enhancing the phagocytic activity of macrophages and by augmenting specific cytotoxicity of lymphocytes for target cells.

ONSET, PEAK, DURATION
Onset and duration unknown. Serum levels peak in 3 to 12 hours.

INDICATIONS & DOSAGE
Hairy-cell leukemia—
Adults: 2 million IU/m^2 I.M. or S.C., three times a week.
Condylomata acuminata (genital or venereal warts)—
Adults: 1 million IU for each lesion intralesionally three times a week for 3 weeks.
AIDS-related Kaposi's sarcoma—
Adults: 30 million IU/m^2 S.C. or I.M. three times a week.
Chronic hepatitis B—
Adults: 30 to 35 million IU weekly I.M. or S.C., administered either as 5 million IU daily or 10 million IU three times a week for 16 weeks.
Chronic hepatitis non A, non B/C (NANB/C)—
Adults: 3 million IU I.M. or S.C. three

---

*Liquid contains alcohol.   **May contain tartrazine.   †Canada only.   ‡Australia only.   ◇OTC.

times a week.

✳ **New indication:** *Adjunct to surgical treatment in patients with malignant melanoma who are asymptomatic postsurgery but at high risk for systemic recurrence for up to 8 weeks after surgery—*
Adults: initially, 20 million IU/m² by I.V. infusion 5 consecutive days a week for 4 weeks, followed by maintenance dose of 10 million IU/m² S.C. three times a week for 48 weeks.

ADVERSE REACTIONS
CNS: *dizziness, confusion, paresthesia,* lethargy, *depression, difficulty in thinking or concentrating, insomnia,* anxiety, *fatigue, hypoesthesia, amnesia,* nervousness, *somnolence,* weakness, *malaise.*
CV: hypotension, *chest pain.*
EENT: visual disturbances, hearing disorders, pharyngitis, *nasal congestion, sinusitis,* rhinitis, stye.
GI: *anorexia, nausea, diarrhea, vomiting,* abdominal pain, *dyspepsia,* constipation, loose stools, eructation, *dry mouth,* dysgeusia, stomatitis, gingivitis.
GU: transient impotence, gynecomastia.
Hematologic: *leukopenia,* anemia, ***thrombocytopenia.***
Respiratory: *dyspnea, coughing.*
Skin: *rash, dryness, pruritus, alopecia,* moniliasis, flushing, dermatitis.
Other: *flulike symptoms (fever, fatigue, headache, chills, muscle aches), arthralgia, asthenia, rigors, back pain, increased diaphoresis.*

INTERACTIONS
Aminophylline, theophylline: may reduce theophylline clearance. Monitor serum concentrations.
CNS depressants: enhanced CNS effects. Avoid concomitant use.
Live virus vaccines: risk of enhanced adverse reactions to vaccine or decreased antibody response. Postpone immunization.
Zidovudine: may be synergistic adverse effects (higher incidence of neutrope-

nia). Carefully monitor WBC count.

EFFECTS ON DIAGNOSTIC TESTS
Drug therapy may cause mild and transient changes in blood pressure (hypotension is likely). Interferons may decrease hemoglobin, hematocrit, leukocyte counts, platelets, and neutrophils (dose-related; recovery occurs within several days or weeks after drug withdrawal). Drug may increase PT and partial thromboplastin time (dose-related); ALT, AST, lactic dehydrogenase, and alkaline phosphatase levels (dose-related; reversibile on drug withdrawal); and serum calcium, serum phosphorous, and fasting blood glucose levels.

CONTRAINDICATIONS
Contraindicated in patients hypersensitive to the drug.

NURSING CONSIDERATIONS
● Use cautiously in patients with a history of CV disease, pulmonary disease, diabetes mellitus, coagulation disorders, and severe myelosuppression.
● Use S.C. administration route in patients whose platelet count is below 50,000/mm³.
● Administer at bedtime to minimize daytime drowsiness.
● When administering interferon for condylomata acuminata, use only 10-million-IU vial because dilution of other strengths required for intralesional use results in a hypertonic solution. Do not reconstitute 10-million-IU vial with more than 1 ml of diluent. Use tuberculin or similar syringe and 25G to 30G needle. Do not inject too deeply beneath lesion or too superficially. As many as five lesions can be treated at one time. To ease discomfort, administer in evening with acetaminophen.
● Make sure patients are well hydrated, especially during initial treatment.
● At the beginning of treatment, monitor most patients for flulike symptoms, which tend to diminish with continued therapy. Premedicate with acetamino-

---

phen to minimize flulike symptoms.
● Periodically monitor for adverse CNS reactions, such as decreased mental status and dizziness, during therapy.
● For patients who develop thrombocytopenia: exercise extreme care in performing invasive procedures; inspect injection site and skin frequently for signs of bruising; limit frequency of I.M. injections; test urine, emesis fluid, stool, and secretions for occult blood.
● Keep in mind that severe adverse reactions may require dosage reduction to one-half or discontinuation of therapy until reactions subside.
Alert: Be aware that neurotoxicity and cardiotoxicity are more common in elderly patients, especially those with underlying CNS or cardiac impairment.
● Be alert that use with blood dyscrasiaↁcausing medications, bone marrow suppressants, or radiation therapy may increase bone marrow suppressant effects. Dosage reduction may be required.
● Refrigerate the drug.
● Keep in mind that maximum response usually occurs 4 to 8 weeks after initiation of therapy. If results are not satisfactory after 12 to 16 weeks, a second course may be instituted. Patients with 6 to 10 condylomata may receive a second course of treatment; patients with more than 10 condylomata may receive additional courses.

☑ PATIENT TEACHING
● Advise patient to avoid contact with persons with viral illness. The patient is at increased risk for infection during therapy.
● Advise patient that laboratory tests will be performed before and periodically during therapy. Tests include a CBC with differential, platelet count, blood chemistry and electrolyte studies, liver function tests, and, if he has a pre-existing cardiac disorder or advanced stages of cancer, ECGs.
● Instruct patient in proper oral hygiene during treatment because the bone mar-

row suppressant effects of interferon may lead to microbial infection, delayed healing, and gingival bleeding. This drug may also decrease salivary flow.
● Advise patient to check with the doctor for instructions after missing a dose.
● Emphasize need to follow the doctor's instructions about taking and recording temperature and how and when to take acetaminophen.
● If patient will be self-administering drug, teach him how to prepare the injection and how to use a disposable syringe. Give him information on drug stability.
● Tell patient drug may cause temporary loss of some hair, which should return when drug is withdrawn.

---

interferon alfa-n3
Alferon N

Pregnancy Risk Category: C

HOW SUPPLIED
Injection: 5 million units/ml in 1-ml vials

ACTION
A naturally occurring antiviral agent derived from human leukocytes. It attaches to membrane receptors and causes cellular changes, including increased protein synthesis.

ONSET, PEAK, DURATION
Unknown.

INDICATIONS & DOSAGE
Condylomata acuminata (genital or venereal warts)—
Adults: 0.05 ml for each wart by intralesional injection. Treatment usually continues twice weekly for up to 8 weeks. Dosage should not exceed 0.5 ml (2.5 million units) per session.

ADVERSE REACTIONS
CNS: dizziness, light-headedness, insomnia, depression.

CV: hypotension.
GI: dyspepsia, heartburn, vomiting, nausea, diarrhea.
Other: *acute hypersensitivity reactions with mild to moderate flulike syndrome (myalgia, fever, chills, fatigue, headache), arthralgia, back pain, malaise, soreness at injection site, chest pains.*

INTERACTIONS
None significant.

EFFECTS ON DIAGNOSTIC TESTS
Drug therapy may cause mild and transient changes in blood pressure (hypotension is likely). Interferon may decrease hemoglobin and hematocrit levels and leukocyte, platelet, and neutrophil counts. Drug may increase PT and PTT (dose-related) and ALT, AST, lactate dehydrogenase, and alkaline phosphatase levels (dose-related; reversible on drug withdrawal).

CONTRAINDICATIONS
Contraindicated in patients hypersensitive to interferon alfa and in those with a history of anaphylactic reactions to murine (mouse) immunoglobulin, egg protein, or neomycin.

NURSING CONSIDERATIONS
● Use cautiously in patients with debilitating illnesses (uncontrolled CHF, unstable angina, severe pulmonary disease, coagulation disorders, seizure disorders, severe myelosuppression, or diabetes mellitus with ketoacidosis) because of the association of interferon with a flulike syndrome.
● Although anaphylaxis hasn't been reported, be prepared to treat acute hypersensitivity reactions.
● Inject each lesion at the base of the wart, using a 30G needle.
● Administer acetaminophen for flulike symptoms.

☑ **PATIENT TEACHING**
● Teach patient how to recognize symptoms of hypersensitivity: urticaria, tight-

ness of the chest, wheezing, shortness of breath. Tell him to report such symptoms immediately.
● Explain to patient that warts will continue to disappear after completion of 8 weeks of therapy and discontinuation of drug.

▼ *NEW DRUG*

interferon beta-1a
Avonex

Pregnancy Risk Category: C

HOW SUPPLIED
Lyophilized powder for injection: 33 mcg (6.6 million IU)

ACTION
Mechanisms by which interferon beta-1a exerts its actions in multiple sclerosis are not clearly understood. The biological response-modifying properties of interferon beta-1a are mediated through its interactions with specific cell receptors found on the surface of human cells. The binding of these receptors induces the expression of a number of interferon-induced gene products believed to be the mediators of the biological actions of interferon beta-1a.

ONSET, PEAK, DURATION
Onset and duration unknown. Peak occurs within 3 to 15 hours.

INDICATIONS & DOSAGE
Treatment of relapsing forms of multiple sclerosis to slow the accumulation of physical disability and decrease the frequency of clinical exacerbation—
Adults: 30 mcg I.M. once weekly.

ADVERSE REACTIONS
CNS: *headache, sleep difficulty, dizziness,* syncope, suicidal tendency, seizure, speech disorder, ataxia.
CV: chest pain, vasodilation.
Respiratory: *upper respiratory tract in-*

Reactions may be *common*, uncommon, *life-threatening*, or COMMON AND LIFE-THREATENING.

fection, sinusitis, dyspnea.
EENT: otitis media, decreased hearing.
GI: *nausea, diarrhea, dyspepsia,* anorexia, abdominal pain.
GU: ovarian cyst, vaginitis.
Hematologic: anemia, elevated eosinophil levels, decreased hematocrit.
Musculoskeletal: *muscle ache,* muscle spasm, arthralgia.
Skin: ecchymosis at injection site, urticaria, alopecia, nevus, herpes zoster, herpes simplex.
Other: *flulike symptoms, pain, fever, asthenia, chills, infection,* injection site reaction, malaise, hypersensitivity reaction, elevated AST levels.

INTERACTIONS
None reported.

EFFECTS ON DIAGNOSTIC TESTS
None reported.

CONTRAINDICATIONS
Contraindicated in patients with history of hypersensitivity to natural or recombinant interferon beta, human albumin, or any other component of the formulation.

NURSING CONSIDERATIONS
● Use cautiously in patients with depression, seizure disorders, or severe cardiac conditions.
● Be aware that safety and efficacy of interferon beta-1a in chronic progressive multiple sclerosis or in children under age 18 have not been established.
● Monitor patients closely for depression and suicidal ideation. It is not known if these symptoms are related to the underlying neurologic basis of multiple sclerosis or to interferon beta-1a.
● Monitor WBC counts, platelet counts, and blood chemistries, including liver function tests.
● To reconstitute drug, inject 1.1 ml of the supplied diluent (sterile water for injection) into vial and gently swirl to dissolve drug. Do not shake.
● Interferon beta-1a should be used as

soon as possible but may be used within 6 hours after being reconstituted if stored at 36° to 46° F (2° to 8° C.).
● Vials should be stored in the refrigerator. If a refrigerator is unavailable, drug can be stored at 77° F (25° C) for up to 30 days. Drug should not be exposed to high temperatures or frozen.
● It is not known whether interferon beta-1a is excreted in breast milk. Because of the potential for serious adverse reactions in breast-fed infants, a decision whether to discontinue breastfeeding or the drug must be made.

☑ **PATIENT TEACHING**
● Teach patient and family member how to reconstitute the drug and administer I.M.
● Caution patient not to change dosage or the schedule of administration. If a dose is missed, tell him to take it as soon as he remembers. The regular schedule may then be resumed. Two injections should not be administered within 2 days of each other.
● Instruct patient how to store the drug.
● Inform patient that flulike symptoms are not uncommon following initiation of therapy. Acetaminophen 650 mg P.O. may be taken immediately prior to injection and for an additional 24 hours after each injection, as ordered, to lessen the severity of flulike symptoms.
● Advise patient to report depression, suicidal ideation, or other adverse reactions.
● Instruct patient to keep syringes and needles away from children. Also instruct patient not to reuse needles or syringes and to discard them in a syringe-disposal unit.
● Advise women of childbearing age not to become pregnant while taking interferon beta-1a because of the potential of the drug to cause spontaneous abortion. If pregnancy occurs, instruct patient to notify the doctor immediately and to discontinue the drug, as ordered.

interferon beta-1b, recombinant
Betaseron

Pregnancy Risk Category: C

HOW SUPPLIED
Powder for injection: 9.6 million IU (0.3 mg)

ACTION
A naturally occurring antiviral and immunoregulatory agent derived from human fibroblasts. It attaches to membrane receptors and causes cellular changes, including increased protein synthesis.

ONSET, PEAK, DURATION
Unknown.

INDICATIONS & DOSAGE
To reduce the frequency of exacerbations in patients with relapsing-remitting multiple sclerosis—
Adults: 8 million IU (0.25 mg) S.C. every other day.

ADVERSE REACTIONS
CNS: depression, anxiety, emotional lability, depersonalization, ***suicidal tendencies,*** confusion, somnolence, *hypertonia, asthenia, migraine,* **seizures,** *headache,* dizziness.
CV: palpitations, hypertension, tachycardia, peripheral vascular disorder, hemorrhage.
EENT: laryngitis, *sinusitis, conjunctivitis,* abnormal vision.
GI: *diarrhea, constipation, abdominal pain,* vomiting.
GU: *menstrual disorders (bleeding or spotting, early or delayed menses, fewer days of menstrual flow, menorrhagia).*
Hematologic: *decreased WBC and absolute neutrophil counts.*
Respiratory: dyspnea.
Other: *flulike symptoms (fever, chills, malaise, myalgia, diaphoresis), elevated ALT levels, elevated bilirubin levels,* breast pain, *pelvic pain; inflammation, pain, and necrosis at injection site, lymphadenopathy, pain,* generalized edema, *myasthenia, diaphoresis,* alopecia.

INTERACTIONS
None significant.

EFFECTS ON DIAGNOSTIC TESTS
None reported.

CONTRAINDICATIONS
Contraindicated in patients hypersensitive to interferon beta or human albumin.

NURSING CONSIDERATIONS
● Use cautiously in women of childbearing age. Inconclusive evidence exists about the drug's teratogenic effects, but it may be an abortifacient.
● To reconstitute, inject 1.2 ml of the supplied diluent (0.54% sodium chloride injection) into the vial and gently swirl to dissolve drug. Do not shake. Reconstituted solution will contain 8 million IU (0.25 mg)/ml. Discard vials that contain particulate material or discolored solution.
● Inject immediately after preparation.
● Rotate injection sites to minimize local reactions.
● Refrigerate the drug or reconstituted product (up to 3 hours) at 36° to 46° F (2° to 8° C). Do not freeze.
● Monitor patient for signs of depression.

☑ PATIENT TEACHING
● Warn patient of childbearing age about dangers to the fetus. If a patient becomes pregnant during therapy, tell her to notify the doctor and stop taking the drug.
● Teach the patient how to self-administer S.C. injections, including solution preparation, use of aseptic technique, rotation of injection sites, and equipment disposal. Periodically reevaluate the patient's technique.
● Advise patient to take this drug at

bedtime to minimize the mild flulike symptoms that commonly occur.

interferon gamma-1b
Actimmune

Pregnancy Risk Category: C

HOW SUPPLIED
Injection: 100 mcg (3 million units)/0.5-ml vial

ACTION
Acts as an interleukin-type lymphokine. It has potent phagocyte-activating properties and enhances the oxidative metabolism of tissue macrophages.

ONSET, PEAK, DURATION
Onset and duration unknown. Peak levels occur within 7 hours after S.C. use.

INDICATIONS & DOSAGE
Chronic granulomatous disease—
Adults with a body surface area 0.5 m^2: 50 mcg/m^2 (1.5 million units/ m^2) S.C. three times weekly, preferably h.s. The preferred injection site is the deltoid or anterior thigh muscle.
Adults with a body surface area 0.5 m^2 or below: 1.5 mcg/kg three times weekly.

ADVERSE REACTIONS
CNS: *fatigue,* decreased mental status, gait disturbance, dizziness.
GI: *nausea, vomiting, diarrhea,* abdominal pain.
Hematologic: neutropenia, ***thrombocytopenia.***
Metabolic: elevated liver enzyme levels (at high doses).
Skin: *rash, erythema or tenderness at the injection site.*
Other: flulike syndrome (headache, fever, chills, myalgia, arthralgia), weight loss, back pain, proteinuria.

INTERACTIONS
Myelosuppressive agents: possible additive myelosuppression. Monitor closely.
Zidovudine: increased plasma levels of zidovudine. Dosage adjustments are necessary when used concurrently.

EFFECTS ON DIAGNOSTIC TESTS
None reported.

CONTRAINDICATIONS
Contraindicated in patients hypersensitive to the drug or to genetically engineered products derived from *Escherichia coli.*

NURSING CONSIDERATIONS
● Use cautiously in patients with cardiac disease, including arrhythmias, ischemia, or CHF. The flulike syndrome commonly seen at high doses of the drug can exacerbate these conditions.
● Use cautiously in patients with compromised CNS function or seizure disorders. CNS adverse reactions that may occur at high doses of the drug can exacerbate these conditions.
● Use myelosuppressive agents together with caution.
● Premedicate with acetaminophen to minimize symptoms at the beginning of therapy. Flulike symptoms tend to diminish with continued therapy.
● Discard unused portion. Each vial is for single-dose use only and does not contain a preservative.
● Refrigerate drug immediately. Vials must be stored at 36° to 46° F (2° to 8° C); do not freeze. Do not shake the vial; avoid excessive agitation. Discard vials that have been left at room temperature for more than 12 hours.

☑ PATIENT TEACHING
● If patient will be self-administering drug, teach him how to administer it and how to dispose of used needles, syringes, containers, and unused medication.
● Instruct patient how to manage flulike symptoms that commonly occur.

---

*Liquid contains alcohol.   **May contain tartrazine.   †Canada only.   ‡Australia only.   ◇OTC.

levamisole hydrochloride
Ergamisol

Pregnancy Risk Category: C

HOW SUPPLIED
Tablets: 50 mg (base)

ACTION
Unknown. It appears to restore depressed immune function and may potentiate the actions of monocytes and macrophages and enhance T-cell responses.

ONSET, PEAK, DURATION
Onset and duration unknown. Plasma levels peak in 1½ to 2 hours.

INDICATIONS & DOSAGE
Adjuvant treatment of Dukes' stage C colon cancer (with fluorouracil) after surgical resection—
Adults: 50 mg P.O. q 8 hours for 3 days, beginning no sooner than 7 days and no later than 30 days after surgery, provided that the patient is out of the hospital, ambulating, and maintaining normal oral nutrition; has well-healed wounds; and has recovered from any postoperative complications. Fluorouracil (450 mg/m²/day I.V.) is given for 5 days with a 3-day course of levamisole starting 21 to 34 days after surgery.

Maintenance dosage is 50 mg P.O. q 8 hours for 3 days q 2 weeks for 1 year. Given in conjunction with fluorouracil maintenance therapy (450 mg/m²/day by rapid I.V. push once a week, beginning 28 days after the initial 5-day course) for 1 year.

ADVERSE REACTIONS
CNS: *dizziness, headache, paresthesia, somnolence, depression, nervousness, insomnia, anxiety, fatigue, fever.*
CV: chest pain, edema.
EENT: blurred vision, conjunctivitis, *stomatitis, dysgeusia, altered sense of smell.*

GI: *nausea, diarrhea, vomiting, anorexia, abdominal pain, constipation, flatulence, dyspepsia.*
Hematologic: *agranulocytosis, leukopenia, thrombocytopenia,* anemia.
Skin: *dermatitis, exfoliative dermatitis, pruritus, urticaria.*
Other: hyperbilirubinemia, rigors, *alopecia, infection, arthralgia, myalgia.*

INTERACTIONS
Ethanol: may precipitate a disulfiram-like reaction. Avoid concomitant use.
Phenytoin: plasma levels may be elevated when administered with levamisole and fluorouracil. Monitor phenytoin plasma levels.

EFFECTS ON DIAGNOSTIC TESTS
No information available.

CONTRAINDICATIONS
Contraindicated in patients hypersensitive to the drug.

NURSING CONSIDERATIONS
Alert: Use cautiously and with close hematologic monitoring because agranulocytosis, which is sometimes fatal, may occur. Neutropenia is usually reversible when therapy is discontinued.
• Obtain baseline CBC with differential, platelet count, and electrolyte levels, and liver function studies, as ordered, immediately before starting therapy.
• Be aware that if levamisole therapy begins 7 to 20 days after surgery, fluorouracil should be started with the second course of levamisole therapy. It should begin no sooner than 21 days and no later than 35 days after surgery. If levamisole is deferred until 21 to 30 days after surgery, fluorouracil therapy should begin with the first course of levamisole.
• Know that dosage modifications are based on hematologic parameters. If WBC count is 2,500/mm³ to 3,500/mm³, don't administer fluorouracil as ordered until WBC count is above 3,500/mm³. When fluorouracil is restarted, reduce

dosage by 20% as ordered. If WBC count stays below 2,500/mm³ for over 10 days after fluorouracil is withdrawn, discontinue levamisole, as ordered.

• Know that recommended doses should not be exceeded. Higher doses are associated with greater incidence of agranulocytosis.

• Obtain CBC with differential and platelet count at weekly intervals, as ordered, before treatment with fluorouracil. Obtain electrolyte levels and liver function studies every 3 months for 1 year, as ordered.

• If platelet count is below 100,000/mm³, know that therapy with both fluorouracil and levamisole should be discontinued and doctor notified.

☑ **PATIENT TEACHING**
• Tell patient to promptly report the development of stomatitis or diarrhea. If either of these reactions occur during the initial course of fluorouracil therapy, drug is discontinued and then weekly fluorouracil therapy is begun 28 days after the start of the initial course. If stomatitis or diarrhea develops during the weekly doses of fluorouracil, fluorouracil therapy is deferred until these symptoms subside. Then fluorouracil therapy is started at reduced dosages (decrease dose by 20%).

• Advise patient to immediately report flulike symptoms.

**sargramostim
(granulocyte-macrophage colony-stimulating factor, GM-CSF)**
Leukine

Pregnancy Risk Category: C

HOW SUPPLIED
Powder for injection: 250 mcg, 500 mcg

ACTION
A glycoprotein containing 127 amino acids manufactured by recombinant DNA technology in a yeast expression system. It differs from the natural human granulocyte-macrophage colony-stimulating factor by substitution of leucine for arginine at position 23. The carbohydrate moiety may also be different. Sargramostim induces cellular responses by binding to specific receptors on cell surfaces of target cells.

ONSET, PEAK, DURATION
Onset occurs within 30 minutes. Peak levels occur in 2 hours. Duration unknown.

INDICATIONS & DOSAGE
Acceleration of hematopoietic reconstitution after autologous bone marrow transplantation in patients with malignant lymphoma or acute lymphoblastic leukemia or during autologous bone marrow transplantation in patients with Hodgkin's disease—
Adults: 250 mcg/m² daily for 21 consecutive days given as a 2-hour I.V. infusion beginning 2 to 4 hours after bone marrow transplantation.
Bone marrow transplantation failure or engraftment delay—
Adults: 250 mcg/m²/day for 14 days as a 2-hour I.V. infusion. Dose may be repeated after 7 days of no therapy. If engraftment still has not occurred, a third course of 500 mcg/m²/day I.V. for 14 days may be tried after another 7 days of no therapy.

ADVERSE REACTIONS
CNS: *malaise, CNS disorders, asthenia.*
CV: *blood dyscrasias, edema,* hemorrhage, supraventricular arrhythmia, pericardial effusion.
GI: *nausea, vomiting, diarrhea, anorexia,* hemorrhage, GI disorders, stomatitis.
GU: *urinary tract disorder,* abnormal kidney function.
Hepatic: *liver damage.*
Respiratory: *dyspnea, lung disorders,* pleural effusion.

Skin: *alopecia, rash.*
Other: *fever, mucous membrane disorder, peripheral edema, sepsis.*

INTERACTIONS
Corticosteroids, lithium: may potentiate myeloproliferative effects of sargramostim. Use cautiously.

EFFECTS ON DIAGNOSTIC TESTS
No interference reported. Because hematopoiesis is stimulated, effects on CBC and differential blood counts will occur.

CONTRAINDICATIONS
Contraindicated in patients with excessive leukemic myeloid blasts in bone marrow or peripheral blood and in those with hypersensitivity to the drug or any of its components or to yeast-derived products.

NURSING CONSIDERATIONS
• Use cautiously in patients with preexisting cardiac disease, hypoxia, preexisting fluid retention, pulmonary infiltrates, CHF, or impaired renal or hepatic function because these conditions may be exacerbated.
• **I.V. use:** Reconstitute with 1 ml of sterile water for injection. Direct stream of sterile water against side of vial and *gently swirl* contents to minimize foaming. Avoid excessive or vigorous agitation or shaking. Dilute in 0.9% sodium chloride solution. If final concentration is below 10 mcg/ml, add human albumin at a final concentration of 0.1% to the sodium chloride solution *before* adding sargramostim to prevent adsorption to components of the delivery system. For a final concentration of 0.1% human albumin, add 1 mg human albumin/1 ml sodium chloride. Administer as soon as possible after mixing and no later than 6 hours after reconstituting.
• Don't add other medications to infusion solution because no data exist regarding solution compatibility and stability.

• Refrigerate the sterile powder, reconstituted solution, and diluted solution for injection. Don't freeze or shake.
• Anticipate reducing dose by half or temporarily discontinue if severe adverse reactions occur and notify doctor. Therapy may be resumed when reactions abate. Transient rashes and local reactions at the injection site may occur; no serious allergic or anaphylactic reactions have been reported.
• Do not administer within 24 hours of last dose of chemotherapy or within 12 hours of last dose of radiotherapy because rapidly dividing progenitor cells may be sensitive to these cytotoxic therapies and drug would be ineffective.
• Monitor CBC with differential, including examination for presence of blast cells biweekly, as ordered. Stimulation of marrow precursors may result in rapid rise of WBC count. If blast cells appear or increase to 10% or more of the WBC count or if progression of the underlying disease occurs, know that therapy should be discontinued. If the absolute neutrophil count is above 20,000/mm^3 or if platelet count is above 50,000/mm^3, know that drug is temporarily discontinued or dose is reduced by half.
• Be aware that sargramostim is effective in accelerating myeloid recovery in patients receiving bone marrow purged from monoclonal antibodies.
• Keep in mind that the drug can act as a growth factor for any tumor type, particularly myeloid malignant disease.

☑ **PATIENT TEACHING**
• Review administration schedule with patient and caregivers, and address their concerns.
• Instruct patient to report adverse reactions promptly.

Reactions may be *common*, uncommon, *life-threatening*, or COMMON AND LIFE-THREATENING.

bacitracin
chloramphenicol
ciprofloxacin hydrochloride
erythromycin
gentamicin sulfate
idoxuridine
natamycin
norfloxacin
ofloxacin 0.3%
polymyxin B sulfate
silver nitrate 1%
sulfacetamide sodium 10%
sulfacetamide sodium 15%
sulfacetamide sodium 30%
sulfisoxazole diolamine
tobramycin
trifluridine
vidarabine

COMBINATION PRODUCTS

AK-POLY-BAC: polymyxin B sulfate 10,000 units and bacitracin zinc 500 units.

BLEPHAMIDE S.O.P. STERILE OPHTHALMIC OINTMENT: sulfacetamide sodium 10% and prednisolone acetate 0.2%.

CETAPRED OINTMENT: sulfacetamide sodium 10% and prednisolone acetate 0.25%.

CORTISPORIN OPHTHALMIC OINTMENT: polymyxin B sulfate 10,000 units, bacitracin zinc 400 units, neomycin sulfate 0.35%, and hydrocortisone 1%.

CORTISPORIN OPHTHALMIC SUSPENSION: polymyxin B sulfate 10,000 units, neomycin sulfate 0.35%, and hydrocortisone 1%.

ISOPTO CETAPRED: sulfacetamide sodium 10% and prednisolone acetate 0.25%.

MAXITROL OINTMENT OPHTHALMIC SUSPENSION: dexamethasone 0.1%, neomycin sulfate 0.35%, and polymyxin B sulfate 10,000 units.

METIMYD OPHTHALMIC OINTMENT SUS-PENSION: sulfacetamide sodium 10% and prednisolone acetate 0.5%.

MYCITRACIN OPHTHALMIC OINTMENT: polymyxin B sulfate 5,000 units, neomycin sulfate 3.5 mg, and bacitracin 500 units.

NEOSPORIN OPHTHALMIC: polymyxin B sulfate 10,000 units, neomycin sulfate 1.75 mg, and gramicidin 0.025 mg.

NEOSPORIN OPHTHALMIC: OINTMENT: polymyxin B sulfate 10,000 units, neomycin sulfate 3.5 mg, and bacitracin zinc 400 units/g.

NEOTAL: polymyxin B sulfate 5,000 units, neomycin sulfate 5 mg, and bacitracin zinc 400 units.

OPHTHOCORT: chloramphenicol 1.0%, polymyxin B sulfate 10,000 units, and hydrocortisone acetate 0.5%.

OPTIMYD: prednisolone phosphate 0.5% and sulfacetamide sodium 10%.

POLYSPORIN OPHTHALMIC OINTMENT: polymyxin B sulfate 10,000 units and bacitracin zinc 500 units.

POLYTRIM OPHTHALMIC: trimethoprim sulfate 1 mg and polymyxin B sulfate 10,000 units/ml.

PRED-G S.O.P.: prednisolone acetate 0.6%, gentamicin sulfate equivalent to gentamicin base 0.3%, chlorobutanol 0.5%, petrolatum, white petrolatum, mineral oil, and lanolin alcohol.

STATROL: neomycin sulfate 3.5 mg and polymyxin B sulfate 10,000 units.

TOBRA DEX: dexamethasone 0.1%, tobramycin 0.3%, chlorobutanol 0.5%, mineral oil, and white petrolatum.

VASOCIDIN OPHTHALMIC OINTMENT: sulfacetamide sodium 10% and prednisolone acetate 0.5%.

VASOCIDIN OPHTHALMIC SOLUTION: sulfacetamide sodium 10% and prednisolone phosphate 0.25%.

VASOSULF: sulfacetamide sodium 15%

---

*Liquid contains alcohol.   **May contain tartrazine.   †Canada only.   ‡Australia only.   ◇OTC.

and phenylephrine hydrochloride
0.125%.

bacitracin
AK-Tracin

Pregnancy Risk Category: NR

HOW SUPPLIED
Ophthalmic ointment: 500 units/g

ACTION
Inhibits bacterial cell wall synthesis.
Bactericidal or bacteriostatic, depending
on concentration and infection.

ONSET, PEAK, DURATION
Unknown. Systemic absorption is negligible.

INDICATIONS & DOSAGE
*Surface bacterial infections involving
conjunctiva and cornea—*
Adults and children: small amount of
ointment applied into conjunctival sac
one or more times daily or p.r.n. until
favorable response is observed.

ADVERSE REACTIONS
EENT: slowed corneal wound healing,
temporary visual haze.
Other: overgrowth of nonsusceptible
organisms.

INTERACTIONS
Heavy metals (for example, silver nitrate): inactivation of bacitracin. Don't
use together.

EFFECTS ON DIAGNOSTIC TESTS
Urinary sediment tests may show increased protein and cast excretion.
Serum creatinine and BUN levels may
increase during drug therapy.

CONTRAINDICATIONS
Contraindicated in hypersensitive and
atopic patients.

NURSING CONSIDERATIONS
● Ophthalmic ointment may be stored at
room temperature.
● Clean eye area of excessive exudate
before application.

☑ PATIENT TEACHING
● Teach patient how to apply; tell him
only a small amount of ointment is
needed and that it may cause blurred vision. Advise patient to wash hands before and after administering and not to
touch tip of tube to eye or surrounding
tissue.
● Advise patient to watch for and report
signs of sensitivity (itching lids,
swelling, or constant burning).
● Tell patient not to share medication,
washcloths, or towels with family members and to notify doctor if anyone develops same symptoms.
● Stress importance of compliance with
recommended therapy.

chloramphenicol
AK-Chlor, Chloromycetin Ophthalmic,
Chloroptic, Chloroptic S.O.P., Chlorsig‡, Fenicol†, Isopto Fenicol†, Ophthoclor Ophthalmic, Pentamycetin†,
Sopamycetin†

Pregnancy Risk Category: NR

HOW SUPPLIED
Ophthalmic ointment: 1%
Ophthalmic solution: 0.5%
Powder for ophthalmic solution: 25 mg

ACTION
Inhibits protein synthesis. Bacteriostatic
or bactericidal, depending on concentration.

ONSET, PEAK, DURATION
Unknown. Systemic absorption occurs,
but has not been characterized; higher
levels occur with ophthalmic ointment.

INDICATIONS & DOSAGE
Surface bacterial infection involving

conjunctiva or cornea—
Adults and children: 1 or 2 drops of solution instilled in eye q 3 to 6 hours or more frequently, if necessary. Or, a small amount of ointment applied to lower conjunctival sac q 3 to 6 hours or more frequently, if necessary. Continued for at least 48 hours after eye appears normal.

ADVERSE REACTIONS
EENT: optic atrophy in children, stinging or burning of eye after instillation, blurred vision (with ointment).
Hematologic: *bone marrow hypoplasia with prolonged use, aplastic anemia.*
Skin: dermatitis.
Other: overgrowth of nonsusceptible organisms; hypersensitivity reactions, including itching and burning eye, angioedema.

INTERACTIONS
None significant.

EFFECTS ON DIAGNOSTIC TESTS
False elevation of urinary PABA levels will result if drug is administered during a bentiromide test for pancreatic function. Drug therapy will cause false-positive results on tests for urine glucose level using cupric sulfate (Clinitest). Platelet, RBC, and WBC counts in the blood and possibly the bone marrow may decrease during drug therapy (from reversible or irreversible bone marrow depression). Hemoglobinuria or lactic acidosis may also occur.

CONTRAINDICATIONS
Contraindicated in patients hypersensitive to the drug.

NURSING CONSIDERATIONS
● If chloramphenicol drops are to be given every hour and then tapered, follow order closely to ensure adequate anterior chamber levels.
● Reconstitute powder for ophthalmic solution with supplied diluent. Use 5 ml of diluent to make a 0.5% solution, 10 ml of diluent to make a 0.25% solution,

or 15 ml to make a 0.16% solution.
● Store in tightly closed, light-resistant container.
● If patients have more than a superficial infection, anticipate using systemic therapy as well.

☑ **PATIENT TEACHING**
● Teach patient how to instill drops or apply ointment. Advise him to wash hands before and after administering ointment or solution, and warn him not to touch tip of applicator to eye or surrounding tissue.
● Tell patient to clean eye area of excessive exudate before application.
● Instruct patient to apply light finger pressure on lacrimal sac for 1 minute after drops are instilled.
● Tell patient not to share medication, washcloths, or towels with family members and to notify doctor if anyone develops same symptoms.
● Tell patient to watch for and report signs of sensitivity (itching lids, swelling, or constant burning).
● Tell patient to notify the doctor if no improvement occurs in 3 days.
● Stress importance of compliance with recommended therapy.

ciprofloxacin hydrochloride
Ciloxan

Pregnancy Risk Category: C

HOW SUPPLIED
Ophthalmic solution: 0.3% (base) in 2.5- and 5-ml containers

ACTION
Inhibits bacterial DNA gyrase, an enzyme necessary for bacterial replication. Bacteriostatic or bactericidal, depending on concentration.

ONSET, PEAK, DURATION
Unknown. Systemic absorption is negligible.

INDICATIONS & DOSAGE
Corneal ulcers caused by Pseudomonas aeruginosa, Staphylococcus aureus, S. epidermidis, Streptococcus pneumoniae, *and possibly* Serratia marcescens *and* Streptococcus viridans—
Adults and children over 12 years: 2 drops in the affected eye q 15 minutes for the first 6 hours; then 2 drops q 30 minutes for the remainder of the first day. On day 2, 2 drops hourly. On days 3 to 14, 2 drops q 4 hours.
Bacterial conjunctivitis caused by Staphylococcus aureus *and* S. epidermidis *and possibly* Streptococcus pneumoniae—
Adults and children over 12 years: 1 or 2 drops into the conjunctival sac of the affected eye q 2 hours while awake for the first 2 days. Then 1 or 2 drops q 4 hours while awake for the next 5 days.

ADVERSE REACTIONS
EENT: *local burning or discomfort, white crystalline precipitate* (in the superficial portion of the corneal defect in patients with corneal ulcers), *margin crusting, crystals or scales, foreign body sensation, itching, conjunctival hyperemia,* bad or bitter taste in mouth, corneal staining, allergic reactions, keratopathy, lid edema, tearing, photophobia, decreased vision.
GI: nausea.

INTERACTIONS
None significant.

EFFECTS ON DIAGNOSTIC TESTS
None reported.

CONTRAINDICATIONS
Contraindicated in patients with a history of hypersensitivity to ciprofloxacin or other fluoroquinolone antibiotics.

NURSING CONSIDERATIONS
● Be aware that it's unknown if drug is excreted in breast milk after application to the eye; however, systemically administered ciprofloxacin has been de-tected in human milk. Use caution.
Alert: Discontinue drug at the first sign of hypersensitivity reactions, such as rash, and notify doctor. Serious hypersensitivity reactions, including anaphylaxis, have occurred in patients receiving systemic fluoroquinolone therapy.
● If corneal epithelium is still compromised after 14 days of treatment, continue therapy, as ordered.
● Institute appropriate therapy if superinfection occurs. Prolonged use may result in overgrowth of nonsusceptible organisms, including fungi.

☑ PATIENT TEACHING
● Tell patient to clean eye area of excessive exudate before instilling.
● Teach patient how to instill drops. Advise him to wash hands before and after administering solution and not to touch tip of dropper to eye or surrounding tissues.
● Instruct patient to apply light finger pressure on lacrimal sac for 1 minute after drops are instilled.
● Tell patient not to share medication, washcloths, or towels with family members and to notify doctor if anyone develops same symptoms.
● Stress importance of compliance with recommended therapy.

---

erythromycin
Ilotycin Ophthalmic Ointment

Pregnancy Risk Category: NR

HOW SUPPLIED
Ophthalmic ointment: 0.5%

ACTION
Inhibits protein synthesis. Bacteriostatic, but may be bactericidal in high concentrations or against highly susceptible organisms.

ONSET, PEAK, DURATION
Unknown. Systemic absorption is negligible.

INDICATIONS & DOSAGE
Acute and chronic conjunctivitis, trachoma, other eye infections—
Adults and children: 1 cm in length applied directly to the infected eye up to six times daily, depending on severity of infection.
Prophylaxis of ophthalmia neonatorum due to Neisseria gonorrhoeae *or* Chlamydia trachomatis—
Neonates: a ribbon of ointment approximately 1 cm long applied in the lower conjunctival sac of each eye shortly after birth.

ADVERSE REACTIONS
EENT: slowed corneal wound healing, blurred vision.
Skin: urticaria, dermatitis.
Other: overgrowth of nonsusceptible organisms with long-term use; hypersensitivity reactions, including itching and burning eyes.

INTERACTIONS
None significant.

EFFECTS ON DIAGNOSTIC TESTS
Drug may interfere with fluorometric determinations of urinary catecholamines. Liver function test results may become abnormal during drug therapy (rare).

CONTRAINDICATIONS
Contraindicated in patients hypersensitive to the drug.

NURSING CONSIDERATIONS
• For prophylaxis of ophthalmia neonatorum, ointment should be applied no later than 1 hour after birth. Used in neonates born either by vaginal delivery or by cesarean section. Gently massage the eyelids for 1 minute to spread the ointment.
• Be aware that drug has a limited antibacterial spectrum.
• To be used only when sensitivity studies show it is effective against infecting organisms. Not for use in infections of unknown etiology.
• Store at room temperature in tightly closed, light-resistant container.

☑ PATIENT TEACHING
• Tell patient to clean eye area of excessive exudate before application.
• Teach patient how to apply. Advise him to wash hands before and after administering ointment, and warn him not to touch tip of applicator to eye or surrounding tissue.
• Instruct patient to apply light finger pressure on lacrimal sac for 1 minute after administering.
• Warn patient that ointment may cause blurred vision.
• Advise patient to watch for and report signs of sensitivity (itching lids, swelling, or constant burning).
• Tell patient not to share medication, washcloths, or towels with family members and to notify doctor if anyone develops same symptoms.
• Stress importance of compliance with recommended therapy.

---

gentamicin sulfate
Garamycin Ophthalmic, Genoptic, Gentacidin, Gentak, Ocu-Mycin

Pregnancy Risk Category: C

HOW SUPPLIED
Ophthalmic ointment: 0.3% (base)
Ophthalmic solution: 0.3% (base)

ACTION
Unknown. Thought to inhibit protein synthesis and is usually bactericidal.

ONSET, PEAK, DURATION
Unknown. Only small amounts of the drug are absorbed systemically.

INDICATIONS & DOSAGE
External ocular infections (conjunctivitis, keratoconjunctivitis, corneal ulcers, blepharitis, blepharoconjunctivitis, meibomianitis, and dacryocystitis) caused

---

by susceptible organisms, especially Pseudomonas aeruginosa, Proteus, Klebsiella pneumoniae, Escherichia coli, *and other gram-negative organisms—*

Adults and children: 1 to 2 drops instilled in eye q 4 hours. In severe infections, up to 2 drops q hour. Alternatively, ointment applied to lower conjunctival sac b.i.d. or t.i.d.

ADVERSE REACTIONS
EENT: burning, stinging, or blurred vision (with ointment), transient irritation (from solution), conjunctival hyperemia.
Other: hypersensitivity reactions; overgrowth of nonsusceptible organisms with long-term use.

Systemic absorption from excessive use may cause systemic toxicities.

INTERACTIONS
None significant.

EFFECTS ON DIAGNOSTIC TESTS
Drug-induced nephrotoxicity may elevate BUN, nonprotein nitrogen, or serum creatinine levels and increase urinary excretion of casts.

CONTRAINDICATIONS
Contraindicated in patients hypersensitive to the drug.

NURSING CONSIDERATIONS
● Use cautiously in patients with history of sensitivity to aminoglycosides because cross-sensitivity may occur.
● Have culture taken before giving drug. Therapy may begin before culture results are known.
● If ophthalmic gentamicin is given concomitantly with systemic gentamicin, monitor serum gentamicin levels.
● Know that solution is not for injection into the conjunctiva or anterior chamber of the eye.
● Store away from heat.

☑ PATIENT TEACHING
● Tell patient to clean eye area of excessive exudate before instilling.
● Teach patient how to instill drops or apply ointment. Advise him to wash hands before and after administering ointment or solution and not to touch tip of dropper or tube to eye or surrounding tissues.
● Instruct patient to apply light finger pressure on lacrimal sac for 1 minute after drops are instilled.
● Tell patient to watch for and report signs of sensitivity (itching lids, swelling, or constant burning).
● Tell patient not to share medication, washcloths, or towels with family members and to notify doctor if anyone develops same symptoms.
Alert: Stress importance of following recommended therapy. *Pseudomonas* infections can cause complete vision loss within 24 hours if infection is not controlled.

---

idoxuridine (IDU)
Herplex

Pregnancy Risk Category: C

HOW SUPPLIED
Ophthalmic solution: 0.1%

ACTION
Interferes with DNA synthesis.

ONSET, PEAK, DURATION
Unknown. Systemic absorption is unlikely.

INDICATIONS & DOSAGE
Herpes simplex keratitis—
Adults and children: 1 drop of solution instilled into conjunctival sac q hour during day and q 2 hours at night. Continue until definite improvement occurs, usually 7 days or less.

ADVERSE REACTIONS
EENT: temporary visual haze; irritation, burning, or inflammation of eye; mild edema of eyelid or cornea; photo-

phobia; small punctate defects in corneal epithelium; corneal ulceration.
Other: hypersensitivity reactions.

INTERACTIONS
Boric acid: precipitate formation; increased risk of ocular toxicity. Avoid concomitant use.

EFFECTS ON DIAGNOSTIC TESTS
None reported.

CONTRAINDICATIONS
Contraindicated in patients with hypersensitivity to the drug.

NURSING CONSIDERATIONS
• Do not mix idoxuridine with other topical eye medications.
• Keep in mind that drug is not for long-term use. Therapy should not continue longer than 21 days.
• Keep idoxuridine 0.1% solution in a tightly closed, light-resistant container at room temperature.

☑ PATIENT TEACHING
• Advise patient not to use old solution; causes ocular burning and has no antiviral activity.
• Tell patient to clean eye area of excessive exudate before application.
• Teach patient how to instill drops or apply ointment. Advise him to wash hands before and after administering, and warn him not to touch tip of dropper to eye or surrounding tissue.
• Instruct patient to apply light finger pressure on lacrimal sac for 1 minute after drops are instilled.
• Advise patient to watch for and report signs of sensitivity (itching lids, swelling, or constant burning).
• Also instruct patient to notify his doctor if symptoms do not diminish in 7 days; drug will need to be discontinued and alternative therapy begun.
• Tell patient not to share medication, washcloths, or towels with family members and to notify doctor if anyone develops same symptoms.

• Tell patient to minimize photophobia by wearing sunglasses and avoiding prolonged exposure to sunlight.
• Stress importance of compliance with recommended therapy.

---

natamycin
Natacyn

Pregnancy Risk Category: C

HOW SUPPLIED
Ophthalmic suspension: 5%

ACTION
Increases fungal cell-membrane permeability.

ONSET, PEAK, DURATION
Unknown.

INDICATIONS & DOSAGE
Fungal keratitis—
Adults: initially, 1 drop instilled in conjunctival sac q 1 to 2 hours. After 3 to 4 days, dosage reduced to 1 drop six to eight times daily.
Blepharitis or fungal conjunctivitis—
Adults: 1 drop instilled q 4 to 6 hours.

ADVERSE REACTIONS
EENT: ocular edema, hyperemia, conjunctival chemosis.

INTERACTIONS
None significant.

EFFECTS ON DIAGNOSTIC TESTS
None reported.

CONTRAINDICATIONS
Contraindicated in patients hypersensitive to the drug.

NURSING CONSIDERATIONS
• Administer drug as ordered for 14 to 21 days or until active disease subsides. Be prepared to reduce dosage gradually at 4- to 7-day intervals, as ordered, to ensure that organism has been eliminat-

---

*Liquid contains alcohol.   **May contain tartrazine.   †Canada only.   ‡Australia only.   ◇OTC.

ed. If infection does not improve within 7 to 10 days of therapy, clinical and laboratory reevaluation is recommended.

● Shake well before use. Refrigerate or store at room temperature.

● Drug is the only antifungal available as ophthalmic preparation.

☑ **PATIENT TEACHING**

● Tell patient to clean eye area of excessive exudate before application.

● Teach patient how to instill drops. Advise him to wash hands before and after administering solution and not to touch tip of dropper to eye or surrounding tissue.

● Instruct patient to apply light finger pressure on lacrimal sac for 1 minute after drops are instilled.

● Tell patient not to share medication, washcloths, or towels with family members and to notify doctor if anyone develops same symptoms.

● Stress importance of compliance with recommended therapy.

---

norfloxacin
Chibroxin

Pregnancy Risk Category: C

HOW SUPPLIED
Ophthalmic solution: 0.3% in 5-ml containers

ACTION
Inhibits bacterial DNA gyrase, an enzyme necessary for bacterial replication. Bacteriostatic or bactericidal, depending on concentration.

ONSET, PEAK, DURATION
Unknown. Systemic absorption is negligible.

INDICATIONS & DOSAGE
Conjunctivitis caused by susceptible strains of bacteria—
Adults and children 1 year and over: 1 drop in the affected eye q.i.d. for up to

7 days. In severe infections, 1 or 2 drops q 2 hours while awake for the first 1 to 2 days of treatment.

ADVERSE REACTIONS
EENT: local burning or discomfort, itching, chemosis, photophobia, conjunctival hyperemia, white crystallin precipitates, lid margin crusting, bad or bitter taste in mouth, nausea, hypersensitivity reactions.
GI: nausea.

INTERACTIONS
Caffeine, cyclosporine, theophylline: impaired metabolism of these drugs with systemic norfloxacin. It's unknown if ophthalmic norfloxacin will have this effect. Monitor closely.
Oral anticoagulants: enhanced activity with systemic norfloxacin. It's unknown if ophthalmic norfloxacin will have this effect. Monitor closely.

EFFECTS ON DIAGNOSTIC TESTS
None reported.

CONTRAINDICATIONS
Contraindicated in patients with a history of hypersensitivity to norfloxacin or other fluoroquinolone antibiotics. Drug shouldn't be injected into eye.

NURSING CONSIDERATIONS
● Be aware that drug is indicated for treating conjunctivitis when caused by susceptible bacteria. Known susceptible strains include *Acinetobacter calcoaceticus, Aeromonas hydrophila, Haemophilus influenzae, Proteus mirabilis, Serratia marcescens, Staphylococcus aureus, S. epidermidis, S. warnerii,* and *Streptococcus pneumoniae.*
Alert: Discontinue drug at the first sign of hypersensitivity, such as rash, and notify doctor. Serious hypersensitivity reactions, including anaphylaxis, have occurred in patients receiving systemic fluoroquinolone therapy.
● Institute appropriate therapy if superinfection occurs. Prolonged use may re-

sult in overgrowth of nonsusceptible organisms, including fungi.

● Know that although systemically administered fluoroquinolones have been shown to cause arthropathy in young animals, ophthalmic norfloxacin has not produced this adverse effect.

☑ **PATIENT TEACHING**

● Tell patient to clean eye area of excessive exudate before application.

● Teach patient how to instill drops. Advise him to wash hands before and after administering and not to touch the tip of the tube or dropper to eye or surrounding tissue.

● Tell patient not to share medication, washcloths, or towels with family members and to notify doctor if anyone develops same symptoms.

● Stress the importance of compliance with recommended therapy.

---

ofloxacin 0.3%
Ocuflox

Pregnancy Risk Category: C

HOW SUPPLIED
Ophthalmic solution: 0.3%

ACTION
Bactericidal; inhibits bacterial DNA gyrase, an enzyme necessary for bacterial replication.

ONSET, PEAK, DURATION
Unknown.

INDICATIONS & DOSAGE
Conjunctivitis caused by Staphylococcus aureus, S. epidermidis, Streptococcus pneumoniae, Enterobacter cloacae, Haemophilus influenzae, Proteus mirabilis, *and* Pseudomonas aeruginosa—
Adults and children older than 1 year: 1 to 2 drops in the conjunctival sac q 2 to 4 hours daily, while awake, for the first 2 days and then four times daily for up to 5 additional days.

ADVERSE REACTIONS
CNS: dizziness (rare).
EENT: *transient ocular burning or discomfort,* stinging, redness, itching, photophobia, lacrimation, eye dryness.

INTERACTIONS
None significant.

EFFECTS ON DIAGNOSTIC TESTS
Drug may increase blood glucose levels.

CONTRAINDICATIONS
Contraindicated in patients with history of hypersensitivity to ofloxacin, to other fluoroquinolones, or to any of the components of this drug; and in breast-feeding women.

NURSING CONSIDERATIONS
Alert: Know that the drug should not be injected into the conjunctiva or introduced directly into the anterior chamber of the eye.

● Be aware that drug should be discontinued if improvement does not occur within 7 days. Prolonged use may result in overgrowth of nonsusceptible organisms, including fungi.

☑ **PATIENT TEACHING**

● If an allergic reaction occurs, tell patient to discontinue the drug and call the doctor. Serious acute hypersensitivity reactions may require emergency treatment.

● Teach patient how to instill drops. Advise him to wash hands before and after instilling solution, and warn him not to touch tip of the dropper to eye or surrounding tissue.

● Advise patient to apply light finger pressure on lacrimal sac for 1 minute after drug instillation.

● Stress the importance of compliance with recommended therapy.

● Warn patient not to use leftover medication for a new eye infection.

● Remind patients to discard drug when no longer needed.

---

*Liquid contains alcohol.   **May contain tartrazine.   †Canada only.   ‡Australia only.   ◇OTC.

polymyxin B sulfate

Pregnancy Risk Category: C

HOW SUPPLIED
Ophthalmic sterile powder for solution:
500,000-unit vials to be reconstituted to
20 to 50 ml

ACTION
Bactericidal. Alters the osmotic barrier
of the bacteria cell membrane.

ONSET, PEAK, DURATION
Unknown. Systemic absorption is negligible.

INDICATIONS & DOSAGE
*Used alone or in combination with oth-
er agents to treat superficial eye infections involving the conjunctiva and
cornea resulting from infection with*
Pseudomonas *or other gram-negative
organism—*
Adults and children: 1 to 3 drops of
0.1% to 0.25% (10,000 to 25,000
units/ml) instilled q hour. Interval increased according to patient response;
or up to 10,000 units injected subcon-
junctivally daily.

ADVERSE REACTIONS
EENT: eye irritation, conjunctivitis.
Other: overgrowth of nonsusceptible
organisms, hypersensitivity reactions
(local burning, itching).

INTERACTIONS
None significant.

EFFECTS ON DIAGNOSTIC TESTS
BUN and serum creatinine levels may
increase during drug therapy.

CONTRAINDICATIONS
Contraindicated in patients hypersensitive to the drug.

NURSING CONSIDERATIONS
● Reconstitute carefully to ensure cor-

rect drug concentration in solution.
● Know that drug is often used in com-
bination with neomycin sulfate.
● Be aware that drug is one of the most
effective antibiotics against gram-nega-
tive organisms, especially
Pseudomonas.
● In severe, life-threatening *Pseudo-
monas* infections, know that polymyxin
B may be used as an ocular irrigant.

☑ PATIENT TEACHING
● Tell patient to clean eye area of excessive exudate before application.
● Teach patient how to instill drops .
Advise him to wash hands before and
after administering solution, and warn
him not to touch tip of dropper to eye or
surrounding tissue.
● Instruct patient to apply light finger
pressure on lacrimal sac for 1 minute after drops are instilled.
● Advise patient to watch for and report
signs of sensitivity (itching lids,
swelling, or constant burning).
● Tell patient not to share medication,
washcloths, or towels with family members and to notify doctor if anyone develops same symptoms.
● Stress importance of compliance with
recommended therapy.

silver nitrate 1%

Pregnancy Risk Category: NR

HOW SUPPLIED
Ophthalmic solution: 1%

ACTION
Causes protein denaturation, which prevents gonorrheal ophthalmia neonatorum. Bacteriostatic, germicidal, astringent, caustic, and escharotic.

ONSET, PEAK, DURATION
Unknown. Systemic absorption is negligible.

INDICATIONS & DOSAGE
Prevention of gonorrheal ophthalmia neonatorum—
Neonates: clean eyelids thoroughly; 2 drops of 1% solution instilled into the lower conjunctival sac of each eye at the angle of the nasal bridge and eyes, preferably immediately after delivery but no later than 1 hour after delivery.

ADVERSE REACTIONS
EENT: periorbital edema, temporary staining of lids and surrounding tissue, *conjunctivitis.*

INTERACTIONS
Bacitracin: inactivation of silver nitrate. Don't use together.
Sulfonamides: Incompatible with silver preparations. Don't use together.

EFFECTS ON DIAGNOSTIC TESTS
None reported.

CONTRAINDICATIONS
None known.

NURSING CONSIDERATIONS
● Always wash hands before instilling solution.
● Apply within 1 hour of birth, as ordered. Used in neonates born either by vaginal delivery or by cesarean section.
● Be aware that instillation may be delayed slightly to allow neonate to bond with mother.
● Don't use repeatedly.
● Don't irrigate eyes after instillation.
● Never use concentrations greater than 1% in the eye.
● If a concentrated solution is accidentally used in eye, promptly irrigate with 0.9% sodium chloride solution to prevent severe eye irritation or blindness.
● Handle carefully. Solution may stain skin and utensils.
● Know that prophylaxis against gonococcal ophthalmia neonatorum is legally required for neonates in most states. Because of a high incidence of conjunctivitis (more than 90%), many clinicians

prefer antibiotic ointments, such as erythromycin, as an alternative.
● Store wax ampules away from light and heat. Do not freeze or use when cold.

☑ PATIENT TEACHING
● Inform parents of need for drug and explain how it is administered.
● Answer questions and address their concerns.

---

sulfacetamide sodium 10%
Bleph-10 Liquifilm Ophthalmic, Cetamide Ophthalmic, Ocu-Sul-10, Sodium Sulamyd 10% Ophthalmic, Sulf-10 Ophthalmic

sulfacetamide sodium 15%
Isopto Cetamide Ophthalmic, Ocu-Sul-15

sulfacetamide sodium 30%
Ocu-Sul-30, Sodium Sulamyd 30% Ophthalmic

Pregnancy Risk Category: C

HOW SUPPLIED
Ophthalmic ointment: 10%
Ophthalmic solution: 10%, 15%, 30%

ACTION
Bacteriostatic although, in high concentrations, may be bactericidal. Prevents uptake of PABA, a metabolite of bacterial folic acid synthesis.

ONSET, PEAK, DURATION
Unknown. Systemic absorption is negligible.

INDICATIONS & DOSAGE
Inclusion conjunctivitis, corneal ulcers, chlamydial infection—
Adults and children: 1 to 2 drops of 10% solution instilled into lower conjunctival sac q 2 to 3 hours during day, less often at night; or 1 to 2 drops of 15% solution instilled into lower con-

---

junctival sac q 1 to 2 hours initially. Interval increased as condition responds; or 1 drop of 30% solution instilled into lower conjunctival sac q 2 hours. 1.25 to 2.5 cm 10% ointment applied into conjunctival sac q.i.d. and h.s. Ointment may be used at night along with drops during the day.
Trachoma—
Adults and children: 2 drops of 30% solution instilled into lower conjunctival sac q 2 hours in conjunction with systemic sulfonamide or tetracycline therapy.

ADVERSE REACTIONS
EENT: slowed corneal wound healing (ointment), pain (on instillation of eyedrops), headache or brow pain, photophobia, periorbital edema.
Other: hypersensitivity reactions (including itching or burning), overgrowth of nonsusceptible organisms, ***Stevens-Johnson syndrome.***

INTERACTIONS
Gentamicin (ophthalmic): in vitro antagonism. Avoid using together.
Local anesthetics (procaine, tetracaine), PABA derivatives: decreased sulfacetamide sodium action. Wait ½ to 1 hour after instilling anesthetic or PABA derivative before instilling sulfacetamide.
Silver preparations: precipitate formation. Avoid using together.

EFFECTS ON DIAGNOSTIC TESTS
None reported.

CONTRAINDICATIONS
● Contraindicated in patients hypersensitive to sulfonamides. Not recommended for children under 2 months.

NURSING CONSIDERATIONS
● Be aware that drug is often used with oral tetracycline in treating trachoma and inclusion conjunctivitis.
● Store in tightly closed, light-resistant container away from heat.

☑ **PATIENT TEACHING**
● Tell patient to clean eye area of excessive exudate before instilling.
● Teach patient how to instill drops or apply ointment. Advise him to wash hands before and after administering ointment or solution and not to touch tip of dropper to eye or surrounding tissues.
● Instruct patient to apply light finger pressure on lacrimal sac for 1 minute after drops are instilled.
● Warn patient that eyedrops burn slightly.
● Advise patient to watch for and report signs of sensitivity (itching lids, swelling, or constant burning).
● Tell patient to wait at least 5 minutes before administering other eyedrops.
● Warn patient that solution may stain clothing.
● Tell patient to minimize photophobia by wearing sunglasses and avoiding prolonged exposure to sunlight.
● Advise patient not to use discolored solution.
● Tell patient not to share eye medication, washcloths, or towels. If anyone develops the same symptoms, the doctor should be notified.
● Stress importance of compliance.

---

sulfisoxazole diolamine
Gantrisin Ophthalmic Solution

Pregnancy Risk Category: C

HOW SUPPLIED
Ophthalmic solution: 4%

ACTION
Inhibits bacterial synthesis of dihydrofolic acid by competing with PABA, thus exerting a bacteriostatic effect.

ONSET, PEAK, DURATION
Unknown.

INDICATIONS & DOSAGE
Conjunctivitis, corneal ulcers, and other superficial ocular infections; adjunct in

systemic sulfonamide therapy of trachoma—
Adults and children: 2 to 3 drops instilled in the conjunctival sac three or more times daily.

ADVERSE REACTIONS
CNS: *headache.*
EENT: *ocular irritation, itching, chemosis, periorbital edema.*
Other: ***Stevens-Johnson syndrome,*** overgrowth of nonsusceptible organisms.

INTERACTIONS
Gentamicin sulfate: antagonism may occur. Do not administer together.
Silver-containing preparations: incompatible. Do not administer together.

EFFECTS ON DIAGNOSTIC TESTS
Drug alters results of urine glucose tests using cupric sulfate (Benedict's reagent or Clinitest). Drug therapy may elevate liver function test results; it may decrease serum levels of erythrocytes, platelets, or leukocytes.

CONTRAINDICATIONS
Contraindicated in patients with hypersensitivity to this drug or other sulfonamides, in infants under age 2 months, during pregnancy at full term, and in breast-feeding women.

NURSING CONSIDERATIONS
● Use with caution in patients with severe dry eye.
● Drug should be discarded when patient's infection is eliminated.

☑ PATIENT TEACHING
● Teach patient how to instill drops. Advise him to wash hands before and after instilling solution, and warn him not to touch tip of the dropper to the eye or surrounding tissue.
● Advise patient to apply light finger pressure on lacrimal sac for 1 minute after drug instillation.
● Stress the importance of compliance.

tobramycin
Aktob, Tobrex

Pregnancy Risk Category: B

HOW SUPPLIED
Ophthalmic ointment: 0.3%
Ophthalmic solution: 0.3%

ACTION
Unknown. Thought to inhibit protein synthesis. Usually bactericidal.

ONSET, PEAK, DURATION
Unknown. Systemic absorption is negligible.

INDICATIONS & DOSAGE
External ocular infections caused by susceptible bacteria—
Adults and children: in mild to moderate infections, 1 or 2 drops instilled into the affected eye q 4 hours, or a thin strip (1 cm long) of ointment applied q 8 to 12 hours. In severe infections, 2 drops instilled into the infected eye q 30 to 60 minutes until condition improves; then frequency reduced. Or, a thin strip (1 cm long) of ointment applied q 3 to 4 hours until improvement; then frequency reduced.

ADVERSE REACTIONS
EENT: burning or stinging on instillation, lid itching or swelling, conjunctival erythema, blurred vision (with ointment).
Other: hypersensitivity reactions, overgrowth of nonsusceptible organisms.

INTERACTIONS
None significant.

EFFECTS ON DIAGNOSTIC TESTS
Drug may elevate BUN, nonprotein nitrogen, or serum creatinine levels and increase urinary excretion of casts.

CONTRAINDICATIONS
Contraindicated in patients hypersensi-

tive to the drug or other aminoglycosides.

NURSING CONSIDERATIONS
• When two different ophthalmic solutions are used, allow at least 5 minutes
before instillation.
Alert: Know that tobramycin ophthalmic
solution is not for injection.
• If topical ocular tobramycin is administered with systemic tobramycin, carefully monitor serum levels.
• Know that prolonged use may result
in overgrowth of nonsusceptible organisms, including fungi.

☑ PATIENT TEACHING
• Tell patient to clean eye area of excessive exudate before application.
• Teach patient how to instill drops or
apply ointment. Advise him to wash
hands before and after administering
and to avoid touching tip of dropper to
eye or surrounding tissue.
• Instruct patient to apply light finger
pressure on lacrimal sac for 1 minute after drops are instilled.
• Advise patient to watch for itching
lids, swelling, or constant burning. Tell
patient who develops these signs to discontinue drug and notify the doctor immediately.
• Tell patient not to share medication,
washcloths, or towels and to notify doctor if anyone develops same symptoms.
• Stress importance of compliance.

---

trifluridine
Viroptic Ophthalmic Solution 1%

Pregnancy Risk Category: C

HOW SUPPLIED
Ophthalmic solution: 1%

ACTION
Unknown. Thought to interfere with
DNA synthesis.

ONSET, PEAK, DURATION
Unknown.

INDICATIONS & DOSAGE
*Primary keratoconjunctivitis and recur-
rent epithelial keratitis caused by herpes simplex virus, types I and II—*
Adults: 1 drop of solution into the affected eye q 2 hours while patient is
awake to a maximum of 9 drops daily
until corneal ulcer reepithelialization
occurs; then 1 drop q 4 hours (minimum
5 drops daily) for an additional 7 days.

ADVERSE REACTIONS
EENT: *stinging on instillation,* edema
of eyelids, increased intraocular pressure, epithelial keratopathy, superficial
punctate keratopathy, stromal edema, irritation, keratitis sicca.
Other: hypersensitivity reactions.

INTERACTIONS
None significant.

EFFECTS ON DIAGNOSTIC TESTS
None reported.

CONTRAINDICATIONS
Contraindicated in patients hypersensitive to the drug.

NURSING CONSIDERATIONS
• Be aware that doctor should consider
another form of therapy if improvement
doesn't occur after 7 days' treatment or
complete reepithelialization after 14
days' treatment. Know that trifluridine
should not be used for more than 21
days continuously due to potential ocular toxicity.
• Watch for signs of increased intraocular pressure.
• Continue trifluridine for several days
after steroid therapy, as ordered.
• Keep refrigerated.

☑ PATIENT TEACHING
• Tell patient to clean eye area of exces-
sive exudate before application.
• Teach patient how to instill drops. Ad-

---

vise him to wash hands before and after administering, and warn him not to touch tip of dropper to eye or surrounding tissue.

● Instruct patient to apply light finger pressure on lacrimal sac for 1 minute after drops are instilled.

● Reassure patient that the mild local irritation that occurs when solution is instilled is usually temporary.

● Tell patient not to share eye medications, washcloths, or towels. If anyone develops the same symptoms, the doctor should be notified.

● Stress importance of complying with recommended therapy.

---

vidarabine
Vira-A

Pregnancy Risk Category: C

HOW SUPPLIED
Ophthalmic ointment: 3% in 3.5-g tube (equivalent to 2.8% vidarabine)

ACTION
Unknown. Thought to interfere with DNA synthesis.

ONSET, PEAK, DURATION
Unknown. Systemic absorption is negligible.

INDICATIONS & DOSAGE
Acute keratoconjunctivitis, superficial keratitis, and recurrent epithelial keratitis caused by herpes simplex—
Adults and children: 1 cm of ointment applied into lower conjunctival sac five times daily at 3-hour intervals.

ADVERSE REACTIONS
EENT: temporary burning, itching, mild irritation, pain, lacrimation, foreign body sensation, conjunctival injection, punctal occlusion, sensitivity, superficial punctate keratitis, photophobia.
Other: hypersensitivity reactions.

INTERACTIONS
None significant.

EFFECTS ON DIAGNOSTIC TESTS
None known.

CONTRAINDICATIONS
Contraindicated in patients hypersensitive to the drug.

NURSING CONSIDERATIONS
● Use cautiously and with close monitoring with steroids. Vidarabine continued for several days after steroid therapy.

● Be aware that drug is not effective against RNA virus, adenoviral ocular infections, or bacterial, fungal, or chlamydial infections.

● Store in tightly closed, light-resistant container.

☑ **PATIENT TEACHING**
● Tell patient to clean eye area of excessive exudate before application.

● Teach patient how to apply. Advise him to wash hands before and after administering ointment and to avoid touching tip of tube to eye or surrounding tissue.

● Instruct patient to apply light finger pressure on lacrimal sac for 1 minute after drops are instilled.

● Explain to patient that the ointment may produce a temporary visual haze.

● Advise patient to watch for signs of sensitivity, such as itching lids, swelling, or constant burning. Tell patient who develops such signs to stop drug and notify the doctor immediately.

● Tell patient to minimize photophobia by wearing sunglasses and avoiding prolonged exposure to sunlight.

● Tell patient not to share eye medication, washcloths, or towels with family members. If anyone develops the same symptoms, notify the doctor.

---

*Liquid contains alcohol.   **May contain tartrazine.   †Canada only.   ‡Australia only.   ◇OTC.

dexamethasone
dexamethasone sodium
   phosphate
diclofenac sodium 0.1%
fluorometholone
flurbiprofen sodium
ketorolac tromethamine
medrysone
prednisolone acetate (suspension)
prednisolone sodium phosphate
   (solution)
rimexolone
suprofen

COMBINATION PRODUCTS
Corticosteroids for ophthalmic use are
commonly combined with antibiotics
and sulfonamides. See Chapter 79, ophthalmic anti-infectives.

---

dexamethasone
Maxidex Ophthalmic Suspension

dexamethasone sodium
phosphate
Decadron Phosphate Ophthalmic,
Maxidex Ophthalmic

Pregnancy Risk Category: C

HOW SUPPLIED
dexamethasone
Ophthalmic suspension: 0.1%
dexamethasone sodium phosphate
Ophthalmic ointment: 0.05%
Ophthalmic solution: 0.1%

ACTION
Unknown. Thought to decrease the infiltration of WBCs at the site of inflammation.

ONSET, PEAK, DURATION
Unknown.

INDICATIONS & DOSAGE
Uveitis; iridocyclitis; inflammatory conditions of eyelids, conjunctiva, cornea, anterior segment of globe; corneal injury from chemical or thermal burns, or penetration of foreign bodies; allergic conjunctivitis; suppression of graft rejection after keratoplasty—
Adults and children: 1 to 2 drops of suspension or solution instilled or 1.25 to 2.5 cm of ointment applied into conjunctival sac. In severe disease, drops may be used hourly, tapering to discontinuation as condition improves. In mild conditions, drops may be used up to four to six times daily or ointment applied t.i.d. or q.i.d. As condition improves, dosage tapered to b.i.d., then once daily. Treatment may extend from a few days to several weeks.

ADVERSE REACTIONS
EENT: increased intraocular pressure; thinning of cornea, interference with corneal wound healing, increased susceptibility to viral or fungal corneal infection, corneal ulceration; with excessive or long-term use— glaucoma exacerbation, cataracts, defects in visual acuity and visual field, optic nerve damage; mild blurred vision; burning, stinging, or redness of eyes; watery eyes, discharge, discomfort, ocular pain, foreign body sensation.
Other: systemic effects and adrenal suppression with excessive or long-term use.

INTERACTIONS
None significant.

EFFECTS ON DIAGNOSTIC TESTS
None reported.

CONTRAINDICATIONS
Contraindicated in patients with acute

Reactions may be *common*, uncommon, ***life-threatening***, or COMMON AND LIFE-THREATENING.

superficial herpes simplex (dendritic keratitis), vaccinia, varicella, or other fungal or viral diseases of cornea and conjunctiva; ocular tuberculosis; any acute, purulent, untreated infection of the eye; or hypersensitivity to any component of the formulation and after uncomplicated removal of a superficial corneal foreign body

NURSING CONSIDERATIONS
● Use cautiously in patients with corneal abrasions that may be infected (especially with herpes).
● Use cautiously in patients with glaucoma (any form), because intraocular pressure may increase. Glaucoma medications may need to be increased to compensate.
● Drug is not for long-term use.
● Watch for corneal ulceration; may require stopping drug.
● Be aware that corneal viral and fungal infections may be exacerbated by steroid application.

☑ **PATIENT TEACHING**
● Tell patient to shake suspension well before use.
● Teach patient how to instill drops or apply ointment. Advise him to wash hands before and after administering ointment or solution, and warn him not to touch tip of dropper to eye or surrounding tissue.
● Tell patient to apply light finger pressure on lacrimal sac for 1 minute after instillation.
● Advise patient that he may use eye pad with ointment.
● Warn patient not to use leftover medication for a new eye inflammation; may cause serious problems.
Alert: Warn patient to call the doctor immediately and to stop drug if visual acuity changes or visual field diminishes.
● Tell patient not to share medication, washcloths, or towels with family members and to notify doctor if anyone develops symptoms.
● Stress the importance of compliance

with recommended therapy.

diclofenac sodium 0.1%
Voltaren Ophthalmic

Pregnancy Risk Category: B

HOW SUPPLIED
Ophthalmic solution: 0.1%

ACTION
Unknown. Thought to inhibit the enzyme cyclooxygenase, which is essential in the biosynthesis of prostaglandins; prostaglandins may be mediators of certain kinds of intraocular inflammation.

ONSET, PEAK, DURATION
Unknown.

INDICATIONS & DOSAGE
Postoperative inflammation following removal of cataract—
Adults: 1 drop in the conjunctival sac q.i.d., beginning 24 hours after surgery and continuing throughout the first 2 weeks of the postoperative period.

ADVERSE REACTIONS
EENT: *transient stinging and burning, increased intraocular pressure, keratitis,* anterior chamber reaction, ocular allergy.
Systemic: nausea, vomiting, viral infection.

INTERACTIONS
None significant.

EFFECTS ON DIAGNOSTIC TESTS
Drug increases platelet aggregation time but does not affect bleeding time, plasma thrombin clotting time, plasma fibrinogen, or factors V and VII to XII.

CONTRAINDICATIONS
Contraindicated in patients with hypersensitivity to any component of the drug and in those wearing soft contact lenses.

---

*Liquid contains alcohol.   **May contain tartrazine.   †Canada only.   ‡Australia only.   ◊ OTC.

Because of the known effects of prostaglandin-inhibiting drugs on the fetal CV system (closure of the ductus arteriosus), the use of this drug during late pregnancy should be avoided.

NURSING CONSIDERATIONS
● Use cautiously in patients with hypersensitivity to acetylsalicylic acid, phenylacetic acid derivatives, and other NSAIDs; the potential for cross-sensitivity exists. It should also be used cautiously in surgical patients with known bleeding tendencies and in those receiving medications that may prolong bleeding time.
● Drug may slow or delay healing.
● Most cases of increased intraocular pressure have occurred postoperatively and before drug administration.

☑ PATIENT TEACHING
● Teach patient how to instill drops. Advise him to wash hands before and after instilling solution, and warn him not to touch tip of the dropper to eye or surrounding tissue.
● Advise patient to apply light finger pressure on lacrimal sac for 1 minute after drug instillation.
● Stress the importance of compliance with recommended therapy.
● Warn patient not to use leftover medication for a new eye inflammation.
● Remind patient to discard drug when no longer needed.

---

fluorometholone
Flarex, FML Forte, FML Liquifilm Ophthalmic, FML S.O.P.

Pregnancy Risk Category: C

HOW SUPPLIED
Ophthalmic ointment: 0.1%
Ophthalmic suspension: 0.1%, 0.25%

ACTION
Unknown. Thought to decrease the infiltration of WBCs at inflammation site.

ONSET, PEAK, DURATION
Unknown.

INDICATIONS & DOSAGE
Inflammatory and allergic conditions of cornea, conjunctiva, sclera, anterior uvea—
Adults and children: 1 to 2 drops instilled in conjunctival sac b.i.d. to q.i.d. May be given q 2 hours during first 1 to 2 days if needed. Alternatively, 1.25-cm ribbon of ointment applied to conjunctival sac q 4 hours, decreased to one to three times a day as inflammation subsides.

ADVERSE REACTIONS
EENT: increased intraocular pressure, thinning of cornea, interference with corneal wound healing, corneal ulceration, increased susceptibility to viral or fungal corneal infections; with excessive or long-term use—glaucoma exacerbation, discharge, discomfort, ocular pain, foreign body sensation, cataracts, decreased visual acuity, diminished visual field, optic nerve damage.
Other: systemic effects and adrenal suppression in excessive or long-term use.

INTERACTIONS
None significant.

EFFECTS ON DIAGNOSTIC TESTS
None reported.

CONTRAINDICATIONS
Contraindicated in patients with vaccinia, varicella, acute superficial herpes simplex (dendritic keratitis), or other fungal or viral eye diseases; ocular tuberculosis; or any acute, purulent, untreated eye infection.

NURSING CONSIDERATIONS
● Use cautiously in patients with corneal abrasions that may be contaminated (especially with herpes).
● Safety and efficacy in children under age 2 have not been established.
● Drug is not for long-term use.

Reactions may be *common*, uncommon, *life-threatening*, or COMMON AND LIFE-THREATENING.

● Shake well before using.
● Be aware that drug is less likely to cause increased intraocular pressure with long-term use than other ophthalmic anti-inflammatory drugs (except medrysone).
● Store in tightly covered, light-resistant container.

☑ **PATIENT TEACHING**
● Teach patient how to instill drops or apply ointment. Advise him to wash hands before and after administering ointment or solution, and warn him not to touch tip of dropper to eye or surrounding tissue.
● Advise patient to apply light finger pressure on lacrimal sac for 1 minute after instillation.
● Advise patient to call the doctor immediately and to stop drug if visual acuity decreases or visual field diminishes.
● Warn patient not to use leftover medication for a new eye inflammation; may cause serious problems.
● Tell patient not to share eye medication, washcloths, or towels with family members. If anyone develops similar symptoms, the doctor should be notified.

---

flurbiprofen sodium
Ocufen Liquifilm

Pregnancy Risk Category: C

HOW SUPPLIED
Ophthalmic solution: 0.03%

ACTION
Unknown. An NSAID that's thought to inhibit the cyclooxygenase enzyme essential in the biosynthesis of prostaglandin.

ONSET, PEAK, DURATION
Unknown.

INDICATIONS & DOSAGE
Inhibition of intraoperative miosis—

Adults: 1 drop instilled into the affected eye approximately every ½ hour, beginning 2 hours before surgery. A total of 4 drops is given.

ADVERSE REACTIONS
EENT: transient burning and stinging on instillation, ocular irritation.

INTERACTIONS
Acetylcholine, carbachol: may be rendered ineffective. Avoid concomitant use.
Anticoagulants: increased risk of bleeding if significant systemic absorption occurs. Monitor closely.

EFFECTS ON DIAGNOSTIC TESTS
None reported.

CONTRAINDICATIONS
Contraindicated in patients with hypersensitivity to the drug.

NURSING CONSIDERATIONS
● Use cautiously in patients who may be allergic to aspirin and other NSAIDs.
● Use cautiously in patients with bleeding tendencies and those who are receiving medications that may prolong clotting times.
● Be aware that wound healing may be delayed.

☑ **PATIENT TEACHING**
● Advise patient to alert the doctor immediately if visual acuity decreases or visual field diminishes.
● Urge him to take drug as prescribed.

---

ketorolac tromethamine
Acular

Pregnancy Risk Category: C

HOW SUPPLIED
Ophthalmic solution: 0.5%

ACTION
Unknown. An NSAID that is thought to

---

*Liquid contains alcohol.   **May contain tartrazine.   †Canada only.   ‡Australia only.   ◇ OTC.

inhibit the action of cyclooxygenase, an enzyme responsible for prostaglandin synthesis. Prostaglandins mediate the inflammatory response and also cause miosis.

ONSET, PEAK, DURATION
Unknown. Systemic absorption is negligible.

INDICATIONS & DOSAGE
Relief of ocular itching caused by seasonal allergic conjunctivitis—
Adults: 1 drop into the conjunctival sac instilled in each eye q.i.d.

ADVERSE REACTIONS
EENT: *transient stinging and burning on instillation,* superficial keratitis, superficial ocular infections, ocular irritation.
Other: hypersensitivity reactions.

INTERACTIONS
None significant.

EFFECTS ON DIAGNOSTIC TESTS
None reported.

CONTRAINDICATIONS
Contraindicated in patients hypersensitive to any component of the formulation and in wearers of soft contact lenses.

NURSING CONSIDERATIONS
● Use cautiously in patients hypersensitive to other NSAIDs or aspirin and in patients with bleeding disorders.
● Store drug away from heat in a dark, tightly closed container and protect from freezing.

☑ **PATIENT TEACHING**
● Teach patient how to instill drops. Advise him to wash hands before and after instilling solution, and warn him not to touch tip of dropper to eye or surrounding tissue.
● Advise patient to apply light finger pressure on lacrimal sac for 1 minute after instillation.

● Remind patient to discard drug when it's no longer needed.
● Stress the importance of compliance with recommended therapy.

---

medrysone
HMS Liquifilm Ophthalmic

Pregnancy Risk Category: C

HOW SUPPLIED
Ophthalmic suspension: 1%

ACTION
Unknown. Thought to decrease the infiltration of WBCs at the site of inflammation.

ONSET, PEAK, DURATION
Unknown. Although systemic absorption occurs, plasma levels are very low and systemic effects are negligible.

INDICATIONS & DOSAGE
Allergic conjunctivitis, vernal conjunctivitis, episcleritis, ophthalmic epinephrine sensitivity reaction—
Adults and children: 1 drop instilled into conjunctival sac q 4 hours.

ADVERSE REACTIONS
EENT: thinning of cornea, interference with corneal wound healing, increased susceptibility to viral or fungal corneal infection, corneal ulceration; with excessive or long-term use—discharge, discomfort, ocular pain, foreign body sensation, glaucoma exacerbation, cataracts, visual acuity and visual field defects, optic nerve damage.
Other: systemic effects and adrenal suppression with excessive or long-term use.

INTERACTIONS
None significant.

EFFECTS ON DIAGNOSTIC TESTS
None reported.

Reactions may be *common*, uncommon, *life-threatening*, or COMMON AND LIFE-THREATENING.

CONTRAINDICATIONS

Contraindicated in patients with vaccinia, varicella, acute superficial herpes simplex (dendritic keratitis), viral diseases of conjunctiva and cornea, ocular tuberculosis, fungal or viral eye diseases, iritis, uveitis, or any acute, purulent, untreated eye infection.

NURSING CONSIDERATIONS

• Use cautiously in patients with corneal abrasions that may be contaminated (especially with herpes).
• Using leftover medication for a new eye inflammation may cause serious problems.

☑ PATIENT TEACHING

• Teach patient how to instill drops. Advise him to wash hands before and after instilling solution, and warn him not to touch tip of dropper to eye or surrounding tissue.
• Tell patient to shake well before using. Don't freeze.
• Advise patient to apply light finger pressure on lacrimal sac for 1 minute after instillation.
• Tell patient not to share medication, washcloths, or towels with family members and to notify doctor if anyone develops symptoms.
• Stress the importance of compliance with recommended therapy.

---

prednisolone acetate (suspension)

Econopred Ophthalmic, Econopred Plus Ophthalmic, Pred-Forte, Pred Mild Ophthalmic

prednisolone sodium phosphate (solution)

AK-Pred, Inflamase Forte, Inflamase Ophthalmic, Predsol Eye Drops‡

Pregnancy Risk Category: C

HOW SUPPLIED

prednisolone acetate
Ophthalmic suspension: 0.12%, 0.125%, 1%
prednisolone sodium phosphate
Ophthalmic solution: 0.125%, 1%

ACTION

Unknown. Thought to decrease the infiltration of WBCs at the site of inflammation.

ONSET, PEAK, DURATION

Unknown. Although systemic absorption occurs, plasma levels are very low and systemic effects are negligible.

INDICATIONS & DOSAGE

Inflammation of palpebral and bulbar conjunctiva, cornea, and anterior segment of globe—
Adults and children: 1 to 2 drops instilled into eye. In severe conditions, may be used hourly, tapering to discontinuation as inflammation subsides. In mild conditions, may be used two to four times daily.

ADVERSE REACTIONS

EENT: increased intraocular pressure; thinning of cornea, interference with corneal wound healing, increased susceptibility to viral or fungal corneal infection, corneal ulceration; with excessive or long-term use—discharge, discomfort, foreign body sensation, glaucoma exacerbation, cataracts, visual acuity and visual field defects, optic nerve damage.
Other: systemic effects and adrenal suppression with excessive or long-term use.

INTERACTIONS

None significant.

EFFECTS ON DIAGNOSTIC TESTS

None reported.

CONTRAINDICATIONS

Contraindicated in patients with acute, untreated, purulent ocular infections; acute superficial herpes simplex (den-

---

dritic keratitis); vaccinia, varicella, or other viral or fungal eye diseases; or ocular tuberculosis.

NURSING CONSIDERATIONS
● Use cautiously in patients with corneal abrasions that may be contaminated (especially with herpes).
● Shake suspension and check dosage before administering to ensure using the correct strength. Store in tightly covered container.

☑ PATIENT TEACHING
● Teach patient how to instill drops. Advise him to wash hands before and after applying, and warn him not to touch tip of dropper to eye or surrounding area.
● Advise patient to apply light finger pressure on lacrimal sac for 1 minute after instillation.
● Tell patient on long-term therapy to have frequent tonometric examinations.
● Warn patient not to use leftover medication for a new eye inflammation; may cause serious problems.
● Tell patient not to share eye medication, washcloths, or towels with family members. If anyone develops similar symptoms, the doctor should be notified.
● Stress the importance of compliance with recommended therapy.

---

rimexolone
Vexol 1% Ophthalmic Suspension

Pregnancy Risk Category: C

HOW SUPPLIED
Ophthalmic suspension: 1%

ACTION
Exact mechanism unknown. A corticosteroid, it inhibits edema, cellular infiltration, capillary dilation, fibroblastic proliferation, and deposition of collagen and scar formation associated with inflammation.

ONSET, PEAK, DURATION
Unknown.

INDICATIONS & DOSAGE
Postoperative inflammation following ocular surgery—
Adults: 1 to 2 drops instilled into the conjunctival sac q.i.d., beginning 24 hours after surgery and continuing throughout the first 2 weeks of the postoperative period.
Anterior uveitis—
Adults: 1 to 2 drops in the conjunctival sac q hour during waking hours for the first week, 1 drop q 2 hours during waking hours of the second week, and then tapered until uveitis is resolved.

ADVERSE REACTIONS
EENT: *blurred vision, ocular discharge, ocular pain or discomfort, increased intraocular pressure, foreign-body sensation, ocular hyperemia, ocular pruritus,* sticky sensation, increased fibrin formation, eye dryness, conjunctival edema, corneal staining, keratitis, lacrimation, photophobia, edema, irritation, corneal ulcer, brow pain, crusting at margin of eyelid, corneal edema, infiltrate, corneal erosion.
Other: headache, hypotension, rhinitis, pharyngitis, taste perversion.

INTERACTIONS
None significant.

EFFECTS ON DIAGNOSTIC TESTS
None reported.

CONTRAINDICATIONS
Contraindicated in patients with hypersensitivity to any component of the drug. Also contraindicated in those with epithelial herpes simplex keratitis, vaccinia, varicella, and most other viral diseases of the cornea and conjunctiva; mycobacterial infection of the eye; and fungal disease of the eye or acute purulent untreated infections that may be masked or enhanced by the presence of a steroid.

NURSING CONSIDERATIONS
● Monitor patient's blood pressure throughout therapy.
● Never use leftover medication for a new eye inflammation.

☑ PATIENT TEACHING
● Teach patient how to instill drops. Advise him to shake the dispenser well before using. Also advise him to wash hands before and after instilling suspension, and warn him not to touch tip of the dropper to eye or surrounding tissue.
● Advise patient to apply light finger pressure on lacrimal sac for 1 minute after drug instillation.
● Stress the importance of compliance with recommended therapy.
● Remind patient to discard drug when no longer needed.
● Advise patient to have intraocular pressure checked frequently.

---

suprofen
Profenal

Pregnancy Risk Category: C

HOW SUPPLIED
Ophthalmic solution: 1%

ACTION
Unknown. An NSAID that inhibits the action of cyclooxygenase, an enzyme responsible for the synthesis of prostaglandins. Prostaglandins mediate the inflammatory response and also cause miosis.

ONSET, PEAK, DURATION
Unknown. Systemic absorption is negligible.

INDICATIONS & DOSAGE
Inhibition of intraoperative miosis—
Adults: 2 drops instilled into the conjunctival sac q 4 hours the day before surgery. On the day of surgery, 2 drops instilled 3 hours, 2 hours, and 1 hour before surgery.

ADVERSE REACTIONS
EENT: *transient stinging and burning on instillation,* discomfort, itching, redness, iritis, pain, chemosis, photophobia, irritation, punctate epithelial staining.
Other: hypersensitivity reactions.

INTERACTIONS
Acetylcholine, carbachol: may be ineffective in patients treated with suprofen.

EFFECTS ON DIAGNOSTIC TESTS
None reported.

CONTRAINDICATIONS
Contraindicated in patients hypersensitive to any component of the formulation and in patients with epithelial herpes simplex keratitis.

NURSING CONSIDERATIONS
● Use cautiously in patients hypersensitive to other NSAIDs or aspirin.
● Use cautiously in patients with bleeding disorders.
Alert: Drug may be absorbed into breast milk following topical ocular administration. It is recommended that breastfeeding be discontinued during administration.

☑ PATIENT TEACHING
● Teach patient how to instill drops. Advise him to wash hands before and after administering solution and not to touch tip of dropper to eye or surrounding tissues.
● Tell patient to apply light finger pressure on lacrimal sac for 1 minute after drops are instilled.
● Tell him to store drug away from heat in a dark, tightly closed container and to protect drug from freezing.
● Remind patient to discard drug when it's no longer needed.

---

acetylcholine chloride
carbachol (intraocular)
carbachol (topical)
demecarium bromide
echothiophate iodide
isoflurophate
physostigmine sulfate
pilocarpine
pilocarpine hydrochloride
pilocarpine nitrate

COMBINATION PRODUCTS

E-PILO: epinephrine bitartrate 1% and pilocarpine hydrochloride 1%, 2%, 3%, 4%, or 6%.

ISOPTO P-ES: pilocarpine hydrochloride 2% and physostigmine salicylate 0.25%.

P_1E_1, P_2E_1, P_3E_1, P_4E_1, P_6E_1: epinephrine bitartrate 1% and pilocarpine hydrochloride 1%, 2%, 3%, 4%, or 6%.

---

acetylcholine chloride
Miochol

Pregnancy Risk Category: NR

HOW SUPPLIED
Ophthalmic injection: 1%

ACTION
A cholinergic that causes contraction of the sphincter muscles of the iris, resulting in miosis, and that produces ciliary spasm, deepening of the anterior chamber, and vasodilation of conjunctival vessels of the outflow tract.

ONSET, PEAK, DURATION
Onset occurs within seconds. Peak unknown. Effects persist for about 10 minutes.

INDICATIONS & DOSAGE
Anterior segment surgery—
Adults and children: before or after se-

curing sutures, the doctor gently instills 0.5 to 2 ml into anterior chamber.

ADVERSE REACTIONS
CV: bradycardia, hypotension.
EENT: corneal edema, clouding, or decompensation.
Respiratory: breathing difficulties.
Other: flushing, diaphoresis.

INTERACTIONS
None significant.

EFFECTS ON DIAGNOSTIC TESTS
None significant.

CONTRAINDICATIONS
Contraindicated in patients with hypersensitivity to the drug or any of its components.

NURSING CONSIDERATIONS
● Reconstitute immediately before using, shaking vial gently until clear solution is obtained.
● Discard any unused solution.
● Don't gas-sterilize vial. Ethylene oxide may produce formic acid.

☑ PATIENT TEACHING
● Inform patient about need for drug during surgical procedure, and answer any questions and address concerns.
● Instruct patient to report breathing difficulties immediately.

---

carbachol (intraocular)
Miostat

carbachol (topical)
Isopto Carbachol

Pregnancy Risk Category: C

Reactions may be *common*, uncommon, *life-threatening*, or COMMON AND LIFE-THREATENING.

HOW SUPPLIED
Intraocular injection: 0.01%
Topical ophthalmic solution: 0.75%,
1.5%, 2.25%, 3%

ACTION
A cholinergic that causes contraction of
the sphincter muscles of the iris, resulting in miosis, and that produces ciliary
spasm, deepening of the anterior chamber, and vasodilation of conjunctival
vessels of the outflow tract.

ONSET, PEAK, DURATION
Onset occurs in 10 to 20 minutes. Peak
effect occurs 4 hours after topical application, 2 to 5 minutes after intraocular
injection. Effects persist about 8 hours
after topical application, 24 hours after
intraocular injection.

INDICATIONS & DOSAGE
*To produce pupillary miosis in ocular
surgery—*
Adults: before or after securing sutures,
the doctor gently instills 0.5 ml (intraocular form) into anterior chamber.
Open-angle glaucoma—
Adults: 1 to 2 drops instilled (topical
form) q 4 to 8 hours.

ADVERSE REACTIONS
CNS: headache, syncope.
CV: arrhythmia, hypotension.
EENT: spasm of eye accommodation,
conjunctival vasodilation, eye and brow
pain, transient stinging and burning,
corneal clouding, bullous keratopathy,
salivation.
GI: abdominal cramps, diarrhea.
GU: urinary urgency.
Respiratory: asthma.
Other: diaphoresis, flushing.

INTERACTIONS
Pilocarpine: additive effect. Use together cautiously.

EFFECTS ON DIAGNOSTIC TESTS
None significant.

CONTRAINDICATIONS
Contraindicated in patients with hypersensitivity to drug or in patients where
cholinergic effects such as constriction
are undesirable (for example, acute iritis, some forms of secondary glaucoma,
pupillary block glaucoma, or acute inflammatory disease of the anterior
chamber).

NURSING CONSIDERATIONS
● Use cautiously in patients with acute
heart failure, bronchial asthma, peptic
ulcer, hyperthyroidism, GI spasm,
Parkinson's disease, and urinary tract
obstruction.
● In case of toxicity, give atropine parenterally as ordered.
● The drug is used in open-angle glaucoma, especially when patients are resistant or allergic to pilocarpine hydrochloride or nitrate.
Alert: Keep in mind that patients with
dark eyes (hazel or brown irises) may
require stronger solutions or more frequent instillation because eye pigment
may absorb the drug.
● If tolerance to the drug develops,
know that the doctor may switch to another miotic for a short time.

☑ PATIENT TEACHING
● Teach patient how to instill. Advise
him to wash hands before and after and
to apply light finger-pressure on lacrimal sac for 1 minute after drops are instilled. Warn him not to exceed recommended dosage.
● Warn patient to avoid hazardous activities, such as operating machinery or driving, until temporary blurring subsides.
Reassure patient that blurred vision usually diminishes with prolonged use.
● Tell glaucoma patient that long-term
use may be necessary. Stress compliance. Tell him to remain under medical
supervision for periodic tonometric
readings.
● Warn patient to use caution during
night driving and other hazardous activities in poor light.

---

*Liquid contains alcohol.   **May contain tartrazine.   †Canada only.   ‡Australia only.   ◇OTC.

demecarium bromide
Humorsol

Pregnancy Risk Category: X

HOW SUPPLIED
Ophthalmic solution: 0.125%, 0.25%

ACTION
An anticholinesterase drug that inhibits the enzymatic destruction of acetylcholine by inactivating cholinesterase, leaving acetylcholine free to act on the effector cells of the iridic sphincter and ciliary muscles, causing pupillary constriction and spasm of accommodation.

ONSET, PEAK, DURATION
Onset occurs in 15 to 60 minutes. Miotic effect peaks within 2 hours; intraocular pressure (IOP) reduction occurs within 24 hours. Miosis persists for 3 to 10 days; IOP reduction, about 9 days.

INDICATIONS & DOSAGE
Acute angle-closure glaucoma after iridectomy, primary open-angle glaucoma—
Adults: 1 drop instilled once or twice daily.
Treatment of convergent strabismus (uncomplicated)—
Adults: 1 drop instilled daily for 2 to 3 weeks, then reduced to 1 drop q 2 days for 3 to 4 weeks. After reevaluation, 1 drop instilled once or twice weekly to once q 2 days as determined by the patient's condition. Reevaluated q 4 to 12 weeks; dosage adjusted as needed. Discontinued after 4 months if dosage required is 1 drop q 2 days.
Diagnosis of convergent strabismus—
Adults: 1 drop instilled daily for 2 weeks, then 1 drop q 2 days for 2 to 3 weeks.

ADVERSE REACTIONS
CNS: brow ache, unusual fatigue or weakness, headache.
CV: bradycardia, palpitations.

EENT: retinal detachment, iris cysts, conjunctival thickening, lens opacities, paradoxical increase in IOP, *lacrimation,* obstruction of nasolacrimal canals; eye pain, burning, redness, stinging and irritation; twitching eyelids; *blurred vision;* visual disturbances.
GI: nausea, vomiting, diarrhea, abdominal cramps or pain.
GU: loss of bladder control.

INTERACTIONS
Anticholinergics, antimyasthenics, other cholinesterase inhibitors: potential for additive toxicity. Monitor closely.
Carbamate or organophosphate-type insecticides (parathion, malathion): increased risk of systemic effects through respiratory tract or skin. Warn patients to protect themselves.
Cocaine: increased risk of cocaine toxicity; anticholinesterase effects may last weeks or months. Avoid concomitant use.
Epinephrine: additive effect, resulting in better control and lower dosages of both drugs.
Local anesthetics, ophthalmic tetracaine: increased risk of systemic toxicity and prolonged ocular anesthetic effect. Monitor closely.
Ophthalmic adrenocorticoids: increased IOP and decreased antiglaucoma effectiveness. Avoid concomitant use.
Ophthalmic belladonna alkaloids, cyclopentolate: may antagonize miotic effects. Avoid concomitant use.
Succinylcholine: enhanced neuromuscular blockade, possible CV collapse and prolonged respiratory depression or apnea may occur for several weeks or months after demecarium is discontinued. Advise the anesthesiologist that the patient has received demecarium.

EFFECTS ON DIAGNOSTIC TESTS
No information available.

CONTRAINDICATIONS
Contraindicated in patients with hypersensitivity to drug, acute angle-closure

Reactions may be *common,* uncommon, *life-threatening,* or COMMON AND LIFE-THREATENING.

glaucoma before iridectomy, and other forms of glaucoma (except for primary open-angle glaucoma).

NURSING CONSIDERATIONS
● Use with extreme caution, if at all, in patients with history or risk of retinal detachment, marked vagotonia, bronchial asthma, spastic GI conditions, urinary tract obstruction, peptic ulcer, severe bradycardia, hypotension, hypertension, hyperthyroidism, acute cardiac failure, recent MI, epilepsy, marked vasomotor instability, or parkinsonism.
● Use with caution in patients with corneal abrasion.
● Administer phenylephrine concurrently, as ordered, to reduce incidence of iris cyst formation.
● If tolerance to the drug develops after prolonged use, know that the doctor may switch to another miotic for a short time.
● Know that toxicity is cumulative; toxic systemic symptoms may not appear for weeks or months after start of therapy. Atropine sulfate S.C., I.M., or I.V. is antidote of choice.

☑ PATIENT TEACHING
● Teach patient how to instill demecarium. Advise him to wash hands before and after instilling drug, to avoid touching applicator tip to any surface, and to remove excess solution around eyes with clean tissue and without touching eye. Warn him not to exceed recommended dosage.
● If dose is missed, instruct patient not to double dose. If schedule is every other day, tell patient to instill as soon as possible if remembered same day; if remembered later, tell him not to instill until next day, then skip a day and resume regular schedule. If schedule is once a day, tell patient to instill as soon as possible. If not remembered until next day, tell him to skip missed dose and resume regular schedule. If schedule is more than once daily, tell patient to instill as soon as possible. If close to time

for next dose, tell him to skip missed dose and resume regular schedule.
● Tell patient that regular medical supervision is required to check ocular pressure.
● Advise patient to carry medical identification card at all times during therapy.

---

echothiophate iodide (ecothiopate iodide)
Phospholine Iodide

Pregnancy Risk Category: C

HOW SUPPLIED
Ophthalmic powder for solution: for reconstitution to make 0.03%, 0.06%, 0.125%, and 0.25% solutions

ACTION
An anticholinesterase drug that inhibits the enzymatic destruction of acetylcholine by inactivating cholinesterase, leaving acetylcholine free to act on the effector cells of the iridic sphincter and ciliary muscles, causing pupillary constriction and spasm of accommodation.

ONSET, PEAK, DURATION
Miosis occurs in 10 to 30 minutes; intraocular pressure (IOP) reduction, 4 to 8 hours. Miotic effect peaks within 30 minutes; IOP reduction occurs within 24 hours. Effects persist for several days to 4 weeks.

INDICATIONS & DOSAGE
Primary open-angle glaucoma, conditions obstructing aqueous outflow—
Adults and children: 1 drop of 0.03% to 0.125% solution instilled into conjunctival sac daily. Maximum dosage is 1 drop b.i.d. Lowest possible dosage used for continuous control of IOP.
Diagnosis of convergent strabismus—
Adults: 1 drop of 0.125% solution instilled daily h.s. for 2 to 3 weeks.
Treatment of convergent strabismus—
Adults: initially, 1 drop of 0.125% solution instilled into each eye daily h.s. for

2 to 3 weeks. Dosage decreased to 1 drop of 0.125% solution every other day or 1 drop of 0.06% solution daily. The 0.03% solution may be used instead for some patients.

ADVERSE REACTIONS
CNS: fatigue, muscle weakness, paresthesia, headache.
CV: bradycardia, hypotension.
EENT: ciliary spasm or spasm of eye accommodation, ciliary or circumcorneal injection, nonreversible cataract formation (time- and dose-related), reversible iris cysts, pupillary block, blurred or dimmed vision, eye or brow pain, twitching of eyelids, hyperemia, photophobia, lens opacities, lacrimation, retinal detachment.
GI: diarrhea, nausea, vomiting, abdominal pain, intestinal cramps, salivation.
GU: frequent urination.
Respiratory: *bronchoconstriction.*
Other: diaphoresis, flushing.

INTERACTIONS
Anticholinergics, ophthalmic belladonna alkaloids (such as atropine), cyclopentolate: antagonized miotic effects. Avoid concomitant use.
Cocaine: increased risk of cocaine toxicity. Avoid concomitant use.
Local anesthetics, ophthalmic tetracaine: increased rate of systemic toxicity and prolonged ocular anesthesia. Monitor closely.
Ophthalmic adrenocorticoids: increased intraocular pressure and decreased antiglaucoma effectiveness. Avoid concomitant use.
Other cholinesterase inhibitors, organophosphate insecticides (parathion, malathion): possible additive effect causing systemic effects. Warn patients exposed to insecticides to protect themselves.
Succinylcholine: respiratory and CV collapse. Don't use together.
Systemic anticholinesterase agents for myasthenia gravis, pilocarpine: effects may be additive. Monitor patients for signs of toxicity.

EFFECTS ON DIAGNOSTIC TESTS
Drug therapy decreases plasma cholinesterase activity.

CONTRAINDICATIONS
Contraindicated in patients with hypersensitivity to drug or iodine, uveal inflammation, acute angle-closure glaucoma before iridectomy, and other forms of glaucoma (except for primary open-angle glaucoma).

NURSING CONSIDERATIONS
● Use with extreme caution, if at all, in patients with seizure disorders, vasomotor instability, parkinsonism, bronchial asthma, spastic GI conditions, urinary tract obstruction, peptic ulcer, severe bradycardia or hypotension, vascular hypertension, MI, or history or risk of retinal detachment.
● Use with caution in patients with corneal abrasion.
● Reconstitute powder, using only diluent provided to avoid contamination. Discard refrigerated, reconstituted solution after 6 months; solution stored at room temperature, after 1 month.
● Stop drug, as ordered, at least 2 weeks preoperatively if succinylcholine is to be used in surgery.
● Know that toxicity is cumulative; toxic systemic symptoms may not appear for weeks or months after start of therapy. Atropine sulfate S.C., I.M., or I.V. is antidote of choice.

☑ PATIENT TEACHING
● Advise patient to carry medical identification card at all times during therapy. Drug is a potent, long-acting, and irreversible.
● Teach patient how to instill drug. Advise him to wash hands before and after instilling drug, to avoid touching applicator tip to any surface and to apply light finger pressure on lacrimal sac for 1 minute after instillation.
● Tell patient to instill drug at bedtime because it causes transient blurred vision. Warn him that transient brow pain

or dimmed or blurred vision is common at first but usually disappears within 5 to 10 days.

• Warn patient to report salivation, diarrhea, profuse diaphoresis, urinary incontinence, or muscle weakness to the doctor.

• Tell patient to remain under constant medical supervision and not to exceed recommended dosage.

isoflurophate
Floropryl

Pregnancy Risk Category: X

HOW SUPPLIED
Ophthalmic ointment: 0.025%

ACTION
An anticholinesterase drug that inhibits the enzymatic destruction of acetylcholine by inactivating cholinesterase, leaving acetylcholine free to act on the effector cells of the iridic sphincter and ciliary muscles, causing pupillary constriction and spasm of accommodation.

ONSET, PEAK, DURATION
Unknown.

INDICATIONS & DOSAGE
Glaucoma—
Adults: 0.5-cm ribbon of ointment applied to conjunctiva q 8 to 72 hours.
Diagnosis of convergent strabismus (uncomplicated)—
Adults: 0.5-cm ribbon of ointment applied to conjunctiva h.s. for 2 weeks.
Treatment of convergent strabismus—
Adults: 0.5-cm ribbon of ointment applied to each eye h.s. for 2 weeks, then once every 2 to 7 days, depending on the patient's condition, for 2 months. If the patient cannot be maintained on a dosage interval of at least 48 hours, the drug should be discontinued.

ADVERSE REACTIONS
CNS: headache, brow ache, unusual fatigue or weakness.
CV: slow or irregular heartbeat.
EENT: retinal detachment, iris cysts, conjunctival thickening, lens opacities, obstruction of nasolacrimal canals, paradoxical increase in intraocular pressure (IOP); *eye burning,* redness, pain, stinging or irritation; twitching of eyelids; *blurred vision;* visual disturbances.
GI: nausea, vomiting, diarrhea, abdominal cramps or pain.
GU: loss of bladder control.
Other: diaphoresis, flushing.

INTERACTIONS
Anticholinergics, antimyasthenics, other cholinesterase inhibitors: potential for additive toxicity. Monitor closely.
Carbamate or organophosphate-type insecticides (parathion, malathion): increased risk of systemic effects through respiratory tract or skin. Warn patients to protect themselves.
Cocaine: increased risk of cocaine toxicity; anticholinesterase effects may last weeks or months. Avoid concomitant use.
Epinephrine: additive effect, resulting in better control and lower dosages of both drugs.
Local anesthetics, ophthalmic tetracaine: increased risk of systemic toxicity, prolonged ocular anesthesia. Monitor closely.
Ophthalmic adrenocorticoids: increased IOP and decreased antiglaucoma effectiveness. Avoid concomitant use.
Ophthalmic belladonna alkaloids, cyclopentolate: may antagonize miotic effects. Avoid concomitant use.
Ophthalmic physostigmine: may shorten duration of action. Avoid concomitant use.
Succinylcholine: enhanced neuromuscular blockade, possible CV collapse, prolonged respiratory depression, or apnea may occur for several weeks or months after demecarium is discontinued. Advise the anesthesiologist that the patient has received demecarium.

---

*Liquid contains alcohol.   **May contain tartrazine.   †Canada only.   ‡Australia only.   ◊ OTC.

EFFECTS ON DIAGNOSTIC TESTS
No information available.

CONTRAINDICATIONS
Contraindicated in pregnant patients and in those with hypersensitivity to drug, active uveal inflammation, glaucoma associated with iridocyclitis, or acute angle-closure glaucoma before iridectomy.

NURSING CONSIDERATIONS
● Use with extreme caution, if at all, in patients with bronchial asthma, pronounced bradycardia and hypotension, seizure disorders, spastic GI disturbances, Parkinson's disease, marked vagotonia, MI, or history of retinal detachment.
● Use with caution in patients with corneal abrasion.
● Administer phenylephrine concurrently, as ordered, to reduce incidence of iris cyst formation.
● If tolerance to the drug develops after prolonged use, know that the doctor may switch to another miotic for a short time.
● Know that toxicity is cumulative; toxic systemic symptoms may not appear for weeks or months after therapy is discontinued. Atropine sulfate S.C., I.M., or I.V. is antidote of choice.

☑ **PATIENT TEACHING**
● Teach patient how to apply drug. Advise him to wash hands before and after application, to avoid touching applicator tip to any surface and to wipe tip with clean tissue. Warn him not to exceed recommended dosage.
● If dose is missed, instruct patient not to double dose. If schedule is every other day, tell patient to apply as soon as possible if remembered same day; if remembered later, tell him not to apply until next day, then skip a day and resume regular schedule. If schedule is once a day, tell patient to apply as soon as possible. If not remembered until next day, tell him to skip missed dose and resume schedule. If schedule is more than once daily, tell him to apply as soon as possible. If close to time for next dose, tell patient to skip missed dose and resume regular schedule.
● Tell patient that regular medical supervision is required to check ocular pressure.
● Advise patient to carry medical identification card at all times during therapy.

---

physostigmine sulfate
Eserine Sulfate

Pregnancy Risk Category: C

HOW SUPPLIED
Ophthalmic ointment: 0.25%

ACTION
Causes contraction of iris sphincter muscles resulting in miosis, and contraction of ciliary muscle, increasing outflow of aqueous humor and decreasing intraocular pressure.

ONSET, PEAK, DURATION
Onset occurs within 30 minutes. Peak unknown. Effects persist for 12 to 48 hours.

INDICATIONS & DOSAGE
Open-angle glaucoma—
Adults and children: apply a thin strip of ointment once daily to t.i.d.

ADVERSE REACTIONS
CNS: headache, weakness.
CV: slow or irregular heartbeat.
EENT: blurred vision, eye pain, burning, redness, stinging, eye irritation, twitching of eyelids, watering of eyes.
GI: nausea, vomiting, diarrhea.
GU: loss of bladder control.
Other: diaphoresis, muscle weakness, shortness of breath.

INTERACTIONS
Echothiophate, isoflurophate: duration of action may be shortened. Monitor closely.

Reactions may be *common,* uncommon, *life-threatening,* or COMMON AND LIFE-THREATENING.

Ophthalmic belladonna alkaloids: may antagonize miotic actions. Avoid concomitant use.

EFFECTS ON DIAGNOSTIC TESTS
None reported.

CONTRAINDICATIONS
Contraindicated in patients with intolerance to physostigmine, active uveitis, or corneal injury.

NURSING CONSIDERATIONS
● Be aware that ointment may be used at night because of its longer duration of action.
● If tolerance to the drug develops, know that the doctor may switch to another miotic for a short time.

☑ **PATIENT TEACHING**
● Warn patient not to exceed recommended dosage.

pilocarpine
Ocusert Pilo

pilocarpine hydrochloride
Adsorbocarpine, Akarapine, E-Pilo, Isopto Carpine, Miocarpine†, Ocusert Pilo, Pilocar, Pilocel, Pilopine HS, Pilopt‡

pilocarpine nitrate
Pilagan, P.V.

Pregnancy Risk Category: C

HOW SUPPLIED
pilocarpine
Extended-release insert: 20 mcg/hour, 40 mcg/hour for 7 days
pilocarpine hydrochloride
Ophthalmic solution: 0.25%, 0.5%, 1%, 2%, 3%, 4%, 5%, 6%, 8%, 10%
Ophthalmic gel: 4%
pilocarpine nitrate
Ophthalmic solution: 1%, 2%, 4%

ACTION
A cholinergic that causes contraction of iris sphincter muscles, resulting in miosis and that produces ciliary spasm, deepening of the anterior chamber, and vasodilation of conjunctival vessels of the outflow tract.

ONSET, PEAK, DURATION
Onset of miosis occurs within 10 to 30 minutes; intraocular pressure (IOP) reduction, within 60 minutes. Miotic effect peaks within 30 minutes; IOP reduction occurs within 75 minutes. Miosis effects persist up to 8 hours; IOP reduction, 4 to 14 hours with topical solution, up to 24 hours with gel, and up to 7 days with extended-release ocular system.

INDICATIONS & DOSAGE
Primary open-angle glaucoma—
Adults and children: 1 drop instilled up to q.i.d. or 1-cm ribbon of 4% gel (Pilopine HS) applied h.s. Alternatively, one Ocusert Pilo system (20 or 40 mcg/hour) applied q 7 days.
Emergency treatment of acute angle-closure glaucoma—
Adults and children: 1 drop of 2% solution instilled q 5 to 10 minutes for three to six doses, followed by 1 drop q 1 to 3 hours until pressure is controlled.
Mydriasis caused by mydriatic or cycloplegic agents—
Adults and children: 1 drop of 1% solution.

ADVERSE REACTIONS
CV: hypertension, tachycardia.
EENT: periorbital or supraorbital headache, *myopia,* ciliary spasm, *blurred vision,* conjunctival irritation, transient stinging and burning, keratitis, lens opacity, retinal detachment, lacrimation, changes in visual field, *brow pain.*
GI: nausea, vomiting, diarrhea, salivation.
Respiratory: *bronchoconstriction, pulmonary edema.*

Other: hypersensitivity reactions, diaphoresis.

INTERACTIONS
Carbachol, echothiophate: additive effect. Don't use together.
Ophthalmic belladonna alkaloids (such as atropine and scopolamine), cyclopentolate: decreased pilocarpine antiglaucoma effectiveness and blocked mydriatic effects of these agents. Avoid concomitant use.
Phenylephrine: decreased dilation by phenylephrine. Don't use together.

EFFECTS ON DIAGNOSTIC TESTS
None reported.

CONTRAINDICATIONS
Contraindicated in patients with hypersensitivity to drug or when cholinergic effects such as constriction are undesirable (for example, acute iritis, some forms of secondary glaucoma, pupillary block glaucoma, acute inflammatory disease of the anterior chamber).

NURSING CONSIDERATIONS
● Use cautiously in patients with acute cardiac failure, bronchial asthma, peptic ulcer, hyperthyroidism, GI spasm, urinary tract obstruction, and Parkinson's disease.
Alert: Keep in mind that patients with dark eyes may require stonger solutions.

☑ PATIENT TEACHING
● Instruct patient to apply gel at bedtime because it will blur vision. Warn him to avoid hazardous activities, such as operating machinery or driving, until temporary blurring subsides.
● Teach patient how to instill pilocarpine. Advise him to wash hands before and after instilling drug and to apply light finger pressure on lacrimal sac for 1 minute after drops are instilled. Warn patient not to touch applicator tip to eye or surrounding tissue.
● If the Ocusert Pilo system falls out of the eye during sleep, tell patient to wash hands, rinse the insert in cool tap water, and reposition it in the eye. Also tell him not to use a deformed insert.
● Warn patient that transient brow pain and myopia are common at first but usually disappear within 10 to 14 days.

82
Mydriatics

atropine sulfate
cyclopentolate hydrochloride
epinephrine hydrochloride
epinephryl borate
homatropine hydrobromide
phenylephrine hydrochloride
scopolamine hydrobromide
tropicamide

COMBINATION PRODUCTS
CYCLOMYDRIL OPHTHALMIC: cyclopentolate hydrochloride 0.2% and phenylephrine hydrochloride 1%.
MUROCOLL-2: scopolamine hydrobromide 0.3% and phenylephrine hydrochloride 10%.

---

atropine sulfate
Atropisol, Atropt‡, BufOpto Atropine, Isopto Atropine

Pregnancy Risk Category: C

HOW SUPPLIED
Ophthalmic ointment: 0.5%, 1%
Ophthalmic solution: 0.5%, 1%, 2%

ACTION
A potent mydriatic and cycloplegic whose anticholinergic action leaves the pupil under unopposed adrenergic influence, causing it to dilate.

ONSET, PEAK, DURATION
Onset unknown. Mydriatic effect peaks within 30 to 40 minutes; cycloplegic, within 1 to 3 hours. Effects of mydriasis persist for 7 to 12 days; of cycloplegia, 6 to 12 days.

INDICATIONS & DOSAGE
Acute iritis; uveitis—
Adults: 1 to 2 drops instilled into the eyes up to four times daily or a small strip of ointment applied to the conjunc-tival sac up to three times daily.
Children: 1 to 2 drops of 0.5% solution instilled into the eyes up to three times daily or a small strip of ointment applied to the conjunctival sac up to three times daily.
Cycloplegic refraction—
Adults: 1 to 2 drops of 1% solution in-stilled 1 hour before refraction.
Children: 1 to 2 drops of 0.5% solution instilled in each eye b.i.d. for 1 to 3 days before eye examination and 1 hour be-fore refraction.

ADVERSE REACTIONS
CNS: confusion, somnolence, headache.
CV: tachycardia.
EENT: ocular congestion with long-term use, conjunctivitis, contact dermatitis of eye, ocular edema, *blurred vision,* eye dryness, photophobia, in-creased intraocular pressure (IOP), transient stinging and burning, irritation, hyperemia, blurred vision.
GI: dry mouth, abdominal distention in infants.
Skin: dryness.

INTERACTIONS
None significant.

EFFECTS ON DIAGNOSTIC TESTS
None reported.

CONTRAINDICATIONS
Contraindicated in patients with glauco-ma, hypersensitivity to drug or bella-donna alkaloids, or who have adhesions between the iris and lens. Atropine should not be used during the first 3 months of life because of the possible association between cycloplegia pro-duced and development of amblyopia.

NURSING CONSIDERATIONS
● Use cautiously in elderly patients and

in those where increased IOP may be encountered. Excessive use in children or in certain susceptible patients, including those with spastic paralysis, brain damage, or Down syndrome, may produce systemic symptoms of atropine poisioning.

Alert: Treat drops and ointment as poison (not for internal use); signs of poisoning are disorientation and confusion. Antidote of choice is physostigmine salicylate I.V. or I.M.

• Watch for signs of glaucoma: increased intraocular pressure, ocular pain, headache, progressive blurring of vision. If present, notify the doctor

☑ PATIENT TEACHING

• Teach patient how to instill atropine. Advise him to wash hands before and after instilling drug and to apply light finger pressure on lacrimal sac for 1 minute after instillation. Warn him not to touch tip of dropper or tube to eye or surrounding tissue.

• Warn patient to avoid hazardous activities, such as operating machinery or driving, until temporary blurring subsides.

• Advise patient to ease photophobia by wearing dark glasses.

---

cyclopentolate hydrochloride
AK-Pentolate, Cyclogyl

Pregnancy Risk Category: NR

HOW SUPPLIED
Ophthalmic solution: 0.5%, 1%, 2%

ACTION
A potent mydriatic and cycloplegic whose anticholinergic action leaves the pupil under unopposed adrenergic influence, causing it to dilate.

ONSET, PEAK, DURATION
Onset rapid. Mydriatic effect peaks within 30 to 60 minutes; cycloplegic, within 25 to 75 minutes. Effects of mydriasis persist for 1 day; of cycloplegia,

0.25 to 1 day.

INDICATIONS & DOSAGE
Diagnostic procedures requiring mydriasis and cycloplegia—
Adults: 1 or 2 drops of 0.5%, 1%, or 2% solution instilled into the eyes followed by 1 or 2 drops in 5 to 10 minutes, if needed.
Children: 1 drop of 0.5%, 1%, or 2% solution instilled into each eye, followed in 5 to 10 minutes with 1 drop 0.5% or 1% solution, if necessary.

ADVERSE REACTIONS
CNS: irritability, confusion, somnolence, hallucinations, ataxia, *seizures,* behavioral disturbances in children.
CV: tachycardia.
EENT: eye burning on instillation, blurred vision, eye dryness, *photophobia,* ocular congestion, contact dermatitis in eye, conjunctivitis, increased intraocular pressure (IOP), transient stinging and burning, irritation, hyperemia.
GU: urine retention.
Skin: dryness.

INTERACTIONS
Carbachol, pilocarpine: may counteract mydriatic effect. Avoid concomitant use.
Long-acting cholinergic antiglaucoma agents: miotic actions may be inhibited. Avoid concomitant use.

EFFECTS ON DIAGNOSTIC TESTS
None reported.

CONTRAINDICATIONS
Contraindicated in patients with glaucoma, hypersensitivity to drug or belladonna alkaloids, or who have adhesions between the iris and lens.

NURSING CONSIDERATIONS
• Use with extreme caution in infants and young children.
• Use cautiously in elderly patients and others where increased IOP may be encountered.
• Know that drug is superior to homat-

---

ropine hydrobromide, and has a shorter duration of action. Physostigmine is antidote of choice.

☑ PATIENT TEACHING
● Teach patient how to instill drug. Advise him to wash hands before and after instilling drug and to apply light finger pressure on lacrimal sac for 1 minute after drops are instilled. Warn him not to touch tip of dropper to eye or surrounding tissue and that drug will burn when instilled.
● Warn patient to avoid hazardous activities, such as operating machinery or driving, until temporary blurring subsides.
● Advise patient to ease photophobia by wearing dark glasses.

---

epinephrine hydrochloride
Epifrin, Glaucon

epinephryl borate
Epinal, Eppy/N

Pregnancy Risk Category: C

HOW SUPPLIED
epinephrine hydrochloride
Ophthalmic solution: 0.1%, 0.25%, 0.5%, 1%, 2%
epinephryl borate
Ophthalmic solution: 0.5%, 1%, 2%

ACTION
An adrenergic that dilates the pupil by contracting the dilator muscle.

ONSET, PEAK, DURATION
Onset of mydriasis occurs within a few minutes; of intraocular pressure (IOP) reduction, within 1 hour. IOP reduction peaks within 4 to 8 hours. Effects of mydriasis persist for several hours; of IOP reduction, 12 to 24 hours.

INDICATIONS & DOSAGE
Open-angle glaucoma—
Adults: 1 or 2 drops of 1% or 2% solution once or twice daily. Dosage is ad-

justed according to tonometric readings.

ADVERSE REACTIONS
CNS: brow ache, headache, light-headedness.
CV: palpitations, tachycardia, arrhythmia, hypertension.
EENT: corneal or conjunctival pigmentation or corneal edema in long-term use; follicular hypertrophy; chemosis; conjunctivitis; iritis; hyperemic conjunctiva; maculopapular rash; eye stinging, burning, and tearing on instillation; eye pain; allergic lid reaction; ocular irritation.

INTERACTIONS
Cyclopropane, halogenated hydrocarbons: arrhythmias, tachycardia. Use together cautiously, if at all.
Digitalis glycosides: increased risk of arrhythmias. Monitor closely.
Local or systemic sympathomimetics: additive toxic effects. Avoid concomitant use.
MAO inhibitors: exaggerated adrenergic effects. Adjust dose of epinephrine carefully.
Topical miotics, beta-adrenergic blockers, osmotic agents, systemic carbonic anhydrase inhibitors: additive lowering of IOP. Use together cautiously.
Tricyclic antidepressants, antihistamines (diphenhydramine, dexchlorpheniramine): potentiated cardiac effects of epinephrine. Monitor closely.

EFFECTS ON DIAGNOSTIC TESTS
Epinephrine therapy alters blood glucose and serum lactic acid levels (both may be increased), increases BUN levels, and interferes with tests for urinary catecholamines.

CONTRAINDICATIONS
Contraindicated in patients with angle-closure glaucoma or when nature of the glaucoma has not been established. Also contraindicated in patients with hypersensitivity to the drug or sulfites and in those with hypertensive CV disease or

---

*Liquid contains alcohol.   **May contain tartrazine.   †Canada only.   ‡Australia only.   ◇OTC.

coronary artery disease.

NURSING CONSIDERATIONS
● Use cautiously in elderly patients and in those with diabetes mellitus, hypertension, Parkinson's disease, hyperthyroidism, aphakia (eye without lens), cardiac disease, cerebral arteriosclerosis, or bronchial asthma.
● Be aware that drug can also can be injected into anterior chamber to produce rapid mydriasis during cataract removal or can be used to control local bleeding during surgery.
Alert: Don't substitute one salt if another one is ordered; epinephrine salts are not interchangeable.
● Monitor blood pressure and other vital signs.

☑ PATIENT TEACHING
● Teach patient how to instill drug. Advise him to wash hands before and after instilling drug and to apply light finger pressure on lacrimal sac for 1 minute after drops are instilled. Warn him not to touch tip of dropper to eye or surrounding tissue.
● Advise patient not to use while wearing soft contact lenses because discoloration of lenses may occur.
● Tell patient not to use darkened solution.

homatropine hydrobromide
Homatrine, Homatropine, Isopto Homatropine

Pregnancy Risk Category: C

HOW SUPPLIED
Ophthalmic solution: 2%, 5%

ACTION
Anticholinergic action leaves the pupil under unopposed adrenergic influence, causing it to dilate.

ONSET, PEAK, DURATION
Onset rapid. Mydriatic effect peaks within 40 to 60 minutes; cycloplegic, within 30 to 60 minutes. Effects of mydriasis persist for 1 to 3 days; of cycloplegia, 1 to 3 days.

INDICATIONS & DOSAGE
Cycloplegic refraction—
Adults and children: 1 to 2 drops instilled into the eyes; if needed, repeated in 5 to 10 minutes for two or three doses.
Uveitis—
Adults and children: 1 to 2 drops instilled into the eyes q 3 to 4 hours.
   Note: Use only 2% solution with children. Patients with heavily pigmented irises may require larger doses.

ADVERSE REACTIONS
CNS: confusion, somnolence, headache.
CV: tachycardia.
EENT: eye irritation, *blurred vision, photophobia,* increased intraocular pressure (IOP), transient stinging and burning, conjunctivitis, vascular congestion, edema.
GI: dry mouth.
Skin: dryness, rash.

INTERACTIONS
None significant.

EFFECTS ON DIAGNOSTIC TESTS
None significant.

CONTRAINDICATIONS
Contraindicated in patients with hypersensitivity to the drug or to other belladonna alkaloids, such as atropine, and in those with glaucoma or who have adhesions between the iris and lens.

NURSING CONSIDERATIONS
● Use cautiously in elderly patients and others where increased IOP may be encountered.
Alert: Be aware that homatropine is similar to atropine but weaker, with a shorter duration of action. May produce symptoms of atropine poisoning, such as severe dryness of mouth or tachycardia.

Reactions may be *common*, uncommon, *life-threatening*, or COMMON AND LIFE-THREATENING.

☑ **PATIENT TEACHING**
● Teach patient how to instill drug. Advise him to wash hands before and after instilling drug and to apply light finger pressure on lacrimal sac for 1 minute after drops are instilled. Warn him not to touch tip of dropper to eye or surrounding tissue.
● Warn patient to avoid hazardous activities, such as operating machinery or driving, until temporary blurring subsides.
● Advise patient to ease photophobia by wearing dark glasses.

---

phenylephrine hydrochloride
AK-Dilate, AK-Nefrin Ophthalmic ◊, I-Phrine 2.5%, Isopto Frin ◊, Mydfrin, Neo-Synephrine, Prefrin Liquifilm

Pregnancy Risk Category: C

HOW SUPPLIED
Ophthalmic solution: 0.12% ◊, 2.5%, 10%

ACTION
An adrenergic that dilates the pupil by contracting the dilator muscle.

ONSET, PEAK, DURATION
Onset is rapid. Mydriatic effect peaks within 15 to 60 minutes after using the 2.5% solution; 10 to 90 minutes after using the 10% solution. Effects of 2.5% solution persist for about 3 hours; of 10% solution, 3 to 7 hours.

INDICATIONS & DOSAGE
Mydriasis without cycloplegia—
Adults and children: 1 drop of 2.5% or 10% solution instilled before examination. May be repeated in 1 hour, if needed.
Mydriasis and vasoconstriction—
Adults and adolescents: 1 drop of 2.5% or 10% solution
Children: 1 drop of 2.5% solution.
Chronic mydriasis—
Adults and adolescents: 1 drop of

2.5% or 10% solution instilled b.i.d. or t.i.d.
Children: 1 drop of 2.5% solution instilled b.i.d. or t.i.d.
Posterior synechia (adhesion of iris)—
Adults and children: 1 drop of 2.5% or 10% solution.
    Do not use 10% concentration in infants.

ADVERSE REACTIONS
CNS: brow ache, headache.
CV: *hypertension* (with 10% solution), tachycardia, palpitations, *PVCs, MI.*
EENT: transient eye burning or stinging on instillation, blurred vision, increased intraocular pressure, keratitis, lacrimation, reactive hyperemia of eye, allergic conjunctivitis, rebound miosis.
Skin: pallor, dermatitis.
Other: trembling, diaphoresis.

INTERACTIONS
Guanethidine: increased mydriatic and pressor effects of phenylephrine. Use together cautiously.
Levodopa (systemic): reduced mydriatic effect of phenylephrine. Use together cautiously.
MAO inhibitors, beta blockers: may cause arrhythmias because of increased pressor effect. Use together cautiously.
Topically applied atropine, cyclopentolate, homatropine, scopolamine: may increase dilation of pupil. Use together cautiously.
Tricyclic antidepressants: potentiated cardiac effects of epinephrine. Use together cautiously.

EFFECTS ON DIAGNOSTIC TESTS
Drug may lower intraocular pressure in normal eyes or in open-angle glaucoma; it may also cause false-normal tonometry readings.

CONTRAINDICATIONS
Contraindicated in patients with hypersensitivity to drug or angle-closure glaucoma and in those who wear soft contact lenses.

---

*Liquid contains alcohol.   **May contain tartrazine.   †Canada only.   ‡Australia only.   ◊ OTC.

NURSING CONSIDERATIONS
● Use cautiously in patients with marked hypertension, cardiac disorders, advanced arteriosclerotic changes, Type I diabetes, or hyperthyroidism; in children of low body weight; and in elderly patients.
● Know that systemic adverse reactions are least likely with 2.5% solution and greatest with 10% solution.

☑ PATIENT TEACHING
● Teach patient how to instill drug. Advise him to wash hands before and after instilling drug and to apply light finger pressure on lacrimal sac for 1 minute after drops are instilled. Warn him not to touch tip of dropper to eye or surrounding tissue.
● Warn patient not to exceed recommended dosage because systemic effects can result. Monitor blood pressure and pulse rate.
● Advise patient to contact the doctor if condition persists longer than 12 hours after discontinuation of the drug.
● Warn patient to avoid hazardous activities, such as operating machinery or driving, until temporary blurring subsides.
● Advise patient to ease photophobia by wearing dark glasses.
● Tell patient not to use brown solutions or solutions that contain precipitate.

---

scopolamine hydrobromide
Isopto Hyoscine

Pregnancy Risk Category: NR

HOW SUPPLIED
Ophthalmic solution: 0.25%

ACTION
Anticholinergic action leaves the pupil under unopposed adrenergic influence, causing it to dilate.

ONSET, PEAK, DURATION
Onset is rapid. Mydriatic effect peaks within 15 to 30 minutes; cycloplegic ef-

fect, within 30 to 45 minutes. Effects persist up to 1 week.

INDICATIONS & DOSAGE
Cycloplegic refraction—
Adults: 1 to 2 drops of 0.25% solution 1 hour before refraction.
Children: 1 drop of 0.25% solution b.i.d. for 2 days before refraction.
Iritis, uveitis—
Adults: 1 to 2 drops of 0.25% solution once daily to q.i.d.
Children: 1 drop once daily to q.i.d.

ADVERSE REACTIONS
CNS: confusion, delirium, somnolence, acute psychotic reactions, headache, hallucinations.
CV: tachycardia.
EENT: ocular congestion with prolonged use, conjunctivitis, *blurred vision,* eye dryness, increased intraocular pressure, *photophobia,* transient stinging and burning, edema.
GI: dry mouth.
Skin: dryness, contact dermatitis.

INTERACTIONS
None significant.

EFFECTS ON DIAGNOSTIC TESTS
None reported.

CONTRAINDICATIONS
Contraindicated in patients with shallow anterior chamber and angle-closure glaucoma, hypersensitivity to the drug, adhesions (synechia) between the iris and lens, and in children who have previously had a severe systemic reaction to atropine.

NURSING CONSIDERATIONS
● Use with extreme caution (if at all) in infants and small children.
● Use cautiously in patients with cardiac disease and in elderly patients.
● Observe patients closely for adverse CNS effects (such as disorientation and delirium).
● Know that scopolamine may be used

Reactions may be *common,* uncommon, *life-threatening,* or COMMON AND LIFE-THREATENING.

in patients sensitive to atropine because it's faster acting and has a shorter duration of action and fewer adverse reactions.

☑ **PATIENT TEACHING**
● Teach patient how to instill drug. Advise him to wash hands before and after instilling drug and to apply light finger pressure on lacrimal sac for 1 minute after drops are instilled. Warn him to avoid touching tip of dropper to eye or surrounding tissue.
● Warn patient to avoid hazardous activities, such as operating machinery or driving, until temporary blurring subsides.
● Advise patient to ease photophobia by wearing dark glasses.

---

tropicamide
Mydriacyl, Tropicacyl

Pregnancy Risk Category: NR

HOW SUPPLIED
Ophthalmic solution: 0.5%, 1%

ACTION
The shortest-acting cycloplegic available, whose anticholinergic action leaves the pupil under unopposed adrenergic influence, causing it to dilate.

ONSET, PEAK, DURATION
Onset rapid. Mydriatic effect peaks within 20 to 40 minutes; cycloplegic effect, within 20 to 35 minutes. Effects persist up to 7 hours.

INDICATIONS & DOSAGE
Cycloplegic refraction—
Adults: 1 drop of 1% solution; repeated in 5 minutes. If needed, additional drop in 20 to 30 minutes.
Children: 1 drop of 0.5% or 1% solution; repeated in 5 minutes, if needed.
Fundus examinations—
Adults and children: 1 to 2 drops of 0.5% solution in each eye 15 to 20 minutes before examination; instillation may be repeated q 30 minutes as needed.

ADVERSE REACTIONS
CNS: confusion, somnolence, hallucinations, behavioral disturbances in children.
EENT: *transient eye stinging on instillation,* increased intraocular pressure, hyperemia, irritation, conjunctivitis, edema, *blurred vision, photophobia; dry throat.*
GI: dry mouth.
Skin: dryness.

INTERACTIONS
None significant.

EFFECTS ON DIAGNOSTIC TESTS
None reported.

CONTRAINDICATIONS
Contraindicated in patients with shallow anterior chamber and angle-closure glaucoma or hypersensitivity to drug.

NURSING CONSIDERATIONS
● Use cautiously in elderly patients.
● Know that tropicamide's mydriatic effect is greater than its cycloplegic effect.

☑ **PATIENT TEACHING**
● Teach patient how to instill drug. Advise him to wash hands before and after instilling drug and to apply light finger pressure on lacrimal sac for 1 minute after drops are instilled. Warn him not to touch tip of dropper to eye or surrounding tissue.
● Warn patient that drug causes transient stinging.
● Warn patient to avoid hazardous activities until blurring subsides.
● Advise patient to ease photophobia by wearing dark glasses.

---

naphazoline hydrochloride
oxymetazoline hydrochloride
tetrahydrozoline hydrochloride

COMBINATION PRODUCTS
ALBALON-A LIQUIFILM: naphazoline hydrochloride 0.05% and antazoline phosphate 0.5%.

BLEPHAMIDE LIQUIFILM SUSPENSION: phenylephrine hydrochloride 0.12%, sulfacetamide sodium 10%, and prednisolone acetate 0.2%.

PREFRIN-A: phenylephrine hydrochloride 0.12%, pyrilamine maleate 0.1%, and antipyrine 0.1%.

VASOCIDIN OPHTHALMIC OINTMENT: phenylephrine hydrochloride 0.125%, sulfacetamide sodium 10%, and prednisolone acetate 0.5%.

VASOCIDIN OPHTHALMIC SOLUTION: phenylephrine hydrochloride 0.125%, sulfacetamide sodium 10%, and prednisolone sodium phosphate 0.25%.

VASOCON-A OPHTHALMIC SOLUTION: naphazoline hydrochloride 0.05% and antazoline phosphate 0.5%.

ZINCFRIN ◊ : phenylephrine hydrochloride 0.12% and zinc sulfate 0.25%.

---

naphazoline hydrochloride
AK-Con, Albalon Liquifilm, Allerest ◊ ,
Clear Eyes ◊ , Degest 2 ◊ , Estivin II,
Naphcon ◊ , Naphcon Forte, Opta-
zine‡, Vasoclear ◊ , Vasocon Regular

Pregnancy Risk Category: C

HOW SUPPLIED
Ophthalmic solution: 0.012% ◊ ,
0.02% ◊ , 0.03% ◊ , 0.1%

ACTION
Unknown. Thought to cause vasoconstriction by local adrenergic action on the blood vessels of the conjunctiva.

ONSET, PEAK, DURATION
Local vasoconstriction usually occurs within 10 minutes. Peak unknown. Effects persist for 2 to 6 hours.

INDICATIONS & DOSAGE
Ocular congestion, irritation, itching—
Adults: 1 drop of 0.1% solution instilled q 3 to 4 hours or 1 drop of 0.012% to 0.03% solution up to q.i.d.

ADVERSE REACTIONS
CNS: headache, dizziness, nervousness, weakness.
EENT: transient eye stinging, pupillary dilation, eye irritation, photophobia, blurred vision, increased intraocular pressure, keratitis, lacrimation.
GI: nausea.
Other: diaphoresis.

INTERACTIONS
Tricyclic antidepressants, MAO inhibitors, maprotiline: hypertensive crisis if naphazoline is systemically absorbed. Use together cautiously.

EFFECTS ON DIAGNOSTIC TESTS
None reported.

CONTRAINDICATIONS
Contraindicated in patients with hypersensitivity to any of drug's ingredients and in patients with acute angle-closure glaucoma. Use of 0.1% solution is contraindicated in children.

NURSING CONSIDERATIONS
● Use cautiously in patients with hyperthyroidism, cardiac disease, hypertension, or diabetes mellitus.
● Know that drug is most widely used ocular decongestant.
● Be aware that drug can produce marked sedation and coma in children, especially infants.

Reactions may be *common*, uncommon, *life-threatening*, or COMMON AND LIFE-THREATENING.

● Store in tightly closed container.

● Teach patient how to instill drug. Advise him to wash hands before and after instilling drug and to apply light finger pressure on lacrimal sac for 1 minute after drops are instilled. Warn him not to touch tip of dropper to eye or surrounding tissue.
● Warn patient not to exceed recommended dosage. Rebound congestion and conjunctivitis may occur with frequent or prolonged use.
● Tell patient to notify the doctor if photophobia, blurred vision, pain, or lid edema develops.
● Instruct patient not to use OTC preparations longer than 72 hours without consulting a doctor.

---

oxymetazoline hydrochloride
OcuClear ◇ , Visine L.R. ◇

Pregnancy Risk Category: C

HOW SUPPLIED
Ophthalmic solution: 0.025%

ACTION
A direct-acting sympathomimetic amine that acts on alpha-adrenergic receptors in the arterioles of the conjunctiva to produce vasoconstriction, resulting in decreased conjunctival congestion.

ONSET, PEAK, DURATION
Onset occurs within 5 minutes. Peak unknown. Effects persist for approximately 6 hours.

INDICATIONS & DOSAGE
Relief of eye redness due to minor eye irritations—
Adults and children 6 years and over: 1 to 2 drops in the conjunctival sac two to four times daily (spaced at least 6 hours apart).

ADVERSE REACTIONS
CNS: headache, light-headedness, nervousness, insomnia.
CV: palpitations, tachycardia, irregular heartbeat.
EENT: *transient stinging upon initial instillation,* blurred vision, reactive hyperemia with excessive dosage or prolonged use, keratitis, lacrimation, increase in intraocular pressure.
Other: trembling.

INTERACTIONS
Tricyclic antidepressants, maprotiline, MAO inhibitors: if significant systemic absorption of oxymetazoline occurs, concurrent use may potentiate the pressor effect of oxymetazoline.

EFFECTS ON DIAGNOSTIC TESTS
None reported.

CONTRAINDICATIONS
Contraindicated in patients hypersensitive to any component of the drug and in those with angle-closure glaucoma.

NURSING CONSIDERATIONS
● Use cautiously in patients with hyperthyroidism, cardiac disease, hypertension, and eye disease, infection, or injury.
● Don't use if solution has become cloudy or changes color.

● Teach patient how to instill drops. Advise him to wash hands before and after instilling solution, and warn him not to touch tip of dropper to eye or surrounding tissue.
● Advise patient to apply light finger pressure on lacrimal sac for 1 minute after drug instillation.
● Advise patient to stop the drug and see a doctor if eye pain occurs, if vision changes, or if redness or irritation continues, worsens, or lasts for more than 72 hours.

---

tetrahydrozoline hydrochloride
Murine Plus◊, Optigene◊,
Soothe◊, Tetrasine◊, Visine◊

Pregnancy Risk Category: C

HOW SUPPLIED
Ophthalmic solution: 0.05%◊

ACTION
Unknown. Thought to cause vasoconstriction by local adrenergic action on
the blood vessels of the conjunctiva.

ONSET, PEAK, DURATION
Onset occurs within a few minutes.
Peak unknown. Effects persist for 4 to 8
hours.

INDICATIONS & DOSAGE
*Conjunctival congestion, irritation, and
allergic conditions—*
Adults and children over 2 years: 1 to
2 drops of 0.05% solution instilled up to
four times daily or as directed by the
doctor.

ADVERSE REACTIONS
CNS: headache, drowsiness, insomnia,
dizziness, tremor.
CV: *cardiac arrhythmias.*
EENT: transient eye stinging, pupillary
dilation, increased intraocular pressure,
keratitis, lacrimation, eye irritation.

INTERACTIONS
*Guanethidine, MAO inhibitors, tricyclic
antidepressants:* hypertensive crisis if
tetrahydrozoline is systemically absorbed. Don't use together.

EFFECTS ON DIAGNOSTIC TESTS
None reported.

CONTRAINDICATIONS
Contraindicated in patients hypersensitive to the drug or any of its components, and in those with angle-closure
glaucoma or other serious eye diseases.

NURSING CONSIDERATIONS
● Use cautiously in patients with hyperthyroidism, heart disease, hypertension,
or diabetes mellitus.
● Rebound congestion may occur with
frequent or prolonged use.

☑ PATIENT TEACHING
● Teach patient how to instill drug. Advise him to wash hands before and after
instilling drug and to apply light finger
pressure on lacrimal sac for 1 minute after drops are instilled. Warn him not to
touch tip of dropper to eye or surrounding tissue.
● Warn patient not to exceed recommended dosage.
● Tell patient to stop drug and notify the
doctor if redness or irritation persists or
increases or if no relief occurs within 2
days.
● Caution patient not to share eye medications with others.

apraclonidine hydrochloride
betaxolol hydrochloride
botulinum toxin type A
carteolol hydrochloride
dipivefrin
dorzolamide hydrochloride
fluorescein sodium
isosorbide
latanoprost
levobunolol hydrochloride
levocabastine hydrochloride
lodoxamide tromethamine
metipranolol hydrochloride
sodium chloride, hypertonic
timolol maleate

COMBINATION PRODUCTS
FLURESS: fluorescein sodium 0.25% and benoxinate hydrochloride 0.4%.

---

apraclonidine hydrochloride
Iopidine

Pregnancy Risk Category: C

HOW SUPPLIED
Ophthalmic solution: 0.5%, 1%

ACTION
Unknown; an alpha-adrenergic agonist that reduces intraocular pressure (IOP), possibly by decreasing production of aqueous humor.

ONSET, PEAK, DURATION
Onset occurs within 1 hour. Peak effect occurs within 3 to 5 hours. Effects persist at least 12 hours.

INDICATIONS & DOSAGE
Prevention or control of IOP elevation before and after ocular laser surgery—
Adults: 1 drop of 1% solution instilled 1 hour before initiation of laser surgery on the anterior segment, followed by 1 drop immediately after surgery.
Short-term adjunct therapy in patients who require additional IOP reduction—
Adults: 1 or 2 drops of 0.5% solution instilled into affected eyes t.i.d.

ADVERSE REACTIONS
CNS: insomnia, irritability, dream disturbances, headache, irritability, paresthesia.
CV: bradycardia, vasovagal attack, palpitations, hypotension, orthostatic hypotension.
EENT: upper eyelid elevation, conjunctival blanching and microhemorrhage, mydriasis, eye burning or discomfort, foreign body sensation in eye, eye dryness, or *itching, hyperemia,* conjunctivitis, blurred vision, nasal burning or dryness, or increased pharyngeal secretions.
GI: abdominal pain, discomfort, diarrhea, vomiting, taste disturbances, dry mouth.
Skin: pruritus not associated with rash, sweaty palms.
Other: body heat sensation, decreased libido, extremity pain or numbness, allergic response.

INTERACTIONS
Topical pilocarpine or beta-adrenergic blockers: additive effects in lowering IOP. Use together cautiously.

EFFECTS ON DIAGNOSTIC TESTS
None reported.

CONTRAINDICATIONS
Contraindicated in patients hypersensitive to apraclonidine or clonidine or on concurrent MAO inhibitor therapy.

NURSING CONSIDERATIONS
● Use cautiously in patients with severe cardiac disease including hypertension

---

or history of vasovagal attack.
● Closely monitor patients who tend to develop exaggerated decreases in IOP after drug therapy.
● Observe patients closely for vasovagal attack during laser surgery.
● Closely monitor patients with severe systemic disease, including hypertension, even though drug's systemic effects (altered heart rate and blood pressure) are uncommon after usual dose.

☑ **PATIENT TEACHING**
● Teach patient how to instill 0.5% solution. Advise him to wash hands before and after instilling drug and to apply light finger pressure on lacrimal sac for 1 minute after instillation.
● Warn patient not to touch tip of dropper to eye or surrounding tissue.
● Tell patient to separate intervals between each ophthalmic product instillation by at least 5 minutes to avoid washing away the previous dose.
● Encourage patient to comply with the three-times-daily dosage regimen.

---

betaxolol hydrochloride
Betoptic

Pregnancy Risk Category: C

HOW SUPPLIED
Ophthalmic solution: 0.5%
Ophthalmic suspension: 0.25%

ACTION
Unknown, although as a cardioselective beta blocker it reduces formation and possibly increases outflow of aqueous humor.

ONSET, PEAK, DURATION
Onset occurs in ½ to 1 hour. Intraocular pressure (IOP) reduction peaks after a single dose within about 2 hours. Effects persist for 12 or more hours.

INDICATIONS & DOSAGE
Chronic open-angle glaucoma and ocu-

lar hypertension—
Adults: 1 or 2 drops of 0.5% solution or 0.25% suspension b.i.d.

ADVERSE REACTIONS
CNS: insomnia, depressive neurosis.
CV: *arrhythmias, heart block, CHF,* palpitations, CVA.
EENT: *eye stinging on instillation causing brief discomfort,* photophobia, erythema, itching, keratitis, occasional tearing.
Respiratory: asthma, *bronchospasm.*

INTERACTIONS
Calcium channel blockers: AV conduction disturbances, ventricular failure, and hypotension if significant systemic absorption occurs. Monitor closely.
Cocaine: may inhibit betaxolol's effects. Avoid concomitant use.
Digitalis glycosides: excessive bradycardia; patients may require ECG monitoring if significant systemic absorption occurs.
Inhalation hydrocarbon anesthetics: prolonged severe hypotension if significant systemic absorption occurs. Tell the anesthesiologist that the patient is receiving ophthalmic betaxolol.
Ophthalmic epinephrine, dipivefrin: may produce mydriasis. Use together cautiously.
Oral antidiabetic agents, insulin: risk of hypoglycemia or hyperglycemia if significant systemic absorption occurs. Dosage adjustments of antidiabetic agents or hypoglycemic medication may be necessary.
Phenothiazines: additive hypotensive effects; increased risk of adverse effects if significant systemic absorption occurs. Monitor closely.
Reserpine: excessive beta blockade. Monitor closely.
Systemic beta blockers: additive effects. Monitor closely.

EFFECTS ON DIAGNOSTIC TESTS
None reported.

Reactions may be *common*, uncommon, *life-threatening*, or COMMON AND LIFE-THREATENING.

CONTRAINDICATIONS
Contraindicated in patients with hypersensitivity to drug, sinus bradycardia, greater-than-first-degree AV block, cardiogenic shock, or overt heart failure.

NURSING CONSIDERATIONS
• Use cautiously in patients with restricted pulmonary function, diabetes mellitus, hyperthyroidism, or a history of heart failure.
• Keep in mind that some patients may need a few weeks' treatment to stabilize IOP-lowering response. Determine IOP after 4 weeks of treatment.

☑ PATIENT TEACHING
• Teach patient how to instill drug. Advise him to wash hands before and after instilling drug and to apply light finger pressure on lacrimal sac for 1 minute after instillation. Warn him not to touch tip of dropper to eye or surrounding tissue. He should shake suspension well before instilling.
• Encourage patient to comply with twice-daily dosage regimen.
• Advise patient to ease photophobia by wearing dark glasses.

---

botulinum toxin type A
Botox

Pregnancy Risk Category: C

HOW SUPPLIED
Powder for injection: 100-unit vial

ACTION
A protein that produces a neuromuscular paralysis by binding to acetylcholine receptors on the motor end-plate and that may inhibit the release of acetylcholine from presynaptic nerve endings.

ONSET, PEAK, DURATION
Onset occurs in 1 or 2 days after injection. Peak occurs within 1 to 2 weeks. Effects persist for 2 to 6 weeks.

INDICATIONS & DOSAGE
Strabismus—
Adults and children 12 years and over: injections should be made only by doctors familiar with the technique, which involves surgical exposure of the region as well as electromyographic guidance of the injection needle.

Dosage varies with the degree of deviation (lower doses are used for small deviations). For vertical muscles and for horizontal strabismus of less than 20 prism diopters, the usual dosage is 1.25 to 2.5 units injected into any one muscle. For horizontal strabismus of 20 to 50 prism diopters, dosage is 2.5 to 5 units into any one muscle. For persistent (greater than 1 month's duration) palsy of the sixth cranial nerve, dosage is 1.25 to 2.5 units into the medial rectus muscle.

Subsequent injections for recurrent or residual strabismus should not be made until 7 to 14 days after the initial dose and unless substantial function has returned to the injected and adjacent muscles. Dosage may be increased up to twice the initial dose for patients experiencing incomplete paralysis; subsequent doses in patients with adequate response should not be increased. The maximum single dose for any one muscle is 25 units.
Blepharospasm—
Adults: initially, 1.25 to 2.5 units injected into the medial and lateral pretarsal orbicularis oculi of the upper lid and into the lateral pretarsal orbicularis oculi of the lower lid. Effects should be apparent within 3 days and peak within 1 to 2 weeks. Dosage may be doubled if inadequate paralysis is achieved; however, exceeding 5 units per site produces no apparent benefit. Each treatment lasts about 3 months and can be repeated indefinitely.

Cumulative dosage should not exceed 200 units/month.

ADVERSE REACTIONS
EENT: *ptosis, vertical deviation* (after

---

treatment of strabismus), *eye irritation, photophobia* (after treatment of blepharospasm), *swelling of eyelid.*
Skin: diffuse rash, ecchymoses.

INTERACTIONS
Aminoglycoside antibiotics, other drugs that interfere with neuromuscular transmission: may potentiate effect of botulinum toxin. Use caution when administered concomitantly.

EFFECTS ON DIAGNOSTIC TESTS
None reported.

CONTRAINDICATIONS
Contraindicated in patients hypersensitive to the drug or any of its components.

NURSING CONSIDERATIONS
● Reconstitute the drug with preservative-free 0.9% sodium chloride solution. The vacuum in the vial should be noticeable when reconstituting. Inject the diluent into the vial gently because severe agitation can denature the protein.
● Keep in mind reconstituting with 1 ml of 0.9% sodium chloride solution produces a concentration of 10 units/0.1 ml; adding 2 ml yields 5 units/0.1 ml. Adding more diluent (such as 4 ml to produce 2.5 units/0.1 ml or 8 ml to yield 1.25 units/0.1 ml) or using different injection volumes may also be used to adjust dosage.
● Reconstituted drug should be clear, colorless, and free of particulate matter. Record the date and time of reconstitution. Keep reconstituted drug in the refrigerator until use. Drug should be administered within 4 hours of removal from the freezer.
● Prepare the injection by drawing slightly more volume than needed into a sterile 1-ml syringe. Expel air bubbles in the barrel of the syringe and attach an electromyographic injection needle (if treating strabismus), such as a 1½" 27G needle. Expel leftover drug into an appropriate waste container while check-

ing for leakage around the needle. Be sure to use a new needle and syringe for each injection.
Alert: Have epinephrine available in case of an anaphylactic reaction.
● Apply several drops of an ocular decongestant and a topical anesthetic as ordered before treating strabismus.
● Freeze at or below 23° F (-5° C).

☑ PATIENT TEACHING
● Explain use and how drug is administered to patient and family. Answer questions and address concerns.
● Inform patient about the adverse reactions associated with drug. Instruct him to report persistent or severe adverse reactions promptly.

---

carteolol hydrochloride
Ocupress Ophthalmic Solution, 1%

Pregnancy Risk Category: C

HOW SUPPLIED
Ophthalmic solution: 1%

ACTION
A nonselective beta-adrenergic blocking agent that reduces intraocular pressure, although the exact mechanism of action has not been definitely demonstrated.

ONSET, PEAK, DURATION
Unknown.

INDICATIONS & DOSAGE
Chronic open-angle glaucoma, intraocular hypertension—
Adults: 1 drop in the conjunctival sac of the affected eye b.i.d.

ADVERSE REACTIONS
EENT: *transient eye irritation, burning, tearing, conjunctival hyperemia, ocular edema,* blurred and cloudy vision, photophobia, decreased night vision, ptosis, blepharoconjunctivitis, abnormal corneal staining, corneal sensitivity.
Systemic: bradycardia, hypotension, ar-

rhythmias, palpitations, dyspnea, asthenia, headache, dizziness, insomnia, sinusitis, taste perversion.

INTERACTIONS
Oral beta-adrenergic blockers, catecholamine-depleting agents (such as reserpine): may cause additive effects and the development of hypotension or bradycardia. Monitor patient closely.

EFFECTS ON DIAGNOSTIC TESTS
None reported.

CONTRAINDICATIONS
Contraindicated in patients hypersensitive to any component of the drug and in those with bronchial asthma, severe COPD, sinus bradycardia, second- or third-degree AV block, overt cardiac failure, or cardiogenic shock.

NURSING CONSIDERATIONS
● Use with caution in patients with non-allergic bronchospastic disease, diabetes mellitus, hyperthyroidism, hypersensitivity to other beta-adrenergic agents, or decreased pulmonary function and in breast-feeding patients.
Alert: Discontinue drug at the first sign of cardiac failure and notify the doctor.
● Be aware that when the drug is used to reduce elevated intraocular pressure in angle-closure glaucoma, it should be used in combination with a miotic and should not be used alone.

☑ PATIENT TEACHING
● Tell patient that if more than one topical ophthalmic drug is being used, the drugs should be administered at least 10 minutes apart.
● Teach patient how to instill drops. Advise him to wash hands before and after instilling solution, and warn him not to touch tip of the dropper to eye or surrounding tissue.
● Also teach patient to keep bottle tightly closed when not in use and to protect it from light.
● Tell patient that drug is a beta-adren-

ergic blocker and, although it is administered topically, it has the potential to be absorbed systemically. Advise patient to apply light finger pressure on lacrimal sac for 1 minute after drug instillation to minimize systemic absorption.
● Also tell patient that the same types of adverse reactions that are attributable to beta-adrenergic agent therapy may occur with topical administration. If signs of serious adverse reactions or hypersensitivity occur, tell the patient to discontinue the drug and notify the doctor immediately.
● Advise patient to ease photophobia by wearing dark glasses.
● Stress the importance of compliance with recommended therapy.

---

dipivefrin
Propine

Pregnancy Risk Category: B

HOW SUPPLIED
Ophthalmic solution: 0.1%

ACTION
A prodrug of epinephrine, dipivefrin is converted to epinephrine in the eye. The liberated epinephrine appears to decrease aqueous production and increase aqueous outflow.

ONSET, PEAK, DURATION
Onset occurs within 30 minutes. Peak effect occurs within 1 hour. Effects persist for 12 hours or more.

INDICATIONS & DOSAGE
Intraocular pressure (IOP) reduction in chronic open-angle glaucoma—
Adults: for initial glaucoma therapy, 1 drop of 0.1% solution q 12 hours. Adjustments in dosage then made based on patient response as determined by tonometric readings.

ADVERSE REACTIONS
CV: tachycardia, hypertension, arrhythmias.
EENT: eye burning or stinging, conjunctival injection, conjunctivitis, mydriasis, allergic reaction, photophobia, *macular edema*.

INTERACTIONS
Digitalis glycosides, inhalation hydrocarbon anesthetics, tricyclic antidepressants: increased risk of adverse cardiac effects if significant systemic absorption occurs. Monitor closely.
Ophthalmic beta blockers, osmotic agents, systemically administered carbonic anhydrase inhibitors: additive lowering of IOP. Use together cautiously. Monitor for potential adverse effects.
Systemic sympathomimetics: possible additive effects if significant systemic absorption occurs. Monitor closely.

EFFECTS ON DIAGNOSTIC TESTS
None reported.

CONTRAINDICATIONS
Contraindicated in patients with angle-closure glaucoma or hypersensitivity to drug.

NURSING CONSIDERATIONS
● Use cautiously in patients with aphakia or CV disease, history of hypersensitivity to epinephrine, and asthma.
● Be aware that drug is often used concomitantly with other antiglaucoma drugs.
● Know that drug may have fewer adverse reactions than conventional epinephrine therapy.

☑ **PATIENT TEACHING**
● Teach patient how to instill dipivefrin. Advise him to wash hands before and after instilling drug and to avoid touching tip of dropper to eye or surrounding tissue.
● Instruct patient to report persistent or serious adverse reactions promptly.

dorzolamide hydrochloride
Trusopt

Pregnancy Risk Category: C

HOW SUPPLIED
Ophthalmic solution: 2%

ACTION
Inhibits carbonic anhydrase in the ciliary processes of the eye, which decreases aqueous humor secretion, presumably by slowing the formation of bicarbonate ions with a subsequent reduction in sodium and fluid transport. The result is a reduction in intraocular pressure (IOP).

ONSET, PEAK, DURATION
Unknown.

INDICATIONS & DOSAGE
Treatment of increased IOP in patients with ocular hypertension or open-angle glaucoma—
Adults: 1 drop in the conjunctival sac of the affected eye t.i.d.

ADVERSE REACTIONS
EENT: *ocular burning, stinging, or discomfort; superficial punctate keratitis; ocular allergic reaction; blurred vision; lacrimation; dryness; photophobia;* iridocyclitis.
Systemic: *bitter taste,* headache, nausea, asthenia, fatigue, rash, urolithiasis.

INTERACTIONS
Oral carbonic anhydrase inhibitors: may cause additive effects. Do not administer concomitantly.

EFFECTS ON DIAGNOSTIC TESTS
None reported.

CONTRAINDICATIONS
Contraindicated in patients hypersensitive to any component of the drug.

NURSING CONSIDERATIONS
● Use with caution in patients with hepatic or renal impairment.
● If more than one topical ophthalmic drug is being used, the drugs should be administered at least 10 minutes apart.

☑ PATIENT TEACHING
● Teach patient how to instill drops. Advise him to wash hands before and after instilling solution, and warn him not to touch tip of the dropper to eye or surrounding tissue.
● Tell patient that the drug is a sulfonamide and, although it is administered topically, it can be absorbed systemically. Advise patient to apply light finger pressure on lacrimal sac for 1 minute after drug instillation to minimize systemic absorption.
● Tell patient that the same types of adverse reactions that are attributable to sulfonamides may occur with topical administration. If signs of serious adverse reactions or hypersensitivity occur, tell the patient to discontinue the drug and notify the doctor immediately.
● Advise patient to discontinue the drug and notify the doctor if any ocular reactions, particularly conjunctivitis and eyelid reactions, occur.
● Tell patient not to wear soft contact lenses while using this drug.
● Stress the importance of compliance with recommended therapy.

---

fluorescein sodium
Fluorescite, Fluor-I-Strip, Fluor-I-Strip A.T., Ful-Glo, Funduscein Injections

Pregnancy Risk Category: C

HOW SUPPLIED
Ophthalmic solution: 2%
Ophthalmic strips: 0.6 mg, 1 mg, 9 mg
Parenteral injection: 10%, 25%

ACTION
A water-soluble dye that produces an intense green fluorescence in alkaline solution (pH 5.0 or less) or a bright yellow one when viewed under cobalt blue illumination.

ONSET, PEAK, DURATION
Onset immediate. Peak and duration unknown.

INDICATIONS & DOSAGE
Diagnostic in corneal abrasions and foreign bodies; fitting hard contact lenses; lacrimal patency; fundus photography; applanation tonometry—
Adults and children: 1 or 2 drops of 2% solution followed by irrigation; or strip moistened with sterile water, then conjunctiva or fornix touched with moistened tip, and eye flushed with irrigating solution. Patient should blink several times after application.
Retinal angiography—
Adults: 5 ml of 10% solution (500 mg) or 3 ml of 25% solution (750 mg) rapidly injected into antecubital vein.
Children: 7.5 mg/kg injected rapidly into antecubital vein.

ADVERSE REACTIONS
Topical use:
EENT: eye stinging or burning, yellow tears.
I.V. use:
CNS: headache, dizziness, syncope, *seizures.*
CV: hypotension, *shock, cardiac arrest, thrombophlebitis.*
GI: nausea, vomiting, GI distress.
GU: bright yellow urine (persists for 24 to 36 hours).
Respiratory: transient dyspnea, bronchospasm.
Skin: yellow skin discoloration (fades in 6 to 12 hours), urticaria, pruritus.
Other: hypersensitivity reactions, including urticaria and *anaphylaxis;* extravasation at injection site; fever; angioedema.

INTERACTIONS
None significant.

EFFECTS ON DIAGNOSTIC TESTS
Bright yellow discoloration of urine may interfere with routine urinalysis.

CONTRAINDICATIONS
Contraindicated in patients with hypersensitivity to drug; do not use with soft contact lenses (lenses may become discolored).

NURSING CONSIDERATIONS
● Use cautiously in patients with history of allergy or bronchial asthma.
● Always use aseptic technique. Easily contaminated by *Pseudomonas aeruginosa.*
● **I.V. use:** Keep an antihistamine, epinephrine, and oxygen available when giving parenterally. Avoid extravasation during injection.
● Use topical anesthetic as ordered before instilling to relieve burning and irritation.
● Never instill dye while patients are wearing soft contact lenses; fluorescein will ruin them.
● Be aware that defects appear green under normal light or bright yellow under cobalt blue illumination. Foreign bodies are surrounded by a green ring. Similar lesions of the conjunctiva are delineated in orange-yellow.
● Don't freeze; store below 80° F (26.7° C).

☑ **PATIENT TEACHING**
● Tell patient to report persistent or serious adverse reactions promptly.

---

isosorbide
Ismotic

Pregnancy Risk Category: B

HOW SUPPLIED
Oral solution: 45% (100 g/225 ml) in 220-ml containers

ACTION
Acts as an osmotic agent by promoting redistribution of water and thereby producing diuresis.

ONSET, PEAK, DURATION
Onset occurs within 30 minutes. Peak effects occur in 1 to 1½ hours. Duration unknown.

INDICATIONS & DOSAGE
Short-term reduction of intraocular pressure (IOP) caused by glaucoma—
Adults: initially, 1.5 g/kg P.O. Usual dosage range is 1 to 3 g/kg b.i.d. to q.i.d., as indicated.

ADVERSE REACTIONS
CNS: vertigo, light-headedness, lethargy, headache, confusion, disorientation, irritability, syncope, dizziness.
GI: gastric discomfort, nausea, vomiting.
Other: hypernatremia, hyperosmolality, thirst.

INTERACTIONS
None significant.

EFFECTS ON DIAGNOSTIC TESTS
None reported.

CONTRAINDICATIONS
Contraindicated in patients with anuria caused by severe renal disease, severe dehydration, acute pulmonary edema, severe cardiac decompensation, and hemorrhagic glaucoma.

NURSING CONSIDERATIONS
● Know that additional doses should be used cautiously, especially in patients with diseases associated with sodium retention, such as CHF.
● To improve palatability, pour medication over cracked ice and tell patients to sip it.
● Monitor patients closely for 5 to 10 minutes after administration for adverse effects.
● Keep in mind that isosorbide is especially useful for rapid reduction of IOP. May be used to interrupt acute attack of

glaucoma before laser surgery.
• In patients with diseases associated with sodium retention, carefully monitor fluid and electrolyte balance.

☑ **PATIENT TEACHING**
• Tell patient that this drug may induce thirst.
• Caution patient not to perform hazardous activities if adverse CNS reactions occur.

▼ *NEW DRUG*

latanoprost
Xalatan

Pregnancy Risk Category: C

HOW SUPPLIED
Ophthalmic solution: 0.005% (50 mcg/ml)

ACTION
Although the exact mechanism of latanoprost's ability to lower intraocular pressure (IOP) is unknown, it is believed to reduce it by increasing the outflow of aqueous humor.

ONSET, PEAK, DURATION
Peak concentrations of the drug in aqueous humor is reached in 2 hours after topical administration. Reduction in IOP starts 3 to 4 hours after administration; maximum effect is reached after 8 to 12 hours.

INDICATIONS & DOSAGE
Treatment of increased IOP in patients with ocular hypertension or open-angle glaucoma who are intolerant of other IOP-lowering medications or insufficiently responsive to other IOP-lowering medications—
Adults: 1 drop in the conjunctival sac of the affected eye once daily in the evening.

ADVERSE REACTIONS
EENT: *blurred vision, burning, stinging,* conjunctival hyperemia, foreign body sensation, itching, increased brown pigmentation of the iris, dry eye, punctate epithelial keratopathy, lid crusting or edema, lid discomfort, excessive tearing, eye pain, photophobia.
Systemic: upper respiratory tract infection, cold, or flu; muscle, joint, back, or chest pain; angina pectoris; rash; allergic skin reaction.

INTERACTIONS
Eyedrops containing thimerosal: precipitation occurs when mixed with latanoprost. If used concomitantly, administer at least 5 minutes apart.

EFFECTS ON DIAGNOSTIC TESTS
None reported.

CONTRAINDICATIONS
Contraindicated in patients with hypersensitivity to latanoprost, benzalkonium chloride, or other ingredients in the product.

NURSING CONSIDERATIONS
• Use cautiously when administering to patients with impaired renal or hepatic function.
• Know that latanoprost should not be administered while patients are wearing contact lenses.
• Be aware that more frequent administration than that recommended may decrease the IOP-lowering effects of drug.
• Latanoprost may gradually change eye color, increasing the amount of brown pigment in the iris. This change in iris color occurs slowly and may not be noticeable for months or years. Increased pigmentation may be permanent.
• Do not allow the tip of the dispenser to contact the eye or surrounding structures may cause ocular infections. Be aware that serious damage to the eye and subsequent loss of vision may result from using contaminated solutions.

☑ **PATIENT TEACHING**
● Inform the patient about the potential for change in iris color. Patients receiving treatment in only one eye should be told about the potential for increased brown pigmentation in the treated eye.
● Teach patient how to instill drops. Advise him to wash his hands before and after instilling solution, and warn him not to touch the dropper or its tip to the eye or surrounding tissue.
● Advise patient to apply light finger pressure on the lacrimal sac for 1 minute after instillation to minimize systemic absorption.
● Instruct patient to report ocular reactions, especially conjunctivitis and lid reactions.
● Tell a patient who wears contact lenses to remove them before administering the solution and not to reinsert the lenses until 15 minutes have elapsed.
● Advise patient that if more than one topical ophthalmic drug is being used, the drugs should be administered at least 5 minutes apart.
● If patient develops another ocular condition (such as trauma or infection) or needs ocular surgery, advise him to contact the doctor about continued use of the multidose container.
● Stress the importance of compliance with recommended therapy.
● Safety and effectiveness in children have not been established.
● It is not known if latanoprost is excreted into breast milk; caution should be exercised when administering drug to breast-feeding women.

---

levobunolol hydrochloride
Betagan

Pregnancy Risk Category: C

HOW SUPPLIED
Ophthalmic solution: 0.25%, 0.5%

ACTION
Unknown. A nonselective beta blocker that is thought to reduce formation and possibly increase outflow of aqueous humor.

ONSET, PEAK, DURATION
Onset occurs within 1 hour. Intraocular pressure (IOP) reduction peaks within 2 to 6 hours after a single dose. Effects persist up to 24 hours.

INDICATIONS & DOSAGE
Chronic open-angle glaucoma and ocular hypertension—
Adults: 1 to 2 drops once daily (0.5%) or b.i.d. (0.25%).

ADVERSE REACTIONS
CNS: headache, depression, insomnia.
CV: slight reduction in resting heart rate.
EENT: *transient eye stinging and burning,* tearing, erythema, itching, keratitis, corneal punctate staining, photophobia; decreased corneal sensitivity with long-term use.
GI: nausea.
Skin: urticaria.
Other: evidence of beta blockade and systemic absorption *(hypotension, bradycardia, syncope, **asthmatic attacks in patients with a history of asthma,** and **CHF**).*

INTERACTIONS
Propranolol, metoprolol, and other oral beta-adrenergic blockers: increased ocular and systemic effects. Use together cautiously.
Reserpine and other catecholamine-depleting drugs: enhanced hypotensive and bradycardiac effects. Monitor closely.
Topical miotics, dipivefrin, epinephrine; systemically administered carbonic anhydrase inhibitors: additive lowered IOP. Use together cautiously.

EFFECTS ON DIAGNOSTIC TESTS
None reported.

CONTRAINDICATIONS
Contraindicated in patients with hypersensitivity to drug, bronchial asthma, history of bronchial asthma or severe COPD, sinus bradycardia, second- or third-degree AV block, cardiac failure, and cardiogenic shock.

NURSING CONSIDERATIONS
● Use cautiously in patients with chronic bronchitis and emphysema, diabetes mellitus, hyperthyroidism, and myasthenia gravis.
● Avoid letting dropper touch the patient's eye or surrounding tissue.

☑ PATIENT TEACHING
● Teach patient how to instill levobunolol. Advise him to wash hands before and after instilling drug and to apply light finger pressure on lacrimal sac for 1 minute after drops are instilled.
● Warn patient not to touch dropper to eye or surrounding tissue.

---

levocabastine hydrochloride
Livostin

Pregnancy Risk Category: C

HOW SUPPLIED
Ophthalmic suspension: 0.05%

ACTION
Selectively blocks ophthalmic histamine H_1 receptors.

ONSET, PEAK, DURATION
Unknown.

INDICATIONS & DOSAGE
Temporary relief of seasonal allergic conjunctivitis—
Adults and children 12 years and over: 1 drop q.i.d. for up to 2 weeks.

ADVERSE REACTIONS
CNS: headache, fatigue, somnolence.
EENT: *transient eye discomfort upon instillation (burning, stinging), eye dis-*charge, *dryness, pain, or redness; lacrimation; eyelid edema; visual disturbances; pharyngitis.*
GI: dry mouth, nausea.
Respiratory: cough, dyspnea.
Skin: rash.

INTERACTIONS
None significant.

EFFECTS ON DIAGNOSTIC TESTS
None reported.

CONTRAINDICATIONS
Contraindicated in patients hypersensitive to the drug or any of its components and while soft contacts are worn.

NURSING CONSIDERATIONS
● Know that drug is for ophthalmic use only; it should never be injected.

☑ PATIENT TEACHING
● Teach patient how to instill levocabastine. Advise him to wash hands before and after instilling drug and to avoid touching tip of dropper to eye or surrounding tissue. He should shake suspension well before instilling.
● Warn patient that he may experience transient discomfort or burning upon instillation. Tell him to contact the doctor if pain persists.
● Tell patient not to wear soft contact lenses during therapy.
● Tell patient to store drug at room temperature and to avoid freezing. He should not use a discolored solution.

---

lodoxamide tromethamine
Alomide

Pregnancy Risk Category: B

HOW SUPPLIED
Ophthalmic solution: 0.1%

ACTION
Stabilizes mast cells and prevents the release of inflammation mediators.

---

*Liquid contains alcohol. **May contain tartrazine. †Canada only. ‡Australia only. ◇OTC.

ONSET, PEAK, DURATION
Unknown.

INDICATIONS & DOSAGE
Vernal conjunctivitis, vernal keratoconjunctivitis, vernal keratitis—
Adults and children 2 years and over: 1 to 2 drops in affected eye q.i.d. for up to 3 months.

ADVERSE REACTIONS
CNS: headache, dizziness, somnolence.
EENT: *transient eye discomfort upon instillation (burning, stinging);* anterior chamber cells; blepharitis; blurred vision; chemosis; corneal erosion, ulcer, or abrasion; crystalline deposits; epitheliopathy; sensation of foreign body, stickiness, or warmth; hyperemia; keratitis; keratopathy; ocular edema, discharge, swelling, fatigue, itching, or allergy; pruritus; scales on eyelids or eyelash; tearing; dry nose.
GI: nausea, stomach discomfort.
Skin: rash, heat sensation.

INTERACTIONS
None significant.

EFFECTS ON DIAGNOSTIC TESTS
None reported.

CONTRAINDICATIONS
Contraindicated in patients hypersensitive to the drug or any of its components.

NURSING CONSIDERATIONS
• Know that drug is for ophthalmic use only; it should never be injected.
• Check expiration date before using.

☑ **PATIENT TEACHING**
• Teach patient how to instill lodoxamide. Advise him to wash hands before and after instilling drug and to avoid touching tip of dropper to eye or surrounding tissue.
• Tell him to contact the doctor if discomfort or burning persists upon instillation.

• Advise patient not to wear soft contact lenses during therapy.

metipranolol hydrochloride
OptiPranolol

Pregnancy Risk Category: C

HOW SUPPLIED
Ophthalmic solution: 0.3% in 5- or 10-ml dropper bottles

ACTION
Unknown. A noncardioselective beta-adrenergic blocker that appears to reduce aqueous production and to reduce elevated and normal intraocular pressure (IOP), with or without glaucoma, with little or no effect on pupil size or accommodation. IOP above 24 mm Hg is reduced an average of 20% to 26%.

ONSET, PEAK, DURATION
Onset occurs within 30 minutes. Peak effect occurs within about 2 hours. Effects persist about 12 to 24 hours.

INDICATIONS & DOSAGE
IOP reduction in ocular conditions, including ocular hypertension and chronic open-angle glaucoma—
Adults: 1 drop into affected eye b.i.d. If IOP is not at a satisfactory level, concomitant therapy to lower it may be instituted.

ADVERSE REACTIONS
CNS: headache, anxiety, dizziness, depression, somnolence, nervousness, asthenia, brow ache.
CV: hypertension, *MI,* atrial fibrillation, angina, palpitation, bradycardia.
EENT: transient local eye discomfort, tearing, conjunctivitis, eyelid dermatitis, blurred vision, blepharitis, abnormal vision, photophobia, eye edema, rhinitis, epistaxis.
GI: nausea.
Respiratory: dyspnea, bronchitis, cough.

Skin: rash.
Other: hypersensitivity reactions, myalgia.

INTERACTIONS
Calcium channel blockers, digitalis glycosides, quinidine: increased risk of adverse cardiac effects if significant amount of drug is systemically absorbed. Use together cautiously.
Fentanyl, general anesthetics: excessive hypotension. Monitor closely.
Metoprolol tartrate, propranolol, other oral beta-adrenergic blockers: increased ocular and systemic effects. Use together cautiously.
Reserpine and other catecholamine-depleting drugs: enhanced hypotensive and bradycardia-induced effects. Avoid concurrent use.

EFFECTS ON DIAGNOSTIC TESTS
None reported.

CONTRAINDICATIONS
Contraindicated in patients hypersensitive to the drug or any of its components and in patients with bronchial asthma, history of bronchial asthma or severe COPD, sinus bradycardia, second- or third-degree AV block, cardiac failure, and cardiogenic shock.

NURSING CONSIDERATIONS
● Use cautiously in patients with nonallergic bronchospasm, chronic bronchitis, emphysema, diabetes mellitus (especially in those subject to spontaneous hypoglycemia), hyperthyroidism, or cerebrovascular insufficiency.
● Anticipate using pilocarpine, other miotics, or systemic carbonic anhydrase inhibitors concomitantly if IOP is not adequately controlled.
● Check expiration date on bottle before use. Do not use if eyedrops have changed color.
● Be aware that a slight increase in outflow facility has been demonstrated with metipranolol. Like other noncardioselective beta-adrenergic blockers,

metipranolol does not have significant local anesthetic (membrane-stabilizing) actions or intrinsic sympathomimetic activity.

☑ PATIENT TEACHING
● Teach patient how to instill metipranolol. Instruct him to first wash hands thoroughly and then tilt head back or lie down and gaze upward. Tell patient to gently grasp lower eyelid below eyelashes and pull eyelid away from eye to form a pouch. Then have him place dropper directly over eye, avoiding contact with eye or any surface; look up just before applying drop; and look down for several seconds after instillation and slowly release eyelid.
● Tell patient to close eyes gently for 1 to 2 minutes and to apply gentle pressure to inside corner of eye at bridge of nose to retard draining of solution from intended area. Warn him not to rub eye or rinse dropper.

---

sodium chloride, hypertonic
Adsorbonac Ophthalmic Solution, Muro-128 Ointment, Sodium Chloride Ointment 5%

Pregnancy Risk Category: NR

HOW SUPPLIED
Ophthalmic ointment: 5%
Ophthalmic solution: 2%, 5%

ACTION
An osmotic agent that removes excess fluid from the cornea.

ONSET, PEAK, DURATION
Unknown.

INDICATIONS & DOSAGE
Temporary relief of corneal edema—
Adults and children: 1 to 2 drops q 3 to 4 hours, or ointment applied q 3 to 4 hours.

ADVERSE REACTIONS
EENT: slight eye stinging.
Other: hypersensitivity reactions.

INTERACTIONS
None significant.

EFFECTS ON DIAGNOSTIC TESTS
No information available.

CONTRAINDICATIONS
Contraindicated in patients hypersensitive to the drug or any of its components.

NURSING CONSIDERATIONS
• Know that ophthalmic solution is for topical use only; never inject.
• Check expiration date before using.

☑ **PATIENT TEACHING**
• Teach patient how to instill drug. Advise him to wash hands before and after instilling drug and to apply light finger pressure on lacrimal sac for 1 minute after drops are instilled. Warn patient not to touch dropper to eye or surrounding tissue.
• Tell patient to prevent caking on dropper bottle tip by putting a few drops of sterile irrigation solution inside bottle cap.
• Warn patient that ointment may cause blurred vision.
• If patient experiences severe headache, pain, rapid change in vision, acute redness of eyes, sudden appearance of floating spots, pain on exposure to light, or double vision, tell him to discontinue the drug and notify doctor.
• Advise patient to store drug in tightly closed container.

---

timolol maleate
Timoptic Solution, Timoptic-XE

Pregnancy Risk Category: C

HOW SUPPLIED
Ophthalmic solution: 0.25%, 0.5%
Ophthalmic gel: 0.25%, 0.5%

ACTION
Unknown. A beta blocker that is thought to reduce aqueous formation and possibly increase aqueous outflow.

ONSET, PEAK, DURATION
Onset occurs within 30 minutes. Peak effects occur within 1 to 2 hours. Effects persist for 12 to 24 hours.

INDICATIONS & DOSAGE
Chronic open-angle, secondary, and aphakic glaucomas; ocular hypertension—
Adults: initially, 1 drop of 0.25% solution in each affected eye b.i.d.; maintenance dosage is 1 drop daily. If no response, 1 drop of 0.5% solution in each affected eye b.i.d. If intraocular pressure (IOP) is controlled, dosage reduced to 1 drop daily. Alternatively, 1 drop of gel in each affected eye once daily.

ADVERSE REACTIONS
CNS: depression, fatigue, dizziness, lethargy, hallucinations, confusion.
CV: slight reduction in resting heart rate, arrhythmia, *CVA, cardiac arrest,* heart block, palpitations.
EENT: minor eye irritation, decreased corneal sensitivity with long-term use, conjunctivitis, blepharitis, keratitis, visual disturbances, diplopia, ptosis.
Other: *evidence of beta blockade and systemic absorption (hypotension, bradycardia, syncope, **asthmatic attacks in patients with a history of asthma,** and **CHF**).*

INTERACTIONS
Calcium channel blockers, digitalis glycosides, quinidine: increased risk of adverse cardiac effects if significant amounts of timolol are systemically absorbed. Use together cautiously.
Fentanyl, general anesthetics: excessive hypotension. Monitor closely.
Metoprolol tartrate, propranolol, other oral beta-adrenergic blockers: in-

creased ocular and systemic effects. Use together cautiously.
Reserpine and other catecholamine-depleting drugs: enhanced hypotensive and bradycardia-induced effects. Avoid concurrent use.

EFFECTS ON DIAGNOSTIC TESTS
Drug therapy may slightly increase BUN, serum potassium, uric acid, and blood glucose levels and may slightly decrease hemoglobin and hematocrit levels.

CONTRAINDICATIONS
Contraindicated in patients hypersensitive to the drug and in patients with bronchial asthma, history of bronchial asthma or severe COPD, sinus bradycardia, second- or third-degree AV block, cardiac failure, and cardiogenic shock.

NURSING CONSIDERATIONS
● Use cautiously in patients with nonallergic bronchospasm, chronic bronchitis, emphysema, diabetes mellitus, hyperthyroidism, or cerebrovascular insufficiency.
● Administer other ophthalmic agents at least 10 minutes before administering gel form of drug.
● Monitor diabetic patients carefully. Systemic beta-blocking effects can mask some signs of hypoglycemia in diabetic patients.
● Be aware that some patients may need a few weeks' treatment to stabilize pressure-lowering response. Determine IOP after 4 weeks of treatment.
● Know that the drug can be used safely in patients with glaucoma who wear conventional hard contact lenses.

☑ **PATIENT TEACHING**
● Teach patient how to instill timolol. Advise him to wash hands before and after instilling drug and to apply light finger pressure on lacrimal sac for 1 minute after drops are instilled. Warn patient not to touch dropper to eye or surrounding tissue.
● Instruct patient using gel form of drug to invert the container and shake once before each use. Also tell him to administer other ophthalmic agents at least 10 minutes before administering the gel drop.

acetic acid
boric acid
carbamide peroxide
chloramphenicol
triethanolamine polypeptide
   oleate-condensate

COMBINATION PRODUCTS
BOROFAIR OTIC: acetic acid 2% and aluminum acetate 2%.

acetic acid
Domeboro Otic, VoSol Otic

Pregnancy Risk Category: NR

HOW SUPPLIED
Otic solution: 2% acetic acid in aluminum acetate solution (Domeboro Otic), 2% acetic acid with 3% propylene glycol diacetate (VoSol Otic)

ACTION
Inhibits or destroys bacteria in the ear canal.

ONSET, PEAK, DURATION
Unknown.

INDICATIONS & DOSAGE
External ear canal infection—
Adults and children: 4 to 6 drops into ear canal q 2 to 3 hours; or insert saturated wick for first 24 hours, then continue with instillations.

ADVERSE REACTIONS
EENT: ear irritation or itching.
Skin: urticaria.
Other: overgrowth of nonsusceptible organisms.

INTERACTIONS
None significant.

EFFECTS ON DIAGNOSTIC TESTS
None significant.

CONTRAINDICATIONS
Contraindicated in patients with perforated eardrum.

NURSING CONSIDERATIONS
● Reculture any persistent drainage.
● Be aware that drug has anti-infective, anti-inflammatory, and antipruritic effects. *Pseudomonas aeruginosa* is particularly sensitive to this drug.

☑ **PATIENT TEACHING**
● Instruct patient or caregiver how to administer drug.
● Warn patient to avoid touching ear with dropper to prevent reinfection.

boric acid
Aurocaine 2◇, Auro-Dri◇, Dri/Ear◇

Pregnancy Risk Category: NR

HOW SUPPLIED
Otic solution: 2.75% boric acid in isopropyl alcohol

ACTION
Weak bacteriostatic that inhibits or destroys bacteria in the ear canal; also is a fungistatic agent.

ONSET, PEAK, DURATION
Unknown.

INDICATIONS & DOSAGE
External ear canal infection—
Adults and children: 3 to 6 drops into ear canal; plug with cotton. Repeated t.i.d. or q.i.d.

ADVERSE REACTIONS
EENT: ear irritation or itching.

Reactions may be *common*, uncommon, *life-threatening*, or COMMON AND LIFE-THREATENING.

Skin: urticaria.
Other: overgrowth of nonsusceptible organisms.

INTERACTIONS
None significant.

EFFECTS ON DIAGNOSTIC TESTS
None reported.

CONTRAINDICATIONS
Contraindicated in patients with a perforated eardrum or excoriated membranes.

NURSING CONSIDERATIONS
● Watch for signs of superinfection.

☑ **PATIENT TEACHING**
● Instruct patient or caregiver how to administer drug.
● Warn patient to avoid touching ear with dropper to prevent reinfection.
● Tell patient using cotton plug to always moisten with medication.

carbamide peroxide
Debrox ◇

Pregnancy Risk Category: NR

HOW SUPPLIED
Otic solution: 6.5% carbamide in glycerin or glycerin and propylene glycol

ACTION
A ceruminolytic that emulsifies and disperses accumulated cerumen.

ONSET, PEAK, DURATION
Onset and peak unknown. Duration is 15 to 30 minutes.

INDICATIONS & DOSAGE
Impacted cerumen—
Adults and children: 5 to 10 drops into ear canal b.i.d. for up to 4 days. Allow solution to remain in ear canal for 15 to 30 minutes; remove with warm water.

ADVERSE REACTIONS
None reported.

INTERACTIONS
None significant.

EFFECTS ON DIAGNOSTIC TESTS
None significant.

CONTRAINDICATIONS
Contraindicated in patients with a perforated eardrum.

NURSING CONSIDERATIONS
● Use in children under 12 years only under a doctor's direction.

☑ **PATIENT TEACHING**
● Instruct patient or caregiver how to administer drug.
● Warn patient to avoid touching ear with dropper to prevent reinfection.
● Tell patient to flush ear gently with warm water, using a rubber bulb syringe.
● Tell patient to call the doctor if redness, pain, or swelling persists.

chloramphenicol
Chloromycetin Otic, Sopamycetin†

Pregnancy Risk Category: NR

HOW SUPPLIED
Otic solution: 0.5%

ACTION
Inhibits or destroys bacteria in the ear canal.

ONSET, PEAK, DURATION
Unknown.

INDICATIONS & DOSAGE
External ear canal infection—
Adults and children: 2 to 3 drops into ear canal t.i.d.

ADVERSE REACTIONS
EENT: ear itching or burning.
Skin: pruritus, urticaria.

Other: overgrowth of nonsusceptible organisms, burning, bone marrow hypoplasia, *aplastic anemia.*

INTERACTIONS
None significant.

EFFECTS ON DIAGNOSTIC TESTS
False elevation of urinary PABA levels will result if drug is given during a bentiromide test for pancreatic function. Drug treatment will cause false-positive results on tests for urine glucose level using cupric sulfate (Clinitest). RBC, WBC, and platelet counts in the blood, and possibly the bone marrow, may decrease during drug therapy (from reversible to irreversible bone marrow depression). Hemoglobinuria or lactic acidosis may also occur.

CONTRAINDICATIONS
Contraindicated in patients with a perforated eardrum or hypersensitivity to any component of drug.

NURSING CONSIDERATIONS
• Obtain history of use and reactions.
• Watch for signs of superinfection. Avoid prolonged use.
• Reculture any persistent drainage.
• Watch for signs of sore throat (early sign of toxicity).

☑ PATIENT TEACHING
• Instruct patient or caregiver how to administer drug.
• Warn patient to avoid touching ear with dropper to avoid reinfection.

---

triethanolamine polypeptide oleate-condensate
Cerumenex

Pregnancy Risk Category: NR

HOW SUPPLIED
Otic solution: 10% in 6-ml, 12-ml bottles with droppers

ACTION
A ceruminolytic that emulsifies and disperses accumulated cerumen.

ONSET, PEAK, DURATION
Onset and peak unknown. Duration is 15 to 30 minutes.

INDICATIONS & DOSAGE
Impacted cerumen—
Adults and children: fill ear canal with solution and insert cotton plug. After 15 to 30 minutes, flush with warm water.

ADVERSE REACTIONS
EENT: ear erythema or itching.
Skin: severe eczema.

INTERACTIONS
None significant.

EFFECTS ON DIAGNOSTIC TESTS
None reported.

CONTRAINDICATIONS
Contraindicated in perforated eardrum, otitis media, and otitis externa.

NURSING CONSIDERATIONS
Alert: If hypersensitivity is suspected, anticipate patch test: Place 1 drop of drug on inner forearm; cover with bandage. Read results in 24 hours. If reaction occurs, drug should not be used.

☑ PATIENT TEACHING
• Teach patient to moisten cotton plug with medication before insertion, leave cotton in place for a maximum of 30 minutes, and flush ear gently with warm water, using a rubber bulb syringe.
• Tell patient not to use drops more often than prescribed.
• Warn patient that this medication is for use only in the ears.
• Advise patient to discontinue the drug if adverse reactions occur and to contact the doctor immediately.
• Tell patient to keep container tightly closed and away from moisture.

---

azelastine hydrochloride
beclomethasone dipropionate
budesonide
dexamethasone sodium
  phosphate
ephedrine sulfate
epinephrine hydrochloride
flunisolide
fluticasone propionate
naphazoline hydrochloride
oxymetazoline hydrochloride
phenylephrine hydrochloride
tetrahydrozoline hydrochloride
triamcinolone acetonide
xylometazoline hydrochloride

COMBINATION PRODUCTS
4-Way Nasal Spray ◊ : phenylephrine
hydrochloride 0.5%, naphazoline hydrochloride 0.05%, and pyrilamine
maleate 0.2%.

▼ NEW DRUG

azelastine hydrochloride
Astelin

Pregnancy Risk Category: C

HOW SUPPLIED
Nasal spray: 137 mcg/metered spray

ACTION
Exhibits histamine H_1-receptor antagonist activity.

ONSET, PEAK, DURATION
Onset and duration unknown. Plasma
levels peak within 2 to 3 hours.

INDICATIONS & DOSAGE
Seasonal allergic rhinitis—
**Adults and children 12 years and old-
er:** 2 sprays per nostril b.i.d.

ADVERSE REACTIONS
CNS: *headache, somnolence,* dizziness.
EENT: *bitter taste,* nasal burning, dry
mouth, epistaxis.
GI: nausea.
Musculoskeletal: myalgia.
Respiratory: pharyngitis, paroxysmal
sneezing, rhinitis.
Other: fatigue, weight increase.

INTERACTIONS
Cimetidine: may increase plasma levels
of azelastine. Avoid concomitant use.
CNS depressants, ethanol: increased sedation. Avoid concomitant use.

EFFECTS ON DIAGNOSTIC TESTS
None reported.

CONTRAINDICATIONS
Contraindicated in patients with known
hypersensitivity to the drug.

NURSING CONSIDERATIONS
• Know that azelastine should be used in
pregnancy only if the benefit justifies the
potential risk to the fetus. Breast-feeding
women should not take the drug.
• Be aware that safety and effectiveness
in patients under 12 years have not been
established.

☑ **PATIENT TEACHING**
• Warn patient not to drive or perform
hazardous activities if somnolence occurs.
• Advise patient not to use alcohol,
CNS depressants, or other antihistamines while taking the drug.
• Teach the patient proper usage of the
nasal spray. Instruct patient to replace
the child-resistant screw top on the bottle with the pump unit. Prime the delivery system with 4 sprays or until a fine
mist appears. Reprime the system with
2 sprays or until a fine mist appears if 3

or more days have elapsed since the last use. The bottle should be stored upright at room temperature with the pump closed tightly. Keep unit away from children.
• Tell patient to avoid getting the spray in the eyes.

---

beclomethasone dipropionate
Beconase AQ Nasal Spray, Beconase Nasal Inhaler, Vancenase AQ Nasal Spray, Vancenase Nasal Inhaler

Pregnancy Risk Category: C

HOW SUPPLIED
Nasal aerosol: 42 mcg/metered spray, 50 mcg/metered spray‡
Nasal spray: 42 mcg/metered spray, 50 mcg/metered spray‡

ACTION
A corticosteroid that decreases nasal inflammation, mainly by stabilizing leukocyte lysosomal membranes.

ONSET, PEAK, DURATION
Onset occurs within 5 to 7 days. Time to maximal benefit is up to 3 weeks for some patients. Duration unknown.

INDICATIONS & DOSAGE
Relief of symptoms of seasonal or perennial rhinitis; prevention of recurrence of nasal polyps after surgical removal—
Adults and children over 12 years: usual dosage is 1 or 2 sprays in each nostril, b.i.d., t.i.d., or q.i.d.

ADVERSE REACTIONS
CNS: headache.
EENT: *mild transient nasal burning and stinging,* nasal congestion, sneezing, burning, stinging, dryness, epistaxis, nasopharyngeal fungal infections.

INTERACTIONS
None significant.

EFFECTS ON DIAGNOSTIC TESTS
None reported.

CONTRAINDICATIONS
Contraindicated in patients hypersensitive to the drug.

NURSING CONSIDERATIONS
• Use cautiously, if at all, in patients with active or quiescent respiratory tract tubercular infections or untreated fungal, bacterial, or systemic viral or ocular herpes simplex infections. Also use cautiously in patients who have recently had nasal septal ulcers, nasal surgery, or trauma.
• Observe the patient for fungal infections.
• Be aware that beclomethasone is not effective for acute exacerbations of rhinitis. Decongestants or antihistamines may be needed.

☑ PATIENT TEACHING
• To instill, instruct the patient to shake the container before using; to blow nose to clear nasal passages; and to tilt head slightly forward and insert nozzle into nostril, pointing away from septum. Tell him to hold the other nostril closed and then to inspire gently and spray. Next, have him shake the container again and repeat in the other nostril.
• Advise the patient to pump the nasal spray three or four times before the first use, and once or twice before first use each day. The cap and nosepiece of the activator should be cleaned in warm water every day, then allowed to air-dry.
• Advise the patient to use drug regularly, as prescribed, because its effectiveness depends on regular use.
• Explain that the drug's therapeutic effects, unlike those of decongestants, are not immediate. Most patients achieve benefit within a few days, but some may require 2 to 3 weeks.
• Warn the patient not to exceed recom-

Reactions may be *common*, uncommon, *life-threatening*, or COMMON AND LIFE-THREATENING.

mended dosages because of the risk of hypothalamic-pituitary-adrenal function suppression.

● Tell the patient to notify the doctor if symptoms don't improve within 3 weeks or if nasal irritation persists.

● Teach the patient good nasal and oral hygiene.

---

budesonide
Rhinocort

Pregnancy Risk Category: C

HOW SUPPLIED
Nasal spray: 32 mcg/metered spray (7-g canister)

ACTION
Unknown. A corticosteroid that probably decreases nasal inflammation, mainly by inhibiting the activities of specific cells and the mediators involved in the allergic response.

ONSET, PEAK, DURATION
Not clearly defined.

INDICATIONS & DOSAGE
Symptoms of seasonal or perennial allergic rhinitis—
Adults and children 6 years and older: 2 sprays in each nostril in the morning and evening or 4 sprays in each nostril in the morning. Maintenance dosage should be the fewest number of sprays needed to control symptoms.

ADVERSE REACTIONS
CNS: nervousness.
EENT: *nasal irritation, epistaxis, pharyngitis,* reduced sense of smell, nasal pain, hoarseness.
GI: bad taste, dry mouth, dyspepsia, nausea.
Respiratory: *cough,* moniliasis, wheezing, dyspnea.
Skin: facial edema, rash, pruritus, contact dermatitis.
Other: myalgia, hypersensitivity

reactions.

INTERACTIONS
None significant.

EFFECTS ON DIAGNOSTIC TESTS
None reported.

CONTRAINDICATIONS
Contraindicated in patients hypersensitive to the drug or any of its components and in those who have had recent septal ulcers, nasal surgery, or nasal trauma until total healing has occurred.

NURSING CONSIDERATIONS
● Use cautiously in patients with tuberculous infections; untreated fungal, bacterial, or systemic viral infections; or ocular herpes simplex.

☑ **PATIENT TEACHING**
● Tell patient to avoid exposure to chickenpox or measles.

● To instill, instruct the patient to shake the container before using; to blow nose to clear nasal passages; and to tilt head slightly forward and insert nozzle into nostril, pointing away from septum. Tell him to hold the other nostril closed and then to inspire gently and spray. Next, have him shake container again and repeat in the other nostril.

● Instruct the patient that the product should be used by one person only to prevent the spread of infection.

● Advise the patient not to break, incinerate, or store canister in extreme heat; contents under pressure.

● Warn the patient not to exceed prescribed dosage or use for long periods of time because of the risk of hypothalamic-pituitary-adrenal axis suppression.

● Tell the patient to contact the doctor if symptoms do not improve in 3 weeks or if condition worsens.

● Teach the patient good nasal and oral hygiene.

---

dexamethasone sodium phosphate
Dexacort Phosphate Turbinaire

Pregnancy Risk Category: C

HOW SUPPLIED
Nasal aerosol: 84 mcg/metered spray, 170 doses/12.6-g canister

ACTION
Decreases nasal inflammation, mainly by stabilizing leukocyte lysosomal membranes.

ONSET, PEAK, DURATION
Not clearly defined.

INDICATIONS & DOSAGE
Allergic or inflammatory conditions, nasal polyps—
Adults: 2 sprays in each nostril b.i.d. or t.i.d. Maximum dosage is 12 sprays daily.
Children 6 to 12 years: 1 or 2 sprays in each nostril b.i.d. Maximum 8 sprays daily.
 Each spray delivers 0.1 mg dexamethasone sodium phosphate equal to 0.084 mg dexamethasone.

ADVERSE REACTIONS
EENT: nasal irritation, dryness, rebound nasal congestion.
Other: hypersensitivity reactions, systemic effects with prolonged use (pituitary-adrenal suppression, sodium retention, *CHF,* hypertension, peptic ulceration, ecchymoses, petechiae, masking of infection).

INTERACTIONS
None significant.

EFFECTS ON DIAGNOSTIC TESTS
None reported.

CONTRAINDICATIONS
Contraindicated in patients with hypersensitivity to drug, systemic fungal infections, tuberculosis, viral and fungal nasal conditions, or ocular herpes simplex and in those who have had recent septal ulcers, nasal surgery, or nasal trauma until total healing has occurred.

NURSING CONSIDERATIONS
● Use cautiously in patients with diabetes mellitus, peptic ulcer, ulcerative colitis, abscess or other pyrogenic infection, diverticulitis, fresh intestinal anastomosis, renal insufficiency, hypertension, osteoporosis, and myasthenia gravis.
● Frequently monitor blood pressure and serum potassium level. Hypertension and hypokalemia can occur with systemic absorption.
● Monitor for fluid retention which can occur from systemic absorption.
● Be prepared to gradually reduce dosage as nasal condition improves.
● Notify the doctor if you suspect underlying bacterial infection that should be controlled with anti-infectives.
● Know that irritation or sensitivity may require stopping drug.

☑ PATIENT TEACHING
● Tell patient to avoid exposure to chickenpox or measles.
● To instill, instruct the patient to shake the container before using; to blow nose to clear nasal passages; and to tilt head slightly forward and insert nozzle into nostril, pointing away from septum. Tell him to hold the other nostril closed and then to inspire gently and spray. Next, have him shake container again and repeat in the other nostril.
● Teach the patient good nasal and oral hygiene.
● Warn the patient that product should be used by only one person to prevent spread of infection.
● Warn the patient to avoid prolonged use because of the risk of hypothalamic-pituitary-adrenal–axis suppression.
● Advise the patient to contact the doctor if he experiences fever, joint or muscle aches, or extreme tiredness.

● Advise the patient not to break, incinerate, or store canister in extreme heat; contents under pressure.

ephedrine sulfate
Vicks Vatronol Nose Drops ◇

Pregnancy Risk Category: NR

HOW SUPPLIED
Nasal solution: 0.5% ◇

ACTION
Causes local vasoconstriction of dilated arterioles, reducing blood flow and nasal congestion.

ONSET, PEAK, DURATION
Unknown.

INDICATIONS & DOSAGE
Nasal congestion—
Adults and children: 2 to 3 drops of 0.5% solution into each nostril. Used no more frequently than q 4 hours.

ADVERSE REACTIONS
CNS: nervousness, excitation.
CV: *tachycardia.*
EENT: rebound nasal congestion with long-term or excessive use, mucosal irritation.

INTERACTIONS
MAO inhibitors: hypertensive crisis if ephedrine is absorbed. Don't use together.

EFFECTS ON DIAGNOSTIC TESTS
None reported.

CONTRAINDICATIONS
Contraindicated in patients with angle-closure glaucoma, psychoneurosis, angina pectoris, substantial organic heart disease, cardiovascular disease, and hypersensitivity to the drug or other sympathomimetics.

NURSING CONSIDERATIONS
● Use cautiously in patients with hyperthyroidism, hypertension, diabetes mellitus, or prostatic hyperplasia.

☑ PATIENT TEACHING
● Teach patient how to instill nosedrops.
● Instruct patient that product should be used by only one person to prevent spread of infection.
● Tell patient not to exceed recommended dosage and to use only when needed.

epinephrine hydrochloride
Adrenalin Chloride

Pregnancy Risk Category: NR

HOW SUPPLIED
Nasal solution: 0.1%

ACTION
Causes local vasoconstriction of dilated arterioles, reducing blood flow and nasal congestion.

ONSET, PEAK, DURATION
Onset occurs within 1 minute. Peak and duration unknown.

INDICATIONS & DOSAGE
Nasal congestion, local superficial bleeding—
Adults and children 6 years and older: instill 1 or 2 drops of solution.

ADVERSE REACTIONS
CNS: nervousness, excitation.
CV: *tachycardia.*
EENT: rebound nasal congestion, slight sting upon application.

INTERACTIONS
None significant.

EFFECTS ON DIAGNOSTIC TESTS
Drug therapy may increase blood glucose and serum lactic acid levels; increases BUN levels; and interferes with tests for urinary catecholamines.

---

*Liquid contains alcohol.   **May contain tartrazine.   †Canada only.   ‡Australia only.   ◇OTC.

CONTRAINDICATIONS
Contraindicated in patients with hypersensitivity to the drug.

NURSING CONSIDERATIONS
● Use cautiously in patients with hyperthyroidism, coronary artery disease, hypertension, or diabetes mellitus.

☑ PATIENT TEACHING
● Teach patient how to instill nosedrops.
● Instruct patient that product should be used by only one person to prevent spread of infection.
● Tell patient not to exceed recommended dosage and to use only when needed.

---

flunisolide
Nasalide, Rhinalar Nasal Mist‡

Pregnancy Risk Category: C

HOW SUPPLIED
Nasal inhalant: 25 mcg/metered spray, 200 doses/bottle‡
Nasal solution: 0.25 mg/ml in pump spray bottle

ACTION
Decreases nasal inflammation, mainly by stabilizing leukocyte lysosomal membranes by unknown mechanism.

ONSET, PEAK, DURATION
Unknown.

INDICATIONS & DOSAGE
Symptoms of seasonal or perennial rhinitis—
Adults: starting dose is 2 sprays (50 mcg) in each nostril b.i.d. Total daily dosage is 200 mcg. If necessary, dosage may be increased to 2 sprays in each nostril t.i.d. Maximum total daily dosage is 8 sprays in each nostril (400 mcg daily).
Children 6 to 14 years: starting dose is 1 spray (25 mcg) in each nostril t.i.d. or 2 sprays (50 mcg) in each nostril b.i.d. Total daily dosage is 150 to 200 mcg.

Maximum total daily dosage is 4 sprays in each nostril (200 mcg daily).

ADVERSE REACTIONS
CNS: headache.
EENT: *mild, transient nasal burning and stinging,* nasal congestion, nasopharyngeal fungal infection, burning, stinging, dryness, sneezing, epistaxis, watery eyes.
GI: nausea, vomiting.

INTERACTIONS
None significant.

EFFECTS ON DIAGNOSTIC TESTS
None reported.

CONTRAINDICATIONS
Contraindicated in patients hypersensitive to the drug. Also, drug should not be used in the presence of untreated localized infection involving nasal mucosa.

NURSING CONSIDERATIONS
● Use cautiously, if at all, in patients with active or quiescent respiratory tract tubercular infections or in untreated fungal, bacterial, or systemic viral or ocular herpes simplex infections. Also use cautiously in patients who have recently had nasal septal ulcers, nasal surgery, or nasal trauma.
● Be aware that flunisolide is not effective for acute exacerbations of rhinitis. Decongestants or antihistamines may be needed.

☑ PATIENT TEACHING
● Tell patient to avoid exposure to chickenpox or measles.
● To instill, instruct patient to shake the container before using; to blow nose to clear nasal passages; and to tilt head slightly forward and insert nozzle into nostril, pointing away from septum. Tell him to hold the other nostril closed, and then to inspire gently and spray. Have him repeat the above in the other nostril. Tell him to clean nosepiece with warm

water if it becomes clogged.
• Explain that the drug's therapeutic effects are not immediate. Most achieve benefit within a few days, but some may require 2 to 3 weeks.
• Advise patient to use drug regularly, as prescribed.
• Warn patient not to exceed recommended dosage to avoid suppression of hypothalamic-pituitary-adrenal function.
• Tell him to stop drug and notify doctor if symptoms don't diminish in 3 weeks or if nasal irritation persists.

---

fluticasone propionate
Flonase

Pregnancy Risk Category: C

HOW SUPPLIED
Nasal spray: 50 mcg/metered spray (9-g, 16-g bottles)

ACTION
Decreases nasal inflammation; exact mechanism unknown.

ONSET, PEAK, DURATION
Unknown.

INDICATIONS & DOSAGE
Seasonal and perennial allergic rhinitis—
Adults: initially, 2 sprays (50 mcg each spray) in each nostril once daily. Alternatively, 1 spray in each nostril b.i.d. After a few days, dosage may be re-. duced to 1 spray in each nostril daily. Maximum daily dosage is 2 sprays in each nostril.
Children 12 years and older: initially, 1 spray (50 mcg) in each nostril once daily. If patient doesn't respond or symptoms are severe, increase to 2 sprays in each nostril. Depending on patient's response, may decrease dosage to 1 spray in each nostril daily. Maximum daily dosage is 2 sprays in each nostril.

ADVERSE REACTIONS
CNS: headache.
EENT: epistaxis, nasal burning, blood in nasal mucus, pharyngitis, nasal irritation.

INTERACTIONS
None reported.

EFFECTS ON DIAGNOSTIC TESTS
None significant.

CONTRAINDICATIONS
Contraindicated in patients with hypersensitivity to drug or any component.

NURSING CONSIDERATIONS
• Use cautiously, if at all, in patients with active or quiescent tuberculous infections; glaucoma; untreated fungal, bacterial, or systemic viral infections; or ocular herpes simplex. Also use cautiously in patients already receiving systemic corticosteroids and in breast-feeding women.
• Do not use in patients with recent nasal septal ulcers, nasal surgery, or nasal trauma until healing has occurred.
• Although they rarely occur, monitor for signs of immediate hypersensitivity reactions or contact dermatitis after intranasal administration.

☑ **PATIENT TEACHING**
• Urge patient to read instruction sheet before using drug for first time.
• Explain how to instill drug. Tell patient to shake container gently before use; to blow nose to clear nasal passages; and to tilt head slightly forward and insert nozzle into nostril, pointing away from the septum. Tell him to hold the other nostril closed and then to inspire gently and spray. Next, have patient shake container again and repeat this procedure in the other nostril.
• Stress importance of adhering to a schedule for instillation because drug effectiveness depends on regular use. Caution patient not to exceed recommended dose; doing so may lead to hy-

percorticism, suppression of HPA function, or suppression of growth in children or teenagers.

● Tell patient to notify the doctor if symptoms do not improve or condition worsens.

● Warn patient to avoid exposure to chickenpox and measles and, if exposed, to obtain medical advice.

● Instruct patient to watch for and report signs and symptoms of nasal infection.

---

naphazoline hydrochloride
Privine◇

Pregnancy Risk Category: NR

HOW SUPPLIED
Nasal drops: 0.05% solution
Nasal spray: 0.05% solution

ACTION
Causes local vasoconstriction of dilated arterioles, reducing blood flow and nasal congestion.

ONSET, PEAK, DURATION
Onset occurs within 10 minutes. Peak unknown. Effects persist 2 to 6 hours.

INDICATIONS & DOSAGE
Nasal congestion—
Adults and children 12 years and older: 2 drops or sprays instilled in each nostril q 3 to 4 hours (drops) or 3 to 6 hours (spray).
Children 6 to 12 years: 1 to 2 drops or sprays instilled in each nostril q 3 to 6 hours, p.r.n. Not to be used longer than 3 to 5 days.

ADVERSE REACTIONS
EENT: rebound nasal congestion with excessive or long-term use, sneezing, stinging, dryness of mucosa.
Other: systemic effects in children after excessive or long-term use, marked sedation.

INTERACTIONS
None significant.

EFFECTS ON DIAGNOSTIC TESTS
None reported.

CONTRAINDICATIONS
Contraindicated in patients with hypersensitivity to drug.

NURSING CONSIDERATIONS
● Use cautiously in patients with hyperthyroidism, heart disease, hypertension, or diabetes mellitus and in those with difficulty in urination due to enlargement of the prostate gland.

☑ PATIENT TEACHING
● Teach patient how to use drug. For nasal drops, instruct patient to tilt head back as far as possible, instill drops, then lean head forward while inhaling and to repeat procedure for other nostril. For nasal spray, instruct him to hold spray container and head upright. Tell patient not to shake the container.
● Tell patient that product should be used by only one person to prevent spread of infection.
● Warn patient not to exceed recommended dosage.
● Tell patient to contact the doctor if nasal congestion persists after 5 days.

---

oxymetazoline hydrochloride
Afrin◇, Afrin Children's Strength Nose Drops◇, Allerest 12-Hour Nasal◇, Chlorphed-LA◇, Coricidin Nasal Mist◇, Dristan Long Lasting◇, Drixine Nasal‡, Duramist Plus◇, Duration◇, 4-Way Long-Acting Nasal, Genasal Spray◇, Neo-Synephrine 12 Hour◇, Nostrilla◇, NTZ Long Acting Nasal◇, Sinarest 12-Hour◇, Sinex Long-Acting◇, Twice-A-Day Nasal◇

Pregnancy Risk Category: NR

HOW SUPPLIED
Nasal solution: 0.025% ◇, 0.05% ◇

ACTION
Unknown. Thought to cause local vaso-constriction of dilated arterioles, reducing blood flow and nasal congestion.

ONSET, PEAK, DURATION
Onset occurs in 5 to 10 minutes. Peak effect occurs within 6 hours. Effects persist less than 12 hours.

INDICATIONS & DOSAGE
Nasal congestion—
Adults and children 6 years and over: 2 to 3 drops or sprays of 0.05% solution in each nostril b.i.d.
Children 2 to 6 years: 2 to 3 drops of 0.025% solution in each nostril b.i.d. Use no longer than 3 to 5 days.

ADVERSE REACTIONS
CNS: headache, drowsiness, dizziness, insomnia, possible sedation.
CV: palpitations, *CV collapse,* hypertension.
EENT: rebound nasal congestion or irritation with excessive or long-term use, dryness of nose and throat, increased nasal discharge, stinging, sneezing.
Other: systemic effects in children with excessive or long-term use.

INTERACTIONS
None significant.

EFFECTS ON DIAGNOSTIC TESTS
None reported.

CONTRAINDICATIONS
Contraindicated in patients with hypersensitivity to drug.

NURSING CONSIDERATIONS
● Use cautiously in patients with hyperthyroidism, cardiac disease, hypertension, or diabetes mellitus.

☑ PATIENT TEACHING
● Teach patient how to apply oxymeta-

zoline. Tell him to hold head upright to minimize swallowing of medication, then sniff spray briskly.
● Tell patient that product should be used by only one person to prevent spread of infection.
● Tell patient not to exceed recommended dosage and to use only when needed.
Alert: Warn patient that excessive use may cause bradycardia, hypotension, dizziness, and weakness.

phenylephrine hydrochloride
Alconefrin 12 ◇, Alconefrin 25 ◇, Alconefrin 50 ◇, Doktors ◇, Duration ◇, Neo-Synephrine ◇, Nostril ◇, Rhinall ◇, Rhinall-10 ◇, Sinex ◇, St. Joseph Measured Dose Nasal Decongestant ◇

Pregnancy Risk Category: NR

HOW SUPPLIED
Nasal jelly: 0.5%
Nasal solution: 0.125%, 0.16%, 0.2%, 0.25%, 0.5%, 1%

ACTION
Causes local vasoconstriction of dilated arterioles, reducing blood flow and nasal congestion.

ONSET, PEAK, DURATION
Onset is rapid. Peak unknown. Effects persist for ½ to 4 hours.

INDICATIONS & DOSAGE
Nasal congestion—
Adults and children 12 years and over: 2 to 3 drops or 1 to 2 sprays instilled in each nostril or small amount of jelly to nasal mucosa q 4 hours, p.r.n. Do not use for more than 3 to 5 days.
Children 6 to 12 years: 2 to 3 drops or 1 to 2 sprays of a 0.25% solution instilled in each nostril q 4 hours, p.r.n.
Children under 6 years: 2 to 3 drops of 0.125% solution q 4 hours, p.r.n.

ADVERSE REACTIONS
CNS: headache, tremor, dizziness, nervousness.
CV: *palpitations, tachycardia, PVCs,* hypertension, pallor.
EENT: transient burning or stinging, dryness of nasal mucosa, rebound nasal congestion with continued use.
GI: nausea.

INTERACTIONS
None significant.

EFFECTS ON DIAGNOSTIC TESTS
Drug may lower intraocular pressure in normal eyes or in open-angle glaucoma. It may also cause false-normal tonometry readings.

CONTRAINDICATIONS
Contraindicated in patients with hypersensitivity to drug.

NURSING CONSIDERATIONS
● Use cautiously in patients with hyperthyroidism, marked hypertension, Type I diabetes mellitus, cardiac disease, or advanced arteriosclerotic changes; in children of low body weight; and in elderly patients.

☑ **PATIENT TEACHING**
● Teach patient how to apply phenylephrine. Tell him to hold head upright to minimize swallowing of medication, then to sniff spray briskly.
● Tell patient that product should be used by only one person to prevent spread of infection.
● Tell patient not to exceed recommended dosage and to use only when needed.
● Advise patient to contact the doctor if symptoms persist beyond 3 days.

---

tetrahydrozoline hydrochloride
Tyzine Drops, Tyzine Pediatric Drops

Pregnancy Risk Category: C

HOW SUPPLIED
Nasal solution: 0.05%, 0.1%

ACTION
Unknown. Thought to cause local vasoconstriction of dilated arterioles, reducing blood flow and nasal congestion.

ONSET, PEAK, DURATION
Onset occurs within a few minutes. Peak unknown. Effects persist for 4 to 8 hours.

INDICATIONS & DOSAGE
Nasal congestion—
Adults and children over 6 years: 2 to 4 drops of 0.1% solution or spray into each nostril q 4 to 6 hours, p.r.n.
Children 2 to 6 years: 2 to 3 drops of 0.05% solution into each nostril q 4 to 6 hours, p.r.n.

ADVERSE REACTIONS
EENT: transient burning, stinging; sneezing, rebound nasal congestion with excessive or long-term use.

INTERACTIONS
None significant.

EFFECTS ON DIAGNOSTIC TESTS
None reported.

CONTRAINDICATIONS
Contraindicated in patients with hypersensitivity to drug and in those with angle-closure glaucoma or other serious eye diseases. Also contraindicated in children under 2 years. The 0.1% solution is contraindicated in children under 6 years.

NURSING CONSIDERATIONS
● Use cautiously in patients with hyperthyroidism, hypertension, and diabetes mellitus.

☑ **PATIENT TEACHING**
● Teach patient how to apply tetrahydrozoline. Tell him to hold head upright to minimize swallowing of medication,

---

then sniff spray briskly.
• Instruct patient that product should be used by only one person to prevent spread of infection.
• Tell patient not to exceed recommended dosage and to use only as needed for 3 to 5 days.

---

triamcinolone acetonide
Nasacort

Pregnancy Risk Category: C

HOW SUPPLIED
Nasal aerosol: 55 mcg/metered spray

ACTION
Unknown. A glucocorticoid with anti-inflammatory properties.

ONSET, PEAK, DURATION
A decrease in symptoms may occur within 12 hours after therapy is started. Effects peak within 3 to 4 days and may last for several days after drug is discontinued.

INDICATIONS & DOSAGE
Relief of symptoms of seasonal or perennial allergic rhinitis—
Adults and children 12 years and over: initially, 2 sprays (110 mcg) in each nostril once daily. Increased as needed up to 440 mcg daily either as once-daily dosage or in divided doses up to four times daily. After desired effect is obtained, dosage decreased, if possible, to as little as one spray (55 mcg) in each nostril daily.

ADVERSE REACTIONS
EENT: *nasal irritation,* dry mucous membranes, nasal and sinus congestion, irritation, burning, stinging, throat discomfort, sneezing, epistaxis.
Other: *headache.*

INTERACTIONS
None significant.

EFFECTS ON DIAGNOSTIC TESTS
None reported.

CONTRAINDICATIONS
Contraindicated in patients hypersensitive to any component of the drug.

NURSING CONSIDERATIONS
• Use with extreme caution, if at all, in patients with active or quiescent tuberculosis infection of the respiratory tract and in patients with untreated fungal, bacterial, or systemic viral infection or ocular herpes simplex.
• Use cautiously in patients who are already receiving systemic corticosteroids because of the increased likelihood of hypothalamic-pituitary-adrenal suppression compared with a therapeutic dosage of either one alone. Also use cautiously in patients with recent nasal septal ulcers, nasal surgery, or trauma because of the inhibitory effect on wound healing. Also use with caution in breast-feeding women.
Alert: Be aware that when excessive doses are used, signs and symptoms of hyperadrenocorticism and adrenal suppression may occur; the drug should be discontinued slowly.

☑ PATIENT TEACHING
• Urge the patient to read the patient-instruction sheet contained in each package before using drug for the first time.
• To instill, instruct the patient to shake the container before using; to blow nose to clear nasal passages; and to tilt head slightly forward and insert nozzle into nostril, pointing away from the septum. Tell him to hold the other nostril closed and then to inspire gently and spray. Next, have the patient shake container and repeat procedure in other nostril.
• Tell the patient to discard the canister after 100 actuations.
• Stress the importance of using the drug on a regular schedule because its effectiveness depends on regular use. However, caution the patient not to exceed the dosage prescribed because seri-

---

ous adverse reactions may occur.
• Tell the patient to notify the doctor if symptoms do not diminish within 2 to 3 weeks or if condition worsens.
• Warn the patient to avoid exposure to chickenpox or measles and, if exposed to either, to obtain medical advice.
• Instruct the patient to watch for signs and symptoms of nasal infection. If symptoms occur, tell the patient to notify the doctor because the drug may need to be discontinued and appropriate local therapy given.
• Advise the patient not to break canister, to incinerate canister, or to store canister in extreme heat; contents are under pressure and may explode.

xylometazoline hydrochloride
4-Way Long Acting, Neo-Synephrine II, Otrivin, Sine-Off Nasal Spray, Sinex-L.A.

Pregnancy Risk Category: NR

HOW SUPPLIED
Nasal solution: 0.05%, 0.1%

ACTION
Unknown. Thought to cause local vasoconstriction of dilated arterioles, reducing blood flow and nasal congestion.

ONSET, PEAK, DURATION
Onset in 5 to 10 minutes. Peak unknown. Effects persist for 5 to 6 hours.

INDICATIONS & DOSAGE
Nasal congestion—
Adults and children 12 years and over: 2 to 3 drops or sprays of 0.1% solution in each nostril q 8 to 10 hours.
Children 2 to 12 years: 2 to 3 drops of 0.05% solution in each nostril q 8 to 10 hours.
Children 6 months to 2 years: 1 drop of 0.05% solution instilled into each nostril q 6 hours, p.r.n.

ADVERSE REACTIONS
EENT: transient burning, stinging; dryness or ulceration of nasal mucosa; sneezing; rebound nasal congestion or irritation with excessive or long-term use.

INTERACTIONS
None significant.

EFFECTS ON DIAGNOSTIC TESTS
None reported.

CONTRAINDICATIONS
Contraindicated in patients with hypersensitivity to drug or angle-closure glaucoma.

NURSING CONSIDERATIONS
• Use cautiously in patients with hyperthyroidism, cardiac disease, hypertension, diabetes mellitus, and advanced arteriosclerosis.

✓ PATIENT TEACHING
• Teach patient how to apply xylometazoline. Have patient hold head upright to minimize swallowing of medication, then sniff spray briskly.
• Tell patient that product should be used by only one person.
• Tell patient not to exceed recommended dose and to use only as needed for 3 to 5 days.

87

Local anti-infectives

acyclovir
amphotericin B
azelaic acid cream
bacitracin
butoconazole nitrate
ciclopirox olamine
clindamycin phosphate
clotrimazole
econazole nitrate
erythromycin
gentamicin sulfate
ketoconazole
mafenide acetate
metronidazole (topical)
miconazole nitrate
mupirocin
naftifine
neomycin sulfate
nitrofurazone
nystatin
oxiconazole nitrate
silver sulfadiazine
sulconazole nitrate
terbinafine hydrochloride
terconazole
tetracycline hydrochloride
tioconazole
tolnaftate

COMBINATION PRODUCTS

BENZAMYCIN GEL: erythromycin 3% and benzoyl peroxide 5%.
LANABIOTIC ◊ : polymyxin B sulfate 5,000 units, neomycin sulfate 5 mg, bacitracin 500 units, and lidocaine 40 mg/g.
LOTRISONE CREAM: clotrimazole 1% and betamethasone dipropionate 0.05%.
MYCITRACIN OINTMENT ◊ : polymyxin B sulfate 5,000 units, bacitracin 500 units, and neomycin sulfate 3.5 mg/g.
MYCOLOG II CREAM, OINTMENT: triamcinolone acetonide 0.1% and nystatin 100,000 units/g.
NEO-CORTEF OINTMENT: hydrocortisone acetate 1% and neomycin sulfate 0.5%.

NEO DECADRON CREAM: dexamethasone phosphate 0.1% and neomycin sulfate 0.5%.
NEOSPORIN CREAM† ◊ : polymyxin B sulfate 10,000 units and neomycin sulfate 5 mg.
NEOSPORIN OINTMENT ◊ : polymyxin B sulfate 5,000 units, bacitracin zinc 400 units, and neomycin sulfate 5 mg/g.
POLYSPORIN OINTMENT ◊ : polymyxin B sulfate 10,000 units and bacitracin zinc 500 units/g.
VIOFORM-HYDROCORTISONE MILD CREAM: iodochlorhydroxyquin 3% and hydrocortisone 0.5%.

---

acyclovir
Zovirax

Pregnancy Risk Category: C

HOW SUPPLIED
Ointment: 5%

ACTION
Inhibits herpes simplex and varicella-zoster viral DNA synthesis by inhibiting viral DNA polymerase action.

ONSET, PEAK, DURATION
Not applicable.

INDICATIONS & DOSAGE
Initial herpes genitalis; limited, non–life-threatening mucocutaneous herpes simplex virus infections in immunocompromised patients—
Adults and children: cover all lesions q 3 hours six times daily for 7 days. Although dosage will vary depending on the total lesion area, use about a ½″ ribbon of ointment on each 4″ square of surface area.

ADVERSE REACTIONS
Skin: transient burning and stinging, rash, pruritus, vulvitis.

INTERACTIONS
None significant.

EFFECTS ON DIAGNOSTIC TESTS
Serum creatinine and BUN levels may increase during drug therapy.

CONTRAINDICATIONS
Contraindicated in patients with hypersensitivity or chemical intolerance to the drug.

NURSING CONSIDERATIONS
● As ordered, start therapy as early as possible after onset of symptoms.
● Apply with a finger cot or rubber glove to prevent autoinoculation of other body sites and transmission of infection to other persons.
● Know that the drug is for cutaneous use only; don't apply to the eye.

☑ **PATIENT TEACHING**
● Teach the patient that virus transmission can occur during treatment.
● Emphasize importance of compliance for successful therapy.

amphotericin B
Fungizone

Pregnancy Risk Category: B

HOW SUPPLIED
Cream: 3%
Lotion: 3%
Ointment: 3%

ACTION
Usually fungistatic; binds to sterols in the fungal cell membrane, resulting in increased membrane permeability and subsequent cell leakage.

ONSET, PEAK, DURATION
Not applicable.

INDICATIONS & DOSAGE
Cutaneous or mucocutaneous candidal infections—
Adults and children: apply liberally b.i.d. to q.i.d. for 1 to 3 weeks; interdigital lesions and paronychias treated for 2 to 4 weeks, and onychomycoses for several months because relapses are common.

ADVERSE REACTIONS
Skin: possible dryness, contact sensitivity, erythema, burning, pruritus.

INTERACTIONS
None significant.

EFFECTS ON DIAGNOSTIC TESTS
Drug therapy may increase BUN, serum creatinine, alkaline phosphatase, and bilirubin levels. Drug may cause hypokalemia and hypomagnesemia and may decrease WBC, RBC, and platelet counts.

CONTRAINDICATIONS
Contraindicated in patients hypersensitive to the drug.

NURSING CONSIDERATIONS
● Clean area before applying.
● Report local irritation. Cream may dry skin; ointment may irritate if applied to moist, hairy areas.
● Avoid using occlusive dressings.
● Be aware that cream or lotion is preferred for such areas as groin folds, armpit, and neck creases.
● Stop drug if irritation or hypersensitivity occurs, and notify doctor.
● Store at room temperature.

☑ **PATIENT TEACHING**
● Tell patient to use drug for full treatment period, even if condition has improved.
● Inform patient that cream discolors skin slightly when rubbed in; lotion or ointment may stain nail lesions but not skin if thoroughly rubbed in.
● Tell patient that fabric discoloration

Reactions may be *common*, uncommon, *life-threatening*, or COMMON AND LIFE-THREATENING.

caused by cream or lotion can be removed by washing; discoloration by ointment, by cleaning fluid.

---

azelaic acid cream
Azelex

Pregnancy Risk Category: B

HOW SUPPLIED
Cream: 20%

ACTION
Unknown. May inhibit microbial cellular protein synthesis.

ONSET, PEAK, DURATION
Not applicable.

INDICATIONS & DOSAGE
Mild to moderate inflammatory acne vulgaris—
Adults: Apply a thin film and gently but thoroughly massage into affected areas b.i.d, in morning and evening.

ADVERSE REACTIONS
Skin: pruritus, burning, stinging, tingling.

INTERACTIONS
None reported.

EFFECTS ON DIAGNOSTIC TESTS
None reported.

CONTRAINDICATIONS
Contraindicated in patients with hypersensitivity to any drug component.

NURSING CONSIDERATIONS
● Monitor the patient for early signs of hypopigmentation, especially a patient with dark complexion.
● If sensitivity or severe irritation occurs, notify the doctor, who may discontinue drug and order appropriate treatment.

☑ **PATIENT TEACHING**
● Instruct the patient to wash and pat dry affected areas before applying drug and to wash hands well after application. Warn him not to apply occlusive dressings or wrappings to affected areas.
● Warn him that skin irritation may occur when drug is applied to broken or inflamed skin, usually at start of therapy. Tell him to notify the doctor if irritation persists.
● Advise him to keep drug away from mouth, eyes, and other mucous membranes. If contact occurs, tell him to rinse thoroughly with water and consult a doctor if irritation persists.
● Advise him to report abnormal changes in skin color.
● Urge him to use drug for the full treatment period.

---

bacitracin
Baciguent ◇, Bacitin†

Pregnancy Risk Category: C

HOW SUPPLIED
Ointment: 500 units/g

ACTION
Bactericidal or bacteriostatic, depending on organism and concentration of drug; inhibits bacterial cell wall synthesis.

ONSET, PEAK, DURATION
Not applicable.

INDICATIONS & DOSAGE
Topical infections, abrasions, cuts, and minor burns or wounds—
Adults and children: apply thin film once daily to t.i.d, depending on severity of condition. Drug should not be used for more than 1 week.

ADVERSE REACTIONS
Skin: stinging, rashes, other allergic reactions; pruritus, burning, swelling of lips or face.

Systemic: tightness in chest, hypotension.

INTERACTIONS
None significant.

EFFECTS ON DIAGNOSTIC TESTS
Urinary sediment tests may show increased protein and cast excretion. Serum creatinine and BUN levels may increase during therapy.

CONTRAINDICATIONS
Contraindicated in patients hypersensitive to the drug and in atopic patients.

NURSING CONSIDERATIONS
• Clean area before applying, especially if crusted or suppurative.
• Anticipate alternative treatment for burns that cover more than 20% of body surface, especially if the patient suffers impaired renal function.
• Prolonged use may result in overgrowth of nonsusceptible organisms, particularly *Candida* species.

☑ **PATIENT TEACHING**
• If no improvement occurs or condition worsens, tell the patient to stop using and notify the doctor.
• Instruct patient to report systemic and skin adverse reactions that persist or are severe.
• Tell patient to not use drug for more than 1 week, except on doctor's advice.

---

butoconazole nitrate
Femstat

Pregnancy Risk Category: C

HOW SUPPLIED
Vaginal cream: 2% with applicators supplied

ACTION
Unknown. Thought to control or destroy fungus by disrupting cell membrane permeability, causing osmotic instability.

ONSET, PEAK, DURATION
Unknown.

INDICATIONS & DOSAGE
Vulvovaginal mycotic infections caused by Candida *species—*
Adults: for nonpregnant patient, 1 applicatorful intravaginally h.s. for 3 days. If needed, treat for another 3 days. For pregnant patient during second or third trimester, 1 applicatorful intravaginally h.s. for 6 days.

ADVERSE REACTIONS
GU: vulvovaginal burning and itching, soreness, and swelling.
Skin: finger itching.

INTERACTIONS
None significant.

EFFECTS ON DIAGNOSTIC TESTS
None reported.

CONTRAINDICATIONS
Contraindicated in patients hypersensitive to the drug.

NURSING CONSIDERATIONS
• Confirm diagnosis by smears or cultures, as ordered.
• Know that drug should be used in the second and third trimesters of pregnancy only when the potential benefits outweigh the possible risks to the fetus.
• Drug may be used with oral contraceptive and antibiotic therapy.

☑ **PATIENT TEACHING**
• Teach the patient how to apply drug, and tell her not to use tampons during treatment.
• Advise the patient to keep affected area cool and dry, wear loose-fitting cotton clothing, avoid feminine hygiene sprays, wash daily with unscented soap, dry thoroughly with clean towel, and prevent reinfection by wiping perineum from front to back.
• Tell the patient's sexual partner to wear a condom during intercourse until

treatment is complete. He should consult the doctor if he experiences penile itching, redness, or discomfort.

ciclopirox olamine
Loprox

Pregnancy Risk Category: B

HOW SUPPLIED
Cream: 1%
Lotion: 1%

ACTION
Unknown. Thought to deplete essential fungal intracellular substrates by blocking amino acid transport and altering cell membrane integrity.

ONSET, PEAK, DURATION
Not applicable.

INDICATIONS & DOSAGE
Tinea pedis, cruris, corporis, and versicolor; cutaneous candidiasis—
Adults and children over 10 years: massage gently into the affected and surrounding areas b.i.d., in the morning and evening for 2 to 4 weeks.

ADVERSE REACTIONS
Skin: pruritus, burning, irritation, redness, pain.

INTERACTIONS
None significant.

EFFECTS ON DIAGNOSTIC TESTS
None reported.

CONTRAINDICATIONS
Contraindicated in patients hypersensitive to the drug.

NURSING CONSIDERATIONS
● Cleanse with soap and water, then dry thoroughly.
● Don't use occlusive dressings.
● Avoid drug contact with eyes.

☑ PATIENT TEACHING
● Reassure patient that hypopigmentation from tinea versicolor will resolve gradually.
● If hypersensitivity reaction occurs, advise patient to discontinue treatment and notify the doctor.
● Tell patient to continue using drug for prescribed period even if symptoms have improved.
● Tell patient to call doctor if no improvement occurs in 4 weeks.

clindamycin phosphate
Cleocin T Gel, Lotion, Solution;
Cleocin Vaginal Cream

Pregnancy Risk Category: B

HOW SUPPLIED
Gel: 1%
Lotion: 1%
Topical solution: 1%
Vaginal cream: 2%

ACTION
Bacteriostatic or bactericidal, based on drug concentration and susceptibility of organism; suppresses growth of susceptible organisms in sebaceous glands by blocking protein synthesis.

ONSET, PEAK, DURATION
Not applicable for gel, lotion, or solution. Unknown for vaginal cream.

INDICATIONS & DOSAGE
Inflammatory acne vulgaris—
Adults and adolescents: apply to skin b.i.d., morning and evening.
Bacterial vaginosis—
Adults: 1 applicatorful intravaginally h.s. for 7 consecutive days.

ADVERSE REACTIONS
GI: upset, diarrhea, bloody diarrhea, abdominal pain, colitis (including pseudomembranous colitis).
GU: *cervicitis or vaginitis,* Candida albicans overgrowth, *vulvar irritation.*

---

*Liquid contains alcohol.   **May contain tartrazine.   †Canada only.   ‡Australia only.   ◇OTC.

Skin: *dryness,* rash, *redness,* pruritus, swelling, irritation, contact dermatitis, burning.

INTERACTIONS
Abrasive or medicated soaps or cleansers; acne preparations or other preparations containing peeling agents (benzoyl peroxide, resorcinol, salicylic acid, sulfur, tretinoin); alcohol-containing products (after-shave, cosmetics, perfumed toiletries, shaving creams or lotions); astringent soaps or cosmetics; isotretinoin; medicated cosmetics or cover-ups: potential cumulative dryness, resulting in excessive skin irritation. Use cautiously.
Erythromycin: may antagonize clindamycin's effect.

EFFECTS ON DIAGNOSTIC TESTS
Liver function test results may become abnormal in some patients during drug therapy.

CONTRAINDICATIONS
Contraindicated in patients hypersensitive to the drug and in those with history of ulcerative colitis, regional enteritis, or antibiotic-associated colitis.

NURSING CONSIDERATIONS
• For treating acne, know that drug may be used concurrently with tretinoin or benzoyl peroxide as well as systemic antibiotics.
• Know that drug can cause excessive dryness.

☑ PATIENT TEACHING
• Tell the patient to wash area with warm water and soap, rinse, and pat dry and to wait 30 minutes after washing or shaving to apply.
• Warn the patient to avoid too-frequent washing of area. Tell him to cover entire affected area but to avoid contact with eyes, nose, mouth, and other mucous membranes.
• Tell the patient to use only as prescribed.

• Tell the patient to dab, not roll, applicator-tipped bottle. If tip becomes dry, he should invert bottle and depress tip several times to moisten.
• Warn the patient not to smoke while applying topical solution.
• When used intravaginally, make sure the patient knows how to use applicators that come with the drug.
• If diarrhea occurs, tell the patient to check with the doctor or pharmacist before using antidiarrheal medication because it may worsen the condition.

---

clotrimazole
Canesten†, Gyne-Lotrimin ◊, Lotrimin, Mycelex, Mycelex-7 ◊, Mycelex-G, Mycelex-OTC ◊

Pregnancy Risk Category: B

HOW SUPPLIED
Troches: 10 mg
Cream: 1%
Topical lotion: 1%
Topical solution: 1%
Vaginal cream: 1% ◊
Vaginal tablets: 100 mg ◊, 500 mg
Combination pack: vaginal inserts 100 mg and vulvar cream 1% ◊

ACTION
Fungistatic but may be fungicidal, depending on concentration. Alters fungal cell wall permeability and produces osmotic instability.

ONSET, PEAK, DURATION
For lozenges, onset and peak unknown; effects persist for 3 hours. Not applicable for other forms.

INDICATIONS & DOSAGE
Superficial fungal infections (tinea pedis, tinea cruris, tinea corporis, or tinea versicolor; candidiasis)—
Adults and children: apply thinly and massage into affected and surrounding area, morning and evening, for 2 to 4 weeks. If no improvement occurs after 4

weeks, patient should be reevaluated.
Vulvovaginal candidiasis—
Adults: two 100-mg vaginal tablets inserted daily h.s. for 7 consecutive days, or one 500-mg vaginal tablet daily h.s. for 1 day; or 1 applicatorful vaginal cream daily h.s. for 7 days.
Oropharyngeal candidiasis treatment—
Adults and children 3 years and older: dissolve lozenge over 15 to 30 minutes in mouth five times daily for 14 consecutive days.
Prevention of oropharyngeal candidiasis in patients immunocompromised by such conditions as chemotherapy, radiotherapy, or steroid therapy in the treatment of leukemia, solid tumors, or renal transplantation—
Adults and children: dissolve lozenge over 15 to 30 minutes in mouth three times daily for duration of chemotherapy or until steroid is reduced to maintenance levels.

ADVERSE REACTIONS
GI: nausea and vomiting (with lozenges), lower abdominal cramps.
GU: *mild vaginal burning or irritation* (with vaginal use), cramping, urinary frequency.
Skin: blistering, *erythema,* edema, pruritus, burning, stinging, peeling, urticaria, skin fissures, general irritation.
Systemic: *increased liver function tests.*

INTERACTIONS
None significant.

EFFECTS ON DIAGNOSTIC TESTS
Abnormal liver function test results have been reported in patients receiving lozenges.

CONTRAINDICATIONS
Contraindicated in patients hypersensitive to the drug. Also contraindicated for ophthalmic use.

NURSING CONSIDERATIONS
● Clean area before applying.
● Watch for and report irritation or sensitivity; discontinue if irritation occurs and notify doctor.
● Know that improvement usually demonstrated within a week; if no improvement occurs in 4 weeks, diagnosis should be reviewed.
● When compliance is a problem, be aware that mild to moderate vaginal candidiasis may be treated with a single 500-mg tablet.

☑ PATIENT TEACHING
● Reassure the patient that hypopigmentation from tinea versicolor will resolve gradually.
● Warn the patient not to use occlusive wrappings or dressings.
● Ensure that the patient understands that frequent or persistent yeast infections may be a symptom of a more serious medical problem such as AIDS.
● Warn the patient that topical preparation may stain clothing.
● Emphasize the need to continue treatment for full course.

---

econazole nitrate
Ecostatin†, Spectazole

Pregnancy Risk Category: C

HOW SUPPLIED
Cream: 1%

ACTION
Fungistatic; may be fungicidal, depending on concentration. Alters fungal cell wall permeability and promotes osmotic instability.

ONSET, PEAK, DURATION
Not applicable.

INDICATIONS & DOSAGE
Tinea pedis, tinea cruris, tinea corporis and tinea versicolor; cutaneous candidiasis—
Adults and children: rub into affected areas once daily for at least 2 weeks.
Cutaneous candidiasis—

---

*Liquid contains alcohol.   **May contain tartrazine.   †Canada only.   ‡Australia only.   ◇OTC.

Adults and children: rub into affected areas b.i.d.

ADVERSE REACTIONS
Skin: burning, pruritus, stinging, erythema.

INTERACTIONS
Topical corticosteroids: may inhibit antifungal effect.

EFFECTS ON DIAGNOSTIC TESTS
None reported.

CONTRAINDICATIONS
Contraindicated in patients hypersensitive to the drug.

NURSING CONSIDERATIONS
● Clean affected area before applying.
● Don't use occlusive dressings.

☑ **PATIENT TEACHING**
● Tell patient to use drug for entire treatment period, even if symptoms improve. Instruct him to notify the doctor if no improvement occurs after 2 weeks (tinea cruris, tinea corporis, and tinea versicolor) or 4 weeks (tinea pedis).
● Reassure patient that hypopigmentation from tinea versicolor will resolve gradually.
● If condition persists or worsens or if irritation occurs, tell patient to stop use and call doctor.
● Warn that drug may stain clothing.

---

erythromycin
Akne-mycin, A/T/S, Del-Mycin, Emgel, Erycette, EryDerm, EryGel, Ery-Sol†, ETS†, Sans-Acne†, Staticin, T-Stat†

Pregnancy Risk Category: C

HOW SUPPLIED
Ointment: 2%
Topical gel: 2%
Topical solution: 1.5%*, 2%*
Pledgets: 2%

ACTION
Usually bacteriostatic but may be bactericidal in high concentrations or against highly susceptible organisms. Disrupts protein synthesis in susceptible bacteria.

ONSET, PEAK, DURATION
Not applicable.

INDICATIONS & DOSAGE
Inflammatory acne vulgaris—
Adults and children: apply to affected areas b.i.d.

ADVERSE REACTIONS
Skin: sensitivity reactions, erythema, burning, *dryness, pruritus,* irritation, peeling, oily skin.

INTERACTIONS
Abrasive or medicated soaps or cleansers; acne preparations or other preparations containing peeling agents (benzoyl peroxide, resorcinol, salicylic acid, sulfur, tretinoin); alcohol-containing products (after-shave, cosmetics, perfumed toiletries, shaving creams or lotions); astringent soaps or cosmetics; isotretinoin; medicated cosmetics or cover-ups: may cause cumulative dryness, resulting in excessive skin irritation. Use cautiously.

EFFECTS ON DIAGNOSTIC TESTS
Drug may interfere with fluorometric determinations of urinary catecholamines. Liver function test results may become abnormal during drug therapy (rare).

CONTRAINDICATIONS
Contraindicated in patients hypersensitive to the drug.

NURSING CONSIDERATIONS
● Wash, rinse, and dry affected areas before application.
● Know that prolonged use may be necessary when treating acne vulgaris; such use may result in overgrowth of nonsusceptible organisms.

Reactions may be *common*, uncommon, *life-threatening*, or COMMON AND LIFE-THREATENING.

☑ **PATIENT TEACHING**
● Advise patient not to use near eyes, nose, mouth, or other mucous membranes.
● If no improvement occurs or if condition worsens, tell patient to stop using and notify the doctor.

---

gentamicin sulfate
Garamycin, G-Myticin

Pregnancy Risk Category: C

HOW SUPPLIED
Cream: 0.1%
Ointment: 0.1%

ACTION
A bactericidal agent that disrupts bacterial protein synthesis by binding to ribosomes although its exact mechanism is unknown.

ONSET, PEAK, DURATION
Not applicable.

INDICATIONS & DOSAGE
Treatment and prophylaxis of superficial infections of the skin caused by susceptible bacteria—
Adults and children over 1 year: rub in small amount gently t.i.d. or q.i.d., with or without gauze dressing.

ADVERSE REACTIONS
Skin: minor skin irritation, possible photosensitivity, allergic contact dermatitis.

INTERACTIONS
None significant.

EFFECTS ON DIAGNOSTIC TESTS
Drug-induced nephrotoxicity may elevate BUN, nonprotein nitrogen, or serum creatinine levels and increase urinary excretion of casts.

CONTRAINDICATIONS
Contraindicated in patients hypersensitive to the drug or in those who may exhibit cross-sensitivity with other aminoglycosides, such as neomycin.

NURSING CONSIDERATIONS
Alert: Avoid use on large skin lesions or over a wide area because of possible systemic toxic effects.
● Know that use should be restricted to selected patients; widespread use may lead to resistant organisms.
● Prolonged use may result in overgrowth of nonsusceptible organisms.

☑ **PATIENT TEACHING**
● Tell patient to clean affected area before applying. Have him remove crusts before application for impetigo contagiosa to enhance absorption.
● Tell patient to store in cool place.
● If no improvement occurs or if condition worsens, tell patient to stop using and notify the doctor.

---

ketoconazole
Nizoral

Pregnancy Risk Category: C

HOW SUPPLIED
Cream: 2%
Shampoo: 2%

ACTION
Unknown. An imidazole that probably inhibits yeast growth by altering the permeability of the cell membrane.

ONSET, PEAK, DURATION
Not applicable.

INDICATIONS & DOSAGE
Tinea corporis, tinea cruris, tinea pedis, and tinea versicolor caused by susceptible organisms; seborrheic dermatitis; cutaneous candidiasis—
Adults: cover the affected and immediate surrounding area once daily for at least 2 weeks; for seborrheic dermatitis, apply b.i.d. for 4 weeks. When using

shampoo, wet hair, lather, and massage for 1 minute. Rinse and repeat, but leave drug on scalp for 3 minutes before rinsing. Shampoo twice weekly for 4 weeks, with at least 3 days between shampoos and then intermittently p.r.n. to maintain control.

ADVERSE REACTIONS
Skin: severe irritation, pruritus, stinging.

INTERACTIONS
None significant.

EFFECTS ON DIAGNOSTIC TESTS
Drug has been reported to cause transient elevations in AST, ALT, and alkaline phosphatase; it has also been reported to cause transient alterations in serum cholesterol and triglyceride levels.

CONTRAINDICATIONS
Contraindicated in patients hypersensitive to the drug.

NURSING CONSIDERATIONS
• Be aware that most patients show improvement soon after treatment begins.
• Keep in mind that treatment of tinea cruris or tinea corporis should continue for at least 2 weeks to reduce the possibility of recurrence.

☑ **PATIENT TEACHING**
• Tell patient to discontinue drug and notify doctor if hypersensitivity reaction occurs.
• Advise patient to check with the doctor if condition worsens; drug may have to be discontinued and diagnosis redetermined.

---

mafenide acetate
Sulfamylon

Pregnancy Risk Category: C

HOW SUPPLIED
Cream: 8.5%

ACTION
Unknown, although it interferes with bacterial cellular metabolism.

ONSET, PEAK, DURATION
Not applicable.

INDICATIONS & DOSAGE
Adjunctive treatment of second- and third-degree burns to prevent infection caused by susceptible organisms (especially Pseudomonas aeruginosa)—
Adults and children: apply ¹⁄₁₆″ thickness of cream daily or b.i.d. to clean debrided wounds. Reapply p.r.n. to keep burned area covered.

ADVERSE REACTIONS
Hematologic: eosinophilia.
Respiratory: tachypnea.
Skin: pain, *burning sensation,* rash, pruritus, swelling, urticaria, blisters, erythema.
Other: *metabolic acidosis,* facial edema.

INTERACTIONS
None significant.

EFFECTS ON DIAGNOSTIC TESTS
None reported.

CONTRAINDICATIONS
Contraindicated in patients with hypersensitivity to the drug.

NURSING CONSIDERATIONS
• Use cautiously in patients with acute renal failure and in those with known hypersensitivity to the drug or to sulfonamides.
• Clean area before applying, bathing patient daily, if possible.
• Use sterile gloves and instruments when applying cream to minimize risk of further wound contamination.
• Keep burn areas medicated at all times.

Alert: Closely monitor acid-base balance, especially in patients with pulmonary and renal dysfunction. If acidosis occurs, discontinue use for 24 to 48 hours and notify doctor.

● Be aware that sometimes it is difficult to distinguish between adverse reactions and effects of severe burn.

☑ **PATIENT TEACHING**
● Tell patient purpose of drug and importance of keeping burned areas covered with the drug at all times. Tell patient to alert nurse if drug rubs off in any area visible to patient.

● Tell patient to report adverse reactions, especially pain or burning when drug is applied; these symptoms may indicate allergy. Tell patient to notify doctor if pain is severe or prolonged; treatment may need to be temporarily stopped.

---

metronidazole (topical)
MetroGel, MetroGel-Vaginal

Pregnancy Risk Category: B

HOW SUPPLIED
Topical gel: 0.75%
Vaginal gel: 0.75%

ACTION
Unknown; may cause bactericidal effect by interacting with bacterial DNA. Active against many anaerobic gram-negative bacilli, anaerobic gram-positive cocci, *Gardnerella vaginalis,* and *Campylobacter fetus.*

ONSET, PEAK, DURATION
Not applicable for topical gel. Onset and duration unknown for vaginal gel; peak effects occur in 6 to 12 hours after intravaginal use.

INDICATIONS & DOSAGE
Acne rosacea—
Adults: apply a thin film to affected area b.i.d., morning and evening. Frequency and duration of therapy is adjusted after response is seen.
Bacterial vaginosis—
Adults: 1 applicatorful b.i.d., morning and evening, for 5 days.

ADVERSE REACTIONS
Topical gel
EENT: lacrimation (if drug applied around the eyes).
Vaginal form
CNS: dizziness, light-headedness, headache.
GI: cramps, pain, nausea, diarrhea, constipation, metallic or bad taste in mouth.
GU: *cervicitis, vaginitis.*
Skin: rash, *transient redness, dryness, mild burning, stinging.*
Other: overgrowth of nonsusceptible organisms, decreased appetite.

INTERACTIONS
Ethanol: a disulfiram-like reaction may occur.
Oral anticoagulants: may potentiate anticoagulant effect. Monitor the patient for potential adverse reactions.

EFFECTS ON DIAGNOSTIC TESTS
None reported.

CONTRAINDICATIONS
Contraindicated in patients hypersensitive to drug or its ingredients (such as parabens) and other nitromidazole derivatives.

NURSING CONSIDERATIONS
● Use cautiously in patients with history or evidence of blood dyscrasia; chemically related compounds are associated with blood dyscrasia.
● Use vaginal gel cautiously in patients with history of CNS diseases; a theoretical risk of seizures and peripheral neuropathy exist because these adverse reactions are associated with the oral form.
● Topical metronidazole therapy has not been linked with the adverse effects observed with parenteral or oral metron-

---

idazole therapy (including disulfiram-like reactions after alcohol ingestion). However, some drug may be absorbed after topical use.

● Instruct the patient using topical gel to avoid use of drug around the eyes. Also advise the patient to clean area thoroughly before use, but wait 15 to 20 minutes after cleaning the skin before applying drug to minimize risk of local irritation. Cosmetics may be used after applying drug.
● If local reactions occur, advise the patient to apply less frequently or to discontinue and contact the doctor.

---

miconazole nitrate
Micatin ◇ , Monistat-Derm Cream and Lotion, Monistat 3 Vaginal Suppository, Monistat 7 Vaginal Cream ◇ , Monistat 7 Vaginal Suppository ◇

Pregnancy Risk Category: C

HOW SUPPLIED
Cream: 2% ◇
Powder: 2% ◇
Spray: 2% ◇
Vaginal cream: 2% ◇
Vaginal suppositories: 100 mg ◇ , 200 mg

ACTION
A fungicidal imidazole that disrupts fungal cell membrane permeability.

ONSET, PEAK, DURATION
Not applicable for spray or cream form. Onset, peak, and duration unknown for suppositories.

INDICATIONS & DOSAGE
Tinea pedis, tinea cruris, tinea corporis; cutaneous candidiasis (moniliasis); common dermatophyte infections—
Adults and children: apply or spray sparingly b.i.d. for 2 to 4 weeks.
Tinea versicolor—

Adults and children: apply sparingly once daily for 2 weeks.
Vulvovaginal candidiasis—
Adults: 1 applicatorful or 100 mg suppository (Monistat 7) inserted intravaginally h.s. for 7 days; course repeated if necessary. Alternatively, 200 mg suppository (Monistat 3) intravaginally h.s. for 3 days.

ADVERSE REACTIONS
CNS: headache.
GU: vulvovaginal burning, pruritus, or irritation with vaginal cream; pelvic cramps.
Skin: irritation, burning, maceration, allergic contact dermatitis.

INTERACTIONS
None significant.

EFFECTS ON DIAGNOSTIC TESTS
Drug may cause a transient decrease in hematocrit levels and an increase or decrease in platelet counts; it frequently causes RBC aggregation. Drug also may cause hyponatremia, hyperlipidemia, and hypertriglyceridemia; abnormalities in lipoprotein and immunoelectrophoretic patterns are from the polyoxyl 35 castor oil vehicle.

CONTRAINDICATIONS
Contraindicated in patients hypersensitive to the drug.

NURSING CONSIDERATIONS
● Know that concurrent use of intravaginal forms and certain latex products, such as vaginal contraceptive diaphragms, are not recommended because of possible interaction.
● Don't use occlusive dressings.

☑ **PATIENT TEACHING**
● Advise patient that drug is for perineal or intravaginal use only. Keep out of eyes.
● Ensure that patient understands that frequent or persistent yeast infections may be a symptom of a more serious

medical problem such as AIDS.
● Tell patient to cautiously insert intravaginal forms high into the vagina with applicator provided.
● Tell patient drug may stain clothing.
● Warn patient to discontinue if sensitivity or chemical irritation occurs.
● Tell patient to continue using for full treatment period prescribed.
● Advise patient to avoid sexual intercourse during vaginal treatment.

---

mupirocin
Bactroban

Pregnancy Risk Category: B

HOW SUPPLIED
Ointment: 2%

ACTION
Unknown. Thought to inhibit bacterial protein and RNA synthesis.

ONSET, PEAK, DURATION
Not applicable.

INDICATIONS & DOSAGE
Impetigo—
Adults and children: apply to affected areas t.i.d. for 1 to 2 weeks.

ADVERSE REACTIONS
Skin: burning, pruritus, stinging, rash, pain, erythema.

INTERACTIONS
None significant.

EFFECTS ON DIAGNOSTIC TESTS
None reported.

CONTRAINDICATIONS
Contraindicated in patients hypersensitive to the drug.

NURSING CONSIDERATIONS
● Use cautiously in patients with burns or impaired renal function.
● Drug is not for ophthalmic use.

● Prolonged use may cause overgrowth of nonsusceptible bacteria and fungi.
● Local reactions appear to be caused by the polyethylene glycol vehicle.

☑ **PATIENT TEACHING**
● If no improvement occurs in 3 to 5 days or if condition worsens, tell patient to notify the doctor immediately.
● Warn patient about local adverse reactions associated with drug application.

---

naftifine
Naftin

Pregnancy Risk Category: B

HOW SUPPLIED
Cream: 1%
Gel: 1%

ACTION
Unknown. A broad-spectrum fungicidal agent that is thought to inhibit sterol biosynthesis in susceptible fungi by blocking the enzyme squalene 2,3 epoxidase.

ONSET, PEAK, DURATION
Not applicable.

INDICATIONS & DOSAGE
Tinea corporis, tinea cruris, and tinea pedis—
Adults: apply to affected area once daily with the cream, or b.i.d. in the morning and evening with the gel.

ADVERSE REACTIONS
Skin: *burning, stinging,* dryness, pruritus, local irritation, erythema.

INTERACTIONS
None significant.

EFFECTS ON DIAGNOSTIC TESTS
No information available.

CONTRAINDICATIONS
Contraindicated in patients hypersensi-

---

*Liquid contains alcohol.   **May contain tartrazine.   †Canada only.   ‡Australia only.   ◊ OTC.*

tive to the drug.

NURSING CONSIDERATIONS
● Therapy should be reevaluated if no improvement occurs after 4 weeks.
● Keep cream away from mucous membranes. Not for ophthalmic use.

☑ PATIENT TEACHING
● Tell the patient not to use occlusive dressings unless directed otherwise by the doctor.
● Instruct the patient to wash hands after application.
● Instruct the patient to discontinue therapy and notify the doctor if irritation or sensitivity develops.

---

neomycin sulfate
Mycifradin†, Myciguent◇, Neo-Rx

Pregnancy Risk Category: C

HOW SUPPLIED
Cream: 0.5%◇
Ointment: 0.5%◇

ACTION
Unknown. Thought to disrupt bacterial protein synthesis by binding to bacterial ribosomes.

ONSET, PEAK, DURATION
Not applicable.

INDICATIONS & DOSAGE
Prevention or treatment of superficial bacterial infections—
Adults and children: rub into affected area one to three times daily.

ADVERSE REACTIONS
Skin: *rash, contact dermatitis,* urticaria.
Systemic: *possible nephrotoxicity, ototoxicity,* **neuromuscular blockade.**

INTERACTIONS
None significant.

EFFECTS ON DIAGNOSTIC TESTS
Drug-induced nephrotoxicity may elevate levels of BUN, nonprotein nitrogen, or serum creatinine; it may increase urinary excretion of casts, if systemic absorption occurs.

CONTRAINDICATIONS
Contraindicated in patients hypersensitive to the drug.

NURSING CONSIDERATIONS
● Use cautiously in patients with extensive dermatologic conditions. Don't use on more than 20% of the body surface.
● Prolonged use may result in overgrowth of nonsusceptible organisms.
● In combination products containing corticosteroids, be aware that use of occlusive dressings increases corticosteroid absorption and the likelihood of systemic effects.
● Keep in mind that enhanced systemic absorption occurs on denuded or abraded areas.
● Watch for signs of hypersensitivity and contact dermatitis.
Alert: Watch for signs of ototoxicity with prolonged or extended use.

☑ PATIENT TEACHING
● If no improvement occurs or if condition worsens, tell patient to stop using and notify the doctor.
● Tell patient to report adverse reactions, especially systemic reactions.

---

nitrofurazone
Furacin

Pregnancy Risk Category: C

HOW SUPPLIED
Cream: 0.2%
Ointment: 0.2% (soluble dressing)
Topical solution: 0.2%

ACTION
Unknown. A broad-spectrum antibiotic that probably inhibits bacterial enzymes

---

Reactions may be *common*, uncommon, *life-threatening*, or COMMON AND LIFE-THREATENING.

involved in carbohydrate metabolism.

ONSET, PEAK, DURATION
Not applicable.

INDICATIONS & DOSAGE
Adjunctive treatment of second- and third-degree burns (especially when resistance to other antibiotics and sulfonamides occurs); prevention of skin allograft rejection—
Adults and children: apply directly to lesion daily or every few days, depending on severity of burn. May also be applied to dressings used to cover affected area.

ADVERSE REACTIONS
Skin: *erythema, pruritus,* burning, edema, *allergic contact dermatitis.*

INTERACTIONS
None significant.

EFFECTS ON DIAGNOSTIC TESTS
None reported.

CONTRAINDICATIONS
Contraindicated in patients hypersensitive to the drug.

NURSING CONSIDERATIONS
● Use cautiously in patients with known or suspected renal impairment. Monitor serum creatinine levels regularly, as ordered.
● Clean wound, as indicated by the doctor, before reapplying dressings.
● Use sterile application technique to prevent further wound contamination.
● When using wet dressing, protect skin around wound with zinc oxide ointment.
● Be aware that drug may discolor in light but still retains its potency.
● Discard cloudy solutions if warming to 55° to 60° C (131° to 140° F) does not restore clarity.
● Store solution in tight, light-resistant containers (brown bottles). Avoid exposure to direct light, prolonged heat, and alkaline materials.

☑ **PATIENT TEACHING**
● Tell patient to report irritation, sensitization, or infection.
● Explain all procedures to patient.

---

nystatin
Mycostatin, Nadostine†, Nilstat

Pregnancy Risk Category: NR

HOW SUPPLIED
Cream: 100,000 units/g
Ointment: 100,000 units/g
Powder: 100,000 units/g
Vaginal tablets: 100,000 units

ACTION
Disrupts integrity of fungal cell wall, promoting osmotic instability.

ONSET, PEAK, DURATION
Not applicable for cream, ointment, or powder. Unknown for tablets.

INDICATIONS & DOSAGE
Cutaneous and mucocutaneous infections caused by Candida albicans—
Adults and children: apply to affected area up to several times a day.
Vulvovaginal candidiasis—
Adults: 1 vaginal tablet daily for 14 days.

ADVERSE REACTIONS
Skin: occasional contact dermatitis from preservatives in some forms.

INTERACTIONS
None significant.

EFFECTS ON DIAGNOSTIC TESTS
None reported.

CONTRAINDICATIONS
Contraindicated in patients hypersensitive to the drug.

NURSING CONSIDERATIONS
● Do not use occlusive dressings.
● Keep in mind that preparation does

---

not stain skin or mucous membranes.
● Cream is recommended for intertriginous areas; powder, for moist areas; ointment, for dry areas.

☑ **PATIENT TEACHING**
● Instruct female patient how to administer vaginal tablets, and tell her to continue using the vaginal tablets during her menstrual period. Instruct her to refrigerate the tablets.
● Tell patient to use drug for full prescribed period, even if condition improves. Immunosuppressed patients may use the drug chronically.
● Instruct patient not to use occlusive dressings with skin application.

---

oxiconazole nitrate
Oxistat

Pregnancy Risk Category: B

HOW SUPPLIED
Cream: 1%
Lotion: 1%

ACTION
Unknown. May inhibit ergosterol synthesis in fungal cell walls, causing osmotic instability and cell lysis.

ONSET, PEAK, DURATION
Not applicable.

INDICATIONS & DOSAGE
Tinea pedis, cruris, and tinea corporis caused by Trichophyton rubrum *or* T. mentagrophytes—
Adults: apply to affected area once or twice daily. Treat tinea cruris and tinea corporis for 2 weeks and tinea pedis for 1 month to minimize risk of recurrence.

ADVERSE REACTIONS
Skin: pruritus, burning, stinging, contact dermatitis, irritation, scaling, tingling, pain, eczema.

INTERACTIONS
None significant.

EFFECTS ON DIAGNOSTIC TESTS
None reported.

CONTRAINDICATIONS
Contraindicated in patients hypersensitive to the drug.

NURSING CONSIDERATIONS
● Know that drug is not for ophthalmic or vaginal administration.
● Know that drug is for external use only.

☑ **PATIENT TEACHING**
● Inform patient that drug shouldn't touch the eyes or vagina.
● Tell patient to stop drug and call doctor if local irritation occurs.

---

silver sulfadiazine
Flamazine†, Flint SSD, Silvadene, SSD-AF, Thermazene

Pregnancy Risk Category: B

HOW SUPPLIED
Cream: 1%

ACTION
Broad-spectrum sulfonamide that acts on cell membrane and cell wall; bactericidal for many gram-positive and gram-negative organisms.

ONSET, PEAK, DURATION
Not applicable.

INDICATIONS & DOSAGE
Prevention and treatment of wound infection in second- and third-degree burns—
Adults: apply $^1/_{16}$" thickness to clean debrided burn wound daily or b.i.d.

ADVERSE REACTIONS
Hematologic: *leukopenia.*
Skin: pain, burning, rashes, pruritus,

---

skin necrosis, erythema multiforme, skin discoloration.

INTERACTIONS
Topical proteolytic enzymes: inactivation of enzymes. Do not use together.

EFFECTS ON DIAGNOSTIC TESTS
If used on extensive areas of body surface, systemic absorption may result in a decreased neutrophil count, indicating a reversible leukopenia.

CONTRAINDICATIONS
Contraindicated in premature and full-term neonates during first 2 months of life. Drug may increase possibility of kernicterus. Also contraindicated in patients with hypersensitivity to the drug or G6PD deficiency and in pregnant women at or near term.

NURSING CONSIDERATIONS
● Use with caution in patients hypersensitive to sulfonamides.
● Use sterile application technique to prevent wound contamination.
● Use only on affected areas. Keep these areas medicated at all times.
● Bathe the patient daily, if possible.
● Inspect the patient's skin daily, and note any changes. Notify the doctor if burning or excessive pain develops.
● Monitor serum sulfadiazine concentrations and renal function, as ordered, and check urine for sulfa crystals in patients with extensive burns.
● Tell doctor if hepatic or renal dysfunction occurs; drug may need to be stopped.
● Discard darkened cream, which indicates drug is ineffective.

☑ **PATIENT TEACHING**
● Instruct patient to report adverse reactions promptly, especially burning or excessive pain with application.
● Inform patient of need for frequent blood and urine tests to monitor for adverse effects.

sulconazole nitrate
Exelderm

Pregnancy Risk Category: C

HOW SUPPLIED
Topical solution: 1%
Cream: 1%

ACTION
Unknown. A broad-spectrum antifungal imidazole derivative that inhibits the growth of both fungi and yeast.

ONSET, PEAK, DURATION
Not applicable.

INDICATIONS & DOSAGE
Tinea cruris, tinea corporis, tinea pedis, or tinea versicolor—
Adults: massage a small amount of drug into affected area daily to b.i.d. for 3 weeks. Treat tinea pedis with cream b.i.d. for 4 weeks.

ADVERSE REACTIONS
Skin: pruritus, burning, stinging, redness.

INTERACTIONS
None significant.

EFFECTS ON DIAGNOSTIC TESTS
None reported.

CONTRAINDICATIONS
Contraindicated in patients hypersensitive to any component of the drug.

NURSING CONSIDERATIONS
● Use only cream for tinea pedia. Efficacy against tinea pedis (athlete's foot) has not been proven with the topical solution.
● Know that if no improvement occurs after 4 weeks, diagnosis should be reconsidered.

☑ **PATIENT TEACHING**
● Tell the patient to avoid touching the

---

eyes with the drug and to wash hands thoroughly after applying.
● Explain to the patient the necessity of completing the full course of therapy to prevent recurrence. Clinical improvement is usually apparent within 1 week, with symptomatic relief in just a few days.
● If irritation develops during treatment, tell the patient to discontinue drug and contact the doctor.

terbinafine hydrochloride
Lamisil

Pregnancy Risk Category: B

HOW SUPPLIED
Cream: 1%

ACTION
Fungicidal; selectively inhibits an early step in synthesis of sterols used by fungi for cell wall synthesis.

ONSET, PEAK, DURATION
Not applicable.

INDICATIONS & DOSAGE
Interdigital tinea pedis, tinea cruris, and tinea corporis—
Adults: cover affected area and immediate surrounding area b.i.d. for at least 1 week.

ADVERSE REACTIONS
Skin: irritation, burning, pruritus, dryness.

INTERACTIONS
None significant.

EFFECTS ON DIAGNOSTIC TESTS
Drug may cause liver enzyme abnormalities at least twice the upper limit of normal range.

CONTRAINDICATIONS
Contraindicated in patients hypersensitive to the drug.

NURSING CONSIDERATIONS
● Observe patients for 2 to 4 weeks after therapy is complete to determine if treatment was successful; review the diagnosis if the condition persists beyond this observation period.
● Be aware that therapy shouldn't exceed 4 weeks.

☑ **PATIENT TEACHING**
● Teach the patient proper use of drug. Tell the patient to use only as directed for the full recommended course, even if symptoms disappear and not to apply near the eyes, mouth, or mucous membranes or use occlusive dressings unless so directed.
● Tell the patient to discontinue drug and contact the doctor if irritation or sensitivity develops.

terconazole
Terazol 3 Vaginal Suppositories, Terazol 7 Vaginal Cream

Pregnancy Risk Category: C

HOW SUPPLIED
Vaginal cream: 0.4%, 0.8%
Vaginal suppositories: 80 mg

ACTION
Unknown; may increase fungal cell membrane permeability (*Candida* species only).

ONSET, PEAK, DURATION
Unknown.

INDICATIONS & DOSAGE
Vulvovaginal candidiasis—
Adults: 1 applicatorful of cream or 1 suppository inserted into vagina h.s. 0.4% cream used for 7 consecutive days; 0.8% cream or 80-mg suppository for 3 consecutive days. Course repeated, if necessary, after reconfirmation by smear or culture.

Reactions may be *common,* uncommon, *life-threatening,* or COMMON AND LIFE-THREATENING.

ADVERSE REACTIONS
CNS: *headache.*
GU: dysmenorrhea, pain of the female genitalia, vulvovaginal burning.
Skin: irritation, *pruritus,* photosensitivity.
Other: fever, chills, body aches.

INTERACTIONS
None significant.

EFFECTS ON DIAGNOSTIC TESTS
None reported.

CONTRAINDICATIONS
Contraindicated in patients with known sensitivity to terconazole or any inactive ingredients in drug.

NURSING CONSIDERATIONS
● Discontinue if the patient develops fever, chills, other flulike symptoms, or sensitivity and notify doctor
● Keep in mind that therapeutic effect of drug is unaffected by menstruation.

☑ **PATIENT TEACHING**
● Advise patient to continue treatment during the menstrual period. However, tell her not to use tampons.
● Tell patient to use for full treatment period prescribed. Explain how to prevent reinfection.
● Tell patient to refrain from sexual intercourse during treatment.

---

tetracycline hydrochloride
Achromycin, Topicycline

Pregnancy Risk Category: B

HOW SUPPLIED
Ointment: 3%
Topical solution: 2.2 mg/ml

ACTION
Unknown. A broad-spectrum antibiotic that probably disrupts bacterial protein synthesis; usually bacteriostatic.

ONSET, PEAK, DURATION
Unknown.

INDICATIONS & DOSAGE
Acne vulgaris—
Adults and children over 11 years: rub solution into affected areas b.i.d. until skin is thoroughly covered.
Prevention or treatment of superficial skin infections caused by susceptible bacteria—
Adults: apply to affected area b.i.d. in morning and evening or t.i.d.

ADVERSE REACTIONS
Skin: temporary stinging or burning on application; slight yellowing of treated skin, especially in patients with light complexions; severe dermatitis.

INTERACTIONS
Abrasive or medicated soaps or cleansers; acne preparations or other preparations containing peeling agents (benzoyl peroxide, resorcinol, salicylic acid, sulfur, tretinoin); alcohol-containing products (after-shave, cosmetics, perfumed toiletries, shaving creams or lotions); astringent soaps or cosmetics; isotretinoin; medicated cosmetics or cover-ups: may cause cumulative dryness, resulting in excessive skin irritation. Use cautiously.

EFFECTS ON DIAGNOSTIC TESTS
Drug causes false-negative results in urine tests using glucose oxidase reagent (Clinistix or Tes-Tape) and false elevations in fluorometric tests for urinary catecholamines. Drug may elevate BUN levels in patients with decreased renal function.

CONTRAINDICATIONS
Contraindicated in patients hypersensitive to the drug.

NURSING CONSIDERATIONS
● Use cautiously in patients with hepatic or renal impairment.
● Prolonged use may result in over-

---

growth of nonsusceptible organisms.
• Store at room temperature, away from excessive heat.
• Be aware that ointment form should not be used to treat acne vulgaris.

☑ **PATIENT TEACHING**
• Tell the patient to wash area before applying.
• Explain that floating plug in bottle of Topicycline—an inert and harmless result of proper reconstitution of the preparation—shouldn't be removed.
• Tell the patient how to increase or decrease applicator pressure against skin to control flow rate of solution.
• Tell the patient that she may continue normal use of cosmetics.
• Tell the patient not to share medication with family members.
• Advise the patient to use or discard the drug within 2 months.
• If no improvement occurs or if condition worsens, advise the patient to stop using and notify the doctor.

---

tioconazole
Vagistat

Pregnancy Risk Category: C

HOW SUPPLIED
Vaginal ointment: 6.5%

ACTION
A fungicidal imidazole that alters cell wall permeability.

ONSET, PEAK, DURATION
Unknown.

INDICATIONS & DOSAGE
Vulvovaginal candidiasis—
Adults: 1 applicatorful (about 4.6 g) inserted intravaginally h.s. one time only.

ADVERSE REACTIONS
GU: *burning, pruritus,* discharge, vaginal pain, dysuria, dyspareunia, vulvar edema, irritation.

INTERACTIONS
None significant.

EFFECTS ON DIAGNOSTIC TESTS
None reported.

CONTRAINDICATIONS
Contraindicated in patients hypersensitive to the drug or other imidazole antifungal agents (miconazole, ketoconazole).

NURSING CONSIDERATIONS
• Know that if patient is breast-feeding, she should temporarily stop doing so because it is not known if drug is excreted in breast milk.
• Notify the doctor if patient reports irritation or sensitivity.

☑ **PATIENT TEACHING**
• Review proper use of the drug with the patient. Written instructions for the patient are available with the product. Tell the patient to insert drug high into the vagina.
• To avoid contamination of the ointment, tell the patient to open the applicator just before using it.
• Tell the patient to use a sanitary napkin to avoid staining her clothing.
• Advise the patient to avoid sexual intercourse on the night after insertion, or advise her partner to use a condom to prevent reinfection.
• Emphasize the need to complete the full course of therapy, even after symptoms have improved. The patient should continue using the drug during her menstrual period.

---

tolnaftate
Aftate for Athlete's Foot ◊, Aftate for Jock Itch ◊, Dr. Scholl's Athlete's Foot Powder ◊, Dr. Scholl's Athlete's Foot Spray ◊, Footwork ◊, Fungatin ◊, Genaspor ◊, NP-27 ◊, Tinactin ◊, Ting ◊, Zeasorb-AF ◊

Pregnancy Risk Category: C

Reactions may be *common*, uncommon, ***life-threatening***, or COMMON AND LIFE-THREATENING.

HOW SUPPLIED
Aerosol liquid: 1% (36% alcohol) ◊
Aerosol powder: 1% (14% alcohol) ◊
Cream: 1% ◊
Gel: 1% ◊
Powder: 1% ◊
Pump spray liquid: 1% (36% alcohol) ◊
Topical solution: 1% ◊

ACTION
Unknown, although drug has been demonstrated to distort the hyphae and stunt mycelial growth in susceptible fungi.

ONSET, PEAK, DURATION
Not applicable.

INDICATIONS & DOSAGE
Superficial fungal infections of the skin; infections due to common pathogenic fungi; tinea pedis, tinea cruris, tinea corporis, and tinea versicolor—
Adults and children: apply ¼″ to ½″ ribbon of cream or 2 to 3 drops of solution to cover area; same amount of cream or 2 to 3 drops of solution to cover toes and interdigital webs of one foot; or gel, powder, or spray to cover affected area. Apply and massage gently into skin b.i.d. for 2 to 6 weeks.

ADVERSE REACTIONS
Skin: possible irritation.

INTERACTIONS
None significant.

EFFECTS ON DIAGNOSTIC TESTS
No information available.

CONTRAINDICATIONS
Contraindicated in patients hypersensitive to the drug.

NURSING CONSIDERATIONS
● Be aware that drug is not used to treat fungal infections of the hair or nails; tolnaftate is ineffective against these fungi.
● Know that drug is odorless and greaseless; it won't stain or discolor skin, hair, nails, or clothing.
● Know that powder or aerosol may be used inside socks and shoes of persons susceptible to tinea infections.

☑ PATIENT TEACHING
● Tell patient to cleanse area and dry thoroughly before applying drug.
● Tell patient to continue using for full treatment period prescribed, even if condition has improved. Treatment should continue for at least 2 weeks after symptoms have resolved.
● Advise patient to use only a small quantity of cream or lotion; treated area should not be wet with solution.
● If no improvement occurs after 10 days, tell patient to call doctor.
● Tell patient to discontinue if condition worsens and to check with the doctor.

88

Scabicides and pediculicides

benzyl benzoate lotion
crotamiton
lindane
permethrin
pyrethrins

COMBINATION PRODUCTS
None.

---

benzyl benzoate lotion
Ascabiol‡

Pregnancy Risk Category: C

HOW SUPPLIED
Lotion: 14% (with benzocaine 2%)‡
Emulsion: 50%‡

ACTION
Unknown.

ONSET, PEAK, DURATION
Unknown.

INDICATIONS & DOSAGE
Parasitic infestation (scabies, Phthirus
pubis, Pediculus humanus capitis)—
Adults and children: scrub entire body
with soap and water. Remove scales or
crusts. Then apply the lotion undiluted
over affected area (include whole body
for scabies), except the face and scalp,
while still damp. Be sure to apply
around nails. Let dry. Apply second coat
on the most involved areas. Bathe after
24 hours.
　　Treatment may be repeated in 7 to 10
days if mites appear or new lesions develop.

ADVERSE REACTIONS
Skin: *irritation, pruritus; contact dermatitis* (with repeated applications).

INTERACTIONS
None significant.

EFFECTS ON DIAGNOSTIC TESTS
No information available.

CONTRAINDICATIONS
Contraindicated when skin is raw or inflamed or in patients hypersensitive to
drug.

NURSING CONSIDERATIONS
● Do not apply to face, eyes, mucous
membranes, or urethral meatus. If accidental contact with eyes occurs, flush
with water and notify the doctor.
● Apply topical corticosteroids as prescribed if dermatitis develops from
scratching.
● Do not apply to infants' or small children's hands because they put their
hands into their mouths.
● Make sure hospitalized patients are
placed in isolation, with linen-handling
precautions, until treatment is completed.
● Store drug in light-resistant container;
avoid exposure to excessive heat.

☑ **PATIENT TEACHING**
● Teach the patient how to administer
drug.
● Tell the patient to discontinue drug
and to wash it off skin and notify the
doctor immediately if skin irritation or
hypersensitivity develops.
● Instruct the patient to change and sterilize (boil, launder, dry clean, or apply
very hot iron) all clothing and bed linen
after drug is washed off.
● Instruct the patient to reapply drug if
it is washed off during treatment time.
● After application for lice infestation,
tell the patient to use a fine-tooth comb
dipped in white vinegar to remove nits
from hairy areas.

Reactions may be *common,* uncommon, *life-threatening,* or COMMON AND LIFE-THREATENING.

• Tell the patient to warn other family members and sexual contacts about infestation. Sexual contacts should be treated simultaneously.

• Reassure the patient that although itching may continue for several weeks, it will stop; continued itching does not indicate that therapy is ineffective.

---

crotamiton
Eurax

Pregnancy Risk Category: C

HOW SUPPLIED
Cream: 10%
Lotion: 10%

ACTION
Unknown.

ONSET, PEAK, DURATION
Unknown.

INDICATIONS & DOSAGE
Parasitic infestation (scabies)—
Adults and children: scrub entire body with soap and water. Remove scales or crusts. Then apply a thin layer of cream over entire body, from chin down (with special attention to folds, creases, interdigital spaces, and genital area). Apply second coat in 24 hours. Wait additional 48 hours, then wash off. Treatment is repeated in 7 to 10 days if mites reappear or new lesions develop.
Itching—
Adults and children: applied locally and repeated p.r.n.

ADVERSE REACTIONS
Skin: *irritation,* allergic skin sensitivity.

INTERACTIONS
None significant.

EFFECTS ON DIAGNOSTIC TESTS
None reported.

CONTRAINDICATIONS
Contraindicated when skin is raw or inflamed and in patients hypersensitive to drug.

NURSING CONSIDERATIONS
• Estimate amount of cream needed per application; most patients have a tendency to overuse scabicides. For most adults, a single tube of cream provides a sufficient amount for two applications.

• Apply topical corticosteroids, as prescribed, if dermatitis develops from scratching.

• Make sure hospitalized patients are placed in isolation, with special linen-handling precautions, until treatment is completed.

• Be aware that monthly maintenance treatments may be necessary in long-term care facilities, where infestation is a problem.

☑ PATIENT TEACHING
• Teach the patient how to apply drug. Tell the patient not to apply to face, eyes, mucous membranes, or urethral meatus. If accidental contact with eyes occurs, flush with water and notify the doctor.

• Tell the patient to discontinue drug and to wash it off skin and to notify the doctor immediately if skin irritation or hypersensitivity develops.

• Instruct the patient to change and sterilize (boil, launder, dry clean, or apply very hot iron) all clothing and bed linen after drug is washed off.

• Instruct the patient to reapply drug if it is washed off during treatment time.

• Tell the patient to warn other family members and sexual contacts about infestation. Sexual contacts should be treated simultaneously.

• Reassure the patient that although itching may continue for several weeks, it will stop; continued itching does not indicate that therapy is ineffective.

---

lindane
gBH†, G-Well, Kwell, Kwellada†,
Scabene

Pregnancy Risk Category: B

HOW SUPPLIED
Cream: 1%
Lotion: 1%
Shampoo: 1%

ACTION
Unknown. Appears to inhibit neuronal membrane function in arthropods, causing neuronal hyperactivity, seizures, and death after penetrating the parasites' exoskeleton.

ONSET, PEAK, DURATION
Unknown.

INDICATIONS & DOSAGE
Parasitic infestation (scabies, pediculosis)—
Adults and children: Centers for Disease Control and Prevention recommends avoiding bathing before application on skin. If the patient does bathe, let skin dry and cool thoroughly before using. Apply thin layer of cream or lotion over entire skin surface (with special attention to folds, creases, interdigital spaces, and genital area) for scabies, or to hairy areas for pediculosis. After 8 to 12 hours, wash off drug. Repeat process in 1 week if mites appear or new lesions develop.

Apply shampoo undiluted to affected area and work into lather for 4 to 5 minutes; small amounts of water may enhance formation of lather. Apply 30 ml of shampoo for short hair, 45 ml for medium-length hair, or 60 ml for long hair. Rinse thoroughly and rub dry with towel.

ADVERSE REACTIONS
CNS: *dizziness, seizures.*
Skin: *irritation* (with repeated use).

INTERACTIONS
None significant.

EFFECTS ON DIAGNOSTIC TESTS
None reported.

CONTRAINDICATIONS
Contraindicated in patients hypersensitive to the drug, when skin is raw or inflamed, or in patients with seizure disorders. The lotion form is contraindicated in premature infants.

NURSING CONSIDERATIONS
● Use cautiously in infants and young children, who are at greater risk for CNS toxicity.
● Apply topical corticosteroids or administer oral antihistamines, as prescribed, for pruritus.
● Make sure that hospitalized patients are placed in isolation, with special linen-handling precautions, until treatment is completed.
● Know that modest amounts (6% to 13%) are absorbed through intact skin. Absorption is increased if used with creams, oils, or lotions or if applied to face, scalp, axillae, neck, scrotum, or irritated or broken skin.

☑ **PATIENT TEACHING**
● Teach patient how to administer drug; inform him that drug may be poisonous if misused. Warn patient not to apply to open areas, acutely inflamed skin, or to face, eyes, mucous membranes, or urethral meatus. If accidental contact with eyes occurs, flush with water and notify the doctor. Avoid inhaling vapors.
● Tell patient to wash it off skin and to notify the doctor immediately if skin irritation or hypersensitivity develops.
● Discourage repeated use, which can lead to skin irritation, systemic toxicity, or seizures. Repeat use only if live lice or nits are found after 1 week.
● Instruct patient to change and sterilize (boil, launder, dry clean, or apply very hot iron) all clothing and bed linen after drug is washed off.

● After application for lice infestation, tell patient to use a fine-tooth comb dipped in white vinegar to remove nits from hairy areas.

● Advise patient to use lindane shampoo to clean combs or brushes; wash them thoroughly afterward. Warn the patient not to use routinely.

● Warn patient that itching may continue for several weeks after effective treatment, especially in scabies.

● Instruct patient to reapply drug if it is washed off during treatment time.

● Tell patient to warn other family members and sexual contacts about infestation. Sexual contacts should be treated simultaneously.

---

permethrin
Elimite, Nix

Pregnancy Risk Category: B

HOW SUPPLIED
Topical liquid (cream-rinse): 1%
Cream: 5%

ACTION
Acts on the parasites' nerve cells to disrupt the sodium channel current, causing paralysis of the parasite.

ONSET, PEAK, DURATION
Onset and peak unknown. Residual activity persists for about 10 days.

INDICATIONS & DOSAGE
Infestation with Pediculus humanus capitis *(head lice) and its nits—*
Adults and children: use after hair has been washed with shampoo, rinsed with water, and towel-dried. Apply 25 to 50 ml of liquid to saturate the hair and scalp. Allow to remain on hair for 10 minutes before rinsing off with water.
Treatment of Sarcoptes scabiei—
Adults and children: thoroughly massage into the skin from the head to the soles. Infants should be treated on the hairline, neck, scalp, temple, and fore-

head. Cream should be removed after 8 to 14 hours by washing.

ADVERSE REACTIONS
Skin: pruritus, *burning, stinging,* edema, tingling, numbness or scalp discomfort, mild erythema, scalp rash.

INTERACTIONS
None significant.

EFFECTS ON DIAGNOSTIC TESTS
None reported.

CONTRAINDICATIONS
Contraindicated in patients hypersensitive to pyrethrins or chrysanthemums.

NURSING CONSIDERATIONS
● Be aware that a single treatment is usually all that is necessary. Combing of nits is not required for effectiveness, but drug package supplies a fine-tooth comb for cosmetic use as desired.

● Retreat for lice, as prescribed, if lice are observed 7 days after the initial application.

☑ PATIENT TEACHING
● Explain to the patient that treatment with permethrin may temporarily worsen the symptoms of head lice infestation, such as pruritus, erythema, and edema.

● Tell the patient that headgear, scarves, coats, and bed linens should be disinfected by machine washing with hot water and machine drying for at least 20 minutes, using the hot cycle. Nonwashable items should be sealed in a plastic bag for 2 weeks, or sprayed with a product designed to eliminate lice and their nits.

● Tell the patient to warn other family members and sexual contacts about infestation. Sexual contacts should be treated simultaneously.

---

pyrethrins
A-200 Pyrinate ◇ , Barc ◇ , Blue Gel,
Pronto, Pyrinyl ◇ , R&C, RID ◇ ,
TISIT ◇ , Triple X ◇

Pregnancy Risk Category: C

HOW SUPPLIED
Shampoo: pyrethrins 0.17% and piperonyl butoxide 2%; pyrethrins 0.3% and
piperonyl butoxide 3%
Topical gel: pyrethrins 0.18% and piperonyl butoxide 2.2%; pyrethrins 0.33%
and piperonyl butoxide 3%; pyrethrins
0.3% and piperonyl butoxide 4%
Topical solution: pyrethrins 0.18% and
piperonyl butoxide 2%; pyrethrins
0.2%, piperonyl butoxide 2%, and de-
odorized kerosene 0.8%; pyrethrins
0.3% and piperonyl butoxide 3%

ACTION
Acts as contact poison that disrupts parasite's nervous system, causing parasite
paralysis and death.

ONSET, PEAK, DURATION
Not applicable.

INDICATIONS & DOSAGE
*Infestations of head, body, and pubic
(crab) lice and their eggs—*
Adults and children: apply to hair,
scalp, or other infested areas until en-
tirely wet. Allow to remain for 10 minutes but no longer. Wash thoroughly
with warm water and soap or shampoo.
Remove dead lice and eggs with fine-
tooth comb. Treatment repeated, if necessary, in 7 to 10 days to kill newly
hatched lice. Not to exceed two applications within 24 hours.

ADVERSE REACTIONS
Skin: *irritation* (with repeated use).

INTERACTIONS
None significant.

EFFECTS ON DIAGNOSTIC TESTS
No information available.

CONTRAINDICATIONS
Contraindicated in patients hypersensitive to the drug, ragweed, or crysanthe-
mums.

NURSING CONSIDERATIONS
● Use cautiously in infants and small
children.
● Apply topical corticosteroids or oral
antihistamines as prescribed if dermatitis develops from scratching.
● Be aware that drug is not effective
against scabies.

☑ PATIENT TEACHING
● Instruct the patient not to apply to
open areas or acutely inflamed skin or
to face, eyes, mucous membranes, or
urethral meatus. If accidental contact
with eyes occurs, flush with water and
notify the doctor.
● Discourage repeated use, which can
lead to skin irritation and possible systemic toxicity.
● Tell the patient to discontinue drug
and to wash it off skin and to notify the
doctor immediately if skin irritation develops. All preparations contain petroleum distillates.
● Instruct the patient to change and sterilize all clothing and bed linen after
drug is washed off.
● Teach the patient to remove dead parasites with a fine-tooth comb.
● Tell the patient to warn other family
members and sexual contacts about infestation. Sexual contacts should be
treated simultaneously.

89

Topical corticosteroids

amcinonide
betamethasone dipropionate
betamethasone valerate
clobetasol propionate
clocortolone pivalate
desonide
desoximetasone
dexamethasone
dexamethasone sodium phosphate
diflorasone diacetate
fluocinolone acetonide
fluocinonide
flurandrenolide
fluticasone propionate
halcinonide
halobetasol propionate
hydrocortisone
hydrocortisone acetate
hydrocortisone butyrate
hydrocortisone valerate
mometasone furoate
triamcinolone acetonide

COMBINATION PRODUCTS
Corticosteroids for topical use are commonly combined with antibiotics and antifungals. (See Chapter 87, LOCAL ANTI-INFECTIVES.)

---

amcinonide
Cyclocort

Pregnancy Risk Category: C

HOW SUPPLIED
Cream: 0.1%
Lotion: 0.1%
Ointment: 0.1%

ACTION
Unknown. Diffuses across cell membranes to form complexes with specific cytoplasmic receptors. Exhibits anti-inflammatory, antipruritic, vasoconstrictive, and antiproliferative activity. Considered a group II (high-potency) agent according to vasoconstrictive properties.

ONSET, PEAK, DURATION
Onset and duration unknown. Plasma levels are highest when applied to inflamed or damaged skin, eyelids, or scrotal area; lowest when applied to intact normal skin, palms of hands, or soles of feet.

INDICATIONS & DOSAGE
Inflammation associated with corticosteroid-responsive dermatoses—
Adults and children: apply a light film to affected areas b.i.d. or t.i.d. Rub in gently until it disappears.

ADVERSE REACTIONS
Skin: burning, pruritus, irritation, dryness, erythema, folliculitis, striae, acneiform eruptions, perioral dermatitis, hypopigmentation, hypertrichosis, allergic contact dermatitis; *secondary infection, maceration, atrophy, striae, miliaria* (with occlusive dressings).
Systemic: *hypothalamic-pituitary-adrenal axis suppression,* Cushing's syndrome, hyperglycemia, glucosuria.

INTERACTIONS
None significant.

EFFECTS ON DIAGNOSTIC TESTS
None reported.

CONTRAINDICATIONS
Contraindicated in patients hypersensitive to the drug.

NURSING CONSIDERATIONS
● Gently wash skin before applying. To prevent skin damage, rub medication in gently, leaving a thin coat. Part hair and apply directly to lesion when treating

---

*Liquid contains alcohol.   **May contain tartrazine.   †Canada only.   ‡Australia only.   ◊ OTC.

hairy sites.
• Avoid application near eyes or mucous membranes. Do not use on face, armpits, groin, in ear canal, or under breasts unless specifically ordered.
• For patients with eczematous dermatitis whose skin may be irritated by adhesive material, hold dressing in place with gauze, elastic bandages, stockings, or stockinette.
• Change dressings as ordered. Discontinue drug and notify the doctor if skin infection, striae, or atrophy occurs.
• Notify the doctor and remove occlusive dressing if fever develops.
• If antifungal agents or antibiotics are used concomitantly, stop drug until infection is controlled, as ordered.
• Avoid using plastic pants or tight-fitting diapers on treated areas in young children. Children may absorb larger amounts of drug and be more prone to systemic toxicity.
• Systemic absorption likely with use of occlusive dressings, prolonged treatment, or extensive body-surface treatment. Watch for symptoms.
• Continue treatment for a few days after lesions clear, as ordered.

☑ **PATIENT TEACHING**
• Teach patient how to apply drug.
• If an occlusive dressing is ordered, advise patient not to leave it in place longer than 16 hours each day or use it on infected or exudative lesions.
• Tell patient to stop drug and report signs of systemic absorption, skin irritation or ulceration, hypersensitivity, or infection.

---

betamethasone dipropionate
Alphatrex, Diprolene, Diprolene AF, Diprosone, Maxivate, Psorion

betamethasone valerate
Betatrex, Beta-Val, Betnovate†‡, Valisone

Pregnancy Risk Category: C

HOW SUPPLIED
betamethasone dipropionate
Aerosol: 0.1%
Cream: 0.05%
Lotion: 0.05%
Ointment: 0.05%
betamethasone valerate
Cream: 0.01%, 0.1%
Lotion: 0.1%
Ointment: 0.1%

ACTION
Unknown. Diffuses across cell membranes to form complexes with specific cytoplasmic receptors. Exhibits anti-inflammatory, antipruritic, vasoconstrictive, and antiproliferative activity. Considered a group III (medium-potency) agent according to vasoconstrictive properties.

ONSET, PEAK, DURATION
Onset and duration unknown. Plasma levels are highest when applied to inflamed or damaged skin, eyelids, or scrotal area; lowest when applied to intact normal skin, palms of hands, or soles of feet.

INDICATIONS & DOSAGE
Inflammation associated with corticosteroid-responsive dermatoses—
Adults and children: clean area; apply cream, ointment, lotion, aerosol spray, or gel sparingly. Dipropionate products are given once or twice daily; valerate products are given once daily to q.i.d. Maximum dosage for Diprolene cream is 45 g/week and 50 ml/week for Diprolene lotion.

ADVERSE REACTIONS
Skin: burning, pruritus, irritation, dryness, erythema, folliculitis, striae, acneiform eruptions, perioral dermatitis, hypopigmentation, hypertrichosis, allergic contact dermatitis; *secondary infection, maceration, atrophy, striae, miliaria* (with occlusive dressings).

Reactions may be *common*, uncommon, *life-threatening*, or COMMON AND LIFE-THREATENING.

Systemic: *hypothalamic-pituitary-adrenal axis suppression,* Cushing's syndrome, hyperglycemia, and glucosuria (with betamethasone dipropionate).

INTERACTIONS
None significant.

EFFECTS ON DIAGNOSTIC TESTS
None reported.

CONTRAINDICATIONS
Contraindicated in patients hypersensitive to corticosteroids.

NURSING CONSIDERATIONS
• Gently wash skin before applying. To prevent skin damage, rub medication in gently, leaving a thin coat. When treating hairy sites, part hair and apply directly to lesions.
• Avoid application near eyes, mucous membranes, or in ear canal.
• Because of alcohol content of vehicle, gel preparations may cause mild, transient stinging, especially when used on or near excoriated skin.
• For patients with eczematous dermatitis whose skin may be irritated by adhesive material, hold dressing in place with gauze, elastic bandages, stockings, or stockinette.
• Change dressings as ordered. Discontinue drug and notify the doctor if infection, striae, or atrophy occurs.
• Notify the doctor and remove occlusive dressing if fever develops.
• If antifungal agents or antibiotics are used concomitantly, stop drug until infection is controlled, as ordered.
• Systemic absorption likely with use of prolonged or extensive body-surface treatment. Watch for symptoms.
• Avoid using plastic pants or tight-fitting diapers on treated areas in young children. Children may absorb larger amounts of drug and be more prone to systemic toxicity.

• Continue drug for a few days after lesions clear.
• Diprolene and Diprolene AF may not be substituted generically because other products have different potencies.

☑ **PATIENT TEACHING**
• Teach patient how to apply drug.
• If an occlusive dressing is ordered, advise patient not to leave it in place longer than 16 hours each day and not to use occlusive dressings on infected or exudative lesions.
• Tell patient to stop drug and report signs of systemic absorption, skin irritation or ulceration, hypersensitivity, or infection.

clobetasol propionate
Dermovate†, Temovate

Pregnancy Risk Category: C

HOW SUPPLIED
Cream: 0.05%
Lotion: 0.05%
Ointment: 0.05%

ACTION
Unknown. Diffuses across cell membranes to form complexes with specific cytoplasmic receptors. Exhibits anti-inflammatory, antipruritic, vasoconstrictive, and antiproliferative activity. Considered a group I (very high-potency) agent according to vasoconstrictive properties.

ONSET, PEAK, DURATION
Onset and duration unknown. Plasma levels are highest when applied to inflamed or damaged skin, eyelids, or scrotal area; lowest when applied to intact normal skin, palms of hands, or soles of feet.

INDICATIONS & DOSAGE
Inflammation associated with corticosteroid-responsive dermatoses—
Adults: apply a thin layer to affected

skin areas b.i.d., in the morning and evening for a maximum of 14 days. Total dosage should not exceed 50 g weekly.

ADVERSE REACTIONS
Skin: burning, pruritus, irritation, dryness, erythema, folliculitis, perioral dermatitis, allergic contact dermatitis, hypopigmentation, hypertrichosis, acneiform eruptions.
Systemic: *hypothalamic-pituitary-adrenal (HPA) axis suppression,* Cushing's syndrome, hyperglycemia, glucosuria.

INTERACTIONS
None significant.

EFFECTS ON DIAGNOSTIC TESTS
None significant.

CONTRAINDICATIONS
Contraindicated in patients hypersensitive to corticosteroids.

NURSING CONSIDERATIONS
● Gently wash skin before applying. To prevent skin damage, rub medication in gently, leaving a thin coat. When treating hairy sites, part hair and apply directly to lesions.
● Avoid application near eyes, mucous membranes, or in ear canal.
Alert: Don't use occlusive dressings or bandage, cover, or wrap treated areas.
● If antifungal agents or antibiotics are used concomitantly, stop drug until infection is controlled, as ordered.
● Know that repeated application can result in diminished effectiveness.
● Discontinue drug and notify the doctor if skin infection, striae, or atrophy occurs.
● Do not refrigerate.

☑ **PATIENT TEACHING**
● Teach patient how to apply drug.
● Tell patient to stop drug and report signs of systemic absorption, skin irritation or ulceration, hypersensitivity, or infection.
● Warn patient not to use for longer than 14 consecutive days.

---

clocortolone pivalate
Cloderm

Pregnancy Risk Category: C

HOW SUPPLIED
Cream: 0.1%

ACTION
Unknown. Diffuses across cell membranes to form complexes with specific cytoplasmic receptors. Exhibits anti-inflammatory, antipruritic, vasoconstrictive, and antiproliferative activity. Considered a group III (medium-potency) agent according to vasoconstrictive properties.

ONSET, PEAK, DURATION
Onset and duration unknown. Plasma levels are highest when applied to inflamed or damaged skin, eyelids, or scrotal area; lowest when applied to intact normal skin, palms of hands, or soles of feet.

INDICATIONS & DOSAGE
Inflammation associated with corticosteroid-responsive dermatoses—
Adults and children: apply cream sparingly to affected areas one to four times daily and rub in gently.

ADVERSE REACTIONS
Skin: burning, pruritus, irritation, dryness, erythema, folliculitis, striae, acneiform eruptions, perioral dermatitis, hypertrichosis, hypopigmentation, allergic contact dermatitis; *secondary infection, maceration, atrophy, striae, miliaria* (with occlusive dressings).
Systemic: *hypothalamic-pituitary-adrenal axis suppression,* Cushing's syndrome, hyperglycemia, glucosuria.

Reactions may be *common,* uncommon, *life-threatening,* or COMMON AND LIFE-THREATENING.

INTERACTIONS
None significant.

EFFECTS ON DIAGNOSTIC TESTS
None reported.

CONTRAINDICATIONS
Contraindicated in patients hypersensitive to the drug.

NURSING CONSIDERATIONS
● Gently wash skin before applying. To prevent skin damage, rub medication in gently, leaving a thin coat. When treating hairy sites, part hair and apply directly to lesions.
● Avoid application near eyes or mucous membranes.
● For patients with eczematous dermatitis whose skin may be irritated by adhesive material, hold dressing in place with gauze, elastic bandages, or stockinette.
● Change dressings as ordered. Stop drug and tell the doctor if skin infection, striae, or atrophy occurs.
● Notify the doctor and remove occlusive dressing if fever develops.
● If antifungal agents or antibiotics are used concomitantly, stop drug until infection is controlled, as ordered.
● Systemic adverse reactions. Systemic absorption likely with use of occlusive dressings, prolonged treatment, or extensive body-surface treatment. Watch for symptoms.
● Avoid using plastic pants or tight-fitting diapers on treated areas in young children. Children may absorb larger amounts of drug and be more prone to systemic toxicity.
● Continue drug for a few days after lesions clear, as ordered.

☑ **PATIENT TEACHING**
● Teach patient how to apply drug.
● If an occlusive dressing is ordered, advise patient not to leave it in place longer than 16 hours each day and not to use occlusive dressings on infected or exudative lesions.

● Tell patient to stop drug and report signs of systemic absorption, skin irritation or ulceration, hypersensitivity, or infection.

desonide
DesOwen, Tridesilon

Pregnancy Risk Category: C

HOW SUPPLIED
Cream: 0.05%
Ointment: 0.05%
Lotion: 0.05%

ACTION
Unknown. Diffuses across cell membranes to form complexes with specific cytoplasmic receptors. Exhibits anti-inflammatory, antipruritic, vasoconstrictive, and antiproliferative activity. Considered a group IV (low-potency) agent according to vasoconstrictive properties.

ONSET, PEAK, DURATION
Onset and duration unknown. Plasma levels are highest when applied to inflamed or damaged skin, eyelids, or scrotal area; lowest when applied to intact normal skin, palms of hands, or soles of feet.

INDICATIONS & DOSAGE
Inflammation associated with corticosteroid-responsive dermatoses—
Adults and children: clean area; apply sparingly b.i.d. to q.i.d.

ADVERSE REACTIONS
Skin: burning, pruritus, irritation, dryness, erythema, folliculitis, perioral dermatitis, allergic contact dermatitis, hypertrichosis, hypopigmentation, acneiform eruptions; *maceration of skin, secondary infection, atrophy, striae, miliaria* (with occlusive dressings).
Systemic: *hypothalamic-pituitary-adrenal axis suppression,* Cushing's syndrome, hyperglycemia, glucosuria.

INTERACTIONS
None significant.

EFFECTS ON DIAGNOSTIC TESTS
None reported.

CONTRAINDICATIONS
Contraindicated in patients hypersensitive to the drug.

NURSING CONSIDERATIONS
• Gently wash skin before applying. To prevent skin damage, rub medication in gently, leaving a thin coat. When treating hairy sites, part hair and apply directly to lesions.
• Avoid application near eyes, mucous membranes, or in ear canal.
• For patients with eczematous dermatitis whose skin may be irritated by adhesive material, hold dressing in place with gauze, elastic bandages, stockings, or stockinette.
• Change dressing as ordered. Stop drug and tell doctor if skin infection, striae, or atrophy occurs.
• Notify the doctor and remove occlusive dressing if fever develops.
• If antifungal agents or antibiotics are used concomitantly, stop drug until infection is controlled, as ordered.
• Systemic absorption likely with use of occlusive dressings, prolonged treatment, or extensive body-surface treatment. Watch for symptoms.
• Avoid using plastic pants or tight-fitting diapers on treated areas in young children. Children may absorb larger amounts of drug and be more prone to systemic toxicity.
• Continue treatment for a few days after lesions clear, as ordered.

☑ **PATIENT TEACHING**
• Teach patient how to apply drug.
• If an occlusive dressing is ordered, advise patient not to leave dressing in place longer than 16 hours each day and not to use occlusive dressings on infected or exudative lesions.
• Tell patient to stop drug and report

signs of systemic absorption, skin irritation or ulceration, hypersensitivity, or infection.

---

desoximetasone
Topicort

Pregnancy Risk Category: C

HOW SUPPLIED
Cream: 0.05%, 0.25%
Gel: 0.05%
Ointment: 0.25%

ACTION
Unknown. Diffuses across cell membranes to form complexes with specific cytoplasmic receptors. Exhibits anti-inflammatory, antipruritic, vasoconstrictive, and antiproliferative activity. Considered a group III (medium-potency) agent according to vasoconstrictive properties.

ONSET, PEAK, DURATION
Onset and duration unknown. Plasma levels are highest when applied to inflamed or damaged skin, eyelids, or scrotal area; lowest when applied to intact, normal skin, palms of hands, or soles of feet.

INDICATIONS & DOSAGE
Inflammation associated with corticosteroid-responsive dermatoses—
Adults and children: clean area; apply sparingly b.i.d.

ADVERSE REACTIONS
Skin: burning, pruritus, irritation, dryness, erythema, folliculitis, hypertrichosis, acneiform eruptions, perioral dermatitis, hypopigmentation, allergic contact dermatitis; *maceration, secondary infection, atrophy, striae, miliaria* (with occlusive dressings).
Systemic: *hypothalamic-pituitary-adrenal axis suppression,* Cushing's syndrome, hyperglycemia, glucosuria.

Reactions may be common, uncommon, *life-threatening*, or **COMMON AND LIFE-THREATENING**.

INTERACTIONS
None significant.

EFFECTS ON DIAGNOSTIC TESTS
None reported.

CONTRAINDICATIONS
Contraindicated in patients hypersensitive to the drug.

NURSING CONSIDERATIONS
● Gently wash skin before applying. To prevent skin damage, rub medication in gently, leaving a thin coat. When treating hairy sites, part hair and apply directly to lesions.
● Avoid application near eyes, mucous membranes, or in ear canal.
● For patients with eczematous dermatitis whose skin may be irritated by adhesive material, hold dressing in place with gauze, elastic bandages, stockings, or stockinette.
● Change dressing as ordered. Stop drug and tell doctor if skin infection, striae, or atrophy occurs.
● Notify the doctor and remove occlusive dressing if fever develops.
● If antifungal agents or antibiotics are used concomitantly, stop drug until infection is controlled, as ordered.
● Systemic absorption likely with use of occlusive dressings, prolonged treatment, or extensive body-surface treatment. Watch for symptoms.
● Avoid using plastic pants or tight-fitting diapers on treated areas in young children. Children may absorb larger amounts of drug and be more prone to systemic toxicity.
● Continue drug for a few days after lesions clear, as ordered.
● Gel contains alcohol and may cause burning or irritation in open lesions.
● Store in tightly sealed containers.

☑ **PATIENT TEACHING**
● Teach patient how to apply drug.
● If an occlusive dressing is ordered, advise patient not to leave dressing in place longer than 16 hours each day and not to use occlusive dressings on infected or exudative lesions.
● Tell patient to stop drug and report signs of systemic absorption, skin irritation or ulceration, hypersensitivity, or infection.

---

dexamethasone
Aeroseb-Dex, Decaderm, Decaspray

dexamethasone sodium phosphate
Decadron Phosphate

Pregnancy Risk Category: C

HOW SUPPLIED
dexamethasone
Aerosol: 0.01%, 0.04%
Gel: 0.1%
dexamethasone sodium phosphate
Cream: 0.1%

ACTION
Unknown. Diffuses across cell membranes to form complexes with specific cytoplasmic receptors. Exhibits anti-inflammatory, antipruritic, vasoconstrictive, and antiproliferative activity. Considered a group IV (low-potency) agent according to vasoconstrictive properties.

ONSET, PEAK, DURATION
Onset and duration unknown. Plasma levels are highest when applied to inflamed or damaged skin, eyelids, or scrotal area; lowest when applied to intact normal skin, palms of hands, or soles of feet.

INDICATIONS & DOSAGE
Inflammation associated with corticosteroid-responsive dermatoses—
Adults and children: clean area; apply cream, gel, or aerosol sparingly t.i.d. to q.i.d.
For aerosol use on scalp, shake can well but gently, and apply to dry scalp after shampooing. Hold can upright. Slide applicator tube under hair so that it

---

touches scalp. Spray while moving tube to all affected areas, keeping tube under hair and in contact with scalp throughout spraying, which should take about 2 seconds. Spot spray inadequately covered areas by sliding applicator tube through hair to touch scalp, then pressing and immediately releasing spray button. Don't massage medication into scalp or spray forehead or near eyes.

ADVERSE REACTIONS
Skin: burning, pruritus, irritation, dryness, erythema, folliculitis, hypertrichosis, acneiform eruptions, perioral dermatitis, hypopigmentation, allergic contact dermatitis; *maceration, secondary infection, atrophy, striae, miliaria* (with occlusive dressings).
Systemic: *hypothalamic-pituitary-adrenal axis suppression,* Cushing's syndrome, hyperglycemia, glucosuria.

INTERACTIONS
None significant.

EFFECTS ON DIAGNOSTIC TESTS
None reported.

CONTRAINDICATIONS
Contraindicated in patients hypersensitive to the drug.

NURSING CONSIDERATIONS
● Gently wash skin before applying. To prevent skin damage, rub medication in gently, leaving a thin coat. When treating hairy sites, part hair and apply directly to lesions.
● Avoid application near eyes, mucous membranes, or in ear canal.
● For patients with eczematous dermatitis whose skin may be irritated by adhesive material, hold dressing in place with gauze, elastic bandages, stockings, or stockinette.
● Change dressing as ordered. Stop drug and tell doctor if skin infection, striae, or atrophy occurs.
● Notify the doctor and remove occlusive dressing if fever develops.

● When using aerosol around the face, cover the patient's eyes and warn against inhalation of the spray. Aerosol preparation contains alcohol and may produce irritation or burning in open lesions. To avoid freezing tissues, do not spray longer than 1 to 2 seconds or closer than 6″ (15 cm).
● If antifungal agents or antibiotics are used concomitantly, stop drug until infection is controlled, as ordered.
● Systemic absorption likely with use of occlusive dressings, prolonged treatment, or extensive body-surface treatment. Watch for symptoms.
● Avoid using plastic pants or tight-fitting diapers on treated areas in young children. Children may absorb larger amounts of drug and be more prone to systemic toxicity.
● Continue treatment for a few days after lesions clear, as ordered.

☑ **PATIENT TEACHING**
● Teach patient how to apply drug.
● If an occlusive dressing is ordered, advise patient not to leave it in place longer than 16 hours each day and not to use occlusive dressings on infected or exudative lesions.
● Tell patient to stop drug and report signs of systemic absorption, skin irritation or ulceration, hypersensitivity, or infection.

---

diflorasone diacetate
Florone, Flutone, Maxiflor, Psorcon

Pregnancy Risk Category: C

HOW SUPPLIED
Cream: 0.05%
Ointment: 0.05%

ACTION
Unknown. Diffuses across cell membranes to form complexes with specific cytoplasmic receptors. Exhibits anti-inflammatory, antipruritic, vasoconstrictive, and antiproliferative activity. Con-

sidered a group II (high-potency) agent according to vasoconstrictive properties.

ONSET, PEAK, DURATION
Onset and duration unknown. Plasma levels are highest when applied to inflamed or damaged skin, eyelids, or scrotal area; lowest when applied to intact normal skin, palms of hands, or soles of feet.

INDICATIONS & DOSAGE
Inflammation associated with corticosteroid-responsive dermatoses—
Adults and children: clean area; apply sparingly in a thin film. Apply cream b.i.d. to q.i.d. and emoliant cream and ointment once daily to t.i.d.

ADVERSE REACTIONS
Skin: burning, pruritus, irritation, dryness, erythema, folliculitis, perioral dermatitis, hypertrichosis, hypopigmentation, acneiform eruptions; *maceration, secondary infection, atrophy, striae, miliaria* (with occlusive dressings).
Systemic: *hypothalamic-pituitary-adrenal axis suppression,* Cushing's syndrome, hyperglycemia, glucosuria.

INTERACTIONS
None significant.

EFFECTS ON DIAGNOSTIC TESTS
None reported.

CONTRAINDICATIONS
Contraindicated in patients hypersensitive to the drug.

NURSING CONSIDERATIONS
● Before applying, gently wash skin. To prevent skin damage, rub medication in gently, leaving a thin coat. When treating hairy sites, part hair and apply directly to lesions.
● Avoid application near eyes, mucous membranes, or in ear canal.
● For patients with eczematous dermatitis whose skin may be irritated by adhesive material, hold dressing in place

with gauze, elastic bandages, stockings, or stockinette.
● Change dressing as ordered. Stop drug and tell doctor if skin infection, striae, or atrophy occurs.
● Notify the doctor and remove occlusive dressing if fever develops.
● If antifungal agents or antibiotics are used concomitantly, stop drug until infection is controlled, as ordered.
● Systemic absorption likely with use of occlusive dressings, prolonged treatment, or extensive body-surface treatment. Watch for symptoms.
● Avoid using plastic pants or tight-fitting diapers on treated areas in young children. Children may absorb larger amounts of drug and be more prone to systemic toxicity.

☑ **PATIENT TEACHING**
● Teach patient how to apply drug.
● If an occlusive dressing is ordered, advise patient not to leave it in place longer than 16 hours each day and not to use occlusive dressings on infected or exudative lesions on in combination with Psorcon.
● Tell patient to stop drug and report signs of systemic absorption, skin irritation or ulceration, hypersensitivity, or infection.

---

fluocinolone acetonide
Fluocet, Fluonid, Flurosyn, Synalar, Synemol

Pregnancy Risk Category: C

HOW SUPPLIED
Cream: 0.01%, 0.025%, 0.2%
Ointment: 0.025%
Topical solution: 0.01%

ACTION
Unknown. Diffuses across cell membranes to form complexes with specific cytoplasmic receptors. Exhibits anti-inflammatory, antipruritic, vasoconstrictive, and antiproliferative activity. Con-

---

sidered a group III (medium-potency) agent according to vasoconstrictive properties.

ONSET, PEAK, DURATION
Onset and duration unknown. Plasma levels are highest when applied to inflamed or damaged skin, eyelids, or scrotal area; lowest when applied to intact normal skin, palms of hands, or soles of feet.

INDICATIONS & DOSAGE
Inflammation associated with corticosteroid-responsive dermatoses—
Adults and children: clean area; apply cream, ointment, or topical solution sparingly b.i.d. to q.i.d.

ADVERSE REACTIONS
Skin: burning, pruritus, irritation, dryness, erythema, folliculitis, hypertrichosis, hypopigmentation, acneiform eruptions, perioral dermatitis, allergic contact dermatitis; *maceration, secondary infection, atrophy, striae, miliaria* (with occlusive dressings).
Systemic: *hypothalamic-pituitary-adrenal axis suppression,* Cushing's syndrome, hyperglycemia, glucosuria.

INTERACTIONS
None significant.

EFFECTS ON DIAGNOSTIC TESTS
None significant.

CONTRAINDICATIONS
Contraindicated in patients hypersensitive to the drug.

NURSING CONSIDERATIONS
● Gently wash skin before applying. To prevent skin damage, rub medication in gently, leaving a thin coat. When treating hairy sites, part hair and apply directly to lesions.
● Avoid application near eyes, mucous membranes, or in ear canal.
● For patients with eczematous dermatitis whose skin may be irritated by adhesive material, hold dressing in place with gauze, elastic bandages, stockings, or stockinette.
● Change dressing as ordered. Stop drug and tell doctor if skin infection, striae, or atrophy occurs.
● Notify the doctor and remove occlusive dressing if fever develops.
● If antifungal agents or antibiotics are used concomitantly, stop drug until infection is controlled, as ordered.
● Systemic absorption likely with use of occlusive dressings, prolonged treatment, or extensive body-surface treatment. Watch for symptoms.
● In young children, avoid using plastic pants or tight-fitting diapers on treated areas. Children may absorb larger amounts of drug and be more prone to systemic toxicity.
● Fluonid solution on dry lesions may increase dryness, scaling, or pruritus; on denuded or fissured areas, may produce burning or stinging. If either of these persists and dermatitis has not improved, discontinue use of solution and notify doctor.

☑ PATIENT TEACHING
● Teach patient how to apply drug.
● If an occlusive dressing is ordered, advise patient not to leave it in place longer than 16 hours each day and not to use occlusive dressings on infected or exudative lesions.
● Tell patient to stop drug and report signs of systemic absorption, skin irritation or ulceration, hypersensitivity, or infection.

---

fluocinonide
Lidemol†, Lidex, Lidex-E, Topsyn

Pregnancy Risk Category: C

HOW SUPPLIED
Cream: 0.05%
Gel: 0.05%
Ointment: 0.05%
Topical solution: 0.05%

ACTION
Unknown. Diffuses across cell membranes to form complexes with specific cytoplasmic receptors. Exhibits anti-inflammatory, antipruritic, vasoconstrictive, and antiproliferative activity. Considered a group II (high-potency) agent according to vasoconstrictive properties.

ONSET, PEAK, DURATION
Onset and duration unknown. Plasma levels are highest when applied to inflamed or damaged skin, eyelids, or scrotal area; lowest when applied to intact, normal skin, palms of hands, or soles of feet.

INDICATIONS & DOSAGE
Inflammation associated with corticosteroid-responsive dermatoses—
Adults and children: clean area; apply cream, gel, ointment, or topical solution sparingly b.i.d. or q.i.d.

ADVERSE REACTIONS
Skin: burning, pruritus, irritation, dryness, erythema, folliculitis, hypertrichosis, hypopigmentation, acneiform eruptions, perioral dermatitis, allergic contact dermatitis; *maceration, secondary infection, atrophy, striae, miliaria* (with occlusive dressings).
Systemic: *hypothalamic-pituitary-adrenal axis suppression,* Cushing's syndrome, hyperglycemia, glucosuria.

INTERACTIONS
None significant.

EFFECTS ON DIAGNOSTIC TESTS
None reported.

CONTRAINDICATIONS
Contraindicated in patients hypersensitive to the drug.

NURSING CONSIDERATIONS
● Gently wash skin before applying. To prevent skin damage, rub medication in gently, leaving a thin coat. When treating hairy sites, part hair and apply directly to lesion.
● Avoid application near eyes, mucous membranes, or in ear canal.
● For patients with eczematous dermatitis whose skin may be irritated by adhesive material, hold dressing in place with gauze, elastic bandages, stockings, or stockinette.
● Change dressing as ordered. Stop drug and call doctor if skin infection, striae, or atrophy occurs.
● Notify the doctor and remove occlusive dressing if fever develops.
● If antifungal agents or antibiotics are used concomitantly, stop drug until infection is controlled, as ordered.
● Systemic absorption likely with use of occlusive dressings, prolonged treatment, or extensive body-surface treatment. Watch for symptoms.
● In young children, avoid using plastic pants or tight-fitting diapers on treated areas. Children may absorb larger amounts of drug and be more prone to systemic toxicity.
● Continue treatment for a few days after lesions clear, as ordered.

☑ **PATIENT TEACHING**
● Teach patient how to apply drug.
● If an occlusive dressing is ordered, advise patient not to leave it in place longer than 16 hours each day; don't use occlusive dressings on infected or exudative lesions.
● Tell patient to stop drug and report signs of systemic absorption, skin irritation or ulceration, hypersensitivity, or infection.

---

flurandrenolide
Cordran, Cordran SP, Cordran Tape, Drenison†, Drenison 1/4†, Drenison Tape†

Pregnancy Risk Category: C

HOW SUPPLIED
Cream: 0.025%, 0.05%
Lotion: 0.05%

Ointment: 0.025%, 0.05%
Tape: 4 mcg/cm^2

ACTION

Unknown. Diffuses across cell membranes to form complexes with specific cytoplasmic receptors. Exhibits anti-inflammatory, antipruritic, vasoconstrictive, and antiproliferative activity. Considered a group III (medium-potency) agent according to vasoconstrictive properties.

ONSET, PEAK, DURATION

Onset and duration unknown. Plasma levels are highest when applied to inflamed or damaged skin, eyelids, or scrotal area; lowest when applied to intact normal skin, palms of hands, or soles of feet.

INDICATIONS & DOSAGE

Inflammation associated with corticosteroid-responsive dermatoses—
Adults and children: clean area; apply cream, lotion, or ointment sparingly b.i.d. or t.i.d.

Apply Cordran tape q 12 to 24 hours. Before applying tape, clean skin carefully, removing scales, crust, and dried exudate. Let skin dry for 1 hour before applying new tape. Shave or clip hair to allow good contact with skin and comfortable removal. If tape ends loosen prematurely, trim off and replace with fresh tape.

ADVERSE REACTIONS

Skin: burning, pruritus, irritation, dryness, erythema, folliculitis, hypertrichosis, hypopigmentation, acneiform eruptions, allergic contact dermatitis; *maceration, secondary infection, atrophy, striae, miliaria* (with occlusive dressings); purpura, stripping of epidermis, furunculosis (with tape).
Systemic: *hypothalamic-pituitary-adrenal axis suppression,* Cushing's syndrome, hyperglycemia, glucosuria.

INTERACTIONS

None significant.

EFFECTS ON DIAGNOSTIC TESTS

None significant.

CONTRAINDICATIONS

Contraindicated in patients hypersensitive to the drug.

NURSING CONSIDERATIONS

● Gently wash skin before applying. To prevent skin damage, rub medication in gently, leaving a thin coat. When treating hairy sites, part hair and apply directly to lesions.
● Avoid application near eyes, mucous membranes, or in ear canal.
Alert: Know that tape not advised for exudative lesions or lesions in intertriginous areas. Replace tape every 12 hours or, if well tolerated and adherence is satisfactory, every 24 hours. Do not tear Cordran tape; cut it with scissors.
● For patients with eczematous dermatitis whose skin may be irritated by adhesive material, hold dressing in place with gauze, elastic bandages, stockings, or stockinette.
● Stop drug and tell doctor if skin infection, striae, or atrophy occurs.
● Notify the doctor and remove occlusive dressing if fever develops.
● If antifungal agents or antibiotics are used concomitantly, stop drug until infection is controlled, as ordered.
● Systemic absorption likely with use of occlusive dressings, prolonged treatment, or extensive body-surface treatment. Watch for symptoms.
● Avoid using plastic pants or tight-fitting diapers on treated areas in young children. Children may absorb larger amounts of drug and be more prone to systemic toxicity.
● Continue treatment for a few days after lesions clear, as ordered.

☑ PATIENT TEACHING

● Teach patient how to apply drug.
● If an occlusive dressing is ordered, ad-

vise patient not to leave it in place longer than 16 hours each day and not to use occlusive dressings on infected or exudative lesions.
● Tell patient to stop drug and report signs of systemic absorption, skin irritation or ulceration, hypersensitivity, or infection.

---

fluticasone propionate
Cutivate

Pregnancy Risk Category: C

HOW SUPPLIED
Cream: 0.05%
Ointment: 0.005%

ACTION
Exact mechanism unknown. Exhibits anti-inflammatory, antipruritic, and vasoconstrictive activity. Considered a medium-potency agent.

ONSET, PEAK, DURATION
Onset, peak and duration unknown.

INDICATIONS & DOSAGE
Inflammatory and pruritic manifestations associated with corticosteroid-responsive dermatoses—
Adults: apply sparingly to affected area b.i.d.; rub in gently and completely.

ADVERSE REACTIONS
CNS: light-headedness.
Skin: hives, burning, hypertrichosis, pruritus, irritation, erythema.
Systemic: *HPA axis suppression,* Cushing's syndrome, hyperglycemia, glucosuria.

INTERACTIONS
None significant.

EFFECTS ON DIAGNOSTIC TESTS
None significant.

CONTRAINDICATIONS
Contraindicated in patients hypersensi-
tive to the drug or its components and in patients with viral, fungal, herpetic, or tubercular skin lesions.

NURSING CONSIDERATIONS
● Do not mix drug with other bases or vehicles; this may affect potency.
● Safety in children has not been established.
● If adverse reactions occur, the doctor may order a less potent agent.
● One-time coverage of the adult body requires 12 to 26 g. Do not use more than 50 g weekly.
● Discontinue drug if local irritation or systemic infection, absorption, or hypersensitivity occurs, as ordered.
● Know that generally, absorption of corticosteroids is enhanced when applied to inflamed or damaged skin, eyelids, or scrotal area; lowest when applied to intact normal skin, palms of hands, or soles of feet.

☑ PATIENT TEACHING
● Teach the patient how to apply drug.
● Tell the patient to avoid prolonged use and contact with eyes. Warn him not to apply around eyes, genitals, or rectum; on face; and in skin creases.
● Tell him to notify the doctor if condition persists or worsens or if burning or irritation develops.

---

halcinonide
Halciderm, Halog

Pregnancy Risk Category: C

HOW SUPPLIED
Cream: 0.025%, 0.1%
Ointment: 0.1%
Topical solution: 0.1%

ACTION
Unknown. Diffuses across cell membranes to form complexes with cytoplasmic receptors. Exhibits anti-inflammatory, antipruritic, vasoconstrictive, antiproliferative activity. Considered

---

group II (high-potency) drug due to vasoconstrictive properties.

ONSET, PEAK, DURATION
Onset and duration unknown. Plasma levels are highest when applied to inflamed or damaged skin, eyelids, or scrotal area; lowest when applied to intact normal skin, palms of hands, or soles of feet.

INDICATIONS & DOSAGE
Inflammation associated with corticosteroid-responsive dermatoses—
Adults and children: clean area; apply cream, ointment, or topical solution sparingly b.i.d. or t.i.d.

ADVERSE REACTIONS
Skin: burning, pruritus, irritation, dryness, erythema, folliculitis, hypertrichosis, hypopigmentation, acneiform eruptions, allergic contact dermatitis; *maceration, secondary infection, atrophy, striae, miliaria* (with occlusive dressings).
Systemic: *hypothalamic-pituitary-adrenal axis suppression,* Cushing's syndrome, hyperglycemia, glucosuria.

INTERACTIONS
None significant.

EFFECTS ON DIAGNOSTIC TESTS
None reported.

CONTRAINDICATIONS
Contraindicated in patients hypersensitive to the drug.

NURSING CONSIDERATIONS
● Gently wash skin before applying. To prevent skin damage, rub medication in gently, leaving a thin coat. When treating hairy sites, part hair and apply directly to lesions.
● Avoid application near eyes, mucous membranes, or in ear canal.
● Gently rub small amount of cream into lesion until it disappears. Reapply, leaving a thin coating on lesion, and cover with occlusive dressing, if ordered. Apply ointment to lesion and cover with occlusive dressing, if ordered. Do not leave dressing in place longer than 16 hours each day.
● Don't use occlusive dressings on infected or exudative lesions.
● For patients with eczematous dermatitis whose skin may be irritated by adhesive material, hold dressing in place with gauze, elastic bandages, stockings, or stockinette.
● Change dressing as ordered. Stop drug and tell doctor if skin infection, striae, or atrophy occurs.
● Be aware that good results have been obtained by applying occlusive dressings in the evening and removing them in the morning, providing 12-hour occlusion. Drug should then be reapplied and no occlusive dressings applied during the day.
● Notify the doctor and remove occlusive dressing if fever develops.
● If antifungal agents or antibiotics are used concomitantly, stop drug until infection is controlled, as ordered.
● Systemic absorption especially likely with use of occlusive dressings, prolonged treatment, or extensive body-surface treatment. Watch for symptoms.
● Avoid using plastic pants or tight-fitting diapers on treated areas in young children. Children may absorb larger amounts of drug and be more prone to systemic toxicity.
● Continue treatment for a few days after lesions clear, as ordered.

☑ PATIENT TEACHING
● Teach patient how to apply drug.
● If an occlusive dressing is ordered, advise patient not to leave it in place longer than 16 hours each day and not to use occlusive dressings on infected or exudative lesions.
● Tell patient to stop drug and report signs of systemic absorption, skin irritation or ulceration, hypersensitivity, or infection.

halobetasol propionate
Ultravate

Pregnancy Risk Category: C

HOW SUPPLIED
Cream: 0.05%
Ointment: 0.05%

ACTION
Unknown. Diffuses across cell membranes to form complexes with specific cytoplasmic receptors. Exhibits anti-inflammatory, antipruritic, vasoconstrictive, and antiproliferative activity. Considered a group I (very high-potency) agent according to vasoconstrictive properties.

ONSET, PEAK, DURATION
Onset and duration unknown. Plasma levels are highest when applied to inflamed or damaged skin, eyelids, or scrotal area; lowest when applied to intact normal skin, palms of hands, or soles of feet.

INDICATIONS & DOSAGE
Inflammation associated with corticosteroid-responsive dermatoses—
Adults: apply cream or ointment sparingly to affected area once daily or b.i.d., and rub in gently and completely. Treatment beyond 2 consecutive weeks is not recommended. Total dosage should not exceed 50 g weekly.

ADVERSE REACTIONS
Skin: stinging, burning, pruritus, irritation, dryness, erythema, folliculitis, skin atrophy, leukoderma, vesicles, rash, hypertrichosis, acneiform eruptions, hypopigmentation, perioral dermatitis, allergic contact dermatitis, secondary infection, striae, miliaria.
Systemic: *hypothalamic-pituitary-adrenal (HPA) axis suppression,* Cushing's syndrome, hyperglycemia, glucosuria, fluid retention.

INTERACTIONS
None significant.

EFFECTS ON DIAGNOSTIC TESTS
None significant.

CONTRAINDICATIONS
Contraindicated in patients hypersensitive to the drug or any of its components.

NURSING CONSIDERATIONS
Alert: Do not use occlusive dressings with this drug.
● Avoid use on face, groin, or axilla.
● Be alert that some systemic absorption usually occurs and may cause HPA axis suppression, Cushing's syndrome, hyperglycemia, and glucosuria, which are reversible after discontinuation of therapy.
● Corticotropin stimulation, morning plasma cortisol, and urinary cortisol tests are useful in determining the extent of HPA axis suppression.
● If HPA axis suppression occurs, discontinue drug, reduce frequency of application, or substitute a less potent corticosteroid, as prescribed.
● Discontinue if infection occurs and notify the doctor.

☑ PATIENT TEACHING
● Teach the patient how to apply drug.
● Tell the patient that drug is for external use only, as directed by the doctor. Tell him to avoid contact with eyes and not to cover, bandage, or wrap treated area unless directed by the doctor. Tell the patient not to use more often or for any condition other than prescribed.
● Tell the patient to report any signs of stinging, burning, or irritation.

hydrocortisone
Acticort, Aeroseb-HC, Bactine HC ◇, CaldeCort, Carmol HC, Cetacort, Cort-Dome, Cortef ◇, Cortenema, Cortinal, Cortizone 5 ◇, Cortril, Cremesone, Delacort, DermaCort ◇,

Dermolate◊, Dermtex HC, Durel-Cort, Ecosone, HC Cream, HI-Cor-2.5, Hycortole, Hydrocortex, Hydro-Tex, Hytone, Ivocort, Maso-Cort, Microcort, Nutracort, Orabase HCA, Penecort, Proctocort, Rhus Tox HC, Rocort, Squibb-HC‡, Synacort, T/Scalp, Unicort

hydrocortisone acetate
CortaGel, Cortaid◊, Cortamed†, Cortef, Corticaine, Corticreme†, Cortifoam, Dermacort‡, Dermacort Ointment‡, Epifoam, Gynecort, Hydrocortisone Acetate, Lanacort, MyCort Lotion, Proctofoam-HC

hydrocortisone butyrate
Locoid

hydrocortisone valerate
Westcort Cream

Pregnancy Risk Category: C

HOW SUPPLIED
hydrocortisone
Aerosol: 0.5%
Cream: 0.25%◊, 0.5%◊, 1%◊, 2.5%
Gel: 0.5%, 1%
Lotion: 0.125%, 0.25%, 0.5%◊, 1%, 2%, 2.5%
Ointment: 0.5%◊, 1%◊, 2.5%
Pledgets: 0.5%, 1%
Rectal cream: 1%◊
Topical solution: 0.5%, 1%, 2.5%
hydrocortisone acetate
Cream: 0.5%◊
Lotion: 0.5%◊
Ointment: 0.5%◊, 1%
Paste: 0.5%
Solution: 1%
Rectal foam: 90 mg per application
hydrocortisone butyrate
Cream: 0.1%
Ointment: 0.1%
Solution: 0.1%
hydrocortisone valerate
Cream: 0.2%
Ointment: 0.2%

ACTION
Unknown. Diffuses across cell membranes to form complexes with specific cytoplasmic receptors. Exhibits anti-inflammatory, antipruritic, vasoconstrictive, and antiproliferative activity. Considered a group IV (low-potency) agent according to vasoconstrictive properties.

ONSET, PEAK, DURATION
Onset and duration unknown. Plasma levels are highest when applied to inflamed or damaged skin, eyelids, or scrotal area; lowest when applied to intact normal skin, palms of hands, or soles of feet.

INDICATIONS & DOSAGE
Inflammation associated with corticosteroid-responsive dermatoses; adjunctive topical management of seborrheic dermatitis of scalp—
Adults and children: clean area; apply cream, gel, lotion, ointment, or topical solution sparingly daily to q.i.d. Spray aerosol onto affected area daily to q.i.d. until acute phase is controlled; then reduce dosage to one to three times weekly as needed.
Inflammation associated with proctitis—
Adults: 1 applicatorful of rectal foam P.R. daily or b.i.d. for 2 to 3 weeks, then every other day as necessary.

ADVERSE REACTIONS
Skin: burning, pruritus, irritation, dryness, erythema, folliculitis, hypertrichosis, hypopigmentation, acneiform eruptions, allergic contact dermatitis; *maceration, secondary infection, atrophy, striae, miliaria* (with occlusive dressings).
Systemic: *hypothalamic-pituitary-adrenal axis suppression,* Cushing's syndrome, hyperglycemia, glucosuria.

INTERACTIONS
None significant.

EFFECTS ON DIAGNOSTIC TESTS
None reported.

CONTRAINDICATIONS
Contraindicated in patients hypersensitive to the drug.

NURSING CONSIDERATIONS
• Gently wash skin before applying. To prevent skin damage, rub medication in gently, leaving a thin coat. When treating hairy sites, part hair and apply directly to lesions.

• Avoid application near eyes, mucous membranes, or in ear canal; may be safely used on face, groin, armpits, and under breasts.

• For patients with eczematous dermatitis whose skin may be irritated by adhesive material, hold dressing in place with gauze, elastic bandages, stockings, or stockinette.

• Notify the doctor, and remove occlusive dressing if fever develops.

• Change dressing as ordered. Stop drug and tell doctor if skin infection, striae, or atrophy occurs.

• When using aerosol around the face, cover the patient's eyes and warn against inhalation of the spray. Aerosol preparation contains alcohol and may produce irritation or burning in open lesions. Do not spray longer than 3 seconds or closer than 6″ (15 cm) to avoid freezing tissues. Apply to dry scalp after shampooing; no need to massage medication into scalp after spraying.

• If antifungal agents or antibiotics are used concomitantly, stop drug until infection is controlled, as ordered.

• Systemic absorption likely with use of occlusive dressings, prolonged treatment, or extensive body-surface treatment. Watch for symptoms.

• Avoid using plastic pants or tight-fitting diapers on treated areas in young children. Children may absorb larger amounts of drug and be more prone to systemic toxicity.

• Continue treatment for a few days after lesions clear, as ordered.

☑ PATIENT TEACHING
• Teach patient how to apply drug.

• If an occlusive dressing is ordered, advise patient not to leave it in place longer than 16 hours each day and not to use occlusive dressings on infected or exudative lesions.

• Tell patient to stop drug and report signs of systemic absorption, skin irritation or ulceration, hypersensitivity, or infection.

---

mometasone furoate
Elocon

Pregnancy Risk Category: C

HOW SUPPLIED
Cream: 0.1%
Ointment: 0.1%
Lotion: 0.1%

ACTION
Unknown. Diffuses across cell membranes to form complexes with specific cytoplasmic receptors. Exhibits anti-inflammatory, antipruritic, vasoconstrictive, and antiproliferative activity. Considered a group III (medium-potency) agent according to vasoconstrictive properties.

ONSET, PEAK, DURATION
Onset and duration unknown. Plasma levels are highest when applied to inflamed or damaged skin, eyelids, or scrotal area; lowest when applied to intact normal skin, palms of hands, or soles of feet.

INDICATIONS & DOSAGE
Inflammation associated with corticosteroid-responsive dermatoses—
Adults: apply to affected areas once daily.

ADVERSE REACTIONS
Skin: burning, erythema, pruritus, atrophy, irritation, acneiform eruptions, hypopigmentation, allergic contact der-

---

matitis.
Systemic: *hypothalamic-pituitary-adrenal axis suppression,* Cushing's syndrome, hyperglycemia, glucosuria.

INTERACTIONS
None significant.

EFFECTS ON DIAGNOSTIC TESTS
No information available.

CONTRAINDICATIONS
Contraindicated in patients hypersensitive to the drug or to other corticosteroids.

NURSING CONSIDERATIONS
• Use cautiously in young children.
• Gently wash skin before applying. To prevent skin damage, rub medication in gently, leaving a thin coat. When treating hairy sites, part hair and apply directly to lesions.
• Don't apply near eyes, mucous membranes, or in ear canal.
Alert: Do not use occlusive dressings with this drug.
• If antimicrobial agents are used concomitantly, stop drug until infection is controlled, as ordered.
• Systemic absorption likely with use of occlusive dressings, prolonged treatment, or extensive body-surface treatment. Watch for symptoms.
• Children may absorb larger amounts of drug and be more prone to systemic toxicity. Avoid using plastic pants or tight-fitting diapers on treated areas in young children.

☑ **PATIENT TEACHING**
• Teach patient how to apply drug.
• Tell patient to stop drug and report signs of systemic absorption, skin irritation or ulceration, hypersensitivity, or infection.

triamcinolone acetonide
Aristocort, Flutex, Kenalog, Kenalone‡, Triacet

Pregnancy Risk Category: C

HOW SUPPLIED
Aerosol: 0.2 mg/2-second spray
Cream: 0.02%‡, 0.025%, 0.1%, 0.5%
Lotion: 0.025%, 0.1%
Ointment: 0.02%‡, 0.025%, 0.1%, 0.5%
Paste: 0.1%
Solution: 0.1%

ACTION
Unknown. Diffuses across cell membranes to form complexes with specific cytoplasmic receptors. Exhibits anti-inflammatory, antipruritic, vasoconstrictive, and antiproliferative activity. Considered a group III (medium-potency) agent according to vasoconstrictive properties.

ONSET, PEAK, DURATION
Onset and duration unknown. Plasma levels are highest when applied to inflamed or damaged skin, eyelids, or scrotal area; low levels result when applied to intact, normal skin, palms of hands, or soles of feet.

INDICATIONS & DOSAGE
Inflammation associated with corticosteroid-responsive dermatoses—
Adults and children: clean area; apply aerosol, cream, lotion, or ointment sparingly b.i.d. to q.i.d.
Inflammation associated with oral lesions—
Adults and children: apply paste h.s. and, if needed, two or three times daily, preferably after meals. Apply a small amount without rubbing, and press to lesion in mouth until a thin film develops.

ADVERSE REACTIONS
Skin: burning, pruritus, irritation, dryness, erythema, folliculitis, hypertrichosis, hypopigmentation, acneiform

eruptions, perioral dermatitis, allergic contact dermatitis; *maceration, secondary infection, atrophy, striae, miliaria* (with occlusive dressings).
Systemic: *hypothalamic-pituitary-adrenal axis suppression,* Cushing's syndrome, hyperglycemia, glucosuria.

INTERACTIONS
None significant.

EFFECTS ON DIAGNOSTIC TESTS
None reported.

CONTRAINDICATIONS
Contraindicated in patients hypersensitive to the drug.

NURSING CONSIDERATIONS
● Gently wash skin before applying. To avoid skin damage, rub medication in gently, leaving a thin coat. When treating hairy sites, part hair and apply directly to lesions.
● Don't apply near eyes or in ear canal.
● Change dressing as ordered. Stop drug and tell doctor if skin infection, striae, or atrophy occurs.
● When using aerosol about the face, cover the patient's eyes and warn against inhalation of the spray. Aerosol preparation contains alcohol and may produce irritation or burning in open lesions. Do not spray longer than 3 seconds or closer than 6″ (15 cm) to avoid freezing tissues.
● If antifungal agents or antibiotics are used concomitantly, stop corticosteroids until infection is controlled, as ordered.
● Systemic absorption likely with use of occlusive dressings, prolonged treatment, or extensive body-surface treatment. Watch for symptoms.
● Avoid using plastic pants or tight-fitting diapers on treated areas in young children. Children may absorb larger amounts of drug and be more prone to systemic toxicity.

☑ **PATIENT TEACHING**
● Instruct patient how to apply drug.

● If an occlusive dressing is ordered, advise patient not to leave it in place longer than 16 hours each day; and not to use occlusive dressings on infected or exudative lesions.
● Tell patient to stop drug and report signs of systemic absorption, skin irritation or ulceration, hypersensitivity, or infection.

90

Vitamins and minerals

vitamin A
vitamin B complex
  cyanocobalamin
  hydroxocobalamin
  folic acid
  leucovorin calcium
  niacin
  niacinamide
  pyridoxine hydrochloride
  riboflavin
  thiamine hydrochloride
vitamin C
vitamin D
  cholecalciferol
  ergocalciferol
vitamin E
vitamin K analogue
  phytonadione
sodium fluoride
sodium fluoride, topical
trace elements
  chromium
  copper
  iodine
  manganese
  selenium
  zinc

TRACE ELEMENT COMBINATION PRODUCTS

M.T.E.-4: zinc sulfate 1 mg, copper sulfate 0.4 mg, manganese sulfate 0.1 mg, and chromium chloride 4 mcg per ml.

M.T.E.-4 CONCENTRATED: zinc sulfate 5 mg, copper sulfate 1 mg, manganese sulfate 0.5 mg, and chromium chloride 10 mcg per ml.

M.T.E.-5: zinc sulfate 1 mg, copper sulfate 0.4 mg, manganese sulfate 0.1 mg, chromium chloride 4 mcg, and selenium (as selenious acid) 20 mcg per ml.

M.T.E.-5 CONCENTRATED: zinc sulfate 5 mg, copper sulfate 1 mg, manganese sulfate 0.5 mg, chromium chloride 10 mcg, and selenium (as selenious acid) 60 mcg per ml.

M.T.E.-6: zinc sulfate 1 mg, copper sulfate 0.4 mg, manganese sulfate 0.1 mg, chromium chloride 4 mcg, selenium (as selenious acid) 20 mcg, and sodium iodide 25 mcg per ml.

M.T.E.-6 CONCENTRATED: zinc sulfate 5 mg, copper sulfate 1 mg, manganese sulfate 0.5 mg, chromium chloride 10 mcg, selenium (as selenious acid) 60 mcg, and sodium iodide 75 mcg per ml.

M.T.E.-7: zinc sulfate 1 mg, copper sulfate 0.4 mg, manganese sulfate 0.1 mg, chromium chloride 4 mcg, selenium (as selenious acid) 20 mcg, and sodium iodide 25 mcg per ml.

MULTIPLE TRACE ELEMENT CONCENTRATED: zinc sulfate 5 mg, copper sulfate 1 mg, manganese sulfate 0.5 mg, and chromium chloride 10 mcg per ml.

MULTIPLE TRACE ELEMENT NEONATAL: zinc sulfate 0.5 mg, copper sulfate 0.1 mg, manganese sulfate 0.025 mg, chromium chloride 0.85 mcg.

MULTIPLE TRACE ELEMENT WITH SELENIUM: zinc sulfate 1 mg, copper sulfate 0.4 mg, manganese sulfate 0.1 mg, chromium chloride 4 mcg, and selenious acid 20 mcg.

MULTITRACE 5 CONCENTRATE: zinc chloride 5 mg, copper chloride 1 mg, manganese chloride 0.5 mg, chromium chloride 10 mcg per ml, and selenious acid 60 mcg.

NEOTRACE-4: zinc sulfate 1.5 mg, copper sulfate 0.1 mg, manganese sulfate 0.025 mg, and chromium chloride 0.85 mcg per ml.

PEDIATRIC MULTIPLE TRACE ELEMENT: zinc sulfate 0.5 mg, copper sulfate 0.1 mg, manganese sulfate 0.03 mg, and chromium chloride 1 mcg per ml.

PEDTRACE-4: zinc sulfate 0.5 mg, copper sulfate 0.1 mg, manganese sulfate 0.025 mg, and chromium chloride 0.85 mcg per ml.

P.T.E.-4: zinc sulfate 1 mg, copper sul-

Reactions may be *common*, uncommon, *life-threatening*, or COMMON AND LIFE-THREATENING.

fate 0.1 mg, manganese sulfate 0.025 mg, and chromium chloride 1 mcg per ml.

P.T.E.-5: zinc sulfate 1 mg, copper sulfate 0.1 mg, manganese sulfate 0.025 mg, chromium chloride 1 mcg, and selenium (as selenious acid) 15 mcg per ml. TRACE METALS ADDITIVE: zinc chloride 0.8 mg, copper chloride 0.2 mg, manganese chloride 0.16 mg, and chromium chloride 2 mcg per ml.

VITAMIN COMBINATION PRODUCTS
B complex vitamins ◇
B complex vitamins with iron ◇
B complex with vitamin C ◇
B vitamin combinations ◇
Calcium and vitamin products ◇
Fluoride with vitamins ◇
Geriatric supplements with multivitamins and minerals ◇
Miscellaneous vitamins and minerals ◇
Multivitamins ◇
Multivitamins and minerals with hormones ◇
Multivitamins with B_{12} ◇
Vitamin A and D combinations ◇

---

vitamin A (retinol)
Acon, Aquasol A, Del-Vi-A

Pregnancy Risk Category: C

HOW SUPPLIED
Tablets: 10,000 IU
Capsules: 10,000 IU ◇ , 25,000 IU, 50,000 IU
Drops: 30 ml with dropper (50,000 IU/ 0.1 ml)
Injection: 2-ml vials (50,000 IU/ml with 0.5% chlorobutanol, polysorbate 80, butylated hydroxyanisol, and butylated hydroxytoluene)

ACTION
Coenzyme that stimulates retinal function, bone growth, reproduction, and integrity of epithelial and mucosal tissues.

ONSET, PEAK, DURATION
Onset and duration unknown. Peak levels occur in 3 to 5 hours.

INDICATIONS & DOSAGE
Recommended daily allowance (RDA)—
Note: RDAs have been converted to retinol equivalents (RE). One RE has the activity of 1 mcg all-*trans* retinol, 6 mcg beta carotene.
Neonates and infants to 1 year: 375 mcg RE or 1,250 IU.
Children 1 to 3 years: 400 mcg RE or 1,330 IU.
Children 4 to 6 years: 500 mcg RE or 1,665 IU.
Children 7 to 10 years: 700 mcg RE or 2,330 IU.
Males over 11 years: 1,000 mcg RE or 3,330 IU.
Females over 11 years: 800 mcg RE or 2,665 IU.
Pregnant women: 800 mcg RE or 2,665 IU.
Breast-feeding women (first 6 months): 1,300 mcg RE or 4,330 IU.
Breast-feeding women (second 6 months): 1,200 mcg RE or 4,000 IU.
Severe vitamin A deficiency—
Adults and children over 8 years: 100,000 IU I.M. or 100,000 to 500,000 IU P.O. for 3 days, followed by 50,000 IU I.M. or P.O. for 2 weeks; then 10,000 to 20,000 IU P.O. for 2 months. Follow with adequate dietary nutrition and RDA vitamin A supplements.
Infants under 1 year: 7,500 to 15,000 IU I.M. daily for 10 days.
Children 1 to 8 years: 17,500 to 35,000 IU I.M. daily for 10 days.
Maintenance dosage to prevent recurrence of vitamin A deficiency—
Children 1 to 8 years: 5,000 to 10,000 IU P.O. daily for 2 months, then adequate dietary nutrition and RDA vitamin A supplements.

ADVERSE REACTIONS
Adverse reactions usually occur only with toxicity.
CNS: irritability, headache, *increased*

---

intracranial pressure, fatigue, lethargy, malaise.

EENT: papilledema, exophthalmos.

GI: anorexia, epigastric pain, vomiting, polydipsia.

GU: hypomenorrhea, polyuria.

Hepatic: jaundice, hepatomegaly, *cirrhosis,* elevated liver enzymes.

Skeletal: slow growth, decalcification, hypercalcemia, periostitis, premature closure of epiphyses, migratory arthralgia, cortical thickening over the radius and tibia.

Skin: alopecia; dry, cracked, scaly skin; pruritus; lip fissures; erythema; inflamed tongue, lips, and gums; massive desquamation; increased pigmentation; night sweats.

Other: splenomegaly, *anaphylactic shock.*

INTERACTIONS

Cholestyramine resin, mineral oil: reduced GI absorption of fat-soluble vitamins.

Isotretinoin, multivitamins containing vitamin A: increased risk of toxicity. Avoid concomitant use.

Oral contraceptives: may increase plasma vitamin A levels.

Warfarin: increased risk of bleeding. Monitor PT closely.

EFFECTS ON DIAGNOSTIC TESTS

Vitamin A therapy may falsely increase serum cholesterol level readings by interfering with the Zlatkis-Zak reaction. Vitamin A also has been reported to falsely elevate bilirubin determinations.

CONTRAINDICATIONS

Contraindicated orally in patients with malabsorption syndrome; if malabsorption is from inadequate bile secretion, oral route may be used with concurrent administration of bile salts (dehydrocholic acid). Also contraindicated in hypervitaminosis A and hypersensitivity to any ingredient in product. I.V. route contraindicated except for special water-miscible forms intended for infusion with large parenteral volumes. I.V. push of vitamin A of any type also contraindicated (anaphylaxis or anaphylactoid reactions and death have resulted).

NURSING CONSIDERATIONS

● Use cautiously in pregnant patients, avoiding doses exceeding RDA.

● Assess the patient's vitamin A intake from all sources.

● Liquid preparations available for nasogastric route. Preparation may be mixed with cereal or fruit juice.

● Know that adequate vitamin A absorption requires suitable protein, vitamin E, and zinc intake and bile secretion; give supplemental salts as ordered. Zinc supplements may be needed in patients receiving long-term total parenteral nutrition.

● Monitor for adverse reactions if dosage is high.

● Acute toxicity has resulted from single doses of 25,000 IU/kg of body weight; 350,000 IU in infants and over 2 million IU in adults have also proved acutely toxic. Doses that do not exceed the RDA are usually nontoxic.

● Chronic toxicity in infants (3 to 6 months) has resulted from doses of 18,500 IU daily for 1 to 3 months. In adults, chronic toxicity has resulted from doses of 50,000 IU daily for over 18 months, 500,000 IU daily for 2 months, and 1 million IU daily for 3 days.

● Watch for skin disorders; high dosages may induce chronic toxicity.

☑ PATIENT TEACHING

● To avoid toxicity, tell patient not to take megadoses of vitamins without specific indications.

● Stress that patient should not share prescribed vitamins with others.

● Tell patient to protect drug from light.

---

cyanocobalamin (vitamin B$_{12}$)
Anacobin†, Bedoz†, Bioglan B$_{12}$Plus‡, Crystamine, Crysti-12,

Cyanabin†, Cyanocobalamin, Cyano-ject, Cyomin, Rubesol-1000, Rubion†, Rubramin

hydroxocobalamin (vitamin B₁₂)
Codroxomin, Hydrobexan, Hydro-Cobex, Hydro-Crysti-12, LA-12

Pregnancy Risk Category: NR

HOW SUPPLIED
cyanocobalamin
Tablets: 25 mcg ◇, 50 mcg ◇, 100 mcg ◇, 250 mcg ◇, 500 mcg ◇, 1,000 mcg ◇
Injection: 1,000 mcg/ml
hydroxocobalamin
Injection: 1,000 mcg/ml

ACTION
Coenzyme that stimulates metabolic functions. Necessary for cell replication, hematopoiesis, and nucleoprotein and myelin synthesis.

ONSET, PEAK, DURATION
Onset and duration unknown. Time to peak plasma levels after oral administration is 8 to 12 hours; after I.M. administration, 1 hour.

INDICATIONS & DOSAGE
Recommended daily allowance (RDA) for cyanocobalamin—
Neonates and infants to 6 months: 0.3 mcg.
Infants 6 months to 1 year: 0.5 mcg.
Children 1 to 3 years: 0.7 mcg.
Children 4 to 6 years: 1 mcg.
Children 7 to 10 years: 1.4 mcg.
Adults and children 11 years and over: 2 mcg.
Pregnant women: 2.2 mcg.
Breast-feeding women: 2.6 mcg.
Vitamin B₁₂ deficiency caused by inadequate diet, subtotal gastrectomy, or any other condition, disorder, or disease except malabsorption related to pernicious anemia or other GI disease—
Adults: 30 mcg hydroxocobalamin I.M.

daily for 5 to 10 days, depending on severity of deficiency. Maintenance dosage is 100 to 200 mcg I.M. once monthly. For subsequent prophylaxis, advise adequate nutrition and daily RDA vitamin B₁₂ supplements.
Children: 1 to 5 mg hydroxocobalamin spread over 2 or more weeks in doses of 100 mcg I.M., depending on severity of deficiency. Maintenance dosage is 30 to 50 mcg/month I.M. For subsequent prophylaxis, advise adequate nutrition and daily RDA vitamin B₁₂ supplements.
Pernicious anemia or vitamin B₁₂ malabsorption—
Adults: initially, 100 mcg cyanocobalamin I.M. or S.C. daily for 6 to 7 days, then 100 mcg I.M. or S.C. once monthly.
Children: 30 to 50 mcg I.M. or S.C. daily over 2 or more weeks; then 100 mcg I.M. or S.C. monthly for life.
Methylmalonic aciduria—
Neonates: 1,000 mcg cyanocobalamin I.M. daily.
Schilling test flushing dose—
Adults and children: 1,000 mcg hydroxocobalamin I.M. in a single dose.

ADVERSE REACTIONS
CV: peripheral vascular thrombosis, pulmonary edema, CHF.
GI: transient diarrhea.
Skin: itching, transitory exanthema, urticaria.
Other: *anaphylaxis, anaphylactoid reactions* (with parenteral administration), pain or burning at S.C. or I.M. injection sites.

INTERACTIONS
Aminoglycosides, chloramphenicol, colchicine, alcohol, para-aminosalicylic acid and salts: malabsorption of vitamin B₁₂. Don't use concomitantly.

EFFECTS ON DIAGNOSTIC TESTS
Vitamin B₁₂ therapy may cause false-positive results for intrinsic factor antibodies, which are present in the blood of half of all patients with pernicious

anemia. Methotrexate, pyrimethamine, and most anti-infectives invalidate diagnostic blood assays for vitamin B_{12}.

CONTRAINDICATIONS
Contraindicated in patients hypersensitive to vitamin B_{12} or cobalt and in patients with early Leber's disease.

NURSING CONSIDERATIONS
● Use cautiously in anemic patients with coexisting cardiac, pulmonary, or hypertensive disease; and in patients with severe vitamin B_{12}–dependent deficiencies.
● Use cautiously in premature infants. May contain benzyl alcohol, which may cause a "gasping syndrome."
● Determine reticulocyte count, hematocrit, B_{12}, iron, and folate levels before beginning therapy, as ordered.
● Don't mix parenteral liquids in same syringe with other medications.
● Drug is physically incompatible with dextrose solutions, alkaline or strongly acidic solutions, oxidizing or reducing agents, heavy metals, chlorpromazine, phytonadione, prochlorperazine, and many other drugs.
● Hydroxocobalamin is approved for I.M. use only. Its only advantage over cyanocobalamin is its longer duration.
● Don't give large oral doses of B_{12} routinely; drug is lost through excretion.
● Closely monitor serum potassium levels for first 48 hours. Give potassium supplement if ordered.
● Be aware that drug may cause false-positive intrinsic factor antibody test.
● Infection, tumors, or renal, hepatic, and other debilitating diseases may reduce therapeutic response.
● Keep in mind that deficiencies are more common in strict vegetarians and their breast-fed infants.
● Be aware B_{12} deficiency may suppress symptoms of polycythemia vera.
● Protect vitamin B_{12} from light. Do not refrigerate or freeze.

☑ PATIENT TEACHING
● Stress need for patient with pernicious anemia to return for monthly injections. Although total body stores may last 3 to 6 years, anemia will recur if not treated monthly.
● Stress importance of follow-up visits and laboratory studies.

---

folic acid (vitamin B₉)
Folvite, Novofolacid†

Pregnancy Risk Category: NR

HOW SUPPLIED
Tablets: 0.4 mg, 0.8 mg, 1 mg
Injection: 10-ml vials (5 mg/ml with 1.5% benzyl alcohol or 10 mg/ml with 1.5% benzyl alcohol and 0.2% EDTA)

ACTION
Stimulates normal erythropoiesis and nucleoprotein synthesis.

ONSET, PEAK, DURATION
Onset and duration unknown. Serum levels peak in 30 to 60 minutes.

INDICATIONS & DOSAGE
Recommended daily allowance (RDA)—
Neonates and infants to 6 months: 25 mcg.
Infants 6 months to 1 year: 35 mcg.
Children 1 to 3 years: 50 mcg.
Children 4 to 6 years: 75 mcg.
Children 7 to 10 years: 100 mcg.
Children 11 to 14 years: 150 mcg.
Males 15 years and over: 200 mcg.
Females 15 years and over: 180 mcg.
Pregnant women: 400 mcg.
Breast-feeding women (first 6 months): 280 mcg.
Breast-feeding women (second 6 months): 260 mcg.
Megaloblastic or macrocytic anemia secondary to folic acid or other nutritional deficiency, hepatic disease, alcoholism, intestinal obstruction, excessive hemolysis—
Adults and children over 4 years: 0.4

mg to 1 mg P.O., S.C., or I.M. daily. After anemia secondary to folic acid deficiency is corrected, proper diet and RDA supplements are necessary to prevent recurrence.

Children under 4 years: up to 0.3 mg P.O., S.C., or I.M. daily.

Pregnant and breast-feeding women: 0.8 mg P.O., S.C., or I.M. daily.

Prevention of megaloblastic anemia during pregnancy to prevent fetal damage—

Adults: up to 1 mg P.O., S.C., or I.M. daily throughout pregnancy.

Nutritional supplement—

Adults: 0.1 mg P.O., S.C., or I.M. daily.

Children: 0.05 mg P.O. daily.

To test for folic acid deficiency in patients with megaloblastic anemia without masking pernicious anemia—

Adults and children: 0.1 to 0.2 mg P.O. or I.M. for 10 days while maintaining a diet low in folate and vitamin B_{12}.

Tropical sprue—

Adults: 3 to 15 mg P.O. daily.

ADVERSE REACTIONS

Respiratory: *bronchospasm.*

Skin: allergic reactions (rash, pruritus, erythema).

Other: general malaise.

INTERACTIONS

Aminosalicylic acid, chloramphenicol, methotrexate, oral contraceptives, sulfasalazine, trimethoprim: antagonism of folic acid effect. Monitor for decreased folic acid effect. Use together cautiously.

Anticonvulsants, such as phenobarbital and phenytoin: increased anticonvulsant metabolism and decreased blood levels of the anticonvulsants. Monitor closely.

EFFECTS ON DIAGNOSTIC TESTS

Drug therapy alters serum and RBC folate concentrations; falsely low serum and RBC folate levels may occur with the *Lactobacillus casei* assay in patients receiving anti-infectives, such as tetracycline, which suppress the growth of this organism.

CONTRAINDICATIONS

Contraindicated in patients with undiagnosed anemia because it may mask pernicious anemia. Also contraindicated in those with B_{12} deficiency.

NURSING CONSIDERATIONS

● Safety in pregnancy has not been established but pregnant women are more prone to develop folate deficiency. Folate-deficient mothers may be more prone to pregnancy-related complications and fetal abnormalities.

● Don't mix with other medications in same syringe for I.M. injections.

● Patients with small-bowel resections and intestinal malabsorption may require parenteral administration.

● Protect from light and heat; store at room temperature.

☑ PATIENT TEACHING

● Teach patient about proper nutrition to prevent recurrence of anemia.

● Stress importance of follow-up visits and laboratory studies.

---

leucovorin calcium (citrovorum factor, folinic acid)
Wellcovorin

Pregnancy Risk Category: C

HOW SUPPLIED

Tablets: 5 mg, 10 mg, 15 mg, 25 mg

Injection: 1-ml ampule (3 mg/ml with 0.9% benzyl alcohol)

Powder for injection: 50-mg vial, 100-mg vial, 350-mg vial

ACTION

A reduced form of folic acid that is readily converted to other folic acid derivatives.

ONSET, PEAK, DURATION

Onset occurs in 5 minutes after I.V. administration, 10 to 20 minutes after I.M. administration, 20 to 30 minutes after

---

oral administration. Levels peak within 10 minutes after I.V. administration, less than 1 hour after I.M. administration, or 2 to 3 hours after oral administration. Effects persist for 3 to 6 hours for all routes.

INDICATIONS & DOSAGE
Overdose of folic acid antagonist—
Adults and children: P.O., I.M., or I.V. dose equivalent to weight of antagonist given.
Leucovorin rescue after high methotrexate dose in treatment of malignant disease—
Adults and children: 10 mg/m^2 P.O., I.M., or I.V. q 6 hours until methotrexate levels fall below 5×10^{-8} M.
Megaloblastic anemia caused by congenital enzyme deficiency—
Adults and children: 3 to 6 mg I.M., then 1 mg P.O. or I.M. daily for life.
Folate-deficient megaloblastic anemia—
Adults and children: up to 1 mg of leucovorin I.M daily. Duration of treatment depends on hematologic response.
Prevention of hematologic toxicity caused by pyrimethamine or trimethoprim therapy—
Adults and children: 400 mcg to 5 mg I.M. with each dose of the folic acid antagonist.
Treatment of hematologic toxicity caused by pyrimethamine or trimethoprim therapy—
Adults and children: 5 to 15 mg I.M. daily.
Palliative treatment of advanced colorectal cancer—
Adults: 20 mg/m^2 I.V., followed by fluorouracil 425 mg/m^2 I.V. daily for 5 consecutive days. Repeated at 4-week intervals for two additional courses; then at intervals of 4 to 5 weeks if tolerated.

ADVERSE REACTIONS
Skin: hypersensitivity reactions (urticaria and anaphylactoid reactions).

INTERACTIONS
Anticonvulsants: may decrease effectiveness of these agents.
Fluorouracil: may enhance fluorouracil toxicity.
Methotrexate: may decrease efficacy of intrathecal methotrexate.

EFFECTS ON DIAGNOSTIC TESTS
Leucovorin may mask the diagnosis of pernicious anemia.

CONTRAINDICATIONS
Contraindicated in patients with pernicious anemia and other megaloblastic anemias secondary to the lack of vitamin B_{12}.

NURSING CONSIDERATIONS
● **I.V. use:** When using powder for injection, reconstitute 50-mg vial with 5 ml, 100-mg vial with 10 ml, or 350-mg vial with 17 ml of sterile or bacteriostatic water for injection. When doses are more than 10 mg/m^2, don't use diluents containing benzyl alcohol.
Alert: Don't exceed 160 mg/minute when giving by direct injection.
● Do not confuse leucovorin (folinic acid) with folic acid.
● Follow leucovorin rescue schedule and protocol closely.
● Do not administer leucovorin simultaneously with systemic methotrexate.
● Protect from light and heat, especially reconstituted parenteral drug.

☑ PATIENT TEACHING
● Explain need for drug use to patient and family, and answer any questions or concerns.
● Tell patient to report symptoms of hypersensitivity promptly.

---

niacin (vitamin B$_3$, nicotinic acid)
Niac, Niacor, Nico-400, Nicobid ◇, Nicolar**, Nicotinex

niacinamide (nicotinamide) ◊

Pregnancy Risk Category: C

HOW SUPPLIED
niacin
Tablets: 25 mg ◊ , 50 mg ◊ , 100 mg ◊ ,
250 mg ◊ , 500 mg
Tablets (timed-release): 150 mg ◊ , 250
mg ◊ , 500 mg ◊ , 750 mg ◊
Capsules (timed-release): 125 mg ◊ ,
250 mg ◊ , 300 mg ◊ , 400 mg ◊ , 500
mg
Elixir: 50 mg/5 ml ◊
Injection: 100 mg/ml in 30-ml vials
niacinamide
Tablets: 50 mg ◊ , 100 mg ◊ , 125
mg ◊ , 250 mg ◊ , 500 mg ◊

ACTION
Niacin and niacinamide stimulate lipid
metabolism, tissue respiration, and
glycogenolysis; niacin decreases synthesis of low-density lipoproteins and
inhibits lipolysis in adipose tissue.

ONSET, PEAK, DURATION
Onset unknown. Triglyceride levels decrease within hours; cholesterol levels,
within days. Serum levels peak 45 minutes after oral use. Duration unknown.

INDICATIONS & DOSAGE
Recommended daily allowance (RDA)—
Neonates and infants to 6 months: 5
mg.
Infants 6 months to 1 year: 6 mg.
Children 1 to 3 years: 9 mg.
Children 4 to 6 years: 12 mg.
Children 7 to 10 years: 13 mg.
Males 11 to 14 years: 17 mg.
Males 15 to 18 years: 20 mg.
Males 19 to 50 years: 19 mg.
Males 51 years and over: 15 mg.
Females 11 to 50 years: 15 mg.
Females 51 years and over: 13 mg.
Pregnant women: 17 mg.
Breast-feeding women: 20 mg.
Pellagra—
Adults: 300 to 500 mg P.O., S.C., I.M.,
or I.V. daily in divided doses, depending
on severity of deficiency.
Children: up to 300 mg P.O. or 100 mg
I.V. daily, depending on severity of
niacin deficiency.
   After symptoms subside, advise ade-
quate nutrition and RDA supplements to
prevent recurrence.
Hartnup disease—
Adults: 50 to 200 mg P.O. daily
Niacin deficiency—
Adults: up to 100 mg P.O. daily.
*Hyperlipidemias, especially with hyper-
cholesterolemia—*
Adults: 1 to 2 g P.O. three times a day
with or after meals, increased at inter-
vals to 6 g daily.

ADVERSE REACTIONS
Most reactions are dose-dependent.
CV: *excessive peripheral vasodilation
(especially niacin),* hypotension, atrial
fibrillation, cardiac arrhythmias.
GI: *nausea, vomiting, diarrhea,* possible activation of peptic ulceration, epigastric or substernal pain.
Hepatic: *hepatic dysfunction.*
Skin: *flushing,* pruritus, dryness, tingling.
Other: hyperglycemia, hyperuricemia,
toxic amblyopia.

INTERACTIONS
*Antihypertensive drugs (sympathetic or
ganglionic blockers):* potential additive
vasodilating effect, causing postural hypotension. Use together cautiously; also
warn the patient about postural hypotension.
Lovastatin (statin class): concurrent use
may lead to rhabdomyolysis.
Sulfinpyrazone: uricosuric effects may
be decreased by niacin.

EFFECTS ON DIAGNOSTIC TESTS
Niacin therapy alters fluorometric test
results for urine catecholamines and results for urine glucose tests that use
cupric sulfate (Benedict's reagent).

CONTRAINDICATIONS
Contraindicated in patients with hepatic dysfunction, active peptic ulcers, severe hypotension, arterial hemorrhage, or drug hypersensitivity.

NURSING CONSIDERATIONS
● Use cautiously in patients with gallbladder disease, diabetes mellitus, or coronary artery disease and in patients with a history of liver disease, peptic ulcer, allergy, or gout.
● **I.V. use:** Give slow I.V. (no faster than 2 mg/minute). Explain harmlessness of flushing syndrome.
● To minimize adverse GI effects, give niacin with meals.
● Administer aspirin (325 mg P.O. 30 minutes before niacin dose), as ordered, to possibly reduce the flushing response to niacin.
● Timed-release niacin or niacinamide may prevent excessive flushing that occurs with large doses. However, timed-release niacin is linked with hepatic dysfunction, even at very low doses.
● Monitor hepatic function and blood glucose early in therapy, as ordered.

☑ **PATIENT TEACHING**
● Stress that this substance is a potent medication, not just a vitamin, and may cause serious adverse effects. Explain importance of adhering to therapeutic regimen.
● Advise patient against self-medicating for hyperlipidemia.

pyridoxine hydrochloride (vitamin B₆)
Beesix, Hexa-Betalin, Nestrex ◊, Rodex

Pregnancy Risk Category: A

HOW SUPPLIED
Tablets: 10 mg ◊, 25 mg ◊, 50 mg ◊, 100 mg ◊, 200 mg ◊, 250 mg ◊, 500 mg ◊
Capsules (timed-release): 100 mg
Capsules: 500 mg
Tablets (timed-release): 100 mg
Injection: 100 mg/ml

ACTION
Acts as a coenzyme that stimulates various metabolic functions, including amino acid metabolism.

ONSET, PEAK, DURATION
Unknown.

INDICATIONS & DOSAGE
Recommended daily allowance (RDA)—
Neonates and infants to 6 months: 0.3 mg.
Infants 6 months to 1 year: 0.6 mg.
Children 1 to 3 years: 1 mg.
Children 4 to 6 years: 1.1 mg.
Children 7 to 10 years: 1.4 mg.
Males 11 to 14 years: 1.7 mg.
Males 15 years and over: 2 mg.
Females 11 to 14 years: 1.4 mg.
Females 15 to 18 years: 1.5 mg.
Females 19 years and over: 1.6 mg.
Pregnant women: 2.2 mg.
Breast-feeding women: 2.1 mg.
Dietary vitamin B₆ deficiency—
Adults: 10 to 20 mg P.O., I.M., or I.V. daily for 3 weeks, then 2 to 5 mg daily as a supplement to a proper diet.
Seizures related to vitamin B₆ deficiency or dependency—
Adults and children: 100 mg I.M. or I.V. in single dose.
Vitamin B₆-responsive anemias or dependency syndrome (inborn errors of metabolism)—
Adults: up to 600 mg P.O., I.M., or I.V. daily until symptoms subside, then 30 mg daily for life.
Prevention of vitamin B₆ deficiency during drug therapy—
Adults: 10 to 50 mg P.O. daily.
Antidote for isoniazid poisoning—
Adults: 4 g I.V., followed by 1 g I.M. q 30 minutes until the amount of pyridoxine administered equals the amount of isoniazid ingested.

ADVERSE REACTIONS
CNS: paresthesia, unsteady gait, numbness, somnolence.

INTERACTIONS
Levodopa: decreased levodopa effect. Avoid concomitant use.
Phenobarbital, phenytoin: decreased anticonvulsant serum levels, increasing risk of seizures. Avoid concomitant use.

EFFECTS ON DIAGNOSTIC TESTS
Pyridoxine therapy alters determinations of urobilinogen in the spot test using Ehrich's reagent, resulting in a false-positive reaction.

CONTRAINDICATIONS
Contraindicated in patients hypersensitive to pyridoxine.

NURSING CONSIDERATIONS
● **I.V. use:** Inject undiluted drug into I.V. line of a free-flowing compatible solution. Or, infuse diluted drug over prescribed duration for intermittent infusion. Don't use for continuous infusion.
● Protect from light. Do not use solution if it contains a precipitate, although slight darkening is acceptable.
● When used to treat isoniazid toxicity, expect to also give anticonvulsants.
● If sodium bicarbonate is needed to control acidosis in isoniazid toxicity, don't mix in same syringe with pyridoxine.
● Patients taking high doses (2 to 6 g/day) may experience difficulty walking because of diminished proprioceptive and sensory function.
● Carefully monitor the patient's diet. Excessive protein intake increases daily pyridoxine requirements.

☑ PATIENT TEACHING
● Stress importance of compliance and of good nutrition if prescribed for maintenance therapy to prevent recurrence of deficiency. Explain that pyridoxine, in combination therapy with isoniazid, has

a specific therapeutic purpose and is not just a vitamin.
● Advise patient taking levodopa alone to avoid multivitamins containing pyridoxine because of decreased levodopa effect.

---

riboflavin (vitamin B₂) ◇

Pregnancy Risk Category: NR

HOW SUPPLIED
Tablets: 10 mg ◇, 25 mg ◇, 50 mg ◇, 100 mg ◇
Tablets (sugar-free): 50 mg ◇, 100 mg ◇

ACTION
Converts to two other coenzymes necessary for normal tissue respiration.

ONSET, PEAK, DURATION
Unknown.

INDICATIONS & DOSAGE
Recommended daily allowance (RDA)—
Neonates and infants to 6 months: 0.4 mg.
Infants 6 months to 1 year: 0.5 mg.
Children 1 to 3 years: 0.8 mg.
Children 4 to 6 years: 1.1 mg.
Children 7 to 10 years: 1.2 mg.
Males 11 to 14 years: 1.5 mg.
Males 15 to 18 years: 1.8 mg.
Males 19 to 50 years: 1.7 mg.
Males 51 years and over: 1.4 mg.
Females 11 to 50 years: 1.3 mg.
Females 51 years and over: 1.2 mg.
Pregnant women: 1.6 mg.
Breast-feeding women (first 6 months): 1.8 mg.
Breast-feeding women (second 6 months): 1.7 mg.
Riboflavin deficiency or adjunct to thiamine treatment for polyneuritis or cheilosis secondary to pellagra—
Adults and children over 12 years: 5 to 30 mg P.O. daily, depending on severity.
Children under 12 years: 3 to 10 mg

---

*Liquid contains alcohol. **May contain tartrazine. †Canada only. ‡Australia only. ◇OTC.

P.O. daily, depending on severity.

For maintenance, increase nutritional intake and supplement with vitamin B complex.

ADVERSE REACTIONS
GU: bright yellow urine.

INTERACTIONS
Probenecid: reduces urinary excretion of riboflavin.
Propantheline, other anticholinergics: decreased rate and extent of absorption. Avoid concomitant use.

EFFECTS ON DIAGNOSTIC TESTS
Drug therapy alters urinalysis based on spectrophotometry or color reactions. Large doses of drug result in bright yellow urine. Riboflavin produces fluorescent substances in urine and plasma, which can falsely elevate fluorometric determinations of catecholamines and urobilinogen.

CONTRAINDICATIONS
None known.

NURSING CONSIDERATIONS
● Drug may be given I.M. or I.V. as a component of multiple vitamins.
● Know that riboflavin deficiency usually accompanies other vitamin B complex deficiencies and may require multivitamin therapy.
● Protect from air and light.

☑ **PATIENT TEACHING**
● Tell patient to take riboflavin with meals; food increases its absorption.
● Stress proper nutritional habits to prevent recurrence of deficiency.

thiamine hydrochloride (vitamin B₁)
Betamin‡, Beta-Sol‡, Biamine, Thiamilate

Pregnancy Risk Category: A

HOW SUPPLIED
Tablets: 5 mg ◊ , 10 mg ◊ , 25 mg ◊ , 50 mg ◊ , 100 mg ◊ , 250 mg ◊ , 500 mg ◊
Tablet (enteric-coated): 20 mg
Elixir†: 250 mcg/5 ml
Injection: 100 mg/ml, 200 mg/ml

ACTION
Combines with adenosine triphosphate to form a coenzyme necessary for carbohydrate metabolism.

ONSET, PEAK, DURATION
Unknown.

INDICATIONS & DOSAGE
Recommended daily allowance (RDA)—
Neonates and infants to 6 months: 0.3 mg.
Infants 6 months to 1 year: 0.4 mg.
Children 1 to 3 years: 0.7 mg.
Children 4 to 6 years: 0.9 mg.
Children 7 to 10 years: 1 mg.
Males 11 to 14 years: 1.3 mg.
Males 15 to 50 years: 1.5 mg.
Males 51 years and over: 1.2 mg.
Females 11 to 50 years: 1.1 mg.
Females 51 years and over: 1 mg.
Pregnant women: 1.5 mg.
Breast-feeding women: 1.6 mg.
Beriberi—
Adults: depending on severity, 10 to 20 mg I.M. t.i.d. for 2 weeks, followed by dietary correction and multivitamin supplement containing 5 to 10 mg thiamine daily for 1 month.
Children: depending on severity, 10 to 50 mg I.M. daily for several weeks with adequate diet.
Wet beriberi with myocardial failure—
Adults and children: 10 to 30 mg I.V. t.i.d.
Wernicke's encephalopathy—
Adults: initially, 100 mg I.V., followed by 50 to 100 mg I.V. or I.M. daily until patient is consuming a regular balanced diet.

ADVERSE REACTIONS
CNS: restlessness.
CV: *angioedema,* cyanosis, *CV col-*

lapse.
EENT: tightness of throat (allergic reaction).
GI: nausea, hemorrhage.
Respiratory: pulmonary edema.
Skin: feeling of warmth, pruritus, urticaria, diaphoresis.
Other: weakness; tenderness and induration following I.M. administration.

INTERACTIONS
None significant.

EFFECTS ON DIAGNOSTIC TESTS
Thiamine therapy may produce false-positive results in the phosphotungstate method for determination of uric acid and in the urine spot tests with Ehrich's reagent for urobilinogen. Large doses of drug interfere with the Schack and Waxler spectrophotometric determination of serum theophylline concentrations.

CONTRAINDICATIONS
Contraindicated in patients hypersensitive to thiamine products.

NURSING CONSIDERATIONS
• Know that parenteral administration should be used only when P.O. route is not feasible.
• **I.V. use:** Dilute before giving.
Alert: Administer large I.V. doses cautiously; give the patient a skin test before therapy if he has a history of hypersensitivity reactions. Have epinephrine on hand to treat anaphylaxis.
• Do not use with materials that yield alkaline solutions. Thiamine is unstable in alkaline solutions.
• Know that thiamine malabsorption is most likely in alcoholism, cirrhosis, or GI disease.
• Clinically significant deficiency can occur in approximately 3 weeks of totally thiamine-free diet. Thiamine deficiency usually requires concurrent treatment for multiple deficiencies.
• Keep in mind that doses larger than 30 mg t.i.d. may not be fully utilized. After

tissue saturation with thiamine, it is excreted in urine as pyrimidine.

☑ **PATIENT TEACHING**
• Inform breast-feeding patient that if beriberi occurs in infant, both she and her child should be treated with thiamine.
• Stress proper nutritional habits to prevent recurrence of deficiency.

vitamin C (ascorbic acid)
Ascorbicap◇, Cebid Timecelles◇, Cecon◇, Cee-1000 T.D.◇, Cenolate◇, Cetane◇, Cevalin◇, Cevi-Bid◇, Ce-Vi-Sol*, Cevita◇, C-Span◇, Dull-C◇, Flavettes‡, Flavorcee◇, N'ice Vitamin C Drops◇, Redoxon†, Vita C Crystals◇

Pregnancy Risk Category: C

HOW SUPPLIED
Tablets: 25 mg◇, 50 mg◇, 100 mg◇, 250 mg◇, 500 mg◇, 1,000 mg◇
Tablets (chewable): 50 mg, 100 mg◇, 250 mg◇, 500 mg◇, 1,000 mg◇
Tablets (effervescent): 1,000 mg sugar-free◇
Tablets (timed-release): 500 mg◇, 1,000 mg◇, 1,500 mg
Capsules (timed-release): 500 mg◇
Crystals: 100 g (4 g/tsp)◇, 500 g (4 g/tsp)◇
Lozenges: 60 mg◇
Oral liquid: 50 ml (35 mg/0.6 ml)*◇
Oral solution: 60 mg/ml◇, 100 mg/ml◇
Powder: 100 g (4 g/tsp)◇, 500 g (4 g/tsp)◇
Syrup: 20 mg/ml in 120 ml, 480 ml◇; 500 mg/5 ml in 5 ml◇, 120 ml◇, 480 ml◇
Injection: 100 mg/ml; 250 mg/ml; 500 mg/ml

ACTION
Stimulates collagen formation and tissue repair; involved in oxidation-reduction reactions.

*Liquid contains alcohol.   **May contain tartrazine.   †Canada only.   ‡Australia only.   ◇OTC.

ONSET, PEAK, DURATION
Unknown.

INDICATIONS & DOSAGE
Recommended daily allowance (RDA)—
Neonates and infants to 6 months: 30 mg.
Infants 6 months to 1 year: 35 mg.
Children 1 to 3 years: 40 mg.
Children 4 to 10 years: 45 mg.
Children 11 to 14 years: 50 mg.
Adults and children 15 years and over: 60 mg.
Pregnant women: 70 mg.
Breast-feeding women (first 6 months): 95 mg.
Breast-feeding women (second 6 months): 90 mg.
Frank and subclinical scurvy—
Adults: depending on severity, 300 mg to 1 g P.O., S.C., I.M., or I.V. daily, then 70 to 150 mg daily for maintenance.
Children: depending on severity, 100 to 300 mg P.O., S.C., I.M., or I.V. daily, then at least 30 mg daily for maintenance.
Premature infants: 75 to 100 mg P.O., I.M., I.V., or S.C. daily.
Extensive burns, delayed fracture or wound healing, postoperative wound healing, severe febrile or chronic disease states—
Adults: 300 to 500 mg S.C., I.M., or I.V. daily for 7 to 10 days. 1 to 2 g daily for extensive burns.
Children: 100 to 200 mg P.O., S.C., I.M., or I.V. daily.
Prevention of vitamin C deficiency in patients with poor nutritional habits or increased requirements—
Adults: 70 to 150 mg P.O., S.C., I.M., or I.V. daily.
Pregnant and breast-feeding women: at least 70 to 150 mg P.O., S.C., I.M., or I.V. daily.
Children: at least 40 mg P.O., S.C., I.M., or I.V. daily.
Infants: at least 35 mg P.O., S.C., I.M., or I.V. daily.
Potentiation of methenamine in urine acidification—

Adults: 4 to 12 g P.O. daily in divided doses.

ADVERSE REACTIONS
CNS: faintness or dizziness with too-rapid I.V. administration.
GI: diarrhea.
GU: acid urine, oxaluria, renal calculi.
Other: discomfort at injection site.

INTERACTIONS
Aspirin (high doses): increased risk of salicylate toxicity. Monitor the patient closely.
Contraceptives, estrogen: increased serum levels of estrogen.
Oral iron supplements: increased iron absorption (a beneficial interaction).
Warfarin: decreased anticoagulant effect. Monitor closely.

EFFECTS ON DIAGNOSTIC TESTS
Ascorbic acid is a strong reducing agent; it alters results of tests that are based on oxidation-reduction reactions. Large doses (over 500 mg) may cause false-negative glucose determinations using the glucose oxidase method or false-positive results using the copper reduction method or Benedict's reagent.

Ascorbic acid should not be used for 48 to 72 hours before an amine-dependent test for occult blood in the stool is conducted; a false-negative test may occur. Depending on the reagents used, it may also interact with other diagnostic tests.

CONTRAINDICATIONS
None known.

NURSING CONSIDERATIONS
● **I.V. use:** Infuse cautiously in patients with renal insufficiency.
Alert: Avoid too-rapid I.V. administration.
● When giving for urine acidification, check urine pH to ensure efficacy.
● Protect solution from light, and refrigerate ampules.

☑ **PATIENT TEACHING**
● For patient receiving vitamin C I.M., explain that I.M. route may promote better utilization.
● Stress proper nutritional habits to prevent recurrence of deficiency.

---

vitamin D
cholecalciferol (vitamin D₃)
Delta-D ◊ , Vitamin D₃ ◊

ergocalciferol (vitamin D₂)
Calciferol, Deltalin Gelseals, Drisdol, Radiostol†, Radiostol Forte†, Vitamin D

Pregnancy Risk Category: C

HOW SUPPLIED
Tablets: 1.25 mg (50,000 IU)
Capsules: 1.25 mg (50,000 IU)
Oral liquid: 8,000 IU/ml in 60-ml dropper bottle ◊
Injection: 12.5 mg (500,000 IU)/ml

ACTION
Promotes absorption and utilization of calcium and phosphate, helping to regulate calcium homeostasis.

ONSET, PEAK, DURATION
According to metabolites formed or derivative, onset is as follows: oral calcitriol, 2 to 6 hours; dihydrotachysterol, several hours to 1 day; ergocalciferol, 12 to 24 hours although therapeutic onset may take 10 to 14 days. Time to peak as follows: alfacalcidol, about 12 hours; calcifediol, about 4 hours; calcitriol, about 3 to 6 hours. Duration as follows: alfacalcidol, up to 48 hours; calcifediol, 15 to 20 days; calcitriol, 3 to 5 days; dihydrotachysterol, up to 9 weeks; ergocalciferol, up to 6 months.

INDICATIONS & DOSAGE
Recommended daily allowance (RDA) for cholecalciferol—
Neonates and infants to 6 months: 300 IU.

Infants 6 months to adults 24 years: 400 IU.
Adults 25 years and over: 200 IU.
Pregnant or lactating women: 400 IU.
Rickets and other vitamin D deficiency diseases; renal osteodystrophy—
Adults: initially, 12,000 IU P.O. or I.M. daily, usually increased based on response up to 500,000 IU daily.
Children: 1,500 to 5,000 IU P.O. or I.M. daily for 2 to 4 weeks, repeated after 2 weeks, if necessary. Alternatively, give single dose of 600,000 IU.

After correction of deficiency, maintenance includes adequate diet and RDA supplements.
Hypoparathyroidism—
Adults and children: 50,000 to 200,000 IU P.O. or I.M. daily, with calcium supplement.
Familial hypophosphatemia—
Adults: 1 to 2 mg P.O. daily with phosphorus supplement, increased in 250- to 500-mcg increments at 3- to 4-month intervals.

ADVERSE REACTIONS
Adverse reactions listed usually occur only in vitamin D toxicity.
CNS: headache, weakness, somnolence, decreased libido, overt psychosis, irritability.
CV: *calcification of soft tissues, including the heart,* hypertension, cardiac arrhythmias.
EENT: rhinorrhea, conjunctivitis (calcific), photophobia.
GI: anorexia, nausea, vomiting, constipation, dry mouth, metallic taste, polydipsia.
GU: polyuria, albuminuria, hypercalciuria, nocturia, *impaired renal function,* reversible azotemia.
Skin: pruritus.
Other: bone and muscle pain, bone demineralization, weight loss, *hypercalcemia,* hyperthermia.

INTERACTIONS
Cholestyramine resin, mineral oil: inhibited GI absorption of oral vitamin D.

Space doses. Use together cautiously.
Corticosteroids: antagonized effect of vitamin D. Monitor vitamin D levels closely.
Digitalis glycosides: increased risk of arrhythmias. Monitor serum calcium levels.
Magnesium-containing antacids: possible hypermagnesemia, especially in patients with chronic renal failure. Monitor serum magnesium levels.
Phenobarbital, phenytoin: increased vitamin D metabolism and decreased effectiveness. Monitor closely.
Thiazide diuretics: may cause hypercalcemia in patients with hypoparathyroidism. Monitor closely.
Verapamil: atrial fibrillation has occurred due to increased calcium.

EFFECTS ON DIAGNOSTIC TESTS
Ergocalciferol may falsely increase serum cholesterol levels and may elevate AST and ALT levels.

CONTRAINDICATIONS
Contraindicated in patients with hypercalcemia, hypervitaminosis A, or renal osteodystrophy with hyperphosphatemia.

NURSING CONSIDERATIONS
● Ergocalciferol should be given with extreme caution, if at all, to patients with impaired renal function, heart disease, renal stones, or arteriosclerosis.
● Use cautiously in cardiac patients, especially those taking digitalis glycosides, as well as in patients with increased sensitivity to these drugs.
● Use I.M. injection of vitamin D dispersed in oil for patients unable to absorb the oral form, as ordered.
Alert: Monitor the patient's eating and bowel habits; dry mouth, nausea, vomiting, metallic taste, and constipation may be early signs of toxicity.
● Monitor serum and urine calcium, potassium, and urea levels when high therapeutic dosages are used.
● Dosages of 60,000 IU/day can cause hypercalcemia.
● Be aware that malabsorption from inadequate bile or hepatic dysfunction may require addition of exogenous bile salts to oral form.
● Patients with hyperphosphatemia require dietary phosphate restrictions and binding agents to avoid metastatic calcifications and renal calculi.

☑ **PATIENT TEACHING**
● Warn patient of the dangers of increasing dosage without asking the doctor. This vitamin is fat-soluble.
● Tell the patient taking vitamin D to restrict intake of magnesium-containing antacids.

---

vitamin E (tocopherol)
Amino-Opti-E ◇ , Aquasol E ◇ , E-Complex-600 ◇ , E-200 I.U. Softgels ◇ , E-400 I.U. Softgels ◇ , E Vitamin Succinate ◇ , Vita-Plus E Softgels ◇

Pregnancy Risk Category: NR

HOW SUPPLIED
Tablets (chewable): 200 IU ◇ , 400 IU ◇
Capsules: 200 IU ◇ , 400 IU ◇ , 500 IU ◇ , 600 IU ◇ , 1,000 IU ◇ , 330 mg, 147 mg, 73.5 mg
Oral solution: 50 mg/ml ◇

ACTION
Unknown. Thought to act as an antioxidant and protect RBC membranes against hemolysis.

ONSET, PEAK, DURATION
Unknown.

INDICATIONS & DOSAGE
Recommended daily allowance (RDA)—Note: RDAs for vitamin E have been converted to alpha-tocopherol equivalents (α-TE). One α-TE equals 1 mg of D-alpha tocopherol or 1.49 IU.
Neonates and infants to 6 months: 3 α-TE or 4 IU.

Infants 6 months to 1 year: 4 α-TE or 6 IU.
Children 1 to 3 years: 6 α-TE or 9 IU.
Children 4 to 10 years: 7 α-TE or 10 IU.
Males 11 years and over: 10 α-TE or 15 IU.
Females 11 years and over: 8 α-TE or 12 IU.
Pregnant women: 10 α-TE or 15 IU.
Breast-feeding women (first 6 months): 12 α-TE or 18 IU.
Breast-feeding women (second 6 months): 11 α-TE or 16 IU.
Vitamin E deficiency in premature neonates and in patients with impaired fat absorption—
Adults: depending on severity, 60 to 75 IU P.O. daily.
Children: 1 IU/kg daily.

ADVERSE REACTIONS
None reported with recommended dosages. Hypervitaminosis E symptoms include fatigue, weakness, nausea, headache, blurred vision, flatulence, diarrhea.

INTERACTIONS
Anticoagulants (oral): hypoprothrombinemic effects may be increased, possibly causing bleeding. Monitor closely.
Cholestyramine resin, mineral oil: inhibited GI absorption of oral vitamin E. Space doses. Use together cautiously.
Vitamin K: antagonized effects of vitamin K possible with large doses of vitamin E. Avoid concurrent use.

EFFECTS ON DIAGNOSTIC TESTS
None reported.

CONTRAINDICATIONS
None known.

NURSING CONSIDERATIONS
● Monitor the patient with liver or gallbladder disease for response to therapy. Adequate bile is essential for vitamin E absorption.
● Be aware that water-miscible forms

more completely absorbed in GI tract.
● Requirements increase with rise in dietary polyunsaturated acids.

☑ **PATIENT TEACHING**
● Tell patient that he shouldn't crush tablets or open capsules. An oral solution and chewable tablets are commercially available.
● Discourage the patient from self-medication with megadoses, which can cause thrombophlebitis. This vitamin is fat-soluble.

phytonadione (vitamin K₁)
AquaMEPHYTON, Konakion, Mephyton

Pregnancy Risk Category: C

HOW SUPPLIED
Tablets: 5 mg
Injection (aqueous colloidal solution): 2 mg/ml, 10 mg/ml
Injection (aqueous dispersion): 2 mg/ml, 10 mg/ml

ACTION
An antihemorrhagic factor that promotes hepatic formation of active prothrombin.

ONSET, PEAK, DURATION
Onset occurs in 6 to 12 hours after oral administration, 1 to 2 hours (with hemorrhage controlled in 3 to 6 hours) after parenteral administration. Peak unknown. Normal prothrombin concentrations are often obtained in 12 to 14 hours.

INDICATIONS & DOSAGE
Recommended daily allowance (RDA)—
Neonates and infants to 6 months: 5 mcg.
Infants 6 months to 1 year: 10 mcg.
Children 1 to 3 years: 15 mcg.
Children 4 to 6 years: 20 mcg.
Children 7 to 10 years: 30 mcg.
Children 11 to 14 years: 45 mcg.

Males 15 to 18 years: 65 mcg.
Males 19 to 24 years: 70 mcg.
Males 25 years and over: 80 mcg.
Females 15 to 18 years: 55 mcg.
Females 19 to 24 years: 60 mcg.
Females 25 years and over and pregnant or breast-feeding women: 65 mcg.

Hypoprothrombinemia secondary to vitamin K malabsorption, drug therapy, or excessive vitamin A dosage—
Adults: depending on severity, 2.5 to 10 mg P.O., S.C., or I.M. repeated and increased up to 50 mg if necessary.
Infants: 2 mg P.O. or parenterally.
Children: 5 to 10 mg P.O. or parenterally.

I.V. injection rate for infants and children should not exceed 3 mg/m^2/minute or a total of 5 mg.
Hypoprothrombinemia secondary to effect of oral anticoagulants—
Adults: 2.5 to 10 mg P.O., S.C., or I.M. based on PT, repeated if necessary within 12 to 48 hours after oral dose or within 6 to 8 hours after parenteral dose. In emergency, 10 to 50 mg slow I.V., rate not to exceed 1 mg/minute, repeated q 4 hours, p.r.n.
Prevention of hemorrhagic disease of newborn—
Neonates: 0.5 to 1 mg I.M. within 1 hour after birth.
Treatment of hemorrhagic disease of newborn—
Neonates: 1 mg S.C. or I.M. Higher doses may be necessary if mother has been receiving oral anticoagulants.
Prevention of hypoprothrombinemia related to vitamin K deficiency in long-term parenteral nutrition—
Adults: 5 to 10 mg I.M. weekly.
Children: 2 to 5 mg I.M. weekly.
Prevention of hypoprothrombinemia in infants receiving less than 0.1 mg/liter vitamin K in breast milk or milk substitutes—
Infants: 1 mg I.M. monthly.

ADVERSE REACTIONS
CNS: dizziness.

CV: transient hypotension after I.V. administration, rapid and weak pulse.
Skin: diaphoresis, flushing, erythema.
Other: *anaphylaxis and anaphylactoid reactions* (usually after too-rapid I.V. administration); pain, swelling, and hematoma at injection site.

INTERACTIONS
Anticoagulants: temporary resistance to prothrombin-depressing anticoagulants may result, especially when larger doses of phytonadione are used. Monitor closely.
Cholestyramine resin, mineral oil: inhibited GI absorption of oral vitamin K. Space doses. Use together cautiously.

EFFECTS ON DIAGNOSTIC TESTS
Phytonadione may falsely elevate urine steroid levels.

CONTRAINDICATIONS
Contraindicated in patients with hypersensitivity to drug.

NURSING CONSIDERATIONS
● Check brand name labels for administration route restrictions.
● Effects of I.V. injection are more rapid but shorter-lived than S.C. or I.M. injections.
● **I.V. use:** Dilute with 0.9% sodium chloride for injection, D$_5$W, or D$_5$W in 0.9% sodium chloride for injection. Give I.V. by slow infusion over 2 to 3 hours. Rate shouldn't exceed 1 mg/minute in adults or 3 mg/m^2/minute in children.
● Protect parenteral products from light. Wrap infusion container with aluminum foil.
● For I.M. administration in adults and older children, administer in upper outer quadrant of buttocks; for infants, administer in the anterolateral aspect of the thigh or deltoid region.
● Anticipate order of weekly addition of 5 to 10 mg of phytonadione to total parenteral nutrition solutions.
● Monitor PT to determine dosage ef-

Reactions may be *common*, uncommon, *life-threatening*, or COMMON AND LIFE-THREATENING.

fectiveness, as ordered.
- If severe bleeding occurs, don't delay other measures, such as fresh frozen plasma or whole blood.

Alert: Watch for signs of flushing, weakness, tachycardia, and hypotension; may progress to shock.
- Be aware that phytonadione therapy for hemorrhagic disease in infants causes fewer adverse reactions than do other vitamin K analogues.
- Failure to respond to vitamin K may indicate coagulation defects.

☑ **PATIENT TEACHING**
- Explain the drug's purpose.
- Tell patient to avoid hazardous activities if dizziness occurs.

---

sodium fluoride

Fluor-A-Day†, Fluoritab, Fluorodex, Fluotic†, Flura, Flura-Drops, Flura-Loz, Karidium, Luride, Luride Lozi-Tabs, Luride-SF, Luride-SF Lozi-Tabs, Pediaflor, Pedi-Dent†, Pharmaflur, Pharmaflur df, Pharmaflur 1.1, Phos-Flur, Solu-Flur†

sodium fluoride, topical

ACT◇, Fluorigard◇, Fluorinse, Gel Kam, Gel-Tin◇, Karigel, Karigel-N, Listermint with Fluoride, Minute Gel, Point-Two, PreviDent, Stop◇, Thera-Flur, Thera-Flur-N

Pregnancy Risk Category: NR

HOW SUPPLIED
sodium fluoride
Tablets: 1 mg
Tablets (chewable): 0.5 mg, 1 mg
Drops: 0.125 mg/drop, 0.25 mg/drop, 0.2 mg/ml, 0.5 mg/ml
Lozenges: 1 mg
sodium fluoride, topical
Gel: 0.1%, 0.5%, 1.23%
Gel drops: 0.5%
Rinse: 0.01%◇, 0.02%◇, 0.09%

ACTION
Stabilizes the apatite crystal of bone and teeth.

ONSET, PEAK, DURATION
Onset and duration unknown. Peaks in 30 to 60 minutes.

INDICATIONS & DOSAGE
Prevention of dental caries—
Adults and children over 6 years: 5 to 10 ml of rinse or thin ribbon of gel applied to teeth with toothbrush or mouth trays for at least 1 minute h.s.
Children under 2 years: 0.25 mg P.O. (tablet or drops) daily.
Children 2 to 3 years: 0.5 mg P.O. (tablet or drops) daily.
Children 3 to 13 years: 1 mg P.O. (tablet or lozenge) daily.

ADVERSE REACTIONS
CNS: headache, weakness.
GI: gastric distress.
Skin: hypersensitivity reactions, such as atopic dermatitis, eczema, and urticaria.
Other: staining of teeth.

INTERACTIONS
Dairy products: incompatibility may occur due to formation of calcium fluoride, which is poorly absorbed.

EFFECTS ON DIAGNOSTIC TESTS
None reported.

CONTRAINDICATIONS
Contraindicated in patients hypersensitive to fluoride or when intake from drinking water exceeds 0.7 ppm.

NURSING CONSIDERATIONS
- Administer oral drops undiluted or mixed with fluids or food. Avoid simultaneous ingestion of dairy products.
- Know that chronic toxicity (fluorosis) may result from prolonged use of higher-than-recommended doses.

☑ **PATIENT TEACHING**
- Tell patient that tablets may be dis-

---

solved in mouth, chewed, or swallowed whole.

• Advise patient that topical rinses and gels should not be swallowed by children under 3 years or used if water supply is fluorinated. Most effective when used right after brushing teeth. Tell patient to rinse around and between teeth for 1 minute, then spit out.

• Tell patient not to eat, drink, or rinse mouth for 30 minutes after application.

• Tell patient to dilute drops or rinses in plastic, not glass, containers.

• Advise patient to notify the dentist if tooth mottling occurs.

---

trace elements

chromium (chromic chloride)
Chroma-Pak, Chromic Chloride, Chromium Chloride

copper (cupric chloride, cupric sulfate)
Cupric Sulfate

iodine (sodium iodide)
Iodopen

manganese (manganese chloride, manganese sulfate)

selenium (selenious acid)
Sele-Pak, Selepen

zinc (zinc chloride, zinc sulfate)
Zinca-Pak

Pregnancy Risk Category: C

HOW SUPPLIED
chromium
Injection: 4 mcg/ml, 20 mcg/ml
copper
Injection: 0.4 mg/ml, 2 mg/ml
iodine
Injection: 100 mcg/ml
manganese
Injection: 0.1 mg/ml

selenium
Injection: 40 mcg/ml
zinc
Injection: 1 mg/ml, 5 mg/ml

ACTION
Participates in synthesis and stabilization of proteins and nucleic acids in subcellular and membrane transport systems.

ONSET, PEAK, DURATION
Onset and peak occur right after an I.V. infusion. Duration unknown.

INDICATIONS & DOSAGE
Prevention of individual trace element deficiencies in patients receiving long-term total parenteral nutrition (TPN)—
Chromium—
Adults: 10 to 15 mcg I.V. daily.
Children: 0.14 to 0.20 mcg/kg I.V. daily.
Copper—
Adults: 0.5 to 1.5 mg I.V. daily.
Children: 20 mcg/kg I.V. daily.
Iodine—
Adults: 1 to 2 mcg/kg I.V. daily.
Manganese—
Adults: 0.15 to 0.8 mg I.V. daily.
Children: 2 to 10 mcg/kg I.V. daily.
Selenium—
Adults: 20 to 40 mcg I.V. daily.
Children: 3 mcg/kg I.V. daily.
Zinc—
Adults: 2.5 to 4 mg I.V. daily.
Full-term infants to 5 years: 100 mcg/kg/day.
Neonates under 1,500 g to 3 kg: 300 mcg/kg/day.

ADVERSE REACTIONS
None reported when used at recommended dosages except for hypersensitivity to iodides.

INTERACTIONS
None significant at recommended dosages.

EFFECTS ON DIAGNOSTIC TESTS
No information available.

CONTRAINDICATIONS
None known.

NURSING CONSIDERATIONS
● **I.V. use:** Cautiously infuse diluted solution through a patent I.V. line over the ordered duration.
● Do not administer undiluted due to potential for phlebitis.
● Check serum levels of trace elements in patients who have received TPN for 2 months or longer, as ordered. Give supplement, if ordered. Report low serum levels of these elements.
● Normal serum levels are 1 to 5 mcg/L chromium; 80 to 163 mcg/dl copper; 6 to 12 mcg/dl manganese; 0.1 to 0.19 mcg/ml selenium; and 88 to 112 mcg/dl zinc.
● Be aware that solutions of trace elements are compounded by the pharmacist for addition to TPN solutions according to various formulas. One common trace element solution is Shil's solution, which contains copper 1 mg/ml, iodide 0.06 mg/ml, manganese 0.4 mg/ml, and zinc 2 mg/ml.

☑ **PATIENT TEACHING**
● Explain need for zinc administration to patient and family.
● Tell patient to report signs of hypersensitivity promptly.

91
Calorics

amino acid infusions, crystalline
amino acid infusions in dextrose
amino acid infusions with
  electrolytes
amino acid infusions with
  electrolytes in dextrose
amino acid infusions for hepatic
  failure
amino acid infusions for high
  metabolic stress
amino acid infusions for renal
  failure
dextrose
fat emulsions
medium-chain triglycerides

COMBINATION PRODUCTS
Various products contain dextrose or invert sugar in combination with electrolytes.

amino acid infusions, crystalline
Aminosyn, Aminosyn II, Aminosyn-PF, FreAmine III, Novamine, Travasol, TrophAmine

amino acid infusions in dextrose
Aminosyn II with dextrose

amino acid infusions with electrolytes
Aminosyn with electrolytes, Aminosyn II with electrolytes, FreAmine III with electrolytes, ProcalAmine with electrolytes, Travasol with electrolytes

amino acid infusions with electrolytes in dextrose
Aminosyn II with electrolytes in dextrose

amino acid infusions for hepatic failure
HepatAmine

amino acid infusions for high metabolic stress
Aminosyn-HBC, BranchAmin, FreAmine HBC

amino acid infusions for renal failure
Aminess, Aminosyn-RF, NephrAmine, RenAmin

Pregnancy Risk Category: C

HOW SUPPLIED
Injection: 250 ml, 500 ml, 1,000 ml, 2,000 ml containing amino acids in various concentrations
amino acid infusions, crystalline
Aminosyn: 3.5%, 5%, 7%, 8.5%, 10%
Aminosyn II: 3.5%, 5%, 7%, 8.5%, 10%
Aminosyn-PF: 7%, 10%
FreAmine III: 8.5%, 10%
Novamine: 11.4%, 15%
Travasol: 5.5%, 8.5%, 10%
TrophAmine: 6%, 10%
amino acid infusions in dextrose
Aminosyn II: 3.5% in 5% dextrose, 3.5% in 25% dextrose, 4.25% in 10% dextrose, 4.25% in 20% dextrose, 4.25% in 25% dextrose, 5% in 25% dextrose
amino acid infusions with electrolytes
Aminosyn: 3.5%, 7%, 8.5%
Aminosyn II: 3.5%, 7%, 8.5%, 10%
FreAmine III: 3%, 8.5%
ProcalAmine: 3%
Travasol: 3.5%, 5.5%, 8.5%
amino acid infusions with electrolytes in dextrose
Aminosyn II: 3.5% with electrolytes in 5% dextrose, 4.25% with electrolytes in 10% dextrose

Reactions may be *common*, uncommon, *life-threatening*, or COMMON AND LIFE-THREATENING.

amino acid infusions for hepatic failure
HepatAmine: 8%
amino acid infusions for high metabolic stress
Aminosyn-HBC: 7%
BranchAmin: 4%
FreAmine HBC: 6.9%
amino acid infusions for renal failure
Aminess: 5.2%
Aminosyn-RF: 5.2%
NephrAmine: 5.4%
RenAmin: 6.5%

ACTION
Provides a substrate for protein synthesis or enhances conservation of existing body protein. Formulations for hepatic failure and high metabolic stress contain essential and nonessential amino acids, with high concentrations of the branched chain amino acids isoleucine, leucine, and valine. Formulations for patients with renal failure contain histidine and minimal amounts of essential amino acids; nonessential amino acids are synthesized from excess ammonia in the blood of the uremic patient, thus lowering azotemia.

ONSET, PEAK, DURATION
Onset and peak occur immediately after an I.V. infusion. Duration unknown.

INDICATIONS & DOSAGE
Total parenteral nutrition in patients who cannot or will not eat—
Adults: 1 to 1.5 g/kg I.V. daily.
Children under 10 kg: 2 to 4 g/kg I.V. daily.
Children over 10 kg: 20 to 25 g/kg I.V. daily for the first 10 kg, then 1 to 1.25 g/kg I.V. daily for each kg over 10 kg.
Nutritional support in patients with cirrhosis, hepatitis, and hepatic encephalopathy—
Adults: 80 to 120 g of amino acids (12 to 18 g of nitrogen) I.V. daily of the formulation for hepatic failure.
Nutritional support in patients with high metabolic stress—

Adults: 1.5 g/kg I.V. daily of the formulation for high metabolic stress.
Nutritional support in patients with renal failure—
Adults: 0.3 to 0.5 g/kg I.V. daily (up to total of 26 g daily). Patients on dialysis may require 1 to 1.2 g/kg daily.

ADVERSE REACTIONS
CV: thrombophlebitis, edema, thrombosis.
GI: nausea.
GU: glycosuria, osmotic diuresis.
Hepatic: elevated liver enzyme levels.
Skin: flushing.
Other: hypersensitivity reactions, tissue sloughing at infusion site caused by extravasation, *catheter sepsis, rebound hypoglycemia* (when long-term infusions are abruptly stopped), hyperglycemia, osteoporosis, metabolic acidosis, alkalosis, hypophosphatemia, *hyperosmolar nonketotic syndrome,* hyperammonemia, *electrolyte imbalances,* fever, weight gain.

INTERACTIONS
Tetracycline: may reduce the protein-sparing effects of infused amino acids because of its antianabolic activity.

EFFECTS ON DIAGNOSTIC TESTS
None reported.

CONTRAINDICATIONS
Contraindicated in patients with anuria and in patients with inborn errors of amino acid metabolism, such as maple syrup urine disease and isovaleric acidemia.

NURSING CONSIDERATIONS
● Use with extreme caution in pediatric patients and in neonates, especially those with low birth weight.
● Use cautiously in patients with renal insufficiency or failure, cardiac disease, or hepatic impairment.
● Administer cautiously to diabetic patients; insulin may be required to prevent hyperglycemia. Administer cau-

tiously in cardiac insufficiency; may cause circulatory overload. Patients with fluid restriction may tolerate only 1 to 2 liters.
● Obtain baseline serum electrolytes, glucose, BUN, calcium and phosphorus levels before therapy, as ordered, and then monitor these levels periodically throughout therapy.
● Know that safe and effective use of parenteral nutrition requires a knowledge of nutrition as well as clinical expertise in the recognition and treatment of potential complications. Frequent evaluation of the patient and laboratory studies are necessary.
● **I.V. use:** Control infusion rate carefully with infusion pump. If infusion rate falls behind, notify the doctor; do not increase the rate to catch up.
● Know that peripheral infusions should be limited to 2.5% amino acids and dextrose 10%. Check infusion site frequently for erythema, inflammation, irritation, tissue sloughing, necrosis, and phlebitis. Change peripheral I.V. sites routinely to prevent irritation and infection. If a subclavian catheter is used, administer solution into the midsuperior vena cava.
● Add vitamins, electrolytes, and trace elements, as ordered.
● Check fractional urine every 6 hours for glycosuria initially, then every 12 to 24 hours in stable patients. Abrupt onset of glycosuria may be an early sign of impending sepsis.
● Assess body temperature every 4 hours; elevation may indicate sepsis or infection.
● Monitor for extraordinary electrolyte losses that may occur during nasogastric suction, vomiting, diarrhea, or drainage from GI fistula.
● Be prepared to individualize dosage to metabolic and clinical response as determined by nitrogen balance and body weight corrected for fluid balance.
● If the patient has chills, fever, or other signs of sepsis, replace I.V. tubing and bottle and send them to the laboratory to

be cultured.

☑ **PATIENT TEACHING**
● Explain need for use to patient and family, and answer any questions.
● Tell patient to report adverse reactions promptly.

dextrose (d-glucose)

Pregnancy Risk Category: C

HOW SUPPLIED
Injection: 3-ml ampule (10%); 5-ml ampule (10%); 10 ml (25%); 50 ml (5% and 50% available in vial, ampule, and Bristoject); 70-ml pin-top vial (70% for additive use only); 100 ml (5%); 250 ml (5%, 10%); 400 ml (5%); 500 ml (5%, 10%, 20%, 30%, 40%, 50%, 60%, 70%); 650 ml (38.5%); 1,000 ml (2.5%, 5%, 10%, 20%, 30%, 40%, 50%, 60%, 70%)

ACTION
A simple water-soluble sugar that minimizes glyconeogenesis and promotes anabolism in patients whose oral caloric intake is limited.

ONSET, PEAK, DURATION
Onset and serum levels peak immediately after I.V. infusion. Duration unknown.

INDICATIONS & DOSAGE
Fluid replacement and caloric supplementation in patients who can't maintain adequate oral intake or who are restricted from doing so—
Adults and children: dosage depends on fluid and caloric requirements. Peripheral I.V. infusion of 2.5%, 5%, or 10% solution or central I.V. infusion of 20% solution is used for minimal fluid needs. A 25% solution is used to treat acute hypoglycemia in neonate or older infant. A 50% solution is used to treat insulin-induced hypoglycemia. Solutions of 10%, 20%, 30%, 40%, 50%,

60%, and 70% are diluted in admixtures, usually amino acid solutions, for total parenteral nutrition (TPN) given through a central vein.

ADVERSE REACTIONS

CNS: confusion, *unconsciousness in hyperosmolar nonketotic syndrome.*
CV: with fluid overload—*pulmonary edema, exacerbated hypertension, and CHF* in susceptible patients. Prolonged or concentrated infusions may cause *phlebitis, venous sclerosis,* and tissue necrosis, especially when administered peripherally.
GU: glycosuria, osmotic diuresis.
Skin: sloughing and tissue necrosis, if extravasation occurs with concentrated solutions.
Other: with rapid infusion of concentrated solution or prolonged infusion—hyperglycemia, hypervolemia, hypovolemia, dehydration, fever, hyperosmolarity. Rapid termination of long-term infusions may cause hypoglycemia from rebound hyperinsulinemia.

INTERACTIONS
Corticosteroids: monitor glucose, sodium, and potassium.

EFFECTS ON DIAGNOSTIC TESTS
None reported.

CONTRAINDICATIONS
Contraindicated in patients in diabetic coma while blood glucose remains excessively high. Use of concentrated solutions contraindicated in patients with intracranial or intraspinal hemorrhage, or in dehydrated patients with delirium tremens or in patients with severe dehydration, anuria, hepatic coma, or glucose-galactose malabsorption syndrome.

NURSING CONSIDERATIONS
● Use cautiously in patients with cardiac or pulmonary disease, hypertension, renal insufficiency, urinary obstruction, or hypovolemia.

● **I.V. use:** Control infusion rate carefully; maximum rate is 0.5 g/kg/hour. Use infusion pump when infusing with amino acids for TPN. Never infuse concentrated solutions rapidly, which may cause hyperglycemia and fluid shift.
● Monitor serum glucose levels carefully. Prolonged therapy with D_5W can cause depletion of pancreatic insulin production and secretion.
Alert: Never stop hypertonic solutions abruptly. If necessary, have dextrose 10% in water solution available to treat hypoglycemia if rebound hyperinsulinemia occurs.
● Use central veins to infuse dextrose solutions with concentrations greater than 10%.
● Take care to prevent extravasation. Check injection site frequently to prevent irritation, tissue sloughing, necrosis, and phlebitis.
● Check vital signs frequently. Report adverse effects promptly.
● Monitor fluid intake and output and weight carefully, especially patients with renal function impairment.
● Watch closely for signs of fluid overload, especially if fluid intake is restricted.

☑ **PATIENT TEACHING**
● Explain need for drug to patient and family, and answer any questions.
● Tell patient to report adverse reactions promptly.

fat emulsions
Intralipid 10%, Intralipid 20%, Liposyn II 10%, Liposyn II 20%, Liposyn III 10%, Liposyn III 20%

Pregnancy Risk Category: C

HOW SUPPLIED
Injection: 50 ml (10%, 20%), 100 ml (10%, 20%), 200 ml (10%, 20%), 250 ml (10%, 20%), 500 ml (10%, 20%)

ACTION
Provides neutral triglycerides, predominantly unsaturated fatty acids; acts as a source of calories; and prevents fatty acid deficiency. When substituted for dextrose as a source of calories, fat emulsions decrease carbon dioxide production.

ONSET, PEAK, DURATION
Onset and serum levels peak immediately after I.V. infusion. Duration unknown.

INDICATIONS & DOSAGE
Intralipid:
Source of calories as adjunct to total parenteral nutrition (TPN)—
Adults: 1 ml/minute I.V. for 15 to 30 minutes (10% emulsion); 0.5 ml/minute I.V. for 15 to 30 minutes (20% emulsion). If no adverse reactions occur, rate increased to deliver 500 ml over 4 to 8 hours; total daily dosage should not exceed 3 g/kg.
Children: 0.1 ml/minute for 10 to 15 minutes (10% emulsion), 0.05 ml/minute I.V. for 10 to 15 minutes (20% emulsion). If no adverse reactions occur, rate increased to deliver 1 g/kg over 4 hours; daily dosage should not exceed 3 g/kg. Equals 40% of daily caloric intake; protein-carbohydrate TPN should supply remaining 60%.
Fatty acid deficiency—
Adults and children: 8% to 10% of total caloric intake I.V.
Liposyn:
Prevention of fatty acid deficiency—
Adults: 500 ml (10% emulsion) I.V. twice weekly. Infused initially at a rate of 1 ml/minute for 30 minutes. Rate may be increased to, but should not exceed, 500 ml over 4 to 6 hours.
Children: 5 to 10 ml/kg (10% emulsion) I.V. daily. Initially infused at a rate of 0.1 ml/minute for 30 minutes. Rate may be increased to, but should not exceed, 100 ml/hour.

ADVERSE REACTIONS
Early reactions to fat overload:
CNS: headache, sleepiness, dizziness.
EENT: pressure over eyes.
GI: nausea, vomiting.
Hematologic: hypercoagulability, thrombocytopenia in neonates (rare).
Respiratory: dyspnea, cyanosis.
Skin: flushing, diaphoresis.
Other: hyperlipidemia, fever, chest and back pains, hypersensitivity reactions, irritation at infusion site.
Delayed reactions:
CNS: focal seizures.
Hematologic: *thrombocytopenia,* leukopenia, leukocytosis.
Hepatic: transient increases in liver function test values, hepatomegaly.
Other: fever, splenomegaly.

INTERACTIONS
None significant.

EFFECTS ON DIAGNOSTIC TESTS
Abnormally high mean corpuscular hemoglobin and mean corpuscular hemoglobin concentration values may be found in blood samples drawn during or shortly after fat emulsion infusion. Fat emulsions may cause transient abnormalities in liver function and may alter results of serum bilirubin tests (especially in infants).

CONTRAINDICATIONS
Contraindicated in hyperlipidemia, lipid nephrosis, or acute pancreatitis accompanied by hyperlipidemia; and in patients with severe egg allergies.

NURSING CONSIDERATIONS
● Use cautiously in patients with severe hepatic disease; pulmonary disease; anemia; or blood coagulation disorders, including thrombocytopenia; and in patients at risk for fat embolism.
● Also use cautiously in jaundiced or premature infants.
● **I.V. use:** Avoid rapid infusion, and use an infusion pump to regulate rate.
● Be aware that drug may be mixed

Reactions may be *common*, uncommon, *life-threatening*, or COMMON AND LIFE-THREATENING.

with amino acid solution, dextrose, electrolytes, and vitamins in the same I.V. container. Check with the pharmacist for acceptable proportions and compatibility information.
- Know that an in-line filter with pores of 1.2 microns or larger is sometimes used to remove particulate matter.
- Do not use fat emulsion if it separates or becomes oily.
- Lipids support bacterial growth, so change all I.V. tubing before each infusion. Check injection site daily. Report signs of inflammation or infection promptly.
- Watch for adverse reactions, especially during first half of infusion.
- Monitor serum lipid levels closely when the patient is receiving fat emulsion therapy. Lipemia must clear between dosing.
- Monitor hepatic function carefully in long-term therapy.
- Check platelet count frequently in neonates receiving fat emulsions I.V.
- Carefully monitor serum triglycerides and free fatty acids in infants.
- Refrigeration is not necessary.
- Intralipid and Liposyn differ mainly by their fatty acid components.

☑ **PATIENT TEACHING**
- Explain need for fat emulsion therapy, and answer any questions.
- Tell patient to report adverse reactions promptly.

---

medium-chain triglycerides
M.C.T. ◊

Pregnancy Risk Category: NR

HOW SUPPLIED
Oil: 960 ml (115 calories/15 ml) ◊

ACTION
Source of rapidly hydrolyzable lipid.

ONSET, PEAK, DURATION
Unknown.

INDICATIONS & DOSAGE
Inadequate digestion or absorption of food fats—
Adults: 15 ml P.O. t.i.d. or q.i.d.

ADVERSE REACTIONS
CNS: reversible *coma* in susceptible patients (such as those with advanced hepatic cirrhosis).
GI: *nausea, vomiting, diarrhea, abdominal distention, cramps.*

INTERACTIONS
None significant.

EFFECTS ON DIAGNOSTIC TESTS
None reported.

CONTRAINDICATIONS
None known.

NURSING CONSIDERATIONS
- Use cautiously in patients with hepatic cirrhosis and complications such as portacaval shunts or tendency to encephalopathy.
- To minimize GI adverse reactions, give smaller, more frequent doses with meals, mixed with salad dressing, or in chilled fruit juice.
- Know that drug is more easily absorbed than long-chain fats; not dependent on bile salts for emulsification.
- Know that drug's rapid metabolism provides quick energy.
- Drug provides 7.7 calories/ml. No essential fatty acids are provided.

☑ **PATIENT TEACHING**
- Instruct patient when and how to take drug to minimize GI adverse reactions.
- Tell patient to report persistent or severe adverse reactions promptly.
- Tell patient not to use plastic containers or utensils to give the drug.

---

allopurinol
colchicine
probenecid
sulfinpyrazone

COMBINATION PRODUCTS
COLBENEMID, PROBEN-C, PROBENECID
WITH COLCHICINE: probenecid 500 mg
and colchicine 0.5 mg.

---

allopurinol
Alloremed‡, Apo-Allopurinol†, Capu-
rate‡, Lopurin, Purinol†, Zyloprim

Pregnancy Risk Category: C

HOW SUPPLIED
Tablets (scored): 100 mg, 300 mg
Capsules: 100 mg‡, 300 mg‡

ACTION
Reduces uric acid production by inhibiting the biochemical reactions preceding
its formation.

ONSET, PEAK, DURATION
Onset occurs within 2 or 3 days. Allopurinol levels peak in ½ to 2 hours; oxy-
purinol (active metabolite) levels in 4½
to 5 hours. Effects persist for 1 to 2
weeks.

INDICATIONS & DOSAGE
*Gout, primary or secondary to hyper-
uricemia; secondary to diseases such as
acute or chronic leukemia, polycythemia vera, multiple myeloma, and psoriasis—*
Dosage varies with severity of disease;
can be given as single dose or divided,
but doses larger than 300 mg should be
divided.
Adults: mild gout, 200 to 300 mg P.O.
daily; severe gout with large tophi, 400
to 600 mg P.O. daily. Same dosage for

maintenance in secondary hyperuricemia. Maximum dosage is 800
mg/day.
*Hyperuricemia secondary to malignan-
cies—*
Children under 6 years: 50 mg P.O.
t.i.d.
Children 6 to 10 years: 300 mg P.O.
daily or divided t.i.d.
Prevention of acute gouty attacks—
Adults: 100 mg P.O. daily; increase at
weekly intervals by 100 mg without exceeding maximum dose (800 mg), until
serum uric acid falls to 6 mg/dl or less.
*Prevention of uric acid nephropathy
during cancer chemotherapy—*
Adults: 600 to 800 mg P.O. daily for 1
to 2 days, with high fluid intake.
Recurrent calcium oxalate calculi—
Adults: 200 to 300 mg P.O. daily in single or divided doses.
In impaired renal function in adults:
200 mg P.O. daily if creatinine clearance is 10 to 20 ml/minute; 100 mg P.O.
daily if less than 10 ml/minute; 100 mg
P.O. more than 24 hours apart if less
than 3 ml/minute.

ADVERSE REACTIONS
CNS: drowsiness, headache, paresthe-
sia, peripheral neuropathy, neuritis.
CV: hypersensitivity vasculitis, necrotizing angiitis.
EENT: epistaxis.
GI: nausea, vomiting, diarrhea, abdominal pain, gastritis, dyspepsia.
GU: *renal failure,* uremia.
Hematologic: *agranulocytosis,* anemia,
aplastic anemia, thrombocytopenia,
leukopenia, leukocytosis, eosinophilia.
Hepatic: altered liver function studies,
hepatitis, hepatic necrosis, hepatomegaly, cholestatic jaundice.
Skin: *rash,* (usually maculopapular);
*exfoliative, urticarial, and purpuric le-
sions; erythema multiforme;* severe fu-

runculosis of nose; ichthyosis, *toxic epidermal necrolysis.*
Other: arthralgia, ecchymoses, fever, myopathy, taste loss or perversion, alopecia, chills.

INTERACTIONS

Amoxicillin, ampicillin, bacampicillin: increased possibility of rash. Avoid concomitant use.

Anticoagulants (except warfarin): potentiation of anticoagulant effect. Dosage adjustments may be necessary.

Antineoplastic agents: increased potential for bone marrow suppression. Monitor the patient carefully.

Chlorpropamide: possible increased hypoglycemic effect. Avoid concomitant use.

Diazoxide, diuretics, ethanol, mecamylamine, pyrazinamide: increased serum acid concentration. Adjust dosage of allopurinol.

Ethacrynic acid, thiazide diuretics: increased risk of allopurinol toxicity. Reduce dosage of allopurinol, and closely monitor renal function.

Uricosuric agents: additive effect. May enhance therapy.

Urine-acidifying agents (ammonium chloride, ascorbic acid, potassium or sodium phosphate): may increase the possibility of kidney stone formation. Monitor the patient carefully.

Xanthines: increased serum theophylline levels. Adjust dosage of theophyllines.

EFFECTS ON DIAGNOSTIC TESTS

Increased alkaline phosphatase, AST, and ALT levels have been reported.

CONTRAINDICATIONS

Contraindicated in patients with hypersensitivity to the drug and in those with idiopathic hemochromatosis.

NURSING CONSIDERATIONS

● Monitor serum uric acid levels to evaluate drug's effectiveness.
● Monitor fluid intake and output; daily

urine output of at least 2 liters and maintenance of neutral or slightly alkaline urine are desirable.
● Periodically monitor CBC and hepatic and renal function, especially at start of therapy, as ordered.
● If renal insufficiency occurs at any time during treatment, be prepared to reduce dosage, as ordered.
● Optimal benefits may require 2 to 6 weeks of therapy. Because acute gouty attacks may occur during this time, concurrent use of colchicine may be prescribed prophylactically.

☑ PATIENT TEACHING

● To minimize GI adverse reactions, tell patient to take with or immediately after meals.
● Encourage the patient to drink plenty of fluids while taking this drug unless otherwise contraindicated.
● Drug may cause drowsiness; tell patient not to drive or perform hazardous tasks requiring mental alertness until CNS effects of the drug are known.
● If the patient is taking allopurinol for treatment of recurrent calcium oxalate stones, advise him to also reduce his dietary intake of animal protein, sodium, refined sugars, oxalate-rich foods, and calcium.
● Tell patient to discontinue at first sign of rash, which may precede severe hypersensitivity or other adverse reaction. Rash is more common in patient taking diuretics and in those with renal disorders. Tell the patient to report all adverse reactions.

colchicine

Colchicine MR‡, Colgout‡, Colsalide, Novocolchicine†

Pregnancy Risk Category: C (oral), D (I.V.)

HOW SUPPLIED

Tablets: 0.5 mg (1/120 grain), 0.6 mg (1/100 grain) as sugar-coated granules

Injection: 1 mg (1/60 grain)/2 ml

ACTION
Unknown. As antigout agent, apparently decreases WBC motility, phagocytosis, and lactic acid production, decreasing urate crystal deposits and reducing inflammation. As antiosteolytic agent, apparently inhibits mitosis of osteoprogenitor cells and decreases osteoclast activity.

ONSET, PEAK, DURATION
Onset is 6 to 12 hours after I.V. administration; within 12 hours after oral administration. Levels peak in 0.5 to 2 hours after oral administration; unknown after I.V. administration. Duration unknown.

INDICATIONS & DOSAGE
Prevention of acute gout attacks as prophylactic or maintenance therapy—
Adults: 0.5 or 0.6 mg P.O. daily. Patients who normally have one attack per year or less should receive drug only 1 to 4 days per week; patients who have more than one attack per year should receive drug daily. In severe cases, 1.5 to 1.95 mg P.O. daily.
Prevention of gout attacks in patients undergoing surgery—
Adults: 0.5 to 0.6 mg P.O. t.i.d. 3 days before and 3 days after surgery.
Acute gout, acute gouty arthritis—
Adults: initially, 0.5 to 1.3 mg P.O., then 0.5 or 0.6 mg q 1 to 2 hours until pain is relieved; nausea, vomiting, or diarrhea ensues; or the maximum dosage of 8 mg is reached. Alternatively, 2 mg I.V., followed by 0.5 mg I.V. q 6 hours if necessary. (Note that some clinicians prefer to give a single I.V. injection of 3 mg.) Total I.V. dosage over 24 hours (one course of treatment) should not exceed 4 mg.

ADVERSE REACTIONS
CNS: peripheral neuritis.
GI: *nausea, vomiting, abdominal pain, diarrhea.*

Hematologic: *aplastic anemia, thrombocytopenia, and agranulocytosis* (with long-term use); nonthrombocytopenic purpura.
Skin: urticaria, dermatitis, hypersensitivity reactions.
Other: alopecia, severe local irritation if extravasation occurs, myopathy, reversible azoospermia.

INTERACTIONS
Cyclosporine: increased GI toxicity with concurrent use. Adjust doses if toxicity occurs.
Erythromycin: increased serum colchicine levels. Observe patient; may need to reduce colchicine dosage.
Ethanol: may impair efficacy of colchicine prophylaxis. Don't use together.
Loop diuretics: may decrease efficacy of colchicine prophylaxis. Avoid concomitant use.
Phenylbutazone: may increase risk of leukopenia or thrombocytopenia. Avoid concomitant use.
Vitamin B_{12}: impaired absorption of oral vitamin B_{12}. Avoid concomitant use.

EFFECTS ON DIAGNOSTIC TESTS
Drug therapy may increase alkaline phosphatase, AST, and ALT levels and may decrease serum carotene, cholesterol, and thrombocyte values. It may cause false-positive results of urine tests for RBCs or hemoglobin.

CONTRAINDICATIONS
Contraindicated in patients with hypersensitivity to drug, blood dyscrasias, or serious CV disease, renal disease, or GI disorders.

NURSING CONSIDERATIONS
• Use cautiously in elderly or debilitated patients or in those with early signs of CV, renal, or GI disease.
• Obtain baseline laboratory studies, including CBC, prior to therapy, as ordered, and then periodically throughout therapy.

Reactions may be *common,* uncommon, *life-threatening,* or COMMON AND LIFE-THREATENING.

● **I.V. use:** Give by slow I.V. push over 2 to 5 minutes. Avoid extravasation because colchicine irritates tissues. Don't dilute colchicine injection with dextrose 5% injection or any other fluid that might change pH of colchicine solution. If lower concentration of colchicine injection is needed, dilute with 0.9% sodium chloride solution or sterile water for injection and give over 2 to 5 minutes by direct injection. Preferably, inject into the tubing of a free-flowing I.V. solution. Don't inject if diluted solution becomes turbid.

● Do not administer I.M. or S.C.; severe local irritation occurs.

● Give with meals to reduce GI effects as maintenance therapy. May be used with uricosuric agents, as ordered.

● Monitor fluid intake and output, and keep output at 2,000 ml daily.

Alert: Know that after a full course of I.V. colchicine (4 mg), no more colchicine should be given by any route for at least 7 days. Colchicine is a toxic drug and fatalities have resulted from overdose.

● The first sign of acute overdose may be GI symptoms, followed by vascular damage, muscle weakness, and ascending paralysis. Delirium and seizures may occur without the patient losing consciousness.

● Discontinue drug as soon as gout pain is relieved or at the first sign of GI symptoms, as ordered.

● Be aware that colchicine has no effect on non-gouty arthritis.

● Store in tightly closed, light-resistant container.

☑ PATIENT TEACHING

● Teach the patient how to take the drug and tell him to drink extra fluids.

● Tell the patient to report adverse reactions, especially signs of acute overdose.

probenecid
Benemid, Benn, Benuryl†, Probalan, Robenecid

Pregnancy Risk Category: NR

HOW SUPPLIED
Tablets: 500 mg

ACTION
Blocks renal tubular reabsorption of uric acid, increasing excretion, and inhibits active renal tubular secretion of many weak organic acids, such as penicillins and cephalosporins.

ONSET, PEAK, DURATION
Onset unknown. Serum levels peak in 2 to 4 hours; peak effects occur in 30 minutes for uricosuric effects and 2 hours for suppression of penicillin excretion. Duration unknown for uricosuric effects; effects persist for about 8 hours for suppression of penicillin excretion.

INDICATIONS & DOSAGE
Adjunct to penicillin therapy—
Adults and children over 50 kg: 500 mg P.O. q.i.d.
Children 2 to 14 years or 50 kg or under: initially, 25 mg/kg P.O., then 40 mg/kg/day in divided doses q.i.d.
Gonorrhea—
Adults: 3.5 g ampicillin P.O. with 1 g probenecid P.O. given together; or 1 g probenecid P.O. 30 minutes before dose of 4.8 million units of aqueous penicillin G procaine I.M., injected at two different sites.
Hyperuricemia of gout, gouty arthritis—
Adults: 250 mg P.O. b.i.d. for 1st week, then 500 mg b.i.d., to maximum of 2 g daily. Maintenance dosage should be reviewed every 6 months and reduced by increments of 500 mg if indicated.

ADVERSE REACTIONS
CNS: *headache,* dizziness.
GI: anorexia, nausea, vomiting, sore

---

*Liquid contains alcohol.   **May contain tartrazine.   †Canada only.   ‡Australia only.   ◇OTC.

gums.
GU: urinary frequency, renal colic, nephrotic syndrome.
Hematologic: *hemolytic anemia,* anemia, *aplastic anemia.*
Skin: dermatitis, pruritus.
Other: flushing, fever, exacerbation of gout, *hepatic necrosis,* hypersensitivity reactions (including *anaphylaxis,* fever).

INTERACTIONS
Acyclovir: when used I.V., may increase acyclovir levels.
Ethanol: increased urate levels. Avoid use.
Indomethacin: decreased indomethacin excretion. Lower indomethacin dosages may be required.
Ketoprofen: increased toxicity. Avoid use.
Methotrexate: decreased methotrexate excretion. Lower methotrexate dosage may be required. Serum levels should be determined.
Nitrofurantoin: increased toxicity and reduced effectiveness. Reduce probenecid dose.
Oral antidiabetic agents: enhanced hypoglycemic effect. Monitor blood glucose levels closely. Dosage adjustment may be required.
Salicylates: inhibited uricosuric effect of probenecid, causing urate retention. Do not use together.
Zidovudine: may increase zidovudine levels and toxicity symptoms. Monitor patient.

EFFECTS ON DIAGNOSTIC TESTS
Drug causes false-positive test results for urinary glucose with tests using cupric sulfate reagent (Benedict's reagent, Clinitest, and Fehling's test); perform tests with glucose oxidase reagent (Clinistix, Tes-Tape) instead. Drug also decreases urinary excretion of 17-ketosteroids, Bromsulphalein (BSP), aminohippuric acid, and iodine-related organic acids, interfering with laboratory procedures.

CONTRAINDICATIONS
Contraindicated in patients with hypersensitivity to drug, uric acid kidney stones, or blood dyscrasias; in acute gout attack; and in children under 2 years.

NURSING CONSIDERATIONS
● Use cautiously in patients with peptic ulcer or renal impairment.
● To minimize GI distress, give with milk, food, or antacids. Continued disturbances might indicate need to lower dosage.
● Monitor periodic BUN and renal function tests in long-term therapy.
● Force fluids to maintain minimum daily output of 2 to 3 liters. Alkalinize urine with sodium bicarbonate or potassium citrate, as ordered. These measures will prevent hematuria, renal colic, urate stone development, and costovertebral pain.
● Keep in mind that therapy is not initiated until acute attack subsides. Contains no analgesic or anti-inflammatory agent, and is of no value during acute gout attacks.
● Be aware that drug is suitable for long-term use; no cumulative effects or tolerance reported.
● Drug is ineffective in patients with chronic renal insufficiency (glomerular filtration rate less than 30 ml/minute).
● Drug may increase frequency, severity, and length of acute gout attacks during first 6 to 12 months of therapy. Prophylactic colchicine or another anti-inflammatory agent is given during first 3 to 6 months.

☑ **PATIENT TEACHING**
● Instruct patient and family that drug must be taken regularly as ordered or gout attacks may result.
● Tell him to visit the doctor regularly so that uric acid can be monitored and dosage adjusted, if necessary. Lifelong therapy may be required in patients with hyperuricemia.
● Advise patient with gout to avoid all

medications that contain aspirin, which may precipitate gout. Acetaminophen may be used for pain.
● Tell patient with gout to avoid alcohol; it increases urate level.
● Tell patient with gout to limit intake of foods high in purine: anchovies, liver, sardines, kidneys, sweetbreads, peas, and lentils. Also tell patient to force fluids.

---

sulfinpyrazone
Anturan†, Anturane

Pregnancy Risk Category: NR

HOW SUPPLIED
Tablets: 100 mg
Capsules: 200 mg

ACTION
Blocks renal tubular reabsorption of uric acid, increasing excretion, and inhibits platelet aggregation.

ONSET, PEAK, DURATION
Onset unknown. Serum levels peak 1 to 2 hours after administration. Effects persist for 4 to 6 hours.

INDICATIONS & DOSAGE
Intermittent or chronic gouty arthritis—
Adults: 200 to 400 mg P.O. b.i.d. 1st week, then 400 mg P.O. b.i.d. Maximum dosage is 800 mg daily.

ADVERSE REACTIONS
GI: *nausea, dyspepsia,* epigastric pain, reactivation of peptic ulcerations.
Hematologic: *blood dyscrasias* (for example, anemia, leukopenia, *agranulocytosis, thrombocytopenia, aplastic anemia*).
Respiratory: bronchoconstriction in patients with aspirin-induced asthma.
Skin: rash.

INTERACTIONS
Oral anticoagulants: increased anticoagulant effect and risk of bleeding. Use

together cautiously.
Oral antidiabetic agents: increased effects. Monitor closely.
Probenecid: inhibited renal excretion of sulfinpyrazone. Use together cautiously.
Salicylates, aspirin: inhibited uricosuric effect of sulfinpyrazone. Do not use together.

EFFECTS ON DIAGNOSTIC TESTS
Drug decreases urinary excretion of aminohippuric acid and phenolsulfonphthalein and may alter renal function test results.

CONTRAINDICATIONS
Contraindicated in patients with hypersensitivity to pyrazole derivatives (including oxyphenbutazone and phenylbutazone), blood dyscrasias, active peptic ulcer, or symptoms of GI inflammation or ulceration.

NURSING CONSIDERATIONS
● Use cautiously in patients with healed peptic ulcer and in pregnant patients.
● To minimize GI disturbances, give with milk, food, or antacids.
● Monitor periodic BUN, CBC, and renal function studies advised during long-term use, as ordered.
● Monitor fluid intake and output closely. Therapy, especially at start, may lead to renal colic and formation of uric acid stones until acid levels are normal (about 6 mg/dl).
● Force fluids to maintain minimum daily output of 2 to 3 liters. Alkalinize urine with sodium bicarbonate or other agent, as ordered.
● Drug contains no analgesic or anti-inflammatory agent and is of no value during acute gout attacks.
● Drug may increase frequency, severity, and length of acute gout attacks during first 6 to 12 months of therapy. Prophylactic colchicine or another anti-inflammatory agent is given during first 3 to 6 months.
● Lifelong therapy may be required in patients with hyperuricemia.

• Keep in mind that alkalinizing agents are used therapeutically to increase sulfinpyrazone activity, preventing urolithiasis.

☑ **PATIENT TEACHING**

• Instruct patient and family that drug must be taken regularly as ordered or gout attacks may result.

• Tell patient to visit the doctor regularly so blood levels can be monitored and dosage adjusted if necessary.

• Warn patient with gout not to take any aspirin-containing medications because these may precipitate gout. Acetaminophen may be used for pain.

• Tell patient with gout to avoid foods high in purine: anchovies, liver, sardines, kidneys, sweetbreads, peas, and lentils. Tell him to force fluids.

93

Enzymes

chymopapain
fibrinolysin and desoxyribonu-
    clease
hyaluronidase

COMBINATION PRODUCTS
None.

---

chymopapain
Chymodiactin

Pregnancy Risk Category: C

HOW SUPPLIED
Powder for injection: 4,000 units/vial,
10,000 units/vial; each unit of chymopapain also known as 1 picoKatal (pKat)

ACTION
Hydrolyzes noncollagenous proteins in
the chondromucoprotein of the nucleus
pulposus.

ONSET, PEAK, DURATION
Onset and peak unknown. Effects persist for at least 1 week.

INDICATIONS & DOSAGE
Herniated lumbar disk—
Adults: 2,000 to 4,000 units (pKat)/disk
injected intradiskally. Maximum dosage
for multiple disk herniation is 8,000
units.

ADVERSE REACTIONS
Systemic: *anaphylaxis, anaphylactoid
reaction; paraplegia, subarachnoid and
intracerebral hemorrhage, seizures,
acute transverse myelitis,* nausea, headache, dizziness, leg weakness, paresthesia, numbness of legs and toes, various
GI disturbances.
Other: *back pain, stiffness, back spasm,
soreness,* erythema, rash, pruritic urticaria, conjunctivitis, vasomotor

rhinitis, angioedema.

INTERACTIONS
Radiographic contrast media: potential
adverse reactions when injected concomitantly with chymopapain. Avoid
concurrent use.

EFFECTS ON DIAGNOSTIC TESTS
None reported.

CONTRAINDICATIONS
Contraindicated in patients with history
of allergy to the drug, papaya, or papaya
derivatives (such as meat tenderizers);
in patients who have previously received an injection of chymopapain; and
in those with severe spondylolisthesis in
addition to spinal stenosis, severe progressing paralysis, or evidence of spinal
cord tumor or a cauda equina lesion.

NURSING CONSIDERATIONS
• A ChymoFAST test can detect hypersensitivity to this drug. Giving histamine receptor antagonists prior to drug
may lessen the severity of anaphylactoid
reactions.
• Drug should be used only by doctors
qualified and experienced to perform
laminectomy, diskectomy, or other
spinal procedures, and who have received specialized training in chemonu-
cleolysis. It shouldn't be injected in any
region other than the lumbar spine; extremely toxic if injected into the subarachnoid space.
• Do not use bacteriostatic water for injection to reconstitute the drug. Use
within 1 hour after reconstitution. Discard unused drug.
• Watch very closely for anaphylactoid
reaction (0.5% of patients). Reaction
may be immediate or delayed up to 1
hour after injection and last for minutes
to several hours. Watch for hypotension

---

and bronchospasm, possibly leading to laryngeal edema, arrhythmias, cardiac arrest, coma, and death. Other signs of allergic response include erythema, pilomotor erection, rash, pruritic urticaria, conjunctivitis, vasomotor rhinitis, angioedema, or various GI disturbances.
• Keep an I.V. line open to manage anaphylaxis quickly, if needed. Keep epinephrine and steroids also available.

☑ **PATIENT TEACHING**
• Instruct the patient to anticipate delayed allergic reactions, such as rash, urticaria, or pruritus, which may occur up to 15 days after injection. He should report these at once.
• Warn the patient that he may experience back pain or involuntary muscle spasm in the lower back for several days after injection. Reassure him that this is common and not chronic.

---

fibrinolysin and desoxyribonuclease
Elase

Pregnancy Risk Category: NR

HOW SUPPLIED
Powder for solution: 25 units fibrinolysin and 15,000 units desoxyribonuclease in 30-ml vial
Ointment: 30 units fibrinolysin and 20,000 units desoxyribonuclease in 30-g tube (with applicator)

ACTION
Fibrinolysin attacks fibrin of blood clots and fibrinous exudates; desoxyribonuclease attacks DNA. Combined enzymatic action debrides wound surfaces and promotes healing.

ONSET, PEAK, DURATION
Unknown.

INDICATIONS & DOSAGE
Debridement of inflammatory and infected lesions—

Adults and children: ointment applied to lesions daily to t.i.d. for as long as enzyme action is desired. Alternatively, solution prepared from powder applied topically as a liquid, spray, or wet dressing.
For wet-to-dry dressing, mix 1 vial of Elase powder with 10 to 50 ml of 0.9% sodium chloride solution; saturate strips of fine gauze with solution. Pack ulcerated area with Elase gauze. Let gauze dry in contact with ulcerated lesion for 6 to 8 hours. Remove dried gauze and repeat t.i.d. or q.i.d.
Mild-to-moderate cervicitis or vaginitis—
Adults: 5 g of ointment inserted intravaginally using applicator once daily h.s. for 5 days or until tube is empty.
Irrigation of infected wounds, empyema cavities, abscesses, otorhinolaryngologic wounds, subcutaneous hematomas—
Adults and children: dilute prepared solution and irrigate wound p.r.n., depending on extent and severity.
For solution as irrigating agent, drain cavity and replace Elase every 6 to 10 hours to reduce amount of by-product accumulation and to minimize loss of enzyme activity.

ADVERSE REACTIONS
Systemic: hyperemia with high doses, hypersensitivity reactions.

INTERACTIONS
None significant.

EFFECTS ON DIAGNOSTIC TESTS
None reported.

CONTRAINDICATIONS
Contraindicated in patients with hypersensitivity to the drug or to bovine products; not for parenteral use.

NURSING CONSIDERATIONS
• Dense, dry eschar is surgically removed before enzymatic debridement. Enzyme must be in constant contact with substrate. Necrotic debris is re-

moved periodically; the enzyme is replenished at least once daily.
● Prepare solution just before use and discard after 24 hours.
● Clean and dry wound; cover with thin layer of Elase and nonadherent dressing.
● Ensure that aseptic wound-dressing techniques are used and that antibiotic therapy is instituted, as ordered.
● Change dressing up to three times daily. Flush away necrotic debris and reapply ointment. Frequency of application may be more important than the amount of drug used.

☑ PATIENT TEACHING
● Explain drug use and administration to patient and family.
● Tell patient to report hypersensitivity reactions promptly.

hyaluronidase
Wydase

Pregnancy Risk Category: C

HOW SUPPLIED
Injection: 150 units/ml in 1-ml, 10-ml vials

ACTION
Hydrolyzes hyaluronic acid, promoting diffusion of fluids in tissues.

ONSET, PEAK, DURATION
Unknown.

INDICATIONS & DOSAGE
Adjunct to increase absorption and dispersion of other injected drugs—
Adults and children: 150 units added to solution containing other drug.
Hypodermoclysis—
Adults and children over 3 years: 150 units injected S.C. before clysis or injected into clysis tubing near needle for each 1,000 ml clysis solution.
Excretory urography when contrast medium is given S.C.—
Adults and children: with the patient

in a prone position, 75 units S.C. over each scapula, followed by injection of contrast medium at same sites.

ADVERSE REACTIONS
Skin: allergic reactions (rare).

INTERACTIONS
Local anesthetics: increased potential for toxic local reaction. Use together cautiously.

EFFECTS ON DIAGNOSTIC TESTS
None reported.

CONTRAINDICATIONS
Contraindicated in patients with hypersensitivity to drug.

NURSING CONSIDERATIONS
● Perform a skin test (0.02 ml of solution) for sensitivity. Don't inject into diseased areas. Watch for local reactions (wheal and pseudopods within 5 minutes and persisting, with itching, for 20 to 30 minutes). Erythema alone is *not* considered positive reaction.
● Do not inject into acutely inflamed or cancerous areas.
● Drug not recommended for I.V. use.
● For children, add 15 units to each 100 ml of solution. The drip rate should not exceed 2 ml/minute.
● Don't add to solutions containing epinephrine and heparin.
● In patients with hypodermoclysis, adjust dosage, rate of injection, and type of solution according to the patient's response, as ordered.
● If solution does gets in eyes, flush with water.
● Protect from heat. Don't use cloudy or discolored solution. Store reconstituted solution below 30° C (86° F), and use within 14 days.

☑ PATIENT TEACHING
● Explain need for drug to patient and family, and describe how drug is given.
● Inform patient about possible adverse skin reactions.

---

carboprost tromethamine
dinoprostone
methylergonovine maleate
oxytocin, synthetic injection
oxytocin, synthetic nasal
    solution

COMBINATION PRODUCTS
None.

---

carboprost tromethamine
Hemabate

Pregnancy Risk Category: C

HOW SUPPLIED
Injection: 250 mcg/ml

ACTION
A prostaglandin that produces strong,
prompt contractions of uterine smooth
muscle, possibly mediated by calcium
and cAMP.

ONSET, PEAK, DURATION
Onset unknown. Serum levels peak in
15 to 60 minutes. Average time to abortion, 16 hours; elimination complete in
24 hours.

INDICATIONS & DOSAGE
*To abort pregnancy between 13th and
20th weeks of gestation—*
Adults: initially, 250 mcg deep I.M.
Subsequent doses of 250 mcg administered at intervals of 1½ to 3½ hours, depending on uterine response. Dosage
may be increased in increments to 500
mcg if contractility is inadequate after
several 250-mcg doses. Total dosage
should not exceed 12 mg.
*Postpartum hemorrhage caused by uter-
ine atony not managed by conventional
methods—*
Adults: 250 mcg by deep I.M. injec-

tion. Repeat doses administered at 15-
to 90-minute intervals, as necessary.
Maximum total dosage is 2 mg.

ADVERSE REACTIONS
CNS: headache, anxiety, hot flashes,
paresthesia, syncope, weakness.
CV: chest pain, arrhythmias.
EENT: blurred vision, eye pain.
GI: *vomiting, diarrhea, nausea.*
GU: endometritis, uterine rupture, uter-
ine or vaginal pain.
Respiratory: coughing, wheezing.
Skin: flushing, rash.
Other: *fever,* chills, backache, breast
tenderness, diaphoresis, leg cramps.

INTERACTIONS
None significant.

EFFECTS ON DIAGNOSTIC TESTS
None reported.

CONTRAINDICATIONS
Contraindicated in patients with hypersensitivity to drug, acute pelvic inflammatory disease, or active cardiac, pulmonary, renal, or hepatic disease.

NURSING CONSIDERATIONS
● Use cautiously in patients with history
of asthma; hypotension; hypertension;
CV, adrenal, renal, or hepatic disease;
anemia; jaundice; diabetes; seizure disorders; or previous uterine surgery.
● Unlike other prostaglandin abortifa-
cients, carboprost is administered by
I.M. injection. Injectable form avoids
risk of expelling vaginal suppositories,
which may occur in the presence of profuse vaginal bleeding.
● Know that carboprost should be used
only by trained personnel in a hospital
setting.

Reactions may be *common*, uncommon, *life-threatening*, or COMMON AND LIFE-THREATENING.

☑ PATIENT TEACHING
● Explain to patient and family how drug works and how it is administered.
● Instruct patient to report adverse reactions promptly.

dinoprostone
Prepidil, Prostin E₂

Pregnancy Risk Category: C

HOW SUPPLIED
Vaginal suppositories: 20 mg
Endocervical gel: 0.5 mg per application (2.5-ml syringe)

ACTION
A prostaglandin that produces strong, prompt contractions of uterine smooth muscle, possibly mediated by calcium and cAMP.

ONSET, PEAK, DURATION
Onset occurs within 10 minutes for suppositories, 15 to 30 minutes for gel. Peak unknown. Contractions persist for 2 to 6 hours following insertion of suppository. Average time to abortion is 17 hours for suppositories; unknown for gel.

INDICATIONS & DOSAGE
To abort second-trimester pregnancy; to evacuate uterus in missed abortion, intrauterine fetal deaths up to 28 weeks of gestation, or benign hydatidiform mole (suppository only)—
Adults: 20-mg suppository inserted high into posterior vaginal fornix. Repeated q 3 to 5 hours until abortion is complete.
Ripening of an unfavorable cervix in pregnant patients at or near term (gel only)—
Adults: contents of one syringe administered intravaginally; if cervix remains unfavorable after 6 hours, dosage repeated. No more than 1.5 mg (three applications) should be given within 24-hour period.

ADVERSE REACTIONS
CNS: *headache, dizziness,* anxiety, hot flashes, paresthesia, weakness, syncope.
CV: chest pain, arrhythmias.
EENT: blurred vision, eye pain.
GI: *nausea, vomiting, diarrhea.*
GU: vaginal pain, vaginitis, endometritis.
Respiratory: coughing, dyspnea.
Skin: rash.
Other: *nocturnal leg cramps, fever, shivering, chills,* backache, breast tenderness, diaphoresis, muscle cramps.

INTERACTIONS
Ethanol: inhibited effectiveness of dinoprostone with high doses. Avoid concomitant use.
Other oxytocics: may potentiate action. Avoid concomitant use.

EFFECTS ON DIAGNOSTIC TESTS
None reported.

CONTRAINDICATIONS
The gel form is contraindicated where prolonged contractions of the uterus are considered inappropriate and in patients with hypersensitivity to prostaglandins or constituents of the gel. Also contraindicated in patients with placenta previa or unexplained vaginal bleeding during this pregnancy and in whom vaginal delivery is not indicated (that is, because of vasa previa or active herpes genitalia). The suppository form is contraindicated in patients with hypersensitivity to the drug, acute pelvic inflammatory disease, and active cardiac, pulmonary, renal, or hepatic disease.

NURSING CONSIDERATIONS
● Use suppository form cautiously in patients with asthma; seizure disorders; anemia; diabetes; hypertension or hypotension; jaundice; CV, renal, or hepatic disease; scarred uterus; cervicitis; or acute vaginitis.
● Use gel form cautiously in patients with asthma or history of asthma, glaucoma or raised intraocular pressure, re-

---

nal or hepatic dysfunction, and in patients with ruptured membranes.

● Administer only when critical care facilities are available.

● Just before use, warm dinoprostone suppositories in their wrapping to room temperature. After administration, patient should remain supine for 10 minutes.

● When used as an abortifacient, be prepared to pretreat the patient with an antiemetic and an antidiarrheal agent.

● When used for cervical ripening, have the patient lying on her back, with the cervix visualized using a speculum. Assist with insertion: using aseptic technique, catheter provided with the drug is used to administer the gel into the cervical canal just below the level of the internal os.

● Be aware that when gel form is used, contents of the syringe are used for one patient only. Discard the syringe, catheter, and any unused drug after administration; do not attempt to administer the small amount of drug remaining in the catheter.

● Treat dinoprostone-induced fever (self-limiting and transient and occurs in approximately 50% of all patients) with water or alcohol sponging and increased fluid intake, not with aspirin.

● Check vaginal discharge regularly.

● Keep in mind that abortion should be complete within 30 hours when suppository form is used.

● Freeze suppositories at –20° C (–4° F).

☑ **PATIENT TEACHING**
● Explain to patient and family how drug works and how it is administered.
● Instruct patient to report adverse reactions promptly.

---

methylergonovine maleate
Methergine

Pregnancy Risk Category: C

HOW SUPPLIED
Tablets: 0.2 mg
Injection: 0.2 mg/ml

ACTION
Increases motor activity of the uterus by direct stimulation.

ONSET, PEAK, DURATION
Onset occurs in 2 to 5 minutes after I.M. use, 5 to 10 minutes after oral use, immediately after I.V. use. Serum levels peak 30 minutes after oral use; unknown for other forms of administration. Effects persist for 3 hours or more after oral or I.M. use; 45 minutes after I.V. administration.

INDICATIONS & DOSAGE
Prevention and treatment of postpartum hemorrhage caused by uterine atony or subinvolution—
Adults: 0.2 mg I.M. q 2 to 4 hours; for excessive uterine bleeding or other emergencies, 0.2 mg I.V. over 1 minute while blood pressure and uterine contractions are monitored. After initial I.M. or I.V. dose, 0.2 mg P.O. q 6 to 8 hours for 2 to 7 days. Dosage decreased if severe cramping occurs.

ADVERSE REACTIONS
CNS: dizziness, headache, *seizures, CVA* (with I.V. use), hallucinations.
CV: hypertension, transient chest pain, palpitations, hypotension.
EENT: tinnitus, nasal congestion, foul taste.
GI: *nausea, vomiting,* diarrhea.
GU: hematuria.
Respiratory: dyspnea.
Other: diaphoresis, thrombophlebitis, leg cramps.

INTERACTIONS
Dopamine, I.V. oxytocin, regional anesthetics, vasoconstrictors: excessive vasoconstriction. Use together cautiously.

EFFECTS ON DIAGNOSTIC TESTS
Drug therapy may decrease serum pro-

---

lactin concentrations.

CONTRAINDICATIONS
Contraindicated in patients with hypertension, toxemia, or sensitivity to ergot preparations and in pregnant patients.

NURSING CONSIDERATIONS
• Use cautiously in patients with sepsis, obliterative vascular disease, or hepatic or renal disease and during last stage of labor.
Alert: **I.V. use:** Keep in mind that drug should not be routinely administered I.V. because of the risk of severe hypertension and CVA. If it must be given by this route, administer slowly over 1 minute with careful blood pressure monitoring. I.V. dose may be diluted to 5 ml with 0.9% sodium chloride solution prior to administration. Contractions begin immediately after I.V. use and continue for up to 45 minutes.
• Monitor and record blood pressure, pulse rate, and uterine response; report any sudden change in vital signs, frequent periods of uterine relaxation, and character and amount of vaginal bleeding.
• Monitor contractions which may continue 3 hours or more after P.O. or I.M. administration.
• Store tablets in tightly closed, light-resistant containers. Discard if discolored.
• Store I.V. solutions below 8° C (46.4° F). Daily stock may be kept at room temperature for 60 to 90 days.

☑ PATIENT TEACHING
• Explain to patient and family how drug works and how it is administered.
• Instruct patient to report adverse reactions promptly.

---

oxytocin, synthetic injection
Oxytocin, Pitocin, Syntocinon

Pregnancy Risk Category: NR

HOW SUPPLIED
Injection: 10 units/ml ampule, vial, or tubex

ACTION
Causes potent and selective stimulation of uterine and mammary gland smooth muscle.

ONSET, PEAK, DURATION
Onset occurs 3 to 5 minutes after I.M. use, immediately after I.V. use. Peak unknown. Effects persist 1 hour after I.V. use, 2 to 3 hours after I.M. use.

INDICATIONS & DOSAGE
Induction or stimulation of labor—
Adults: initially, 1-ml (10 units) ampule in 1,000 ml of dextrose 5% injection or 0.9% sodium chloride solution I.V. infused at 1 to 2 milliunits/minute. Rate increased in increments of no more than 1 to 2 milliunits/minute at 15- to 30-minute intervals until normal contraction pattern is established. Rate decreased when labor is firmly established.
Reduction of postpartum bleeding after expulsion of placenta—
Adults: 10 to 40 units added to 1,000 ml of D_5W or 0.9% sodium chloride solution infused at rate necessary to control bleeding, usually 20 to 40 milliunits/minute. Also, 1 ml (10 units) can be given I.M. after delivery of the placenta.
Incomplete or inevitable abortion—
Adults: 10 units of oxytocin I.V. in 500 ml of 0.9% sodium chloride solution or dextrose 5% in 0.9% sodium chloride solution. Infuse at rate of 10 to 20 milliunits (20 to 40 drops)/minute.

ADVERSE REACTIONS
Maternal—
CNS: *subarachnoid hemorrhage* (from hypertension); *seizures or coma* (from water intoxication).
CV: *hypertension;* increased heart rate, systemic venous return, and cardiac output; *arrhythmias.*
GI: nausea, vomiting.

Hematologic: *afibrinogenemia* (may be related to postpartum bleeding).
Other: hypersensitivity reactions *(anaphylaxis)*, tetanic uterine contractions, *abruptio placentae, impaired uterine blood flow,* pelvic hematoma, *increased uterine motility, uterine rupture, postpartum hemorrhage.*
Fetal—
CV: bradycardia, *PVCs,* arrhythmias.
Respiratory: *anoxia, asphyxia.*
Other: *infant brain damage, low Apgar scores at 5 minutes,* neonatal jaundice, neonatal retinal hemorrhage.

INTERACTIONS
Cyclopropane anesthetics: less pronounced bradycardia and hypotension. Use together cautiously.
Thiopental anesthetics: possible delayed induction. Use together cautiously.
Vasoconstrictors: severe hypertension if oxytocin is given within 3 to 4 hours of vasoconstrictor in patients receiving caudal block anesthetic. Avoid concomitant use.

EFFECTS ON DIAGNOSTIC TESTS
None reported.

CONTRAINDICATIONS
Contraindicated when cephalopelvic disproportion is present or when delivery requires conversion, as in transverse lie; in fetal distress when delivery isn't imminent, prematurity, and other obstetric emergencies; and in patients with severe toxemia, hypertonic uterine patterns, hypersensitivity to drug, total placenta previa, and vasoprevia.

NURSING CONSIDERATIONS
● Use with extreme caution during first and second stages of labor because cervical laceration, uterine rupture, and maternal and fetal death have been reported.
● Use with extreme caution, if at all, in patients with history of cervical or uterine surgery (including cesarean section), grand multiparity, uterine sepsis, trau-matic delivery, or overdistended uterus and in invasive cervical cancer.
● **I.V. use:** Don't give by I.V. bolus injection. Administer by infusion only; give by piggyback infusion so the drug may be discontinued without interrupting the I.V. line. Use an infusion pump.
● Know that drug is not recommended for routine I.M. use. However, 10 units may be given I.M. after delivery of placenta to control postpartum uterine bleeding.
● Never give oxytocin simultaneously by more than one route.
● Be aware that drug is used to induce or reinforce labor only when pelvis is known to be adequate, when vaginal delivery is indicated, when fetal maturity is assured, and when fetal position is favorable. Should be used only in hospital where critical care facilities and doctor are immediately available.
● Monitor fluid intake and output. Antidiuretic effect may lead to fluid overload, seizures, and coma.
● Monitor and record uterine contractions, heart rate, blood pressure, intrauterine pressure, fetal heart rate, and character of blood loss every 15 minutes.
● Have magnesium sulfate (20% solution) available for relaxation of the myometrium.
● If contractions occur less than 2 minutes apart and if contractions above 50 mm Hg are recorded, or if contractions last 90 seconds or longer, stop infusion, turn the patient on her side, and notify the doctor.
● Oxytocin is not known to present a risk of fetal abnormalities when used as indicated.

☑ **PATIENT TEACHING**
● Explain to patient and family how drug works and how it is administered.
● Instruct patient to report adverse reactions promptly.

oxytocin, synthetic nasal solution
Syntocinon

Pregnancy Risk Category: X

HOW SUPPLIED
Nasal solution: 40 units/ml

ACTION
Stimulates smooth muscle to facilitate ejection of milk from breasts.

ONSET, PEAK, DURATION
Onset occurs within a few minutes. Peak unknown. Effects persist for 20 minutes.

INDICATIONS & DOSAGE
Promotion of initial milk ejection—
Adults: 1 spray into one or both nostrils 2 or 3 minutes before breast-feeding or pumping breasts.

ADVERSE REACTIONS
EENT: nasal irritation, rhinorrhea, lacrimation.
Other: uterine bleeding, uterine contractions.

INTERACTIONS
None significant.

EFFECTS ON DIAGNOSTIC TESTS
None reported.

CONTRAINDICATIONS
Contraindicated in patients with hypersensitivity to the drug and during pregnancy.

NURSING CONSIDERATIONS
● Inspect nasal cavity for signs of irritation.

☑ PATIENT TEACHING
● Teach patient how to administer drug. Instruct her to clear nasal passages first, then hold her head in a vertical position and, holding squeeze bottle upright, eject solution into nostril.
● Inform patient of adverse reactions associated with drug and to notify doctor if severe.

flavoxate hydrochloride
oxybutynin chloride
phenazopyridine hydrochloride

COMBINATION PRODUCTS
None.

---

flavoxate hydrochloride
Urispas

Pregnancy Risk Category: B

HOW SUPPLIED
Tablets: 100 mg

ACTION
Produces direct spasmolytic effect on smooth muscles of the urinary tract and provides some local anesthesia and analgesia.

ONSET, PEAK, DURATION
Onset and duration unknown. Levels peak within 2 hours.

INDICATIONS & DOSAGE
Symptomatic relief of dysuria, urinary frequency and urgency, nocturia, incontinence, and suprapubic pain associated with urologic disorders—
Adults and children over 12 years:
100 to 200 mg P.O. t.i.d. to q.i.d. Dosage may be reduced with improvement of symptoms.

ADVERSE REACTIONS
CNS: *confusion* (especially in elderly patients), nervousness, dizziness, headache, drowsiness.
CV: tachycardia, palpitations.
EENT: *blurred vision,* disturbed eye accommodation, increased ocular tension.
GI: dry mouth, nausea, vomiting.
GU: dysuria.
Hematologic: eosinophila, leukopenia.

Skin: urticaria, dermatoses.
Other: fever.

INTERACTIONS
None significant.

EFFECTS ON DIAGNOSTIC TESTS
None reported.

CONTRAINDICATIONS
Contraindicated in patients with pyloric or duodenal obstruction, obstructive intestinal lesions or ileus, achalasia, GI hemorrhage, or obstructive uropathies of lower urinary tract.

NURSING CONSIDERATIONS
● Use cautiously in patients suspected of having glaucoma.
● Know that safety and effectiveness in children 12 years and under is unknown.
● Check history for other drug use before giving drugs with anticholinergic adverse reactions. Such reactions may be intensified by flavoxate.

☑ **PATIENT TEACHING**
● Warn patient to avoid hazardous activities, such as operating machinery or driving, until CNS effects of the drug are known.
● Tell patient to contact the doctor if he experiences adverse reactions to the drug or if symptoms don't diminish.

---

oxybutynin chloride
Ditropan

Pregnancy Risk Category: B

HOW SUPPLIED
Tablets: 5 mg
Syrup: 5 mg/5 ml

Reactions may be *common,* uncommon, *life-threatening,* or COMMON AND LIFE-THREATENING.

ACTION
Produces a direct spasmolytic effect and an antimuscarinic (atropine-like) effect on urinary tract smooth muscles, increasing urinary bladder capacity and providing some local anesthesia and mild analgesia.

ONSET, PEAK, DURATION
Onset occurs in 30 to 60 minutes. Levels peak within 3 to 4 hours. Effects persist for 6 to 10 hours.

INDICATIONS & DOSAGE
Antispasmodic for uninhibited or reflex neurogenic bladder—
Adults: 5 mg P.O. b.i.d. to t.i.d., to maximum of 5 mg q.i.d.
Children over 5 years: 5 mg P.O. b.i.d., to maximum of 5 mg t.i.d.

ADVERSE REACTIONS
CNS: dizziness, insomnia, restlessness, hallucinations, asthenia.
CV: *palpitations, tachycardia,* vasodilation.
EENT: mydriasis, cycloplegia, decreased lacrimation, amblyopia.
GI: nausea, vomiting, *constipation, dry mouth,* decreased GI motility.
GU: *urinary hesitancy or urine retention.*
Skin: rash.
Other: decreased diaphoresis, fever, impotence, suppression of lactation.

INTERACTIONS
None significant.

EFFECTS ON DIAGNOSTIC TESTS
None reported.

CONTRAINDICATIONS
Contraindicated in patients with hypersensitivity to drug, myasthenia gravis, GI obstruction, untreated narrow-angle glaucoma, adynamic ileus, megacolon, severe colitis, ulcerative colitis when megacolon is present, or obstructive uropathy; in elderly or debilitated patients with intestinal atony; and in hem-

orrhaging patients with unstable CV status.

NURSING CONSIDERATIONS
● Use cautiously in elderly patients and in patients with autonomic neuropathy, reflux esophagitis, and hepatic or renal disease.
● Before giving oxybutynin, anticipate confirmation of neurogenic bladder by cystometry and rule out partial intestinal obstruction in patients with diarrhea, especially those with colostomy or ileostomy.
● If urinary tract infection is present, administer antibiotics, as ordered.
● Be aware that drug may aggravate symptoms of hyperthyroidism, coronary artery disease, CHF, arrhythmias, tachycardia, hypertension, or prostatic hyperplasia.
● Periodically prepare patient for cystometry to evaluate response to therapy.
● To minimize tendency toward tolerance, be prepared to stop therapy periodically to determine tolerance.

☑ PATIENT TEACHING
● Warn patient to avoid hazardous activities, such as operating machinery or driving, until CNS effects of the drug are known.
● Caution patient that using oxybutynin during very hot weather may precipitate fever or heatstroke because it suppresses diaphoresis.
● Advise patient to store the drug in tightly closed containers at 59° to 86° F (15° to 30° C).

---

phenazopyridine hydrochloride (phenylazo diamino pyridine hydrochloride)
Azo-Standard◇, Baridium◇, Di-Azo◇, Eridium◇, Geridium◇, Phenazo†, Phenazodine◇, Prodium◇, Pyrazodine◇, Pyridiate◇, Pyridin◇, Pyridium,

---

Pyronium†, Urodine◇, Urogesic◇, Viridium◇

Pregnancy Risk Category: B

HOW SUPPLIED
Tablets: 100 mg◇, 200 mg

ACTION
Unknown. Exerts local anesthetic action on urinary mucosa through unknown mechanism.

ONSET, PEAK, DURATION
Unknown.

INDICATIONS & DOSAGE
Pain with urinary tract irritation or infection—
Adults: 200 mg P.O. t.i.d. after meals for 2 days.
Children: 12 mg/kg P.O. daily in three equally divided doses after meals for 2 days.

ADVERSE REACTIONS
CNS: headache.
GI: nausea, GI disturbances.
Hematologic: hemolytic anemia.
Skin: rash, pruritus.
Other: *anaphylactoid reactions,* methemoglobinemia.

INTERACTIONS
None significant.

EFFECTS ON DIAGNOSTIC TESTS
Drug may alter results of Clinistix, Tes-Tape, Acetest, and Ketostix. Clinitest should be used to obtain accurate urine glucose test results. Drug may also interfere with Ehrlich's test for urine urobilinogen; phenolsulfonphthalein (PSP) excretion tests of kidney function; sulfobromophthalein (BSP) excretion tests of liver function; and urine tests for protein, steroids, or bilirubin.

CONTRAINDICATIONS
Contraindicated in patients with hypersenstivity to drug, glomerulonephritis, severe hepatitis, uremia, pyelonephritis during pregnancy, or renal insufficiency.

NURSING CONSIDERATIONS
● Know that when drug is used with an antibacterial agent, therapy should not extend beyond 2 days.

☑ PATIENT TEACHING
● Advise patient that taking the drug with meals may minimize GI distress.
● Caution patient to stop taking drug and to notify the doctor immediately if skin or sclera becomes yellow-tinged. These signs may indicate drug accumulation caused by impaired renal excretion.
● Alert patient that drug colors urine red or orange. May stain fabrics or contact lenses.
● Tell diabetic patient that drug may alter Clinistix or Tes-Tape results. He should use Clinitest for accurate urine glucose test results. Also tell patient drug may interfere with urinary ketone tests (Acetest or Ketostix).

---

auranofin
aurothioglucose
gold sodium thiomalate

COMBINATION PRODUCTS
None.

---

auranofin
Ridaura

Pregnancy Risk Category: C

HOW SUPPLIED
Capsules: 3 mg

ACTION
Unknown. Anti-inflammatory effects in rheumatoid arthritis are probably caused by inhibition of sulfhydryl systems, which alters cellular metabolism. Auranofin may also alter enzyme function and immune response and suppress phagocytic activity.

ONSET, PEAK, DURATION
Onset occurs in 1 to 3 months, possibly 6 months. Serum levels peak within 2 hours. Effects may last for months after drug is discontinued.

INDICATIONS & DOSAGE
Rheumatoid arthritis—
Adults: 6 mg P.O. daily, either as 3 mg b.i.d. or 6 mg once daily. After 6 months, may be increased to 9 mg daily.

ADVERSE REACTIONS
CNS: confusion, hallucinations, *seizures.*
EENT: conjunctivitis.
GI: *diarrhea, abdominal pain, nausea, stomatitis,* glossitis, anorexia, metallic taste, dyspepsia, flatulence, constipation, dysgeusia, *ulcerative colitis.*
GU: proteinuria, hematuria, nephrotic syndrome, glomerulonephritis, *acute renal failure.*
Hematologic: *thrombocytopenia* (with or without purpura), *aplastic anemia, agranulocytosis,* leukopenia, eosinophilia, anemia.
Hepatic: jaundice, elevated liver enzymes.
Respiratory: interstitial pneumonitis.
Skin: *rash, pruritus, dermatitis, exfoliative dermatitis,* urticaria, erythema, alopecia.

INTERACTIONS
Phenytoin: may increase phenytoin blood levels. Monitor for toxicity.

EFFECTS ON DIAGNOSTIC TESTS
Serum protein-bound iodine test, especially when done by the chloric acid digestion method, gives false readings during and for several weeks after gold therapy.

CONTRAINDICATIONS
Contraindicated in patients with history of severe gold toxicity, necrotizing enterocolitis, pulmonary fibrosis, exfoliative dermatitis, bone marrow aplasia, severe hematologic disorders or history of severe toxicity caused by previous exposure to other heavy metals. Also contraindicated in patients with urticaria, eczema, colitis, severe debilitation, hemorrhagic conditions, or systemic lupus erythematosus and in patients who have recently received radiation therapy.

NURSING CONSIDERATIONS
● Use cautiously with other drugs that cause blood dyscrasias. Also use cautiously in patients who have preexisting renal, hepatic, or inflammatory bowel disease; skin rash; or a history of bone marrow depression.
● Monitor patient's platelet count

---

monthly. Auranofin should be stopped if platelet count falls below 100,000/mm^3, if hemoglobin drops suddenly, if granulocytes are below 1,500/mm^3, or if leukopenia (WBC count below 4,000/mm^3) or eosinophilia (eosinophils greater than 75%) is present.

● Monitor patient's urinalysis results. If proteinuria or hematuria is detected, stop drug because it can cause nephrotic syndrome or glomerulonephritis, and notify doctor.

☑ **PATIENT TEACHING**
● Encourage patient to take drug as prescribed.
● Tell patient to continue concomitant drug therapy if prescribed.
● Remind patient to see the doctor for monthly platelet counts.
● Suggest patient have regular urinalysis.
● Tell patient to keep taking drug if mild diarrhea occurs but to immediately report blood in stool. Diarrhea is the most common adverse reaction.
● Advise patient to report rashes or other skin problems and stop drug until reaction subsides. Pruritus may precede dermatitis; any pruritic skin eruption while patient is receiving auranofin should be considered a reaction until proven otherwise.
● Advise patient that stomatitis may be preceded by a metallic taste, which he should report. Promote careful oral hygiene during therapy.
● Inform patient that beneficial effect may be delayed as long as 3 months. If response is inadequate and maximum dose has been reached, expect the doctor to discontinue drug.
● Warn patient not to give the drug to others. Auranofin should be prescribed only for selected rheumatoid arthritis patients.

aurothioglucose
Gold-50‡, Solganal

gold sodium thiomalate
Myochrysine

Pregnancy Risk Category: C

HOW SUPPLIED
aurothioglucose
Injection (suspension): 50 mg/ml in sesame oil in 10-ml vial
gold sodium thiomalate
Injection: 25 mg/ml, 50 mg/ml with benzyl alcohol

ACTION
Unknown. Anti-inflammatory effects in rheumatoid arthritis are probably caused by inhibition of sulfhydryl systems, which alters cellular metabolism. Gold salts may also alter enzyme function and immune response and suppress phagocytic activity.

ONSET, PEAK, DURATION
Onset and duration unknown. Serum levels peak within 3 to 6 hours.

INDICATIONS & DOSAGE
Rheumatoid arthritis—
aurothioglucose
Adults: initially, 10 mg I.M., followed by 25 mg for second and third doses at weekly intervals. Then, 50 mg weekly until 800 mg to 1 g has been given. If improvement occurs without toxicity, 25 to 50 mg is continued at 3- to 4-week intervals indefinitely.
Children 6 to 12 years: one-fourth the usual adult dosage. Do not exceed 25 mg per dose.
gold sodium thiomalate
Adults: initially, 10 mg I.M., followed by 25 mg in 1 week. Then, 25 to 50 mg weekly to total dose of 1 g. If improvement occurs without toxicity, 25 to 50 mg q 2 weeks for 2 to 20 weeks; then, 25 to 50 mg q 3 to 4 weeks as maintenance therapy. If relapse occurs, injections are resumed at weekly intervals.
Children: initially, 10 mg I.M., followed by 1 mg/kg I.M. weekly. Follow

adult spacing of doses.

ADVERSE REACTIONS
CNS: confusion, hallucinations, *seizures.*
CV: bradycardia, hypotension.
EENT: corneal gold deposition, corneal ulcers.
GI: *metallic taste, stomatitis, diarrhea,* anorexia, abdominal cramp, nausea, vomiting, ulcerative enterocolitis.
GU: albuminuria, proteinuria, *nephrotic syndrome,* nephritis, acute tubular necrosis, hematuria, *acute renal failure.*
Hematologic: *thrombocytopenia* (with or without purpura), *aplastic anemia, agranulocytosis,* leukopenia, eosinophilia, anemia.
Hepatic: hepatitis, jaundice, elevated liver function tests.
Skin: photosensitivity, *rash, dermatitis,* erythema, exfoliative dermatitis.
Other: *anaphylaxis, angioedema,* diaphoresis.

INTERACTIONS
None significant.

EFFECTS ON DIAGNOSTIC TESTS
Serum protein-bound iodine test, especially when done by chloric acid digestion method, gives false readings during and for several weeks after therapy.

CONTRAINDICATIONS
Contraindicated in patients with hypersensitivity to the drug; in those with a history of severe toxicity from previous exposure to gold or other heavy metals, hepatitis, or exfoliative dermatitis; and in patients with severe uncontrollable diabetes, renal disease, hepatic dysfunction, uncontrolled heart failure, systemic lupus erythematosus, colitis, or Sjögren's syndrome. Also contraindicated in patients with urticaria, eczema, hemorrhagic conditions, or severe hematologic disorders and in those who have recently received radiation therapy.

NURSING CONSIDERATIONS
● Use with extreme caution, if at all, in patients with rash, marked hypertension, compromised cerebral or CV circulation, or history of renal or hepatic disease, drug allergies, or blood dyscrasias.
● Give only under constant supervision of doctor thoroughly familiar with drug's toxicities and benefits.
● Give gold salts I.M., as ordered, preferably intragluteally. Drug is pale yellow; don't use if it darkens.
● Immerse aurothioglucose vial in warm water; shake vigorously before injecting.
● When injecting gold sodium thiomalate, have patient lie down for 10 to 20 minutes to minimize hypotension.
● Watch for anaphylactoid reaction for 30 minutes after administration.
Alert: Keep dimercaprol on hand to treat acute toxicity.
● Analyze urine for protein and sediment changes before each injection.
● Monitor CBC, including platelet count, before every second injection.
● Monitor platelet counts if patients develop purpura or ecchymoses.
● Know that gold therapy may alter liver function studies.
● If adverse reactions are mild, some rheumatologists resume gold therapy after 2 to 3 weeks' rest.

☑ PATIENT TEACHING
● Advise patient that increased joint pain may occur for 1 to 2 days after injection but usually subsides.
● Advise patient to report rashes or skin problems and stop drug until reaction subsides. Pruritus may precede dermatitis; any pruritic skin eruption while patient is receiving gold therapy should be considered a reaction until proven otherwise.
● Advise patient to report a metallic taste. Promote careful oral hygiene.
● Tell patient to avoid sunlight and artificial ultraviolet light.
● Tell patient that benefits may not appear for 3 to 4 months.
● Stress need for medical follow-up.

Miscellaneous antagonists and antidotes

activated charcoal
aminocaproic acid
ammonia, aromatic spirits
deferoxamine mesylate
digoxin immune FAB
dimercaprol
disulfiram
d-penicillamine
edetate calcium disodium
edetate disodium
flumazenil
ipecac syrup
naloxone hydrochloride
naltrexone hydrochloride
pralidoxime chloride
protamine sulfate
sodium polystyrene sulfonate
succimer
trientine hydrochloride

(See also Chapter 38, anticholinergics.)
(See also Chapter 40, adrenergic blockers [sympatholytics].)

COMBINATION PRODUCTS
None.

---

activated charcoal
Actidose ◇, Actidose-Aqua ◇, Charcoaide ◇, Charcocaps ◇, LiquiChar ◇, Superchar ◇

Pregnancy Risk Category: C

HOW SUPPLIED
Tablets: 200 mg‡ ◇, 300 mg‡ ◇, 325 mg ◇, 650 mg ◇
Capsules: 260 mg ◇
Powder: 30 g ◇, 50 g ◇
Oral suspension: 0.625 g/5 ml ◇, 0.83 g/5 ml ◇, 1 g/5 ml ◇, 1.25 g/5 ml ◇

ACTION
An adsorbent that adheres to many drugs and chemicals, inhibiting their absorption from the GI tract.

ONSET, PEAK, DURATION
Onset immediate upon contact. Peak and duration not applicable because drug is not absorbed.

INDICATIONS & DOSAGE
Flatulence or dyspepsia—
Adults: 600 mg to 5 g P.O. as a single dose or 0.975 g to 3.9 g P.O. t.i.d. after meals.
Poisoning—
Adults and children: initially, 1 to 2 g/kg (30 to 100 g) P.O. or 10 times the amount of poison ingested as a suspension in 120 to 240 ml (4 to 8 oz) of water.

Commonly used for treating poisoning or overdosage with acetaminophen, aspirin, atropine, barbiturates, dextropropoxyphene, digitalis glycosides, poisonous mushrooms, oxalic acid, parathion, phenol, phenylpropanolamine, phenytoin, propantheline, propoxyphene, strychnine, or tricyclic antidepressants.

Check with poison control center for use in other types of poisonings or overdoses.

ADVERSE REACTIONS
GI: *black stools,* nausea, constipation, ***intestinal obstruction.***

INTERACTIONS
Acetylcysteine, ipecac: agents inactivated by charcoal. Administer charcoal after vomiting has been induced by ipecac; remove charcoal by nasogastric tube before giving acetylcysteine.

EFFECTS ON DIAGNOSTIC TESTS
None reported.

Reactions may be *common,* uncommon, *life-threatening,* or COMMON AND LIFE-THREATENING.

CONTRAINDICATIONS
None known.

NURSING CONSIDERATIONS
• Know that although there are no contraindications for the drug, it is not effective in the treatment of all acute poisonings.
• Give after emesis is complete because activated charcoal absorbs and inactivates syrup of ipecac.
• Mix powder form (most effective) with tap water to form consistency of thick syrup. Adding a small amount of fruit juice or flavoring will make mix more palatable. Do not mix with ice cream, milk, or sherbet because these will decrease the absorptive capacity of activated charcoal.
• Give by large bore nasogastric tube after lavage if necessary.
• If patient vomits shortly after administration, be prepared to repeat dose.
• Space doses at least 1 hour apart from other drugs if treatment is for any indication other than poisoning.
• Follow treatment with stool softener or laxative, as ordered, to prevent constipation unless sorbitol is part of product ingredients.
• Be aware that preparations made with sorbitol have a laxative effect that lessens the risk of severe constipation or fecal impaction.
• Do not use charcoal with sorbitol in fructose-intolerant patients or in children under 1 year.
• Ineffective for poisoning or overdose of cyanide, mineral acids, caustic alkalis, and organic solvents; not very effective with ethanol, lithium, methanol, and iron salts.

☑ **PATIENT TEACHING**
• Explain to patient (if awake) and family purpose of drug and how it will be administered.
• Warn patient that stools will be black.

aminocaproic acid
Amicar

Pregnancy Risk Category: C

HOW SUPPLIED
Tablets: 500 mg
Syrup: 250 mg/ml
Injection: 250 mg/ml

ACTION
Inhibits plasminogen activator substances and, to a lesser degree, blocks antiplasmin activity by inhibiting fibrinolysis.

ONSET, PEAK, DURATION
Onset occurs within 1 hour. Levels peak within 2 hours after oral administration; unknown after I.V. administration. Effects persist for less than 3 hours after I.V. administration, unknown for oral administration.

INDICATIONS & DOSAGE
Excessive bleeding resulting from hyperfibrinolysis—
Adults: initially, 5 g P.O. or slow I.V. infusion, followed by 1 to 1.25 g hourly until bleeding is controlled. Maximum dosage is 30 g daily.

ADVERSE REACTIONS
CNS: dizziness, malaise, headache, delirium, *seizures,* hallucinations, weakness.
CV: hypotension, bradycardia, *arrhythmias* (with rapid I.V. infusion).
EENT: tinnitus, nasal congestion, conjunctival suffusion.
GI: nausea, cramps, diarrhea.
Hematologic: generalized thrombosis.
Skin: rash.
Other: malaise, myopathy, *acute renal failure.*

INTERACTIONS
Estrogens, oral contraceptives: increased probability of hypercoagulability. Use together cautiously.

EFFECTS ON DIAGNOSTIC TESTS
Drug may elevate serum potassium level in some patients with decreased renal function; it may increase CK, AST, and ALT levels.

CONTRAINDICATIONS
Contraindicated in patients with active intravascular clotting or presence of disseminated intravascular coagulation unless heparin is used concomitantly. Injectable form is contraindicated in newborns.

NURSING CONSIDERATIONS
• Use cautiously in patients with cardiac, hepatic, or renal disease.
• **I.V. use:** Dilute solution with sterile water for injection, 0.9% sodium chloride for injection, D₅W, or Ringer's injection. Infuse slowly. Don't give by direct or intermittent injection.
Alert: Monitor coagulation studies as ordered and heart rhythm and blood pressure. Notify the doctor of any change immediately.

☑ **PATIENT TEACHING**
• Explain drug use and how it will be administered to patient and family.
• Instruct patient to report adverse reactions promptly.

___

ammonia, aromatic spirits◇

Pregnancy Risk Category: NR

HOW SUPPLIED
Solution: 30 ml ◇, 60 ml ◇, 120 ml ◇; pints ◇; gallons ◇
Inhalant: 0.33 ml ◇, 0.4 ml ◇

ACTION
Irritates the sensory receptors in the nasal membranes, producing reflex stimulation of the respiratory centers.

ONSET, PEAK, DURATION
Onset immediate. Peak and duration unknown.

INDICATIONS & DOSAGE
Treatment or prevention of fainting—
Adults and children: inhale 1 broken capsule until awake or no longer faint. Oral: 2 to 4 ml P.O., diluted in at least 30 ml of water.

ADVERSE REACTIONS
EENT: irritation.

INTERACTIONS
None significant.

EFFECTS ON DIAGNOSTIC TESTS
No information available.

CONTRAINDICATIONS
None known.

NURSING CONSIDERATIONS
• Avoid inhaling vapors when administering drug.
• Monitor patient closely for response.

☑ **PATIENT TEACHING**
• Instruct patient how to use drug.
• Tell patient to store in refrigerator.

___

deferoxamine mesylate
Desferal

Pregnancy Risk Category: C

HOW SUPPLIED
Powder for injection: 500 mg

ACTION
Chelates iron by binding ferric ions.

ONSET, PEAK, DURATION
Unknown.

INDICATIONS & DOSAGE
Adjunctive treatment of acute iron intoxication—
Adults and children: 1 g I.M., followed by 500 mg I.M. for two doses q 4 hours; then 500 mg I.M. q 4 to 12 hours. Maximum dosage is 6 g in 24 hours. Give I.V. by slow infusion (15 mg/kg/

hour or less) only in CV collapse.
Chronic iron overload from multiple transfusions—
Adults and children: 500 mg to 1 g I.M. daily and 2 g by slow I.V. infusion in separate solution along with each unit of blood transfused. Maximum dosage is 6 g daily. Alternatively, 20 to 40 mg/kg via S.C. infusion pump daily.

ADVERSE REACTIONS
CV: tachycardia with long-term use.
EENT: blurred vision, cataracts, hearing loss.
GI: diarrhea and abdominal discomfort with long-term use.
GU: dysuria with long-term use.
Other: hypersensitivity reactions (cutaneous wheal formation, pruritus, rash, *anaphylaxis*); pain and induration at injection site; leg cramps, fever; after too-rapid I.V. administration—*erythema, urticaria, hypotension, shock.*

INTERACTIONS
Ascorbic acid: may enhance the effects of deferoxamine and increase tissue toxicity of iron. Use together with extreme caution and close monitoring.

EFFECTS ON DIAGNOSTIC TESTS
None reported.

CONTRAINDICATIONS
Contraindicated in patients with severe renal disease or anuria.

NURSING CONSIDERATIONS
● Use cautiously in patients with impaired renal function.
● To reconstitute, add 2 ml of sterile water for injection to each ampule. Make sure drug is completely dissolved. Reconstituted solution is good for 1 week at room temperature. Protect from light.
● After reconstitution, administer I.M. or add to 0.9% sodium chloride solution, D₅W, or lactated Ringer's solution and infuse at a rate not exceeding 15 mg/kg hour.
● Have epinephrine 1:1,000 available to

treat hypersensitivity reaction.
● Monitor fluid intake and output carefully.

☑ PATIENT TEACHING
● Warn patient that urine may be red. Tell patient to report persistent or serious adverse reactions promptly.
● Advise patient to have regular eye examinations during long-term therapy because cataract formation has been reported.

---

digoxin immune FAB (ovine)
Digibind

Pregnancy Risk Category: C

HOW SUPPLIED
Injection: 38-mg vial

ACTION
Binds molecules of unbound digoxin and digitoxin, making them unavailable for binding at site of action on cells.

ONSET, PEAK, DURATION
Onset variable but thought to occur within 30 minutes. Peak occurs at completion of I.V. infusion. Effects persist for 2 to 6 hours.

INDICATIONS & DOSAGE
Potentially life-threatening digoxin or digitoxin intoxication—
Adults and children: I.V. dosage varies according to the amount of digoxin or digitoxin to be neutralized. Each vial binds about 0.5 mg of digoxin or digitoxin. Average dosage is 6 vials (228 mg). However, if the toxicity resulted from acute digoxin ingestion and neither a serum digoxin level nor an estimated ingestion amount is known, 20 vials (760 mg) may be required. See package insert for complete, specific dosage instructions.

ADVERSE REACTIONS
CV: *CHF* and rapid ventricular rate

---

*Liquid contains alcohol.   **May contain tartrazine.   †Canada only.   ‡Australia only.   ◇OTC.

(both caused by reversal of the digitalis glycoside's therapeutic effects).
Other: hypersensitivity reactions, hypokalemia, *anaphylaxis*.

INTERACTIONS
None significant.

EFFECTS ON DIAGNOSTIC TESTS
Therapy alters standard cardiac glycoside determinations by radioimmunoassay procedures. Results may be falsely increased or decreased, depending on separation method used. Serum potassium levels may decrease rapidly.

CONTRAINDICATIONS
None known.

NURSING CONSIDERATIONS
● Use cautiously in patients known to be allergic to ovine proteins or those who have previously received antibodies. In these high-risk patients, skin testing is recommended because the drug is derived from digoxin-specific antibody fragments obtained from immunized sheep.
● Know that drug is used only for life-threatening overdose in patients in shock or cardiac arrest; with ventricular arrhythmias, such as ventricular tachycardia or fibrillation; with progressive bradycardia, such as severe sinus bradycardia; or with second- or third-degree AV block not responsive to atropine.
● **I.V. use:** Reconstitute 38-mg vial with 4 ml of sterile water for injection. Gently roll vial to dissolve the powder. Reconstituted solution contains 9.5 mg/ml. Drug may be given by direct injection if cardiac arrest seems imminent. Alternatively, dilute with 0.9% sodium chloride for injection to an appropriate volume and give by intermittent infusion over 30 minutes.
● Infuse the drug through a 0.22-micron membrane filter.
● Refrigerate powder for injection. Reconstitute drug immediately before use. Reconstituted solutions may be refriger-

ated for 4 hours.
● Monitor potassium level closely, as ordered.
● Know that in most patients, signs of digitalis toxicity disappear within a few hours.
● Be aware that because drug will interfere with digitalis immunoassay measurements, standard serum digoxin levels will be misleading until drug is cleared from body (about 2 days).

☑ **PATIENT TEACHING**
● Explain need for drug and how drug is administered to patient and family.
● Instruct patient to report adverse reactions promptly.

dimercaprol
BAL in Oil

Pregnancy Risk Category: NR

HOW SUPPLIED
Injection: 100 mg/ml

ACTION
Forms complexes with heavy metals.

ONSET, PEAK, DURATION
Onset unknown. Levels peak within 30 to 60 minutes. Effects persist for 4 hours.

INDICATIONS & DOSAGE
Severe arsenic or gold poisoning—
Adults and children: 3 mg/kg deep I.M. q 4 hours for 2 days, then q.i.d. on 3rd day, then b.i.d. for 10 days.
Mild arsenic or gold poisoning—
Adults and children: 2.5 mg/kg deep I.M. q.i.d. for 2 days, then b.i.d. on 3rd day, then once daily for 10 days.
Mercury poisoning—
Adults and children: initially, 5 mg/kg deep I.M., then 2.5 mg/kg daily or b.i.d. for 10 days.
Acute lead encephalopathy or lead level greater than 100 mcg/ml—
Adults and children: 4 mg/kg deep

I.M., then q 4 hours with edetate calcium disodium for 2 to 7 days. Use separate sites.

ADVERSE REACTIONS
CNS: pain or tightness in throat, chest, or hands; headache; paresthesia; muscle pain or weakness, anxiety.
CV: *transient increase in blood pressure* (returns to normal in 2 hours), *tachycardia.*
EENT: blepharospasm, conjunctivitis, lacrimation, rhinorrhea, excessive salivation.
GI: *nausea; vomiting; burning sensation in lips, mouth, and throat; abdominal pain.*
Other: *fever* (especially in children).

INTERACTIONS
Iodine 131 uptake thyroid tests: decreased. Don't schedule patient for this test during course of dimercaprol therapy.
Iron: toxic metal complex formed; concurrent therapy contraindicated. Wait 24 hours after last dimercaprol dose.

EFFECTS ON DIAGNOSTIC TESTS
Drug therapy blocks thyroid uptake of ^{131}I, causing decreased values.

CONTRAINDICATIONS
Contraindicated in patients with hepatic dysfunction (except postarsenical jaundice); iron, cadmium, or selenium poisoning; and in those allergic to peanuts.

NURSING CONSIDERATIONS
● Use cautiously in patients with hypertension, G6PD deficiency, or oliguria.
● Know that safe use in pregnancy has not been established and drug should not be used unless judged by doctor to be necessary to treat a life-threatening acute poisoning.
● Don't give I.V.; give by deep I.M. route only.
● Be careful not to let drug come in contact with skin because it may cause a skin reaction.

● Be aware that drug has an unpleasant, garlic-like odor.
● Know that solution with slight sediment is usable.
● Use antihistamine, as ordered, to prevent or relieve mild adverse reactions.
● Keep urine alkaline to prevent renal damage.

☑ PATIENT TEACHING
● Explain need for drug and how drug is administered to patient and family.
● Instruct patient to report adverse reactions promptly.

disulfiram
Antabuse

Pregnancy Risk Category: NR

HOW SUPPLIED
Tablets: 250 mg, 500 mg

ACTION
Blocks oxidation of ethanol at the acetaldehyde stage. Excess acetaldehyde produces a highly unpleasant reaction in the presence of even small amounts of ethanol.

ONSET, PEAK, DURATION
Onset occurs in 1 to 2 hours. Peak unknown. Effects persist for 14 days after drug discontinuation.

INDICATIONS & DOSAGE
Adjunct in management of chronic alcoholism—
Adults: 250 to 500 mg P.O. as a single dose in the morning for 1 to 2 weeks or in evening if drowsiness occurs. Maintenance dosage is 125 to 500 mg P.O. daily (average dosage 250 mg) until permanent self-control is established. Treatment may continue for months or years.

ADVERSE REACTIONS
CNS: drowsiness, headache, fatigue, delirium, depression, neuritis, peripheral

neuritis, polyneuritis, restlessness, psychotic reactions.
EENT: optic neuritis.
GI: metallic or garlic aftertaste.
GU: impotence.
Skin: acneiform or allergic dermatitis, occasional eruptions.
Other: disulfiram reaction (precipitated by ethanol use), which may include flushing, throbbing headache, dyspnea, nausea, copious vomiting, diaphoresis, thirst, chest pain, palpitations, hyperventilation, hypotension, syncope, anxiety, weakness, blurred vision, confusion, arthropathy.
*In severe reactions—**respiratory depression, CV collapse, arrhythmias, MI, acute CHF, seizures, unconsciousness, or death.***

INTERACTIONS
Alfentanil: prolonged duration of effect. Closely monitor patient.
Anticoagulants: increased anticoagulant effect. Adjust dosage of anticoagulant.
Bacampicillin, ethanol, alcohol (all sources, including cough syrups, liniments, shaving lotion, and back-rub preparations): may precipitate disulfiram reaction. Don't use concomitantly. Alcohol reaction may occur as long as 2 weeks after single disulfiram dose; the longer patient remains on drug, the more sensitive he becomes to alcohol.
CNS depressants: increased CNS depression. Use together cautiously.
Isoniazid: ataxia or marked change in behavior. Do not use concomitantly.
Metronidazole: psychotic reaction. Do not use concomitantly.
Midazolam: increased plasma levels of midazolam. Use together cautiously.
Paraldehyde: toxic levels of acetaldehyde. Do not use concomitantly.
Phenytoin: increased blood levels of phenytoin. Monitor phenytoin blood levels, and expect the doctor to adjust phenytoin dosages.
Tricyclic antidepressants, especially amitriptyline: transient delirium. Closely monitor the patient.

EFFECTS ON DIAGNOSTIC TESTS
Drug may decrease urinary vanillylmandelic acid excretion and increase urinary concentrations of homovanillic acid. Decrease of radioactive iodine (^{131}I); uptake or protein-bound iodine levels may occur rarely. Serum cholesterol levels may be elevated.

CONTRAINDICATIONS
Contraindicated during alcohol intoxication and within 12 hours of alcohol ingestion; in patients with hypersensitivity to disulfiram or to other thiuram derivatives used in pesticides and rubber vulcanization; and in patients with psychoses, myocardial disease, or coronary occlusion; and in patients receiving metronidazole, paraldehyde, alcohol, or alcohol-containing preparations.

NURSING CONSIDERATIONS
● Know that drug should not be administered during pregnancy.
● Use with extreme caution in patients with diabetes mellitus, hypothyroidism, seizure disorder, cerebral damage, nephritis or hepatic cirrhosis or insufficiency and with concurrent phenytoin therapy.
● Use only under close medical and nursing supervision. Never administer until the patient has abstained from alcohol for at least 12 hours. Patients should clearly understand consequences of disulfiram therapy and give permission for its use. Use drug only in patients who are cooperative, well motivated, and receiving supportive psychiatric therapy.
● Know that complete physical examination and laboratory studies, including CBC, SMA-12, and transaminase level, should precede therapy and be repeated regularly, as ordered.

☑ PATIENT TEACHING
Alert: Caution patient's family that disulfiram should never be given to the patient without his knowledge; severe reaction or death could result if patient

---

Reactions may be *common*, uncommon, ***life-threatening***, or COMMON AND LIFE-THREATENING.

ingests alcohol.
• Tell patient to wear a bracelet or carry a card supplied by drug manufacturer identifying him as disulfiram user. *Note:* Mild reactions may occur in sensitive patient with blood alcohol levels of 5 to 10 mg/100 ml; symptoms are fully developed at 50 mg/100 ml; unconsciousness typically occurs at 125 to 150 mg/100 ml level. Reaction may last from 30 minutes to several hours or as long as alcohol remains in blood.
• Reassure patient that disulfiram-induced adverse reactions (unrelated to concomitant alcohol use), such as drowsiness, fatigue, impotence, headache, peripheral neuritis, and metallic or garlic taste, subside after about 2 weeks of therapy.

---

d-penicillamine
Cuprimine, Depen, D-Penamine‡

Pregnancy Risk Category: NR

HOW SUPPLIED
Tablets: 125 mg‡, 250 mg
Capsules: 125 mg, 250 mg

ACTION
Chelates heavy metals and may inhibit collagen formation. Unknown for rheumatoid arthritis.

ONSET, PEAK, DURATION
Onset and duration unknown. Peak levels occur in 1 hour.

INDICATIONS & DOSAGE
Wilson's disease—
Adults and children: 250 mg P.O. q.i.d. 30 to 60 minutes before meals. Dosage adjusted to achieve urinary copper excretion of 0.5 to 1 mg daily.
Cystinuria—
Adults: 250 mg to 1 g P.O. q.i.d. before meals. Dosage adjusted to achieve urinary cystine excretion of less than 100 mg daily when renal calculi are present, or 100 to 200 mg daily when no calculi

are present. Maximum dosage is 4 g daily.
Children: 30 mg/kg P.O. daily, divided q.i.d. before meals. Dosage adjusted to achieve urinary cystine excretion of less than 100 mg daily when renal calculi are present, or 100 to 200 mg daily when no calculi are present.
Rheumatoid arthritis—
Adults: initially, 125 to 250 mg P.O. daily, with increases of 125 to 250 mg q 1 to 3 months, if necessary. Maximum dosage is 1.5 g daily.

ADVERSE REACTIONS
EENT: tinnitus, *optic neuritis.*
GI: *anorexia, epigastric pain, nausea, vomiting, diarrhea, loss of or altered taste perception, stomatitis.*
GU: *nephrotic syndrome, glomerulonephritis,* proteinuria, hematuria.
Hematologic: *leukopenia, eosinophilia,* **thrombocytopenia,** *monocytosis,* **agranulocytosis, aplastic anemia,** lupus-like syndrome.
Hepatic: hepatotoxicity.
Skin: friability, especially at pressure spots; wrinkling; erythema; urticaria; ecchymoses.
Other: hair loss, myasthenia gravis syndrome with long-term use, allergic reactions *(rash, pruritus, fever), arthralgia, lymphadenopathy, or pneumonitis.*

INTERACTIONS
Antacids, oral iron: decreased effectiveness of d-penicillamine. Give at least 2 hours apart.

EFFECTS ON DIAGNOSTIC TESTS
Drug therapy may cause positive test results for antinuclear antibody with or without clinical systemic lupus erythematosus-like syndrome.

CONTRAINDICATIONS
Contraindicated in pregnant patients with cystinuria, in patients with penicillamine-related aplastic anemia or granulocytosis, and in rheumatoid arthritis patients with renal insufficiency.

NURSING CONSIDERATIONS
● Use with extreme caution, if at all, in patients with hypersensitivity to penicillin.
● Give dose on empty stomach to facilitate absorption, preferably 1 hour before or 3 hours after meals.
● Keep in mind patients should receive supplemental pyridoxine daily.
● If patients have a skin reaction, give antihistamines as prescribed. Handle patients carefully to avoid skin damage.
● Monitor CBC and renal and hepatic function every 2 weeks for the first 6 months, then monthly, as ordered.
● Monitor urinalysis regularly for protein loss.
Alert: Report rash and fever (important signs of toxicity) to the doctor immediately.
● Withhold drug and notify the doctor if WBC count falls below 3,500/mm³ or platelet count falls below 100,000/mm³. A progressive decline in platelet or WBC count in three successive blood tests may necessitate temporary cessation of therapy, even if such counts are within normal limits.

☑ PATIENT TEACHING
● Tell patient that therapeutic effect may be delayed up to 3 months in treatment of rheumatoid arthritis.
● Tell patient to take drug on an empty stomach and to maintain adequate fluid intake, especially at night.
● Advise patient to report early signs of granulocytopenia: fever, sore throat, chills, bruising, and prolonged bleeding time.
● Reassure patient that taste impairment usually resolves in 6 weeks without changes in dosage.

---

edetate calcium disodium
Calcium Disodium Versenate, Calcium EDTA

Pregnancy Risk Category: NR

HOW SUPPLIED
Injection: 200 mg/ml

ACTION
Forms stable, soluble complexes with metals, particularly lead.

ONSET, PEAK, DURATION
Onset occurs in 1 hour. Effects peak after 24 to 48 hours. Duration unknown.

INDICATIONS & DOSAGE
Acute lead encephalopathy or blood lead levels above 70 mcg/dl—
Adults and children: 1 to 1.5 g/m² I.V. or I.M. daily in two divided doses at 12-hour intervals for 3 to 5 days, usually in conjunction with dimercaprol. A second course may be administered after at least a 2-day drug-free interval.
Lead poisoning without encephalopathy or asymptomatic with blood levels less than 70 mcg/dl—
Children: 1 g/m² I.V. or I.M. daily in divided doses for 5 days.

ADVERSE REACTIONS
GU: proteinuria, hematuria; *nephrotoxicity with renal tubular necrosis leading to fatal nephrosis.*

INTERACTIONS
None significant.

EFFECTS ON DIAGNOSTIC TESTS
None reported.

CONTRAINDICATIONS
Contraindicated in patients with anuria, hepatitis, and acute renal disease.

NURSING CONSIDERATIONS
● Use with extreme caution in patients with mild renal disease. Expect dosages to be reduced.
● **I.V. use:** Dilute with D₅W or 0.9% sodium chloride for injection to a concentration of 2 to 4 mg/ml. Infuse one-half of the daily dose over 1 hour in asymptomatic patients or 2 hours in symptomatic patients. Give the rest of

the infusion at least 12 hours later. Alternatively, give by slow infusion over at least 6 hours.
● Add procaine hydrochloride, as ordered, to I.M. solution to minimize pain. Watch for local reactions.
● Because rapid I.V. use may increase intracranial pressure, know that I.M. route is preferred for treating lead encephalopathy.
● Know that I.M. route preferred, especially for children and patients with lead encephalopathy.
● Monitor fluid intake and output, urinalysis, BUN level, and ECGs daily, as ordered.
● To avoid toxicity, use with dimercaprol, as ordered.
● Do not confuse with edetate disodium, which is used to treat hypercalcemia.

☑ **PATIENT TEACHING**
● Explain need for drug and how drug is administered to patient and family.
● Tell patients with lead encephalopathy to avoid excess fluids.

---

edetate disodium
Disodium EDTA, Disotate, Endrate

Pregnancy Risk Category: NR

HOW SUPPLIED
Injection: 150 mg/ml

ACTION
Chelates with metals, such as calcium, to form a stable, soluble complex.

ONSET, PEAK, DURATION
Unknown.

INDICATIONS & DOSAGE
Hypercalcemic crisis—
Adults: 50 mg/kg/day by slow I.V. infusion added to 500 ml of D_5W or 0.9% sodium chloride solution administered over 3 or more hours. Maximum dosage is 3 g/day.
Children: 40 to 70 mg/kg/day by slow

I.V. infusion, diluted to a maximum concentration of 30 mg/ml in D_5W or 0.9% sodium chloride solution administered over 3 or more hours. Maximum dosage is 70 mg/kg/day.

ADVERSE REACTIONS
CNS: circumoral paresthesia, numbness, headache.
CV: hypotension.
EENT: erythema.
GI: nausea, vomiting, diarrhea.
GU: in excessive doses—nephrotoxicity with urinary urgency, nocturia, dysuria, polyuria, proteinuria, renal insufficiency, *renal failure, tubular necrosis.*
Skin: exfoliative dermatitis.
Other: *severe hypocalcemia,* decreased magnesium, pain at site of infusion, thrombophlebitis.

INTERACTIONS
None significant.

EFFECTS ON DIAGNOSTIC TESTS
Drug lowers serum calcium concentrations (when measured by oxalate or other precipitation methods and by colorimetry) and blood glucose concentration in diabetic patients. Drug-induced hypomagnesemia decreases serum alkaline phosphatase levels.

CONTRAINDICATIONS
Contraindicated in patients with hypersensitivity to drug, anuria, known or suspected hypocalcemia, significant renal disease, active or healed tubercular lesions, or history of seizures or intracranial lesions.

NURSING CONSIDERATIONS
● Use cautiously in patients with limited cardiac reserve, CHF, or hypokalemia.
● **I.V. use:** Dilute before use. Avoid rapid I.V. infusion; profound hypocalcemia may occur, leading to tetany, seizures, arrhythmias, and respiratory arrest. Not recommended for direct or intermittent injection. Avoid extravasation.

---

*Liquid contains alcohol.   **May contain tartrazine.   †Canada only.   ‡Australia only.   ◊ OTC.

● Record I.V. site used, and avoid repeated use of the same site, which increases likelihood of thrombophlebitis.

● Keep I.V. calcium available to treat hypocalcemia.

● Keep patients in bed for 15 minutes after infusion to avoid orthostatic hypotension. Monitor blood pressure closely.

● Monitor ECG and renal function tests frequently, as ordered.

● Obtain serum calcium after each dose, as ordered.

● Don't use to treat lead toxicity; know that edetate calcium disodium should be used instead.

☑ **PATIENT TEACHING**

● Explain need for drug and how drug is administered to patient and family.

● Instruct patient to report adverse reactions promptly.

---

flumazenil
Romazicon

Pregnancy Risk Category: C

HOW SUPPLIED
Injection: 0.1 mg/ml in 5- and 10-ml multiple-dose vials

ACTION
Benzodiazepine antagonist that competitively inhibits the actions of benzodiazepines on the gamma-aminobutyric acid–benzodiazepine receptor complex.

ONSET, PEAK, DURATION
Onset occurs in 1 to 2 minutes after completion of injection. Peak levels are obtained in 6 to 10 minutes. Duration of drug is related to plasma concentration of the sedating benzodiazepin and the dose of flumazenil given.

INDICATIONS & DOSAGE
Complete or partial reversal of sedative effects of benzodiazepines after anesthesia or short diagnostic procedures (conscious sedation)—

Adults: initially, 0.2 mg I.V. over 15 seconds. If patient does not reach the desired level of consciousness after 45 seconds, dose is repeated. Repeated at 1-minute intervals until a cumulative dose of 1 mg has been given (initial dose plus four additional doses), if needed. Most patients respond after 0.6 to 1 mg of drug. In case of resedation, dosage may be repeated after 20 minutes; however, no more than 1 mg should be given at any one time and no more than 3 mg/hour.

Suspected benzodiazepine overdose—
Adults: initially, 0.2 mg I.V. over 30 seconds. If patient does not reach the desired level of consciousness after 30 seconds, 0.3 mg is administered over 30 seconds. If patient still does not respond adequately, 0.5 mg is administered over 30 seconds; 0.5-mg doses are repeated as needed at 1-minute intervals until a cumulative dose of 3 mg has been given. Most patients suffering from benzodiazepine overdose respond to cumulative doses between 1 and 3 mg; rarely, patients who respond partially after 3 mg may require additional doses, up to 5 mg total. If patient does not respond in 5 minutes after receiving 5 mg, sedation is unlikely to be caused by benzodiazepines. In case of resedation, dosage may be repeated after 20 minutes; however, no more than 1 mg should be given at any one time and no more than 3 mg/hour.

ADVERSE REACTIONS
CNS: *dizziness, abnormal or blurred vision, headache, seizures,* agitation, emotional lability, tremor, insomnia.
CV: *arrhythmias,* cutaneous vasodilation, palpitations.
GI: *nausea, vomiting.*
Respiratory: dyspnea, hyperventilation.
Other: *diaphoresis, pain at injection site.*

INTERACTIONS
Antidepressants; drugs that can cause

Reactions may be *common,* uncommon, *life-threatening,* or COMMON AND LIFE-THREATENING.

seizures or arrhythmias: seizures or ar-rhythmias can develop after effect of benzodiazepine overdose is removed. Flumazenil should not be used in mixed overdose, especially in cases where seizures (from any cause) are likely to occur.

EFFECTS ON DIAGNOSTIC TESTS
None reported.

CONTRAINDICATIONS
Contraindicated in patients hypersensitive to flumazenil or benzodiazepines; in patients who show evidence of serious tricyclic antidepressant overdose; and in those who received benzodiazepine to treat a potentially life-threatening condition (such as status epilepticus).

NURSING CONSIDERATIONS
• Use cautiously in patients at high risk for developing seizures; patients who have recently received multiple doses of a parenteral benzodiazepine; patients displaying some signs of seizure activity; patients who may be at risk for unrecognized benzodiazepine dependence, such as intensive care unit patients; patients with head injury; psychiatric patients; and alcohol-dependent patients.
• Be aware that safety and efficacy in children have not been established.
• **I.V. use:** Administer by direct injection or dilute with a compatible solution. Discard unused drug that has been drawn into a syringe or diluted within 24 hours.
• Administer drug into an I.V. line in a large vein with a free-flowing I.V. solution to minimize pain at the injection site. Compatible solutions include D_5W, lactated Ringer's injection, and 0.9% sodium chloride.
• Monitor patients closely for resedation that may occur after reversal of benzodiazepine effects because flumazenil's duration of action is shorter than that of all benzodiazepines. Duration of monitoring period depends on

specific drug being reversed. Monitor closely after long-acting benzodiazepines, such as diazepam, or after high doses of short-acting benzodiazepines, such as 10 mg of midazolam. In most cases, severe resedation is unlikely in patients who fail to show signs of resedation 2 hours after a 1-mg dose of flumazenil.

☑ **PATIENT TEACHING**
• Warn patient not to perform hazardous activities within 24 hours of procedure because of resedation risk.
• Tell patient to avoid alcohol, CNS depressants, and OTC drugs for 24 hours.
• Give family members necessary instructions or provide patient with written instructions. The patient will not recall information given in the postprocedure period; drug does not reverse amnesic effects of benzodiazepines.

---

ipecac syrup

Pregnancy Risk Category: C

HOW SUPPLIED
Syrup*: 70 mg powdered ipecac/ml (contains glycerin 10% and alcohol 1% to 2.5%) ◊

ACTION
Induces vomiting by acting locally on the gastric mucosa and centrally on the chemoreceptor trigger zone.

ONSET, PEAK, DURATION
Onset occurs in 20 to 30 minutes. Peak unknown. Effects persist for 20 to 25 minutes.

INDICATIONS & DOSAGE
To induce vomiting in poisoning—
Adults and children over 12 years: 15 to 30 ml P.O., followed by 3 to 4 glasses of water.
Children 6 months to 1 year: 5 to 10 ml P.O., followed by 120 to 240 ml of water.

Children 1 to 12 years: 15 ml P.O., followed by 240 to 480 ml of water.

Dose may be repeated in patients older than 1 year if vomiting doesn't occur within 20 minutes. If no vomiting occurs within 30 to 35 minutes after second dose, gastric lavage should be performed.

ADVERSE REACTIONS
CNS: depression, *drowsiness*.
CV: *arrhythmias*, bradycardia, hypotension, atrial fibrillation or *fatal myocarditis* after ingestion of excessive dose.
GI: *diarrhea*.

INTERACTIONS
Activated charcoal: neutralized emetic effect. Don't give together; may give activated charcoal after vomiting.

EFFECTS ON DIAGNOSTIC TESTS
None reported.

CONTRAINDICATIONS
Contraindicated in semicomatose or unconscious patients, or those with severe inebriation, seizures, shock, or loss of gag reflex.

NURSING CONSIDERATIONS
● Unless advised otherwise by a poison control center, don't give after ingestion of petroleum distillates (for example, kerosene, gasoline) or volatile oils; retching and vomiting may cause aspiration and lead to bronchospasm, pulmonary edema, or aspiration pneumonitis. Vegetable oil will delay absorption of these substances. Don't give after ingestion of caustic substances, such as lye; additional injury to the esophagus and mediastinum can occur.
● Keep in mind that stomach is usually emptied completely; vomitus also may contain some intestinal material.
● If two doses do not induce vomiting, be prepared for gastric lavage.
● Know that ipecac syrup usually induces vomiting within 20 to 30 minutes.

● In antiemetic toxicity, know that ipecac syrup is usually effective if less than 1 hour has passed since ingestion of antiemetic.
● Be aware that no systemic toxicity occurs with doses of 30 ml (1 oz) or less.
● Be aware that ipecac syrup is now commonly abused by bulimics who binge and then purge.

☑ **PATIENT TEACHING**
● Recommend to parents that 1 oz (30 ml) of syrup be available in the home when child becomes 1 year old for immediate use in case of emergency.
● Instruct parents how to administer the drug and what to do in case of accidental poisoning.

naloxone hydrochloride
Narcan

Pregnancy Risk Category: B

HOW SUPPLIED
Injection: 0.02mg/ml, 0.4 mg/ml, 1 mg/ml

ACTION
Unknown. Thought to displace previously administered narcotic analgesics from their receptors (competitive antagonism). Has no pharmacologic activity of its own.

ONSET, PEAK, DURATION
Onset occurs in 1 to 2 minutes after I.V. use, 2 to 5 minutes after S.C. or I.M. use. Peak unknown. Duration depends on dose and route of administration. I.M. administration provides a more prolonged duration.

INDICATIONS & DOSAGE
Known or suspected narcotic-induced respiratory depression, including that caused by pentazocine and propoxyphene—
Adults: 0.4 to 2 mg I.V., S.C., or I.M.

repeated q 2 to 3 minutes, p.r.n. If no response is observed after 10 mg has been administered, the diagnosis of narcotic-induced toxicity should be questioned.

Children: 0.01 mg/kg I.V., followed by a second dose of 0.1 mg/kg I.V., if needed. If I.V. route is not available, drug may be administered I.M. or S.C. in divided doses.

Neonates: 0.01 mg/kg I.V., I.M., or S.C. Dose may be repeated q 2 to 3 minutes p.r.n.

Postoperative narcotic depression—
Adults: 0.1 to 0.2 mg I.V. q 2 to 3 minutes p.r.n. Dosage may be repeated within 1 to 2 hours, if needed.

Children: 0.005 to 0.01 mg I.V. Repeated q 2 to 3 minutes p.r.n.

Neonates (asphyxia neonatorum): 0.01 mg/kg I.V. into umbilical vein. May be repeated q 2 to 3 minutes.

ADVERSE REACTIONS

CV: tachycardia and hypertension with higher-than-recommended doses, hypotension, *ventricular fibrillation.*

GI: nausea and vomiting with higher-than-recommended doses.

Other: tremors and withdrawal symptoms in narcotic-dependent patients with higher-than-recommended doses, diaphoresis, *seizures,* pulmonary edema.

INTERACTIONS
None reported.

EFFECTS ON DIAGNOSTIC TESTS
None reported.

CONTRAINDICATIONS
Contraindicated in patients with hypersensitivity to the drug.

NURSING CONSIDERATIONS
● Use cautiously in patients with cardiac irritability and opiate addiction. Abrupt reversal of opiate-induced CNS depression may result in nausea, vomiting, diaphoresis, tachycardia, CNS excitement, and increased blood pressure.

● **I.V. use:** Be prepared to administer continuous I.V. infusion (necessary in many instances to control adverse effects of epidurally administered morphine). If 0.02 mg/ml is not available know that the adult concentration (0.4 mg) may be diluted by mixing 0.5 ml with 9.5 ml of sterile water or sodium chloride for injection to make neonatal concentration (0.02 mg/ml).

● Keep in mind that duration of action of the narcotic may exceed that of naloxone and patients may relapse into respiratory depression.

● Know that respiratory rate increases within 1 to 2 minutes.

● Be aware that drug is effective only in reversing respiratory depression caused by opiates, not against other drug-induced respiratory depression.

● Be aware that patients who receive naloxone to reverse opioid-induced respiratory depression may exhibit tachypnea.

● Monitor respiratory depth and rate. Be prepared to provide oxygen, ventilation, and other resuscitation measures.

☑ PATIENT TEACHING
● Inform family of need for drug and explain how it is administered.

● Reassure family that patient will be monitored closely until effects of narcotic are alleviated.

---

naltrexone hydrochloride
ReVia

Pregnancy Risk Category: C

HOW SUPPLIED
Tablets: 50 mg

ACTION
Unknown. Probably reversibly blocks the subjective effects of opioids administered I.V. by occupying opiate receptors in the brain.

ONSET, PEAK, DURATION
Onset occurs in 15 to 30 minutes. Effects peak after 12 hours. Effects persist about 24 hours.

INDICATIONS & DOSAGE
Adjunct for maintenance of opioid-free state in detoxified individuals—
Adults: initially, 25 mg P.O. If no withdrawal signs occur within 1 hour, an additional 25 mg is given. Once patient has been started on 50 mg q 24 hours, flexible maintenance schedule may be used. From 50 to 150 mg may be given daily, depending on the schedule prescribed.
Treatment of alcohol dependence—
Adults: 50 mg P.O. once daily.

ADVERSE REACTIONS
CNS: *insomnia, anxiety, nervousness, headache,* depression, dizziness, fatigue, somnolence, ***suicide ideation.***
GI: *nausea, vomiting,* anorexia, *abdominal pain,* constipation, increased thirst.
GU: delayed ejaculation, decreased potency.
Hepatic: hepatotoxicity.
Skin: rash.
Other: *muscle and joint pain,* chills.

INTERACTIONS
Thioridazine: causes increased somnolence and lethargy.

EFFECTS ON DIAGNOSTIC TESTS
Because of its hepatotoxicity, drug may alter liver function test results. Lymphocytosis also may occur.

CONTRAINDICATIONS
Contraindicated in patients receiving opioid analgesics, in opioid-dependent patients, in patients in acute opioid withdrawal, and in those with positive urine screen for opioids or in acute hepatitis or liver failure. Also contraindicated in patients with hypersensitivity to drug.

NURSING CONSIDERATIONS
● Use cautiously in patients with mild hepatic disease or history of recent hepatic disease.
● Be aware that treatment for opioid dependency shouldn't begin until patients receive naloxone challenge, a provocative test of opioid dependency. If signs of opioid withdrawal persist after naloxone challenge, don't administer naltrexone.
● Keep in mind that patients must be completely free of opioids before taking naltrexone or severe withdrawal symptoms may occur. Patients who have been addicted to short-acting opioids, such as heroin and meperidine, must wait at least 7 days after the last opioid dose before starting naltrexone. Patients who have been addicted to longer-acting opioids, such as methadone, should wait at least 10 days.
● In an emergency, anticipate that patients receiving naltrexone may be given an opioid analgesic, but the dose must be higher than usual to surmount naltrexone's effect. Monitor for respiratory depression from the opioid; it may be longer and deeper.
● For patients being treated because of a history of opioid dependency and who are expected to be noncompliant, be prepared to try a flexible maintenance dosage regimen of 100 mg on Monday and Wednesday and 150 mg on Friday, as ordered.
● Know that naltrexone should be used only as part of a comprehensive rehabilitation program.

☑ PATIENT TEACHING
● Advise patient to carry a medical identification card. Warn him about telling medical personnel that he takes naltrexone.
● Give patient names of nonopioid drugs that they can continue to take for pain, diarrhea, or cough.

Reactions may be *common,* uncommon, ***life-threatening,*** or COMMON AND LIFE-THREATENING.

pralidoxime chloride (pyridine-2-aldoxime methochloride; 2-PAM)

Protopam Chloride

Pregnancy Risk Category: C

HOW SUPPLIED
Injection: 1 g/20 ml in 20-ml vial without diluent or syringe; 1 g/20 ml in 20-ml vial with diluent, syringe, needle, and alcohol swab (emergency kit); 600 mg/2 ml auto-injector, parenteral

ACTION
Reactivates cholinesterase that has been inactivated by organophosphorus pesticides and related compounds, permitting degradation of accumulated acetylcholine and facilitating normal functioning of neuromuscular junctions.

ONSET, PEAK, DURATION
Onset and duration unknown. Levels peak within 5 to 15 minutes after I.V. administration; 10 to 20 minutes after I.M. administration; unknown after S.C. administration.

INDICATIONS & DOSAGE
Antidote for organophosphate poisoning—
Adults: 1 to 2 g in 100 ml of sodium chloride solution by I.V. infusion over 15 to 30 minutes. If pulmonary edema is present, give by slow I.V. push over 5 minutes. Repeated in 1 hour if muscle weakness persists. Additional doses may be given cautiously. I.M. or S.C. injection may be used if I.V. is not feasible.
Children: 20 to 40 mg/kg I.V., administered as for adults.
Cholinergic crisis in myasthenia gravis—
Adults: 1 to 2 g I.V., followed by 250 mg I.V. q 5 minutes as needed.

ADVERSE REACTIONS
CNS: dizziness, headache, drowsiness.

CV: tachycardia.
EENT: blurred vision, diplopia, impaired accommodation.
GI: nausea.
Other: muscular weakness, hyperventilation, mild to moderate pain at injection site, transient elevation of liver enzymes.

INTERACTIONS
None significant.

EFFECTS ON DIAGNOSTIC TESTS
AST and ALT levels are elevated but return to normal in 2 weeks; transient elevation in CK levels.

CONTRAINDICATIONS
Contraindicated in patients hypersensitive to pralidoxime.

NURSING CONSIDERATIONS
● Use with extreme caution in patients with myasthenia gravis (overdose may trigger myasthenic crisis).
● Initially, remove secretions, maintain patent airway, and institute mechnical ventilation if needed. After dermal exposure to organophosphate, remove the patient's clothing and wash his skin and hair with sodium bicarbonate, soap, water, and alcohol as soon as possible. A second washing may be necessary. When washing the patient, wear protective gloves and clothes to avoid exposure.
● Draw blood for cholinesterase levels before giving pralidoxime.
● Drug should be used in hospitalized patients only; have respiratory and other supportive measures available. If possible, obtain accurate medical history and chronology of poisoning. Drug should be given as soon as possible after poisoning; treatment is most effective if initiated within 24 hours after exposure.
● **I.V. use:** Give I.V. preparation slowly as diluted solution. Dilute with sterile water without preservatives.
● To ameliorate muscarinic effects and block accumulation of acetylcholine as-

---

*Liquid contains alcohol.   **May contain tartrazine.   †Canada only.   ‡Australia only.   ◇OTC.

sociated with organophosphate poisoning, give atropine 2 to 4 mg I.V. with pralidoxime if cyanosis is not present, as ordered. (If cyanosis is present, give atropine I.M.) Give atropine every 5 to 6 minutes, as ordered, until signs of atropine toxicity (flushing, tachycardia, dry mouth, blurred vision, excitement, delirium, and hallucinations) appear; atropinization should be maintained for at least 48 hours.

● Observe patient for 48 to 72 hours if poison was ingested. Delayed absorption may occur from lower bowel. It is difficult to distinguish between toxic effects produced by atropine or by organophosphate compounds and those resulting from pralidoxime.

● Watch the patient with myasthenia gravis treated for overdose of cholinergic drugs for signs of rapid weakening. He can pass quickly from cholinergic crisis to myasthenic crisis and requires more cholinergic drugs to treat myasthenia. Keep edrophonium (Tensilon) available for establishing differential diagnosis.

● Drug is not effective against poisoning due to phosphorus, inorganic phosphates, or organophosphates with no anticholinesterase activity.

☑ **PATIENT TEACHING**
● Explain need for drug and how it is administered to patient and family.
● Tell patient to report adverse effects.
● Caution patient treated for organophosphate poisoning to avoid contact with insecticides for several weeks.

---

protamine sulfate

Pregnancy Risk Category: C

HOW SUPPLIED
Injection: 10 mg/ml

ACTION
A heparin antagonist that forms a physi-ologically inert complex with heparin sodium.

ONSET, PEAK, DURATION
Onset within 30 seconds to 1 minute. Peak unknown. Effects last 2 hours.

INDICATIONS & DOSAGE
Heparin overdose—
Adults: dosage based on venous blood coagulation studies, usually 1 mg for each 90 to 115 units of heparin. Give by slow I.V. injection over 10 minutes in doses not to exceed 50 mg.

ADVERSE REACTIONS
CV: fall in blood pressure, bradycardia, *circulatory collapse.*
GI: nausea, vomiting.
Respiratory: dyspnea, *pulmonary edema, acute pulmonary hypertension.*
Other: transitory flushing, feeling of warmth, *anaphylaxis, anaphylactoid reactions,* lassitude.

INTERACTIONS
None significant.

EFFECTS ON DIAGNOSTIC TESTS
Drug shortens heparin-prolonged PTT.

CONTRAINDICATIONS
Contraindicated in patients with hypersensitivity to drug.

NURSING CONSIDERATIONS
● Use cautiously after cardiac surgery.
● Calculate dosage carefully. One mg of protamine neutralizes 90 to 115 units of heparin depending on salt (heparin calcium or heparin sodium) and source of heparin (beef or pork).
● **I.V. use:** Administer slowly by direct I.V. injection. Have emergency equipment available to treat shock.
● Know that risk of a hypersensitivity reaction is increased in patients with known hypersensitivity to fish, vasectomized or infertile males, or patients taking protamine-insulin products.
● Monitor patient continually.

Reactions may be *common*, uncommon, *life-threatening*, or COMMON AND LIFE-THREATENING.

• Watch for spontaneous bleeding (heparin "rebound"), especially in dialysis patients and in those who have undergone cardiac surgery.
• Protamine sulfate may act as anticoagulant in very high doses.

☑ **PATIENT TEACHING**
• Explain need for drug and how it is administered to patient and family.
• Tell patient to report adverse effects.

---

sodium polystyrene sulfonate
Kayexalate, Resonium A, SPS

Pregnancy Risk Category: C

HOW SUPPLIED
Powder: 1-lb jar (3.5 g/tsp)
Suspension: 15 g/60 ml*

ACTION
Potassium-removing resin exchanges sodium ions for potassium ions in the intestine: 1 g of sodium polystyrene sulfonate is exchanged for 0.5 to 1 mEq of potassium. The resin is then eliminated. Much of the exchange capacity is used for cations other than potassium (calcium and magnesium) and possibly for fats and proteins.

ONSET, PEAK, DURATION
Unknown.

INDICATIONS & DOSAGE
Hyperkalemia—
Adults: 15 g P.O. daily to q.i.d. in water or sorbitol (3 to 4 ml/g of resin). Alternatively, mix powder with appropriate medium—aqueous suspension or diet appropriate for renal failure—and instill through a nasogastric (NG) tube.
Or 30 to 50 g/100 ml of sorbitol q 6 hours as warm emulsion deep into sigmoid colon (20 cm).
Children: 1 g/kg of body weight/dose P.O. or P.R. as needed to correct hyperkalemia.

Oral administration preferred because drug should remain in intestine for at least 30 minutes.

ADVERSE REACTIONS
GI: *constipation,* fecal impaction (in elderly patients), anorexia, gastric irritation, nausea, vomiting, *diarrhea* (with sorbitol emulsions).
Other: *hypokalemia,* hypocalcemia, sodium retention.

INTERACTIONS
Antacids and laxatives (nonabsorbable cation-donating types, including magnesium hydroxide): systemic alkalosis and reduced potassium exchange capability. Don't use together.

EFFECTS ON DIAGNOSTIC TESTS
Drug therapy may alter serum magnesium and calcium levels.

CONTRAINDICATIONS
Contraindicated in patients with hypokalemia or hypersensitivity to drug.

NURSING CONSIDERATIONS
• Use cautiously in patients with severe CHF, severe hypertension, or marked edema.
• Don't heat resin; this impairs drug's effect. Mix resin only with water or sorbitol for P.O. administration. *Never* mix with orange juice (high potassium content) to disguise taste.
• Chill oral suspension for greater palatability.
• If sorbitol is given, mix with resin suspension.
• Consider solid form. Resin cookie and candy recipes are available; ask pharmacist or dietitian to supply.
• Know that premixed forms are available (SPS and others). If preparing manually, mix polystyrene resin only with water and sorbitol for rectal use. Do not use mineral oil for rectal administration to prevent impaction; ion exchange requires aqueous medium. Sorbitol content prevents impaction.

● Prepare rectal dose at room temperature. Stir emulsion gently during administration.

● Use #28 French rubber tube for rectal dose; insert 20 cm into sigmoid colon. Tape tube in place. Or, consider an indwelling urinary catheter with a 30-ml balloon inflated distal to anal sphincter to aid in retention. This is especially helpful for patients with poor sphincter control. Use gravity flow. Drain returns constantly through Y-tube connection. Place patient in knee-chest position or with hips on pillow for a while if backleakage occurs.

● After rectal administration, flush tubing with 50 to 100 ml of nonsodium fluid to ensure delivery of all drug. Flush rectum to remove the resin.

● Prevent fecal impaction in elderly patients by administering resin rectally, as ordered. Give cleansing enema before rectal administration. Have patients retain enema—for 6 to 10 hours if possible, but 30 to 60 minutes is acceptable.

● Watch for constipation in oral or NG administration. Use sorbitol (10 to 20 ml of 70% syrup every 2 hours as needed) to produce one or two watery stools daily.

● Monitor serum potassium levels at least once daily. Treatment may result in potassium deficiency and is usually stopped when potassium is reduced to 4 or 5 mEq/L.

● Watch for signs of hypokalemia: irritability, confusion, arrhythmias, ECG changes, severe muscle weakness and sometimes paralysis, and digitalis toxicity in digitalized patients.

● If hyperkalemia is severe, know that doctor does not depend solely on polystyrene resin to lower serum potassium. Dextrose 50% with regular insulin I.V. push may be given.

● Monitor for symptoms of other electrolyte deficiencies (magnesium, calcium) because drug is nonselective. Monitor serum calcium in patients receiving sodium polystyrene therapy for more than 3 days. Supplementary calcium

may be needed.

● Watch for sodium overload. Drug contains about 100 mg sodium/g. About one-third of resin's sodium is retained.

☑ **PATIENT TEACHING**
● Explain need for drug and how it is to be administered to patient.
● Instruct patient to report adverse reactions promptly.

succimer
Chemet

Pregnancy Risk Category: C

HOW SUPPLIED
Capsules: 100 mg

ACTION
A chelating agent that forms water-soluble complexes with lead and increases its excretion in urine.

ONSET, PEAK, DURATION
Onset and duration unknown. Serum levels peak in 1 to 2 hours.

INDICATIONS & DOSAGE
Lead poisoning in children with blood lead levels above 45 mcg/dl—
Children: initially, 10 mg/kg or 350 mg/m^2 q 8 hours for 5 days. Dosage rounded as appropriate to nearest 100 mg (see chart). Then, frequency of administration decreased to q 12 hours for an additional 2 weeks of therapy.

Weight (kg)	Dose (mg)
8 to 15	100
16 to 23	200
24 to 34	300
35 to 44	400
> 45	500

ADVERSE REACTIONS
CNS: *drowsiness, dizziness, sensory motor neuropathy, sleepiness, paresthesia, headache.*
CV: *arrhythmias.*

EENT: plugged ears, cloudy film in eyes, otitis media, watery eyes, sore throat, rhinorrhea, nasal congestion.
GI: *nausea, vomiting, diarrhea, loss of appetite, abdominal cramps, hemorrhoidal symptoms, metallic taste in mouth, loose stools.*
GU: decreased urination, difficult urination, proteinuria.
Hematologic: increased platelet count, intermittent eosinophilia.
Respiratory: cough, head cold.
Skin: papular rash, herpetic rash, mucocutaneous eruptions, pruritus.
Other: *leg, kneecap, back, stomach, rib, or flank pain; flulike symptoms;* moniliasis; *elevated serum AST, ALT, alkaline phosphatase, or cholesterol levels.*

INTERACTIONS
None significant.

EFFECTS ON DIAGNOSTIC TESTS
False-positive results for urinary ketones in tests using nitroprusside reagents (Ketostix) and false decreased levels of serum uric acid and CK have been reported, as well as transient mild elevations of serum transaminase levels.

CONTRAINDICATIONS
Contraindicated in patients with hypersensitivity to the drug.

NURSING CONSIDERATIONS
● Use cautiously in patients with compromised renal function.
● Measure severity by initial blood lead level and by rate and degree of rebound of blood lead level. Severity should be used as a guide for more frequent blood lead monitoring.
● Monitor serum transaminase before and at least weekly during therapy. Transient mild elevations of serum transaminases have been observed. Patients with history of hepatic disease need close monitoring.
● Monitor patients at least once weekly for rebound blood lead levels. Elevated levels and associated symptoms may re-

turn rapidly after drug is stopped because of redistribution of lead from bone to soft tissues and blood.
● Be aware that course of treatment lasts 19 days. Repeated courses may be necessary if indicated by weekly monitoring of blood lead levels.
● Know that a minimum of 2 weeks between courses is recommended unless high blood lead levels indicate need for immediate therapy.
● Know that false-positive results for ketones in urine using nitroprusside reagents (Ketostix) and falsely decreased levels of serum uric acid and CK have been reported.
● Know that concurrent administration of succimer with other chelating agents is not recommended. Patients who have received edetate calcium disodium with or without dimercaprol may use succimer as subsequent therapy after a 4-week interval.

☑ PATIENT TEACHING
● Explain to parents and child need for drug and how it will be given. Stress importance of complying with frequently ordered blood tests.
● Tell parents of young child who cannot swallow capsules that capsule can be opened and its contents sprinkled on a small amount of soft food. Alternatively, medicated beads from capsule may be poured on a spoon; follow with flavored beverage.
● Assist parents with identifying and removing sources of lead in child's environment. Chelation therapy is not a substitute for preventing further exposure and should not be used to permit continued exposure.
● Tell patients to consult the doctor if rash occurs. Consider possibility of allergic or other mucocutaneous reactions each time drug is used.

---

trientine hydrochloride
Syprine

Pregnancy Risk Category: C

HOW SUPPLIED
Capsules: 250 mg

ACTION
Chelates copper and increases its urinary excretion.

ONSET, PEAK, DURATION
Unknown.

INDICATIONS & DOSAGE
Wilson's disease in patients who cannot tolerate penicillamine—
Adults: 750 to 1,250 mg P.O. daily in two, three, or four divided doses. Dosage may then be increased up to 2,000 mg daily.
Children 12 years and younger: 500 to 750 mg P.O. daily in two, three, or four divided doses. Dosage may then be increased up to 1,500 mg daily.

Long-term maintenance dosage should be determined q 6 to 12 months, based on serum copper analysis.

ADVERSE REACTIONS
Hematologic: iron-deficiency anemia.
Other: hypersensitivity reactions (rash), systemic lupus erythematosus.

INTERACTIONS
Mineral supplements, including iron: may block trientine absorption. Administer at least 2 hours apart.

EFFECTS ON DIAGNOSTIC TESTS
None reported.

CONTRAINDICATIONS
Contraindicated in patients with hypersensitivity to the drug, cystinuria, rheumatoid arthritis, or biliary cirrhosis.

NURSING CONSIDERATIONS
● Monitor patients (especially women) closely for signs of iron-deficiency anemia throughout therapy.
● Watch for signs of hypersensitivity reactions, such as rash.

☑ PATIENT TEACHING
● Tell patient to take drug on an empty stomach at least 1 hour before or 2 hours after meals, and at least 1 hour apart from other drugs, food, or milk.
● Tell patient to swallow capsules whole with water.
● If capsule is accidentally opened and contents spilled on skin, tell patient to wash site thoroughly. Exposure to capsule contents may cause contact dermatitis.
● Tell patient to take his temperature every night and report any fevers or skin eruptions, especially during the first month of therapy.
● Urge patients to follow regimen and low-copper diet as prescribed.

98
Uncategorized drugs

abciximab
acetohydroxamic acid
alendronate sodium
alglucerase
alprostadil
aminoglutethimide
aprotinin
calcipotriene
capsaicin
cisapride
clomiphene citrate
cysteamine bitartrate
etretinate
finasteride
gallium nitrate
imiglucerase
isotretinoin
levocarnitine
levomethadyl acetate
   hydrochloride
mesalamine
mesna
methoxsalen
minoxidil (topical)
nimodipine
olsalazine sodium
pamidronate disodium
pilocarpine hydrochloride
riluzole
ritodrine hydrochloride
strontium 89 (^{89}SR) chloride
sulfasalazine
tiopronin
tretinoin
trilostane

COMBINATION PRODUCTS
None.

---

abciximab
ReoPro

Pregnancy Risk Category: C

HOW SUPPLIED
Injection: 2 mg/ml

ACTION
Binds to the glycoprotein 11b/111a
(GP11b/111a) receptor of human
platelets and inhibits platelet aggregation.

ONSET, PEAK, DURATION
Onset and peak occur almost immediately after I.V. infusion. Effects on
platelet aggregation persist for about 48
hours.

INDICATIONS & DOSAGE
*Adjunct to percutaneous transluminal
coronary angioplasty (PTCA) or
atherectomy for the prevention of acute
cardiac ischemic complications in patients at high risk for abrupt closure of
the treated coronary vessel—*
Adults: 0.25 mg/kg as an I.V. bolus administered 10 to 60 minutes before start
of PTCA or atherectomy, followed by a
continuous I.V. infusion of 10 mcg/
minute for 12 hours.

ADVERSE REACTIONS
CNS: hyperesthesia, hypoesthesia, con-
fusion.
CV: *hypotension,* bradycardia, periph-
eral edema.
EENT: abnormal vision.
GI: *nausea, vomiting.*
Hematologic: *bleeding,* **thrombocy-
topenia,** anemia, leukocytosis.
Respiratory: pleural effusion, pleurisy,
pneumonia.
Other: pain.

INTERACTIONS
*Antiplatelet agents, heparin, NSAIDs,
other anticoagulants, thrombolytics:* increased risk of bleeding. Monitor patient closely.

---

*Liquid contains alcohol.   **May contain tartrazine.   †Canada only.   ‡Australia only.   ◇OTC.

EFFECTS ON DIAGNOSTIC TESTS
None reported.

CONTRAINDICATIONS
Contraindicated in patients with hypersensitivity to any component of the drug or to murine proteins; in those with active internal bleeding, recent (within 6 weeks) GI or GU bleeding of clinical significance, history of CVA within past 2 years or CVA with significant residual neurologic deficit, bleeding diathesis, thrombocytopenia (less than 100,000/mm^2), recent (within 6 weeks) major surgery or trauma, intracranial neoplasm, intracranial arteriovenous malformation, intracranial aneurysm, severe uncontrolled hypertension, or history of vasculitis; when oral anticoagulants have been administered within past 7 days unless PT is equal to or less than 1.2 times control; or with use of I.V. dextran before PTCA or intent to use it during PTCA.

NURSING CONSIDERATIONS
● Use with caution in patients at increased risk for bleeding. Patients at risk include those who weigh less than 75 kg, are over age 65, have a history of GI disease, or are receiving thrombolytic agents. Conditions that also increase the patient's risk of bleeding include PTCA within 12 hours of onset of symptoms for acute MI, prolonged PTCA (lasting more than 70 minutes), or failed PTCA. Heparin used in conjunction with abciximab also may contribute to the risk of bleeding.
● Know that patients who are at risk for abrupt closure and thus would be candidates for abciximab therapy include those undergoing PTCA with at least one of the following conditions: unstable angina or a non–Q–wave MI, an acute Q-wave MI within 12 hours of onset of symptoms, the presence of two type B lesions in the artery to be dilated, the presence of one type B lesion in the artery to be dilated in a woman over age 65 or in a patient with diabetes, the

presence of one type C lesion in the artery to be dilated, or angioplasty of an infarct-related lesion within 7 days of MI.
● Be aware that abciximab is intended for use with aspirin and heparin.
● Keep epinephrine, dopamine, theophylline, antihistamines, and corticosteroids readily available in case anaphylaxis occurs.
● **I.V. use:** Inspect solution for particulate matter before administration. If any visibly opaque particles are found, discard solution and obtain new vial. Withdraw the necessary amount of abciximab for I.V. bolus injection through a sterile, nonpyrogenic, low-protein-binding 0.2- or 0.22-micron filter into a syringe. The I.V. bolus should be administered 10 to 60 minutes before the procedure.
● Withdraw 4.5 ml of abciximab for continuous I.V. infusion through a sterile, nonpyrogenic, low-protein-binding 0.2-or 0.22-micron filter into a syringe. Inject into 250 ml of sterile 0.9% sodium chloride solution or 5% dextrose, and infuse at a rate of 10 mcg/minute for 12 hours via a continuous infusion pump equipped with an in-line filter. Discard the unused portion at the end of the 12-hour infusion.
● Administer abciximab in a separate I.V. line; no other medication should be added to the infusion solution.
● Monitor the patient closely for bleeding. Bleeding associated with therapy falls into two broad categories: that observed at the arterial access site used for cardiac catheterization and internal bleeding involving the GI or GU tract, or retroperitoneal sites.
● Institute bleeding precautions. Maintain patient on bed rest for 6 to 8 hours following sheath removal or discontinuation of abciximab infusion, whichever is later. Minimize or avoid, if possible, arterial and venous punctures; I.M. injections; use of urinary catheters, nasogastric tubes, or automatic blood pressure cuffs; and nasotracheal intubation.

PATIENT TEACHING
● Explain need for drug and how it is administered to patient and family.
● Instruct patient to report adverse reactions immediately.

---

acetohydroxamic acid
Lithostat

Pregnancy Risk Category: X

HOW SUPPLIED
Tablets (scored): 250 mg

ACTION
Prevents formation of renal stones by inhibiting bacterial urease activity.

ONSET, PEAK, DURATION
Onset and duration unknown. Serum levels peak within 15 to 60 minutes.

INDICATIONS & DOSAGE
Urinary tract infection caused by kidney stones—
Adults: 250 mg P.O. t.i.d. or q.i.d. at 6- to 8-hour intervals when the stomach is empty. Maximum daily dosage is 1.5 g.
Children: 10 mg/kg/day P.O. in two or three divided doses.

ADVERSE REACTIONS
CNS: *mild headache, depression, anxiety, nervousness, malaise, tremulousness.*
CV: phlebitis, palpitations.
GI: *nausea, vomiting, diarrhea, constipation, anorexia.*
Hematologic: *hemolytic anemia,* negative Coombs' test results, reticulocytosis.
Skin: *nonpruritic, macular rash on arms and face.*
Other: alopecia, deep vein thrombosis.

INTERACTIONS
Methenamine: may produce synergistic effects.
Oral iron supplements: reduced absorption of acetohydroxamic acid and iron.

Consult the doctor, who may prescribe I.M. administration of iron.

EFFECTS ON DIAGNOSTIC TESTS
None reported.

CONTRAINDICATIONS
Contraindicated in patients whose physical state and disease are amenable to surgery and appropriate antibiotics, in patients whose urine is infected by nonurease-producing organisms, during pregnancy, and in patients with poor renal function.

NURSING CONSIDERATIONS
● Monitor CBC, including reticulocyte count, after 2 weeks of therapy, then at 3-month intervals for duration of treatment, as ordered. If laboratory findings indicate hemolytic anemia, discontinue drug and notify doctor.
● Anticipate using a reduced dosage in renal impairment.
● Be aware that a negative Coombs' test for hemolytic anemia has occurred in patients receiving acetohydroxamic acid.
● Keep in mind that patients may also be given methenamine to enhance response to acetohydroxamic acid.
● Monitor for skin rash, more common during prolonged use and with concomitant use of alcoholic beverages. The rash appears 30 to 45 minutes after ingestion of alcoholic beverages and disappears spontaneously in 30 to 60 minutes.

☑ PATIENT TEACHING
● Instruct patient to take drug on an empty stomach.
● Although rash doesn't usually require treatment, advise patient to avoid drinking alcoholic beverages.
● Instruct women of childbearing age to use an effective method of birth control while taking the drug.

---

alendronate sodium
Fosamax

Pregnancy Risk Category: C

HOW SUPPLIED
Tablets: 10 mg, 40 mg

ACTION
Suppresses osteoclast activity on newly formed resorption surfaces, which reduces bone turnover. Bone formation exceeds resorption at remodeling sites, leading to progressive gains in bone mass.

ONSET, PEAK, DURATION
Decreased rate of bone resorption is evident in 1 month; in 3 to 6 months, it reaches a plateau that is maintained for duration of therapy.

INDICATIONS & DOSAGE
Osteoporosis in postmenopausal women—
Adults: 10 mg P.O. daily, taken with plain water only, at least 30 minutes before first food, beverage, or medication of day.
Paget's disease of bone—
Adults: 40 mg P.O. daily for 6 months, taken with plain water only, at least 30 minutes before first food, beverage, or medication of day.

ADVERSE REACTIONS
CNS: headache.
GI: abdominal pain, nausea, dyspepsia, constipation, diarrhea, flatulence, acid regurgitation, esophageal ulcer, vomiting, dysphagia, abdominal distention, gastritis.
Other: musculoskeletal pain, taste perversion.

INTERACTIONS
Antacids, calcium supplements: may interfere with absorption of alendronate. Have patient wait at least 30 minutes after taking alendronate before taking any other drug.
Aspirin, NSAIDs: increased risk of upper GI adverse reactions with alendronate doses greater than 10 mg/day. Monitor patient closely.
Hormone replacement therapy: not recommended for use with alendronate in treating osteoporosis; evidence of effectiveness is lacking.

EFFECTS ON DIAGNOSTIC TESTS
None reported.

CONTRAINDICATIONS
Contraindicated in patients with hypersensitivity to drug, hypocalcemia, or severe renal insufficiency.

NURSING CONSIDERATIONS
● Use cautiously in patients with active upper GI problems (dysphagia, symptomatic esophageal diseases, gastritis, duodenitis, ulcers) or mild to moderate renal insufficiency.
● Hypocalcemia and other disturbances of mineral metabolism (such as vitamin D deficiency) should be corrected before therapy begins.
● When drug is used to treat osteoporosis in postmenopausal women, osteoporosis may be confirmed by findings of low bone mass on diagnostic studies or by history of osteoporotic fracture.
● When used to treat Paget's disease, drug is indicated for patients with alkaline phosphatase level at least two times the upper limit of normal, in those who are symptomatic, and in those at risk for future complications from the disease.
● Monitor patient's serum calcium and phosphate levels throughout therapy, as ordered.

☑ PATIENT TEACHING
● Stress importance of taking tablet with a glass of plain water at least 30 minutes before ingesting anything else, including food, beverages, and other medications. Tell the patient that waiting longer than 30 minutes will improve absorption.

Reactions may be *common*, uncommon, **life-threatening**, or COMMON AND LIFE-THREATENING.

• Warn the patient not to lie down for at least 30 minutes after taking drug to facilitate delivery to stomach and to reduce potential for esophageal irritation.
• Advise the patient to take supplemental calcium and vitamin D, if dietary intake is inadequate.
• Tell the patient about the benefits of weight-bearing exercises in increasing bone mass. If applicable, explain the importance of reducing or eliminating cigarette smoking and alcohol use.

alglucerase (glucocerebrosidase, glucosylceramidase, glucocerebrosidase-beta-glucosidase)
Ceredase

Pregnancy Risk Category: C

HOW SUPPLIED
Injection: 10 IU/ml in 5-ml bottles, 80 IU/ml in 5-ml bottles

ACTION
Reduces glycolipid accumulation by acting as a catalyst for the hydrolysis of glucocerebroside to glucose and ceramide—part of the normal degradation pathway for lipids.

ONSET, PEAK, DURATION
Onset of activity within 60 minutes following I.V. administration.

INDICATIONS & DOSAGE
Long-term endogenous enzyme (glucosylceramidase) replacement therapy in confirmed type I Gaucher's disease—
Adults and children: individualized dosage; initially, 2.5 units/kg I.V. three times weekly up to as much as 60 units/kg once a week or as infrequently as q 4 weeks. Infusion should run over 1 to 2 hours. Once response is established, dosage reduced for maintenance at 3- to 6-month intervals.

ADVERSE REACTIONS
GI: abdominal discomfort, nausea, vomiting.
Other: chills, slight fever, discomfort, burning, swelling at injection site.

INTERACTIONS
None significant.

EFFECTS ON DIAGNOSTIC TESTS
None reported.

CONTRAINDICATIONS
None known.

NURSING CONSIDERATIONS
• Use cautiously in patients with symptoms of hypersensitivity to drug. Know that pretreatment with antihistamines may be required. Also use cautiously in patients with androgen-sensitive malignant disease such as prostate cancer and patients with known prior allergies to human chorionic gonadotropin.
• **I.V. use:** To prepare solution, dilute appropriate amount of alglucerase with 0.9% sodium chloride solution to a final volume not to exceed 100 ml. Use an in-line particulate filter during administration. Because alglucerase is preservative-free, use immediately.
• Do not shake bottle. Shaking may denature the glycoprotein and render it biologically inactive.
• Monitor response parameters to use lowest effective dose.
• Be aware that alglucerase is purified from a large pool of human placental tissue collected from selected donors. Although the risk of viral contamination from slow-acting or latent viruses is believed to be remote, the risks and benefits of therapy must be carefully assessed before treatment.
• Keep in mind that hemoglobin levels may normalize after 6 months of therapy. Improved mineralization may also occur after prolonged treatment.
• Store at 39° F (4° C). Do not use solution that is discolored or that contains particles.

☑ **PATIENT TEACHING**

● Explain to patient and family how drug works and is administered. Stress importance of compliance with administration schedule.

● Tell patient to report discomfort at I.V. site promptly.

---

alprostadil
Caverject

Pregnancy Risk Category: NR

HOW SUPPLIED
Injections: 10 mcg/vial and 20 mcg/vial, mcg/ml and 20 mcg/ml after reconstitution

ACTION
A prostaglandin derivative that induces erection by relaxing trabecular smooth muscle and dilating cavernosal arteries. This leads to expansion of lacunar spaces and entrapment of blood by compressing venules against the tunica albuginea, a process referred to as the corporal veno-occlusive mechanism.

ONSET, PEAK, DURATION
Onset and peak occur in 5 to 20 minutes. Duration is preferably no longer than 1 hour but can last longer than 6 hours.

INDICATIONS & DOSAGE
Erectile dysfunction due to vasculogenic, psychogenic, or mixed etiology—
Adults: dosages are highly individualized, with initial dose of 2.5 mcg intracavernously. If partial response occurs, second dose of 2.5 mcg is given, then increased further in increments of 5 to 10 mcg until patient achieves erection (one suitable for intercourse and not exceeding 1 hour's duration). If no response occurs to initial dose, second dose may be increased to 7.5 mcg within 1 hour, then increased further in increments of 5 to 10 mcg until patient achieves suitable erection. Patient must

remain in doctor's office until complete detumescence occurs. Procedure should not be repeated for at least 24 hours.
Erectile dysfunction of neurogenic etiology (spinal cord injury)—
Adults: dosages are highly individualized, with initial dose of 1.25 mcg intracavernously. If partial response occurs, second dose of 1.25 mcg is given, followed by an increment of 2.5 mcg, to a dose of 5 mcg, and then in increments of 5 mcg until patient achieves erection (one suitable for intercourse and not exceeding 1 hour's duration). If no response occurs to initial dose, the next higher dose may be given within 1 hour. Patient must remain in doctor's office until complete detumescence occurs. If there is a response, procedure should not be repeated for at least 24 hours.

ADVERSE REACTIONS
CNS: headache, dizziness.
CV: hypertension.
GU: *penile pain;* prolonged erection; penile fibrosis, rash, or edema; penis disorder; prostatic disorder.
Respiratory: upper respiratory infection, flu syndrome, sinusitis, nasal congestion, cough.
Other: injection site hematoma or ecchymosis, back pain, localized trauma or pain.

INTERACTIONS
Anticoagulants: increased risk of bleeding from intracavernosal injection site. Monitor patient closely.
Vasoactive agents: safety and efficacy of concomitant use have not been studied. Avoid concomitant use.

EFFECTS ON DIAGNOSTIC TESTS
None reported.

CONTRAINDICATIONS
Contraindicated in patients with hypersensitivity to drug, conditions associated with predisposition to priapism (sickle cell anemia or trait, multiple myelo-

ma, leukemia), or penile deformation (angulation, cavernosal fibrosis, Peyronie's disease). Drug also should not be used in men who have penile implants or for whom sexual activity is inadvisable or contraindicated. Drug is not given to women or children.

NURSING CONSIDERATIONS
● Know that regular follow-up care, with thorough examination of the penis, is strongly recommended to detect signs of penile fibrosis. Drug should be discontinued in patients who develop penile angulation, cavernosal fibrosis, or Peyronie's disease.

☑ PATIENT TEACHING
● Teach the patient how to prepare and administer drug before he begins treatment at home. Stress importance of reading and following patient instructions in each package insert.
● Tell him not to shake contents of reconstituted vial, and remind him that vial is designed for single use only. Tell him to discard vial if solution is discolored or contains precipitate.
● Inform the patient that he can expect an erection 5 to 20 minutes after administration, with a preferable duration of no more than 1 hour. If his erection lasts longer than 6 hours, tell him to seek medical attention immediately.
● Remind him to take drug as prescribed (generally, no more than 3 times weekly, with at least 24 hours between each use). Warn him not to change dosage without consulting the doctor.
● Review possible adverse reactions. Tell him to inspect his penis daily and to report redness, swelling, tenderness, curvature, priapism, unusual pain, nodules, or hard tissue.
● Urge him not to reuse or share needles, syringes, or medication.
● Warn him that drug does not protect against sexually transmitted diseases. Also caution him that bleeding at injection site can increase risk of transmitting blood-borne diseases to his partner.

● Remind the patient to keep regular follow-up appointments so the doctor can evaluate drug effectiveness and safety.

aminoglutethimide
Cytadren

Pregnancy Risk Category: D

HOW SUPPLIED
Tablets: 250 mg

ACTION
Blocks conversion of cholesterol to delta-5-pregnenolone in the adrenal cortex, inhibiting the synthesis of adrenal steroids.

ONSET, PEAK, DURATION
Suppression of adrenal function occurs in 3 to 5 days. Time to peak concentration occurs in 1½ hours. Adrenal function usually returns to normal 1½ to 3 days after discontinuing drug, although recovery may take a year or longer after prolonged therapy.

INDICATIONS & DOSAGE
Suppression of adrenal function in Cushing's syndrome and adrenal cancer—
Adults: 250 mg q.i.d. at 6-hour intervals. Dosage may be increased in increments of 250 mg daily q 1 to 2 weeks to a maximum daily dosage of 2 g.

ADVERSE REACTIONS
CNS: *drowsiness,* headache, dizziness.
CV: hypotension, tachycardia.
GI: *nausea, anorexia,* vomiting.
Hematologic: transient leukopenia, *agranulocytosis, thrombocytopenia.*
Skin: *morbilliform rash,* pruritus, urticaria.
Other: fever, myalgia, adrenal insufficiency, masculinization, hirsutism, hypothyroidism.

INTERACTIONS

Dexamethasone, medroxyprogesterone: increased hepatic metabolism of these agents. Monitor patient closely.
Ethanol: may potentiate the effects of aminoglutethimide. Avoid concomitant use.
Oral anticoagulants: decreased anticoagulant effect. Monitor P.T.

EFFECTS ON DIAGNOSTIC TESTS

Drug therapy may decrease plasma cortisol, serum thyroxine, and urinary aldosterone levels, and may increase serum alkaline phosphatase, AST, and thyroid-stimulating hormone concentrations.

CONTRAINDICATIONS

Contraindicated in patients hypersensitive to the drug or to glutethimide.

NURSING CONSIDERATIONS

● Perform baseline hematologic studies, as ordered.
● Monitor blood pressure frequently.
● Monitor CBC periodically, as ordered.
● Be aware that drug may cause adrenal hypofunction, especially under stressful conditions, such as surgery, trauma, or acute illness. Patients may need mineralocorticoid supplements to treat hyponatremia and orthostatic hypotension. Glucocorticoid replacement may also be necessary, especially in patients with breast cancer. Monitor such patients carefully.
● Know that drug may cause a decrease in thyroid hormone production. Monitor thyroid function studies.

☑ PATIENT TEACHING

● Warn patient to watch for signs of infection (fever, sore throat, fatigue) and bleeding (easy bruising, nosebleeds, bleeding gums, melena). He should take his temperature daily.
● Warn patient to avoid activities that require alertness and good motor coordination until CNS effects of the drug are known.

● Advise patient to stand up slowly to minimize orthostatic hypotension.
● Tell patient to report rash that persists for more than 8 days. Reassure patient that drowsiness, nausea, and loss of appetite usually diminish within 2 weeks after start of aminoglutethimide therapy, but advise him to notify the doctor if these symptoms persist.

aprotinin
Trasylol

Pregnancy Risk Category: B

HOW SUPPLIED

Injection: 10,000 KIU (kallikrein inactivator units)/ml (1.4 mg/ml) in 100-ml and 200-ml vials

ACTION

A naturally occurring protease inhibitor that acts as a systemic hemostatic agent, decreasing bleeding and turnover of coagulation factors. It inhibits fibrinolysis by affecting kallikrein and plasmin, prevents triggering of the contact phase of the coagulation pathway, and increases the resistance of platelets to damage from mechanical injury and high plasmin levels that occur during cardiopulmonary bypass.

ONSET, PEAK, DURATION

Unknown.

INDICATIONS & DOSAGE

To reduce blood loss or the need for transfusion in patients undergoing coronary artery bypass grafts—
Adults: started with 10,000 units (1 ml) test dose at least 10 minutes before the loading dose. If no allergic reaction is evident, anesthesia may be induced while the loading dose of 2 million units is given slowly over 20 to 30 minutes. When the loading dose is complete, sternotomy may be performed. Before bypass is initiated, the cardiopulmonary bypass circuit is primed with 2 million

units of the drug by replacing an aliquot of the priming fluid with the drug. A continuous infusion at a rate of 500,000 units/hour is then given until the patient leaves the operating room. This is known as *regimen A*. Alternatively, a second regimen known as *regimen B* may be given which is half the dosage of *regimen A* (except for test dose).

ADVERSE REACTIONS
CV: *cardiac arrest, CHF,* **heart failure, ventricular tachycardia, MI,** heart block, *atrial fibrillation,* atrial flutter, hypotension, supraventricular tachycardia.
GU: nephrotoxicity, **renal failure.**
Respiratory: pneumonia, respiratory disorder, apnea, asthma, dyspnea.
Other: hypersensitivity reactions, **anaphylaxis,** fever, **shock,** sepsis.

INTERACTIONS
None significant.

EFFECTS ON DIAGNOSTIC TESTS
Because aprotinin inhibits contact activation of the intrinsic clotting system, drug therapy prolongs the results of coagulation assays that depend on contact activation, including the partial thromboplastin time (PTT) and celite- activation clotting time (ACT) assays.

Aprotinin has resulted in elevated serum creatine levels postoperatively. In most cases, renal dysfunction was not severe and was reversible.

Aprotinin may alter liver function studies and may block the acute hypotensive effect of captopril.

CONTRAINDICATIONS
Contraindicated in patients hypersensitive to beef because the drug is prepared from bovine lung.

NURSING CONSIDERATIONS
Alert: Use drug cautiously and monitor patients closely for hypersensitivity reaction. Patients may experience anaphylaxis after the full therapeutic dose even

if they remained asymptomatic after the test dose. If symptoms of hypersensitivity occur (skin eruptions, itching, dyspnea, nausea, tachycardia), discontinue the infusion immediately, make doctor aware, and provide supportive treatment.
● Obtain history of possible allergies. Patients with a history of allergies to drugs or other substances may be at higher risk of developing an allergic reaction to aprotinin.
● Be prepared to administer a test dose. Test dose is particularly important in patients who have previously received the drug because they have a higher risk of anaphylaxis. In such patients, pretreat with an antihistamine, as ordered.
● **I.V. use:** Keep in mind that aprotinin is incompatible with amino acids, corticosteroids, fat emulsions, heparin, and tetracyclines. Don't add any drugs to the I.V. container and use a separate I.V. line.
● Administer all doses through a central line.
● To avoid hypotension, make sure patients are supine when the loading dose is given.
● Monitor laboratory studies, as ordered. Aprotinin will prolong activated clotting time and PTT. It may increase CK and transaminase levels and may falsely prolong whole blood clotting times when determined by surface activation methods, such as the Hemachron method.
● Monitor patients for increased serum creatinine levels and other signs of nephrotoxicity. If nephrotoxicity occurs, it is usually mild and reversible.
● Store between 36° and 77° F (2° and 25° C). Protect from freezing.

☑ **PATIENT TEACHING**
● Explain need for drug and how drug is administered to patient and family.
● Reassure patient and family that patient will be monitored continuously throughout drug administration for adverse reactions.

---

*Liquid contains alcohol.   **May contain tartrazine.   †Canada only.   ‡Australia only.   ◇OTC.

calcipotriene
Dovonex

Pregnancy Risk Category: C

HOW SUPPLIED
Ointment: 0.005%

ACTION
A synthetic vitamin D_3 analogue that regulates the development and production of skin cells.

ONSET, PEAK, DURATION
Unknown.

INDICATIONS & DOSAGE
Moderate plaque psoriasis—
Adults: apply a thin layer to the affected area b.i.d. Rub in gently and completely.

ADVERSE REACTIONS
Skin: *burning, pruritus, irritation,* atrophy, dermatitis, dry skin, erythema, folliculitis, hyperpigmentation, peeling, rash, worsening of psoriasis.
Other: hypercalcemia.

INTERACTIONS
None significant.

EFFECTS ON DIAGNOSTIC TESTS
None reported.

CONTRAINDICATIONS
Contraindicated in patients hypersensitive to the drug or any components in the preparation. Also contraindicated in patients with hypercalcemia or evidence of vitamin D toxicity.

NURSING CONSIDERATIONS
● Use cautiously in breast-feeding patients.
● Use cautiously in elderly patients; they may experience more severe adverse skin reactions.

☑ PATIENT TEACHING
● Advise patients to apply only a thin layer of ointment. Transient elevations of serum calcium can occur, especially when applied excessively.
● Advise patients not to use the drug on the face, in the eyes, orally, or vaginally. Tell them to wash their hands after applying the ointment.
● Tell patients discontinue drug and call doctor if drug irritates lesions or surrounding uninvolved skin.

capsaicin
Axsain ◇, Zostrix ◇, Zostrix-HP 0.075%, Capzacin-P

Pregnancy Risk Category: NR

HOW SUPPLIED
Cream: 0.025% ◇ (Zostrix ◇), 0.075% ◇ (Axsain ◇)

ACTION
Unknown. May deplete substance P, the principal neurotransmitter for pain, in peripheral type C sensory fibers.

ONSET, PEAK, DURATION
Unknown.

INDICATIONS & DOSAGE
Temporary relief of pain after herpes zoster infections, neuralgias, such as postoperative pain and painful diabetic neuropathy; pain associated with osteoarthritis or rheumatoid arthritis—
Adults and children over 2 years: applied to affected areas not more than q.i.d.

ADVERSE REACTIONS
Respiratory: cough, irritation.
Skin: redness, *stinging or burning on application.*

INTERACTIONS
None significant.

EFFECTS ON DIAGNOSTIC TESTS
None reported.

CONTRAINDICATIONS
Contraindicated in patients hypersensitive to the drug.

NURSING CONSIDERATIONS
● Know that drug is for external use only.

☑ PATIENT TEACHING
● Warn patient to avoid getting drug in eyes or on broken skin.
● Advise patient not to bandage area tightly after applying drug.
● Tell patient to wash hands after applying drug.
● Inform patient that transient burning or stinging is usually evident at initial therapy but decreases with cautious use. This effect persists in patient who uses drug less often than three times a day.
● Tell patient who is self-medicating with capsaicin to contact the doctor if symptoms persist beyond 2 to 4 weeks or resolve and shortly reappear.

---

cisapride
Propulsid

Pregnancy Risk Category: C

HOW SUPPLIED
Tablets: 10 mg, 20 mg
Suspension: 1 mg/ml

ACTION
Stimulates serotonin-4 (5-HT$_4$) receptors, enhancing the release of acetylcholine at the myenteric plexus and increasing GI motility.

ONSET, PEAK, DURATION
Onset occurs in 30 to 60 minutes. Plasma levels peak within 1 to 2 hours. Duration unknown.

INDICATIONS & DOSAGE
Symptoms of nocturnal heartburn caused by gastroesophageal reflux disease—
Adults: initially, 10 mg P.O. q.i.d. 15 minutes before meals and h.s. If response is inadequate, increased to 20 mg q.i.d.

ADVERSE REACTIONS
CNS: *headache,* insomnia, anxiety, nervousness.
EENT: abnormal vision.
GI: *diarrhea, abdominal pain,* nausea, constipation, flatulence, dyspepsia.
GU: frequency, urinary tract infection, vaginitis.
Respiratory: rhinitis, sinusitis, cough, upper respiratory tract infections.
Skin: rash, pruritus.
Other: pain, fever, viral infections, arthralgia.

INTERACTIONS
Anticholinergics: decreased effectiveness of cisapride. Avoid concomitant use.
Anticoagulants: may increase clotting times. Monitor closely.
Benzodiazepines, ethanol: enhanced sedation. Avoid concomitant use.
Cimetidine, ranitidine: increased absorption of these agents; cimetidine increases cisapride levels. Use together cautiously.
Itraconazole, ketoconazole, fluconazole, erythromycin, clarithromycin, I.V. miconazole, troleandomycin: increased cisapride levels which may cause ventricular arrhythmias. Avoid concomitant use.

EFFECTS ON DIAGNOSTIC TESTS
None reported.

CONTRAINDICATIONS
Contraindicated in patients hypersensitive to the drug. Also contraindicated in patients in whom increased GI motility may be harmful, such as those with mechanical obstruction, hemorrhage, or perforation of the GI tract.

---

*Liquid contains alcohol.   **May contain tartrazine.   †Canada only.   ‡Australia only.   ◇OTC.

NURSING CONSIDERATIONS
• Use cautiously in breast-feeding patients because small amounts of the drug are excreted in breast milk.
• Protect 20-mg tablets from light; protect all products from moisture.

☑ PATIENT TEACHING
• Remind patient to avoid alcohol and sedatives while using this drug.
• Advise patient to immediately report any adverse effects to the doctor.

---

clomiphene citrate
Clomid, Milophene, Serophene

Pregnancy Risk Category: NR

HOW SUPPLIED
Tablets: 50 mg

ACTION
Unknown. Appears to stimulate release of pituitary gonadotropins, follicle-stimulating hormone, and luteinizing hormone. This results in maturation of the ovarian follicle, ovulation, and development of the corpus luteum.

ONSET, PEAK, DURATION
Not clearly defined although ovulation usually occurs 4 to 10 days after last day of treatment; this period of time may vary among patients and for each cycle.

INDICATIONS & DOSAGE
To induce ovulation—
Adults: 50 mg P.O. daily for 5 days starting on day 5 of the menstrual cycle (first day of menstrual flow is day 1) if bleeding occurs or at any time if patient has not had recent uterine bleeding. If ovulation does not occur, may increase dose to 100 mg P.O. daily for 5 days as soon as 30 days after previous course. Repeated until conception occurs or until three courses of therapy are completed.

ADVERSE REACTIONS
CNS: headache, restlessness, insomnia, dizziness, light-headedness, depression, fatigue.
EENT: blurred vision, diplopia, scotoma, photophobia.
GI: nausea, vomiting, bloating, distention, weight gain.
GU: urinary frequency and polyuria; abnormal uterine bleeding; *ovarian enlargement* and cyst formation, which regress spontaneously when drug is stopped.
Skin: urticaria, rash, dermatitis.
Other: *hot flashes,* reversible alopecia, *breast discomfort.*

INTERACTIONS
None significant.

EFFECTS ON DIAGNOSTIC TESTS
Drug therapy may increase levels of serum thyronine, thyroxine-binding globulin, and sex hormone-binding globulin. It may also increase sulfobromophthlein retention and follicle-stimulating hormone and luteinizing hormone secretion.

CONTRAINDICATIONS
Contraindicated during pregnancy and in patients with undiagnosed abnormal genital bleeding, ovarian cyst not due to polycystic ovarian syndrome, hepatic disease or dysfunction, uncontrolled thyroid or adrenal dysfunction, or presence of organic intracranial lesion (such as a pituitary tumor).

NURSING CONSIDERATION
Know that patient must be monitored closely because of potentially serious adverse reactions.

☑ PATIENT TEACHING
• Tell patient there is a possibility of multiple births with this drug. Risk increases with higher doses.
• Teach patient to take and chart basal body temperature to ascertain whether ovulation has occurred.

Reactions may be *common,* uncommon, *life-threatening,* or COMMON AND LIFE-THREATENING.

• Reassure patient that ovulation generally occurs after the first course of therapy. If pregnancy does not occur, course of therapy may be repeated twice.
• Advise patient to stop drug and contact the doctor immediately if pregnancy is suspected because the drug may have teratogenic effect.

Alert: Advise patient to stop drug and contact the doctor immediately if abdominal symptoms or pain occurs because these may indicate ovarian enlargement or ovarian cyst. Also tell patient to report signs of impending visual toxicity—blurred vision, diplopia, scotoma, or photophobia—to the doctor immediately.

• Warn patient to avoid hazardous activities, such as driving or operating machinery, until CNS effects are known. Drug may cause dizziness or visual disturbances.

---

cysteamine bitartrate
Cystagon

Pregnancy Risk Category: C

HOW SUPPLIED
Capsules: 50 mg, 150 mg

ACTION
Reacts with cystine, thereby decreasing the cystine level in cells.

ONSET, PEAK, DURATION
Unknown.

INDICATIONS & DOSAGE
Management of nephropathic cystinosis—

Adults and children over age 12 and weighing more than 50 kg: initially, one-fourth to one-sixth of the maintenance dosage, then increased gradually over 4 to 6 weeks to achieve maintenance dosage. Maintenance dosage is 2 g (free base) P.O. in four divided doses.
Children 12 years and under: initially, one-fourth to one-sixth of the mainte-

nance dosage, then increased gradually over 4 to 6 weeks to achieve maintenance dosage. Maintenance dosage is 1.3 g/m^2 (free base) P.O. daily in four divided doses.

ADVERSE REACTIONS
CNS: *lethargy,* somnolence, encephalopathy, headache, *seizures,* ataxia, confusion, tremor, hyperkinesis, decreasing hearing, dizziness, jitteriness, nervousness, abnormal thinking, depression, emotional lability, hallucinations, nightmares.
CV: hypertension.
GI: *vomiting, anorexia, diarrhea,* nausea, abdominal pain, dyspepsia, constipation, gastroenteritis, duodenitis, duodenal ulcer.
Hepatic: abnormal liver function.
Hematologic: anemia, leukopenia.
Skin: *rash,* urticaria.
Other: *fever,* dehydration, bad breath.

INTERACTIONS
None significant.

EFFECTS ON DIAGNOSTIC TESTS
None reported.

CONTRAINDICATIONS
Contraindicated in patients with hypersensitivity to the drug, cysteamine, or penicillamine.

NURSING CONSIDERATIONS
• Know that drug therapy should begin as soon as the diagnosis of nephropathic cystinosis has been confirmed by increased level of cystine in increased WBCs.
• Monitor patient for a rash. If one develops, notify the doctor because the drug will need to be withheld until the rash clears. The doctor may then restart the drug at a lower dosage and slowly titrate dosage to achieve therapeutic effect. However, if a severe rash (such as erythema multiforme bullosa or toxic epidermal necrolysis) develops, know that the drug should not be restarted.

---

*Liquid contains alcohol.   **May contain tartrazine.   †Canada only.   ‡Australia only.   ◊ OTC.

• Monitor patient closely for adverse CNS or GI reactions. If any develop, notify the doctor because the dosage will need to be adjusted or the drug temporarily withheld.

• Monitor patient's CBC and liver function studies, as ordered, to detect adverse hematologic reactions. Notify the doctor if any laboratory abnormalities are present.

• Be aware that measurements of cystine level in leukocytes may be ordered because they are useful in determining adequate dosage and compliance. When the drug is well tolerated, the goal of therapy is to keep leukocyte cystine levels below 1 mmol/^{1}/$_{2}$ cystine/mg protein 5 to 6 hours after administration of the drug. Measurements should be done at least every 3 months.

• Know that patients with cystinosis taking cysteamine hydrochloride or phosphocysteamine solutions may be transferred to equimolar doses of the drug.

☑ **PATIENT TEACHING**
• Inform the patient and parents that dosage of cysteamine is based on the patient's weight and that patient must follow doctor's directions exactly.

• Instruct the patient and parents that if a dose of the drug is missed, it should be taken as soon as possible. However, if within 2 hours of the next dose, patient should skip the missed dose and resume the regular dosing schedule. Tell patient not to double the dose.

• Tell parents of a child under age 6 not to give the child the capsule to swallow because the child may choke or aspirate it. Instead, the capsule may be opened and the contents sprinkled on food or mixed in formula.

• Inform the patient or parents that supplements also will be given to replace electrolytes lost through the kidneys and that periodic blood tests will need to be performed to help determine the correct dosage of the drug. Compliance with these measures is extremely important for maximal effectiveness of the drug.

• Instruct the patient not to engage in hazardous activities (such as driving) until the drug's CNS effects are known.

• Advise patient and parents to store the drug in a dry place, away from light.

---

etretinate
Tegison

Pregnancy Risk Category: X

HOW SUPPLIED
Capsules: 10 mg, 25 mg

ACTION
Unknown. Thought to inhibit ornithine decarboxylase, an enzyme that regulates cell growth and differentiation. May also block neutrophil migration into the epidermis.

ONSET, PEAK, DURATION
Onset and duration unknown. Peak concentration occurs in 2 to 6 hours.

INDICATIONS & DOSAGE
Severe recalcitrant psoriasis, including erythrodermia and generalized pustular types in patients unresponsive to standard therapy (topical tar plus UVB light, psoralens plus UVA light, systemic corticosteroids, and methotrexate)—
Adults: initially, 0.75 to 1 mg/kg P.O. daily in divided doses. Maximum initial dosage is 1.5 mg/kg daily. After initial response, maintenance dosage is 0.5 to 0.75 mg/kg daily.

ADVERSE REACTIONS
CNS: *benign intracranial hypertension (pseudotumor cerebri), fatigue, headache,* dizziness, lethargy, pain, rigors.
CV: thrombosis, edema.
EENT: *eye pain, blurred vision, dry eyes,* photosensitivity, decreased night vision, *conjunctivitis, diplopia, dry nose, sore mouth,* gingival bleeding.
GI: *appetite change, nausea, sore tongue, chapped lips, dry mouth, thirst,*

abdominal pain.
GU: *WBCs in urine,* proteinuria, hematuria, glycosuria.
Hematologic: *blood dyscrasia,* anemia, altered PT, *thrombocytopenia.*
Hepatic: *hepatitis,* elevated liver enzymes.
Respiratory: dyspnea.
Skin: *peeling, pruritus, alopecia, dry skin, rash, red scaly face, bruising, sunburn, nail disorders.*
Other: *bone pain, hypokalemia or hyperkalemia, hyperlipidemia, hyperostosis, muscle cramps, myalgia, fever.*

INTERACTIONS

Ethanol: increased risk of hypertriglyceridemia. Avoid concomitant use.
Hepatotoxic medications (including methotrexate): increased risk of hepatotoxicity. Monitor closely.
Tetracyclines: increased risk of pseudotumor cerebri. Avoid concomitant use.
Vitamin A: additive toxic effects. Avoid concomitant use.

EFFECTS ON DIAGNOSTIC TESTS

Hypertriglyceridemia, hypercholesterolemia, and decreased high-density lipoprotein levels have been reported in some patients. Drug may elevate AST, ALT, and low-density lipoprotein levels.

CONTRAINDICATIONS

Contraindicated in patients who are pregnant, who intend to become pregnant, or who may not use reliable contraception during and after treatment (drug causes severe birth defects).

NURSING CONSIDERATIONS

● Be aware that women of childbearing age must not receive etretinate unless pregnancy is excluded by a pregnancy test within 2 weeks before initiating therapy. Therapy may begin on 2nd or 3rd day of next normal menstrual period.
● Monitor liver function tests every 1 to 2 weeks for the first 1 to 2 months of therapy, and every 1 to 3 months there-

after, as ordered. Suspected hepatotoxicity requires discontinuation of drug.
● Monitor blood lipids every 1 to 2 weeks during treatment, as ordered.
Alert: Monitor patient for pseudotumor cerebri. If symptoms occur, immediately check for papilledema. If present, discontinue drug immediately and notify doctor.

☑ PATIENT TEACHING

● Warn patient to use effective contraception for 1 month before therapy begins, during treatment, and for an indefinite time after treatment is discontinued. Know that significant residual blood levels of etretinate have been reported as long as 3 years after discontinuation of treatment. Consequently, the period after treatment during which pregnancy must be avoided to prevent teratogenicity is unknown.
● Advise patient to take drug with milk or fatty food to enhance absorption.
● Advise patient never to double the dose but to take a missed dose as soon as possible. If it's nearly time for the next dose, the missed dose should be skipped and the schedule resumed.
● Warn patient not to take vitamin A supplements to avoid possible additive adverse reactions.
● Reassure patient that transient exacerbation of psoriasis is common during beginning of therapy.
● Advise patient to expect dry skin and possible difficulty tolerating contact lenses during treatment.
● Tell patient to avoid bright sun and to use a sunblock to prevent photosensitivity reactions.
● Advise patient to use ice or sugarless hard candy or gum for dry mouth and to check with the dentist if this continues beyond 2 weeks.
● Advise patient to report visual difficulties.
● Advise diabetic patient to monitor blood glucose closely. Adjustments of hypoglycemic medications may be necessary.

● Tell patient to report possible early signs of pseudotumor cerebri—headache, nausea and vomiting, and visual disturbances—to the doctor promptly.

---

finasteride
Proscar

Pregnancy Risk Category: X

HOW SUPPLIED
Tablets: 5 mg

ACTION
Competitively inhibits steroid 5 alpha-reductase, an enzyme responsible for formation of the potent androgen 5 alpha-dihydrotestosterone (DHT) from testosterone. Because DHT influences development of the prostate gland, decreasing levels of this hormone in adult males should relieve the symptoms associated with benign prostatic hyperplasia (BPH).

ONSET, PEAK, DURATION
Onset unknown. Serum levels peak in 1 to 2 hours. Effects persist for 24 hours after single dose; about 2 weeks after withdrawal of therapy.

INDICATIONS & DOSAGE
Symptomatic BPH—
Adults: 5 mg P.O. daily.

ADVERSE REACTIONS
GU: impotence, decreased volume of ejaculate.
Other: decreased libido.

INTERACTIONS
Theophylline: may increase theophylline clearance and decrease theophylline half-life. Monitor theophylline levels.

EFFECTS ON DIAGNOSTIC TESTS
Finasteride will decrease levels of prostate-specific antigen (PSA) even in prostate cancer. This does not indicate a beneficial effect.

CONTRAINDICATIONS
Contraindicated in patients hypersensitive to the drug. Know that although drug is not used in women, manufacturer indicates pregnancy as a contraindication.

NURSING CONSIDERATIONS
● Before therapy, know that patient should be evaluated for conditions that might mimic BPH, including hypotonic bladder; prostate cancer, infection, or stricture; or relevant neurologic conditions.
● Anticipate baseline and periodic digital rectal examinations. Although drug decreases serum PSA levels, even in prostate cancer, in clinical trials it didn't appear to decrease the rate of prostate cancer detection.
● Carefully monitor patients who have a large residual urine volume or severely diminished urine flow. Know that these patients may not be candidates for finasteride therapy.
● Carefully evaluate sustained increases in serum PSA levels, which could indicate noncompliance with therapy.
● Be aware that although drug's elimination rate is decreased in elderly patients, dosage adjustments aren't necessary.
● Because it's impossible to identify which patients will respond to finasteride, know that a minimum of 6 months of therapy may be necessary.
● Keep in mind that the long-term effects on the complications of BPH, including acute urinary obstruction, and incidence of surgery are unknown.

☑ PATIENT TEACHING
● Warn woman who is or may become pregnant not to handle crushed tablets because of risk of adverse effects on a male fetus.
● Caution patient whose sexual partner is or may become pregnant to discontinue drug or take precautions to avoid exposing her to his semen.
● Reassure patient that finasteride may decrease volume of ejaculate but

---

Reactions may be *common*, uncommon, *life-threatening*, or COMMON AND LIFE-THREATENING.

doesn't appear to impair normal sexual function. However, impotence and decreased libido have occurred in less than 4% of patients.

gallium nitrate
Ganite

Pregnancy Risk Category: C

HOW SUPPLIED
Injection: 25 mg/ml

ACTION
Unknown. Appears to reduce hypercalcemia by inhibiting resorption of bone and reducing bone turnover in patients with increased bone turnover.

ONSET, PEAK, DURATION
Onset and peak unknown. Effects persist for 6 days.

INDICATIONS & DOSAGE
Symptomatic, unresponsive hypercalcemia caused by cancer—
Adults: 200 mg/m^2 as a continuous I.V. infusion daily for 5 consecutive days or until serum calcium is normal. Lower doses (100 mg/m^2) may be given to patients with mild hypercalcemia.

ADVERSE REACTIONS
CNS: lethargy, confusion, paresthesia.
CV: tachycardia, lower extremity edema, decreased mean systolic and diastolic blood pressures.
EENT: visual or hearing impairment, acute optic neuritis.
GI: nausea and vomiting, diarrhea, constipation.
GU: *acute renal failure, increased BUN and creatinine levels.*
Hematologic: anemia, leukopenia.
Respiratory: dyspnea, rales and rhonchi, pulmonary infiltrates, pleural effusion.
Skin: rash.
Other: *hypophosphatemia, hypocalcemia, decreased serum bicarbonate,* fever, hypothermia.

INTERACTIONS
Nephrotoxic drugs, such as aminoglycosides or amphotericin B: increased risk of nephrotoxicity. Avoid concomitant use.

EFFECTS ON DIAGNOSTIC TESTS
Drug elevates serum creatinine and BUN levels; it may also alter serum calcium levels.

CONTRAINDICATIONS
Contraindicated in patients with severe renal impairment.

NURSING CONSIDERATIONS
● Make sure that patients are adequately hydrated, either with oral fluids or I.V. sodium chloride solution, as ordered, before using drug. Establish adequate urine flow (2 liters/day) before treatment. Diuretic therapy is not recommended before correction of hypovolemia. Avoid overhydration, especially in patients with decreased CV function.
● **I.V. use:** Dilute daily dose in 1 liter of 0.9% sodium chloride for injection or D$_5$W. Discard unused portion (drug contains no preservatives).
● Know that rapid I.V. infusion or dosage over 200 mg/m^2 may increase risk of nephrotoxicity or cause nausea and vomiting.
● Monitor BUN and serum creatinine levels, as ordered, during therapy. Discontinue drug if serum creatinine rises above 2.5 mg/dl, and notify doctor.
● Carefully monitor fluid intake and output and renal function, as ordered. Short-term therapy with I.V. calcium may also be needed. Overdosage is usually treated with vigorous hydration, sometimes with diuretics, for 2 to 3 days.
● In patients who require treatment with a potentially nephrotoxic drug, such as an aminoglycoside, be prepared to discontinue gallium nitrate therapy and continue hydration for several days after

administration of the nephrotoxic drug, as ordered. Monitor renal function closely.

● Monitor serum calcium levels, as ordered, and assess patients for signs of hypocalcemia, including a positive Chvostek's sign. If hypocalcemia occurs, discontinue drug and notify doctor. Treatment of hypocalcemia may be required.

● Be aware that transient hypophosphatemia is common. Patients may require oral phosphorus supplements.

☑ **PATIENT TEACHING**
● Stress importance of forcing fluids as directed throughout therapy.

● Advise patient to report hearing or vision problems. In early clinical trials, a few patients experienced hearing loss and optic neuritis after high-dose gallium nitrate therapy when combined with investigational antineoplastic agents.

---

imiglucerase
Cerezyme

Pregnancy Risk Category: C

HOW SUPPLIED
Injection: 200 units/vial

ACTION
Catalyzes the hydrolysis of glucocerebroside to glucose and ceramide (part of the normal degradation pathway for lipids) and thus prevents the sequelae of Gaucher's disease, which normally occur as a result of the accumulation of glucocerebroside.

ONSET, PEAK, DURATION
Onset and duration unknown. Levels peak in 1 hour.

INDICATIONS & DOSAGE
Long-term endogenous enzyme (glucosylceramidase) replacement therapy in confirmed type I Gaucher's disease—
Adults and children: dosage individu-

alized; initially, 2.5 to 60 U/kg I.V. administered over 1 to 2 hours. Frequency of dosing typically is once q 2 weeks, but may range from three times weekly to once monthly, depending on severity of the disease. Dosage may be reduced for maintenance therapy, at intervals of 3 to 6 months, while response parameters are carefully monitored.

ADVERSE REACTIONS
CNS: headache, dizziness.
CV: mild hypotension.
GI: nausea, abdominal discomfort.
GU: decreased urinary frequency.
Skin: pruritus, rash.
Other: hypersensitivity reactions.

INTERACTIONS
None significant.

EFFECTS ON DIAGNOSTIC TESTS
None reported.

CONTRAINDICATIONS
None known.

NURSING CONSIDERATIONS
● Use with caution in patients who have exhibited symptoms of hypersensitivity to the product and in those who have previously been treated with alglucerase and who have developed antibody to alglucerase or exhibited symptoms of hypersensitivity to alglucerase.
● **I.V. use:** Reconstitute each vial with 5.1 ml of sterile water for injection USP. Inspect solution for particulate matter and discoloration before use; if either is present, do not use. Withdraw 5 ml (amount in vial after reconstitution is 5.3 ml) of the reconstituted solution and dilute solution further with 0.9% sodium chloride solution to a final volume of 100 to 200 ml. Because imiglucerase is preservative-free, use immediately. Administer by I.V. infusion over 1 to 2 hours.
● Know that when diluted to 50 ml, imiglucerase has been shown to be stable for up to 24 hours when stored at 2°

---

to 8° C (36° to 46° F).
● Monitor response parameters for doctor to determine lowest effective dosage.

☑ **PATIENT TEACHING**
● Explain to patient and family how drug works and how it is administered. Stress importance of compliance with administration schedule.
● Tell patient to report persistent or severe adverse reactions promptly.

---

isotretinoin
Accutane, Roaccutane‡

Pregnancy Risk Category: X

HOW SUPPLIED
Capsules: 10 mg, 20 mg, 40 mg

ACTION
Unknown. Thought to normalize keratinization, reversibly decrease size of sebaceous glands, and alter composition of sebum to a less viscous form that is less likely to cause follicular plugging.

ONSET, PEAK, DURATION
Onset and duration unknown. Plasma levels peak in about 3 hours.

INDICATIONS & DOSAGE
Severe recalcitrant nodular acne unresponsive to conventional therapy—
Adults and adolescents: 0.5 to 2 mg/kg P.O. daily in two divided doses for 15 to 20 weeks.

ADVERSE REACTIONS
CNS: headache, fatigue, *pseudotumor cerebri* (benign intracranial hypertension).
EENT: *conjunctivitis,* corneal deposits, dry eyes, visual disturbances, *epistaxis, dry nose.*
GI: nonspecific GI symptoms, gum bleeding and inflammation, *nausea, vomiting,* anorexia, *dry mouth, abdominal pain.*
Hematologic: anemia, elevated platelet count.
Hepatic: elevated AST, ALT, and alkaline phosphatase levels.
Skin: *cheilosis, rash, dry skin, facial skin desquamation,* peeling of palms and toes, skin infection, photosensitivity, *cheilitis, pruritus, fragility.*
Other: *hypertriglyceridemia, musculoskeletal pain (skeletal hyperostosis), drying of mucous membranes, petechiae, nail brittleness,* thinning of hair, hyperglycemia.

INTERACTIONS
Ethanol: increased risk of hypertriglyceridemia. Avoid concomitant use.
Tetracyclines: increased risk of pseudotumor cerebri. Avoid concomitant use.
Vitamin A, products containing vitamin A: increased toxic effects of isotretinoin. Don't use together without the doctor's permission.

EFFECTS ON DIAGNOSTIC TESTS
The physiologic effects of the drug may alter liver function tests, blood counts, and blood glucose, uric acid, cholesterol, and triglyceride levels. May cause elevation of erythrocyte sedimentation rate.

CONTRAINDICATIONS
Contraindicated in women of childbearing age unless patient has had a negative serum pregnancy test within 2 weeks before beginning therapy; will begin drug therapy on 2nd or 3rd day of next menstrual period; and will comply with stringent contraceptive measures for 1 month before therapy, during therapy, and for at least 1 month after therapy. *Severe fetal abnormalities may occur if used during pregnancy.* Also contraindicated in patients hypersensitive to parabens, which are used as preservatives.

NURSING CONSIDERATIONS
● Monitor baseline serum lipid studies and liver function tests prior to therapy, as ordered.
● Monitor serum lipid studies and liver

---

function tests at regular intervals until response to drug is established, usually about 4 weeks.

• Monitor blood glucose level regularly.

• Monitor CK levels in patients who participate in vigorous physical activity, as ordered.

• Know that most adverse reactions appear to be dose-related, occurring at dosages greater than 1 mg/kg daily. They are generally reversible when therapy is discontinued or dosage is reduced.

Alert: Be aware that patients who experience headache, nausea and vomiting, or visual disturbances should be screened for papilledema. Signs and symptoms of pseudotumor cerebri require immediate discontinuation of therapy and prompt neurologic intervention.

• Anticipate a second course of therapy, if needed, not to start for at least 8 weeks after completion of first course because improvement may continue after withdrawal of drug.

☑ **PATIENT TEACHING**

• Advise patient to take drug with or shortly after meals to ensure adequate absorption.

• Tell patient to immediately report any visual disturbances and bone, muscle, or joint pain.

• Warn patient that contact lenses may feel uncomfortable during isotretinoin therapy.

• Warn patient against using abrasives, medicated soaps and cleansers, acne preparations containing peeling agents, and topical alcohol preparations (including cosmetics, after-shave, cologne) because these agents cause cumulative irritation or excessive drying of skin.

• Tell patient to avoid prolonged exposure to the sun and to use sunblock. Drug may have additive effect if used with other agents that cause photosensitivity.

• Advise patient of childbearing age to use two reliable forms of contraception simultaneously, unless abstinence is the chosen method of birth control, for 1

month prior to, during, and 1 month after treatment.

• Advise patient not to donate blood during or for 30 days after therapy; severe fetal abnormalities may occur if a pregnant patient receives blood containing isotretinoin.

---

levocarnitine (L-carnitine)
Carnitor, VitaCarn

Pregnancy Risk Category: B

HOW SUPPLIED
Tablets: 330 mg
Capsules: 250 mg ◊
Oral liquid: 100 mg/ml
Injection: 1 g/5 ml

ACTION
Facilitates transport of fatty acids into cellular mitochondria. The fatty acids are then used to produce energy.

ONSET, PEAK, DURATION
Unknown.

INDICATIONS & DOSAGE
Primary and secondary systemic carnitine deficiency—
Adults: 990 mg P.O. b.i.d. or t.i.d. Alternatively, 10 to 30 ml (1 to 3 g) of oral liquid daily.
Children: 50 to 100 mg/kg/day P.O. in divided doses.
   All dosages depend on the clinical response. Higher dosages may be given. However, for children, maximum dosage is 3 g/day.
Acute and chronic treatment of secondary carnitine deficiency—
Adults: 50 mg/kg I.V. slowly over 2 to 3 minutes q 3 to 4 hours.

ADVERSE REACTIONS
GI: *nausea, vomiting, cramps, diarrhea.*
Other: *body odor.*

INTERACTIONS
D,L-carnitine (sold as vitamin B$_T$): inhi-

bition of levocarnitine and possible deficiency. Avoid concomitant use.
Valproic acid: increased requirement for carnitine. Adjust dosage as ordered.

EFFECTS ON DIAGNOSTIC TESTS
None reported.

CONTRAINDICATIONS
None known.

NURSING CONSIDERATIONS
● Give enteral liquid alone or dissolved in drinks or liquid food.
● Space doses evenly every 3 to 4 hours and give drug with or after meals, if possible.
● Use entire or partial contents of containers of liquid immediately after opening; discard any unused contents.
● Do not refrigerate solution.
● Monitor patient's tolerance during 1st week of therapy and after increasing dosage, as ordered.
● Monitor blood chemistry results and plasma carnitine concentrations periodically, as ordered, as well as vital signs and patient's overall clinical condition.

☑ **PATIENT TEACHING**
● Tell patient to consume oral liquid slowly to minimize GI distress. If GI intolerance persists, dosage may have to be reduced.
● Warn patient to avoid "vitamin B_T" in health food stores. This will interact with the drug and render it ineffective.
● Caution patient not to share drug with others. Some people have used it to improve athletic performance.
● Warn patient about possible body odor.

---

levomethadyl acetate hydrochloride
ORLAAM

Controlled Substance Schedule II
Pregnancy Risk Category: C

HOW SUPPLIED
Oral solution: 10 mg/ml

ACTION
A synthetic opiate agonist structurally similar to methadone that suppresses symptoms of withdrawal in opiate-tolerant persons by cross-substituting for opiate agonists. Long-term administration may produce sufficient tolerance to block the euphoric effects of opiate agonists.

ONSET, PEAK, DURATION
Onset unknown. Peak $1\frac{1}{2}$ to 4 hours. Effects persist for 48 to 72 hours.

INDICATIONS & DOSAGE
Opiate addiction—
Adults: dosage is highly individualized. Initially, 20 to 40 mg q 48 to 72 hours. Subsequent doses increased in increments of 5 to 10 mg at 48 to 72 hour intervals until steady state is reached, usually within 1 to 2 weeks. Most patients are stable on 60 to 90 mg three times a week.

ADVERSE REACTIONS
CNS: drowsiness, sedation.
CV: bradycardia, edema, prolonged QT interval.
EENT: blurred vision, rhinitis.
GI: *abdominal pain, diarrhea, constipation, dry mouth, nausea, vomiting.*
GU: *impotence, difficulty with ejaculation.*
Respiratory: *cough.*
Skin: *rash, diaphoresis.*
Other: yawning, arthralgia, asthenia, back pain, chills, flulike syndrome, malaise, abstinence syndrome with sudden withdrawal.

INTERACTIONS
Carbamazepine, phenobarbital, phenytoin, rifampin: increased hepatic enzyme activity; may increase levomethadyl's peak activity or shorten its duration of action. Monitor closely.
Cimetidine, erythromycin, ketoconazole:

---

decreased hepatic enzyme activity; may decrease levomethadyl's peak activity or prolong its duration of action. Monitor closely.

Naloxone, pentazocine or other opioid agonist-antagonists: may precipitate abstinence syndrome. Don't use together.

EFFECTS ON DIAGNOSTIC TESTS
None reported.

CONTRAINDICATIONS
Contraindicated in patients hypersensitive to the drug.

NURSING CONSIDERATIONS
● Use cautiously in patients with cardiac conduction defects or with hepatic or renal failure.
● Be aware that levomethadyl is to be used only by certain licensed and approved clinics. There are no recognized clinical uses for the drug outside of addiction treatment programs. Levomethadyl may only be dispensed by treatment programs approved by the FDA, DEA, and designated state authority. By law, take-home doses are forbidden. Also by law, oral solutions must be diluted before being administered to the patient. The diluent should be a different color than the one used to dilute the methadone oral solution in the same clinic setting.
● If administering to women of childbearing age, anticipate monthly pregnancy tests. Patients should be switched to methadone if pregnancy occurs.
Alert: Know that this drug should never be administered on a daily basis because of the risk of fatal overdose.
● Know that most patients can tolerate the 72-hour interval between weekly regimens. If withdrawal is a problem during the 72-hour interval, be prepared to increase the preceding dose or switch to an alternate-day schedule as ordered. Never give levomethadyl on 2 consecutive days; instead, give small supplemental doses of methadone. Consider the risk of drug diversion before giving

patients take-home methadone.
● When used to replace methadone, keep in mind that the suggested initial dose is 1.2 to 1.3 times the daily methadone dose three times a week, not to exceed 120 mg. Adjust dosage according to clinical response as ordered. The crossover to methadone should be done in a single dose rather than decreasing doses of methadone and increasing doses of levomethadyl.

☑ **PATIENT TEACHING**
● Explain how drug is administered, and review administration schedule with patient and family.
● Inform female patient of need for monthly pregnancy tests. Advise patient to avoid pregnancy but if pregnancy is suspected to call doctor immediately because drug will need to be discontinued.

mesalamine
Asacol, Salofalk, Mesasal, Pentasa, Rowasa

Pregnancy Risk Category: B

HOW SUPPLIED
Tablets (delayed-release): 400 mg
Extended-release tablets: 250 mg
Capsules (controlled-release): 250 mg
Rectal suspension: 4 g/60 ml
Suppositories: 500 mg

ACTION
Unknown. An active metabolite of sulfasalazine; probably acts topically by inhibiting prostaglandin production in the colon. Exact mechanism unknown.

ONSET, PEAK, DURATION
Onset and duration unknown. Peak levels occur within 3 to 12 hours.

INDICATIONS & DOSAGE
Active mild to moderate distal ulcerative colitis, proctitis, or proctosigmoiditis—
Adults: 800 mg P.O. (tablets) t.i.d. for

total dose of 2.4 g/day for 6 weeks; 1 g P.O. (capsules) 4 times daily for a total dose of 4 g up to 8 weeks; 500 mg P.R. (suppository) b.i.d., or 4 g as a retention enema once daily (preferably h.s.). Rectal dosage form should be retained overnight (for about 8 hours). Usual course of therapy for rectal form is 3 to 6 weeks.

ADVERSE REACTIONS
CNS: headache, dizziness, fatigue, malaise, asthenia, chills.
GI: abdominal pain, cramps, discomfort, flatulence, diarrhea, rectal pain, bloating, nausea, *pancolitis*, vomiting, constipation, eructation.
Respiratory: wheezing.
Skin: itching, rash, urticaria, hair loss.
Other: *anaphylaxis* (rare), fever, arthralgia, chest pain, myalgia, back pain, hypertonia.

INTERACTIONS
Lactolose: may impair release of delayed or extended release preparations.
Omeprazole: increases absorption of mesalamine.

EFFECTS ON DIAGNOSTIC TESTS
None reported.

CONTRAINDICATIONS
Contraindicated in patients hypersensitive to the drug, its components, or salicylates.

NURSING CONSIDERATIONS
● Use cautiously in patients with renal impairment. Problems have not been documented, but nephrotoxic potential from absorbed mesalamine exists.
● Monitor periodic renal function studies in patients on long-term therapy, as ordered.
● Because it contains potassium metabisulfite, keep in mind that mesalamine may cause hypersensitivity reactions in patients sensitive to sulfites.

☑ PATIENT TEACHING
● Instruct patient to carefully follow instructions supplied with medication.
● Instruct patient to discontinue drug if he experiences a fever or rash. Patient intolerant of sulfasalazine may also be hypersensitive to mesalamine.

---

mesna
Mesnex, Dromitexan

Pregnancy Risk Category: B

HOW SUPPLIED
Injection: 100 mg/ml

ACTION
Prevents ifosfamide-induced hemorrhagic cystitis by reacting with urotoxic ifosfamide metabolites.

ONSET, PEAK, DURATION
Unknown.

INDICATIONS & DOSAGE
Prophylaxis of hemorrhagic cystitis in patients receiving ifosfamide—
Adults: dosage varies with amount of ifosfamide administered; calculated as 20% (w/w) of the ifosfamide dose at time of ifosfamide administration. Usual dosage is 240 mg/m^2 as an I.V. bolus with administration of ifosfamide; repeated at 4 and 8 hours after administration of ifosfamide.

ADVERSE REACTIONS
CNS: *headache, fatigue.*
GI: *soft stools, nausea, vomiting, diarrhea, dysgeusia.*
Other: *limb pain, hypotension, allergy.*
Note: Because mesna is used concomitantly with ifosfamide and other chemotherapeutic agents, it is difficult to determine adverse reactions attributable solely to mesna.

INTERACTIONS
None significant.

EFFECTS ON DIAGNOSTIC TESTS
Mesna may produce a false-positive test for urinary ketones. A red-violet color will return to violet with the addition of acetic acid.

CONTRAINDICATIONS
Contraindicated in patients hypersensitive to mesna or thiol-containing compounds.

NURSING CONSIDERATIONS
• **I.V. use:** Prepare I.V. solution by diluting commercially available ampules with D_5W solution, dextrose 5% and 0.9% sodium chloride for injection, 0.9% sodium chloride for injection, or lactated Ringer's solution to obtain a final solution of 20 mg mesna/ml.
• Mesna I.V. is incompatible with cisplatin; do not mix them.
• Diluted solutions are stable for 24 hours at room temperature, but it is recommended that they be refrigerated and used within 6 hours. After opening ampule, discard any unused drug.
• Monitor urine samples daily in patients receiving mesna for hematuria.
• Know that mesna is not effective in preventing hematuria from other causes (such as thrombocytopenia).
• Although formulated to prevent hemorrhagic cystitis from ifosfamide, be aware that drug will not protect against other toxicities associated with ifosfamide therapy.
• Keep in mind that up to 6% of patients may not respond to drug's protective effects.

☑ **PATIENT TEACHING**
• Explain need for drug and how it is administered to patient and family.
• Instruct patient to report persistent or severe adverse reactions.

---

methoxsalen (topical)
Oxsoralen

Pregnancy Risk Category: C

HOW SUPPLIED
Lotion: 1%

ACTION
Unknown. May enhance melanogenesis, either directly or secondarily, to an inflammatory process.

ONSET, PEAK, DURATION
Unknown.

INDICATIONS & DOSAGE
To induce repigmentation in vitiligo; psoriasis—
Adults and children over 12 years: lotion applied to small, well-defined vitiliginous lesions. For optimum effect, the lotion should be applied about 1 to 2 hours before exposure to UV light. The treated area may be exposed to UV light for a limited time.
   After exposure, wash lesions with soap and water, and protect area with sunblock. Manufacturer recommends weekly treatment.

ADVERSE REACTIONS
Skin: edema, erythema, painful blistering, burning, peeling, pruritus.

INTERACTIONS
Photosensitizing agents: may increase methoxsalen toxicity. Don't use together.

EFFECTS ON DIAGNOSTIC TESTS
Abnormal liver function test results have been reported, but the exact relationship is unknown.

CONTRAINDICATIONS
Contraindicated in patients sensitive to psoralen compounds and in patients with diseases associated with photosensitivity (such as porphyria, acute lupus erythematosus, xerodoma, or hydromorphic and polymorphic light eruptions). Also contraindicated in patients with melanoma, invasive squamous cell carcinoma, and aphakia.

Reactions may be *common*, uncommon, *life-threatening*, or COMMON AND LIFE-THREATENING.

NURSING CONSIDERATIONS

• Use cautiously in patients with familial history of sunlight allergy, GI diseases, or chronic infection.

• Be prepared to regulate therapy carefully. Overdosage or overexposure to light can cause serious burning or blistering.

• Protect patient's eyes and lips during light exposure treatments.

• Obtain monthly liver function tests for patients with vitiligo (especially at beginning of therapy), as ordered.

☑ PATIENT TEACHING

• Tell patient to avoid excessive sunlight during therapy.

• Inform patient of need for monthly blood tests, and stress importance of compliance to test schedule.

---

minoxidil (topical)
Rogaine

Pregnancy Risk Category: C

HOW SUPPLIED
Topical solution: 2%

ACTION
Unknown. Stimulates hair growth, possibly by dilating arterial microcapillaries around hair follicles.

ONSET, PEAK, DURATION
Unknown.

INDICATIONS & DOSAGE
Androgentic alopecia—
Adults: 1 ml of 2% solution applied to affected area b.i.d. Maximum daily dosage is 2 ml.

ADVERSE REACTIONS
CNS: headache, dizziness, faintness, light-headedness.
CV: edema, chest pain, hypertension, hypotension, palpitations, increased or decreased pulse rate.
EENT: sinusitis.

GI: diarrhea, nausea, vomiting.
GU: urinary tract infection, renal calculi, urethritis.
Respiratory: bronchitis, upper respiratory infection.
Skin: irritant dermatitis, allergic contact dermatitis, eczema, hypertrichosis, local erythema, pruritus, dry skin or scalp, flaking, alopecia, exacerbation of hair loss.
Other: back pain, tendinitis, edema, weight gain.

INTERACTIONS
Topical corticosteroids, petrolatum, topical retinoids, or other drugs that may enhance skin absorption: increased risk of systemic effects of minoxidil. Do not apply minoxidil with other drugs.

EFFECTS ON DIAGNOSTIC TESTS
None reported.

CONTRAINDICATIONS
Contraindicated in patients hypersensitive to the drug or any component of the solution.

NURSING CONSIDERATIONS
• Use cautiously in individuals over 50 years, and in those with cardiac, renal, or hepatic disease.

• Know that patients need to have normal, healthy scalps before beginning therapy, because absorption of drug through irritated skin may cause adverse systemic effects.

• Be aware that treatment is most likely to succeed in patients with balding area smaller than 4″ (10 cm) that developed within the past 10 years.

☑ PATIENT TEACHING
• Teach patient how to apply topical minoxidil. Hair and scalp should be thoroughly dry before application, and drug should not be applied to any other body areas. Tell patient not to use drug on irritated or sunburned scalp or with any other medication on scalp. Tell him to thoroughly wash hands after application.

• Warn patient to avoid inhaling any spray or mist from drug. He should avoid spraying around eyes because solution contains alcohol and may be irritating.
• Teach patient to monitor pulse rate and body weight.
• Advise patient of need for medical follow-ups 1 month after therapy starts and every 6 months thereafter.
• Advise patient that therapy will be prolonged and will continue for at least 4 months before clinical effects appear. About 40% of patients will see moderate to dense hair growth.
• Tell patient that discontinuing drug may result in loss of new hair growth. New hair growth is usually fine and may be colorless, but will resemble existing hair after continued treatment.

nimodipine
Nimotop

Pregnancy Risk Category: C

HOW SUPPLIED
Capsules: 30 mg

ACTION
Inhibits calcium ion influx across cardiac and smooth muscle cells, decreasing myocardial contractility and oxygen demand, and dilates coronary and cerebral arteries and arterioles.

ONSET, PEAK, DURATION
Onset and duration unknown. Peak effect occurs within 1 hour.

INDICATIONS & DOSAGE
Improvement of neurologic deficits in patients after subarachnoid hemorrhage from ruptured congenital aneurysms—
Adults: 60 mg P.O. q 4 hours for 21 days. Therapy begun within 96 hours after subarachnoid hemorrhage.
  In patients with hepatic failure, 30 mg P.O. q 4 hours for 21 days.

ADVERSE REACTIONS
CNS: headache, psychic disturbances.
CV: decreased blood pressure, flushing, edema, tachycardia.
GI: nausea, diarrhea, abdominal discomfort.
Respiratory: dyspnea.
Skin: dermatitis, rash.
Other: muscle cramps.

INTERACTIONS
Antihypertensives: possible enhanced hypotensive effect. Monitor patient closely.
Calcium channel blockers: possible enhanced CV effects. Monitor patient closely.

EFFECTS ON DIAGNOSTIC TESTS
None reported.

CONTRAINDICATIONS
None known.

NURSING CONSIDERATIONS
• Use cautiously in patients with hepatic failure.
• Know that nimodipine should be reserved for patients who are in good neurologic condition (for example, Hunt and Hess grades I to III).
• Monitor blood pressure and heart rate in all patients, especially at start of therapy.
• If the capsule cannot be swallowed, make a hole in each end of the capsule with an 18-gauge needle, and extract the contents into a syringe. Empty the syringe into patient's naso-gastric tube. Flush tube with 30 ml of normal (0.9%) saline solution.

☑ PATIENT TEACHING
• Explain need for drug, and review administration schedule with patient and family. Stress importance of compliance for maximum drug effectiveness.
• Instruct patient to report persistent or severe adverse reactions promptly.

olsalazine sodium
Dipentum

Pregnancy Risk Category: C

HOW SUPPLIED
Capsules: 250 mg

ACTION
Unknown. After oral administration, converts to 5-aminosalicylic acid (5-ASA or mesalamine) in the colon, where it has a local anti-inflammatory effect.

ONSET, PEAK, DURATION
Onset and duration unknown. Time to peak concentration is 1 hour.

INDICATIONS & DOSAGE
Maintenance of remission of ulcerative colitis in patients intolerant of sulfasalazine—
Adults: 500 mg P.O. b.i.d. with meals.

ADVERSE REACTIONS
CNS: headache, depression, vertigo, dizziness, fatigue.
GI: *diarrhea,* nausea, *abdominal pain,* dyspepsia, bloating, anorexia.
Skin: rash, itching.
Other: arthralgia.

INTERACTIONS
Anticoagulants, coumarin derivatives: prolonged PT.

EFFECTS ON DIAGNOSTIC TESTS
None known.

CONTRAINDICATIONS
Contraindicated in patients hypersensitive to salicylates.

NURSING CONSIDERATIONS
● Use cautiously in patients with preexisting renal disease. Although problems have not been reported with this drug, the possibility of renal tubular damage from absorbed mesalamine or its metabolites must be considered.

● Regularly monitor BUN and creatinine levels and urinalysis in patients with preexisting renal disease, as ordered.
● Be aware that in clinical trials, 17% of all patients reported diarrhea during therapy. Although diarrhea appears dose-related, it is difficult to distinguish from worsening of disease symptoms. Exacerbation of disease has been noted with similar drugs.

☑ **PATIENT TEACHING**
● Teach patient to take drug in evenly divided doses and with food to minimize adverse GI reactions.
● Instruct patient to report persistent or severe adverse reactions promptly.

pamidronate disodium
Aredia

Pregnancy Risk Category: C

HOW SUPPLIED
Injection: 30-mg, 60-mg, 90-mg vials

ACTION
An antihypercalcemic agent that inhibits resorption of bone. Adsorbs to hydroxyapatite crystals in bone and may directly block dissolution of calcium phosphate. Blocks mature osteoclast formation. Drug apparently doesn't inhibit bone formation or mineralization.

ONSET, PEAK, DURATION
Unknown.

INDICATIONS & DOSAGE
Moderate to severe hypercalcemia associated with cancer (with or without bone metastases)—
Adults: dosage depends on severity of hypercalcemia. Serum calcium levels should be corrected for serum albumin:

$$\text{Corrected serum calcium (CCa) (in mg/dl)} = \text{serum calcium (in mg/dl)} + 0.8 \, (4 - \text{serum albumin (in g/dl)})$$

Patients with moderate hypercalcemia (CCa levels of 12 to 13.5 mg/dl) may re-

ceive 60 to 90 mg by I.V. infusion over 4 hours for 60-mg dose and over 24 hours for 90-mg dose. Patients with severe hypercalcemia (CCa levels over 13.5 mg/dl) may receive 90 mg by I.V. infusion over 24 hours. A minimum of 7 days should elapse before retreatment to allow for full response to the initial dose.
Moderate to severe Paget's disease—
Adults: 30 mg I.V. as a 4-hour infusion on 3 consecutive days for total dose of 90 mg. Cycle repeated, as needed.
✳ *New indication: Osteolytic bone metastases of breast cancer in combination with standard antineoplastic therapy—*
Adults: 90 mg I.V. infusion over 2 hours q 3 to 4 weeks.

ADVERSE REACTIONS
CNS: *seizures, fatigue,* somnolence.
CV: atrial fibrillation, syncope, tachycardia, *hypertension.*
GI: *abdominal pain, anorexia, constipation, nausea, vomiting,* GI hemorrhage.
Hematologic: leukopenia, ***thrombocytopenia,*** anemia.
Other: *hypophosphatemia, hypokalemia, hypomagnesemia, hypocalcemia, fever, infusion-site reaction.*

INTERACTIONS
None significant.

EFFECTS ON DIAGNOSTIC TESTS
Pamidronate therapy may alter serum electrolyte levels, including serum calcium, potassium, magnesium, and phosphate.

CONTRAINDICATIONS
Contraindicated in patients hypersensitive to the drug or to other biphosphonates, such as etidronate.

NURSING CONSIDERATIONS
• Use with extreme caution, and consider the risks versus benefits in patients with renal impairment.
• Assess hydration status prior to treatment. Know that drug should be used only after patients have been vigorously hydrated with sodium chloride solution. In patients with mild to moderate hypercalcemia, hydration alone may be sufficient.
• **I.V. use:** Reconstitute vial with 10 ml of sterile water for injection. After drug is completely dissolved, add to 1,000 ml of 0.45% or 0.9% sodium chloride for injection or D_5W. Do not mix with infusion solutions that contain calcium, such as Ringer's injection or lactated Ringer's injection. Visually inspect for precipitate before administering.
• Give only by I.V. infusion. Animal studies have shown evidence of nephropathy when drug is given as a bolus.
• Because drug can cause electrolyte disturbances, carefully monitor serum electrolytes, especially calcium, phosphate, and magnesium, as ordered. Short-term administration of calcium may be necessary in patients with severe hypocalcemia. Also monitor creatinine level, CBC and differential count, and hematocrit and hemoglobin levels, as ordered.
• Carefully monitor patients with preexisting anemia, leukopenia, or thrombocytopenia during first 2 weeks of therapy.
• Monitor patient's temperature. In clinical trials, 27% of patients experienced an elevation of 1° C (1.8° F) for 24 to 48 hours after therapy.
• Solution is stable for 24 hours at room temperature.

☑ PATIENT TEACHING
• Explain need for drug and how it is administered to patient and family.
• Instruct patient to report adverse reactions promptly.

---

pilocarpine hydrochloride
Salagen

Pregnancy Risk Category: C

HOW SUPPLIED
Tablets: 5 mg

ACTION
A cholinergic parasympathomimetic agent that increases secretion of salivary glands, eliminating dryness.

ONSET, PEAK, DURATION
Onset is 20 minutes. Time to peak effect is 1 hour. Duration of action is 3 to 5 hours.

INDICATIONS & DOSAGE
Treatment of xerostomia from salivary gland hypofunction caused by radiotherapy for cancer of head and neck—
Adults: 5 mg P.O. t.i.d.; may be increased to 10 mg P.O. t.i.d, as needed.

ADVERSE REACTIONS
CNS: *dizziness, headache,* tremor.
CV: hypertension, tachycardia.
EENT: *rhinitis,* lacrimation, amblyopia, pharyngitis, voice alteration, conjunctivitis, epistaxis, *sinusitis, abnormal vision.*
GI: *nausea,* dyspepsia, diarrhea, abdominal pain, vomiting, dysphagia.
GU: *urinary frequency.*
Skin: *flushing,* rash, pruritus.
Other: *sweating, chills, asthenia,* edema, taste perversion, myalgia.

INTERACTIONS
Beta-adrenergic antagonists: may increase risk of conduction disturbances. Use together cautiously.
Drugs with parasympathomimetic effects: may result in additive pharmacologic effects. Monitor patient closely.
Drugs with anticholinergic effects: may antagonize anticholinergic effects. Use together cautiously.

EFFECTS ON DIAGNOSTIC TESTS
None reported.

CONTRAINDICATIONS
Contraindicated in patients with uncontrolled asthma or hypersensitivity to pilocarpine and when miosis is undesirable, such as in acute iritis or narrow-angle glaucoma.

NURSING CONSIDERATIONS
● Use cautiously in patients with cardiovascular disease, controlled asthma, chronic bronchitis, chronic obstructive pulmonary disease, cholelithiasis, biliary tract disease, nephrolithiasis, or cognitive or psychiatric disturbances.
● Drug should not be used in breast-feeding women.
● Safety and efficacy in children have not been established.
● Because retinal detachment has been reported with pilocarpine use in patients with retinal disease, examine the patient's fundus carefully before therapy begins.
● Monitor the patient for signs of toxicity: headache, visual disturbance, lacrimation, sweating, respiratory distress, gastrointestinal spasm, nausea, vomiting, diarrhea, atrioventricular block, tachycardia, bradycardia, hypotension, hypertension, shock, mental confusion, arrhythmia, and tremors. Immediately notify the doctor of suspected toxicity.

☑ **PATIENT TEACHING**
● Warn the patient that driving ability may be impaired by drug-induced visual disturbances, especially at night.
● Advise the patient to drink plenty of fluids to prevent dehydration.

---

riluzole
Rilutek

Pregnancy Risk Category: C

HOW SUPPLIED
Tablets: 50 mg

ACTION
Unknown.

ONSET, PEAK, DURATION
Unknown.

INDICATIONS & DOSAGE
Amyotrophic lateral sclerosis—
Adults: 50 mg P.O. q 12 hours, taken on empty stomach.

ADVERSE REACTIONS
CNS: headache, aggravation reaction, hypertonia, depression, dizziness, insomnia, somnolence, vertigo, circumoral paresthesia.
CV: hypertension, tachycardia, palpitation, postural hypotension.
GI: abdominal pain, *nausea,* vomiting, dyspepsia, anorexia, diarrhea, flatulence, stomatitis.
GU: urinary tract infection, dysuria.
Respiratory: *decreased lung function,* rhinitis, increased cough, sinusitis.
Skin: pruritus, eczema, alopecia, exfoliative dermatitis.
Other: *asthenia,* back pain, malaise, dry mouth, tooth disorder, oral moniliasis, phlebitis, weight loss, peripheral edema, arthralgia.

INTERACTIONS
No clinical trials have studied riluzole's interaction with other drugs. Closely monitor patients receiving concomitant therapy, and use caution when giving potentially hepatotoxic drugs (allopurinol, methyldopa, sulfasalazine) concomitantly. Potential inhibitors of CVP 1AZ (caffeine, phenacetin, theophylline, amitriptyline, and quinolones) could decrease riluzole's elimination. Inducers of CVP 1AZ (cigarette smoke, charbroiled foods, rifampicin, and omeprazole) could increase riluzole's elimination.

EFFECTS ON DIAGNOSTIC TESTS
None reported.

CONTRAINDICATIONS
Contraindicated in patients with history of severe hypersensitivity to riluzole or any component of drug.

NURSING CONSIDERATIONS
● Use cautiously in patients with hepatic or renal dysfunction, in elderly patients, and in females and Japanese patients (who may have a lower metabolic capacity to eliminate riluzole than do males and Caucasians, respectively).
● Be aware that elevations in baseline liver function studies (especially bilirubin) preclude use of riluzole. Liver function studies should be done periodically during therapy, as ordered. In many patients, drug may increase serum aminotransferase; if level exceeds 5 times the upper limit of normal or if clinical jaundice develops, notify the doctor.
● Give drug at least 1 hour before or 2 hours after a meal to avoid decreased bioavailability.

☑ PATIENT TEACHING
● Tell the patient to take drug at same time each day. If a dose is missed, tell him to take next tablet when planned.
● Instruct him to report fever to the doctor, who will want to order a WBC count.
● Warn him to avoid hazardous activities until CNS effects of drug are known and to limit alcohol use while taking drug.
● Tell him to store drug at room temperature, protected from bright light, and to keep it out of children's reach.

---

ritodrine hydrochloride
Yutopar

Pregnancy Risk Category: B

HOW SUPPLIED
Injection: 10 mg/ml, 15 mg/ml
Injection for I.V. infusion: 0.3 mg/ml (150 mg in 500 ml D_5W)

ACTION
A beta-receptor agonist that stimulates the $beta_2$-adrenergic receptors in uterine smooth muscle, inhibiting contractility.

ONSET, PEAK, DURATION
Onset occurs in 30 to 60 minutes after oral administration, 5 minutes after I.V. administration. Serum levels peak 30 to 60 minutes after oral administration in nonpregnant women; 60 minutes after I.V. administration in nonpregnant women. Duration unknown.

INDICATIONS & DOSAGE
Preterm labor—
Adults: dilute 150 mg in 500 ml of fluid, yielding a final concentration of 0.3 mg/ml. Usual initial dose is 0.05 mg/minute I.V., gradually increased by 0.05 mg/minute q 10 minutes until desired result is obtained or until maternal heart rate reaches 130 beats/ minute. Effective dosage usually ranges from 0.15 to 0.35 mg/minute.
Note: I.V. infusion should be continued for 24 hours after contractions have stopped. Recurrence of preterm labor may be treated with repeated infusion of ritodrine.

ADVERSE REACTIONS
CNS: nervousness, anxiety, *headaches, tremors,* emotional upset, malaise.
CV: dose-related alterations in blood pressure, palpitations, ***pulmonary edema,*** tachycardia.
GI: *nausea, vomiting.*
Hematologic: leukopenia, **agranulocytosis.**
Other: *erythema, hyperglycemia,* hypokalemia, ***anaphylactic shock.***

INTERACTIONS
Atropine: may potentiate systemic hypertension.
Beta-adrenergic blockers: may inhibit ritodrine's action. Avoid concurrent use.
Corticosteroids: may produce pulmonary edema in mother. Monitor patient closely.
Inhalation anesthetics, magnesium sulfate, diazoxide, and meperidine: potentiated adverse cardiac effects, arrhythmias, and hypotension. Monitor patient closely.

Sympathomimetics: additive sympathomimetic effects. Use together cautiously.

EFFECTS ON DIAGNOSTIC TESTS
I.V. administration of ritodrine elevates the plasma insulin and glucose levels and decreases plasma potassium concentrations (values usually return to normal within 24 hours after drug is stopped).

CONTRAINDICATIONS
Contraindicated in pregnant women before 20th week of pregnancy and in women with antepartum hemorrhage, eclampsia and severe preeclampsia, intrauterine fetal death, chorioamnionitis, maternal cardiac disease, pulmonary hypertension, maternal hyperthyroidism, or uncontrolled maternal diabetes mellitus. Also contraindicated in patients hypersensitive to the drug or with pre-existing maternal medical conditions that would seriously be affected by the known pharmacologic properties of this drug, such as hypovolemia, pheochromocytoma, or uncontrolled hypertension.

NURSING CONSIDERATIONS
● Use cautiously in patients with a sulfite sensitivity.
● **I.V. use:** Don't use ritodrine I.V. if solution is discolored or contains a precipitate.
Alert: Because CV responses are common and more pronounced during I.V. administration, closely monitor CV effects—including maternal pulse rate and blood pressure, and fetal heart rate. Maternal tachycardia of over 140 beats/minute or persistent respiratory rate of over 20 breaths/minute may be a sign of impending pulmonary edema. Discontinue drug if pulmonary edema develops and notify doctor.
● Monitor blood glucose concentrations during infusion, especially in diabetic mother.
● Monitor amount of fluids adminis-

tered I.V. to prevent circulatory overload. These patients may require diuretics.
• Patient should be in left lateral position to minimize risks of hypotension.

• Explain need for drug and how drug is administered to patient and family.
• Instruct patient to report adverse reactions promptly.

---

strontium 89 (⁸⁹Sr) chloride
Metastron

Pregnancy Risk Category: D

HOW SUPPLIED
Injection: 4 millicuries (mCi)/10 ml

ACTION
Acts as a calcium analogue that is actively taken up by bone, particularly in areas of active osteogenesis such as metastatic bone tumors. The drug locally irradiates tissue with beta radiation.

ONSET, PEAK, DURATION
Rapidly taken up by bone within hours of injection. Pain relief typically takes 7 to 20 days. Effects persist for 4 to 12 months.

INDICATIONS & DOSAGE
Relief of bone pain in patients with painful metastatic lesions—
Adults: 4 mCi by slow I.V. injection over 1 to 2 minutes.

ADVERSE REACTIONS
CV: cutaneous flushing with rapid injection.
Hematologic: *bone marrow suppression.*
Other: transient increase in pain ("flare" reaction).

INTERACTIONS
Calcium supplements: decreased effectiveness of ⁸⁹Sr. Discontinue calcium supplements about 2 weeks before ⁸⁹Sr administration.
Cytotoxic agents: additive bone marrow suppression. Monitor closely.

EFFECTS ON DIAGNOSTIC TESTS
None reported.

CONTRAINDICATIONS
None known.

NURSING CONSIDERATIONS
• Use cautiously in patients with platelet counts below 60,000/mm³ or WBC counts below 2,400/mm³.
Alert: Follow institutional safety measures to minimize radiation exposure. Urinary excretion of radiation is greatest during the first 2 days after administration.
• Consider placing an indwelling urinary catheter in incontinent patients to minimize contamination of the environment with radiation.
• Frequently assess the degree of pain relief after administration of the drug. During the lst week, a transient increase in pain may necessitate a dosage increase in concomitantly administered analgesics. Pain relief from ⁸⁹SR usually occurs after 2 to 3 weeks. In clinical trials, over 75% of patients received substantial pain relief, allowing a reduction or elimination of opioid analgesics.
• Because the drug is a potential carcinogen, know that use should be restricted to patients with documented metastatic bone cancer.
• Because of the delayed onset of pain relief, be aware that this drug should not be used in patients with a short life expectancy.

• Teach patient proper radiation precautions; during the first few days of treatment, patient should flush the toilet twice, wipe any spilled urine with a tissue that is subsequently flushed, and immediately launder any linens soiled with blood or urine. Tell the patient to wash hands after using the toilet. Make

sure patient understands that the drug has a low level of radioactivity and that he will pose no risk to family members.
● Advise female patient of childbearing age to avoid becoming pregnant while taking this drug.

---

sulfasalazine (salazosulfapyridine, sulphasalazine)
Azulfidine, Azulfidine EN-Tabs, PMS Sulfasalazine E.C.†, Salazopyrin†‡, Salazopyrin EN-Tabs†‡, S.A.S., S.A.S.-Enteric

Pregnancy Risk Category: B

HOW SUPPLIED
Tablets: 500 mg with or without enteric coating
Oral suspension: 250 mg/5 ml

ACTION
Unknown.

ONSET, PEAK, DURATION
Onset and duration unknown. Peak serum levels of parent drug occur within 3 to 12 hours; peak levels of metabolites, within 12 to 24 hours.

INDICATIONS & DOSAGE
Mild to moderate ulcerative colitis, adjunctive therapy in severe ulcerative colitis, Crohn's disease—
Adults: initially, 3 to 4 g P.O. daily in evenly divided doses; usual maintenance dosage is 2 g P.O. daily in divided doses q 6 hours. Dosage may be started with 1 to 2 g, with a gradual increase in dosage to minimize adverse effects.
Children over 2 years: initially, 40 to 60 mg/kg P.O. daily, divided into three to six doses; then 30 mg/kg daily in four doses. Dosage may be started at lower dose if GI intolerance occurs.
✳ *New indication: Rheumatoid arthritis in patients who have responded inadequately to salicylates or NSAIDs—*
Adults: 2 g P.O. daily in evenly divided

doses. Dosage may be started at 0.5 to 1 g daily to reduce possible GI intolerance.

ADVERSE REACTIONS
CNS: headache, depression, *seizures,* hallucinations.
GI: *nausea, vomiting, diarrhea,* abdominal pain, anorexia, stomatitis.
GU: *toxic nephrosis with oliguria and anuria,* crystalluria, hematuria, oligospermia, infertility.
Hematologic: *agranulocytosis, aplastic anemia,* megaloblastic anemia, *thrombocytopenia,* leukopenia, *hemolytic anemia.*
Hepatic: jaundice, hepatotoxicity.
Skin: *erythema multiforme (Stevens-Johnson syndrome),* generalized skin eruption, *epidermal necrolysis, exfoliative dermatitis,* photosensitivity, urticaria, pruritus.
Other: hypersensitivity reactions (*serum sickness, drug fever, anaphylaxis*).

INTERACTIONS
Antibiotics: may alter action of sulfasalazine by altering internal flora. Monitor closely.
Digoxin: may reduce absorption of digoxin. Monitor closely.
Folic acid: absorption may be decreased. No intervention necessary.
Iron: lowered blood concentrations of sulfasalazine caused by iron chelation. Monitor closely.
Oral anticoagulants: increased anticoagulant effect. Monitor for bleeding.
Oral antidiabetic agents: increased hypoglycemic effect. Monitor blood glucose levels.
Oral contraceptives: decreased contraceptive effectiveness and increased risk of breakthrough bleeding. Suggest a nonhormonal form of contraception.

EFFECTS ON DIAGNOSTIC TESTS
Drug alters results of urine glucose tests that use cupric sulfate (Benedict's reagent or Clinitest). It may elevate liver function test results and may decrease

---

serum levels of RBCs, WBCs, or platelets.

CONTRAINDICATIONS
Contraindicated in patients with hypersensitivity to the drug or its metabolites, porphyria, or intestinal and urinary obstruction and in infants under 2 years.

NURSING CONSIDERATIONS
● Use cautiously and in reduced dosages in patients with impaired hepatic or renal function, severe allergy, bronchial asthma, and G6PD deficiency.
● Although therapeutic response in rheumatoid arthritis has been noted as soon as 4 weeks after starting therapy, it may take 12 weeks of therapy before some patients show benefit.
● Be aware that drug colors alkaline urine orange-yellow.
Alert: Discontinue immediately if the patient shows signs and symptoms of hypersensitivity and notify doctor.

☑ PATIENT TEACHING
● Instruct patient to take drug after food intake and to space doses evenly.
● Warn patient to avoid ultraviolet light.
● Advise patient to make sure fluid intake is adequate.

---

tiopronin
Thiola

Pregnancy Risk Category: C

HOW SUPPLIED
Tablets: 100 mg

ACTION
Forms a water-soluble chemical complex with cysteine in the urine, increasing cysteine solubility and preventing formation of urinary cysteine stones.

ONSET, PEAK, DURATION
Onset rapid. Peak unknown. Effects persist less than 10 hours.

INDICATIONS & DOSAGE
Prevention of urinary cysteine stone formation in patients with severe homozygous cysteinuria unresponsive to or intolerant of other therapies—
Adults: 800 mg P.O. daily, divided t.i.d.
Children: initially, 15 mg/kg P.O. daily, divided t.i.d. Maintenance dosage may be individualized.

ADVERSE REACTIONS
GI: hypogeusia.
Skin: rash, pruritus, wrinkling, friability.
Other: drug fever, lupus erythematosus–like reaction.

INTERACTIONS
None significant.

EFFECTS ON DIAGNOSTIC TESTS
None reported.

CONTRAINDICATIONS
Contraindicated in patients with a history of agranulocytosis, aplastic anemia, or thrombocytopenia.

NURSING CONSIDERATIONS
● Institute conservative measures to treat cysteinuria before tiopronin is administered. Patients should drink at least 3 liters of fluid daily, including at least two 8-oz glasses of water at each meal and at bedtime. Urine output should be at least 3 liters daily, and urine pH should be 6.5 to 7. Excessive alkalization may precipitate calcium stones. Urine pH should not exceed 7.
● Monitor CBC, platelet counts, hemoglobin, serum albumin, liver function tests, 24-hour urine protein, and routine urinalysis at 3- to 6-month intervals during treatment, as ordered.
● Frequently monitor urine cysteine during first 6 months of treatment to identify optimal dosage level and then at least every 6 months, as ordered.
● Inspect skin for rash. Generalized rash with mild pruritus that develops may be controlled with antihistamines and will

---

Reactions may be *common*, uncommon, *life-threatening*, or COMMON AND LIFE-THREATENING.

disappear after stopping drug. A rash accompanied by intense pruritus may appear on the trunk after 6 months of therapy. This rash disappears slowly after stopping drug.
● Drug fever may develop, especially during 1st month of therapy. Expect drug to be stopped until fever subsides and to be restarted at lower dosages.
● Know that dosage is usually adjusted to keep urine cysteine levels below 250 mg/L.
● Be aware about two-thirds of patients who cannot tolerate penicillamine will tolerate tiopronin.

☑ **PATIENT TEACHING**
● Tell patient to take tiopronin at least 1 hour before or 2 hours after meals.
● Advise patient to have annual abdominal X-ray to assess for presence of stones.
● Tell patient to report any signs or symptoms of hematologic abnormalities, including fever, sore throat, bleeding or bruising, and chills. Blood dyscrasias have been reported in patients receiving other drugs for cysteinuria.

---

tretinoin (vitamin A acid, retinoic acid)
Renova, Retin-A, StieVAA†

Pregnancy Risk Category: C

HOW SUPPLIED
Cream: 0.025%, 0.05%, 0.1%
Gel: 0.025%, 0.01%
Solution: 0.05%

ACTION
Inhibits comedones by increasing epidermal cell mitosis and turnover.

ONSET, PEAK, DURATION
Unknown.

INDICATIONS & DOSAGE
Acne vulgaris—
Adults and children: clean affected

area and lightly apply once daily h.s.
Adjunct therapy to skin care and sun avoidance program—
Adults: apply to affected area once daily h.s.

ADVERSE REACTIONS
Skin: *feeling of warmth, slight stinging, local erythema, peeling,* chapping, swelling, blistering, crusting, temporary hyperpigmentation or hypopigmentation.

INTERACTIONS
Abrasive cleansers, skin preparations containing alcohol, medicated cosmetics, topical minoxidil, or photosensitizing medications: increased risk of skin irritation. Don't use together.
Topical agents containing sulfur, resorcinol, or salicylic acid: increased risk of skin irritation. Don't use together.

EFFECTS ON DIAGNOSTIC TESTS
None reported.

CONTRAINDICATIONS
Contraindicated in patients hypersensitive to any tretinoin component.

NURSING CONSIDERATIONS
● Use cautiously in patients with eczema.
● Know that relapses generally occur within 3 to 6 weeks after therapy is stopped.

☑ **PATIENT TEACHING**
● Instruct patient to clean area thoroughly before application and to avoid getting drug in eyes, mouth, or mucous membranes.
● Tell patient to wash face with mild soap no more than two or three times a day. Warn against using strong or medicated cosmetics, soaps, or other skin cleansers. Also advise patient to avoid topical products containing alcohol, astringents, spices, and lime because they may interfere with drug.
● Advise patient not to discontinue the

drug if it causes transient exacerbation of inflammatory lesions. If severe local irritation develops, advise patient to discontinue temporarily and notify doctor. Dosage will be readjusted when application is resumed. Some redness and scaling are normal reactions.
• Warn patient that he may experience increased sensitivity to wind or cold temperatures.
• Instruct patient to minimize exposure to sunlight or ultraviolet rays during treatment. If patient become sunburned, he should delay therapy until sunburn subsides. Tell patient who can't avoid exposure to sunlight to use SPF-15 sunblock and to wear protective clothing.
• Warn patient that he may have a temporary increase in lesions, which will improve in 2 to 3 weeks.

---

trilostane
Modrastane

Pregnancy Risk Category: X

HOW SUPPLIED
Capsules: 30 mg, 60 mg

ACTION
Reversibly lowers elevated circulating levels of glucocorticoids by inhibiting the enzyme system essential for their production in the adrenal gland.

ONSET, PEAK, DURATION
Unknown.

INDICATIONS & DOSAGE
Adrenocortical hyperfunction in Cushing's syndrome—
Adults: 30 mg P.O. q.i.d. initially. May be increased at intervals of 3 to 4 days to maximum of 480 mg/day. Most patients respond to doses below 360 mg/day.

ADVERSE REACTIONS
CNS: headache, dizziness, light-headedness.

CV: *orthostatic hypotension.*
EENT: burning of oral and nasal membranes.
GI: *diarrhea, upset stomach,* nausea, flatulence, cramps, bloating.
Skin: flushing, rash.
Other: fever, fatigue, hot flashes, muscle aches, hyperkalemia.

INTERACTIONS
Aminoglutethimide, mitotane: may cause severe adrenocortical hypofunction.
Loop diuretics, thiazides: decreased potassium loss because trilostane inhibits aldosterone production.

EFFECTS ON DIAGNOSTIC TESTS
None reported.

CONTRAINDICATIONS
Contraindicated in patients with severe renal or hepatic disease.

NURSING CONSIDERATIONS
• Use cautiously in patients receiving drugs that suppress adrenal function.
• Monitor blood pressure regularly in all patients.
• Be aware that trilostane may prevent normal response to physiologically stressful situation. Therefore, patients who develop a severe illness or need surgery may need to have this drug temporarily discontinued. Supplemental corticosteroids may be necessary.

☑ PATIENT TEACHING
• Explain to patient that the drug does not cure the underlying disease.
• Tell patient to seek medical attention if stressful situation arises.

Reactions may be *common*, uncommon, *life-threatening*, or COMMON AND LIFE-THREATENING.

Appendices and Index

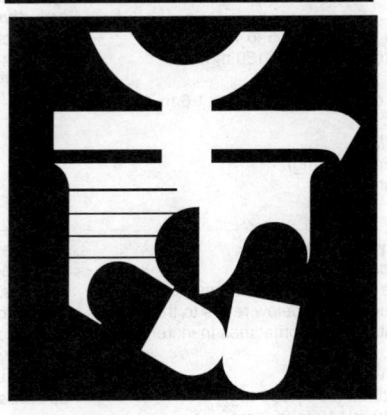

Selected local and topical anesthetics

DRUG, INDICATIONS, DOSAGE	ADVERSE REACTIONS

Local

bupivacaine hydrochloride
(Marcain‡, Marcaine, Sensorcaine)
Dosages given are for the drug without epinephrine and for adults. Volume listed below refers to the total volume of anesthetic given, sometimes in incremental doses of 2 to 6 ml.
Epidural block—
0.25% solution: 10 to 20 ml (25 to 50 mg)
0.5% solution: 10 to 20 ml (50 to 100 mg)
0.75% solution: 10 to 20 ml (75 to 150 mg), single-dose only
Caudal block—
0.25% solution: 15 to 30 ml (37.5 to 75 mg)
0.5% solution: 15 to 30 ml (75 to 150 mg)
Spinal block—
0.75% solution: (in dextrose 8.25%): 1 to 1.6 ml (7.5 to 12 mg)
Peripheral nerve block—
0.25% solution: 5 ml (12.5 mg)
0.5% solution: 5 ml (25 mg)

Skin: dermatologic reactions.
Other: edema, *status asthmaticus, anaphylaxis, anaphylactoid reactions.* Systemic effects from high blood levels of the drug—
CNS: anxiety, nervousness, *seizures* followed by drowsiness.
CV: myocardial depression, hypotension, *bradycardia, arrhythmias, cardiac arrest.*
EENT: blurred vision, tinnitus.
GI: nausea, vomiting
Respiratory: *respiratory arrest.*

chloroprocaine hydrochloride
(Nesacaine, Nesacaine MPF)
Dosages given are for the drug without epinephrine and for adults. Volume listed below refers to the total volume of anesthetic given, sometimes in incremental doses of 2 to 6 ml.
Infiltration and nerve block—
1% solution: 3 to 20 ml (30 to 200 mg)
2% solution: 2 to 40 ml (40 to 800 mg)
Caudal and epidural block—
2% to 3% solution: 15 to 25 ml (300 to 750 mg)
   May be repeated with smaller doses q 40 to 50 minutes. Dose and interval may be increased when combined with epinephrine. Maximum adult dosage is 800 mg or 11 mg/kg; when combined with epinephrine, maximum dosage is 1 g.

Skin: dermatologic reactions.
Other: edema, *status asthmaticus, anaphylaxis, anaphylactoid reactions.* Systemic effects from high blood levels of the drug—
CNS: anxiety, nervousness, *seizures* followed by drowsiness.
CV: myocardial depression, bradycardia, hypotension, *arrhythmias, cardiac arrest.*
EENT: blurred vision, tinnitus.
GI: nausea, vomiting.
Respiratory: *respiratory arrest.*

etidocaine hydrochloride
(Duranest)
Dosages given are for the drug without epinephrine and for adults.
   Dose limit is 4 mg/kg or 300 mg per injection. When combined with epinephrine, dose limit is 5.5 mg/kg or 400 mg per injection. May be repeated q 2 to 3 hours.
Peripheral nerve block—
1% solution: 5 to 40 ml (50 to 400 mg)

Skin: dermatologic reactions.
Other: edema, *status asthmaticus, anaphylaxis, anaphylactoid reactions.* Systemic effects from high blood levels of the drug—
CNS: anxiety, apprehension, nervousness, *seizures* followed by drowsiness.

Reactions may be *common*, uncommon, *life-threatening*, or COMMON AND LIFE-THREATENING.

INTERACTIONS	NURSING CONSIDERATIONS

Beta-adrenergic blockers: enhanced sympathomimetic effects when used with bupivacaine and epinephrine.
Chloroprocaine: may lessen bupivacaine's action. Don't use together.
Cyclic antidepressants, MAO inhibitors: severe, sustained hypertension when used with bupivacaine and epinephrine. Use with extreme caution.
Enflurane, halothane, isoflurane, related drugs: arrhythmias when used with bupivacaine and epinephrine. Use with extreme caution.
Phenothiazines, butyrophenones: may reduce or reverse the pressor effect of epinephrine.

- Contraindicated in children under 12 years and for spinal or topical anesthesia or paracervical block.
- Some solutions contain sulfites and should be avoided in patients with sulfite hypersensitivity.
- Should not be used for I.V. regional anesthesia (Bier block, Bier's anesthesia).
- The 0.75% solution should not be used for obstetrical surgery; lower concentrations are effective and less hazardous.
- Use cautiously in debilitated, elderly, or acutely ill patients and in patients with severe hepatic disease or drug allergies.
- Use solutions with epinephrine cautiously in patients with CV disorders and in body areas with limited blood supply (ears, nose, fingers, toes).
- Keep resuscitation equipment and drugs available.
- Don't use solution with preservatives for caudal or epidural block.
- Discard partially used vials without preservatives.
- Check solution for particles.
- Protect solutions containing epinephrine from light.

Bupivacaine: chloroprocaine may lessen bupivacaine's action.

- Contraindicated in patients with hypersensitivity to procaine, tetracaine, or other PABA derivatives and for spinal or topical anesthesia. Epidural and caudal blocks are contraindicated in patients with CNS disease.
- Use cautiously in debilitated, elderly, or acutely ill patients; in children; and in patients with drug allergies, paracervical block, or CV disease.
- Keep resuscitation equipment and drugs available.
- Don't use solution with preservatives for caudal or epidural block.
- Don't use discolored solution.
- Check solution for particles.
- Discard partially used vials without preservatives.

Cyclic antidepressants, MAO inhibitors, phenothiazines: severe, sustained hypertension or hypotension with etidocaine and epinephrine. Use with extreme caution.
Enflurane, halothane, isoflurane, related drugs: arrhythmias when used with etidocaine and epinephrine. Use with extreme caution.

- Contraindicated in patients with inflammation or infection in puncture region, septicemia, severe hypertension, spinal deformities, or neurologic disorders; in children under 14 years; and for spinal anesthesia.
- Some solutions contain sulfites and should be avoided in patients with sulfite hypersensitivity.
- Use cautiously in debilitated, elderly, or acutely ill patients; in patients with severe shock, heart block, general drug allergies, or hepatic and renal disease; and as epidural block in obstetric patients.

---

*Liquid contains alcohol.   **May contain tartrazine.   †Canada only.   ‡Australia only.   ◊ OTC.

Selected local and topical anesthetics *(continued)*

DRUG, INDICATIONS, DOSAGE	ADVERSE REACTIONS

Local *(continued)*

etidocaine hydrochloride *(continued)*
Central neural block (lower limbs, cesarean section, lumbar, epidural)—
1% solution: 10 to 30 ml (100 to 300 mg)
1.5% solution: 10 to 20 ml (150 to 300 mg)
Transvaginal block—
1% solution: 5 to 20 ml (50 to 200 mg)
Caudal block—
1% solution: 10 to 30 ml (100 to 300 mg)

CV: myocardial depression, bradycardia, hypotension, *arrhythmias, cardiac arrest.*
EENT: blurred vision, tinnitus.
GI: nausea, vomiting.
Respiratory: *respiratory arrest.*

---

lidocaine hydrochloride
[lignocaine hydrochloride]
(Dilocaine, Lidoject-1, Lidoject-2, Xylocaine)
Dosages given are for the drug without epinephrine and for adults. Volume listed below refers to the total volume of anesthetic given, sometimes in incremental doses of 2 to 6 ml.
For anesthesia other than spinal—
Maximum single dose is 4.5 mg/kg or 300 mg. With epinephrine, maximum dose is 7 mg/kg or 500 mg.
Caudal (obstetric) or epidural (thoracic) block—
1% solution: 20 to 30 ml (200 to 300 mg)
Epidural (lumbar anesthesia) block—
1% solution: 25 to 30 ml (250 to 300 mg)
1.5% solution: 15 to 20 ml (225 to 300 mg)
2% solution: 10 to 15 ml (200 to 300 mg)
Spinal surgical anesthesia—
5% (with 7.5% dextrose): 1.5 to 2 ml (75 to 100 mg)
Caudal (surgery) block—
1.5% solution: 15 to 20 ml (225 to 300 mg)

Skin: dermatologic reactions.
Other: edema, *status asthmaticus, anaphylaxis, anaphylactoid reactions.*
Systemic effects from high blood levels of the drug—
CNS: anxiety, nervousness, *seizures* followed by drowsiness.
CV: myocardial depression, bradycardia, hypotension, *arrhythmias, cardiac arrest.*
EENT: blurred vision, tinnitus.
GI: nausea, vomiting.
Respiratory: *respiratory arrest.*

---

procaine hydrochloride
(Novocain)
Spinal anesthesia—
Adults: initial dose should not exceed 1 g.
   Before using, dilute 10% solution with 0.9% sodium chloride injection, sterile distilled water, or CSF. For hyperbaric technique, use dextrose solution.
Perineum: 0.5 ml 10% solution and 0.5 ml diluent injected at the L4 interspace
Perineum and lower extremities: 1 ml 10% solution and 1 ml diluent injected at the L3 or L4 interspace
Up to costal margin: 2 ml 10% solution and 1 ml diluent injected at the L2, L3, or L4 interspace
Peripheral nerve block—
1% solution: 50 ml (500 mg)
2% solution: 25 ml (500 mg)
Infiltration—
350 to 600 mg in a 0.25% to 0.5% solution. Maximum initial dose is 1 g.

Skin: dermatologic reactions.
Other: edema, *status asthmaticus, anaphylaxis, anaphylactoid reactions.*
Systemic effects from high blood levels of the drug—
CNS: anxiety, nervousness, *seizures* followed by drowsiness.
CV: myocardial depression, bradycardia, hypotension, *arrhythmias, cardiac arrest.*
EENT: blurred vision, tinnitus.
GI: nausea, vomiting.
Respiratory: *respiratory arrest.*

Reactions may be *common*, uncommon, *life-threatening*, or COMMON AND LIFE-THREATENING.

INTERACTIONS	NURSING CONSIDERATIONS
	• Use solutions with epinephrine cautiously in patients with CV disease and in body areas with limited blood supply (ears, nose, fingers, toes). • Don't use solution with preservatives for caudal or epidural block. • Keep resuscitation equipment and drugs available. • Check solution for particles.
Beta-adrenergic blockers: enhanced sympathomimetic effects. Avoid concomitant use with lidocaine and epinephrine. *Cyclic antidepressants, MAO inhibitors:* severe, sustained hypertension when used with lidocaine and epinephrine. Use with extreme caution. *Enflurane, halothane, isoflurane, related drugs:* arrhythmias when used with lidocaine and epinephrine. Use with extreme caution. *Phenothiazines, butyrophenones:* may reduce or reverse the pressor effect of epinephrine.	• Contraindicated in patients with inflammation or infection in puncture region, septicemia, severe hypertension, spinal deformities, and neurologic disorders. • Use cautiously in debilitated, elderly, or acutely ill patients; in patients with severe shock, heart block, general drug allergies; in obstetric patients; and for paracervical block. • Dose and interval are increased with epinephrine. • Use solutions with epinephrine cautiously in patients with CV disorders and in body areas with limited blood supply (ears, nose, fingers, toes). • Don't use solution with preservatives for spinal, epidural, or caudal block. • Keep resuscitation equipment and drugs available. • Discard partially used vials without preservatives. • Check solution for particles.
Echothiophate iodide: reduced hydrolysis of procaine. Use together cautiously. *Succinylcholine:* prolonged neuromuscular blockade. Use cautiously together.	• Contraindicated in patients with traumatized urethras and in those with hypersensitivity to chloroprocaine, tetracaine, or other PABA derivatives. • Contraindicated for obstetric use in patients with cephalopelvic disproportion, placenta previa, abruptio placentae, floating fetal head, and intrauterine manipulation. • Use cautiously in hyperexcitable patients; in those with CNS disease, infection at puncture site, shock, profound anemia, cachexia, sepsis, hypertension, hypotension, GI hemorrhage, bowel perforation or strangulation, peritonitis, cardiac decompensation, massive pleural effusion, or increased intra-abdominal pressure; and in obstetric patients. • Keep resuscitation equipment and drugs available. • Use solution without preservatives for epidural block. • Discard partially used vials without preservatives.

Selected local and topical anesthetics *(continued)*

DRUG, INDICATIONS, DOSAGE	ADVERSE REACTIONS

Local *(continued)*

tetracaine hydrochloride
(Pontocaine)
Dosage for adults varies according to the extent of the block as follows:
Low spinal (saddle) block in vaginal delivery—
2 to 5 mg as hyperbaric solution (in 10% dextrose)
Perineum and lower extremities: 5 to 10 mg
Up to costal margin: 15 to 20 mg

Skin: dermatologic reactions.
Other: edema, *status asthmaticus, anaphylaxis, anaphylactoid reactions.*
Systemic effects from high blood levels of the drug—
CNS: anxiety, nervousness, *seizures* followed by drowsiness.
CV: bradycardia, hypotension, myocardial depression, *arrhythmias, cardiac arrest.*
EENT: blurred vision, tinnitus.
GI: nausea, vomiting.
Respiratory: *respiratory arrest.*

Topical

proparacaine hydrochloride
(AK-taine, Alcaine, Ophthaine, Ophthetic)
Anesthesia for tonometry, gonioscopy—
Adults and children: 1 or 2 drops of 0.5% solution instilled in eye just before procedure.
Anesthesia for cataract extraction, glaucoma surgery—
Adults and children: 1or 2 drops of 0.5% solution instilled in eye q 5 to 10 minutes for five to seven doses.
Removal of foreign bodies or sutures—
Adults and children: 1 or 2 drops 2 to 3 minutes before procedure or q 5 to 10 minutes for one to three doses.

EENT: conjunctival redness, transient eye pain.
Other: hypersensitivity reactions.

tetracaine
(Pontocaine Eye Ointment, Solution)
tetracaine hydrochloride
(Pontocaine)
Anesthesia for tonometry, gonioscopy; removal of corneal foreign bodies, suture removal from cornea; other diagnostic and minor surgical procedures—
Adults and children: 1 to 2 drops of 0.5% solution or a small strip ½" to 1" [1.25 to 2.5 cm] of ointment in eye just before procedure.

EENT: transient stinging in eye 30 seconds after initial instillation, epithelial damage in excessive or long-term use.
Other: sensitization with repeated use (allergic skin rash, urticaria).

Reactions may be *common*, uncommon, *life-threatening*, or COMMON AND LIFE-THREATENING.

INTERACTIONS	NURSING CONSIDERATIONS
None significant.	• Safety and efficacy in children have not been established. • Contraindicated in patients with infection at injection site or CNS disease and in those with hypersensitivity to procaine or related agents. • Saddle block is contraindicated in patients with cephalopelvic disproportion, placenta previa, abruptio placentae, intrauterine manipulation, and floating fetal head. • Use cautiously in patients with shock, profound anemia, cachexia, hypertension, hypotension, peritonitis, cardiac decompensation, massive pleural effusion, increased intracranial pressure, and infection. • Keep resuscitation equipment and drugs available. • When CSF is added to powdered drug or drug solution during spinal anesthesia, solution may be cloudy. Don't use discolored or crystallized solutions. • Protect from light; store in refrigerator.
None significant.	• Use cautiously in patients with cardiac disease and hyperthyroidism. • Not for long-term use; may delay wound healing. • Warn patients not to rub or touch eye while cornea is anesthetized. This may cause corneal abrasion and greater discomfort when anesthesia wears off. • Warn patients with corneal abrasion that pain is relieved only temporarily. • Don't use discolored solution. • Store in tightly closed container. Refrigerate opened containers. • Check solution for particles.
Cholinesterase inhibitors: prolonged ocular anesthesia and increased risk of toxicity. *Sulfonamides:* interference with sulfonamide antibacterial activity. Wait ½ hour after anesthesia before instilling sulfonamide.	• Contraindicated in patients with hypersensitivity to the drug. • Avoid long-term use. • Does not dilate the pupil, paralyze accommodation, or increase intraocular pressure. • Don't use discolored solution. Keep container tightly closed. • Warn patient not to touch or rub eye while cornea is anesthetized. This may cause corneal abrasion and greater discomfort when anesthesia wears off.

Cancer chemotherapy: Acronyms and protocols

Combination chemotherapy is well established for treatment of cancer. The chart below lists commonly used acronyms and protocols, including standard dosages for specific cancers.

ACRONYM & INDICATION	DRUG		DOSAGE
	Generic name	Trade name	
ABVD (Hodgkin's disease)	doxorubicin	Adriamycin	25 mg/m^2 I.V., days 1 and 15
	bleomycin	Blenoxane	10 U/m^2 I.V., days 1 and 15
	vinblastine	Velban	6 mg/m^2 I.V., days 1 and 15
	dacarbazine	DTIC-Dome	350 to 375 mg/m^2 I.V., days 1 and 15 *Repeat cycle q 28 days.*
AC (Bony sarcoma)	doxorubicin	Adriamycin	75 to 90 mg/m^2 (total dose) by 96-hour continuous I.V. infusion
	cisplatin	Platinol	90 to 120 mg/m^2 I.A. or I.V., day 6 *Repeat cycle q 28 days.*
AC (Breast cancer)	doxorubicin	Adriamycin	60 mg/m^2 I.V., day 1
	cyclophosphamide	Cytoxan	400 to 600 mg/m^2 I.V., day 1 *Repeat cycle q 21 days.*
ACE (CAE) (Small-cell lung cancer)	doxorubicin	Adriamycin	45 mg/m^2 I.V., day 1
	cyclophosphamide	Cytoxan	1,000 mg/m^2 I.V., day 1
	etoposide (VP-16)	VePesid	50 mg/m^2 I.V., days 1 to 5 *Repeat cycle q 21 days.*
AP (Endometrial cancer)	doxorubicin	Adriamycin	60 mg/m^2 I.V., day 1
	cisplatin	Platinol	50 to 60 mg/m^2 I.V., day 1 *Repeat cycle q 21 days.*
BEP (Testicular cancer)	bleomycin	Blenoxane	30 U I.V., days 2, 9, and 16
	etoposide (VP-16)	VePesid	100 mg/m^2, days 1 to 5
	cisplatin	Platinol	20 mg/m^2 I.V., days 1 to 5 *Repeat cycle q 21 days.*
CAF (FAC) (Breast cancer)	cyclophosphamide	Cytoxan	100 mg/m^2 P.O., days 1 to 14
	doxorubicin	Adriamycin	30 mg/m^2 I.V., days 1 (and day 8, optional)
	fluorouracil (5-FU)	Adrucil	400 to 500 mg/m^2 I.V., days 1 and 8 *Repeat cycle q 28 days.*
or	cyclophosphamide	Cytoxan	500 mg/m^2 I.V., day 1
	doxorubicin	Adriamycin	50 mg/m^2 I.V., day 1
	fluorouracil (5-FU)	Adrucil	500 mg/m^2 I.V., day 1 *Repeat cycle q 21 days.*

Cancer chemotherapy: Acronyms and protocols (continued)

ACRONYM & INDICATION	DRUG		DOSAGE
	Generic name	Trade name	
CAMP (Non-small-cell lung cancer)	cyclophosphamide	Cytoxan	300 mg/m² I.V., days 1 and 8
	doxorubicin	Adriamycin	20 mg/m² I.V., days 1 and 8
	methotrexate	Folex	15 mg/m² I.V., days 1 and 8
	procarbazine	Matulane	100 mg/m² P.O., days 1 to 10 *Repeat cycle q 28 days.*
CAP (Non-small-cell lung cancer)	cyclophosphamide	Cytoxan	400 mg/m² I.V., day 1
	doxorubicin	Adriamycin	40 mg/m² I.V., day 1
	cisplatin	Platinol	60 mg/m² I.V., day 1 *Repeat cycle q 28 days.*
CAV (VAC) (Small-cell lung cancer)	cyclophosphamide	Cytoxan	750 to 1,000 mg/m² I.V, day 1
	doxorubicin	Adriamycin	40 to 50 mg/m² I.V., day 1
	vincristine	Oncovin	1.4 mg/m² (2 mg maximum) I.V., day 1 *Repeat cycle q 21 days.*
CC (Ovarian cancer, epithelial)	carboplatin	Paraplatin	300 mg/m² I.V., day 1
	cyclophosphamide	Cytoxan	600 mg/m² I.V., day 1 *Repeat cycle q 28 days.*
CF (Head and neck cancer)	cisplatin	Platinol	100 mg/m² I.V., day 1
	fluorouracil (5-FU)	Adrucil	1,000 mg/m² daily by continuous I.V. infusion, days 1 to 5 *Repeat cycle q 21 to 28 days.*
or	carboplatin	Paraplatin	400 mg/m² I.V., day 1
	fluorouracil (5-FU)	Adrucil	1,000 mg/m² daily by continuous I.V. infusion, days 1 to 5 *Repeat cycle q 21 to 28 days.*
CFM (CNF, FNC) (Breast cancer)	cyclophosphamide	Cytoxan	500 mg/m² I.V., day 1
	fluorouracil (5-FU)	Adrucil	500 mg/m² I.V., day 1
	mitoxantrone	Novantrone	10 mg/m² I.V., day 1 *Repeat cycle q 21 days.*
CHAP (Ovarian cancer, epithelial)	cyclophosphamide	Cytoxan	300 to 500 mg/m², day P.O., day 1
	altretamine	Hexalen	150 mg/m² P.O., days 1 to 7
	doxorubicin	Adriamycin	30 to 50 mg/m² I.V., day 1
	cisplatin	Platinol	50 mg/m² I.V., day 1 *Repeat cycle q 28 days.*

Cancer chemotherapy: Acronyms and protocols *(continued)*

ACRONYM & INDICATION	DRUG		DOSAGE
	Generic name	Trade name	
ChlVPP (Hodgkin's disease)	chlorambucil	Leukeran	6 mg/m^2 (10 mg/day maximum) P.O., days 1 to 14
	vinblastine	Velban	6 mg/m^2 (10 mg/day maximum) I.V., days 1 and 8
	procarbazine	Matulane	100 mg/m^2 P.O., days 1 to 14
	prednisone	Deltasone	40 mg/m^2 P.O., days 1 to 14 *Repeat cycle q 28 days.*
CHOP (Malignant lymphoma)	cyclophosphamide	Cytoxan	750 mg/m^2 I.V., day 1
	doxorubicin	Adriamycin	50 mg/m^2 I.V., day 1
	vincristine	Oncovin	1.4 mg/m^2 (2 mg maximum) I.V., day 1
	prednisone	Deltasone	100 mg P.O., days 1 to 5 *Repeat cycle q 21 days.*
CHOP-Bleo (Malignant lymphoma)	cyclophosphamide	Cytoxan	750 mg/m^2 I.V., day 1
	doxorubicin	Adriamycin	50 mg/m^2 I.V., day 1
	vincristine	Oncovin	2 mg I.V., days 1 and 5
	prednisone	Deltasone	100 mg P.O., days 1 to 5
	bleomycin	Blenoxane	15 U I.V., days 1 and 5 *Repeat cycle q 14 to 21 days.*
CISCA (Genitourinary cancer)	cisplatin	Platinol	70 to 100 mg/m^2 I.V., day 2
	cyclophosphamide	Cytoxan	650 mg/m^2 I.V., day 1
	doxorubicin	Adriamycin	50 mg/m^2 I.V., day 1 *Repeat cycle q 21 to 28 days.*
CMF (Breast cancer)	cyclophosphamide	Cytoxan	100 mg/m^2 P.O., days 1 to 14, or 400 to 600 mg/m^2 I.V., day 1
	methotrexate	Folex	40 mg/m^2 I.V., days 1 and 8
	fluorouracil (5-FU)	Adrucil	400 to 600 mg/m^2 I.V., days 1 and 8 *Repeat cycle q 28 days.*
CMFVP (Breast cancer)	cyclophosphamide	Cytoxan	100 mg/m^2 P.O., days 1 to 14, or 400 to 600 mg/m^2 I.V., day 1
	methotrexate	Folex	40 mg/m^2 I.V., days 1 and 8
	fluorouracil (5-FU)	Adrucil	400 to 600 mg/m^2 I.V., days 1 and 8
	vincristine	Oncovin	1 mg I.V., days 1 and 8
	prednisone	Deltasone	40 mg to 40 mg/m^2/day P.O., days 1 to 7 or 14 *Repeat cycle q 28 days.*

Cancer chemotherapy: Acronyms and protocols (continued)

ACRONYM & INDICATION	DRUG		DOSAGE
	Generic name	Trade name	
COB (Head and neck cancer)	cisplatin	Platinol	100 mg/m^2 I.V., day 1
	vincristine	Oncovin	1 mg I.V., days 2 and 5
	bleomycin	Blenoxane	30 U/day by continuous I.V. infusion, days 2 to 5 *Repeat cycle q 21 days.*
COMLA (Malignant lymphoma)	cyclophosphamide	Cytoxan	1,500 mg/m^2 I.V., day 1
	vincristine	Oncovin	1.4 mg/m^2 (2 mg maximum) I.V., days 1, 8, and 15
	methotrexate	Folex	120 mg/m^2 I.V., days 22, 29, 36, 43, 50, 57, 64, and 71
	leucovorin calcium	Wellcovorin	25 mg/m^2 P.O. q 6 hours for four doses, beginning 24 hours after each methotrexate dose
	cytarabine (ara-C)	Cytosar-U	300 mg/m^2 I.V., days 22, 29, 36, 43, 50, 57, 64, and 71 *Repeat cycle q 91 days or 12 weeks.*
COP (Malignant lymphoma)	cyclophosphamide	Cytoxan	750 to 1,000 mg/m^2 I.V., day 1
	vincristine	Oncovin	1.4 mg/m^2 (2 mg maximum) I.V., day 1
	prednisone	Deltasone	60 mg/m^2 P.O., days 1 to 5 *Repeat cycle q 21 days.*
COPE (Small-cell lung cancer)	cyclophosphamide	Cytoxan	750 mg/m^2 I.V., day 1
	cisplatin	Platinol	20 mg/m^2 I.V., days 1 to 3
	etoposide (VP-16)	VePesid	100 mg/m^2 I.V., days 1 to 3
	vincristine	Oncovin	1.4 mg/m^2 (2 mg maximum) I.V., day 3 *Repeat cycle q 21 days.*
COPP (Hodgkin's disease and malignant lymphoma)	cyclophosphamide	Cytoxan	500 to 650 mg/m^2 I.V., days 1 and 8
	vincristine	Oncovin	1.4 mg/m^2 (2 mg maximum) I.V., days 1 and 8
	procarbazine	Matulane	100 mg/m^2 P.O., days 1 to 10 or 1 to 14
	prednisone	Deltasone	40 mg/m^2 P.O., days 1 to 14 *Repeat cycle q 28 days.*
CP (Ovarian cancer)	cyclophosphamide	Cytoxan	600 to 1,000 mg/m^2 I.V., day 1
	cisplatin	Platinol	50 to 100 mg/m^2 I.V., day 1 *Repeat cycle q 21 days.*

Cancer chemotherapy: Acronyms and protocols (continued)

ACRONYM & INDICATION	DRUG		DOSAGE
	Generic name	Trade name	
CVI (VIC) (Non-small-cell lung cancer)	carboplatin	Paraplatin	300 mg/m² I.V., day 1
	etoposide (VP-16)	VePesid	60 to 100 mg/m² I.V., days 1, 3, and 5
	ifosfamide	Ifex	1.5 g/m² I.V., days 1, 3, and 5
	mesna	MESNEX	Dosage is 20% of ifosfamide dose, given immediately before and at 4 and 8 hours after ifosfamide infusion *Repeat cycle q 28 days.*
CVP (Leukemia— CLL)	cyclophosphamide	Cytoxan	400 mg/m² P.O., days 1 to 5
	vincristine	Oncovin	1.4 mg/m² (2 mg maximum) I.V., day 1
	prednisone	Deltasone	100 mg/m² P.O., days 1 to 5 *Repeat cycle q 21 days.*
CVP (Malignant lymphoma)	cyclophosphamide	Cytoxan	400 mg/m² P.O., days 1 to 5
	vincristine	Oncovin	1.4 mg/m² (2 mg maximum) I.V., day 1
	prednisone	Deltasone	100 mg/m² P.O., days 1 to 5 *Repeat cycle q 21 days.*
CVPP (Hodgkin's disease)	lomustine (CCNU)	CeeNU	75 mg/m² P.O., day 1
	vinblastine	Velban	4 mg/m² I.V., days 1 and 8
	procarbazine	Matulane	100 mg/m² P.O., days 1 to 14
	prednisone	Deltasone	30 mg/m² P.O., days 1 to 14 (cycles 1 and 4 only) *Repeat cycle q 28 days.*
CYVADIC (Soft-tissue sarcoma)	cyclophosphamide	Cytoxan	500 to 600 mg/m² I.V., day 1
	vincristine	Oncovin	1.4 mg/m² (2 mg maximum) I.V., days 1 and 5
	doxorubicin	Adriamycin	50 mg/m² I.V., day 1
	dacarbazine	DTIC-Dome	250 mg/m² I.V., days 1 to 5 *Repeat cycle q 21 days.*
DCT (DAT, TCD) (Leukemia— AML, adult induction)	daunorubicin	Cerubidine	60 mg/m² I.V., days 1 to 3
	cytarabine (ara-C)	Cytosar-U	200 mg/m² daily by continuous I.V., days 1 to 5
	thioguanine (6-TG)	Lanvis	100 mg/m² P.O. q 12 hours, days 1 to 5

Cancer chemotherapy: Acronyms and protocols (continued)

ACRONYM & INDICATION	DRUG		DOSAGE
	Generic name	Trade name	
DHAP (Malignant lymphoma)	dexamethasone	Decadron	40 mg P.O. or I.V., days 1 to 4
	cisplatin	Platinol	100 mg/m² by continuous I.V. infusion over 24 hours, day 1
	cytarabine (ara-C)	Cytosar-U	2 g/m² I.V. q 12 hours for two doses (total dose of 4 g/m²), day 2. Administer with saline, methylcellulose, or steroid eyedrops to both eyes q 2 to 4 hours, starting on day 2 and continuing 48 to 72 hours after last dose. *Repeat cycle q 21 to 28 days.*
DVP (Leukemia—ALL, adult induction)	daunorubicin	Cerubidine	45 mg/m² I.V., days 1 to 3 and day 14
	vincristine	Oncovin	2 mg/m² I.V., days 1, 8, 15, and 22
	prednisone	Deltasone	45 mg/m² P.O., for 28 to 35 days
EP (Small-cell or non-small-cell lung cancer)	cisplatin	Platinol	75 to 100 mg/m² I.V., day 1
	etoposide (VP-16)	VePesid	75 to 100 mg/m² I.V., days 1 to 3 *Repeat cycle q 21 to 28 days.*
ESHAP (Malignant lymphoma)	etoposide (VP-16)	VePesid	40 to 60 mg/m² I.V. over 30 to 60 minutes, days 1 to 4
	cisplatin	Platinol	25 mg/m² daily by continuous I.V., days 1 to 4
	cytarabine (ara-C)	Cytosar-U	2 g/m² I.V. on day 5 after completion of etoposide and cisplatin therapy
	methylpredniso-lone	Solu-Medrol	500 mg I.V. daily, days 1 to 4 *Repeat cycle q 21 to 28 days.*
EVA (Hodgkin's disease)	etoposide (VP-16)	VePesid	100 mg/m² I.V., days 1 to 3
	vinblastine	Velban	6 mg/m² I.V., day 1
	doxorubicin	Adriamycin	50 mg/m² I.V., day 1 *Repeat cycle q 28 days.*
FAC (CAF) (Breast cancer)	fluorouracil (5-FU)	Adrucil	500 mg/m² I.V., days 1 and 8
	doxorubicin	Adriamycin	50 mg/m² I.V., day 1
	cyclophosphamide	Cytoxan	500 mg/m² I.V., day 1 *Repeat cycle q 21 days.*
FAM (Adenocarcinoma, gastric cancer)	fluorouracil (5-FU)	Adrucil	600 mg/m² I.V., days 1, 8, 29, and 36
	doxorubicin	Adriamycin	30 mg/m² I.V., days 1 and 29
	mitomycin	Mutamycin	10 mg/m² I.V., day 1 *Repeat cycle q 8 weeks.*

Cancer chemotherapy: Acronyms and protocols (continued)

ACRONYM & INDICATION	DRUG		DOSAGE
	Generic name	Trade name	
FAMe (Gastric cancer)	fluorouracil (5-FU)	Adrucil	350 mg/m² I.V., days 1 to 5 and 36 to 40
	doxorubicin	Adriamycin	40 mg/m² I.V., days 1 and 36
	semustine (methyl CCNU)		150 mg/m² P.O., day 1 *Repeat cycle q 10 weeks.*
F-CL (Colorectal cancer)	fluorouracil (5-FU)	Adrucil	600 mg/m² I.V., 1 hour after initiating leucovorin infusion weekly for 6 weeks
	leucovorin calcium	Wellcovorin	500 mg/m² over 2 hours weekly for 6 weeks *Repeat cycle after 2-week break.*
or	fluorouracil (5-FU)	Adrucil	370 to 400 mg/m² I.V., days 1 to 5, following leucovorin
	leucovorin calcium	Wellcovorin	200 mg/m² daily I.V., days 1 to 5 *Repeat cycle q 28 to 35 days.*
or	fluorouracil (5-FU)	Adrucil	425 mg/m² I.V., days 1 to 5, following leucovorin
	leucovorin calcium	Wellcovorin	20 mg/m² I.V., days 1 to 5 *Repeat q 28 to 35 days.*
5 + 2 (Leukemia— AML, induction)	cytarabine (ara-C)	Cytosar-U	100 to 200 mg/m² by continuous I.V. infusion, days 1 to 5
	daunorubicin	Cerubidine	45 mg/m² I.V., days 1 and 2
FL (Prostate cancer)	flutamide	Eulexin	250 mg P.O. t.i.d.
	leuprolide acetate	Lupron	1 mg S.C. daily
or	flutamide	Eulexin	250 mg P.O. t.i.d.
	leuprolide acetate	Lupron Depot	7.5 mg I.M. q 28 days *Repeat cycle q 28 days.*
Fle (Colorectal cancer)	levamisole	Ergamisol	50 mg P.O. q 8 hours for days 1 to 3, repeated q 2 weeks for 1 year
	fluorouracil (5-FU)	Adrucil	450 mg/m² I.V. for days 1 to 5 and day 28; weekly thereafter for 48 weeks
FZ (Genitourinary, prostate cancer)	flutamide	Eulexin	250 P.O. q 8 hours
	goserelin acetate	Zoladex	3.6 mg implant S.C. q 28 days
HDMTX (high-dose methotrexate) (Bony sarcoma)	methotrexate	Folex	8 to 12 g/m² I.V. weekly for 2 to 12 weeks
	leucovorin calcium	Wellcovorin	15 to 25 mg/m² I.V. or P.O. q 6 hours for 10 doses, beginning 24 hours after methotrexate dose (serum methotrexate levels must be monitored) *Repeat cycle q 7 days for 2 to 4 weeks.*

Cancer chemotherapy: Acronyms and protocols *(continued)*

ACRONYM & INDICATION	DRUG		DOSAGE
	Generic name	Trade name	
MACOP-B (Malignant lymphoma)	methotrexate	Folex	100 mg/m² I.V., weeks 2, 6, and 10
	leucovorin calcium	Wellcovorin	15 mg/m² P.O. q 6 hours for six doses, beginning 24 hours after methotrexate dose
	doxorubicin	Adriamycin	50 mg/m² I.V., weeks 1, 3, 5, 7, 9, and 11
	cyclophosphamide	Cytoxan	350 mg/m² I.V., weeks 1, 3, 5, 7, 9, and 11
	vincristine	Oncovin	1.4 mg/m² (2 mg maximum) I.V., weeks 2, 4, 6, 8, 10, and 12
	bleomycin	Blenoxane	10 U/m² I.V., weeks 4, 8, and 12
	prednisone	Deltasone	75 mg P.O. daily for 12 weeks; taper dose over last 2 weeks *Repeat cycle as indicated in protocol.*
MAID (Soft-tissue sarcoma)	mesna	MESNEX	Uroprotection 1.5 to 2.5 g/m²/day by continuous I.V. infusion, days 1 to 3
	doxorubicin	Adriamycin	15 to 20 mg/m² by continuous I.V. infusion, days 1 to 3
	ifosfamide	Ifex	1.5 to 2.5 g/m² I.V., days 1 to 3
	dacarbazine	DTIC-Dome	250 to 300 mg/m² by continuous I.V. infusion days 1 to 3 *Repeat cycle q 28 days.*
m-BACOD (Malignant lymphoma)	bleomycin	Blenoxane	4 U/m² I.V., day 1
	doxorubicin	Adriamycin	45 mg/m² I.V., day 1
	cyclophosphamide	Cytoxan	600 mg/m² I.V., day 1
	vincristine	Oncovin	1 mg/m² (2 mg maximum) I.V., day 1
	dexamethasone	Decadron	6 mg/m² I.V., days 1 to 5
	methotrexate	Folex	200 mg/m² I.V., days 8 and 15
	leucovorin calcium	Wellcovorin	10 mg/m² P.O. q 6 hours for eight doses, beginning 24 hours after each methotrexate dose *Repeat cycle q 21 days.*
MBC (Head and neck cancer)	methotrexate	Folex	40 mg/m² I.V., days 1 and 15
	bleomycin	Blenoxane	10 U/m² I.M. or I.V., days 1, 8, and 15
	cisplatin	Platinol	50 mg/m² I.V., day 4 *Repeat cycle q 21 days.*
MC (Leukemia—AML, induction)	mitoxantrone	Novantrone	12 mg/m² I.V. daily, days 1 to 3
	cytarabine (ara-C)	Cytosar-U	100 to 200 mg/m² daily by continuous I.V. infusion, days 1 to 7 *Repeat cycle q 28 days.*

Cancer chemotherapy: Acronyms and protocols (continued)

ACRONYM & INDICATION	DRUG		DOSAGE
	Generic name	Trade name	
MICE (ICE) (Non-small-cell lung cancer)	mesna	MESNEX	Dosage is 20% of ifosfamide dose given I.V. immediately before and at 4 and 8 hours after ifosfamide infusion
	ifosfamide	Ifex	2,000 mg/m² I.V., days 1 to 3
	carboplatin	Paraplatin	300 to 350 mg/m² I.V., day 1
	etoposide (VP-16)	VePesid	60 to 100 mg/m² I.V., days 1 to 3 *Repeat cycle q 28 days.*
MOPP (Hodgkin's disease)	mechlorethamine (nitrogen mustard)	Mustargen	6 mg/m² I.V., days 1 and 8
	vincristine	Oncovin	1.4 mg/m² (2 mg maximum) I.V., days 1 and 8
	procarbazine	Matulane	100 mg/m² P.O., days 1 to 14
	prednisone	Deltasone	40 mg/m² P.O., days 1 to 14 *Repeat cycle q 28 days.*
MP (Multiple myeloma)	melphalan (L-phenylalanine mustard)	Alkeran	8 to 10 mg/m² P.O., days 1 to 4
	prednisone	Deltasone	40 to 60 mg/m² P.O., days 1 to 7 *Repeat cycle q 28 to 42 days.*
MVAC (Genitourinary cancer)	methotrexate	Folex	30 mg/m² I.V., days 1, 15, and 22
	vinblastine	Velban	3 mg/m² I.V., days 2, 15, and 22
	doxorubicin	Adriamycin	30 mg/m² I.V., day 2
	cisplatin	Platinol	70 mg/m² I.V., day 2 *Repeat cycle q 28 days.*
MVP (Non-small-cell lung cancer)	mitomycin	Mutamycin	8 mg/m² I.V., days 1, 29, and 71
	vinblastine	Velban	4.5 mg/m² I.V., days 15, 22, and 29, then q 2 weeks
	cisplatin	Planitol	120 mg/m² I.V., days 1 and 29, then q 6 weeks
MVPP (Hodgkin's-disease)	mechlorethamine (nitrogen mustard)	Mustargen	6 mg/m² I.V., days 1 and 8
	vinblastine	Velban	6 mg/m² I.V., days 1 and 8
	procarbazine	Matulane	100 mg/m² P.O., days 1 to 14
	prednisone	Deltasone	40 mg/m² P.O., days 1 to 14 *Repeat cycle q 4 to 6 weeks.*
PCV (Brain tumors)	procarbazine	Matulane	60 mg/m² P.O., days 8 to 21
	lomustine (CCNU)	CeeNu	110 mg/m² P.O., day 1
	vincristine	Oncovin	1.4 mg/m² (2 mg maximum) I.V., days 8 and 29 *Repeat cycle q 6 to 8 weeks.*

Cancer chemotherapy: Acronyms and protocols (continued)

ACRONYM & INDICATION	DRUG		DOSAGE
	Generic name	Trade name	
ProMACE (Malignant lymphoma)	prednisone	Deltasone	60 mg/m² P.O., days 1 to 14
	methotrexate	Folex	1.5 g/m² I.V., day 14
	leucovorin calcium	Wellcovorin	50 mg/m² I.V. q 6 hours for five to six doses, beginning 24 hours after methotrexate dose
	doxorubicin	Adriamycin	25 mg/m² I.V., days 1 and 8
	cyclophosphamide	Cytoxan	650 mg/m² I.V., days 1 and 8
	etoposide (VP-16)	VePesid	120 mg/m² I.V., days 1 and 8
ProMACE/ cytaBOM (Malignant lymphoma)	cyclophosphamide	Cytoxan	650 mg/m² I.V., day 1
	doxorubicin	Adriamycin	25 mg/m² I.V., day 1
	etoposide (VP-16)	VePesid	120 mg/m² I.V., day 1
	prednisone	Deltasone	60 mg/m² P.O., days 1 to 14
	cytarabine (ara-C)	Cytosar-U	300 mg/m² I.V., day 8
	bleomycin	Blenoxane	5 U/m² I.V., day 8
	vincristine	Oncovin	1.4 mg/m² (2 mg maximum) I.V., day 8
	methotrexate	Folex	120 mg/m² I.V., day 8
	leucovorin calcium	Wellcovorin	25 mg/m² P.O. q 6 hours for six doses beginning 24 hours after methotrexate dose *Repeat cycle q 21 to 28 days.*
7 + 3 (A + D) (Leukemia— AML, induction)	cytarabine (ara-C)	Cytosar-U	100 or 200 mg/m²/day by continuous I.V. infusion, days 1 to 7
	daunorubicin	Cerubidine	45 mg/m² I.V., days 1 to 3
VAC Standard (soft-tissue sarcoma)	vincristine	Oncovin	2 mg/m² (2 mg/week maximum) I.V. weekly for 12 weeks
	dactinomycin (actinomycin D)	Cosmegen	0.015 mg/kg/day (0.5 mg/day maximum) I.V., days 1 to 5 q 3 months
	cyclophosphamide	Cytoxan	2.5 mg/kg daily P.O. for 2 years
VAD (Multiple myeloma)	vincristine	Oncovin	0.4 mg by continuous I.V. infusion, days 1 to 4
	doxorubicin	Adriamycin	9 to 10 mg/m² by continuous I.V. infusion, days 1 to 4
	dexamethasone	Decadron	40 mg P.O. on days 1 to 4, 9 to 12, and 17 to 20 *Repeat cycle q 4 to 5 weeks.*
VATH (Breast cancer)	vinblastine	Velban	4.5 mg/m² I.V., day 1
	doxorubicin	Adriamycin	45 mg/m² I.V., day 1
	thiotepa	Thioplex	12 mg/m² I.V., day 1
	fluoxymesterone	Halotestin	30 mg P.O. daily (through each course) *Repeat cycle q 21 days.*

Cancer chemotherapy: Acronyms and protocols (continued)

ACRONYM & INDICATION	DRUG		DOSAGE
	Generic name	Trade name	
VBAP (Multiple myeloma)	vincristine	Oncovin	1 mg I.V., day 1
	carmustine	BiCNU	30 mg/m² I.V., day 1
	doxorubicin	Adriamycin	30 mg/m² I.V., day 1
	prednisone	Deltasone	60 mg/m²/day P.O., days 1 to 4 *Repeat cycle q 21 days.*
VBP (Genitourinary, testicular cancer)	vinblastine	Velban	6 mg/m² I.V., days 1 and 2
	bleomycin	Blenoxane	30 U I.V., days 1, 8, 15, and (optional) 22
	cisplatin	Platinol	20 mg/m² I.V., days 1 to 5 *Repeat cycle q 21 to 28 days.*
VC (Non-small-cell lung cancer)	vinorelbine	Navelbine	30 mg/m² I.V. weekly
	cisplatin	Platinol	120 mg/m² I.V., days 1 and 29 *Repeat cycle q 6 weeks.*
VCAP (Multiple myeloma)	vincristine	Oncovin	1 mg/m² (2 mg maximum) I.V., day 1
	cyclophosphamide	Cytoxan	100 to 125 mg/m² P.O., days 1 to 4
	doxorubicin	Adriamycin	25 to 30 mg/m² I.V., day 2
	prednisone	Deltasone	60 mg/m² P.O., days 1 to 4 *Repeat cycle q 28 days.*
VDP (Malignant melanoma)	vinblastine	Velban	5 mg/m² I.V., days 1 and 2
	dacarbazine	DTIC-Dome	150 mg/m² I.V., days 1 to 5
	cisplatin	Platinol	75 mg/m² I.V., day 5 *Repeat cycle q 21 to 28 days.*
VIP (Genitourinary, testicular cancer)	vinblastine	Velban	0.11 mg/kg I.V., days 1 and 2
	ifosfamide	Ifex	1.2 g/m²/day continuous I.V. infusion, days 1 to 5
	cisplatin	Platinol	20 mg/m² I.V. over 1 hour, days 1 to 5
	mesna	MESNEX	400 mg I.V. 15 minutes before ifosfamide day 1, then 1.2 g daily by continuous I.V. infusion, days 1 to 5 *Repeat cycle q 21 days.*
or	etoposide (VP-16)	VePesid	75 mg/m² I.V., days 1 to 5
	ifosfamide	Ifex	1.2 g/m²/day continuous I.V. infusion, days 1 to 5
	cisplatin	Platinol	20 mg/m², days 1 to 5
	mesna	MESNEX	400 mg I.V. 15 minutes before ifosfamide day 1, then 1.2 g daily by continuous I.V. infusion, days 1 to 5 *Repeat cycle q 21 days.*
VM (Breast cancer)	vinblastine	Velban	5 mg/m² I.V., days 1, 14, 28, and 42 for first two cycles; then 5 mg/m² I.V., days 1 and 21
	mitomycin	Mutamycin	10 mg/m² I.V., days 1 and 28 for first two cycles; then 10 mg/m² I.V., day 1

Table of equivalents

Metric system equivalents

Metric weight

1 kilogram (kg or Kg)	=	1,000 grams (g or gm)
1 gram	=	1,000 milligrams (mg)
1 milligram	=	1,000 micrograms (µg or mcg)
0.6 g	=	600 mg
0.3 g	=	300 mg
0.1 g	=	100 mg
0.06 g	=	60 mg
0.03 g	=	30 mg
0.015 g	=	15 mg
0.001 g	=	1 mg

Metric volume

1 liter (l or L)	=	1,000 milliliters (ml)*
1 milliliter	=	1,000 microliters (µl)

Household		Metric
1 teaspoon (tsp)	=	5 ml
1 tablespoon (T or tbs)	=	15 ml
2 tablespoons	=	30 ml
1 measuring cupful	=	240 ml
1 pint (pt)	=	473 ml
1 quart (qt)	=	946 ml
1 gallon (gal)	=	3,785 ml

Temperature conversions

FAHRENHEIT DEGREES	CENTIGRADE DEGREES	FAHRENHEIT DEGREES	CENTIGRADE DEGREES	FAHRENHEIT DEGREES	CENTIGRADE DEGREES
106.0	41.1	100.6	38.1	95.2	35.1
105.8	41.0	100.4	38.0	95.0	35.0
105.6	40.9	100.2	37.9	94.8	34.9
105.4	40.8	100.0	37.8	94.6	34.8
105.2	40.7	99.8	37.7	94.4	34.7
105.0	40.6	99.6	37.6	94.2	34.6
104.8	40.4	99.4	37.4	94.0	34.4
104.6	40.3	99.2	37.3	93.8	34.3
104.4	40.2	99.0	37.2	93.6	34.2
104.2	40.1	98.8	37.1	93.4	34.1
104.0	40.0	98.6	37.0	93.2	34.0
103.8	39.9	98.4	36.9	93.0	33.9
103.6	39.8	98.2	36.8	92.8	33.8
103.4	39.7	98.0	36.7	92.6	33.7
103.2	39.6	97.8	36.5	92.4	33.6
103.0	39.4	97.6	36.4	92.2	33.4
102.8	39.3	97.4	36.3	92.0	33.3
102.6	39.2	97.2	36.2	91.8	33.2
102.4	39.1	97.0	36.1	91.6	33.1
102.2	39.0	96.8	36.0	91.4	33.0
102.0	38.9	96.6	35.9	91.2	32.9
101.8	38.8	96.4	35.8	91.0	32.8
101.6	38.7	96.2	35.7	90.8	32.7
101.4	38.6	96.0	35.6	90.6	32.6
101.2	38.4	95.8	35.4	90.4	32.4
101.0	38.3	95.6	35.3	90.2	32.3
100.8	38.2	95.4	35.2	90.0	32.2

Weight conversions

1 oz = 30 g	1 lb = 453.6 g	2.2 lb = 1 kg

*1 ml = 1 cubic centimeter (cc); however, ml is the preferred measurement term today.

Diagnostic skin tests

DRUG, INDICATIONS, DOSAGE

coccidioidin
BioCox, Spherulin

Suspected coccidioidomycosis—
Adults and children: 0.1 ml of 1:100 dilution intradermally into flexor surface of forearm. In persons nonreactive to this form, test is repeated using 1:10 dilution.
Use 1:1,000 or 1:10,000 dilution if erythema nodosum is evident.

histoplasmin
Histolyn-CYL, Histoplasmin Diluted

To differentiate histoplasmosis from coccidioidomycosis, tuberculosis, sarcoidosis, and other mycotic or bacterial infections—
Adults and children: 0.1 ml intradermally into flexor surface of forearm.

mumps skin test antigen
MSTA

To assess T-cell-mediated immunity—
Adults and children: 0.1 ml intradermally into flexor surface of forearm.

tuberculin purified protein derivative (PPD)
Aplisol, PPD-stabilized Solution (Mantoux test), Selavo-PPD Solution, Tubersol

Diagnosis of tuberculosis—
Adults and children: initially, 1 TU (for patients suspected of being highly sensitized) or 5 TU (for patients not expected to be highly sensitized) intradermally into flexor surface of forearm. If negative, patient is retested with 250 TU.

tuberculosis multiple-puncture tests
Aplitest (dried purified protein derivative [PPD]), Mono-Vacc Test (liquid Old Tuberculin [OT]), Sclavo Test (dried PPD), Tine Test (dried OT, dried PPD)

Screening for tuberculosis—
Adults and children: clean skin thoroughly with alcohol; make skin taut on flexor surface of forearm and press points firmly into selected site. Hold device at injection site for about 3 seconds to ensure depositing of dried tuberculin B in tissue lymph.

Reactions may be *common*, uncommon, *life-threatening*, or COMMON AND LIFE-THREATENING.

ADVERSE REACTIONS	SPECIAL CONSIDERATIONS
Systemic: hypersensitivity reactions (vesiculation, ulceration, necrosis), ***anaphylaxis,*** Arthus reaction.	• Pregnancy risk category: C. • Contraindicated in patients with hypersensitivity to thimerosal or erythema nodosum. • Read test at 24 and 48 hours.
Skin: urticaria, ulceration, or necrosis in highly sensitive patients. **Systemic:** ***anaphylaxis.***	• Pregnancy risk category: C. • Contraindicated in patients known to be positive reactors. • Read test within 24 to 48 hours.
Systemic: hypersensitivity reactions (vesiculation, ulceration), ***anaphylaxis,*** Arthus reaction.	• Pregnancy risk category: C. • Contraindicated in patients with hypersensitivity to eggs, egg products, or thimerosal. • Read test at 48 and 72 hours.
Skin: pruritus, vesiculation. **Systemic:** hypersensitivity reactions, ***anaphylaxis,*** Arthus reaction. **Other:** pain, ulceration, necrosis.	• Pregnancy risk category: C. • Contraindicated in known tuberculin-positive reactors; severe reactions may occur. • Read test within 48 to 72 hours. If repeat test using 250 TU shows no response, patient is nonreactive.
Systemic: hypersensitivity reactions (vesiculation, ulceration, necrosis), ***anaphylaxis.***	• Pregnancy risk category: C. • Contraindicated in known tuberculin-positive reactors. • Read test within 48 to 72 hours. Verify questionable or positive reactions with the Mantoux test.

Nomogram for estimating surface area in children

The surface area (S.A.) is indicated below where the S.A. column intersects the straight line that connects height and weight; or for a child of average size, opposite the child's weight.

FOR CHILDREN OF NORMAL HEIGHT AND WEIGHT   **NOMOGRAM**

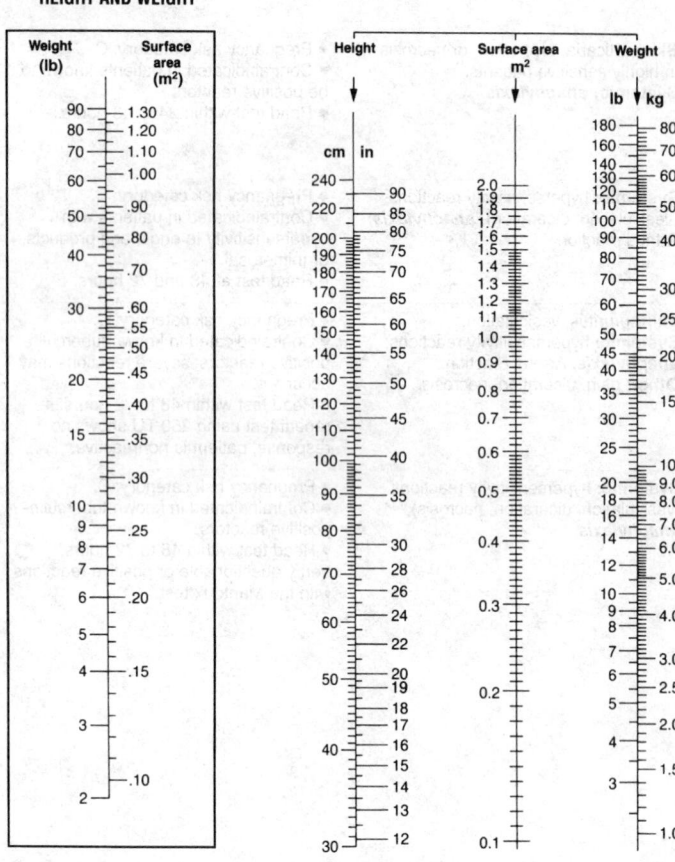

Behrman, R.E., ed., *Nelson Textbook of Pediatrics*, 15th ed, Philadelphia; W.B. Saunders Co., 1996.

Index

A

Abbocillin VK, 97
Abbokinase, 881
Abbokinase Open-Cath, 881
abciximab, 1225-1227
Abdominal distention
    neostigmine for, 528-529
    vasopressin for, 800-801
Abenol, 330
Abortion
    carboprost for, 1192-1193
    dinoprostone for,
        1193-1194
    oxytocin, synthetic injec-
        tion, for, 1195-1196
Absorption of drug, 6
    in children, 13
acarbose, 761-762
A.C. & C., 366
Accolate, 639
Accupril, 303, C1
Accurbron, 618
Accutane, 1243
acebutolol, 265-266
Acel-Imune, 981
Aceta Elixir, 330
Acet-Am, 618
acetaminophen, 330-333
acetaminophen and codeine,
    C1
Acetaminophen toxicity,
    acetylcysteine for,
    624-625
Acetaminophen Uniserts, 330
Aceta Tablets, 330
Aceta with Codeine, 366
Acetazolam, 808
acetazolamide, 808-810
acetazolamide sodium,
    808-810
acetic acid, 1096
acetohexamide, 762-764
acetohydroxamic acid, 1227
acetylcholine chloride, 1062
acetylcysteine, 624-625
acetylsalicylic acid, 333-335
Aches-N-Pain, 348
Achromycin, 1129
Achromycin V, 143
Acidifier, 847-848
Aclin, 363
Acne
    azelaic acid cream for, 1113
    clindamycin for, 1115-1116
    erythromycin for,
        1118-1119
    isotretinoin for, 1243-1244
    tetracycline for, 143-145,
        1129-1130
    tretinoin for, 1259-1260
Acne rosacea, metronidazole
    for, 1121-1122
Acon, 1157

Acromegaly
    bromocriptine for, 505-506
    octreotide for, 659-660
ACT, 1173
ACT-3, 348
Actamin, 330
Actamin Extra, 330
ACTH, 794-796
Acthar, 794
Acthar Gel (H.P.), 794
ACTH Gel, 794
ActHIB/DTP, 978
Acticort, 1151
Actidose, 1204
Actidose-Aqua, 1204
Actidil, 595
Actifed, 597
Actigall, 654
Actimmune, 1035
Actimol, 330
Actinic keratoses, fluorouracil
    for, 907-909
actinomycin D, 916-917
activated charcoal, 1204-1205
Actraphane HM, 771
Actraphane HM Penfill, 771
Actraphane MC, 771
Actrapid HM, 771
Actrapid HM Penfill, 771
Actrapid MC, 771
Actrapid MC Penfill, 771
Actron, 352
Acular, 1057
Acute renal failure, mannitol
    for, 822-824
acyclovir, 1111-1112
acyclovir sodium, 166-168
Adalat, 254, C1
Adalat CC, 254
Adalat FT, 254
Adalat P.A., 254
Adenocard, 221
adenosine, 221-222
ADH, 800-801
Adipex-P, 501
Adrenal cancer, aminog-
    lutethimide for,
    1231-1232
Adrenalin, 604
Adrenalin Chloride, 604, 1103
adrenaline, 604-607
Adrenal insufficiency
    cortisone for, 701-703
    hydrocortisone for, 706-709
Adrenergic blockers, 552-555
Adrenergics, 541-551
Adrenocortical cancer, mi-
    totane for, 950-951
Adrenocortical function, diag-
    nosis of
    corticotropin for, 794-796
    cosyntropin for, 796

adrenocorticotropic hormone,
    794-796
Adrenogenital syndrome, flu-
    drocortisone for, 705-706
Adriamycin, 919
Adriamycin PFS, 919
Adriamycin RDF, 919
Adrucil, 907
Adsorbents, 642-649
Adsorbocarpine, 1069
Adsorbonac Ophthalmic Solu-
    tion, 1093
Adverse reactions, 9-10
    in elderly patients, 19-20
Advil, 348
Advil Cold and Sinus, 342
AeroBid, 636
AeroBid-M, 636
Aerolone, 609
Aeroseb-Dex, 1143
Aeroseb-HC, 1151
Aerosporin, 210
Afko-Lube, 666
Afrin, 550, 1106
Afrin Children's Strength Nose
    Drops, 1106
Afrinol Repetabs, 550
Aftate for Athlete's Foot, 1130
Aftate for Jock Itch, 1130
Agammaglobulinemia,
    immune globulin for,
    1014-1015
Agon, 279
Agon SR, 279
Agoral, 662
Agoral Plain, 671
AHF, 867-868
A-hydroCort, 706
AIDS. See also HIV infection.
    cidofovir for, 169-171
    foscarnet for, 173-175
    ganciclovir for, 175-176
    megestrol for, 933-934
    zidovudine for, 188-190
Airbron, 624
Akarapine, 1069
AK-Chlor, 200, 1040
AK-Con, 1078
AK-Dilate, 1075
Akineton, 504
Akineton Lactate, 504
AK-Nefrin Ophthalmic, 1075
Akne-mycin, 1118
AK-Pentolate, 1072
AK-Poly-Bac, 1039
AK-Pred, 1059
AK-taine, 1266t
Aktob, 1051
AK-Tracin, 1040
AK-Zol, 808
Ala-Tet, 143
Albalon-A Liquifilm, 1078
Albalon Liquifilm, 1078

t refers to a table; **boldface** refers to full-color photographs

albumin 5%, 866-867
albumin 25%, 866-867
Albuminar 5%, 866
Albuminar 25%, 866
Albutein 5%, 866
Albutein 25%, 866
albuterol, 597-599
albuterol sulfate, 597-599
Alcaine, 1266t
Alclox, 84
Alcoholism
  disulfiram for, 1209-1211
  mesoridazine for, 472-474
  naltrexone for, 1217-1218
Alcohol withdrawal symptoms
  chloral hydrate for, 391-393
  chlordiazepoxide for,
    451-452
  clorazepate for, 452-453
  diazepam for, 453-456
  oxazepam for, 461
Alconefrin 12, 1107
Alconefrin 25, 1107
Alconefrin 50, 1107
Aldactazide 25/25, 808
Aldactazide 50/50, 808
Aldactone, 826
Aldazine, 482
Aldecin Inhaler, 626
aldesleukin, 1022-1024
Aldoclor-150, 263
Aldoclor-250, 263
Aldomet, 291
Aldomet Ester Injection, 291
Aldomet M, 291
Aldoril-15, 263
Aldoril-25, 263
Aldoril D30, 263
Aldoril D50, 263
alendronate sodium,
  1228-1229
Alepam, 461
Aleve, 359
Alexan, 903
Alfenta, 367
alfentanil hydrochloride,
  367-368
Alferon N, 1031
alglucerase, 1229-1230
Alkaban-AQ, 963
Alkalinizers, 848-850
Alka-Mints, 645
Alka-Seltzer with Aspirin, 642
Alka-Seltzer without Aspirin,
  642
Alkeran, 896
Alkylating drugs, 883-901
Allegra, 593
Allegron, 438
Alleract, 595
Aller-Chlor, 587
Allerdryl, 591
Allerest, 1078

Allerest Maximum Strength
  Tablets, 583
Allerest No Drowsiness
  Tablets, 330
Allerest 12-Hour Nasal, 1106
Allergex, 587
Allergic reactions
  cortisone for, 701-703
  dexamethasone for,
    703-705
Allergy symptoms
  astemizole for, 584
  azatadine for, 584-585
  brompheniramine for,
    585-586
  cetirizine for, 586-587
  chlorpheniramine for,
    587-588
  clemastine for, 588-589
  cyproheptadine for,
    589-590
  dexchlorpheniramine for,
    590-591
  diphenhydramine for,
    591-593
  promethazine for, 594-595
  triprolidine for, 595-596
Allerid, 550
AllerMax Caplets, 591
Allermed, 550
Aller-med, 591
Allograft rejection
  lymphocyte immune globu-
    lin for, 972-973
  muromonab-CD3 for,
    973-974
  mycophenolate for, 974-975
  nitrofurazone for,
    1124-1125
  tacrolimus for, 975-977
allopurinol, 1182-1183
Alloremed, 1182
Alomide, 1091
Alopecia, minoxidil for,
  1249-1250
Alophen, 672
Alpha₁-antitrypsin deficiency,
  alpha₁ proteinase in-
  hibitor for, 625-626
Alphamox, 77
Alphamul, 665
AlphaNine, 871
AlphaNine SD, 871
Alphapress, 285
alpha₁ proteinase inhibitor
  (human), 625-626
Alpha-Tamoxifen, 935
Alphatrex, 1138
alprazolam, 449-450
alprostadil, 322-323,
  1230-1231
Altace, 304, C1
alteplase, 874-875
AlternaGEL, 644
altretamine, 937-938

Alu-Cap, 644
Aludrox Suspension, 642
aluminum carbonate, 642-643
aluminum hydroxide, 644-645
Aluminum Hydroxide Gel, 644
Aluminum Hydroxide Gel Concentrated, 644
aluminum-magnesium com-
  plex, 647-648
aluminum phosphate, 645
Alupent, 611
Alu-Tab, 644
Alzapam, 457
Alzheimer's disease
  donepezil for, 514-515
  tacrine for, 522-523
amantadine hydrochloride,
  168
Amaphen, 330
Amaryl, 765
ambenonium chloride,
  524-525
Ambien, 402, C1
amcinonide, 1137-1138
Amebiasis
  chloroquine for, 45-46
  erythromycin for, 195-197
  iodoquinol for, 25-26
  metronidazole for, 26-28
  paromomycin for, 28-29
Amebicides, 25-30
Amen, 751
Amenorrhea
  bromocriptine for, 505-506
  gonadorelin for, 756-757
  hydroxyprogesterone for,
    748-749
  medroxyprogesterone for,
    751-752
  norethindrone for, 752-753
  progesterone for, 754-755
Amersol, 348
A-methaPred, 709
amethopterin, 911-914
Amicar, 1205
amifostine, 938-939
Amigesic, 340
amikacin sulfate, 65-66
Amikin, 65
amiloride hydrochloride,
  810-811
Aminess, 1176
amino acid infusions, crystalline, 1176-1178
amino acid infusions for hepatic failure, 1176-1178
amino acid infusions for high
  metabolic stress,
  1176-1178
amino acid infusions for renal
  failure, 1176-1178
amino acid infusions in dextrose, 1176-1178
amino acid infusions with
  electrolytes, 1176-1178

t refers to a table; **boldface** refers to full-color photographs

amino acid infusions with electrolytes in dextrose, 1176-1178
aminocaproic acid, 1205-1206
Aminofen, 330
Aminofen Max, 330
aminoglutethimide, 1231-1232
Aminoglycosides, 65-74
Amino-Opti-E, 1170
Aminophyllin, 599
aminophylline, 599-602
aminosalicylate sodium, 52-53
Aminosyn, 1176
Aminosyn II, 1176
Aminosyn II with dextrose, 1176
Aminosyn II with electrolytes, 1176
Aminosyn II with electrolytes in dextrose, 1176
Aminosyn-HBC, 1176
Aminosyn-PF, 1176
Aminosyn-RF, 1176
Aminosyn with electrolytes, 1176
amiodarone hydrochloride, 222-224
Amitone, 645
amitriptyline hydrochloride, 423-424, **C1**
amitriptyline pamoate, 423-424
amlodipine besylate, 246-247
ammonia, aromatic spirits, 1206
ammonium chloride, 847-848
amoxapine, 424-426
amoxicillin/clavulanate potassium, 75-76
amoxicillin trihydrate, 77-78, **C1**
Amoxil, 77, **C2**
amoxyclllin/clavulanate potassium, 75-76
amphetamine sulfate, 488-489
Amphocin, 34
Amphojel, 644
amphotericin B, 34-36, 1112-1113
Amphotericin B for injection, 34
ampicillin, 78-80
ampicillin sodium, 78-80
ampicillin sodium/sulbactam sodium, 80-81
ampicillin trihydrate, 78-80
Ampicin, 78-80
Ampicyn Injection, 78
Ampicyn Oral, 78
Amprace, 277
amrinone lactate, 216-217

amyl nitrite, 247
Amyotrophic lateral sclerosis, riluzole for, 1253-1254
Anabolin IM, 723
Anabolin LA, 722
Anacin-3, 330
Anacin-3 Children's Elixir, 330
Anacin-3 Children's Tablets, 330
Anacin-3 Extra Strength, 330
Anacin-3 Infants', 330
Anacin-3 Maximum Strength Caplets, 330
Anacin with Codeine, 366
Anacobin, 1158
Anafranil, 427
Anaphylaxis, epinephrine for, 604-607
Anaprox, 359
Anaprox DS, 359
Anaspaz, 536
anastrozole, 927
Anatensol, 467
Ancalixir, 414
Ancasal, 333
Ancasal 8, 366
Ancasal 15, 366
Ancasal 30, 366
Ancef, 107
Ancobon, 37
Ancolan, 681
Ancotil, 37
Andro 100, 726
Andro-Cyp 100, 726
Andro-Cyp 200, 726
Androgyn L.A., 718
Android, 721
Android-F, 719
Androlone, 723
Androlone-D, 722
Andronaq-50, 726
Andronaq-LA, 726
Andronate 100, 726
Andronate 200, 726
Andrumin, 678
Anectine, 578
Anectine Flo-Pack, 578
Anemia
    antithymocyte globulin for, 972-973
    epoetin alfa for, 1024-1026
    folic acid for, 1160-1161
    leucovorin for, 1161-1162
    nandrolone for, 722-724
Anergan 25, 594
Anergan 50, 594
Anesthesia
    alfentanil for, 367-368
    butorphanol for, 369-371
    epinephrine for, 604-607
    fentanyl for, 372-375
    meperidine for, 376-378
    midazolam for, 459-460
    nalbuphine for, 381-383
    sufentanil for, 387-388

Anesthetics, 1262-1267t
Anexia 5/500, 366
Angina
    amlodipine for, 246-247
    amyl nitrite for, 247
    atenolol for, 266-268
    bepridil for, 248
    diltiazem for, 249-250
    isosorbide for, 250-252
    metoprolol for, 293-294
    nadolol for, 252-253
    nicardipine for, 253-254
    nifedipine for, 254-255
    nitroglycerin for, 255-258
    papaverine for, 326-327
    propranolol for, 258-260
    sotalol for, 242-244
    verapamil for, 260-262
Anginine, 255
anisoylated plasminogen-streptokinase activator complex, 875-877
anistreplase, 875-877
Ankylosing spondylitis
    diclofenac for, 342-344
    indomethacin for, 349-352
    naproxen for, 359-360
    sulindac for, 363-364
Anoquan, 330
Anorexia, dronabinol for, 680-681
Anovulation
    clomiphene for, 1236-1237
    gonadorelin for, 756-757
    menotropins for, 758-760
Anpec, 260
Anpine, 254
Ansaid, 346, **C2**
Antacids, 642-649
Antadine, 168
Antagonists, miscellaneous, 1204-1224
Anthelmintics, 31-33
Antianginals, 246-262
Antianxiety drugs, 449-461
Antiarrhythmics, 221-245
Antibiotic antineoplastic drugs, 915-926
Anticholinergics, 533-540
Anticholinesterase insecticide poisoning, atropine for, 224-225
Anticoagulant overdose, factor IX for, 871-872
Anticoagulants, 857-865
Anticonvulsants, 403-422
Antidepressants, 423-448
Antidiabetic drugs, 761-780
Antidiarrheals, 656-661
Antiemetics, 678-688
Antiflatulents, 642-649
Antiflux, 647
Antifungals, 34-44
Antigout drugs, 1182-1191

antihemophilic factor, 867-868
Antihistamines, 583-596
Antihypertensives, 263-311
Anti-infectives, local, 1111-1131
Anti-infectives, miscellaneous, 198-215
anti-inhibitor coagulant complex, 869-870
Antileprotics, 52-64
Antilipemics, 312-321
Antilirium, 529
Antimalarials, 45-51
Antimetabolites, 902-914
Antiminth, 31
Anti-Naus, 685
Antineoplastic drugs, miscellaneous, 937-968
Antineoplastics that alter hormone balance, 927-936
Antiparkinsonian drugs, 503-513
Antiprotozoals, 25-30
Antipsychotics, 462-487
Antipyretics, 330-341
Antispas, 533
antithrombin III, human, 870-871
antithymocyte globulin (equine), 972-973
Antitoxins, 1008-1011
Antituberculars, 52-64
Anti-Tuss, 623
Anti-Tuss DM Expectorant, 622
Antitussives, 621-623
Antiulcer drugs, 689-698
Antivenin (Latrodectus mactans), 1008
Antivenins, 1008-1011
Antivert, 681
Antivert/25, 681
Antivert/50, 681
Antivirals, 166-190
Anturan, 1187
Anturane, 1187
Anxanil, 456
Anxiety
alprazolam for, 449-450
buspirone for, 450-451
chlordiazepoxide for, 451-452
clorazepate for, 452-453
diazepam for, 453-456
doxepin for, 430-431
hydroxyzine for, 456-457
lorazepam for, 457-458
mephobarbital for, 413-414
meprobamate for, 458-459
mesoridazine for, 472-474
oxazepam for, 461
prochlorperazine for, 685-687
Apacet Capsules, 330

Apacet Elixir, 330
Apacet Extra Strength Caplets, 330
Apacet Extra Strength Tablets, 330
Apacet Infants', 330
Apacet Regular Strength Tablets, 330
APAP, 330-333
Aparkane, 512
Aplisol, 1280t
Aplitest (dried purified protein derivative), 1280t
Apo-Acetaminophen, 330
Apo-Acetazolamide, 808
Apo-Allopurinol, 1182
Apo-Alpraz, 449
Apo-Amitriptyline, 423
Apo-Amoxi, 77
Apo-Ampi, 78
Apo-Atenolol, 266
Apo-Benztropine, 503
Apo-Cal, 832
Apo-Capto, 271
Apo-Carbamazepine, 403
Apo-Cephalex, 130
Apo-Chlordiazepoxide, 451
Apo-Chlorpropamide, 764
Apo-Chlorthalidone, 814
Apo-Clorazepate, 452
Apo-Cloxi, 84
Apo-Diazepam, 453
Apo-Diltiaz, 249
Apo-Dimenhydrinate, 678
Apo-Dipyridamole, 323
Apo-Doxy, 137
Apo-Erythro, 195
Apo-Erythro-ES, 195
Apo-Erythro-S, 195
Apo-Ferrous Sulfate, 853
Apo-Fluphenazine, 467
Apo-Flurazepam, 395
Apo-Flurbiprofen, 346
Apo-Furosemide, 817
Apo-Guanethidine, 283
Apo-Haloperidol, 469
Apo-Hydro, 819
Apo-Hydroxyzine, 456
Apo-Ibuprofen, 348
Apo-Imipramine, 432
Apo-Indomethacin, 350
Apo-ISDN, 250
Apo-Keto, 352
Apo-Keto-E, 352
Apo-Lorazepam, 457
Apo-Meprobamate, 458
Apo-Methyldopa, 291
Apo-Metoclop, 682
Apo-Metoprolol, 293
Apo-Metoprolol (Type L), 293
Apo-Metronidazole, 26
Apo-Minocycline, 140
Apo-Napro-Na, 359
Apo-Naproxen, 359
Apo-Nifed, 254

Apo-Nitrofurantoin, 208
Apo-Oxazepam, 461
Apo-Pen-VK, 97
Apo-Perphenazine, 476
Apo-Pindol, 301
Apo-Piroxicam, 362
Apo-Prednisone, 714
Apo-Primidone, 419
Apo-Propranolol, 258
Apo-Quinidine, 240
Apo-Ranitidine, 696
Apo-Sulfamethoxazole, 149
Apo-Sulfatrim, 146
Apo-Sulfatrim DS, 146
Apo-Sulin, 363
Apo-Tetra, 143
Apo-Thioridazine, 482
Apo-Timol, 308
Apo-Tolbutamide, 778
Apo-Triazo, 401
Apo-Trifluoperazine, 485
Apo-Trihex, 512
Apo-Trimip, 446
Apo-Verap, 260
Apo-Zidovudine, 188
Appendicitis
meropenem for, 205-207
piperacillin and tazobactam for, 100-101
Applanation tonometry, fluorescein for, 1087-1088
Apprehension
chlordiazepoxide for, 451-452
mephobarbital for, 413-414
midazolam for, 459-460
apraclonidine hydrochloride, 1081-1082
Apresazide 25/25, 263
Apresazide 50/50, 263
Apresazide 100/50, 263
Apresodex, 263
Apresoline, 285
Apresoline-Esidrix, 263
aprotinin, 1232-1233
APSAC, 875-877
A-200 Pyrinate, 1136
Aquachloral Supprettes, 391
AquaMEPHYTON, 1171
Aquaphyllin, 618
Aquasol A, 1157
Aquasol E, 1170
Aquazide-H, 819
ara-C, 903-905
Aralen HCl, 45
Aralen Phosphate, 45
Aralen Phosphate with Primaquine Phosphate, 45
Aramine, 545
Aratac, 222
Arduan, 575
Aredia, 1251
Argesic-SA, 340
Aricept, 514
Arimidex, 927

t refers to a table; **boldface** refers to full-color photographs

Aristocort, 716, 1154
Arm-a-Med Isoetharine, 608
Arm-A-Med Metaproterenol, 611
Arm and Hammer Pure Baking Soda, 848
Armour Thyroid, 785
Arrestin, 688
Arrhythmias
  acebutolol for, 265-266
  adenosine for, 221-222
  amiodarone for, 222-224
  atropine for, 224-225
  bretylium for, 225-227
  digoxin for, 217-219
  diltiazem for, 249-250
  disopyramide for, 227-228
  esmolol for, 228-230
  flecainide for, 230-231
  ibutilide for, 231-232
  isoproterenol for, 609-611
  lidocaine for, 232-234
  magnesium salts for, 412-413, 838-840
  mexiletine for, 234-235
  moricizine for, 235-237
  phenylephrine for, 548-550
  procainamide for, 237-239
  propafenone for, 239-240
  propranolol for, 258-260
  quinidine for, 240-242
  sotalol for, 242-244
  tocainide for, 244-245
  verapamil for, 260-262
  warfarin for, 863-865
Arsenic poisoning, dimer-caprol for, 1208-1209
Artane, 512
Artane Sequels, 512
Arteriosclerosis obliterans, isoxsuprine for, 324
Arteriovenous cannula occlusion
  streptokinase for, 878-881
  urokinase for, 881-882
Arthra-G, 340
Arthrexin, 349
Arthrinol, 333
Arthritis
  ibuprofen for, 348-349
  magnesium salicylate for, 339-340
  salsalate for, 340-341
Arthritis Pain Formula Aspirin Free, 330-331
Arthropan, 337
Artria S.R., 333
ASA, 333
Asacol, 1246
ASA Enseals, 333
Ascabiol, 1132
ascorbic acid, 1167-1169
Ascorbicap, 1167
Ascriptin, 330
Ascriptin A/D, 330

Asendin, 424
Asig, 303
Asmalix, 618
Asmol, 597
asparaginase, 939-941
A-Spas, 533
Aspergillosis
  amphotericin B for, 34-36
  itraconazole for, 39-40
Aspergum, 333
aspirin, 333-335
Aspro, 333
Astelin, 1099
astemizole, 584
Asthma
  aminophylline for, 599-602
  beclomethasone for, 626-627
  bitolterol for, 602-603
  cromolyn sodium for, 631-632
  dexamethasone for, 632-633
  epinephrine for, 604-607
  flunisolide for, 636-637
  isoetharine for, 608-609
  isoproterenol for, 609-611
  metaproterenol for, 611-613
  nedocromil for, 637-638
  oxtriphylline for, 613-614
  pirbuterol for, 614-615
  salmeterol for, 615-616
  triamcinolone for, 638-639
  zafirlukast for, 639-640
  zileuton for, 640-641
AsthmaHaler, 604
Asthma-Nefrin, 604
Astramorph PF, 379
Astrin, 333
AT-10, 805
Atarax, 456
Atasol Caplets, 331
Atasol Drops, 331
Atasol Elixir, 331
Atasol Forte Caplets, 331
Atasol Forte Tablets, 331
Atasol Tablets, 331
Atelectasis, acetylcysteine for, 624-625
Atenex, 453
atenolol, 266-268, **C2**
ATG, 972-973
Atgam, 972
Atherectomy, abciximab for, 1225-1227
AT-III, 870-871
AT-III deficiency, antithrombin III, human, for, 870-871
Ativan, 457, **C2**
ATnativ, 870
Atolone, 716
atorvastatin calcium, 312-313
atovaquone, 25
Atozine, 456
atracurium besylate, 565-566

Atrophic vaginitis
  chlorotrianisene for, 729-731
  dienestrol for, 731-732
  esterified estrogens for, 734-736
  estradiol for, 736-738
  estrogens, conjugated, for, 738-741
atropine sulfate, 224-225, 1071-1072
Atropisol, 1071
Atropt, 1071
Atrosept, 198
Atrovent, 607
A/T/S, 1118
attapulgite, 656-657
Attention deficit hyperactivity disorder
  amphetamine for, 488-489
  dextroamphetamine for, 493-494
  methamphetamine for, 498-499
  methylphenidate for, 499-500
  pemoline for, 500-501
Attenuvax, 993
Augmentin, 75, **C2**
auranofin, 1201-1202
Aurocaine 2, 1096
Auro-Dri, 1096
aurothioglucose, 1202-1203
Austramycin V, 143
Austrastaph, 84
Autoplex T, 869
Aventyl, 438
Avirax, 166
Avlosulfon, 56
Avomine, 594
Avonex, 1032
Axid, 694, **C2**
Axotal, 330
Axsain, 1234
Ayercillin, 94
Aygestin, 752
Aygestin Cycle Pack, 752
Azactam, 198
azatadine maleate, 584-585
azathioprine, 969-970
azelaic acid cream, 1113
azelastine hydrochloride, 1099-1100
Azelex, 1113
Azide, 812
azidothymidine, 188-190
azithromycin, 191-192
Azmacort, 638
Azo Gantanol, 146
Azo Gantrisin, 146
Azo-Standard, 1199
Azo Sulfamethoxazole, 146
Azo Sulfisoxazole, 146, 150
AZT, 188-190
aztreonam, 198-199

Azulfidine, 1257
Azulfidine EN-Tabs, 1257

B
bacampicillin hydrochloride,
    81-82
Baciguent, 199, 1113
Baci-IM, 199
bacillus Calmette-Guérin, live
    intravesical, 941-943
Bacitin, 199, 1113
bacitracin, 199-200, 1040,
    1113-1114
baclofen, 556-557
Bacteremia
    cefoperazone for, 114-115
    cefotaxime for, 115-117
    ceftazidime for, 122-124
    ceftizoxime for, 125-126
    ceftriaxone for, 126-128
    chloramphenicol for,
        200-202
Bacterial infections
    amikacin for, 65-66
    ceftriaxone for, 126-128
    clindamycin for, 202-203
    demeclocycline for,
        136-137
    doxycycline for, 137-140
    gentamicin for, 66-68
    kanamycin for, 68-69
    metronidazole for, 26-28
    minocycline for, 140-141
    neomycin for, 1124
    netilmicin for, 70-72
    oxytetracycline for, 142-143
    tetracycline for, 143-145
    tobramycin for, 73-74
    vancomycin for, 214-215
Bactine HC, 1151
Bactocill, 89
Bactrim, 146
Bactrim DS, 146
Bactrim I.V. Infusion, 146
Bactroban, 1123
BAL in Oil, 1208
Balminil D.M., 622
Balminil Expectorant, 623
Banesin, 331
Banophen, 591
Banophen Caplets, 591
Barbidonna Elixir, 533
Barbidonna No. 2 Tablets, 533
Barbidonna Tablets, 533
Barbita, 414
Barbloc, 301
Barc, 1136
Baridium, 1199
Basal cell carcinoma, fluo-
    rouracil for, 907-909
Basaljel, 642
Bayer Aspirin, 333
Bayer Select Pain Relief, 348
Baytussin, 623
Baytussin DM, 622

BCG, 941-943
BCG vaccine, 978-979
BCNU, 886-887
Bebulin VH Immuno, 871
Beclodisk, 626
Becloforte Inhaler, 626
beclomethasone dipropionate,
    626-627, 1100-1101
Beclovent, 626
Beclovent Rotacaps, 626
Beconase AQ Nasal Spray,
    1100
Beconase Nasal Inhaler, 1100
Bedoz, 1158
Beepen-VK, 97
Beesix, 1164
Beldin, 591
Belix, 591
Bell/ans, 848
Bellaspaz, 536
Bellergal-S, 552
Bel-phen-ergot-S, 552
Bemote, 533
Bena-D 10, 591
Bena-D 50, 591
Benadryl, 591
Benadryl 25, 591
Benadryl 50, 591
Benadryl Kapseals, 591
Benahist 10, 591
Benahist 50, 591
Ben-Allergin-50, 591
benazepril hydrochloride,
    268-269
Benemid, 1185
Benign prostatic hyperplasia
    doxazosin for, 276-277
    finasteride for, 1240-1241
Benn, 1185
Benoject-10, 591
Benoject-50, 591
Bensylate, 503
Bentyl, 533
Bentylol, 533
Benuryl, 1185
Benylin Cough, 591
Benylin DM, 622
Benylin Expectorant Cough
    Formula, 622
Benzacot, 688
Benzamycin Gel, 1111
benzonatate, 621
benzphetamine hydrochloride,
    489-490
benztropine mesylate,
    503-504
benzyl benzoate lotion,
    1132-1133
benzylpenicillin benzathine,
    91-92
benzylpenicillin potassium,
    92-94
benzylpenicillin procaine,
    94-95
benzylpenicillin sodium,
    95-97

Bepadin, 248
bepridil hydrochloride, 248
beractant, 627-629
Beriberi, thiamine for,
    1166-1167
Betachron E-R, 258
Betagan, 1090
Betaloc, 293
Betaloc Durules, 293
betamethasone, 699-701
betamethasone acetate and
    betamethasone sodium
    phosphate, 699-701
betamethasone dipropionate,
    1138-1139
betamethasone sodium phos-
    phate, 699-701
betamethasone valerate,
    1138-1139
Betamin, 1166
Betapace, 242
Betapen-VK, 97
Betaseron, 1034
Beta-Sol, 1166
Betatrex, 1138
Beta-Val, 1138
betaxolol hydrochloride,
    269-270, 1082-1083
bethanechol chloride,
    525-526
Betnelan, 699
Betnesol, 699
Betnovate, 1138
Betoptic, 1082
Bex, 333
Biamine, 1166
Biavax II, 1001
Biaxin, 192, **C2**
bicalutamide, 927-928
Bicillin L-A, 91
BiCNU, 886
Bile obstruction, cholestyra-
    mine for, 313-314
Biliary colic, papaverine hy-
    drochloride for, 326-327
BioCal, 832
Bio-cef, 130
BioCox, 1280t
Bio-Gan, 688
Bioglan B₁₂ Plus, 1158
Bioglan Panazyme, 651
Biological response modifiers,
    1022-1038
biperiden hydrochloride,
    504-505
biperiden lactate, 504-505
Biquin Durules, 240
Bisac-Evac, 662
bisacodyl, 662-663
Bisacolax, 662
Bisalax, 662
Bisco-Lax, 662
Bismatrol, 657
Bismatrol Extra Strength, 657
bismuth subsalicylate, 657

bisoprolol fumarate, 270-271
bitolterol mesylate, 602-603
Black-Draught, 675
black widow spider antivenin, 1008
Bladder cancer
  bacillus Calmette-Guérin for, 941-943
  cisplatin for, 888-890
  doxorubicin for, 919-921
  thiotepa for, 899-900
Blastomycosis
  amphotericin B for, 34-36
  itraconazole for, 39-40
Bleeding, excessive, aminocaproic acid for, 1205-1206
Blenoxane, 915
bleomycin sulfate, 915-916
Bleph-10 Liquifilm Ophthalmic, 1049
Blephamide Liquifilm Suspension, 1078
Blephamide S.O.P. sterile Ophthalmic Ointment, 1039
Blepharitis
  gentamicin for, 1043-1044
  natamycin for, 1045-1046
Blepharospasm, botulinum toxin type A for, 083-1084
Blocadren, 308
Blood derivatives, 866-873
Bloodstream infections, cefoxitin sodium for, 118-119
Blue Gel, 1136
Bonamine, 681
Bone and joint infections
  cefazolin for, 107-108
  cefonicid for, 113-114
  cefotaxime for, 115-117
  cefotetan for, 117-118
  cefoxitin for, 118-119
  ceftizoxime for, 125-126
  ceftriaxone for, 126-128
  cefuroxime for, 128-130
  cephalexin for, 130-131
  cephapirin for, 131-133
  cephradine for, 133-134
  ciprofloxacin for, 153-154
  imipenem/cilastatin for, 204-205
  ticarcillin/clavulanate for, 103-104
Bone disease, calcifediol for, 802-803
Bone marrow transplantation
  immune globulin for, 1014-1015
  sargramostim for, 1037-1038
Bone pain, strontium 89 for, 1256-1257
Bonine, 681

boric acid, 1096-1097
Borofair Otic, 1096
Botox, 1083
botulinum toxin type A, 1083-1084
Bowel examination, preparation for
  bisacodyl for, 662-663
  cascara sagrada for, 664-665
  castor oil for, 665-666
  mineral oil for, 671-672
  senna for, 675-676
Bowel management, psyllium for, 674-675
Bowel sterilization, kanamycin for, 68-69
Brain tumor
  carmustine for, 886-887
  lomustine for, 894-895
BranchAmin, 1176
Breast cancer
  anastrozole for, 927
  cyclophosphamide for, 890-892
  diethylstilbestrol for, 732-734
  esterified estrogens for, 734-736
  docetaxel for, 944-946
  doxorubicin for, 919-921
  estradiol for, 736-738
  estrogens, conjugated, for, 738-741
  ethinyl estradiol for, 742-744
  fluorouracil for, 907-909
  fluoxymesterone for, 719-721
  goserelin for, 930-932
  megestrol for, 933-934
  methyltestosterone for, 721-722
  nandrolone for, 722-724
  pamidronate for, 1251-1252
  tamoxifen for, 935-936
  testolactone for, 936
  testosterone for, 726-728
  thiotepa for, 899-900
  vinblastine for, 963-965
Breast engorgement
  methyltestosterone for, 721-722
  testosterone for, 726-728
Breonesin, 623
Brethaire, 616
Brethine, 616
Bretylate, 225
bretylium tosylate, 225-227
Bretylol, 225
Brevibloc, 228
Brevicon, 744
Bricanyl, 616
bromocriptine mesylate, 505-506

Bromphen, 585
brompheniramine maleate, 585-586
Bronchial Capsules, 597
Bronchitis
  acetylcysteine for, 624-625
  cefixime for, 110-111
  cefpodoxime proxetil for, 120-121
  cefprozil for, 121-122
  ceftibuten for, 124-125
  clarithromycin for, 192-193
  co-trimoxazole for, 146-148
  dirithromycin for, 193-194
  levofloxacin for, 156-158
  lomefloxacin for, 158-159
  loracarbef for, 134-135
  sparfloxacin for, 163-165
Broncho-Grippol-DM, 622
Bronchodilators, 597-620
Bronchospasm
  albuterol for, 597-599
  aminophylline for, 599-602
  bitolterol for, 602-603
  cromolyn for, 631-632
  epinephrine for, 604-607
  ipratropium for, 607-608
  isoetharine for, 608-609
  isoproterenol for, 609-611
  metaproterenol for, 611-613
  oxtriphylline for, 613-614
  pirbuterol for, 614-615
  salmeterol for, 615-616
  terbutaline for, 616-618
  theophylline for, 618-620
Broniten Mist, 604
Bronkaid Mist, 604
Bronkaid Mistometer, 604
Bronkaid Mist Suspension, 604
Bronkodyl, 618
Bronkometer, 608
Bronkosol, 608
Brucellosis
  oxytetracycline for, 142-143
  tetracycline for, 143-145
Brufen, 348
budesonide, 1101
Buff-A-Comp No. 3, 366
Bufferin AF Nite Time, 330
BufOpto Atropine, 1071
Bulimia, fluoxetine for, 431-432
bumetanide, 811-812
Bumex, 811, **C2**
Buminate 5%, 866
Buminate 25%, 866
bupivacaine hydrochloride, 1262-1263t
Buprenex, 368
buprenorphine hydrochloride, 368-369
bupropion hydrochloride, 426-427
Burinex, 811

t refers to a table; **boldface** refers to full-color photographs

Burkitt's lymphoma, methotrexate for, 911-914
Burns
bacitracin for, 1113-1114
mafenide for, 1120-1121
nitrofurazone for, 1124-1125
silver sulfadiazine for, 1126-1127
vitamin C for, 1167-1169
Bursitis
indomethacin for, 349-352
naproxen for, 359-360
sulindac for, 363-364
Buscospan, 538
BuSpar, 450, **C3**
buspirone hydrochloride, 450-451
busulfan, 883-884
butabarbital sodium, 390-391
butabarbitone sodium, 390-391
Butace, 330
Butalan, 390
Butisol, 390
butoconazole nitrate, 1114-1115
butorphanol tartrate, 369-371
Byclomine, 533
Bydramine Cough, 591

C

Cafatin Suppositories, 552
Cafergot, 552
Cafergot Suppositories, 552
Cafetrate Suppositories, 552
Caffedrine Caplets, 490
caffeine, 490-491
Calan, 260, **C3**
Calan SR, 260
Calcarb 600, 832
Cal-Carb-HD, 832
Calci-Chew, 832
Calciday 667, 832
calcifediol, 802-803
Calciferol, 1169
Calciject, 832
Calcijex, 804
Calcilac, 645, 832
Calcilean, 860
Calcimar, 803
Calcimax, 645
Calci-Mix, 832
Calciparine, 860
calcipotriene, 1234
Calcite 500, 832
calcitonin (human), 803-804
calcitonin (salmon), 803-804
calcitriol, 804-805
Calcium 500, 832
Calcium 600, 832
calcium acetate, 832-835
calcium carbonate, 645-646, 832-835
calcium chloride, 832-835

calcium citrate, 832-835
Calcium Disodium Versenate, 1212
Calcium EDTA, 1212
calcium glubionate, 832-835
calcium glucepate, 832-835
calcium gluconate, 832-835
calcium lactate, 832-835
calcium phosphate, dibasic, 832-835
calcium phosphate, tribasic, 832-835
calcium polycarbophil, 663-664
Calcium-Sandoz, 832
Calcium supplementation, calcium carbonate for, 645-646
Calculi formation
allopurinol for, 1182-1183
tiopronin for, 1258-1259
CaldeCort, 1151
Calderol, 802
Calglycine, 645, 832
Cal-Guard Softgels, 832
Calmazine, 485
Calm X, 678
Calorics, 1176-1181
Caloric supplementation, dextrose for, 1178-1179
Cal-Plus, 832
Calsan, 832
Cal-Sup, 645
Caltrate 300, 832
Caltrate 600, 832
Caltrate Chewable, 832
Cama Arthritis Pain Reliever, 330
Camalox Tablets, 642
Cam-ap-es, 263
Camptosar, 948-950
Candidal infections
amphotericin B for, 34-36, 1112-1113
butoconazole for, 1114-1115
ciclopirox for, 1115
econazole for, 1117-1118
fluconazole for, 36-37
flucytosine for, 37-38
ketoconazole for, 40-42, 1119-1120
miconazole for, 42-43, 1122-1123
nystatin for, 43-44, 1125-1126
terconazole for, 1128-1129
tioconazole for, 1130
Canesten, 1116
Capastat Sulfate, 53
Capital with Codeine, 366
Capoten, 271, **C3**
Capozide 25/15, 263
Capozide 25/25, 263
Capozide 50/15, 264

Capozide 50/25, 264
capreomycin sulfate, 53-54
Caprin, 860
capsaicin, 1234-1235
captopril, 271-273
Capurate, 1182
Capzacin-P, 1234
Carafate, 697, **C3**
carbachol (intraocular), 1062-1063
carbachol (topical), 1062-1063
carbamazepine, 403-405
carbamide, 830-831
carbamide peroxide, 1097
carbenicillin indanyl sodium, 83-84
carbidopa-levodopa, 506-508
Carbolith, 516
carboplatin, 884-886
carboprost tromethamine, 1192-1193
Carbrital, 396
Cardene, 253
Cardene IV, 253
Cardene SR, 253
Cardiac arrest
calcium salts for, 832-835
epinephrine for, 604-607
sodium bicarbonate for, 848-849
tromethamine for, 850
Cardiac output, increasing
dobutamine for, 541-542
dopamine for, 542-544
Cardiac pump failure, nitroprusside for, 298-299
Cardiac surgery, dobutamine for, 541-542
Cardiac vagal reflexes, blockage of
atropine for, 224-225
glycopyrrolate for, 534-536
hyoscyamine for, 536-537
Cardiogenic shock, nitroprusside for, 298-299
Cardioquin, 240
Cardiovascular drugs, miscellaneous, 322-329
Cardioversion, diazepam for, 453-456
Cardizem, 249, **C3**
Cardizem CD, 249, **C3**
Cardizem SR, 249, **C3**
Cardophyllin, 599
Cardura, 276, **C3**
carisoprodol, 557-558
Carmol HC, 1151
carmustine, 886-887
Carnitine deficiency, levocarnitine for, 1244-1245
Carnitor, 1244
carteolol, 273-274
carteolol hydrochloride, 1084-1085

t refers to a table; **boldface** refers to full-color photographs

Carter's Little Pills, 662
Cartrol, 273
cascara sagrada, 664-665
cascara sagrada aromatic
    fluidextract, 664-665
cascara sagrada fluidextract,
    664-665
Casodex, 927-928
castor oil, 665-666
Castor Oil Capsules, 665
Castration
    esterified estrogens for,
        734-736
    estradiol for, 736-738
    estrogens, conjugated, for,
        738-741
    estropipate for, 741-742
Cataflam, 342
Catapres, 274
Catapres-TTS, 274
Cataract removal, diclofenac
    sodium 0.1% for,
    1055-1056
Caverject, 1230
CCNU, 894-895
CdA, 902-903
CDDP, 888-890
Cebid Timecelles, 1167
Ceclor, 105, **C3**
Cecon, 1167
Cedax, 124
Cedocard-SR, 250
CeeNU, 894
Cee-1000 T.D., 1167
cefaclor, 105-106
cefadroxil monohydrate,
    106-107
Cefadyl, 131
Cefanex, 130
cefazolin sodium, 107-108
cefepime hydrochlodride,
    108-110
cefixime, 110-111
cefmetazole sodium, 111-113
cefmetazone, 111-113
Cefobid, 114
cefonicid sodium, 113-114
cefoperazone sodium,
    114-115
Cefotan, 117
cefotaxime sodium, 115-117
cefotetan disodium, 117-118
cefoxitin sodium, 118-119
cefpodoxime proxetil,
    120-121
cefprozil, 121-122
ceftazidime, 122-124
ceftibuten, 124-125
Ceftin, 128, **C4**
ceftizoxime sodium, 125-126
Ceftizox, 125
ceftriaxone sodium, 126-128
cefuroxime axetil, 128-130
cefuroxime sodium, 128-130
Cefzil, 121, **C4**

Celestone, 699
Celestone Chronodose, 699
Celestone Phosphate, 699
Celestone Soluspan, 699
CellCept, 974
Cenafed, 550
Cena-K, 842
Cenocort A-40, 716
Cenolate, 1167
cephalexin hydrochloride,
    130-131, **C4**
cephalexin monohydrate,
    130-131
Cephalosporins, 105-135
cephapirin sodium, 131-133
cephradine, 133-134
Cephulac, 668
Ceporex, 130
Ceptaz, 122
Cerebral edema, dexametha-
    sone for, 703-705
Cerebral palsy, dantrolene for,
    560-561
Cerebrovascular accident,
    ticlopidine for, 327-329
Cerebrovascular insufficiency,
    isoxsuprine for, 324
Cerebyx, 407
Ceredase, 1229
Cerespan, 326
Cerezyme, 1242
Cerubidin, 917
Cerubidine, 917
Cerumen impaction
    carbamide peroxide for,
        1097
    triethanolamine polypeptide
        oleate-condensate for,
        1098
Cerumenex, 1098
Cervical ripening, dinopros-
    tone for, 1193-1194
Cervicitis
    azithromycin for, 191-192
    fibrinolysin and desoxyri-
        bonuclease for,
        1190-1191
    ofloxacin for, 162-163
    spectinomycin hydrochlo-
        ride for, 211-212
C.E.S., 738
Cetacort, 1151
Cetamide Ophthalmic, 1049
Cetane, 1167
Cetapred Ointment, 1039
cetirizine hydrochloride,
    586-587
Cevalin, 1167
Cevi-Bid, 1167
Ce-Vi-Sol, 1167
Cevita, 1167
Chancroid, azithromycin for,
    191-192
Charcoaids, 1204
Charcocaps, 1204

Cheilosis, riboflavin for,
    1165-1166
Chemet, 1222
Chemotherapy acronyms and
    protocols, 1268-1278t
Cheracol D Cough, 622
Cherapas, 264
Chibroxin, 1046
Children, drug therapy in,
    13-17
Children's Advil, 348
Children's Congestion Relief,
    550
Children's Dramamine, 678
Children's Hold, 622
Children's Kaopectate, 656
Children's Motrin, 348
Children's Sudafed Liquid,
    550
Chlamydial infections
    erythromycin for, 195-197
    sulfacetamide for,
        1049-1050
    sulfamethoxazole for,
        149-150
    sulfisoxazole for, 150-152
Chlo-Amine, 587
Chlor-100, 587
chloral hydrate, 391-393
chlorambucil, 887-888
chloramphenicol, 200-202,
    1040-1041, 1097-1098
chloramphenicol palmitate,
    200-202
chloramphenicol sodium
    succinate, 200-202
Chlorate, 587
chlordiazepoxide, 451-452
chlordiazepoxide hydrochlo-
    ride, 451-452
Chloride replacement, ammo-
    nium chloride for,
    847-848
Chlor-Niramine, 587
2-chlorodeoxyadenosine,
    902-903
Chloromycetin, 200
Chloromycetin-Hydrocorti-
    sone Ophthalmic, 1039
Chloromycetin Kapseals, 200
Chloromycetin Ophthalmic,
    1040
Chloromycetin Otic, 1097
Chloromycetin Palmitate, 200
Chloromycetin Sodium
    Succinate, 200
chloroprocaine hydrochloride,
    1262-1263t
Chloroptic, 200, 1040
Chloroptic S.O.P., 1040
chloroquine hydrochloride,
    45-46
chloroquine phosphate, 45-46
chloroquine sulfate, 45-46
chlorothiazide, 812-814

chlorothiazide sodium, 813-814
chlorotrianisene, 729-731
Chlorphed, 585
Chlorphed-LA, 1106
chlorpheniramine maleate, 587-588
Chlor-Pro, 587
Chlor-Pro 10, 587
Chlorpromanyl-5, 462
Chlorpromanyl-20, 462
Chlorpromanyl-40, 462
chlorpromazine hydrochloride, 462-465
chlorpropamide, 764-765
Chlorquin, 45
Chlorsig, 1040
Chlorspan-12, 587
Chlortab-4, 587
Chlortab-8, 587
chlorthalidone, 814-816
Chlor-Trimeton, 587
Chlor-Trimeton Allergy Decongestant, 583
Chlor-Trimeton Decongestant Repetabs, 583
Chlor-Trimeton 12 Hour Allergy, 587
Chlor-Tripolon, 587
chlorzoxazone, 558-559
Chlotride, 812
Cholac, 668
cholecalciferol, 1169-1170
Choledyl, 613
Cholera, tetracycline for, 143-145
cholera vaccine, 979-980
cholestyramine, 313-314
choline magnesium trisalicylate, 335-337
Cholinergic adverse effects, glycopyrrolate for, 534-536
Cholinergic crisis
edrophonium for, 526-528
pralidoxime for, 1219-1220
Cholinergics, 524-532
choline salicylate, 337-338
choline salicylate and magnesium salicylate, 335-337
choline salt of theophyllinate, 613-614
Cholybar, 313
Chooz, 645, 832
Choriocarcinoma
methotrexate for, 911-914
vinblastine for, 963-965
Chroma-Pak, 1174
Chromic Chloride, 1174
chromic chloride, 1174-1175
chromium, 1174-1175
Chromium Chloride, 1174
Chronic obstructive pulmonary disease, azithromycin for, 191-192

Chronulac, 668
Chymodiactin, 1189
chymopapain, 1189-1190
Cibacalcin, 803
Cibalith-S, 516
ciclopirox olamine, 1115
cidofovir, 169-171
Cidomycin, 66
Cilamox, 77
Cilicane VK, 97
Cillium, 674
Ciloxan, 1041
cimetidine, 689-691, **C4**
Cinonide 40, 716
Cin-Quin, 240
Cipro, 153, **C4**
ciprofloxacin, 153-154
ciprofloxacin hydrochloride, 1041-1042
Cipro I.V., 153
Ciproxin, 153
cisapride, 1235-1236
cisatracurium besylate, 566-568
cisplatin, 888-890
cis-platinum, 888-890
citrate of magnesia, 669-670
Citrical, 832
Citrical Liquitabs, 832
Citrocarbonate, 848
Citroma, 669
Citro-Mag, 669
Citro-Nesia, 669
citrovorum factor, 1161-1162
Citrucel, 670
Citrucel Orange Flavor, 670
Citrucel Sugar-Free Orange Flavor, 670
cladribine, 902-903
Claforan, 115
Claratyne, 593
clarithromycin, 192-193
Claritin, 593, **C4**
Claritin-D, 583
Clavulin, 75
Clear Eyes, 1078
clemastine fumarate, 588-589
Cleocin HCl, 202
Cleocin Pediatric, 202
Cleocin Phosphate, 202
Cleocin T, 202
Cleocin T Gel, Lotion, Solution, 1115
Cleocin Vaginal Cream, 1115
C-Lexin, 130
Climara, 736
Climara Patch, 736
clindamycin hydrochloride, 202-203
clindamycin palmitate hydrochloride, 202-203
clindamycin phosphate, 202-203, 1115-1116
Clinoril, 363

clobetasol propionate, 1139-1140
clocortolone pivalate, 1140-1141
Cloderm, 1140
clofazimine, 54-55
Clofen, 556
Clomid, 1236
clomiphene citrate, 1236-1237
clomipramine hydrochloride, 427-428
clonazepam, 405-406
clonidine, 274-275
clonidine hydrochloride, 274-275
Clopra, 682
clorazepate dipotassium, 452-453
clotrimazole, 1116-1117
cloxacillin sodium, 84-85
Cloxapen, 84
clozapine, 465-467
Clozaril, 465
CMV-IGIV, 1012-1013
CNS depression, drug-induced, doxapram for, 495-497
CNS drugs, miscellaneous, 514-523
CNS infections
cefotaxime for, 115-117
ceftazidime for, 122-124
CNS stimulants, 488-502
CNS stimulation, caffeine for, 490-491
CNS toxicity, physostigmine for, 529-530
coccidioidin, 1280-1281t
codeine phosphate, 371-372
codeine sulfate, 371-372
Codimal-A, 585
Codistan No. 1, 622
Codroxomin, 1159
Cogentin, 503
Cognex, 522
Colace, 666
Co-Lav, 673
Colbenemid, 1182
colchicine, 1183-1185
Colchicine MR, 1183
Coldrine, 330
Colestid, 314
colestipol hydrochloride, 314-316
colfosceril palmitate, 629-631
Colgout, 1183
Cologel, 670
Colorectal cancer
fluorouracil for, 907-909
irinotecan for, 948-950
leucovorin for, 1161-1162
levamisole for, 1036-1037
Colovage, 673
Coloxyl, 666

Coloxyl Enema Concentrate, 666
Colsalide, 1183
CoLyte, 673
Combantrin, 31
Combipres 0.1, 264
Combipres 0.2, 264
Compa-Z, 685
Compazine, 685, **C4**
Compazine Spansule, 685, **C4**
Compazine Syrup, 685
Compoz, 591
Comvax, 978
Condrin-LA, 583
Condylomata acuminata
    interferon alfa-2b, recombinant, for, 1029-1031
    interferon alfa-n3 for, 1031-1032
Congespirin, 597
Congestac N.D. Caplets, 550
Congestion Relief, 550
Congestive heart failure
    amrinone lactate for, 216-217
    captopril for, 271-273
    digoxin for, 217-219
    fosinopril sodium for, 280-281
    lisinopril for, 289-290
    milrinone lactate for, 219-220
    nitroglycerin for, 255-258
    quinapril hydrochloride for, 303-304
    ramipril for, 304-306
Conjec-B, 585
Conjunctivitis
    bacitracin for, 1040
    chloramphenicol for, 1040-1041
    ciprofloxacin for, 1041-1042
    cromolyn for, 631-632
    dexamethasone for, 1054-1055
    erythromycin for, 195-197, 1042-1043
    gentamicin for, 1043-1044
    ketorolac for, 1057-1058
    levocabastine for, 1091
    lodoxamide for, 1091-1092
    medrysone for, 1058-1059
    natamycin for, 1045-1046
    norfloxacin for, 1046-1047
    ofloxacin 0.3% for, 1047
    polymyxin B sulfate for, 1048
    sulfacetamide for, 1049-1050
    sulfisoxazole for, 1050-1051
Constant-T, 618
Constilac, 668

Constipation
    bisacodyl for, 662-663
    calcium polycarbophil for, 663-664
    cascara sagrada for, 664-665
    glycerin for, 667-668
    lactulose for, 668-669
    magnesium citrate for, 669-670
    magnesium hydroxide for, 669-670
    magnesium sulfate for, 669-670
    methylcellulose for, 670-671
    mineral oil for, 671-672
    phenolphthalein for, 672-673
    psyllium for, 674-675
    senna for, 675-676
    sodium phosphates for, 677
Constulose, 668
Contac capsules, 583
Contac 12-hour caplets, 583
Contact dermatitis, dexchlorpheniramine for, 590-591
Contact lens, fitting, fluorescein for, 1087-1088
Contraception
    ethinyl estradiol combinations for, 744-748
    levonorgestrel for, 749-751
    medroxyprogesterone for, 751-752
    norethindrone for, 752-753
    norgestrel for, 753-754
Cope, 330
Cophene-B, 585
copper, 1174-1175
Coptin, 148
Coradur, 250
Coral snake bite, *Micrurus fulvius* antivenin for, 1010-1011
Cordarone, 222
Cordarone X, 222
Cordilox, 260
Cordilox SR, 260
Cordran, 1147
Cordran SP, 1147
Cordran Tape, 1147
Corgard, 252
Coricidin "D" Tablets, 583
Coricidin Nasal Mist, 1106
Corneal edema, sodium chloride, hypertonic, for, 1093-1094
Corneal infections
    bacitracin for, 1040
    chloramphenicol for, 1040-1041
    polymyxin B sulfate for, 1048

Corneal injury
    dexamethasone for, 1054-1055
    fluorescein for, 1087-1088
Corneal ulcers
    ciprofloxacin for, 1041-1042
    gentamicin for, 1043-1044
    sulfacetamide for, 1049-1050
    sulfisoxazole for, 1050-1051
Coronary artery bypass grafting, aprotinin for, 1232-1233
Coronary insufficiency, dipyridamole for, 323-324
Coronex, 250
Coro-Nitra, 255
Corophyllin, 599
Cort-Dome, 1151
CortaGel, 1152
Cortaid, 1152
Cortalone, 711
Cortamed, 1152
Cortate, 701
Cortef, 706, 1151, 1152
Cortenema, 706, 1151
Corticaine, 1152
Corticosteroids, 699-717
Corticosteroids, topical, 1137-1155
corticotropin, 794-796
Corticreme, 1152
Cortifoam, 706, 1152
Cortinal, 1151
cortisone acetate, 701-703
Cortisporin Ophthalmic Ointment, 1039
Cortisporin Ophthalmic Suspension, 1039
Cortizone 5, 1151
Cortone Acetate, 701
Cortril, 1151
Cortrosyn, 796
Corvert, 231
Coryphen, 333
Corzide, 264
Cosmegen, 916
cosyntropin, 796
Cotazym Capsules, 652
Cotazym-S Capsules, 652
Cotranzine, 685
Cotrim, 146, **C4**
Cotrim D.S., 146
co-trimoxazole, 146-148
Cough
    benzonatate for, 621
    codeine for, 371-372
    dextromethorphan for, 622-623
    diphenhydramine for, 591-593
    hydromorphone hydrochloride for, 375-376

Coumadin, 863, **C4**
Cozaar, 290
Cremacoat 2, 623
Cremesone, 1151
Creon, 651
Creon 10 Capsules, 652
Creon 20 Capsules, 652
Cretinism, levothyroxine for, 781-782
Critifib, 225
Crixivan, 176
Crohn's disease, sulfasalazine for, 1257-1258
Crolom, 631
cromolyn sodium, 631-632
Crotalidae antivenin, polyvalent, 1008-1009
crotamiton, 1133
Cryptorchidism, methyltestosterone for, 721-722
crystalline zinc insulin, 771-774
Crystamine, 1158
Crystapen, 95
Crysti-12, 1158
Crysticillin 300 A.S., 94
C-Span, 1167
cupric chloride, 1174-1175
cupric sulfate, 1174-1175
Cupric Sulfate, 1174
Cuprimine, 1211
Curretab, 751
Cushing's syndrome
aminoglutethimide for, 1231-1232
trilostane for, 1260
Cutivate, 1149
C2 with Codeine, 366
Cyanabin, 1159
cyanocobalamin, 1158-1160
Cyanocobalamin, 1159
Cyanoject, 1159
Cyclidox, 137
cyclobenzaprine hydrochloride, 559-560, **C4**
Cyclocort, 1137
Cyclogyl, 1072
Cyclomen, 718
Cyclomydril Ophthalmic, 1071
cyclopentolate hydrochloride, 1072-1073
cyclophosphamide, 890-892
Cycloplegic refraction
atropine for, 1071-1072
cyclopentolate for, 1072-1073
homatropine for, 1074-1075
scopolamine for, 1076-1077
tropicamide for, 1077
cycloserine, 55-56
cyclosporin, 970-972
cyclosporine, 970-072
Cycoblastin, 890
Cycrin, 751
Cylert, 500

Cylert Chewable, 500
Cynadide poisoning, amyl nitrite for, 247
Cyomin, 1159
cyproheptadine hydrochloride, 589-590
Cyronine, 782
Cystagon, 1237
cysteamine bitartrate, 1237-1238
Cystex, 198
Cystic fibrosis
acetylcysteine for, 624-625
dornase alfa for, 633-634
pancreatin for, 651-652
pancrelipase for, 652-654
Cystinosis, cysteamine for, 1237-1238
Cystinuria, d-penicillamine for, 1211-1212
Cystitis
fosfomycin for, 203-204
lomefloxacin for, 158-159
loracarbef for, 134-135
mesna for, 1247-1248
norfloxacin for, 160-162
ofloxacin for, 162-163
Cystospaz, 536
Cystospaz-M, 536
Cytadren, 1231
cytarabine, 903-905
CytoGam, 1012
Cytomegalovirus disease prevention, ganciclovir for, 175-176
cytomegalovirus immune globulin (human), intravenous, 1012-1013
Cytomegalovirus retinitis
cidofovir for, 169-171
foscarnet for, 173-175
ganciclovir for, 175-176
Cytomel, 782
Cytosar, 903
Cytosar-U, 903
cytosine arabinoside, 903-905
Cytotec, 693
Cytovene, 175
Cytoxan, 890
Cytoxan Lyophilized, 890

D
dacarbazine, 943-944
Dacodyl, 662
Dacryocystitis, gentamicin for, 1043-1044
dactinomycin, 916-917
Dalacin C, 202
Dalacin C, 202
Dalacin C Palmitate, 202
Dalacin C Phosphate, 202
Dalalone, 703
Dalalone D.P., 703
Dalalone L.A., 703
Dalmane, 395

dalteparin sodium, 857-858
D-Amp, 78
danaparoid sodium, 858-859
danazol, 718-719
Danocrine, 718
Dantrium, 560
Dantrium Intravenous, 560
dantrolene sodium, 560-561
Dapa, 331
Dapa X-S, 331
dapsone, 56-57
Dapsone 100, 56
Daraprim, 50
Darvocet-N 50, 366
Darvocet-N 100, 366, **C4**
Darvon, 386
Darvon Compound, 366
Darvon Compound-65, 366
Darvon Compound with A.S.A., 366
Darvon-N, 386
Darvon NC-Compound, 366
Datril Extra-Strength, 331
daunorubicin hydrochloride, 917-919
Daypro, 360, **C4**
Dazamide, 808
DC Softgels, 666
DC 240, 666
DDAVP, 797
ddC, 187-188
ddI, 171-172
Debridement, fibrinolysin and desoxyribonuclease for, 1190-1191
Debrox, 1097
Decaderm, 1143
Decadron, 703
Decadron-LA, 703
Decadron Phosphate, 703, 1143
Decadron Phosphate Ophthalmic, 1054
Decadron Phosphate Respihaler, 632-633
Decadron Phosphate with Xylocaine, 699
Deca-Durabolin, 722
Decaject, 703
Decaject-L.A., 703
Decaspray, 1143
Declomycin, 136
Decofed, 550
Decolone, 722
Deconamine, 583
Deep vein thrombosis
dalteparin for, 857-858
danaparoid for, 858-859
enoxaparin for, 859-860
heparin for, 860-863
De-Fed-60, 550
deferoxamine mesylate, 1206-1207
Deficol, 662
Degest 2, 1078

Dehist, 585
Delacort, 1151
Deladumone, 718
Delaxin, 561
Delestrogen, 736
Delirium, scopolamine for,
   538-540
Del-Mycin, 1118
Delta-Cortef, 711
Delta D, 804, 1169
delta-g-tetrahydrocannabinol,
   680-681
Deltalin Gelseals, 1169
Delta-Lutin, 748
Deltasolone, 711
Deltasone, 714, **C5**
Del-Vi-A, 1157
Demadex, 827
demecarium bromide,
   1064-1065
demeclocycline hydrochloride,
   136-137
Demerol, 376
Demi-Regroton, 264
Demulen 1/35, 744
Demulen 1/50, 744
Dental caries prevention,
   sodium fluoride for,
   1173-1174
2'-deoxycoformycin, 923-925
Depakene, 420
Depakene Syrup, 420
Depakote, 420, **C5**
Depakote Sprinkle, 420, **C5**
depAndro 100, 726
depAndro 200, 726
Depandrogen, 718
Depen, 1211
depGynogen, 736
depMedalone-40, 709
depMedalone-80, 709
Depo-Estradiol, 736
Depoject-40, 709
Depoject-80, 709
Depo-Medrol, 709
Deponit, 255
Depopred-40, 709
Depopred-80, 709
Depo-Predate 40, 709
Depo-Predate 80, 709
Depo-Provera, 751
Depotest, 726
Depo-testadiol, 718
Depotestogen, 718
Depo-Testosterone, 726
Depression
   amitriptyline for, 423-424
   amoxapine for, 424-426
   bupropion for, 426-427
   desipramine for, 428-430
   doxepin for, 430-431
   fluoxetine for, 431-432
   imipramine for, 432-434
   maprotiline for, 434-435
   mirtazapine for, 435-436

Depression *(continued)*
   nefazodone for, 436-438
   nortriptyline for, 438-439
   paroxetine for, 439-440
   phenelzine for, 440-441
   protriptyline for, 441-443
   sertraline for, 443-444
   thioridazine for, 482-484
   tranylcypromine for,
      444-445
   trazodone for, 445-446
   trimipramine for, 446-447
   venlafaxine for, 447-448
Deptran, 430
Deralin, 258
DermaCort, 1151
Dermacort, 1152
Dermacort Ointment, 1152
Dermatitis herpetiformis,
   dapsone for, 56-57
Dermolate, 1152
Dermovate, 1139
Dermtex HC, 1152
Deronil, 703
DES, 732
Deseril, 554
Desferal, 1206
desipramine hydrochloride,
   428-430
desmopressin acetate,
   797-798
Desogen, 744
desonide, 1141-1142
DesOwen, 1141
desoximetasone, 1142-1143
Desoxyn, 498
Desoxyn Gradumet, 498
Desyrel, 445
Detensol, 258
Detoxification, naltrexone for,
   1217-1218
Dexacen-4, 703
Dexacen LA-8, 703
Dexacort Phosphate
   Turbinaire, 1102
Dexameth, 703
dexamethasone, 703-705,
   1054-1055, 1143-1144
dexamethasone acetate,
   703-705
Dexamethasone Intensol, 703
dexamethasone sodium phosphate, 703-705,
   1054-1055, 1102-1103,
   1143-1144
dexamethasome sodium
   phosphate inhalation,
   632-633
Dexamethasone suppression
   test, 703-705
Dexasone, 703
Dexasone-LA, 703
Dexchlor, 590
dexchlorpheniramine maleate,
   590-591

Dexedrine, 493
Dexedrine Spansule, 493
dexfenfluramine hydrochloride, 491-493
Dexitac, 490
Dexone, 703
Dexone 0.5, 703
Dexone 0.75, 703
Dexone 1.5, 703
Dexone 4, 703
Dexone LA, 703
dextran 40, 835-836
Dextran 40, 835
dextran 70, 836-837
dextran 75, 836-837
Dextran 75, 836
dextran, high molecular
   weight, 836-837
dextran, low molecular
   weight, 835-836
dextroamphetamine sulfate,
   493-494
dextromethorphan hydrobromide, 622-623
dextropropoxyphene
   hydrochlride, 386-387
dextropropoxyphene
   napsylate, 386-387
dextrose, 1178-1179
Dey-Dose Isoetharine, 608
Dey-Dose Isoetharine S/F, 608
Dey-Dose Isoproterenol, 609
Dey-Dose Metaproterenol,
   611
Dey-Lute Isoetharine S/F, 608
Dey-Lute Metaproterenol, 611
d-glucose, 1178-1179
D.H.E. 45, 552
DHT Intensol, 805
DiaBeta, 769, **C5**
Diabetes insipidus
   desmopressin for, 797-798
   vasopressin for, 800-801
Diabetes mellitus
   acarbose for, 761-762
   acetohexamide for, 762-764
   chlorpropamide for,
      764-765
   glimepiride for, 765-767
   glipizide for, 767-768
   glyburide for, 769-771
   insulins for, 771-774
   metformin for, 774-776
   tolazamide for, 776-778
   tolbutamide for, 778-779
   troglitazone for, 779-780
Diabetic ketoacidosis, insulins
   for, 771-774
Diabetic nephropathy,
   captopril for, 271-273
Diabinese, 764
Diagnostic skin tests,
   1280-1281t
Dialose, 666
Dialose Plus, 662

t refers to a table; **boldface** refers to full-color photographs

Dialume, 644
Diamine T.D., 585
Diamox, 808
Diamox Parenteral, 808
Diamox Sequels, 808
Diamox Sodium, 808
Diaqua, 819
Diarrhea
    attapulgite for, 656-657
    bismuth subsalicylate for,
        657
    calcium polycarbophil for,
        663-664
    ciprofloxacin for, 153-154
    co-trimoxazole for, 146-148
    kaolin and pectin mixtures
        for, 657-658
    loperamide for, 658-659
    neomycin for, 69-70
    octreotide for, 659-660
    opium tincture for, 660-661
Diasorb, 656
Diazemuls, 453
diazepam, 453-456
Diazepam Intensol, 453
Di-Azo, 1199
diazoxide, 275-276
Dibent, 533
Dicarbosil, 645, 832
Dichlotride, 819
diclofenac potassium,
    342-344
diclofenac sodium, 342-344
diclofenac sodium 0.1%,
    1055-1056
dicloxacillin sodium, 85-86
dicyclomine hydrochloride,
    533-534, **C5**
didanosine, 171-172
2,3 didehydro-3-deoxythymi-
    dine, 185-186
dideoxycytidine, 187-188
Didrex, 489
Didronel, 806
dienestrol, 731-732
dienoestrol, 731-732
diethylpropion hydrochloride,
    494-495
diethylstilbestrol, 732-734
diethylstilbestrol diphosphate,
    732-734
diflorasone diacetate,
    1144-1145
Diflucan, 36, **C5**
diflunisal, 338-339
Di-Gel Liquid, 642
Digestive enzymes, 650-655
Digibind, 1207
Digitoxin intoxication, digoxin
    immune FAB (ovine) for,
    1207-1208
digoxin, 217-219
Digoxin, 217
digoxin immune FAB (ovine),
    1207-1208

Digoxin intoxication, digoxin
    immune FAB (ovine) for,
    1207-1208
Dihydergot, 552
dihydroergotamine mesylate,
    552-553
Dihydroergotamine-Sandoz,
    552
dihydromorphinone hy-
    drochloride, 375-376
dihydrotachysterol, 805-806
dihydroxyaluminum sodium
    carbonate, 646-647
1,25-dihydroxycholecalciferol,
    804-805
diiodohydroxyquin, 25-26
Dilacor XR, 249, **C5**
Dilantin, 417, **C5**
Dilantin-125, 417
Dilantin Infatabs, 417
Dilantin Kapseals, 417, **C5**
Dilantin-30 Pediatric, 417
Dilantin with Phenobarbital
    Kapseals, 403
Dilatrate-SR, 250
Dilaudid, 375
Dilaudid-HP, 375
Dilocaine, 1264t
Dilomine, 533
Dilor-G Tablets, 597
diltiazem hydrochloride,
    249-250
Dimelor, 762
dimenhydrinate, 678-679
dimercaprol, 1208-1209
Dimetabs, 678
Dimetane, 585
Dimetane Extentabs, 585
Dimetapp Extentabs, 583
Dimetapp Sinus, 342
Dinate, 678
dinoprostone, 1193-1194
Diochloram, 200
Diocto, 666
Dioctocal, 666
dioctyl calcium sulfosucci-
    nate, 666-667
dioctyl sodium sulfosuccinate,
    666-667
Diodoquin, 25
Dioeze, 666
Dionex, 666
Diosuccin, 666
Dio-Sul, 666
Dioval, 736
Diovan, 310
Dipentum, 1251
Diphenacen-50, 591
Diphenadryl, 591
Diphen Cough, 591
Diphenhist, 591
Diphenhist Captabs, 591
diphenhydramine hydrochlo-
    ride, 591-593

diphenidol hydrochloride,
    679-680
diphenylhydantoin, 417-419
diphtheria and tetanus tox-
    oids, adsorbed, 980-981
diphtheria and tetanus toxoids
    and acellular pertussis
    vaccine, 981-982
diphtheria and tetanus toxoids
    and whole-cell pertussis
    vaccine, 981-982
diphtheria antitoxin, equine,
    1009-1010
dipivefrin, 1085-1086
Dipridacot, 323
Diprolene, 1138
Diprolene AF, 1138
Diprosone, 1138
dipyridamole, 323-324
Diquinol, 25
dirithromycin, 193-194
Disalcid, 340
disalicylic acid, 340-341
Disodium EDTA, 1213
Disonate, 666
disopyramide, 227-228
disopyramide phosphate,
    227-228
Di-Sosul, 666
Disotate, 1213
Di-Spaz, 533
Dispos-a-Med Isoetharine,
    608
Dispos-a-Med Isoproterenol,
    609
Disseminated intravascular
    coagulation, heparin for,
    860-863
Distribution of drug, 6-7
    in children, 13
disulfiram, 1209-1211
Ditropan, 1198
Diuchlor H, 819
Diulo, 824
Diupres-250, 264
Diupres-500, 264
Diurese-R, 264
Diuresis
    chlorothiazide for, 812-814
    mannitol for, 822-824
    torsemide for, 827-829
Diuret, 812
Diuretics, 808-831
Diurigen, 812
Diurigen with reserpine, 264
Diuril, 812
Diutensen-R, 264
divalproex sodium, 420-422
Dixarit, 274
Dizmiss, 681
Dizymes Tablets, 651
DM Syrup, 622
Doan's Extra-Strength, 339
Doan's P.M., 339

Doan's P.M. Extra Strength, 330
dobutamine hydrochloride, 541-542
Dobutrex, 541
docetaxel, 944-946
docusate calcium, 666-667
docusate sodium, 666-667
Doktors, 1107
Dolanex, 331
Dolene, 386
Dolene-AP-65, 366-367
Dolobid, 338
Dolophine, 378
Doloxene, 386
Doloxene Co, 386
Dolsed, 198
Domeboro Otic, 1096
Dommanate, 678
donepezil hydrochloride, 514-515
Donnagel, 656
Donnatal Elixir, 533
Donnatal Extentabs, 533
Donnatal No. 2 Tablets, 533
Donnatal Tablets and Capsules, 533
Donnazyme Tablets, 650
Dopamet, 291
dopamine hydrochloride, 542-544
Dopar, 508
Dopram, 495
Doral, 398
Dorcol Children's Decongestant Liquid, 550
Dorcol Children's Fever and Pain Reducer, 331
Dormarex 2, 591
Dormel, 391
dornase alfa, 633-634
Doryx, 137
dorzolamide hydrochloride, 1086-1087
DOS, 666
Doss, 666
Dovonex, 1234
doxacurium chloride, 568-570
Doxapap-N, 366
doxapram hydrochloride, 495-497
doxazosin mesylate, 276-277
doxepin hydrochloride, 430-431, **C5**
Doxidan, 662
Doxinate, 666
doxorubicin hydrochloride, 919-921
Doxy-Caps, 137
Doxy 100, 137
Doxy 200, 137
Doxycin, 137
doxycycline calcium, 137-140
doxycycline hyclate, 137-140

doxycycline hydrochloride, 137-140
doxycycline monohydrate, 137-140
Doxylin, 137
D-Penamine, 1211
d-penicillamine, 1211-1212
DPT, 981-982
Dramamine, 678
Dramamine Chewable, 678
Dramamine Liquid, 678
Dramanate, 678
Dramilin, 678
Dramocen, 678
Dramoject, 678
Drenison, 1147
Drenison 1/4, 1147
Drenison Tape, 1147
D-Rex-65, 366-367
Dri/Ear, 1096
Drisdol, 1169
Dristan, 597
Dristan Long Lasting, 1106
Dristan Sinus Caplets, 342
Drixine Nasal, 1106
Drixoral, 550
Drixoral Non-Drowsy Formula, 550
Drize, 583
Dromitexan, 1247
dronabinol, 680-681
Dr. Scholl's Athlete's Foot Powder, 1130
Dr. Scholl's Athlete's Foot Spray, 1130
Drug action, 6
 factors that affect, 6-7, 18
Drug administration, considerations for, 7-8
Drug interactions, 8-9
Drug therapy
 in children, 13-17
 in elderly patients, 18-20
 nursing process and, 21-24
Drug use guidelines, 11-12
D-S-S, 666
D-S-S plus, 662
d4T, 185-186
DTaP, 981
DTIC, 943-944
DTIC-Dome, 943
DTP, 981-982
DTwP, 981
Ducene, 453
Dulcagen, 662
Dulcolax, 662
Dull-C, 1167
Duo-cyp, 718
Duodenal ulcer
 cimetidine for, 689-691
 famotidine for, 691-692
 lansoprazole for, 692-693
 nizatidine for, 694-695
 omeprazole for, 695-696
 ranitidine for, 696-697

Duodenal ulcer *(continued)*
 sucralfate for, 697-698
Duo-Medihaler, 597
Duosol, 666
Duphalac, 668
Durabolin, 723
Dura-Estrin, 736
Duragen-10, 736
Duragen-20, 736
Duragen-40, 736
Duragesic-25, 372
Duragesic-50, 372
Duragesic-75, 372
Duragesic-100, 372
Duralith, 516
Duralone-40, 709
Duralone-80, 709
Duralutin, 748
Duramist Plus, 1106
Duramorph, 379
Duramorph PF, 379
Duranest, 1262t
Duraphyl, 618
Duratest-100, 726
Duratest-200, 726
Duratestrin, 718
Duration, 1106, 1107
Durel-Cort, 1152
Duricef, 106, **C5**
Durolax, 662
Duromine, 501
Durrax, 456
Duvadilan, 324
Duvoid, 525
DV, 731
D-Vert 15, 681
D-Vert 30, 681
Dyazide, 808, **C5**
Dycill, 85
Dyclone, 1262t
Dyflex-G Tablets, 597
Dyline-GG Tablets, 597
Dymadon, 331
Dymadon P, 331
Dymelor, 762
Dymenate, 678
Dynabac, 193
Dynacin, 140
DynaCirc, 286, **C6**
Dynapen, 85
Dyrenium, 829
Dyslipidemia, atorvastatin for, 312-313
Dysmenorrhea
 diclofenac for, 342-344
 ibuprofen for, 348-349
 ketoprofen for, 352-353
 meclofenamate for, 355-356
 mefenamic acid for, 356-357
 naproxen for, 359-360
Dyspepsia, activated charcoal for, 1204-1205
Dystonic reaction, benztropine mesylate for, 503-504

t refers to a table; **boldface** refers to full-color photographs

Dysuria
  flavoxate for, 1198
  phenazopyridine for,
    1199-1200
Dytac, 829

E

Ear infection
  acetic acid for, 1096
  boric acid for, 1096-1097
  chloramphenicol for,
    1097-1098
Earwax. *See* Cerumen
    impaction.
Easprin, 333
echothiophate iodide,
    1065-1067
Eclampsia, magnesium salts
    for, 412-413, 838-840
EC-Naprosyn, 359
E-Complex-600, 1170
econazole nitrate, 1117-1118
Econopred Ophthalmic, 1059
Econopred Plus Ophthalmic,
    1059
Ecosone, 1152
Ecostatin, 1117
ecothiopate iodide,
    1065-1067
Ecotrin, 333
Ectasule, 603
E-Cypionate, 736
Edecril, 816
Edecrin, 816
Edema
  acetazolamide for, 808-810
  amiloride for, 810-811
  bumetanide for, 811-812
  chlorothiazide for, 812-814
  chlorthalidone for, 814-816
  ethacrynate for, 816-817
  furosemide for, 817-819
  hydrochlorothiazide for,
    819-821
  indapamide for, 821-822
  metolazone for, 824-826
  spironolactone for, 826-827
  triamterene for, 829-830
edetate calcium disodium,
    1212-1213
edetate disodium, 1213-1214
edrophonium chloride,
    526-528
EEG Dulcets, 195
EEG premedication, chloral
    hydrate for, 391-393
E.E.S., 195, **C6**
EES-400, 195
EES granules, 195
Efedron, 603
Effercal-600, 645
Effer-Syllium Instant Mix, 674
Effexor, 447, **C6**
Efficol Cough Whip, 622
Efidac/24, 550

Efudex, 907
E-200 I.U. Softgels, 1170
E-400 I.U. Softgels, 1170
E-L, 366-367
Elase, 1190
Elavil, 423
Eldepryl, 511
Elderly patients, drug therapy
    in, 18-20
Electrolytes, 832-844
Elimite, 1135
Elixicon, 618
Elixomin, 618
Elixophyllin, 618
Elixophylline KI Elixir, 597
Elixophyllin SR, 618
Elocon, 1153
Elspar, 939
Eltor 120, 550
Eltroxin, 781
Emcyt, 928
Emex, 682
Emgel, 1118
Eminase, 875
Emitrip, 423
Emotional emergencies, hy-
    droxyzine for, 456-457
Emphysema
  acetylcysteine for, 624-625
  alpha$_1$ proteinase inhibitor
    for, 625-626
Empirin, 333
Empirin with Codeine No. 2,
    367
Empirin with Codeine No. 3,
    367
Empirin with Codeine No. 4,
    367
Empracet-30, 366
Empracet-60, 367
Empyema, bacitracin for,
    199-200
Emtec-30, 366
Emulsoil, 665
EMU-V, 195
E-Mycin, 195, **C6**
enalaprilat, 277-279
enalapril maleate, 277-279
Encephalopathy, magnesium
    sulfate for, 412-413
Endep, 423
Endocan, 367
Endocarditis
  cefazolin for, 107-108
  cephapirin for, 131-133
  cephradine for, 133-134
  imipenem/cilastatin for,
    204-205
Endocarditis prophylaxis
  amoxicillin for, 77-78
  ampicillin for, 78-80
  clindamycin for, 202-203
  erythromycin for, 195-197
  gentamicin for, 66-68

Endocarditis prophylaxis
    (continued)
  penicillin G sodium for,
    95-97
  penicillin V for, 97-98
  streptomycin for, 72-73
  vancomycin for, 214-215
Endocervical infections
  doxycycline for, 137-140
  enoxacin for, 155-156
  erythromycin for, 195-197
  minocycline for, 140-141
  sulfisoxazole for, 150-152
  tetracycline for, 143-145
Endocet, 367
Endolor, 330
Endometrial cancer
  hydroxyprogesterone for,
    748-749
  medroxyprogesterone for,
    751-752
  megestrol for, 933-934
Endometriosis
  danazol for, 718-719
  ethinyl estradiol combina-
    tions for, 744-748
  goserelin for, 930-932
  leuprolide for, 932-933
  nafarelin for, 760
  norethindrone for, 752-753
Endometritis, piperacillin and
    tazobactam for, 100-101
Endone, 383
Endotracheal intubation
  atracurium for, 565-566
  cisatracurium for, 566-568
  metocurine for, 570-571
  mivacurium for, 571-573
  pancuronium for, 573-575
  rocuronium for, 576-578
  succinylcholine for,
    578-580
  tubocurarine for, 580-581
  vecuronium for, 581-582
Endoxan-Asta, 890
Endrate, 1213
Engerix-B, 985
Enlon, 526
Enovid 5 mg, 745
Enovid 10 mg, 745
Enovil, 423
enoxacin, 155-156
enoxaparin sodium, 859-860
Enterocolitis, vancomycin for,
    214-215
Entex, 541
Entex Liquid, 541
Entex PSE, 541
Entozyme, 651
Entozyme Tablets, 650
Entrophen, 333
Enulose, 668
Enuresis
  desmopressin for, 797-798
  imipramine for, 432-434

Enzymes, 1189-1191
ephedrine sulfate, 603-604, 1103
Ephedsol, 603
Epididymitis, ofloxacin for, 162-163
Epifoam, 1152
Epifrin, 1073
Epilepsy. *See* Seizure disorders.
Epilim, 420
E-pilo, 1062
E-Pilo, 1069
Epimorph, 379
Epinal, 1073
epinephrine, 604-607
epinephrine bitartrate, 604-607
epinephrine hydrochloride, 604-607, 1073-1074, 1103-1104
epinephryl borate, 1073-1074
Epi-Pen, 604
Epi-Pen Jr., 604
Epistaxis, epinephrine for, 1103-1104
Epitol, 403
Epival, 420
Epivir, 177
epoetin alfa, 1024-1026
Epogen, 1024
epoprostenol sodium, 634-636
Eppy/N, 1073
epsom salts, 669-670
eptastatin, 319-320
Equagesic, 449
Equalactin, 663
Equanil, 458
Equilet, 645
Eramycin, 195
Ercaf, 552
Erectile dysfunction, alprostadil for, 1230-1231
Ergamisol, 1036
ergocalciferol, 1169-1170
Ergodryl Mono, 553
Ergomar, 553
Ergostat, 553
ergotamine tartrate, 553-554
Eridium, 1199
Erybid, 195
ERYC, 195
Erycette, 1118
EryDerm, 1118
EryGel, 1118
EryPed, 195
EryPed 200, 195
EryPed 400, 195
Ery-Sol, 1118
Ery-Tab, **C6**
Erythema nodosum leprosum, clofazimine for, 54-55
Erythrasma, erythromycin for, 195-197
Erythrocin, 195

Erythrocin Stearate, 195, **C6**
Erythromid, 195
erythromycin, 1042-1043, 1118-1119
erythromycin base, 195-197
Erythromycin Base Filmtab, 195, **C6**
Erythromycin Delayed-Release, 195
erythromycin estolate, 195-197
erythromycin ethylsuccinate, 195-197
Erythromycin Lactobionate, 195
erythromycin lactobionate, 195-197
erythromycin stearate, 195-197
erythropoietin, 1024-1026
Eryzole, 146
eserine salicylate, 529-530
Eserine Sulfate, 1068
Esgic, 330
Esidrix, 819
Esimil, 264
Eskalith, 516
Eskalith CR, 516
esmolol hydrochloride, 228-230
Esophageal cancer, porfimer for, 956-958
Esophagitis
  lansoprazole for, 692-693
  omeprazole for, 695-696
  ranitidine for, 696-697
Espotabs, 672
estazolam, 393-394
esterified estrogens, 734-736
Estinyl, 742
Estivin II, 1078
Estrace, 736, **C6**
Estrace Vaginal Cream, 736
Estracyst, 928
Estraderm, 736
estradiol, 736-738
estradiol cypionate, 736-738
Estradiol L.A., 736
estradiol valerate, 736-738
Estra-L 20, 736
Estra-L 40, 736
estramustine phosphate sodium, 928-929
Estratab, 734
Estratest, 718
Estratest H.S., 718
Estraval, 736
Estraval P.A., 736
Estro-Cyp, 736
Estrofem, 736
estrogenic substances, conjugated, 738-741
Estrogens, 729-755
estrogens, conjugated, 738-741

Estroject-L.A., 736
estropipate, 741-742
ethacrynate sodium, 816-817
ethacrynic acid, 816-817
ethambutol hydrochloride, 57-58
ethchlorvynol, 394-395
ethinyl estradiol, 742-744
ethinyl estradiol and desogestrel, 744-748
ethinyl estradiol and ethynodiol diacetate, 744-748
ethinyl estradiol and levonorgestrel, 744-748
ethinyl estradiol and norethindrone, 744-748
ethinyl estradiol and norethindrone acetate, 745-748
ethinyl estradiol and norgestimate, 745-748
ethinyl estradiol and norgestrel, 745-748
ethinyl estradiol, norethindrone acetate, and ferrous fumarate, 745-748
ethinyloestradiol, 742-744
ethionamide, 58-59
Ethmozine, 235
ethosuximide, 406-407
Ethyol, 938
Etibi, 57
etidocaine hydrochloride, 1262-1265t
etidronate sodium, 806-807
etodolac, 344-345
Etopophos, 946
etoposide, 946-947
etoposide phosphate, 946-947
Etrafon, 423
Etrafon 2-10, 423, 462
Etrafon-A, 423, 462
Etrafon-Forte, 423, 462
etretinate, 1238-1240t
ETS, 1118
Euflex, 929
Euglucon, 769
Euhypnos 10, 400
Euhypnos 20, 400
Eulexin, 929
Eurax, 1133
Eustachian tube congestion, pseudoephedrine for, 550-551
Euthroid, 784
Evac-Q-Mag, 669
Evac-U-Gen, 672
Evac-U-Lax, 672
Evalose, 668
E-Vista, 456
E Vitamin Succinate, 1170
Ewing's sarcoma, dactinomycin for, 916-917
Excedrin Extra Strength, 330
Excedrin IB Caplets, 348

Excedrin IB Tablets, 348
Excedrin P.M., 330
Exchange transfusions, calcium salts for, 832-835
Excretion of drug, 7
    in children, 14
Excretory urography, hyaluronidase for, 1191
Exdol, 331
Exdol Strong, 331
Exelderm, 1127
Ex-Lax, 672
Ex-Lax Chocolated, 672
Ex-Lax Maximum Relief Formula, 672
Ex-Lax Pills, 672
Exna-R Tablets, 264
Exosurf Neonatal, 629
Expectorants, 621-623
Extra Action Cough, 622
Extracorporeal circulation, dextran, low molecular weight, for, 835-836
Extrapyramidal disorders, drug-induced
    benztropine for, 503-504
    biperiden for, 504-505
Extra Strength Gas-X, 649
Extravasation, phentolamine for, 300-301
Eye infections
    erythromycin for, 1042-1043
    gentamicin for, 1043-1044
    polymyxin B sulfate for, 1048
    sulfisoxazole for, 1050-1051
    tobramycin for, 1051-1052
Eye inflammation
    dexamethasone for, 1054-1055
    fluorometholone for, 1056-1057
    prednisolone for, 1059-1060
Eye irritation
    ketorolac for, 1057-1058
    naphazoline for, 1078-1079
    oxymetazoline for, 1079-1080
    tetrahydrozoline for, 1080
Eye surgery
    acetylcholine for, 1062
    carbachol for, 1062-1063
    rimexolone for inflammation after, 1060-1061
Ezide, 819

F

factor IX complex, 871-872
factor IX (human), 871-872
Fainting, ammonia, aromatic spirits, for, 1206
famciclovir, 172-173

famotidine, 691-692
Famvir, 172
Fansidar, 50
Fastin, 501
fat emulsions, 1179-1181
Fats, inadequate digestion of, medium-chain triglycerides for, 1181
Fatty acid deficiency, fat emulsions for, 1179-1181
5-FC, 37-38
Fedahist, 583
Feen-A-Mint, 672
Feen-A-Mint Chocolated, 672
Feen-A-Mint Gum, 672
Feiba VH Immuno, 869
Feldene, 362
felodipine, 279-280
Femcet, 330
Feminate, 736
Feminone, 742
Femiron, 851
Femogex, 736
Femstat, 1114
Fenac, 342
fenfluramine hydrochloride, 497-498
Fenicol, 1040
fenoprofen calcium, 345-346
fentanyl citrate, 372-375
Fentanyl Oralet, 372
fentanyl transdermal system, 372-375
fentanyl transmucosal, 372-375
Feosol, 853
Feostat, 851
Feostat Drops, 851
Fergon, 852
Fergon Plus, 851
Fer-In-Sol, 853
Fer-In-Sol Drops, 853
Fer-In-Sol Syrup, 853
Fer-Iron Drops, 853
Feritard, 853
Ferocyl, 851
Fero-Grad, 853
Fero-Gradumet, 853
Ferospace, 853
Ferralyn Lanacaps, 853
Ferra-TD, 853
Ferro-Docusate-T.R., 851
Ferro-Dok TR, 851
Ferro-Dss, 851
Ferro-Sequels, 851
ferrous fumarate, 851-852
ferrous gluconate, 852-853
ferrous sulfate, 853-854
ferrous sulfate, dried, 853-854
Fertinic, 852
Fever
    acetaminophen for, 330-333
    aspirin for, 333-335

Fever (continued)
    choline magnesium trisalicylate for, 335-337
    choline salicylate for, 337-338
    ketoprofen for, 352-353
    magnesium salicylate for, 339-340
Feverall, Children's, 331
Feverall Junior Strength, 331
Feverall Sprinkle Caps, Children's, 331
Feverall Sprinkle Caps, Junior Strength, 331
fexofenadine hydrochloride, 593
Fiberall, 663, 674
FiberCon, 663
FiberLax, 663
FiberNorm, 663
Fibrepur, 674
fibrinolysin and desoxyribonuclease, 1190-1191
Fibrocystic breast disease, danazol for, 718-719
filgrastim, 1026-1027
finasteride, 1240-1241
Fiorgen PF, 330
Fioricet, 330
Fioricet with Codeine, 367
Fiorinal, 330
Fiorinal with Codeine, 367, **C6**
Flagyl, 26
Flagyl I.V. RTU, 26
Flamazine, 1126
Flarex, 1056
Flatulence
    activated charcoal for, 1204-1205
    simethicone for, 649
Flatulex, 642
Flavettes, 1167
Flavorcee, 1167
flavoxate hydrochloride, 1198
flecainide acetate, 230-231
Fleet Babylax, 667
Fleet Bisacodyl, 662
Fleet Bisacodyl Prep, 662
Fleet Flavored Castor Oil, 665
Fleet Laxative, 662
Fleet Mineral Oil Enema, 671
Fleet Phospho-Soda, 677
Fletcher's Castoria, 675
Flexeril, 559
Flint SSD, 1126
Flolan, 634
Flonase, 1105
Florinef, 705
Florone, 1144
Floropryl, 1067
Floxin, 162, **C7**
Floxin I.V., 162
floxuridine, 905-906
fluconazole, 36-37
flucytosine, 37-38

Fludara, 906
fludarabine phosphate, 906-907
fludrocortisone acetate, 705-706
Fluid and electrolyte replacement
Ringer's injection, lactated, for, 845
Ringer's injection for, 844-845
sodium chloride for, 845-846
Fluid replacement, dextrose for, 1178-1179
Flumadine, 181
flumazenil, 1214-1215
flunisolide, 636-637, 1104-1105
Fluocet, 1145
fluocinolone acetonide, 1145-1146
fluocinonide, 1146-1147
Fluonid, 1145
Fluor-A-Day, 1173
fluorescein sodium, 1087-1088
Fluorescite, 1087
Fluorigard, 1173
Fluorinse, 1173
Fluor-I-Strip, 1087
Fluor-I-Strip A.T., 1087
Fluoritab, 1173
5-fluorocytosine, 37-38
Fluorodex, 1173
fluorometholone, 1056-1057
Fluoroplex, 907
Fluoroquinolones, 153-165
fluorouracil, 907-909
5-fluorouracil, 907-909
Fluotic, 1173
fluoxetine hydrochloride, 431-432
fluoxymesterone, 719-721
fluphenazine decanoate, 467-469
fluphenazine enanthate, 467-469
fluphenazine hydrochloride, 467-469
Flura, 1173
Flura-Drops, 1173
Flura-Loz, 1173
flurandrenolide, 1147-1149
flurazepam hydrochloride, 395-396
flurbiprofen, 346-348
flurbiprofen sodium, 1057
Fluress, 1081
Flurosyn, 1145
flutamide, 929-930
Flutex, 1154
fluticasone propionate, 1105-1106, 1149
Flutone, 1144

fluvastatin sodium, 316-317
Fluvirin, 987
fluvoxamine maleate, 515-516
Fluzone (Whole), 988
FML Forte, 1056
FML Liquifilm Ophthalmic, 1056
FML S.O.P., 1056
Folex, 911
Folex PFS, 911
folic acid, 1160-1161
folinic acid, 1161-1162
Folvite, 1160
Footwork, 1130
Formulex, 533
Fortaz, 122
Fortral, 385
Fosamax, 1228
foscarnet sodium, 172-175
Foscavir, 173
fosfomycin tromethamine, 203-204
fosinopril sodium, 280-281
fosphenytoin sodium, 407-409
4-Way Long Acting, 1110
4-Way Long-Acting Nasal, 1106
4-Way Nasal Spray, 1099
4X Pancreatin 600 mg, 651
Fowler's, 656
Fragmin, 857
FreAmine HBC, 1176
FreAmine III, 1176
FreAmine III with electrolytes, 1176
Froben, 346
Froben SR, 346
frusemide, 817-819
5-FU, 907-909
FUDR, 905
Fungizone, 1112
Fulcin, 38
Ful-Glo, 1087
Fulvicin P/G, 38
Fulvicin-U/F, 38
Fumasorb, 851
Fumerin, 851
Funduscein Injections, 1087
Fundus examination, tropicamide for, 1077
Fungal infections
amphotericin B for, 34-36
clotrimazole for, 1116-1117
flucytosine for, 37-38
itraconazole for, 39-40
ketoconazole for, 40-42
miconazole for, 42-43
tolnaftate for, 1130-1131
Fungatin, 1130
Fungilin Oral, 34
Fungizone Intravenous, 34
Furacin, 1124
Furadantin, 208
Furalan, 208

Furan, 208
Furanite, 208
furosemide, 817-819, C7
Furoside, 817
Fynex, 591

G
gabapentin, 410-411
Galactorrhea, bromocriptine for, 505-506
gallium nitrate, 1241-1242
Gallstones, dissolving
monoctanoin for, 650-651
ursodiol for, 654-655
Gallstone solubilizers, 650-655
Gamimune N, 1014
Gammagard S/D, 1014
gamma globulin, 1014-1015
Gammar, 1014
Gammar-P IV, 1014
Gamulin Rh, 1017
ganciclovir, 175-176
Ganite, 1241
Gantanol, 149
Gantrisin, 150
Gantrisin Ophthalmic Solution, 1050-1051
Garamycin, 66, 1119
Garamycin Ophthalmic, 1043
Gas expulsion, vasopressin for, 800-801
Gas-Relief, 649
Gastric bloating, simethicone for, 649
Gastric emptying, delayed, metoclopramide for, 682-683
Gastric ulcer
cimetidine for, 689-691
famotidine for, 691-692
misoprostol for, 693-694
nizatidine for, 694-695
omeprazole for, 695-696
ranitidine for, 696-697
Gastrocrom, 631
Gastroesophageal reflux disease
cimetidine for, 689-691
cisapride for, 1235-1236
famotidine for, 691-692
metoclopramide for, 682-683
nizatidine for, 694-695
omeprazole for, 695-696
ranitidine for, 696-697
Gastrosed, 536
Gas-X, 649
Gaucher's disease
alglucerase for, 1229-1230
imiglucerase for, 1242-1243
Gaviscon, 642
gBH, 1134
G-CSF, 1026-1027

2/G-DM Cough, 622
Gee-Gee, 623
Gel Kam, 1173
Gel-Tin, 1173
Gelusil, 642
Gelusil-II, 642
gemcitabine hydrochloride, 947-948
gemfibrozil, 317-318, **C7**
Gemzar, 947
Genabid, 326
Genagesic, 366-367
Genahist, 591
GenAllerate, 587
Genapap, Infants', 331
Genapap Children's Elixir, 331
Genapap Extra Strength Caplets, 331
Genapap Extra Strength Tablets, 331
Genapap Regular Strength Tablets, 331
Genaphed, 550
Genasal Spray, 1106
Genasoft, 666
Genaspor, 1130
Gencalc, 645
Gencalc 600, 832
Gendex 75, 836
Gen-D-phen, 591
Genebs Extra Strength Caplets, 331
Genebs Regular Strength Tablets, 331
Genebs X-Tra, 331
Generlac, 668
Genfiber, 674
Genital herpes
 acyclovir for, 166-168
 famciclovir for, 172-173
 valacyclovir for, 186-187
Genital ulcer disease, azithromycin for, 191-192
Genital warts. See Condylomata acuminata.
Genitourinary tract infections. See also Urinary tract infections.
 cefoxitin for, 118-119
 cephapirin for, 131-133
 cephradine for, 133-134
Genoptic, 1043
Genora 0.5/35, 744
Genora 1/35, 744
Genora 1/50, 745
Genpril Caplets, 348
Genpril Tablets, 348
Gentacidin, 1043
Gentak, 1043
gentamicin sulfate, 66-68, 1043-1044, 1119
Gentamicin Sulfate ADD-Vantage, 66
Gentran 40, 835
Gentran 70, 836

Gentran 75, 836
Gen-XENE, 452
Geocillin, 83
Geopen Oral, 83
Geridium, 1199
Gesterol 50, 754
Gesterol L.A. 250, 748
GG-CEN, 623
GI adenocarcinoma
 floxuridine for, 905-906
 mitomycin for, 922-923
Giardiasis, metronidazole for, 26-28
GI bleeding, cimetidine for, 689-691
GI colic, papaverine for, 326-327
GI disorders
 atropine for, 224-225
 dicyclomine for, 533-534
 glycopyrrolate for, 534-536
 hyoscyamine for, 536-537
GI examination, polyethylene glycol and electrolyte solution for, 673-674
GI tract infections
 amphotericin B for, 34-36
 cephalexin for, 130-131
 cephapirin for, 131-133
 cephradine for, 133-134
 nystatin for, 43-44
Glaucoma
 acetazolamide for, 808-810
 betaxolol for, 1082-1083
 carbachol for, 1062-1063
 carteolol for, 1084-1085
 demecarium for, 1064-1065
 dipivefrin for, 1085-1086
 dorzolamide for, 1086-1087
 echothiophate for, 1065-1067
 epinephrine for, 1073-1074
 isoflurophate for, 1067-1068
 isosorbide for, 1088-1089
 latanoprost for, 1089-1090
 levobunolol for, 1090-1091
 methazolamide for, 824
 metipranolol for, 1092-1093
 physostigmine for, 1068-1069
 pilocarpine for, 1069-1070
 timolol for, 1094-1095
 urea for, 830-831
Glaucon, 1073
glibenclamide, 769-771
glimepiride, 765-767
glipizide, 767-768, **C7**
glucagon, 768-769
Glucamide, 764
glucocerebrosidase, 1229-1230
glucocerebrosidase-beta-glucosidase, 1229-1230
Glucophage, 774

glucosylceramidase, 1229-1230
Glucotrol, 767, **C7**
Glucotrol XL, 767, **C7**
Glu-K, 843
Glyate, 623
glyburide, 769-771
glycerin, 667-668
glyceryl guaiacolate, 623
Glyceryl-T Capsules, 597
glyceryl trinitrate, 255-258
Glycoprep, 673
glycopyrrolate, 534-536
Glycotuss, 623
Glycotuss dM, 622
Glynase PresTab, 769, **C7**
Glytuss, 623
GM-CSF, 1037-1038
G-Myticin, 1119
Go-Evac, 673
Goiter, liothyronine for, 782-784
Gold-50, 1202
Gold poisoning, dimercaprol for, 1208-1209
Gold salts, 1201-1203
gold sodium thiomalate, 1202-1203
GoLYTELY, 673
gonadorelin acetate, 756-757
Gonadotropins, 756-760
Gonorrhea
 amoxicillin for, 77-78
 ampicillin for, 78-80
 bacampicillin for, 81-82
 cefixime for, 110-111
 cefotaxime for, 115-117
 cefpodoxime for, 120-121
 cefuroxime for, 128-130
 demeclocycline for, 136-137
 doxycycline for, 137-140
 minocycline for, 140-141
 norfloxacin for, 160-162
 ofloxacin for, 162-163
 oxytetracycline for, 142-143
 penicillin G procaine for, 94-95
 probenecid for, 1185-1187
 tetracycline for, 143-145
goserelin acetate, 930-932
Gout
 allopurinol for, 1182-1183
 colchicine for, 1183-1185
 naproxen for, 359-360
Gouty arthritis
 colchicine for, 1183-1185
 indomethacin for, 349-352
 probenecid for, 1185-1187
 sulfinpyrazone for, 1187-1188
 sulindac for, 363-364
granisetron hydrochloride, 681

granulocyte colony-stimulating factor, 1026-1027
granulocyte-macrophage colony-stimulating factor, 1037-1038
Granuloma inguinale
demeclocycline hydrochloride for, 136-137
doxycycline for, 137-140
minocycline hydrochloride for, 140-141
oxytetracycline hydrochloride for, 142-143
tetracycline hydrochloride for, 143-145
Granulomatous disease, interferon gamma-1b for, 1035
Gravol, 678
Gravol L/A, 678
Grifulvin V, 38
Grisactin, 38
Grisactin Ultra, 38
griseofulvin microsize, 38-39
griseofulvin ultramicrosize, 38-39
Griseostatin, 38
Grisovin, 38
Grisovin 500, 38
Grisovin-FP, 38
Gris-PEG, 38
Growth failure
somatrem for, 798-799
somatropin for, 799-800
GTN-Pohl, 255
guaifenesin, 623
guanabenz acetate, 281-282
guanadrel sulfate, 282-283
guanethidine monosulfate, 283-284
guanfacine hydrochloride, 284-285
Guiamid D.M. Liquid, 622
Guiatuss, 623
Guiatuss-DM, 622
G-Well, 1134
Gynecologic infections
aztreonam for, 198-199
cefoperazone for, 114-115
cefotaxime for, 115-117
cefotetan for, 117-118
ceftazidime for, 122-124
ceftizoxime for, 125-126
ceftriaxone for, 126-128
imipenem/cilastatin for, 204-205
Gynecort, 1152
Gyne-Lotrimin, 1116
Gynergen, 553
Gynogen L.A., 736

H

Habitrol, 519

Haemophilus b conjugate vaccine, diphtheria CRM$_{197}$ protein conjugate, 982-984
Haemophilus b conjugate vaccine, diphtheria toxoid conjugate, 982-984
Haemophilus b conjugate vaccine, meningococcal protein conjugate, 983-984
Haemophilus influenzae type b, rifampin for, 63-64
Halciderm, 1149
halcinonide, 1149-1150
Halcion, 401, **C7**
Haldol, 469
Haldol Decanoate, 469
Haldol LA, 469
Halenol Children's, 331
Haley's M-O, 662
Halfprin, 333
halobetasol propionate, 1151
Halodrin, 718
Halofed, 550
Halofed Adult Strength, 550
Halog, 1149
haloperidol, 469-471
haloperidol decanoate, 469-471
haloperidol lactate, 469-471
Halotestin, 719
Halotussin, 623
Halotussin-DM Expectorant, 622
Haltran, 348
Hansen's disease. *See* Leprosy.
Hartmann's solution, 845
Hartnup disease, niacin for, 1162-1164
Havrix, 984
H-BIG, 1013
HbOC, 982-984
HC Cream, 1152
HDCV, 1000-1001
Head and neck cancers, hydroxyurea for, 909-910
Head lice
benzyl benzoate lotion for, 1132-1133
permethrin for, 1135
pyrethrins for, 1136
Heart attack, reducing risk of, aspirin for, 333-335
Heartburn
cimetidine for, 689-691
famotidine for, 691-692
ranitidine for, 696-697
Heart transplantation, cyclosporine for, 970-972
Heat cramp, sodium chloride for, 845-846
Helicobacter pylori infection
clarithromycin for, 192-193
omeprazole for, 695-696

H. pylori infection *(continued)*
tetracycline for, 143-145
Hemabate, 1192
Hematinics, 851-856
Hematologic toxicity, leucovorin for, 1161-1162
Hemocyte, 851
Hemodialysis, gentamicin sulfate for, 66-68
Hemodynamic imbalances, dopamine hydrochloride for, 542-544
Hemofil M, 867
Hemophilia
antihemophilic factor for, 867-868
anti-inhibitor coagulant complex for, 869-870
desmopressin for, 797-798
factor IX for, 871-872
Hemorrhagic disease of newborn, phytonadione for, 1171-1173
Hemostasis, epinephrine for, 604-607
Hepalean, 860
heparin calcium, 860-863
heparin cofactor I, 870-871
Heparin Leo, 860
Heparin Lock Flush Solution (with Tubex), 860
Heparin overdose, protamine sulfate for, 1220-1221
heparin sodium, 860-863
HepatAmine, 1176
Hepatic coma
kanamycin for, 68-69
neomycin for, 69-70
Hepatic disease
bumetanide for, 811-812
lactulose for, 668-669
metronidazole for, 26-28
Hepatic encephalopathy, lactulose for, 668-669
Hepatitis A exposure, immune globulin for, 1014-1015
hepatitis A vaccine, inactivated, 984-985
Hepatitis B, interferon alfa-2b, recombinant, for, 1029-1031
Hepatitis B exposure, hepatitis B immune globulin, human, for, 1013-1014
hepatitis B immune globulin, human, 1013-1014
hepatitis B vaccine, recombinant, 985-987
Hepatitis non A, non B/C, interferon alfa-2b, recombinant, for, 1029-1031
Hep-B-Gammagee, 1013
Hep-Lock, 860
Heptalac, 668

Hereditary angioedema
    danazol for, 718-719
    stanozolol for, 724-726
Herniated disk, chymopapain
    for, 1189-1190
Herpes genitalis. *See* Genital
    herpes.
Herpes simplex virus infec-
    tions, acyclovir for,
    166-168, 1111-1112
Herpes zoster infection
    acyclovir for, 166-168
    famciclovir for, 172-173
    valacyclovir for, 186-187
Herplex, 1044
Hespan, 838
hetastarch, 838
Hexa-Betalin, 1164
Hexadrol, 703
Hexadrol Phosphate, 703
Hexalen, 937
hexamethylmelamine,
    937-938
H.H.R., 264
HibTITER, 982
Hiccups, intractable, chlorpro-
    mazine for, 462-465
HI-Cor-2.5, 1152
Hiprex, 207
Hip-Rex, 207
Hismanal, 584, **C7**
Histaject Modified, 585
Histantil, 594
Histerone-50, 726
Histerone-100, 726
Histiocytosis, vinblastine for,
    963-965
Histolyn-CYL, 1280t
histoplasmin, 1280-1281t
Histoplasmin Diluted, 1280t
Histoplasmosis
    amphotericin B for, 34-36
    itraconazole for, 39-40
histrelin acetate, 757-758
Hi-Vegi-Lip Tablets, 651
Hivid, 187
HIV infection
    didanosine for, 171-172
    ganciclovir for, 175-176
    immune globulin for,
        1014-1015
    indinavir for, 176-177
    lamivudine for, 177-179
    nevirapine for, 179-180
    ritonavir for, 182-184
    saquinavir for, 184-185
    stavudine for, 185-186
    zalcitabine for, 187-188
    zidovudine for, 188-190
HMM, 937-938
HMS Liquifilm Ophthalmic,
    1058
Hodgkin's disease
    bleomycin for, 915-916
    carmustine for, 886-887

Hodgkin's disease *(continued)*
    chlorambucil for, 887-888
    cyclophosphamide for,
        890-892
    dacarbazine for, 943-944
    doxorubicin for, 919-921
    lomustine for, 894-895
    mechlorethamine for,
        895-896
    procarbazine for, 958-959
    thiotepa for, 899-900
    uracil mustard for, 901
    vinblastine for, 963-965
    vincristine for, 965-966
Hold, 622
Homatrine, 1074
Homatropine, 1074
homatropine hydrobromide,
    1074-1075
Honvol, 732
Hookworm, mebendazole for,
    31
Hostacycline P, 143
H.P. Acthar Gel, 794
Human immunodeficiency
    virus infection. *See* HIV
    infection.
Humate-P, 867
Humatin, 28
Humatrope, 799
Humibid L.A., 623
Humorsol, 1064
Humulin 50/50, 761, 771
Humulin 70/30, 761, 771
Humulin L, 771
Humulin N, 771
Humulin NPH, 771
Humulin R, 771
Humulin U, 771
Hyaline membrane disease,
    beractant for, 627-629
hyaluronidase, 1191
Hyate:C, 867
Hybolin Decanoate, 722
Hybolin Improved, 723
Hycamtin, 960
Hycortole, 1152
Hydatidiform mole,
    methotrexate for, 911-914
Hydeltrasol, 711
Hydeltra-TBA, 712
Hydergine, 552
Hydopa, 291
hydralazine hydrochloride,
    285-286
Hydramine, 591
Hydramine Cough, 591
Hydramyn, 591
Hydrate, 678
Hydrea, 909
Hydril, 591
Hydrobexan, 1159
hydrochlorothiazide, 819-821
Hydrocil Instant, 674
Hydro-Cobex, 1159

hydrocodone bitartrate and
    acetaminophen, **C7**
Hydrocortex, 1152
hydrocortisone, 706-709,
    1151-1153
hydrocortisone acetate,
    706-709, 1152-1153
Hydrocortisone Acetate, 1152
hydrocortisone butyrate,
    1152-1153
hydrocortisone sodium
    phosphate, 706-709
hydrocortisone sodium
    succinate, 706-709
hydrocortisone valerate,
    1152-1153
Hydrocortone, 706
Hydrocortone Acetate, 706
Hydrocortone Phosphate, 706
Hydro-Crysti-12, 1159
Hydro-D, 819
HydroDIURIL, 819
hydromorphone hydrochlo-
    ride, 375-376
Hydromox-R, 264
Hydro-Par, 819
Hydropine, 264
Hydropine HP, 264
Hydropres-25, 264
Hydro-Reserp, 264
Hydro-serp, 264
Hydroserpine, 264
Hydrotensin-25 Tablets, 264
HydroTex, 1152
Hydroxacen, 456
hydroxocobalamin,
    1159-1160
hydroxychloroquine sulfate,
    46-48
hydroxyprogesterone
    caproate, 748-749
hydroxyurea, 909-910
hydroxyzine embonate,
    456-457
hydroxyzine hydrochloride,
    456-457
hydroxyzine pamoate,
    456-457
Hy/Gestrone, 748
Hygroton, 814
Hylorel, 282
Hylutin, 748
hyoscine, 538-540
hyoscine butylbromide,
    538-540
hyoscine hydrobromide,
    538-540
hyoscyamine, 536-537
hyoscyamine sulfate, 536-537
Hy-Pam, 456
Hyperab, 1015
Hyperaldosteronism, spirono-
    lactone for, 826-827
Hyperbilirubinemia, albumin
    for, 866-867

Hypercalcemia
  calcitonin for, 803-804
  etidronate for, 806-807
  gallium for, 1241-1242
  pamidronate for, 1251-1252
  plicamycin for, 925-926
Hypercalcemic crisis, edetate
  disodium for, 1213-1214
Hypercalciuria, plicamycin for,
  925-926
Hypercholesterolemia
  atorvastatin for, 312-313
  cholestyramine for, 313-314
  colestipol for, 314-316
  fluvastatin for, 316-317
  lovastatin for, 318-319
  pravastatin for, 319-320
  simvastatin for, 320-321
HyperHep, 1013
Hyperkalemia, sodium polystyrene sulfonate for,
  1221-1222
Hyperlipidemia
  cholestyramine for, 313-314
  gemfibrozil for, 317-318
  niacin for, 1162-1164
Hyperphosphatemia, calcium
  salts for, 832-835
Hyperprolactinemia,
  bromocriptine for,
  505-506
Hypersecretory conditions
  cimetidine for, 689-691
  famotidine for, 691-692
  lansoprazole for, 692-693
  omeprazole for, 695-696
  ranitidine for, 696-697
Hypersensitivity reactions, epinephrine for, 604-607
Hyperstat IV, 275
Hypertension
  acebutolol for, 265-266
  amiloride for, 810-811
  amiodipine for, 246-247
  atenolol for, 266-268
  benazepril for, 268-269
  betaxolol for, 269-270
  bisoprolol for, 270-271
  captopril for, 271-273
  carteolol for, 273-274
  chlorothiazide for, 812-814
  chlorthalidone for, 814-816
  clonidine for, 274-275
  diltiazem for, 249-250
  doxazosin for, 276-277
  enalaprilat for, 277-279
  enalapril for, 277-279
  esmolol for, 228-230
  felodipine for, 279-280
  fosinopril for, 280-281
  furosemide for, 817-819
  guanabenz for, 281-282
  guanadrel for, 282-283
  guanethidine for, 283-284
  guanfacine for, 284-285

Hypertension (continued)
  hydralazine for, 285-286
  hydrochlorothiazide for,
    819-821
  indapamide for, 821-822
  isradipine for, 286-287
  labetalol for, 287-289
  lisinopril for, 289-290
  losartan for, 290-291
  magnesium sulfate for,
    412-413
  methyldopa for, 291-293
  metolazone for, 824-826
  metoprolol for, 293-294
  minoxidil for, 294-295
  moexipril for, 295-297
  nadolol for, 252-253
  nicardipine for, 253-254
  nifedipine for, 254-255
  nisoldipine for, 297-298
  nitroglycerin for, 255-258
  nitroprusside for, 298-299
  penbutolol for, 299-300
  phentolamine for, 300-301
  pindolol for, 301-302
  prazosin for, 302-303
  propranolol for, 258-260
  quinapril for, 303-304
  ramipril for, 304-306
  reserpine for, 306-307
  sotalol for, 242-244
  spironolactone for, 826-827
  terazosin for, 307
  timolol for, 308-309
  torsemide for, 827-829
  trandolapril for, 309-310
  valsartan for, 310-311
  verapamil for, 260-262
Hypertensive crisis
  diazoxide for, 275-276
  labetalol for, 287-289
  methyldopa for, 291-293
  nitroprusside for, 298-299
Hyper-Tet, 1019
Hyperthyroidism
  methimazole for, 788-789
  propylthiouracil for,
    790-791
  radioactive iodine for,
    791-793
Hypertrophic subaortic stenosis, propranolol for,
  258-260
Hyperuricemia
  allopurinol for, 1182-1183
  probenecid for, 1185-1187
Hypnotics. See Sedative-
  hypnotics.
Hypnovel, 459
Hypocalcemia
  calcifediol for, 802-803
  calcitriol for, 804-805
  calcium salts for, 832-835
  dihydrotachysterol for,
    805-806

Hypocalcemic tetany, dihydrotachysterol for, 805-806
Hypodermoclysis,
  hyaluronidase for, 1191
Hypogammaglobulinemia, immune globulin for,
  1014-1015
Hypoglycemia, glucagon for,
  768-769
Hypogonadism
  chlorotrianisene for,
    729-731
  esterified estrogens for,
    734-736
  estradiol for, 736-738
  estrogens, conjugated, for,
    738-741
  estropipate for, 741-742
  ethinyl estradiol for,
    742-744
  fluoxymesterone for,
    719-721
  methyltestosterone for,
    721-722
  testosterone for, 726-728
  testosterone transdermal
    system for, 728
Hypokalemia
  potassium acetate for,
    840-841
  potassium bicarbonate for,
    841-842
  potassium chloride for,
    842-843
  potassium gluconate for,
    843-844
  spironolactone for, 826-827
Hypomagnesemia
  magnesium oxide for,
    648-649
  magnesium salts for,
    838-840
  magnesium sulfate for,
    412-413
Hypoparathyroidism
  calcitriol for, 804-805
  vitamin D for, 1169-1170
Hypophosphatemia, vitamin D
  for, 1169-1170
Hypoproteinemia
  albumin for, 866-867
  plasma protein fraction for,
    872-873
Hypoprothrombinemia, phy-
  tonadione for, 1171-1173
Hypotension
  controlled, during anesthe-
    sia, nitroprusside for,
    298-299
  dopamine for, 542-544
  ephedrine for, 603-604
  mephentermine for,
    544-545
  metaraminol for, 545-547
  norepinephrine for, 547-548

Hypotension *(continued)*
  phenylephrine for, 548-550
  producing, nitroglycerin for,
    255-258
Hypothyroidism
  liothyronine for, 782-784
  liotrix for, 784-785
  thyroid for, 785-787
  thyrotropin for, 787
Hypovolemic shock, albumin
    for, 866-867
HypRho-D, 1017
HypRho D-MiniDose, 1017
Hyprogest 250, 748
Hypurin Isophane, 771
Hypurin Neutral, 771
Hyrexin-50, 591
Hytakerol, 805
Hytinic, 856
Hytone, 1152
Hytrin, 307, **C7**
Hytuss, 623
Hytuss-2X, 623
Hyzaar, 264
Hyzine-50, 456

I
^{131}I, 791-793
Ibiamox, 77
Ibu-Cream, 348
Ibuprin, 348
ibuprofen, 348-349, **C8**
Ibuprohm Caplets, 348
Ibuprohm Tablets, 348
Ibu-Tab, 348
ibutilide fumarate, 231-232
Idamycin, 921
idarubicin hydrochloride,
    921-922
Idiopathic thrombocytopenic
    purpura, immune globulin
    for, 1014-1015 idoxuri-
    dine, 1044-1045
IDU, 1044-1045
IFEX, 892
IFN-alpha 2, 1029-1031
ifosfamide, 892-894
IG, 1014-1015
IGIM, 1014-1015
IGIV, 1014-1015
IL-2, 1022-1024
Ilosone, 195
Ilosone pulvules, 195
Ilotycin Ophthalmic Ointment,
    1042
Ilozyme Tablets, 652
I.M. administration, children
    and, 16
Imdur, 250
Imferon, 854
imiglucerase, 1242-1243
imipenem/cilastatin sodium,
    204-205
imipramine hydrochloride,
    432-434

imipramine pamoate, 432-434
Imiprin, 432
Imitrex, 521
ImmuCyst, 941
immune globulin intramuscu-
    lar, 1014-1015
immune globulin intravenous,
    1014-1015
Immune serums, 1012-1021
Immune thrombocytopenic
    purpura, Rh$_0$(D) immune
    globulin, human, for,
    1017-1019
Immunization
  cholera vaccine for,
    979-980
  diphtheria and tetanus tox-
    oids, adsorbed, for,
    980-981
  diphtheria and tetanus tox-
    oids and acellular per-
    tussis vaccine for,
    981-982
  diphtheria and tetanus
    toxoids and whole-cell
    pertussis vaccine for,
    981-982
  Haemophilus b conjugate
    vaccines for, 982-984
  hepatitis A vaccine, inacti-
    vated, for, 984-985
  hepatitis B vaccine, recom-
    binant, for, 984-987
  influenza virus vaccine,
    1995-1996 trivalent
    types A and B (purified
    surface antigen), for,
    987-989
  influenza virus vaccine,
    1995-1996 trivalent
    types A and B (split or
    purified split virus), for,
    987-989
  influenza virus vaccine,
    1995-1996 trivalent
    types A and B (whole
    virion), for, 988-989
  Japanese encephalitis virus
    vaccine, inactivated,
    for, 989-991
  measles, mumps, and
    rubella virus vaccine,
    live, for, 991-992
  measles and rubella virus
    vaccine, live attenuated,
    for, 992-993
  measles virus vaccine, live
    attenuated, for,
    993-994
  meningococcal polysaccha-
    ride vaccine for,
    994-995
  mumps virus vaccine, live,
    for, 995-996
  plague vaccine for, 996-997

Immunization *(continued)*
  pneumococcal vaccine,
    polyvalent, for, 997-998
  poliovirus vaccine, inacti-
    vated, for, 998-999
  poliovirus vaccine, live,
    oral, trivalent, for,
    998-999
  rabies vaccine, adsorbed,
    for, 999-1000
  rabies vaccine, human
    diploid cell, for,
    1000-1001
  rubella and mumps virus
    vaccine, live, for,
    1001-1002
  rubella virus vaccine, live
    attenuated, for,
    1002-1003
  tetanus toxoid for,
    1003-1004
  typhoid vaccine for,
    1004-1005
  typhoid Vi polysaccharide
    vaccine for, 1005-1006
  varicella virus vaccine for,
    1006-1007
  yellow fever vaccine for,
    1007
Immunodeficiencies, immune
    globulin for, 1014-1015
Immunosuppressants, 969-977
Immunosuppression
  betamethasone for, 699-701
  methylprednisolone for,
    709-711
  prednisolone for, 711-714
  prednisone for, 714-715
  triamcinolone for, 716
Imodium, 658
Imodium A-D, 658
Imogam Rabies, 1015
Imovax Rabies, 1000
Imovax Rabies I.D., 1000
Impetigo
  loracarbef for, 134-135
  mupirocin for, 1123
Impril, 432
Imuran, 969
Inborn errors of metabolism,
    pyridoxine for, 1164-1165
indapamide, 821-822
Inderal, 258, **C8**
Inderal LA, 258
Inderide 40/25, 264
Inderide 80/25, 264
Inderide LA 80/50, 264
Inderide LA 120/50, 264
Inderide LA 160/50, 264
indinavir sulfate, 176-177
Indochron E-R, 349
Indocid, 349
Indocid PDA, 350
Indocid SR, 349-350
Indocin, 350

Indocin I.V., 350
Indocin SR, 350
indomethacin, 349-352
indomethacin sodium trihy-
    drate, 350-352
Infections, bacitracin for,
    1113-1114. *See also
    specific type.*
InFeD, 854
Infertility
    bromocriptine for, 505-506
    menotropins for, 758-760
Inflam, 348
Inflamase Forte, 1059
Inflamase Ophthalmic, 1059
Inflammation
    amcinonide for, 1137-1138
    aspirin for, 333-335
    betamethasone for,
        699-701, 1138-1139
    choline magnesium trisali-
        cylate for, 335-337
    choline salicylate for,
        337-338
    clobetasol for, 1139-1140
    clocortolone for, 1140-1141
    cortisone for, 701-703
    desonide for, 1141-1142
    desoximetasone for,
        1142-1143
    dexamethasone for,
        703-705, 1143-1144
    diflorasone for, 1144-1145
    fluocinolone for, 1145-1146
    fluocinonide for, 1146-1147
    flurandrenolide for,
        1147-1148
    fluticasone for, 1149
    halcinonide for, 1149-1150
    hydrocortisone for,
        706-709, 1151-1153
    methylprednisolone for,
        709-711
    mometasone for, 1153-1154
    prednisolone for, 711-714
    prednisone for, 714-715
    triamcinolone for, 716,
        1154-1155
Influenza
    amantadine for, 168
    rimantadine for, 181-182
influenza virus vaccine,
    1995-1996 trivalent types
    A and B (purified surface
    antigen), 987-989
influenza virus vaccine,
    1995-1996 trivalent types
    A and B (split or purified
    split virus), 987-989
influenza virus vaccine,
    1995-1996 trivalent types
    A and B (whole virion),
    988-989
Infumorph 200, 379
Infumorph 500, 379

INH, 59-61
Innovar Injection, 367
Inocor, 216
Inotropics, 216-220
Insomnal, 591
Insomnia
    butabarbital for, 390-391
    chloral hydrate for, 391-393
    estazolam for, 393-394
    ethchlorvynol for, 394-395
    flurazepam for, 395-396
    lorazepam for, 457-458
    pentobarbital for, 396-398
    phenobarbital for, 414-416
    quazepam for, 398
    secobarbital for, 398-400
    temazepam for, 400-401
    triazolam for, 401-402
    zolpidem for, 402
Insulatard, 771
Insulatard Human, 771
Insulin 2, 771
insulin injection, 771-774
insulins, 771-774
insulin zinc suspension,
    extended (ultralente),
    771-774
insulin zinc suspension,
    prompt (semilente),
    771-774
insulin zinc suspension
    (lente), 771-774
Intal, 631
Intal Aerosol Spray, 631
Intal Nebulizer Solution, 631
interferon alfa-2a, recombi-
    nant, 1027-1029
interferon alfa-2b, recombi-
    nant, 1029-1031
interferon alfa-n3, 1031-1032
interferon beta-1a, 1032-1033
interferon beta-1b, recombi-
    nant, 1034-1035
interferon gamma-1b, 1035
interleukin-2, 1022-1024
Intermittent claudication,
    pentoxifylline for, 327
Intra-abdominal infections
    aztreonam for, 198-199
    cefmetazole for, 111-113
    cefoperazone for, 114-115
    cefotaxime for, 115-117
    cefotetan for, 117-118
    cefoxitin for, 118-119
    ceftazidime for, 122-124
    ceftizoxime for, 125-126
    ceftriaxone for, 126-128
    ciprofloxacin for, 153-154
    imipenem/cilastatin for,
        204-205
Intracranial pressure, increased
    mannitol for, 822-824
    urea for, 830-831
Intralipid 10%, 1179
Intralipid 20%, 1179

Intraocular pressure, reducing
    apraclonidine for,
        1081-1082
    dipivefrin for, 1085-1086
    dorzolamide for, 1086-1087
    metipranolol for, 1092-1093
Intraperitoneal irrigation,
    kanamycin for, 68-69
Intron A, 1029
Intropin, 542
Invirase, 184
Inza-250, 359
Inza-500, 359
iodine, 1174-1175
Iodopen, 1174
iodoquinol, 25-26
Iodotope Therapeutic, 791
Iopidine, 1081
Iosopan, 647
Iostat, 789
ipecac syrup, 1215-1216
I-Phrine 2.5%, 1075
IPOL, 998
ipratropium bromide, 607-608
IPV, 998-999
Ircon, 851
Iridocyclitis, dexamethasone
    for, 1054-1055
irinotecan hydrochloride,
    948-950
Iris, adhesion of, phenyl-
    ephrine for, 1075-1076
Iritis
    atropine for, 1071-1072
    scopolamine for, 1076-1077
Iron deficiency
    ferrous fumarate for,
        851-852
    ferrous gluconate for,
        852-853
    ferrous sulfate, dried, for,
        853-854
    ferrous sulfate for, 853-854
Iron deficiency anemia
    iron dextran for, 854-856
    iron sorbitol for, 854-856
    polysaccharide iron com-
        plex for, 856
iron dextran, 854-856
Iron intoxication, deferox-
    amine for, 1206-1207
iron sorbitol, 854-856
Irritable bowel syndrome
    atropine for, 224-225
    dicyclomine for, 533-534
Ismelin, 283
ISMO, 250
Ismotic, 1088
isoetharine hydrochloride,
    608-609
isoetharine mesylate, 608-609
isoflurophate, 1067-1068
Isollyl Improved, 330
Isonate, 250
isoniazid, 59-61

Isoniazid poisoning, pyridoxine for, 1164-1165
isonicotinic acid hydride,
59-61
Isopap, 330
isophane insulin suspension,
771-774
isophane insulin suspension
with insulin injection,
771-774
isoprenaline, 609-611
isoproterenol, 609-611
isoproterenol hydrochloride,
609-611
isoproterenol sulfate, 609-611
Isoptin, 260
Isoptin SR, 260
Isopto Atropine, 1071
Isopto Carbachol, 1062
Isopto Carpine, 1069
Isopto Cetamide Ophthalmic,
1049
Isopto Cetapred, 1039
Isopto Fenicol, 1040
Isopto Frin, 1075
Isopto Homatropine, 1074
Isopto Hyoscine, 1076
Isopto P-ES, 1062
Isorbid, 250
Isordil, 250
Isordil Tembids, 250
Isordil Titradose, 250
isosorbide, 1088-1089
isosorbide dinitrate, 250-252
isosorbide mononitrate,
250-252
Isotamine, 59
Isotard MC, 771
Isotrate, 250
isotretinoin, 1243-1244
isoxsuprine hydrochloride,
324
isradipine, 286-287
Isuprel, 609
Isuprel Glossets, 609
Isuprel Mistometer, 609
itraconazole, 39-40
I.V. administration, children
and, 15-16
I.V. indwelling catheter,
heparin for, 860-863
Ivocort, 1152
I.V. Persantine, 323

J

Janimine, 432
Japanese encephalitis virus
vaccine, inactivated,
989-991
Jenamicin, 66
Jenset-28, 744
JE-VAX, 989-991
Joint infections. *See* Bone and
joint infections.

K

K⁺10, 842
Kabikinase, 878
Kabolin, 722
Kalcinate, 832
Kaluril, 810
kanamycin sulfate, 68-69
Kanasig, 68
Kantrex, 68
Kaochlor 10%, 842
Kaochlor S-F 10%, 842
Kaochlor-Cl, 842
Kaon-Cl 20%, 842
Kaon Liquid, 843
Kaon Tablets, 843
Kaopectate Advanced
Formula, 656
Kaopectate II Caplets, 658
Kaopectate Maximum
Strength, 656
Kao-Spen, 657
Kapectolin, 657
Kaposi's sarcoma
interferon alfa-2a, recombi-
nant, for, 1027-1029
interferon alfa-2b, recombi-
nant, for, 1029-1031
vinblastine for, 963-965
Karacil, 674
Karidium, 1173
Karigel, 1173
Karigel-N, 1173
Kato Powder, 842
Kawasaki syndrome, aspirin
for, 333-335
Kay Ciel, 842
Kayexalate, 1221
Kaylixir, 843
K-C, 656, 657
K+Care, 842
K+Care ET, 841
K-Dur, 842, **C8**
Keflex, 130
Keftab, 130
Kefurox, 128
Kefzol, 107
K-Electrolyte Effervescent
Tablets, 841
Kellogg's Tasteless Castor Oil,
665
Kenacort, 716
Kenaject-40, 716
Kenalog, 1154
Kenalog-10, 716
Kenalog-40, 716
Kenalone, 1154
Keratitis
idoxuridine for, 1044-1045
Iodoxamide for, 1091-1092
natamycin for, 1045-1046

Keratitis *(continued)*
trifluridine for, 1052-1053
vidarabine for, 1053
Keratoconjunctivitis
gentamicin for, 1043-1044
Iodoxamide for, 1091-1092
trifluridine for, 1052-1053
vidarabine for, 1053
Kerlone, 269
ketoconazole, 40-42,
1119-1120
ketoprofen, 352-353
ketorolac tromethamine,
354-355, 1057-1058
Key-Pred-SP, 711
K-G Elixir, 843
K-Gen ET, 841
K-Ide, 841
Kidney cancer, medroxyprog-
esterone for, 751-752
Kidney disease, bumetanide
for, 811-812
Kidney transplantation
azathioprine for, 969-970
cyclosporine for, 970-972
cytomegalovirus immune
globulin (human), intra-
venous, for, 1012-1013
Kidrolase, 939
Kinesed Tablets, 533
Kinidin Durules, 240
K-Lease, 842
Klonopin, 405, **C8**
K-Lor, 842
Klor-10%, 842
Klor-Con, 842
Klor-Con/EF, 841
Klorvess, 832, 842
Klotrix, 842
K-Lyte, 841
K-Lyte-CL, 832
K-Lyte/Cl, 842
K-Norm, 842
Koate-HP, 867
Koate-HS, 867
Koffex, 622
Kolephrin GG/DM, 622
Konakion, 1171
Kondremul, 671
Kondremul Plain, 671
Kondremul with Phenolph-
thalein, 662
Konsyl, 674
Konsyl-D, 674
Konyne-80, 871
K-Pek, 656
Kraurosis vulvae
chlorotrianisene for,
729-731
dienestrol for, 731-732
estradiol for, 736-738
estrogens, conjugated, for,
738-741
K-Tab, 842
Ku-Zyme HP Capsules, 652

Kwell, 1134
Kwellada, 1134
Kytril, 681

L
LA-12, 1159
labetalol hydrochloride, 287-289
Labor
  butorphanol for, 369-371
  oxymorphone for, 384-385
  oxytocin, synthetic injection, for induction of, 1195-1196
  pentazocine for, 385-386
Labor, premature
  albuterol for prevention of, 597-599
Labor, preterm
  ritodrine for, 1254-1256
Lactation, drugs and, 11
Lactulax, 668
lactulose, 668-669
Lactulose PSE, 668
L.A.E., 736
Lamictal, 411
Lamisil, 1128
lamivudine, 177-179
lamotrigine, 411-412
Lamprene, 54
Lanabiotic, 1111
Lanacort, 1152
Laniazid, 59
Lanophyllin, 618
Lanorinal, 330
Lanoxicaps, 217
Lanoxin, 217, **C8**
Lansooyl, 671
lansoprazole, 692-693
Lanvis, 914
Largactil, 462
Lariam, 48
Larodopa, 508
Larotid, 97
Larva migrans infestation, thiabendazole for, 32-33
Lasix, 817, **C8**
Lasix Special, 817
L-asparaginase, 939-941
latanoprost, 1089-1090
Laxative, magnesium oxide for, 648-649. *See also* Laxatives.
Laxatives, 662-676
Laxinate 100, 666
Laxit, 662
Lax-Pills, 672
L-carnitine, 1244-1245
L-deprenyl hydrochloride, 511-512
Lead encephalopathy
  dimercaprol for, 1208-1209
  edetate calcium disodium for, 1212-1213

Lead poisoning
  edetate calcium disodium for, 1212-1213
  succimer for, 1222-1223
Ledercillin VK, 97
Ledermycin, 136
Legionnaire's disease, erythromycin for, 195-197
Lennox-Gastaut syndrome, clonazepam for, 405-406
Lenoltec with Codeine No. 1, 367
Lente Iletin II, 771
Lente Insulin, 771
Lente MC, 771
Lente Purified Pork Insulin, 771
Leprosy
  clofazimine for, 54-55
  dapsone for, 56-57
Lescol, 316
leucovorin calcium, 1161-1162
Leukemia
  asparaginase for, 939-941
  busulfan for, 883-884
  chlorambucil for, 887-888
  cladribine for, 902-903
  cyclophosphamide for, 890-892
  cytarabine for, 903-905
  daunorubicin for, 917-919
  doxorubicin for, 919-921
  fludarabine for, 906-907
  hydroxyurea for, 909-910
  idarubicin for, 921-922
  immune globulin for, 1014-1015
  interferon alfa-2a, recombinant, for, 1027-1029
  interferon alfa-2b, recombinant, for, 1029-1031
  mechlorethamine for, 895-896
  mercaptopurine for, 910-911
  methotrexate for, 911-914
  mitoxantrone for, 951
  pegaspargase for, 954-956
  pentostatin for, 923-925
  teniposide for, 959-960
  thioguanine for, 914
  tretinoin for, 962-963
  uracil mustard for, 901
  vincristine for, 965-966
Leukeran, 887
Leukine, 1037
leuprolide acetate, 932-933
Leustatin, 902
levamisole hydrochloride, 1036-1037
Levaquin, 156
levarterenol bitartrate, 547-548
Levate, 423

Levatol, 299
Levlen, 744
levobunolol hydrochloride, 1090-1091
levocabastine hydrochloride, 1091
levocarnitine, 1244-1245
levodopa, 508-510
levofloxacin, 156-158
levomethadyl acetate hydrochloride, 1245-1246
levonorgestrel, 749-751
Levophed, 547
Levo-T, 781
Levothroid, 781
levothyroxine sodium, 781-782
Levoxine, 781
Levoxyl, 781, **C8**
Levsin, 536
Levsin Drops, 536
Levsinex Timecaps, 536
Levsin S/L, 536
Librax, 449
Libritabs, 451
Librium, 451
Lice infestation
  benzyl benzoate lotion for, 1132-1133
  permethrin for, 1135
  pyrethrins for, 1136
Lidemol, 1146
Lidex, 1146
Lidex-E, 1146
lidocaine hydrochloride, 232-234, 1264-1265t
Lidoject-1, 1264t
Lidoject-2, 1264t
LidoPen Auto-Injector, 232
lignocaine hydrochloride, 232-234, 1264-1265t
Limbitrol DS, 423, 449
lindane, 1134-1135
Lioresal, 556
Lioresal Intrathecal, 556
liothyronine sodium, 782-784
liotrix, 784-785
Lipex, 320
Lipitor, 312
Liposyn II 10%, 1179
Liposyn II 20%, 1179
Liposyn III 10%, 1179
Liposyn III 20%, 1179
Liquaemin Sodium, 860
Liqui-Char, 1204
Liqui-Doss, 671
liquid petrolatum, 671-672
Liquid Pred, 714
Liquiprin Infants' Drops, 331
lisinopril, 289-290
Listeria infection, erythromycin for, 195-197
Listermint with Fluoride, 1173
Lithane, 516
Lithicarb, 516

lithium carbonate, 516-518
lithium citrate, 516
Lithizine, 516
Lithobid, 516
Lithonate, 516
Lithostat, 1227
Lithotabs, 516
Liver transplantation, cyclo-
    sporine for, 970-972
Livostin, 1091
Lixolin, 618
10% LMD, 835
Lobeta, 299
Local anesthetics, 1262-1267t
Locoid, 1152
Lodine, 344, **C9**
Iodoxamide tromethamine,
    1091-1092
Loestrin 21, 1/20, 745
Loestrin 21 1.5/30, 745
Loestrin Fe 1/20, 745
Loestrin Fe 1.5/30, 745
lomefloxacin hydrochloride,
    158-159
Lomine, 533
lomustine, 894-895
Loniten, 294
Lo/Ovral, 745
loperamide, 658-659
Lopid, 317, **C9**
Lopresor, 293
Lopresor SR, 293
Lopressor, 293
Lopressor HCT 50/25, 264
Lopressor HCT 100/25, 264
Lopressor HCT 100/50, 264
Loprox, 1115
Lopurin, 1182
Lorabid, 134, **C9**
loracarbef, 134-135
loratadine, 593-594
lorazepam, 457-458
Lorazepam Intensol, 457
Lorcet 10/650, 367, **C9**
Lorcet Plus, 367
Lortab 2.5/500, 367
Lortab 5/500, 367
Lortab 7.5/500, 367
losartan potassium, 290-291
Losec, 695
Lotensin, 268
Lotrimin, 1116
Lotrisone Cream, 1111
lovastatin, 318-319
Lovenox, 859
Lowsium, 647
Loxapac, 471
loxapine hydrochloride,
    471-472
loxapine succinate, 471-472
Loxitane, 471
Loxitane C, 471
Loxitane IM, 471
Lozide, 821
Lozol, 821, **C9**

L-phenylalanine mustard,
    896-898
L-thyroxine sodium, 781-782
Lucrin, 932
Ludiomil, 434
Lugol's solution, 789-790
Luminal Sodium, 414
Lung cancer
    amifostine for, 938-939
    doxorubicin for, 919-921
    etoposide for, 946-947
    mechlorethamine for,
        895-896
    vinorelbine for, 966-968
Lupron, 932
Lupron Depot, 932
Lupron Depot-Ped, 932
Lupron Depot-3 Month, 932
Lupus erythematosus, hy-
    droxychloroquine for,
    46-48
Luride, 1173
Luride Lozi-Tabs, 1173
Luride-SF, 1173
Luride-SF Lozi-Tabs, 1173
Lutrepulse, 756
Luvox, 515
Lyme disease
    ceftriaxone for, 126-128
    cefuroxime for, 128-130
    doxycycline for, 137-140
lymphocyte immune globulin,
    972-973
Lymphogranuloma, chloram-
    phenicol for, 200-202
Lymphogranuloma venereum
    sulfamethoxazole for,
        149-150
    sulfisoxazole for, 150-152
Lymphoma
    carmustine for, 886-887
    chlorambucil for, 887-888
    cyclophosphamide for,
        890-892
    doxorubicin for, 919-921
    thiotepa for, 899-900
    uracil mustard for, 901
    vinblastine for, 963-965
    vincristine for, 965-966
Lymphosarcoma
    bleomycin for, 915-916
    chlorambucil for, 887-888
    mechlorethamine for,
        895-896
    methotrexate for, 911-914
    vinblastine for, 963-965
Lyphocin, 214
Lysodren, 950

M

Maalox, 642
Maalox Anti-Diarrheal Caplets,
    658
Maalox Daily Fiber Therapy,
    674

Maalox Extra Strength Tablets,
    642
Maalox Plus Tablets, 642
Maalox TC Tablets, 642
Macrobid, 198, 208, **C9**
Macrodantin, 208
Macrodex, 836
Macrolide anti-infectives,
    191-197
Madopar, 503
Madopar HBS, 503
Madopar Q, 503
mafenide acetate, 1120-1121
magaldrate, 647-648
Magan, 339
Magnaprin, 330
Magnaprin Arthritis Strength,
    330
magnesium chloride, 838-840
magnesium citrate, 669-670
magnesium hydroxide,
    669-670
Magnesium intoxication, cal-
    cium salts for, 832-835
magnesium oxide, 648-649
magnesium salicylate,
    339-340
magnesium sulfate, 412-413,
    669-670, 838-840
Mag-Ox 400, 648
Malaria
    chloroquine for, 45-46
    doxycycline for, 137-140
    hydroxychloroquine for,
        46-48
    mefloquine for, 48-49
    primaquine for, 49-50
    pyrimethamine for, 50-51
    pyrimethamine with sulfa-
        doxine for, 50-51
    quinidine for, 240-242
    sulfadiazine for, 148-149
    tetracycline for, 143-145
Malignant hyperthermia,
    dantrolene for, 560-561
Mallamint, 645, 832
Malogen, 726
manganese, 1174-1175
manganese chloride,
    1174-1175
manganese sulfate,
    1174-1175
Mania
    divalproex sodium for,
        420-422
    lithium for, 516-518
mannitol, 822-824
Mantoux test, 1280t
Maox-420, 648
Mapap with Codeine, 366
maprotiline hydrochloride,
    434-435
Marax, 597
Marax DF Syrup, 597

Marbaxin-750, 561
Marcain, 1262t
Marcaine, 1262t
Marinol, 680
Marmine, 678
Marnel, 330
Maso-Cort, 1152
Mastocytosis
    cimetidine for, 689-691
    cromolyn for, 631-632
Matulane, 958
Mavik, 309
Maxair, 614
Maxair Autohaler, 614
Maxaquin, 158
Maxenal, 550
Maxeran, 682
Maxidex Ophthalmic, 1054
Maxidex Ophthalmic Suspen-
    sion, 1054
Maxiflor, 1144
Maximum Strength Pepto-
    Bismol Liquid, 657
Maximum Strength Phazyme
    125 Softgels, 649
Maxipime, 108
Maxitrol Ointment Ophthalmic
    Suspension, 1039
Maxivate, 1138
Maxolon, 682
Maxolon High Dose, 682
Maxzide, 264, 808
Maxzide-25mg, 808
Mazepine, 403
M.C.T., 1181
measles, mumps, and rubella
    virus vaccine, live,
    991-992
measles and rubella virus vac-
    cine, live attenuated,
    992-993
Measles exposure, immune
    globulin for, 1014-1015
measles virus vaccine, live
    attenuated, 993-994
Measurin, 333
Mebaral, 413
mebendazole, 31
mechlorethamine hydrochlo-
    ride, 895-896
meclizine hydrochloride,
    681-682
meclofenamate, 355-356
Meclomen, 355
meclozine hydrochloride,
    681-682
Meda Cap, 331
Medigesic, 330
Medihaler-Epi, 604
Medihaler Ergotamine, 553
Medihaler Iso, 609
Medihaler-Iso, 609
Medilax, 672
Medipren Caplets, 348
Medipren Tablets, 348

Mediquell, 622
medium-chain triglycerides,
    1181
Medralone-40, 709
Medralone-80, 709
Medrol, 709
medroxyprogesterone acetate,
    751-752
medrysone, 1058-1059
mefenamic acid, 356-357
Mefic, 356
mefloquine hydrochloride,
    48-49
Mefoxin, 118
Mega-Cal, 832
Megace, 933
Megacillin, 92
megestrol acetate, 933-934
Megostat, 933
Meibomianitis, gentamicin for,
    1043-1044
Melanoma
    dacarbazine for, 943-944
    hydroxyurea for, 909-910
    interferon alfa-2b, recombi-
        nant, for, 1029-1031
Melipramine, 432
Mellaril, 482
Mellaril Concentrate, 482
melphalan, 896-898
Menadol, 348
Menaval, 736
Menest, 734
Meni-D, 681
Meningitis
    amphotericin B for, 34-36
    ampicillin for, 78-80
    ceftizoxime for, 125-126
    ceftriaxone for, 126-128
    cefuroxime for, 128-130
    chloramphenicol for,
        200-202
    fluconazole for, 36-37
    flucytosine for, 37-38
    gentamicin for, 66-68
    meropenem for, 205-207
    miconazole for, 42-43
    polymyxin B sulfate for,
        210-211
Meningococcal carriers
    minocycline for, 140-141
    rifampin for, 63-64
    sulfadiazine for, 148-149
meningococcal polysaccha-
    ride vaccine, 994-995
Menomune-A/C/Y/W-135, 994
Menopausal symptoms
    chlorotrianisene for,
        729-731
    esterified estrogens for,
        734-736
    estradiol for, 736-738
    estrogens, conjugated, for,
        738-741
    estropipate for, 741-742

Menopausal symptoms
    (continued)
    ethinyl estradiol for,
        742-744
Menorrhagia, meclofenamate
    for, 355-356
menotropins, 758-760
Menrium 5-2, 729
Menrium 5-4, 729
Menrium 10-4, 729
meperidine hydrochloride,
    376-378
mephentermine sulfate,
    544-545
mephobarbital, 413-414
Mephyton, 1171
meprobamate, 458-459
Mepron, 25
Meprospan 200, 458
Meprospan-400, 458
Merbentyl, 533
mercaptopurine, 910-911
6-mercaptopurine, 910-911
Mercury poisoning, dimer-
    caprol for, 1208-1209
meropenem, 205-207
Merrem I.V., 205
Meruvax II, 1002
mesalamine, 1246-1247
Mesasal, 1246
mesna, 1247-1248
Mesnex, 1247
mesoridazine besylate,
    472-474
Mestinon, 530
Mestinon Timespans, 530
mestranol and norethindrone,
    745-748
mestranol and norethynodrel,
    745-748
Metabolic acidosis
    sodium bicarbonate for,
        848-849
    sodium lactate for, 849-850
    tromethamine for, 850
Metabolic alkalosis, ammoni-
    um chloride for, 847-848
Metabolism of drug, 7
    in children, 14
Metamucil, 674
Metamucil Effervescent Sugar
    Free, 674
Metamucil Instant Mix, 674
Metandren, 721
Metaprel, 611
metaproterenol sulfate,
    611-613
metaraminol bitartrate,
    545-547
Metastron, 1256
Metatensin Tablets #2 or #4,
    264
metformin hydrochloride,
    774-776

t refers to a table; **boldface** refers to full-color photographs

methadone hydrochloride, 378-379
Methadose, 378
methamphetamine hydrochloride, 498-499
methazolamide, 824
methenamine hippurate, 207-208
methenamine mandelate, 207-208
Methergine, 1194
methimazole, 788-789
methocarbamol, 561-563
methotrexate, 911-914
Methotrexate overdose, leucovorin rescue for, 1161-1162
methotrexate sodium, 911-914
methoxsalen (topical), 1248-1249
methylcellulose, 670-671
methyldopa, 291-293
methyldopate hydrochloride, 291-293
methylergonovine maleate, 1194-1195
Methylmalonic aciduria, cyanocobalamin for, 1159
methylphenidate hydrochloride, 499-500, **C9**
methylprednisolone, 709-711
methylprednisolone acetate, 709-711
methylprednisolone sodium succinate, 709-711
methyltestosterone, 721-722
methysergide maleate, 554-555
Meticorten, 714
Metimyd Ophthalmic Ointment Suspension, 1039
metipranolol hydrochloride, 1092-1093
metoclopramide hydrochloride, 682-683
metocurine iodide, 570-571
metolazone, 824-826
metoprolol succinate, 293-294
metoprolol tartrate, 293
Metric-21, 26
Metric system equivalents, 1279t
MetroGel, 1121
MetroGel-Vaginal, 1121
Metrogyl, 26
Metro I.V., 26
metronidazole, 26-28
metronidazole hydrochloride, 26-28
metronidazole (topical), 1121-1122
Metrozine, 26
Metubine Iodide, 570

Mevacor, 318, **C9**
mevinolin, 318-319
Mexate-AQ, 911
mexiletine hydrochloride, 234-235
Mexitil, 234
Mezlin, 86
mezlocillin sodium, 86-88
Miacalcin, 803
Miacalcin Nasal Spray, 803
Micatin, 1122
miconazole, 42-43
miconazole nitrate, 1122-1123
MICRhoGAM, 1017
Microcort, 1152
Micro-K Extencaps, 842, **C9**
Micronase, 769, **C10**
Micro-Nefrin, 604
Micronor, 752
Microsulfon, 148
Micrurus fulvius antivenin, 1010-1011
Mictrin, 819
Midamor, 810
midazolam hydrochloride, 459-460
midodrine hydrochloride, 324-325
Midol-200, 348
Midol IB, 348
Midrin, 330
Migraine headache
dihydroergotamine for, 552-553
divalproex sodium for, 420-422
ergotamine for, 553-554
methysergide for, 554-555
propranolol for, 258-260
sumatriptan for, 521-522
timolol for, 308-309
Milk ejection, oxytocin, synthetic nasal solution, for, 1197
Milkinol, 671
milk of magnesia, 669-670
Milk of Magnesia, 669
Milk of Magnesia Concentrate, 669
Milontin, 416
Milophene, 1236
milrinone lactate, 219-220
Miltown-200, 458
Miltown-400, 458
Miltown-600, 458
Minax, 293
mineral oil, 671-672
Minerals, 1173-1175
Minidiab, 767
Mini-Gamulin Rh, 1017
Minims Castor Oil, 665
Minipress, 302
Minirin, 797
Minitran, 255

Minizide 1, 264
Minizide 2, 264
Minizide 5, 264
Minocin, 140
minocycline hydrochloride, 140-141
Minodyl, 294
Minomycin, 140
Minomycin IV, 140
minoxidil, 294-295
minoxidil (topical), 1249-1250
Mintezol, 32
Minute Gel, 1173
Miocarpine, 1069
Miochol, 1062
Miosis
flurbiprofen for inhibition of, 1057
suprofen for inhibition of, 1061
Miostat, 1062
Miotics, 1062-1070
mirtazapine, 435-436
misoprostol, 693-694
Mithracin, 925
mithramycin, 925-926
mitomycin, 922-923
mitomycin-C, 922-923
mitotane, 950-951
mitoxantrone hydrochloride, 951-952
Mitrolan, 663
Mivacron, 571
mivacurium chloride, 571-573
Mixtard Human, 761
M-M-R II, 991
Moban, 474
Mobenol, 778
Mobidin, 339
Moctanin, 650
Modane, 672
Modane Bulk, 674
Modane Plus, 662
Modane Soft, 666
Modecate, 467
Modecate Concentrate, 467
ModiCon, 744
Moditen Enanthate, 467
Moditen HCl, 467
Moditen HCl-H.P., 467
Modrastane, 1260
Moduretic, 808
moexipril hydrochloride, 295-297
Molatoc, 666
molindone hydrochloride, 474-475
Mol-Iron, 853
mometasone furoate, 1153-1154
Monistat-Derm Cream and Lotion, 1122
Monistat I.V., 42
Monistat 3 Vaginal Suppository, 1122

Monistat 7 Vaginal Cream, 1122
Monistat 7 Vaginal Suppository, 1122
Monitan, 265
Monocid, 113
Monoclate, 867
Monoclate-P, 867
monoctanoin, 650-651
Monodox, 137
Mono-Gesic, 340
Monoket, 250
Mononine, 871
Monopril, 280
Monotard HM, 771
Monotard MC, 771
Mono-Vacc Test (liquid Old Tuberculin), 1280t
Monurol, 203
M-Orexic, 494
moricizine hydrochloride, 235-237
Morphine H.P., 379
morphine hydrochloride, 379-381
morphine sulfate, 379-381
morphine tartrate, 379-381
Morphitec, 379
M.O.S., 379
M.O.S.-S.R., 379
Motion sickness
    dimenhydrinate for, 678-679
    diphenhydramine for, 591-593
    meclizine for, 681-682
    promethazine for, 594-595
    scopolamine for, 538-540
Motrin, 348, **C10**
Motrin IB Caplets, 348
Motrin IB Sinus, 342
Motrin IB Tablets, 348
Mountain sickness, acetazolamide for, 808-810
Moxacin, 77
6-MP, 910-911
M-R-Vax II, 992
MS Contin, 379
MSIR, 379
MS/L, 379
MSTA, 1280t
M.T.E.-4, 1156
M.T.E.-4 Concentrated, 1156
M.T.E.-5, 1156
M.T.E.-5 Concentrated, 1156
M.T.E.-6, 1156
M.T.E.-6 Concentrated, 1156
M.T.E.-7, 1156
MTX, 911-914
Muci-Lax, 674
Mucocutaneous lymph node syndrome, aspirin for, 333-335
Mucomyst, 624
Mucomyst-10, 624

Mucosil-10, 624
Mucosil-20, 624
Multipax, 456
Multiple myeloma
    carmustine for, 886-887
    cyclophosphamide for, 890-892
    melphalan for, 896-898
Multiple sclerosis
    baclofen for, 556-557
    dantrolene for, 560-561
    interferon beta-1a for, 1032-1033
    interferon beta-1b, recombinant, for, 1034-1035
Multiple Trace Element Concentrated, 1156
Multiple Trace Element Neonatal, 1156
Multiple Trace Element with Selenium, 1156
Multitrace 5 Concentrate, 1156
mumps skin test antigen, 1280-1281t
Mumpsvax, 995
mumps virus vaccine, live, 995-996
mupirocin, 1123
Murelax, 461
Murine Plus, 1080
Murocoll-2, 1071
muromonab-CD3, 973-974
Muro-128 Ointment, 1093
Muscle spasm
    cyclobenzaprine for, 559-560
    diazepam for, 453-456
Musculoskeletal conditions
    carisoprodol for, 557-558
    chlorzoxazone for, 558-559
    methocarbamol for, 561-563
Mustargen, 895
Mutamycin, 922
Myambutol, 57
Myapap Elixir, 331
Myapap, Infants', 331
Myasthenia gravis
    ambenonium for, 524-525
    edrophonium for diagnosis of, 526-528
    neostigmine for, 528-529
    pyridostigmine for, 530-532
    tubocurarine for diagnosis of, 580-581
Myasthenic crisis, edrophonium for, 526-528
Mycelex, 1116
Mycelex-7, 1116
Mycelex-G, 1116
Mycelex-OTC, 1116
Mycifradin, 69, 1124
Myciguent, 1124
Mycitracin Ointment, 1111

Mycitracin Ophthalmic Ointment, 1039
Mycobacterium avium complex
    azithromycin for, 191-192
    clarithromycin for, 192-193
    rifabutin for, 62-63
Mycobutin, 62
Mycolog II Cream, Ointment, 1111
mycophenolate mofetil, 974-975
MyCort Lotion, 1152
Mycosis fungoides
    cyclophosphamide for, 890-892
    mechlorethamine for, 895-896
    methotrexate for, 911-914
    uracil mustard for, 901
    vinblastine for, 963-965
Mycostatin, 43, 1125
Mydfrin, 1075
Mydriacyl, 1077
Mydriasis
    cyclopentolate for, 1072-1073
    phenylephrine for, 1075-1076
    pilocarpine for, 1069-1070
Mydriatics, 1071-1077
Myfedrine, 550
Myidyl, 595
Mykrox, 824
Mylanta Gas, 649
Mylanta Gas Maximum Strength, 649
Mylanta Gas Regular Strength, 649
Mylanta-II Tablets, 642
Mylanta Natural Fiber Supplement, 674
Mylanta Tablets, 642
Myleran, 883
Mylicon, 649
Mymethasone, 703
Myocardial infarction
    alteplase for, 874-875
    anistreplase for, 875-877
    atenolol for, 266-268
    captopril for, 271-273
    heparin for, 860-863
    lisinopril for, 289-290
    metoprolol for, 293-294
    papaverine for, 326-327
    propranolol for, 258-260
    reteplase, recombinant, for, 877-878
    streptokinase for, 878-881
    timolol for, 308-309
Myochrysine, 1202
Myotonachol, 525
Myproic Acid, 420
Myproic Acid Syrup, 420
Myrosemide, 817

Mysoline, 419
Mytelase Caplets, 524
Mytussin DM, 622
Myxedema, liothyronine for, 782-784
Myxedema coma, levothyroxine for, 781-782

N

nabumetone, 358
nadolol, 252-253
Nadopen-V-200, 97
Nadopen-V-400, 97
Nadopen-VK, 97
Nadostine, 43, 1125
Nafcil, 88
nafcillin sodium, 88-89
naftifine, 1123-1124
Naftin, 1123
nalbuphine hydrochloride, 381-383
Nalcrom, 631
Naldecon, 583, 597
Naldecon Senior DX, 622
Naldecon Senior EX, 623
Nalfon, 345
Nalfon 200, 345
nalidixic acid, 159-160
Nallpen, 88
naloxone hydrochloride, 1216-1217
naltrexone hydrochloride, 1217-1218
Nandrobolic, 723
Nandrobolic L.A., 722
nandrolone decanoate, 722-724
nandrolone phenpropionate, 723-724
naphazoline hydrochloride, 1078-1079, 1106
Naphcon, 1078
Naphcon Forte, 1078
Naprelan, 359
Naprogesic, 359
Naprosyn, 359, **C10**
Naprosyn-E, 359
Naprosyn SR, 359
naproxen, 359-360, **C10**
naproxen sodium, 359-360
Naquival, 264
Narcan, 1216
Narcolepsy
    amphetamine for, 488-489
    dextroamphetamine for, 493-494
    methylphenidate for, 499-500
Narcotic analgesics, 366-389
Narcotic depression, naloxone for, 1216-1217
Narcotic withdrawal syndrome, methadone for, 378-379

Nardil, 440
Nasacort, 1109
Nasahist B, 585
Nasal congestion
    ephedrine for, 603-604, 1103
    epinephrine for, 1103-1104
    naphazoline for, 1106
    oxymetazoline for, 1106-1107
    phenylephrine for, 1107-1108
    pseudoephedrine for, 550-551
    tetrahydrozoline for, 1108-1109
    xylometazoline for, 1110
Nasalcrom, 631
Nasal drugs, 1099-1110
Nasalide, 1104
Nasal inflammation, dexamethasone for, 1102-1103
Nasal polyps
    beclomethasone for, 1100-1101
    dexamethasone for, 1102-1103
Natacyn, 1045
natamycin, 1045-1046
Natrilix, 821
Natulan, 958
Naturacil, 674
natural lung surfactant, 627-629
Nausea
    chlorpromazine for, 462-465
    diphenidol for, 679-680
    dronabinol for, 680-681
    granisetron for, 681
    hydroxyzine for, 456-457
    metoclopramide for, 682-683
    ondansetron for, 684-685
    perphenazine for, 476-478
    prochlorperazine for, 685-687
    promethazine for, 594-595
    thiethylperazine for, 687-688
    trimethobenzamide for, 688
Nauseatol, 678
Navane, 484
Navelbine, 966
Naxen, 359
ND-Stat Revised, 585
Nebcin, 73
NebuPent, 29
nedocromil sodium, 637-638
N.E.E. 1/35, 744
nefazodone hydrochloride, 436-438
NegGram, 159
Nelova 0.5/35 E, 744
Nelova 1/35 E, 744

Nelova 1/50 M, 745
Nelova 10/11, 744
Nemasol Sodium, 52
Nembutal, 396
Nembutal Sodium, 396
Neo-Calglucon, 832
Neo-Codema, 819
Neo-Cortef Ointment, 1111
Neo-Cultol, 671
Neo Decadron Cream, 1111
Neo-DM, 622
Neo-Durabolic, 722
Neo-Estrone, 734
NeoFed, 550
Neo-fradin, 69
Neoloid, 665
Neo-Metric, 26
neomycin sulfate, 69-70, 1124
Neopap, 331
Neoplasias, dexamethasone for, 703-705
Neoplastic effusions
    mechlorethamine for, 895-896
    thiotepa for, 899-900
Neoquess, 533, 536
Neoral, 970
Neo-Rx, 1124
Neosar, 890
Neo-Spec, 623
Neosporin Cream, 1111
Neosporin G.U. Irrigant, 65
Neosporin Ointment, 1111
Neosporin Ophthalmic Ointment, 1039
neostigmine methylsulfate, 528-529
Neosulf, 69
Neo-Synephrine, 548, 1075, 1107
Neo-Synephrine 12 Hour, 1106
Neo-Synephrine II, 1110
Neo-Tabs, 69
Neotal, 1039
Neothylline-GG Tablets, 597
Neotrace-4, 1156
NephrAmine, 1176
Nephro-Calci, 832
Nephro-Fer, 851
Nephron, 604
Nephronex, 208
Nephrox, 644
Neptazane, 824
Nervine Nighttime Sleep-Aid, 591
Nesacaine, 1262t
Nesacaine MPF, 1262t
Nestrex, 1164
netilmicin sulfate, 70-72
Netromycin, 70
Neupogen, 1026

t refers to a table; **boldface** refers to full-color photographs

Neuroblastoma
cyclophosphamide for, 890-892
doxorubicin for, 919-921
vincristine for, 965-966
Neurogenic bladder
bethanechol for, 525-526
neostigmine for, 528-529
oxybutynin for, 1198-1199
Neuromuscular blockade, maintenance of, doxacurium for, 568-570
Neuromuscular blockers, 565-582
Neuromuscular blocking action, reversal of
edrophonium for, 526-528
neostigmine for, 528-529
pyridostigmine for, 530-532
Neurontin, 410
neutral protamine Hagedorn insulin, 771-774
Neutra-phos, 832
Neutrexin, 213
Neutropenia, filgrastim for, 1026-1027
nevirapine, 178-180
Niac, 1162
niacin, 1162-1164
niacinamide, 1163-1164
Niacor, 1162
nicardipine, 253-254
N'ice Vitamin C Drops, 1167
Nico-400, 1162
Nicobid, 1162
Nicoderm, 519
Nicolar, 1162
Nicorette, 518
Nicorette DS, 518
nicotinamide, 1163-1164
nicotine polacrilex, 518-519
nicotine-polacrilin resin complex, 518-519
nicotine transdermal system, 519-521
Nicotine withdrawal symptoms
nicotine polacrilex for, 518-519
nicotine transdermal system for, 519-521
Nicotinex, 1162
nicotinic acid, 1162-1164
Nicotrol, 519
Nico-Vert, 678
Nidryl, 591
nifedipine, 254-255
Niferex, 856
Niferex-150, 856
Nilandron, 934
Nilstat, 43, 1125
nilutamide, 934-935
Nimbex, 566
nimodipine, 1250
Nimotop, 1250

Nipent, 923
nisoldipine, 297-298
Nitradisc, 255
Nitro-Bid, 255
Nitro-Bid I.V., 255
Nitrocine, 255
Nitrodisc, 255
Nitro-Dur, 255
nitrofurantoin macrocrystals, 208-210
nitrofurantoin microcrystals, 208-210
nitrofurazone, 1124-1125
Nitrogard, 255
Nitrogard-SR, 255
nitrogen mustard, 895-896
nitroglycerin 255-258
Nitroglyn, 255
Nitroject, 255
Nitrol, 255
Nitrolate, 255
Nitrolingual, 255
Nitrong, 255
Nitropress, 29
nitroprusside sodium, 298-299
Nitro-Spray, 250
Nitrostat, 255, **C10**
Nitro-Time, 255
Nitrotym-plus, 246
Nivaquine, 45
Nix, 1135
nizatidine, 694-695
Nizoral, 40, 1119
Nobesine, 494
Nobesine-75, 494
Nocardiosis, sulfadiazine for, 148-149
Noctec, 391
NoDoz, 490
Nolamine, 583
Nolvadex, 935, **C10**
Nolvadex-D, 935
Nonnarcotic analgesics, 330-341
Nonsteroidal anti-inflammatory drugs, 342-365
noradrenaline acid tartrate, 547-548
Noradryl, 591
Norcept-E 1/35, 744
Norcuron, 581
Nordette, 744
Nordryl, 591
Nordryl Cough, 591
norepinephrine bitartrate, 547-548
Norethin 1/35 E, 744
Norethin 1/50 M, 745
norethindrone, 752-753
norethindrone acetate, 752-753
norfloxacin, 160-162, 1046-1047
Norfranil, 432

Norgesic, 556
Norgesic Forte, 556
norgestrel, 753-754
Norinyl 1+35, 744
Norinyl 1+50, 745
Norisodrine Aerotrol, 609
Norlestrin 21 1/50, 745
Norlestrin 21 2.5/50, 745
Norlestrin Fe 1/50, 745
Norlestrin Fe 2.5/50, 745
Norlutate, 752
Norlutin, 752
Normison, 400
Normodyne, 287
Normozide 100/25, 264
Normozide 200/25, 264
Normozide 300/25, 264
Noroxin, 160
Norpace, 227
Norpace CR, 227
Norplant System, 749
Norpramin, 428
Nor-Pred TBA, 712
Nor-Q.D., 752
Nortab, 438
Nor-Tet, 143
nortriptyline hydrochloride, 438-439, **C10**
Nortussin, 623
Norvasc, 246, **C10**
Norvir, 182
Norwich Aspirin Extra Strength, 333
Norzine, 687
Nosebleed, epinephrine for, 1103-1104
Nostril, 1107
Nostrilla, 1106
Noten, 266
Novafed, 550
Novafed A, 583
Novahistine Elixir, 583, **C10**
Novamine, 1176
Novamoxin, 77
Novantrone, 951
Nova Rectal, 396
Novasen, 333
Novo-Alprazol, 449
Novo Ampicillin, 78
Novo-AZT, 188
Novo-Butamide, 778
Novocain, 1264t
Novo-Captopril, 271
Novocarbamaz, 403
Novo-Chlorhydrate, 391
Novochlorocap, 200
Novo-Chlorpromazine, 462
Novoclopate, 452
Novo-Cloxin, 84
Novocolchicine, 1183
Novodigoxin, 217
Novo-Dimenate, 678
Novodipam, 453
Novodipiradol, 323
Novo-Doxepin, 430

Novo-Doxylin, 137
Novoferrogluc, 852
Novoferrosulfa, 853
Novoflupam, 395
Novo-Flurazine, 485
Novofolacid, 1160
Novofumar, 851
Novo-Furan, 208
Novogesic C8, 367
Novohexidyl, 512
Novo-Hydrazide, 819
Novohydroxyzin, 456
Novo-Hylazin, 285
Novo-Keto-EC, 352
Novo-Lexin, 130
Novolin 70/30, 761, 771
Novolin 70/30 PenFill, 771
Novolin L, 771
Novolin N, 771
Novolin N PenFill, 771
Novolin R, 771
Novolin R PenFill, 771
Novo-Lorazem, 457
Novomedopa, 291
Novomethacin, 350
Novo-Methacin, 350
Novometoprol, 293
Novo-Naprox, 359
Novo-Naprox Sodium, 359
Novonidazol, 26
Novonifedin, 254
Novopentobarb, 396
NovoPen-VK, 97
Novo-Peridol, 469
Novopheniram, 587
Novo-Pindol, 301
Novo-Pirocam, 362
Novopoxide, 451
Novopramine, 432
Novopranol, 258
Novo-prednisone, 714
Novo-Profen, 348
Novo-Propamide, 764
Novopropoxyn, 386
Novoquinidin, 240
Novoreserpine, 306
Novo-Ridazine, 482
Novo-rythro, 195
Novosecobarb, 398
Novosemide, 817
Novosorbide, 250
Novo-Soxazole, 150
Novospiroton, 826
Novo-Sundac, 363
Novo-Tamoxifen, 935
Novo-Tetra, 143
Novo-Thalidone, 814
Novotrimel DS, 146
Novo-Triolam, 401
Novo-Tripramine, 446
Novotriptyn, 423
Novo-Veramil, 260
Novoveramil, 260
Novoxapam, 461

NP-27, 1130
NPH, 771-774
NPH Insulin, 771
NPH Purified Pork, 771
NTS, 255
NTZ Long Acting Nasal, 1106
Nu-Alpraz, 449
Nu-Amoxi, 77
Nu-Ampi, 78
Nu-Atenol, 266
Nubain, 381
Nu-Cal, 832
Nu-Cephalex, 130
Nu-Cloxi, 84
Nu-Cotrimox, 146
Nuelin, 618
Nuelin-SR, 618
Nu-Iron, 856
Nu-Iron-150, 856
Nu-Loraz, 457
Nulytely, 673
Nu-Medopa, 291
Nu-Metop, 293
Nu-Naprox, 359
Nu-Nifed, 254
Nu-Pen VK, 97
Nuprin Caplets, 348
Nuprin Tablets, 348
Nurofen, 348
Nuromax, 568
Nursing process, drug therapy
    and, 21-24
Nu-Tetra, 143
Nutracort, 1152
Nu-Triazo, 401
Nutritional support, amino
    acid solutions for,
    1176-1178
Nutropin, 799
Nu-Verap, 260
Nydrazid, 59
nystatin, 43-44, 1125-1126
Nystat-Rx, 43
Nystex, 43
Nytol Maximum Strength, 591
Nytol with DPH, 591

O
Obe-Mar, 501
Obe-Nix, 501
Obephen, 501
Obesity
    amphetamine for, 488-489
    benzphetamine for, 489-490
    dexfenfluramine for,
        491-493
    dextroamphetamine for,
        493-494
    diethylpropion for, 494-495
    fenfluramine for, 497-498
    methamphetamine for,
        498-499
    phentermine for, 501-502

Obsessive-compulsive
    disorder
    clomipramine for, 427-428
    fluoxetine for, 431-432
    fluvoxamine for, 515-516
    sertraline for, 443-444
Obstetric amnesia, scopo-
    lamine for, 538-540
Oby-Trim, 501
OCL, 673
Octamide, 682
Octamide PFS, 682
octreotide acetate, 659-660
OcuClear, 1079
Ocufen Liquifilm, 1057
Ocuflox, 1047
Ocular hypertension
    betaxolol for, 1082-1083
    carteolol for, 1084-1085
    dorzolamide for, 1086-1087
    latanoprost for, 1089-1090
    levobunolol for, 1090-1091
    metipranolol for, 1092-1093
    timolol for, 1094-1095
Ocu-Mycin, 1043
Ocupress Ophthalmic Solution
    1%, 1084
Ocusert Pilo, 1069
Ocu-Sul-10, 1049
Ocu-Sul-15, 1049
Ocu-Sul-30, 1049
oestradiol, 736-738
oestradiol valerate, 736-738
oestrogens, conjugated,
    738-741
ofloxacin, 162-163
ofloxacin 0.3%, 1047
Ogen, 741, **C10**
olanzapine, 475-476
Oliguria, mannitol for,
    822-824
olsalazine sodium, 1251
omeprazole, 695-696
Omnipen, 78
Omnipen-N, 78
OMS Concentrate, 379
Oncaspar, 954
Oncovin, 965
ondansetron hydrochloride,
    684-685
Onychomycosis, itraconazole
    for, 39-40
o,p'-DDD, 950-951
Open-heart surgery, heparin
    for, 860-863
Ophthaine, 1266t
Ophthalmia neonatorum
    erythromycin for,
        1042-1043
    silver nitrate 1% for,
        1048-1049
Ophthalmic anti-infectives,
    1039-1053
Ophthalmic anti-inflammatory
    drugs, 1054-1061

Ophthalmics, miscellaneous, 1081-1095
Ophthalmic vasoconstrictors, 1078-1080
Ophthetic, 1266t
Ophthoclor Ophthalmic, 1040
Opiate addiction, lev-omethadyl for, 1245-1246
Opioid analgesics, 366-389
opium tincture, 660-661
opium tincture, camphorated, 660-661
Optazine, 1078
Optigene, 1080
Optimine, 584
Optimyd, 1039
OptiPranolol, 1092
Orabase HCA, 1152
Oral medications, children and, 15
Oramide, 778
Oraminic II, 585
Oramorph SR, 379
Orap, 478
Oraphen-PD, 331
Orasone, 714, **C11**
Orbenin, 84
Orbenin Injection, 84
Oretic, 819
Oreton Methyl, 721
Organic mental syndrome, mesoridazine for, 472-474
Organophosphate poisoning, pralidoxime for, 1219-1220
Orgaran, 858
Orimune, 998
Orinase, 778
ORLAAM, 1245
Ormazine, 462
Ornade Spansules, 583
Ornex Cold, 550
Ornex-DM 15, 622
Ornex-DM 30, 622
Ornex No Drowsiness Caplets, 330
Oroxine, 781
Ortho-Cept, 744
Orthoclone OKT3, 973
Ortho Cyclen, 745
Ortho Dienestrol, 731
OrthoEST, 741
Ortho-Novum 1/35, 744
Ortho-Novum 1/50, 745
Ortho-Novum 7/7/7, 745
Ortho-Novum 10/11, 744
Orthopedic manipulations, tubocurarine for, 580-581
Orthostatic hypotension, midodrine for, 324-325
Ortho Tri-Cyclen, 745
Or-Tyl, 533
Orudis, 352

Orudis-E, 352
Orudis KT, 352
Orudis-SR, 352
Oruvail, 352, **C11**
Os-Cal, 832
Os-Cal 500, 832
Os-Cal Chewable, 832
Osmitrol, 822
Osteitis deformans. See Paget's disease of bone.
Osteoarthritis
  aspirin for, 333-335
  choline magnesium trisalicylate for, 335-337
  choline salicylate for, 337-338
  diclofenac for, 342-344
  diflunisal for, 338-339
  etodolac for, 344-345
  fenoprofen calcium for, 345-346
  flurbiprofen for, 346-348
  ibuprofen for, 348-349
  indomethacin for, 349-352
  ketoprofen for, 352-353
  meclofenamate for, 355-356
  nabumetone for, 358
  naproxen for, 359-360
  oxaprozin for, 360-362
  piroxicam for, 362-363
  sulindac for, 363-364
  tolmetin for, 364-365
Osteoporosis
  alendronate for, 1228-1229
  calcitonin for, 803-804
  estrogens, conjugated, for, 738-741
  estropipate for, 741-742
Osteosarcoma, methotrexate for, 911-914
Otics, 1096-1098
Otitis media
  amoxicillin/clavulanate for, 75-76
  bacampicillin for, 81-82
  cefaclor for, 105-106
  cefixime for, 110-111
  cefpodoxime for, 120-121
  cefprozil for, 121-122
  ceftibuten for, 124-125
  cefuroxime for, 128-130
  cephalexin for, 130-131
  cephradine for, 133-134
  clarithromycin for, 192-193
  co-trimoxazole for, 146-148
  loracarbef for, 134-135
Otrivin, 1110
Ovarian cancer
  altretamine for, 937-938
  amifostine for, 938-939
  carboplatin for, 884-886
  cisplatin for, 888-890
  cyclophosphamide for, 890-892
  doxorubicin for, 919-921

Ovarian cancer (continued)
  hydroxyurea for, 909-910
  melphalan for, 896-898
  paclitaxel for, 952-954
  thiotepa for, 899-900
  topotecan for, 960-962
Ovcon-35, 744
Ovcon-50, 744
Ovol, 649
Ovol-40, 649
Ovol-80, 649
Ovral, 745
Ovrette, 753
Ovulation induction, clomiphene for, 1236-1237
oxacillin sodium, 89-90
oxaprozin, 360-362
oxazepam, 461
oxiconazole nitrate, 1126
Oxistat, 1126
Ox-Pam, 461
Oxsoralen, 1248
oxtriphylline, 613-614
oxybutynin chloride, 1198-1199
Oxycocet, 367
Oxycodan, 367
oxycodone hydrochloride, 383-384
oxycodone pectinate, 383-384
Oxydess II, 493
oxymetazoline hydrochloride, 1079-1080, 1106-1107
oxymorphone hydrochloride, 384-385
oxytetracycline hydrochloride, 142-143
Oxytocics, 1192-1197
Oxytocin, 1195
oxytocin, synthetic injection, 1195-1196
oxytocin, synthetic nasal solution, 1197
Oysco, 832
Oysco 500 Chewable, 832
Oyst-Cal 500, 832
Oyst-Cal 500 Chewable, 832
Oystercal 500, 832
Oyster Shell Calcium-500, 832

P
paclitaxel, 952-954
P-A-C Tablets, 330
Paget's disease of bone
  alendronate for, 1228-1229
  calcitonin for, 803-804
  etidronate for, 806-807
  pamidronate for, 1251-1252
Pain
  acetaminophen for, 330-333
  aspirin for, 333-335
  buprenorphine for, 368-369
  butorphanol for, 369-371
  capsaicin for, 1234-1235

Pain *(continued)*
  choline magnesium trisalicylate for, 335-337
  choline salicylate for, 337-338
  codeine for, 371-372
  diflunisal for, 338-339
  etodolac for, 344-345
  fentanyl for, 372-375
  hydromorphone for, 375-376
  ibuprofen for, 348-349
  ketoprofen for, 352-353
  ketorolac for, 354-355
  magnesium salicylate for, 339-340
  meclofenamate for, 355-356
  mefenamic acid for, 356-357
  meperidine for, 376-378
  methadone for, 378-379
  morphine for, 379-381
  nalbuphine for, 381-383
  naproxen for, 359-360
  oxycodone for, 383-384
  oxymorphone for, 384-385
  pentazocine for, 385-386
  propoxyphene for, 386-387
  tramadol for, 388-389
Palafer, 851
Palafer Pediatric Drops, 851
2-PAM, 1219-1220
Pamelor, 438, **C11**
pamidronate sodium, 1251-1252
Pamprin-IB, 348
Panadol, 331
Panadol, Children's, 331
Panadol Extra Strength, 331
Panadol, Infants', 331
Panadol Junior Strength Caplets, 331
Panadol Maximum Strength Caplets, 331
Panadol Maximum Strength Tablets, 331
Panafcort, 714
Panafcortelone, 711
Panamax, 331
Panasol, 714
Pancrease Capsules, 650
Pancrease Capsules, 652
Pancrease MT 4, 652
Pancrease MT 10, 652
Pancrease MT 16, 652
Pancrease MT 20, 652
Pancreatic cancer
  fluorouracil for, 907-909
  gemcitabine for, 947-948
  streptozocin for, 898-899
Pancreatic enzyme deficiency
  pancreatin for, 651-652
  pancrelipase for, 652-654
Pancreatic insufficiency
  pancreatin for, 651-652
  pancrelipase for, 652-654

pancreatin, 651-652
pancrelipase, 652-654
Pancrelipase Capsules, 652
Pancrezyme 4X Tablets, 651
pancuronium bromide, 573-575
Panex, 331
Panex-500, 331
Panic disorder
  alprazolam for, 449-450
  paroxetine for, 439-440
Panmycin, 143
Panmycin P, 143
Panshape M, 501
Pantheline, 537
Panwarfin, 863
papaverine hydrochloride, 326-327
para-amino salicylate, 52-53
paracetamol, 330-333
Paraflex, 558
Parafon Forte DSC, 558
Paralgin, 331
Paraplatin, 884
Paraplatin-AQ, 884
Paraspen, 331
Parasympathomimetics, 524-532
Parathyroid-like drugs, 802-807
paregoric, 660-661
Parenteral nutrition, children and, 16-17
Parepectolin, 656
Parkinsonism
  benztropine for, 503-504
  biperiden for, 504-505
  bromocriptine for, 505-506
  carbidopa-levodopa for, 506-508
  diphenhydramine for, 591-593
  levodopa for, 508-510
  pergolide for, 510-511
  selegiline for, 511-512
  trihexyphenidyl for, 512-513
Parlodel, 505
Parnate, 444
paromomycin sulfate, 28-29
paroxetine hydrochloride, 439-440
Parvolex, 624
PAS, 52-53
Patent ductus arteriosus
  alprostadil for, 322-323
  indomethacin for, 349-352
Pathocil, 85
Patient noncompliance, 20
Patient teaching, drug use and, 11-12
Pavabid, 326
Pavabid HP, 326
Pavabid Plateau, 326
Pavacels, 326
Pavagen, 326

Pavarine, 326
Pavased, 326
Pavasule, 326
Pavatine, 326
Pavatym, 326
Paveral, 371
Paverolan Lanacaps, 326
Pavulon, 573
Paxil, 439, **C11**
PCE Dispertab, 195, **C11**
P$_1$E$_1$, 1062
P$_2$E$_1$, 1062
P$_3$E$_1$, 1062
P$_4$E$_1$, 1062
P$_6$E$_1$, 1062
PediaCare Infants' Decongestant, 550
PediaCare Infants' Oral Decongestant Drops, 550
Pediaflor, 1173
Pediapred, 711
PediaProfen, 348
Pediatric dosages, calculating, 14-15
Pediatric Multiple Trace Element, 1156
Pediazole, 146
Pediculicides, 1132-1136
Pediculosis
  benzyl benzoate lotion for, 1132-1133
  lindane for, 1134-1135
Pedi-Dent, 1173
Pedtrace-4, 1156
PedvaxHIB, 983
pegaspargase, 954-956
PEG-L-asparaginase, 954-956
Pellagra, niacin for, 1162-1164
Pelvic inflammatory disease
  clindamycin for, 202-203
  doxycycline for, 137-140
  erythromycin for, 195-197
  ofloxacin for, 162-163
  piperacillin and tazobactam for, 100-101
pemoline, 500-501
Penbritin, 78
penbutolol sulfate, 299-300
Penecort, 1152
Penetrex, 155
Penglobe, 81
penicillin G benzathine, 91-92
penicillin G potassium, 92-94
penicillin G procaine, 94-95
penicillin G sodium, 95-97
Penicillins, 75-104
penicillin V, 97-98
penicillin V potassium, 97-98
Pentacarinat, 29
Pentam 300, 29
pentamidine isethionate, 29-30
Pentamycetin, 200, 1040
Pentasa, 1246

Pentazine, 594
pentazocine hydrochloride, 385-386
pentazocine hydrochloride and naloxone hydrochloride, 385-386
pentazocine lactate, 385-386
pentobarbital, 396-398
pentobarbital sodium, 396-398
pentobarbitone, 396-398
pentostatin, 923-925
pentoxifylline, 327
Pen Vee, 97
Pen Vee K, 97
Pepcid, 691, **C11**
Pepcid AC, 691
Pepcidine, 691
Peptic ulcer disease
    atropine for, 224-225
    glycopyrrolate for, 534-536
    hyoscyamine for, 536-537
    propantheline for, 537-538
Pepto-Bismol, 657
Pepto Diarrhea Control, 658
Percocet, 367, **C11**
Percodan, 367
Percodan-Demi, 367
Percodan-Roxiprin, 367
Percutaneous transluminal coronary angioplasty, abciximab for, 1225-1227
Perdiem Fiber, 674
pergolide mesylate, 510-511
Pergonal, 758
Periactin, 589
Peri-Colace-Capsules, 662
Peri-Colace-Syrup, 662
Peridol, 469
Peripheral vascular disease
    isoxsuprine for, 324
    papaverine for, 326-327
Peritonitis
    meropenem for, 205-207
    piperacillin and tazobactam for, 100-101
Permapen, 91
Permax, 510
permethrin, 1135
Permitil, 467
Permitil Concentrate, 467
Pernicious anemia, cyanocobalamin for, 1158-1160
perphenazine, 476-478
Persantin, 323
Persantin 100, 323
Persantine, 323
Pertofran, 428
Pertofrane, 428
Pertussin All-Night CS, 622
Pertussin Cough Suppressant, 622
Pertussin CS, 622
Pertussin ES, 622

pethidine hydrochloride, 376-378
Petrogalar Plain, 671
Pfeiffer's Allergy, 587
Pfizerpen, 92
Pharmaflur, 1173
Pharmaflur 1.1, 1173
Pharmaflur df, 1173
Pharyngitis
    azithromycin for, 191-192
    cefadroxil for, 106-107
    cefixime for, 110-111
    cefpodoxime for, 120-121
    cefprozil for, 121-122
    ceftibuten for, 124-125
    cefuroxime for, 128-130
    clarithromycin for, 192-193
    dirithromycin for, 193-194
    loracarbef for, 134-135
Phazyme, 649
Phazyme 55, 649
Phazyme 95, 649
Phenameth, 594
Phenaphen-650 with Codeine, 367
Phenazine 25, 594
Phenazo, 1199
Phenazodine, 1199
phenazopyridine hydrochloride, 1199-1200
Phencen-50, 594
Phendry, 591
Phendry Children's Allergy Medicine, 591
phenelzine sulfate, 440-441
Phenerbel-S, 552
Phenergan, 594
Phenergan Fortis, 594
Phenergan Plain, 594
Phenetron, 587
phenobarbital, 414-416
phenobarbital sodium, 414-416
phenobarbitone, 414-416
phenobarbitone sodium, 414-416
Phenoject-50, 594
Phenolax Wafers, 672
phenolphthalein, white, 672-673
phenolphthalein, yellow, 672-673
phenoxymethylpenicillin, 97-98
phenoxymethylpenicillin potassium, 97-98
phensuximide, 416-417
Phentercot, 501
phentermine hydrochloride, 501-502
phentolamine mesylate, 300-301
Phentride, 501
Phentride Caplets, 501
Phentrol, 501

Phentrol-2, 501
Phentrol-4, 501
Phentrol-5, 501
phenylazo diamino pyridine hydrochloride, 1199-1200
phenylephrine hydrochloride, 548-550, 1075-1076, 1107-1108
Phenytex, 417
phenytoin, 417-419
phenytoin sodium, 417-419
phenytoin sodium (extended), 417-419
Pheochromocytoma
    phentolamine for, 300-301
    propranolol for, 258-260
Phillips' Milk of Magnesia, 669
Phos-Ex, 832
Phos-Flur, 1173
Phos-Lo, 832
Phosphaljel, 645
Phospholine Iodide, 1065
phosphonoformic acid, 173-175
Phosphorus, reducing fecal elimination of, aluminum phosphate for, 645
Photofrin, 956
Phrenilin, 330
Phrenilin Forte, 330
Phyllocontin, 599
Phyllocontin-350, 599
Physeptone, 378
physostigmine salicylate, 529-530
physostigmine sulfate, 1068-1069
phytonadione, 1171-1173
Pilagan, 1069
Pilocar, 1069
pilocarpine, 1069-1070
pilocarpine hydrochloride, 1069-1070, 1252-1253
pilocarpine nitrate, 1069-1070
Pilocel, 1069
Pilopine HS, 1069
Pilopt, 1069
Pima, 789
pimozide, 478-479
pindolol, 301-302
Pink Bismuth, 657
Pinworm
    mebendazole for, 31
    pyrantel for, 31-32
pipecuronium bromide, 575-576
piperacillin sodium, 98-100
piperacillin sodium and tazobactam sodium, 100-101
piperazine estrone sulfate, 741-742
Pipracil, 98
Pipril, 98

pirbuterol, 614-615
Piriton, 587
piroxicam, 362-363
Pitocin, 1195
Pitressin, 800
Pituitary hormones, 794-801
Pituitary trauma, desmopressin for, 797-798
Placidyl, 394
plague vaccine, 996-997
Plaquenil, 46
Plasbumin 5%, 866
Plasbumin 25%, 866
Plasmanate, 872
Plasma-Plex, 872
plasma protein fraction, 872-873
Plasmatein, 872
Plasma volume expansion
  dextran, high molecular weight, for, 836-837
  dextran, low molecular weight, for, 835-836
  hetastarch for, 838
Platamine, 888
Platinol, 888
Platinol AQ, 888
Plendil, 279
Plendil ER, 279
Pleural effusion, bleomycin for, 915-916
plicamycin, 925-926
PMB-200, 729
PMB-400, 729
PMS-Amitriptyline, 423
PMS Benztropine, 503
PMS-Carbamazepine, 403
PMS-Diazepam, 453
PMS-Dimenhydrinate, 678
PMS Ferrous Sulfate, 853
PMS Isoniazid, 59
PMS-Methylphenidate, 499
PMS Metronidazole, 26
PMS Perphenazine, 476
PMS Primidone, 419
PMS Prochlorperazine, 685
PMS-Promethazine, 594
pms Propranolol, 258
PMS Sulfasalazine E.C., 1257
PMS Thioridazine, 482
pneumococcal vaccine, polyvalent, 997-998
Pneumocystis carinii pneumonia
  atovaquone for, 25
  clindamycin for, 202-203
  pentamidine for, 29-30
  trimetrexate for, 213-214
Pneumonia
  acetylcysteine for, 624-625
  azithromycin for, 191-192
  bacitracin for, 199-200
  cefepime for, 108-110
  cefpodoxime for, 120-121
  clarithromycin for, 192-193

Pneumonia *(continued)*
  dirithromycin for, 193-194
  erythromycin for, 195-197
  levofloxacin for, 156-158
  loracarbef for, 134-135
  penicillin G procaine for, 94-95
  piperacillin and tazobactam for, 100-101
  sparfloxacin for, 163-165
Pneumopent, 29
Pneumovax 23, 997
Pnu-Imune 23, 997
Point-Two, 1173
Poisoning, activated charcoal for, 1204-1205
Poladex, 590
Poladex T.D., 590
Polaramine, 590
Polaramine Repetabs, 590
Polargen, 590
Poliovax, 998
poliovirus vaccine, inactivated, 998-999
poliovirus vaccine, live, oral, trivalent, 998-999
Polycillin, 78
Polycillin-N, 78
Polycillin-PRB, 75
Polycythemia vera
  mechlorethamine for, 895-896
  uracil mustard for, 901
polyethylene glycol and electrolyte solution, 673-674
Polymox, 77
polymyxin B sulfate, 210-211, 1048
Polyneuritis, riboflavin for, 1165-1166
polysaccharide iron complex, 856
Polysporin Ointment, 1111
Polysporin Ophthalmic Ointment, 1039
Polytrim Ophthalmic, 1039
Ponderal, 497
Ponderal Pacaps, 497
Ponderax, 497
Ponderax Pacaps, 497
Pondimin, 497
Pondimin Extentabs, 497
Ponstan, 356
Ponstel, 356
Pontocaine, 1266t
Pontocaine Eye Ointment, Solution, 1266t
porfimer sodium, 956-958
Pork NPH Iletin II, 771
Pork Regular Iletin II, 771
Porphyria, chlorpromazine for, 462-465
Portalac, 668

Postanesthesia respiratory stimulation, doxapram for, 495-497
Postpartum bleeding
  carboprost for, 1192-1193
  methylergonovine for, 1194-1195
  oxytocin, synthetic injection, for, 1195-1196
Posture, 832
potassium acetate, 840-841
potassium bicarbonate, 841-842
potassium chloride, 842-843, **C11**
potassium gluconate, 843-844
potassium iodide, 789-790
potassium iodide, saturated solution, 789-790
Potassium-Rougier, 843
PPD, 1280-1281t
PPD-stabilized Solution, 1280t
pralidoxime chloride, 1219-1220
Pramin, 682
Pravachol, 319, **C11**
pravastatin sodium, 319-320
prazosin hydrochloride, 302-303
Precocious puberty
  histrelin for, 757-758
  leuprolide for, 932-933
  nafarelin for, 760
Precose, 761
Predalone TBA, 712
Predate-S, 711
Predate TBA, 712
Predcor TBA, 712
Pred-Forte, 1059
Pred-G S.O.P., 1039
Predicort RP, 711
Pred Mild Ophthalmic, 1059
Prednicen-M, 714
prednisolone, 711-714
Prednisolone Acetate and Prednisolone Sodium Phosphate, 699
prednisolone acetate (suspension), 1059-1060
prednisolone sodium phosphate, 711-714
prednisolone sodium phosphate (solution), 1059-1060
prednisolone steaglate, 712-714
prednisolone tebutate, 712-714
prednisone, 714-715
Prednisone Intensol, 714
Predsol Eye Drops, 1059
Predsol Retention Enema, 711-712

Predsol Suppositories, 712
Preeclampsia, magnesium
  salts for, 412-413,
  838-840
Prefrin-A, 1078
Prefrin Liquifilm, 1075
Pregnancy
  drugs and, 10-11
  Rh₀(D) immune globulin
    for, 1017-1019
Prelone, 711
Premarin, 738, **C12**
Premarin Intravenous, 738
Premarin with Methyltestos-
  terone, 718
Prepidil, 1193
Presolol, 287
Prevacid, 692
Prevalite, 313
PreviDent, 1173
Priadel, 516
Prilosec, 695, **C12**
Primacor, 219
primaquine phosphate, 49-50
Primary ovarian failure
  esterified estrogens for,
    734-736
  estradiol for, 736-738
  estrogens, conjugated, for,
    738-741
  estropipate for, 741-742
Primatene Mist, 604
Primatene Mist Suspension,
  604
Primaxin IM, 204
Primaxin IV, 204
Primazine, 479
primidone, 419-420
Primogyn Depot, 736
Principen, 78
Principen-250, 78
Principen-500, 78
Principen with Probenecid, 75
Prinivil, 289, **C12**
Prinzide 10-12.5, 264
Prinzide 20-12.5, 264
Prinzide 20-25, 264
Priscoline, 329
Privine, 1106
Pro-50, 594
ProAmatine, 324
Probalan, 1185
Pro-Banthine, 537
Probate, 458
Proben-C, 1182
probenecid, 1185-1187
Probenecid with Colchicine,
  1182
Procainamide Durules, 237
procainamide hydrochloride,
  237-239
procaine hydrochloride,
  1264-1265t
ProcalAmine with electrolytes,
  1176

Pro-Cal-Sof, 666
Procanbid, 237
Procan SR, 237
procarbazine hydrochloride,
  958-959
Procardia, 254
Procardia XL, 254, **C12**
prochlorperazine, 685-687
prochlorperazine edisylate,
  685-687
prochlorperazine maleate,
  685-687
Procrit, 1024
Proctitis
  hydrocortisone for, 706-709
  mesalamine for, 1246-1247
  prednisolone for, 711-714
  spectinomycin for, 211-212
Proctocort, 1152
Proctofoam-HC, 1152
Procytox, 890
Pro-Depo, 748
Prodiem Plain, 674
Prodium, 1199
Prodrox 250, 748
Profenal, 1061
Profilate OSD, 867
Profilnine Heat-Treated, 871
progesterone, 754-755
Progestilin, 754
Progestins, 729-755
Prograf, 975
ProHIBIT, 982
Proladone, 383
Prolastin, 625
Pro-Lax, 674
Proleukin, 1022
Prolixin, 467
Prolixin Concentrate, 467
Prolixin Decanoate, 467
Prolixin Enanthate, 467
Proloprim, 212
promazine hydrochloride,
  479-481
Prometh-25, 594
Prometh-50, 594
promethazine hydrochloride,
  594-595
promethazine theoclate,
  594-595
Promethegan, 594
Promine, 237
Pronestyl, 237
Pronestyl-SR, 237
Pronto, 1136
propafenone hydrochloride,
  239-240
Propanthel, 537
propantheline bromide,
  537-538
proparacaine hydrochloride,
  1266-1267t
Propine, 1085
Propion, 494
Proplex T, 871

Pro Pox with APAP, 366-367
propoxyphene hydrochloride,
  386-387
propoxyphene napsylate,
  386-387
propoxyphene napsylate with
  acetaminiophen, **C12**
propranolol hydrochloride,
  258-260
Propulsid, 1235, **C12**
propylthiouracil, 790-791
Propyl-Thyracil, 790
Prorazin, 685
Prorex-25, 594
Prorex-50, 594
Proscar, 1240
Prosed/DS, 198
Pro-Sof, 666
Pro-Sof Liquid Concentrate,
  666
Pro-Sof Liquid Plus, 666
ProSom, 393
Pro-Span, 748
Prostaphlin, 89
Prostate cancer
  bicalutamide for, 927-928
  chlorotrianisene for,
    729-731
  diethylstilbestrol for,
    732-734
  esterified estrogens for,
    734-736
  estradiol for, 736-738
  estrogens, conjugated, for,
    738-741
  ethinyl estradiol for,
    742-744
  flutamide for, 929-930
  goserelin for, 930-932
  leuprolide for, 932-933
  mitoxantrone for, 951
  nilutamide for, 934-935
Prostatitis
  carbenicillin indanyl sodium
    for, 83-84
  ciprofloxacin for, 153-154
  ofloxacin for, 162-163
ProStep, 519
Prosthetic heart valves,
  platelet adhesion in,
  dipyridamole for, 323-324
Prostigmin, 528
Prostin E₂, 1193
Prostin VR Pediatric, 322
protamine sulfate, 1220-1221
Protamine Zinc Insulin MC,
  771
protamine zinc suspension,
  771-774
Protaphane HM, 771
Protaphane HM Penfill, 771
Protaphane MC, 771
Protenate, 872
Prothazine, 594
Prothazine Plain, 594

t refers to a table; **boldface** refers to full-color photographs

Protilase Capsules, 652
Protopam Chloride, 1219
Protostat, 26
Protrin, 146
Pro-Trin, 146
Protrin DF, 146
protriptyline hydrochloride, 441-443
Protropin, 798
Proventil, 597
Proventil Repetabs, 597
Provera, 751, **C12**
Prozac, 431, **C12**
Prozac-20, 431
Prozine-50, 479
PRP-D, 982-984
PRP-OMP, 983-984
Prulet, 672
Pruritus
    cyproheptadine for, 589-590
    dexchlorpheniramine for, 590-591
    fluticasone for, 1149
    hydroxyzine for, 456-457
Pseudo, 550
pseudoephedrine hydrochloride, 550-551
pseudoephedrine sulfate, 550-551
Pseudofrin, 550
Pseudo-gest, 550
Pseudohypoparathyroidism, calcitriol for, 804-805
Psittacosis
    chloramphenicol for, 200-202
    demeclocycline for, 136-137
    doxycycline for, 137-140
    minocycline for, 140-141
    oxytetracycline for, 142-143
    tetracycline for, 143-145
Psorcon, 1144
Psoriasis
    calcipotriene for, 1234
    etretinate for, 1238-1240
    methotrexate for, 911-914
    methoxsalen for, 1248-1249
Psorion, 1138
Psychiatric emergencies, hydroxyzine for, 456-457
Psychotic disorders
    chlorpromazine for, 462-465
    fluphenazine for, 467-469
    haloperidol for, 469-471
    loxapine for, 471-472
    molindone for, 474-475
    olanzapine for, 475-476
    perphenazine for, 476-478
    prochlorperazine for, 685-687
    promazine for, 479-481
    risperidone for, 481-482

Psychotic disorders (continued)
    thioridazine for, 482-484
    thiothixene for, 484-485
    trifluoperazine for, 485-487
psyllium, 674-675
P.T.E.-4, 1156-1157
P.T.E.-5, 1157
PTU, 790-791
Puberty, delayed, fluoxymesterone for, 719-721
Pulmonary complications, acetylcysteine for, 624-625
Pulmonary disease, hypercapnia-associated, doxapram for, 495-497
Pulmonary edema
    ethacrynate for, 816-817
    furosemide for, 817-819
Pulmonary embolism
    alteplase for, 874-875
    enoxaparin for, 859-860
    heparin for, 860-863
    papaverine for, 326-327
    streptokinase for, 878-881
    urokinase for, 881-882
    warfarin for, 863-865
Pulmonary hypertension
    epoprostenol for, 634-636
    tolazoline for, 329
Pulmozyme, 633
Purge, 665
Purinethol, 910
Purinol, 1182
P.V., 1069
PVF K, 97
PVK, 97
P-V-Tussin Syrup, 583
Pyelonephritis
    cefepime for, 108-110
    levofloxacin for, 156-158
    loracarbef for, 134-135
Pyranistan, 587
pyrantel pamoate, 31-32
pyrazinamide, 61-62
Pyrazinamide, 61
Pyrazodine, 1199
pyrethrins, 1136
Pyridiate, 1199
Pyridin, 1199
pyridine-2-aldoxime methochloride, 1219-1220
Pyridium, 1199
pyridostigmine bromide, 530-532
pyridoxine hydrochloride, 1164-1165
pyrimethamine, 50-51
pyrimethamine with sulfadoxine, 50-51
Pyrinyl, 1136
Pyronium, 1200
PZI, 771-774

Q
quazepam, 398
Quelicin, 578
Questran, 313
Questran Light, 313
Questran Lite, 313
Quibron Capsules, 597
Quibron-T/SR, 618
Quick Pep, 490
Quiess, 456
Quinaglute Dura-Tabs, 240
Quinalan, 240
quinapril hydrochloride, 303-304
Quinate, 240
Quinidex Extentabs, 240
quinidine bisulfate, 240-242
quinidine gluconate, 240-242
quinidine polygalacturonate, 240-242
quinidine sulfate, 240-242
Quinora, 240

R
RA 27/3, 1002-1003
Rabies exposure, rabies immune globulin, human, for, 1015-1016
rabies immune globulin, human, 1015-1016
rabies vaccine, adsorbed, 999-1000
rabies vaccine, human diploid cell, 1000-1001
Racepinephrine, 604
radioactive iodine, 791-793
Radiologic examination, glucagon for, 768-769
Radiostol, 1169
Radiostol Forte, 1169
Rafen, 348
Ramace, 304
ramipril, 304-306
ranitidine hydrochloride, 696-697
Rattlesnake bite, Crotalidae antivenin, polyvalent, for, 1008-1009
Rauzide, 264-265
Raynaud's disease, isoxsuprine for, 324
R&C, 1136
Reclomide, 682
Recombivax HB, 985
Recommended daily allowances. See specific vitamin.
Rectal examination
    bisacodyl for, 662-663
    cascara sagrada for, 664-665
    castor oil for, 665-666
    senna for, 675-676

Rectal infections
doxycycline for, 137-140
erythromycin for, 195-197
minocycline for, 140-141
sulfisoxazole for, 150-152
tetracycline for, 143-145
Redoxon, 1167
Redutemp, 331
Redux, 491
Reese's Pinworm Medicine,
31
Regional anesthesia, phenyle-
phrine for, 548-550
Regitine, 300
Reglan, 682
Regonol, 530
Regroton, 265
Regular (Concentrated) Iletin
II, 771
Regular Iletin I, 771
regular insulin, 771-774
Regular Purified Pork Insulin,
771
Regulax SS, 666
Regulex, 666
Reguloid Natural, 674
Regutol, 666
Rela, 557
Relafen, 358, **C12**
Remeron, 435
Remular-S, 558
Renal calculi formation,
preventing, aluminum
carbonate for, 642-643
Renal cell carcinoma,
aldesleukin for,
1022-1024
Renal osteodystrophy, vitamin
D for, 1169-1170
RenAmin, 1176
Renedil, 279
Renese-R, 265
Renitec, 277
Renova, 1259
ReoPro, 1225
Repan, 330
Replacement solutions,
844-846
repository corticotropin,
794-796
Rep-pred 40, 709
Rep-pred 80, 709
reserpine, 306-307
Resonium A, 1221
Respbid, 618
RespiGam, 1016
Respiratory distress
syndrome
beractant for, 627-629
colfosceril for, 629-631
Respiratory drugs, miscella-
neous, 624-641
Respiratory syncytial virus,
ribavirin for, 180-181

respiratory syncytial virus
immune globulin intra-
venous, human,
1016-1017
Respiratory tract infections
amoxicillin/clavulanate for,
75-76
aztreonam for, 198-199
bacampicillin for, 81-82
cefaclor for, 105-106
cefazolin for, 107-108
cefmetazole for, 111-113
cefonicid for, 113-114
cefoperazone for, 114-115
cefotaxime for, 115-117
cefotetan for, 117-118
cefoxitin for, 118-119
ceftazidime for, 122-124
ceftizoxime for, 125-126
ceftriaxone for, 126-128
cefuroxime for, 128-130
cephalexin for, 130-131
cephapirin for, 131-133
cephradine for, 133-134
ciprofloxacin for, 153-154
co-trimoxazole for, 146-148
erythromycin for, 195-197
imipenem/cilastatin for,
204-205
ofloxacin for, 162-163
penicillin G benzathine for,
91-92
respiratory syncytial virus
immune globulin intra-
venous, human, for
prevention of,
1016-1017
ticarcillin/clavulanate for,
103-104
Respolin, 597
Respolin Autohaler Inhalation
Device, 597
Respolin Inhaler, 597
Respolin Respirator Solution,
597
Resprim, 146
Restore, 674
Restoril, 400
Resyl, 623
reteplase, recombinant,
877-878
Retavase, 877
Reticulum cell carcinoma,
bleomycin for, 915-916
Retin-A, 1259
Retinal angiography, fluores-
cein for, 1087-1088
retinoic acid, 1259-1260
retinol, 1157-1158
Retrovir, 188
Reversol, 526
ReVia, 1217
Revimine, 542
Rezide, 265
Rezulin, 779

Rhabdomyosarcoma
dactinomycin for, 916-917
vincristine for, 965-966
R-HCTZ-H, 265
Rheaban Maximum Strength,
656
Rheomacrodex, 835
Rheumacin, 350
Rheumatic fever
erythromycin for, 195-197
penicillin G benzathine for,
91-92
sulfadiazine for, 148-149
Rheumatoid arthritis. See also
Arthritis.
aspirin for, 333-335
auranofin for, 1201-1202
aurothioglucose for,
1202-1203
azathioprine for, 969-970
choline magnesium trisalicylate for, 335-337
choline salicylate for,
337-338
diclofenac for, 342-344
diflunisal for, 338-339
d-penicillamine for,
1211-1212
fenoprofen for, 345-346
flurbiprofen for, 346-348
gold sodium thiomalate for,
1202-1203
hydroxychloroquine for,
46-48
ibuprofen for, 348-349
indomethacin for, 349-352
ketoprofen for, 352-353
meclofenamate for, 355-356
methotrexate for, 911-914
nabumetone for, 358
naproxen for, 359-360
oxaprozin for, 360-362
piroxicam for, 362-363
sulfasalazine for, 1257-1258
sulindac for, 363-364
tolmetin for, 364-365
Rheumatrex, 911
Rh exposure, Rh$_o$(D) immune
globulin for, 1017-1019
Rhinalar Nasal Mist, 1104
Rhinall, 1107
Rhinall-10, 1107
Rhinitis
astemizole for, 584
azatadine for, 584-585
azelastine for, 1099-1100
beclomethasone for,
1100-1101
brompheniramine for,
585-586
budesonide for, 1101
cetirizine for, 586-587
chlorpheniramine for,
587-588
clemastine for, 588-589

Rhinitis *(continued)*
  cromolyn for, 631-632
  dexchlorpheniramine for, 590-591
  diphenhydramine for, 595-593
  fexofenadine for, 593
  flunisolide for, 1104-1105
  fluticasone for, 1105-1106
  ipratropium for, 607-608
  loratadine for, 593-594
  promethazine for, 594-595
  triamcinolone for, 1109-1110
Rhinocort, 1101
Rhinorrhea, ipratropium for, 607-608
Rhinosyn-DMX Expectorant, 622
$Rh_o(D)$ immune globulin, human, 1017-1019
$Rh_o(D)$ immune globulin intravenous, human, 1017-1019
Rhodis, 352
Rhodis-E, 352
Rhodis-EC, 352
RhoGAM, 1017
Rhotrimine, 446
Rhus Tox HC, 1152
ribavirin, 180-181
riboflavin, 1165-1166
Rickets, vitamin D for, 1169-1170
Rickettsial infections, chloramphenicol for, 200-202
RID, 1136
Ridaura, 1201
Ridenol Caplets, 331
rifabutin, 62-63
Rifadin, 63
Rifadin IV, 63
Rifamate, 52
rifampicin, 63-64
rifampin, 63-64
Rifater, 52
Rilutek, 1253
riluzole, 1253-1254
Rimactane, 63
Rimactane/INH Dual Pack, 52
rimantadine hydrochloride, 181-182
rimexolone, 1060-1061
Rimycin, 63
Ringer's injection, 844-845
Ringer's injection, lactated, 845
Ringer's lactate solution, 845
Ringworm infections, griseofulvin for, 38-39
Riopan, 647
Riopan Plus Chewable Tablets, 642
Riopan Plus Suspension, 642
Riphen-10, 333

Risperdal, 481
risperidone, 481-482
Ritalin, 499
Ritalin-SR, 499
ritodrine hydrochloride, 1254-1256
ritonavir, 182-184
rIFN-A, 1027-1029
RMS Uniserts, 379
Roaccutane, 1243
Robafen, 623
Robaxin, 561
Robaxin-750, 561
Robaxisal, 556
Robenecid, 1185
Robese, 493
Robicillin VK, 97
Robidex, 622
Robidrine, 550
Robigesic, 331
Robimycin, 195
Robinul, 534
Robinul Forte, 534
Robitet, 143
Robitussin, 623
Robitussin-DM, 622
Robitussin Pediatric, 622
Robomol-500, 561
Robomol-750, 561
Rocaltrol, 804
Rocephin, 126
Rocort, 1152
rocuronium bromide, 576-578
Rodex, 1164
Rofact, 63
Roferon-A, 1027
Rogaine, 1249
Rogitine, 300
Rolaids, 646
Rolaids Calcium Rich, 645, 832
Romazicon, 1214
Roubac, 146
Roubac DS, 146
Roundworm
  mebendazole for, 31
  pyrantel pamoate for, 31-32
  thiabendazole for, 32-33
Rounox, 331
Rounox and Codeine 15, 367
Rounox and Codeine 30, 367
Rounox and Codeine 60, 367
Rowasa, 1246
Roxanol, 379
Roxanol 100, 379
Roxanol Rescudose, 379
Roxanol SR, 379
Roxanol UD, 379
Roxicet, 367, **C12**
Roxicet 5/500, 367
Roxicet Oral Solution, 367
Roxicodone, 383
Roxicodone Intensol, 383
RSV-IGIV, 1016-1017

rubella and mumps virus vaccine, live, 1001-1002
rubella virus vaccine, live attenuated, 1002-1003
Rubesol-1000, 1159
Rubex, 919
Rubion, 1159
Rubramin, 1159
Ru-Est-Span 20, 736
Ru-Est-Span 40, 736
Rufen, 348
Rum-K, 842
Ru-Vert M, 681
Rynacrom, 631
Rythmodan, 227
Rythmodan LA, 227
Rythmol, 239

S

Sal-Adult, 333
Salagen, 1252
Salazopyrin, 1257
Salazopyrin EN-Tabs, 1257
salazosulfapyridine, 1257-1258
salbutamol, 597-599
salbutamol sulphate, 597-599
Saleto-200, 348
Saleto-400, 348
Saleto-600, 348
Saleto-800, 348
Salflex, 340
Salgesic, 340
salicylsalicylic acid, 340-341
Sal-Infant, 333
salmeterol xinafoate, 615-616
Salmonella infection, chloramphenicol for, 200-202
Salmonine Osteocalcin, 803
Salofalk, 1246
salsalate, 340-341
Salsitab, 340
Salutensin, 265
Salutensin Demi, 265
Sandimmun, 970
Sandimmune, 970
Sandoglobulin, 1014
Sandostatin, 659
Sandril, 306
Sanery, 390
Sani-Supp, 667
Sans-Acne, 1118
Sansert, 554
saquinavir mesylate, 184-185
Sarcoma
  cyclophosphamide for, 890-892
  dactinomycin for, 916-917
  doxorubicin for, 919-921
sargramostim, 1037-1038
Sarisol No. 2, 390
S.A.S., 1257
S.A.S.-Enteric, 1257
Scabene, 1134
Scabicides, 1132-1136

Scabies
  benzyl benzoate lotion for, 1132-1133
  crotamiton for, 1133
  lindane for, 1134-1135
  permethrin for, 1135
SCF, 697
Schilling test flushing dose, hydroxocobalamin for, 1158-1160
Schizophrenia
  clozapine for, 465-467
  mesoridazine for, 472-474
Sclavo Test (dried purified protein derivative), 1280t
Scoline, 578
Scop, 538
scopolamine, 538-540
scopolamine butylbromide, 538-540
scopolamine hydrobromide, 538-540, 1076-1077
Scot-Tussin DM Cough Chaser, 622
Scurvy, vitamin C for, 1167-1169
Seborrheic dermatitis
  hydrocortisone for, 1151-1153
  ketoconazole for, 1119-1120
secobarbital sodium, 398-400
Seconal Sodium, 398
Sectral, 265
Sedation
  butabarbital for, 390-391
  chloral hydrate for, 391-393
  diazepam for, 453-456
  diphenhydramine for, 591-593
  lorazepam for, 457-458
  midazolam for, 459-460
  pentobarbital for, 396-398
  phenobarbital for, 414-416
  promethazine for, 594-595
  scopolamine for, 538-540
  secobarbital for, 398-400
Sedative effects, reversal of, flumazenil for, 1214-1215
Sedative-hypnotics, 390-402
Sedatuss, 622
Seizure disorders
  acetazolamide for, 808-810
  carbamazepine for, 403-405
  clonazepam for, 405-406
  clorazepate for, 452-453
  diazepam for, 453-456
  ethosuximide for, 406-407
  fosphenytoin for, 407-410
  gabapentin for, 410-411
  lamotrigine for, 411-412
  magnesium salts for, 838-840
  magnesium sulfate for, 412-413

Seizure disorders *(continued)*
  mephobarbital for, 413-414
  phenobarbital for, 414-416
  phensuximide for, 416-417
  phenytoin for, 417-419
  primidone for, 419-420
  pyridoxine for, 1164-1165
  valproic acid for, 420-422
Selavo-PPD Solution, 1280t
Seldane, **C13**
Seldane-D, **C13**
selegiline hydrochloride, 511-512
selenious acid, 1174-1175
selenium, 1174-1175
Sele-Pak, 1174
Selepen, 1174
Selestoject, 799
Semilente MC, 771
Semprex-D, 541, 597
Senexon, 675
senna, 675-676
Senna-Gen, 675
Senokot, 675
Senokot-S, 662
SenokotXTRA, 675
Senolax, 675
Sensorcaine, 1262t
Septicemia
  aztreonam for, 198-199
  cefazolin for, 107-108
  cefonicid for, 113-114
  cefoperazone for, 114-115
  cefotaxime for, 115-117
  ceftazidime for, 122-124
  ceftizoxime for, 125-126
  ceftriaxone for, 126-128
  cefuroxime for, 128-130
  cephapirin for, 131-133
  cephradine for, 133-134
  imipenem/cilastatin for, 204-205
  ticarcillin/clavulanate for, 103-104
Septra, 146
Septra DS, 146
Septra I.V. Infusion, 146
Septrin, 146
Ser-A-Gen, 265
Seralazide, 265
Ser-Ap-Es, 265
Serax, 461
Sereen, 451
Serenace, 469
Serentil, 472
Serentil Concentrate, 472
Serepax, 461
Serevent, 615
Seromycin, 55
Serophene, 1236
Serpalan, 306
Serpasil, 306
Serpasil-Apresoline #1, 265
Serpasil-Apresoline #2, 265
Serpasil-Esidrix #1, 265

Serpasil Esidrix #2, 265
Serpasil-Esidrix 25, 265
Serpazide, 265
Sertan, 419
sertraline hydrochloride, 443-444
Serutan, 674
Serzone, 436
Setamol-500, 331
Seudotabs, 550
Shigellosis, co-trimoxazole for, 146-148
Shingles. *See* Herpes zoster infection.
Shock
  dexamethasone for, 703-705
  dopamine for, 542-544
  hydrocortisone for, 706-709
  methylprednisolone for, 709-711
  phenylephrine for, 548-550
  plasma protein fraction for, 872-873
Siblin, 674
Silexin Cough, 622
Silvadene, 1126
silver nitrate 1%, 1048-1049
silver sulfadiazine, 1126-1127
simethicone, 649
Simron, 852
simvastatin, 320-321
Sinarest 12-Hour, 1106
Sine-Aid IB, 342
Sinemet, 506, **C13**
Sinemet 10-100, 503
Sinemet 25-100, 503
Sinemet 25-250, 503
Sinemet CR, 503, 506, **C13**
Sine-Off Nasal Spray, 1110
Sinequan, 430
Sinex, 1107
Sinex-L.A., 1110
Sinex Long-Acting, 1106
Sintisone, 712
Sinufed, 550
Sinus Excedrin Extra Strength, 330
Sinusitis
  amoxicillin/clavulanate for, 75-76
  cefprozil for, 121-122
  clarithromycin for, 192-193
  levofloxacin for, 156-158
  loracarbef for, 134-135
Sinusol-B, 585
Sinus Relief Tablets, 330
Sinustat, 550
Sinustop Pro, 550
Sinutab, 330
Sinutab Maximum Strength, 330
Sinutab without Drowsiness, 330
642, 386

692, 366
Skeletal muscle relaxants, 556-564
Skeletal muscle relaxation
  atracurium for, 565-566
  cisatracurium for, 566-568
  doxacurium for, 568-570
  metocurine for, 570-571
  mivacurium for, 571-573
  pancuronium for, 573-575
  pipecuronium for, 575-576
  rocuronium for, 576-578
  succinylcholine for, 578-580
  tubocurarine for, 580-581
  vecuronium for, 581-582
Skin infections
  amoxicillin/clavulanate for, 75-76
  ampicillin/sulbactam for, 80-81
  azithromycin for, 191-192
  aztreonam for, 198-199
  bacampicillin for, 81-82
  cefaclor for, 105-106
  cefadroxil for, 106-107
  cefazolin for, 107-108
  cefepime for, 108-110
  cefmetazole for, 111-113
  cefonicid for, 113-114
  cefoperazone for, 114-115
  cefotaxime for, 115-117
  cefotetan for, 117-118
  cefoxitin for, 118-119
  cefpodoxime for, 120-121
  cefprozil for, 121-122
  ceftazidime for, 122-124
  ceftizoxime for, 125-126
  ceftriaxone for, 126-128
  cefuroxime for, 128-130
  cephalexin for, 130-131
  cephapirin for, 131-133
  cephradine for, 133-134
  ciprofloxacin for, 153-154
  clarithromycin for, 192-193
  dirithromycin for, 193-194
  erythromycin for, 195-197
  gentamicin for, 1119
  imipenem/cilastatin for, 204-205
  levofloxacin for, 156-158
  loracarbef for, 134-135
  ofloxacin for, 162-163
  piperacillin and tazobactam for, 100-101
  tetracycline for, 1129-1130
  ticarcillin/clavulanate for, 103-104
  tolnaftate for, 1130-1131
Skin tests, diagnostic, 1280-1281t
Sleep aid, diphenhydramine for, 591-593
Sleep-Eze 3, 591
Slo-bid Gyrocaps, 618, C13

Slo-Phyllin, 618
Slophyllin GG Syrup, 597
Slow-Fe, 853
Slow-K, 842
Slow-Mag, 838
Small-bowel intubation, meto-clopramide for, 682-683
SMZ-TMP, 146
Snaplets-FR, 331
Soda Mint, 848
sodium bicarbonate, 848-849
sodium chloride, 845-846
sodium chloride, hypertonic, 1093-1094
Sodium Chloride Ointment 5%, 1093
sodium cromoglycate, 631-632
Sodium Diuril, 813
Sodium Edecrin, 816
sodium fluoride, 1173-1174
sodium fluoride, topical, 1173-1174
sodium iodide, 791-793, 1174-1175
Sodium Iodide 131I Thera-peutic, 791
sodium lactate, 849-850
Sodium P.A.S., 52
sodium phosphates, 677
sodium polystyrene sulfonate, 1221-1222
Sodium Sulamyd 10% Ophthalmic, 1049
Sodium Sulamyd 30% Ophthalmic, 1049
Sodol, 557
Sofarin, 863
Soft-tissue infections
  cefaclor for, 105-106
  cefadroxil for, 106-107
  cefazolin for, 107-108
  cefoxitin for, 118-119
  cephalexin for, 130-131
  cephapirin for, 131-133
  cephradine for, 133-134
  erythromycin for, 195-197
  imipenem/cilastatin for, 204-205
Solazine, 485
Solfoton, 414
Solganal, 1202
Solium, 451
Solone, 711
Solprin, 333
Solu-Cortef, 706
Solu-Flur, 1173
Solu-Medrol, 709
Solurex, 703
Solurex-LA, 703
Soma, 557
Soma Compound, 556
Soma Compound with Codeine, 556
somatrem, 798-799

somatropin, 799-800
Sominex Formula 2, 591
Somophyllin, 599
Somophyllin-CRT, 618
Somophyllin-DF, 599
Somophyllin-T, 618
Sone, 714
Soothe, 1080
Sopamycetin, 200, 1040, 1097
Soprodol, 557
Sorbitrate, 250
Soridol, 557
Sotacor, 242
sotalol, 242-244
Spancap #1, 493
Span-FF, 851
sparfloxacin, 163-165
Sparine, 479
Spasmoban, 533
Spasmoject, 533
Spasmolytics, 1198-1200
Spasticity
  baclofen for, 556-557
  dantrolene for, 560-561
  scopolamine for, 538-540
  tizanidine for, 563-564
Spectazole, 1117
spectinomycin hydrochloride, 211-212
Spectrobid, 81
Spherulin, 1280t
Spinal anesthesia
  mephentermine for, 544-545
  metaraminol for, 545-547
  phenylephrine for, 548-550
Spinal cord injury
  baclofen for, 556-557
  dantrolene for, 560-561
  etidronate for, 806-807
spironolactone, 826-827
Spirotone, 826
Spirozide, 826
Sporanox, 39
SPS, 1221
S-P-T, 785
Squamous cell carcinoma, bleomycin for, 915-916
Squibb-HC, 1152
89Sr, 1256-1257
SSD-AF, 1126
SSKI, 789-790
Stadol, 369
Stadol NS, 369
Stanback AF Extra Strength Powder, 331
stanozolol, 724-726
Statex, 379
Staticin, 1118
Statrol, 1039
Status epilepticus
  clonazepam for, 405-406
  diazepam for, 453-456
  fosphenytoin for, 407-410

Status epilepticus *(continued)*
  phenobarbital for, 414-416
  phenytoin for, 417-419
  secobarbital for, 398-400
stavudine, 185-186
Steatorrhea, pancrelipase for, 652-654
Stelazine, 485
Stelazine Concentrate, 485
Stemetic, 688
Stemetil, 685
Sterapred, 714
Sterine, 207
S-T Expectorant, 623
StieVAA, 1259
stilboestrol, 732-734
Stilphostrol, 732
Stimate, 797
St. Joseph Aspirin-Free Fever Reducer for Children, 331
St. Joseph Cough Suppressant for Children, 622
St. Joseph Measured Dose Nasal Decongestant, 1107
Stomach acid, neutralizing
  aluminum carbonate for, 642-643
  aluminum hydroxide for, 644-645
  calcium carbonate for, 645-646
  dihydroxyaluminum sodium carbonate for, 646-647
  magaldrate for, 647-648
  magnesium hydroxide for, 669-670
  magnesium oxide for, 648-649
  sodium bicarbonate for, 848-849
Stomach cancer
  doxorubicin for, 919-921
  fluorouracil for, 907-909
Stool softening, docusate for, 666-667
Stop, 1173
Strabismus
  botulinum toxin type A for, 1083-1084
  demecarium for, 1064-1065
  echothiophate for, 1065-1067
  isoflurophate for, 1067-1068
Streptase, 878
streptokinase, 878-881
streptomycin sulfate, 72-73
streptozocin, 898-899
Stroke, alteplase for, 874-875
strong iodine solution, 789-790
strontium 89 chloride, 1256-1257
Stulex, 666

Subarachnoid hemorrhage, nimodipine for, 1250
Sublimaze, 372
succimer, 1222-1223
succinylcholine chloride, 578-580
Sucostrin, 578
sucralfate, 697-698
Sucrets Cough Control Formula, 622
Sudafed, 550
Sudafed Plus, 583
Sudafed-60, 550
Sudafed 12 Hour, 550
Sudrin, 550
Sufedrin, 550
Sufenta, 387
sufentanil citrate, 387-388
Sular, 297
sulconazole nitrate, 1127-1128
Sulcrate, 697
sulfacetamide sodium 10%, 1049-1050
sulfacetamide sodium 15%, 1049-1050
sulfacetamide sodium 30%, 1049-1050
sulfadiazine, 148-149
sulfafurazole, 150-152
Sulfalax Calcium, 666
sulfamethoxazole, 149-150
sulfamethoxazole-trimethoprim, 146-148
Sulfamylon, 1120
sulfasalazine, 1257-1258
Sulfatrim, 146
Sulfineycin, 146
sulfinpyrazone, 1187-1188
sulfisoxazole, 150-152
sulfisoxazole acetyl, 151-152
sulfisoxazole diolamine, 1050-1051
Sulfonamides, 146-152
Sulf-10 Ophthalmic, 1049
sulindac, 363-364
sulphafurazole, 150-152
sulphamethoxazole, 149-150
sulphasalazine, 1257-1258
sumatriptan succinate, 521-522
Sumycin, 143, **C13**
Supasa, 333
Super Calcium 1200, 832
Superchar, 1204
Supeudol, 383
Suppap-120, 331
Suppap-325, 331
Suppap-650, 331
Supprelin, 757
Suppression therapy, nitrofurantoin for, 208-210
Suprax, 110, **C13**
Supres, 285
suprofen, 1061

Surfak, 666
Surgery preparation
  bisacodyl for, 662-663
  chlorpromazine for, 462-465
  magnesium citrate for, 669-670
  magnesium hydroxide for, 669-670
  magnesium sulfate for, 669-670
  mineral oil for, 671-672
  neomycin for, 69-70
  piperacillin for, 98-100
Surgical prophylaxis
  cefmetazole for, 111-113
  cefonicid for, 113-114
  cefotaxime for, 115-117
  cefotetan for, 117-118
  cefoxitin for, 118-119
  ceftriaxone for, 126-128
  cefuroxime for, 128-130
  cephapirin for, 131-133
  cephradine for, 133-134
Surmontil, 446
Survanta, 627
Sus-Phrine, 604
Sustaire, 618
suxamethonium chloride, 578-580
Syllact, 674
Symadine, 168
Symmetrel, 168
Sympatholytics, 552-555
Sympathomimetics, 541-551
Synacort, 1152
Synalar, 1145
Synarel, 760
Syn-Captopril, 271
Synemol, 1145
Synflex, 359
Syn-Mynocycline, 140
Synophylate-GG Syrup, 597
Syn-Pindolol, 301
Synthroid, 781, **C13**
Syntocinon, 1195, 1197
Syphilis
  doxycycline for, 137-140
  erythromycin for, 195-197
  minocycline for, 140-141
  oxytetracycline for, 142-143
  penicillin G benzathine for, 91-92
  tetracycline for, 143-145
Syprine, 1224
Systemic infections
  amoxicillin for, 77-78
  ampicillin for, 78-80
  cloxacillin for, 84-85
  dicloxacillin for, 85-86
  mezlocillin for, 86-88
  nafcillin for, 88-89
  oxacillin for, 89-90
  penicillin G potassium for, 92-94

Systemic infections
   (continued)
  penicillin G procaine for,
     94-95
  penicillin G sodium for,
     95-97
  penicillin V for, 97-98
  piperacillin for, 98-100
  sulfamethoxazole for,
     149-150
  sulfisoxazole for, 150-152
  ticarcillin for, 101-103
syvinolin, 320-321

T
T₃, 782-784
T₄, 781-782
Tac-3, 716
TACE, 729
tacrine hydrochloride,
   522-523
tacrolimus, 975-977
Tagamet, 689, **C14**
Tagamet HB, 689
Tagamet HCl, 689
Tagamet Tiltab, 689
Talacen, 367
Talwin, 385
Talwin Compound, 367
Talwin-Nx, 385
Tambocor, 230
Tamofen, 935
Tamone, 935
Tamoplex, 935
tamoxifen citrate, 935-936
Tapanol Extra Strength
     Caplets, 331
Tapanol Extra Strength
     Tablets, 331
Tapazole, 788
Tapeworm, paromomycin for,
     28-29
Tavist, 588
Tavist-1, 588
Tavist-D, 583
Taxol, 952
Taxotere, 944
Tazac, 694
Tazicef, 122
Tazidime, 122
T-Cypionate, 726
T-Diet, 501
Tebamide, 688
Tebrazid, 61
Tecnal, 330
Teejel, 337
Tegamide, 688
Tega-Vert, 678
Tegison, 1238
Tegopen, 84
Tegretol, 403
Tegretol Chewable Tablets,
     403
Tegretol CR, 403
Telachlor, 587

Teldrin, 587
Teline, 143
Temaze, 400
temazepam, 400-401
Temgesic Injection, 368
Temovate, 1139
Temperature conversions,
     1279t
Tempra, 331
Tempra, Infants', 331
Tempra Caplets, 331
Tempra Chewable Tablets, 331
Tempra Drops, 331
Tempra D.S., 331
Tempra Syrup, 331
Tencet, 330
Tendinitis
  indomethacin for, 349-352
  naproxen for, 359-360
  sulindac for, 363-364
Tenex, 284
teniposide, 959-960
Ten-K, 842
Tenol, 331
Tenoretic 50, 265
Tenoretic 100, 265
Tenormin, 266, **C14**
Tensilon, 526
Tension, mephobarbital for,
     413-414
Tenuate, 494
Tenuate Dospan, 494
Tepanil, 494
Tepanil Ten-Tab, 494
Terazol 3 Vaginal Supposi-
     tories, 1128
Terazol 7 Vaginal Cream, 1128
terazosin hydrochloride, 307
terbinafine hydrochloride,
     1128
terbutaline sulfate, 616-618
terconazole, 1128-1129
Teril, 403
Terramycin, 142
Tertroxin, 782
Tesamone 100, 726
Teslac, 936
TESPA, 899-900
Tessalon, 621
Testa-C, 726
Testaqua, 726
Test Est Cyp (oil), 718
Testex, 726
Testicular cancer
  bleomycin for, 915-916
  cisplatin for, 888-890
  dactinomycin for, 916-917
  etoposide for, 946-947
  ifosfamide for, 892-894
  plicamycin for, 925-926
  vinblastine for, 963-965
Testoderm, 728
Testoject-50, 726

Testoject-LA, 726
testolactone, 936
Testomet, 721
testosterone, 726-728
testosterone cypionate,
     726-728
testosterone propionate,
     726-728
testosterone transdermal
     system, 728
Testred, 721
Testred Cypionate 200, 726
Tetanus
  chlorpromazine for,
     462-465
  methocarbamol for,
     561-563
Tetanus exposure, tetanus
     immune globulin, human,
     for, 1019-1020
tetanus immune globulin,
     human, 1019-1020
Tetanus seizure, secobarbital
     for, 398-400
tetanus toxoid, adsorbed,
     1003-1004
tetanus toxoid, fluid,
     1003-1004
tetracaine, 1266-1267t
tetracaine hydrochloride,
     1266-1267t
Tetracap, 143
tetracycline hydrochloride,
     143-145, 1129-1130
Tetracyclines, 136-145
Tetracyn 143
tetrahydrozoline hydrochlo-
     ride, 1080, 1108-1109
Tetralan, 143
Tetram, 143
Tetramune, 978
Tetrasine, 1080
6-TG, 914
T-Gen, 688
Thalfed, 597
Thalitone, 814
Thallium scintigraphy, dipyri-
     damole for, 323-324
Tham, 850
Theo-24, 618
Theobid Duracaps, 618
Theobid Jr. Duracaps, 618
Theochron, 618
Theo-Dur, 618, **C14**
Theo-Dur Sprinkle, 618
Theolair Liquid, 618
Theolair-SR, 618
Theon, 618
theophylline, 618-620
theophylline ethylenediamine,
     599-602
theophylline sodium glycinate,
     618-620
Theospan-SR, 618
Theo-Time, 618

Theovent Long-Acting, 618
TheraCys, 941
Thera-Flur, 1173
Thera-Flur-N, 1173
Theralax, 662
Therevac Plus, 666
Therevac-SB, 666
Thermazene, 1126
thiabendazole, 32-33
Thiamilate, 1166
thiamine hydrochloride,
    1166-1167
thiethylperazine maleate,
    687-688
thioguanine, 914
6-thioguanine, 914
Thiola, 1258
Thioplex, 899
Thioprine, 969
thioridazine hydrochloride,
    482-484
thiotepa, 899-900
thiothixene, 484-485
thiothixene hydrochloride,
    484-485
Thorazine, 462
Thor-Prom, 462
Threadworm, thiabendazole
    for, 32-33
Thrombate III, 870
Thromboangiitis obliterans,
    isoxsuprine for, 324
Thrombolytic enzymes,
    874-882
Thrombosis
    aspirin for, 333-335
    dextran, low molecular
        weight, for, 835-836
    streptokinase for, 878-881
    urokinase for, 881-882
Thyrar, 785
Thyro-Block, 789
thyroid, 785-787
Thyroid cancer
    doxorubicin for, 919-921
    radioactive iodine for,
        791-793
    thyrotropin for, 787
Thyroidectomy, strong iodine
    solution for, 789-790
Thyroid gland, radiation
    protection for, potassium
    iodide for, 789-790
Thyroid hormone antagonists,
    788-793
Thyroid hormone replacement
    levothyroxine for, 781-782
    liothyronine for, 782-784
Thyroid hormones, 781-787
thyroid-stimulating hormone,
    787
Thyroid Strong, 785
Thyroid USP Enseals, 785
Thyrolar, 784
Thyro-Teric, 785

Thyrotoxic crisis
    potassium iodide for,
        789-790
    propylthiouracil for,
        790-791
thyrotropin, 787
Thytropar, 787
Ticar, 101
ticarcillin disodium, 101-103
ticarcillin disodium/clavu-
    lanate potassium,
    103-104
TICE BCG, 941, 978
Ticillin, 101
Ticlid, 327
ticlopidine hydrochloride,
    327-329
Ticon, 688
Tigan, 688
Tilade, 637
Timentin, 103
Timolide 10/25, 265
timolol maleate, 308-309,
    1094-1095
Timoptic Solution, 1094
Timoptic-XE, 1094
Tinactin, 1130
Tinea infections
    ciclopirox for, 1115
    clotrimazole for, 1116-1117
    econazole for, 1117-1118
    griseofulvin for, 38-39
    ketoconazole for, 40-42,
        1119-1120
    miconazole for, 1122-1123
    naftifine for, 1123-1124
    oxiconazole for, 1126
    sulconazole for, 1127-1128
    terbinafine for, 1128
    tolnaftate for, 1130-1131
Tine Test (dried Old Tuber-
    culin, dried purified pro-
    tein derivative), 1280t
Ting, 1130
tioconazole, 1130
tiopronin, 1258-1259
Tipramine, 432
TISIT, 1136
tissue plasminogen activator,
    recombinant, 874-875
Titracid, 645
Titralac, 645, 832
Titralac Extra Strength, 645
Titralac Plus, 645
Titralac Plus Suspension, 642
Titralac Tablets, 642
tizanidine hydrochloride,
    563-564
Tobra Dex, 1039
tobramycin, 1051-1052
tobramycin sulfate, 73-74
Tobrex, 1051
tocainide hydrochloride,
    244-245
tocopherol, 1170-1171

Tofranil, 432
Tofranil-PM, 432
Tolamide, 776
tolazamide, 776-778
tolazoline hydrochloride, 329
tolbutamide, 778-779
Tolectin 200, 364
Tolectin 400, 364
Tolectin 600, 364
Tolectin DS, 364
Tolinase, 776
tolmetin sodium, 364-365
tolnaftate, 1130-1131
Tolu-Sed DM, 622
Tonocard, 244
Tonsillitis
    azithromycin for, 191-192
    cefadroxil for, 106-107
    cefixime for, 110-111
    cefpodoxime for, 120-121
    cefprozil for, 121-122
    ceftibuten for, 124-125
    cefuroxime for, 128-130
    clarithromycin for, 192-193
    dirithromycin for, 193-194
    loracarbef for, 134-135
Topical anesthetics,
    1266-1267t
Topicort, 1142
Topicycline, 1129
topotecan hydrochloride,
    960-962
Toprol XL, 293, C14
Topsyn, 1146
TOPV, 998-999
Toradol, 354, C14
Torecan, 687
Tornalate, 602
torsemide, 827-829
Totacillin, 78
Totacillin-N, 78
Total hip replacement,
    etidronate for, 806-807
Total parenteral nutrition
    amino acid solutions for,
        1176-1178
    fat emulsions for,
        1179-1181
Tourette syndrome, pimozide
    for, 478-479
Toxic reactions, 10
Toxoids, 978-1007
Toxoplasmosis
    pyrimethamine for, 50-51
    sulfadiazine for, 148-149
tPA, 874-875
T-Quil, 453
Trace Metals Additive, 1157
Trachoma
    erythromycin for,
        1042-1043
    sulfisoxazole for,
        1050-1051
Tracrium, 565
Trac Tabs 2X, 198

tramadol hydrochloride, 388-389
Trancot, 458
Trandate, 287
trandolapril, 309-310
Transdermal-NTG, 255
Transderm-Nitro, 255
Transderm-Scōp, 538
Transderm-V, 538
Transfusion accidents, Rh₀(D) immune globulin for, 1017-1019
Transiderm-Nitro, 255
Transrectal prostate biopsy, lomefloxacin for, 158-159
Transurethral resection of prostate gland, mannitol for, 822-824
Transurethral surgery prophylaxis, lomefloxacin for, 158-159
Tranxene, 452
Tranxene-SD, 452
Tranxene-T-Tab, 452
tranylcypromine sulfate, 444-445
Trasylol, 1232
Travamine, 678
Travasol, 1176
Travasol with electrolytes, 1176
Travs, 678
trazodone hydrochloride, 445-446
Trazon, 445
Trecator-SC, 58
Tremor, propranolol for, 258-260
Trendar, 348
Trental, 327, **C14**
tretinoin, 962-963, 1259-1260
Triacet, 1154
Triad, 330
Triadapin, 430
Trialodine, 445
Triam-A, 716
triamcinolone, 716-717
triamcinolone acetonide, 638-639, 716-717, 1109-1110, 1154-1155
Triaminic-12, 583
Triamonide 40, 716
triamterene, 829-830
Triaphen-10, 333
Triavil 2-10, 423, 462
Triavil 2-25, 423, 462
Triavil 4-10, 423, 462
Triavil 4-25, 423, 462
Triavil 4-50, 423, 462
triazolam, 401-402
Triban, 688
Tri-Barbs Capsules, 390
Tribenzagan, 688
Trichinosis, thiabendazole for, 32-33

Trichomoniasis, metronidazole for, 26-28
Tricosal, 335
Tridesilon, 1141
Tridil, 255
trientine hydrochloride, 1224
triethanolamine polypeptide oleate-condensate, 1098
triethylenethiophosphoramide, 899-900
trifluoperazine hydrochloride, 485-487
trifluridine, 1052-1053
Trigeminal neuralgia, carbamazepine for, 403-405
Trihexane, 512
Trihexy-2, 512
Trihexy-5, 512
trihexyphenidyl hydrochloride, 512-513
Tri-Hydroserpine, 265
Tri-Immunol, 981
Trikacide, 26
Tri-Kort, 716
Trilafon, 476
Trilafon Concentrate, 476
Tri-Levlen, 744
Trilisate, 335
Trilog, 716
trilostane, 1260
Trimazide, 688
trimethobenzamide hydrochloride, 688
trimethoprim, 212-213
trimetrexate glucuronate, 213-214
trimipramine maleate, 446-447
Trimox, 77, **C14**
Trimpex, 212
Trinalin Repetabs, 583
Tri-Norinyl, 745
Triostat, 782
Tripedia, 981
Triphasil, 744
Triple X, 1136
Triprim, 212
triprolidine hydrochloride, 595-596
Triptil, 441
Triptone Caplets, 678
Tritace, 304
Trobicin, 211
Trocal, 622
troglitazone, 779-780
tromethamine, 850
TrophAmine, 1176
Trophoblastic tumors dactinomycin for, 916-917 methotrexate for, 911-914
Tropicacyl, 1077
Tropical sprue, folic acid for, 1160-1161
tropicamide, 1077
Truphylline, 599

Trusopt, 1086
Trymegen, 587
Tryptanol, 423
T/Scalp, 1152
TSH, 787
TSPA, 899-900
T-Stat, 1118
T₃ suppression test, 782
Tubarine, 580
tuberculin purified protein derivative, 1280-1281t
Tuberculosis
  acetylcysteine for, 624-625
  aminosalicylate for, 52-53
  capreomycin for, 53-54
  cycloserine for, 55-56
  ethambutol for, 57-58
  ethionamide for, 58-59
  isoniazid for, 59-61
  pyrazinamide for, 61-62
  rifampin for, 63-64
  streptomycin for, 72-73
Tuberculosis exposure, BCG vaccine for, 978-979
tuberculosis multiple-puncture tests, 1280-1281t
Tubersol, 1280t
tubocurarine chloride, 580-581
Tuinal 50 mg Pulvules, 390
Tuinal 100 mg Pulvules, 390
Tuinal 200 mg Pulvules, 390
Tularemia, streptomycin sulfate for, 72-73
Tums, 645, 832
Tums E-X, 645, 832
Tums Liquid Extra Strength, 645
Tuss-DM, 622
Tusstat, 591
Twice-A-Day Nasal, 1106
Twilite Caplets, 591
Twin-K, 832
Two-Dyne, 330
222, 366
222 Forte, 366
282, 366
292, 366
293, 366
Tylenol Caplets, 331
Tylenol Chewable Tablets, 331
Tylenol Children's Elixir, 331
Tylenol Children's Tablets, 331
Tylenol Drops, 331
Tylenol Elixir, 331
Tylenol Extended Relief, 331
Tylenol Extra Strength Adult Liquid Pain Reliever, 331
Tylenol Extra Strength Caplets, 331
Tylenol Extra Strength Gelcaps, 331
Tylenol Extra Strength Tablets, 331
Tylenol Infants', 331

Tylenol Junior Strength Caplets, 331
Tylenol Junior Strength Tablets, 331
Tylenol Regular Strength Caplets, 331
Tylenol Regular Strength Tablets, 331
Tylenol Tablets, 331
Tylenol with Codeine Elixir, 366
Tylenol with Codeine No. 1, 367
Tylenol with Codeine No. 2, 367
Tylenol with Codeine No. 3, 367, **C15**
Tylenol with Codeine No. 4, 367
Tylox, 367
Ty-Pap, 331
Ty-Pap, Infants', 331
Ty-Pap Syrup, 331
Ty-Pap with Codeine Elixir, 366
Typhim Vi, 1005
Typhoid fever, ciprofloxacin for, 153-154
typhoid vaccine, oral, 1004-1005
typhoid vaccine, parenteral, 1004-1005
typhoid Vi polysaccharide vaccine, 1005-1006
Ty-Tab, Children's, 331
Ty-Tab Caplets, 331
Ty-Tab Capsules, 331
Ty-Tab Tablets, 331
Tyzine Drops, 1108
Tyzine Pediatric Drops, 1108

U
UAA, 198
Ukidan, 881
Ulcerative colitis
  hydrocortisone for, 706-709
  mesalamine for, 1246-1247
  olsalazine for, 1251
  prednisolone for, 711-714
  sulfasalazine for, 1257-1258
Ultracef, 106
ultradol, 344-345
Ultralente Insulin, 771
Ultram, 388, **C15**
Ultrase MT 12, 652
Ultrase MT 20, 652
Ultrase MT 24, 652
Ultratard HM, 771
Ultratard MC, 771
Ultravate, 1151
Ultrazine-10, 685
Unasyn, 80
Uncategorized drugs, 1225-1260
Uni-Bent Cough, 591

Unicort, 1152
Uni Laxative, 674
Unilax Softgel, 662
Uniparin, 860
Uniparin-Ca, 860
Unipen, 88
Uniphyl, 618
Unipres, 265
Univasc, 295
Univol, 642
Unproco, 622
Urabeth, 525
uracil mustard, 901
Uracil Mustard Capsules, 901
urea, 830-831
Ureaphil, 830
Urecholine, 525
Ureteral colic, papaverine for, 326-327
Urethral infections
  doxycycline for, 137-140
  enoxacin for, 155-156
  erythromycin for, 195-197
  minocycline hydrochloride for, 140-141
  sulfisoxazole for, 150-152
  tetracycline hydrochloride for, 143-145
Urethritis
  azithromycin for, 191-192
  erythromycin for, 195-197
  esterified estrogens for, 734-736
  minocycline hydrochloride for, 140-141
  ofloxacin for, 162-163
  spectinomycin for, 211-212
Urex, 207, 817
Urex-M, 817
Uridon, 814
Uridon Modified, 198
Urimar-T, 198
Urinary alkalinization
  sodium bicarbonate for, 848-849
  sodium lactate for, 849-850
Urinary Aseptic No. 2, 198
Urinary frequency and urgency, flavoxate for, 1198
Urinary tract infections. See also Genitourinary tract infections.
  acetohydroxamic acid for, 1227
  amikacin for, 65-66
  amoxicillin for, 77-78
  amoxicillin/clavulanate for, 75-76
  ampicillin for, 78-80
  aztreonam for, 198-199
  bacampicillin for, 81-82
  carbenicillin indanyl sodium for, 83-84
  cefaclor for, 105-106
  cefadroxil for, 106-107

Urinary tract infections (continued)
  cefepime for, 108-110
  cefixime for, 110-111
  cefmetazole for, 111-113
  cefonicid for, 113-114
  cefotaxime for, 115-117
  cefotetan for, 117-118
  cefpodoxime for, 120-121
  ceftazidime for, 122-124
  ceftizoxime for, 125-126
  ceftriaxone for, 126-128
  cefuroxime for, 128-130
  ciprofloxacin for, 153-154
  co-trimoxazole for, 146-148
  enoxacin for, 155-156
  flucytosine for, 37-38
  fosfomycin for, 203-204
  imipenem/cilastatin for, 204-205
  levofloxacin for, 156-158
  lomefloxacin for, 158-159
  methenamine for, 207-208
  nalidixic acid for, 159-160
  netilmicin for, 70-72
  nitrofurantoin for, 208-210
  norfloxacin for, 160-162
  ofloxacin for, 162-163
  sulfamethoxazole for, 149-150
  sulfisoxazole for, 150-152
  ticarcillin/clavulanate for, 103-104
  trimethoprim for, 212-213
Urine retention, bethanechol for, 525-526
Urised, 198
Urisedamine, 198
Uri-Tet, 142
Uritin, 198
Uritol, 817
Urobiotic-250, 136
Urocarb Liquid, 525
Urocarb Tablets, 525
Urodine, 1200
Uro Gantanol, 146
Urogesic, 1200
Urogesic Blue, 198
urokinase, 881-882
Uro-Mag, 648
Uro Phosphate, 198
Uroplus DS, 146
Uroplus SS, 146
Uroquid-Acid No. 2, 198
Urozide, 819
ursodiol, 654-655
Urticaria
  astemizole for, 584
  azatadine for, 584-585
  cetirizine for, 586-587
Uterine bleeding, abnormal
  estrogens, conjugated, for, 738-741
  hydroxyprogesterone for, 748-749

Uterine bleeding, abnormal *(continued)*
  medroxyprogesterone for, 751-752
  norethindrone for, 752-753
  progesterone for, 754-755
Uveitis
  atropine for, 1071-1072
  dexamethasone for, 1054-1055
  homatropine for, 1074-1075
  rimexolone for, 1060-1061
  scopolamine for, 1076-1077

V
Vaccines, 978-1007
Vaginal atrophy, estropipate for, 741-742
Vaginal infections, nystatin for, 43-44
Vaginitis
  fibrinolysin and desoxyribonuclease for, 1190-1191
Vaginosis
  clindamycin for, 1115-1116
  metronidazole for, 1121-1122
valacyclovir hydrochloride, 186-187
Valcote, 420
Valergen-10, 736
Valergen-20, 736
Valergen-40, 736
Valertest No. 1, 718
Valisone, 1138
Valium, 453, **C15**
Valorin, 331
Valorin Extra, 331
valproate sodium, 420-422
valproic acid, 420-422
Valrelease, 453
valsartan, 310-311
Valtrex, 186
Vamate, 456
Vancenase AQ Nasal Spray, 1100
Vancenase Nasal Inhaler, 1100
Vanceril, 626
Vancocin, 214
Vancoled, 214
vancomycin hydrochloride, 214-215
Vanquish, 330
Vantin, 120
Vapo-Iso, 609
Vaponefrine, 604
Vaqta, 984
Varicella exposure, varicella-zoster immune globulin for, 1020-1021
Varicella infections, acyclovir sodium for, 166-168

varicella virus vaccine, 1006-1007
varicella-zoster immune globulin, 1020-1021
Varivax, 1006
Vascor, 248
Vascular headaches
  dihydroergotamine for, 552-553
  ergotamine for, 553-554
  methysergide for, 554-555
  propranolol for, 258-260
Vaseretic, 265
Vasocardol SR, 249
Vasocidin Ophthalmic Ointment, 1039, 1078
Vasocidin Ophthalmic Solution, 1039, 1078
Vasoclear, 1078
Vasocon-A Ophthalmic Solution, 1078
Vasocon Regular, 1078
Vasodilan, 324
vasopressin, 800-801
Vasosulf, 1039-1040
Vasotec, 277, **C15**
Vasotec I.V., 277
Vazepam, 453
V-Cillin K, 97
VCR, 965-966
vecuronium bromide, 581-582
Veetids, 97, **C15**
Velban, 963
Velbe, 963
Velosef, 133
Velosulin Human, 771
Velosulin Insuject, 771
Velsar, 963
Veltane, 585
Venereal warts. *See* Condylomata acuminata.
venlafaxine hydrochloride, 447-448
Venoglobulin-I, 1014
Venoglobulin-S, 1014
Ventilation, mechanical
  atracurium for, 565-566
  cisatracurium for, 566-568
  mivacurium for, 571-573
  pancuronium for, 573-575
  rocuronium for, 576-578
  succinylcholine for, 578-580
  tubocurarine for, 580-581
  vecuronium for, 581-582
Ventolin, 597
Ventolin Obstetric Injection, 597
Ventolin Rotacaps, 597
VePesid, 946
Veracaps SR, 260
verapamil, 260-262
verapamil hydrochloride, 260-262, **C15**

Verelan, 260, **C15**
Vergon, 681
Vermox, 31
Versabran, 674
Versed, 459
Vertigo, meclizine for, 681-682
Vesanoid, 962
Vexol 1% Ophthalmic Suspension, 1060
V-Gan-25, 594
V-Gan-50, 594
Vibramycin, 137
Vibra-Tabs, 137
Vibra-Tabs 50, 137
Vicks Formula 44 Pediatric Formula, 622
Vicks Pediatric Formula 44E, 622
Vicks Vatronol, 603
Vicks Vatronol Nose Drops, 1103
Vicodin, 367, **C15**
Vicodin ES, 367, **C15**
vidarabine, 1053
Videx, 171
vinblastine sulfate, 963-965
Vincasar PFS, 965
Vincent's Powders, 333
vincristine sulfate, 965-966
vinorelbine tartrate, 966-968
Vioform-Hydrocortisone Mild Cream, 1111
Viokase Powder, 652
Viokase Tablets, 652
Vira-A, 1053
Viramune, 178
Virazole, 180
Viridium, 1200
Virilon, 721
Virilon IM, 726
Viroptic Ophthalmic Solution 1%, 1052
Visine, 1080
Visine L.R., 1079
Visken, 301
Vistacon-50, 456
Vistaject-25, 456
Vistaject-50, 456
Vistaquel, 456
Vistaril, 456
Vistazine 50, 456
Vistide, 169
VitaCarn, 1244
Vita C Crystals, 1167
vitamin A, 1157-1158
vitamin A acid, 1259-1260
vitamin B$_1$, 1166-1167
vitamin B$_2$, 1165-1166
vitamin B$_3$, 1162-1164
vitamin B$_6$, 1164-1165
vitamin B$_9$, 1160-1161
vitamin B$_{12}$, 1158-1160
vitamin C, 1167-1169
Vitamin D, 1169

vitamin D, 1169-1170
vitamin D₂, 1169-1170
vitamin D, 1169-1170
Vitamin D, 1169
Vitamin deficiencies. See specific vitamin.
vitamin E, 1170-1171
vitamin K₁, 1171-1173
Vitamins, 1156-1173
Vita-Plus E Softgels, 1170
Vitiligo, methoxsalen for, 1248-1249
Vivactil, 441
Vivarin, 490
Vivol, 453
Vivotif Berna Vaccine, 1004
V-Lax, 674
VLB, 963-965
VM-26, 959-960
Volmax, 597
Voltaren, 342
Voltaren Ophthalmic, 1055
Voltaren SR, 342
Vomiting
    chlorpromazine for, 462-465
    diphenidol for, 679
    dronabinol for, 680-681
    granisetron for, 681
    hydroxyzine for, 456-457
    ipecac syrup for induction of, 1215-1216
    metoclopramide for, 682-683
    ondansetron for, 684-685
    perphenazine for, 476-478
    prochlorperazine for, 685-687
    thiethylperazine for, 687-688
    trimethobenzamide for, 688
Vontrol, 679
von Willebrand's disease, desmopressin for, 797-798
VoSol Otic, 1096
VP-16, 946-947
Vulval atrophy, estropipate for, 741-742
Vulvovaginitis, ceftriaxone for, 126-128
Vumon, 959
VZIG, 1020-1021

W

warfarin sodium, 863-865
Warfilone Sodium, 863
Wehamine, 678
Wehdryl-10, 591
Wehdryl-50, 591
Weight conversions, 1279t
Weight loss, dronabinol for, 680-681

Weight loss management, dexfenfluramine for, 491-493
Wellbutrin, 426
Wellcovorin, 1161
Wernicke's encephalopathy, thiamine for, 1166-1167
Westcort Cream, 1152
Westhroid, 785
Whipworm
    mebendazole for, 31
    thiabendazole for, 32-33
Wigraine, 552
Wigraine Suppositories, 552
Wilms' tumor
    dactinomycin for, 916-917
    doxorubicin for, 919-921
    vincristine for, 965-966
Wilson's disease
    d-penicillamine for, 1211-1212
    trientine for, 1224
WinGel, 642
Winpred, 714
WinRho SD, 1017-1019
Winsprin Capsules, 333
Winstrol, 724
Wound healing, vitamin C for, 1167-1169
Wound irrigation
    fibrinolysin and desoxyribonuclease for, 1190-1191
    kanamycin for, 68-69
Wounds, bacitracin for, 1113-1114
Wyamine, 544
Wycillin, 94
Wydase, 1191
Wygesic, 366-367
Wymox, 77
Wytensin, 281

X

Xalatan, 1089
Xanax, 449, C16
Xerostomia, pilocarpine for, 1252-1253
X-Prep Liquid, 675
Xylocaine, 232, 1264t
Xylocard, 232
xylometazoline hydrochloride, 1110

Y

yellow fever vaccine, 1007
YF-Vax, 1007
Yodoquinol, 25
Yodoxin, 25
Yutopar, 1254

Z

Zadine, 584
zafirlukast, 639-640
Zagam, 163

zalcitabine, 187-188
Zanaflex, 563
Zanosar, 898
Zantac, 696, C16
Zantac 75, 696
Zantac 150, 696
Zantac 150 EFFERdose, 696, C16
Zantac 300, 696
Zantac 300 GELdose, 696
Zantac-C, 696
Zantac 150 GELdose, 696
Zapex, 461
Zarontin, 406
Zaroxolyn, 824
Zeasorb-AF, 1130
Zebeta, 270
Zefazone, 111
Zemuron, 576
Zerit, 185
Zestoretic 20-12.5, 265
Zestoretic 20-25, 265
Zestril, 289, C16
Zetran, 453
Ziac, 265
Ziac 2.5, 808
Ziac 5, 808
Ziac 10, 808
zidovudine, 188-190
zileuton, 640-641
Zinacef, 128
Zinamide, 61
zinc, 1174-1175
Zinca-Pak, 1174
zinc chloride, 1174-1175
Zincfrin, 1078
zinc sulfate, 1174-1175
Zithromax, 191, C16
Zocor, 320, C16
Zofran, 684
Zoladex, 930
Zolicef, 107
Zollinger-Ellison syndrome
    cimetidine for, 689-691
    famotidine for, 691-692
    lansoprazole for, 692-693
    omeprazole for, 695-696
    ranitidine for, 696-697
Zoloft, 443, C16
zolpidem tartrate, 402
ZORprin, 333
Zostrix, 1234
Zostrix-HP 0.075%, 1234
Zosyn, 100
Zovirax, 166, 1111, C16
Zyflo, 640
Zyloprim, 1182
Zymase Capsules, 652
Zyprexa, 475
Zyrtec, 5866